W9-BDD-896

Analyte	Expected adult reference or therapeutic range					Clinical correlation range (page)	Methods of analysis* (page)
	Conventional units			SI units			
	Parameter	Arterial	Venous	Arterial	Venous		
Blood gases and oxygen saturation (B)	pH	7.35-7.45	7.33-7.43	7.35-7.45	7.33-7.43	464	477
	P_{CO_2}	35-45 mm Hg	38-50 mm Hg	263-338	285-375 kPa		
	P_{O_2}	80-100 mm Hg	30-50 mm Hg	600-750	225-375 kPa		
	O_2 saturation	95%-100%	60%-80%				
Caffeine (S, P)	5-20 µg/mL			25-100 µmol/L		1086	1108
Calcium (S)	80-105 mg/L			2.0-2.6 mmol/L		528	549
(U)	<275 mg/24 hr males			<6.87 mmol/24 hr males			
	<250 mg/24 hr females			<6.25 mmol/24 hr females			
Carbohydrate screen (U)	Undetectable			—		939	965
Carbon dioxide total (S, P)	21-31 mmol/L			21-31 mmol/L		464	480
Carcinoembryonic antigen (S)	<2.5 ng/mL (method dependent)			—		983	995
	<5.0 ng/mL smokers			—			
Ceruloplasmin (S)	250-630 mg/L			1.5-4 µmol/L		939	966
Chloride (S)	97-107 mEq/L			97-107 mmol/L		439	458
(U)	110-250 mEq/L (or 24 hr)			110-250 mmol/24 hr			
Cholesterol total (S)	Age, sex, and risk dependent			pp. 669-672		642	672
High-density lipoprotein, HDL	Age, sex, and risk dependent			pp. 669-672		642	674
Low-density lipoprotein, LDL	Age, sex, and risk dependent			pp. 669-672		642	
Cholinesterase	Age, sex, and phenotype dependent					939	967
Chorionic gonadotropin, human (hCG)	<20 mIU/mL					793	815
Creatine kinase total (S)	130-253 U/L (method dependent)			2.17×10^{-6} katal/L		593	603
Creatine kinase isoenzymes (S)	<10 µg/L for CK-MB			—		593	605
	<3% of total CK activity for CK-MB						
Creatinine (S)	6.4-10.4 mg/L male			57-92 µmol/L		484	497
	5.7-9.2 mg/L female			50-81 µmol/L			
(U)	1.0-2.0 g/day male			8.8-17.7 mmol/day			
	0.8-1.8 g/day female			7.1-15.9 mmol/day			
Creatinine clearance	97-137 mL/min male					484	497
	88-128 mL/min female						
Cyclosporin A (B)	Dependent on organ and time after transplant					1086	1103
	150-225 µg/L renal <3 mo			0.12-0.18 µmol/L			
	100-150 µg/L renal >3 mo			0.08-0.12 µmol/L			
Digoxin (S, P)	0.9-2.0 ng/mL			1.1-2.4 nmol/L		593	607
Drug screen (U)	Not present					1017	1026
Folic acid (S)	1.9-14 ng/mL			4.3-31.7 nmol/L		760	787
Glucose (S)	700-1050 mg/L			3.9-5.8 mmol/L		613	634
Glycosylated hemoglobin (A_{1c}) (B)	4.1%-5.3% (method dependent)					613	635
Haptoglobin (S)	600-2000 mg/L			7.0-31.8 µmol/L		716	731
Hemoglobin F (B)	0.6-1.0% of total hemoglobin					716	731
Hemoglobin separation and quantitation (B)	(see p. 733)					716	732

(see p. 733)

B, Whole blood; P, plasma; S, serum; U, urine.
*A more complete list and description of methods of analysis can be found in
Clinical chemistry: a managerial and scientific infobase, Cincinnati, 1996, Pesce-Kaplan Publishers.

Continued on back endpaper.

Clinical Chemistry

Theory, analysis, and correlation

The Publisher regrets the following changes could not be made before press time.

Dr. Shaw's name and affiliation should read as follows:

Dr. Leslie M. Shaw, Ph.D.
Professor, Director of Therapeutic Drug Monitoring & Clinical Toxicology Lab,
University of Pennsylvania Medical Center,
Philadelphia, Pennsylvania

In Table 56-3 under "comments" for Method 1 the statement "Not suitable for stat analysis" should be deleted.

On page 1105, column 1 beginning with line 4, "Newer immunoassays that . . ." should read "Newer immunoassays that employ monoclonal antibodies have somewhat improved specificity. The mean overestimation of CsA concentrations compared with HPLC ranged from 8% to 30% with EMIT, 24% to 48% with mFPIA, and 22% to 30% with the INCSTAR mRIA.[16]"

On page 1105, column 2 under *Specimen:* The second sentence says, "CsA is found . . ." should read "CsA is found predominantly in erythrocytes (58%) and leukocytes in whole blood.[61]"

On page 1105, column 2 under *Therapeutic range:* This entire subsection should read: "It has been difficult to establish a therapeutic range for CsA for the following reasons: (1) there are no simple parameters for assessment for the immunosuppressive effect; (2) the methods for measurement of CsA have different degrees of specificity for the parent drug; (3) different immunosuppression protocols are used including center-specific preferences for the degree of initial exposure of patients to CsA. Overall, the incidence of organ rejection is higher at low CsA concentrations, whereas toxicity occurs more frequently at high CsA concentrations . . ." [remainder as in the text].

Clinical Chemistry

Theory, analysis, and correlation

THIRD EDITION

Lawrence A. Kaplan, Ph.D.

Director, Clinical Chemistry and Toxicology
Laboratories,
Bellevue Hospital;
Department of Pathology,
New York University
New York, New York

Amadeo J. Pesce, Ph.D.

Director, Clinical Toxicology Laboratory,
Department of Pathology and Laboratory
Medicine,
University of Cincinnati Hospital
Cincinnati, Ohio

Methods editor:

Steven C. Kazmierczak, Ph.D.

Scientific Director, Clinical Chemistry,
Department of Pathology and Laboratory Medicine,
East Carolina University School of Medicine
Greenville, North Carolina

with 527 illustrations

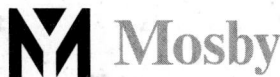 Mosby

St. Louis Baltimore Boston Carlsbad Chicago Naples New York Philadelphia Portland
London Madrid Mexico City Singapore Sydney Tokyo Toronto Wiesbaden

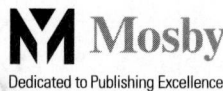

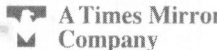

Editors: James F. Shanahan, Jennifer Roche
Developmental Editor: Sandra J. Parker
Editorial Assistant: Jennifer McCartney
Project Manager: Dana Peick
Production Editors: Carl Masthay, Blair Woodcock
Manuscript Editor: Judith E. Kaplan
Designer: Amy Buxton
Cover Designer: Frank Loose/Frank Loose Design
Manufacturing Supervisor: Betty Richmond

THIRD EDITION
Copyright © 1996 by Mosby–Year Book, Inc.

Previous editions copyrighted 1984, 1989

Printed in the United States of America
Composition by Clarinda Company
Printing/binding by Maplevail Press

Mosby–Year Book, Inc.
11830 Westline Industrial Drive
St. Louis, Missouri 63146

Library of Congress Cataloging-in-Publication Data
Clinical chemistry: theory, analysis, and correlation / [edited by]
  Lawrence A. Kaplan, Amadeo J. Pesce.—3rd ed.
      p.   cm.
   Includes bibliographical references and index.
   ISBN 0-8151-5243-4
   1. Clinical chemistry.   I. Kaplan, Lawrence A., 1944-
II. Pesce, Amadeo J.
   [DNLM: 1. Chemistry, Clinical.   QY 90 C6415 1996]
RB40.C58   1996
616.07′56—dc20
DNLM/DLC
for Library of Congress   95-47197
                                                        CIP

96 97 98 99 00 / 9 8 7 6 5 4 3 2 1

Contributors

Nancy W. Alcock, Ph.D.
Director, Nutrition Laboratory,
Department of Preventive Medicine
  and Community Health,
University of Texas Medical Branch,
Galveston, Texas
Chapter 37 Human nutrition
Chapter 38 Trace elements

David J. Anderson, Ph.D.
Associate Professor,
Director of Clinical Chemistry,
Department of Chemistry,
Cleveland State University,
Cleveland, Ohio
Chapter 6 Liquid chromatography

F. Phillip Anderson, M.S.
Department of Pathology,
Medical College of Virginia,
Richmond, Virginia
Methods: Chapter 24

Victor W. Armstrong
Georg-August-Universität
  Göttingen,
Göttingen, Federal Republic of
  Germany
Chapter 56 Therapeutic drug
monitoring (TDM): Practical aspects
of TDM

Susan Bassion, Ph.D.
[affiliations unavailable]
Chapter 11 Immunological reactions

Larry D. Bowers, Ph.D.
Professor,
Department of Pathology,
Indiana University Medical Center,
Indianapolis, Indiana
Chapter 6 Liquid chromatography

John M. Brewer, Ph.D.
Professor of Biochemistry,
Department of Biochemistry,
University of Georgia,
Athens, Georgia
Chapter 10 Electrophoresis

Marge A. Brewster, Ph.D.
Professor, Departments of
  Pathology and Pediatrics,
University of Arkansas for Medical
  Sciences;
Clinical Biochemist, Arkansas
  Children's Hospital,
Little Rock, Arkansas
Chapter 39 Vitamins

Elizabeth Ann Byrne, M.S., C.L.S.
Assistant Professor, Biology
  Department,
College of Mount St. Joseph,
Mount St. Joseph, Ohio
Chapter 1 Basic laboratory principles
and techniques (Part II: Calculations in
clinical chemistry)

R. Neill Carey, Ph.D.
Clinical Chemist,
Department of Pathology,
Peninsula Regional Medical Center,
Salisbury, Maryland
Chapter 22 Evaluation of methods

John F. Chapman, Dr.P.H.
Associate Professor of Pathology,
University of North Carolina at
  Chapel Hill;
Director, Clinical Chemistry
  Laboratories,
University of North Carolina
  Hospitals,
Chapel Hill, North Carolina
Chapter 31 Cardiac and muscle
disease
Chapter 40 Pregnancy and fetal
development
Chapter 55 Isoenzymes and isoforms

I-Wen Chen, Ph.D.
Professor,
Department of Pathology and
  Laboratory Medicine,
University of Cincinnati Medical
  Center,
Cincinnati, Ohio
Chapter 9 Radioisotopes in clinical
chemistry
Methods: Chapters 31, 39, 44

Kee Cheung, Ph.D.
University of Queensland,
Woolloongabba, Queensland,
  Australia
Methods: Chapter 27

David Chou, M.D.
Division of Pathology and
  Laboratory Medicine,
The Cleveland Clinic Foundation,
Cleveland, Ohio
Chapter 18 Laboratory information
system

Robert H. Christenson, Ph.D.
Associate Professor of Pathology,
University of Maryland School of
  Medicine;
Director, Clinical Chemistry
  Laboratories,
University of Maryland Medical
  Center,
Baltimore, Maryland
Chapter 31 Cardiac and muscle
diseases
Chapter 55 Isoenzymes and isoforms

Lawrence J. Crolla, Ph.D.
Managing Director,
World-Wide Health Care
  Consulting,
Surprise, Arizona
Chapter 2 Laboratory Management

Donald Davis, Ph.C.
Department of Clinical
  Pharmacology,
Princess Alexandra Hospital,
Woolloongabba, Queensland,
  Australia
Methods: Chapter 51

Laurence M. Demers, Ph.D.
Department of Pathology,
Milton S. Hershey Medical Center,
Pennsylvania State University,
Hershey, Pennsylvania
Chapter 43 General endocrinology

Joseph R. DiPersio, Ph.D.
Microbiologist,
Akron City Hospital,
Akron, Ohio
Methods: Chapter 56

Helen M. Dodds,
Department of Clinical
  Pharmacology,
Princess Alexandra Hospital,
Woolloongabba, Queensland,
  Australia
Methods: Chapter 51

Richard F. Dods, Ph.D.
Chemistry Team Leader for
  Curriculum Development,
Illinois Mathematics and Science
  Academy,
Palatine, Illinois
Chapter 32 Diabetes mellitus

David R. Dufour, M.D.
Chief, Laboratory Services,
Department of Pathology,
Veterans Affairs Medical Center,
Washington, D.C.
Chapter 3 Sources and control of
preanalytical variation

Carolyn S. Feldkamp, Ph.D.
Pathology Department,
Henry Ford Hospital,
Detroit, Michigan
Chapter 12 Immunochemical
techniques

Mariano Fernández-Ulloa, M.D.
Department of Radiation/Nuclear
  Medicine,
University of Cincinnati,
Cincinnati, Ohio
Chapter 44 Thyroid

M. Roy First, M.D.
Professor,
Department of Internal Medicine,
University of Cincinnati Medical
  Center,
Cincinnati, Ohio
Chapter 26 Renal function
Chapter 50 Laboratory evaluation of
the transplant recipient and donor

Donald T. Forman, Ph.D.
Professor,
Division of Laboratory Medicine,
Department of Pathology,
University of North Carolina
Chapel Hill, North Carolina
Methods: Chapter 49

Christopher S. Frings, Ph.D.
President, Chris Frings and
  Associates;
Clinical Professor,
Departments of Pathology and
  Allied Health Sciences,
University of Alabama at
  Birmingham,
Birmingham, Alabama
Chapter 4 Spectral techniques

Carl C. Garber, Ph.D.
Laboratory Administration,
MetPath,
Teterboro, New Jersey
Chapter 22 Evaluation of methods

Jack Gauldie, Ph.D.
Associate Professor,
Department of Pathology,
McMaster University,
Hamilton, Ontario, Canada
Chapter 4 Spectral techniques

Lewis Glasser, M.D.
Chief, Hematopathology
  Laboratories,
Department of Pathology,
Arizona Health Sciences Center,
University of Arizona,
Tucson, Arizona
Chapter 41 Extravascular biological
fluids

R. Jeffrey Goldsmith, Ph.D.
Associate Professor,
Department of Psychiatry,
University of Cincinnati Medical
  Center,
Cincinnati, Ohio
Chapter 52 Addiction and substance
abuse

F. Michael Hassan, M.T.(ASCP)
Assistant Director of Toxicology,
Department of Pathology and
  Laboratory Medicine,
University of Cincinnati Medical
  Center,
Cincinnati, Ohio
Methods: Chapter 51

William R. Heineman, Ph.D.
Distinguished Research Professor,
Department of Chemistry,
University of Cincinnati,
Cincinnati, Ohio
Chapter 15 Electrochemistry:
principles and measurements

Linda A. Heminger, B.S.(CNMT)
Department of Pathology and
  Laboratory Medicine,
University of Cincinnati Medical
  Center,
Cincinnati, Ohio
Methods: Chapters 27, 31

Peter Hickman, Ph.D.
Clinical Associate Professor of
  Pathology,
University of Queensland;
Director of Chemical Pathology,
Princess Alexandra Hospital,
Woolloongabba, Queensland,
  Australia
Methods: Chapters 27, 31

W. Edward Highsmith, Jr., Ph.D.
Director, Molecular Diagnostics
  Laboratory,
Department of Pathology,
School of Medicine,
University of Maryland at
  Baltimore,
Baltimore, Maryland
Chapter 48 Molecular biology in the
clinical laboratory

Gregory A. Hobbs, Ph.D.
Department of Pathology,
University of Louisville School of
  Medicine,
Louisville, Kentucky
Methods: Chapter 49

David C. Hohnadel, Ph.D.
Director, Clinical Chemistry,
Department of Pathology,
The Genesee Hospital,
Rochester, New York
Chapter 54 Clinical enzymology

Oussama Itani, M.D.
Instructor in Pediatrics,
Department of Pediatrics,
University of Cincinnati,
Cincinnati, Ohio;
Director of Nurseries,
St. Luke's Hospital,
Ft. Thomas, Kentucky
Chapter 28 Bone disease

Gayle Jackson, M.S.
Supervisor, Clinical Laboratory,
Children's Hospital Medical Center,
Cincinnati, Ohio
Methods: Chapter 49

Ellis Jacobs, Ph.D.
Department of Pathology,
Director, Stat Laboratory,
Mt. Sinai School of Medicine,
Mt. Sinai Hospital,
New York, New York
Chapter 17   Point-of-care (near-patient)
testing

Mark A. Jandreski, Ph.D.
Assistant Professor, Department of
  Pathology,
Loyola University of Chicago,
Director, Special Chemistry and
  Immunoserology,
Foster G. McGaw Hospital,
Loyola University Medical Center,
Maywood, Illinois
Chapter 19   Laboratory statistics

Sarah H. Jenkins, Ph.D.
Assistant Professor,
Director of Primary Services
  Laboratory,
Department of Pathology and
  Laboratory Medicine,
University of Cincinnati,
Cincinnati, Ohio
Chapter 15   Electrochemistry:
principles and measurements

William R. Johnson, Ph.D.
Department of Pathology,
University of Louisville School of
  Medicine,
Louisville, Kentucky
Methods: Chapter 49

Saeed A. Jortani, Ph.D.
Department of Pathology,
University of Louisville,
School of Medicine,
Louisville, Kentucky
Methods: Chapter 56

Stephen E. Kahn, Ph.D.
Associate Professor, Pathology and
  Biochemistry,
Loyola University of Chicago;
Associate Director, Clinical Chemistry,
Foster G. McGaw Hospital,
Loyola University Medical Center,
Maywood, Illinois
Chapter 19   Laboratory statistics

Lawrence A. Kaplan, Ph.D.
Associate Professor,
Director, Clinical Chemistry and
  Toxicology Laboratories,
Bellevue Hospital;
Department of Pathology
New York University,
New York, New York

Chapter 14   Measurement of colligative
properties
Chapter 23   Interferences in chemical
analysis
Chapter 53   Classifications and
description of proteins, lipids, and
carbohydrates (Part I: Proteins;
Part III: Carbohydrates)
Methods: Chapter 24

Steven C. Kazmierczak, Ph.D.
Associate Professor,
Scientific Director, Clinical
  Chemistry,
Department of Pathology and
  Laboratory Medicine,
East Carolina University School of
  Medicine,
Greenville, North Carolina
*Methods: Chapters 24, 25, 26, 27, 28,
29, 30, 32, 35, 36, 39, 47, 56*

Thaddeus E. Kelly, M.D., Ph.D.
Professor, Department of Pediatrics,
University of Virginia Medical
  Center,
Charlottesville, Virginia
Chapter 47   Diseases of genetic origin

Jon R. Kirchhoff, Ph.D.
Associate Professor,
Department of Chemistry,
University of Toledo,
Toledo, Ohio
Chapter 15   Electrochemistry:
principles and measurements

Leonard I. Kleinman, M.D.
Professor and Director of Newborn
  Services,
Department of Pediatrics,
State University of NY at Stony
  Brook School of Medicine,
Stony Brook, New York
Chapter 24   Physiology and
pathophysiology of body water
and electrolytes

Christian Kohler, M.D.
Department of Psychiatry,
Mental Health Clinical Research
  Center,
University of Pennsylvania,
Philadelphia, Pennsylvania
Chapter 42   Nervous system

William J. Korzum, Ph.D.
Department of Pathology,
Medical College of Virginia,
Richmond, Virginia
Methods: Chapters 24, 25

**Robert W. Lang, M.T.(ASCP),
M.B.A., C.L.S.(NCA)**
Administrative Director of
  Laboratory Services,
LaGrange Memorial Hospital,
LaGrange, Illinois
Chapter 2   Laboratory management

Michael Lehrer, Ph.D.
Chief, Division of Biochemistry,
Department of Pathology,
Long Island Jewish Medical Center,
New Hyde Park, New York
Chapter 8   Mass spectrometry

Mark W. Linder, Ph.D.
Department of Pathology,
University of Louisville,
School of Medicine,
Louisville, Kentucky
Methods: Chapter 42

John M. Lorenz, M.D.
Associate Professor of Pediatrics,
Director, Division of Neonatology,
Department of Pediatrics and
  Human Development,
Michigan State University;
Medical Director, Regional
  Newborn Intensive Care Services,
Sparrow Hospital,
Lansing, Michigan
Chapter 24   Physiology and
pathophysiology of body water
and electrolytes

John A. Lott, Ph.D.
Professor of Pathology,
The Ohio State University;
Director, Clinical Chemistry,
The Ohio State University Hospitals,
Columbus, Ohio
Chapter 29   The pancreas: function
and chemical pathology
Methods: Chapters 27, 31, 49

Marvin H. Lucas, M.D.
Internal Medicine,
Premier Medical Associates,
Cincinnati, Ohio
Chapter 44   Thyroid

Michael D.D. McNeely, M.D.
Head, Chemistry and Immunology,
Metro-McNair Clinical Laboratories,
Victoria, British Columbia, Canada
Chapter 30   Gastrointestinal function
and digestive disease

Craig E. Lunte, Ph.D.
Associate Professor,
Department of Chemistry,
University of Kansas,
Lawrence, Kansas
Chapter 15   Electrochemistry:
principles and measurements

Charles L. Mendenhall, M.D.
Director of Hepatic Research,
Department of Digestive Diseases,
Veterans Affairs Medical Center,
Cincinnati, Ohio
Chapter 34 Alcoholism

M. Gregory Miller, Ph.D.
Associate Professor,
Department of Pathology,
Medical College of Virginia,
Richmond, Virginia
Methods: Chapters 24, 25

Patricia A. Miller-Canfield, M.D.
Staff Pathologist,
Department of Pathology,
Terra Haute Medical Labs,
Terra Haute, Indiana
Chapter 36 Hemoglobin

Herbert K. Naito, Ph.D.
Director, Clinical Chemistry,
Department of Laboratory Services,
Department of Veterans Affairs
  Medical Center,
Cleveland, Ohio
Chapter 33 Coronary artery disease
and disorders of lipid metabolism
Chapter 53 Classifications and
descriptions of proteins, lipids, and
carbohydrates (Part II: Lipids)

Karen L. Nickel, Ph.D.
Chief, Laboratory Field Services,
California State Department of
  Health Services,
Berkeley, California
Chapter 45 Gonads

Steven A. Noel, Ph.D.
Department of Pathology,
Greater Baltimore Medical Center,
Baltimore, Maryland
Methods: Chapter 49

Ross L.G. Norris
Chief Scientist,
Department of Clinical
  Pharmacology,
Princess Alexandra Hospital,
Woolloongabba, Queensland,
  Australia
Methods: Chapter 51

Michael Oellerich, Ph.D.
Professor,
Georg-August-Universität Göttingen,
Göttingen, Federal Republic of
  Germany
Chapter 56 Therapeutic drug
monitoring (TDM): Practical aspects
of TDM

Kalpana Panigrahi, Ph.D.
Fellow, Clinical Chemistry,
Department of Pathology,
University of Maryland,
Baltimore, Maryland
Chapter 55 Isoenzymes and isoforms

K. Michael Parker, Ph.D.
Professor, Department of
  Pathology,
Oklahoma Medical Center
Oklahoma City, Oklahoma
Methods: Chapter 34

Richard B. Passey, Ph.D.
Professor of Pathology,
Director, Clinical Chemistry
  Laboratory,
University of Oklahoma;
Director, Clinical Chemistry,
University Hospital,
Oklahoma City, Oklahoma
Chapter 21 Quality control for the
clinical chemistry laboratory

Monika Payne, M.T.
Technologist,
Midwestern Regional Medical
  Center,
Zion, Illinois
Formerly in Department of
  Chemical Pharmacology,
Princess Alexandra Hospital,
Woolloongabba, Queensland,
  Australia
Methods: Chapter 31

Gerardo Perrotta, M.T.(ASCP), S.H.,
Coordinator, Primary Service
  Laboratory,
Department of Pathology and
  Laboratory Medicine,
University of Cincinnati Hospital,
Cincinnati, Ohio
Methods: Chapters 35, 36

Amadeo J. Pesce, Ph.D.
Professor,
Department of Pathology and
  Laboratory Medicine,
University of Cincinnati Medical
  Center,
Cincinnati, Ohio
Chapter 4 Spectral techniques
Chapter 23 Interferences in chemical
analysis
Chapter 51 Toxicology
Methods: Chapter 31

Michael A. Pesce, Ph.D.
Professor,
Director of Laboratories,
Department of Pathology,
Columbia Presbyterian Medical
  Center,
New York, New York
Chapter 16 Automation

Alphonse Poklis, Ph.D.
Associate Professor, Department of
  Pathology,
Affiliate Professor, Department of
  Pharmacology and Toxicology,
Medical College of Virginia;
Director, Toxicology Laboratory,
Medical College of Virginia Hospitals,
Richmond, Virginia
Chapter 7 Gas chromatography
Chapter 51 Toxicology

Julia M. Potter, Ph.D.
Department of Chemical Pathology,
Royal Brisbane Hospital,
Herston, Queensland, Australia
Methods: Chapters 51, 56

Michael D. Privitera, M.D.
Associate Professor, Department of
  Neurology,
University of Cincinnati Medical
  Center;
Staff Neurologist,
Director, Epilepsy Treatment
  Center,
University of Cincinnati Hospital,
Cincinnati, Ohio
Chapter 42 Nervous system

Morris R. Pudek, Ph.D.
Clinical Professor, Department of
  Pathology,
University of British Columbia;
Clinical Chemist,
Vancouver General Hospital,
Vancouver, British Columbia,
  Canada
Chapter 46 Adrenal hormones and
hypertension

Wolfgang A. Ritschel, M.D., Ph.D.
Professor of Pharmacokinetics and
  Biopharmaceutics;
Head, Division of Pharmaceutics
  and Drug Delivery Systems,
University of Cincinnati Medical
  Center,
Cincinnati, Ohio
Chapter 56 Therapeutic drug
monitoring (TDM): Basic overview
of principles

Andrea Rose, Ph.D.
Department of Pathology,
University of Louisville School of
  Medicine,
Louisville, Kentucky
Methods: Chapter 32

Stephen J. Rossi, Pharm.D.
Division of Nephrology,
University of Michigan Medical
  Center,
Ann Arbor, Michigan
Chapter 50 Laboratory evaluation of
the transplant recipient and donor

Donald L. Rucknagel, Ph.D.
Director, Sickle Center,
Children's Hospital Medical Center,
Cincinnati, Ohio
Chapter 47 Diseases of genetic origin

Paul Salm
Department of Clinical
  Pharmacology,
Princess Alexandra Hospital,
Woolloongabba, Queensland,
  Australia
Methods: Chapter 56

Edward A. Sasse, Ph.D.
Associate Professor, Department of
  Pathology,
Medical College of Wisconsin;
Chief, Chemistry Section,
  Pathology and Laboratory
  Medicine Service,
Milwaukee Veterans Affairs Medical
  Center,
Milwaukee, Wisconsin
Chapter 20 Reference intervals and
clinical decision limits

Kevin T. Schleuter, Ph.D.
Department of Pathology and
  Laboratory Medicine,
University of Cincinnati,
Cincinnati, Ohio
Chapter 50 Laboratory evaluation of
the transplant recipient and donor

William E. Schreiber, M.D.
Associate Professor, Department of
  Pathology and Laboratory
  Medicine,
University of British Columbia,
Vancouver, British Columbia,
  Canada
Chapter 35 Iron, porphyrin, and
bilirubin metabolism

Timothy J. Schroeder, M.S.
Associate Professor,
Director, Transplant Division,
Department of Pathology and
  Laboratory Medicine,
University of Cincinnati Medical
  Center,
Cincinnati, Ohio
Chapter 50 Laboratory evaluation of
the transplant recipient and donor

Arnold L. Schultz, Ph.D.
Associate Professor,
Department of Pathology,
University of Colorado Health
  Sciences Center,
Denver, Colorado
Methods: Chapter 26

Harold R. Schumacher, M.D.
Professor,
Director, Hematology Division,
Department of Pathology and
  Laboratory Medicine,
University of Cincinnati Medical
  Center,
Cincinnati, Ohio
Chapter 36 Hemoglobin

G. Berry Schumann, M.D.
Dianon Systems,
Stratford, Connecticut
Chapter 57 Examination of urine

**Susan C. Schweitzer, M.S.,
M.T.(ASCP)**
Department of Pathology,
University of Colorado Health
  Science Center,
Denver, Colorado
Chapter 57 Examination of urine

Bette Seamonds, Ph.D.
Assistant Professor, Department of
  Laboratory Sciences,
Thomas Jefferson University,
Philadelphia, Pennsylvania
Chapter 1 Basic laboratory principles
and techniques (Part I: Basic laboratory
principles)

Lester Shaw, Ph.D.
Professor,
Department of Pathology and
  Laboratory Medicine,
University of Pennsylvania;
William Pepper Laboratory,
Hospital of the University of
  Pennsylvania,
Philadelphia, Pennsylvania
Methods: Chapter 56

John E. Sherwin, Ph.D.
Consultant,
Westlake Village, California
Chapter 25 Acid-base control and
acid-base disorders
Chapter 27 Liver function
Methods: Chapter 31

Lawrence M. Silverman, Ph.D.
Professor,
Director, Special Chemistry,
Department of Pathology,
North Carolina Memorial Hospital,
Chapel Hill, North Carolina
Chapter 31 Cardiac and muscle
disease
Chapter 48 Molecular biology in the
clinical laboratory
Chapter 55 Isoenzymes and isoforms

David A. Smith, M.S., Captain
Laboratory Science Officer,
United States Army Medical Service
  Corps,
Fort Sam Houston, San Antonio,
  Texas
Methods: Chapter 49

Juan R. Sobenes, M.D.
Associate Clinical Professor,
Department of Laboratory
  Medicine and Pathology,
Valley Medical Center, Fresno,
University of California,
Fresno, California
Chapter 27 Liver function

Bernard E. Statland, M.D.
National Reference Laboratories,
Nashville, Tennessee
Chapter 49 Neoplasia

Paul W. Stiffler, Ph.D.
Microbiology Consultant,
LaGrange Memorial Hospital,
LaGrange, Illinois
Chapter 2 Laboratory management

Jay Stoerker, Ph.D.
Applied Technology Genetics
  Corporation,
Malvern, Pennsylvania
Chapter 48 Molecular biology in the
clinical laboratory

M. Wilson Tabor, Ph.D.
Associate Professor of
  Environmental Health,
Director of Environmental
  Analytical Chemistry,
Institute of Environmental Health,
University of Cincinnati Medical
  Center,
Cincinnati, Ohio
Chapter 5 Chromatography: theory
and practice
Methods: Chapter 51

Paul J. Taylor
Department of Clinical
  Pharmacology,
Princess Alexandra Hospital,
Woolloongabba, Queensland,
  Australia
Methods: Chapter 56

Stephan G. Thompson, Ph.D.
Staff Scientist,
Coulter Corporation,
Hialeah, Florida
Chapter 13 Principles for
competitive-binding assays

Reginald C. Tsang, M.D.
Gamble Professor of Neonatology,
  Obstetrics, and Gynecology,
University of Cincinnati Medical
  Center;
Director of Neonatology,
Associate Chairman of Pediatrics,
Children's Hospital Medical Center,
Cincinnati, Ohio
Chapter 28 Bone disease

Gregory J. Tsongalis, Ph.D.
Department of Pathology and
  Laboratory Medicine,
Hartford Hospital,
Hartford, Connecticut
Chapter 40 Pregnancy and fetal
development

Kory M. Ward, Ph.D.
Associate Professor, Division of
  Medical Technology,
School of Allied Medical
  Professions,
Ohio State University,
Columbus, Ohio
Methods: Chapters 31, 54, 55

Robert E. Weesner, M.D.
Assistant Professor, Department of
  Internal Medicine,
University of Cincinnati Medical
  Center;
Director, GI Endoscopy Services,
Veterans Affairs Medical Center,
  Cincinnati, Ohio
Chapter 34 Alcoholism

John F. Wheeler, Ph.D.
Assistant Professor,
Department of Chemistry,
Furman University,
Greenville, South Carolina
Chapter 15 Electrochemistry:
principles and measurements

Per Winkel, M.D., Doc. Med. Sci.
Clinical Chemistry Department,
Rigshospitalet,
Copenhagen, Denmark
Chapter 49 Neoplasia

Delores Wishart, M.T.(ASCP)
Laboratory Administrative Director,
Alexian Brothers Medical Center,
Elk Grove Village, Illinois
Chapter 2 Laboratory management

Steven H.Y. Wong, Ph.D.
Professor, Pathology and Psychiatry
  & Behavioral Medicine,
Director, Clinical Toxicology and
  Therapeutic Drug Monitoring,
Department of Pathology,
Medical College of Wisconsin,
Milwaukee, Wisconsin
Chapter 51 Toxicology

To our wives

Judith E. Kaplan and **Anna Pesce**
whose love and support have
not diminished in these years

and our mentors

Samuel Natelson and **George F. Grannis**
whose imparted knowledge continues
to serve us and future generations

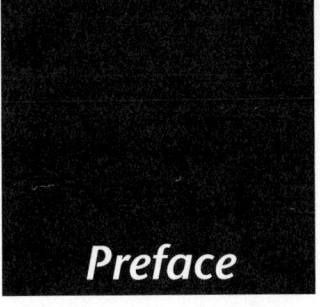

Preface

It has been more than a decade since the first edition of the textbook was published. In the ensuing time we have been very gratified by the response from our readership. We have changed the text of this edition of *Clinical Chemistry* in response to both the constructive criticisms that we have received and the continued evolution of the field. Recent changes in clinical chemistry reflect both the economic pressures for continuing the historic trends for increased automation and laboratory consolidation, and the strong effect of regulatory forces, which requires clinical chemists to have expertise as managers.

Therefore we have added a new chapter on *Laboratory Management* (Chapter 2) and upgraded all the text to reflect CLIA '88 regulations. The management chapter can be used by all readers, at all levels, to better cope with the increasing regulatory nature of the profession. The new chapter on *Mass Spectrometry* (Chapter 8) reflects the more widespread use of this technique. The new chapters reviewing *Laboratory Evaluation of the Transplant Recipient and Donor* (Chapter 50) and *Addiction and Substance Abuse* (Chapter 52) will help readers understand the changes and growth of these clinical disciplines. Readers will find that almost all the chapters have been revised to incorporate the latest clinical and technical advances. We would like to point out the chapters on *Liquid Chromatography* (Chapter 6), *Immunochemical Techniques* (Chapter 12), and *Automation* (Chapter 16), which have been extensively revised to incorporate the many technical changes that have occurred in these areas since the second edition. Chapter 19, on *Laboratory Statistics*, has been rewritten to provide students with practical examples of statistics as applied in the clinical laboratory. Chapter 20, *Reference Intervals and Clinical Decision Limits*, has been revised to incorporate NCCLS guidelines.

In a major change from the previous edition, we have deleted the separate "methods" section and placed the description of individual methods in the clinical chapters where the use of these analytes are discussed. This change allowed more space to be allotted to updating the clinical and technical chapters and allowed us to add the new chapters noted above. To facilitate ready access by students to the method reviews, we have placed each review at the end of the appropriate clinical chapter in a new, discrete chapter section, Methods of Analysis. We believe that educators will appreciate that this modification of *Clinical Chemistry*, responding to the continued change in laboratories toward the use of prepackaged reagents, will allow them to focus on what is important for students entering the field of clinical chemistry.

We would like to recognize the important contribution of Dr. Steven C. Kazmierczak, who served as the editor of the methods areas of the text, to this edition. With his help, we have tried to choose methods for review that will be most useful for teaching the modern principles of analysis.

We continue the liberal use throughout the text of summary tables and boxes and figures in the belief that these are useful aids to the learning process. The chapter outlines and glossary of key terms, to which our educator colleagues have responded so favorably, are continued and expanded to all new chapters.

The result of these changes is, on one hand, a textbook that will be very familiar to those who have used the previous editions. This will allow educators to reuse current teaching plans. On the other hand, the changes ensure that students will be learning from a textbook that will reflect the most recent changes in the field. We believe, therefore, that more than ever, this text can continue to take its place as both a teaching text for students in medical technology and an up-to-date reference book for advanced students and for individuals already practicing clinical chemistry.

We would like to thank the directors of our academic departments of pathology (Drs. Vittorio Defendi and John Pearson, New York University, and Dr. Fenoglio-Priser, University of Cincinnati) for providing an atmosphere in which this work could be completed. We cannot give enough thanks to our many authors who have provided the reader with their expertise. We thank Judith E. Kaplan, for once again ensuring that the text would be most readable, and to our editor, Mr. James F. Shanahan for his forbearance over the past years. We acknowledge Dr. Myer Horowitz for his help in reviewing manuscripts and the expert word processing of Georgia Coddington and Diane Gorman.

Lawrence A. Kaplan
Amadeo J. Pesce

Contents

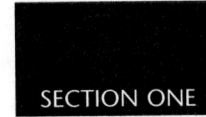
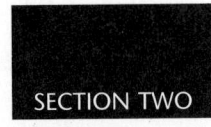

Appendixes

SECTION ONE

Laboratory Techniques

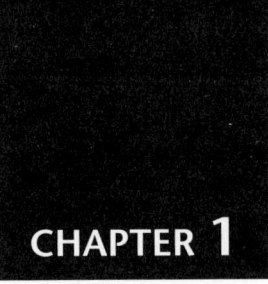

CHAPTER 1

Basic laboratory principles and techniques

Bette Seamonds
Elizabeth Ann Byrne

OBJECTIVES

- Describe the methods used for water purification and the specifications, uses, and storage and handling procedures associated with the different grades of reagent water.

- Describe the quality control and impurity testing procedures used for different grades of reagent water.

- List commonly used laboratory supplies and describe their proper use, quality control, cleaning, and maintenance procedures.

- Compare and contrast the use and care of glass and plastic supplies.

- Describe the specifications associated with the quality of reagent chemicals and solvents.
- Know the proper procedures for using pipets.
- Describe the operation and maintenance of balances, centrifuges, and water baths and heating blocks in the clinical laboratory.
- Describe the use and calibration of thermometers.
- Know general laboratory safety regulations, the components of the OSHA-mandated Chemical Hygiene Plan, and the plan for protection against blood-borne pathogens.

KEY TERMS

balances Mechanical or electronic instruments used to measure weight accurately.

beakers Laboratory utensils used to contain liquids or solids.

blood-borne pathogens Potentially infectious agents in blood and body fluids.

buret (burette) Laboratory utensil used to deliver a wide range of volumes accurately.

centrifuge Instrument used to separate materials from solution by application of increased gravitational force by rotating or spinning samples rapidly.

Chemical Hygiene Plan A laboratory plan that follows OSHA-mandated regulations, to protect employees against chemical hazards.

chemical purity Degree of purity or homogeneity as designated by various scientific agencies, such as the American Chemical Society and National Institute of Standards and Technology (NIST).

desiccant Material used in a desiccator to absorb water from the air.

desiccator Large container used to store material in a water-free environment.

dilution Process of preparing less concentrated solutions from a solution of greater concentration.

Erlenmeyer flask Laboratory utensil used to contain liquids.

funnel Laboratory utensil used to transfer liquids or solids into a container; also used for extraction of liquids.

graduated cylinder Laboratory utensil used to measure a volume of liquid.

heating block A temperature-controlled device used to warm and maintain materials at a specified temperature.

metric system A system of measurement of weights, distances, and volumes.

Occupational Safety and Health Administration (OSHA) Government agency responsible for mandating regulations to ensure safety in the workplace.

pipet (pipette) Laboratory utensil used to transfer a specific or varying volume of liquid.

sanitization The process used to maintain cleanliness in a water-purification system.

syringe A device used for drawing up a specified quantity of liquid and then dispensing it volumetrically.

Système International d'Unités (SI) An internationally accepted system of measurements.

thermometer A device, physical, electronic, or optical, that is used to measure temperature.

volumetric flask Laboratory utensil used to contain a specific volume of liquid.

water bath A temperature-controlled device filled with water, used to warm and maintain materials at a specified temperature.

water purification A treatment process (distillation, deionization, reverse osmosis, ultraviolet irradiation, ultrafiltration, or ozonolysis) used to remove water contaminants.

water purity Three levels of purity are defined, based on the amount of biological and dissolved organic and inorganic material present in the water.

Part I: Basic laboratory principles and techniques
BETTE SEAMONDS

To provide accurate and precise clinical data, the clinical chemistry laboratory must be concerned with the analytical components of the test methods used to determine this information. Familiarity with the purity of chemicals, solvents, and reagent water is essential. In addition, selection and use of appropriate analytical equipment and safe work practices are essential.

WATER AS A REAGENT

Water is one of the most important and commonly used reagents in the clinical laboratory. Because of its importance as a laboratory reagent and because it is often "produced" within each laboratory, water is discussed more fully in the following section.

Reagent-grade water

Impurities, both organic and inorganic, in the reagent water can introduce significant error into an analysis. Some impurities are easy to detect, but others are far more difficult. The need for high-purity reagent water in the clinical laboratory cannot be overemphasized.

Water systems that are improperly designed or inadequately maintained may actually add contaminants not originally found in the feedwater. Thus the quality of reagent water produced by different purification systems can differ greatly. In general, systems that continually recirculate the water provide protection against stagnation and consequently minimize bacterial growth. It is always, however, necessary to decontaminate the system at regular intervals. The material used for the construction of pipes is important; plastics such as polyvinyl chloride (PVC) are commonly used but are not necessarily the best choice. PVC, in particular, leaches organic impurities into the purified water. In addition, it has a porous surface that tends to harbor bacteria and other biologic impurities. For more detailed information, refer to the guideline *Preparation and Testing of Reagent Water in the Clinical Laboratory,* published by the National Committee for Clinical Laboratory Standards (NCCLS).[1]

Water quality is *not* synonymous with the purification process used. Different types of purification processes may be employed, and in many laboratories multiple processes are often used. The quality of the source water (feedwater) is of major importance, often dictating what purification processes should be used and ultimately what types of contaminants are likely to remain. Many of the characteristics of source water will be affected by geographical and seasonal variations. The seasonal variability is dependent on parameters such as rainfall, ground drainage, sewage, and industrial waste, whereas geographic locale will determine the hardness (mineral content) of the feedwater. Table 1-1 summarizes the effectiveness of seven purification processes in removing contaminants from feedwater. The laboratory should work closely with a reputable manufacturer to design a water-purification system that will meet its specific needs.

Purification process

Distillation. Distillation of water in glass effectively removes bacteria, pyrogens, particulate matter, dissolved ionized solids, and to a lesser extent dissolved organic contaminants. It is not useful for elimination of dissolved ionized gases such as ammonia, carbon dioxide, and chlorine or low-boiling-point organic compounds.

Deionization. In the deionization process, water is passed through a bed of mixed cation- and anion-exchange resins. Hydrogen and hydroxyl ions on the surface of the resins are displaced by cationic and anionic impurities. This process is excellent for removal of dissolved ionized gases and solids but is ineffective for all other contaminants. In addition, the binding capacity of the resin is quickly exhausted, and the resin must be frequently replaced or regenerated. Deionization is used with **carbon adsorption,** which is very effective in removal of dissolved organic compounds. The characteristics of the carbon employed dictate the efficacy of removal of the different organic contaminants. Neither deionization nor carbon adsorption will remove particulate matter, bacteria, or pyrogens.

Reverse osmosis. In reverse osmosis, water is forced under pressure through a semipermeable membrane leaving behind remnants of the dissolved organic, ionic, and suspended impurities, including microbial and viral contaminants. Reverse osmosis, however, does not remove dissolved gases effectively. This method is frequently used to pretreat water before purification by deionization.

Ultrafiltration. In ultrafiltration, water is passed through semipermeable membranes of pore size ≤ 0.22 μm, removing particulate matter, emulsified solids, most bacteria, and pyrogens. Increasingly, 0.1 μm postmembrane filters are being used to achieve an improved bacteria-free and pyrogen-free product. Ultrafiltration does not effectively remove dissolved ionized solids, gases, and most organic contaminants.

Ultraviolet oxidation and sterilization. UV oxidation and sterilization are used after other purification processes to remove trace amounts of organic contaminants

Table 1-1   A comparison of water-purification processes

Purification process	Major classes of contaminants					
	Dissolved ionized solids	Dissolved ionized gases	Dissolved organics*	Particulates	Bacteria*	Pyrogens/ endotoxins
Distillation	E/G†	P	G	E	E	E
Deionization	E	E	P	P	P	P
Reverse osmosis	G‡	P	G	E	E	E
Carbon adsorption	P	P§	E/G‖	P	P	P
Filtration	P	P	P	E	E	P
Ultrafiltration	P	P	G¶	E	E	E
Ultraviolet oxidation	P	P	E/G#	P	G**	P

NOTE: This chart is offered only as a general guideline. Because of the variability of performance within each process and feedwater supply, potential users are urged to contact a reputable manufacturer of pure water equipment for applications assistance before selecting a system for the laboratory.
E, Excellent (capable of complete or near-total removal); *G*, Good (capable of removing large percentages); *P*, Poor (little or no removal).
*Treatment with ozone, though currently not commonly used in clinical laboratory water-purification systems, has been shown preliminarily to be very effective in oxidizing bacteria, viruses, and their organic metabolites.
†The resistivity of water purified by distillation is an order of magnitude less than that of water purified by deionization because of the presence of CO_2 and sometimes H_2S, NH_3, and other ionized gases if present in the feedwater.
‡The residual concentration of dissolved ionized solids is partly dependent on the original concentration in the feedwater.
§Activated carbon will remove chlorine by adsorption.
‖When used in combination with other purification processes, special grades of activated carbon and other synthetic adsorbents exhibit excellent capabilities for removing organic contaminants. Their use, however, is targeted toward specific compounds and applications; consult with the manufacturer before use.
¶Ultrafilters are useful for reducing specific feedwater organic contaminants based on the rated molecular weight cutoff of the membrane.
#185 nm UV oxidation (batch process systems) is effective in removing trace organic contaminants when used after treatment. Feedwater makeup plays a critical role in the performance of these batch processors. They should not be confused with in-line UV sterilizers which use 254 nm UV radiation to inactivate bacteria.
**254 nm UV sterilizers, though not physically removing bacteria, may have bactericidal or bacteriostatic capabilities limited by intensity, contact, time, and flow rate.

(oxidation) and bacteria (sterilization). Different wavelengths are used for these processes: 185 nm for oxidation and 254 nm for sterilization. UV treatment is limited by intensity, contact time, and flow rate.

Ozone. Ozone treatment, used primarily in industrial settings, effectively removes organic contaminants. However, smaller, less expensive ozone generators are becoming available and undoubtedly will begin finding their way into clinical laboratory settings. Once introduced into the pretreated water, the ozone kills bacteria by rupturing the cell membrane almost instantaneously ($\sim$2 sec). Chlorine, on the other hand, simply diffuses into the cell and requires approximately a half hour to achieve its effect. The actual rate of lysis is dependent on the ozone level: higher ozone concentrations are used for highly contaminated systems, whereas lower concentrations are used for maintenance. After the microorganisms are lysed, the cytoplasmic constituents are oxidized by the ozone. The ozone is then removed by UV irradiation at 254 nm. Removal is critical, since ozone is incompatible with the deionization resins.

Ozone treatment can be effectively used to combat microbial contamination in pipes and purified water.

Grades of water purity

Three levels of water purity (types I, II, and III) plus a special reagent water category have been defined by the NCCLS. The College of American Pathologists (CAP) has also defined three grades of reagent water, which are essentially equivalent to those of the NCCLS. Table 1-2 summarizes the NCCLS specifications for the three levels of water. Waters falling into the "Special" category may require additional treatment to meet more specific requirements and applications.

Water conforming to specifications published by other agencies such as the American Society for Testing and Materials (ASTM), the American Chemical Society (ACS), and the United States Pharmacopeia (USP) may or may not be equivalent to water conforming to NCCLS specifications. ASTM water most closely resembles NCCLS type II water, whereas USP specifications are designed to ensure safe

in vivo and in vitro applications. USP water must pass a series of designated tests, such as those that document the absence of pyrogens, rather than meet requirements for maximum contaminant concentrations.

Storage and handling of reagent water

Type I water should be used immediately after it is produced. It cannot be stored because its resistivity will rapidly decrease as carbon dioxide is absorbed. In addition, ionic and organic contaminants will be leached from the storage container, and microbial contamination will occur.[2] Type II water can be stored for short periods. The storage and distribution systems should be constructed of materials that will minimize bacterial and chemical contamination. When water is drawn from a storage tank into a secondary vessel for routine use, the secondary vessel and the water must be replaced at least daily. Water should not be stored in carboys for routine use, since this leads to the degradation of the water quality.[2]

Under some conditions purchased stored water may be used. One example is water that is provided as a diluent by the manufacturer of a specific analytic system. In this case the water has been validated by the manufacturer for use as stated in the product insert. *Under no conditions can such a product be substituted for reagent water.* Similarly, sterile water is not equivalent to reagent-grade water and therefore is not an acceptable substitute. As already stated, USP water meets specifications for particular tests and not for specific contaminants. Other purchased products may include those for use in high-performance liquid chromatographic (HPLC) procedures in facilities where the quality of in-house reagent water is not satisfactory for that purpose.

If water must be purchased, there are several issues of importance. The purchased product should define silica content, bacterial contamination, and conductivity at the time of manufacture. The water should be purchased in quantities appropriate to usage. The packaged water should be protected from environmental contamination and from the leaching effects of the container. When the container is

Table 1-2 Reagent water specifications

	Type I	Type II	Type III
Maximum bacterial content, colony-forming units per milliliter (CFU/mL)	10*	1000	N.S.
pH	N.S.	N.S.	5.0-8.0
Minimum resistivity, megaohm-centimeter (megaohm-cm 25° C)	10 (in line)	1.0	0.1
Maximum silicate, mg/L of SiO_2	0.05	0.1	1.0
Particulate matter†	0.22 μm filter†	N.S.	N.S.
Organic contaminants‡	Activated carbon†	N.S.	N.S.

N.S., Not specified.
*Preferably, type I water should be bacteria free.
†This specification is a process specification and is not measured by the end user.
‡At a minimum, some form of activated carbon should be included in a reagent water system as pretreatment to help remove organic contaminants found in raw water supplies. Furthermore, additional treatment with special grades of carbon may be indicated for applications requiring extremely low levels of organic contaminants. Because the performance of carbon used in pretreatment and posttreatment is site specific, it is necessary to consult with the manufacturer for recommended replacement intervals. (See also footnote ‖, Table 1-1.)

opened, the bacterial count and conductivity should be measured for assessment of quality degradation since manufacture. The limits of acceptability should be similar to those of type II water. When required analytically, the water should be poured into an appropriate secondary container from which it will be sampled. Care must be taken to avoid touching the inside lid or dipping a pipet directly into the primary vessel. Unused portions of water must not be returned to the primary container. Water from the primary container should be discarded after a period of no longer than 1 week.

Purchased water provides an ideal supply of feedwater for benchtop purification systems. Many such systems are now available and allow even the smallest laboratory to produce limited quantities of type I water.

Suggested uses

Table 1-3 summarizes some suggested uses of the three grades of water. There is little documentation in the literature of the analytical difficulties caused by poor quality water. However many users of the NCCLS document on reagent water have reported specific instances of analytic problems attributed to water quality. These include difficulty with spectrophotometric hormonal assays, difficulty with coagulation and hematologic analyses, interference with some immunoassay procedures, instrumentation problems including background absorbance difficulties, leaching of contaminants from improperly regenerated deionization resins, and absorption of perfume into highly purified water causing difficulty with cell culture procedures. In addition, bacteria as well as silicate and other ion contamination have been shown to interfere with enzyme and bilirubin analyses.[3] Undoubtedly as techniques become more sensitive, more definitive information will become available.

Type I water should be used in all quantitative and most qualitative laboratory procedures, for electrophoretic analyses, for toxicology screening procedures, and in the preparation of buffers, standards, and controls. Further treatment of type I water may be necessary for trace element and

heavy metal analyses. Type II water is acceptable for use in reagents with preservatives or reagents that are sterilized, and in most stains. Type III water is acceptable for washing and preliminary rinsing of glassware. It may also serve as source water for further purification.

Special-purpose reagent water may be necessary for specific procedures such as High Performance Liquid Chromatography (HPLC), chromosome analyses, HLA testing and in vitro fertilization, and gamete intrafallopian transfer (IVF/GIFT) procedures. Systems can be designed to produce water that meets specific requirements, or type I water can be purified further.

Quality control and impurity testing

Water must be monitored at regular intervals to evaluate the performance of a water-purification system. Because of the variety of contaminants found in water, no single test can measure water purity. The time schedule for regular evaluations may vary with the season and with the contaminants found. In addition to ensuring that the purification system is functioning acceptably under routine conditions, monitoring ensures the purity of the water after a component or components of the system have been changed. As a minimum, bacterial surveillance and resistivity determinations are necessary on a frequent basis. The monitoring of other parameters such as pH, silicate content, pyrogens, organic contamination, and particulate matter will depend on many factors. Each laboratory will have to determine frequency guidelines based on the history, system design, and use of its water-purification system. In general, if the source water and the purification system produce a product that is consistently negative for a particular contaminant, the laboratory may test for that contaminant on an infrequent basis. Some of the tests must be performed by the laboratory, and other tests may be referred out.

Microbial monitoring. Bacteria can inactivate reagents by metabolizing certain reagent components. In addition, they contribute to the total organic contamination

Table 1-3   Suggested uses of reagent water

Special*	Type I	Type II	Type III
HPLC	Assays of trace elements and heavy metals†	Bacteriological media preparation	Glassware washing and preliminary rinse
Tissue/cell culture (pyrogen free)	Enzyme assays	Stains and dyes (histology/ parasitology)	
	Ligand assays		
	Reagents without preservatives		
Chromosome analysis	Quantitative (immuno)- fluorescent assays	Reagents that will be sterilized	
IVF/GIFT‡	Preparation of standard solutions	Reagents with preservatives	
HLA testing (with ultrafilter)	Electrophoretic procedures		

NOTE: The specifications of reagent water defined in this table are those for the water at the time of production. Type I water cannot be stored because its resistivity will decrease and metals or organic contaminants will be leached from the storage container. Bacterial contamination may also occur.

*For certain purposes, additional requirements beyond those specified for type I water may be necessary. This column lists several of those purposes.

†When accurate determinations of chemical species (trace elements or heavy metals) at the level of μg/L (parts per billion) are required, the water used must be tested for the trace species under consideration. If present, such trace species may be tolerated only at a concentration that is not significant for the concentration level at which the analysis is to be performed.

‡In vitro fertilization/gamete intrafallopian transfer.

and can alter optical properties of test solutions. Although microbial monitoring is retrospective, it provides the laboratory with useful information and may be helpful in detecting impending problems. Testing should be performed on a weekly basis. Several acceptable methods are available, though no single method can be assumed to quantitate all bacteria in a water sample. Thus the number of viable bacteria may be higher than the number of colony-forming units determined in any given method. Several criteria may be applied to choosing a method, but no matter which method is selected, the first step in obtaining a reliable result is the collection of an appropriate sample.

Before collection, the spigot should be fully opened for at least 1 minute. This procedure will flush the system adequately. The system must also be flushed before one draws water for use in reagent preparation. One of the most common causes of bacterial contamination in water is inadequate flushing. The volume of water collected for analysis will vary with the procedure used. Anywhere from 1 mL (for bacteriologic samplers) to 100 mL (standard plate count or filtration methods) may be collected. After collection, the sample should be processed as soon as possible. The sample may not be stored more than 1 hour at room temperature, or 6 hours in the refrigerator. For certain procedures the sample must be vortexed vigorously to ensure distribution of organisms within the sample. The most commonly found organisms are gram-negative rods.

Resistivity. Resistivity measurements are used to assess the ionic content of purified water. The higher the ion concentration, the lower the resistivity. Ion-exchange tanks should be equipped with an in-line "resistivity" light that is calibrated to go off when the resistivity falls below 2 $M\Omega$·cm, at which point the capacity of the tanks is exhausted. Systems that supply type I water *must* have an in-line resistivity meter that is capable of reading to 18 $M\Omega$·cm. The resistivity must be at least 10 $M\Omega$·cm (preferably 15 to 18 $M\Omega$·cm) in order to meet type I specifications. Off-line measurements may be used for resistivity monitoring of type II and type III water; however, in-line measurements are easier and more accurate and are recommended for systems producing type II water. Procedures for off-line measurements are available.[1] The frequency of monitoring is daily.

pH. It is generally not necessary to monitor the pH of purified (particularly type I) water. Methods are available in the event that a pH problem is suspected.[1] Anecdotal reports have suggested that in some facilities' source-water pH problems have led to product-water pH problems. There are now some systems that allow in-line pH measurements. These systems, however, are not yet used in clinical laboratories.

Pyrogens. Pyrogens are not monitored routinely in the clinical laboratory. However, anecdotal reports from manufacturers indicate that some immunoassay reagents are affected by interference from pyrogens. Thus testing for this contaminant may become more important with time. Procedures for such testing are readily available.[4,5]

Silica. Silica in the water supply can be a major problem in some geographical areas. Silica can interfere with trace metal and electrolyte analyses, enzyme determinations, and some spectrophotometric assays. Colloidal silica is readily removed by distillation and certain reverse osmosis membranes. Soluble silica may be measured by spectrophotometric analysis.[1] However the procedure requires the use of a narrow-bandpass instrument, preferably capable of reading at ~800 nm. Frequently the reagent blanks generate absorbances higher than those of the water being tested. For this reason it may be preferable to refer samples for analysis by inductively coupled plasma spectrometry.

Organic contaminants. Bacteria can multiply in the resin beds, significantly increasing the organic contamination of water. Methods for assessing contamination on a routine basis, though plentiful, are either not sufficiently specific (permanganate) or not practical (requiring research-grade spectrophotometers and HPLC). If the laboratory has access to HPLC, the measurement is easily accomplished.[6] The best approach to dealing with organic contamination is to design and maintain the system optimally. *Sanitization* at least on a semiannual basis (or more frequently if quality control data dictate) will help control bacteria levels. Use of carbon adsorption and UV treatment will help remove organic contaminants. Constant surveillance of the system will ensure the production of reagent water of the desired quality.

System documentation and record keeping

A procedure manual should be developed for the water-purification system that includes: (1) a quality assurance plan defining responsibilities of personnel, (2) procedures for preventive maintenance, (3) quality control checklists, (4) worksheets for documenting daily, weekly, monthly, and other testing, and (5) documentation of all corrective action taken.[1,7]

CHEMICAL LABORATORY SUPPLIES
Chemicals

Chemicals are available in varying degrees of purity, and, in many instances, the types and concentrations of impurities are known. Less pure grades of chemicals include *chemically pure, practical grade, technical grade,* and *commercial grade.* Such chemicals are unsuitable for use in analytical work. Certain chemicals, especially pharmaceuticals, are produced to meet the specifications that are given in *The United States Pharmacopeia (USP), The National Formulary,* and *The Food Chemical Index.* These specifications define impurity tolerances that will not be injurious to health.

Most qualitative and quantitative analyses in the clinical laboratory require the use of chemicals that meet the specifications of the ACS; such chemicals are described as either analytical grade or reagent grade. ACS specifications establish the maximum quantities of impurities allowable in each chemical or provide impurity contents on a lot-to-lot basis. Some manufacturers sell certified or very pure materials when specifications have not been established by the ACS.

Additional standards of purity for certain chemicals have been specified by the *International Union for Pure and Applied Chemistry (IUPAC)*. These include atomic weight standards (grade A), ultimate standards (grade B), primary standards (grade C), which are commercially available and have less than 0.002% impurities, working standards (grade D), which are commercially available and have less than 0.05% impurities, and secondary substances (grade E), which are defined or standardized by an acceptable reference method using a primary standard (grade C) as the reference material.

Primary standards

Primary standards are supplied with certificates of analysis for each lot. These preparations must be stable, nonhygroscopic substances of definite composition that can be dried without changing composition.

Standard reference materials

Standard reference materials (SRMs) are available from the *National Institute for Standards and Technology (NIST)*. Not all SRMs are as pure as primary standards; however, NIST defines their chemical and physical properties and provides a certificate documenting results of characterization. These standards may then be used to characterize other materials. SRMs are available in solid, liquid, or gaseous form. The solids may be crystalline, powder, or lyophilized products.

Organic solvents

Classification of organic solvents follows the same guidelines as those used for other chemicals. Thus for many analyses, in particular those involving spectroscopy and chromatography, reagents of even higher purity than reagent grade are required. These solvents frequently are referred to as *spectrograde*, *nanograde*, or *HPLC grade*, and information about the presence of contaminants is supplied with the solvent. The purity ensures minimal spectral interference and minimal residual contamination after extraction and evaporation of the solvent in the analytic procedure. In general these solvents are more than 99% pure (as determined by gas chromatography) and no single impurity exceeds 0.2%.

Gases

Gases, particularly those used in gas chromatography and atomic absorption analyses, must be extremely pure. Helium purity must be 99.9999% for gas chromatographic procedures. As with other reagents, information regarding contaminants and their concentrations is of utmost importance. (See Appendix D for more specific information.)

Chemical safety

Many chemicals and solvents are flammable, teratogenic, or carcinogenic. Thus all chemicals should be handled with great care, and inhalation of fumes or dust should be avoided. Similarly the handling of gas cylinders requires adherence to specific regulations. The specifics of safe practices will be discussed in the laboratory safety section.

Desiccants (Table 1-4)

A desiccant is a material used to absorb and remove water from the air or from another substance. Some desiccants are deliquescent and therefore lose their efficiency after liquefaction occurs. Others produce dust and should therefore be avoided. The most commonly used desiccants are manufactured with a moisture-sensitive indicator salt, such as cobalt chloride, to indicate exhaustion. Silica gel and Drierite (anhydrous calcium sulfate) are examples. These agents can be regenerated by heat, making them cost efficient.

LABORATORY PLASTIC AND GLASSWARE COMPOSITION AND CLEANING

Laboratory supplies that are used for the preparation, measurement, and storage of fluids and other products of reactions include tubing, glassware, and plasticware. Glass must be used for procedures involving HPLC and gas-liquid chromatography (GLC), since solvents readily attack plas-

Table 1-4 Some common drying agents (desiccants)

Desiccant	Properties	Uses
Anhydrous $CaCl_2$	High capacity, slow acting, works well below 30° C	Most conditions, very inexpensive
Anhydrous $MgSO_4$	Neutral, rapid action	Most conditions, inexpensive
Anhydrous Na_2SO_4	Neutral, high capacity, works only below 32° C, slow action	Can remove large volumes of water
Anhydrous $CaSO_4$	Extremely rapid in action, chemically inert, limited capacity to absorb water (6% to 10% weight in water)	More expensive than $MgSO_4$ and Na_2SO_4; sold commercially as Drierite; can be easily regenerated by heating at 230° to 240° C for 3 hours
Al_2O_3 (activated alumina)	Can absorb 15% to 20% of its weight in water	Can be repeatedly reactivated by heating at 175° C for 7 hours

tics. On the other hand, many solutions with a pH above 6.0 can attack glassware, and alkaline solutions should be stored in plastic.[8] Glass also tends to adsorb metal ions, possibly altering significantly the concentrations of standard solutions.

Tubing. Natural latex rubber tubing is durable and can be used for glass connections. It is, however, affected by contact with oils, alkalis, corrosives, and hot water. Neoprene (synthetic) rubber tubing may be substituted for latex tubing in most situations. It should not be used with chlorinated or aromatic hydrocarbons.

More expensive than rubber tubing, synthetic plastic Tygon tubing is the most useful. Tygon is resistant to chemicals and is chemically inert to chemicals. It can be used in many applications such as peristaltic pumps; it can also be joined to other tubing using a heat welding process. Over time it tends to discolor and become slightly brittle. Polytetrafluoroethylene (Teflon) tubing is also available; it is more expensive than Tygon tubing but serves as a substitute in certain situations.

Types of glass. There are many types of glass commercially available. They differ in their tensile strength, resistivity to certain agents, and heat or light resistance. Most reusable glassware in the clinical laboratory is made from borosilicate glass, which is available under the brand names of Pyrex (Corning Glass Works, Corning, N.Y.) and Kimax (Kimble Glass Company, Vineland, N.J.). Borosilicate glass has a low alkaline earth content and is free of contaminants such as heavy metals. Thus liquids can be heated in borosilicate glass with minimal contamination. This type of glass can be safely heated to approximately 600° C for short periods. Table 1-5 lists additional types of glass and their uses.

Types of plastic. Plastic laboratory utensils are made from polymerized organic monomers. The properties of the plastics depend on the nature of the monomer and the final polymer forms used to prepare the plastic materials. The most commonly used plastics include the polyolefins (polyethylene, polypropylene), polystyrene, polycarbonate, polytetrafluoroethylene (Teflon), and polyvinyl chloride.

Polyolefins, which are relatively chemically inert, are resistant to most acids, alkalis, and salt solutions. Organic acids and other hydrocarbons cause swelling and penetration of the plastic. Concentrated sulfuric acid attacks polyethylene at room temperature. Polyethylene is used in most disposable plasticware and cannot be sterilized. Polypropylene may be sterilized.

Polycarbonate is stronger than polypropylene and has better temperature tolerances. Its chemical resistance is not as good as that of the polyolefins. Its primary advantages are its clarity and resistance to shatter, making it the material of choice for items such as centrifuge tubes.

Teflon is an extremely inert plastic with excellent temperature tolerance (-270 to $+255°$ C) and chemical resistivity. Because of its nonwettable surface and antiadhesive properties, it is an excellent material for stir bars, bottle-cap liners, stopcocks, and tubing. It is one of the most desirable materials for use in water distribution systems; however, it is considerably more costly than other plastics used for this purpose. Although it is easy to clean and dry, it scratches and warps readily.

Table 1-5   Types of commonly used glass and their properties

Glass	Properties	Purpose
Kimax/Pyrex	Relatively inert borosilicate glass, high resistance to heat and cold shock	All purpose
Vycor	Good resistance to drastic conditions of heat, shock, chemical treatment, and high temperature; acid and alkali resistant	Ashing, ignition techniques
Corex	Aluminosilicate glass, about six-fold stronger than borosilicate glass; scratch resistant; resistant to alkaline etching	Used under conditions of stress
High silica	>96% silicate; comparable to fused quartz; heat, chemical, and electrical tolerance; excellent optical properties	For high-precision analytical work, optical reflectors, and mirrors
Boron-free	Alkali resistant; poor heat resistance; soft; <0.2% boron	Highly alkaline solutions
Low actinic	Amber or red color reduces light exposure of contents	For use with light-sensitive materials in range of 300 to 500 nm (e.g., bilirubin, vitamin A, carotene)
Flint	Soda-lime glass containing oxides of sodium, silicon, and calcium; poor resistance to high temperature or temperature changes, poor chemical resistance; may also leach organic contaminants	Used for disposable glassware items (e.g., pipets)
Coated	Thin, metallic oxide fire-bonded to glass surface	Conducts electricity, acts as electrostatic shield; protects against infrared
Optical	Made of soda lime, lead, and borosilicate	Prisms, lenses, and optical mirrors
Pyroceram	High thermal resistance, chemically stable, corrosion resistant	Hot plates, heat exchangers

Polyvinyl chloride plastic is soft and flexible but porous. It is used frequently in the form of tubing, particularly in reagent water systems. Its drawbacks have been discussed in the section on reagent water.

Table 1-6 reviews the characteristics of some plastics commonly encountered in laboratory products.

In many instances plastic utensils should be used instead of glass because plastic utensils do not release ions into solution, and they are unbreakable. However, some plastics such as polyethylene are porous, and evaporation may be a problem. Thus long-term storage in partially filled plastic containers is undesirable. In addition, polyethylene and other plastics can adsorb proteins and other compounds such as dyes, stains, and some salts, resulting in analytical

Table 1-6 Summary of the chemical resistance (at 20° C) and physical properties of various plastics

Classes of substances	Types of resins*									
	LDPE	HDPE	PP, PA	PMP	FEP, TFE, ETFE	PC	PSF	PVC bottles†	PS	Nylon
Chemical resistance										
Acids, dilute or weak	E	E	E	E	E	E	E	E	E	F
Acids,‡ strong and concentrated	E	E	E	E	E	N	G	E	F	N
Alcohols, aliphatic	E	E	E	E	E	G	G	E	E	G
Aldehydes	G	G	G	G	E	F	F	N	N	F
Bases	E	E	E	E	E	N	E	E	E	F
Esters	G	G	G	G	E	N	N	N	N	E
Hydrocarbons, aliphatic	F	G	G	F	E	F	G	E	N	E
Hydrocarbons, aromatic	F	G	F	F	E	N	N	N	N	E
Hydrocarbons, halogenated	N	F	F	N	E	N	N	N	N	G
Ketones	G	G	G	F	E	N	N	N	N	E
Oxidizing agents, strong	F	F	F	F	E	N	G	G	N	N
Physical properties										
Maximum-use temperature (° C)	80	120	135 (PP) 130 (PA)	175	205 (FEP) 150 (ETFE)	135	165	70¶	—	—
Brittleness temperature (° C)	−100	−100	0 (PP) −40 (PA)	20	−270 (FEP) −100 (ETFE)	−135	−100	−30	—	—
Sterilization§										
Autoclaving	No	No	Yes	Yes	Yes	Yes‖	Yes	No¶	—	—
Gas	Yes	Yes	Yes	Yes	Yes	Yes	Yes	Yes	—	—
Dry heat	No	No	No	Yes‖	Yes	No	Yes	No	—	—
Chemical	Yes	Yes	Yes	Yes	Yes	Yes	Yes	Yes	—	—

Modified from *1983-1984 Nalgene Labware Catalog,* Nalge Co., Division of Sybron Corp., Rochester, N.Y.
Resin codes: *ETFE,* Tefzel ETFE (ethylene tetrafluoroethylene); *FEP,* Teflon FEP (fluorinated ethylene propylene); *HDPE,* high-density polyethylene; *LDPE,* low-density polyethylene; *PA,* polyallomer; *PC,* polycarbonate; *PMP,* polymethylpentene ("TPX"); *PP,* polypropylene; *PS,* polystyrene; *PSF,* polysulfone; *PVC,* polyvinyl chloride; *TFE,* Teflon TFE (tetrafluoroethylene).
Chemical resistance classification: *E,* 30 days of constant exposure cause no damage. Plastic may even tolerate it for years. *G,* Little or no damage after 30 days of constant exposure to the reagent. *F,* Some effect after 7 days of constant exposure to the reagent. Depending on the plastic, the effect may be crazing, cracking, loss of strength, or discoloration. Solvents may cause softening, swelling, and permeation losses with LDPE, HDPE, PP, PA, and PMP. The solvent effects on these five resins are normally reversible; the part will usually return to its normal condition after evaporation. *N,* Not recommended for continuous use. Immediate damage may occur. Depending on the plastic, the effect will be a more severe crazing, cracking, loss of strength, discoloration, deformation, dissolution, or permeation loss.
†For polyvinyl chloride tubing, see the current *Nalgene Labware Catalog.*
‡Except for oxidizing acids. For oxidizing acids, see "Oxidizing agents, strong."
§Sterilization: Autoclaving: Clean and rinse item with distilled water before autoclaving. Certain chemicals that have no appreciable effect on resin at room temperature may cause deterioration at autoclaving temperatures unless removed with distilled water beforehand. *Gas:* Ethylene oxide. *Dry heat:* At 160° C. *Chemical:* Benzalkonium chloride, formalin, ethanol, and so on.
‖Sterilizing reduces mechanical strength. Do not use polycarbonate vessels for vacuum applications if they have been autoclaved.
¶Except for the polyvinyl chloride in tubing, which will withstand temperatures to 121° C and can be autoclaved. Refer to "The Use and Care of Plastic Labware" in the current *Nalgene Labware Catalog* for detailed information on sterilization.
Interpretation of chemical resistance. This summary is a general guide only. Because so many factors can affect the chemical resistance of a given product, you should test under your own conditions. If any doubt exists about specific applications of Nalgene products, please contact Technical Service, Nalgene Labware Department, Nalge Company, 75 Panorama Creek Drive, Rochester, NY 14602, or call (716) 586-3985, Fax (716) 264-3707.
Effects of chemicals on plastics. Chemicals can affect the strength, flexibility, surface appearance, color, dimensions, or weight of plastics. The basic modes of interaction that cause these changes are (1) chemical attack on the polymer chain, resulting in reduction in physical properties, including oxidation; reaction of functional groups in or on the chain; and depolymerization; (2) physical change, including absorption of solvents, resulting in softening and swelling of the plastic; permeation of solvent through the plastic; dissolution in a solvent; and (3) stress cracking from the interaction of a "stress-cracking agent" with molded-in or external stresses. The reactive combination of compounds of two or more classes may cause a synergistic or undesirable chemical effect. Other factors affecting chemical resistance include temperature, pressure, and internal or external stresses (such as centrifugation), length of exposure, and concentration of the chemical. As temperature increases, resistance to attack decreases.
CAUTION. Do not store strong oxidizing agents in plastic labware except that made of Teflon FEP. Prolonged exposure causes embrittlement and failure. Although prolonged storage may not be intended at the time of filling, a forgotten container will fail in time and result in leakage of contents. Do not place plastic labware in a flame or on a hot plate.

problems. Nevertheless, plastic containers are preferable for use in trace-metal analyses. One can remove the small quantities of trace metals in the plastic by soaking the plastic in 1 M HCl and rinsing with water purified to eliminate trace-metal contamination. For even more sensitive analytical analyses, the plastic is then soaked in 1 M HNO_3 (highest purity) and rinsed with purified water. Long-term soaking (>8 hr) in acid should be avoided, since it makes the plastic brittle. Plastic can also be cleaned with alcohol, alkalis, or alcoholic alkalis to remove trace organic contaminants that contribute to trace-metal adsorption.

Cleaning of glass and plastic utensils. Glassware must be thoroughly clean before it is used in any analytical procedure. Unclean glassware will result in chemical contamination. In addition, if glassware is not clean, the surface of the glass will not wet uniformly, and volume errors, caused by incomplete drainage of dispensing devices or distortion of the meniscus, will result.

Dirty utensils should be rinsed immediately after use and soaked in either a weak detergent solution or in a tenfold dilution of household bleach. Any vessels in which hazardous materials were contained should be handled separately to prevent unintentional exposure to the hazardous agent. Numerous effective cleaning agents are available for washing laboratory glassware and plasticware. Some items, such as pipets, will require additional soaking before washing. In many institutions washing is done by an automatic glassware washer. The manufacturers of automatic washers usually recommend or require specific detergents. In general, metal-free, nonionic detergents that are not highly alkaline are used. The washer must be equipped with the appropriate purified water rinse cycles to prevent contamination. If utensils are washed manually, they must be thoroughly rinsed with tap water and then rinsed three to five times with purified, preferably type I, water. When glassware is clean, purified water drains as a continuous film; whereas unclean vessels will have small drops of water clinging to the surface. After drying, the appearance of spots indicates unclean glassware, possibly the result of inadequate rinsing. This procedure is not appropriate for nonwettable plastics.

One can detect incomplete detergent removal by rinsing a vessel with a dilute (20 mg/L) aqueous solution of sulfobromophthalein (Bromsulphalein) dye or some other acid-base indicator, or by measuring the pH of purified water added to the glassware.

As previously mentioned acid washing may be necessary in some instances. Dilute HCl (1 M) or dilute HNO_3 (1 M) is preferred. Chromic acid is no longer used for this procedure because of residual contamination and the hazards of handling and preparing the solutions.

Ultrasonic cleaners can be used to supplement the action of detergents. These may be particularly helpful in cleaning protein-coated utensils.

Both glassware and plasticware should be dried either at room temperature or at temperatures below 100° C. This procedure will prevent degradation of the plastic and changes in the volume designations of glassware. If solvents are used to assist in drying, they should be of high quality and water miscible. Any gases used should also be of high purity.

LABORATORY UTENSILS

Beakers. Beakers (Fig. 1-1,*D*) are wide-mouthed, straight-sided, cylindrical vessels available in both glass and plastic. Beaker volumes vary from 5 mL to several liters. They are used for general mixing and preparation of nonvolumetric liquid reagents.

Funnels. Funnels are most commonly used to transfer liquids or solids into containers. *Filtering funnels* (Fig. 1-1,*G*) are usually 58- or 60-degree angled funnels with either short or long, thin stems. They are used with filter paper to remove particles from solution. Many funnels have ridges to increase the surface area available for filtering purposes. *Powder funnels* for use in transferring solids (Fig. 1-1,*H*) have wide-mouthed stems to allow easy passage of solids. The inner surface of these funnels is smooth. Both filtering and powder funnels are available in plastic and glass. *Separatory funnels* (Fig. 1-1,*B*) are constructed with a ground-glass stoppered opening at one end and a stopcock opening at the other end. These devices are used for manual liquid-liquid extractions of relatively large volumes of samples. The lower phase is separated from the upper phase through the stopcock, allowing salvage of one or both phases.

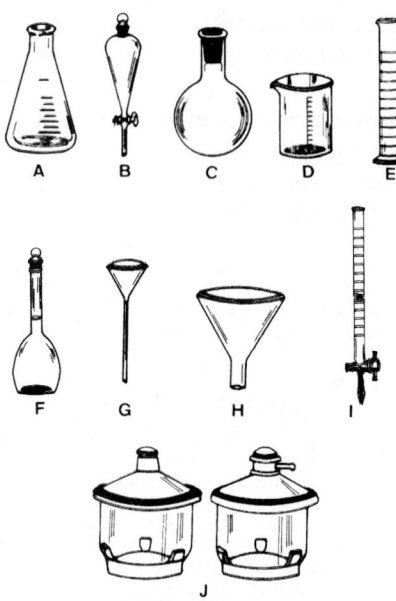

Fig. 1-1 Examples of commonly used laboratory utensils. **A,** Ehrlenmeyer flask. **B,** Separatory funnel. **C,** Round-bottom flask. **D,** Beaker. **E,** Graduated cylinder. **F,** Volumetric flask. **G,** Long-stem funnel (filtering). **H,** Powder funnel. **I,** Buret. **J,** Desiccators.

Desiccators. Desiccators (Fig. 1-1,*J*) are used to dry, or keep dry, solid or liquid materials. The desiccant is usually placed in the bottom of the desiccator and a shelf placed above the desiccant. The material is then stored on top of the shelf. The top of the desiccator has a wide, flat, ground-glass lip that fits snugly against an opposing lip on the bottom part of the desiccator. Stopcock grease is usually placed on the surface of the lips to provide an airtight seal. Many desiccators also have a stopcock outlet on the upper portion to allow the desiccator to be evacuated. A laboratory will often have several desiccators to allow for storage at different temperatures including ambient, refrigerator, and freezer temperatures. The types of desiccants available are described in Table 1-4.

Graduated cylinders. Graduated cylinders are narrow, straight-sided vessels that are used to measure specific volumes (Fig. 1-1,*E*). Graduated cylinders are available in plastic and glass in sizes ranging from 5 mL to several liters. They may be calibrated *to deliver (TD)* or *to contain (TC)* the volume indicated at specific temperatures, and they are graduated into subdivisions of approximately 100 portions of the total volume of the cylinder. Sometimes they are equipped with stoppers and are used to prepare solutions requiring less accuracy than those prepared volumetrically.

Burets. Traditional burets are long, graduated glass tubes with a stopcock at one end (Fig. 1-1,*I*). These devices are used to deliver, accurately, known amounts of liquid into a container. By measurement from graduated line to graduated line, fractional volumes of less than 1 mL may be dispensed with a high degree of accuracy. There are now available automatic burets that are microprocessor-controlled devices with an accuracy as high as 0.1%. The dispensed volumes are monitored on a digital display capable of reading to 0.001 mL.

Flasks. Flasks of many types are used in the clinical laboratory; the most commonly used are the volumetric and Erlenmeyer flasks shown in Fig. 1-1,*F* and *A*. Round-bottom flasks are often used to evaporate a sample to

Table 1-7   Accuracies of volumetric flasks

Capacity (mL)	Limit of error (mL)	Percent error
25	0.03	0.1
50	0.05	0.1
100	0.08	0.08
250	0.11	0.04
500	0.15	0.03
1000	0.30	0.03

dryness. The sizes of laboratory flasks vary from 1 mL to several liters.

Volumetric flasks. Volumetric flasks are essential for the accurate preparation of solutions of known concentration. Class A specifications for volumetric flasks are defined by the NIST and imprinted on the glass (Fig. 1-2). These specifications are accurate only at the temperature specified on the flask (Table 1-7). Volumetric flasks are used to contain (TC) an exact volume when the flask is filled to the indicator line. Such flasks therefore do not deliver an exact volume and cannot be used as transfer devices. The top of the volumetric flask is capped by a tight-fitting ground-glass or Teflon stopper. This allows the flask to be inverted without loss of liquid. Under no circumstances should a volumetric flask be heated because heating can distort the shape and volume of the flask. **Volumetric flasks should not be used for reagent storage.**

Syringes. Syringes may be used for accurate volumetric work such as the injection of small volumes of liquid for chromatographic analysis. Syringes are available in a range of sizes from 1 to 500 μL. They are constructed of glass and have a precision-bore hole into which is placed a tight-fitting plunger. The dispensing tip of the syringe is a very fine diameter metal needle that is able to pierce the septum of the injection port. For syringes of greater than 5 μL volume, manufacturers claim that inaccuracy will not exceed 1% of the total syringe volume and repeated measurements will not differ by more than 1% of the dispensed

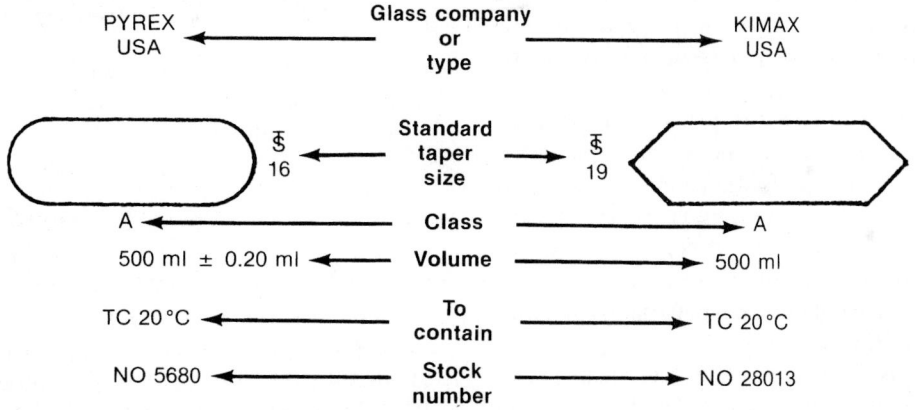

Fig. 1-2   Example of NIST (National Institute of Science and Technology) specifications found imprinted on class A volumetric flasks.

volume. For devices of less than 5 μL volume, 2% inaccuracy is the best that is achievable. In general, syringes are not calibrated because internal standards are employed in chromatographic procedures, allowing for correction of transfer errors. For gas chromatographic work with volatile samples, the syringes must be airtight.

Pipets

Most pipets are made of glass, though plastic serological pipets are available. Two general categories of manual pipets are defined: transfer (volumetric) and measuring. Within these categories, there are three further subclassifications: to contain (TC), to deliver (TD), and to deliver/ blow-out (TD/blow-out) designations.

TC or *rinse-out* pipets must be refilled or rinsed with the appropriate solvent after the initial liquid has been drained from the pipet. These pipets contain or hold an exact amount of liquid that must be completely transferred for accurate measurement. Some examples of TC pipets are Sahli hemoglobin, transfer micro, and Lang-Levy pipets. None of these devices meets class A specifications.

TD/blow-out pipets are filled and allowed to drain, after which the remaining fluid in the tip is blown out. These devices thus transfer or deliver an exact amount of liquid and are not rinsed out. Pipets belonging to this group include Ostwald-Folin and serological devices. They are easily identified by the two frosted bands near the mouthpiece of the pipet (Fig. 1-3). Serological pipets are long glass (or plastic) tubes of uniform diameter. They have volume graduations extending to the delivery tip of the pipet. Thus the last drop of liquid blown out is included in the delivery volume. These pipets come with long tapered tips and variable tip openings to allow for controlled delivery. Pipets with large tipped openings are used for delivery of viscous fluids.

TD pipets are filled and allowed to drain by gravity. To ensure complete drainage, the flow rates are set to specifications defined by the NIST. The pipet must be held vertically and the tip placed against the side of the accepting vessel but not touching the liquid in it. Pipets classified in this group include volumetric transfer, Mohr, and serological pipets (Figs. 1-3 and 1-4). TD pipets meet class A standards.

Volumetric (TD) pipets (Figs. 1-3 and 1-4) have an open-ended bulb, which holds the bulk of the liquid, a long glass tube at one end with a line (mark) indicating the extent to which the pipet is to be filled, and a tapered delivery portion. After draining, these devices deliver the volume specified with a high degree of accuracy (Table 1-8). *Ostwald-Folin* (TD) pipets are similar in appearance to volumetric pipets but have their bulbs closer to the delivery tip. They are used for accurate measurement of viscous liquids such as blood or serum and require that the contents be blown out. Thus they have etched bands near the top. To ensure complete delivery of the viscous fluid, the liquid is blown

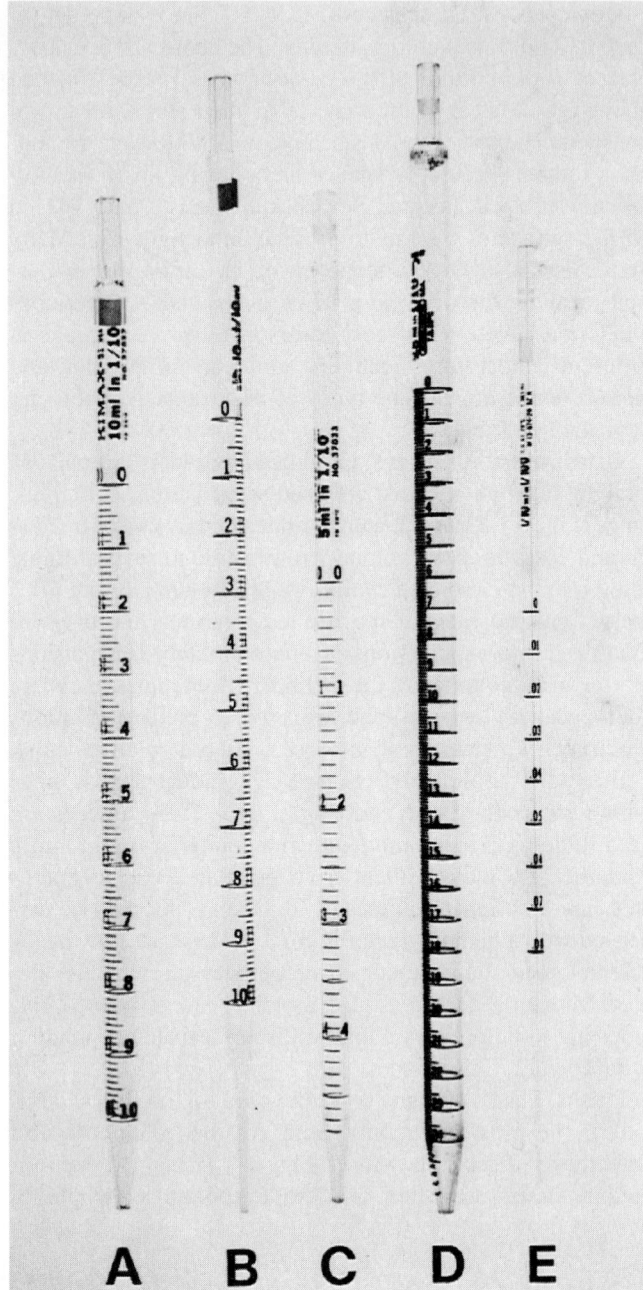

Fig. 1-3 Examples of transfer to deliver (TD) pipets. **A,** Mohr. **B,** Mohr long tip. **C,** Serological. **D,** Serological large opening. **E,** Serological long tip.

out after the pipet is allowed to drain freely to the last drop.

Mohr (TD) pipets are uniform in diameter with tapered delivery tips. Graduations are incised on the stem at uniform intervals so that the calibration occurs above but not on the tip. The accuracy listed for these pipets is valid only when the pipet is filled. If smaller volumes are dispensed, the accuracy decreases proportionally. Mohr pipets with long tips are used for dispensing liquids into small vials.

Table 1-8 Accuracies (in mL) of manual pipets

Type of pipet	1.0 mL	5.0 mL	10.0 mL	25.0 mL
NBS standard	—	0.01	0.02	0.025
Class A volumetric	0.006	0.01	0.02	0.03
Mohr	0.01	0.02	0.03	0.10
Mohr long tip	0.02	0.04	0.06	—
Serological	0.01	0.02	0.03	0.10
Serological large opening	0.05	0.10	0.10	0.20
Serological long tip	0.02	0.04	0.06	—

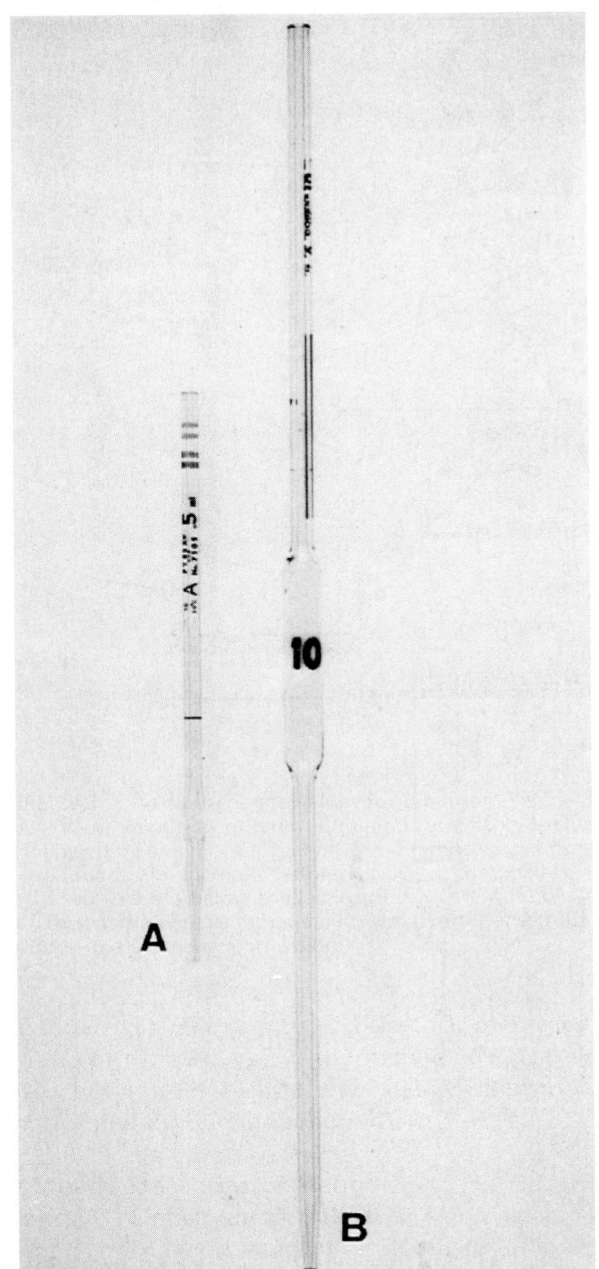

Fig. 1-4 Examples of to deliver (TD) pipets. **A,** Ostwald-Folin. **B,** Class A volumetric.

They are less accurate than the standard tapered-tip variety. Mohr pipets are never used as blow-out devices. The accuracy of Mohr and other pipets is summarized in Table 1-8.

Micropipets

Micropipets contain or deliver small volumes of liquid ranging from 1 to 1000 μL. Reusable glass micropipets are no longer used in the clinical laboratory; however, their characteristics are described elsewhere.[9] Inexpensive disposable tubes with specific volume demarcations are available. They are filled by capillary action, and the liquid is blown out of the tube by a device that is similar to a medicine dropper.

The most common type of micropipet is a semiautomated device that uses either air displacement or positive displacement to dispense the contained liquid. Some models with a digital volume adjustment are also available. There are many brands of *air-displacement* pipets, but all are piston-operated devices. A disposable and exchangeable polypropylene tip is attached to the pipet barrel, and liquid is drawn into and dispensed from this disposable tip (Fig. 1-5). Some instruments can automatically eject the used pipet tip and reload a new one, minimizing analytical contamination. There are also several brands of *positive-displacement* pipets available. The capillary tips, which may be made of siliconized glass, glass, or plastic, can be reused. These devices are particularly useful for handling reagents that will react with plastics. Positive-displacement pipettors deliver liquid by means of a Teflon-tipped plunger that fits snugly inside the capillary. Carryover of liquid is negligible in properly maintained instruments. In some instances, a washing step is used between samples.

The precision and accuracy of these devices are excellent if they are properly maintained. Sample recovery is at least 99%, with reproducibility errors of 0.6% to 0.3% for volumes between 10 and 500 μL. For volumes less than 10 μL the errors are significantly larger. For this reason manual procedures involving small volumes should be avoided.

Dilutors and dispensers

Manual dispensers and pipettors are frequently used in the laboratory to add repeatedly a specified volume of reagent or diluent to a solution (Fig. 1-6). Several types are commercially available, but all consist of a reagent bottle to which a plunger with a valve system is attached. The dispenser is fitted with a tube or straw that essentially reaches to the bottom of the bottle. The device must be primed with liquid to ensure removal of any air bubbles. Once primed, depression of the plunger delivers a selected amount of liquid. Return of the plunger to the raised position refills the dispenser chamber. Manufacturers claim an error of 1% and a reproducibility of 0.1% for these devices at full deflection of the plunger. Manual dispensers require frequent cleaning to remove material that can hamper piston action.

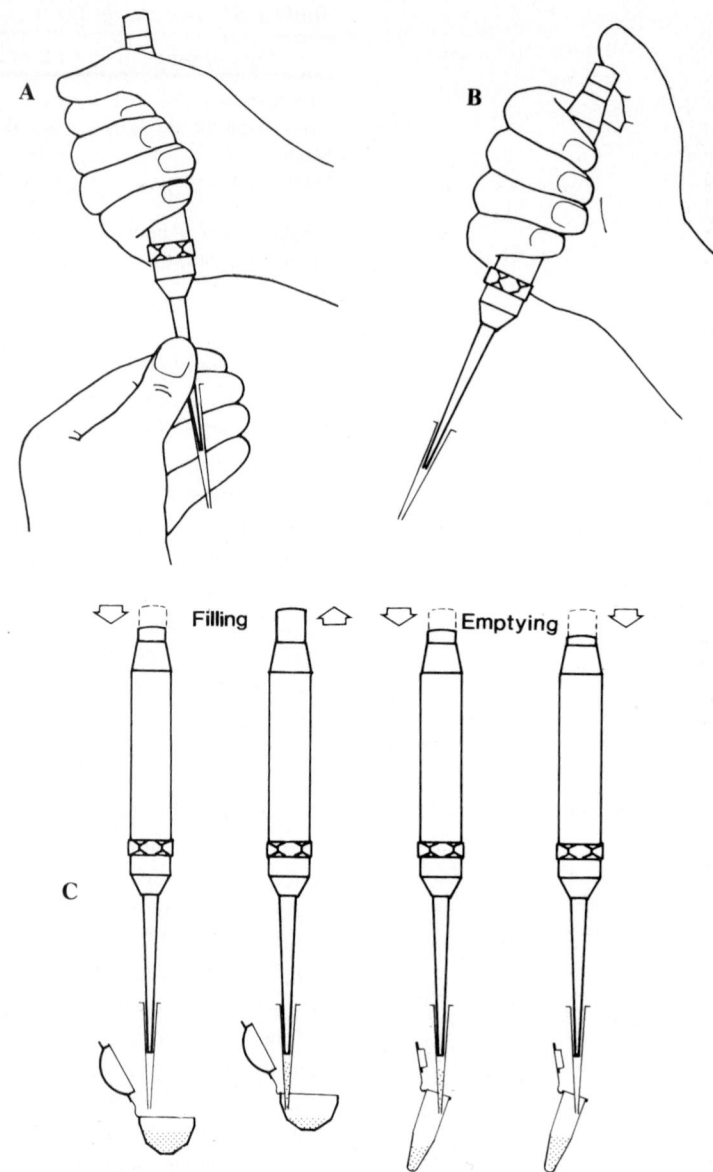

Fig. 1-5 Steps in using Eppendorf type of micropipet. **A,** Attaching proper tip size for range of pipet volume and twisting tip as it is pushed onto pipet to give an airtight, continuous seal. **B,** Holding pipet before use. **C,** Detailed instructions for filling and emptying pipet tip. Follow manufacturer's complete instructions for care and use of micropipets.

Repetitive dispensing pipettors are useful for the serial dispensing of relatively small volumes of the same liquid. The volume dispensed is determined by the pipettor setting and by the size of the disposable syringe type of tip, which also acts as the liquid reservoir.

Automated dilutor-dispensers are frequently used to prepare many samples for analysis. Such devices can be an integral part of an automated chemistry analyzer. The dispensers pipet a preset volume of sample and diluent into a receiving vessel or instrument. The frequently used dual-piston dispenser allows adjustment of both sample and diluent volumes (Fig. 1-7). One motor-driven syringe processes the sample, the other the diluent. The syringes are activated by a microprocessor allowing each piston to fill the syringes simultaneously. A second signal repositions the valves to allow diluent to flow through the sample syringe. This displaces the sample, forcing it through the pipet tip and rinsing it in preparation for the next sample. Variable ratios of sample to diluent can be selected. However, a tenfold volume of diluent will ensure adequate rinsing and negligible carryover. The inaccuracy is considered to be less than 0.5% of dispensed volume, and reproducibility is on the order of 0.05% of full-syringe volume, or 0.1% when at least 10% of the syringe volume is dispensed.

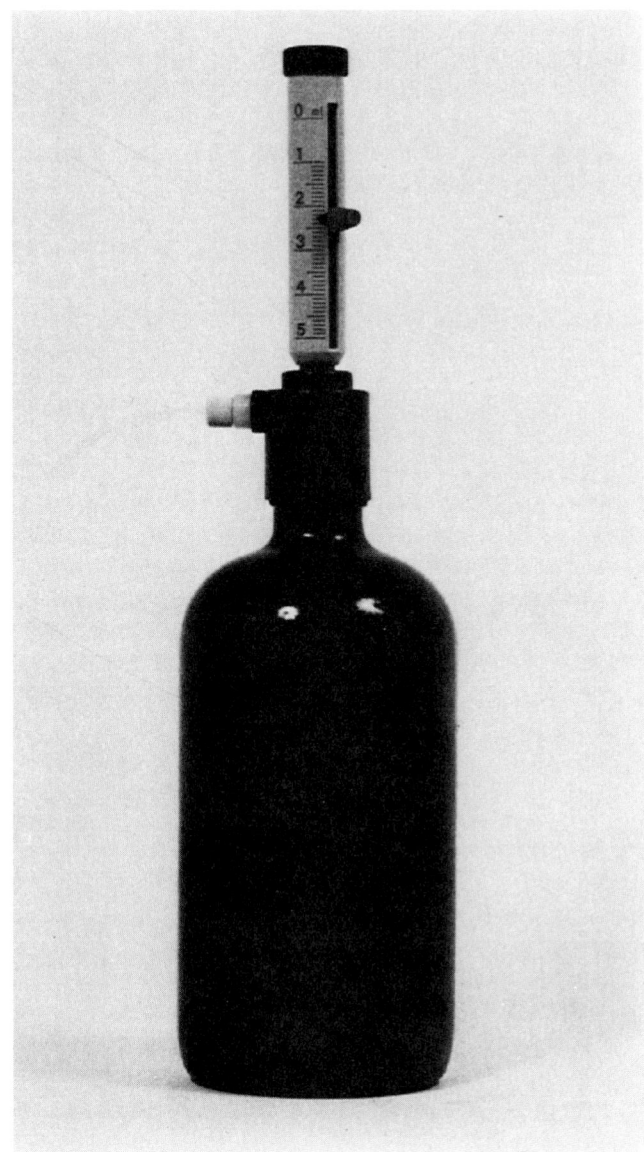

Fig. 1-6 Example of manual dispenser or repipettor.

VOLUMETRIC TECHNIQUES
Class A pipets

Clinical chemistry analytical procedures require exact volumetric measurements and transfers to ensure accurate results, and class A glassware is thus required. In fact, the College of American Pathologists specifies that volumetric pipets must be of certified accuracy (class A) or the volumes of the devices must be verified (for example, by a gravimetric procedure). In addition, automatic pipets and diluting devices must be periodically checked for accuracy and precision. Therefore most laboratories utilize class A glassware on a routine basis. In addition, glassware must be scrupulously clean or beads of liquid will cling to the sides of the dirty vessels and pipets and volume measurements will be inaccurate. Borosili-

cate glass pipets must be inspected frequently. If the tips are broken or the glass is etched, pipets should be discarded.

Class A pipets are filled with the aid of a rubber bulb or similar device. **Under no circumstances is mouth pipetting permissible.** The bulb is used to fill the pipet above the calibration mark. The pipet is grasped by the thumb and middle finger, with the index finger placed over the upper opening, controlling the flow of liquid (Fig. 1-8). Once the pipet is filled above the mark, the tip is wiped with a lint-free tissue to remove excess fluid. The liquid is then allowed to drain so that the lowest part of the meniscus, sighted at eye level, is lined up with the mark. Next the pipet is held in a vertical position, with the tip against the side of the receiving vessel, and the liquid is drained as the index finger is removed from the pipet orifice. TD pipets must be held in position long enough (~2 sec) to permit delivery of the specified volume. With TC or blow-out pipets, the rubber bulb is used to blow out the last remaining solution after drainage is complete.

Micropipets

Air-displacement micropipets may be used in either of two modes, the *forward mode* or the *reverse mode*. The reverse mode is used with two-component stroke mechanism systems only. The precision of these devices in the forward mode depends on the precise draining caused by the air pressure, and they are relatively sensitive to the physical characteristics of the liquid being pipetted. Reverse-mode operation, on the other hand, is considerably less sensitive to the type of liquid being dispensed. In the forward mode the piston is depressed to the first stop on a two-stroke device, the tip is placed in the liquid, and the piston is slowly allowed to rise back to the original position. This fills the tip with the designated volume of liquid. The pipet tip is then drawn up the sidewall of the vessel so that any adhering liquid is removed. If there are any extraneous droplets, the tip is wiped carefully with a lint-free tissue, with care being taken not to "wick" out any sample from the pipet tip. The tip is then placed on the wall of the receiving vessel, and the piston is depressed smoothly to the first stop on a two-stroke device, allowing the liquid to drain. Then one should allow 1 second to elapse before depressing the piston to the second stop, blowing out the remaining liquid. When the reverse mode is used, the liquid is aspirated after depressing to the second stop position. This overfills the pipet with sample. To dispense the liquid, one then depresses the piston to the first stop and removes it after waiting 1 second.

Positive-displacement micropipets are used in the same manner as forward-mode air-displacement devices. Again careful wiping of the tip is crucial in order not to "wick" out a sample from the tip. The need for maintenance of the Teflon tip cannot be overemphasized. More detailed information on this technique is published elsewhere.[10]

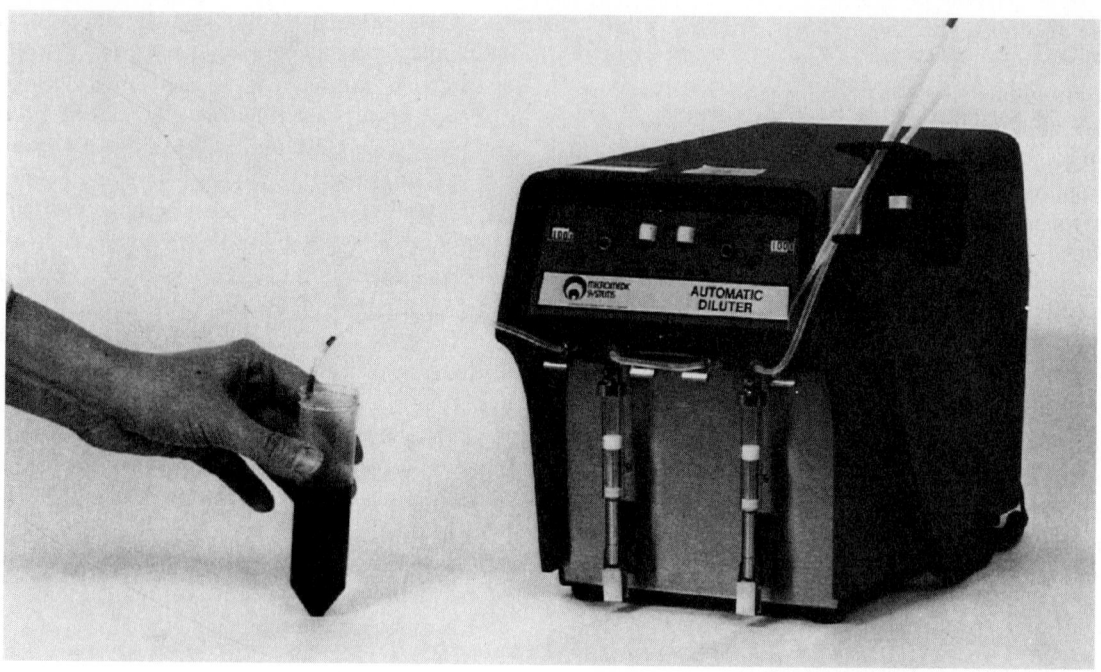

Fig. 1-7   Example of dual-syringe type of dilutor-dispenser.

General procedures for solution preparation

Solution preparation requires accurate measurements of the solute and solvent. The degree of accuracy required will dictate what specific glassware should be used.

1. Measure the solute by weighing, pipetting, or dispensing from a graduated cylinder or pipettor (as examples).

2. Prepare volumetric solutions by quantitatively transferring the solute to the receiving flask. If the solute exists as a stock solution, a volumetric pipet is used for the transfer.

3. Add sufficient solvent to dissolve the solute where necessary.

4. When the receiving flask is a volumetric flask, the solids or liquids are added to the flask and the diluent is added to approximately two thirds the volume of the flask. Dissolution of the solid or liquid can be effected by swirling of the liquid. After dissolution, diluent is added until the meniscus, sighted at eye level, reaches the line etched into the neck of the flask. Completely mix the solution by placing a cover on the opening of the flask, holding the neck of the flask in one's hand, and swirling the liquid while simultaneously inverting the flask. Alternatively the dilution or dissolving of a solid in diluent can be achieved in an Erlenmeyer flask. The solution is then transferred to a volumetric flask, followed by several washes of the Erlenmeyer flask with diluent, transferring the liquid used for the washes to the volumetric flask.

5. Bring the solution to volume after the solute is completely dissolved.

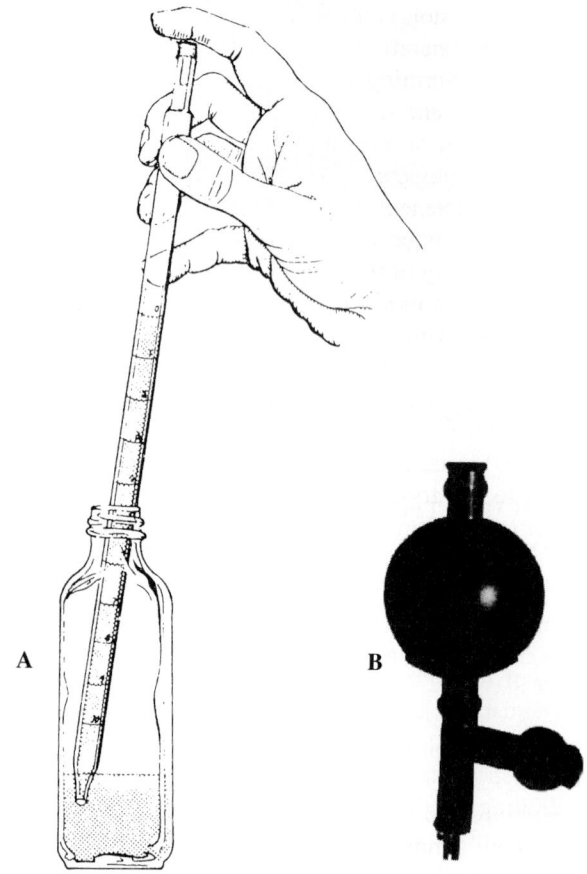

Fig. 1-8   **A,** Proper pipetting technique as described in text. **B,** Example of rubber pipetting bulb used to aspirate sample into pipet.

6. If the use of a magnetic stir bar is necessary, remove the bar and rinse it with solvent before bringing the solution to volume.
7. Bring the solution to volume at room temperature **only.**
8. Mix the solution well to ensure homogeneity.
9. Transfer to an appropriate reagent-storage container (amber/clear, plastic/glass).

Quality control of micropipets, dispensers, and dilutors

General. The accuracy and precision of each manual micropipet should be verified on acquisition and monitored during the course of the year. The frequency of verification will depend on the amount of use. Heavily used devices may need monthly verification, whereas rarely used devices may need to be checked only once or twice per year unless more frequent validation is mandated by an inspection agency. Manufacturers of newer micropipets are claiming a 2-year calibration stability. Whether these claims are accepted by inspection agencies remains to be seen.

Routine maintenance is critical. Air-displacement pipets have a fixed stroke length that must be maintained. In addition, there are seals to prevent air from leaking into the pipet when the piston is moved. These must be greased to maintain proper operation. The manufacturer will provide guidelines for performing this maintenance. Any worn parts must be replaced and devices that do not meet specifications for precision or accuracy will generally require servicing by the manufacturer.

Positive-displacement pipets, in general, require similar maintenance with regard to spring checks and replacement of Teflon tips. Many of these devices also are supplied with a slide wire that is used to quickly check the plunger setting. This device cannot be used in place of routine performance checks. Again the manufacturer provides guidelines for performing routine maintenance.

Quality control validation. The primary method for validating performance of micropipets is a gravimetric technique.[10] A secondary method is a spectrophotometric procedure with potassium dichromate. The latter method is unacceptable for volumes of less than 10 μL. The following protocol describes the gravimetric method of verification and is based on the procedure described in the NCCLS guideline, *Determining Performance of Volumetric Equipment.*[10]

1. Make sure all items used (water, weighing vials, and pipets) are at room temperature.
2. All measurements require the use of type I water.
3. Measure and record the barometric pressure and the ambient temperature (*t*) of the water to 0.1° C.
4. To minimize evaporation errors, place a small amount of water in the weighing vial (between 2 and 30 sample volumes, or a minimum of 0.5 mL). Cover (for example, with a square of Parafilm or with a stopper). Ensure that all manipulations are performed without handling the vial directly.
5. Weigh the vial (water and cover) and record the weight to the nearest 0.1 mg (W_v), or preferably set to zero the weight of the vial, water, and cover.
6. Transfer the aliquot of water to be measured to the weighing vial using the pipet to be tested. Recover the vial.
7. Reweigh the vial to the nearest 0.1 mg and record the weight (W_t).
8. Repeat these measurements (W_v and W_t) to obtain 10 readings in order to evaluate both accuracy and precision. (A "quick check" method using 4 samplings allows rough assessment of precision.)
9. Refer to the *Handbook of Chemistry and Physics*[11] to obtain the correction factor for the water temperature. Assess the conversion factor *z* (μL/mg) incorporating the density of water at the test temperature and pressure.
10. Calculate the volume measured as follows:

$$\text{Mean volume, } \overline{V}_t = \text{Mean weight, } \overline{W}_t \cdot z$$
$$\text{where } \overline{W}_t = W_t$$

11. The *accuracy* is then computed by evaluating the difference between the actual mean volume measured and the nominal volume as stated by the manufacturer, expressed as %:

$$\frac{\text{Mean volume}}{\text{Nominal volume}} \times 100\%$$

12. The *precision* is derived from the distribution of the individual weighings about their mean and expressed as percent coefficient of variation (%CV).

In general, an error of 0.1% or less in the accuracy may be ignored when one is using the pipet. Larger errors may have to be evaluated more critically and the pipet adjusted, if necessary, to achieve a more accurate volume. Manufacturers may use mercury in place of water to assess performance. This practice is discouraged in a routine laboratory setting.

The practice of using radioisotopes and enzymes is unacceptable because of large inherent errors and poor standardization. Other methods such as acid-base titration, flame photometry, and coulometry have been suggested, but there is not yet sufficient documentation to validate these methods.

The accuracy of a dispenser can also be evaluated by a gravimetric procedure. The volume to be tested is set and the device is primed to ensure that no air bubbles are present. The water is then carefully dispensed into a preweighed test tube or other container and the near volume is determined by use of the same equation used for pipet testing. A graduated cylinder can be used to make a rough assessment of the dispenser performance. This procedure is helpful when one is making adjustments to the dispenser volume and provides a mechanism for daily verification. The gravimetric procedure should be performed at regular intervals (monthly, quarterly), depending on the use of the pipettor.

Automatic dilutors are best evaluated by use of a potassium dichromate spectrophotometric method. A series of dilutions ($n = 20$) are prepared by the dilutor, measured spectrophotometrically, and then compared with a manual dilution made in the same volume ratios. The manual dilution must be prepared in volumetric flasks with sufficiently large volumes of sample (no less than 1 mL) to ensure accuracy. The absorbance of the sample prepared using the automatic dilutor is then compared with that of the sample diluted manually, and the accuracy of the automatic dilutor is computed as previously described. Agreement should be within 2%. Similarly the precision is computed by use of the distribution of individual absorbances about the mean, expressed as %CV. The %CV should be no more than 1%. This procedure can be used to evaluate some dilutor systems that are incorporated into automated instruments. Again procedures involving the use of enzymes are unacceptable. The frequency of verification will be determined by the amount of use. Monthly determinations will be sufficient for most devices, including dilutors incorporated into automated equipment.

Pipets, dilutors, and dispensers must be reevaluated whenever the devices are serviced or repaired. All procedures must be documented and records maintained according to federal, state, and local inspection agency guidelines.

UNITS OF MEASUREMENT
SI units

There are seven basic units of the SI system[12] (Table 1-9). Two or more basic units may be combined by multiplication or division to form SI-derived units (Table 1-10). Basic and derived units may be too large or too small for convenient use. Prefixes that form decimal multiples or submultiples of the units are permissible (Table 1-11). A few non-SI units have been retained because of difficulties encountered in converting them to SI units or because of their widespread use. Non-SI units relevant to clinical chemistry and their symbols are time, expressed in minutes (min), hours (h), or days (d), and volume, expressed as liters (L) or deciliters (dL). The General Conference of Weights and Measures (*Conférence Générale des Poids et Mésures,* CGPM) has approved l, *l,* or L as the volume designation; however, L is the official abbreviation accepted in the United States.

SI units in the clinical laboratory[12-15]

The SI unit describes the concentration of body constituents in terms of the number of dissolved molecules, measured in moles (mol, μmol, and so on) rather than the amount of dissolved mass (mg, g, and so on). A *mole* of a chemical contains the number of grams equivalent to its formula mass (see below, p. 36). The SI unit of enzyme activity is the *katal,* which is defined as the amount of enzyme that will catalyze the transformation of 1 mole of substrate per second in an assay system. This terminology has been approved by the Joint Commission on Biochemical Nomenclature of the International Union of Biochemistry and the IUPAC but has not been approved by CGPM. Thus the use of International Units (IU) for describing enzyme activity will undoubtedly continue (see Chapter 54). There is a constant relationship between the katal and IU (1 katal = 16.67 IU) when measured under identical conditions of temperature, pH, and substrate and coenzyme concentration.

Often SI units are not used when the molecular weight of a protein is uncertain. However, even under these conditions it is possible to express substance concentration rather than mass concentration, provided that the approximate molecular weight is included in the documentation. Such an approach also applies to hormones. IU are used to express enzyme activity while SI units are used for reporting osmolality. The SI unit for reporting pressure is the *pascal.* However, the numerical values expressed in pascals for blood pressure and blood gas partial pressures are too large, and therefore the kilopascal is the preferred unit. For further information regarding the SI unit system, refer to the NIST publication *Guide for the Use of the International System of Units.*[13]

Table 1-9 Basic quantities and units of the SI (Système International d'Unités)

Quantity	Basic unit	Symbol
Length	Meter	m
Mass	Kilogram	kg
Time	Second	s
Electric current	Ampere	A
Temperature	Kelvin	K
Luminous intensity	Candela	cd
Amount of substance	Mole	mol

Table 1-10 SI-derived units used in medicine

Derived quantity	Derived unit	Symbol
Area	Square meter	m^2
Volume	Cubic meter	m^3
Speed	Meter per second	m/s, or $m \cdot s^{-1}$
Substance concentration	Mole per cubic meter	mol/m^3, or $mol \cdot m^{-3}$
Pressure	Pascal	Pa
Work energy or quantity of heat	Joule	J
Celsius temperature	Celsius degree	°C
Activity (radionuclide)	Becquerel	Bq
Power	Watt	W
Electric charge or quantity	Coulomb	C
Electric potential	Volt	V
Resistance		Ω
Conductance	Siemens	S

Table 1-11   SI prefixes

Prefix*	Factor	Symbol	Prefix*	Factor	Symbol
atto	10^{-18}	a	deka	10^1	da
femto	10^{-15}	f	hecto	10^2	h
pico	10^{-12}	p	kilo	10^3	k
nano	10^{-9}	n	mega	10^6	M
micro	10^{-6}	μ	giga	10^9	G
milli	10^{-3}	m	tera	10^{12}	T
centi	10^{-2}	c	peta	10^{15}	P
deci	10^{-1}	d	exa	10^{18}	E

*It is recommended that only one prefix be used.

MEASUREMENT OF MASS

Mass may be defined as the quantity of matter. Weight is a function of mass under the influence of gravity as expressed by the equation:

$$Weight = Mass \times Gravity$$

Thus two objects of equal mass that are subject to the same gravitational force have equal weights. The gram is a unit of mass. Measurement of mass, or weight, is achieved through use of a balance. The type of balance selected will depend on the function being performed. Different balances are required for measuring kilogram weights (for example, for fecal fat analysis) and microgram weights (for example, for preparation of drug standards for toxicology analyses). Thus the laboratory will be equipped with different balances so that all necessary weight measurements can be performed.

Types of balances

Two general types of balances may be found in the clinical laboratory: mechanical and electronic. Mechanical balances include the trip, single pan, torsion, and analytical varieties. Weighings requiring less precision may be made using a trip, or single pan, balance. These balances have been previously described.[9] Most laboratories today have replaced mechanical balances with electronic ones. These are either top loading or analytical in design. The electronic balance is a single pan balance that uses an electromagnetic force instead of weights to counterbalance the load placed on the pan (Fig. 1-9). The pan is attached directly to a coil suspended in the field of a permanent magnet. A current is passed through the coil, producing an electromagnetic force that keeps the pan in a constant position. When a load is placed on the pan, a photoelectric-cell scanning device attached to the lever arm changes position and transmits a

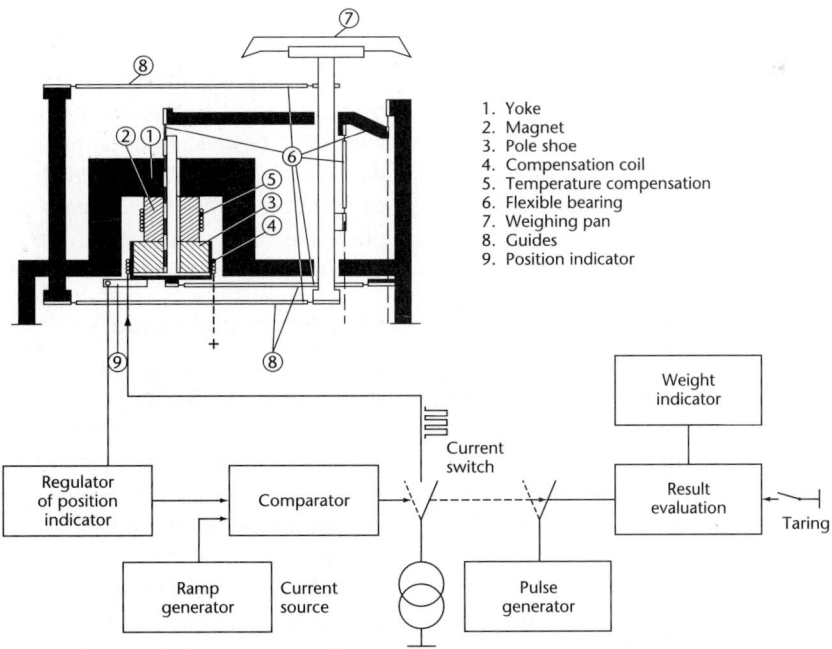

1. Yoke
2. Magnet
3. Pole shoe
4. Compensation coil
5. Temperature compensation
6. Flexible bearing
7. Weighing pan
8. Guides
9. Position indicator

Fig. 1-9   Switching principle of an electronic force compensator balance. (Courtesy of The Mettler Instrument Corp., Hightstown, N.J.)

Table 1-12 Characterization of types of balances in relationship to their operating ranges

Type of balance	Weighing capacity, g	Readability	Reproducibility
Precision balances			
Electronic	32,000	0.1 g	±0.1 g
	16,000	0.1 g	±0.05 g
	6,000	0.01 g	±0.01 g
	2,000	0.01 g	±0.005 g
	1,200	0.001 g	±0.001 g
	110	0.001 g	±0.0005 g
Mechanical	20,000	2	±1 g
	10,000	1	±0.5 g
	5,000	0.1	±0.05 g
	2,200	0.01	±0.01 g
	160	0.001	±0.001 g
Analytical balances			
Electronic	210	0.1 mg	±0.1 mg
	205	0.01 mg	±0.03 mg
	50	0.1 mg	±0.1 mg
	20	2 μg	±3 μg
Mechanical	160	0.1 mg	±0.05 mg
	160	0.01 mg	±0.01 mg
Microbalances			
Electronic	5.1	1 μg	±0.9 μg
	2.1	0.1 μg	±0.25 μg
Mechanical	20	0.001 mg	±0.001 mg

current to an amplifier that increases the current flow through the coil and restores the pan to its original position. This current is proportional to the weight of the load on the pan and produces a measurable voltage that is converted by a microprocessor to a numeric display or data output that gives the mass of the load. The accuracy of an electronic balance is dependent on the linearity of both the torque motor and the digital voltmeter. Some electronic balances have a built-in electronic vibration damper. Excessive vibration can be detected when variation of the pointer or oscillation of numbers in the last decimal place of the digital display is observed. Most electronic balances have built-in taring ability allowing the weight of the weighing vessel to be "zeroed." This is a great convenience when one is performing multiple weighings, such as for pipet calibrations. In addition, electronic balances can be interfaced with data-processing equipment, thus providing calculations such as weight averaging and statistical analysis of multiple weighings. An electronic balance is at least five times faster than a mechanical instrument. Weighings take 5 seconds or less. Table 1-12 summarizes balance types and their performance characteristics.

Requirements for operation

All balances should be located away from direct sunlight and drafts that can interfere with the weighing process. Analytical balances should be placed in a vibration-free location, preferably on an isolated heavy (such as marble) table. The more sensitive the balance, the more critical these re-

quirements are. Before a balance is used, it should be leveled by adjustment of the foot screws and centering of the bubble in the spirit level. The optical zero should also be verified. All weighings must be performed using weighing paper, plastic boats, beakers, or some other container. Under no conditions should chemicals be placed directly on the pan. After completion of the weighing process, all loose chemical crystals must be removed from the balance area. Similarly any liquid spills, particularly of corrosive chemicals, must be cleaned up immediately to prevent permanent damage to the pans. Weights should be handled using forceps, never bare hands. Direct contact with skin deposits oils, salts, and moisture on the weights. The smaller the weight, the more significant the effect.

Maintenance procedures

In addition to the requirements already described, balances should be serviced at least on an annual basis, more frequently if heavily used. Service must be performed by the manufacturer or its representative. Periodic checks to verify weight accuracy are also required, and records must be kept documenting quality control and maintenance procedures. Verification procedures should be performed at least monthly and before any critical analytical procedure. Verification of performance requires the use of NIST class S weights. The College of American Pathologists requires that approved laboratories validate balance performance using class S weights.[16] A 100-g weight should weigh 100 g ±0.5 mg. Class S weights should be checked to

Table 1-13   Individual NIST tolerances for class S weights

Nominal mass	Individual tolerance (mg)	Maintenance tolerance (mg)
1, 2, 3, 4, 10, 20, 30, 50 mg	±0.014	±0.014
100, 200, 300, 500 mg	±0.025	±0.05
1, 2, 3, 5 g	±0.054	±0.11
10, 20, 30 g	±0.074	±0.148
50 g	±0.12	±0.22
100 g	±0.25	±0.5

verify that their apparent weights are within NIST specifications (Table 1-13). Unacceptable performance indicates the need for service. Some newer analytical balances have a single built-in weight for performing this function. Such balances still require verification of the entire measuring range.

THERMOMETRY
Types of thermometers

Water baths and heating blocks must be maintained at constant temperature when temperature-sensitive assays are performed. Refrigerators and freezers must be maintained at constant temperature when used to store temperature-sensitive materials. Liquid-in-glass thermometers, thermistors, and electronic digital thermometers are used to monitor the temperature of these devices.

The temperature of every temperature-controlled device must be checked and recorded, along with any corrective action, every day as part of the quality control procedures performed in the laboratory. The accuracy of the thermometers used to monitor the heating baths should be verified at regular intervals, usually every 6 to 12 months. It has been recommended[17] that the thermometer have an accuracy range of one half that of the desired temperature range. For instance, if the desired accuracy for a heating bath is ±0.1° C, the thermometer should have a maximum uncertainty of ±0.05° C.

Liquid-in-glass thermometers are available for partial or total immersion. Partial immersion thermometers are used to measure the temperature of water baths, heating blocks, and ovens. The immersion depth is engraved on the stem and is usually located about 76 mm from the bulb. Total immersion thermometers are generally used to check refrigerator and freezer temperatures but can be substituted for partial immersion thermometers if they are verified at the same immersion depth that they will be used in the laboratory.

Calibration of liquid-in-glass thermometers

Calibration of thermometers requires the use of an NIST-certified or NIST-traceable thermometer. As part of the NIST Standard Reference Material program, certified thermometers are available that can be used to calibrate thermometers at 0° C and in the range of 24° to 38° C. The NIST-traceable thermometers have wider operating ranges.

The following procedure outlines the necessary steps to validate noncertified thermometers; it is based on the NCCLS standard *Temperature Calibration of Water Baths, Instruments, and Temperature Sensors.*[17]

1. Check the mercury column for separation or gas bubbles. (If any are present, refer to the NCCLS standard for procedures to correct the problem.)
2. Perform an ice-point determination.[17] This will check for changes in bulb volume. After completion set the thermometer aside for a few days to ensure recovery of the bulb.
3. Adjust the heating bath to the temperature required for analysis. It is important that the volume of the bath be at least 100 times greater than the volume of the fluid in which the thermometer being calibrated is placed. This will ensure maintenance of a uniform temperature throughout the bath.
4. Place the reference and noncertified thermometers in test tubes filled with water to the appropriate depth. The thermometers should be placed close to one another but with sufficient space between to ensure adequate circulation in the bath.
5. If a total-immersion thermometer is being calibrated for use as a partial-immersion device, it must be immersed in the heating bath to the same depth used for test applications. Proper immersion of the thermometer is essential.
6. After thermal equilibrium is reached (this will require several minutes for liquid-in-glass thermometers), determine the temperature reading for both thermometers.
7. Electronic thermometers that use thermistor probes may be calibrated similarly. Thermal equilibrium of these devices occurs in a few milliseconds.

Thermometers differing from the reference thermometer by more than 1° C should be discarded or returned to the supplier. Agreement within 0.1° C is required for critical laboratory purposes such as enzyme analyses. If discrepancies are between 0.2° and 1° C, the thermometer can be used for less critical functions such as monitoring ovens, refrigerators, and freezers. Assign each thermometer a log number and list it and the results of the calibration in a thermometer log book; this will be useful for inspection purposes.

Also available from NIST is a gallium–melting point cell, which can be used to calibrate electronic thermistor probes to a temperature of 29.772° C. These probes can then be used to verify the accuracy of liquid-in-glass thermometers in the 20° to 40° C range.[17]

WATER BATHS, HEATING BLOCKS, AND OVENS

Water baths may be either circulating or noncirculating in design. For clinical chemistry applications, noncirculating baths are, in general, unacceptable because temperature control is inadequate (±1° C), and circulating water baths, which have a tighter temperature control, are necessary.

Such baths are equipped with an external or internal circulating pump that maintains adequate thermal equilibrium. In some instances the pump may be coupled to a refrigeration unit to provide temperature control below room temperature. The bath liquid should be type II (or type I) reagent water to which is added a bactericidal agent such as thimerosal (Merthiolate) at a dilution of 1:1000. The bactericidal agent controls bacterial growth, reducing the frequency with which the bath water must be changed. The use of high-quality water is necessary to control salt deposits on the heat exchangers; such deposits interfere with maintenance of adequate temperature control.

Metal heating blocks are somewhat less efficient in maintaining a constant temperature and usually operate within $\pm0.5°$ C. Blocks that are incorporated into the cuvette compartment of a spectrophotometer will operate with greater accuracy, usually $\pm0.2°$ C or better.

The temperature of water baths and heating blocks should be measured daily with a thermometer calibrated against an NIST or NIST-certified thermometer. All measurements must be recorded and any corrective action documented.

Laboratory ovens may be used to dry chemicals, extracts, electrophoretic support media, thin-layer chromatography plates, and glassware. For most purposes, a temperature control of $\pm1°$ C is adequate. Thermometers used to monitor oven temperature should be checked for accuracy at least annually. The temperature of the oven should be measured daily to check for malfunction of the heating elements or thermistor controls. All gaskets should also be checked to verify integrity. Worn gaskets will require replacement to ensure adequate temperature control. All measurements must be recorded and any corrective action documented.

CENTRIFUGES
Types

Three general types of centrifuge are available: *swinging-bucket,* or *horizontal-head, centrifuges; fixed-angle,* or *angle-head, centrifuges;* and *ultracentrifuges.* These are available as floor or table models, allowing the laboratory to purchase the instrument that best suits its needs.

Centrifuges are used in the clinical laboratory to separate substances of significantly different masses or densities. The two substances to be separated can be a solid (particles) and a liquid or two liquids of different densities. Centrifuges are used in the chemistry laboratory primarily to separate clotted blood or cells from serum or plasma and body fluids. Although the choice of a specific relative centrifugal force (RCF) to carry out these separations is not critical, a force of 1000 to 1200 $\times$ g for 10 $\pm$ 5 min is recommended.[18] In some instances, more time may be necessary (see Chapter 3).

Swinging bucket, or horizontal-head, rotors hold the tubes in a vertical position when the centrifuge is at rest; the tubes move to and remain in a horizontal position when the rotor is in motion. During centrifugation, particles constantly move along the tube while it is in the horizontal position, distributing the sediment uniformly against the bottom of the tube. After centrifugation is complete and the rotor has ceased turning, the surface of the sediment is flat with a column of liquid above it.

Fixed-angle rotors keep the tubes at a specified angle, 25 to 52 degrees to the vertical axis of rotation. During centrifugation, particles move along the side of the tube to form a sediment that packs against the side and bottom of the tube. The surface of the sediment in this case is parallel to the shaft of the centrifuge. As the rotor slows and then stops, gravity may cause the sediment to slide down the tube forming a poorly packed pellet. Fixed-angle rotors are used when rapid sedimentation of small particles is required. The design of these rotors is more aerodynamic, allowing operation at speeds higher than those achievable with a swinging-bucket rotor. This capability allows microhematocrit centrifuges to operate at 11,000 to 15,000 revolutions per minute (rpm), with an RCF up to 14,000 $\times$ G.

Ultracentrifuges are high-speed centrifuges that use fixed-angle or swinging-bucket rotors. They are often refrigerated to counter the heat generated as a result of friction. A small air-driven ultracentrifuge, the Airfuge (Beckman Instruments, Spinco Division, Palo Alto, CA 94304) is a miniature air turbine with a small rotor operating at 90,000 to 100,000 rpm, generating a maximum RCF of 178,000 $\times$ g. This type of centrifuge has been used to separate chylomicrons from serum, allowing accurate analyses to be performed on the clear infranatant. It has also been used to fractionate lipoproteins, perform drug-binding assays, and prepare tissue for hormone-receptor assays. Analytical ultracentrifuges are used to determine sedimentation coefficients of proteins, allowing assessment of molecular weights.

Centrifuge components

All centrifuges have a motor, drive shaft, and head or rotor, which may be in the form of a chamber with a cover. A power switch, timer, speed control, tachometer, and brake are the components that control the centrifuge. When necessary, refrigeration units are included. Some centrifuges are equipped with an alarm that sounds when there is a malfunction such as a tube imbalance. Some centrifuges automatically shut down, preventing tube breakage and the potential for exposure to biohazardous agents. All modern centrifuges have a required safety latch that prevents the operator from opening the instrument before the rotor has stopped.

Swinging-bucket rotors use pairs of buckets or carriers that swing freely. The carriers are designed to accept a variety of cushioned inserts allowing centrifugation of small tubes or large bottles. Different fixed-angle rotors are required for different-sized containers.

The motor in a large centrifuge is usually a direct-current, heavy-duty, high-torque, electric motor. In smaller centrifuges, the current is usually alternating. Power is transmitted to the rotor by the commutator and brushes. The rotor shaft is usually driven by a gyro system, and the bearings are, in general, sealed, minimizing vibration and the need for lubrication. Centrifuge speed is controlled by a potentiometer that modulates the voltage that is supplied to the motor. Speed is also determined by the mass of the load in the rotor. The tachometer measures rotor speed in rpm. The brake decelerates the rotor by reversing the polarity of the current to the motor. The timer permits the rotor to reach a preprogrammed speed; the rotor then decelerates without braking after a set time has elapsed.

Refrigerated centrifuges are used when the heat generated during centrifugation could cause evaporation or denaturation of protein or leakage of cellular components in the sample. The temperature can be controlled between $-15°$ and $25°$ C, allowing centrifugation at higher speeds and for prolonged periods.

The selection of centrifuge tubes and bottles is of importance. Plastic tubes (polystyrene, polypropylene) have a higher speed tolerance and can withstand RCFs of up to $5000 \times G$. Tubes with tapered bottoms, which form more compact pellets, may be required under certain conditions such as preparing urine sediment for microscopic analysis and some radioimmunoassay procedures. The tubes must fit snugly in the carriers; small tubes in too large a carrier result in improperly packed pellets. The top of the tube must not protrude so far above the carrier that the rotor is impeded. Balancing of tubes within the carriers is critical. Newer centrifuges automatically decelerate and shut down when carriers are improperly balanced. Fig. 1-10 demonstrates appropriate balancing. Improper balancing can cause the centrifuge to vibrate, disrupting the formed pellet. Whenever possible, tubes containing biohazardous materials should be centrifuged with the caps or stoppers in place to minimize aerosols.

Maintenance and quality assurance

Daily cleaning of the inside surfaces of the centrifuge with a tenfold dilution of household bleach or an equivalent disinfectant is critical. When tube breakage occurs, the portions of the centrifuge in contact with the blood or other potentially infectious agent must be immediately decontaminated. The centrifuge bowl should be cleaned with a germicidal disinfectant, and the rotor heads and buckets should be autoclaved. All broken glass or plastic must be carefully removed and disposed of appropriately.

Centrifuge speeds that are routinely used should be checked periodically using a reliable photoelectric or strobe tachometer, usually every 3 months in accordance with CAP inspection guidelines.[19] The measured and rated speeds should not differ by more than 5% under specified conditions. The accuracy of the centrifuge timer should also be checked and verified quarterly. The temperature of refrig-

erated centrifuges should be checked at least monthly (daily is preferred) under standardized conditions. The agreement between the measured and expected (or programmed) temperature should be within $2°$ C.

Manufacturer's instructions for lubrication, maintenance, and replacement of brushes should be followed. Failure to replace worn brushes may cause the motor to fail and require replacement. All maintenance function checks must be recorded, and all corrective actions documented.

Principles of centrifugation

The speed of a centrifuge is expressed in revolutions per minute, whereas the relative centrifugal force generated is expressed as a number times the gravitational force, G. The relationship between rpm and RCF is expressed by the equation:

$$RCF = 1.12 \times 10^{-5} \times r \times (rpm)^2$$

where r is the radius of the centrifuge expressed in centimeters and is equal to the horizontal distance from the center of the centrifuge bucket to the rotor shaft, and 1.12×10^{-5} is an empirical factor. Fig. 1-11 shows a nomogram for determination of the RCF when the radius and revolutions per minute are known. The RCF applied to a tube in a swinging-bucket rotor may be considerably greater than that applied to the same tube in a fixed-angle rotor because the tube never reaches a horizontal position under the latter conditions. For this reason, it is preferable to process serum separator tubes with swinging-bucket, horizontal rotors, which operate at higher RCFs.

At times it may be necessary to duplicate centrifugation conditions in two different instruments. This may be done by application of the following equations:

Calculation of adjusted speed[20]:

$$rpm \text{ (new rotor)} = 1000 \times \frac{RCF \text{ (original rotor)}}{1.12 \times r \text{ (cm, original rotor)}}$$

Calculation of adjusted time[20]:

$$Time \text{ (new rotor)} = \frac{Time \text{ (old rotor)} \times RCF \text{ (original rotor)}}{RCF \text{ (new rotor)}}$$

These calculations do not take into account the differences between the instruments in the time necessary to reach full speed or to decelerate. Thus some additional adjustments will be necessary.

LABORATORY SAFETY

The Occupational Safety and Health Administration (OSHA) has mandated two programs to ensure the safety of laboratory personnel. The first, which deals with occupational exposure to chemical hazards,[21] became law in January 1991, and the second, which deals with occupational exposure to blood-borne pathogens,[22] became law in March 1992. In addition to these mandated programs, the

Balanced Load

Top view of
Partially-Filled Rotor

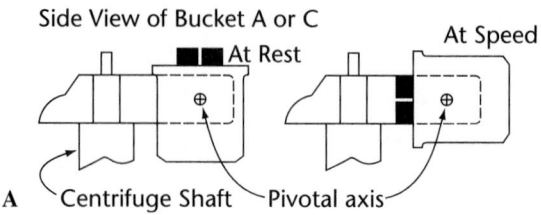

Unbalanced Load

Top view of
Partially-Filled Rotor

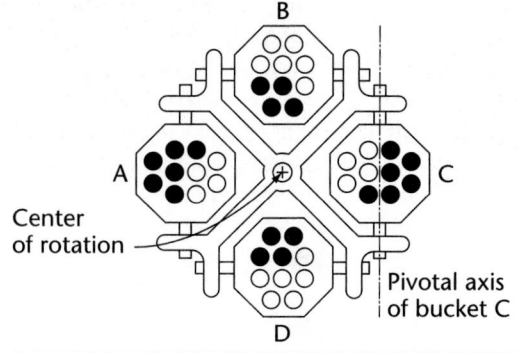

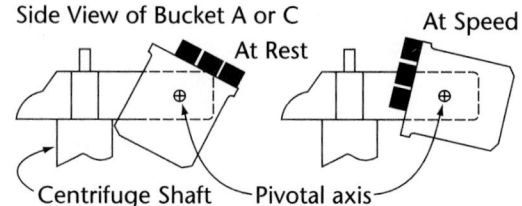

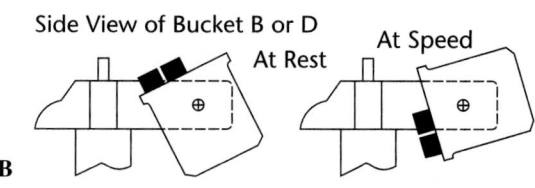

Fig. 1-10 Examples of balanced and unbalanced loads. **A,** Assuming all tubes have been filled with an equal amount of liquid, this rotor load is balanced. The opposing bucket sets A-C and B-D are loaded with an equal number of tubes and are balanced across the center of rotation. Each bucket is also balanced with respect to its pivotal axis. **B,** Even if all the tubes are filled equally, this rotor is improperly loaded. None of the bucket loads are balanced with respect to their pivotal axes. At operating speed, buckets A and C will not reach the horizontal position. Buckets B and D will pivot past the horizontal. Also note that the tube arrangement in the opposing buckets B and D is *not* symmetrical across the center of rotation. (Reprinted from *A Centrifuge Primer,* Spinco Division of Beekman Instruments, Palo Alto, CA, 1980, by permission of Beekman Instruments, Inc.)

laboratory is responsible for the practice of general safety procedures.

Each clinical laboratory is responsible for designating a safety officer. This individual may also function as the chemical hygiene officer and program coordinator for the blood-borne pathogen program. The responsibilities of this employee include the preparation and updating of manuals that address safety policies and procedures, maintenance of records of training and continuing education, and maintenance of records of exposure to hazardous materials. The safety officer may also be responsible for ensuring that protective devices are available and are being properly and consistently used and that the laboratory is functioning as a safe working environment. In a large facility these functions are shared by several employees; however, the safety officer still plays a key role in ensuring that all regulations are followed.

General safety practices

Fire safety is of utmost importance in the clinical laboratory. All equipment used for fire protection should meet the standards set by the National Fire Protection Association (NFPA). The equipment, which should be accessible to laboratory workers, may include fire extinguishers, fire blankets, cabinets for storage of flammable solvents and chemicals, fire alarms, smoke detectors, and sprinkler sys-

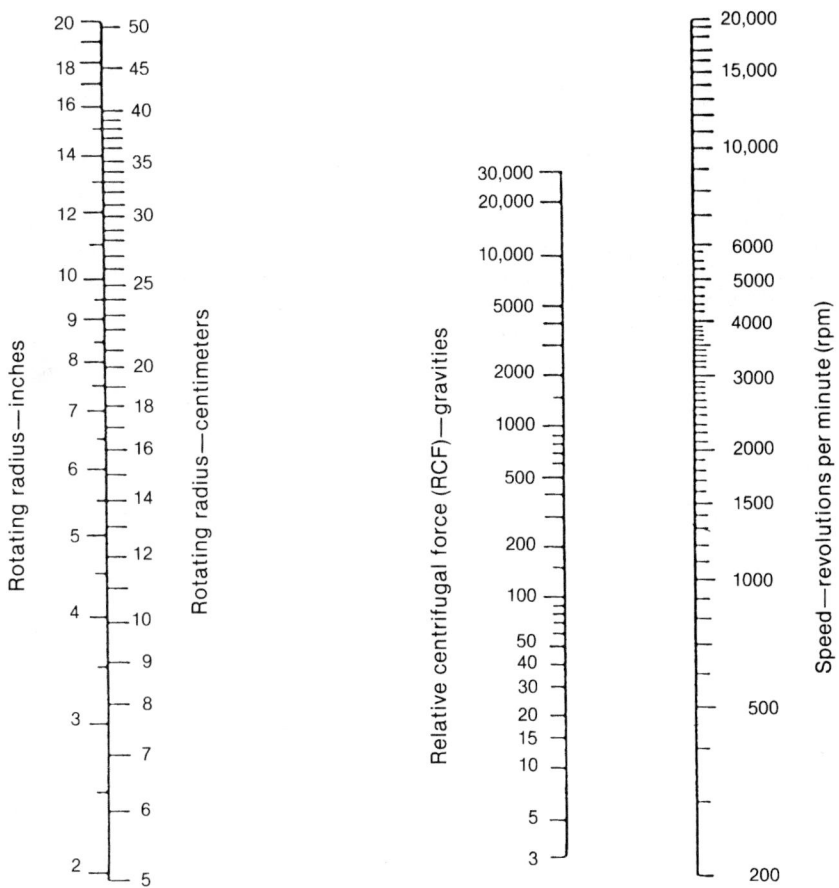

Fig. 1-11   Nomogram for relating relative centrifugal force, *RCF,* to revolutions per minute, *rpm.*

tems. The selection of the appropriate type of extinguisher is important as is frequent inspection to ensure that equipment is in good working order. Tables 1-14 and 1-15 classify types of fires and compare types of fire extinguishers. Halon extinguishers are generally used for areas in which computers are housed. Warning signs must be posted in these areas, and self-contained breathing equipment must be provided. Several extinguishers will be necessary in a larger laboratory, and different types may be appropriate. All employees must be familiar with their use, and annual retraining is mandatory.

Electrical safety is also critical, since the potential for both electrical shock and fire exists. All equipment must be Underwriter Laboratories approved. This includes extension cords, which should be used as temporary solutions only. All electrical outlets and equipment must be grounded and wires checked for fraying or wear. Regular inspection will prevent the likelihood of electrical accidents. Document these inspections.

Any equipment used in an area where organic solvents are present must be equipped with explosion-free fittings such as plugs and outlets.

General safety equipment includes safety showers and eyewashes in each large work area. The safety program must also include measures for routinely verifying that this equipment is operational, and maintenance records must be kept. Asbestos (heat-resistant) gloves will be required for handling hot equipment such as glassware and dry ice. Other personal protective equipment is discussed in the sections involving chemical and biological hazards.

The chemical hygiene plan

OSHA has mandated that as of January 31, 1991, laboratories must develop a chemical hygiene plan for the protec-

Table 1-14   Classes or types of fires

Class	Hazard
A	Cloth, wood, paper, ordinary combustibles
B	Flammable liquids (greases, solvents)
	Flammable gases (natural or manufactured)
C	Operating electrical equipment
	(If electricity is turned off, fire is reclassified as A or B)

Table 1-15 Comparison of fire-extinguisher types

Type	Advantages	Disadvantages	Notes*
Halon (class A, B, C, or B, C)	• Quick fire knockdown • Will reach hidden fires • No damage to equipment • Good discharge range • Heat absorber • Rechargeable	• Requires rapid discharge • More expensive • Personnel hazard (Halon 1211) • Not for deep-seated fires • Environmental hazard	• Most common system for electrical/electronics • Maximum effectiveness requires rapid detection • Less environmental impact when recharged in a closed system
Triclass dry chemical (class A, B, C)	• Good on oil/grease • Good knockdown • Low cost • Rechargeable	• Limited personnel hazard • Equipment damage likely • Clean-up required • Not suitable for hidden fires	• Compatible with other agents • Subject to equipment interference
Carbon dioxide (class B, C)	• Good fire suppression and cooling capability • Will reach hidden fires • No equipment damage • No messy clean-up/odor • Rechargeable	• May be toxic to personnel • May cause thermal/static (shock) damage • Heavy vapor settles out limiting total discharge range	• Secondary choice to Halon when fighting class B and C fires
Dry chemical regular (class B, C)	• Won't bake on • Easy clean-up • Good knockdown • No odor • Nonconductive • Rechargeable	• Not suitable for hidden fires • Slight respiratory hazard	• Secondary choice to Halon when fighting class B and C fires

*From Lab Safety Supply, Janesville, Wisconsin.

tion and education of employees.[21] This plan should contain the elements indicated in the box.

Standard operating procedures

These procedures include protocols for handling accidents and chemical spills. In general, if chemicals have come into contact with eyes or skin, the contact areas require flushing with copious amounts of water followed by medical attention when necessary. The eyewashing procedure requires 15 minutes of washing; portable eyewash stations are therefore unacceptable. Clean-up procedures should be individually defined for specific chemicals when necessary and should specifically designate the protective clothing to be used during the clean-up procedure.

Rules for avoiding unnecessary chemical exposure must also be defined. Smoking, eating, drinking, and applying cosmetics must be prohibited in all work areas. Long hair and loose clothing should be secured; sandals and canvas shoes should be prohibited. Contact lenses should not be worn in the laboratory, since they prevent proper washing of the eyes in the event of a splash. In addition, plastic lenses may be damaged by organic vapors, leading to chronic eye infections. Handwashing after handling chemicals and before leaving the laboratory for the purposes of eating or drinking should be emphasized.

Cracked or chipped glassware should be immediately discarded, since it can break during use. All glassware that has been in contact with a toxic or corrosive substance should be rinsed well with water or alcohol before being placed with other soiled glassware.

Elements of a Chemical Hygiene Plan

1. A description of standard operating procedure.
2. Material Safety Data Sheets (MSDSs).
3. A list of chemicals in inventory.
4. Information on appropriate chemical storage.
5. Labeling requirements.
6. A description of required engineering controls.
7. A list of required personal protective equipment.
8. Information on waste removal and disposal.
9. Information on mandated environmental monitoring where appropriate.
10. Housekeeping requirements.
11. Requirements for employee physicals and medical consultations.
12. Training requirements.
13. Record-keeping requirements.
14. Designation of a chemical hygiene officer and committee.
15. Other information deemed necessary for safety ensurance.

The laboratory is required to maintain an alphabetized, up-to-date file of MSDSs to comply with local, state, and federal Right-to-Know laws. MSDSs are required for all chemicals, reagents, and kits used by the laboratory but not for any pharmaceutical agents such as aspirin.[23] The MSDS contains information about the physical and health hazards of each product. The file must be accessible to all employees and outside contractors working in the laboratory.

Inventory

A *chemical inventory* is performed annually, listing all hazardous agents used or stored in the laboratory. A substance can be classified as hazardous by the Department of Transportation (DOT), the Environmental Protection Agency (EPA), or by the NFPA (see under labeling). The inventory should be arranged alphabetically and should include the following information for each chemical: manufacturer and manufacturing address, physical state, quantity stored, Chemical Abstract Service number, if known, location of storage, and any hazard classification for health risks, fire, reactivity, or corrosivity. A separate list must be maintained for carcinogens or suspected carcinogens.

Storage of chemicals

The quantities of chemicals stored in the laboratory should be as small as practical. All refrigerators used for chemical storage must be clearly marked. Under no conditions may food or drink be stored, even temporarily, in a refrigerator used for chemical storage. Explosion-proof refrigerators, clearly labeled, will be necessary for storage of solvents with a low flash point.

Toxic chemicals, including carcinogens, must be stored in unbreakable, chemically resistant, secondary containers in well-ventilated areas. The containers must be labeled to indicate that the compound is a CANCER SUSPECT AGENT or has HIGH CHRONIC TOXICITY.

Large amounts of volatile solvents must be stored in special safety cabinets approved by the NFPA. Where possible, these cabinets should be vented to the outside. Bench storage of volatile solvents is limited based on the OSHA classification of the solvent. The classification is determined by flash point and boiling point, with class IA and IB solvents being the most combustible. Benchtop storage of such solvents may be limited to as little as 1 pint; however, some local fire departments have more stringent regulations. Larger quantities must be transferred to safety cans with spring-loaded spouts. All cabinets where solvents are kept should be appropriately labeled.

Large cylinders of *compressed gas* are often used in the laboratory. The most commonly used gases are oxygen, hydrogen, nitrogen, helium, carbon dioxide, and, to a lesser extent, acetylene and propane. Usually the tanks are color-coded and the contents labeled by the NFPA diamond system. OSHA regulations governing gas cylinders are based on publications of the Compressed Gas Association, Inc.[24] Cylinders should be stored away from the laboratory in a secure, upright position, preferably in a locked, ventilated, fire-resistant space with the empty cylinders well separated from the full ones. The cylinder must always be secured on a dolly or hand truck during transport. The protective cap must be left in place until the cylinder is connected. Gas cylinders (even when empty) must be securely fastened to a wall or bench or placed in a floor retainer, since a fall can rupture the outlet valve, allowing the cylinder to be pro-

pelled like a torpedo. Mark each cylinder with a tag that lists the date that it was put into use. An exhausted cylinder should be replaced before it is completely empty to avoid contamination with foreign materials; it should be labeled with an EMPTY sign. In general, empty cylinders are recycled by suppliers. Small cylinders containing propane, however, are not. These should be disposed of according to the local fire codes.

Reduction valves for different types of gases are not interchangeable. Never substitute one regulator, with or without an adaptor, for another. Laboratory personnel should never attempt to force or free stuck or frozen regulator valves. All connections should be tested for leaks with soapy water. Very small leaks of oxygen or nitrogen are of little consequence, but leaks of hydrogen, acetylene, or other flammable gases are unacceptable. When a cylinder of flammable gas is shut down, it should be turned off at the main intake valve and the gas allowed to burn out. The reduction valves are then closed. A cylinder valve is not turned on unless the reduction valve is off. It is important to remember that propane is heavier than air, and thus a small quantity of leaking gas can flow along the top of the bench and be ignited by a flame elsewhere. For this reason, small, single-use cylinders of propane are safer to use.

Labeling and handling requirements

OSHA regulation 29 CFR 1910.1450[21] defines specific *labeling* requirements. The labels of chemicals in the original containers must not be removed or defaced. For those not in the original container, the labeling information must include the following: (1) identity of the hazardous chemical, (2) route of body entry (eyes, nose, mouth, skin), (3) health hazard, (4) physical hazard, and (5) target organ affected. Labeling requirements apply to all substances with a rating of 2 or greater, according to the Hazards Identification System developed by the NFPA. This system consists of four small, diamond-shaped symbols grouped into a larger diamond shape (Fig. 1-12). The left diamond is **blue** and represents **health** hazards, the top is **red** and identifies the **flammability** hazard, the right diamond is **yellow** and indicates a reactivity-stability hazard (used for substances that are capable of explosion or violent chemical change), and the bottom **white** diamond is used for provision of special hazard information such as water reactivity. The degree of the hazard is rated using a scale of 0 to 4, with 4 indicating the most severe risk. Such common items as isopropanol (isopropyl alcohol) or diluted bleach in squirt bottles will therefore require regulatory labels. In addition, it may be desirable to use additional warning labels such as those used by the DOT and shown in Fig. 1-13.

The handling of hazardous chemicals requires great care. A discussion of the handling and disposal of radioactive chemicals is presented in Chapter 9. All flammable and toxic liquids must be used in an area with good ventilation, preferably in a fume hood. A properly operating fume hood

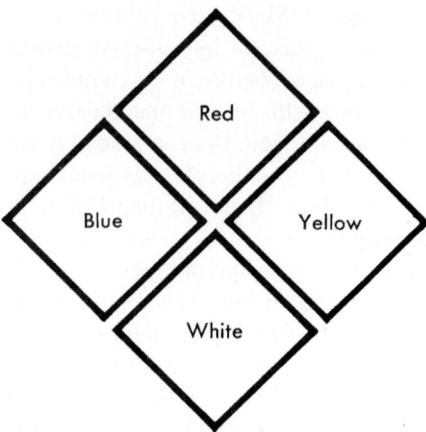

Fig. 1-12 Identification system of the National Fire Protection Association. (From Bauer JD: *Clinical laboratory methods,* ed 9, St. Louis, 1982, Mosby.)

should have a minimum air flow of 150 linear ft^3/min. Corrosive solutions, such as acids, alkalis, and mercury salts, should also be used in a fume hood. Stock bottles of concentrated acids should be transported in acid carriers to prevent and contain breakage. The use of personal protective equipment must be enforced. When reagents are prepared with concentrated acid, the acid must be *slowly* added to the water. Precautions for the handling of powdered carcinogens include the use of disposable equipment and a respirator, in addition to all other standard safety measures. After the compound is handled, the area should be carefully cleaned, and the glassware rinsed with strong acid or an organic solvent, before regular washing.

Engineering controls are an important part of the daily operation of the laboratory. In addition to the provision, inspection, and documentation of functionality of fire extinguishers, eyewashes, and safety showers, other aspects of the laboratory environment must be monitored and validated. The quality and quantity of room ventilation (4 to 12 air changes per hour) must be documented on a quarterly basis and air flow through the laboratory monitored. All areas where hazardous substances are handled or stored, such as storerooms, glove boxes, and cold rooms, must have adequate ventilation and exhaust ducting. All fume hoods must be inspected after installation, and then annually, by a reputable company. The inspection should include an evaluation of flow patterns and a flow-velocity profile. Any hood that fails inspection must be taken out of service immediately. A weekly safety checklist should be maintained that includes the following items: adequate air flow, no unnecessary items in the hood, baffle settings correct, and guard window sash operable. Before a hood is used, acceptable hood performance should be confirmed by the technologist. One can accomplish this by using a permanent flowmeter or observing the disappearance of smoke or fumes produced after carefully bringing together two applicator sticks whose cotton tips have been dipped in strong ammonia and hydrochloric acid respectively. (The tips are drenched with running water before disposal.) Alternatively, a Kimwipe may be firmly held under the baffle while in the down position and the force of the exhaust evaluated. *Care must be taken not to release the tissue into the exhaust system.*

OSHA has defined the *personal protective equipment* required for laboratory operations involving chemical hazards. (Much of this equipment is identical to that required for protection against blood-borne pathogens as will be described in the following section.) Handling of hazardous chemicals requires the use of gloves (the type to be used is dependent on the type of chemical hazard). Laboratory coats protect clothing; if chemical splashes are probable, an impervious, full-body apron offers additional protection. Masks, safety glasses with side shields, or full face shields are necessary when there is potential for eye, nose, or mouth contamination. Respirators must be provided and used according to the requirements listed in 29 CFR 1910.134. All personal protective equipment should be removed before one leaves a work area.

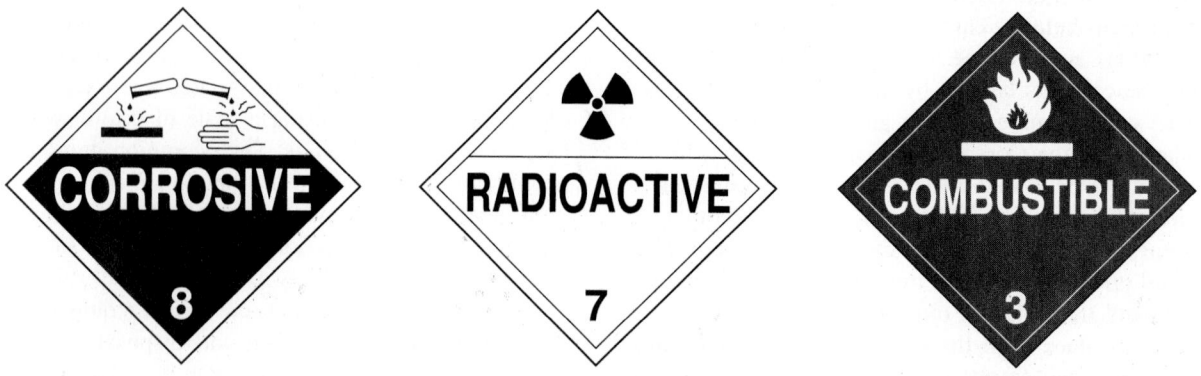

Fig. 1-13 DOT (Department of Transportation) labels.

Waste and chemical control

Chemical waste and hazardous chemical disposal procedures must comply with all local and state regulations. Most laboratories are considered small-quantity generators by the EPA and are required to secure a generation number from the regional EPA office. Certain chemicals can be disposed of in the sanitary sewer system. Specific information must be obtained from local sources, but only those chemicals that are reasonably soluble (at least 3%) in water can be poured down the drain, and these must be flushed with at least 100 volumes of excess water. Compounds that should never be poured down a drain include organic solvents with a boiling point of less than 50° C, hydrocarbons, halogenated hydrocarbons, nitrogen compounds, mercaptans, most oxygenated compounds that contain more than five carbon atoms (such as Freon), organic compounds such as azides and peroxides, concentrated acids and bases, and highly toxic, malodorous, or lacrimatory (tear-producing) compounds.

It is the laboratory's responsibility to determine the disposition of chemical waste that is removed from the premises. The MSDS sheets and other sources may provide useful information for disposal of specific chemicals.[23,25] Incineration in an environmentally acceptable manner is very common for combustible liquids. **Placing volatile chemicals in a hood for the purpose of evaporation is unacceptable.** The laboratory must familiarize itself with the rules and regulations governing storage and disposition of toxic chemicals such as solvents and formaldehyde. Records of disposal must be maintained.

Sodium azide, another troublesome chemical, is still sometimes used as a bacteriostatic agent. Azides form explosive salts with many metals, such as copper and iron. These salts are readily detonated by mechanical shock. Although the amount of sodium azide used as a preservative is relatively small, continued use can result in a buildup of the metallic salts in the sewer pipes. These salts are extremely explosive; even the use of a wrench on a drain line can result in a violent explosion. The removal of azides from pipes is difficult. One method involves closing the lower end of a section of pipe and allowing a 10% solution of sodium hydroxide to remain in contact with the pipe for at least 16 hours. The pipe is then rinsed with copious amounts of water for at least 15 minutes. The use of azides should be avoided or minimized, since in addition to their explosive potential they are carcinogenic.

Some colorimetric methods (such as chloride determination) that use mercury salts in the reagent are still in use, though mercury-free procedures have mostly replaced them. The disposal of large amounts of spent reagent produced by automated analyzers that use those methods may be a problem, since the solution should not be disposed of in the sewer system. The waste material should be collected in large plastic containers and made slightly acidic with acetic acid; if necessary, thioacetamide (about 10 g/L) is added. The solution is then stored in a well-ventilated area (small amounts of hydrogen sulfide may be liberated), and over a period of time the mercury will precipitate as mercuric sulfide. The supernatant may then be decanted and disposed of in the sewer. The mercuric sulfide should be disposed of by burial.

Environmental monitoring may be necessary if the laboratory uses three or more times per week any chemical defined in the OSHA publication 29 CFR 1910 Subpart Z. Included in this list is formaldehyde. The monitoring is performed as semiannual room air monitoring during an 8-hour period as well as individual badge monitoring of one or more employees exposed to the chemical. In the event that permissible exposure limits are exceeded, monitoring is required more frequently (quarterly) until acceptable exposure levels are achieved. Although xylene is not officially included on the list, a similar procedure should be followed for this chemical.

Housekeeping, such as floor cleaning and general laboratory cleaning, should be done regularly according to a defined schedule; housekeeping personnel must be informed of the risks associated with working in the laboratory. It is understood that the laboratory will be maintained as a clutter-free environment. Hallways and stairwells should be free from obstruction, waste must be handled appropriately, laboratory supplies should be stored appropriately, and all spills should be cleaned up appropriately. *Spill clean-up kits* must be readily available for use. Multipurpose products such as sand and soda ash are useful, as are commercial products such as those marketed by chemical companies and safety product suppliers (such as J.T. Baker, Mallinckrodt Chemical Co., and Lab Safety Supply). The laboratory can assemble a kit containing equivalent supplies (rubber gloves, towels, scoop, and various chemicals for neutralizing and absorbing organic solvents and corrosive chemicals). Kits must be labeled and highly accessible. Spills should be cleaned up immediately, using appropriate personal protective equipment. Special clean-up kits are available for handling formaldehyde and mercury spills. The formaldehyde kits neutralize the spill and allow the contents to be disposed of in the regular trash under most conditions. Spilled mercury tends to break up into very small droplets, which are difficult to pick up. Even after collection, disposal tends to be a problem, since metallic mercury must not be incinerated or burned. Many mercury kits are available, such as the Mercury Absorption Disposal Kit (Aldrich Chemical Co., Milwaukee), which contains a material that absorbs mercury droplets, producing a less toxic substance, which may be disposed of by burial. Some kits also include waste disposal through the kit manufacturer (Merc*Clean from H-B Instrument Co.). The benches and floors in older laboratories often contain fine cracks in which mercury droplets can lodge. These droplets are very difficult to remove, but the cracks should be cleaned, if possible, since mercury is somewhat volatile at room temperature. Rubbing powdered sulfur or sodium polysulfide into the cracks may help to change the mercury to the less volatile sulfide salt.

OSHA regulations mandate that personnel who are routinely exposed to hazardous chemicals be provided with *medical consultations* and *examinations* on a regular basis (such as annually). The extent of the physical examination is determined by the amount and type of exposure. In addition to regular examinations, personnel should be medically evaluated whenever there has been a major spill, when environmental monitoring indicates exposure above action levels, or when signs and symptoms of toxicity develop. Employees should then be continuously monitored and counseled until a medical clearance is given. **Medical records must be maintained for 30 years after the employee leaves the workplace.**

Training is a necessary and important part of the Chemical Hygiene Plan. Refresher training sessions must be held at least annually and attendance records documented. Training should ensure that the employee knows the extent of chemical exposure, understands the labeling system, knows the meaning of and location of the laboratory's MSDS book, is familiar with the required personal protective equipment, and knows how to react to and handle spills. Many training methods may be used, such as video tapes, handouts, and demonstrations.

Record keeping is a critical component of the laboratory safety program. One must maintain records of (1) accident and incident reports, (2) inventory and usage records for high-risk substances, (3) environmental monitoring where appropriate, (4) medical consultations, (5) training attendance records, (6) housekeeping procedures, and (7) safety inspections.

Protection against biohazards and medical wastes

Universal precautions. OSHA promulgated a final set of rules on December 6, 1991, that dealt with occupational exposure to blood and other potentially infectious materials. The program for protection against biohazards had to be fully instituted by July 6, 1992.[22] Many of the requirements of the program are similar to those contained in the Chemical Hygiene Plan, including development of a document describing the following: (1) the extent of exposure for all employees, (2) engineering and work practice controls, (3) personal protective equipment, (4) task assessment, (5) housekeeping procedures, (6) spill cleanup procedures, (7) laundry requirements, (8) labeling requirements, (9) waste disposal, (10) provision of vaccinations, (11) medical consultations, (12) training, and (13) record keeping.

Some *occupational exposure* to blood-borne pathogens is probably inherent in every task in the chemistry laboratory. Therefore all personnel are at risk. Even though this is the case, it is necessary to define the extent of exposure.

Universal precautions, as defined by the Centers for Disease Control and Prevention and adopted by OSHA, are observed to prevent contact with blood and other potentially infectious materials.[26] The general recommendations include:

1. All personnel must routinely use barrier precautions to prevent skin and mucous membrane exposure when contact with blood or body fluids from any patient is expected. Gloves must be worn when one is performing venipuncture and when handling blood or body fluids or items soiled with blood or fluids. Protective eyewear or face shields must be worn during procedures that are likely to cause splashing, to prevent exposure of mucous membranes of the mouth, nose, and eyes to droplets of blood or body fluids. Gowns (and aprons) must be worn during procedures that are likely to generate splashing.

2. If the hands or skin become contaminated with blood or other body fluids, they should be washed immediately and thoroughly. Hands should be washed immediately after gloves are removed.

3. Healthcare workers must avoid injuries from needles, scalpels, and other sharp devices. Needles must *not* be recapped, bent, broken, or removed from disposable syringes. After use, disposable syringes, needles, scalpel blades, and other sharp items must be placed in puncture-resistant containers.

4. Healthcare workers who have exudative skin lesions or weeping dermatitis must avoid direct patient care and contact with blood and other potentially infectious materials until the condition is resolved.

5. Pregnant women are particularly cautioned to follow the above rules.

Other work practice controls include the following:

1. Specimens of blood and other potentially infectious materials must be transported in leakproof containers. Care should be taken to avoid contamination of the outside of the container and the accompanying laboratory requisition.

2. Biological safety cabinets should be used for procedures such as blending, sonicating, and vigorous mixing, which can generate droplets.

3. Mouth pipetting is prohibited. Mechanical devices are used to pipet **ALL** liquids.

4. Eating, drinking, smoking, applying cosmetics or lip balm, and handling contact lenses are prohibited in biohazardous work areas, just as they are prohibited in areas where chemicals are used.

5. Only authorized personnel are permitted in the laboratory. Casual visitors are discouraged. Any visitor to the work area, including instrument service personnel, should be provided with personal protective equipment to the extent necessary.

6. Instruments requiring service should be decontaminated before repair.
7. Chemistry analyzers that generate fine sprays of sample from the sample probe should be equipped with shields, if possible.
8. All employees must wash their hands and remove laboratory coats and other personal protective equipment before leaving the work area.

Personal protective equipment. Safety equipment must be provided in the appropriate size by the employer at no cost to the employee. The laboratory coats must be impervious to fluids, offering optimal protection against biohazardous agents. Aprons may be used to provide additional protection. Safety glasses, masks, or full face shields are used to protect the eyes, mouth, and nose.

Task assessment. Safety policies should be established for each task performed by the laboratory. These policies should include engineering and work practice controls and requirements for personal protective equipment. For much of the work performed in the chemistry laboratory, coats, glasses, and gloves will be necessary. For some tasks, additional protection will be required.

Housekeeping procedures. Following a written schedule, one must decontaminate all equipment and work surfaces with a chemical germicide such as a 1 : 10 dilution of household bleach (1) after completing specified procedures, (2) when surfaces are overtly contaminated, (3) immediately after any spill of a potentially infectious material, and (4) at the end of the work shift.

Routine cleaning procedures should be instituted for items such as waste cans and other receptacles. Broken glassware that may be contaminated is handled using mechanical means and disposed of appropriately.

Spills of biological material are decontaminated as soon as possible by absorbing the spilled fluid with disposable absorbent material such as paper towels or gauze, flooding the contaminated area with bleach or wiping it with bleach-soaked towels, and then wiping the area with clean, dry towels or gauze. All contaminated items are placed in a biohazard bag and disposed of according to laboratory policy. Spill clean-up requires the use of personal protective equipment.

Contaminated laundry must be packed in red bags at the location where it is used or labeled with a biohazard sign if placed in another type of bag. All laundering and repair of laboratory coats are provided by the employer. **Under no conditions may employees launder their own laboratory coats.** When handling soiled laundry, personnel must wear gloves. Storage of clean and dirty coats must be well separated.

Warning labels (Fig. 1-14) must be used to identify (1) the entrance to work areas, (2) refrigerators and freezers that contain blood and other potentially infectious agents, (3) all containers used to store, transport, or ship potentially infectious materials, and (4) containers of regulated waste (other than red bags). Areas where food is stored should be labeled as nonbiohazard (clean) areas.

Disposal. Regulated medical waste (infectious waste) must be disposed of in accordance with local and state regulations.[27] Contaminated materials should be segregated at the point of use into categories such as needles or sharp objects and other infectious waste. Containers must be leak-

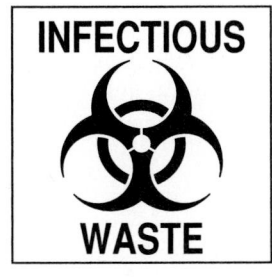

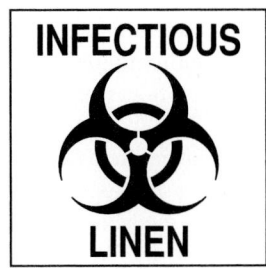

JB-20622

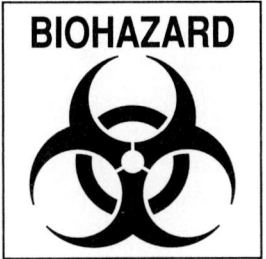

Fig. 1-14 Biohazard labels.

proof and should be disposed of when three fourths full. Any biohazardous waste that is decontaminated by a procedure such as autoclaving is exempt from these regulations and may be disposed of by standard processes. There are now several types of systems available for waste treatment that render the treated product unrecognizable; these include pulverizing or high heat processes. The legality of these devices is determined on a state-by-state basis.

Vaccination. Vaccinations against hepatitis B virus (HBV) must be offered to all employees without cost. Any employee who declines the vaccination must sign a form indicating that the continued risk of exposure to blood-borne pathogens is understood. These employees are at liberty to change their minds at any time. The vaccine is administered in a series of three doses over a 6-month period. Protective levels of antibodies are induced in 90% to 99% of adults; however, follow-up studies 3 to 5 years after vaccination have shown that in many individuals, titers are no longer measurable. These individuals should receive a single booster vaccination. No time frame for further follow-up action has been suggested.

Medical consultations and evaluations must be provided if an employee is exposed to a biohazardous agent through a needlestick, a cut, a mucous membrane exposure (eyes, nose, or mouth), or an exposure involving skin contact with large amounts of blood. The source patient is requested to consent to testing for both HBV and human immunodeficiency virus (HIV), if necessary by law. Where consent is not required, testing is performed and the employee is informed of the results. The employee's blood is collected and tested as soon as possible. If the employee does not consent to HIV testing, the sample must be preserved for at least 90 days to allow for a change of mind.

High-risk exposures from patients known to be HIV positive or patients at risk of being HIV positive are handled as emergencies. Medication such as azidothymidine (AZT) must be administered, preferably within 4 hours of the exposure.

Follow-up study of the exposed employee, including antibody or antigen testing, counseling, and postexposure prophylaxis, is conducted. The employee is retested at 6, 12, and 26 weeks after exposure if the patient is HIV positive or a high-risk subject.

Training. All new employees require specific training sessions to ensure that they understand the epidemiology of blood-borne diseases and the modes of transmission. Explanation of the types and appropriate use of personal protective equipment is essential, as is the explanation of emergency procedures to be followed in the event of exposure. All employees must be familiar with the laboratory's policies for protection against transmission of blood-borne pathogens. Adherence to all policies must be monitored regularly and counseling or retraining provided when failures are evident.

Records of the employee's HBV vaccination status are mandatory. In addition, results of physical examinations and consultations must be maintained. **All such records must be maintained for the duration of employment plus 30 years.**

Documentation of training sessions is kept for 3 years and includes dates of all programs, a summary of each program content, names and qualifications of all instructors, and an attendance list, including names and job titles.

Quality control of all safety procedures as defined by OSHA is a major issue in today's laboratory. All the necessary records covering chemical hygiene and biohazard protection should be readily available and carefully maintained to meet the current government regulations.

Part II: Calculations in clinical chemistry[28]
ELIZABETH ANN BYRNE

DILUTION

In several areas of the medical laboratory, one must dilute blood or body fluids to prepare a measurable concentration. Accurate preparation of these dilutions is mandatory for reporting the actual concentrations of body-fluid constituents. Diagnosis, prognosis, and therapy depend on these test results.

Dilution can be defined as expressions of concentrations. Dilutions express the amount, either volume or weight, of a substance in a specified total final volume. A 1:5 dilution contains 1 volume (weight) in a *total* of 5 volumes (weights), that is, 1 volume and 4 volumes.

Expression of a 1:5 dilution can be stated as the common fraction ⅕. This fraction enables one to calculate the actual concentration of a diluted solution.

Example. A 100 mg/mL nitrogen standard is diluted 1:10. The concentration of the resulting solution is $100 \times 1/10 = 10$ mg/mL.

The most commonly used equation for preparing dilutions is

$$V_1 \times C_1 = V_2 \times C_2 \qquad \textit{Eq. 1-1}$$

V_1 is the volume, C_1 is the concentration of solution 1, and V_2 and C_2 are the volume and concentration of the diluted solution. These may be expressed as % (weight/volume, w/v), or molarity, or normality concentration. Similarly V_2 and C_2 are related. This basic equation can be expressed as

$$\frac{V_1}{V_2} = \frac{C_1}{C_2} \qquad \textit{Eq. 1-2}$$

The most common error in setting up any equation of this type is *not placing* the related volumes or concentrations in the proper place and having the units cancel out, leaving the final, uncanceled units.

One helpful practice for successfully solving laboratory

calculations is to label all numbers in any equation with their respective units of measurement. It may take an extra minute but will save many minutes of reviewing calculations when the final result appears illogical or incorrect. A problem that does *not* properly cancel out units cannot be successfully solved. A second helpful practice is to reduce fractions to their least common denominators before one calculates the results.

Example. Prepare 500 mL of 0.5 M NaCl (molecular weight of NaCl = 58.5 g/mol).

$$500 \text{ mL} \times \frac{\text{Liter}}{1000 \text{ mL}} \times \frac{0.5 \text{ mol}}{\text{Liter}} \times \frac{58.5 \text{ g}}{\text{mol}}$$

$$= \frac{0.5 \times 58.5 \text{ g}}{2} = \frac{29.25 \text{ g}}{2} = 14.6 \text{ g}$$

14.6 g of NaCl diluted to 500 mL = 0.5 M NaCl

Example. Preparation of 250 mL of 0.1 M HCl from stock 1 M HCl.

Using $C_1 \times V_1 = C_2 \times V_2$
Where V_1 is the unknown $V_2 = 250$ mL
    $C_1 = 1.0$ mol/L $C_2 = 0.1$ mol/L

$$1.0 \text{ mol/L} \times V_1 = 250 \text{ mL} \times 0.1 \text{ mol/L}$$
$$V_1 = 25 \text{ mL}$$

Measure 25 mL of 1 M HCl; dilute to 250 mL with distilled water. This diluted solution has a 0.1 M HCl concentration. (Mathematical reasoning indicates that a 1:10 dilution of stock 1 M HCl results in a 0.1 M concentration, and 25 mL diluted to 250 mL equals a 1:10 dilution.)

Another application of dilutions

So that a 24-hour urine creatinine concentration could be assayed, the specimen had to be diluted 1:5 before measurement. Calculate the 24-hour excretion if the 24-hour urine volume is 1800 mL and the measured creatinine concentration is 260 mg/L:

Total excretion = Total urine volume × Concentration × Dilution

$$\text{Total excretion} = 1800 \frac{\text{mL}}{24 \text{ hr}} \times 260 \frac{\text{mg}}{\text{L}} \times 5 \times \frac{1 \text{ L}}{1000 \text{ mL}}$$

Total excretion = 2340 mg/24 hr or 2.34 g/24 hr

Exercises

Calculate the concentrations (answers are in the appendix at the end of this chapter).
1. 10 M NaOH, which is diluted 1:20 = ____ M?
2. 2 M HCl, which is diluted 1:5 = ____ M?
3. 1000 mg/L glucose, diluted 1:10 and then 1:2 = ____ mg/L?

Serial dilutions are those in which all the dilutions after the first one are the same. Exceptions to this general description of preparation of serial dilutions are included with certain techniques in serology, such as the antistreptolysin titer.

Serial dilution example. To determine the anti-Rh$_0$ (D) titer, serum is diluted 1:5 by addition of 0.2 mL of serum to 0.8 mL of saline solution, in tube 1. Tubes 2 through 8 contain 0.5 mL of saline as diluent. Dilution is performed by transferal of 0.5 mL of tube 1 to tube 2, mixing, and then transferring 0.5 mL of tube 2 to tube 3, continuing through the tubes to tube 8, mixing after each transfer. The concentration of serum in the tubes decreases by a factor of 2 with each dilution: 1:5, 1:10, 1:20, 1:40, 1:80, 1:160, 1:320, and 1:640.

4. For an ABO titer, tube 1 contains 0.9 mL of diluent, tubes 2 to 8 contain 0.5 mL of diluent, 0.1 mL of serum is added to tube 1 and serial dilutions using 0.5 mL are carried out in the remaining tubes. If the last tube showing agglutination with A cells is tube 6, what is the anti-A titer of the serum? (This is equal to the dilution in tube 6 = 1:?)
5. All tubes for a serial dilution contain 0.5 mL of saline solution, 0.5 mL of serum is added to tube 1, and 0.5 mL is transferred through the row of tubes. Sheep cells are added to the tubes, and agglutination is demonstrated through tube 7. What is the titer of sheep cell agglutinations?

WEIGHTS AND CONCENTRATIONS
Definitions and examples

Percent concentrations. Percent concentrations are generally expressed as parts of solute per 100 parts of total solution; hence the expression *percent,* or *per one hundred.* The use of percent concentration is derived historically from the early pharmaceutical chemists. Although these terms are still commonly used in the United States, major organizations (AACC, CAP) are attempting to use unified SI units. Concentrations in SI units are described in moles per liter when the molecular weight of the substance is known. If the molecular weight is unknown, weight (mass) per milliliter, or weight per liter, is used. Throughout the text SI units are used where possible.

The three basic forms of concentration are as follows:
Weight per unit weight (w/w). Both solute and solvent are weighed, the total equaling 100 g.

Example. 5% w/w of NaCl contains 50 g of NaCl + 950 g of diluent.

Volume per unit volume (v/v). The volume of liquid solute per total volume of solute and solvent is expressed.

Example. 1% of HCl (v/v) contains 1 mL of HCl per 100 mL (or 1 dL) of solution.

Weight per unit volume (w/v). The most frequently used expression, concentrations of w/v are reported as grams percent (g%) or g/dL, as well as mg/dL and μg/dL. When percent concentration is expressed without specifying the form, it is assumed to be weight per unit volume. The use of weight percent to describe concentration is being discouraged by professional organizations and, with few exceptions, is not used in this book. With SI units this would be in terms of weight per microliters (μL), milliliters (mL), or liters (L).

Example. To prepare 100 mL of 100 g/L of NaCl, weigh 10 g of NaCl and dilute to volume in a 100 mL volumetric flask.

Molarity. Molarity expresses concentration as the number of moles per liter of solution. One mole is the molecular weight of the substance in grams. A millimole is 1/1000 of a mole. A molar solution contains one gram-molecular weight of a substance per liter.

$$1 \text{ mol} = 1000 \text{ mmol}$$
$$1 \text{ mmol} = 1000 \text{ } \mu\text{mol}$$
$$1 \text{ } \mu\text{mol} = 1000 \text{ nmol}$$

Examples. 1 M NaOH (molecular weight, or MW = 40.0 g/mol) contains one gram-equivalent molecular weight per liter, or 40 g diluted to 1000 mL with distilled water. A millimolar (1 mM) solution, or 0.001 molar (0.001 M), contains 1 mmol/L. 1 millimole of NaOH is 1/1000 of 40 g, that is, 0.040 g (or 40 mg). When diluted to 1000 mL, the concentration of the solution will be 0.001 M.

Normality. Normality expresses concentration in terms of equivalent weights of substances. Equivalent weights are determined by the valence, which reflects the number of combining or replaceable units. A 1 normal (1 N) solution contains 1 equivalent weight per liter. The equivalent weight of an element or compound is equal to the molecular weight divided by the valence.

Normality and *molarity* relationships can be readily calculated if their definitions are understood.

Examples

1 M HCl = 1 N HCl, since 1 mole of H^+ or Cl^- reacts for every mole of HCl.

1 M H_2SO_4 = 2 N H_2SO_4, since 2 moles of H^+ (that is, equivalents) react for every mole of H_2SO_4.

1 M H_3PO_4 = 3 N H_3PO_4, since 3 moles of H^+ react for every mole of H_3PO_4.

1 M $CaCl_2$ = 2 N $CaCl_2$, since 2 Cl^- can react for every mole of $CaCl_2$.

1 M $CaSO_4$ = 2 N $CaSO_4$, since 2 mole volume electrons are available for reaction with either Ca^{++} or $SO_4^=$.

Equivalent weights are known as the number of grams of an element (or compound) that will react with another element (or compound). This so-called law of combining weights is operable for all chemical compounds.

To simplify chemistry procedures and reports, factors can be used to express a quantity of one compound as an equivalent quantity of another compound. This process can be termed *equivalency*.

Example. Calculate the amount of urea if a patient's urea nitrogen level is 800 mg/L. The formula for urea is NH_2—CO—NH_2, and its molecular weight is 60 g/mol. The molecular equivalent weight for nitrogen in the mole is 14

g/mol $\times$ 2 molecules = 28. The *urea/nitrogen factor* is determined by the following equation:

$$\frac{\text{MW of urea (60)}}{2 \times \text{MW of nitrogen (28)}} = \frac{x \text{ g of urea}}{1 \text{ g of urea nitrogen}}$$

$$28 x = 60$$

$$x = 2.14 \text{ (factor)}$$

This factor states that 2.14 g of urea would equivalently represent 1 g of urea nitrogen. So 800 mg/L urea nitrogen $\times$ 2.14 equals 1712 mg/L of urea. Laboratory results today are reported as urea nitrogen, since historical methods for this particular test are based on measurement of the urea nitrogen.

Competent laboratory personnel should be able to convert mg/dL to mEq/L. Electrolyte equivalents can be calculated from the equation:

$$\text{mg/dL} \times 10 = 10 \text{ mg/L}$$

Since mg/mEq weight is the millimolar weight in milligrams divided by the valence

$$\frac{\text{mg/L}}{\text{mg/mEq}} = \text{mEq/L}$$

or

$$\frac{\text{mg/dL}}{\text{mg/mEq}} \times 10 \frac{\text{dL}}{\text{L}} = \text{mEq/L}$$

Example. What is the mEq/L concentration of serum chloride reported as 250 mg/dL? Since the millimolecular weight of chloride is 35.5 (that is, 1 mmol = 35.5 mg), the milliequivalent weight of chloride is

$$\frac{\text{MW}}{\text{Valence}} = \frac{35.5 \text{ g/mol}}{1}$$

$$\frac{250 \text{ mg/dL}}{35.5 \text{ mg/mEq}} \times 10 \frac{\text{dL}}{\text{L}} = 70 \text{ mEq/L}$$

Specific gravity. Specific gravity can be used to determine the mass (weight) of solutions. It relates the weight of 1 mL of the solution and the weight of an equal volume of pure water at 4° C (1 g). One particular use of specific gravity is in preparation of dilutions from concentrated commercial acids, the equation being:

Specific gravity $\times$ Percent assay =
Grams of compound per milliliter

Example. Concentrated HCl has a specific gravity of 1.25 g/mL and is assayed as being 38% HCl. What is the amount of HCl per milliliter?

$$1.25 \text{ g/mL} \times 0.38 = 0.475 \text{ g of HCl per mL}$$

One common error is neglecting to change the percent assay to its proper decimal; in the above example, 38% = 0.38!

Exercise

6. How many milliliters of concentrated HCl are needed to prepare 1 L of a 0.1 N HCl solution if the molecular weight of HCl = 36.5?

Water of hydration. Some salts are available in forms both anhydrous (no water) and hydrated (with water molecules). The form of the available salt, including the water of hydration, is listed on the manufacturer's label. To prepare accurate weight concentrations of these salts, calculations must include the molecules of water present in the compound. This is most easily done by calculation of the percentage of the compound that is in the anhydrous form. With this percentage, the weight of the hydrated form can be corrected to that of the anhydrous form.

The advantage of using molar concentrations is that the water of hydration does *not* have to be accounted for in the calculations. For example, 1 mol of $CuSO_4$ = 160 g, and 1 mol of $CuSO_4 \cdot 5H_2O$ = 250 g. One gram-equivalent molecular weight of each compound will contain 1 mol of $CuSO_4$; that is:

$$250 \text{ g } CuSO_4 \cdot 5H_2O = 1 \text{ mol of } CuSO_4 = 160 \text{ g of } CuSO_4$$

Example. How many grams of $MgCl_2$ are there in 1 g of $MgCl_2 \cdot 3H_2O$?

$$
\begin{array}{ll}
\text{Mg } 24 & \text{Mg } 24 \\
\underline{\text{Cl}_2 \ 71} & \text{Cl}_2 \ 71 \\
95 \text{ MW} & \underline{3 \text{ H}_2\text{O } 54} \\
& 149 \text{ MW}
\end{array}
$$

$$\frac{95}{149} = \frac{x}{1}$$

$$149 x = 95$$

$$x = 63.8\%$$

One gram of $MgCl_2 \cdot 3H_2O$ contains 0.637 g of $MgCl_2$.

Mole fraction. Mole fraction refers to the ratio of the amount of a component to the total mixture of components. Mole fraction is a derived unit that is expressed as either a percent or as a decimal.

Example. What percent Mg is contained in $MgCl_2 \cdot 3H_2O$?

$$
\begin{array}{ll}
\text{Mg} = 24 & \\
\text{Cl} = 35.5 & \dfrac{24}{149} = 16.1\% \\
MgCl_2 \cdot 3H_2O = 149 &
\end{array}
$$

Mg is 16.1% of the molecule $MgCl_2 \cdot 3H_2O$.

Example. To determine mole percent calcium in calcium carbonate (MW = 100), 1 mol of $CaCO_3$ contains 100 g, comprising 40 (Ca) + 12 (C) + 48 (3 × O), of which 40 is calcium. The mole fraction of calcium in 1 L of 1 mol of calcium carbonate equals 40%.

Example. How much $CuSO_4 \cdot 5H_2O$ must be weighed to prepare 1 L of a solution containing 80 mg of $CuSO_4$?

$$\text{Total MW of } CuSO_4 \cdot 5H_2O = 250$$

$$\text{MW of } CuSO_4 = 160$$

The proportion of $CuSO_4 \cdot 5H_2O$ that is $CuSO_4$ is 160/250 = 0.64. Thus, 1 g of $CuSO_4 \cdot 5H_2O$ contains 1 g × 0.64 = 0.64 g of $CuSO_4$. The rest, 0.36 g, is water. Therefore

$$\frac{80}{0.64} = 125 \text{ mg of } CuSO_4 \cdot 5H_2O$$

Examples of calculations

a. What is the normality of concentrated HCl that has a specific gravity of 1.19 g/mL and a 38% assay?

$$\text{Specific gravity} \times \text{Percent} = \text{Grams/milliliter}$$

$$1.19 \times 0.38 = 0.452 \text{ g/mL} = 452 \text{ g/L}$$

$$36.5 \text{ g of HCl/L} = 1 \text{ N}$$

$$\frac{452 \text{ g/L}}{36.5 \text{ g/Eq}} = 12.4 \text{ N}$$

b. If 24.5 g of H_2SO_4 (MW = 98 g/mol) are dissolved in a 1 L solution
   (1) What is its molarity?
   (2) What is its normality?
   (Answer 1) 1 mol of H_2SO_4 = 98 g; therefore 24.5 g equals

$$\frac{1 \text{ mol}}{98 \text{ g}} = \frac{x}{24.5 \text{ g}}$$

$$x = 0.25 \text{ mol}$$

$$0.25 \text{ mol in 1 L} = 0.25 \text{ mol/L} = 0.25 \text{ M}$$

   (Answer 2) The valence of H_2SO_4 equals 2; therefore the equivalent weight of H_2SO_4 is expressed as follows:

$$\text{Equivalent weight} = \frac{\text{Molecular weight}}{\text{Valence}} = \frac{98 \text{ g}}{2}$$

$$\text{Equivalent weight} = 49 \text{ g}$$

   To solve for number of equivalents in 24.5 g

$$\frac{1 \text{ equivalent}}{49 \text{ g}} = \frac{x}{24.5 \text{ g}}$$

$$x = 0.5 \text{ equivalent}$$

$$0.5 \text{ equivalent in 1 L} = 0.5 \text{ Eq/L} = 0.5 \text{ N}$$

c. The molecular weight of $CaCO_3$ is 100 g/mol and the atomic weight of calcium is 40 g/mol; how many grams or milligrams of $CaCO_3$ are needed to prepare:
   (1) 1 L of 0.1 M $CaCO_3$?
   (2) 10 mL of 100 mg/dL of Ca^{++} using $CaCO_3$?
   (3) 50 mg/L of $CaCO_3$?
   (4) 0.2 mEq/L of Ca^{++} using $CaCO_3$?
   (Answer 1) 10 grams; 1 mol of $CaCO_3$ = 100 g; therefore 0.1 mol = 10 g, since 0.1 molar = 0.1 mol/L = 10 g/L

(Answer 2) The percentage weight Ca^{++} in $CaCO_3$ is

$$\frac{\text{Atomic weight } Ca^{++}}{\text{Molecular weight } CaCO_3} = \frac{40}{100} = 40\%$$

In 10 mL, 10 mg of Ca^{++} is needed or

$$\frac{10 \text{ mg}}{\% \text{ Ca in } CaCO_3} = \frac{10 \text{ mg}}{40\%} = \frac{10 \text{ mg}}{0.4} = 25 \text{ mg of } CaCO_3$$

Therefore 25 mg of $CaCO_3 = 10$ mg Ca^{++}
(Answer 3) For 1 L, 50 mg of $CaCO_3$ is needed.
(Answer 4) 1 equivalent weight of $CaCO_3$ equals

$$\frac{\text{Molecular weight of } CaCO_3}{\text{Valence}} = \frac{100 \text{ g/mol}}{2 \text{ equivalents/mol}}$$
$$= 50 \text{ g/equivalent}$$

To convert to milliequivalents

$$1 \text{ mEq} = \frac{1 \text{ Eq}}{1000}$$

$$\therefore \frac{50 \text{ g}}{1 \text{ Eq}} \times \frac{1 \text{ Eq}}{1000 \text{ mEq}} = 50 \text{ mg/mEq}$$

To calculate amount to prepare 1 L of 0.2 mEq

$$\frac{1 \text{ mEq wt}}{50 \text{ mg}} = \frac{0.2 \text{ mEq wt}}{x}$$

$$x = 10 \text{ mg of } CaCO_3$$

Exercises

7. 3 M $CaCl_2$ (MW 111.1) = _____ N $CaCl_2$
8. 2 NH_3PO_4 (MW 98) = _____ M H_3PO_4
9. 2 M H_2SO_4 (MW 98) = _____ N H_2SO_4
10. 250 mL of 5% NaCl contains _____ g of NaCl
11. How much $CuSO_4 \cdot 5H_2O$ must be weighed to prepare 100 mL of 5% $CuSO_4$? (MW $CuSO_4 = 159.61$; MW $H_2O = 18$)
12. What percent of $CuSO_4 \cdot 5H_2O$ is water? _____%

CALCULATIONS BASED ON PHOTOMETRIC MEASUREMENTS (BEER'S LAW)

Refer to Chapter 4 for a description of the relationship between percent transmittance, absorbance, and concentration.

Colorimetry

Colorimetry is the measurement of the kind and amount of light absorbed or transmitted by a solution. These measurements of absorbance or transmittance are logarithmically related. Beer's law (see below) reflects the relationships between the absorbance and concentration of a known standard solution with that of solutions with unknown concentrations, the patients' samples. Beer's law states that the absorbance of a solution is directly related to its concentration. If Beer's law is true, then:

$$C_u = \frac{A_u}{A_s} \times C_s \qquad\qquad \textit{Eq. 1-3}$$

C_u and A_u represent concentration and absorbance of the unknown samples, whereas C_s and A_s reflect that of the standard solution. When preparing a colorimetric method for clinical chemistry analysis, one must be sure that Beer's law is followed or this formula cannot be used. In other words, this formula can only be used if the absorbance and concentration are directly related, that is, if the absorbance doubles with a doubling of concentration. A *standard curve* can be used to determine concentration values graphically. Standard-curve preparations are described on p. 41.

Absorbance and transmittance

Absorbance measures the amount of light that is blocked, or absorbed by a solution. Absorbance is also termed "optical density" (OD), a term found in the older literature and not in common use today.

Transmittance measures the amount of light that passes through a solution. The transmittance is usually expressed as a percentage, or %T. The %T scale is linear, as noted on a colorimeter readout scale.

As discussed in Chapter 4, the absorbance and percent transmittance are logarithmically related, since absorbance is a logarithmic function. Interconversion of the absorbance and percent transmittance is commonly expressed by the following formula:

$$A = -\log \frac{\%T}{100} \qquad\qquad \textit{Eq. 1-4}$$

This equation can be algebraically converted to the following form:

$$A = -(\log \%T - \log 100)$$
$$A = -(\log \%T - 2)$$
$$A = -\log \%T + 2$$
$$A = 2 - \log \%T \qquad\qquad \textit{Eq. 1-5}$$

One can obtain absorbance from a hand calculator using this formula by punching in the numbers for %T, converting to the log form, placing a minus sign, and adding 2.

Examples. Determining concentrations using absorbance (A, or OD) readings.

a. If absorbance of an unknown is 0.25 and the concentration of a standard is 4 mg/L with an absorbancy of 0.40, the concentration of the unknown can be calculated using:

$$C_u = \frac{A_u}{A_s} \times C_s$$
$$C_u = \frac{0.25}{0.40} \times 4 \text{ mg/L}$$
$$C_u = 2.5 \text{ mg/L}$$

b. To calculate the concentration of glucose if the following information is known:

$$C_s = 2000 \text{ mg/L}, A_s = 0.40, A_u = 0.25$$

Using the same formula above

$$C_u = \frac{0.25}{0.40} \times 2000 \text{ mg/L}$$

$$C_u = 1250 \text{ mg/L}$$

c. To calculate glucose concentration of unknown (C_u) if the %T is given.

If the 1000 mg/L glucose standard (C_s) reads 49% T, and the unknown reads 55% T, the %T must be converted to absorbance, since only absorbance is linearly proportional to concentration:

$$A_s = 2 - \log \%T \qquad A_u = 2 - \log \%T$$

$$A_s = 2 - 1.690 \qquad A_u = 2 - 1.740$$

$$A_s = 0.31 \qquad A_u = 0.26$$

$$49\% \text{ T} = 0.31 \, A = A_s$$

$$55\% \text{ T} = 0.26 \, A = A_u$$

$$C_s = 1000 \text{ mg/L}, A_u = 0.26, A_s = 0.31$$

Using the formula as in (a) and (b) above:

$$C_u = \frac{0.26}{0.31} \times 1000 \text{ mg/L} = 839 \text{ mg/L}$$

Molar extinction coefficient

Molar extinction coefficients are used in the clinical laboratory to calculate concentrations and activities of enzymes in international units (U) and to determine the purity of dissolved substances. Specific applications are checking standard solutions, such as hemoglobin or bilirubin. The molar extinction coefficient, or molar absorbance coefficient, or ϵ, is defined as the absorbance at a given wavelength of a 1 M solution of the substance in a 1 cm cuvette at 25° C. It is related to absorbance by the formula

$$A = \epsilon c l \qquad\qquad \textbf{Eq. 1-6}$$

where A = absorbance at a specified wavelength, c = concentration of substance being measured, in moles/L, and l = the path length in cm.

A suitable bilirubin standard, as a 1 M solution in chloroform, would have a theoretical absorbance of 60,700 (mean) $\pm$ 800 liters·moles^{-1}·cm^{-1} at 453 nm, when measured in a 1 cm cuvette at 25° C. Logical reasoning suggests that if this standard were diluted to 1:60,700 the absorbance would read 1.

Example. 1 M bilirubin standard is diluted to 1:60,700 and then 1:2, with the final dilution being 1:121,400. The absorbance of this dilution reads 0.495 nm in a 1 cm cuvette. What is the extinction coefficient of this bilirubin standard?

$$\epsilon = \frac{0.495 \, (121,400)}{1 \text{ mol/L} (1 \text{ cm})}$$

$$\epsilon = 60,093 \text{ liters·mol}{-1}\text{·cm}{-1}$$

A major application of ϵ is the measurement of concentrations of substances. If the ϵ of a substance is known and a 1 cm cuvette is used, Beer's law formula is simplified to the following:

$$c = \frac{A}{\epsilon}$$

Example. The ϵ of NADH at 340 nm is 6.22×10^3 liters·mol^{-1}·cm^{-1}. If the absorbance of NADH at 340 nm reads 0.350, what is the concentration?

$$c = \frac{0.350}{6.22 \times 10^3 \text{ L·mol}^{-1}}$$

$$c = 5.6 \times 10^{-5} \text{ mol/L}$$

Exercises

13. NADH has a molar absorptivity of 3.3×10^3 at a wavelength of 366 nm. Calculate the concentration of a solution that has an A (absorbance) of 0.175 at 366 nm.
14. A chemistry technologist is checking a bilirubin standard. What would be the molar absorptivity of a 1 M solution diluted to 1:60,700 and reading 0.70 in a 7 mm cuvette?
15. The chemistry technologist has a solution of NADH with a concentration of 0.05×10^{-3} mol/L. Calculate the molar absorptivity if it measures 0.300 at 334 nm.

BUFFERS

Buffers resist changes in acidity by forming a weakly ionized acid or base with the added H^+ or OH^- ions. For example, when HCl is added to a solution of Na^+Ac^- (sodium acetate) plus H^+Ac^- (acetic acid), the H^+ of HCl will react with the Ac^- forming more HAc, which is only slightly ionized. The acetate-acetic acid effectively buffers by removing H^+ from the solution.

The Henderson-Hasselbalch equation is used to express acid-base relationships. There are several forms of this equation that will not be delineated at this time but can be used for calculating acid-base problems. The simplest equation is

$$pH = pK + \log \frac{\text{Concentration of conjugate base}}{\text{Concentration of weak acid}} \quad \textbf{Eq. 1-7}$$

The pK value depends on a specific set of conditions; these are degree of dissociation, temperature, and pH. The pK for the bicarbonate buffer system in serum or plasma is 6.10 at 37° C. Chemical reference books, such as the *Handbook of Chemistry and Physics*,* contain pK values. As capable medical technologists we should grasp the basic calculations of the Henderson-Hasselbalch equations, even though laboratory instruments provide direct "read-out" values on patients' acid-base tests.

---

*Lide DR, editor: *Handbook of Chemistry and Physics,* Cleveland, Ohio, CRC Press, yearly updated editions.

Examples

a. Calculate the pH of an acetate buffer composed of 0.20 M sodium acetate and 0.05 M acetic acid. (The pK for acetic acid is 4.76.)

$$pH = pK + \log \frac{[Salt]}{[Acid]}$$

$$= 4.76 + \log \frac{0.20}{0.05}$$

$$= 4.76 + \log 4$$

$$= 5.3621$$

$$pH = 5.36$$

b. Now for a complicated example. Prepare IL of an acetate buffer whose acetate concentration is 0.2 M and has a pH of 5.0. (The pK of acetic acid is 4.76; the molecular weight of acetic acid is 60 and is 82 for sodium acetate.)

$$pH = 4.76 + \log \frac{[Salt]}{[Acid]}$$

$$\log \frac{[Salt]}{[Acid]} = 5.0 - 4.76$$

$$[Salt]/[Acid] = antilog\ 0.24$$

$$[Salt]/[Acid] = 1.7$$

The number 1.7 is the ratio of the moles per liter of salt to the moles per liter of acid. Any molar concentrations of salt to acid yielding a ratio of 1.7 will result in a 5.0 pH acetate buffer.

Note. The problem specifies a concentration of 0.2 M solution, or HAc + Ac$^-$ = 0.2 M.

If

$$Ac^-/HAc = 1.7$$

then

$$Ac^- = 1.7\ HAc$$

or

$$HAc + 1.7\ HAc = 0.2\ M$$

and

$$2.7\ HAc = 0.2$$

$$HAc = 0.074\ mol/L\ of\ acid$$

$$MW \times M = g/L$$

$$60 \times 0.074 = 4.44\ g/L\ of\ acid\ needed$$

To calculate the weight of salt needed, for IL use:

$$Moles\ of\ salt = Total\ moles - Moles\ of\ acid$$

$$= 0.2 - 0.074$$

$$= 0.126\ moles\ of\ salt$$

As done for the acid:

$$MW\ of\ salt \times M = Grams\ of\ salt/liter$$

$$82\ g/mol \times 0.126\ mol/L = 10.33\ g\ of\ salt/L$$

When 4.44 g of acid and 10.33 of salt are dissolved in a total volume of 1 L, the resulting buffer concentration is 0.2 M at a pH of 5.0.

ENZYME CALCULATIONS

Expressing enzyme activity in international units has been generally accepted since its recommendation by the International Union of Biochemistry in the early 1960s. One international unit, U, of an enzyme is defined as the amount that will catalyze the transformation of 1 μmole of the substrate per minute under standard conditions. Activity is expressed in terms of enzyme units per liter of serum, or milliunits per milliliter, in the following relationship:

$$1\ U/L = \mu mol/minute/liter\ of\ serum$$

Explanation of the basic equation for the conversion of absorbance data to international units will not be attempted in this portion of laboratory calculation. Suffice it to state that any change in factors such as temperature or volume must be accounted for in the following basic equation (see Chapter 54):

$$U/L = \frac{\Delta A/min \times V_t \times 10^6\ (\mu mol/mol)}{\epsilon \times V_s \times l} \qquad \textit{Eq. 1-8}$$

$\Delta A/min$ = Absorbance change per minute
V_t = Total reaction volume including sample, reagent, and diluent
V_s = Serum volume
l = Cuvette path length
ϵ = Extinction coefficient

The factor of 10^6 μmol/mol is added to convert the answer to μmol/min/L (U/L).

Example. What is the lactate dehydrogenase (LD) activity of 0.1 ml of serum + 3 mL of substrate if the NADH being formed showed a 0.002 $\Delta A/min$ at 340 nm? ϵ for NADH = 6.22×10^3 L·mol^{-1}·cm^{-1}.

Using the above formula:

$$U/L = \frac{0.002\ (10^6\ \mu mol/mol)\ (3.1\ mL)}{1\ min \left(6.22 \times 10^3\ \dfrac{L}{mol \cdot cm}\right)(0.1\ mL)\ (1\ cm)}$$

$$U/L = 9.9$$

Example. Calculation of international units per liter of alkaline phosphatase activity using *p*-nitrophenol standard requires attention to all factors of the formula:

$$U/L = \frac{\Delta A/min \times V_t \times 10^6\ (\mu mol/mol)}{\epsilon \times V_s \times l}$$

If ΔA of sample = 0.070, the ϵ for *p*-nitrophenol is 50,000 L/mol·cm; timing = 15 min; V_t = 5.5 mL; V_s = 0.005 mL.

$$U/L = \frac{0.070 \left(10^6\ \dfrac{\mu mol}{mol}\right)(5.5\ mL)}{15\ min \left(50,000\ \dfrac{L}{mol \cdot cm}\right)(0.005\ mL)\ (1\ cm)}$$

$$U/L = \frac{0.070 \times 5.5 \times 1000}{50 \times 0.075}$$

103 U/L = Alkaline phosphatase activity

STANDARD CURVES

Preparation of standard curves on graph paper is an essential way of examining data for validity. Often calculations or computers do not reveal abnormalities of the system, but calculate averages of results. Therefore graphing of data is a very important way to validate assays.

Previously in this chapter, Beer's law was defined as the direct relationship of the absorbance and concentration of a solution. This means that if a 2% solution reads 0.1 A, then a 4% concentration will read 0.2 A, and an 8% solution will read 0.4 A. To repeat, most solutions obey Beer's law; that is, concentration and absorbance are directly proportional only over specified ranges of concentrations.

Graphs

Fig. 1-15. Absorbances of glucose standard concentrations plotted on linear paper result in a straight line, confirming that Beer's law is followed for the concentrations up to 3000 mg/L.

Fig. 1-16. Plotting the %T values of the same glucose concentrations used in Fig. 1-15 on linear paper produces a semicurved line; %T values are *not* linear versus concentrations. (Recall the logarithmic relationship of absorbance and %T.)

Fig. 1-17. Plotting %T values on semilog paper results in a straight line, which can be used to interpolate the concentrations of glucose from %T values.

Exercises (Figs. 1-15 and 1-17)

Find glucose concentrations for the following readings using Figs. 1-15 and 1-17.
16. 0.3 A = _____ mg/L
17. 0.39 A = _____ mg/L
18. 49% T = _____ mg/L
19. 52% T = _____ mg/L

Exercises using one known standard value to determine concentrations of unknowns

What are the glucose concentrations of the following patients' samples if the 2000 mg/L standard reads 0.32 A?

We can employ either:

$$C_u = \frac{A_u}{A_s} \times C_s$$

or

$$\frac{C_u}{C_s} = \frac{A_u}{A_s}$$

20. 0.22 A = _____ mg/L
21. 0.14 A = _____ mg/L
22. 0.46 A = _____ mg/L

Renal clearance test calculations

Renal clearance tests are used to assess kidney function. Renal clearance is a rate measurement that expresses the volume of blood cleared of the substance being studied (typically creatinine or urea) per unit of time. Therefore the unit for the clearance test is milliliters per minute.

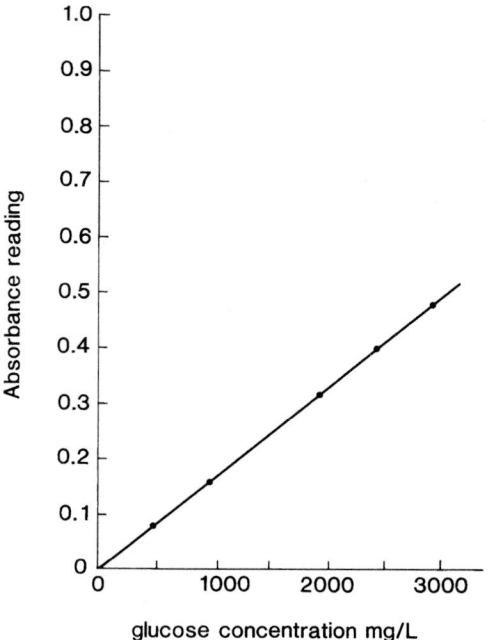

Fig. 1-15 Standard curve for glucose analysis: absorbance versus concentration on linear-linear graph paper.

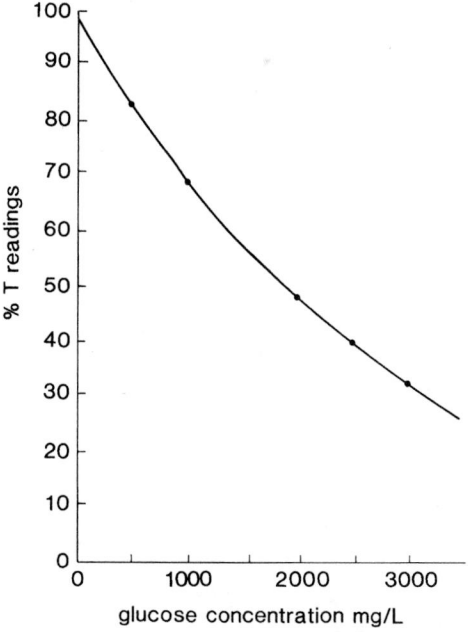

Fig. 1-16 Standard curve for glucose analysis: percent transmittance (%T) versus concentration on linear-linear graph paper.

To calculate creatinine clearance, the following information is required:

Serum concentration (S)

Urine concentration (U) (*Caution:* the serum and urine concentrations must be in the same units, e.g., mg/L or mg/dL.)

Volume of urine excreted per minute (V) (Volume of urine collected divided by time period in minutes)

$$\frac{\text{Clearance}}{\text{(uncorrected)}} = \frac{U \times V}{S}$$

The calculation above does not account for the patient's body surface area. If the physician requests a corrected value, the equation must be multiplied by 1.73/A, where 1.73 equals the average body surface area in square meters and A equals the patient's body surface area.

$$\frac{\text{Clearance}}{\text{(corrected)}} = \frac{U \times V}{S} \times \frac{1.73}{A}$$

The patient body surface area is computed from a nomogram, using the patient height and weight or calculated using the following formula:

$$\log A = (0.425 \times \log W) + (0.725 \times \log H) - 2.144$$

where A is the body surface area in square meters; W is the patient's weight in kilograms; and H is the patient's height in centimeters.

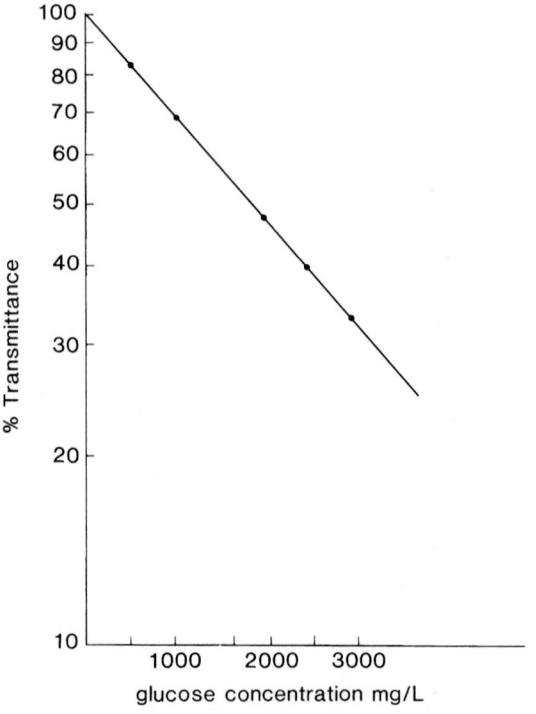

Fig. 1-17 Standard curve for glucose analysis: percent transmittance (%T) versus concentration on log-linear graph paper.

Examples

a. Determine the uncorrected creatinine clearance for a patient with a serum creatinine of 25 mg/L. The urine creatinine was 500 mg/L and the urine volume was 312 mL/4 hr.

$$312 \text{ mL}/240 \text{ min} = 1.3 \text{ mL/min}$$

$$C = \frac{U}{S} \times V = \frac{500}{25} \times 1.3 = 26 \text{ mL/min}$$

b. Calculate the corrected creatinine clearance for a child who weighed 22.7 kg, was 95 cm long, and passed 500 mL of urine during a 24-hour period. Serum and urine creatinine values were 0.14 mmol/L and 4.75 mmol/L respectively.

$$\log A = (0.425 \times \log 22.7)$$
$$+ (0.725 \times \log 95)$$
$$- 2.144$$
$$\log A = 0.576 + 1.434 - 2.144 = 0.134$$
$$A = 0.734$$
$$500 \text{ mL}/1440 \text{ min} = 0.35 \text{ mL/min}$$

$$C = \frac{U}{X} \times V \times \frac{1.73}{A}$$
$$= \frac{4.75}{0.14} \times 0.35 \times \frac{1.73}{0.734}$$
$$= 28.0 \text{ mL/min}$$

Timed urine tests

Results of urine tests may be reported in several ways. Values can be reported as concentration units, quantity per total volume, and quantity per unit of time. The clinical usefulness of urine tests is increased when quantitative results are expressed as amount per total volume or amount excreted in a given time period. Good laboratory practice dictates that the urine total volume and the beginning and end time period of collection be recorded.

When urine test results are reported as quantity per total volume, the concentration is measured and the results are corrected as follows:

$$\frac{\text{Amount}}{\text{Total volume}} = \text{Measured concentration} \times \text{Total volume}$$

This calculation requires that both the urine volume and the instrument concentration be reported using the same units.

Examples

a. Calculate the amount of protein in 2400 mL of urine having a concentration of 30 mg/dL.

$$\frac{\text{Amount}}{\text{Total volume}} = \frac{30 \text{ mg}}{100 \text{ mL}} \times 2400 \text{ mL} = 720 \text{ mg}$$

b. Determine the amount of sodium in 1800 mL of urine with a sodium concentration of 35 mEq/L.

$$\frac{\text{Amount}}{\text{Total volume}} = \frac{35 \text{ mEq}}{1000 \text{ mL}} \times 1800 \text{ mL} = 63 \text{ mEq}$$

When results are reported as quantity per time period of collection, the calculation of amount of substance per total volume must be performed first and the result reported for the length of time instead of for total volume.

ADDITIONAL EXERCISES

23. The hemoglobin standard solution contains 200 g/L. What amounts would be used to prepare 6 mL of the following concentrations?

    200 g/L?   150 g/L?   100 g/L?   50 g/L?

24. a. What fraction of urea is nitrogen? Urea is $CO(NH_2)_2$.

    Atomic weights:
    C = 12
    O = 16
    N = 14
    H = 1

    b. What percent of urea is nitrogen?

25. There is available concentrated HCl having a 38% assay and a specific gravity of 1.170.
    a. What is the weight of HCl present in 1 mL?
    b. For the preparation of 100 mL of 10% wt/vol HCl, _____ mL of HCl would be diluted to total volume of _____ mL.

26. Normal saline solution is 0.85% concentration. What is its molarity? (NaCl molecular weight is 58.5.)

27. If a protein standard reads 0.48 *A*, and a patient's sample reads 0.36 *A*, what is the patient's protein concentration? Select one of the following answers:
    a. Twice the standard concentration
    b. Equal to the standard concentration
    c. Three fourths of the standard concentration
    d. Not enough data for calculation

28. A patient in diabetic coma has high blood glucose levels; so serum from this patient is diluted 1:2 and again 1:2 before it is readable from the glucose chart as 1900 mg/L. What is the actual concentration in (a) mg/L, (b) mg/dL, and (c) g/L?

29. How many mEq/L are there in a solution containing 27.7 mg/dL of potassium? (Atomic weight of K = 39.)

30. How many milliliters of 0.4 N NaOH can be made from 20 mL of 2 N solution?

31. What is the normality of a solution containing 40 mEq of NaOH per 50 mL?

32. What is the dilution of serum in a tube containing 200 μL of serum, 500 μL of saline, and 300 μL of reagent?

33. Calculate the alkaline phosphatase activity in U/L for the following:

    ϵ of standard (*p*-nitrophenol) $= 5 \times 10^4 \text{ L} \cdot \text{mol}^{-1} \cdot \text{cm}^{-1}$

    $$\Delta A_{\text{sample}} = 0.150$$

$$V_{\text{sample}} = 0.2 \text{ mL}$$

$$V_{\text{total}} = 2.2 \text{ mL}$$

$$\text{Timing} = 15 \text{ minutes}$$

34. What is the extinction coefficient for the following:

    Solution concentration = 1.2 molar

    Dilution of solution = 1/121,400

    A reading in a 1 cm cuvette = 0.6

35. A 0.01 M Na_2HPO_4 solution needs to be prepared (MW of Na_2HPO_4 = 141.98). Only the hydrated salt, $Na_2HPO_4 \cdot 7H_2O$ (MW = 267.98) is available. How many grams will be needed to prepare 250 mL?

36. If a 50 mg/mL solution of Na_2HPO_4 needs to be prepared, how many grams of the hydrated salt listed above need to be weighed to make a 1 L solution?

37. A medical technologist desires to prepare 50 mL of a 10 mg/mL solution of NADH (MW = 663.44). To do this accurately, the technologist will first prepare a stock solution containing approximately 50 mg/mL. The absorbance of a 1:1000 dilution of the stock solution will be measured at 340 nm and from the known molar absorbance of NADH at this wavelength (6.22×10^3), the actual concentration will be calculated. A suitable dilution will then be made to prepare the 500 mL of the desired 10 mg/mL solution. Presume that the technologist, following these directions, has prepared a dilution of the stock solution with an absorbance of 0.562. Calculate the concentration of NADH in this stock solution as mmol/L and mg/L. What dilution should be made to prepare the 10 mg/mL of NADH solution?

38. A patient's serum calcium level is 3.5 mEq/L. The expected normal range is 90 to 110 mg/L. Is the patient's calcium level lower than, within, or higher than the expected normal range?

39. A sodium concentration is reported as 3500 mg/L. What is the concentration in mEq/L? (atomic wt. of sodium = eq. wt. = 23 g/mol or 23 mg/mmol)

40. If the cyanmethemoglobin standard, with a concentration of 200 g/L, reads 0.426 *A,* and a patient's blood sample reads 0.297 *A,* what is the concentration of hemoglobin in the sample?

41. A 200 mg/L urea nitrogen standard reads 0.30 *A* and a patient's sample reads 0.40 *A*. The concentration of the standard compared to the patient's level is:
    a. Higher
    b. Twice as much
    c. 3/4 as much
    d. 4/3 as much

42. A glucose standard of 2000 mg/L reads 0.4 *A* and a patient's sample reads 1.0 *A*. The technologist should:
    a. Report result as 500 mg/dL.
    b. Repeat test before reporting.

c. Repeat test on diluted sample.

d. Prepare fresh glucose standard.

APPENDIX: ANSWERS TO PROBLEMS

1. 0.5 M
2. 0.4 M
3. 50 mg/L
4. 1:320
5. 1:128
6. 7.68 mL
7. 6
8. 0.667
9. 4
10. 12.5
11. 7.82
12. 36.05
13. $c = 53 \times 10^{-6}$ mol/L
14. $\epsilon = 60{,}700$ L·mol^{-1}·cm^{-1}
15. 6.0×10^3 L·mol^{-1}·cm^{-1}
16. 1900 mg/L
17. 2400 mg/L
18. 1920 mg/L
19. 1740 mg/L
20. 1375 mg/L
21. 875 mg/L
22. 2875 mg/L
23. 200 g/L = 6 mL + 0 mL of diluent
    150 g/L = 4.5 mL + 1.5 mL of diluent
    100 g/L = 3.0 mL + 3 mL of diluent
    50 g/L = 1.5 mL + 4.5 mL of diluent
24. a. 28/60 = 7/15
    b. 46.6%
25. a. 0.445 g
    b. 22.5 mL will be diluted to 100 mL
26. 0.145 mol/L
27. c
28. a. 7600 mg/L
    b. 760 mg/dL
    c. 7.6 g/L
29. 7.1 mEq/L
30. 100 mL
31. 0.8 N
32. 1:5
33. 2.2 U/L
34. 6.07×10^4
35. 0.67 g
36. 94.4 g
37. Concentration of NADH in stock solution is 90.4 mmol/L or 60 mg/mL. Take 8.3 mL of the stock and dilute to 50 mL to prepare the 10 mg/mL of solution.
38. 70 mg/L: lower than the expected range
39. 152 mEq/L
40. 139 g/L
41. c. 3/4 as much
42. c

REFERENCES

1. *Preparation and testing of reagent water in the clinical laboratory,* ed 2, NCCLS Approved Guideline C3-A2, Villanova, Pa., 1991, National Committee for Clinical Laboratory Standards.
2. Gabler R, Hegde R, Hughes D: Degradation of high purity water on storage, *J Liquid Chromatog* 6:2565-2570, 1983.
3. Winstead M: *Reagent grade water: how, when and why?* American Society of Medical Technologists, Austin, Texas, 1967, Steck Co.
4. Jorgenson JH, Smith, RF: Rapid detection of contaminated intravenous fluids using the *Limulus in vitro* endotoxin assay, *Appl Microbiol* 26:521-524, 1973.
5. Sullivan JD Jr, Valoes FW, Watson SW: Endotoxins: the *Limulus* amebocyte lysate system. In Bernheimer AW, editor: *Mechanisms in bacterial toxicology,* New York, 1976, Wiley & Sons.
6. Bristol DW: Detection of trace organic impurities in binary solvent systems: a solvent purity test, *J Chromatog* 188:193, 1980.
7. *Clinical laboratory technical procedure manuals,* ed 2, NCCLS Approved Standard GP2-A2, Villanova, Pa., 1992, National Committee for Clinical Laboratory Standards.
8. Statement from Quadrennial Symposium on Measurable Properties (Quantities) and Units in Clinical Chemistry, Gaithersburg, Md., August 5 and 6, 1976, *Am J Clin Pathol* 71:465-468, 1979.
9. Kaplan LA, Pesce AJ, editors: *Clinical chemistry: theory, analysis, and correlation,* ed 2, St. Louis, 1989, Mosby.
10. *Determining performance of volumetric equipment,* NCCLS Proposed Standard I8-P, Villanova, Pa., 1984, National Committee for Clinical Laboratory Standards.
11. Lide DR, editor: *Handbook of chemistry and physics,* ed 76, Boca Raton, Fla., 1995, CRC Press.
12. Lashor TW, Macurdy LB: *Precision laboratory standards of mass and laboratory weights,* National Bureau of Standards Circular 547, Washington, D.C., 1954, United States Department of Commerce.
13. McCoubrey AO: *Guide for the use of the international system of units: the modernized metric system,* National Institute of Standards and Technology Spec Publ 811, Washington, D.C., 1991, United States Department of Commerce.
14. The National Committee for Clinical Laboratory Standards Position Paper (PPC-11): quantities and units (SI), *Clin Chem* 25:657-658, 1979.
15. Committee on Hospital Care, American Academy of Pediatrics: Metrication and SI units, *Pediatrics* 65:659-664, 1980.
16. *Laboratory instrument evaluation and verification manual,* Skokie, Ill., 1989, p 99, College of American Pathologists.
17. *Temperature calibration of water baths, instruments, and temperature sensors,* ed 2, NCCLS Approved Standard I2-A2, Villanova, Pa., 1990, National Committee for Clinical Laboratory Standards.
18. *Procedures for the handling and processing of blood specimens,* NCCLS Approved Guideline H18-A, Villanova, Pa., 1990, National Committee for Clinical Laboratory Standards.
19. *Laboratory instrument evaluation and verification manual,* College of American Pathologists, Skokie, Ill., 1989, p 111.
20. *A centrifuge primer,* Palo Alto, Calif., 1980, Spinco Div. Beckman Instruments, Inc.
21. Occupational Safety and Health Administration (Department of Labor): Occupational exposures to hazardous chemicals in laboratories: final rule, *Federal Register* 29 CFR Part 1910.1450, 55(21):300-3335, Jan 31, 1990.
22. Occupational Safety and Health Administration (Department of Labor): Occupational exposure to blood-borne pathogens: final rule, *Federal Register* 29 CFR Part 1910.1030, (235):64003-64182, Dec 6, 1991.
23. *Sigma-Aldrich Library of Chemical Safety Data,* Sigma Chemical Co, St. Louis, Mo. (available in printed or CD-ROM format).
24. Compressed Gas Association, Inc: *Handbook of compressed gases,* ed 2, New York, 1981, Reinhold Publishing Corp.
25. Lan G, Sansone EB: *Destruction of hazardous chemicals in the laboratory,* New York, 1990, Wiley & Sons.
26. United States Department of Health and Human Services: Recommendations for prevention of HIV transmission in health care setting, *Morbidity Mortality Weekly Report* 56(25), Aug 21, 1987.
27. Rutale WA, Weber DJ: Infectious waste—mismatch between science and policy: soundboard, *N Engl J Med* 325:578-581, 1991.
28. Campbell JM and Campbell JP: Laboratory mathematics: medical and biological applications, ed 4, St. Louis, 1990, C.V. Mosby.

CHAPTER 2

Laboratory management

Lawrence J. Crolla
Robert W. Lang
Paul W. Stiffler
Delores Wishart

KEY TERMS

blood-borne pathogens Pathogenic microorganisms that are present in human blood and can cause disease in humans. These pathogens include but are not limited to hepatitis B virus (HBV) and human immunodeficiency virus (HIV).

CAP College of American Pathologists.

CLIA '88 Clinical Laboratory Improvement Amendments of 1988.

complexity model The seven criteria used for categorizing test systems, assays, and examinations based on assigning scores of 1, 2, or 3 within each category.

deemed status Equivalency between accreditation/state requirements and CLIA standards.

demographics Personal data about a specific population.

empowerment When managers create a nurturing environment in which their staff can learn, grow, improve, and function effectively.

Federal Register Provides a uniform system for making available to the public, regulations and legal notices issued by federal agencies.

full-time equivalent (FTE) full-time employee scheduled to work 8 hours per work day for 260 days; or 10 hours per work day for 208 days; or 2080 hours per year.

HCFA Health Care Financing Administration.

HHS Department of Health and Human Services.

high-complexity test One that scores 13 or higher by the complexity model categorization system described in CLIA '88.

hospital information system Miniframe, macroframe, or mainframe computers.

JCAHO Joint Commission on Accreditation of Healthcare Organizations.

laboratory information system (LIS) Miniframe, macroframe, or mainframe computers.

Medicaid A program sponsored by the federal, state, and local governments providing medical benefits to the medically indigent regardless of age.

Medicare A program of medical care and hospital services sponsored by the federal government for persons 65 years and older.

moderate complexity test Test with a score of 12 or less by the complexity model categorization system.

OSHA Occupational Safety and Health Administration.

patient mix The percentage of Medicare, Medicaid, private pay, and charity patients in a hospital's patient population.

productivity Production efficiency expressed as units of work divided by defined hours or defined positions.

quality assurance (QA) program Program designed to (1) monitor and evaluate the ongoing and overall quality of the total testing process and the effectiveness of its policies and procedures; (2) identify and correct problems and assure the accurate, reliable, and prompt reporting of test results; and (3) assure the adequacy and competency of the staff.

quality control (QC) Procedures for monitoring and evaluating the quality of the analytical testing process of each method to assure the accuracy and reliability of patient test results and reports.

service level demands Specimen collection and test turn-around-time requirements for the laboratory.

waived test Test systems or simple laboratory examinations and procedures that are cleared by the FDA for home use; they employ methodologies that are so simple and accurate as to render the likelihood of erroneous results negligible or pose no reasonable risk of harm to the patient if the test is performed incorrectly.

By performing analyses on various biological specimens, the personnel of a clinical chemistry laboratory provide information to physicians that can be used for the diagnosis and treatment of disease. The laboratory must not only comply with legal operating regulations, but it must perform tests in a cost-effective manner as well. The balancing of these requirements is the responsibility of the laboratory management staff. The production of patient results requires a complex infrastructure comprising testing systems (analyzers, reagents, test procedures, and so on), staff to perform the analyses, administrative staff, and systems for the integration of laboratory results with a hospital or other information system.

Much of the way a laboratory must operate is delineated in great detail by federal regulations. The most important of these are found in the Clinical Laboratory Improvement Amendments of 1988 (CLIA '88). The goals of these regulations are to ensure the quality of laboratory test results regardless of where the tests are performed. These regulations cover most aspects of laboratory testing, including proficiency testing, approval of proficiency testing programs, patient test management, quality control, personnel, quality assurance, inspections, and consultations. Other federal and state regulations regulate chemical waste disposal, radioisotope usage, and employee safety, including delineating universal precautions for handling biological specimens.

Because of the great influence of CLIA '88 on laboratory management, much of this chapter refers to sections of these regulations. Therefore we will begin our discussion by first reviewing the regulatory concerns of laboratories.

REGULATIONS

A large part of managing a laboratory today is ensuring that the laboratory is in compliance with all the federal, state, and city regulations that now abound. A hospital laboratory needs to be certified by the Health Care Financing Administration (HCFA), by a private certifying agency, or by a state regulatory agency that has received "deemed status." These certifying agencies inspect laboratories to determine that the laboratories are in compliance with federal regulations, including CLIA '88. The College of American Pathologists (CAP) and the Joint Commission on Accreditation of Healthcare Organizations (JCAHO) are two of the certifying agencies that have received *deemed status* to act on behalf of the federal government. Blood banks require inspections by different certifying agencies.

The CLIA '88 regulations apply to almost every laboratory in the United States that is performing laboratory testing for the assessment of the health of human beings. The regulations are broken into various subparts; the most important subcategories are proficiency testing, quality control, patient test management, and quality assurance.

CLIA '88

The *proficiency testing* (PT) section lists the tests that will be evaluated under federally regulated PT programs. Also listed are the scores necessary for passing such testing and the documentation needed when a laboratory has a PT deficiency.

The patient test management section deals with test requisition and the reporting of test results. This section also specifies how long records must be kept and outlines the documentation necessary for any problems that may have occurred in the reporting process.

The quality control (QC) section specifies how QC is to be done and how often. It also covers procedure manuals (see box, p. 47) and the documentation that is necessary to bring a new test into the laboratory.

The personnel section defines the responsibilities of and the education, training, and experience required for each of the personnel positions at a testing site at which moderate- or high-complexity testing is performed.

The quality assurance section deals with the various *monitors* that should be evaluated to ensure that the laboratory is producing quality work. If all monitors are evaluated in a consistent program, according to the guidelines presented in this section, laboratories will be in compliance with most regulations and should not have to fear unannounced inspections.

The inspection process by the Department of Health and Human Services (HHS) or its designee is described in detail. Failure of an inspection or failure to permit an inspection has severe consequences.

Another federal regulation that is very important to laboratories is the Occupational and Safety Health Act of 1970. Under this act, the Occupational Safety and Health Administration (OSHA) is authorized to implement regulations that ensure the operation of a safe laboratory. OSHA covers all forms of safety, from the physical environment to working with chemicals and blood-borne

---

What Every Procedure Manual Must Include

The procedure manual must include the following, when applicable to the test procedure:

1. Requirements for specimen collection and processing and criteria for specimen rejection.
2. Procedures for microscopic examinations, including the detection of inadequately prepared slides.
3. Step-by-step performance of the procedure, including test calculations and interpretation of results.
4. Preparation of slides, solutions, calibrators, controls, reagents, stains, and other materials used in testing.
5. Calibration and calibration-verification procedures.
6. The reportable range for patient test results as established or verified in CLIA Section 493.1213.
7. Control procedures.
8. Remedial action to be taken when calibration or control results fail to meet the laboratory's criteria for acceptability.
9. Limitations in methodologies, including interfering substances.
10. Reference range (normal values).
11. Imminent life-threatening laboratory results or "panic" (critical) values.
12. Pertinent literature references.
13. Appropriate criteria for specimen storage and preservation to ensure specimen integrity until testing is completed.
14. The laboratory's system for reporting patient results including, when appropriate, the protocol for reporting critical values.
15. Description of the course of action to be taken in the event that a test system becomes inoperable.
16. Criteria for the referral of specimens including procedures for specimen submission and handling as described in CLIA Section 493.1103.

---

pathogens. Chapter 1 discusses many aspects of OSHA regulations.

Several organizations have issued guidelines regarding the length of time that laboratory records must be retained (Table 2-1, p. 50). Because the agencies that issue these guidelines also accredit hospitals and laboratories, these guidelines have the force of law.

The laboratory must devote time to these compliance issues. As an inducement, severe fines can be levied for violation of any of the federal CLIA '88 or OSHA regulations. CLIA '88 certification is also required for Medicare reimbursement, another strong motivation for compliance.

One of the most important actions the laboratory can take to ensure compliance with regulations is to obtain copies of the regulations and make them available to the laboratory personnel. Forming a regulatory committee made up of representatives from each laboratory section also helps to ensure that a laboratory is in compliance with all regulations. The committee can help formulate needed policies and procedures for compliance issues and conduct in-service education and inspections to keep the laboratory

aware of its responsibilities. One can achieve compliance with regulations only by having everyone involved.

HOSPITAL MANAGEMENT STRUCTURE
Organization of a hospital

The size, patient base, market, and affiliations of a hospital affect its organizational structure. Fig. 2-1 illustrates a common organizational structure for a 200- to 300-bed hospital. Larger hospitals will have a similar structure. It is important to note that the vice-presidents each have several departments reporting to them. Since they cannot be experts in all areas, they must work closely with the managers of each reporting department. Each department has its own internal structure, depending on its specific functions. In general, there is a flow of responsibility from least senior managers up through more senior managers up to the department head. The importance of fiscal concerns is so great that most departments have an assumed line of responsibility to the finance department (whether it does or does not officially appear on the organizational chart) to manage billings, research funds, and purchasing. There is usually a discrete section within both the hospital and laboratory for maintaining the computers. The hospital computer processes patient demographic and billing information, whereas the laboratory computer processes laboratory data (see Chapter 18).

Organization of a clinical chemistry laboratory

Departments of pathology should have a generalized organizational chart that shows the reporting relationship between staff member positions in each laboratory or section. This helps everyone to understand the chain of command (authority). This organizational chart should show the lines of "courtesy" reporting, as well as direct reporting, and any outside factors that strongly affect the organizational reporting structure. A typical schema of a department of pathology is illustrated in Fig. 2-2.

Within each clinical laboratory, there should be a detailed organizational chart that shows how each laboratory section is structured. A schema of a "typical" chemistry laboratory is shown in Fig. 2-3. The subdividing of a clinical laboratory into departments, sections or units, and then into shifts should be done in a manner that enables the individual laboratory to use space, equipment, reagents, and personnel efficiently and flexibly to meet the service demands expected of the laboratory. Therefore, the laboratory may not be made up of departments corresponding to the specialties and subspecialties described in the final regulations for CLIA '88, published February 28, 1992, in the *Federal Register*. All laboratory testing must be performed and supervised by qualified and properly trained employees (see below and on p. 50).

Under CLIA '88, the education, certification, and experience requirements for the *laboratory director* of a labora-

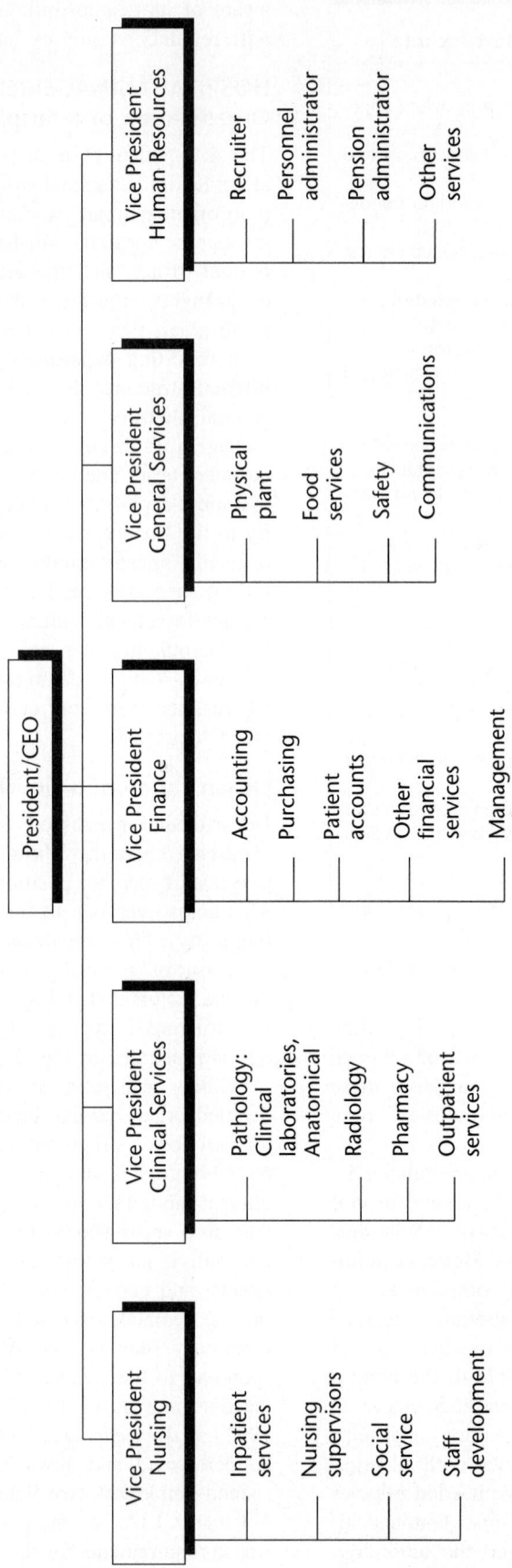

Fig. 2-1 Chart of a hospital organizational structure.

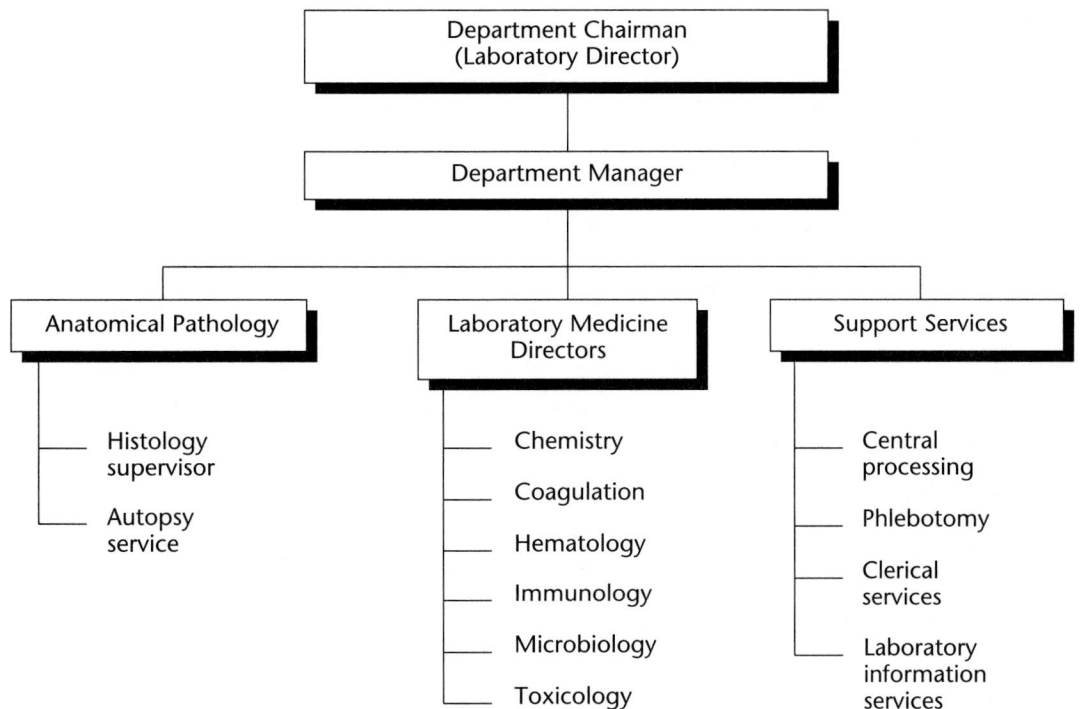

Fig. 2-2   Organizational chart for a department of pathology.

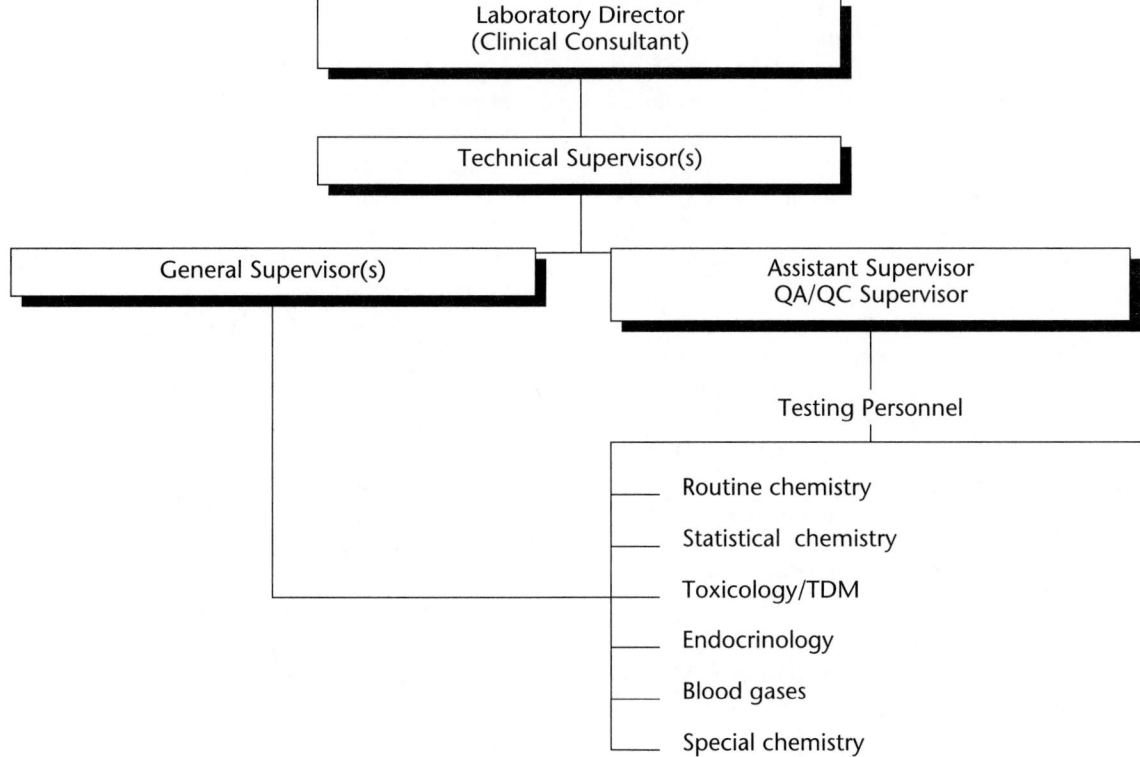

Fig. 2-3   Organizational chart for a chemistry laboratory.

Table 2-1   Guidelines for retaining laboratory records

Type of record	Length of record retention (years)	Note
General§		
Test requisition	2*	
Test records	2†	
Test reports	2†	From date of report, preliminary or final
Quality control	2†	
Laboratory manual test procedures	2*	Two years *after* test is discontinued
Proficiency tests and records of remedial actions	2*	
Instrument maintenance	Life of instrument†	
Personnel	30†	
Clinical laboratory		
Patient accession and test records	2†	
Specimens	24 hours†	
Controlled substances	3†	
Radionucleotides	3†	
Hazardous substances/infectious diseases		
Employee training	3‡	
Employee medical and exposure history	30‡	Thirty years *after* employment
Formaldehyde and benzene exposure	30‡	
Training records	3	From date of training

From Passay R: *Med Lab Observer,* Feb 1993.
*CLIA '88 regulations.
†College of American Pathologists.
‡Occupational Safety and Health Administration.
§CLIA states that records must be kept for 3 years if their retention time is not specifically mentioned in the regulations.

tory performing moderately and highly complex testing are explicitly delineated (sections 493.1405, 493.1406, and 493.1443). These requirements are summarized in Figs. 2-4 and 2-5. A state-licensed M.D., D.O., or D.P.M. or a board-certified Ph.D. can also serve as the laboratory's clinical consultant; that is, interpret laboratory data for the clinical staff for both moderate- and high-complexity testing. If the laboratory performs only moderate-complexity testing, there must be a technical consultant and testing personnel. If high-complexity testing is performed, the laboratory must also have a designated technical supervisor and a general supervisor. CLIA '88 defines a technical supervisor as one who acts as the principal laboratory supervisor, whereas a general supervisor acts as the immediate bench supervisor, reviewing daily work and quality control. Personnel requirements under CLIA are being constantly modified. Please consult the most current regulation for personnel requirements before making any personnel decisions.

Good management skills and personal characteristics

The management skills and personal characteristics of the laboratory manager determine the day-to-day work environment of the clinical laboratory. A motivated professional team is not only able to provide the level of service expected by the medical staff, hospitalized patients, and patients from outpatient and outreach services, but is also able to establish and accomplish its strategic goals.

Many positive management skills and personal characteristics are listed in Table 2-2. Laboratory managers should concentrate on those skills and characteristics that fit their own personalities and the personalities of their employees.

In addition to working with their strengths, good laboratory managers must identify their weaknesses so that these in turn can be strengthened by formal education and training, or by finding the resources (plans and people) that are available to balance these weaknesses. Although the technical staff of laboratories receives training for the specific tasks they will perform, laboratory managers rarely receive management training. It is important to provide both formal and on-the-job training to the laboratory manager. The laboratory manager's personal style, which is the result of the integration of management skills and personal characteristics, will strongly determine how easily and how well the laboratory achieves its goals.

The mix of management skills and personal characteristics will be different for each successful laboratory manager for three basic reasons. The first is that each hospital's administration management team and laboratory staff will have their own unique personalities. The second is that each hospital will have a different strategic plan with specific goals for the laboratory to achieve in addition to maintaining its established service level. The third reason is that the amount and type of resources allocated to the laboratory for maintaining its day-to-day operations will vary from institution to institution.

**Personnel Qualifications
Laboratory Director
Moderate Complexity Testing**
42 CFR 493.1405

A qualified laboratory director must meet the requirements stated in one of the boxes below.

M.D. or D. O.
and
certified by
ABP or AOBP
or
M.D. or D.O. or D.P.M.
and 1 of the following:

- 1 yr. directing or supervising nonwaived lab testing
  - As of 1/19/93, 20 CMEU in lab practice
  - Lab training in Medical Residency equivalent to 20 CMEU

Ph.D. in chemical, physical, biological, or clinical lab sciences and 1 of the following:

- Certified by ABMM, ABCC, ABB, or the ABMLI
- 1 year directing or supervising nonwaived lab testing

Master's degree in chemical, physical, biological, or clinical lab sciences, or medical technology

and

1 year of lab training or experience or both and 1 year supervisory lab experience

Bachelor's degree in chemical, physical, or biological science or medical technology and
2 years of lab training or experience, or both
and
2 years of supervisory lab experience or be serving as a laboratory director and meet qualifications on or before 2/28/92 as laboratory director under CFR 493.1406
or
be qualified on or before 2/28/92 under state law to direct a lab in state in which lab is located

M.D. or D.O. or D.P.M. always needs to be licensed in the state in which the lab is located.

State may require other degrees and experience to be licensed.

All degrees must be from an accredited institution.

This chart is a paraphrased and abridged version of the Code of Federal Regulations, Chapter 42, Section 493. Please consult the Code of Federal Regulations for exact wording. See Federal Register for job responsibilities and more detailed information.

Fig. 2-4 Summary chart of CLIA '88 personnel qualifications for a laboratory director for moderate-complexity testing.

Personnel Qualifications
Laboratory Director
Moderate Complexity Testing
CFR 493.1443

A qualified laboratory director must meet the requirements stated in one of the boxes below.

M.D. or D. O.
and
certified by
ABP or AOBP

or

M.D. or D.O. or D.P.M.
and 1 of the following:

• 2 years directing or supervising
high-complexity testing

• 1 year of lab training
during medical residency

Ph.D. in chemical, physical,
biological, or clinical lab sciences
and 1 of the following:

• Certified by ABMM, ABCC,
ABB, or the ABMLI

• 1 year directing or supervising
nonwaived lab testing

Be serving as a lab director
and must have previously qualified
or been eligible to qualify under
42CFR 493.1415
(published 3/14/90 at 55 FR 9538)
on or before 2/28/92

or

On or before 2/28/92
be qualified under state law
to direct a lab in the state in which
the lab is located

M.D. or D.O. or D.P.M. always needs to be
licensed in the state in which the lab is
located.

State may require other degrees and experience
to be licensed.

All degrees must be from an accredited
institution.

This chart is a paraphrased and abridged
version of the Code of Federal Regulations,
Chapter 42, Section 493. Please consult the
Code of Federal Regulations for exact
wording. See Federal Register for job
responsibilities and more detailed
information.

Fig. 2-5   Summary chart of CLIA '88 personnel qualifications for a laboratory director for high-complexity testing.

Table 2-2   Desirable management skills and personal characteristics for laboratory managers

Analytical	Competent	Compassionate	Trustworthy
Communicative	Articulate	Giving feedback	Financially astute
Fair	Informed	Considerate	LIS literate
Understanding	Political	Listening	Organized
Objective	Punctual	Responsible	Respectful
Accurate	Providing leadership	Rational	Able to delegate
Visionary	Resourceful	Credible	Goal setting

LIS, Laboratory information system.

COMMUNICATION MANAGEMENT
Communication within the total organization

The laboratory manager must communicate effectively and frequently with the appropriate departmental and hospital administrators, hospital departments, hospital committees, and medical staff to keep them informed of the laboratory's progress toward achieving the hospital's goals. This is also a good way for the laboratory manager to keep informed of any changes in the strategic plan or goals, or in the priority of the goals. All interdepartmental communications should be formally documented. When a problem exists, the facts are gathered, and the relative effect of the problem on patients and service level is assessed. Possible solutions are weighed, and a plan of corrective action is developed. The problem, action plan, and outcome must be documented. After an appropriate time, the original problem and solution must be reviewed and reevaluated by everyone involved.

In addition to solving problems as they arise, the lab manager should use frequent, formal communication modes to maintain a professional, cooperative relationship with the medical staff. Modes of communication can include participation in daily medical rounds, participation in departmental and hospital grand rounds, and publication of newsletters. These devices allow the laboratory to keep the medical staff apprised of changes in the field of laboratory science and in the laboratory itself (such as new methods, test availability, or new tests) and allow the medical staff the opportunity to have input into prospective changes. When change in laboratory policy is made without the review and input of the appropriate medical staff that change is at risk for failure.

The laboratory manager must also be adept at using political skills to represent the interests and concerns of the laboratory staff to the entire hospital, especially when resources are limited and additional supplies, space, and staff are needed. Political skill is also required to negotiate agreements and to promote understanding and cooperation in the total organization. It cannot be emphasized strongly enough that the laboratory manager, while being an advocate for the laboratory, is expected to be a loyal member of the administrative staff.

Communication within the laboratory

Two effective tools that can help laboratory managers to be successful are *participative management* and *empower-*

ment. For these tools to be used effectively, the laboratory staff must be kept informed with accurate and timely information.

For participatory management the laboratory staff must have a clear understanding of the level of service it needs to provide (work load), the long-term goals it must achieve (strategic plan), and the resources that have been allocated to accomplish these tasks. With this information, the laboratory staff can actively participate in planning. After clearly communicating the laboratory's goals, the laboratory manager should allow the laboratory staff to participate in setting objectives, planning, and problem solving. The perspective of technologists and supervisors is clearly different from that of a laboratory manager, and each can contribute to overall planning. This is also an effective way for the laboratory manager to establish visibility, accessibility, and credibility with the staff and to gain their trust and respect. Also giving and receiving feedback, positive or negative, help motivate the laboratory staff to achieve its goals.

No manager should assume that the laboratory staff has unlimited capacity and no burn-out threshold. With the use of positive feedback on a regular basis, dedicated staff members can occasionally achieve herculean goals under unusual circumstances. However, a good manager recognizes that there are limitations in operating a laboratory this way. A workable laboratory operation must have an adequate number of testing personnel and the necessary reagents and equipment to process the routine work load and achieve the goals of the strategic plan.

The manager needs to stay in constant touch with the technical staff, either directly or through the supervisory staff, to monitor the progression of assigned tasks. This may take the form of informal meetings in the laboratory or formal meetings with one or more staff members. Formal meetings should always have an agenda. The laboratory manager can communicate with the staff by memorandum, bulletin board posting, computer mail box, telephone, or facsimile transmission. Minutes should be taken when one is meeting with personnel, either individually or in groups. Minutes should clearly state the outcome of the meeting, including goals that have been set or actions that need to be taken. Meeting minutes should be distributed to everyone who attended or usually attends a meeting. Frequent communication shortens the period of time the staff or manager is "off target" for achieving the goals and allows for a constant reassessment of the practicality of the plan of action.

PERSONNEL MANAGEMENT
Staff

CLIA '88 has created job categories for all clinical laboratory technical and testing positions. It has also established uniform requirements that include the minimum education and experience a person must have to direct, consult, supervise, or perform each specific test on human specimens. These job categories are described in the final regulations for CLIA '88, published in the *Federal Register* on February 28, 1992, and in the correction amendments published in the *Federal Register* on January 19, 1993, July 22, 1993, April 24, 1995, and May 15, 1995.

Under CLIA '88 the education and experience requirements for each job category depend on the complexity rating of the tests being performed in the laboratory. The test-complexity model assigns all tests to one of four categories: waived, physician-performed microscopy, moderately complex, or highly complex. The HCFA classifies each test by method, instrument, reagent, and complexity. These test classifications are published periodically in the *Federal Register*. Until a test is classified, it is considered highly complex. There are no education or experience requirements for the personnel who perform and report the results of waived tests. Currently waived tests include some procedures used for home testing. If the tests performed by the laboratory are classified as moderately complex (with no highly complex tests being performed), the laboratory must have a laboratory director, technical consultant, clinical consultant, and testing personnel. The requirements for education and experience or training for each of these positions are less stringent than those for the positions required when highly complex tests are performed.

When highly complex testing is performed (whether or not moderately complex tests are performed too), the laboratory must have a laboratory director, technical supervisor, clinical consultant, general supervisor, and testing personnel. Testing personnel who perform highly complex tests must have at least an associate degree, or they must have a high school diploma or equivalent and have been doing high-complexity testing as of January 19, 1993; the work of personnel in the latter category must be reviewed within 24 hours by a general supervisor. By 1997, individuals without at least an associate degree in laboratory science or meeting other requirements in the April 24, 1995 Federal Register Section 493.1489 will not be permitted to perform high-complexity testing. Anyone who is eligible to perform highly complex testing can also perform moderately complex testing. Laboratory managers must keep abreast of additions, changes, and deletions to these personnel qualifications as HCFA makes them.

The laboratory manager must identify each test performed in house as waived, moderately complex, or highly complex, so that the tests can be performed by adequately trained and supervised personnel. The test mix, test volume, and service level including test frequency, and turnaround time will then determine the actual number and types of supervisory and testing personnel positions needed to be in compliance with CLIA '88 and to provide adequate service.

Job or position description

Every technical and testing staff *position* should have a clearly written three-part job or position description. One part should state, as a minimum, the education and experience or training required by CLIA '88 for the position. Any additional requirements formulated by the laboratory should be included. The second part should document the specific tests to be performed or supervised, showing the classification of each test as waived, moderately complex, or highly complex. The job description must indicate whether the individual holding a specific position will be performing or supervising each analysis. It is essential to verify the credentials of each staff member to be sure that each has the education and experience required by CLIA '88 to perform, direct, or supervise the specified tests. The third part of the job description should contain, as a minimum, the general responsibilities of the specific position, the CLIA '88 requirements that must be met, and the standards for acceptable performance.

According to 493.1425 of the final regulations of CLIA '88, "the testing personnel for moderately complex testing are responsible for specimen processing, test performance, and reporting test results:

a. Each individual performs only those moderate complexity tests that are authorized by the laboratory director and require a degree of skill commensurate with the individual's education, training or experience, and technical abilities.

b. Each individual performing moderate complexity testing must:
(1) Follow the laboratory's procedures for specimen handling and processing, test analyses, reporting and maintaining records of patient test results;
(2) Maintain records that demonstrate that proficiency testing samples are tested in the same manner as patient samples;
(3) Adhere to the laboratory's quality control practices, document all quality control activities, instrument and procedural calibrations and maintenance performed;
(4) Follow the laboratory's established corrective action policies and procedures whenever test systems are not within the laboratory's established acceptable levels of performance;
(5) Be capable of identifying problems that may adversely affect test performance or reporting of test results and either must correct the problems or im-

mediately notify the technical consultant, clinical consultant or director; and

(6) Document all corrective actions taken when test systems deviate from the laboratory's established performance specifications.

According to 493.1495 of the final regulations of CLIA '88, for high-complexity testing, the testing personnel are responsible for specimen processing, test performance, and for reporting test results:

a. Each individual performs only those high-complexity tests that are authorized by the laboratory director and require a degree of skill commensurate with the individual's education, training or experience, and technical abilities.

b. Each individual performing high-complexity testing must follow the six directives listed previously for those performing moderately complex tests. In addition, a seventh directive and an exception apply:

(7) "If qualified under 493.1489(b)(4), [the individual] must perform high complexity testing only under the on-site, direct supervision of a general supervisor qualified under 493.1461."

c. *Exception:* "For individuals qualified under 493. 1489(b)(4), who were performing high complexity testing on or before January 19, 1993, the requirements of paragraph (b)(7) of this section are not effective, provided that all high complexity testing performed by the individual in the absence of a general supervisor is reviewed within 24 hours by a general supervisor qualified under 493.1461."*

A parallel description should be prepared for each testing person listing the person's educational background, the degree of testing complexity the person can perform under CLIA rules, and whether or not the person requires direct supervision or supervisory review. Table 2-3 lists the information that should be kept in each analyst's personnel file.

Work scheduling

The actual staff schedule for a particular laboratory may not conform to the standard three 8-hour shifts per day, with staff members working five 8-hour days per week. Alternative scheduling formats include the use of 10-hour shifts, flex-time, and staggered shifts. Many laboratories will use a combination of all these formats to achieve complete coverage. This provides overlap between shifts and enhances intershift communication and continuity of work flow.

Laboratory managers must take into account the strengths and weaknesses of individual technologists when planning a work schedule, including the balance of weaker and stronger technologists in each shift. By careful review of

Table 2-3   Useful information to keep in each employee's personnel file

- Performance standards
- Employee application including working experience
- Relevant education and certification
- Level of CLIA test complexity employee can perform
- Whether employee requires direct supervision
- Areas of the laboratory employee is competent to staff
- Periodic evaluations for competency
- In-service education record
- Record of training in health and safety measures
- Training courses attended
- Record of vaccinations, such as for hepatitis B, or a signed statement declining the vaccination

CLIA, Clinical Laboratories Improvement Amendments.

work-load statistics, the laboratory manager can determine whether the work-load is distributed equitably within a shift as well as between shifts, and schedule staff accordingly. Some work areas, such as an intensive-care laboratory, are station-filled positions and must always be staffed.

Laboratory staffing must take into account the number of days off allowed for sick leave, personal leave, holiday leave, and vacation leave. Thus, for one station-filled position, between 1.5 and 2.0 individuals must be hired for each shift to provide coverage 7 days a week.

Because the largest single cost for a laboratory is labor, most laboratories will attempt to increase productivity (billable tests/full-time equivalents [FTE]) by automation or by combining work stations to increase efficiency (see Chapter 16). Further discussion of productivity is found on page 57 (resource management).

Continuing education and employee competency

Continuing education. The final regulations of CLIA '88 state that the laboratory director or technical consultant in the moderately complex testing laboratory and the laboratory director or technical supervisor in the highly complex testing laboratory must identify needs for remedial training or continuing education to improve skills. They must also identify the training needs for each work station and assure that each individual performing tests receives regular in-service training and education appropriate for the type and complexity of the laboratory services performed. Therefore the laboratory must maintain a current list of the continuing education programs available both in house and through professional organizations that meet these needs for laboratory personnel.

The laboratory can offer programs on general topics such as laboratory management, laboratory information systems, government regulations for laboratories, OSHA, safety, and technology of the future, and programs on specific technical topics such as pathophysiology, current in-house testing, and instrumentation. Attendance at state, regional, and national meetings should be encouraged when topics and

---

*The CLIA '88 personnel qualifications and regulations are frequently being modified, and so it is advisable to consult with HCFA for the most current information.

exhibits are pertinent. Attendance at all continuing education programs must be documented and a record of attendance maintained in the employee's personnel file.

Employee competency. The laboratory director has the ultimate responsibility for ensuring the competency and continuing education of the testing personnel under the final regulations of CLIA '88. The actual details are specified in sections 493.1413(b)(8,9) and 493.1451(b)(8,9), which state that "the technical consultant in the moderately complex testing laboratory and the technical supervisor in a highly complex testing laboratory, respectively, are responsible for:

(8) Evaluating the competency of all testing personnel and assuring that the staff maintain their competency to perform and report test results promptly, accurately and proficiently. The procedures for evaluation of the competency of the staff must include, but are not limited to:

(i) Direct observations of routine patient test performance, including patient preparations, if applicable, specimen handling, processing and testing;

(ii) Monitoring the recording and reporting of test results;

(iii) Review of intermediate test results or worksheets, quality control records, proficiency testing results, and preventive maintenance records;

(iv) Direct observation of performance of instrument maintenance and function checks;

(v) Assessment of test performance through testing previously analyzed specimens, internal blind testing samples or external proficiency testing samples; and

(vi) Assessment of problem solving skills; and

(9) Evaluating and documenting the performance of individuals responsible for moderate complexity testing (technical consultant) and high complexity testing (technical supervisor) at least semiannually during the first year the individual tests patient specimens. Thereafter, evaluation must be performed at least annually unless test methodology or instrumentation changes, in which case, prior to reporting patient test results, the individual's performance must be reevaluated to include the use of the new test methodology or instrumentation.

The frequency of reviews may be greater, according to local regulations.

Besides evaluating employee competency under CLIA '88, routine assessments of the testing personnel for productivity and general goal achievement must be discussed with each individual employee. Personnel should know why they have performed less well than, as well as, or better than expected, and each should be given positive ways to achieve better performance. The employee must be given an opportunity to comment on the review. The entire assessment process must be documented, with copies sent to the employee and the employee's file. Documentation of fair and frequent assessments is important for the development of the employee (see below), as well as to provide a framework for necessary disciplinary actions.

Career ladders

The process of continuously training and motivating the laboratory staff is a significant part of the manager's job. Routine technical work coupled with limited opportunity for advancement can lead to high staff turnover. The use of a system of career ladders can help to overcome these obstacles to staff retention. In this system the credentials and experience required to advance to the next position (the next rung of the ladder) are clearly delineated. To establish a system of career ladders in the clinical laboratory, an employee planning group, after studying the needs of the laboratory and the workers, should design and prepare a model program and submit it to management for review and approval. Once approved, the steps for implementation must be formally established by management and the laboratory staff. This approach helps enhance employee acceptance and focuses the program on specific worker-identified needs.

The basic career ladder must give all qualified employees the opportunity for advancement. To make this possible, the steps on the career ladder, along with the responsibility and privileges of each step, must be defined. New positions with responsibilities that are intermediate between those of a technologist and those of a supervisor may need to be created. In addition, the laboratory manager, whenever possible, should promote from within. This type of policy tends to develop dedicated and loyal employees who can move both horizontally and vertically within the organization. Once a career ladder plan is accepted, management should meet individually with each employee to set specific goals for that employee, including implementation guidelines, time frames for the tasks to be completed, and the rewards for successful completion. The laboratory manager must regularly monitor the progress of each employee and give feedback and encouragement to keep the employees on track to reach their goals.

The final regulations of CLIA '88 state that anyone with at least a high school diploma or equivalent can be trained to perform moderately complex tests (493.1423). Appropriate training and proficiency must be documented before the staff member is permitted to analyze patient specimens. This makes it possible for certain nontesting personnel like phlebotomists and aides to be trained to function as testers. Criteria should be established for the promotion of testing personnel to supervisory positions within the laboratory. Likewise, management positions or ancillary positions with the laboratory information system, outreach programs, or nonlaboratory positions should be identified. The education and training requirements and job responsibilities for all positions must be written down. The benefits of promotion to the employees are greater job satisfaction, additional education, recognition for achievement by feedback, a basis for a more objective performance appraisal, and monetary compensation.

Cross-training, which allows staff members to be rotated into several departments, is another option for career ladders. Cross-training serves to relieve the monotony of specialization where an analyst performs the same job function day after day. Cross-training can broaden and sharpen a worker's skills, allowing that staff member to work with more people and develop a better understanding of the entire laboratory operation. In some laboratories, cross-training may be a necessity, providing increased staffing flexibility so that the laboratory can meet service demands. A specialist in an area can promote continuity and competently train new staff members. However, specialization can cause staffing problems by decreasing laboratory flexibility.

RESOURCE MANAGEMENT

The laboratory manager is responsible for managing laboratory resources, which include laboratory staff, reagents, supplies, and capital equipment. Using these resources, the laboratory must provide the services expected of it, as defined by the hospital's strategic plan. The laboratory's role is developed during discussions with laboratory users that elucidate their needs and expectations. What services should be provided, for whom, how often, at what cost, and at what time must all be agreed upon.

The laboratory manager must accept the strategic plan on behalf of the laboratory and must use all laboratory resources to fulfill the goals of the plan. The competent manager will motivate and empower the laboratory staff to plan and implement the tasks necessary to achieve the goals of the strategic plan. Therefore the manager must promote an atmosphere of freedom and creativity where employee involvement is valued.

In addition to introducing new diagnostic tests to maintain service levels at the highest possible standards, the laboratory manager, when appropriate, seeks new business for the laboratory. If successful, the manager must motivate the laboratory staff by helping them to realize that these opportunities are in their best professional interest.

Practically speaking, resource management is used to carry out the day-to-day laboratory operation. To manage these responsibilities successfully, the laboratory manager must prepare one set of agenda for the short-term (day-to-day operation) plan and a second set of agenda for the long-term (strategic) plan, which sets goals for the next 5 years.

Resources need to be allocated based upon current data, historical data, and predictions about the effect of current trends as they relate to the laboratory's operation. In the short term, sudden increases in the work load can be ac-

commodated if the laboratory has equipment with the capacity to handle higher volumes or backup equipment and cross-trained staff. Use of overtime, reassigning work to another work station, or sending low-volume testing to a reference laboratory may also help. Moving work to another shift that has the capacity to absorb the extra work is another option. If the trend is sustained and permanent increases are seen in the routine work load, appropriate measures must be taken to obtain additional staff, reagents and supplies, and equipment, if necessary. If the work load suddenly decreases, work stations can be shut down or consolidated with other work stations that have the capacity to handle additional work. In addition, laboratory staff members can be encouraged to use earned vacation time, take personal time off, or cut back on hours.

Long-term planning is concerned with the laboratory operation a year or more into the future. The laboratory manager must closely follow the current day-to-day operation of the laboratory, predicting the effects of current trends on laboratory operation in the future. Specifically the effect of projected changes in test volume and test mix on staffing, reagents, supplies, and equipment must be evaluated so that future service level demands can be adequately met. When planning for the future, one should consider the following significant factors: the possibility of new government regulations, the opportunity for reimbursement, the need for cost control, the existence of markets for laboratory services, customer satisfaction, employee satisfaction, and existing competition. In addition, the laboratory manager must be aware of technological advances that have the possibility of increasing the laboratory's productivity.

It is critical that the laboratory manager communicate regularly with the laboratory staff about those changes that strongly influence the current day-to-day operation of the laboratory and about those changes that may influence the laboratory in the future. All staff members should participate in the process of making provisional or final plans to accommodate these changes.

FINANCIAL MANAGEMENT
Budgeting

The laboratory manager has the responsibility for preparing the laboratory's operating budget and for ensuring that the laboratory operates within that budget. Supervisors and section heads should participate in preparing the budget by taking responsibility for the budgets of their respective sections.

The budget is prepared by using actual figures from the laboratory's current operating expenses, revenues, utilization data, and patient demographics. Any factors that may have a material effect on the financial operation of the laboratory during the current and next budget years must be taken into account when one is preparing the budget. The greater the service level demands, the greater the basic operating expenses will be because more personnel, reagents, and equipment will be needed. Increases in basic expenses must be considered when the profitability of increases in testing volume is analyzed. Once the budget has been approved by the administration, the laboratory manager must verify the budget to be sure that all provisions are accurate. The actual verification of the budget can be done by those in the laboratory most familiar with each component of the operation. The supporting detailed documents that were used to prepare the budget are also used for this process.

The budget should be easy to read and understand so that it can be regularly monitored and variations beyond established limits can be readily identified and investigated. The expense, revenue, and utilization line items for each laboratory unit should be individually defined so that they can be closely monitored to ensure that the budget is being followed. The line items for each financial and operational laboratory unit may include labor and benefits, testing supplies, nontesting supplies, reagents, equipment rental and lease contracts, service contracts, repairs and maintenance, payment for tests sent to reference laboratories, individual test utilization, inpatient/outpatient/other charges and revenue (billed and collected), and bad debt.

The records used to prepare the current budget should be retained so that variations within each line item can be readily investigated. There should be monthly reports comparing each unit's actual performance to that predicted in the budget. The laboratory should establish criteria for investigating variances from the budget. Explanations for each unacceptable line item variance should describe the variance as a trend, a random fluctuation, or an actual change caused by periodic ordering or payment patterns, changes in work load, personnel-related matters, or operational changes. The explanation should include any corrective actions to be taken. Notes kept during the corrective action investigation will help in preparing the next budget.

Comparisons of year-to-date actual performance to both the budget predictions and to last year's actual figures may be used to show trends in specific line items. These trends can sometimes be seen only in the budget of a particular item and not in the budget of the entire laboratory. Monthly and year-to-date comparison studies allow the laboratory

manager to review each unit's specific variances and to take corrective action to adjust the budget for the individual unit or total laboratory. Understanding the reasons for the variances from budget will enable the laboratory manager to prepare future budgets that will reflect revenue and expense items more accurately.

Capital justification

Most laboratories require capital justification for one-time purchases costing over a designated amount, often $500. The level of detail required to justify a purchase may vary with the cost of the purchase. If equipment is purchased for laboratory testing, the justification must clearly detail the costs of the item, installation, supplies, reagents, controls, standards, and a service contract. The laboratory manager should calculate the cost per reportable result, taking into account the frequency and size of runs, frequency of calibrations, whether the equipment will be used for stat. or routine testing, or both, whether single or duplicate samples will be tested, and the number of repeat, control, and standard samples analyzed per run. The labor cost per test must also be accurately calculated. Finally an operational and financial comparison of the proposed method to the existing method should underscore and substantiate the capital justification.

When acquiring a piece of capital equipment, the laboratory manager may wish to maximize flexibility for obtaining "state of the art" technology by minimizing the time period that the laboratory is obligated to use a specific instrument. Therefore the laboratory manager must carefully evaluate the costs of purchasing, leasing, renting, or reagent renting an instrument. When an instrument is acquired through a reagent rental plan, the laboratory is billed for the reagents only (the vendor includes the equipment price in the reagent pricing) at an agreed upon price. The laboratory contracts to purchase a minimum amount of testing materials, based on current and future needs. Table 2-4 shows how to compare reagent rental costs to an outright purchase. The type of buying decisions described in Table 2-4 are based on cash flow. If lump sum capital dollars are not available, reagent rental can be used to acquire a piece

Table 2-4 Comparison of outright purchase* versus reagent rental

Outright purchase	Reagent rental
Instrument price	Reagent cost/test†,‡ × Test volume/year × 5 years
Loss of interest on money for 5 years	Total cost for 5 years
Service contract for 4 years	
Instrument cost for 5 years	
Instrument cost for 5 years	
Reagent cost†/test × Test volume/year × 5 years	
Total cost for 5 years	

*Add individual lines to sum up costs.
†Includes volume of calibrators and controls.
‡Assumes service is included for 5 years.

of equipment. However, buying capital equipment using reagent rental programs may cost the hospital more real dollars than a lump sum purchase. The reason is that the hospital normally gets some reimbursement from Medicare and other payers for capital expenditure. If reagent rental is used, there is no capital reimbursement. If cash flow is an issue, a true lease can be used. In this vehicle, a monthly capital cost is billed along with the reagent cost. This capital cost can usually be submitted for reimbursement.

Additional incentives are sometimes offered by the manufacturer when more than one unit is to be obtained. As stated above, it is necessary to perform a cost analysis for each test being considered and to prepare a pro forma financial statement for the equipment being acquired. Also the cost of evaluating and setting up the method chosen should be taken into account. In all cases, the test cost analysis and pro forma financial statement must be clearly written and carefully documented with supporting data attached to the written report. A copy of the manufacturer's contract should also be included.

Purchasing

Supplies, reagents, and equipment are purchased with funds allocated in the department budget. To stay within this budget, the laboratory manager, staff, and purchasing department must work as a team, securing the lowest prices available from vendors, national contracts, and various buying groups. Price, location of distribution centers, availability of items, and a vendor's customer service should be evaluated before one makes the decision to place a specific or standing order. It may be necessary to purchase a specific, more expensive reagent or supply instead of purchasing a lower-price generic item to be certain that test results are accurate and that test systems function properly. The purchasing department should aid in negotiating volume discounts and in obtaining the same lot numbers over time for longer consistency of results. CLIA '88 stipulates (493.1218) that new lots of reagent, or even new shipments of the same lot, must be verified for usability.

One of the biggest problems most hospitals face is cash flow; that is, collecting sufficient funds in time to pay expenses. For this reason, alternative purchasing options have become common in the laboratory setting. However, when making these transactions, one must always consider the cost of borrowing money.

Cost accounting

Cost accounting is a method by which all costs associated with the production or acquisition of a particular item are identified. In the clinical laboratory, this is primarily applied to calculation of the cost per billable test result. The more detailed and complete the analysis, the more accurate and useful the cost determination will be. Table 2-5 supplies a list of costs to be included in the analysis. Using a complete analysis may highlight overlooked cost factors that

Table 2-5   Direct versus indirect costs

Direct costs	Indirect costs
Reagents	Building depreciation
Labor	Hospital overhead
Equipment costs	Laboratory overhead
Service costs	Accounting expenses
Collection supplies	Regulatory expenses
Testing supplies	Management labor
Quality control material	LIS expenses
Depreciation	

LIS, Laboratory information system.

have a significant influence on calculating the true cost per reportable result. There is a significant advantage in understanding which factors have the greatest effect on test costs and which factors are affected by equipment or methodologies within one's own laboratory. This type of analysis is also advantageous when one is comparing a new test method or procedure to an existing one to calculate more accurately the true cost per reportable test result. The ultimate goal of cost accounting is the determination of the *actual* cost for a billable test. This allows the laboratory manager to price tests aggressively in a competitive marketplace. The simplest way to perform cost accounting is to use software, such as SUMIT™, which is specifically designed for laboratory cost accounting.

Overview of reimbursement issues

Reimbursement in a hospital setting refers to the process by which payments are received from payers such as Medicare and Medicaid, private insurance companies, health maintenance organizations, and patients. Private patient billing is the smallest billing component in most institutions, and these patients are the only ones who pay the full amount of the hospital bill. Most other payers negotiate a discount rate with the hospital or laboratory. Medicare pays a flat rate per diagnosis. This flat rate is based on a 1983 system called the DRG (Diagnosis Related Group). The flat payment is fixed for each diagnosed disease (DRG) and covers all inpatient services, including laboratory tests performed during a patient's hospital stay.

Medicare reimbursement is broken into two categories: Part A and Part B billing. Most simply stated, Part A billings provide payment for inpatient hospital services, whereas Part B billings pay for physician services and outpatient laboratory tests. If outpatient laboratory tests are performed within 72 hours of admission, hospitals are required to include them for coverage under the DRG payment rather than bill separately for them. All outpatient tests are reimbursed according to a code number. These numbers, called CPT codes (Common Procedure Terminology), are constantly updated and modified. The laboratory must always have a current copy of CPT codes for billing.

Medicare currently reimburses hospitals for some capital expenditures using a formula based upon expenses. Medicare is, however, phasing in a 10-year plan that will make a fixed payment for capital expenditure for each Medicare patient treated. This new reimbursement plan will have the effect of forcing a laboratory to operate more like a business. Reimbursement will be based upon a capital payment of approximately $400 per discharge. Fewer patients means less money available for capital expenditures. Also, if a hospital doesn't make a capital purchase, it still receives the same money. This policy could induce laboratories to retain equipment for longer periods of time. The reimbursement could then be accounted for as profit. This plan, however, will eventually put an institution behind in acquiring new, high-efficiency equipment that is needed to maintain competitiveness.

INFORMATION MANAGEMENT

Chapter 18, Laboratory information systems (LIS), reviews the use of an LIS to manage information and increase a laboratory's productivity. Financial and utilization reports generated by the LIS are some of the tools used to manage information. Table 2-6 lists many of the utilization reports that should be routinely reviewed by a laboratory manager. A list of work production reports can be found on p. 332 in Chapter 18.

When one is setting up a management system to evaluate laboratory performance, it is important that the system include monitors for four aspects of operations. These elements include:

Financial performance
Productivity
Utilization
Test-result turnaround time

The following section briefly summarizes several key indicators for each aspect of operations. The monitoring system should evaluate each section individually (such as chemistry, hematology, and microbiology) and the laboratory as a whole.

Financial performance

Financial reports of the LIS should provide accurate, up-to-date, detailed information about how actual laboratory expenses compare with those planned for in the budget. However, these financial reports don't inform the laboratory manager about how well the laboratory is performing compared to hospitals of similar size, acuity, location, and service level. Subscribing to a commercially available database system such as LABTRENDS* allows such comparisons to be made. Comparisons can be made for specific laboratory areas, and significant differences can be evaluated and corrective action can be taken to improve productivity, expenses, or revenue.

The average cost per performed test is an exceptionally important measure of operational performance. Since labor

---

*LABTRENDS is a database service offered by Health Care Development Inc., Northbrook, Illinois.

Table 2-6 Examples of laboratory management reports provided by an LIS

Type of report	Function	Frequency
Total work load	Monitors adequacy of the total number of personnel in the laboratory	Quarterly
	Monitors work-load trends	
Shift work load	Monitors adequacy of the number of staff in each shift	Quarterly
Employee work load	Monitors the work load of one analyst; compares productivity to others in shift and between shifts	Quarterly
Routine quality control	Monitors short-term accuracy and precision	Bimonthly
Turnaround time	Monitors the adequacy of service	Monthly

and supplies usually constitute about 70% to 75% of most laboratories' budgets (including employee benefits, depreciation expense, and pathologist compensation), it is important to monitor these elements of laboratory costs. Repair, preventive maintenance, and referred testing usually represent 3% to 10% of most hospital laboratory budgets. Monitors for these costs are shown in the box on page 61.

Productivity

Measuring the overall productivity of the laboratory and of each laboratory section should be part of any operational performance system developed. The following indicators should be included in the review of productivity:

Number of performed tests/testing FTE (including supervisor time) (assigned to an individual work station)
Number of performed tests/total FTE
Number of performed tests/worked hour
Worked hours as a percentage of paid hours

In the past, laboratories used the CAP work-load units as an indicator of productivity. These units assigned a certain number of work units to every laboratory procedure based on the time required to perform the procedure. Laboratories would then compare their actual productivity values to a calculated number based on the procedures they performed. However, these numbers were believed to be unreliable, and in 1992 the CAP discontinued their work-load plan. It has been replaced by a system that uses some of the parameters listed above.

Using the above parameters and comparing the laboratory to a database such as LABTRENDS™ or the CAP program, LMIP™, the laboratory manager can see how efficient his or her laboratory is compared to similar laboratories. This comparison can then be used to help justify additional personnel if the laboratory is operating with insufficient staff (higher than average productivity) compared to the mean of the comparative database.

Financial Performance Monitors

Cost/On-Site Performed Test
Compensation and Benefit Expense/Performed Test
Compensation and Benefit Expense/Hour
Supply Expense/Performed Test
Cost/Referred Test
Repair and Preventive Maintenance Expense/Performed Test
Pathologist Compensation as a Percentage of Total Laboratory
    Expense

Test utilization

It is widely accepted that a medical staff's utilization of laboratory tests varies greatly from hospital to hospital and is not driven exclusively by patient acuity (a measurement which indicates how sick the patient is) or programmatic demands. Laboratory test utilization at hospitals with similar in-patient acuity and programs (such as organ transplant or acquired immunodeficiency syndrome [AIDS]) have substantially different rates of laboratory utilization. Systems that are used to monitor operational performance should include the key utilization indicators as listed on the next page.

Number of in-patient performed tests/patient day.

Number of in-patient performed tests/patient discharge.
Some hospitals may perform test utilization reviews for individual areas or for individual physicians in an attempt to control overutilization of laboratory resources.

Turnaround time

Test-result turnaround time (TAT) statistics can help laboratory managers better understand and evaluate operational performance. Since service demands can greatly affect staffing patterns, instrumentation choice, and labor costs, it is important to measure actual TATs to determine whether the TAT expectations of the hospital's medical staff are met. The TAT monitoring system should include the 20 to 30 tests most commonly performed in the laboratory, as well as those requiring an especially short TAT (such as Stat. tests and pregnancy tests).

There are several approaches to monitoring TAT by test name. A common methodology identifies and tracks the distribution of TATs based on the length of time elapsed from the time the test was ordered until the time the result was available. It is also important to evaluate three time components of a TAT: the preanalytic, analytic, and postanalytic phases. To monitor TAT in this manner, LIS software needs to identify specimen collection time, specimen accession time (or time that the specimen is received in the laboratory), and the time the result was available to a physician.

CONTINUOUS QUALITY IMPROVEMENT

Continuous quality improvement (CQI) is a process the laboratory uses to ensure that the correct result is recorded

for the right patient at the right time. This process has been required by JCAHO for some time. Recently it has been mandated by HCFA in the CLIA '88 legislation. This process involves evaluating quality assurance (QA) indicators that monitor a level of performance in the laboratory. A target for performance is agreed upon, and if it is not met after auditing of the indicator, a plan of action is put into place to correct the deficiency. The indicator is again monitored to ensure that the problem has been corrected. If not, a new plan and audit are put in place until the performance of the indicator is satisfactory. An example of a form for performance monitoring is found in Fig. 2-6.

In setting up a QA program, one must establish a goal. An example, as described in Fig. 2-6, would be "To monitor, evaluate, and improve, if necessary, the turnaround time for stat. HCG analyses." After a goal has been decided upon by the laboratory director, a QA committee should be established. This committee should be composed of a representative from each laboratory section. The laboratory director must be involved in the CQI process for it to be effective. The committee should set up the parameters to be monitored and the target values for these monitors.

Monitors can vary because of the uniqueness of each laboratory operation, but CLIA '88 demands that, as a minimum, the monitors listed in Quality Assurance Monitors be evaluated. One can obtain copies of the 2/28/92, 1/19/93, and 4/24/95 *Federal Register* for a complete description of the QA process under CLIA '88—Subpart P 493.1701-493.1721.

Quality assurance monitors

1. *Patient test management*

    The laboratory must monitor, evaluate, and revise, if necessary, based on the results of its evaluations, the following:

    a. The criteria established for patient preparation, specimen collection, labeling, preservation, and transportation;

    b. The information solicited and obtained on the laboratory's test requisition for its completeness, relevance, and necessity for the testing of patient specimens;

    c. The use and appropriateness of the criteria established for specimen rejection;

    d. The completeness, usefulness, and accuracy of the test report information necessary for the interpretation or utilization of test results;

    e. The timely reporting of test results based on testing priorities (Stat., routine, etc.); and

    f. The accuracy and reliability of test reporting systems, appropriate storage of records, and retrieval of test results.

2. *QC assessment*

    The laboratory must have an ongoing mechanism to evaluate the corrective actions taken under 493.1219, Remedial Actions. Ineffective policies and procedures

Name of Institution: Sunland Hospital
Name of Laboratory or Section: Chemistry

<u>**Quality Assurance Monitor Report**</u>

Test Name: Stat. pregnancy test, serum
Monitor: Turnaround time
Evaluation criteria and/or threshold:

    95% of stat. serum pregnancy tests are completed within:
    (a)   30 minutes within receipt in the laboratory.
    (b)   90 minutes from the time of collection.

Time period of monitor: Month, Year: July, 1995 OR
                                 Quarter: 1st   <u>2nd</u>   3rd   4th

Status of monitor: <u>MET</u>   NOT MET   (underline)

Data for monitor:

    (a)   96.3% of all requests completed within 30 minutes of receipt in laboratory.
    (b)   95.9% of all requests completed within 90 minutes of collection.

Review of action: There was 1 outlier that was completed 2 hours after collection. Sample lost in accessioning area, clerk was advised.

Further action or comments: Three samples outside laboratory turnaround times. Samples entered laboratory during lunch periods. Will speak with supervisor about maintaining coverage during this time.

Comparison with previous monitors: Give % within limits

Previous: *Two previous:*   :
Date: _____ %: _____   Date: _____ %: _____

Laboratory Director: _____
Technical supervisor: _____

Fig. 2-6   Form for quality assurance monitoring.

must be revised based on the outcome of the evaluation. The mechanism must evaluate and review the effectiveness of corrective actions taken for:

a. Problems identified during the evaluation of calibration and control data for each test method;

b. Problems identified during the evaluation of patient test values for the purpose of verifying the reference range of a test method; and

c. Errors detected in reported results.

3. *Proficiency testing assessment*

Under Subpart H of this part, Proficiency Testing, the corrective actions taken for any unacceptable, unsatis-factory, or unsuccessful proficiency testing result(s) must be evaluated for effectiveness.

4. *Comparison of test results*

a. If a laboratory performs the same test using different methodologies or instruments, or performs the same test at multiple testing sites, the laboratory must have a system that twice a year evaluates and defines the relationship between test results using different methodologies, instruments, or testing sites.

b. If a laboratory performs tests that are not included under Subpart I of this part, Proficiency Testing Programs, the laboratory must have a system for verifying the accuracy of its test results at least twice a year.

5. *Relationship of patient information to patient test results*

For internal QA, the laboratory must have a mechanism to identify and evaluate patient test results that appear inconsistent with clinically relevant criteria, such as:

   a. Patient age;
   b. Sex;
   c. Diagnosis or pertinent clinical data, when provided;
   d. Distribution of patient test results when available; and
   e. Relationship with other test parameters, when available within the laboratory.

6. *Personnel assessment*

The laboratory must have an ongoing mechanism to evaluate the effectiveness of its policies and procedures for assuring employee competence and, if applicable, consultant competence.

7. *Communications*

The laboratory must have a system in place to document problems that occur as a result of breakdowns in communication between the laboratory and the authorized individual who orders or receives the results of test procedures or examinations. Corrective actions must be taken, as necessary, to resolve the problems and minimize communication breakdowns.

8. *Complaint investigation*

The laboratory must have a system in place to assure that all complaints and problems reported to the laboratory are documented. Investigations of complaints must be made when appropriate, and, as necessary, corrective actions instituted.

9. *QA review with staff*

The laboratory must have a mechanism for documenting and assessing problems identified during QA reviews and discussing them with the staff. The laboratory must take corrective actions that are necessary to prevent recurrences.

10. *Standard; QA records*

The laboratory must maintain documentation of all QA activities including problems identified and corrective actions taken. All QA records must be available to HHS and maintained for a period of 2 years.

After the monitors are established, the committee must decide how often these monitors will be examined. Some, such as turnaround time, might be evaluated monthly until the target time is repeatedly met. Others will follow different schedules. For example, proficiency testing documentation may be monitored every 4 months when the laboratory performs proficiency tests. The CQI process, though essential, is time consuming, and the committee must balance the need for thorough CQI monitoring against the fact that the laboratory must also produce a daily work load.

After the monitors are evaluated, the committee must formulate a plan to improve those monitors that do not meet their targets. After the new plan is put in place, the monitoring process is begun again. It is important to review the QA results with the staff and secure their input.

REFERENCES
General
NOTE: *Clinical Laboratory Management Review* is a recent journal published by Williams & Wilkins, Baltimore, Md.
Davidson JP: Are you entrepreneurial material? *Clin Lab Manage Rev* 4(3):192-195, 1990.
Fritz R: I'm your new boss . . . why are you laughing? *Clin Lab Manage Rev* 6(2):162-163, 1992.

Regulations
Federal Register 56(235):64175-64182, Dec 6, 1991.
Federal Register 57(40):7001-7186, Feb 28, 1992.
Federal Register 58(11):5211-5237, Jan 19, 1993.
Federal Register 58(139):39154-39156, July 22, 1993.
Federal Register 60(78):20035, Apr 24, 1995.
Federal Register 60:25944-25976, May 15, 1995.

Hospital management structure communication management
Baytos LM: Launching successful diversity initiatives, *HR Magazine* 37(3):91-97, 1992.
Haynes ME: How to conduct quality meetings, *Clin Lab Manage Rev* 4(1):29-36, 1990.
Hunt LB: Here's how you can harness the positive energy of conflict, *Clin Lab Manage Rev* 6(5):456-459, 1992.
Ketchum SM: Overcoming the four toughest management challenges, *Clin Lab Manage Rev* 5(4):246-263, 1991.
Lussier RN: Assigning tasks effectively using a model, *Clin Lab Manage Rev* 6(2):150-153, 1992.
Miner FC: If two heads are better than one, why do I have bruises on my forehead? *Clin Lab Manage Rev* 5(5):386-393, 1991.
Pfeiffer IL, Dunlap JB: Empowered employees—a good personnel investment, *Clin Lab Manage Rev* 6(2):154-161, 1992.
Rinke WJ: Establishing a shared vision in your organization, *Clin Lab Manage Rev* 3(2):95-99, 1989.
Veninga RL: Crisis management: strategies for building morale in uncertain times, *Clin Lab Manage Rev* 6(5):449-455, 1992.
Young S: Developing your political skills, *Clin Lab Manage Rev* 3(2):100-102, 1989.

Personnel management
Comer DR: Improving group productivity by reducing individual loafing, *Clin Lab Manage Rev* 6(3):232-235, 1992.
Dawson KM, Dawson SN: The cure for employee malaise—motivation, *Clin Lab Manage Rev* 5(4):296-302, 1991.
Fritz R: How to keep your best people for the '90s, *Clin Lab Manage Rev* 4(4):306-310, 1990.
Petrick JA, Manning GE: Work morale and assessment and development for the clinical laboratory manager, *Clin Lab Manage Rev* 6(2):141-149, 1992.
Surber JA, Wallhermfechtel M: A comprehensive career ladder for the clinical laboratory, *Clin Lab Manage Rev* 4(6):441-446, 1991.

Resource management
Hinterhuber HH, Popp W: Are you a strategist or just a manager? *Harvard Business Rev* 70(1):105-113, 1992.
Reeves PN: Strategic planning for every manager, *Clin Lab Manage Rev* 4(4):272-275, 1990.

Financial management
Brase SJ, Matysik MK: Laboratory manager's financial handbook, *Clin Lab Manage Rev* 6(2):164-169, 1992.
Carpenter RB: Laboratory cost analysis: a practical approach, *Clin Lab Manage Rev* 4(3):168-177, 1990.

Getzen TE: Laboratory manager's financial handbook: what is value? *Clin Lab Manage Rev* 6(3):237-240, 1992.

Kisner HJ: Laboratory manager's financial handbook: expense management—supplies, *Clin Lab Manage Rev* 6(4):341-348, 1992.

Melbin JE: One for all, *MT Today,* pp 8-9, Dec 7, 1992.

Patterson PP: Cost accounting in hospitals and clinical laboratories: part II, *Clin Lab Manage Rev* 3(1):26-33, 1989.

Portugal B: Factors influencing relative financial performance of hospital laboratories, *Clin Lab Manage Rev* 3(2):81-87, 1989.

Continuous quality improvement

Bull G, Maffetone MA, Miller SK: As we see it: implementing TQM, *Clin Lab Manage Rev* 6(3):256-261, May/June 1992.

Clark GB: Quality assurance, an administrative means to a managerial end, *Clin Lab Manage Rev* 6(5): Part I, 4(1):7-17, 1990; Part II, 4(4):224-252, 1990; Part III, 5(6):463-475, 1991; Part IV, 6(5): 426-440, 1992.

Westgard JO, Barry PL, Tomar RH: Implementing total quality management (TQM) in health-care laboratories, *Clin Lab Manage Rev* 5(5):353-370, 1991.

GENERAL RESOURCES

Lifshitz MS, De Cresce RP: *Understanding, selecting, and acquiring clinical laboratory analyzers,* New York, 1986, Alan R. Liss.

Martin BG, editor: *The CLMA guide to managing a clinical laboratory,* Pennsylvania, 1991.

Rubenstein NM: *Handbook of clinical laboratory management,* Rockville, Md., 1986, Aspen Publishers.

Sattler J, Smith A: *A practical guide to financial management of the clinical laboratory,* ed 2, Oradell, N.J., 1986, Medical Economics Books.

Snyder JR, Senhauser DA, editors: *Administration and supervision in laboratory medicine,* Philadelphia, 1989, Lippincott.

CHAPTER 3

Sources and control of preanalytical variation

David R. Dufour

Precollection causes of variation
    Cyclic biological variables
    Patient-related physical variables
    Procedures to minimize patient variables

Blood collection causes of variation
    Blood collection technique
    Types of blood samples
    Errors related to preservatives and anticoagulants
    Errors related to serum separator tubes
    Errors related to faulty collection techniques
    Errors related to patient and sample identification
    Chain of custody
    Procedures to minimize phlebotomy-related variation

Postcollection causes of variation
    Sample transportation
    Sample processing
    Sample storage

Other preanalytical collection concerns
    Urine collection: sources of variation
    Specimen collection from infants
    Computer-based aids for error detection
    Criteria for rejection of specimens

OBJECTIVES

- Describe the three major categories of preanalytic variation; for each category, outline the steps that can be taken by laboratories to minimize variation.

- Outline the differences between arterial, capillary, and venous blood, and the common laboratory tests that are significantly affected by these differences.

- Discuss the appropriate uses of anticoagulants and preservatives, and their effects on common laboratory tests. Recognize the causes and pattern of EDTA contamination.

- Categorize the types of tests affected by hemoconcentration, the causes of hemoconcentration, and the control techniques to limit its occurrence.

- Discuss the sequence of changes occurring in specimens after specimen collection and the control techniques to limit the resulting alterations in analyte concentration.

- Define delta checks and summarize their utility in detection of preanalytic errors.

KEY TERMS

additive A chemical added to a specimen that changes one or more of its physical or chemical properties.

adsorb Attachment of a chemical substance to a solid surface.

aerosol A fine mist produced by atomization of a liquid.

aliquot A portion of a specimen smaller than the whole, which has the same chemical composition.

analyte A substance that can be measured by an analytical technique.

anastomotic Connecting two blood vessels.

anticoagulant A substance that can suppress, delay, or prevent coagulation of blood by preventing formation of fibrin.

antiseptic A chemical that reduces the number of bacteria.

arterial Related to or derived from arteries, the vessels delivering blood from the heart to the tissues of the body.

artifactual Changed state of a material resulting from artificial, rather than natural, processes or conditions.

bar code A system of using varying-width bars as a way to provide identification information.

capillary Related to tiny blood vessels in tissues where nutrients are delivered and waste products are removed by the blood.

catheter A hollow plastic or rubber tube that connects a body cavity with the surface of the body.

chelation The process of an organic molecule binding multiple metal ions.

chronobiology The science of study of cyclic variation in living organisms.

circadian variation (pronounced ser-ca-dé-un) Changes in concentration of analytes that occur over the course of a single day.

clot An aggregation of blood cells held together by fibrin, a polymerized protein.

cyclic variation Changes in concentration of analytes that occur repetitively in a predictable fashion over a given period of time.

delta check Comparison of analyte concentration in one specimen from a person with that in the previous specimen from the same person.

EDTA Ethylenediaminetetraacetic acid, a commonly used chemical that chelates calcium. It acts as an anticoagulant and preservative by binding calcium and other cations, which inactivates several enzymes needed for clot formation and for breaking down protein and lipid analytes in blood.

evaporation Transformation of water to vapor.

extracellular Outside of cells.

glycolytic Relating to the process of metabolism of glucose.

hemoconcentration The process of increasing concentration of cells, proteins, and occasionally other analytes in blood through loss of water, either in vitro or in vivo.

hemolysis Rupture of red blood cells, releasing analytes found in cells into the serum or plasma.

heparin An anticoagulant that directly inhibits formation of fibrin.

infradian (pronounced infra-dé-un) Changes in concentration of analytes that occur with less frequency than once a day.

intraindividual Within a single person.

intravenous Within a vein; usually refers to intravenous fluid in which water containing medications, glucose, or electrolytes is given to a patient through a catheter inserted into a vein.

in vitro Literally, 'in glass'; occurring in an artificial situation, as in a test tube.

in vivo Occurring in a living organism.

nonlaminar Not in an orderly, layered fashion with smooth gradations from one layer to another. With liquids, nonlaminar flow produces shearing forces where different layers or laminae come into contact.

phlebotomy Puncturing a vein with a needle for the purpose of obtaining a sample of blood.

plasma The liquid part of blood in the bloodstream; as a specimen obtained by collecting blood with an anticoagulant and centrifugating the specimen.

postprandial After a meal, also postcibal.

preanalytical variables Factors that alter results of a laboratory test and that occur before the process of performing that test.

preservatives Chemicals that prevent a change in the concentration of analytes in a sample of blood, urine, or other body fluid.

proteolysis The process of degradation of proteins, which may occur by chemical reactions or enzymatic processes.

serum The liquid part of blood remaining after a clot has formed.

serum separator A mechanical device that physically separates serum from cells (plasma separators separate plasma from cells), preventing changes in concentration of serum analytes as the result of cell metabolism.

stasis A decrease in flow of blood to or from a part of the body.

TBEP Tris(2-butoxyethyl) phosphate, a chemical found in rubber, which may leak from stoppers and bind to proteins, displacing chemicals and altering their serum (or plasma) concentrations.

tourniquet A mechanical device (such as a wide rubber band) used on the surface of an extremity that compresses veins, enlarging them by preventing the return of blood to the heart and lungs.

ultradian (pronounced ultra-dé-un) Changes in concentration of analytes that occur over a period of time much less than 1 day.

venous Related to veins, the vessels returning blood from tissues to the heart and lungs.

Laboratory tests, which measure an analyte in a specimen of blood or other body fluid, are ordered by physicians to evaluate the status of a patient. It is assumed that the analytical results obtained are representative of the actual analyte concentration in the patient. Unfortunately there are several factors that may invalidate this assumption. Errors may occur because of analytical bias; traditional quality control is aimed at minimizing measurement errors. However, many nonanalytical factors can actually change the concentration of one or more analytes in a specimen so that results do not reflect the patient's physiological condition. These are collectively termed *preanalytical* sources of error. Just as control of temperature, wavelength, and time of incubation will limit analytical error, preanalytical error can also be controlled. The purpose of this chapter is to detail the common sources of preanalytical error and the methods that can be used to control them.

It is the responsibility of laboratories to take steps to minimize sources of error by developing standard procedures that govern patient preparation, sample collection, methods of sample transport, and preservation of samples. Agencies that accredit laboratories, including the College of American Pathologists and the Joint Commission on Accreditation of Health Care Organizations, require each laboratory to provide a detailed manual that documents the proper method for specimen collection. It is advisable to include in such a document the procedures used to minimize errors at each of the points where variation may develop.

PRECOLLECTION CAUSES OF VARIATION
Cyclic biological variables

Cyclic variation refers to changes in concentration of analytes that occur in a predictable fashion at certain times of the day, week, or month. The study of such cyclic changes is termed "chronobiology."[1] Rhythmic variation is typical of many biologic functions; diurnal variation in drug metabolism and incidence of myocardial infarction are but two examples of the importance of this field.[2] The most reproducible cyclic variation is *circadian* variation, which occurs during the course of a single day. Melatonin, a peptide produced by the pineal gland in response to darkness, is known to influence the function of many parts of the hypothalamic-pituitary axis.[3] As a result, the concentration of most pituitary hormones increases at night and falls during the day. Those hormones whose concentrations are affected by pituitary stimulation show a similar diurnal variation. Diurnal changes seem to be influenced by sleeping and waking, rather than simply by the time on the clock. People who work irregular shifts or who have recently arrived in a new time zone typically have some delay in adjusting their diurnal cycle; however, eventually the concentration of pituitary hormones will be highest during sleep, gradually falling after awakening.[4] When one is reporting the time of sample collection for hormonal tests, therefore, it is necessary to indicate the time of waking of the patient. Several other commonly measured substances, such as iron[5] and acid phosphatase,[6] also show a prominent circadian variation. Urinary excretion of most electrolytes, such as sodium, potassium, and phosphate, shows considerable circadian variation.[7] The excretion rates of these analytes determined in specimens obtained at different times of the day may differ by as much as 50%.

Some hormones are not released into the circulation in a constant fashion but are secreted in episodic bursts. This *ultradian* variation is typical of most pituitary hormones, as shown in Fig. 3-1. The concentration during such a burst of secretion may be several times the basal level. A single specimen, therefore, is unlikely to be representative of total hormone production.

Cyclic variation over a period greater than 1 day (*infradian*) may also affect laboratory test results. In women, the menstrual cycle is associated with significant changes in the concentrations of ovarian hormones. Related to this are monthly fluctuations in the concentrations of other analytes such as calcium, magnesium, cholesterol, parathyroid hormone, renin, aldosterone, and antidiuretic hormone.[8] *Circannual* variation, which has been reported for some substances, is related to seasonal changes in the diet or climatic variation. For example, serum 1,25-dihydroxyvitamin D concentration is higher in the summer than in the winter,[9] and urinary oxalate is higher in the summer than in other seasons (oxalate is present in high concentrations in strawberries).[10] For other analytes, such as the higher thyroid-stimulating hormone (TSH) response to thyroid-releasing hormone in summer,[11] the cause of variation is not clear.

In addition to such predictable variability, random fluctuations can cause pronounced changes in concentration from one day to the next. Although many analytes such as electrolytes, proteins, and alkaline phosphatase show less than 5% intraindividual variation, day-to-day variation may be over 20% for substances such as bilirubin, creatine kinase, triglycerides, and most steroid hormones. Urinary ex-

cretion of creatinine varies by approximately 10% in a given individual, but most other substances excreted in the urine show fluctuations of 25% to 50% over relatively short periods of time.[12] Table 3-1 lists the long-term biological variability for many common analytes.

Patient-related physical variables

Exercise is a common, controllable cause for variation in laboratory test results. Among routine chemistry tests potassium, phosphate, creatinine, and serum proteins are significantly altered by a brief period of exercise.[13] With regular exercise, there is an increase in the activity of muscle-related enzymes and an increase of uric acid concentrations in blood (Fig. 3-2). Intensive exercise, such as marathon running, produces rapid increases in potassium, uric acid, bilirubin, and muscle enzymes, whereas glucose and phosphate concentrations fall significantly.[14] In persons training for distance events, serum gonadotropin and sex steroid concentrations are greatly decreased, whereas prolactin concentration is increased.[15]

Diet-related changes in laboratory tests are pronounced for many analytes; most are transient and easily controlled. After food ingestion, there is an increase in concentration of substances absorbed from food, such as glucose and triglycerides. In addition, sodium, uric acid, iron, and lac-

Table 3-1 Intraindividual variation for common laboratory tests

Test serum	Average (%)	Range (%)
Alanine aminotransferase	20	5-30
Albumin	2.5	1.5-4
Alkaline phosphatase	7	5-10
Amylase	9	5-12
Aspartate aminotransferase	8	5-12
Bilirubin, total	19	13-30
Calcium, total	2	1-3
Chloride	1.2	1.1-1.3
Cholesterol, total	6	5-9
Cholesterol, HDL	6	3-9
Creatinine	5	3-8
Ferritin	10	5-18
Glucose, fasting	10	5-13
Iron	15	10-25
Lactate dehydrogenase	10	8-13
Magnesium	4	3-5
Osmolality	1	1-2
Phosphate	8	5-10
Potassium	3	1-5
Protein, total	2	2-3.5
Sodium	0.6	0.5-1
Thyrotropin (TSH)	18	15-20
Thyroxine	5	4-7
Triglycerides	20	15-30
Urea (BUN)	10	5-17
Uric acid	7	5-10

From Rosen JF, Chesney RW: *J Pediatr* 103:1-17, 1983; Fraser CG: *Arch Pathol Lab Med* 116:916-923, 1992; Fraser CG: *Arch Pathol Lab Med* 112:404-415, 1988; Dufour DR, in Becker KL, editor: *Principles and practice of endocrinology*, ed 2, Philadelphia, 1995, Lippincott.

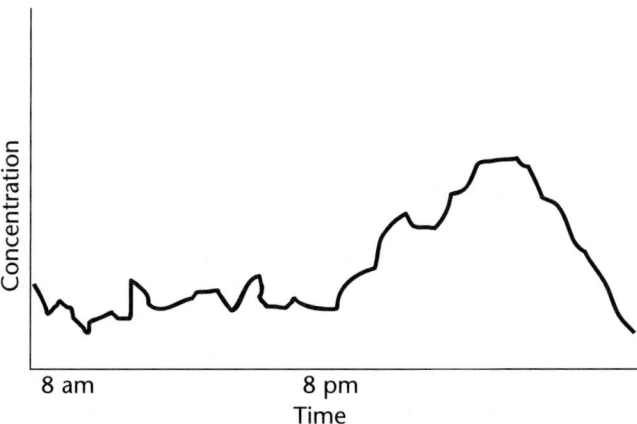

Fig. 3-1 Diurnal and ultradian pattern of hormone release. Most pituitary hormones show pronounced diurnal variation, with levels generally higher during sleep than during the day. Some, such as growth hormone (illustrated here), are released in episodic bursts during the day. A randomly obtained result is difficult to interpret because it may represent a peak, a trough, or some point between.

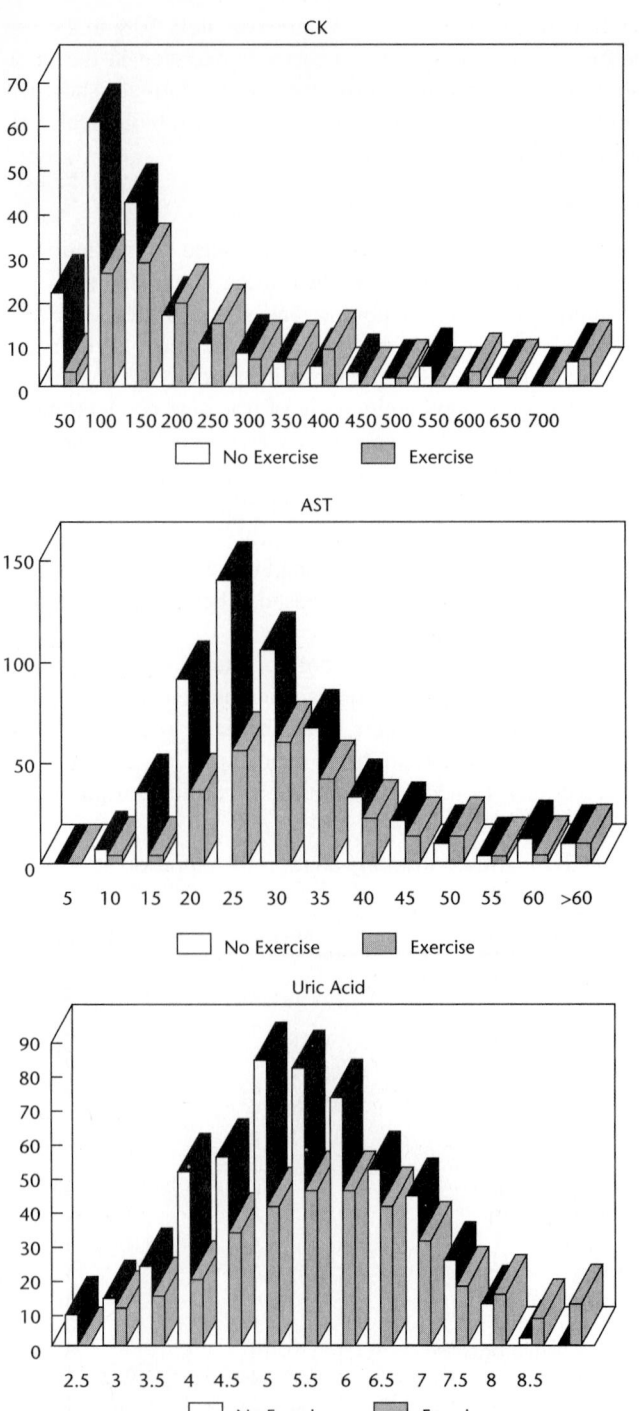

CK

AST

Uric Acid

Fig. 3-2 Effect of exercise on laboratory test results. Data from 750 medical students show that exercise is associated with shifting of the distribution of results to higher values (displayed on *x* axis; *y* axis represents number of students).

tate dehydrogenase concentrations are significantly altered after a meal,[13] showing a postprandial rise. Hormones that are secreted in response to eating, such as gastrin and insulin, will also show a postprandial rise. The plasma concentration of substances, such as potassium and phos-

phate, that shift into cells under the influence of insulin will fall after meals. Substances present in food may interfere chemically with test results. For example, vanillin interferes in chemical assays for vanillylmandelic acid, and dietary serotonin can increase urine concentration of 5-hydroxy-indoleacetic acid (5 HIAA). Stool occult blood tests, which detect heme, are affected by intake of meat and, in some cases, iron and horseradish.[16] Dietary variation can also induce longer-lasting changes in laboratory tests; alteration in dietary protein intake is associated with reversible changes in urine creatinine excretion and in creatinine clearance.[17]

Stress, whether mental or physical, can reversibly alter results of many laboratory tests. It is well known that stress induces production of ACTH, cortisol, and catecholamines. Even mild stress, which can result from a needle stick, preparing for an examination, or an elective hospital admission, may be enough to cause changes. Although total cholesterol may increase with mild stress,[18] high-density-lipoprotein cholesterol falls by about 15%.[19] Preparation of the antecubital fossa for venipuncture will result in a pronounced increase in plasma catecholamines. More severe stress causes more profound changes. After acute myocardial infarction, cholesterol begins to fall by 24 hours and may reach a nadir of 60% of baseline value, returning to typical values for the patient after about 3 months.[20] Patients in intensive care units have suppression of production of many pituitary hormones[21,22] and aldosterone.[23] Because of these changes, elective evaluation of endocrine function and lipid status should not be combined with a hospital admission for some other cause.

Posture is a readily controllable cause of preanalytic variation. In the upright position, increased hydrostatic pressure causes leakage of water and electrolytes from the intravascular fluid compartment, resulting in an increase in concentration of proteins. If phlebotomy is performed before a patient is seated for at least 15 minutes after a period of standing, hemoconcentration as great as 5% to 8% occurs.[24] This increase can produce clinically important differences in concentrations of calcium, cholesterol, and lipoproteins. In the supine position, water and electrolytes return to the vascular space, resulting in a fall in protein concentrations of a similar magnitude. The difference in the measured hemoglobin concentration between the time of admission to a hospital (when the patient may have had phlebotomy performed after a period of standing) and the next morning (when blood may have been drawn while the patient was lying in bed) could lead the physician to suspect that the patient had developed internal hemorrhage or hemolysis.

Procedures to minimize patient variables

Important ways to control patient variables include asking the health care provider to take a good patient history, providing the phlebotomist or patient with clear instructions, and taking steps to determine that all protocols have been followed.

Tests Subject to Diurnal Variation
Acid phosphatase*
ACTH
Catecholamines
Cortisol (and other adrenal steroids)
Gastrin*
Growth hormone*
Glucose tolerance
Iron
Osteocalcin*
Parathyroid hormone*
Prolactin*
Renin/aldosterone
TSH*

*Higher in the afternoon and evening; all others higher in the morning.

Tests Affected by Meals
Chloride*
Gastrin
Glucagon
Glucose
Growth hormone
Insulin
Ionized calcium
Phosphate*
Potassium*
Triglycerides
Urine pH

*Lower after meals; all others higher.

Biological cyclic variables. The laboratory should determine which of the tests performed have significant cyclic or food-related changes in concentration; the two boxes list the most important tests that are affected in this manner. Optimally the specimens for these tests should be collected shortly after the patient awakens, with the patient still in the fasting state. If there is an ultradian pattern of variation, as there is for most pituitary hormones, several specimens should be collected at intervals extending over the usual cycle to provide an accurate picture of hormone production.[25] For example, for gonadotropins, it is advisable to collect three or four specimens with at least a half hour between specimen collections and to pool the serum before analysis. A more sophisticated method is to place an indwelling catheter in the patient and obtain specimens hourly over a day. Each specimen is analyzed separately, and the concentration is plotted against the time of day the specimen was obtained. The area under the curve is reported as an integrated measure of hormone production.

Physical variables. If samples are being collected for analytes that will be affected by exercise, it is prudent to inquire whether the patient has engaged in strenuous exercise in the past 24 to 48 hours. Any history of strenuous exercise should be noted on the requisition form and included in the final report. Alternatively the patient may be asked to return at a later time for specimen collection. Stress before collection is difficult to control; physicians should, however, be apprised of those tests that are thus affected and of the magnitude of change induced by physical and mental stress. It may be advisable for the laboratory to require special consultation before the collection of samples for tests that are severely affected by patient stress, such as adrenal or pituitary function tests, catecholamine metabolites, lipid analysis, and glucose tolerance tests. The effects of posture can be minimized if one requires ambulatory patients to be seated for at least 15 minutes before blood is drawn. For assays that are subject to pronounced dietary effects, including measurements of glucose tolerance, urine

hydroxyproline, 5-HIAA, and catecholamine metabolites, it is advisable to provide the patient with specific guidelines before the day scheduled for sample collection. If a test, such as measurement of renin and aldosterone, glucose tolerance tests, 24-hour urine analysis, or 72-hour fecal fat, requires special patient preparation, it is good practice to schedule the test in advance and to give the patient a printed instruction sheet at that time.

BLOOD COLLECTION CAUSES OF VARIATION
Blood collection technique

The use of improper procedures for obtaining specimens can introduce significant error in the final results of laboratory tests; in the author's laboratory, collection-related errors are the most common cause of erroneous results. Several publications[26-28] detail appropriate procedures for performing phlebotomy to obtain blood specimens, and certification programs in phlebotomy have established standards for the training and education of phlebotomists. In teaching hospitals, phlebotomy is often performed by a variety of individuals (such as nurses, physicians' assistants, and students) who have limited or no formal training in phlebotomy techniques.

In most laboratories, specimens are collected using evacuated tubes and specially designed needles that allow simultaneous puncture of the vein and the tube's stopper. Collection tubes are typically made of glass, though plastic tubes are being used more frequently; plastic and glass tubes are equally suitable for most assays.[29] Many tubes are coated with silicone, which reduces adhesion of clot, allowing better separation of serum and cells. Stoppers are typically made of rubber. In older formulations, tris(2-butoxyethyl) phosphate (TBEP) was used as a plasticizer; this compound is capable of displacing many drugs from their transport proteins. The drugs then diffuse into red cells, lowering the serum concentration of the drug. TBEP has been removed from most currently used stoppers. Some tubes have special protective caps over the stoppers that are not in direct contact with the blood, lowering the risk of transmission of infectious agents.

In some cases, blood is drawn into a syringe and then transferred to tubes for transport to the laboratory. If this procedure is used, there is a risk of infection for the phlebotomist during the specimen transfer. The safest method for preparing sample aliquots is to select the needed tubes containing anticoagulants or preservatives before sample collection, removing the stoppers from the tubes. After sample collection, the needle is removed from the syringe, and the blood is added to the tubes; the stoppers are then replaced. Injection of blood into evacuated tubes increases the risk of skin puncture by the needle and also increases the risk of producing a hemolyzed specimen (p. 110).

In infants and in adults with poor venous access, skin puncture may be used to obtain specimens. Special microtubes, which contain anticoagulants, can be filled by capillary action. If such specimens are to be transported to the laboratory, these capillary tubes should contain a small piece of metal, which should be moved through the specimen by means of a magnet to mix the blood immediately after collection and before centrifugation or analysis (Fig. 3-3). If testing is to be done near the site of collection, as is typical for many near-patient testing instruments, such mixing devices are usually not needed, since the delay between collection and analysis is minimal. Contamination of the sample with fluid from tissue is a potential cause of concern in all capillary blood collection procedures, since tissue fluid contains virtually no protein and therefore no protein-bound analytes. One may minimize such contamination by using only freely flowing blood from puncture sites. It is therefore unacceptable to "milk" blood by applying pressure to the tissue near the puncture site.

Types of blood samples

Differences between arterial, capillary, and venous blood are an occasional cause for misleading test results. *Arterial blood* is the source of nutrients for all body tissues and is the best sample to use for analysis of the delivery of necessary substances such as oxygen to the body tissues. *Venous blood* differs from arterial blood in that it has lower

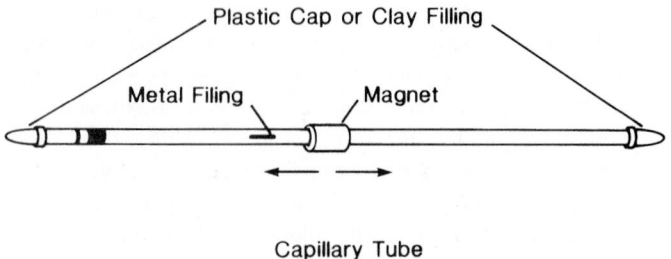

Plastic Cap or Clay Filling

Metal Filing   Magnet

Capillary Tube

Fig. 3-3   Schematic of heparinized capillary tubes. Magnet is used to move metal filing back and forth through the sealed tube to mix the blood sample with heparin and, later, to remix the sample before analysis.

concentrations of substances used in metabolism, such as oxygen and glucose, and higher concentrations of waste products, such as organic acids, ammonia, and carbon dioxide. The extent of the difference in analyte concentration between arterial and venous blood is dependent on tissue perfusion; with poor perfusion, the difference increases. Some have suggested measuring the difference in blood gases between arterial and central venous blood as a measure of generalized tissue perfusion for monitoring patients in shock.[30] *Capillary blood* is, in general, closer in composition to arterial than to venous blood. By warming specific sites, such as the earlobe or the foot, specimens of capillary blood that closely resemble arterial blood are obtained. In states of poor tissue perfusion and in neonates, however, there is a significant difference in the Po_2 of capillary and arterial blood. Fingerstick glucose may be as much as 50% lower than venous plasma glucose in patients in shock[31]; at least some of the difference is caused by the lower Po_2 in capillary blood in shock cases, which affects whole blood glucose oxidase methods. For some substances, the difference between venous and capillary blood concentrations depends on hormonal factors that affect tissue extraction. For example, in the fasting state, the concentration of capillary blood glucose is similar to that of venous glucose. In postprandial specimens, when insulin concentration is increased, the difference between capillary and venous blood glucose concentrations may be as high as 15%.[32]

Errors related to preservatives and anticoagulants

Preservatives and anticoagulants are widely used for collecting specimens of blood, urine, and other body fluids. When blood is removed from the body and allowed to clot, it separates into a solid clot containing blood cells and fibrin and a liquid phase termed *serum*. If an anticoagulant such as heparin is added, the liquid phase is termed *plasma*. Serum and plasma are similar in most respects. Serum differs from plasma in that it lacks fibrinogen, lowering total protein by an average of 3 g/L. In clotting, platelets release potassium into the serum; plasma potassium is typically about 0.2 to 0.3 mmol/L lower than that of serum potassium. For unknown reasons, phosphate concentration is lower in plasma by an average of 2 mg/L.[33] In patients with some hematologic disorders, these differences are exaggerated. With these few exceptions, serum and heparinized plasma are often used interchangeably for laboratory tests. The choice of specimen type is dependent on instrumentation, assay methods, and need for rapid results.

Heparinized plasma can be separated from cells immediately after collection, and thus plasma specimens are suitable for rapid analysis in emergency situations. Although heparin is an effective anticoagulant, in many cases fibrin formation occurs after separation, which may cause coating and plugging of sampling probes and tubing. Heparin can interfere in some analytical systems, such as the dry-slide amylase assay. The cation used in heparin salts (such as lithium or ammonium) will cause contamination of specimens used for these analytes. For these reasons, some laboratories prefer not to use heparinized blood.

In addition to heparin, other anticoagulants and preservatives are often used for various specimens. Table 3-2 lists some of the most commonly used substances and some typical indications for the use of these additives. Although these compounds are essential for certain tests, they may be totally inappropriate for other tests. EDTA, which is used for hematology specimens, is also used for some chemistry assays because chelation of divalent cations inactivates several enzymes that lead to in vitro changes in lipids and peptide hormones. Chelation of cations such as iron, magnesium, and calcium, however, falsely lowers results in most colorimetric assays and reduces the activity of enzymes that require cation activators (including alkaline phosphatase and creatine kinase). Contamination of specimens with anticoagulants, especially EDTA, is a common problem in many laboratories.

In our laboratory, approximately two or three specimens are received each month with EDTA contamination. The pattern of abnormalities seen with EDTA contamination is shown in the following box. To avoid contamination, tubes without anticoagulants or preservatives should be filled first, followed by tubes containing other preservatives and anticoagulants. Because of the potential for EDTA interference in many assays, tubes containing EDTA should be drawn last. If liquid anticoagulants are used, it is important to ensure that the proportion of blood and anticoagulant used is constant. In specimens with inadequate blood volume ("short draw"), there may be significant dilution of blood by the anticoagulant solution. Since most anticoagulants do not enter into cells, alterations in hematocrit will affect the ratio of anticoagulant to plasma. For example, patients with a high hematocrit will have a relative excess of the anticoagulant and a resulting dilution of the plasma,

whereas in anemic individuals there may be insufficient anticoagulant.

Errors related to serum separator tubes

Serum and plasma separator tubes are used by many laboratories to simplify the process of separating serum (or plasma) from cellular elements. If separation does not occur, metabolism continues in the cellular phase, producing a variety of changes that are discussed later in this chapter. Serum and plasma separator tubes contain a relatively inert, impenetrable gel that has a density intermediate between cellular elements and plasma or serum. During centrifugation, the gel rises from the bottom of the tube and forms a mechanical barrier that prevents metabolic changes from affecting plasma concentrations (Fig. 3-4). Tubes containing such gels can be centrifuged and stored without removal of the stopper, reducing the risk of producing infectious aerosols and preventing evaporation. Some therapeutic agents adsorb onto the gel, falsely lowering the concentrations of tricyclic antidepressants and certain antiarrhythmic drugs, such as flecainide. With these exceptions, most substances in plasma are unaffected by the use of separator gels.

Errors related to faulty collection techniques

Tourniquets. Tourniquet use is an important, controllable cause of variation in laboratory test results. Tourniquets are widely used in phlebotomy to block venous return, causing dilatation of the veins and making identifica-

---

Effects of EDTA Contamination

Increased potassium
Reduced calcium, magnesium (colorimetric assays)
Reduced alkaline phosphatase, creatine kinase

Table 3-2   Commonly used anticoagulants and preservatives and indications for their use

Samples	Type of anticoagulant or additive	Chemical basis of anticoagulant or additive	Application
Whole blood	EDTA*	Binds calcium	Hematology
	Na heparin	Lead free	Lead
Plasma	Na citrate	Binds calcium	Coagulation
	Heparin†	Inhibits thrombin	Chemistry
	Oxalates	Binds calcium	Coagulation
Serum	None	None	Chemistry
	None	Contaminant free	Trace elements
	Serum separator	Gel barrier	Chemistry
	Thrombin	Increased rate of clotting	Stat. chemistries
Antiglycolytic agents			
Serum	Iodoacetate	Inhibits glyceraldehyde-3-phosphate dehydrogenase	Glucose, lactic acid
Partial plasma	Fluoride/oxalate	Inhibits enolase	Glucose

*Comes as Na^+ or K^+ salt forms.
†Comes as Na^+, Li^+, or NH_4^+ salt forms.

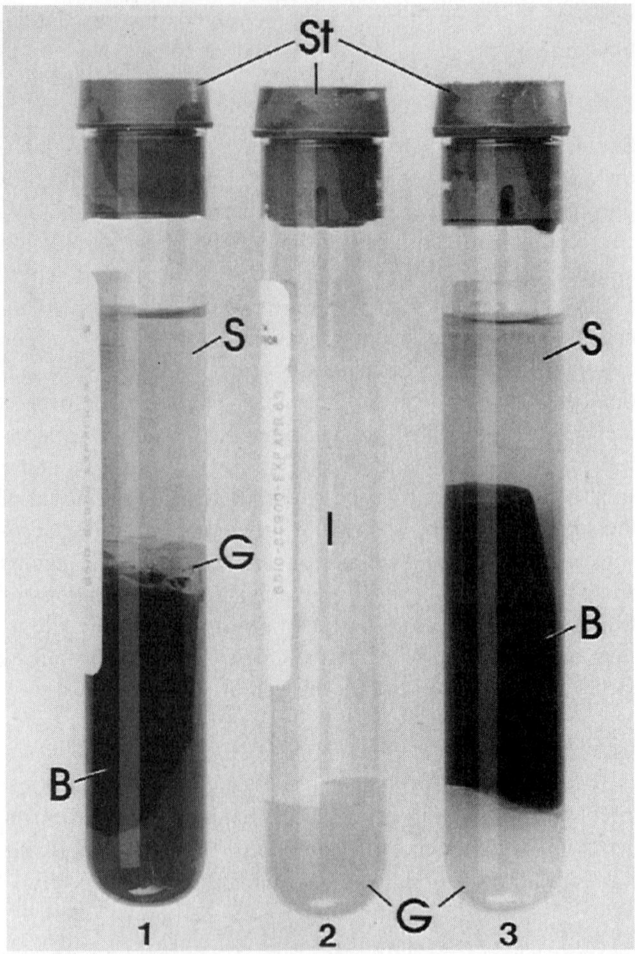

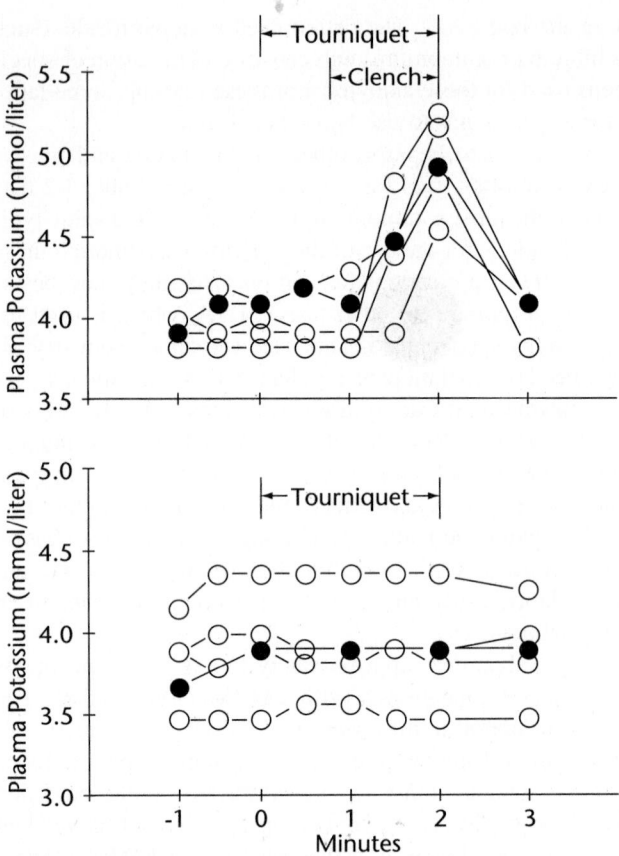

Fig. 3-4   Vacutainer phlebotomy tubes containing barrier gel (red/gray tops). *1*, Tube filled with blood and centrifuged; *2*, unfilled tube; and *3*, tube filled with blood and not centrifuged. Notice positions of gel before *(3)* and after centrifugation *(1)*. *B*, Clotted blood; *St*, red/gray stoppers; *G*, barrier gel; *S*, serum.

Fig. 3-5   Effects of the application of a tourniquet plus fist clenching (*upper panel*) and tourniquet alone (*lower panel*) on Plasma Potassium Concentrations. Solid circles represent the patient, and open circles the control subjects. The application of a tourniquet alone had no effect on plasma potassium levels, whereas clenching the fist as well resulted in a strong increase in these levels in both the patient and the control subjects. (From Don BR Sebastian A, Cheitlin M, et al: *N Engl J Med* 322:1291, 1990.)

tion of an appropriate site for venipuncture easier. Tourniquets are often left on during the process of venipuncture, under the assumption that continued venous dilatation will allow faster specimen collection and prevent "collapse" of the vein. Although tourniquets do make the process of phlebotomy easier, the stasis they induce causes predictable changes in laboratory test results. One minute after applying a tourniquet, the increased pressure causes loss of water and electrolytes from plasma to the extracellular fluid space, producing a rise in the concentration of proteins, cells, and substances bound to cells and proteins. After 3 minutes, there is generally a 5% to 8% increase in concentration of proteins. If a tourniquet is left on for as long as 15 minutes, the increase in concentration may reach 15%. The magnitude of this effect may differ from the first tube to the last tube drawn, with later specimens showing greater hemoconcentration. An additional concern with tourniquet

use is relative stasis of blood flow. Concentrations of metabolic byproducts such as lactate and hydrogen ion increase in tissue, and restoration of blood flow after removal of a tourniquet causes a rise in the venous lactate concentration. When blood is collected by use of a tourniquet, patients are often advised to alternately clench and relax their fist to increase the speed of collection of specimens. Not only is there little evidence of the efficacy of this procedure, but it may also be the cause of artifactual hyperkalemia[34] (Fig. 3-5).

Hemolysis.   Hemolysis occurs whenever there is trauma to the relatively fragile red blood cells, either during collection or, less commonly, after phlebotomy is completed. Failure to allow drying of disinfectants, such as alcohol, before phlebotomy, is an uncommon cause of hemolysis. More frequently, hemolysis is caused by turbulent, nonlaminar flow during the process of collection. Within the range of calibers commonly utilized, hemolysis is not caused by using a needle that is too small or too large. Nonlaminar flow is a common occurrence when blood moves too slowly or too rapidly through a needle. If blood is drawn with a syringe, drawing the plunger back forcefully or injecting blood into evacuated tubes using pressure on the plunger frequently produces hemolysis. Similarly, a slow flow rate into an evacuated tube from a collapsed vein often produces a hemolyzed specimen. Turbulence in a tube containing blood can also cause hemolysis after collection is completed; faulty mechanical transporters and centrifuges are rare causes of hemolysis, as discussed later in the chapter.

Hemolysis alters laboratory test results in two ways. Most importantly, the contents of the red blood cells are released, increasing the concentration of intracellular substances such as lactate dehydrogenase (LD), potassium, and magnesium while lowering the concentration of extracellular solutes such as sodium. Since the activity of LD is approximately 150 times higher and potassium concentration is 30 times higher within red blood cells, hemolysis falsely elevates the serum or plasma levels of these analytes. Because hemoglobin absorbs light over much of the visible and near-ultraviolet spectrum, hemolysis can interfere with results of many spectrophotometric assays. The box gives the tests most commonly affected by hemolysis and the nature of the interference in each assay.

Intravenous fluid contamination. Intravenous fluid contamination can be an important cause of variation in test results. Many inpatients are given intravenous fluids, which typically have higher concentrations of glucose, drugs, and some electrolytes than those found in blood. Intravenous fluid contamination occurs when blood is drawn from a vein connected to the one containing the catheter. Although it may appear that a vein in the forearm is sufficiently distant from the catheter, there are extensive anastomotic connections. Any blood drawn from a vein on the same side of a tourniquet as a catheter runs the risk of fluid contamination. In many cases, blood is drawn through a connector or port in a catheter. It has been shown that, for most analytes, removing and discarding a volume of blood equal to the volume of the catheter is adequate for preventing contamination. In the case of drugs administered through a catheter (including heparin and potassium), it may take a volume of more than five times that of the catheter to prevent incorrect results. In patients receiving intravenous fluids on a long-term basis, a multilumen catheter is commonly used to provide a port for collection of blood. Even if blood is drawn through this separate port, contamination can still occur if intravenous fluid is being administered simultaneously through a different lumen.

The most common pattern of intravenous fluid interference is a sharp increase in the blood concentration of the substances contained in the fluid. Potassium concentration of intravenous fluid can be as much as tenfold higher than that of blood, and the glucose concentration of intravenous

---

Effects of Hemolysis on Chemistry Tests

Increase caused by release from red blood cells
Potassium, magnesium, lactate dehydrogenase, aspartate aminotransferase, total protein, iron, phosphate, ammonium

Increase caused by interference in assay
Cholesterol, triglycerides, creatine kinase, CK-MB (immunoinhibition)

Decrease caused by interference in assay
Bilirubin (direct spectrophotometry), carotene, insulin, albumin

---

fluid is 50,000 mg/L. Drug concentrations are typically over a hundredfold higher than those of blood when fluid is administered as a slow infusion. Less frequently, there may be enough fluid present to actually dilute the concentration of normal blood constituents, including solutes such as urea and creatinine; in most cases of fluid contamination, these are only minimally altered.

Errors related to patient and sample identification

Because there is no way to prove that an unlabeled specimen came from a given patient, proper specimen identification is essential. Although labeling may seem the simplest part of specimen collection, in most laboratories it is the single most common cause of erroneous laboratory results. In our hospital, approximately 1% of the specimens that are not drawn by the laboratory are received with inadequate identification. Approximately 0.05% are received with incorrect patient identification. Although errors can be made when one is labeling the specimens from patients with similar names, the most common cause of inaccurate specimen identification is the phlebotomist's failure to label the specimen before leaving the patient's bedside. In our laboratory, over 99% of mislabeled specimens occur in this setting.

Chain of custody

In certain situations, as in forensic testing, positive specimen identification is required at every step in the process of collection, transport, and analysis. For such specimens, an appropriate chain-of-custody form (Fig. 3-6) should be used. According to guidelines published by the National Institute of Drug Abuse,[36] positive identification begins with placing a tamperproof seal on the specimen container before it leaves the donor's sight; the label is typically initialed by the donor and sometimes by the witness. After the donor certifies on the chain-of-custody form that the specimen was obtained from him, or her, each person who takes possession of the specimen signs the form and notes the date and time the specimen was transferred to the next person in the testing process. Commonly, each person certifies that the specimen was kept in a secure condition during the time

---

TOXICOLOGY LABORATORY

Chain of Evidence Form

SUBJECT NAME _____ SUBJECT SOCIAL SEC. # _____

DATE/TIME OF COLLECTION _____ COLLECTED BY _____

NUMBER OF SPECIMENS _____ TYPE OF SPECIMEN: ___ BLOOD ___ SERUM ___ URINE

WITNESS _____

Sent By Name/Date/Time	Received By Name/Date/Time	Condition of Seals
1.		
2.		
3.		
4.		
5.		

Specimen Opened for Testing Name/Date/Time	Witnessed By Name/Date/Time	Condition of Seals
A. Outside Package 6.		
B. Specimen 7.		

LABORATORY ACCESSION NUMBER: _____

This form must remain with the specimen until line #7 is complete. At that time the form should be turned over to the laboratory supervisor or the designate for filing.

Fig. 3-6 Example of a chain-of-custody form. (From Pesce AJ, Kaplan LA: *Methods in clinical chemistry,* St. Louis, 1987, Mosby)

---

it was in that person's custody. This assures that the result will be legally admissible in court, since it can be traced directly to the person from whom it was obtained.

Procedures to minimize phlebotomy-related variation

Procedures to minimize collection-related variation are generally directly under the control of the laboratory. Therefore the laboratory should work closely with the phlebotomy team, nursing administration, and physicians to produce clear written guidelines to help minimize all errors. Phlebotomy guidelines for *each* test that the laboratory performs should be included in the laboratory manual. Guidelines should specify the type of specimen to collect, the vol-

ume of specimen needed, and, for blood, whether arterial, capillary, or venous blood is required. The frequency of phlebotomy errors should be monitored, as suggested by CLIA '88 regulations (see Chapter 2).

Patient identification. The initial step in preventing collection errors is the accurate identification of the patient before specimen collection. When working with outpatients, ask for a name, including correct spelling of the last name, and any identification number needed (such as patient registration or insurance number). Hospital inpatients should be asked for a name, and identification should be confirmed when the information given by the patient is compared to that written on the hospital arm band. The patient's hospital identification number should be checked against the number on the request slip to ensure that both are the same. If the patient has more than one identification band, all bands should be checked to ensure that they contain the same information; there is a relatively high frequency of errors in patients with more than one band.

With children, or adults with neurologic or mental illnesses, a more positive form of identification, such as a hospital card or picture identification, may be necessary. Handwritten specimen labels should be clearly and legibly written before the phlebotomist leaves the patient's bedside; the label should include the name and identification number of the patient and the date and time of collection.

To assist in making proper identification, laboratory computer systems usually provide preprinted labels along with collection lists (see Chapter 18). Many hospitals have begun to use a bar-code system on these labels to increase the accuracy of positive patient identification.[35] The complexity of bar-coded labels varies. Some simply have the patient's name and hospital number, whereas others contain a list of all tests to be performed on the specimen, the time the specimen was obtained, and the name of the person performing the phlebotomy. Portable bar-code readers may be taken to the patient's bedside to compare the specimen-label code with the patient's wrist-band code to verify specimen identification. Bar codes also reduce clerical error, identifying samples to be introduced onto instruments for analysis. They can also be used to automate test requests on random-access instruments; in addition, bar codes facilitate sampling from the collection tube on many currently used instruments, further reducing the likelihood of specimen identification errors (see Chapter 18). In one study using bar codes, not a single specimen identification error occurred in the analysis of over 300,000 specimens. Because of the many types of bar codes available, laboratories should carefully review manufacturer's specifications before starting to use a bar-code label system. Chapters 16 and 18 discuss the use of bar codes in greater detail.

Preservatives and anticoagulants. Any anticoagulants or preservatives that are needed should be specified, and allowable alternatives should also be itemized. Since many laboratories prefer to use plasma or serum from separator tubes for the majority of chemistry analyses, those tests for which these cannot be used should be clearly listed; a short list is provided in the box. Use of a specific order of specimen collection will prevent specimen contamination; tubes without anticoagulants are always collected first, followed in order by tubes with heparin, other anticoagulants, and finally EDTA.

Sample collection. Guidelines for phlebotomy procedures on patients with indwelling catheters should be included in the phlebotomy manual. If the patient has an intravenous line, blood should not be drawn from the same side of a tourniquet as the intravenous line and preferably not from the same arm. Instructions on the amount of blood

---

Tests for Which Separator Gels Are Inappropriate

Analyte adsorbs to gel
Flecainide, tricyclic antidepressants, haloperidol

Whole blood needed
Red blood cell enzymes, hemoglobin A_{1c}, lead, cyclosporin A

Possible contaminants in gel
Trace metals

Preservatives needed
Most peptide hormones, renin, catecholamines

---

to be withdrawn before sampling from an intravenous or intra-arterial line must be provided. Since removal of a volume of blood equal to the volume of the catheter is adequate for most analytes, the volume of the most commonly used catheters should be provided in the manual. Those tests that are more severely affected by fluid contamination, such as therapeutic drugs, should carry the caution *not* to draw specimens through an indwelling catheter.

Although many veins can be used for venipuncture, the antecubital fossa in the arm is the most widely used site. Because tourniquets are used in most instances of venipuncture, specific instructions on appropriate tourniquet use are needed. The phlebotomist can identify the phlebotomy site and clean the skin before applying the tourniquet; alternatively the tourniquet should be released after a suitable vein is identified. The tourniquet should be kept on for as short a period as possible, preferably less than 1 minute, before phlebotomy is actually performed. Any antiseptic used should be allowed to dry before specimen collection to minimize the likelihood of hemolysis. Specimens should be collected only if blood is free flowing; otherwise venous blood samples may hemolyze, and capillary blood specimens will be diluted with tissue fluid. Because chemistry tests are usually most affected by hemoconcentration, the specimens for these should be the first drawn. The patient should not be advised to clench and loosen his or her fist during collection, since this action will stimulate the release of muscle metabolites into the vein.

POSTCOLLECTION CAUSES OF VARIATION

Postcollection causes of variation are more easily controlled by the laboratory than phlebotomy-related variations, since it is possible to develop criteria for acceptable conditions for storage and handling of specimens after collection, at a time when the specimens are usually in the laboratory's possession. Among the specimen-handling variables that may affect test results are transportation, separation of serum from cellular elements, and storage conditions.

Sample transportation

Errors related to sample transportation. Specimens are usually transported manually by phlebotomists or couriers. A reasonable delay in transportation is usually well tolerated for most analytes, since metabolic changes occur relatively slowly at room temperature. In general, delays of up to an hour will not change the concentration of most analytes. Glucose, often considered one of the more labile substances in blood, falls by approximately 2% to 3% per hour at normal room temperature in tubes without glycolytic inhibitors, such as fluoride.[37] An arterial blood-gas sample is probably the specimen most subject to handling error. Table 3-3 lists the common causes of changes in arterial blood-gas results and the direction and relative magnitude of the changes induced. Products of metabolism (such as lactate, ammonia, and hydrogen ion) accumulate in the sample after collection unless enzymatic reactions are slowed. Other metabolic processes, such as proteolysis, also occur at room temperature. Peptides, which are susceptible to degradation by plasma proteases, will generally decrease in concentration; however, renin precursor (prorenin) will be converted to enzymatically active renin if plasma is allowed to cool slowly.[38]

Procedures to minimize sample-transportation errors

Sample preservation during transportation. To minimize postcollection variation, specimens should be delivered and stored promptly after collection. Analytes that are subject to in vitro change in concentration at room temperature should be promptly transported to the laboratory in an ice slurry. Handling instructions should be clear; in many cases, specimens are improperly placed on top of ice, or are transported protruding from a container of ice or immersed in ice without water. Since a solid conducts heat less rapidly than a liquid, specimens handled in this way will not cool as rapidly and may show artifactual changes. Although cooling samples during transport minimizes many artifactual changes in analyte concentration, cooling increases the release of potassium from cells.

For a substance whose concentration changes with in vitro metabolism, a specific time of delay that can be tolerated should be given. The two most common techniques for preventing metabolism of glucose are the use of glycolytic inhibitors, such as fluoride and iodoacetate, and chilling specimens in ice water. If plain or serum separator tubes are used, at least a half hour should pass before centrifugation to allow clot formation to become complete. Tubes with clot accelerators or anticoagulants can be centrifuged immediately. After centrifugation, specimen collection tubes without barrier gels should have the plasma or serum separated from the cells as quickly as possible to prevent artifacts.

Use of mechanical transporters. Transportation of specimens to the laboratory often significantly delays processing. A College of American Pathologists' Q-Probe on emergency department laboratory tests showed that specimen transport by couriers adds a median of 60% to 100% to the total turnaround time for stat. specimens.[39] Mechanical transport systems, typically using pneumatic tubes, are used by some laboratories to expedite specimen delivery. Carefully designed systems can greatly reduce the time needed for specimens to reach the laboratory. In contrast to the average delay of approximately 30 minutes for manual transport, the average delay with pneumatic tube systems in one hospital system was 2 minutes. Thus pneumatic tube systems have the potential to reduce the need for satellite laboratories and near-patient testing devices. However, the pneumatic tube system may produce trauma to the red blood cells. The risk of hemolysis is increased by use of specimen tubes that are less than fully filled, sudden deceleration, and sharp turns in the tube system. Lack of adequate packing can increase the number of tubes that are broken during transit. Pneumatic tube systems should be periodically monitored to ensure that tube velocity does not increase beyond acceptable limits. Monitoring of the prevalence of hemolyzed samples can be used for this purpose.

Transportation to remote sites. When specimens are transported to remote testing sites, such as reference laboratories, changes can occur in the concentration of many substances. In general, unless the assay specifically calls for whole blood testing, it is best to separate plasma or serum physically from cells before preparing specimens for shipping. To avoid breakage during transit, it is preferable to use tightly capped plastic tubes. Precautions must be taken to prevent the thawing of frozen specimens. Although most referral laboratories suggest the use of insulated containers packed with dry ice, overnight delivery services have become reliable enough that most specimens can be adequately preserved by the use of reusable "ice packs." Specimens must be packaged securely to prevent leakage and labeled as potentially infectious.

Table 3-3 Effect of specimen handling variables on blood-gas measurements

Factor not controlled	pH	Po_2	Pco_2
Not submersing specimen in ice slurry	Decrease up to 0.01 in 10 minutes	Decrease up to 5% in 10 minutes	Minimal change
Air bubbles not removed	Increase if sample agitated	Increase slightly, decrease in patients with high initial Po_2	Decrease
Excess liquid heparin added	Decrease with some forms; usually no effect	Increase slightly, decrease in patients with high initial Po_2	Decrease

Sample processing

Errors arising from incorrect sample processing.

Centrifugation is the method commonly used for the initial separation of serum and cells. The principles of centrifugation are covered in Chapter 1. In general, centrifugation of samples for 5 to 10 minutes at 1000 to 2000 *G* is adequate for complete separation of serum and red blood cells, including specimens containing serum or plasma separator gels. Serum specimens should not be centrifuged until clot formation is completed (at least 20 to 30 minutes after the specimen is collected). When separator gels are used, centrifuges with horizontal rotors produce better mechanical separations. In our laboratory, we store samples with separator gels up to 72 hours with no significant changes in the concentrations of most analytes as long as there were no visible points of contact between the serum and cells. With fixed angle-head centrifuges, occasional gaps occur that allow the serum and cells to remain in contact.

Caution should be taken to ensure that clotting has, in fact, been completed because there can be physiological reasons for extended clotting times. For example, specimens from dialysis patients may continue to clot for hours after collection because of the heparin employed to prepare patients for dialysis. In such cases, recentrifugation, serum filters, and wooden sticks can be used to remove additional fibrin. With tubes that do not contain separator gels, an additional step is necessary to complete the separation. Before centrifugation, substances such as glass beads, plugs, or other mechanical devices may be added to tubes to perform the same function as the gel. After centrifugation, hollow cylinders containing filters or one-way valves at one end can be inserted into the collection tube to provide a physical barrier, and pipets can be used to manually remove the serum. The serum yield when these alternative separation methods are used is often less than that achieved with gels. The use of such alternative procedures instead of serum separator gels increases the risk of spillage and concomitant infection and thus often increases laboratory costs.

As discussed previously, serum must be separated from cells because hematological cells will continue to perform their metabolic functions and alter specimen composition. Although this occurs most rapidly and most dramatically for blood-gas measurements, more subtle changes occur with delayed separation of other specimens. At room temperature, glycolysis continues slowly, with glucose falling by an average of 3% per hour. After approximately 24 hours, the lack of glucose causes leakage of potassium and smaller proteins, such as enzymes, from the cells; and breakdown of organic phosphate compounds causes a rise in inorganic phosphate. After several days, visible hemolysis becomes apparent. If specimens are refrigerated without separation, glycolysis is inhibited, but leakage of potassium and enzymes occurs.

In persons with high white blood cell or platelet counts, dramatic changes can occur following the phlebotomy.

Platelets release potassium from their cytoplasm during clot formation; this causes potassium concentration to be higher in serum than in plasma. Although normal individuals have a difference of 0.2 to 0.3 mmol/L between serum and plasma potassium, this difference increases by an average of 0.15 mmol/L for each increment in the platelet count of 100,000/mm.[39,40] Because white blood cells are more active metabolically than red blood cells, changes resulting from delayed separation are exaggerated in patients with leukemia. Glucose concentration may fall and potassium concentration may begin to rise in as little as 30 minutes,[41] and pH may decrease by as much as 0.6 in 10 minutes if the specimen is not rapidly chilled in an ice slurry. In patients with lymphocytic leukemia, heparin appears to induce degeneration of lymphocytes in vitro, leading to rapid rises in plasma (but not serum) potassium concentration[42] as shown in Fig. 3-7.

Procedure to minimize sample-processing errors.

The most effective way to minimize sample-processing errors is to centrifuge samples requiring separation as soon as possible. If plain tubes are used, centrifugation should not be performed until at least a half hour after blood collection to allow complete clot formation. Tubes with clot accelerators or anticoagulants can be separated immediately. After centrifugation, in specimens without gels, plasma or serum should be separated from the cells as quickly as possible to prevent changes to the sample.

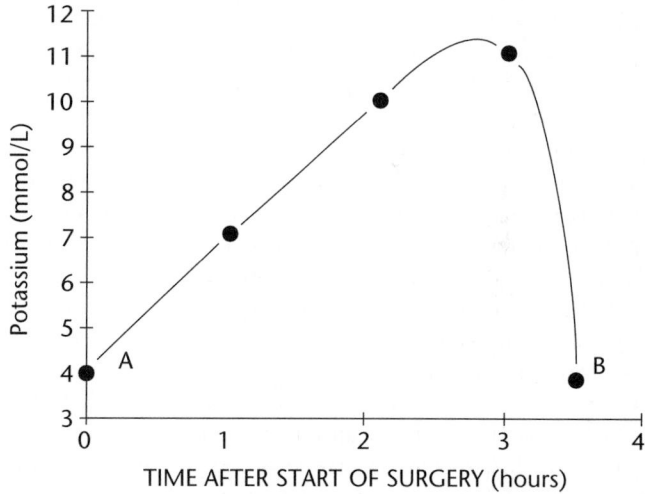

Fig. 3-7 Effect of heparin on potassium in lymphocytic leukemia. The graph represents "serum" potassium concentration obtained during surgery to remove the spleen in a patient with chronic lymphocytic leukemia and white blood count of about 350,000/mm³. *Point A* represents preoperative serum potassium. The next three points represent specimens obtained through an arterial catheter containing heparin at 1, 2, and 3.25 hours into the surgery. *Point B* represents a serum potassium obtained from the arm opposite the arterial catheter 15 minutes after the previous specimen with "serum" potassium of 11.2 mmol/L.

Sample storage

Errors arising from improper sample storage.
Once serum or plasma has been separated from cells, most substances show little change in concentration over a 2- or 3-day period when kept at 4° C. For labile analytes, including enzymes such as creatine kinase and lactate dehydrogenase, most polypeptide hormones, and some other substances, the specimen must be frozen to prevent storage-related changes. Analytes that may be intrinsically stable on storage may change in the presence of other compounds. For example, triglyceride concentration falls in "serum" obtained from patients taking heparin, apparently because of the activation of lipoprotein lipase.[43] Aminoglycoside antibiotics, such as tobramycin and gentamicin, are stable when stored at refrigerator temperatures unless the serum also contains certain synthetic penicillins, most notably piperacillin; aminoglycoside concentrations can fall to less than 50% of baseline value at 72 hours when both drugs are present.[44]

Evaporation can increase sample concentration. When a sample is uncovered, the rate of evaporation is affected by temperature, humidity, air movement, and the surface area of the sample.[45] If humidity is low, a situation often found in air-conditioned laboratories, there is a direct linear relationship between temperature and rate of evaporation; however, at high humidities, temperature changes have a minimal effect on evaporation rate. One of the most important factors affecting evaporation is the rate of air movement over the surface of a liquid. For any given rate of air flow, increasing the height of the column of air over the specimen or decreasing the area of opening in the specimen container will decrease the rate of evaporation by decreasing air movement over the specimen. Small, fully filled sample cups may show as much as 50% loss of water in a few hours. As with any other form of hemoconcentration, this will lead to an increase in concentration of proteins and protein-bound substances; however, evaporation also increases the concentration of other solutes.

Procedures to minimize storage errors. Storage errors can be prevented by the proper selection of time, temperature, and storage conditions. Most analytes are stable when stored at refrigerator temperatures for up to 72 hours. If an analyte is not stable, specimens should be frozen until analysis. Most specimens can be stored at −70° C without affecting analyte concentrations, even when frozen for many years.[46] Alkaline phosphatase activity will increase with freezing, apparently as a result of the destruction of an inhibitor. At standard freezer temperatures of −10° to −20° C, most substances will be stable for shorter periods. Care must be taken to prevent repeated thawing and refreezing of specimens; this is especially problematic with newer "frost-free" freezers, which periodically increase freezer temperature to allow the melting of frost. Analytes that are susceptible to repeated freeze/thaw cycles, such as complement, should be stored in other types of freezers. Frozen samples should be allowed to thaw slowly at room temperature or in a 37° C water bath and should then be mixed thoroughly before analysis.

To prevent specimen evaporation, specimens should be stored covered and kept, if at all possible, away from areas of rapid air flow. Whenever possible, containers with a small surface area and a large column of air over the specimen should be used to minimize evaporation. The identification of each sample should be confirmed at each step of the operation to minimize the likelihood of specimen confusion. Direct sampling from the collection tube is the best way to minimize such errors, especially if bar-coded labels and bar-code readers are available.

OTHER PREANALYTICAL COLLECTION CONCERNS
Urine collection: sources of variation

Biological variables. Preanalytical variation in urine is somewhat difficult to control. Although changes in serum concentration are primarily related to degree of hemoconcentration, urine variation can be caused by several factors. The most important variable in determining urine concentration of a substance is the relative amount of water excreted. The body is capable of greatly altering urine concentration to meet the need for water excretion or water conservation. Since most of the solute in urine is composed of waste products such as urea and creatinine, urine osmolality is a measure of relative water excretion. Normal individuals may have urine osmolality as low as 75 mOsm/kg and as high as 1200 mOsm/kg; the relative concentration of other solutes may thus vary over a fifteenfold range in concentration. As mentioned earlier in the discussion of random variation, intraindividual variation in urinary concentration is, on the average, several times higher than intraindividual variation for the same analytes in serum.[1] Controlling the hydration status of the patient during the urine collection process can minimize this source of variability.

Other causes of preanalytic variation also affect urine measurements. *Diurnal variation* independent of relative concentration is observed for many urine substances, notably protein, sodium and potassium, phosphate, and hormones. Part of the diurnal variation in protein excretion is posture related since the relative concentration of protein compared to creatinine increases in the upright position.[47] *Stress* increases protein excretion; both exercise and fever have been shown to cause transient increase in urinary protein.[48] *Dietary changes* in intake of a substance will often alter urinary excretion. Hydroxyproline, a component of collagen, is often used to measure bone turnover; gelatin, a component of many processed foods, contains collagen and can be a major source of urinary hydroxyproline excretion.[49] Creatinine excretion is often used to evaluate the adequacy of collection of a timed urine. However, short-term fluctuation in dietary protein intake alters the excretion of creatinine in the urine.[17]

Time of collection. Variation in urine measurements can be the result of improperly collected 24-hour urine specimens. Such specimens are among the most difficult to collect properly. As mentioned above, urine creatinine is often used as a measure of the completeness of urine collection, and specimens with too much or too little creatinine are considered to indicate an improperly timed collection. Because excretion of creatinine is relatively reproducible in a given individual on a stable diet (average day-to-day variation of 10% with little diurnal variation), the ratio of the concentration of the substance of interest to that of creatinine has also been advocated as a means to provide an accurate estimate of total urinary excretion.[50,51] This is especially important for pediatric specimens because it is often difficult to get children to cooperate with timed urine collections.

Sample stability. Many compounds stable in serum are unstable in urine. Both bacterial contamination and low pH can produce in vitro changes in the concentration of many analytes. Collection of urine into containers with various preservatives, acids, or bases is commonly needed to prevent such variation; a more complete discussion of urine preservatives is given in Chapter 57. In general, stable substances such as electrolytes, protein, and creatinine can be measured in urine samples without the use of preservatives. Addition of concentrated acids or bases does not usually affect electrolyte or creatinine measurements; however, a specimen containing an appropriate preservative for the measurement of one analyte may be unsuitable for use in the measurement of a different substance. Storage of urine specimens during collection may also alter analyte concentration. For example, porphyrins are unstable when exposed to light, whereas calcium may precipitate at low temperatures. Most formed elements in urine, such as cells and casts, are unstable when stored. Refrigeration is often used to prevent bacterial growth in urine specimens. Refrigeration, however, promotes the formation of crystals that would not have been found at body temperature and lowers the concentrations of those substances that have precipitated.

Preanalytical variation in other body fluids. Preanalytical variation in other body fluids has not been extensively studied. Many factors that affect other samples such as hemoconcentration, tourniquet use, and stress do not affect the composition of cerebrospinal, pleural, peritoneal, and synovial fluids. A delay in transport of specimens to the laboratory usually causes little change in normal fluid composition, since these specimens are virtually cell free. If measurements of unstable analytes such as lactate, glucose, or pH are requested, specimens should be transported to the laboratory in an ice slurry to prevent artifactual change in concentration. For fluids other than cerebrospinal fluid, use of an anticoagulant is advisable to prevent the formation of fibrin clots, which can falsely lower cell counts.

Specimen collection from infants

Capillary sampling. Venipuncture in infants and small children is usually not an acceptable method for obtaining blood, both because of the difficulty in finding a vein and the importance of preserving available veins for use in administration of intravenous fluid. Capillary blood is the specimen usually available for testing in these children. In neonates, the outer aspects of the sole of the foot are the preferred sites for skin puncture whereas earlobes or fingers are acceptable in older infants and small children. The skin surface is often warmed to produce "arterialized" capillary blood; as mentioned earlier, however, agreement with arterial blood gases is poor in neonates, particularly in premature infants. It is essential to allow any topical antiseptics to dry before skin puncture, since the collected blood will freely mix with any remaining liquid on the surface. Contamination with antiseptics can falsely dilute specimens and may cause hemolysis. It may be helpful to apply mild pressure after the skin is punctured, but squeezing or "milking" the puncture site will contaminate the sample with tissue fluid.

Because of the small volume of sample obtained and, in neonates, the high hematocrit, relatively little serum or plasma is available for testing. Special capillary tubes containing appropriate anticoagulants or preservatives are available to facilitate collection of required specimens. Use of pediatric serum separator tubes or heparinized plasma will result in a greater amount of sample for the same amount of blood obtained. However, the small sample size often results in a relatively large surface area, making evaporation an even more important consideration. Control of factors causing evaporation is especially important for pediatric specimens. Hemoconcentration, posture, and diet-related changes are relatively less important for neonates than with older children or adults. The extent of cyclic variations in infants and children is largely unknown.

Blood collection for metabolic diseases. When infants are screened for inborn metabolic errors, specimens are often collected on filter paper and transported to a specialized laboratory as dried blood spots. There is little information on specific preanalytic factors related to dried blood spots; however, some factors do affect results of such tests.[52] Because such specimens are collected as capillary blood, care must be taken to avoid contamination with antiseptics, which may interfere in the assays. The paper must be fully saturated in the area of collection to provide an adequate amount of sample. For many metabolic errors, screening must not be done until at least 24 hours after the infant has begun feeding, since the metabolic product that accumulates is derived from ingested food. Obtaining specimens before this time can produce false-negative results. For tests that require measurement of enzyme activity, care must be taken to prevent exposure of the specimens to excess heat during the shipping process; if specimens are mailed, temperatures in outdoor mail boxes can be high

Table 3-4 Delta checks for analysis

Appropriate	Inappropriate
Electrolytes: Na, K, Cl	Glucose
Total protein	Phosphate
Albumin	Lactate dehydrogenase
Urea	Creatine kinase
Creatinine	Aspartate aminotransferase
Alkaline phosphatase	Alanine aminotransferase
Hemoglobin and hematocrit; mean cell volume and red blood cell distribution width index	

enough to produce falsely low results. All the general precautions discussed previously, such as prevention of evaporation and mislabeling, must be carefully followed.

Computer-based aids for error detection

Computer-based systems that aid in error detection can reduce the number of erroneous results that are reported.[53] In many laboratory and hospital computer systems, it is possible to compare the results from the current specimen with those from previous samples on the same patient (see Chapter 18). Such result comparisons are termed *delta checks*.[54] A delta check can test for results that vary by a set amount or set percentage; on some systems, it is possible to use one type of check for values at a certain level and another for higher or lower concentrations. Tests that are particularly appropriate for monitoring with delta checks are those that normally change little from one day to the next. Some of these are listed in Table 3-4. Measuring the rate of analyte change may also add to the sensitivity of error detection.[55] Delta checks should not be used for substances that are subject to pronounced intraindividual variation (see Table 3-4). A list of delta check values used in our laboratory is given in Table 3-5. Although fluctuations in one test result may be seen in as many as 1% of all specimens, multiple test results that fail delta checks are usually the result of either a significant change in the patient's condition or a nonrepresentative specimen. Selection of tests that typically change in parallel, such as AST and ALT or urea and creatinine, may improve delta check utility (Table 3-4).[56] Common causes of failed delta checks include specimens drawn above intravenous lines, contaminated specimens, and misidentified specimens. Review of such results before release can lead to a significant reduction in the reporting of erroneous results. A method that can be used for the evaluation of specimens failing delta checks is outlined in Fig. 3-8.

Criteria for rejection of specimens

To prevent the reporting of misleading results, each laboratory must establish criteria for specimen rejection. A specimen must be rejected when the results obtained by analysis of that specimen will not be representative of the patient's condition. The most common cause for specimen rejection is inadequate identification. Specimens *must* have the patient's name and identification number on both the sample and the accompanying request slip. Specimens that are not drawn by laboratory personnel should be checked carefully before they are accepted by the laboratory. For specimens requiring special handling, improper collection and transportation are the most common causes for rejection. In most laboratories that process blood-gas specimens, an average of 5% of the specimens have not been collected correctly and must be rejected.[57] Specimens are often collected in the

Table 3-5 Delta check values

Test	Delta check value
Albumin	10 g/L
Anion gap	10 mmol/L
Calcium	10 mg/L
Chloride	5 mmol/L
Cholesterol	±30%
CO_2 content	5 mmol/L
Creatinine	±50%
Direct bilirubin	±50%
Glucose (fasting only)	±30%
Magnesium	0.25 mmol/L
Mean corpuscular volume	4 μm^3
Mean platelet volume	1.5 μm^3
Osmolality	15 mOsm/kg
Potassium	1 mmol/L
Protein	10 g/L
Red blood cell distribution width	2% (absolute change)
Sodium	5 mmol/L
Total bilirubin	±50%
Urea nitrogen	±50%
Uric acid	15 mg/L

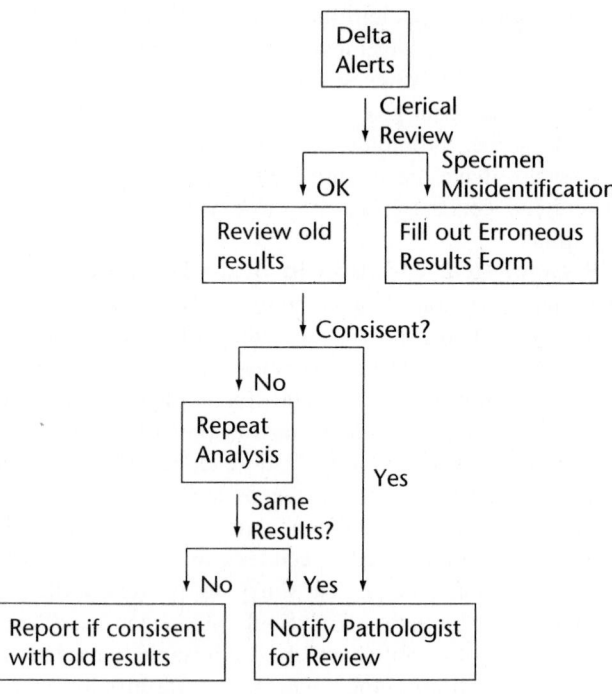

Fig. 3-8 Flow chart for delta alerts.

incorrect tube for the assay requested. Each laboratory must have a list of acceptable alternative specimens for each test; for example, a laboratory manual may suggest collection of serum for a particular test, but heparinized plasma is an acceptable alternative. If the specimen contains another anticoagulant or preservative, it should be rejected (though it may be used for other analyses). For tubes containing preservatives or anticoagulants, there must be a proper ratio of specimen to preservative. This is most critical with liquid solutions of preservatives but may also occur with powdered anticoagulants. Tubes that do not have the appropriate ratio should not be accepted for analysis. For tests that require special patient preparation, its absence should cause rejection. If a test is affected by hemolysis, hemolyzed specimens should be rejected. If a test result is affected by lipemia (and the specimen cannot be cleared by ultracentrifugation before analysis), test results should not be reported. Finally, any specimens that have results that fail delta checks or that are considered to be unlikely to be real (potassium over 10 mmol/L, calcium less than 40 mg/L, and so on) should be reported to the laboratory director for review before the results are reported. Although many physicians complain when the laboratory does not report results for tests ordered for their patients, if there is any question about the validity of a result, it should not be reported. Erroneous results can lead to inappropriate treatment of the patient.

REFERENCES

1. Arendt J, Minors DS, Waterhouse JM, editors: *Biological rhythms in clinical practice*, Boston, 1989, Wright.
2. Liskowsky DR: Biological rhythms and shift work, *JAMA* 268:3047, 1992.
3. Utiger RD: Melatonin—the hormone of darkness, *N Engl J Med* 327:1377-1379, 1992.
4. Fevre-Montage M, Van Cauter E, Refetoff S, et al: Effects of "jet lag" on hormonal patterns. II. Adaptation of melatonin circadian periodicity, *J Clin Endocrinol Metab* 52:642-649, 1978.
5. Tietz NW: *Clinical guide to laboratory tests*, ed 2, Philadelphia, 1990, Saunders.
6. Benvenuti M, Legnaioli M, Melone F, et al: Circadian rhythm in prostatic acid phosphatase (PAP): a potential tumor marker rhythm in prostatic cancer (PCa), *Chronobiologia* 10:383, 1983.
7. Kemp GJ, Blumsohn A, Morris BW: Circadian changes in plasma phosphate concentration, urinary phosphate excretion, and cellular phosphate shifts, *Clin Chem* 38:400-402, 1992.
8. Dufour DR: Reference values in endocrinology. In Becker KL, editor: *Principles and practice of endocrinology*, ed 2, Philadelphia, 1995, Lippincott.
9. Rosen JF, Chesney RW: Circulating calcitriol concentrations in health and disease, *J Pediatr* 103:1-17, 1983.
10. Elomaa I, Karonen S-L, Kairento A-L, Pelkonen R: Seasonal variation of urinary calcium and oxalate excretion, serum 25(OH)D₃, and albumin level in relation to renal stone formation, *Scand J Urol Nephrol* 16:155-161, 1982.
11. Harrup JS, Ashwell K, Hopton MR: Circannual and within-individual variation of thyroid function tests in normal subjects, *Ann Clin Biochem* 22 (pt 4):371-375, 1985.
12. Fraser CG: Biological variation in clinical chemistry—an update: collated data, 1988-1991, *Arch Pathol Lab Med* 116:916-923, 1992.
13. Statland BE, Winkel P, Bokelund H: Factors contributing to intraindividual variation of serum constituents: 2. Effects of exercise and diet on variation of serum constituents in healthy subjects, *Clin Chem* 19:1380-1383, 1973.
14. Stansbie D, Bedley JP: Biochemical consequences of exercise, *JIFCC* 3:87-91, 1991.
15. Ronkainen H: Depressed follicle-stimulating hormone, luteinizing hormone, and prolactin responses to luteinizing hormone-releasing hormone, thyrotropin-releasing hormone, and metoclopramide test in endurance runners in the hard training season, *Fertil Steril* 44:755-759, 1985.
16. Ahlquist DA, McGill DB, Schwartz S, et al: HemoQuant, a new quantitative assay for fecal hemoglobin: comparison with hemoccult, *Ann Intern Med* 101:297-302, 1984.
17. Perrone RD, Madias NE, Levey AS: Serum creatinine as an index of renal function: new insights into old concepts, *Clin Chem* 38:1933-1953, 1992.
18. Muldoon MF, Bachen EA, Mannuck SB, et al: Acute cholesterol responses to mental stress and change in posture, *Arch Intern Med* 152:775-780, 1992.
19. Genest JJ, McNamara JR, Ordovas JM, et al: Effect of elective hospitalization on plasma lipoprotein cholesterol and apolipoproteins AI, B, and LP(a), *Am J Cardiol* 65:677-679, 1990.
20. Gore JM, Goldberg RJ, Matsumoto AS, et al: Validity of serum total cholesterol level obtained within 24 hours of acute myocardial infarction, *Am J Cardiol* 54:722-725, 1984.
21. Gebhart SP, Watts NB, Clark RV, et al: Reversible impairment of gonadotropin secretion in critical illness: observations in postmenopausal women, *Arch Intern Med* 149:1637-1641, 1989.
22. Kaptein EM, Grieb DA, Spencer CA, et al: Thyroxine metabolism in the low thyroxine state of critical nonthyroidal illnesses, *J Clin Endocrinol Metab* 53:764-771, 1981.
23. Davenport MW, Zipser RD: Association of hypotension with hyperreninemic hypoaldosteronism in the critically ill patient, *Arch Intern Med* 143:735-737, 1983.
24. Statland BE, Bokelund H, Winkel P: Factors contributing to intraindividual variation of serum constituents: 4. Effects of posture and tourniquet application on variation of serum constituents in healthy subjects, *Clin Chem* 20:1513-1519, 1974.
25. Van Cauter E: Endocrine rhythms. In Becker KL, editor: *Principles and practice of endocrinology*, Philadelphia, 1990, Lippincott.
26. National Committee for Clinical Laboratory Standards: *Approved standard procedures for the collection of diagnostic blood specimens by skin puncture*, Villanova, Pa., 1982.
27. College of American Pathologists: *So you're going to collect a blood specimen*, ed 5, Danville, Ill., 1992, Interstate Printers.
28. Pendergraph GA: *Handbook of phlebotomy*, ed 2, Philadelphia, 1988, Lea & Febiger.
29. Hill BM, Laessig RH, Koch DD, Hassemer DJ: Comparison of plastic vs. glass evacuated serum-separator (SST) blood-drawing tubes for common clinical chemistry determinations, *Clin Chem* 38:1474-1478, 1992.
30. Adrogue HJ, Rashad MN, Gorin AB, et al: Assessing acid-base status in circulatory failure: differences between arterial and central venous blood, *N Engl J Med* 320:1312-1316, 1989.
31. Atkin S, Dasmahapatra A, Jaker MA, et al: Fingerstick glucose determination in shock, *Ann Intern Med* 114:1020-1024, 1991.
32. Irjala K, Koskinen P, Näntö V, Peltola O: Interpretation of oral glucose tolerance test: capillary-venous difference in blood glucose and the effect of analytical method, *Scand J Clin Lab Invest* 46:307-313, 1986.
33. Doumas BT, Hause LL, Simuncak DM, Breitenfeld D: Differences between values for plasma and serum in tests performed in the Ektachem 700 XR analyzer, and evaluation of "plasma separator tubes (PST)," *Clin Chem* 35:151-153, 1989.
34. Don BR, Sebastian A, Cheitlin M, et al: Pseudohyperkalemia caused by fist clenching during phlebotomy, *N Engl J Med* 322:1290-1292, 1990.
35. Weilert M, Tilzer LL: Putting bar codes to work for improved patient care, *Clin Lab Med* 11:227-238, 1991.
36. National Institute on Drug Abuse: Urinalysis collection handbook for federal drug testing programs, Washington, D.C., 1988, U.S. Department of Health and Human Services.
37. Sazama K, Robertson EA, Chesler RA: Is routine antiglycolysis re-

quired for routine glucose analysis? *Clin Chem* 25:1086-1087, 1979.

38. Sealey JE: Plasma renin activity and plasma prorenin assays, *Clin Chem* 37:1811-1819, 1991.
39. Howanitz PJ, Steindel SJ, Cembrowski GS, Long TA: Emergency department stat test turnaround times: a College of American Pathologists' Q-probes study for potassium and hemoglobin, *Arch Pathol Lab Med* 116:122-128, 1992.
40. Graber M, Subramani K, Corish D, Schwab A: Thrombocytosis elevates serum potassium, *Am J Kidney Dis* 12:116-120, 1988.
41. Ringelhann B, Laszlo E, Vajda L: Pseudohyperkalaemia in acute myeloid leukemia, *Lancet* 1:928, 1974.
42. Dufour DR, Mesonero C, Miller K: Artefactual hyperkalemia induced by heparin in patients with extreme leukocytosis, *Clin Chem* 33:914, 1987.
43. Hortin G, Cole TG, Gibson DW, Kessler G: Decreased stability of triglycerides and increased free glycerol in serum from heparin-treated patients, *Clin Chem* 34:1847-1849, 1988.
44. Pickering LK, Rutherford I: Effect of concentration and time upon inactivation of tobramycin, gentamicin, netilmicin, and amikacin by azlocillin, carbenicillin, mecillinam, mezlocillin and piperacillin, *J Pharmacol Exp Ther* 217:345-349, 1981.
45. Burtis CA: The effects of temperature and evaporation on analytical error in the clinical laboratory, *Clin Lab Annu* 1:1-35, 1982.
46. DiMagno EP, Corle D, O'Brien JF, et al: Effect of long-term freezer storage, thawing, and refreezing on selected constituents of serum, *Mayo Clin Proc* 64:1226-1234, 1989.
47. Howey JEA, Browning MCK, Fraser CG: Selecting the optimum specimen for assessing slight albuminuria, and a strategy for clinical investigation: novel uses of data on biological variation, *Clin Chem* 33:2034-2038, 1987.
48. Clerico A, Giammattei C, Cecchini L, et al: Exercise-induced proteinuria in well-trained athletes, *Clin Chem* 36:562-564, 1990.
49. Yoneyama K, Ishigure S, Ikeda J, Nagata H: The day to day variations of urinary hydroxyproline and creatinine excretions, and dietary protein intake, *Nippon Eiseigaku Zasshi* 39:587-594, 1984.
50. Ginsberg JM, Chang BS, Matarese RE, Garella S: Use of single voided urine samples to estimate quantitative proteinuria, *N Engl J Med* 309:1543-1546, 1983.
51. Huikeshoven FJM, Zuiderhoudt FMJ: Hypocalciuria in hypertensive disorder in pregnancy and how to measure it, *Eur J Obstet Gynecol Reprod Biol* 36:81-85, 1990.
52. Buist NRM: Laboratory aspects of newborn screening for metabolic disorders, *Lab Med* 19:145-150, 1988.
53. Ladenson JH: Patients as their own controls: use of the computer to identify "laboratory error," *Clin Chem* 21:1648-1653, 1975.
54. Sher PP: An evaluation of the detection capacity of a computer-assisted real-time delta check system, *Clin Chem* 25:870-872, 1979.
55. Lacher DA, Connelly DP: Rate and delta checks compared for selected chemistry tests, *Clin Chem* 34:1966-1970, 1988.
56. Lacher DA: Relationship between delta checks for selected chemistry tests, *Clin Chem* 36:2134-2136, 1990.
57. Shapiro BA, Harrison RA, Cane RD, Kozlowski-Templin R: *Clinical application of blood gases,* ed 4, St. Louis, 1989, Mosby, pp 274-275.

CHAPTER 4

Spectral techniques

Amadeo J. Pesce
Christopher S. Frings
Jack Gauldie

———————————————◼———————————————

———————————————◼———————————————

OBJECTIVES

- Describe the relationships among wavelength, frequency, energy, and color of the ultraviolet and visible spectra.
- Describe the relationship between percent transmittance (%T) and absorbance (A) and how this relationship affects the color of a solution.
- Describe the Beer-Lambert law and its limitations.
- Illustrate the construction and operation of photometric monochromators and detectors and explain the advantages or disadvantages associated with the use of each in spectral instruments. Further describe the principles of spectral isolation and band pass.
- Draw a block diagram of the essential components of the atomic absorption spectrophotometer and the fluorometer and state the principle of the operation of each, highlighting similarities and differences. Explain the interferences associated with each.
- Describe how the instrumentation and basic principles of photometry are modified with the applications of turbidity, nephelometry, or fluorometry and identify any unique interferences or sources of error associated with each.
- Describe one of the chemical reactions that results in chemiluminescence.
- Compare and contrast the principles of absorption and emission spectroscopy.

KEY TERMS

absorbance Defined as $2 - \log \%T$, it is directly proportional to concentration of absorbing species if Beer's law is followed.

absorption spectrum The range of electromagnetic energy that is used for spectroanalysis, including both visible light and ultraviolet radiation; also graph of spectrum for a specific compound.

absorptivity Absorbance divided by the product of the concentration of a substance and the sample path length.

angle of detection The angle at which scattered light is measured in nephelometry.

atomic absorption spectrophotometry A quantitative spectroscopic measurement in which the emitted light from a source composed of one element is absorbed by the same element in a vapor phase. The amount of light absorbed is directly related to the concentration of the element in a sample.

band pass The range of wavelengths that reaches the exit slit of a monochromator; usually referred to as the range of wavelengths transmitted at a point equal to half the peak intensity transmitted.

***Beer-Lambert law* (most commonly referred to as *Beer's law*)** The concentration of a substance is directly proportional to the amount of radiant energy absorbed.

bioluminescence An enzyme-catalyzed reaction that uses complex organic molecules and adenosine triphosphate (ATP) to yield light.

blank A solution consisting of all the components including solvents and solutes except the compound to be measured. This solution is used to set I_0, the original light intensity.

chemiluminescence A chemical reaction usually involving oxidation in which one of the products is light.

cuvette The receptacle in a photometer in which the sample is placed.

diode array A two-dimensional matrix of light-sensitive semiconductors the response of which allows recording of a complete absorption spectrum in milliseconds.

electronic transition The change in the orbital position of an electron of an atom or molecule. In the case of the absorption of a photon of light, the electron usually goes from the ground or the lowest energy level to some higher one with a consequent higher energy state (increased energy) of the molecule. Basis of fluorescence phenomena.

emission wavelength The wavelength of light (λ_{em}) that is used to monitor decay of excited molecules into fluorescence; usually refers to the wavelength of output photons measured by a fluorometer.

excitation wavelength The wavelength of radiant energy (λ_{ex}) that is absorbed by a molecule and causes it to be raised to a higher energy state; usually refers to the wavelength of incident energy of a fluorometer.

filter An optical device (usually glass) that allows only a portion of polychromatic, incident light to pass through. The amount of transmitted light is related to the band pass of the filter.

flameless atomic absorption An atomic absorption technique in which the element is converted to a vapor phase without the use of a flame.

fluorescence The light emitted by an atom or molecule after absorption of a photon. This light is at longer wavelengths (less energy) than the absorbed light and is usually emitted in less than 10^{-8} sec. However, some compounds emit the photon at a slower rate.

grating An optical device consisting of a reflecting, ruled surface that disperses polychromatic light into a uniform, continuous spectrum. Dispersion of light is attributable to interference phenomena at the ruled surface.

hollow-cathode lamp A lamp consisting of a metal cathode and an inert gas. When an electric current is passed through the cathode, the metal is sputtered free and, after colliding with the gas in the lamp, emits a line spectrum of specific wavelengths related to the metal of the cathode.

infrared radiation The region of the electromagnetic spectrum extending from about 780 to 300,000 nm.

internal standard An element or compound added in a known amount to yield a signal against which an instrument or an analyte to be measured can be calibrated.

light scattering The interaction of light with particles that cause the light to be bent away from its original path (cause of turbidity).

line spectrum Discontinuous emission spectrum of elements in which the emitted light bands cover a very narrow (0.1 nm) range of energies.

luminescence Light emitted at low temperatures, often as the result of a chemical reaction (*chemiluminescence*).

***molar absorptivity* (ϵ)** The absorbance of light, at a specific wavelength, divided by the product of concentration in moles per liter and the sample path length in centimeters. Molar absorptivity is expressed as L/mol·cm.

monochromatic Light of one color (wavelength). In practice this refers to radiant energy composed of a very narrow range of wavelengths.

monochromator Device used to isolate a certain wavelength or range of wavelengths. Usually refers to prisms or grating.

nephelometry A technique that measures the amount of light scattered by particles suspended in a solution.

phosphorescence Similar to fluorescence, the light emitted by an atom or molecule after absorption of a photon. The light is usually emitted at a time greater than 10^{-3} sec after absorption of the photon.

photodetector A device that responds to light (photons) usually in a manner proportional to the number of photons striking its light-sensitive surface. Commonly a current that is proportional to the incident light intensity is generated.

photometer An instrument that measures light intensity; composed of a source of radiant energy, filter for wavelength selection, cuvette holder, detector, and a readout device.

photon A particle consisting of a discrete packet of radiant energy.

polarized fluorescence The orientation of the emitted fluorescent light, which can be calculated from the polarization formula.

polychromatic Light of many colors (wavelengths), usually referring to white light, or that encompassing a defined portion of the spectrum.

Rayleigh scatter The reflection of light at different angles by particles suspended in a solution. This scattering occurs when the wavelength of light is greater than the size of the particles.

reflectance spectrophotometry A quantitative spectrophotometric technique in which the light reflected from the surface of a colorimetric reaction is used to measure the amount of the reaction product.

refraction A process by which the path of incident light is bent after the light passes obliquely from one medium to another of different density.

refractive index The ratio of the speed of light in two different mediums; usually the reference medium is air.

refractometer An instrument for measuring the refractive index (refractivity) of various substances, especially of solutions.

spectrophotometer An instrument that measures light intensity. It is composed of a source of radiant energy, entrance slit, monochromator, exit slit, cuvette holder, detector, and readout device. Measurements in these instruments can be made over a continuous range of available spectrum.

stray light Radiant energy reaching the detector and consisting of wavelengths other than those defined by the filter or monochromator.

time-delayed fluorescence A technique in which the fluorescence of slowly emitting compounds such as metal chelates is measured. Usually the time between 400 and 1000 msec is monitored.

ultraviolet radiation The region of the electromagnetic spectrum from about 180 to 390 nm.

visible light The radiant energy in the electromagnetic spectrum visible to the human eye (approximately 390 to 780 nm).

wavelength The linear distance traversed by one complete wave cycle of electromagnetic energy.

LIGHT AND MATTER[1-3]
Properties of light and radiant energy

Electromagnetic radiant energy is a form of energy that can be described in terms of its wavelike properties. Electromagnetic waves travel at high velocities and do not require the existence of a supporting medium for propagation.

The wavelength, λ, of a beam of electromagnetic radiant energy is the linear distance traversed by one complete wave cycle and is usually given in nanometers (nm, 10^{-9} meters). The frequency, ν, is the number of cycles occurring per second and is obtained by the relationship

$$\nu = \frac{c}{\lambda}$$

The velocity, c, varies with the medium through which the radiant energy is passing ($c = 3 \times 10^{10}$ cm/sec when measured in a vacuum).

Radiant energy can be shown to behave as if it were composed of discrete packets of energy called *photons*. The energy of a photon is variable and depends on the frequency or wavelength of the radiant energy. The relationship between the energy, E, of a photon and frequency is given by the formula

$$E = h\nu$$

h is Planck's constant and has a numerical value of 6.62×10^{-27} erg·sec. The equivalent expression involving wavelength is

$$E = \frac{hc}{\lambda}$$

This equation shows that shorter wavelengths have a higher energy than longer wavelengths have.

The electromagnetic spectrum covers a very large range of wavelengths, as shown in Table 4-1. The areas of the electromagnetic spectrum that are commonly used in the clinical laboratory are the ultraviolet (UV) and visible regions. The visible region is generally specified as the region between 390 and 780 nm, whereas the ultraviolet spec-

trum usually referred to in the clinical chemistry laboratory falls between 180 and 390 nm. Sunlight or light emitted from a tungsten filament is a mixture of radiant energy of different wavelengths that the eye recognizes as "white." The breakdown of the visible region into color absorbed and color reflected is shown in Table 4-2. If a solution absorbs radiant energy (light) between 400 and 480 nm (blue), it will *transmit* all other colors and appear yellow to the eye. Therefore yellow is the complementary color of blue. If white light is focused on a solution that absorbs energy between 505 and 555 nm (green), the transmitted light and thus the solution will appear purple (blue and red). If a red light is focused on a red solution, red light will be transmitted because this solution cannot absorb red light. On the other hand, if green light is focused on the red solution, no light is transmitted, since the solution absorbs all light but red. The human eye responds to radiant energy between 390 and 700 nm, but laboratory instrumentation permits measurements at both shorter wavelengths, such as UV, and longer wavelengths, such as infrared, of the spectrum.

Interactions of light with matter

Absorption process. When an atom, ion, or molecule absorbs a photon, the added energy results in an alteration of state, and the species is said to be excited. Excitation may involve any of the following processes:

1. Transition of an electron to a higher energy level
2. A change in the mode of vibration of the molecule's covalent bonds
3. Alteration of its mode of rotation about the covalent bonds

Each of these transitions requires a definite quantity of energy; the probability of occurrence for a particular transition is greatest when the photon absorbed supplies this exact quantity of energy.

The energy requirements for these transitions vary widely. Usually elevation of electrons to higher energy levels requires greater energy absorption than is needed to cause vibrational changes. Rotational alterations usually have the lowest energy requirements. Therefore absorption of energy in the microwave and far-infrared regions results in shifts in the rotational energy levels, since the energy of the radiant energy is insufficient to cause other types of transitions. Changes in vibrational levels are caused by absorption in the near-infrared and visible regions. Promotion of an electron to a higher energy level occurs after energy absorption in the visible, ultraviolet, and x-ray regions of the spectrum. The energy content of the electrons of covalent

Table 4-1 Electromagnetic spectrum

	Gamma rays	X rays	Ultraviolet (UV)	Visible	Infrared (IR)	Microwaves
Wavelength (nm)*	0.1	1	180	390	780	400×10^3

*This is the wavelength interval where the lowest type of respective radiant energy occurs.

Table 4-2 Colors and complementary colors of visible spectrum

Wavelength* (nm)	Color absorbed†	Complementary or solution color transmitted
350-430	violet	yellow
430-475	blue	orange
475-495	blue green	red-orange
495-505	blue green	orange-red
505-555	green	red
555-575	yellow green	violet-red
575-600	yellow	violet
600-650	orange	blue
670-700	red	green

From Brown TL, Lemay HE: *Chemistry: the central science,* Englewood Cliffs, N.J., 1977, Prentice-Hall.
*Because of the subjective nature of color, the wavelength ranges are only approximations.
†If a solution absorbs light of the color listed in the second column, the observed color of the solution, that is, the transmitted complementary light, is given in the third column.

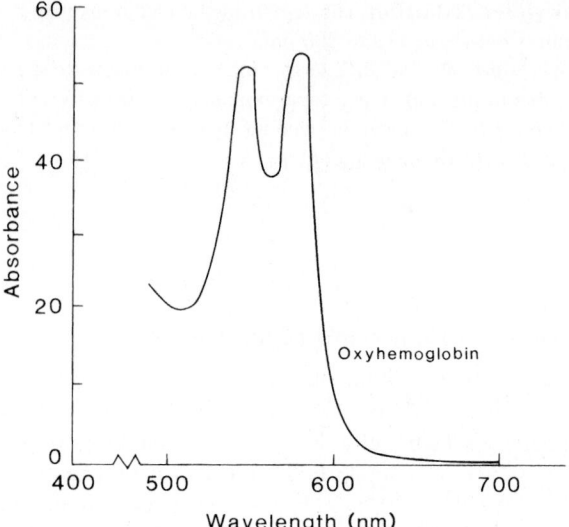

Fig. 4-1 Absorption spectrum of oxyhemoglobin.

bonds varies with the nature of the bonds. The energy of a photon of light needed to excite an electron will therefore vary with the bond, and each type of bond will have its own characteristic pattern of optimum wavelengths of light that can be absorbed by that bond. Table 4-3 gives the electronic absorption bands for many organic groups.[4]

The absorption pattern of a complex organic molecule containing tens of thousands of bonds must therefore describe the cumulative sum of the absorption of *all* the individual covalent bonds.

The absorption of radiant energy by a solution can be described by means of a plot of the absorbance as a function of wavelength. This graph is called an *absorption spectrum* (Fig. 4-1). The absorption spectrum reflects the sum of the energy transitions characteristic for a molecule at each wavelength of light. Absorption spectra are often helpful for qualitative identification purposes. This is particularly true for low-energy absorptions such as those found in the in-

Table 4-3 Electron absorption bands for representative chromophores

Chromophore	System	λ_{max}	ϵ_{max}	λ_{max}	ϵ_{max}	λ_{max}	ϵ_{max}
Ether	—O—	185	1000				
Thioether	—S—	194	4600	215	1600		
Amine	—NH₂	195	2800				
Thiol	—SH	195	1400				
Disulfide	—S—S—	194	5500	255	400		
Sulfone	—SO₂—	180	—				
Ethylene	—C═C—	190	8000				
Ketone	>C═O	195	1000	270-285	18-30		
Esters	—COOR	205	50				
Aldehyde	—CHO	210	strong	280-300	11-18		
Carboxyl	—COOH	200-210	50-70				
Nitro	—NO₂	210	strong				
Azo	—N═N—	285-400	3-25				
Nitrate	—ONO₂	270 (shoulder)	12				
	—(C═C)₂— (acyclic)	210-230	21,000				
	—(C═C)₃—	260	35,000				
	—(C═C)₅—	330	118,000				
	C═C—C≡C	219	6500				
Benzene		184	46,700	202	6900	255	170
Anthracene		252	199,000	375	7900		
Quinoline		227	37,000	270	3600	314	2750
Isoquinoline		218	80,000	266	4000	317	3500

From Willard HH, Merritt LL, Dean JA: *Instrumental methods of analysis,* ed 4, Princeton, N.J., 1965, Van Nostrand.

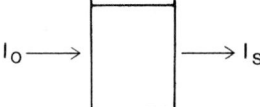

Fig. 4-2 Transmittance of radiant energy through a cuvette. I_0 is the incident radiation; I_s is the transmitted radiation.

frared region. Irrespective of the amount of energy absorbed, an excited species tends to return spontaneously to its unexcited, or ground, state; in the process it releases energy as kinetic (movement), vibrational, or light (see the discussion of fluorescence below) energy.

Emission process. Some elements and compounds can be excited in such a fashion that when the electrons return from the excited state to the ground state, the energy is dissipated as radiant energy. The radiant energy may consist of one or more than one energy level and therefore may consist of different wavelengths. This principle is used in flame photometry and fluorometric methods and is further discussed with these topics.

ABSORPTION SPECTROSCOPY[4-11]
Radiant-energy absorption

Consider a beam of radiant energy with an original intensity, I_0, impinging on and passing through a square cell (whose sides are perpendicular to the beam) containing a solution of a compound that absorbs radiant energy of a certain wavelength (Fig. 4-2). The intensity of the transmitted radiant energy, I_s, will be less than I_0. Some of the incident radiant energy may be reflected by the surface of the cell or absorbed by the cell wall or the solvent. Therefore these factors must be eliminated if one is to consider *only* the absorption of the compound of interest. This is done by use of a blank or reference solution containing everything but the compound to be measured. The amount of light passing through the blank solution is set as the new I_0 (relative to the reference cell and solution). The transmittance for the compound in solution is defined as the proportion of the incident light that is transmitted:

$$\text{Transmittance} = T = I_s/I_0$$

Usually this ratio is described as a percentage:

$$\text{Percent T} = \%T = I_s/I_0 \times 100\%$$

The concept of transmittance is important because only transmitted light can be measured.

As the concentration of the compound in solution increases, more light is absorbed by the solution and less light is transmitted. Percent T varies inversely and logarithmically with concentration. However, it is more convenient to use absorbance, A, which is directly proportional to concentration. Therefore

$$A = -\log I_s/I_0 = -\log T = \log \frac{1}{T}$$

To convert T to %T, the denominator and numerator are multiplied by 100%:

$$A = \log \frac{1}{T} \times \frac{100\%}{100\%} = \log \frac{100\%}{\%T}$$

This can be rearranged to

$$A = \log 100\% - \log \%T$$

or

$$A = 2 - \log \%T$$

It is important to remember that absorbance is not a directly measurable quantity but can be obtained only by mathematical calculation from transmittance data.

The relationship between absorbance and %T is shown in Fig. 4-3, in which the linear %T scale runs from 0 to 100%, whereas the logarithmic absorbance scale runs from infinity to 0.

Beer-Lambert law

The Beer-Lambert law (most commonly referred to simply as *Beer's law*) states that the concentration of a substance is directly proportional to the amount of radiant energy absorbed or inversely proportional to the logarithm of the transmitted radiant energy. If the concentration of a solution is constant and the path length through the solution that the light must traverse is doubled, the effect on the absorbance is the same as doubling the concentration, since twice as many absorbing molecules are now present in the radiant-energy path. Thus the absorbance is also directly proportional to the path length of the radiant energy through the cell.

The mathematical relationship that connects absorbance of radiant energy, concentration of a solution, and path length is shown by Beer's law:

$$A = abc$$

A is absorbance; a, absorptivity; b, light path of the solution in centimeters; and c, concentration of the substance of interest.

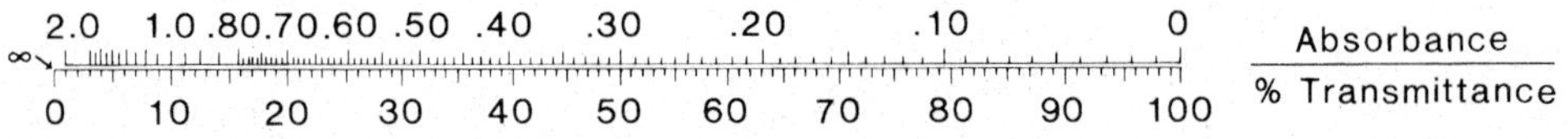

| 2.0 | 1.0 | .80 | .70 | .60 | .50 | .40 | .30 | .20 | .10 | 0 | Absorbance |

| 0 | 10 | 20 | 30 | 40 | 50 | 60 | 70 | 80 | 90 | 100 | % Transmittance |

Fig. 4-3 Scale showing relationship between absorbance and percent transmittance.

This equation forms the basis of quantitative analysis by absorption photometry or absorption spectroscopy. Absorbance values have no units. The absorptivity is a proportionality constant related to the chemical nature of the solute and has units that are reciprocal of those for b and c.

When c is expressed in moles per liter and b is expressed in centimeters, the symbol ϵ, called the molar absorptivity, is used in place of a and is a constant for a given compound at a given wavelength under specified conditions of solvent, pH, temperature, and so on. It has units of L/mole·cm. The higher the molar absorptivity, the higher is the absorbance for the same mass concentration of two compounds. Therefore, in selecting a chromogen for spectrophotometric methods, one should use the chromogen with a higher molar absorptivity, which will impart a greater sensitivity to the measurement.

Once a chromogen is proved to follow Beer's law at a specific wavelength (that is, a linear plot of A versus c with a zero intercept; Fig. 4-4, A), the concentration of an unknown solution can be determined by measurement of its absorbance and interpolation of its concentration from the graph of the standards. In contrast, when %T is plotted versus concentration (on linear graph paper), a curvilinear relationship is obtained (Fig. 4-4, B). Because of the linear relationship between absorbance and concentration, it is possible to relate unknown concentrations to a single standard by a simple proportional equation. Therefore

$$\frac{A_s}{A_u} = \frac{C_s}{C_u}$$

and

$$C_u = \frac{A_u}{A_s} \times C_s$$

where C_u and C_s are the concentration of the unknown and standard respectively and A_u and A_s are the absorbance of the unknown and standard.

The above equation is valid *only* if the chromogen obeys Beer's law and both standard and unknown are measured in the same cell. The concentration range over which a chromogen obeys Beer's law must be determined for each set of analytical conditions.

Beer's law is an ideal mathematical relationship that contains several limitations. Deviations from Beer's law, that is, variations from the linearity of the absorbance versus concentration curve (Fig. 4-5), occur when (1) very elevated concentrations are measured, (2) incident radiant energy is not monochromatic, (3) the solvent absorption is significant compared with the solute absorbance, (4) radiant energy is transmitted by other mechanisms (stray light), and (5) the sides of the cell are not parallel. If two or more chemical species are absorbing the wavelength of incident radiant energy, each with a different absorptivity, Beer's law will not be followed. If the absorbance of a fluorescent solution is being measured, Beer's law may not be followed.

Stray radiation (stray light) is radiant energy that reaches the detector at wavelengths other than those indicated by the monochromator setting. All radiant energy that reaches the detector with or without having passed through the sample will be recorded. Fig. 4-5 shows the effects of stray light on Beer's law. As the amount of stray light increases (or monochromicity decreases), deviation from Beer's law also increases (that is, linearity decreases).

Instrumentation

Single-beam spectrophotometer. The major components of a single-beam spectrophotometer are shown in Fig. 4-6. The apparatus needed can be divided into seven basic components: (1) a stable source of radiant energy; (2) an entrance slit to focus the light; (3) a wavelength selector; (4) an exit slit to focus the light; (5) a device to hold the transparent container (cuvette), which contains the solution to be measured; (6) a radiant-energy detector; and (7)

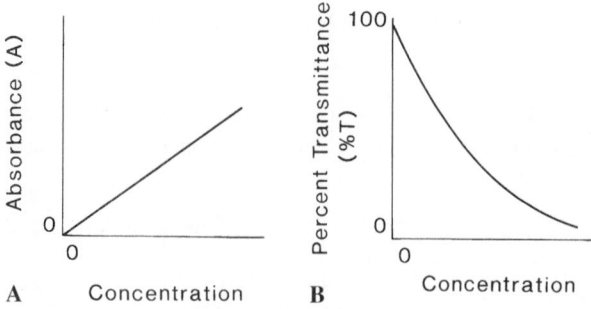

Fig. 4-4 Relationships of absorbance, **A,** and percent transmittance, **B,** to concentration.

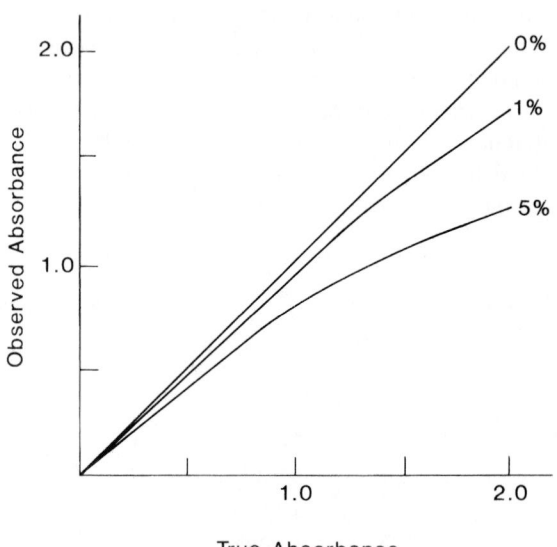

Fig. 4-5 Effect of stray radiation on true absorbance. (From Frings CS, Broussard LA: *Clin Chem* 25:1013-1017, 1979.)

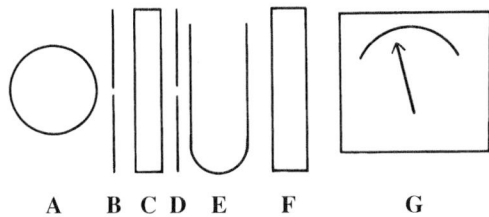

A   B C D E   F   G

Fig. 4-6 Components of a spectrophotometer. **A,** Source of radiant energy; **B,** entrance slit; **C,** wavelength selector; **D,** exit slit; **E,** cuvette and cuvette holder; **F,** detector; **G,** readout device.

a device to read out the electrical signal generated by the detector. If a filter is used as the wavelength selector, monochromatic light at only discrete wavelengths is available, and the instrument is called a *photometer.* If a monochromator is used (that is, a prism or grating, see below) as the wavelength selector, the instrument can provide monochromatic light over a continuous range of wavelengths and is called a *spectrometer* or *spectrophotometer.* Spectrophotometers can be double-beam instruments with two cuvette holders, one for the sample and the other for the blank, or reference sample. Advantages of the double-beam instrument include the capability of making simultaneous corrections for changes in light intensity, grating efficiency, slit-width variation, and so on. It is particularly useful for obtaining spectral curves.

Sources of radiant energy. A tungsten-filament lamp is useful as the source of a continuous spectrum of radiant energy from 360 to 950 nm (Fig. 4-7). Tungsten iodide lamps are often used as sources of visible and near-ultraviolet radiant energy. The tungsten halide filaments are longer lasting, produce more light at shorter wavelengths, and emit a higher intensity radiant energy than tungsten filaments do.

Hydrogen and deuterium discharge lamps emit a continuous spectrum and are used for the ultraviolet region of the spectrum (220 to 360 nm) (Fig. 4-8). The deuterium lamp has more intensity than the hydrogen lamp does. Mercury-vapor lamps emit a discontinuous or line spectrum (313, 365, 405, 436, and 546 nm) (Fig. 4-8). This is useful for wavelength-calibration purposes but is not used in many spectrophotometers. The mercury lamp is used in photometers or spectrophotometers employed for high-performance liquid chromatography. Recently, light-emitting diodes have been employed as light sources.

It is important to understand that the amount of light emitted from a light source is not constant over a continuous range of wavelengths. Thus a typical lamp has a complex transmittance spectrum with maxima and minima (Figs. 4-7 and 4-8). Lamps of different types and even from different manufacturers can vary. Therefore one must take care in choosing a lamp for a particular analysis, since the amount of light emitted at the desired wavelength may be too little or too much. For example, hydrogen or deuterium lamps, used for ultraviolet analysis, have a maximum output of ultraviolet radiation in the 250 to 300 nm range. The output of radiant energy at longer wavelengths (greater than 340 nm) is considerably less and can be too weak for many analyses.

Wavelength selectors. Isolation of the required wavelength or range of wavelengths can be accomplished by use of a filter or monochromator. Filters are the simplest devices, consisting of only a material that selectively transmits the desired wavelengths and absorbs all other wavelengths. In a monochromator, radiant energy from the source lamp is dispersed by a *grating* or *prism* into a spectrum from which the desired wavelength is isolated by mechanical slits.

Filters. There are two types of filters: (1) those with selective transmission characteristics, including glass and

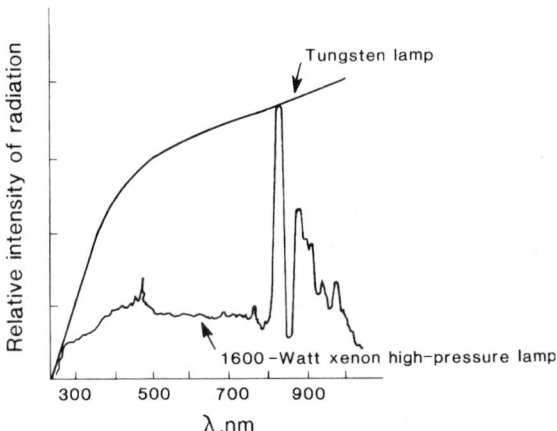

Fig. 4-7 Intensity of radiant energy versus wavelength for a tungsten filament and a 1600-watt xenon light source. Tungsten lamp intensity has been magnified approximately a hundredfold to place it on the same scale as the xenon lamp. (Modified from Brewer JM et al, editors: *Experimental techniques in biochemistry,* Englewood Cliffs, N.J., 1974, Prentice-Hall.)

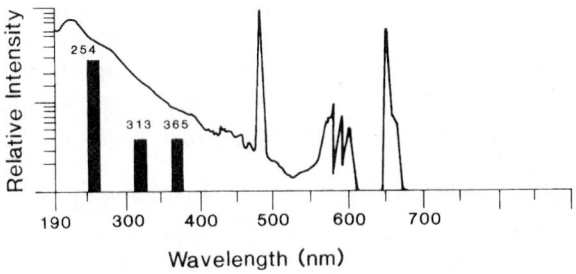

Fig. 4-8 Intensity of radiant energy versus wavelength for a mercury lamp *(solid bars)* and a deuterium lamp *(continuous line).* For illustrative purposes, the intensity of the mercury emission lines has been reduced several hundredfold, and only those lines (wavelengths are *numbers* above bars) in the ultraviolet region of the spectra have been depicted.

Wratten filters, and (2) those based on the principle of interference (interference filters). The Wratten filter consists of colored gelatin between clear glass plates; glass filters are composed of one or more layers of colored glass. Both types of filters transmit more radiant energy in some parts of the spectrum than in others.

Interference filters work on a different principle. The principle is the same as that underlying the play of colors from a soap film, namely, interference. When radiant energy strikes the thin film, some is reflected from the front surface, but some of the radiant energy that penetrates the film is reflected by the surface on the other side. The latter rays of radiant energy have now traveled farther than the first by a distance two times the film thickness. If the two reflected rays are in phase, their resultant intensity is doubled, whereas, if they are out of phase, they destroy each other. Therefore, when white light strikes the film, some reflected wavelengths will be augmented and some destroyed, resulting in colors.

Monochromators. Monochromators can give a much narrower range of wavelength than filters can and are easily adjustable over a wide spectral range. The dispersing element may be a prism or a grating.

Dispersion by a prism is nonlinear, becoming less linear at longer wavelengths (over 550 nm). Therefore, to certify wavelength calibration, one must check three different wavelengths. Prisms give only one order of emerging spectrum and thus provide higher optical efficiency, since the entire incident energy is distributed over the single emerging spectrum.

A grating consists of a large number of parallel, equally spaced lines ruled on a surface. Dispersion by a grating is linear; therefore only two different wavelengths must be checked to certify the wavelength accuracy.

Band pass. Except for laser optical devices, the light obtained by a wavelength selector is not truly monochromatic (that is, of a single wavelength) but consists of a range of wavelengths. The degree of monochromicity is defined by the following terms. *Band pass* is that range of wavelengths that passes through the exit slit of the wavelength-selecting device. The *nominal wavelength* of this light beam is the wavelength at which the peak intensity of light occurs. For a wavelength selector such as a filter or a monochromator whose entrance and exit slits are of equal width, the nominal wavelength is the middle wavelength of the emerging spectrum.

The range of wavelengths obtained by a filter producing a symmetrical spectrum is usually noted by its *half-band width* (or *half-band pass*). This describes the wavelengths obtained between the two sides of the transmittance spectrum at a transmittance equal to one half the peak transmittance (Fig. 4-9). For monochromators, the degree of monochromicity is described by the *nominal band width*, which corresponds to those wavelengths that are centered about

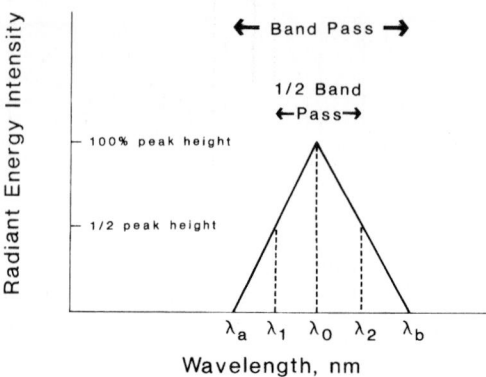

Fig. 4-9   Idealized distribution of radiant energy emerging from exit slit of wavelength selector. For a filter, or a monochromator with entrance and exit slits of equal width, a symmetrical distribution of transmitted energy occurs, as shown.

the peak wavelengths and transmit 75% of the total radiant energy present in the emerging beam of light. For monochromators with variable exit slits, the band pass will also vary.

Slits. There are two types of slits present in monochromators. The first, at the entrance, focuses the light on the grating or prism where it can be dispersed with a minimum of stray light. The second slit, at the exit, determines the band width of light that will be selected from the dispersed spectrum. By increasing the width of the exit slit, the band width of the emerging light is broadened, with a resultant increase in energy intensity but a decrease in spectral purity. In diffraction-grating monochromators, the exit slit may be of fixed width, resulting in a constant band pass. In contrast, prism monochromators have variable exit slits.

The purpose of both slits in filter photometers is to make the light parallel and reduce stray radiation.

Cuvettes. The receptacle in which a sample is placed for spectrophotometric or photometric measurement is called a *cuvette,* or *cell.* Glass cuvettes are satisfactory for use in the range of 320 to 950 nm. For measurement below 320 nm it is necessary to use quartz (silica) cells. Such cells can be used at higher wavelengths also. Fig. 4-10 shows the transmission pattern of several types of cuvettes. Cuvettes with a square cross section and with a circular cross section (that is, test tubes) are available. Greater accuracy is achieved by square cuvettes with parallel sides made of *optical glass.* Although cuvettes usually have internal dimensions (that is, path lengths) of 1 cm, cuvettes with other dimensions are available.

Detectors

Barrier layer (photovoltaic) cells. Barrier layer cells are detectors consisting of a plate of copper or iron on which a semiconducting layer of cuprous oxide or selenium is placed. This layer is covered by a light-transmitting layer of metal that serves as a collector electrode. As illumina-

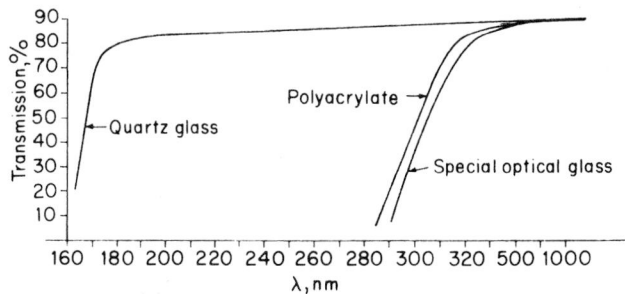

Fig. 4-10 Transmission characteristics of several types of optical materials used for cuvettes. (From Keller H: In Richterich R, Colombo JP, editors: *Clinical chemistry,* New York, 1981, Wiley & Sons.)

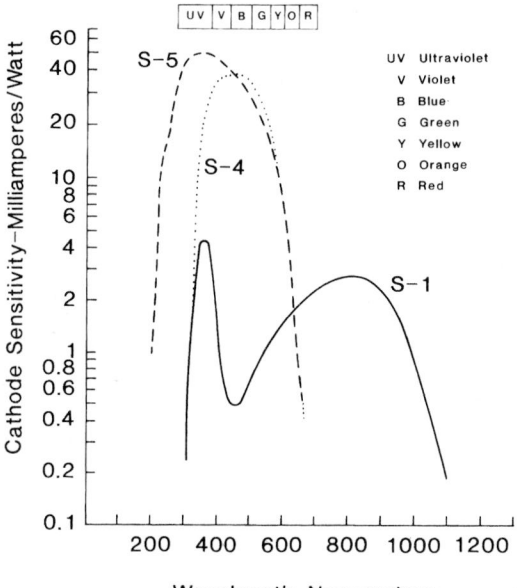

Fig. 4-11 Response of cathode of several photomultiplier tubes to energy of different wavelengths. Sensitivity is expressed as milliamperes of current generated per watt of incident radiation.

tion passes through the transparent electrode to the semiconducting layer, an electron flow is induced in the semiconducting layer, and this flow can be sensed by an ammeter. These detectors are rugged, relatively inexpensive, and sensitive from the ultraviolet region up to about 1000 nm. No external power is required, and the photocurrent produced is essentially directly proportional to the radiant-energy intensity.

Barrier layer cells exhibit the fatigue effect, which means that on illumination, the current rises above the apparent equilibrium value and then gradually decreases.

Photomultiplier tubes. A photomultiplier tube is an electron tube that is capable of significantly amplifying a current. The cathode is made of a light-sensitive metal that can absorb radiant energy and emit electrons in proportion to the radiant energy that strikes the surface of the light-sensitive metal. These surfaces vary in their response to light of different energies (wavelengths) and so also in the sensitivity of the photomultiplier tube (Fig. 4-11). The electrons produced by the first stage go to a secondary surface, where each electron produces between four and six additional electrons. Each of the electrons from the second stage goes on to another stage, again producing four to six electrons. As many as 15 stages (or dynodes) are present in today's photomultiplier tubes (Fig. 4-12). Photomultiplier tubes have rapid response times, do not show as much fatigue as other detectors, and are very sensitive.

Photodiodes. Photodiodes are semiconductors that change their charged voltage (usually 5 V) upon being struck by light. The voltage change is converted to current and is measured. A photodiode array is a two-dimensional matrix composed of hundreds of thin semiconductors spaced very closely together. Light from the instrument is dispersed by either a grating or prism onto the photodiode array. Each position or diode on the array is calibrated to correspond to a specific wavelength. Each diode is scanned, and the resultant electronic change is calculated to be proportional to absorption. The entire spectrum is essentially recorded within milliseconds.

Instrument performance

The sensitivity of response of a spectrophotometer is a combination of lamp output, efficiency of the filter or monochromator in the transmission of light, and response of the photomultiplier. Since these factors are all functions of wavelength, it is clear that the instrument must be reset when one changes wavelengths. This resetting most often takes the form of adjustment of the blank solution to read 100% T (zero absorbance) by changing the photomultiplier gain.

A series of recommendations on instrument specifications that covers many aspects of instrumentation used for photometric analysis has been proposed.[12] These specifications are listed in Table 4-4.

Selection of optimum conditions and limitations

When one is establishing a new spectrophotometric procedure, it is important to record the absorption spectrum of the material that is being measured. This absorption spectrum should be recorded in relation to either water or a reagent blank, depending on the actual method of analysis chosen. Examples of such spectra are presented throughout the sections of this text. This spectrum will help in determining the best wavelength for the spectrophotometric analysis. The optimum wavelength for a specific analysis will depend on several factors, including the absorption maxima of the chromogen, the slope of the absorption peak, and the absorption spectra of possible interfering chromogens.

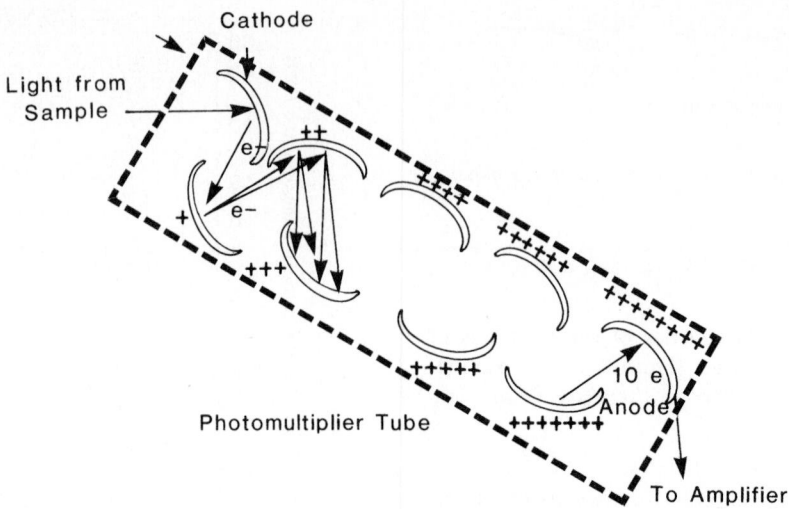

Fig. 4-12 Schema of photomultiplier tube. Each dynode (electrode used to generate secondary emissions of electrons) is represented by a crescent. Light impinges on cathode and frees an electron. Electron is drawn toward first dynode (stage) by applied voltage. Secondary electrons are released and pass on to successive dynodes, which are at increasingly higher voltages, as depicted by the "+" symbols. Increasing numbers of secondary electrons are generated at each stage. In this diagram a tenfold amplification of the initial signal is produced at the anode. A photomultiplier tube may increase the signal several thousandfold. (From Simonson MG: In Kaplan LA, Pesce AJ, editors: *Nonisotopic alternatives to radioimmunoassay*, New York, 1981, Marcel Dekker.)

Table 4-4 Guidelines for photometric enzyme instruments

Parameter	Error or range (95% confidence, ±2 SD)
Carry-over	
Sample to sample	<0.3%
Temperature accuracy	±0.1° C
Equilibration time	20 sec
Sample handling	
Accuracy	1%
Precision	0.5%
Size	50 μL or less
Reagent handling	
Mixing time	≤10 sec
Photometric performance (at a rate of 0.1 A/min)	
Initial absorbance 0-1 A	<3%
Initial absorbance 1-2 A	<5%
Wavelength accuracy	±2 nm
Band width	<8 nm
Wavelength range	Variable
Absorbance range	0-2 A
Linearity	<2%
Cell path/placement	<0.6%
Absorbance drift (10 to 60 min)	<2%
Absorbance accuracy	<2%
Absorbance reproducibility	
Low 0-1 A	±2%
High 1-2 A	±4%

From Instrumentation Guidelines Study Group, Subcommittee on Enzymes: *Clin Chem* 23:2160-2162, 1977.

An example of an absorption spectrum is seen in Fig. 4-13. According to Beer's law, the higher the molar absorptivity, the greater the absorption there is at a given concentration and wavelength and the higher the sensitivity of the analysis will be. In this spectrum there are three peaks of absorption (highest absorption coefficient): λ_1, λ_2, and λ_3 nm. The absorptivity at λ_2 is too low, and the use of λ_2 can be ruled out immediately.

If an absorption peak is too narrow, as it is for λ_1, any small error in the setting of the spectrophotometer at this wavelength will result in a large change in absorbance. With spectrophotometers using manually set wavelengths, this can cause large run-to-run imprecision and analytical error. With filter photometers one would require a high-quality, accurate filter to ensure accuracy when monitoring at a narrow absorption peak.

These problems can be avoided by use of a wider absorption peak (λ_3). With this absorption peak, small changes in wavelength adjustment will result in small changes in absorptivity, and precision and accuracy will be high.

The sensitivity of many methods may be improved by use of absorption bands at shorter wavelengths (such as the ultraviolet), since very often these are more intense. However, often there is additional nonspecific absorption from buffers or other chemical moieties in the solution at shorter wavelengths. Therefore appropriate blanks must be used to obtain accurate measurements. In some techniques the analyte is purified before analysis, and detection at short wave-

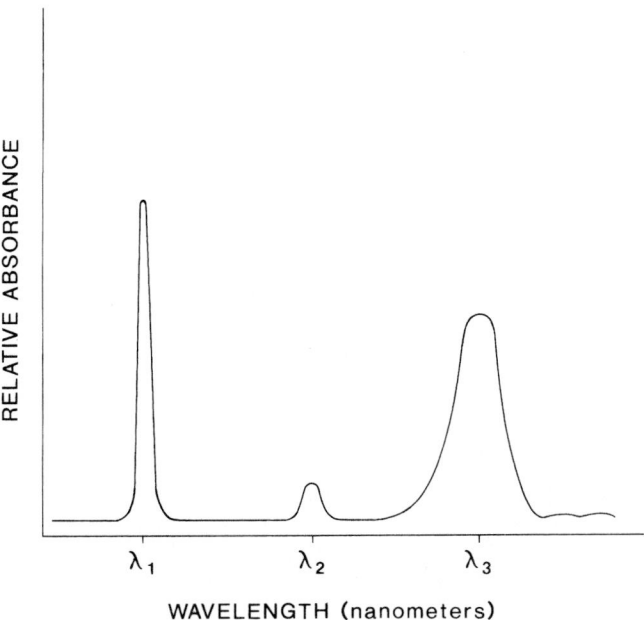

Fig. 4-13 Schema of idealized absorption spectrum. λ_1, λ_2, and λ_3 represent the absorption bands of a chromophore.

lengths (ultraviolet) is feasible and provides optimum sensitivity.

Knowledge of the wavelengths at which the commonly interfering chromogens absorb light will also help determine the wavelength of choice. A general rule for selecting the optimum wavelength at which to monitor a spectrophotometric reaction would include three criteria: (1) Choose an absorption peak with the greatest possible molar absorptivity. (2) Choose a relatively broad peak. (3) Choose a peak that is as far as possible from the absorption peaks of commonly interfering chromogens.

Quality control checks of spectrophotometers[13]

Several quality control checks should be performed to certify that spectrophotometers are functioning within specifications. These checks are wavelength accuracy, linearity of detector response, stray radiation (stray light), and photometric accuracy. Details of the spectrophotometer performance checks can be found in references 5 and 13.

Wavelength accuracy. If the wavelength calibration of an instrument changes, the measured absorbance will change. The magnitude of the absorbance error attributable to inaccurate wavelength calibration depends on the relative location of the point on the absorption spectrum of the chromophore to be measured. That is, the absorbance error relative to the wavelength error is greater when the absorbance measurement is on the slope of the absorbance band than when the absorbance measurement is on or near the peak of the absorbance band. Maintenance of wavelength calibration is especially important for analyses such as spectrophotometric enzyme assays.

The most accurate method of checking the wavelength accuracy involves the replacement of the source lamp with a radiant energy source that has strong emission lines at well-defined wavelengths. Useful radiant energy sources are (1) the mercury vapor lamp, which has strong emission lines at 313, 365, 405, 436, and 546 nm, and (2) the deuterium or hydrogen lamp, which has useful emission lines at 486 and 656 nm (Fig. 4-8). Spectrophotometers equipped with a hydrogen or deuterium radiant-energy lamp have built-in sources for checking wavelength accuracy.

A second method for checking wavelength calibration involves the use of rare-earth glass filters such as holmium oxide and didymium. Holmium oxide has strong absorption lines at approximately 241, 279, 287, 333, 361, 418, 453, 536, and 636 nm. Didymium has much broader absorption bands at approximately 573, 586, 685, 741, and 803 nm. Because of the possibility of filter deterioration, this wavelength accuracy should be periodically checked.

A third method for checking wavelength calibration involves the use of solutions. A solution of a stable chromogen can be used as a secondary wavelength calibration standard to determine whether the wavelength accuracy of an instrument has changed after the wavelength accuracy has been certified by a primary wavelength calibration standard such as a mercury or deuterium lamp. Disadvantages of using chemical solutions for wavelength calibration are that the absorption peaks are generally broad and spectral shifts may result from contamination, aging, or preparation errors.

Irrespective of the method, calibration at two wavelengths is necessary for grating instruments, and calibration at three wavelengths is necessary for prism instruments.

Linearity of detector response. A properly functioning spectrophotometer must exhibit a linear relationship between the radiant energy absorbed and the instrument readout. Instrument linearity is a prerequisite for spectrophotometric accuracy and analytical accuracy. Solid glass filters may be used to check instrument linearity. The most common method for certifying linearity of detector response is through the use of solutions of varying concentrations of a compound known to follow Beer's law. Some compounds used for this purpose are oxyhemoglobin at 415 nm, *p*-nitrophenol at 405 nm, cobalt ammonium sulfate at 512 nm, copper sulfate at 650 nm, and green food coloring at 257, 410, and 630 nm.

The absorbances of solutions containing increasing concentrations of one such compound are plotted against the known concentration. A nonlinear plot of absorbance versus concentration indicates either an error in dilution or an instrument problem. Besides a faulty detector, stray radiation or too wide a slit may cause a nonlinear response.

Stray radiation. An increase in stray radiation is often observed at the extreme ends of the spectral range, where detector response or source energy is at its lowest. Stray radiation usually causes a negative deviation from Beer's law. Methods used to detect stray radiation employ filters or solutions that are highly transmitting over a portion of the spectrum but are essentially opaque below an abrupt "cutoff" wavelength. Several solutions have been used to check for stray radiation, including Li_2CO_3 below 250 nm, NaBr (0.1 mol/L) below 240 nm, and acetone below 320 nm. The exact wavelength at which the cutoff occurs is a function of concentration, cell path length, and temperature; thus the wavelengths reported may vary somewhat. Many filters can detect stray radiation. If solutions or filters that transmit no radiant energy at the measurement wavelength are used, the measured transmittance would be the amount of stray radiation present. Multiplication of this transmittance by 100 would give the percentage of stray radiation. An instrument malfunction is indicated whenever the amount of stray radiation exceeds 1%.

Action taken to eliminate stray radiation includes changing the light source, verifying wavelength calibration, sealing light leaks, realigning instrument components, and cleaning optical surfaces.

Photometric accuracy. When one performs analyses that do not use chemical standards, absorbance accuracy is essential. An absorbance standard should have a constant, stable absorbance at a suitable wavelength that is insensitive to the spectral band width of the instrument and to variations in the configuration of the light beam. Such standards should be easy to use and readily available. The National Institute of Standards and Technology (NIST) has a set of three neutral-density glass filters (SBM 930) that have known absorbances at four wavelengths for each filter. These filters are not completely stable and must be recalibrated by the NIST periodically.

Potassium dichromate solution, cobalt ammonium sulfate solution, and potassium nitrate solution have been used as standards for checking photometric accuracy. Standard solutions are subject to absorbance changes with time, temperature, and pH, which make them unsuitable as long-term calibration standards for photometric accuracy.

Reflectance spectrophotometry

In reflectance spectrophotometry, a beam of light is directed at a flat surface and the reflected light is quantified. The light reflected from the surface is focused onto a photomultiplier tube. The instrumentation can be similar to that of a single-beam filter spectrophotometer (Fig. 4-14). A lamp generates light that passes through a filter and a series of slits and is focused on the test surface. Some of the light incident to a test sample is absorbed by the chromophores on the surface, and the remainder is reflected. (This is analogous to light passing through a solution, for in this case also, some light is absorbed and the remainder passes through.) The reflected light is then passed through a series of slits

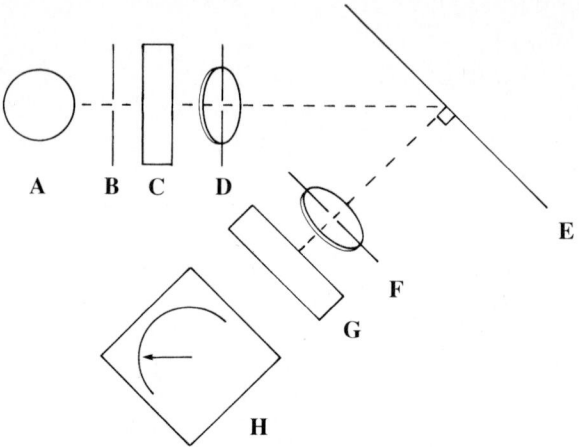

Fig. 4-14 Diagram of reflectance spectrophotometer: **A,** Light source; **B,** slit; **C,** filter or wavelength selector; **D,** collimating lens or slit; **E,** test surface; **F,** collimating lens or slit; **G,** detector; **H,** readout device.

and lenses and on to a photodetector. The signal is then converted to an appropriate readout. The term *reflection density* is used to describe the absorption of light by chromophores at the surface. Reflection density is related to the intensity of light reflected by the sample.[14] The reflection density, D_R, of the test sample is related to the ratio of the light reflected by the standard reflector (usually a barium sulfate–coated surface), R_0, to the light reflected by the test sample (R_{test}), as described by the equation

$$D_R = \log (R_0/R_{test})$$

This is analogous to the equation that relates %T (and thus absorbance) to incidental transmitted light (see equation, p. 87). In general, the optical properties of different surfaces vary considerably. The optical properties of test paper or plastic strips differ from those of dry film. Therefore, to calibrate an instrument for the measurement of reflection density, one must use a standard with the specific surface employed by the test system. The D_R value in the equation above may be corrected for stray reflectance. A black standard with the same surface characteristics as the test sample can be used to give a value for maximum absorbance. Any reflection read by the instrument under these conditions will be stray reflection. This value can be subtracted from the test value to correct for this variable. The use of reflectance allows quantitative measurement of reactions on surfaces such as a dipstick or dry film.

Disadvantages of the procedure include the problem of standardization. The amount of light reflected and subsequently measured is instrument dependent. The angle at which the reflection is measured, the surface area monitored, and so on are variables. In addition, test-surface variations (caused during the manufacturing or handling process) can alter surface reflectance properties.

Recording or spectral spectrophotometry

The recording of the entire absorption spectra is used either for the identification of compounds or to convert the spectra mathematically to their first or second derivative. Recording of spectra can be done by spectrophotometers of the type described above or by diode-array detection systems, where there is a spatial relationship between the spectral lines spread by a prism or grating and the diode light detector. First- and second-derivative spectroscopy are the mathematical conversion of the absorption curve into the derivative function. These derivatives are used to eliminate interference to the observed absorption spectral lines and permit more accurate analyses.

ATOMIC ABSORPTION[15,16]

Atomic absorption spectrophotometry is used in the clinical laboratory for determining calcium, magnesium, lithium, lead, copper, zinc, and other metals.

Principle

Vaporized atoms in the ground state absorb light at very narrowly defined wavelengths. These absorption bands are on the order of 0.001 to 0.01 nm in width, and thus the entire absorption spectrum of atoms is called a *line* spectrum. If these atoms in the vapor state are excited, they can return to the ground state by emitting light of the same discrete wavelengths as the line spectrum. In atomic absorption spectrophotometry the ionic form of the element is not excited in the flame but is dissociated from its chemical bonds and, by attracting free electrons produced by the combustion process, is placed in the atomic ground state. In this form it is capable of absorbing light at the specific wavelengths of its line spectrum.

In atomic absorption a beam of radiant energy containing the line spectrum of the element to be measured is passed through a flame containing the vaporized metal to be determined. The source emitting such radiant energy is called a *hollow-cathode lamp*. The wavelength of the absorbed radiant energy is the same as what would be emitted if the element were excited. With the aid of a monochromator, the attenuation of one of the wavelengths of the incident light is measured. This attenuation is caused by the photons interacting with ground-state atoms in the flame. Beer's law is valid for relating the concentration of atoms in the flame and transmission or absorption of light. Only a small percentage of atoms in the flame are excited, and most atoms are in a form capable of absorbing radiant energy emitted by the hollow-cathode lamp.

Instrumentation

Fig. 4-15 shows the major components of an atomic absorption spectrophotometer.

Hollow-cathode lamp. The hollow-cathode lamp is the most practical means of generating a line spectrum of the required spectral purity. The lamps have a hollow or

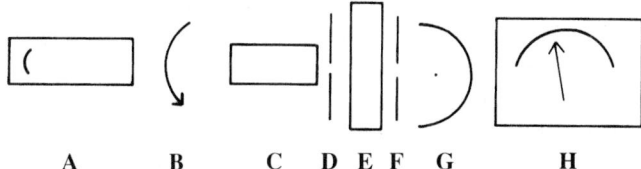

Fig. 4-15 Essential components of atomic absorption spectrophotometer. **A,** Hollow-cathode lamp; **B,** chopper; **C,** flame and burner assembly; **D,** entrance slit; **E,** wavelength selector; **F,** exit slit; **G,** detector; **H,** readout device.

cuplike cathode that is lined with the pure metal of the element to be determined or with an appropriate alloy. A separate lamp is used for each element, except for a few instances in which the cathode can be constructed in such a manner that a single lamp serves for two or three elements (such as calcium and magnesium). The lamp is filled with an inert monatomic gas, usually argon or neon, at low pressure. The inert gas selected for the lamp can vary with the analyte to be measured. For example, lead and iron can be better analyzed with neon-filled lamps, whereas lithium analysis is better performed with argon-filled lamps. For other measured elements, the choice of inert gas is not critical. Quartz or a special glass that allows transmission of the proper wavelength is used as the window. A current is supplied to the cathode, and metal atoms are continually released (sputtered) from the inner surface of the cathode, filling the lamp with an atomic vapor. Atoms in this vapor undergo electronic excitation by collisions with the inert gas, and the resulting excited atoms emit their characteristic radiant energy when returning to the ground-state electron level. This results in a beam of radiant energy with the correct wavelength for absorption by ground-state atoms in the flame.

Burner. In atomic absorption spectrophotometry, the sample solution must be converted into the vapor phase. One technique converts the sample into a fine spray or aerosol while it is being introduced into the flame. This process is called *nebulization*. The nebulizer is usually considered part of the burner. Within the flame, solvent evaporates from the aerosol, leaving microscopic particles that disintegrate under the influence of heat to yield atoms. This phenomenon is termed *atomization*. Acetylene is the commonly used fuel in the burner. Temperatures of 2300° C are usually achieved in flame atomic absorption.

Two kinds of burners have been used in most clinical applications. One is the total-consumption burner. With this burner, the gases and the sample mix within the flame. The flame in this type of burner can be made hotter, causing molecular dissociations, which may be desirable for some chemical systems. The second type of burner is the premix burner (laminar-flow burner), in which larger droplets from the atomization go to waste and not into the flame. The path length through the premix burner is longer than that of the total consumption burner, which provides greater sensitivity. The flame temperature is not so hot as that of the total consumption burner.

Flameless atomic absorption. The purpose of the flame is to convert the sample into an atomic vapor. The flame can be replaced by other atomization processes. One process applicable to mercury analysis uses chemical reactions to convert mercury into an atomic vapor. The sample is decomposed by digestion with acids, then a reducing agent is added to convert mercury to the elemental state, and finally a stream of gas is bubbled through the apparatus pushing mercury vapor into a sealed cell with quartz windows in the path of the optical beam. Absorbance measurements are made at 253.7 nm.

In a more frequently employed atomization technique, the sample is dried on a carbon support platform or tube. The sample is vaporized in an inert atmosphere when an electric current is passed through the support to create instantaneously temperature sufficiently elevated to vaporize the analyte. These atomizers are in the space normally occupied by the flame in flame atomic absorption (AA) instruments. The temperatures achieved by flameless atomic absorption (up to 2700° C) are necessary to vaporize heavier metals. Flameless atomic absorption instruments have a greater sensitivity than flame atomic absorption instruments have.

Monochromator and detector. Monochromators (grating or prisms) and photomultiplier tubes can isolate a pure radiant-energy signal and measure the intensity of that signal, respectively. Extraneous radiant energy, both from other wavelengths of the line spectrum and from light generated by the flame, is kept from reaching the photomultiplier tube by the monochromator. The photomultiplier tube converts the radiant energy that was *not* absorbed in the flame into a signal and amplifies this signal to drive a recorder or meter.

Sources of error

Chemical, ionization, matrix, and burner interferences can occur in atomic absorption measurements. Additional factors that may cause variable behavior from sample to sample or between unknowns and standards include temperature, solvent composition, salt content, viscosity, and surface tension.

Chemical interference. With some elements the presence of certain anions in the sample results in the formation of compounds that are not completely dissociated in the flame. The result is a decrease in the number of ground-state atoms present in the flame. The most common example of chemical interference in atomic absorbance is the formation of a tight complex of calcium with anions, especially phosphate ions. The effect of tightly complexing anions can be minimized or eliminated when lanthanum is added to the sample to displace calcium from the complex. Lanthanum

forms a more stable complex with phosphate than calcium does.

In flameless AA, chemical interference may arise from compounds that vaporize with the element to be measured. The addition of "matrix modifiers" to the sample permits the vaporization of the element to occur at higher temperatures, allowing interfering compounds to be burned off at lower temperatures.

Ionization interference. When atoms in the flame become ionized (A^+) instead of remaining in the ground state (A^0), they will not absorb the incident light. This is termed *ionization interference,* and this effect will result in an apparent decrease in analyte concentration. Ionization interference can be corrected when one adds an excess of a substance that is more easily ionized, thus providing free electrons. The excess free electrons thus shift the reaction:

$$A^+ + e^- \rightarrow A^0$$

to the formation of ground-state atoms. Ionization interference is minimized by operation of the flame at the lower temperatures of acetylene-air combustion.

Matrix interference. Differences in the matrix between the sample and the standard can result in errors. Protein is sometimes included in the standards when the serum dilution factor is small. The matrix effects are minimized as compositional differences between the standard and the sample become negligible. Calcium standards must contain physiological concentrations of sodium, since sodium will cause a negative interference.

The "standard-addition" technique has been employed to minimize matrix differences in the measurement of aluminum and other elements by flameless atomic absorption. In this technique, multiple levels of standard are added to diluted samples, and all are measured by flameless AA. The negative intercept of the regression line of signal versus amount of aluminum added is equal to the amount of aluminum in the sample.

Burner problems. The most critical component in the flame atomic absorption spectrophotometer is the flame and its associated nebulizer. A steady flame is essential, and controlled gas flows are required for both oxidant and fuel. A clean burner head is essential for precise and accurate analysis. Similarly, in flameless atomic absorption, the carbon platform must be changed after some number of firings in order to give reproducible results.

Emission interference. Many analyte atoms introduced into the flame will become excited and emit a photon to return to the ground state. The light emitted is, of course, at the same wavelengths as the incident light being measured. The emitted light enhances the signal being received by the photodetector. The increased signal is translated as a decreased absorption and therefore a falsely lower concentration of analyte. This interference can be eliminated by use of a *chopper* (see Fig. 4-15) to create a pulsed beam of incident light from the hollow-cathode lamp. The light caused by emission interference, however, is a constantly produced beam. This steady emission can be electronically differentiated from the pulsed beam of transmitted light and thus eliminated as a source of interference.

FLAME PHOTOMETRY[17,18]

Flame photometry was widely used in the clinical laboratory to determine sodium, potassium, and lithium concentrations in biological fluids. This technique is now rarely used.

Principle

Atoms of some metals, when given sufficient heat energy as supplied by a hot flame, will become excited and will reemit this energy at wavelengths characteristic for the element as described previously. The reactions undergone by ions in the flame are as follows:

$$A^+ + e^- \rightarrow A^0$$

$$A^0 + \text{Heat} \rightarrow A^*$$

$$A^* \rightarrow A^0 + h\nu$$

A^* represents the excited atom in the flame, A^0 an atom with ground-state electron energy, and $h\nu$ a photon. Alkali metals are relatively easy to excite in a flame. Lithium produces a red emission; sodium, a yellow emission; and potassium, a red-violet color in a flame. These colors are characteristic of the metal atoms that are present as cations in solution.

The intensity of the characteristic wavelength of radiant energy produced by the atoms in the flame is directly proportional to the number of atoms excited in the flame, which is directly proportional to the concentration of the substance of interest in the sample. The actual number of atoms present in the excited state is a small fraction of the total number of atoms present in the flame.

A review of the technique of flame photometry can be found in reference 18.

FLUOROMETRY[19-21]
Principle

Fluorescence may be considered one of the results of the interactions of light with matter. When light impinges on matter, it can simply pass through, as in a transparent solution, it can be scattered by the interaction, or it can be absorbed. When light is transmitted, there is no loss of energy. When light is scattered, there is no change of energy; the light is the same wavelength before and after it interacts with matter. But when light is absorbed, there is conversion of the light energy into any one of a number of forms, including radiationless transitions (converting the energy into heat) and others, such as fluorescence and phosphorescence, where photons are emitted (Fig. 4-16). Absorption of the light can be used, of course, to determine the concentration of compounds as is done in absorption spectroscopy. If the absorbed light is reemitted, the emitted photons can be used to quantitate the amount of the light-emitting compound (fluor). Quantitation is also possible with use of scattered light, since the amount of scattered light is related to the number and size of particles in solution. Methods that use light scattering are termed *nephelometry* and *turbidity* (see p. 100).

Fluorescent light is the result of the absorbance of a photon of radiant energy by a molecule. Once the molecule absorbs a photon, the molecule has an increased energy level, and because the molecular energy is greater than that of its environment, it will seek to eject the excess energy. When the energy is lost as an ejected photon, the result is fluorescence or phosphorescence emission.

For fluorescence to occur, there has to be a good probability that the energy of the excited state can be converted to the ground state by the ejection of a photon. In general, not all compounds fluoresce; indeed, only a very few fluoresce. Of those that do fluoresce, not every single photon absorbed will be converted to fluorescent light. Some excited compounds will lose energy by radiationless transitions, that is, by transfer of the energy to the solvent. For

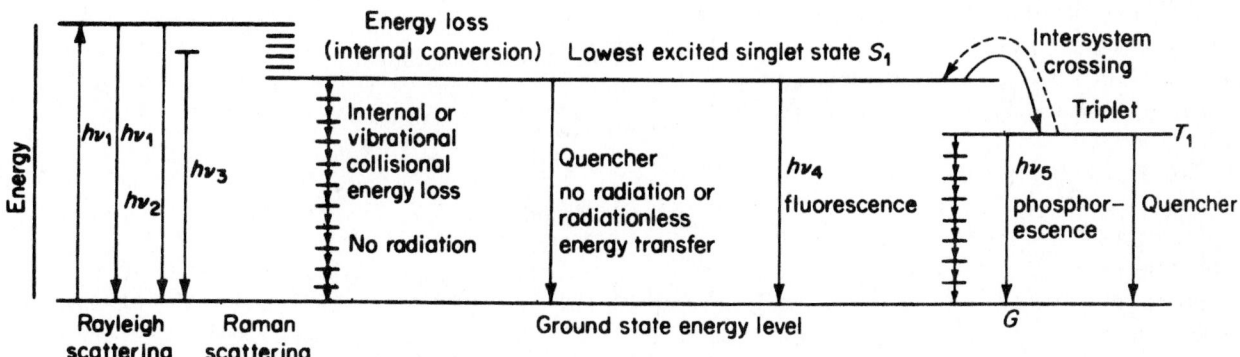

Fig. 4-16 Schema showing conversion of light energy into different forms of molecular and radiant energy. (From Pesce AJ et al, editors: *Fluorescence spectroscopy,* New York, 1971, Marcel Dekker.)

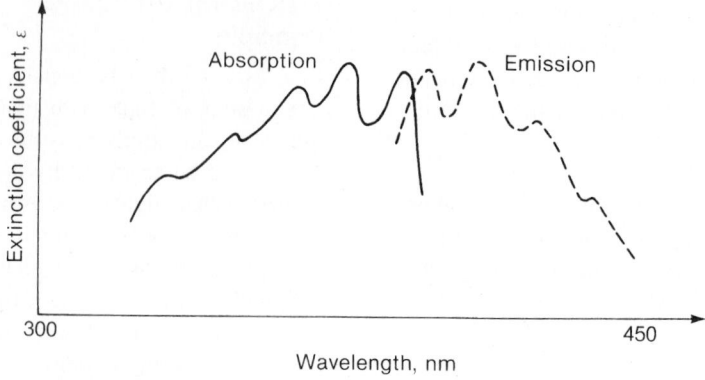

Fig. 4-17   Absorption (excitation) and emission (fluorescence) spectra of a fluorescent compound. (From Pesce AJ et al, editors: *Fluorescence spectroscopy,* New York, 1971, Marcel Dekker.)

the same amount of light absorbed, the molecules with higher fluorescence efficiency will have brighter or more intense fluorescence. In solutions, when a molecule returns to the ground state by emitting a photon, there is less energy in the emitted photon than was present in the one initially absorbed. In other words, the emitted fluorescent light is at a longer wavelength than the exciting or absorbed radiation (Fig. 4-17).

Instrumentation

The basic components of a fluorometer are similar to those of an absorption spectrophotometer. The major difference is the introduction of a set of filters or a monochromator before and after the cell to isolate the emitted light. A diagram of a fluorometer is presented in Fig. 4-18.

The principal components are the exciting light, filters or monochromators to separate the exciting light from the emitted light, and a sensitive detector. Most often, the measurement of fluorescent light is made at an angle of 90 degrees to the exciting light. This is done to maximize the sensitivity of the instrument by minimizing the amount of

excitation light that can reach the photodetector. The detector is a photomultiplier or similar device that can quantitate the very small fluorescent light signal and thus achieve the desired level of sensitivity. Because the spectrum of absorption and emission varies from one compound to another, the instrument must be optimized for every analyte measured. This is done by adjustment of the exciting wavelength to achieve the maximum absorption of photons, which usually means setting the instrument to the absorption maxima of the compound. By the same token, the wavelength of maximum emission of the fluorescent photons must also be ascertained, and this is the wavelength at which the fluorescence signal is most often recorded.

Limitations

The fluorescence signal of a compound is affected by many variables, including (1) solvent, (2) pH, (3) temperature, (4) absorbance of the solution, and (5) presence of interfering or specifically quenching compounds. Standardization is not usually done by an absolute procedure as in absorption spectroscopy because the fluorescence varies depending on

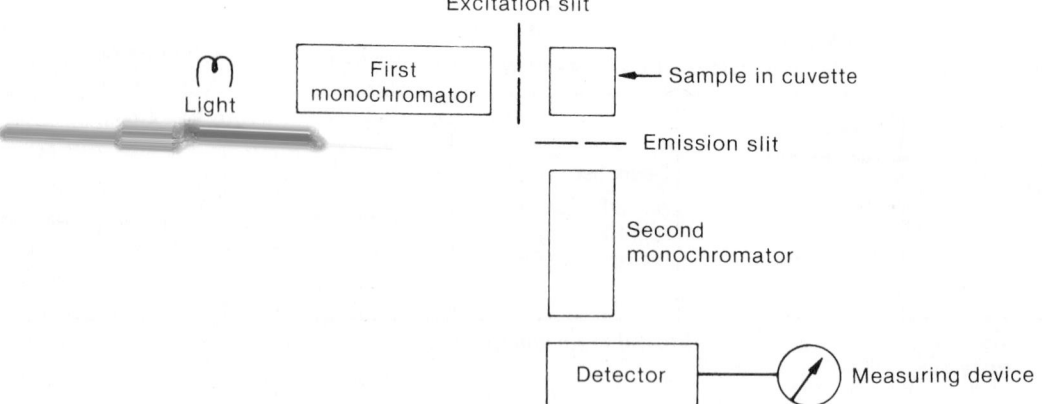

Fig. 4-18   Essential components of fluorometer. (From Brewer JM et al, editors: *Experimental techniques in biochemistry,* Englewood Cliffs, N.J., 1974, Prentice-Hall.)

(1) the intensity of the incident light on the sample, (2) the amount of light intercepted by the detector as controlled by the slits, (3) the band width of light analyzed, and (4) the efficiency of the detector. The quantum yield or efficiency of light emission of a photon is constant if solvent, pH, temperature, and so on are kept constant. But in general the instrument will not be constant on a daily basis. Therefore relative fluorescence yield is used for most measurements. For a reagent blank in a fluorometric assay, only the zero, or null, fluorescence can be set. There is no equivalent to the 100% scale of transmission. Therefore the electronic signal will vary from instrument to instrument for the same concentration of analyte.

To enable a series of fluorescent standards to form a curve that is linear with concentration, the absorbance of the solutions should not exceed 0.1. Above this absorbance, all portions of the solution are not uniformly illuminated; that is, the initially illuminated layer of the solution will absorb more light than the final layer, and thus the initial layer will fluoresce more than the final layer. With dilute solutions, such as those with absorbance of less than 0.1, this does not occur. However, certain assays employ the inverse quantitative relationship between fluorescence intensity and the amount of light absorbed by a solution whose absorbance is greater than 0.1. Such assays are termed *fluorescence attenuation assays*. In these systems a constant amount of fluorescent dye is placed in each test and control solution. In the test solution, the analyte causes a reaction in which a light-absorbing compound is produced. The greater the amount of colored reaction product formed by the analyte, the smaller the amount of light absorbed by the fluorescent dye. Thus the decrease in light passing through the solution results in a proportionate decrease in fluorescence intensity that can be related to the concentration of the analyte.

Time-delayed fluorescence[22]

One approach that can be used to improve the sensitivity of fluorescence techniques is the use of *time-resolved fluorescence*. The fluorescence emission time of most fluorescence molecules, such as fluorescein, is in the range of nanoseconds (nsec); that is, the fluorescence signal decays within 100 nsec. Some compounds such as the metal chelate diketone-europium have very long fluorescence lifetimes, 10 to 1000 microseconds (μsec). By measuring the fluorescence after 400 μsec, over a period of an additional 400 μsec the fluorescence intensity of these compounds can be obtained without interference from light scattering or from any other molecules that may fluoresce. Aside from increasing the specificity of analysis, this technique provides greatly increased sensitivity.

Specialized instruments that use this technique illuminate the sample for a period of time, stop the illumination, and measure the emitted fluorescence over a specified time from 400 to 800 μsec after the illumination (Fig. 4-19). A limi-

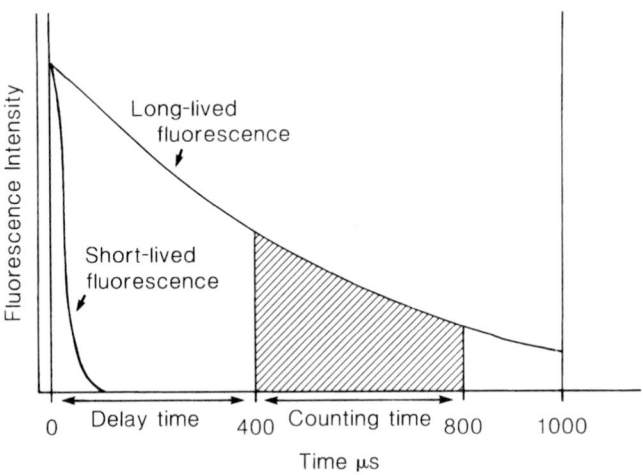

Fig. 4-19 Schema showing difference between short- and long-lived fluorescence.

tation of this technique is the requirement for separation steps because the chelates cannot be measured directly in body fluids (see Chapter 13 for more details).

Chemiluminescence[22-24]

A chemiluminescent reaction is any chemical reaction in which one of the products of the reaction is light. The enzyme peroxidase can react with molecules such as luminol (5-amino-2,3-dihydro-1,4-phthalazinedione) to yield light as part of the reaction product. The luminol reaction results in photon emission in the range of 400 to 450 nm. The low photon yield of this reaction has limited its sensitivity and its application. However, by adding enhancer molecules (luciferin, 6-hydroxybenzothiazole) the reaction can be followed for many minutes (30 or more) with a several thousand–fold increase in photon output. The products of these reactions are not known. A partial reaction may be written as follows:

$$2\ H_2O_2 + \text{Luminol and enhancer} \xrightarrow{\text{Peroxidase}} 2\ H_2O + h\nu + \text{Oxidized luminol}$$

The peroxidase is often part of an enzyme-labeled immunoassay system in which peroxidase is the label. The reaction can be measured by very sensitive photomultiplier tubes. The advantage of this technique is that it can be very sensitive. One molecule of peroxidase can turn over several million molecules of substrate per minute. Thus detection can be more sensitive than that achievable with radioisotopes. A disadvantage of the system is that the reaction is performed in a heterogeneous system in which the peroxidase is attached to a solid phase. The H_2O_2 and luminol must be in a system free from common biological matrices, such as serum, and therefore a separation step is necessary.

Other dye systems resulting in quantitative chemiluminescent reactions use the aromatic acridinium esters and the dioxetanes. The acridinium esters are most often oxidized by hydrogen peroxide to yield light, whereas the dioxetanes are made into stable phosphate ester derivatives that, when hydrolyzed, become spontaneously degraded, yielding light as one of the products.

Bioluminescence, the naturally occurring chemiluminescence phenomenon, has been extensively studied, and the reaction involving the molecule luciferin, adenosine triphosphate (ATP), and luciferase in the presence of oxygen is the best understood.

$$\text{Luciferin} + \text{ATP} + O_2 \xrightarrow{\text{Luciferase}} \text{Oxyluciferin} + \text{Light}$$

The reaction is quantitative in that one photon of light is released for every ATP consumed. The sensitivity of the reaction is limited only by the photodetector's ability to count photons.

Fluorescence polarization[20,25,26]

Light is considered to be composed of an electronic vector and a magnetic vector. If the light is polarized, all the electronic vectors have the same orientation.

When light is absorbed by a fluorescent molecule, it excites the chromophore that has specific orientations, resulting in the transition of an electron to a higher energy level. The excited molecule emits light as the electron (fluorescent oscillator) returns to a lower energy level. Fluorescence polarization measurements require a dye with an electronic orientation such that the emitted light retains the initial orientation of the incident beam. An example of such a molecule is fluorescein. If polarized light is used to excite fluorescein molecules, the reemitted fluorescent light can also be polarized. However, molecules in solution rotate, and so this orientation and the fluorescence polarization can be lost. In fluorescence polarization, the dye must be selected so that its molecular rotation is so great between the times of light absorption and emission that the molecule becomes randomly oriented during this time and the fluorescence is minimally polarized. The quantity that is measured is the intensity of the oriented light or the difference between the oriented and unoriented light.

To measure polarized light, several options are available. One approach is to excite the test solution with light polarized in one dimension and to record the amount of the emitted fluorescence. The polarizer is placed immediately after the first monochromator as shown in the diagram of a fluorometer given in Fig. 4-18. The solution is then excited by light that is polarized at 90 degrees to the light used in the first excitation, and the emitted fluorescence is recorded. Polarization (*P*) can be determined from the following equation:

$$P = \frac{I_{vv} - I_{hv}}{I_{vv} + I_{hv}}$$

where I_{vv} equals the signal recorded when the vertically polarized light is used to excite the sample, and I_{hv} is the re-

sponse when the horizontally polarized light is used to excite the sample. Emitted light is measured from the vertical polarizer at a 90-degree orientation from the incident light by use of a second polarizer that is placed before the second monochromator.

Numerous processes affect the final polarization. For many fluorescent dyes, including the most popular one, fluorescein, orientation of light is retained if the molecule is held rigid. When the molecule randomly rotates by the process of brownian motion, polarization is lost. The ability of a molecule in solution to rotate partially depends on the viscosity of the solution and on the molecular volume of the molecule. When the viscosity of the solution or the molecular volume increases, the fluorescent molecules rotate slower and the polarization increases. In the case of the fluorescence polarization immunoassay, when the drug-fluorescein derivative is bound by antibody, the molecular volume increases. Therefore the polarized fluorescence increases. When the derivative is unbound, the molecular volume is low and the fluorescence polarization is low (see Chapter 13).

Fluorescence polarization measurements can be made very accurately, and they are less affected by variations in fluorescence intensity than standard fluorescence measurements are (see previous equation). Thus precision on the order of 1% or greater of measurement is readily achieved, which translates into more precise assay measurements. An-

A SMALL PARTICLES
-LIGHT SCATTERED SYMMETRICALLY BUT MINIMALLY AT 90° (RAYLEIGH)

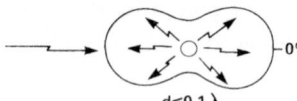

B VERY LARGE PARTICLES
-LIGHT MOSTLY SCATTERED FORWARD (MIE)

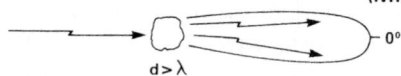

C LARGE PARTICLES
-LIGHT SCATTERED PREFERENTIALLY FORWARD (RAYLEIGH-DEBYE)

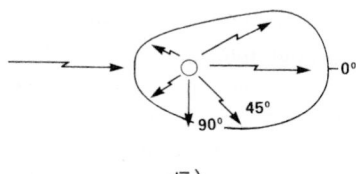

Fig. 4-20 Effect of particle size on scattering of incident light in a homogeneous solution. (From Gauldie J: In Kaplan LA, Pesce AJ, editors: *Nonisotopic alternatives to radioimmunoassay,* New York, 1981, Marcel Dekker.)

other advantage of fluorescence polarization is that the technique can be used as a homogeneous assay. Disadvantages include the fact that the technique is limited to assays that can use fluorescent dyes, the instrumentation required for performing fluorescence polarization measurement is often very specialized and may measure only fluorescence intensity or polarization, and the system is less flexible than absorption spectroscopy. In addition, when one is performing fluorescence polarization measurements, it is crucial to control temperature and viscosity.

NEPHELOMETRY AND TURBIDITY[27-29]
Principle

Interaction of light with particles. To understand the principle of nephelometric or turbidimetric assays, we must first examine the concept of light scattering. When a collimated (that is, parallel, nondivergent) beam of light strikes a particle in suspension, some light is reflected, some is scattered, some is absorbed, and some is transmitted. Nephelometry is the measurement of the light scattered by a particulate solution. Turbidity measures light scattering as a decrease in the light transmitted through the solution.

In considering nephelometry, the question of how light is scattered by a *homogeneous* particle suspension must be examined. Three types of scatter can occur. If the wavelength, λ, of light is much larger than the size of the particle ($d < 0.1 \lambda$), the light is symmetrically scattered around the particle, with a minimum in the intensity of the scatter occurring at 90 degrees to the incident beam, as described by Rayleigh (Fig. 4-20, *A*).

If the wavelength of the incident light is much smaller than the size of the particle ($d > 10 \lambda$), most of the light appears to be scattered forward because of destructive out-of-phase backscatter, as described by the Mie theory (Fig. 4-20, *B*).

If, however, the wavelength of light is approximately equal to the size of the particles, more light appears scattered in a forward direction than in a backward direction (Fig. 4-20, *C*), as described by Rayleigh-Debye scatter.[27]

One of the most common uses of light-scattering analyses is the measurement of antigen-antibody reactions. Since most antigen-antibody complex systems are heterogeneous with particle diameters of 250 to 1500 nm and the wavelengths used in most light-scattering analyzers are 320 to 650 nm, the scatter seen is essentially Rayleigh-Debye, with the blank scatter being primarily described by Rayleigh scatter. Thus the ability to detect light scatter in a forward direction ($\theta = 15$ to 90 degrees) would lead to greater sensitivity for nephelometric determinations. Such is the case in the newer rate and laser nephelometers.

Detection of scattered light

Turbidity. Turbidity is a measure of the reduction in the light transmission caused by particle formation, and it quantifies the residual light transmitted (Fig. 4-21). The instrumentation required for turbidity measurements ranges from a simple manual spectrophotometer available in most laboratories to a sophisticated discrete analyzer. Because this technique measures a decrease in a large signal of transmitted light, the sensitivity of turbidimetry is limited primarily by the photometric accuracy and sensitivity of the instrument. Instruments used for turbidimetry can be used for many other assays, such as enzyme assays and those assays based on color development.

Nephelometry. Nephelometry, on the other hand, detects a portion of the light that is scattered at a variety of angles (Fig. 4-22). The sensitivity of this method primarily depends on the absence of blank or background scatter, because the instruments are detecting a small increment of signal at a scatter angle, θ, on a supposedly black, or null, background. Ideally, no light is detected in the absence of a scattering species, and so subsequent scatter in samples is measured against this black background. The signal is magnified by the use of a photomultiplier, and so the detection range is increased. However, such measurements require the committed use of a nephelometer, which has limited use in other assays.

Instrumentation

Schematic layout of instruments. A schematic layout of the basic components of a nephelometer is shown in Fig. 4-23. Typical systems consist of a light source, a col-

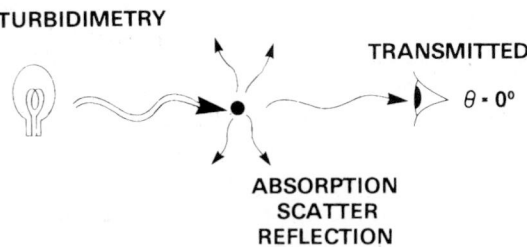

TURBIDIMETRY

TRANSMITTED

$\theta \cdot 0°$

ABSORPTION
SCATTER
REFLECTION

Fig. 4-21 Schema of nephelometric measurement. θ, Angle of detection. (From Gauldie J: In Kaplan LA, Pesce AJ, editors: *Nonisotopic alternatives to radioimmunoassay*, New York, 1981, Marcel Dekker.)

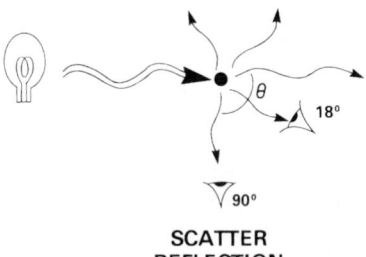

θ

18°

90°

SCATTER
REFLECTION

Fig. 4-22 Schema of turbidity measurements. θ, Angle of detection. (From Gauldie J: In Kaplan LA, Pesce AJ, editors: *Nonisotopic alternatives to radioimmunoassay*, New York, 1981, Marcel Dekker.)

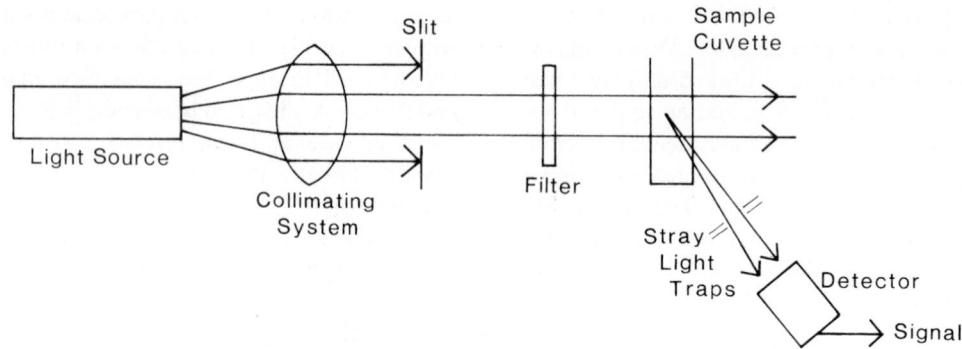

Fig. 4-23 Schema of basic components of a nephelometer.

limating system, a wavelength selector such as a filter (the last two items are unnecessary with laser light sources), a sample cuvette, a stray light trap, and a photodetector.

Light source. Fluoronephelometers use a medium-pressure mercury-arc lamp as a light source, which serves both for nephelometry and fluorometry. The relatively high-intensity light and short-wavelength emission bands make this a good source. Other light sources range from simple low-voltage tungsten-filament lamps and light-emitting diodes to sophisticated low-power lasers. Lasers produce stable, highly collimated, and intense beams of light (typically 1 milliradian divergence) that require no additional optical collimators as other light sources do. In optical systems using laser light, it is easier to reduce stray light, which contributes to background scatter, and to mask the transmitted beam, thus allowing measurement of forward scatter. The increase in light intensity achievable with lasers also results in an improvement of signal-to-noise ratio, but this is limited somewhat by detector saturation. Disadvantages of laser sources include cost, safety problems, and the restricted availability of limited fixed wavelengths. Since particle size may continually change during the course of reaction analysis, as during immune precipitate formation, light scatter at a single wavelength may change while the average light scatter over many wavelengths remains relatively constant. The Beckman Array employs a broad-band filter for selection of a wavelength region from a normal tungsten lamp source to overcome this problem, which is obviously more acute in rate methods when the size of the particle is changing most rapidly.

In all cases, the photodetector system must be matched to the wavelength or wavelengths of the scattered light, which, for nephelometry and turbidimetry, corresponds to the incident light wavelength or wavelengths.

Angle of detection.[30] Since particles the size of antigen-antibody complexes appear to scatter light more in the forward direction, there is an increased signal-to-noise ratio as the detector is placed nearer the transmitted path (0 degrees).

The blank signal, described best by Rayleigh scatter (see

Fig. 4-20, *A*), is not so affected by an altered angle of detection. Thus, although most early nephelometers detected light scattered at 90 degrees for reasons of manufacturing ease, which limited low-angle measurement capability, the detection of forward light scatter should provide theoretically greater sensitivity. The newer instruments tend to operate with lower detection angles, optimized in many cases to give the highest signal-to-noise ratio for the particular instrument's optics. Obviously, detection at 0 degrees is not possible because of the high intensity of the transmitted beam, but some laser-equipped fast analyzers using a mask to block the transmitted beam are able to operate at very low angles. Instruments employing low-angle detectors tend to have greater sensitivity than the 90-degree type of instruments.

Limitations: turbidimetry versus nephelometry

Although the principle of nephelometry—detection of a small signal (amplifiable) on a black background—should lend this method high sensitivity, the sophistication and specifications of the instruments available do not achieve this promise. Turbidimetry—detection of a small decrease in a large signal—should be limited in sensitivity; however, current instruments have excellent discrimination and can quantify small changes in signal, thereby allowing turbidimetric measurements to achieve high sensitivity.

Turbidimetry and nephelometry have similarities to absorption spectrophotometry, and many sources of interference and errors are common to all these systems. Many techniques, discussed in Chapter 23, that can be used to minimize absorption interferences are also applicable to turbidimetry and nephelometry. Nevertheless, sample turbidity can be an interference for both techniques. Because of the uniqueness of nephelometric measurements, especially in the case of antibody-antigen reactions, some specific applications are discussed in this chapter.

Endogenous color and choice of wavelength. Basic light-scattering theory predicts that the intensity of scattered light increases as shorter wavelengths of incident light are used. Most immunological assay reactions employ serum protein reactions requiring the choice of a wavelength

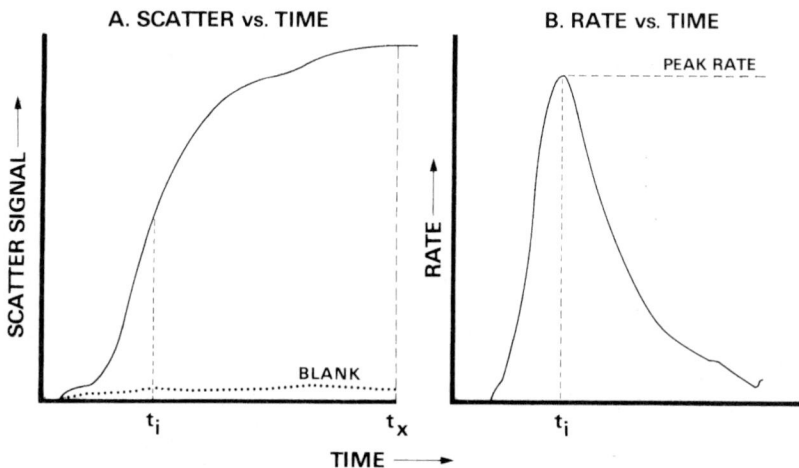

Fig. 4-24 Kinetic analysis of light scattering. *Curve A,* Intensity of scattered light signal versus time; *curve B,* rate of change of scattered light signal versus time.

at which neither the proteins nor the colored serum components absorb appreciably. Since proteins absorb strongly below 300 nm and serum has an absorption peak at 400 to 425 nm because of porphyrins, instruments tend to operate in the 320 to 380 or 500 to 650 nm ranges. Reduction of the protein concentration by dilution will decrease background absorption. Most immunochemical reactions measured by nephelometry use high-affinity antibodies that allow for large dilutions of protein and consequent improvement of sensitivity.

Comparison of sensitivity. Sensitivity in nephelometers is largely controlled by the amount of background scatter from sample and reagents. Since background scatter can be high relative to specific scatter, instruments do not reach their full potential of sensitivity. This limitation, coupled with the higher wavelengths generated in laser instruments, accounts for the fact that laser instruments show no great increase in sensitivity over conventional nephelometers.

Sensitivity in turbidimetric measurements depends on the ability of the detector to resolve small changes in light intensity. Using low wavelengths and high-quality spectrophotometers with their high-precision detection systems, sensitivity in turbidimetry is usually adequate for many measurements and in many cases compares well to nephelometry. Theoretically, with additional refinements, nephelometry ultimately should provide higher sensitivity than turbidimetry does.

End-point versus kinetic analysis. Examination of light scattered as a function of time, after there is mixture of an antibody and antigen, shows that after an initial delay there is an almost linear increase in scatter followed by a slower attainment of plateau scatter. The secondary reaction occurs much more slowly than the first because larger particles form and begin to flocculate, and they

distort the scatter intensity seen at forward angles. Both turbidity and nephelometry measurements behave in this manner.

There are two basic ways of measuring light scatter caused by this reaction, end-point analysis and rate analysis. End-point analysis requires blank (reagent) determinations and a reasonable amount of elapsed time before final measurement. Fig. 4-24 shows the forward scatter developed at 70 degrees of a rate nephelometric analyzer.[29] Comparing the two graphs, one can see the differences between an end-point analysis (blank value versus reading at $t = x$) and a rate or kinetic analysis (increase in scattered intensity over a set time interval). The kinetic approach, which electronically subtracts any blank signal, does not require a separate reagent blank to be run. Both kinetic and end-point analysis can be applied equally to turbidimetry and nephelometry.

REFRACTIVITY
Principle

When a beam of light impinges on a boundary surface, it can be reflected, absorbed, or, if the material is transparent, pass into the boundary and emerge on the other side. When light passes from one medium into another, the path of the light beam will change direction at the boundary surface if its speed in the second medium is different from that in the first (Fig. 4-25). This bending of light is called *refraction.*[31]

Since the degree of refraction of a light beam depends on the difference in the speed of light between two different mediums, the *ratio* of the two speeds has been expressed as the *index of refraction,* or *refractive index.* The relative ability of a substance to bend light is called *refractivity.* The expression of a refractive index, *n,* is always relative to air with the convention that *n* of air = 1. The measurement of the refractive index is the measurement of angles, since the

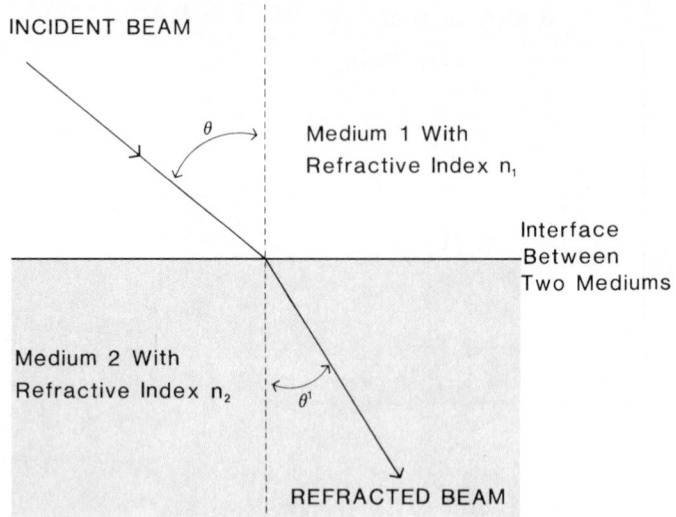

INCIDENT BEAM

θ

Medium 1 With
Refractive Index n_1

Interface
Between
Two Mediums

Medium 2 With
Refractive Index n_2

θ^1

REFRACTED BEAM

Fig. 4-25 Schema illustrating bending of light when it passes from a medium of one density into a medium of a different density, with an angle of deflection, θ^1.

light is bent at an angle proportional to the relationship of *n* in the medium through which the light is passing:

$$\frac{n}{n_1} = \frac{\sin \theta}{\sin \theta_1}$$

The refractivity of a liquid depends on (1) the wavelength of the incident light, (2) the temperature, (3) the nature of the liquid, and (4) the total mass of solid dissolved in the liquid. If the first three factors are held constant, the refractive index of a solution is a direct measure of the total mass of dissolved solids.

Applications

Refractometry has been applied to the measurement of total serum protein concentration.[32] The assumption of this analysis is that the serum matrix (that is, the concentration of electrolytes and small organic molecules) remains essentially the same from patient to patient. Since the mass of protein is normally so much greater than the mass of other serum constituents, small variations of these other substances have no significant effect on the refractive index of serum. Refractometers are calibrated against "normal" serum, and total protein concentrations are read directly from a scale.

Refractometry is also used to estimate the specific gravity of urine samples. The refractive index is linearly related to the total mass of dissolved solids and thus to specific gravity. This remains valid over most of the range normally encountered for urine (that is, up to 1.035 g/mL).

Interference

When the concentration of small molecular weight compounds or particulate matter greatly increases, positive in-

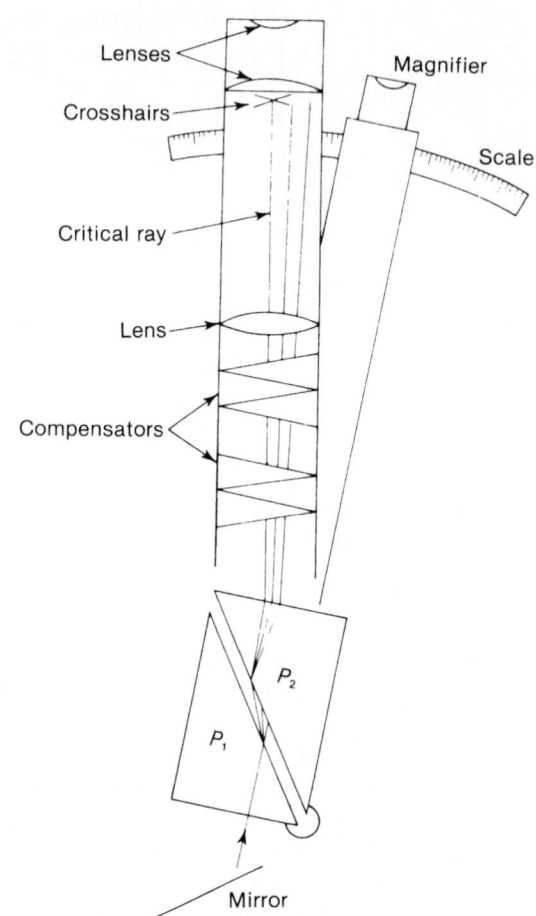

Lenses

Magnifier

Crosshairs

Scale

Critical ray

Lens

Compensators

P_2

P_1

Mirror

Fig. 4-26 Schema of an Abbé refractometer. (From Shugar GJ, Shugar RA, Bauman L: *Chemical technicians' ready reference book,* New York, 1973, McGraw-Hill.)

terference results. This interference occurs in the presence of hyperglycemia, hyperbilirubinemia, azotemia (increased serum urea), lyophilized samples, and hyperlipidemia. Hemolysis will also result in false-positive values for total serum protein.

Instrumentation

Most clinical refractometers are based on the Abbé refractometer (Fig. 4-26), marketed by American Optical Corporation. This refractometer consists of two prisms and a series of lenses. Light passes through the first prism where the light beam is dispersed. The dispersed light passes into and through the thin layer of the liquid sample where it is refracted. The light beam passes through a second prism where the light is again dispersed and on leaving is again refracted. The boundary at the edge of the refracted light beam is aligned perpendicularly to the scale on which serum protein concentrations or specific gravity can be read. The scale for reading serum protein (g/dL or g/L) is established by calibration of the instrument against a "normal" serum solution.

This type of refractometer is extraordinarily simple, having no moving or electrical parts. Thus it is easily reproducible, measuring protein with a precision of $\pm 1\%$ and an accuracy of ± 1 g/L. The sample size is on the order of 50 μL.

More complex refractometers are used to monitor column effluents for high-performance liquid chromatography analysis (see Chapter 6).

REFERENCES

1. Richards WG, Scott RR: *Structure and spectra of molecules,* New York, 1985, Wiley & Sons.
2. Clayton RK: *Light and living matter: the physical part,* New York, 1970, McGraw-Hill.
3. Jaffe HH, Orchin M: *Theory and applications of ultraviolet spectroscopy,* New York, 1966, Wiley & Sons.
4. Willard HH, Merritt LL, Dean JA: *Instrumental methods of analysis,* ed 4, Princeton, N.J., 1965, Van Nostrand.
5. Frings CS, Broussard LA: Calibration and monitoring of spectrometers and spectrophotometers, *Clin Chem* 25:1013-1017, 1979.
6. Brewer JM, Pesce AJ, Ashworth RB, editors: *Experimental techniques in biochemistry,* Englewood Cliffs, N.J., 1974, Prentice-Hall.
7. Keller H: Optical methods of measurement. In Richterich R, Colombo JP, editors: *Clinical chemistry,* New York, 1981, Wiley & Sons.
8. Ward KM, Harris E: Spectrophotometry. In Ward KM, Lehmann CA, Leiken AM, editors: *Clinical laboratory instrumentation and automation: principles, application, and selection,* Philadelphia, 1994, Saunders.
9. Narayanan S: *Principles and applications of laboratory instrumentation,* Chicago, 1989, ASCP Press, pp 8-17.
10. Khazanie P: Spectrophotometry. In Anderson SC, Cockagne S, editors: *Clinical chemistry: concepts and applications,* Philadelphia, 1993, Saunders.
11. *Federal Register* 57(4):7164-7165, 1992.
12. Instrumentation Guidelines Study Group, Subcommittee on Enzymes: *Clin Chem* 23:2160-2162, 1977.
13. Alexander LR, Barnhart ER: *Photometric quality assurance instrument check procedures,* Atlanta, Ga., 1980, U.S. Department of Health and Human Services, Centers for Disease Control, Bureau of Laboratories.
14. Curme HG, Columbus RL, Dappen GM, et al: Multilayer film elements for clinical analysis: general concepts, *Clin Chem* 24:1335-1342, 1978.
15. Rubeska I: *Atomic absorption spectroscopy,* Cleveland, 1969, Chemical Rubber Co. Press.
16. Robinson JW: *Atomic absorption spectroscopy,* ed 2, New York, 1973, Marcel Dekker.
17. Winefordner JD, editor: *Spectrochemical methods of analysis,* New York, 1977, John Wiley & Sons, Inc, Wiley Interscience.
18. Dvorak J, Rubeska I, Rezak Z: *Flame photometry: laboratory practice,* Cleveland, 1971, Chemical Rubber Co. Press.
19. Simonson MG: The application of a photon-counting fluorometer for the immunofluorescent measurement of therapeutic drugs. In Kaplan LA, Pesce AJ, editors: *Nonisotopic alternatives to radioimmunoassay,* New York, 1981, Marcel Dekker.
20. Pesce AJ, Rosen CG, Pasby TL, editors: *Fluorescence spectroscopy,* New York, 1971, Marcel Dekker.
21. Wehry FL, editor: *Modern fluorescence spectroscopy,* New York, 1976, Plenum Press.
22. Hemmilä I: Fluoroimmunoassays and immunofluorometric assays, *Clin Chem* 31:359-370, 1985.
23. *Enhanced luminescence: a practical immunoassay system,* Medicine Publishing Foundation Symposium Series 18, Oxford, 1986, Medicine Publishing Foundation, pp 1-56.
24. Scholmerich J et al, editors: *Bioluminescence and chemiluminescence: new perspectives,* Chichester, 1987, Wiley & Sons.
25. Spencer RD: Fluorescence polarization. In Kaplan LA, Pesce AJ, editors: *Nonisotopic alternatives to radioimmunoassay,* New York, 1981, Marcel Dekker.
26. Jolly MD, Stroupe SD, Wang CJ, et al: Fluorescence polarization immunoassay. I. Monitoring aminoglycoside antibiotics in serum and plasma, *Clin Chem* 27:1190-1197, 1981.
27. Ritchie RF, editor: *Automated immunoanalysis,* parts 1 and 2, New York, 1978, Marcel Dekker.
28. Deverill I, Reeves WG: Light scattering and absorption developments in immunology, *J Immunol Methods* 38:191-204, 1980.
29. Gauldie J: Principles and clinical applications of nephelometry. In Kaplan LA, Pesce AJ, editors: *Nonisotopic alternatives to radioimmunoassay,* New York, 1981, Marcel Dekker.
30. Kusnetz J, Mansberg HP: In Ritchie RF: *Automated immunoanalysis,* part 1, New York, 1978, Marcel Dekker.
31. Glover FA, Gaulden JDS: Relationship between refractive index and concentration of solutions, *Nature* 200:1165-1166, 1963.
32. Rubini MD, Wolf AV: Refractometric determination of total solids and water of serum and urine, *J Biol Chem* 225:868-876, 1957.

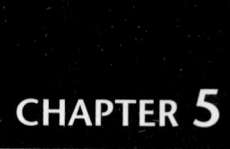

CHAPTER 5

Chromatography: theory and practice

M. Wilson Tabor

Branches of chromatography
General principles
Resolution
  Theoretical plates
  Retention
  Selectivity
  Improving peak resolution
Polarity
  Solvent polarity and solvent strength
  Stationary-phase polarity and selectivity
Mechanisms of chromatography
  Adsorption
  Partition
  Ion exchange
  Gel-permeation (molecular or size exclusion)
    chromatography
Sample preparation for chromatography
  Nature of problem
  Mechanical methods for initial isolation of analyte
  Chromatographic methods for initial isolation of
    analyte
  Extraction methods for analyte isolation
  Processing of sample extracts

OBJECTIVES

- State the general principles of chromatography and describe their application to the divisions and subdivisions of chromatography, supporting each description with an illustration of mechanism.
- State the effect of each of the following chromatographic parameters on the resolution of a chromatographic separation:
  1. Height equivalent to a theoretical plate
  2. Retention time
  3. Mobile phase polarity
  4. R_f
- Describe the separation processes involved with the following types of chromatography and list the class of molecules that can be separated by each type:
  1. Adsorption
  2. Partition
  3. Ion exchange
  4. Gel permeation
- Describe four physicochemical forces that are central to

polarity and explain how polarity affects the chromatographic behavior of compounds in normal-phase and reversed-phase chromatography.

- List three basic techniques for sample preparation for chromatography and provide the basis of purification for each technique.

KEY TERMS

adsorption Process whereby one substance adheres to another because of attractive forces between surface atoms of the two substances. (See Fig. 5-13.)

analyte The substance or component in a sample that is being measured.

band A chromatographic zone; that is, a region where the separated substance is concentrated.

capacity factor The ratio of the elution volume of a substance to the void volume in the column. (See Equation 5-6 and Fig. 5-9, A.)

chromatogram A series of separated bands or zones detected either visually, as in some paper chromatographic or thin-layer chromatographic separations, or indirectly by a detection system. In the latter case, the detection system usually outputs an electrical signal, which is graphically plotted through time, to display the series of separated bands or zones.

chromatography A method of analysis in which the flow of a mobile phase (gas or liquid) containing the sample promotes the separation of sample components, which are differentially distributed between this phase and a stationary phase. The stationary phase may be a solid or a liquid coated or bonded onto a solid.

dipole The attractive force of compounds with centers of both positive and negative charges that are the result of an unequal sharing of bonding electrons between two elements of the compound with large differences in electronegativity. (See Fig. 5-11, B.)

dispersive force The attractive force, sometimes termed *van der Waals forces*, of compounds that results from the induction of a temporary dipole within an individual compound. (See Fig. 5-11, A.)

efficiency A measure of chromatographic performance usually related to the sharpness of the peaks in the chromatogram and quantitated by the number, N, of theoretical plates of a column. (See Equation 5-3, Figs. 5-6 and 5-7, and Table 5-1.)

electrostatic attraction The attractive force between compounds with formal positive or negative charges. (See Fig. 5-11, D.)

eluotropic series Series of solvents or solvent mixtures arranged in the order of their ability to elute a solute from an adsorbent.

elution Removal of a solute from a stationary phase by passage of a suitable mobile phase.

elution volume (Ve) The volume of mobile phase required to elute a solute from a chromatographic column. (See Equation 5-6 and Fig. 5-9, *A*.)

emulsion For a liquid-liquid extraction, a mixture formed when one of the immiscible liquid phases becomes dispersed as fine droplets in the other immiscible liquid phase.

equilibrium concentration distribution coefficient (K_D) The ratio of the concentration of a sample component in one phase to its concentration in a second phase at equilibrium. The two phases may be two immiscible liquids or the mobile phase and the stationary phase. (See Equation 5-1 and Fig. 5-3.)

height equivalent to a theoretical plate (HETP) The number obtained by dividing the column length by the theoretical plate number. (See Equation 5-4 and Fig. 5-7.)

hydrogen bonding The attractive force of compounds formed when a hydrogen atom covalently linked to an electronegative element, like oxygen, nitrogen, or sulfur, has a large degree of positive character relative to the electronegative atom, thereby causing the compound to possess a large dipole. (See Fig. 5-11, *C*.)

pK_a The pK of an acid is the pH at which it is half dissociated.

partition Process by which a solute is distributed between two immiscible phases. (See Fig. 5-15.)

peak A band or zone in a chromatogram showing a maximum of concentration between two minima.

polarity (P') The attractive forces encompassing the total interaction of solvent molecules with sample molecules and of solvent or sample molecules with the stationary phase.

R_f A ratio used in paper chromatography and thin-layer chromatography that is the distance from the origin to the center of the separated zone divided by the distance from the origin to the solvent front. (See Equation 5-9.)

resolution (R or R_s) The degree of separation between two components by chromatography. (See Equations 5-2, 5-8, and 5-10 and Fig. 5-5.)

retention time (t_R) The time that has elapsed from the injection of the sample into the chromatographic system to the recording of the peak maximum of the component in the chromatogram. (See Fig. 5-7.)

selectivity (α) The ratios of the capacity factors for two substances measured under identical chromatographic conditions; sometimes termed *separation factor*, or *chromatographic selectivity*. (See Equation 5-7 and Fig. 5-9, *B*.)

theoretical plate number (N) A number defining the efficiency of the chromatographic column. (See Equation 5-3 and Fig. 5-7.)

void volume (V) The interstitial volume of the chromatographic column, that is, the volume of mobile phase imbibed in the pores and around the stationary phase in a column. (See Equation 5-8 and Fig. 5-9, *A*.)

The need for fast, reproducible, and accurate analyses for many classes of analytes present in small amounts is being met today in the clinical laboratory largely as a result of the developments in chromatography during the past two decades. *Chromatography* is a collective term referring to a group of separation processes whereby a mixture of solutes, dissolved in a common solvent, are separated from one another by a differential distribution of the solutes between two phases. One phase, the solvent, is mobile and carries the mixture of solutes through the other phase, the fixed or stationary phase. Chromatographic methods encompass a great number of variations in technique in which the mobile phase ranges from liquids to gases and the stationary phase ranges from sheets of cellulose paper to capillary glass tubes as fine as a human hair that are internally coated with a covalently bonded complex or complex organic polymers. A cursory examination of the scientific literature shows that both the numbers of chromatographic methods published and their applications have been growing exponentially.[1-4]

Modern chromatography began in 1906, when Michael S. Tswett detailed his separation of chlorophylls using a column of calcium carbonate (chalk)[5] and introduced a system of nomenclature that is now universally applied to chromatography ('color writing,' from the Greek words *khrōma, khrōmatos,* meaning 'color,' and *graphē,* meaning 'drawing, writing'). This is but the first of the many published accounts of the colorful history of chromatography.

BRANCHES OF CHROMATOGRAPHY

Chromatographic methods are generally classified according to the physical state of the solute carrier phase, that is, the mobile phase. These branches are represented in Figs. 5-1 and 5-2 as solution and gas chromatography, referring to the respective liquid and gaseous states of the mobile phase. In Fig. 5-1 these branches are further classified according to how the stationary-phase matrix is contained for a particular chromatographic method. For example, solution chromatography is divided into flat and column methods, depending on whether the stationary phase is a thin layer mechanically supported on a sheet or is packed into a column. The flat method of support may involve use of a sheet of paper, such as cellulose, or a thin layer on a mechanical backing, such as glass or plastic.

Column methods are classically referred to as *liquid chromatography.* Furthermore, *column methods* is a phrase generally used to subdivide solution chromatography wherein the stationary phase is packed into a glass or metal tube. However, it is noted that gas chromatography is strictly a column method because a column must be used for containment of the stationary phase (see Chapter 7).

The main divisions of chromatography, based on mobile phase, may also be subdivided according to the mechanism of solute interaction with the stationary phase (Fig. 5-2). Two mechanisms, adsorption and partition, are the most commonly encountered for both solution and gas mobile-phase separations. Adsorption chromatography (liquid-solid

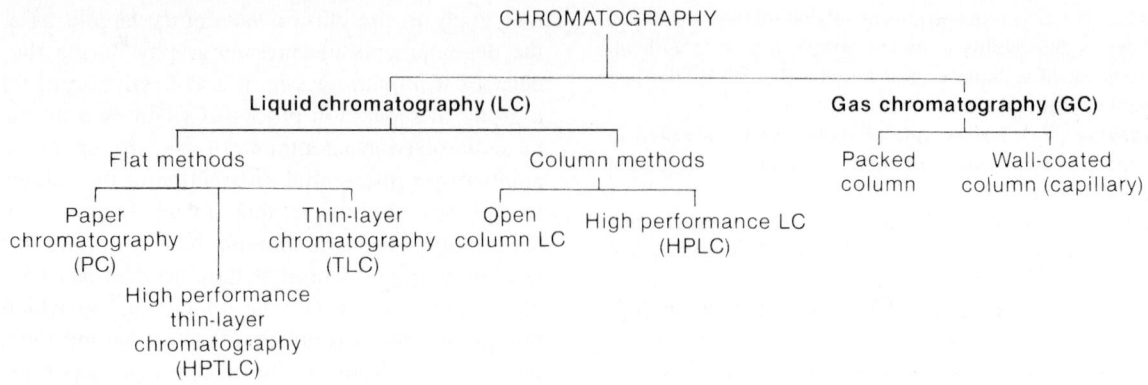

Fig. 5-1 Branches of chromatography according to mobile phase and physical apparatus.

[L/S] or gas-solid [G/S]) is a process whereby solutes of a sample are separated by their differences in *attraction* to the stationary versus the mobile phase. Partition chromatography (liquid-liquid [L/L] or gas-liquid [G/L]) is a process whereby the solutes of a sample are separated by differences in their *distribution* between two liquid phases (L/L) or between a gas and a liquid phase (G/L). In both cases of partition chromatography, the stationary phase is liquid, and the mobile phase is a liquid or a gas.

Other mechanistic divisions of solution chromatography are ion exchange and gel permeation. Ion-exchange chromatography (IE) uses an insoluble matrix containing covalently linked ionic groups for the stationary phase, which can reversibly exchange either cations or anions with the mobile phase. Gel-filtration (GF) chromatography refers to a stationary phase of a solvent-swollen hydrophilic gel in the form of porous beads that is used with an aqueous-solvent mobile phase. Gel-permeation (GP) chromatography refers to a stationary phase of solvent-swollen hydrophobic gel in the form of porous beads that is used with an organic-solvent mobile phase. Both GF and GP chromatography are sometimes referred to as *molecular exclusion (or inclusion) chromatography* (see p. 122).

The boundaries between these mechanistically different types of chromatography are not finite, since for some chromatographic separations more than one mechanism may be operating. For example, in GF chromatography adsorptive interactions between the solute molecules and the stationary phase are common, in addition to the prevailing size-exclusion mechanism. More discussion of these mechanisms is presented below, after a brief discussion of chromatographic theory and principles.

GENERAL PRINCIPLES

The theoretical basis of chromatography is well developed, with both solution and gas-phase methods sharing the same foundation.[11] Only a few general concepts of this theory are discussed in this section. For more extensive discussions and additional reference leads, refer to representative reviews and books[6-8,12-15] and the *Analytical Chemistry* compendium reviews[1-5,9] on specialized chromatographic techniques.

The separation of a mixture containing two or more components is an operation with the goal of producing fractions, with each fraction having an increased concentration of one component relative to the other components contained in the original mixture. The physicochemical basis of chromatographic separation techniques is principally distribution equilibrium.[13] Distribution equilibrium refers to the differences in solubility and adsorption of a component in two immiscible phases.

Separation equilibrium can be visualized as the distribu-

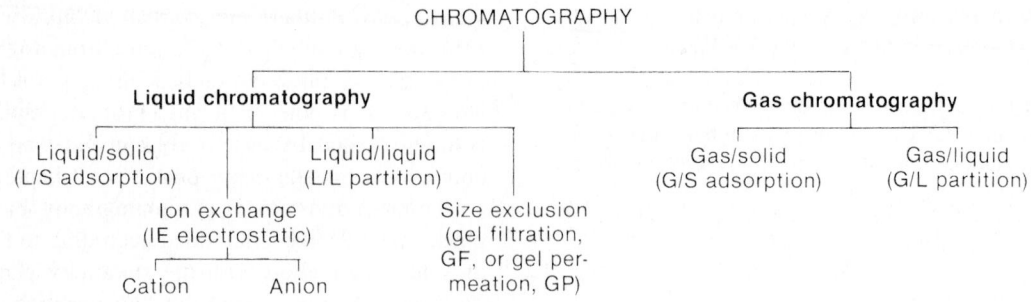

Fig. 5-2 Branches of chromatography according to mechanism of separation on stationary phase.

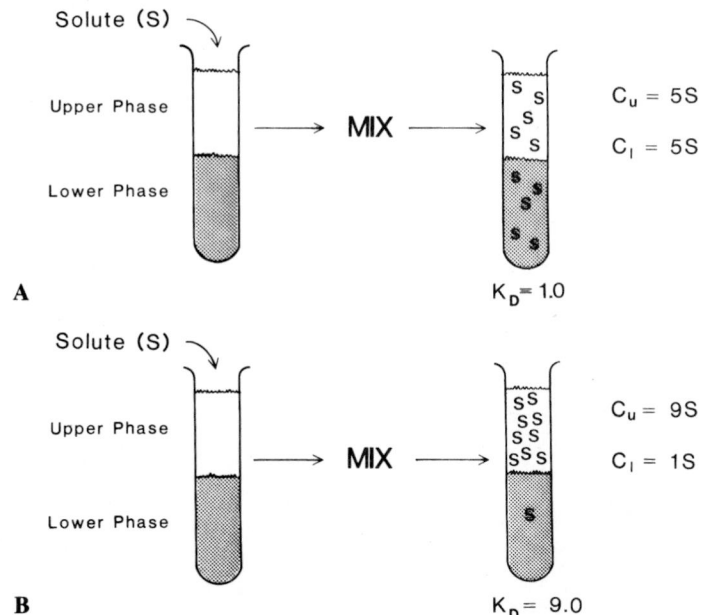

Fig. 5-3 Separation of a solute, *S*, by partition into two different solvent systems. In the first system, **A**, solute has a distribution coefficient, K_D, of 1.0, indicating an equal partitioning between upper and lower phases after mixing. In the second system, **B**, solute has a K_D of 9.0, indicating a partitioning of nine parts of the solute in the upper phase and one part of the solute in the lower phase after mixing. C_u, Upper-phase concentration; C_l, lower-phase concentration.

tion of a solute, *S*, between two immiscible phases, upper phase (u) and lower phase (l), at constant temperature and pressure. The ratio of the solute concentrations in the two phases determines the separation, which can be defined by an equilibrium concentration distribution coefficient, K_D, for the molar concentration, C_u and C_l, of solute in the upper and lower phases respectively:

$$K_D = \frac{C_u}{C_l} \qquad \textit{Eq. 5-1}$$

Molar concentration is defined in the classical sense as the number of moles of solute per unit volume of solvent. The distribution coefficient is sometimes referred to as a *partition ratio*. In practical terms, a K_D of 1.0 means that 50% of the solute is distributed in the upper phase and 50% is distributed in the lower phase (Fig. 5-3, *A*). Likewise, a K_D of 9.0 means that 90% of the solute is distributed in the upper phase and 10% is in the lower phase (Fig. 5-3, *B*).

For a more generalized application of distribution coefficients to chromatography, let $C_l = C_m$, where C_m refers to the amount of the solute distributed into a unit amount of mobile phase, and let $C_u = C_s$, where C_s refers to the amount of the solute distributed into a unit amount of stationary phase. In this more generalized case, the distribution equilibriums for a solute being separated in a given chromatographic system at constant temperature (that is, *isothermal*) can be graphically illustrated by a plot of solute concentration in the mobile phase, C_m, versus the con-

centration in the stationary phase, C_s. This is called an *adsorption-distribution isotherm plot* (Fig. 5-4, *A*). The slope of the isotherm is equal to the distribution equilibrium coefficient, K_D.

The resulting shape of a distribution isotherm plot (Fig. 5-4, *A*) depends on several factors. Since solute movement between the mobile phase and the stationary phase is a thermodynamic equilibrium process, the distribution equilibrium coefficient, K_D, is both temperature and pressure dependent. However, the earlier assumption that temperature and pressure are not contributing factors in the situation under discussion is usually made for most routine chromatographic procedures. This assumption and the overall thermodynamic basis of solute-solvent interaction theory[12,14] hold true only for dilute solutions of the solute in the mobile phase. This type of situation exists in conventional gas chromatography and high-performance liquid chromatography (HPLC). For these separations, the distribution isotherms approach linearity (Fig. 5-4, *A*), and the solute-concentration profiles resemble a discrete circular spot (Fig. 5-4, *B*) or a symmetric bell-shaped (that is, gaussian) elution peak (Fig. 5-4, *C1*). But it must be noted that one cannot predict the behavior of any given sample in any given chromatographic system.

Linearity of distribution isotherms, as in Fig. 5-4, *A1*, is the exception rather than the norm. In most cases, convex or concave distribution isotherms are observed for solute-stationary phase interactions (Fig. 5-4, *A2* and *A3* respec-

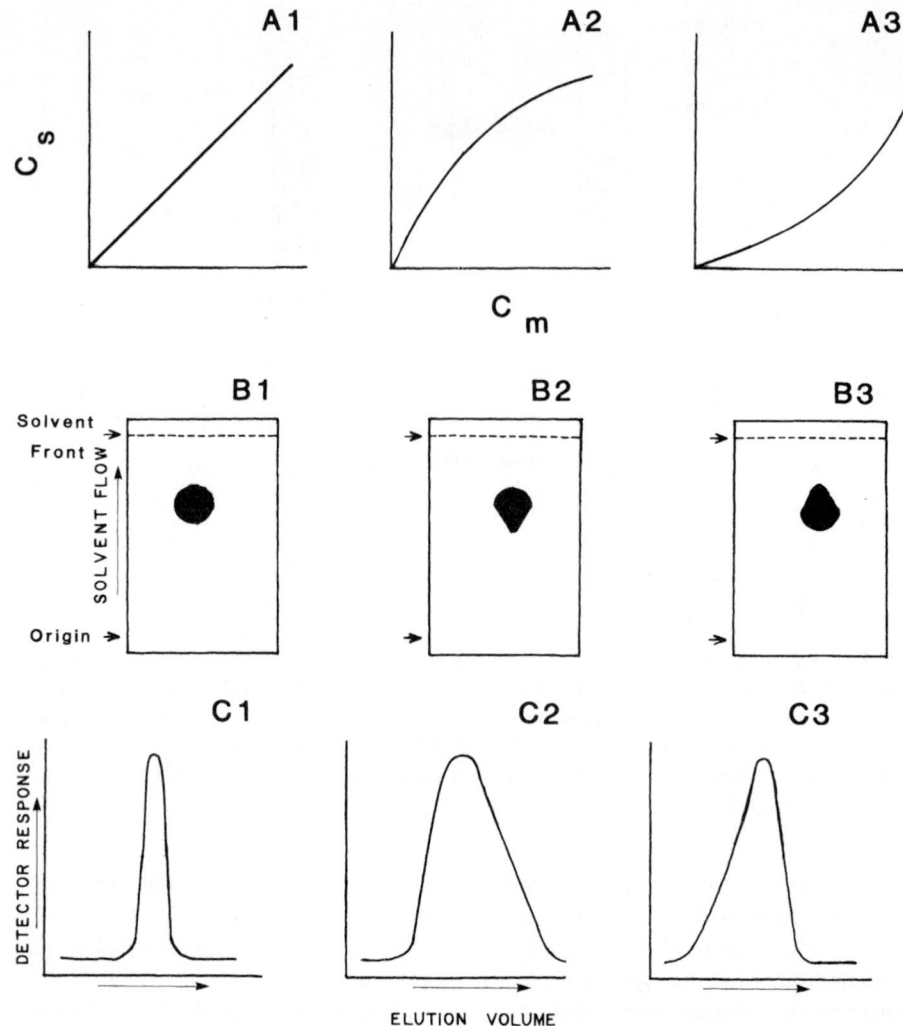

Fig. 5-4   Relationship between equilibrium distribution isotherm *(A1* to *A3)* and solute shape, position, and elution profile in a PC/TLC chromatogram *(B1* to *B3)* or a GC/HPLC chromatogram *(C1* to *C3)*. C_s, Concentration of solute in stationary phase; C_m, concentration of solute in mobile phase.

tively). Several factors influence the degree to which non-linearity is observed. At higher concentrations of solute in the mobile phase, nonlinearity results, since the thermodynamic basis of solute-solvent interactions holds only for dilute solutions. Another factor is the complexity of the sample, that is, the presence of multiple solutes. Interaction of these components with each other will cause a deviation from linearity.

If dilute solutions are used or there are no solute-solute interactions, a Langmuir, or convex, isotherm (Fig. 5-4, *A2*) may be observed. This isotherm shows that the limited number of adsorptive sites on the stationary phase become occupied by solute with increasing solute concentration, thereby losing their capacity to adsorb in proportion to the overall increase in solute concentration. Therefore the resulting solute-elution profile (Fig. 5-4, *B2* and *C2*) is characterized by a sharp front or leading edge, which indicates

a high-solute concentration. The rear boundary of the solute-elution pattern decreases asymmetrically from the peak.

When the solute is poorly adsorbed to the stationary phase, preferring the mobile phase, the anti-Langmuir, or concave, isotherm (Fig. 5-4, *A3*) is observed. In this situation, the resulting solute-elution profile (Fig. 5-4, *B3* and *C3*) is characterized by sloping (that is, low-solute concentration) front boundaries and sharp (that is, high-solute concentration) rear boundaries. Also, the elution volume for the solute is a function of sample size.

RESOLUTION

The ultimate goal of any given chromatographic technique is to separate the components of a given sample within a reasonable time. The purpose of such a separation is to detect or quantitate a particular component or group of com-

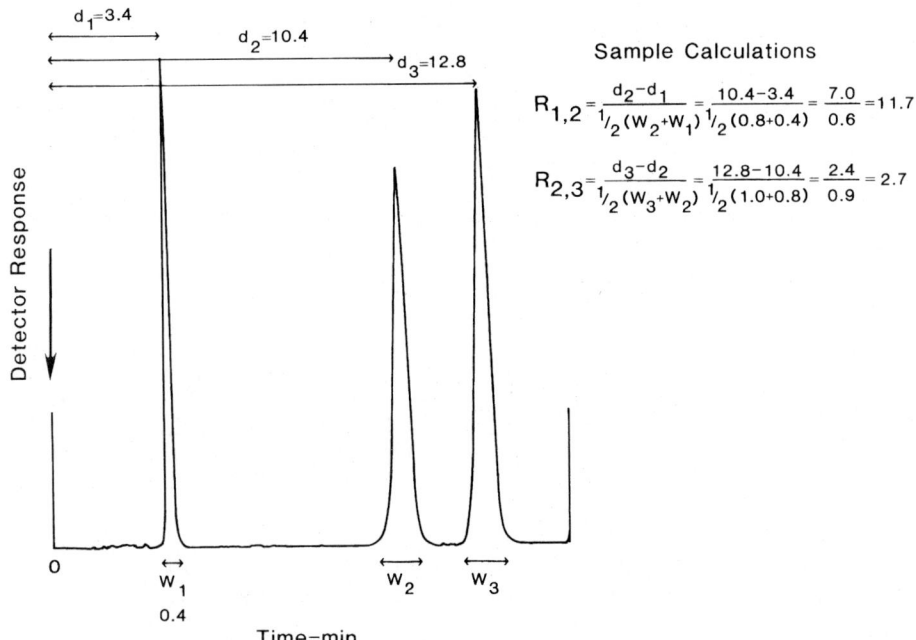

Sample Calculations

$$R_{1,2} = \frac{d_2 - d_1}{\frac{1}{2}(W_2 + W_1)} = \frac{10.4 - 3.4}{\frac{1}{2}(0.8 + 0.4)} = \frac{7.0}{0.6} = 11.7$$

$$R_{2,3} = \frac{d_3 - d_2}{\frac{1}{2}(W_3 + W_2)} = \frac{12.8 - 10.4}{\frac{1}{2}(1.0 + 0.8)} = \frac{2.4}{0.9} = 2.7$$

Fig. 5-5 Calculation of resolution of sample components actually separated by HPLC. The distances, d_1 to d_3, are the actual amounts of time from injection ($\downarrow$) to apex of eluting peak for each component, *1* to *3*, respectively. Peak widths, W_1 to W_3, are measured by triangulation at base of each peak for components *1* to *3*, respectively. Both *d* and *W* must be measured the same way from the time of injection, that is, in units of time (minutes or seconds), length (inches or centimeters), or elution volume (milliliters). Resolution, *R*, is unitless.

ponents of interest in pure form. The ability to resolve the components from one another and the degree to which this resolution is accomplished are measures of the adequacy of the chromatographic separation. The question of what is adequate resolution for a given sample has been detailed by Snyder.[16] One can answer this question by defining the objectives of the chromatographic separation. Generally, objectives for the analyst in a chemical laboratory depend on the following questions. (1) Is a particular substance present in a sample; that is, should a qualitative analysis be followed? (2) How much of a particular substance is present in a sample; that is, should a quantitative analysis be followed?[17] In the following discussion of the theory of resolution, the principal emphasis (and corresponding illustrations) will be on column techniques, gas or liquid, rather than on flat methods.

Note that, by convention, the concentrations of solutes separated in a chromatographic system are plotted out versus time, units of elution volume, or distance. The bands or zones of analytes separated are usually termed a *peak.*

An actual chromatographic separation of a three-component mixture by high-performance liquid chromatography is shown in Fig. 5-5, indicating important parameters for assessment of resolution, *R*. The quantity *R* for any

two components is defined as the distance, *d*, between the peak centers of two peaks divided by the average base width, *W*, of the peaks:

$$R = \frac{d_2 - d_1}{\frac{1}{2}(W_1 + W_2)} \qquad \textit{Eq. 5-2}$$

For this calculation, both the distance, *d*, and the peak width, *W*, are measured in the same units. This method of calculating resolution is based on the assumption that the distribution isotherms for the components being separated approach linearity (Fig. 5-4, *A*) under specified conditions. The set of specified conditions are mobile phase, stationary phase, and solute-concentration range.

A resolution value of 1.25 or greater is required for good quantitative or qualitative chromatographic analyses. If the resolution is 0.4 or less, the peak shape does not clearly show the presence of two or more components. The actual value of the resolution depends on two factors: width of the peak and the distance between the peak maxima for column separations or diameter of the circular spots and the distance between these spots for flat-method separations.

These determinant factors of resolution also are indicative of the efficiency of the chromatographic process. Effi-

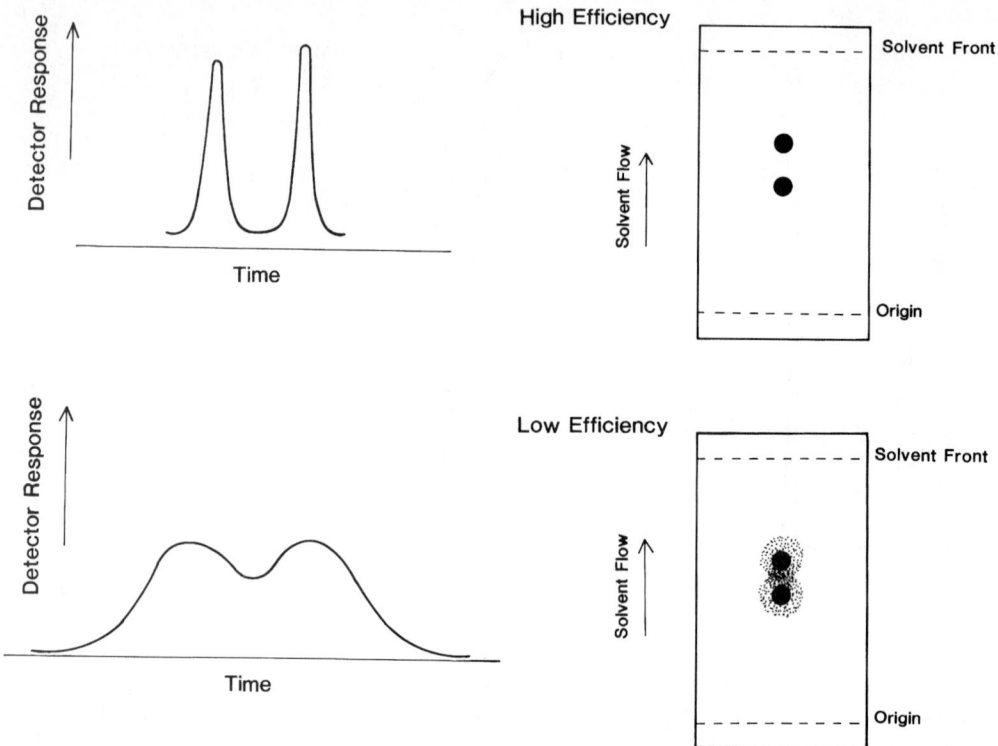

Fig. 5-6 Model chromatograms exemplifying high-efficiency separations and low-efficiency separations.

ciency is decreased by the broadening of a solute band as it migrates through the stationary phase. If broadening occurs to any significant extent during the chromatographic process, the resulting peaks will be wide or the resulting spots will be diffuse. The separation of components is then poor, and the sensitivity with which they can be detected is reduced. An example of high- versus low-efficiency separation is illustrated in Fig. 5-6 for both column and flat-method separations.

Solute-band broadening occurs during the actual chromatographic process and may be described as follows for a column separation. The sample, in a small volume of solvent, is introduced into the mobile phase at a point near the inlet end of the column. Once entering the column, the sample begins to disperse by thermal diffusion processes, which continue as it passes through the column. The longer the time a solute band spends in a column (that is, the longer the retention time), the greater the opportunity for thermal diffusion and the greater the band dispersion. The result is broader but gaussian (symmetrical, as in Fig. 5-4, *C1*) elution peaks for the more retained solutes. This process is similar in flat methods of chromatography, resulting in larger diameter but symmetrical spots, as in Fig. 5-4, *B1*, for the more retained solutes. Several additional factors contribute to solute-band broadening.[18,19] These include nonuniform regions of the stationary phase, nonuniform

particle-size distribution, and nonuniform column packing, which may result in nonuniform passage of solute molecules. In the latter case, some molecules spend more time in the separation system than others do; that is, they have a longer path. These processes result in broader, nongaussian dispersion of solute bands, such as asymmetric eluting peaks or trailing spots, as in Fig. 5-4, *C2* and *B2* respectively.

Therefore one way to maximize column efficiency (that is, decrease the extent of band broadening) is to use a well-packed chromatography column that contains a stationary-phase packing that is not only small but also uniform in size distribution of particles. Columns meeting these criteria are readily obtainable today from numerous commercial sources.

Theoretical plates

One can obtain a numerical assessment of column efficiency by calculating the number of theoretical plates, *N,* for a given column. A theoretical plate is a microscopic segment of a column where a perfect equilibrium is assumed to exist between the solute in the mobile and stationary phases. It is the theoretical, smallest unit of separation in a column. The theory originated with Martin and Synge[20] in their mathematical treatment of the chromatographic process. The number of theoretical plates can be calculated for a column directly from a chromatogram (Fig. 5-7) by the following:

$$N = 16 \left(\frac{t_R}{W} \right)^2 \qquad \textit{Eq. 5-3}$$

In this expression, W is the base width of the chromatographic peak, and t_R is the retention time of the solute, that is, the time from introduction of the sample onto the column to the apex of the eluting solute peak. Both t_R and W must be measured in the same units, such as time or distance. (Note that N is dimensionless.) A larger number of theoretical plates indicates relatively narrow peaks, that is, an efficient column and better resolution.

Related to the number of theoretical plates is the column height equivalent to a theoretical plate (HETP), which can be calculated by the following:

$$\text{HETP} = \frac{L}{N} \qquad \textit{Eq. 5-4}$$

In this equation, L equals the column length, usually in millimeters. Maximum column efficiency is obtained when HETP is as small as possible.

In addition to the factors affecting column efficiency, N is affected by the flow rate of the mobile phase. The mobile-phase linear velocity, μ, can be calculated by:

$$\mu = \frac{L}{t_0} \qquad \textit{Eq. 5-5}$$

In this equation, L is column length, and t_0 is the time it takes a discrete portion of the solvent to flow through the column. A plot of HETP versus μ shows the experimental relationship of these two variables in gas chromatography (GC) (Fig. 5-8, *A*) and in liquid chromatography (LC) (Fig. 5-8, *B*). At the minimum HETP, the optimum flow veloc-

ity, μ_{opt}, is obtained. For gas chromatography (Fig. 5-8, *A*) this plot is the well-known van Deemter plot.[21]

At high mobile-phase velocities, HETP varies linearly with μ for gas chromatography (Fig. 5-8, *A*), but in liquid chromatography (Fig. 5-8, *B*) a minimum in HETP is seldom observed, and the HETP tends to level off at high values for μ. In practice, GC mobile-phase velocities are usually between one and two orders of magnitude greater than those of LC. For LC, lower velocities and column efficiencies are necessary because of the active role the mobile phase plays in the chromatographic separation process. Therefore, to improve separation efficiency in LC, one uses smaller stationary-phase particles, usually one tenth to one hundredth the size of those used in GC.

Retention

Resolution depends on factors in addition to theoretical plates. One of these is the ratio of the volumes of mobile

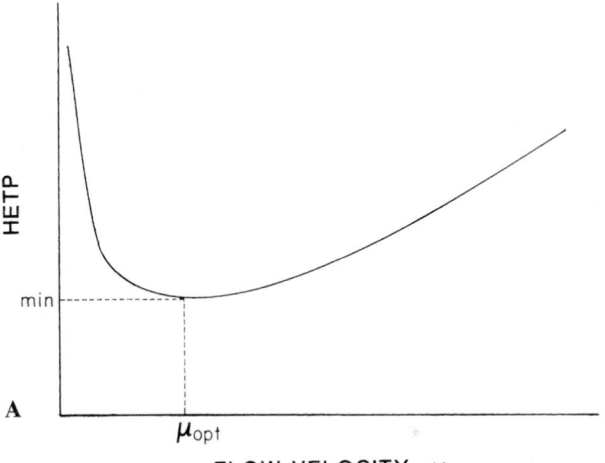

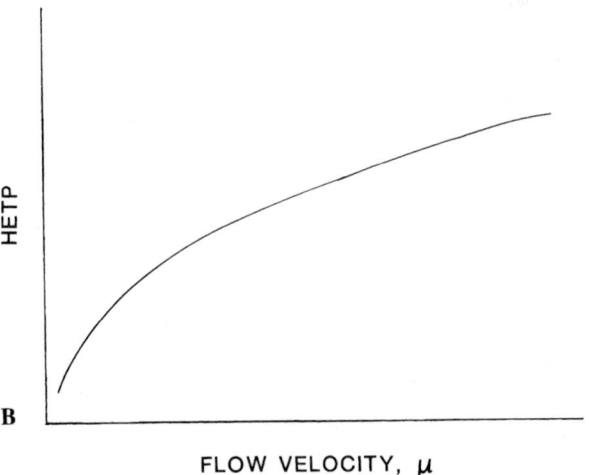

Fig. 5-8 Dependence of theoretical plate height, HETP, on mobile-phase velocity, μ, in gas chromatography, **A,** and in liquid chromatography, **B.**

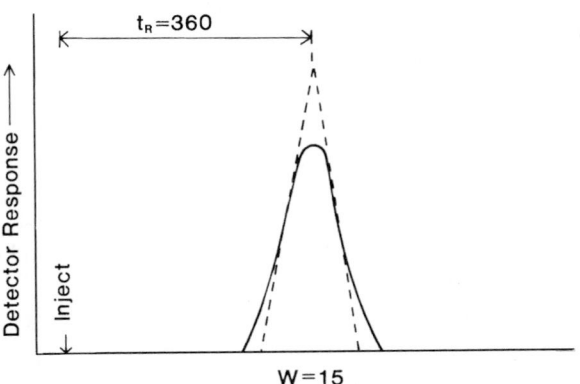

Fig. 5-7 Calculation of number of theoretical plates, *N,* from an HPLC or gas chromatogram. Elution or retention time, t_R, is measured from time of injection to apex of eluting peak for component. Peak width, *W,* is measured at the base of the peak by triangulation, as shown. Both t_R and *W* are measured in the same units.

and stationary phases in the column, that is, the capacity factor, k', which can be calculated from the chromatogram (Fig. 5-9, *A*) by the equation

$$k' = \frac{V_e - V_0}{V_0} = \frac{t_R - t_0}{t_0} \qquad \textit{Eq. 5-6}$$

The volumes in this equation are the void volume, V_0, of the column, that is, the volume of the mobile phase in the column, and the elution volume, V_e, of a solute retained by the stationary phase and undergoing chromatography. The HPLC chromatogram for Fig. 5-9, *A*, was obtained by injection of a sample containing two solutes, the first of which was not retained by the stationary phase and the second of which was retained, undergoing chromatography. The vol-

umes, V_0 and V_e, were then measured from the injection point to the apex of the peak of each component. As indicated previously, the capacity factor can be calculated also by the measurement of the times, t_0 and t_R, from sample injection to the apex of the peak of the component not retained and of the peak of the component retained, respectively.

Small values of k' indicate that the sample components are little retained by the stationary phase and elute close to the unretained peak. Large values of k' indicate that the sample components are well retained by the stationary phase and that long analysis times are required. For this latter situation, one must remember that solute-band broadening increases with residence time on the column because of an increased diffusion of the solute. Therefore the result-

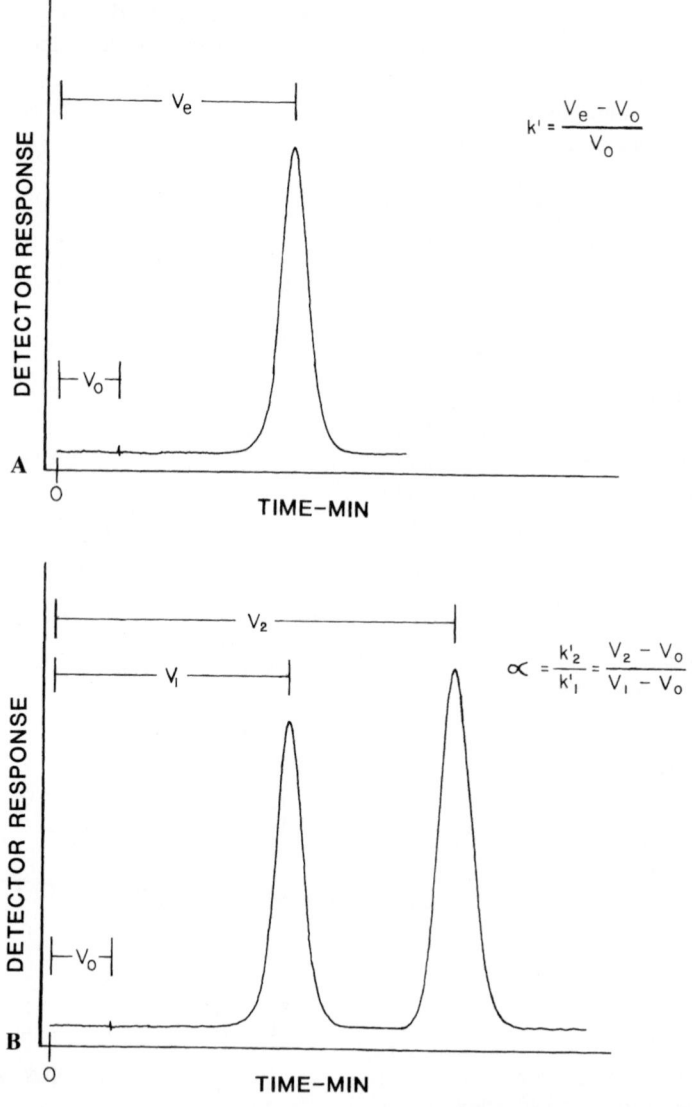

Fig. 5-9   **A,** Calculation of capacity factor, k', from an HPLC chromatogram. Sample was retained by stationary phase and underwent chromatography. **B,** Calculation of selectivity factor, α, from HPLC chromatogram. Solutes *A* and *B* were retained by stationary phase and underwent a chromatographic separation as indicated.

ing peaks on elution will be wide and diffuse, decreasing sensitivity, and making detection difficult.

The k' value for a particular solute is constant for any given chromatography system at constant mobile-phase compositions and stationary-phase size and composition. Within these limits, the capacity factor varies neither with flow rate of the mobile phase nor with column dimensions, that is, length and diameter.

Selectivity

Another parameter on which resolution depends is the selectivity factor, α (alpha), a term that describes the ability of a chromatographic system to separate two solutes. It is the ratio of the capacity factors for two solutes:

$$\alpha = \frac{k'_2}{k'_1} \qquad \textit{Eq. 5-7}$$

The capacity factors for two solutes are determined as shown in Fig. 5-9, *B,* from which the resultant selectivity of the system can be calculated. The selectivity of any given column for the sample is a function of the process of solute exchange between the mobile phase and the stationary phase.[12] Therefore, to affect selectivity, one can change the chemical composition of either the mobile phase or the stationary phase to increase the preference of the solute for one phase or the other. In LC, changes either in the stationary or in the mobile phases are usually made to improve selectivity. However, in GC, changes in stationary-phase chemistry are used for selectivity improvement.

Improving peak resolution

General peak resolution. With the definition of the factors affecting resolution, a more fundamental equation can now be written:

$$R = \left(\frac{N^{0.5}}{4}\right)\left(\frac{\alpha - 1}{\alpha}\right)\left(\frac{k'_2}{1 + k'_1}\right) \qquad \textit{Eq. 5-8}$$

Therefore the resolution of any two solutes in a given chromatographic system is a function of three factors: (1) theoretical plate number N, a column-efficiency factor; (2) a selectivity factor, α; and (3) a capacity factor, k'.

A similar relationship can be derived for flat methods of chromatography.[12] However, a major difference exists between flat and column methods of chromatography. In a column method of chromatography, the solutes in a given sample pass completely through the bed of the stationary phase. But in a flat method of chromatography, the separation process is stopped when the mobile phase has reached the end of the bed of the stationary phase, thereby resulting in the solute bands having migrated through only a portion of the bed (Fig. 5-10). For this type of separation, solute retention is measured in terms of the R_f value, which is the distance, d_2, migrated by the solute divided by the distance, d_1, migrated by the mobile phase, or solvent front. This relationship can be expressed as

$$R_f = \frac{d_2}{d_1} \qquad \textit{Eq. 5-9}$$

In consideration of this major feature of flat methods of chromatography, the resolution equation for the separation of two solutes becomes as follows:

$$R = \left(\frac{N^{0.5}}{4}\right)\left(\frac{\alpha - 1}{\alpha}\right)\left(\frac{k'_2}{(1 + k'_2)^{2/3}}\right) \qquad \textit{Eq. 5-10}$$

The terms of this equation are as previously defined. The question of the practical significance of the resolution equations can now be addressed. Specifically, how do these equations relate resolution to the actual experimental conditions of the chromatographic separation and the physical design of a particular chromatographic device? The three fundamental parameters, N, α, and k', of resolution can be adjusted more or less independently of each other.

Variation of N to optimize resolution. The dynamics or rates of the various physical processes that occur during the separation determine N. Experimentally one can change N by adjusting or varying a variety of parameters or conditions. Remember that a doubling of the value for N will increase the resolution by a factor of 1.4. (Notice that in the resolution equation R is proportional to the square root of N.) Experimental parameters that can be changed to optimize N are summarized in Table 5-1.

Variation of capacity factor k' to optimize resolution. Temperature is one parameter that is varied to effect a change in the capacity factor. Since the solute-stationary phase interactions are temperature dependent, a change in this parameter will affect solute retention. This is especially important in GC, but it is also important, though to a much lesser extent, for other chromatographic techniques.

A second way to vary the capacity factor is by effecting changes in the strength of the stationary phase. For partition chromatography, increasing the percentage of liquid-

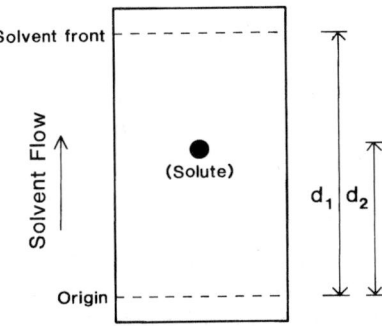

Fig. 5-10 Calculation of R_f (solvent-front ratio) value for a sample component from a paper or thin-layer chromatogram. The distance d_1 from origin to solvent front and distance d_2 from origin to center of spot of separated component are measured, as shown, in terms of same units; that is, length (centimeters or millimeters). Resulting R_f value, d_2 divided by d_1, is unitless.

Table 5-1   Experimental parameters affecting *N*

Parameters	Direction of change necessary to increase *N*
Mobile-phase flow rate	Decrease
Column length	Increase
Average particle size of stationary phase	Decrease
Particle-size distribution	Decrease
Volume of sample introduced	Decrease
Viscosity of sample introduced	Increase
Viscosity of mobile phase	Increase
Temperature (as it controls mobile-phase viscosity)	Decrease
Extracolumnar effects (that is, dead volumes, excessive connective tubing)	Decrease

phase coating on the matrix support will effect an increase in *k'*. Most GLC analyses are done on columns containing 2% to 10% ratios of liquid-phase coating to stationary-phase matrix support.[22,23] Since retention time is proportional to the amount of liquid phase present, lower percentage ratios mean shorter analysis times. However, higher percentages of stationary phase for partition chromatography mean higher resolution. Therefore the final selection of the percentage of stationary phase must be a compromise between analysis time and resolution.

Additionally, one can vary the capacity factor, *k'*, to improve resolution by changing the solvent strength of the mobile phase, but this is applicable only to LC methods (see p. 118). In GC the mobile phase is an inert gas like helium or nitrogen, but in LC the mobile phase is an active component of the chromatographic procedure, ranging from very nonpolar, such as hexane, to polar, such as water, in solvent strength.

For the adsorption and partition modes of LC (Fig. 5-2), the chromatographic process involves a continual distribution of the solute molecules between the mobile and the stationary phases. Any shift in the equilibrium concentration distribution coefficient (K_D) affects the capacity factor; that is, the elution volume per time of a particular solute in the given sample. One way to shift this coefficient is to increase or decrease the polarity of the mobile phase relative to the stationary phase. Numerous examples of mobile-phase alterations could be given. This is a powerful technique for varying the *k'* of solutes being separated (see p. 131, Chapter 6).

Variation of selectivity to optimize resolution. After optimization of the *k'* values, the selectivity, or separation factor, α, then can be adjusted to maximize the resolution. In general, the separation factor is varied by changes in the chemistries of the mobile phase, the stationary phase, or the sample. These changes may be accomplished as follows.

Derivatization. The chemical form of the sample can be altered in a variety of ways to affect selectivity. The most common method is derivatization. Knapp[24] has summarized an extensive variety of derivatization reactions for samples to be separated by GC. Derivatization is not only used in GC to improve sample volatility or solute detection limits, but is also used to improve selectivity.[25] In LC, derivatization techniques are generally used to improve detection,[19,21,26] with the most extensive collection of methods presented in a book by Frei and Lawrence.[27]

Alterations in mobile-phase chemistry. Another method for improving the separation factor in LC is altering the mobile-phase chemistry.[28] Solvent polarity changes can be used to improve the capacity factor, *k'*. For improving the separation factor, solvents of similar polarity (strength) but different chemical natures are interchanged without affecting the overall polarity of the mobile phase, resulting in changes in the solvent selectivity. For example, the resolution of an HPLC separation initially developed with a mobile phase of methylene chloride to hexane, 50/50 by volume, could be improved by substitution of tetrahydrofuran for methylene chloride without changing the solvent strength.[14,29,30] The reason for improvement in resolution would be that tetrahydrofuran has a quite different selectivity toward certain classes of compounds, such as lipids, than methylene chloride does. In this case, with substitution of an ether for an organic halide, the functional groups of the mobile phase have been altered. Changing solvent functionality without changing solvent strength is a powerful technique for improving selectivity and thereby resolution in LC. Depending on the sample and chromatographic and detector requirements, the choice of solvent or solvents that can be used to effect changes in selectivity is extensive, as detailed by Snyder[31] in his compendium of properties of 911 solvents. A further discussion of the properties of solvents is presented in a later section.

Alterations in stationary-phase chemistry. As adjustments in the functionality of the mobile phase are used to improve the separation factor in LC, similar changes in the functionality of the stationary phase are commonly used to improve the separation factor in GC. For example, many polyester stationary phases, such as ethylene glycol succinate, can be replaced by the cyanopropyl silicone stationary phases, such as Silar 10C, allowing for a change in functionality with little or no change in polarity. For relatively nonpolar stationary phases, the hydrocarbon phases, such as Apiezon N, can be readily replaced by the alkyl silicone phases, such as OV-1, for a functionality change. These changes in stationary phase afford an improvement in selectivity, thereby leading to an optimization in resolution. Details as to the initial choice of phase are discussed in the following sections.

POLARITY

In previous sections, the importance of solvent strength and stationary-phase strength was discussed in relationship to their effect on resolution. Both factors affect chromato-

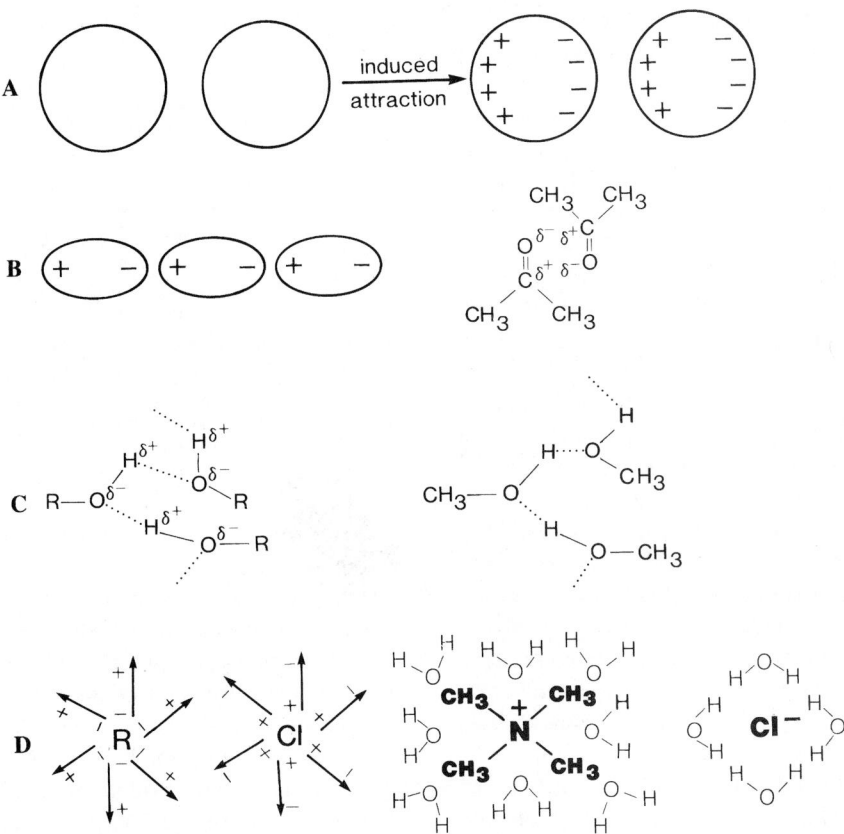

Fig. 5-11 Physicochemical interactions between molecules that constitute concept of polarity. **A,** Dispersive or van der Waals interactions. **B,** Dipole interactions. **C,** Hydrogen bonding. **D,** Electrostatic interactions.

graphic resolution by altering the capacity factor and the separation factor as described earlier in Equations 5-6 and 5-7. These parameters are linked by the *principle of polarity.*

The role of polarity is central to the interaction of molecules in the liquid or gaseous state, and polarity is a major determinant property in the overall chromatographic process. The concept of polarity can be interpreted several ways[19,29,30] but generally is considered to encompass the total interaction of solvent molecules with sample molecules and of solvent or sample molecules with the stationary phase. The physicochemical basis for polarity is the interaction of attractive forces that exist between molecules. These four attractive forces are more specifically referred to as dispersive, dipolar, hydrogen-bonding, and dielectric interactions. As illustrated in Fig. 5-11 and discussed below, all four of these interactions involve the attraction of induced, partial, or formal positive and negative charges.

Dispersion interactions of molecules, sometimes termed *van der Waals forces,* refer to the induced attraction between two molecules. This temporary separation of opposite charges (dipole) in one molecule induces the polarization of electrons in an adjacent molecule, thereby causing the two molecules to be attracted to each other by electrostatic interactions (Fig. 5-11, *A*). The formation of temporary di-

poles in molecules is the physical basis for existence in the liquid state of many compounds composed of elements with small differences in electronegativity, for example, the elements carbon and hydrogen. Generally, dispersive interactions are an important determinant in polarity only when other forces are lacking or when some elemental constituents of molecules are electron-rich species (such as halogens in halohydrocarbons).

Some molecules possess permanent rather than temporary dipoles (Fig. 5-11, *B*). These compounds have centers of positive and negative charge that are the result of an unequal sharing of bonding electrons between two elements with large differences in electronegativity within the same molecule. This overall molecular dipole is enhanced by the presence of elemental nonbonding electron pairs within a compound. These are outer shell electrons within an element that are spin paired. Elements such as oxygen, sulfur, halogens, and nitrogen possess nonbonding electrons when covalently linked to other atoms in compounds. The resulting permanent dipole is directional, with one end of the molecule being partially positive and the other being partially negative.

One special category of dipolar molecules is composed of those with hydrogen covalently linked to an electronegative element such as oxygen, nitrogen, or sulfur. In these molecules the hydrogen has a large degree of positive character relative to the electronegative atom to which it is bonded. Because of the small size of the hydrogen atom compared with other atoms, this positive end of the dipole can approach close to the negative end of a neighboring dipole. The force of attraction between the two is quite large, about 10 times that of normal dipolar interactions. This special case of dipole-dipole interactions is termed *hydrogen bonding* and is one of the most important types of weak attractive forces. This bonding is illustrated in Fig. 5-11, *C*, for the alcohol methanol.

The fourth type of attractive force is the electrostatic or dielectric interaction. In this case, the solute molecule of the stationary phase is a charged ionic species having either a formal positive or a formal negative charge. A small counterion, such as H^+ or Cl^-, is present but is generally separated from the charged solute or stationary phase because of solvation by the mobile phase (Fig. 5-11, *D*). These ionic species increase the dipolar character of the solvent by an enhancement of polarization. Dielectric interactions are quite strong and favor the dissolution of ionic or ionizable sample molecules in strongly dipolar solvents such as water or methanol.

The polarity of a solute molecule is the result of the four attractive forces described above. The polarity of a molecule will affect its interactions with the mobile and stationary phases. The more polar molecules have this property primarily because of strong dipoles, an ionic character, an ability to form strong hydrogen bonds, or a combination of the three forces. The less polar (nonpolar) molecules have dispersive forces as a primary basis of interaction with a very weak ability to interact through dipolar, hydrogen bonding, or dielectric forces. The practical aspects of these interactive forces and the degree of polarity or nonpolarity form the basis for the mechanisms of chromatography. The role of polarity in these mechanisms is discussed below for each of the three chromatographic constituents—the solute, the solvent or mobile phase, and the stationary phase.

Solvent polarity and solvent strength

Solvent strength in liquid chromatography is a measure of the ability of the mobile phase to compete with the solute molecules for active sites (that is, interaction or attraction sites) on the stationary phase. When the stationary phase is silica gel, the active sites are the highly polar hydroxyl groups (Si—OH). Therefore, in this case, solvent strength increases with solvent or mobile-phase polarity. However, when the stationary phase is nonpolar, such as a polydivinylbenzene (such as XAD-2), the solvent strength decreases with increases in solvent or mobile-phase polarity. The strength of a solvent is directly related to its polarity.

Solvent polarity has been described and quantitated in various ways.[29-34] The four most common solvent polarity-classification schemes are (1) the Hildebrand solubility pa-

Table 5-2 Solvent classification by selectivity groups

Solvent group	Representative classes or examples of compounds
0	*n*-Alkanes, cyclohexane, saturated fluorochlorohydrocarbons
1 (I)	Aliphatic ethers, trialkylamines
2 (II)	Aliphatic alcohols
3 (III)	Pyridine derivatives, tetrahydrofuran, amides
4 (IV)	Glycols, benzyl alcohol, acetic acid
5 (V)	Methylene chloride, ethylene chloride, bis(2-ethoxyethyl) ether
6 (VIA)	Aliphatic ketones and esters, nitriles, dioxane, sulfoxides
7 (VIB)	Nitrocompounds, phenyl alkyl ethers, aromatic hydrocarbons, carbon tetrachloride
8 (VII)	Halobenzenes, diphenyl ether
9 (VIII)	Fluoroalkanols, chloroform, water

rameter, which is based on thermodynamic properties of the compound in question[34]; (2) the Rohrschneider polarity scale of P′ values, which is based on the measurement of solvent properties through the use of model solutes[31]; (3) the eluotropic series, which ranks solvents in order of their eluting power for removing solutes from a polar stationary phase, such as alumina[36]; and (4) the solvent selectivity grouping of Snyder and Karger, which is a blend of the three previous approaches and incorporates specific solubility parameters for dispersion, dipole, and hydrogen-bonding interactions. A listing of the solvent selectivity groups is given in Table 5-2 along with representative classes of compounds and specific examples for each group.

Solvents within any one group exhibit the same types of attractive forces. For example, the compounds of group 1 (I) are all strong hydrogen-bonding acceptors and weak hydrogen-bonding donors and have intermediate dipole moments. The solvents in group 5 (V) are compounds whose dipole interactions predominate over any hydrogen-bonding interactions. However, the solvents in group 0 are compounds in which only dispersion interactions (that is, temporary dipoles) are the predominant force. These solvents do not have permanent dipoles, nor do they interact through hydrogen bonding.

The overall degree of the interactive forces of the solvent is quantitated in the polarity index, P′.[29,30] A list of solvents commonly used in chromatography is presented in Table 5-3 with values for their polarity indices and their solvent selectivity group classifications. It is noted that solvents within any one group may vary widely in their overall degree of polarity. For example, the solvents listed for group 6 (VIA) vary more than three polarity units. In group 2 (II), the polarity index varies more than two units. Even though these variations are relatively large, one must remember that solvents within the same group exhibit the same kinds of chemical interactions.

This information can be used as a basis for solvent selections and can be used to vary the mobile-phase selectivity, α, to improve resolution. The first important step in sol-

Table 5-3   Representative solvent polarity indices

Solvent	Polarity index	Solvent group
Isooctane	−0.4	0
Hexane	0.0	0
Carbon tetrachloride	1.7	7
Dibutyl ether	1.7	1
Triethylamine	1.8	1
Toluene	2.3	7
Chlorobenzene	2.7	8
Diphenyl ether	2.8	8
Diethyl ether	2.9	1
Benzene	3.0	7
Ethyl bromide	3.1	6
Methylene chloride	3.4	5
1,2-Dichloroethane	3.7	5
Bis(2-ethoxyethyl) ether	3.9	5
n-Propanol	4.1	2
Tetrahydrofuran	4.2	3
Chloroform	4.3	9
Ethyl acetate	4.3	6
Isopropanol	4.3	2
2-Butanone	4.5	6
Dioxane	4.8	6
Ethanol	5.2	2
Nitroethane	5.3	7
Pyridine	5.3	3
Acetone	5.4	6
Benzyl alcohol	5.5	4
Methoxyethanol	5.7	4
Acetic acid	6.2	4
Acetonitrile	6.2	6
Dimethylformamide	6.4	3
Dimethyl sulfoxide	6.5	6
Methanol	6.6	2
Nitromethane	6.8	7
Water	9.0	9

vent selection is to maximize solute solubility in a given solvent. For a solvent to be an effective mobile phase in chromatography, it should dissolve the sample over the range of expected solute concentrations.

The most significant factor affecting solute solubility is solvent polarity. One can vary liquid mobile-phase polarity systematically over a wide range of P′ values by using a combination of two solvents, since solvent polarities are additive according to:

$$P' \text{ (of combined solvents A+B)} = \phi_A P'_A + \phi_B P'_B \qquad \textit{Eq. 5-11}$$

In this expression, ϕ_A and ϕ_B are the volume fractions of solvents A and B, which have solvent polarities of P'_A and P'_B respectively. The two solvents should differ in P′ values so that maximization of sample solubility can be achieved. It is important that the two solvents are miscible in all proportions. Usually a solvent that is too weak (A) to dissolve the sample is mixed with a solvent that is too strong (B). The two solvents are now chosen from the solvent groups (Table 5-3) according to the compatibility of interactive forces with sample solutes and stationary-phase chemical functionalities. For example, to calculate P′ for solvent mixtures of isooctane (solvent A) and chloroform (solvent B), their individual polarity values are obtained from Table 5-3. Any mixtures of these two solvents would range in polarity from −0.4 to 4.3, that is, weakest (100% isooctane) to strongest (100% chloroform). A 50%:50% mixture of these two solvents would have a P′ of (0.5 × −0.4) + (0.5 × 4.3), or 1.95. Also, for each 10% change in solvent composition, the polarity of the mixture would change by 0.47 unit:

$$0.1(P'_B - P'_A) = 0.1 (4.3 - [-0.4]) = 0.47$$

Once a suitable solvent mixture has been found to dissolve the sample, it is then applied to a chromatographic system such as a silica HPLC column. As previously discussed, the retention index k' for the solutes in the sample is maximized to a value between 2 and 8. This is accomplished by adjustment of the solvent polarity by small changes in the relative proportions of the two solvents.

Resolution is then maximized for the solute separation by adjustments in chromatographic selectivity, α. This is done by exchanging one of the mobile-phase solvents for a solvent in another solvent selectivity group (see Table 5-3) but with the *same polarity* of the overall mixture being kept. For example, chloroform, P′ = 4.3, could be exchanged with isopropanol, P′ = 4.3, in the previously described isooctane-chloroform mixture. The net effect of this exchange would be to go from a solvent that is a strong hydrogen-bonding donor, chloroform, to a solvent that is both a strong hydrogen-bonding donor and hydrogen-bonding acceptor. Other examples of such changes were given earlier in the discussion on selectivity. Further discussions of solvent selection and optimization are given by Snyder and associates.[19,30]

In principle, this approach is a general guide to solvent choice both for dissolving the sample and for optimizing a mobile phase in LC (HPLC, thin-layer chromatography, and so on). It does, however, require knowledge of the forces involved in the chromatographic separation process. The latter is discussed in the following sections on the role of stationary-phase polarity and the mechanisms of chromatography.

Stationary-phase polarity and selectivity

The stationary phase is the fundamental component of the chromatographic separation (Table 5-4). The role of the stationary phase depends on its selectivity, which, in turn, is determined by the polarity of the phase. The forces constituting stationary-phase polarity are the same interactions responsible for mobile-phase (solvent) polarity: dispersion, dipole, hydrogen bonding, and dielectric.

The relative strength of polarity of stationary phases is more difficult to ascertain than the relative strength of polarity of liquid mobile phases, as previously described. Most attention has been directed to the stationary phases used in

Table 5-4 Preferred stationary phases

Phase type	Examples
Dimethylsilicone	OV-1, OV-101, SE-30, SP-2100
50% phenylmethylsilicone	OV-17, SP-2750
Trifluoropropylmethylsilicone	OV-210, SP-2401
Polyethylene glycol	Carbowaxes
Polyesters	DEGS, EGSS-X, EGA
3-Cyanopropylsilicone	Silar 10C, SP-2340, Apolar 10C

From Hawkes S, Grossman D, Hartkopf A, et al: *J Chromatogr Sci* 13:115-117, 1975.

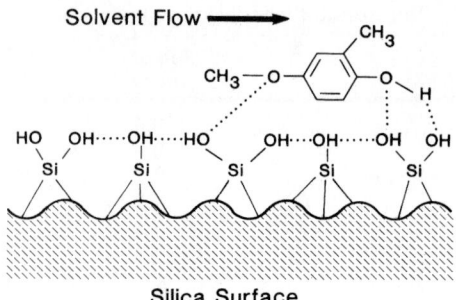

Fig. 5-12 Mechanism of separation of a metabolite of methylanisole by silica gel chromatography. Hydrogen bonds, ...; covalent bonds, ____.

GC wherein the two major variables determining the separation are the stationary phase itself and the temperature of the column. In this mode of chromatography, studies of the affinity of solute molecules of varying polarities have led to a classification system for stationary phase according to polarity. Details on the Rohrschneider[37] and McReynolds[38] classifications can be found in Chapter 7.

MECHANISMS OF CHROMATOGRAPHY

The mechanisms by which a chromatographic method can separate sample components are generally based on polar interactions and physical interactions (interactions resulting from the size and shape of the solute molecules). The latter interaction is principally the mechanism for gel-permeation chromatography, though molecular size plays a minor role in other modes of chromatography. The other broad mechanistic classes of chromatography are adsorption, partition, and ion exchange. Each is briefly discussed in the following sections.

Adsorption

The interactions of solute or mobile-phase molecules at the surface of a solid particle form the basis of the adsorption mechanism. There are fundamentally two types of adsorbents, nonpolar and polar. The latter category includes those that are acidic (that is, having electron-accepting surfaces) and those that are basic (that is, having electron-donating surfaces).

The nonpolar adsorbents have limited application in gas-solid chromatography (GSC)[22] (see Chapter 7). The mechanism for adsorption of the solute to nonpolar stationary phases is principally by dispersive interactions. Retention is determined by the adsorption energy and the surface volume of the stationary phase. A decrease in temperature or an increase in pressure increases adsorption. The converse is also true; that is, an increase in desorption can be accomplished by an increase in temperature or a decrease in pressure.

Polar adsorbents are the most widely used stationary phases in liquid-solid chromatography (LSC), with applications in both flat and column methods. Limited applications are found in GSC. The most common stationary phases are silica and alumina for LSC and silica or porous glass and aluminosilicates (zeolites or molecular sieves) for GSC. This latter group also has application in LC for gel-

permeation chromatography, in which the separation is principally through the mechanism of molecular exclusion. This is discussed later in the section on the mechanism of gel permeation.

The principal polar adsorbents used in LC are silica and alumina, accounting for more than 95% of the applications in HPLC[19] and thin-layer chromatography (TLC).[15,39,40] Both hydrogen bonding and dipole interactions between the solute and the surface hydroxyl (silica and acid-washed alumina) or the oxygen anionic (base-washed alumina) groups of the stationary phases constitute the mechanisms of separation by this method (Fig. 5-12). The number and topographic arrangement of these groups, along with the total surface area, determine the activity and strength of the adsorption. Retention of solutes on these phases increases with increasing polarity of the compound class (Table 5-5). Retention of a solute molecule requires displacement of adsorbed solvent molecules (Fig. 5-13). Adjustments in solvent polarity, as previously described, ultimately determine the strength of adsorption of the solute to the stationary phase and the retention characteristics of the system.

Adsorption chromatography offers many advantages for use in LC separations. First, an extensive literature is available to the investigator for the separation of many types and classes of compounds by TLC. These methods are readily transferable to adsorption HPLC. Second, the flexibility, speed, and low cost of TLC allow its use in experimental development, particularly for selection of mobile phases. Once the optimum separation has been achieved, the transfer of the method to HPLC is straightforward. Third, TLC has a great value for use in the preliminary investigation of samples of unknown constituents, particularly when one considers the advantages noted above. Finally, adsorption chromatography, particularly with silica gel, has been widely used for the separation of drugs in both the HPLC and TLC modes.

Partition

Partition chromatography is based on the separation of solutes by use of differences in their distribution between two

Table 5-5 Selected groups of solutes in order of increased retention in normal-phase and reversed-phase chromatography

Reversed phase	Solute type	Normal phase
Most retained	Fluorocarbons	Least retained
↓	Saturated hydrocarbons	↓
	Unsaturated hydrocarbons	
	Halides and esters	
	Aldehydes and ketones	
	Alcohol and thiols	
Least retained	Acids and bases	Most retained

immiscible phases. In liquid-liquid chromatography (LLC), the phase support is usually coated with a polar substance (normal phase), with separations accomplished by use of an immiscible mobile phase. A normal-phase partition system would consist of silica coated with a monolayer of water or some other polar liquid and a relatively nonpolar solvent system. Separations in this system are based on solute polarity, with the least polar compounds eluting first and the most polar substances retained the longest (Fig. 5-14). A similar separation system operates in paper chromatography, in which the cellulose is coated with an aqueous monolayer, and immiscible solvents are used as the mobile phase.

In 1969 Halasz and Sebastian[41] introduced a variation in the stationary phase for LLC, in which the silica support was chemically modified to produce a monolayer of a nonpolar organic substituent. These chemically bonded stationary-phase supports are available with a variety of functional groups. The most commonly used bonded phases are hydrocarbon phases such as octadecyl or octyl groups bonded to silica (Fig. 5-15). The organic nature of the bonded phases imparts a nonpolar character to the stationary phase. Therefore the mobile phases commonly used are highly polar, such as water, methanol, or acetonitrile (see Table 5-3). Solutes are separated by their relatively nonpolar character (that is, the most polar eluting first), whereas the nonpolar solutes are retained longer. From this type of separation characteristic, the use of bonded phases in LLC is termed *reversed-phase chromatography.* A further discussion and examples of normal-phase and reversed-phase LC are given in Chapter 6.

Another example of chromatography in which a partition mechanism operates is gas-liquid chromatography (GLC). The forces of interaction between solute molecules and the liquid-coated stationary phase are as previously discussed for LLC. However, for GC, the mobile phase serves as an inert carrier for the sample constituents, whereas in LLC the mobile phase is an active, interacting component in the partition mechanism.

Ion exchange

Ion-exchange chromatography uses stationary phases that possess formal positive or negative charges. The most common retention mechanism is the exchange of sample ions,

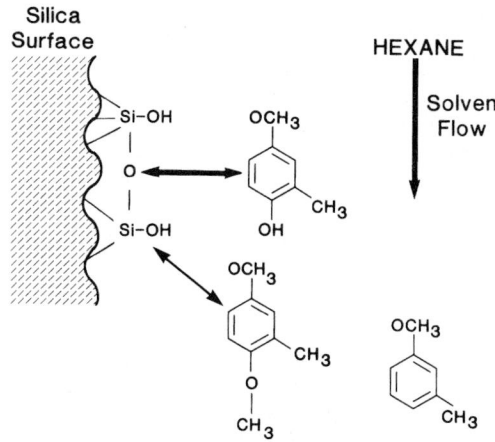

Fig. 5-13 Mechanism of adsorption chromatography by separation of 3-methylanisole and two of its biochemical metabolites. The most polar sample components, such as 3-methyl-4-hydroxyanisole, are retained the most by polar silica gel stationary phase *(heavy arrow)*. Sample components of intermediate polarity, such as 2,5-dimethoxytoluene, are retained to a much lesser degree *(light arrow)*, whereas relatively nonpolar components, such as 3-methylanisole, are not retained and prefer the nonpolar mobile phase, hexane.

A, and mobile-phase ions, *B*, with the charged groups, *R*, of the stationary phase:

$$A^- + R^+B^- \rightarrow B^- + R^+A^- \quad \textit{Anion exchange } \textbf{Eq. 5-12,A}$$
$$A^+ + B^+R^- \rightarrow B^+ + A^+R^- \quad \textit{Cation exchange } \textbf{Eq. 5-12,B}$$

In the first case, anion exchange is occurring, whereas cation exchange is shown for the second; sample ions compete with mobile-phase ions for ionic sites on the stationary phase. The sample ions that interact weakly with the stationary phase will be retained least, whereas those that interact strongly will be retained the most and will be eluted later. The principal force of these interactions is electrostatic, or the attraction of opposite charges.

To effect a separation of sample constituents, the extent of ionization of sample molecules is controlled by variations in pH of the mobile phase. Since the solutes are predominantly weak acids, HA, or weak bases, B, a change in pH will shift the following ionization equilibriums either to the right or to the left:

$$\text{pH↓} \quad \text{pH↑}$$
$$HA \rightleftharpoons H^+ + A^- \qquad \textbf{Eq. 5-13,A}$$
$$BH^+ \rightleftharpoons H^+ + B \qquad \textbf{Eq. 5-13,B}$$

An increase in ionization leads to an increased retention of the sample. Factors other than pH controlling solute retention in ion-exchange chromatography are (1) charge strength of the solute ion, (2) ionic strength of the mobile phase, and (3) charge strength of the counterion on the stationary phase. One can decrease the retardation of solutes

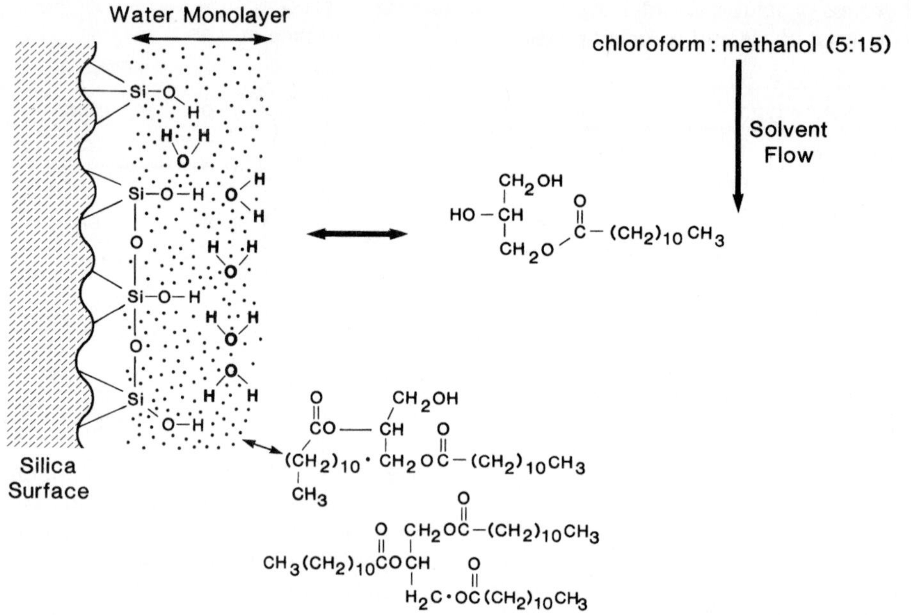

Fig. 5-14 Mechanism of liquid/liquid chromatography as exemplified by the separation of the monoglycerides, diglycerides, and triglycerides of lauric acid. Silica gel stationary phase has a monolayer of water strongly held by hydrogen bonding. Solute molecules are partitioned between the liquid mobile phase (chloroform:methanol) and liquid stationary phase, or water monolayer. The most polar sample components, the monoglycerides, are retained most by the polar stationary phase *(heavy arrow)*. Sample components of intermediate polarity, such as the diglycerides, are retained to a much lesser degree *(light arrow)*, whereas relatively nonpolar components, such as the triglycerides, are not retained and prefer the relatively nonpolar stationary phase.

by increasing the ionic strength of the mobile phase and decreasing the strength of the counterion, such as use of Na^+ instead of H^+ for cation-exchange phases, or by adjusting the pH of the mobile phase in a manner to decrease dissociation of either the solute, the counterion on the packing, or both.

Gel-permeation (molecular or size exclusion) chromatography[43]

In contrast to the previous mechanisms and modes of chromatography, gel-permeation chromatography (GPC) separation is strictly based on molecular size. The stationary phase for GPC contains pores of a particular average size, and if the sample molecules are too large to enter the pores, they are not retained (excluded) by the stationary phase and are eluted from the column first. Small sample molecules permeate deeply into the pores and are retained the longest. They ultimately diffuse from the pores and are swept away by the flow of the mobile phase. Intermediate-sized sample molecules enter the pores to some extent but are not retained as easily as the small sample molecules because they do not penetrate as deeply into the pores. They are eluted from the column in volumes between those needed to elute the largest solute (small V_e) and smallest solutes (large V_e). This mechanism is illustrated in Fig. 5-16.

The major advantage of this mode of chromatography is that the LC method can be used to separate virtually any sample, as long as it is soluble in a mobile phase. Additionally, it is applicable to soluble species with an average molecular weight of 50 to more than 10 million. Since molecular size is the property of interest, representative calibration curves should be obtained by use of calibration standards of known molecular weight. Likewise, stationary phase choice is based on the expected molecular-weight range of the solute molecules in the sample and compatibility with the mobile phase. A mobile phase for GPC should be chosen first on the basis of sample solubility, and then a compatible stationary phase is selected. Most stationary phases are compatible with aqueous or proton-donating (such as methanol) solvents. However, there are available stationary phases that are compatible only with organic solvents. Lists of the available phases for GPC are tabulated in the manufacturers' literature, in reviews,[42] and in books.

SAMPLE PREPARATION FOR CHROMATOGRAPHY
Nature of problem

Few chromatographic analyses are conducted on the sample as submitted to the clinical laboratory. For any given sample, the goal of the chromatographic analysis is either a

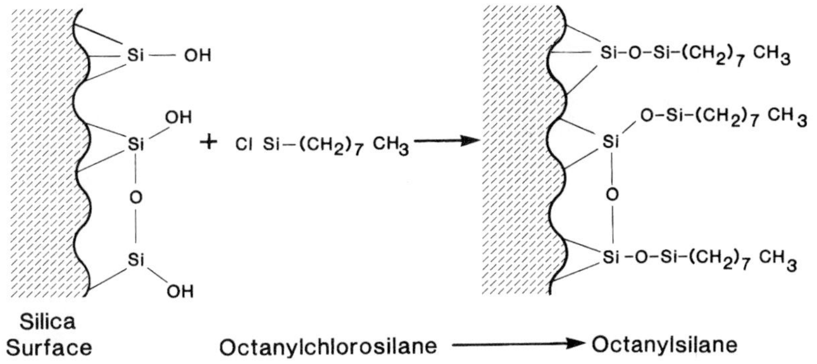

Fig. 5-15 Chemical preparation of bonded, stationary phase (reversed phase). Organo-chlorosilane reacts with nucleophilic hydroxyl (OH) groups of silica gel, forming siloxane covalent bond (Si—O—Si).

qualitative or a quantitative determination of its components. To achieve this objective, one should separate the components of interest as discrete zones with the same peak or spot distributions and k' or R_f values as the standards under identical chromatographic conditions. However, the complexity of a biological sample matrix usually renders the chromatographic separation ineffectual by (1) interaction of sample impurities with the stationary phase, causing a reduction in the resolving power of the system; (2) saturation of most chromatographic detector systems, tending to raise the noise level and thereby decreasing sensitivity; (3) interaction of the component of interest with other matrix components, leading to irreproducibility of the separation from sample to sample; and (4) poorly resolved components that interfere with the analysis. To minimize these sample effects in the chromatographic separation, a strategy for separation of the analyte from interfering components (*sample cleanup*) is required.

Any separation method employed in the laboratory must meet the criteria of yield, separation, capacity, and cost effectiveness. The advantages of having high yield in any sample manipulation step are obvious, but if recovery is quantitative with little purification, the method is unsatisfactory. The corollary is also true: if the separation from impurities is excellent but there is a low yield, the method is of little value. Many separation methods are readily applied on a large scale where large amounts of sample are available, but others are applicable only to small-scale separations. The criterion of cost effectiveness, which includes time, equipment, reagents, and labor, may render a separation method impracticable.

The strategy of sample preparation for chromatographic analysis should include consideration of whether the objective of the analysis is to qualitatively detect or to quantitate the substance under investigation.[44]

Mechanical methods for initial isolation of analyte

The type of sample matrix received by the analyst in a clinical chemistry laboratory varies from a simple homogeneous-appearing liquid such as perspiration to a complex heterogeneous solid such as feces. However, the most commonly received sample matrices are urine and blood (or plasma). The initial step in analyte preparation for chromatography will vary according to matrix.

Solid samples, such as tissues or feces, are first disrupted or treated for preparation of a homogeneous solution or suspension from which the analyte can be isolated. Homogenization of tissues in a blender such as a Polytron (Brinkmann Instruments, Inc., Westbury, N.Y.) with an appropriate solvent may solubilize the desired analyte. The use of a Potter-Elvehjem tissue grinder is also effective. Tissue can also be extracted in a mortar with a pestle and a small amount of solvent. In addition to these grinding or shearing techniques, solid samples can be disrupted by sonication in solvent or hydrolyzed by acid, base, or enzymes. A procedure for preparing homogeneous powders of feces for subsequent extraction has been developed for the investigation of drug metabolism. It involves grinding the sample with a stainless steel ball mill in the presence of anhydrous sodium sulfate.[45]

Liquid samples may also require an initial treatment for removal of analytes sequestered by matrix components. Mild base hydrolysis has been used to release sequestered polychlorinated biphenyls from blood lipid components.[46] Whole blood can be diluted with sterile water to disrupt blood cells osmotically before analyte isolation. Another initial treatment applied to blood or urine samples is to remove proteins and other macromolecules through precipitation. Two of the more commonly used protein-precipitating agents are trichloroacetic acid and barium sulfate.

In other mechanical methods of matrix disruption, such as homogenization in a solvent or buffer, centrifugation is commonly employed to remove cell debris, particulate matter, or other large contaminants. An alternative method for the removal of insolubles is filtration, either through an inert material, such as glass wool, or through a nitrocellulose or nylon membrane.

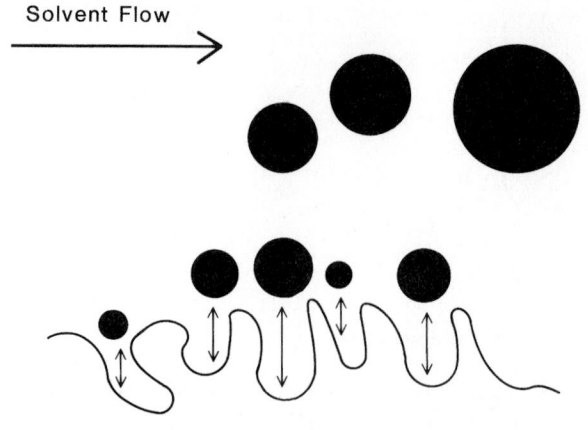

Solvent Flow →

Surface of Stationary Phase

Fig. 5-16 Mechanism of size-exclusion chromatography. Stationary phase, in form of porous beads, contains pores of varying diameter. Mobile phase outside and inside pores is the same, except the liquid inside is immobilized. When a sample containing solutes varying from small to large molecules elutes through column, small molecules penetrate all pores and are retained, thus being eluted later than large molecules, which move only in mobile phase. Molecules of intermediate size penetrate only some pores, thereby being retained to a lesser degree than small molecules.

Chromatographic methods for initial isolation of analyte

A common method for the initial isolation of components of interest from aqueous solutions, such as urine or blood, is the use of XAD-2 resin chromatography.[47] This stationary phase of polydivinylbenzene has a large surface area and is of a nonionic character, making it capable of adsorbing many classes of organic compounds from aqueous solution, principally by dispersive and dipole interactions. The adsorbed organics are eluted from the XAD-2 by organic solvents like methanol, acetone, diethyl ether, hexane, methylene chloride, or combinations of these solvents.[48] The XAD-2 method has been applied most often to urine- or blood-screening methods for drugs of abuse and their metabolites, but it can also be applied to isolate trace amounts of many types of compounds.

Another very common chromatographic technique for initial analyte isolation is the use of small columns of silica or of octadecylsilyl-bonded phase.[49,50] The analytes from a relatively large volume of sample are adsorbed from aqueous solution by forces similar to those operating in the XAD-2 procedure. Desorption is accomplished when a small volume of an appropriate solvent is passed through the silica or reversed-phase cartridge; the sample may then be processed for any mode of chromatography. Many additional resins, of the type just described, are currently available for the isolation of compounds of interest to the clinical chemist.[51]

Other types of chromatographic methods have been used in the preparation of samples for analysis. Ion-exchange chromatography has been widely used to isolate charged analytes. Anion exchange, first suggested by Horning and Horning,[52] has been widely used for the isolation of acidic constituents from biological fluids. Although DEAE-Sephadex is the most widely used ion-exchange stationary phase for sample cleanup, other anion exchangers, such as AGIX and Dowex 3, have been used.

Extraction methods for analyte isolation

Liquid-liquid and liquid-solid partition methods have been widely used for both primary and secondary extraction steps in a wide variety of clinical chemistry analyses before the chromatographic quantitation step. The reasons for the use of extraction procedures are numerous, including the isolation of the analyte from large quantities of contaminating materials and its concentration into a small volume of solvent, making detection easier. Liquid-liquid extraction procedures are easily accomplished, usually permitting the workup of multiple samples simultaneously.

The success of an extraction step depends on knowledge of the polarity of the analyte. This information is used to select an extracting solvent that will effectively remove the analyte from the sample. A general rule of solvent selection is that compounds tend to favor solvents having the same polarity interaction forces. It is critical that the chosen solvent be immiscible with the sample matrix.

There are other points to consider in solvent selection. The solvent must be chemically compatible with the analyte; that is, no chemical reaction should be possible between the two. The solvent must be compatible with all subsequent operations after the extraction. For example, a solvent with a high boiling point would be difficult to remove, and so the analyte solution would be difficult to concentrate by evaporation. The solvent should not introduce any contaminants that would make the analysis difficult. Many laboratory supply companies offer common solvents of high-purity grades, such as (1) *HPLC-grade solvents,* which are compatible with most detector systems and do not contain particulate matter that would foul the HPLC equipment; (2) *pesticide-grade solvents,* which are compatible with electron-capture GC detectors because they do not introduce any contaminating substances; and (3) *lipograde-grade solvents,* which do not contain any greases or other substances that would interfere with the analysis of lipids. These are but a few of the types of quality solvents available. If the solvent is not available in the required purity, a purification of the solvent must be done before use in any sample cleanup procedure. Most commonly, a distillation of the solvent will suffice, but sometimes more extensive purification measures are required. Methods of more rigorous purification procedures for most solvents are described in Weissberger's text.[53] Even with the use of the highest quality solvents commercially available or prior purification of solvents, impurities may still be a problem. The most common contaminant is plasticizers, usually coming from cap liners and other plastic materials.[54] These contaminants, various alkyl phthalates, can interfere with some analyses, particularly when electron-capture gas chromatography is used. Foil-lined screw caps of extraction tubes or sample vials have been shown to be the source of contaminants that interfered with GC.[55] These contamination problems can be eliminated by using screw-cap liners made of Teflon.

Once a decision on the solvents for extraction has been made, the actual operations in extraction must be considered. In general, a repeated series of extractions with smaller volumes of solvent will be more efficient than a single extraction with a large volume. For solid samples, the solvent may be introduced during the mechanical disruption step as previously mentioned. The cycle of grinding, sonication, and so on is repeated several times with several volumes of solvent. However, doing so sometimes does not effectively extract the desired analyte. In this case, the pulverized solid sample may have to be extracted with a Soxhlet extractor or a continuous infusion extractor. Both of these methods are more efficient than manual operations for extracting substances from a solid matrix. However, the requirements for these methods include a reasonably volatile extracting solvent and stability of the analyte at the boiling point of the solvent.

To extract an analyte with ionizable groups, it is best to first solubilize the solid sample in an aqueous solution. The pH of the sample solution is then adjusted below the pK_a of acidic components or above the pK_a of basic components with the addition of acid or base, respectively, to convert the analyte, 95% or greater, into its extractable (nonionized) form. A nomogram relating pK_a values of acids to percent ionization at various pH values has been published by Hopgood.[56] If the pK_a of the analyte is not known, a lowering of the pH of the aqueous solution to a pH of 2.0 by the addition of acid is usually sufficient to permit the extraction of most acidic analytes. Likewise, raising the pH to 12 is usually sufficient to permit the extraction of most basic analytes of unknown pK_a.

For liquid-liquid extraction, an increase in the ionic strength of the aqueous layer will enhance the ease of extraction of the analyte, causing it to favor the extracting solvent. An ionic neutral salt, such as sodium chloride or potassium bromide, is commonly used for this purpose.

One of the problems frequently encountered in liquid-liquid extractions is the formation of emulsions, that is, one of the immiscible phases becomes dispersed as fine droplets in the other. To avoid emulsion formation, several precautions can be taken during the actual extraction process: (1) If the two liquid layers have a large contact surface, avoid vigorous mixing of the phases. The use of gentle agitation will accomplish the extraction. (2) Filter all finely divided particulate matter before extraction. (3) Use solvent pairs with large differences in density.

If an emulsion does form, there are several steps that will possibly break it. First, try to get the dispersed droplets to achieve coalescence by mechanically disrupting their surfaces. Stirring with a glass rod or filtration through a loose bed of glass wool will sometimes break the emulsion. Second, if the densities of the two solvents are sufficiently different, centrifugation will sometimes effect separation. Third, cooling or freezing the mixture sometimes causes a coalescence of droplets. Fourth, an increase in ionic strength, by the addition of salt or a small amount of an alcohol, such as ethanol or 2-ethyl-1-hexanol, may cause a decrease in the forces stabilizing the emulsion. Fifth, a change in the ratio of the two solvents by addition of more extraction solvent or a partial evaporation of solvent may break the emulsion. Finally, filtration through phase-separation filter paper will break many emulsions commonly encountered.

In most cases, one of these procedures will be successful in breaking the emulsion. For examples of the use of solvent extraction techniques, see the procedures for the analysis of drugs in Chapter 51.

Processing of sample extracts

Many analyte extracts are too dilute for direct chromatographic analysis or for derivatization reactions before chromatography and are usually concentrated by evaporation of the extracting solvent.

Any solvent-evaporation procedure must be conducted with care to avoid loss of the analyte. Such a loss of analyte can occur if traces of water are present in the extract. These can be removed by use of an anhydrous salt, such as sodium carbonate or sodium sulfate. Alternative desiccating salts, such as calcium oxide or magnesium sulfate, can also be used. Other purposes for drying an extract may be to conduct subsequently a derivatization procedure, such as acetylation or silylization, or to prevent interference with the chromatography step.

During concentration of an extract, one must take care to avoid losses of the analyte. The analyte may be lost by irreversibly binding to the walls of the concentration vessel during concentration. This can be avoided by prior silylization of the glassware. Some substances are sufficiently volatile to form azeotrope mixtures with the solvent and be lost during evaporation. To avoid this, many gentle concentration methods or apparatuses are available. MicroSynder or Kurderna-Danish concentrators evaporate solvent under mild conditions. If the analyte is heat sensitive or sensitive to oxygen, evaporation of the solvent under a stream of purified inert gas, such as nitrogen or argon, can be employed. In this case, one can warm the vessel to a range of 35° to 50° C to expedite the evaporation process. The use of a rotary evaporator under reduced pressure is also a gentle method for solvent evaporation. A comparison of solvent reduction methods has been made by Constable et al[57] wherein recoveries of analytes varied from 41% to 140%, depending on the method employed. These results emphasize the importance of method validation and the key role that quality assurance samples, such as samples spiked with analyte, play in the use of a specific approach to cleanup.

Another method for concentrating the analyte is the back-extraction of the compound of interest from the solvent. For example, Kossa and associates[58] have published a variety of methods whereby the analyte, in the original extracting solvent, is backextracted into a small volume of analyte-derivatizing solvent before gas chromatography. Methods of this type expedite the analysis, since solvent-evaporation steps are not required. Other examples of analyte cleanup procedures for preparing samples for chromatography are detailed in the review by Ko and Petzold[59] and Sunshine.[60] Additional examples are given in Chapters 6 and 7 on HPLC and GC and for individual analytes.

REFERENCES

1. Anderson DJ, Van Lente F, Apple FS, et al: Clinical chemistry, *Anal Chem* 63:165R-270R, 1991.
2. Eiceman GA, Clement RE, Hill HH Jr: Gas chromatography, *Anal Chem* 64:170R-180R, 1992.
3. Dorsey JG, Foley JB, Cooper WWT, et al: Liquid chromatography: theory and methodology, *Anal Chem* 64:353R-389R, 1992.
4. Sherma J: Planar chromatography, *Anal Chem* 64:134R-147R, 1992.
5. Tswett MS: *Chromatographic absorption analysis: selected works.* In Berezken VG, compiler; Masson MR, translation editor: Ellis Horwood Series in Analytical Chemistry, New York, 1990, E. Horwood Publishing.
6. Heftman E: History of chromatography. In Heftman E, editor: *Chromatography: fundamentals and applications of chromatography and related differential migration methods,* ed 5, Journal of Chromatography Library, vol 51Aa, New York, 1992, Elsevier Science Publishers.
7. Strain HH, Svec WA: Differential methods of analysis. In Heftman E, editor: *Chromatography: a laboratory handbook of chromatography methods,* ed 3, New York, 1975, Van Nostrand Reinhold Co.
8. Kalasz H, Ettre LS: *Chromatography: the state of the art,* Wellingborough, U.K., 1984, Collets.
9. Ettre LS: The development of chromatography, *Anal Chem* 43:20A-21A, 25A, 27A-31A, 1971.
10. Laitinen HA, Ewing GW, editors: *A history of analytical chemistry,* Washington, D.C., 1977, Analytical Chemistry Division of American Chemical Society.
11. Giddings JC: Reduced plate height equation: a common link between chromatographic methods, *J Chromatogr* 13:301-304, 1964.
12. Schoenmakers OJ: *Optimization of chromatographic selectivity: a guide to method development,* New York, 1986, Elsevier.
13. Wong HY: *Therapeutic drug monitoring and toxicology,* Chromatographic Science Series, vol 32, New York, 1985, Marcel Dekker.
14. Snyder LR, Glajch JL, Kirkland JJ: *Practical HPLC method development,* New York, 1988, Wiley & Sons.
15. Sherma J, Fried B, editors: *Thin layer chromatography,* Chromatographic Science Series, vol 55, New York, 1990, Marcel Dekker.
16. Snyder LR: A rapid approach to selecting the best experimental conditions for high speed liquid column chromatography. 1. Estimating initial sample resolution and the final resolution required by a given problem, *J Chromatogr Sci* 10:200-212, 1972.
17. Katz E: *Quantitative analysis using chromatographic techniques,* New York, 1987, Wiley & Sons.
18. Giddings JC: Non-equilibrium and diffusion: a common basis for theories of chromatography, *J Chromatogr* 2:44-52, 1959.
19. Snyder LR, Kirkland JJ: *Introduction of modern liquid chromatography,* ed 2, New York, 1979, Wiley & Sons.
20. Martin AJP, Synge RLM: A new form of chromatogram employing two liquid phases. I. A theory of chromatography. II. Application to the micro-determinations of the higher monoamino-acids in proteins, *Biochem J* 35:1358-1368, 1941.
21. Van Deemter JJ, Zuiderweg FJ, Klinkenberg A: Longitudinal diffusion and resistance to mass transfer as causes of nonideality in chromatography, *Chem Engl Sci* 5:271-289, 1956.
22. Grob RL: *Modern practice of gas chromatography,* ed 2, New York, 1985, Wiley & Sons.
23. Rotzsche H: *Stationary phases in gas chromatography,* Journal of Chromatography Library, vol 48, New York, 1991, Elsevier Science Publishers.
24. Knapp DR: *Handbook of analytical derivatization reactions,* New York, 1979, Wiley & Sons.
25. McMahon DH: Methods development guidelines for chemical derivatization in gas chromatography, *J Chromatogr Sci* 23:426-428, 1985.
26. Lawrence JF: Advantages and limitations of chemical derivatization for trace analysis by liquid chromatography, *J Chromatogr Sci* 23:484-487, 1985.
27. Lingeman H, Underberg WJM, editors: *Detection-oriented derivatization techniques in liquid chromatography,* Chromatographic Science Series, vol 48, New York, 1990, Marcel Dekker.
28. West SD: The prediction of reversed-phase HPLC retention indices and resolution as a function of solvent strength and selectivity, *J Chromatogr Sci* 25:122-129, 1987.
29. Keller RA, Snyder LR: Relation between the solubility parameter and the liquid-solid solvent strength parameter, *J Chromatogr Sci* 9:345-459, 1971.
30. Karger BL, Snyder LR, Eon C: An expanded solubility parameter treatment for classification and use of chromatographic solvents and absorbents: parameters for dispersion, dipole, and hydrogen bonding interactions, *J Chromatogr* 125:71-88, 1976.
31. Snyder LR: Solvent selection for separation processes. In Perry ES, Weissberger A, editors: *Techniques of chemistry: separation and purification,* ed 3, vol 12, New York, 1978, Wiley & Sons.
32. Glajch JL, Kirkland JJ, Squire KM, Minor JM: Optimization of solvent strength and selectivity for reverse-phase liquid chromatography using an interactive mixture-design statistical technique. *J Chromatogr* 199:57-59, 1980.
33. Snyder LR: Classification of the solvent properties of common liquids, *J Chromatogr* 92:223-230, 1974.
34. Hildebrand JH, Scott RI: *The solubility of non-electrolytes,* ed 3, New York, 1964, Dover Publications; and Hildebrand JH, Scott RI: *Regular solutions,* Englewood Cliffs, N.J., 1962, Prentice-Hall.
35. Snyder LR: Solvent selection for separation processes. In Perry ES, Weissberger A, editors: *Techniques of chemistry: separation and purification,* ed 3, vol 12, New York, 1978, Wiley & Sons.
36. Trappe W: Die Trennung von biologischen Fettstoffen aus ihren naturlichen Gemischen durch Anwendung von Adsorptionssäulen. 1. Mitteilung: Die eluotrope Reihe der Lösungsmittel, *Biochem Z* 305:150-161, 1940.
37. Rohrschneider L: Eine Methode zur Charakterisierung von gaschromatographischen Trennflüssigkeiten, *J Chromatogr* 22:6-22, 1966.
38. McReynolds WO: Characterization of some liquid phases, *J Chromatogr Sci* 8:685-691, 1970.
39. Zlatkin A, Kaiser RE: *HPTLC: high performance thin-layer chromatography,* Journal of Chromatography Library Series 9, New York, 1977, Elsevier Scientific Publishing.
40. Touchstone JC: *Practice of thin layer chromatography,* ed 3, New York, 1992, Wiley & Sons.
41. Halasz I, Sebastian I: New stationary phase for chromatography, *Angew Chem, Int Ed* 8:453-454, 1969.
42. Anderson DMW: Gel permeation chromatography. In Simpson CF, editor: *Practical high performance liquid chromatography,* Philadelphia, 1978, Heyden & Sons.

43. Hunt BJ, Holding SR, editors: *Size exclusion chromatography,* New York, 1989, Chapman & Hall.
44. Tabor MW: Chemical analysis for assessment and evaluation of environmental pollutants: fact or artifact, *Environ Sci Res* 38:205-214, 1990.
45. Smith CC, Khalil A, Tabor MW: Fractionation of urinary and fecal metabolites of the antimalarial drug WR-158,122 following oral doses in rats and rhesus monkey, *Toxicologist* 3:52, 1983.
46. Que Hee SS, Ward JA, Tabor MW, Suskind RR: Screening method for Aroclor 1254 in whole blood, *Anal Chem* 55:157-160, 1983.
47. Stolman A, Pranitis PA: XAD-2 resin drug extraction methods for biologic samples, *Clin Toxicol* 10:49-60, 1977.
48. Weissman N, Lowe ML, Beattie JM, Demetriou JA: Screening method for detection of drugs of abuse in human urine, *Clin Chem* 17:875-881, 1971.
49. Shackleton CHL, Whitney JD: Use of Sep-Pak cartridges for urinary steroid extraction: evaluation of the method for use prior to gas chromatographic analysis, *Clin Chim Acta* 107:231-243, 1980.
50. Heikkinen R, Fotsis T, Adlercreutz H: Reversed-phase C18 cartridge for extraction of estrogens from urine and plasma, *Clin Chem* 27:1186-1189, 1981.
51. Tabor MW, Loper JC: Analytical isolation, separation and identification of mutagens from nonvolatile organics of drinking water, *Int J Environ Anal Chem* 19:281-318, 1985.
52. Horning EC, Horning MG: Metabolic profiles: gas-phase methods for analysis of metabolites, *Clin Chem* 17:802-809, 1971.
53. Riddick JA, Bunger WB: Organic solvents. In Weissberger A, editor: *Techniques of chemistry,* vol 2, ed 3, New York, 1978, Wiley & Sons.
54. DeZeeuw RA, Jonkman JHG, van Mansvelt FJW: Plasticizers as contaminants in high purity solvents: a potential source of interference in biological analysis, *Anal Biochem* 67:339-341, 1975.
55. Denney DW, Karsek FW: Detection and identification of contaminants from foil-lined screw-cap sample vials, *J Chromatogr* 151:75-80, 1978.
56. Hopgood MF: Nomogram for calculating percentage ionization of acids and bases, *J Chromatogr* 47:45-50, 1970.
57. Constable DJC, Smith SR, Tanaka J: Comparison of solvent reduction methods for concentration of polycyclic aromatic hydrocarbon solutions, *Environ Sci Technol* 18:975-978, 1984.
58. Kossa WC, MacGee J, Ramachandran S, Webber AJ: Pyrolytic methylation/gas chromatography: a short review, *J Chromatogr Sci* 17:177-187, 1979.
59. Ko H, Petzold EN: Isolation of samples prior to chromatography. In Tsuji K, Morozowich W, editors: *GLC and HPLC determination of therapeutic agents,* part 1, New York, 1978, Marcel Dekker.
60. Sunshine I: *Manual of analytical toxicology,* Boca Raton, Fla, 1971, CRC Press, Inc.

BIBLIOGRAPHY
Books
American Society of Testing Materials: *ASTM standards on chromatography,* ed 2, ASTM Subcommittee E19.07 on Compilation of Chromatographic Methods, Philadelphia, 1989, ASTM.
Grob RL: *Modern practice of gas chromatography,* ed 2, New York, 1985, Wiley & Sons.
Heftman E: *Chromatography: fundamentals and applications of chromatography and related differential migration methods,* ed 5, Journal of Chromatography Library, vol 51 A and B, New York, 1992, Elsevier Science Publishers.
Papadoyannis IN: *HPLC in clinical chemistry,* Chromatographic Science Series, vol 54, New York, 1990, Marcel Dekker.
Sherma J, Fried B, editors: *Thin layer chromatography,* Chromatographic Science Series, vol 55, New York, 1990, Marcel Dekker.
Snyder LR, Glajch JL, Kirkland JJ: *Practical HPLC method development,* New York, 1988, Wiley & Sons.

Comprehensive abstracts, journals, and series in chromatography
Advances in Chromatography, New York, Marcel Dekker, Inc.
Analytical Abstracts, London, Royal Society of Chemistry.
Chemical Abstracts, Columbus, Ohio, American Chemical Society.
Chromatographia, New York, Pergamon Press.
Chromatographic Reviews, Amsterdam, Elsevier Scientific Publishing Co.
Chromatographic Science Series, New York, Marcel Dekker, Inc.
Chromatography Symposium Series, New York, Elsevier Scientific Publishing Co.
Gas and Liquid Chromatography Abstracts, Barking, Essex, Applied Science Publishers.
Gas Chromatography Abstracts, London, Butterworth & Co.
Journal of Chromatography, New York, Elsevier Scientific Publishing Co.
Journal of Chromatography Library, New York, Elsevier Scientific Publishing Co.
Journal of Chromatographic Science, Niles, Ill., Preston Publications.
Journal of High Resolution Chromatography and Chromatography Communications, Heidelberg, N.Y., Muthing Press.
Journal of Liquid Chromatography, New York, Marcel Dekker, Inc.
Progress in Thin-Layer Chromatography and Related Methods, Ann Arbor, Mich., Lewis Publishers.

CHAPTER 6

Liquid chromatography

David J. Anderson
Larry D. Bowers

OBJECTIVES

- Describe the advantage of using peak height or peak area to quantitate an analyte using liquid chromatography.

- Define external standardization, internal standardization, and standard addition; explain how unknown concentrations are determined with each standardization process; state the requirements for internal standard selection and use.

- Discuss the various liquid chromatographic modes used to separate molecules and discuss the factors to consider in choosing the appropriate mode.

- Describe the different types of packing material that are

commercially available, detailing the advantages and disadvantages of each.

- Diagram the basic column liquid chromatographic system; list four basic components of a high-performance liquid chromatography (HPLC) separation system and state the purpose of each.

- List four types of detector systems used in HPLC and, for each, describe the principle of operation, its practical use, and the advantages or disadvantages associated with its use.

- Summarize the applications of HPLC in the analysis of clinically relevant compounds.

KEY TERMS

bonded phase A chromatographic packing material in which the stationary phase is covalently bound to the surface of the support.

efficiency Characteristic of a column or packing material that describes the extent of broadening of the chromatographic peak. Higher efficiencies lead to narrower chromatographic peaks.

effluent Mobile phase that has left the column.

eluate A compound or mixture that has been separated in the column and left it.

eluent Mobile phase.

gradient elution An elution system where the solvent composition is varied during the run.

H Height equivalent to one theoretical plate (HETP).

isocratic elution Elution with a solvent mixture of constant composition.

L Length of the chromatographic column, usually in millimeters.

mobile phase The mixture of solvents that is percolated through the column.

μ Solvent velocity in the column ($\mu = L/t_0$).

N Number of theoretical separating plates in a chromatographic column.

normal phase A chromatographic mode in which the mobile phase is less polar than the stationary phase.

packing material Term referring to the material that is placed ("packed") into the chromatographic column, consisting of both the stationary phase and the support.

permeability A measure of the ease with which the mobile phase can be forced through the column.

R_s Resolution; the degree of separation between two eluates.

reversed phase A chromatographic mode in which the mobile phase is more polar than the stationary phase.

stationary phase The portion of the separation system that is immobilized in the column.

support The particles on which the stationary phase is held.

t_0 Time required to elute an unretained substance.

t_R Retention time; the time required to elute a compound from a chromatographic column.

V_0 Volume of solvent required to elute an unretained compound; also called *void volume*.

V_R Retention volume; the volume of the mobile phase required to elute a compound from a chromatographic column at t_R.

Liquid chromatography is a form of separation science in which a liquid mobile phase is percolated through a column or thin layer of particles. Fig. 6-1 shows a schematic diagram of a column chromatograph used in liquid chromatography. The liquid mobile phase is taken from the reservoir and moved through the column, usually by a pump. A method of introducing the sample into the chromatographic system is also required. The most important constituent of a chromatographic instrument is the column. The column is filled with *packing material,* which consists of small particles *(support)* on which specific sites or a layer of solvent (both referred to as *stationary phase*) is held. The differential equilibration of the analytes between the mobile and the stationary phases results in their separation. All chromatographic modes (see Chapter 5) can be used in liquid chromatography. Finally, we can either collect the column effluent for further analysis or analyze the effluent with an on-line detector, such as a photometer. Aliquots of the liquid phase can be collected if subsequent analysis is de-

sired. The recording of any parameter that allows the analyte or analytes to be monitored as a function of elution volume or time is called a *chromatogram.*

Liquid chromatography is well suited for use in the clinical laboratory. Since the retention of a compound is determined by equilibria, the position of the peak in the chromatogram (that is, the retention volume) can be helpful in analytical identification. If a substance coelutes with a known compound, it may be the same material; an identical retention, however, does not *prove* identity. In addition, quantitative information can be obtained by measurement of the height or area of the peak. Because the components of a mixture are separated, quantitation of several compounds in a single analysis is possible. Such quantitation is useful in the measurement of drugs or intermediates in a metabolic pathway (such as porphyrins). Another advantage of liquid chromatography is that the relatively polar compounds present in body fluids readily dissolve in commonly used mobile-phase solvents. This is in contrast to gas chromatography, which requires volatile analytes. Proteins and peptides are readily separated by liquid chromatography.

Despite the fact that liquid chromatography was discovered before gas chromatography, it was used in only a very small number of analytical applications in the clinical laboratory. Classical liquid chromatography typically required hours or days to complete a separation, whereas gas chromatography required only minutes. With the development of small (10 μm) totally porous particles in the early 1970s, liquid chromatography was able to achieve speed and resolution comparable to packed-column gas chromatography (GC). The introduction of covalently bonded stationary phases resulted in the further popularization of high-performance liquid chromatography (HPLC). Develop-

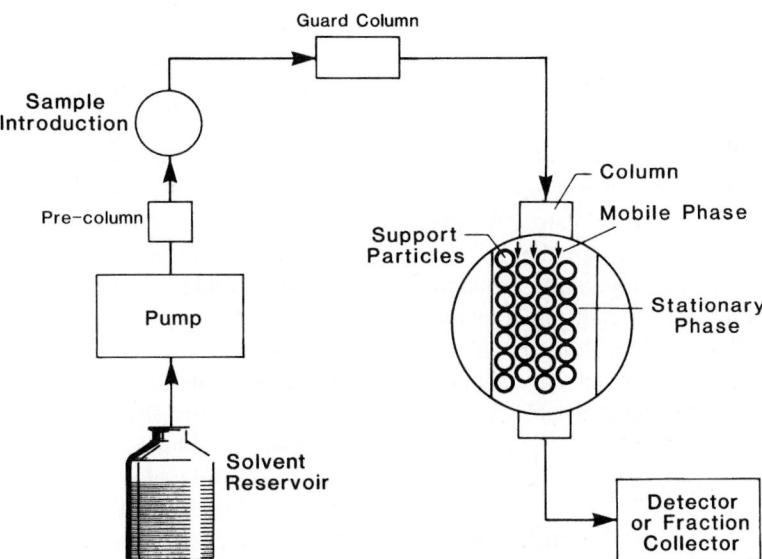

Fig. 6-1   Schematic diagram of a column liquid chromatographic system. (From Bowers LD, Carr PW: *Quantitative aspects of HPLC workshop,* Minneapolis, 1983.)

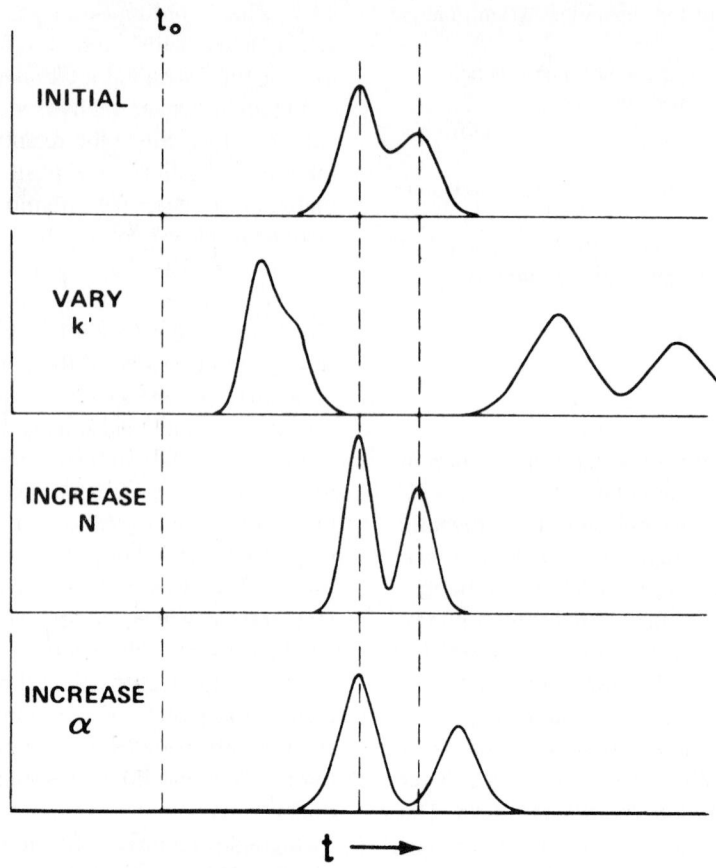

Fig. 6-2   Effect of varying *k'*, *N*, and α on a resolution. *t,* Time. (From Snyder LK, Kirkland JJ: *Introduction to modern liquid chromatography,* ed 2, New York, 1979, Wiley & Sons.)

ments, such as microprocessor automation, have made both analytical and preparative chromatography easier to perform and more appealing. At present, HPLC is recognized as a true complement to GC in chromatographic analysis.

RESOLUTION, EFFICIENCY, AND SPEED OF ANALYSIS

The object of any chromatographic technique is to separate, or resolve, the species of interest from other compounds of interest or from interferences in the sample matrix. As analysts, we must also be concerned about the speed of the analytical scheme, including any sample preparation steps, the separation itself, and the calculation and reporting of results. Not surprisingly, speed of analysis and resolving power are related. The evolution of HPLC was based on an understanding and optimization of the factors that affect resolution.

Resolution

The relative separation of two chromatographic peaks is measured by a parameter known as *resolution,* or, R_s. A further definition of R_s, as well as an example of the calculation of R_s, can be found on p. 111 of Chapter 5. It is depen-

dent on the positions of the centers of the peaks that correspond to each compound and on the width of the peak between the points where it is indistinguishable from the background signal. If the peak tracing reaches the background level before rising for the second peak, baseline resolution has been achieved. If the first peak shown in the bottom panel of Fig. 6-2 were collected up to the minimum in the valley between the two peaks, the compound in that peak would be 100% free of the compound making up the second peak. When the baseline resolution is not achieved (Fig. 6-2, top), some of the compound present in the second peak will be collected along with the compound in the first peak. Table 6-1 shows the relative impurity in the first peak for various resolution values when both peaks are the same size. Snyder and Kirkland have covered this topic more completely.[1] Resolution of peaks will also affect quantitation as discussed later.

Because resolution depends on peak widths, resolution must be controlled by the factors that govern the peak width, namely, efficiency (*N*, number of theoretical plates) and relative peak retention. Peak retention is determined by the capacity factor *(k')* and selectivity (α) as discussed in Chapter 5. Equation 6-1 gives an expression for calculating resolution from these factors.

Table 6-1 Effect of resolution on various peak parameters*

Resolution	Purity†	% error in area‡	% error in peak height‡
0.6	90	>−25	~15
0.8	95	−10	1
1.0	98	−3	<1
1.25	99.5	<−1	0
1.5	100	0	0

*Assuming a peak-height ratio of 1 to 1 for the two components.
†Purity of major peak, assuming collection is stopped at the lowest point of the valley between the peaks.
‡Error for the smaller peak.

$$R_s = \left(\frac{\sqrt{N}}{4}\right)\left(\frac{\alpha - 1}{\alpha}\right)\left(\frac{k'}{1 + k'}\right) \qquad \textit{Eq. 6-1}$$

The effect of changes in each of these parameters on resolution is illustrated in Fig. 6-2.

Chromatographic efficiency

Chromatographic efficiency (p. 112 of Chapter 5) is a characteristic of a column or packing material describing the extent of broadening of the chromatographic peak. Higher efficiencies lead to narrower peaks, increased resolution, and increased sensitivity. The efficiency of a column can be estimated quantitatively from the van Deemter equation:

$$H = A + B/\mu + C\mu \qquad \textit{Eq. 6-2}$$

where H is the height of the theoretical plate, μ is the mobile-phase velocity, and A, B, and C are constants, the values of which depend on fundamental parameters of the chromatographic system as given below:

$$A = 2\lambda d_p \qquad \textit{Eq. 6-3}$$

$$B = 2\lambda D_m \qquad \textit{Eq. 6-4}$$

$$C = \frac{(1 + 6k' + 11k'^2)\, d_p^2}{24\,(1 + k')^2 D_m} + \frac{8k' d_f^2}{\pi^2\,(1 + k')^2 D_s} \qquad \textit{Eq. 6-5}$$

where d_p is the particle diameter of the packing material, d_f is the thickness of the stationary-phase layer, D_m and D_s are diffusion coefficients of the analyte in the mobile and stationary phase respectively, k' is the capacity factor, and λ and γ are correction factors taking into account column packing inhomogeneity. Each term in equation 6-2 is descriptive of different processes in liquid chromatography that lead to band spreading, with the A, B, and C terms giving the contributions of the multipath effect (eddy diffusion), longitudinal diffusion, and mass transfer (both in the mobile and stationary phases) respectively. Other expressions quantitating efficiency have been suggested; however, the van Deemter equation appears to be the most appropriate to use.[2] Several books giving more details on theoretical aspects of efficiency as they apply to chromatography have been published.[2-4]

The important conclusions to be drawn from equations 6-2 to 6-5 are that efficiency increases (H decreases) with (1) decreased particle diameter of the packing material; (2) decreased flow velocity of the mobile phase; and (3) increased diffusion coefficient of the analyte. It should be noted that the role of longitudinal diffusion (B term in equation 6-2) is significant only at low flow velocities, lower than the flow velocities commonly used in HPLC. The major design feature employed for increasing efficiency of HPLC systems has been the use of small-diameter packing materials. HPLC techniques typically utilize packing materials having diameters of 10, 5, and 3 μm. Use of packing materials of particle diameter less than 3 μm is not normally done because of the high pressure that would be generated with the pumping of mobile phase through the column. Also evident from equations 6-2 to 6-5 is the effect of the analyte's diffusion coefficient on efficiency. As seen from equation 6-5, macromolecules, which have smaller diffusion coefficients, will give broader peaks than smaller molecules, which have larger diffusion coefficients. In general, modern HPLC columns have about 10,000 theoretical plates for smaller molecules.

For the practicing chromatographer, four final points about efficiency are worthy of mention. First, a new column should always be tested upon receipt to be sure that reasonable efficiency is obtained with that column. An initial efficiency value also serves as a benchmark for measuring the decline in column performance as it is used. Second, the column should be tested under the manufacturer's flow and mobile-phase conditions. The buyer should be aware that a column tested at 0.1 mL/min to obtain a high number of theoretical plates may not be the best column to use at more practical flow rates. Third, N is in reality a measure of system efficiency. Thus a poorly designed detector can make the best column look bad. To achieve the high efficiencies reported by some column manufacturers, the entire system must be optimized. Finally, remember that to enhance resolution twofold, one must increase N fourfold. Thus adjustment of N is normally used to fine-tune a relatively good separation.

The retention of a compound on a column is often described by using its *capacity factor, k'* (see p. 113 of Chapter 5). The capacity factor is a normalizing factor that allows retention on different-sized columns, or columns operated at different flow rates, to be compared because the k', by definition, is related to the equilibrium of the analyte between the mobile and stationary phases. In terms of resolution, k' values over 5 do not increase resolution much and can, in fact, slow analysis and deteriorate the limit of detection. In liquid chromatography, k' is adjusted primarily by changes in mobile-phase composition, though it is also inversely related to the temperature.

The difference in retention of two compounds as measured by the ratio of their capacity factors is called the *selectivity,* or α (see p. 115 of Chapter 5). Note that if α is large there will be a large difference in the retention volumes of the two compounds, and we can perform the separation with few plates and little column retention. Selectivity is frequently adjusted by changes in mobile-phase composition. One of the major advantages of liquid chromatography is the wide range of selectivity achievable by varying the composition of the mobile phase. For example, an ion-exchange separation depends on the number of charges on the analytes. We can change the selectivity by varying the mobile-phase pH, ionic strength, or salt composition (NaCl versus LiCl). Selection of a mobile-phase system requires an understanding of the separation mechanisms and a great deal of experience. A change in the stationary phase can also be used to adjust selectivity because the equilibrium achieved between the stationary phase and the mobile phase is the basis of any chromatographic separation. If the retention of the analytes is adequate ($1.5 \leq k' \leq 6$), one can improve the resolution most readily by changing the selectivity.

Speed of analysis

So far, we have discussed retention only in terms of mobile-phase volume, V_R, because (1) the volume of mobile phase used is a direct reflection of cost and (2) changes in the flow rate do not affect the V_R. In contrast, the retention time, t_R, is a function of flow rate and retention volume, that is:

$$t_R = \frac{V_R}{F} \qquad \textit{Eq. 6-6}$$

where F is the flow rate in milliliters per minute. For example, if the diameter of the column were doubled, its volume and thus the retention volume would increase by a factor of 4. We could keep t_R constant by increasing the flow rate by a factor of 4, but solvent consumption would increase accordingly.

The optimization of analysis speed depends on several factors. The most important relationships in achieving a rapid separation are given in the box. Guichon has discussed these factors in great detail.[5] The minimum time possible for a separation is the product of the time required for an analyte to pass one plate and the number of plates required

---

Practical Considerations in Speed of Analysis

$$t_R = N \cdot \frac{H}{\mu} \cdot (1 + k')$$

$$L = NH$$

$$\Delta P = NH\mu \cdot \frac{\eta}{K_0}$$

μ, Solvent velocity in the column (= L/t_0); η, solvent viscosity; K_0, column permeability. (See reference 5 for more detail.) ΔP, Column back-pressure.

---

for adequate resolution. The smaller the height of a theoretical plate, H, the faster the separation. Retention time is also increased by the need for more resolution; by small selectivities, α; and by large capacity factors, k'. Again, to obtain the fastest separations, a mobile phase must be selected to maximize α at relatively small values of k'. Under optimal conditions for a separation requiring 3000 plates, an analysis time of 100 seconds is feasible with HPLC. One of the problems in translating theory to practice in the clinical laboratory is that the analyte may have to be separated from an unknown metabolite or interferent, and hence α is not known during the development of the separation. In this case, a slower separation time is acceptable, and the selectivity of the detector must be relied upon to indicate a potential problem.

QUANTITATION
Approaches

Quantitation in liquid chromatography is achieved when one relates either the peak height or the peak area to the concentration of analyte in the sample. The chromatographic trace is a recording of the concentration of the analyte or analytes as sensed by the detector. At the peak height maximum

$$C_{max} = \frac{C_s V_s}{V_R} \sqrt{\frac{N}{2\pi}} \qquad \textit{Eq. 6-7}$$

C_s and V_s are the concentration and volume of sample injected respectively, V_R is the retention volume, and N is the number of theoretical plates. The greater the peak height for any given concentration, the more sensitive is the method. Thus minimizing the retention volume and maximizing the number of theoretical plates will result in the most sensitive assay. The factors that decrease the retention volume are a small column void volume and a small capacity factor. Large plate counts can be achieved by low flow rates and small support-particle diameters. Also note that, unlike the sensitivity of gas chromatography, liquid chromatographic sensitivity is improved by injection of larger sample volumes. The peak height can be related to the concentration in the sample by a sensitivity factor, S. The sensitivity factor will change if the retention volume changes, making day-to-day operation without standardization difficult but not impossible.

Example. If an identical sample were injected onto a 4.6 mm internal diameter (ID) and a 2.1 mm ID column, what would be the relative size of the peaks if all else were unchanged?

$$C_{max} = \frac{1}{V_R}\left[C_s V_s \sqrt{\frac{N}{2\pi}} \right] = \frac{1}{\Phi \pi r^2 L}[\bar{C}] \qquad \textit{Eq. 6-8}$$

where Φ is the void fraction, r is the radius, and L is the length (15 cm) of the column; $\overline{C}$ is the mass injected into the column. If Φ and L are the same for the two columns, then

$$\frac{C_{\max}(2.1)}{C_{\max}(4.6)} = \frac{(2.3)^2}{(1.05)^2} = 4.8 \qquad \textit{Eq. 6-9}$$

Therefore the peak from the 2.1 mm column would be almost five times as large. This sensitivity advantage is causing increased interest in microbore columns.

How much of a decrease in length would be necessary to observe a similar increase in peak height? What would the decrease in length change that the decrease in radius would not (k'; α; *or N*)?

The second approach to quantitation of an analyte is measurement of the peak area. Although other methods of integration are available microprocessor-based integrators have become so inexpensive that they are the most reasonable means of measuring peak areas. Most liquid chromatography detectors are concentration dependent; that is, they measure a concentration in the flow cell. (This is in contrast to most GC detectors, which are mass-flow dependent.) The peak area obtained from a concentration-dependent detector is inversely proportional to flow rate. Therefore significant variation in peak area can occur if the flow rate changes during a chromatographic run. In addition, less resolution is required for an equal degree of accuracy when peak heights rather than peak areas are used because the overlap of peaks, even with a resolution of 1.0, affects peak area but does not affect the peak maximum.[1] A rough rule of thumb is: Use peak *height* when there are interfering peaks or when maximum accuracy is required, but use peak area when precision is the main requirement. For peaks barely above the baseline noise, peak heights should always be used.

Standardization

Standardization in liquid chromatography (LC) can be accomplished in any of three ways: external standardization, internal standardization, or standard addition. For external standardization, a calibration curve is constructed from the peak height (or peak area) values obtained with known concentrations of analyte and a constant injection volume. The slope of the curve is the sensitivity factor, *S,* in peak-height units per concentration unit (such as mm/mM). The concentration of the unknown is then simply its peak height divided by the sensitivity factor. Notice that, if the calibration curve is linear, the sensitivity factor can be obtained from a single standard. It would be important in this case to check several control specimens to verify the validity of the sensitivity factor. The principal sources of error in external calibration are variable losses in the preparative steps before LC analysis and sample-injection variability. It is thus important to treat the standards and samples in the same way. It should be possible to achieve 1% precision with external calibration, but up to 5% is commonly observed.

Internal standardization uses a compound that is usually structurally similar to the analyte to correct for losses during sample preparation and injection imprecision. The same amount of internal standard is added to each sample and standard before sample pretreatment and chromatography. The calibration curve is then constructed from the ratio of the peak heights (or areas) of the standard and the internal standard at various standard concentrations (Fig. 6-3). Again, one can measure unknown concentrations by using the sensitivity factor or interpolating the value from the calibration curve. It is hoped that any losses or variations that occur will affect the analyte and internal standard equivalently. In practice, this is difficult to achieve. An internal standard can be used not only to improve accuracy and precision but also as a quality control check because its peak height should be the same in all chromatograms. Several requirements must be met in the selection of an internal standard. These are summarized in the box on page 134. In some cases internal standards do not improve precision and accuracy and may deteriorate precision because of the imprecision involved in measuring two peaks. The precision that can be attained with HPLC has been studied, and sources of error have been analyzed.[6]

The final calibration method, standard addition, requires two analyses to be performed on each sample and thus is not as popular as the other methods. After a sample is analyzed once, a known amount of the compound of interest is added in a very small amount of liquid so that little dilution occurs, and the sample is reanalyzed. To correct for extraction variability, the addition should be made to the biologi-

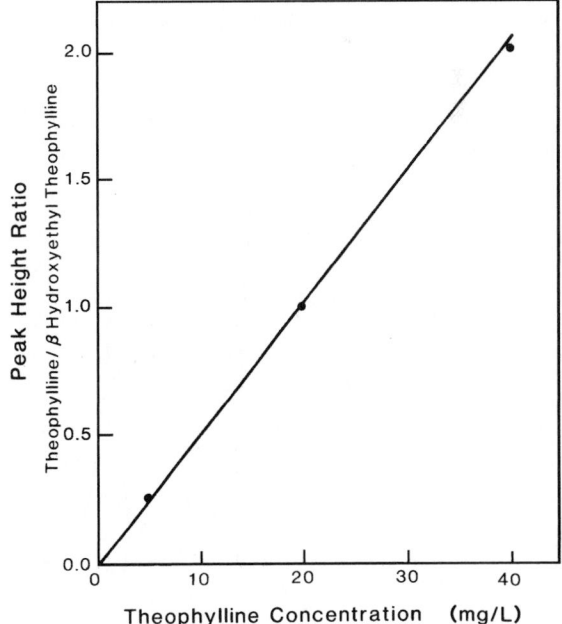

Fig. 6-3 Calibration curve for theophylline using internal standard technique.

Requirements for Internal Standard (IS) Selection and Use

1. The internal standard must be completely resolved from all peaks in the sample.
2. It must be eluted near the analyte, with k' ±30% being preferable.
3. It must behave similarly to the analyte in pretreatment if losses are to be corrected. This may require more than one internal standard.
4. It must have a peak height or area approximately equal to a standard in the concentration range desired.
5. It must not normally be present in the sample.
6. It should be commercially available in pure form.
7. It should be added as a liquid.

---

cal fluid and the entire analytical scheme repeated. Quantitative data can be obtained from the ratio of the peak height (or area) before and after addition of the standard. Addition of the standard can also help to verify the identity of the peak because the standard must coelute for the unknown to be the same compound. The converse is not true, however, because more than one compound may elute at the same retention volume.

GENERAL ELUTION PROBLEM

The chromatographer is sometimes required to separate compounds that, though structurally related, behave quite differently in the separation system. In Fig. 6-4, a separation of bile acid conjugates demonstrates the problem. When the mobile-phase composition is adjusted to achieve resolution of peaks 2 and 3, peak 8 is retained for over 30

minutes. Since there are no other peaks near peak 8, the excessive baseline value present between peaks 7 and 8 is a waste of valuable analysis time. A mobile phase with a constant composition is referred to as *isocratic*. The alternative to this is to change the mobile-phase composition during the chromatographic run. This can be done as a single change from one mobile phase to another (step gradient) or as a continuous change in any of a variety of shapes (such as linear, segmented linear, or exponential gradient). A complete treatment of gradient elution can be found in references 7 to 9. In brief, the peak retention volume, width, and resolution are determined primarily by the rate of solvent-composition change. Thus many of the concepts discussed earlier are not valid in gradient elution. Any quantitative analyses developed using gradient elution should be carefully documented. In HPLC, the ability to vary mobile-phase composition can be purchased as a part of the solvent-delivery system. It generally increases the cost of the system significantly.

A disadvantage of gradient elution is that the column requires equilibration with the original mobile-phase conditions before the next run. This can take considerable time, particularly with reversed-phase analyses. Thus, isocratic techniques are predominantly used in the clinical laboratory.

SELECTION OF A CHROMATOGRAPHIC MODE

In Chapter 5 the various mechanisms of chromatography were discussed, including ion exchange, size exclusion (gel permeation or steric exclusion), adsorption, and partition (reversed and normal phase). As mentioned previously, all these modes are available in liquid chromatography. The selection of the "best" mode is a problem of significant magnitude for the chromatographer. The choice is made based

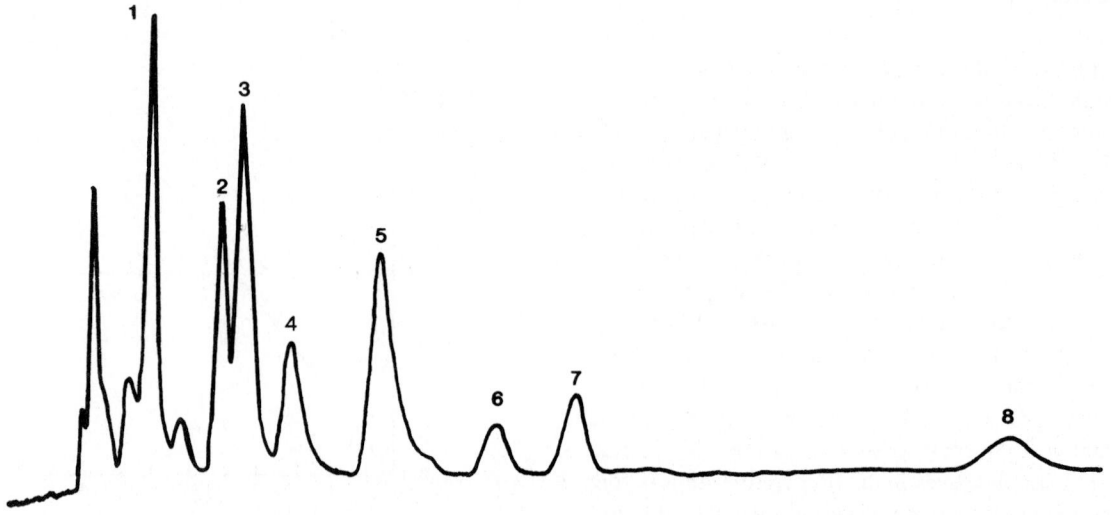

Fig. 6-4 Separation of common human bile acid conjugates by reversed-phase HPLC. Peaks correspond to taurocholate, *1;* taurochenodeoxycholate, *2;* taurodeoxycholate, *3;* taurolithocholate, *4;* glycocholate, *5;* glycochenodeoxycholate, *6;* glycodeoxycholate, *7;* and glycolithocholate, *8.* (From Roberts G, Bowers LD, unpublished data.)

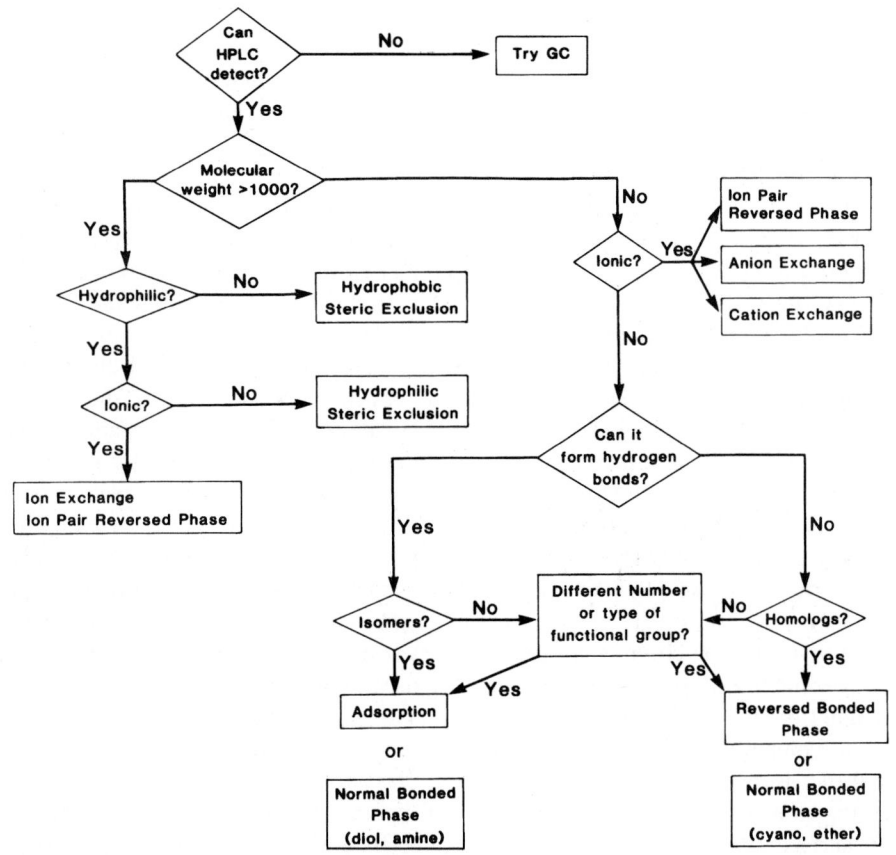

Fig. 6-5   Selection guide for chromatographic modes. (From Bowers LD, Carr PW: *Quantitative aspects of HPLC workshop,* Minneapolis, 1983.)

on an understanding of the mechanism of each mode and its strengths and weaknesses, and frequently it is accomplished by experience. Fig. 6-5 illustrates one method of selecting a chromatographic mode using mechanistic considerations. In addition to these modes, more specialized techniques have been employed, including affinity chromatography and chromatographic techniques for the determination of enantiomers.

Size-exclusion chromatography

One of the chromatographer's first considerations is the size of the molecules to be separated. If the molecules are relatively large (>100,000 daltons), *size* (or *steric*) exclusion (SEC) is a logical first choice (see Chapter 5). If, on the other hand, the molecular weights are less than 1000, steric exclusion is probably not the mode of choice.

Ion-exchange chromatography

Another key factor that affects the choice of a separation mode is if the analyte is an ion or if an ionizable group is present on the molecule. Ion exchange would be a logical choice for molecules that can be charged, regardless of molecular size. Ion exchange is based on the interaction of analyte charges with an oppositely charged group bound to the

chromatographic support. One can vary retention by varying pH or ionic strength. The greater the number of charges on the analyte, the greater is the retention. Increasing ionic strength, and with it the number of charged groups (such as Na^+) competing with the analyte for the exchange sites on the support, reduces retention. *Ion-pair* chromatography, which uses reversed-phase packing materials, can also be used to separate ionic compounds (see p. 139).

Adsorption chromatography

If the molecule has a molecular weight less than 1000 and is not ionizable, another characteristic of the compound must be used to achieve the separation. One such characteristic is the ability of the compound to form hydrogen bonds. Adsorption chromatography is based on the interaction of the analyte with a three-dimensional binding site on the support matrix, which may involve hydrogen bonding. Thus the structure and polarity of the solute are important in determining retention. For example, it would be relatively easy to separate *p*-dinitrobenzene from *o*-dinitrobenzene using adsorption chromatography because of the structural differences between the two compounds. On the other hand, separating caproic acid (with six carbon atoms) from caprylic acid (with eight carbon atoms) would be very difficult because the parts of the molecules that interact with the stationary phase are identical.

In adsorption chromatography, compounds are eluted from the column because of competition between the analyte and the solvent for the binding site. A solvent that elutes compounds more rapidly and therefore competes better for the chromatographic sites is called a "strong solvent." Water would be a strong solvent for silica adsorbents because it interacts strongly with the silanol (SiOH) groups responsible for the adsorption mechanism. A solvent that does not compete well for sites is called a "weak solvent." Hexane would be a weak solvent for silica adsorbents. One can adjust solvent strength by using mixtures of solvents. Snyder[10] has developed a scale of solvent strength called the eluotropic series and has extended the solvent strength theory to binary and ternary[11] mixtures. Interestingly, solvent mixtures of the same strength can show differences in selectivity because Snyder's theory considers only the adsorption process, whereas in reality the solute can also interact with the solvent.

One final consideration in adsorption chromatography is the control of the "activity" of the adsorbent. Silica contains several types of silanol groups, which interact differently with various types of compounds. A small amount of water, methanol, acetonitrile, isopropanol, or other strong solvent is used to block the strongest sites and give a more reproducible adsorption surface. This problem has caused some chromatographers to avoid adsorption systems, probably unnecessarily. A separation that involves nonpolar to intermediate polarity compounds that can form hydrogen bonds or that have isomeric components will probably be easily achieved with adsorption chromatography.

Partition and bonded-phase chromatography

The interactions between solute and stationary phase in partition chromatography are not nearly so well defined as those for adsorption systems. Any chemical forces that exist between molecules can be used in partition-based separations, including hydrogen bonding, van der Waals forces, ion-ion interactions, and so on (see Chapter 5). The basis of partition systems is the distribution of a solute between two liquid solvent layers, one stationary and the other mobile. It is essentially analogous to thousands of liquid extractions taking place in a column. In classical partition chromatography, a polar liquid, such as β,β'-oxydipropionitrile (β,β'-ODPN), was coated onto the support particles, and an immiscible solvent such as hexane was used as the mobile phase. Since solvent-solute interactions involve the entire molecule, a typical partition system as given here would separate a homologous series (C6, C7, and C8 carboxylic acids) and some positional isomers. A partition system with a polar stationary phase and a nonpolar mobile phase is called *normal phase* because it was the first type of system developed. Later, a system with a nonpolar stationary phase, such as squalane, and a polar

mobile phase, such as a water-acetonitrile mixture, was developed and called *reversed phase*. Both types of liquid-liquid partition chromatography had many problems related to the finite solubility of all solvents in each other. For example, the β,β'-ODPN would slowly dissolve in the hexane and slowly change the amount of stationary phase, which in turn would change the retention volumes of the analytes. The temperature had to be very closely controlled, and gradient elution was impossible with partition chromatography. These problems made partition chromatography difficult to use in the clinical laboratory.

All of this changed with the development of chemically bonded stationary phases. These materials are prepared by covalent bonding of an organic moiety onto the surface of the support particle, usually silica. The organic groups include nonpolar functions, such as octadecylsilane (ODS, or C18) or octylsilane (C8), and polar groups, such as cyanopropyl (CN), aminopropyl (NH_2), or glycidoxypropyl (diol) silanes. The advantages of bonded phases are that (1) polar and ionic compounds are readily separated, (2) the stationary phase does not strip off, (3) a gradient elution can be used, and (4) the columns are easy to use and take care of. The main disadvantage of bonded phases is that at pHs below 2 the bonded group is cleaved from the support and at pHs above 8 the silica support particles dissolve. Since most separations for clinical laboratory applications can be performed within this workable pH window, bonded phases are very popular. A separate section below has been included to discuss the variety of separations feasible with reversed-phase systems.

Reversed-phase chromatography

The discussion is expanded below for the reversed-phase chromatographic technique because of its popularity in use. In a recent survey of HPLC users, approximately 50% of the HPLC separations were performed on reversed-phase columns.[12] The most popular reversed-phase packing material is the octadecylsilane (ODS, or C18) packing material. The mobile phase in reversed phase is most commonly water containing an organic modifier such as methanol, acetonitrile, or tetrahydrofuran. In general, retention of an analyte on the reversed-phase column will depend on the relative amounts of polar and nonpolar character of the analyte, as shown in Fig. 6-6, for the amino acid tyrosine. Retention on the reversed-phase packing material is favored by increased nonpolar content of the analyte, whereas residence in the mobile phase leading to early elution from the column is favored by an increased content of polar functionalities present on the analyte. The organic modifier component of the mobile phase competes with the stationary phase for the nonpolar part of the analyte molecule, and thus retention is decreased with an increased organic modifier in the mobile phase. The mechanism of retention for bonded reversed-phase chromatography has been reviewed.[13,14] Although a partition mechanism is proposed by some (in

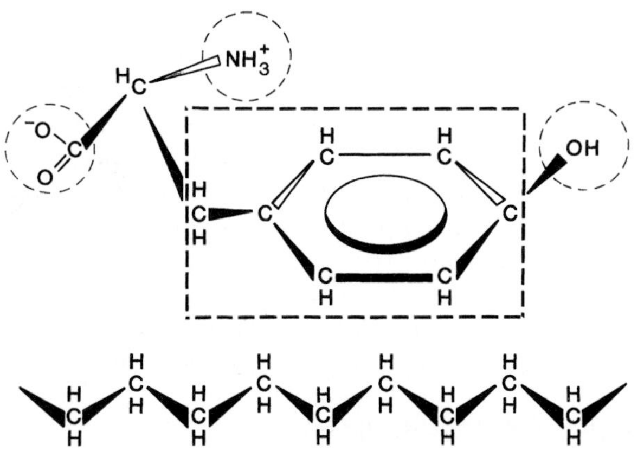

Fig. 6-6 Retention in reversed-phase chromatography is the result of the interaction of the nonpolar portion of the compound such as tyrosine *(enclosed in box)* with the nonpolar stationary phase. Hydrophilic groups *(circled)* tend to decrease retention.

which solute is fully encompassed by the stationary phase), an adsorption mechanism (in which the solute is retained on the stationary phase through surface contact only), or a combination of both, has also been proposed.

Stationary-phase considerations. As noted earlier, the separation obtained for any group of analytes is a function of both the stationary phase and the mobile phase. The analyst has the ability to vary mobile-phase conditions but is dependent on manufacturers for the stationary phase, particularly for bonded-phase packings. If one is to do reproducible chromatography, the behavior of the stationary phase toward nonpolar, polar, and ionic compounds must be the same from column to column and from lot to lot. In addition, the durability of the column is important because of their expense. Significant improvements in these features have occurred in recent years, but there are some limitations in producing a column with absolutely reproducible reversed-phase column packings.

The preparation of an octadecylsilane (ODS) stationary phase is usually accomplished when the silanol (SiOH) groups on the silica gel are reacted with an octadecylsilane such as octadecyldimethylchlorosilane. The resulting surface contains octadecyl groups bound to the surface by siloxone (Si—O—Si) bonds as shown in Fig. 6-7. Most manufacturers of columns use silanes with only one chloride group, and the resulting stationary phase is called *monomeric*. Because of the stereochemistry of the silica gel surface, only about one third of the silanol groups can react with the ODS groups. The remaining silanol groups are polar and can interact with polar analytes, changing the selectivity of the stationary phase. Trimethylchlorosilane can react with about an additional 20% of the surface silanol groups with a resultant increase in the nonpolar character of the support (Fig. 6-7). This process is called *end capping* and is used in many commercially available packing materials. As might be expected, differences in the surface morphology of the silica gel, reaction conditions in the ODS-bonding step, and the presence or absence of end capping make columns purchased from different manufacturers perform differently. In fact, variations from lot to lot of packing material may be quite noticeable in the separations obtained for certain analyses. Thus it is not surprising that in adapting a method to a laboratory one may require significant changes in the mobile phase if a C18 column from a manufacturer other than that named in the original report is used. Choice of a reversed-phase column still requires trial and error. For the novice, use of the brand of column reported in a publication is probably warranted to obtain acceptable chromatograms in a reasonable amount of time. The situation with respect to columns is improving as a better understanding of the silica backbone is achieved.

Mobile-phase considerations. The real power in liquid chromatography arises from the fact that changes in mobile-phase composition can have major effects on selectivity and thus on resolution. In reversed-phase systems, two types of changes can be made: (1) changing the type of organic solvent used and (2) additions to the mobile phase that affect its pH, ionic strength, or complexing ability. It has been recognized for some time that the type of organic solvent used has an effect on retention and selectivity. In some cases, a change from methanol to acetonitrile actually alters the elution order of the compounds. Unfortunately at this time the use of solvents to vary selectivity is

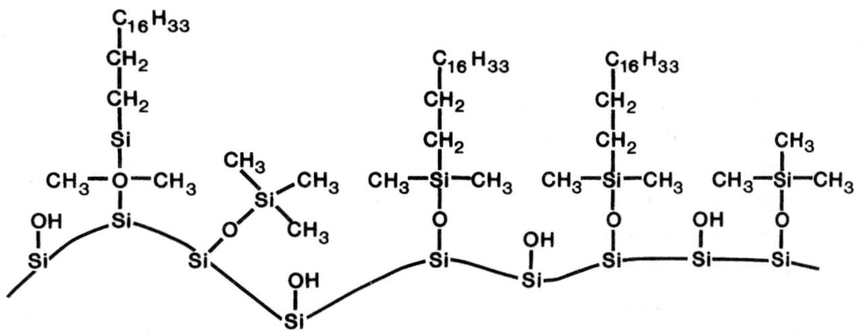

Fig. 6-7 Schematic diagram of a silica-based octadecyl reversed-phase support that has been end capped. Notice presence of residual silanol groups on surface.

largely empirical, and the exact role of each solvent in a separation is poorly defined; however, the relative strength of solvents is well defined with solvent strength and therefore the ability to elute solutes, increasing in the following order: methanol < DMSO < ethanol ≤ acetonitrile < tetrahydrofuran < dioxane < isopropanol. As a rule, when one is adjusting the retention of a solute, a 10% increase in the fraction of organic solvent (such as methanol or acetonitrile) in water causes a twofold or threefold decrease in the k' value.

Ion suppression. Mobile-phase modifications that change retention by introducing a second chemical equilibrium process in the mobile phase have been used since the inception of reversed-phase chromatography.[15] The first approach was control of pH to effect retention. If, for example, ascorbic acid was to be separated by HPLC, there would be a strong influence of pH on retention. At pHs above the pK_a of ascorbic acid, the acid would be deprotonated and charged and therefore would not partition itself strongly into the nonpolar stationary phase. Retention would be relatively low. On the other hand, at pHs below the pK_a, the acid would be protonated and uncharged and so would be much more strongly retained. In the area about one pH unit on either side of the pK_a, the retention changes rapidly as a function of pH, as shown in Fig. 6-8. The use of pH control to increase retention for acids has been termed *ion suppression*. It is a very useful method of adjusting retention behavior. Buffers are normally used to control the pH. It is important to remember that an acid-base pair is a good buffer only within one pH unit of the pK_a. Table 6-2 lists some useful buffers for reversed-phase HPLC.

Chromatography of basic compounds on conventional reversed-phase packing material. Basic compounds can be chromatographed on conventional reversed-phase packing materials by making modifications in the mobile phase. The biggest difficulty in chromatographing basic compounds on silica reversed-phase packing materials is the presence of silanol groups on the silica surface. As mentioned previously, approximately 50% of the silanol groups remain on the silica support after synthesis of the reversed-phase packing material. A small percentage of these remaining silanol groups are strongly reactive, leading to adverse chromatographic effects, including severe tailing and irreversible adsorption of basic compounds and variable retention for different reversed-phase columns. At the mobile phase pHs normally used in reversed-phase analysis (neutral pH) a basic analyte is positively charged. The highly reactive silanol groups on the silica surface, which are acidic and thus negatively charged, interact with the positively charged basic compound through an ion-exchange mechanism. Addition of amine modifiers (such as triethylamine) to the mobile phase prevents adverse chromatographic effects of silanol on basic analytes through a mechanism by which the positively charged amine modifier binds to the silanol ion-exchange sites present on the

reversed-phase packing material, thus blocking the silanol sites from interaction with the basic analyte. Low pH and high ionic-strength mobile phases, which drive the equilibrium of the silanol groups to the protonated or counter ion–associated form (which do not interact with positively charged basic compounds), are additional strategies used in conventional reversed-phase chromatography of basic compounds. In addition to the silanol ion-exchange mechanism mentioned above, silanol hydrogen bonding and metal impurities present within the silica have been implicated in the adverse chromatography effects seen for silica supports.

Ion-pair chromatography[14]

The most popular method for chromatographing ionizable analytes (such as weak bases or weak acids) as well as ionic analytes on a reversed-phase column is by ion-pair chromatography. Ion-pair chromatography has advantages over ion-suppression and ion-exchange chromatography. Use of

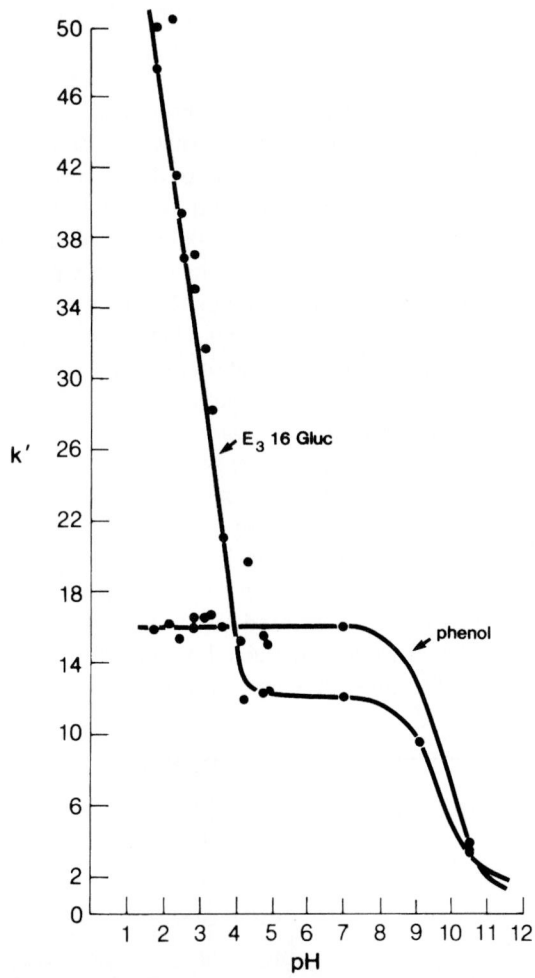

Fig. 6-8 Change in k' as a function of pH for estriol-16α-glucuronide and phenol. Decrease in k' at pH 2 is attributable to ionization of glucuronic acid; decrease at pH 10 is attributable to ionization of phenolic group. (From Oliphant C, Bowers LD, unpublished data.)

Table 6-2 Useful buffers for reversed-phase high-performance liquid chromatography

Buffer pair	pK$_a$
Phosphoric acid/dihydrogen phosphate	2.12
Chloracetic acid/chloracetate	2.87
Succinic acid/monohydrogen succinate	4.23
Acetic acid/acetate	4.77
Piperazine phosphate	5.33
Monohydrogen succinate/succinate	5.65
Tetramethylethylenediamine phosphate	6.13
Dihydrogen phosphate/monohydrogen phosphate	7.20
Tris(hydroxymethyl)aminomethane	8.19

ion suppression employing silica-based, reversed-phase packing material is limited by the range of pH stability of the silica support (which is stable from pH 2 to 8). Thus the requirement of a low-pH mobile phase for the ion-suppression chromatography of weak acids limits the column lifetime, whereas ion suppression of weak bases is not possible on silica-based, reversed-phase materials, since the pH requirement is too high. The advantage of ion-pair chromatography over ion-exchange chromatography is that it can separate both ionic and nonionic compounds simultaneously.

In ion-pair chromatography, a hydrophobic ionic species *(counterion)* that has the opposite charge to the analyte is added to the mobile phase, which is pumped through a reversed-phase column. The complex of the counterion and ionic analyte is called an *ion pair.* Several retention mechanisms have been proposed for ion-pair chromatography with the exact mechanism still being a matter of debate. Retention is most commonly explained by one of two basic models. One model depicts the role of the counterion as a neutralizing agent, combining with the analyte ion in the mobile phase to form a neutral species, which is retained on the reversed-phase column. The other model depicts the role of the counterion in terms of a modifier of the stationary phase, with the adsorption of the counterion on the reversed-phase packing material, changing the packing material into an ion exchanger, which will retain the ionic analyte.

Optimization of the separation in ion-pair chromatography is achieved through the manipulation of several mobile-phase variables, including type and concentration of ion-pair reagent, pH, type and concentration of organic modifier, ionic strength, and temperature.

The most common types of ion-pairing reagents used are alkyl (or aryl) sulfonates (RSO_3^-), alkyl sulfates ($ROSO_3^-$), and perchlorate (ClO_4^-), which are anionic counterions used for the chromatography of cationic species, and quaternary amines (NR_4^+), which are cationic counterions for the chromatography of anionic species. As would be expected, retention of analyte (which binds to the counterion) is increased with increased alkyl chain length of the ion-pairing reagent. Retention is also increased with increased concentration of ion-pair reagent. These two ef-

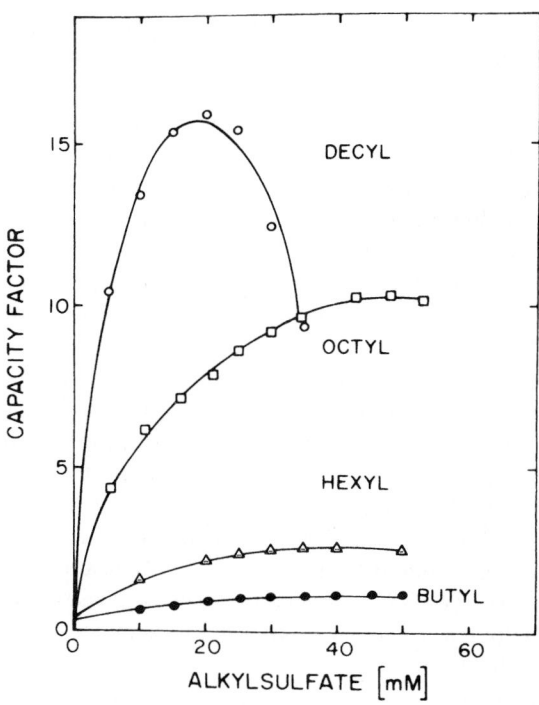

Fig. 6-9 Variation of capacity factor, *k'*, of epinephrine as a function of ion-pairing reagent concentration for several *n*-alkylsulfonates. (From Horvath C et al: *Anal Chem* 49: 2295, 1977.)

fects are shown in Fig. 6-9 in which the retention of epinephrine is shown to increase when (1) the chain length is increased from butyl sulfonate to decyl sulfonate and (2) when the concentration of any ion-pairing reagent is increased (up to a point where there is limited solubility of the ion-pairing reagent or there is a saturation effect, in which the concentration of the ion-pairing agent adsorbed onto the reversed-phase packing material is limited). It should be noted that analytes that do not bind to the counterion have decreased retention with increased concentration of the ion-pairing reagent (neutral species show a slight decrease in retention, whereas ionic analytes having the same charge as the counterion show a pronounced decrease in retention).

Adjustment of pH is also critical to ion-pair chromatography. Mobile-phase pH affects retention by controlling the charge state of analytes and counterions that are weak acids or weak bases. In general, retention is greatest at pH values in which the counterion and analyte are fully charged, which occurs at intermediate pH values. For example, for chromatography of a weak acid compound using a weak base counterion (or vice versa, a weak base analyte and a weak acid counterion), the pH must be between the pK$_a$ of the acid and the base, such that both are charged. For analytes that have different pKs, the separation of analytes can be affected by adjusting the pH.

Retention can also be adjusted through manipulation of

organic modifier (such as acetonitrile) concentration, ionic strength, and temperature. A decreased retention is seen for increased organic modifier content, which is attributable to the decreased strength of adsorption of the ion-pair reagent to the reversed-phase column. Increased ionic strength decreases retention because of reduced formation of ion pairs between the analyte and counterion as the result of competitive binding of the salt component to the counterion or analyte ion, or to both. The effect of temperature on retention is not predictable, being dependent on the particular ion pair.

Selection of the type of reversed-phase column to use is not a critical factor affecting selectivity of separation in ion-pair chromatography. The chain length and carbon content of the packing material are important to the determination of the concentration of the ion-pair reagent and organic modifier required for reasonable retention times. However, there is little to be gained in terms of optimization of separation by changing types of reversed-phase columns. C18 columns are most often employed in ion-pair chromatography.

Affinity chromatography[16,17]

A powerful tool in the analysis of biochemicals is affinity chromatography. In affinity chromatography the principle of specifically interacting biochemical pairs is employed. Examples of biochemical pairs used in affinity chromatography are given in Table 6-3. In affinity chromatography one of the components of the pair (termed the *affinity ligand*) is immobilized onto a support and packed into a column, making it a very specific chromatographic technique for the complementary component of the pair.

There are three stages to the affinity chromatographic separation process. The first stage is the injection of the sample into the aqueous *application buffer* (usually pH 7)

Table 6-3 Biochemical pairs used in affinity chromatography

Affinity ligand	Complementary component
Inhibitors, cofactors, substrate analogs	Enzymes
Immunoglobulins	Antigens, haptens
Receptors	Hormones
Nucleic acid components	Complementary nucleic acid components, Polynucleotide-binding proteins
Lectins	Carbohydrates, glycoproteins
m-Aminophenylboronic acid	*Cis*-diol containing compounds (carbohydrates, nucleic acid components, catecholamines, glycoproteins)
Protein A, protein G	Immunoglobulin G
Heparin	Coagulation proteins
Dye molecules	Various proteins and enzymes
Metal chelators	Proteins, peptides, nucleic acid components

pumped through the column, with all species passing through the column nonretained, except for the complementary analyte, which is retained by the column. After all the nonretained components pass through the column, the second stage of the chromatographic process is initiated and the mobile phase is switched to an aqueous *elution buffer,* which causes disruption of the binding forces between the analyte and affinity ligand, leading to elution of the analyte from the column. There are two categories of elution buffers, biospecific and general. Biospecific elution buffers contain a species that specifically interacts with the affinity ligand or analyte to affect elution. Biospecific elution thus adds a second step of specificity to the chromatographic process because there is specificity not only in retention, but also in elution of the analyte. Examples of biospecific elution include addition of sugars to the mobile phase in affinity chromatography by using lectin supports and enzyme inhibitors to the mobile phase in the affinity chromatography of enzymes. General elution buffers affect elution by nonspecific means, through disruption of the electrostatic, hydrogen bonds, van der Waals, and hydrophobic forces. Strategies for general elution include changing mobile-phase pH or ionic strength, adding organic modifiers to the mobile phase, or using denaturing conditions in the mobile phase (5 to 8 M urea or 6 M guanidine). The disadvantage of general elution schemes is that species that nonspecifically adsorb to the support may elute with the analyte. The third stage of the affinity chromatographic process is reequilibration of the column with application buffer before injection of the next sample.

Traditionally affinity chromatography has been relegated to purification roles, as only large-particle diameter polysaccharide-based hydrophilic supports were available in the past (hydrophilic supports are required in affinity chromatography to minimize nonspecific adsorption or denaturation of biomacromolecules). These low-performance supports have low efficiency and do not have the mechanical strength to withstand the high pressures that are generated from the high flow rates used in HPLC. The broad peaks and long analysis times precluded conventional affinity chromatography from being used as an analytical tool. This changed with the development of high-performance silica supports in which the surface was modified by the covalent attachment of a hydrophilic layer. In addition, hydrophilic high-performance polymeric supports have been developed. *High-performance affinity chromatography* is done by incorporation into normal HPLC setup columns containing high-performance packing material with covalently attached affinity ligands.

Affinity chromatography using *m*-aminophenylboronic acid columns is commonly employed in the clinical laboratory in the determination of glycated hemoglobins, which is used in the assessment of treatment of diabetics. The affinity ligand *m*-aminophenylboronic acid is a general ligand that binds compounds that contain a *cis*-diol functional group, which is present in compounds such as catechols, carbohydrates, and the carbohydrate portion of many glycoproteins. In the determination of glycated hemoglobins, hemolysate of red blood cells is injected onto an *m*-aminophenylboronic acid column, which retains the glycated hemoglobin, allowing the nonglycated hemoglobins to pass through the column. One elutes the glycated hemoglobin by changing the mobile phase to one containing the sugar alcohol sorbitol and monitoring the eluant at 415 nm.

Affinity chromatography has limitless flexibility through the use of antibodies as affinity ligands, a subclassification of affinity chromatography referred to as *immunoaffinity chromatography.*

Chromatography of enantiomers[18,19]

Separation of enantiomers (chiral compounds) has its greatest application in the determination of pharmaceuticals, since approximately 50% of the most frequently used drugs exist as enantiomer pairs. A compound that has one chiral center (which is most commonly a carbon atom that has four different groups bonded) exists in two isomeric forms differing from one another in the spatial arrangement of the atoms around the chiral center. Each of the enantiomer pairs has identical physical properties (making separation difficult) but differs in reactivities toward chiral reagents and in their reactivity in biological systems. The activity, metabolism, and sometimes the toxicity of a drug depend on the enantiomeric form, and thus the separation of drug enantiomers is critical in pharmaceutical analysis. HPLC is the method of choice for the determination of enantiomers.

There are three general ways of determining enantiomers by HPLC: chromatography on conventional columns after derivatization with a chiral reagent, chromatography on conventional columns using mobile phases containing chiral complexing reagents, and chromatography on columns containing a *chiral stationary phase.*

Derivatization of the enantiomer analyte with a chiral reagent leads to the formation of a diastereomer. One diastereomer isomer is formed when a particular enantiomer reacts with the derivatizing agent, whereas a different diastereomer isomer is formed when the other enantiomer reacts. Diastereomer isomers have different physical properties, which facilitate their separation on conventional HPLC columns. In a similar manner, the presence of chiral reagents in the mobile phase leads to the formation of a different diastereomer isomer complex for each component of a particular enantiomer pair. These diastereomer isomer complexes can be readily separated by conventional HPLC columns.

Specialized packing material containing a chiral compound as a stationary phase separates enantiomers as a result of differential spatial interaction of each enantiomer with the chiral support. Determination of enantiomers using chiral stationary-phase columns is advantageous compared to the derivatization or mobile-phase complexation

methods because these previously described methods require reagents that have a high degree of optical purity. Chiral stationary phases include Pirkle type of derivatives of amino acids or dipeptides, cyclodextrin, proteins such as albumin or α1-acid glycoprotein, polymers with helical structures, and chiral ligand exchange (consisting of an immobilized ligand with a bound transition metal). There are many different types of chiral stationary phases that are commercially available, the suitability of which for a particular enantiomer separation must largely be determined empirically. Thus there is not one universal chiral stationary phase applicable to all enantiomer separations; the choice of column is dependent on the enantiomer compound determined.

RECENT ADVANCES IN HPLC PACKING MATERIALS

A useful reference has been published giving information on HPLC packing materials.[20] Tables 6-4 to 6-6 contain a summary of general information and list the types of packing material commercially available for the different HPLC modes. Advances in packing materials have been along three lines: (1) development of packing materials that are designed to alleviate the problems of silica supports; (2) development of packing materials, known as restricted access media, that allow direct chromatography of serum (or plasma); and (3) development of higher efficiency supports for macromolecules. In Table 6-6, adsorption and polar-bonded packing materials are grouped together under normal-phase chromatography, which is consistent with a classification made by others, since both are polar packing materials.

Advances addressing problems with silica supports

Problems associated with the use of silica supports include a limited pH range ($2 < pH < 8$), poor performance in the reversed-phase chromatography of basic compounds, and problems with reproducibility. An ideal support material would have the high performance and pressure capabilities of silica supports but would be able to withstand a larger pH range, be inert, and have reproducible retention characteristics. Supports that are better than silica supports in some aspects but inferior to silica in other aspects have been developed.[21] These are described below.

High-performance polymeric supports.[22,23] Significant advances have been made in the last several years in upgrading polymeric supports from a low-performance status (low-pressure operation; low-efficiency packing materials; purification uses) to a high-performance status (high-pressure operation; high-efficiency packing materials; analytical as well as purification uses). Polymeric supports can be classified as either hydrophobic or hydrophilic. Poly(styrene-divinylbenzene) (PS-DVB) was the first polymeric HPLC support developed and is the predominant hy-

Table 6-4   Reversed-phase HPLC: general information and packing materials

Mode	Reversed phase
General information	
Compounds determined	Low- and medium-polarity compounds
Comments	Most widely used chromatographic mode in clinical analysis
	Mobile-phase ion suppression or ion pairing is required for ionic or ionizable compounds
Commercially available packing materials	
Bonded phase	*n*-Octadecyl (C18), *n*-octyl (C8)
	(Most widely used reversed-phase functionality in clinical analysis)
	n-Butyl (C4)
	(Preferred functionality for protein separations; however, less stable in acidic mobile phases [such as TFA] than C8, C18)
	Phenyl
	(Preferred functionality for compounds containing an aromatic group or groups)
	(These functional groups can be attached to the following supports: silica, polybutadiene modified/PHAM/alumina, PS-DVB, PVA)
Polymer covered	Silica modified with alkyl polysiloxanes, multifunctional alkyl silanes, alkyl PVA
	Alumina modified with polybutadiene (with or without attached alkyl groups)
Base support (native)	PS-DVB
	PAM
	Porous graphite
Nonporous	PS-DVB (native), PHAM silica (reversed-phase-functionalities)
Perfusion	PS-DVB (native and C18 functionality) (from PerSeptive Biosystems)
Restricted access media	Internal surface reversed phase (ISRP) (from Regis Chemical)
	(Glycine-L-phenylalanine-L-phenylalanine [GFF] functionalities)
	Semipermeable surface (SPS) (from Regis Chemical)
	(C8, C18, and phenyl functionalities)
	Shielded hydrophobic phase (SHP) (from Supelco)
	(Phenyl functionality)

PS-DVB, Poly(styrenemethyl divinylbenzene); *PAM*, poly(alkylmethylacrylate); *PHAM*, poly(hydroxyalkyl methacrylate or acrylate); *PVA*, poly(vinyl alcohol); *TFA*, trifluoroacetic acid.

drophobic polymeric support used. Poly(alkyl methacrylate) (PAM) is another hydrophobic support. The major hydrophilic polymeric supports that are commercially available are poly(vinyl alcohol) (PVA) and cross-linked agarose. The uses of these supports are given in Tables 6-4 to 6-6. Ligands are covalently attached to these supports to produce reversed-phase, ion-exchange, and normal-phase packing materials. No modification of the polymer support is required for size-exclusion chromatography. It should be noted that PS-DVB reversed-phase packing materials are most often used without modification of the surface. These native PS-DVB packing materials, however, have selectivities different from those of conventional alkyl-bonded reversed-phase packing materials. PS-DVB supports require hydrophilic surface modification in order to be utilized in modes other than reversed-phase.

Polymeric supports have two advantages over silica supports. The first is the extended pH range of polymeric supports. All polymeric supports listed above have a pH range of at least 2 to 12 (up to 14). This allows reversed-phase determination of a basic compound without the necessity of adding ion-pairing reagents. High-pH mobile phases can be used with polymeric supports, allowing basic compounds

to be chromatographed as neutral species and thus retained on the reversed-phase column. The second advantage of polymeric supports is that they do not have reactive functional groups such as silanols on the surface and thus do not show adverse peak tailing and recovery effects when basic analytes are chromatographed.

The major disadvantage of polymeric supports is that they are less efficient than silica supports (20,000 to 50,000 plates per meter for polymeric supports). PS-DVB supports also require at least 10% to 20% organic content in the mobile phase to prevent shrinkage of the support material. In comparison, the hydrophilic polymeric supports are less susceptible to shrinkage and swelling effects when the concentration of the organic modifier is changed, and these supports are thus compatible with completely aqueous mobile phases. A disadvantage of the hydrophilic polymeric supports is that they are subject to pressure limitations, which can preclude their use at very high flow rates. Upper pressure limits are 4500 to 6000 psi for PS-DVB supports, 2000 to 2900 psi for PHAM and PVA supports, and 200 to 400 psi for the cross-linked agarose supports (compared to a pressure rating of greater than 6000 psi for most silica packing materials). For PHAM and PVA supports, flow rates up

Table 6-5 Ion-exchange HPLC: general information and packing materials

	Ion exchange	
Mode	Anion	Cation
General information		
Compounds determined	Negatively charged compounds, acidic compounds, proteins with pI <8	Positively charged compounds, basic compounds, proteins with pI >6
Comments	The charge of the stationary phase will vary with mobile phase pH (near pK_a of support functionality) for weak ion exchangers but not for strong ion exchangers	
Commercially available packing material		
Bonded phase	*Weak* Primary, secondary, tertiary amines (—NR$_2$, —NHR, —NH$_2$) (Weak base functionalities with pK_a = 5-9; most utilized is DEAE [—O—CH$_2$—CH$_2$—N—(C$_2$H$_5$)$_2$]) *Strong* Quaternary amine [—NR$_3^+$] [Strong base functionality with pK_a >13) (Note that functional groups given above can be attached to silica, PS-DVB, and PHAM)	*Weak* Carboxylic acid [—COO$^-$] (Weak acid functionalities with pK_a = 4–6; most utilized is CM [—CH$_2$—COO$^-$]) *Strong* Sulfonic acid [—SO$_3^-$] (Strong acid functionalities with pK_a <1) *Intermediate* Sulfoalkyl [—(CH$_2$)$_n$—SO$_3^-$] (Most utilized is SE and SP [pK_a for SP = 2.3]) (Note that functional groups given above can be attached to silica, PS-DVB, and PHAM)
Polymer covered	*Weak* Polyethyleneimine (PEI)-coated supports (silica and PS-DVB) *Strong* Latex with quaternary amine functionality coated onto poly(ethylvinyl-divinylbenzene) or PS-DVB supports	*Weak* Latex with carboxylic acid functionality coated onto poly(ethylvinyl-divinylbenzene) or PS-DVB supports Polybutadiene–maleic acid copolymer on silica
Base support (native)	None	None
Nonporous	PHAM (PEI, DEAE, and —NR$_3^+$ functionalities), poly(dimethylaminopropylmethacrylamide) (dimethylaminopropyl functionality)	PHAM (carboxyl and SP functionalities), (SP functionality), silica (cation functionalities), silica (anion functionalities),
Perfusion	PS-DB (DEAE, —NR$_3^+$ functionalities) PS-DVB (PEI and DEAE functionalities)	PS-DVB (SE and CM functionalities)
Restricted access media	None	None

PS-DVB, Poly(styrene-divinylbenzene); *PHAM,* poly(hydroxyalkyl methacrylate or acrylate); *PVA,* poly(vinyl alcohol); *PEI,* polyethyleneimine. *DEAE,* diethylaminoethyl; *SE,* sulfoethyl; *SP,* sulfopropyl.

to 1.5 to 2.0 mL/min can be employed (15 cm × 4.6 mm column). Cross-linked agarose gels have more severe flow rate restrictions.

Polymeric packing materials have yet to be extensively characterized with respect to reproducibility.

Other high-performance packing materials. There have been other packing materials developed, in addition to polymeric packing materials, that address the problems associated with silica supports. Deactivated reversed-phase silica packing materials have been developed by various manufacturers and do not require the presence of amine modifiers in the mobile phase so that chromatography of basic compounds can be performed. These packing materials employ high-purity silica with low trace metal content. One or more of the following strategies may be used to further deactivate the silica: excessive end capping; attaching a dense surface coverage of alkyl ligand; covering the silica surface with a polymer layer; employing proprietary treat-

ments to modify the reactivity and distribution of the silanols on the surface; attaching novel ligands; and electrostatically shielding the silica surface. As with conventional silica packing materials these packing materials are limited to a mobile-phase pH range of 2 to 8, though some manufacturers claim an increase in upper pH limit to pH 10 for some polymer-covered silica supports.

Other packing materials are also commercially available. Alumina-based reversed-phase packing materials have an operating pH range of 2 to 13. Porous graphite is a material that has reversed-phase retention characteristics, with the additional characteristic of being able to separate geometric isomers, and retain hydrophilic compounds, an increased pH range (1-14), and better performance with basic solutes. Porous graphite is considerably more hydrophobic than conventional reversed-phase silica, requiring a higher concentration of organic modifier in the mobile phase.

Table 6-6   Normal-phase and size-exclusion HPLC: general information and packing materials

Mode	Normal phase	Size exclusion
General information		
Compounds determined	Hydrophilic compounds (such as saccharides; complements reversed phase, which does not retain hydrophilic compounds) Isomers (such as steroids) Class separation (Low-performance normal-phase cleanup of sample is often done before HPLC or immunoassay procedure)	Compounds >1000 daltons
Comments	Bonded normal phases compared to silica and alumina: • Sharper peaks, no tailing • Less strength of retention • Faster mobile-phase equilibration, making gradient chromatography possible	Hydrophilic SEC (all packing materials listed below except PS-DVB) is used in clinical analysis
Commercially available packing materials		
Bonded phase	Diol [$-(CH_2)_3OCH_2CH(OH)CH_2(OH)$] Cyano [$-(CH_2)_3CN$] (also referred to as nitrile) Amino [$-(CH_2)_nNH_2$] (where n = 3 or 5) (Polarity: amino > cyano > diol) Almost all bonded phase supports are silica based, with a few exceptions	Diol on silica [$-(CH_2)_3OCH_2CH(OH)CH_2(OH)$]
Polymer covered	None	Polyether and PVA on silica
Base support (native)	Silica Alumina Porous graphite	PHAM, PVA, cross-linked agarose, PS-DVB
Nonporous	None	Not applicable
Perfusion	PS-DVB (diol functionality) (PerSeptive Biosystems)	None
Restricted access media	Semipermeable surface (SPS) (Regis Chemical) (Cyano functionality)	Not applicable

PS-DVB, Poly(styrene-divinylbenzene); *PHAM,* poly(hydroxyalkyl methacrylate or acrylate); *PVA,* poly(vinyl alcohol); *SEC,* size exclusion.

Restricted access media[24]

It is normally necessary to remove proteins from plasma and serum samples before reversed-phase and normal-phase chromatography because the organic composition of the mobile phases used in these modes causes the denaturation and precipitation of proteins, which adsorb onto the packing material, leading to pressure buildup, decreased column efficiency, and decreased column capacity. Packing materials known as *restricted access media* allow direct injection of serum or plasma samples onto the column without any sample pretreatment. The different types of restricted-access media that are commercially available are listed in Tables 6-4 and 6-6. These packing materials consist of the stationary phase of silica covered by a hydrophilic barrier. The hydrophilic barrier allows the passage of small molecules into the interior stationary phase while sterically preventing larger molecules, such as proteins, from interacting with the stationary phase. Because restricted access techniques require no sample preparation, they are simpler and faster than conventional HPLC. Disadvantages include poorer detection limits (µg/mL) and an inherent difficulty in determining compounds that are tightly bound to proteins or other macromolecules.

High-efficiency, high-speed analysis of macromolecules

Conventionally, macromolecules are chromatographed on supports that have pores large enough for the macromolecule to enter them (pore diameters ranging from 30 to 400 nm), and smaller molecules are chromatographed on supports with smaller pore sizes (diameters of 5 to 15 nm). When HPLC analysis is performed on macromolecules, peaks that are broader than those seen with HPLC analysis of smaller molecules are obtained. This decrease in efficiency is seen because macromolecules, which have smaller diffusion coefficients, move more slowly into and out of the pores of the packing material. This phenomenon leads to decreased sensitivity, decreased resolution, and increased analysis time. To deal with this problem two types of packing materials have recently been developed: nonporous and perfusion packing materials.

Nonporous packing materials do not have pores that are accessible to macromolecules and thus have increased efficiency for macromolecules, leading to fast, high-resolution separations. The disadvantages of these packing materials are diminished capacity (1% to 10% of that of conventional supports) and high back-pressures (resulting from the small particle diameter [1 to 3 μm] of the supports). The reason for the diminished capacity of a nonporous packing material is the decreased surface area of the support, since most of the surface area in a chromatographic support is in the pores. Nonporous packing materials that are commercially available are polymeric and silica supports with reversed-phase, ion-exchange, and affinity functionalities.

Perfusion packing materials[25] (from PerSeptive Biosystems), which have a greater loading capacity than that of the nonporous packing materials, consist of a PS-DVB core, a hydrophilic cross-linked copolymer layer bonded to the PS-DVB support and the stationary phase. The support contains two types of pores, suprapores measuring 600 to 800 nm in diameter, and a family of smaller pores measuring 50 to 150 nm in diameter. Analyte transport in these pores occurs through convection in the suprapores (that is, the pores are large enough that the mobile phase actually flows through these pores) and by diffusion in the smaller pores. The higher capacity of the perfusion packing materials (in comparison to that of the nonporous packing materials) results from the increased surface area created by the 50 to 150 nm pores, the pores in which retention of the analyte occurs. The high efficiencies for these supports in the chromatography of macromolecules can be explained by the fact that the 50 to 150 nm pores generally measure 1 μm or less in length, limiting the space that the analyte has to diffuse in the pores. Perfusion packing materials for reversed-phase, ion-exchange, normal-phase, and affinity chromatography have been developed.

INSTRUMENTATION

As mentioned previously, modern HPLC requires relatively sophisticated instrumentation to achieve difficult separations in less than 10 minutes. There are four basic components in the separation system itself: (1) a solvent-delivery system to provide the driving force for the mobile phase, (2) a sample introduction system, (3) the column, and (4) the detector (Fig. 6-1). In addition, a recorder or integrator, often used with computer data acquisition, is used to display or calculate the results. A book detailing proper operation, maintenance, and troubleshooting for all the components of an HPLC has been published.[26]

Solvent-delivery systems

The most common delivery system is based on the reciprocating piston pump. Other types, including pneumatic amplification and diaphragm pumps, are mainly of historical interest.

In the first pumps used in HPLC, solvent delivery occurred during less than half the cycle time. This meant that flow through the column was erratic. The stoppage of flow and the compression of the solvent that occurred when the pump head refilled also resulted in a signal at the detector, which limited the detection of analyte. In the jargon of chromatography, the stoppage is known as a "pulse." Subsequently, manufacturers have used a variety of designs to

minimize pulsation. These range from a very rapid refill stroke relative to the delivery stroke, to two or more pump heads that are out of phase such that one head is always delivering solvent. There are also mechanical devices known as "pulse dampeners" that work quite well under isocratic conditions with all but the most crude pumps. It must be emphasized, however, that although pulses can be minimized in a reciprocating piston pump, they can never be eliminated. Syringe pumps are advantageous in applications that are sensitive to pulsation, such as when electrochemical detection is used, and when very low flow rates (μL/min) are used (microbore LC).

Gradient elution can be attained when the solvents are mixed after they have passed through the pumps or are mixed before they enter the pump. A well-maintained system of either type can function well, and selection of one or the other is based on gradient reproducibility, gradient shapes available, cost, and operator preference.

Sample-introduction systems

The most widely used method of introducing a sample into the chromatographic system is the fixed-loop injection valve. A sample aliquot is loaded into an external loop of stainless steel tubing. The valve is then rotated so that the sample loop is flushed onto the column by the mobile phase from the pump. Returning the valve to the original position allows loading of the next sample. Fixed-loop valves can be used in two ways: partial-fill method and full-loop method. In the latter the entire loop (such as 20 μL) is filled with sample and injected. It is the most precise method. One should recognize, however, that accurate results require flushing of the loop with 5 to 10 loop volumes before loading. In the partial-fill mode, the sample loop is not filled with sample. In this case, the precision of the injection volume is determined by the loading syringe.

In addition to the manual valve injector described above, many automatic sampling devices are also available. These autosamplers allow unattended operation of the HPLC system, making 24-hour-a-day use possible. They are usually quite reliable and precise because of mechanical advances and computerization. The devices may cost $5,000 to $10,000 but play an important role in busy laboratories.

Columns and connectors

The column is of course the most important part of the separation system. The packing material for columns has been discussed at length. The usual HPLC column has an inside or internal diameter of 4.1 or 4.6 mm and a length of 100 to 250 mm. Column-end fittings are required at both ends to connect the column to the other system components and to hold the packing material inside. The frits used should have pores less than one fourth the average diameter of the packing material. In addition to the analytical (or preparative) column, which actually performs the separation, two types of protector columns might be used. A *guard column* (Fig. 6-1) is located between the injector and the analytical column and is $\frac{1}{15}$ to $\frac{1}{25}$ the volume of the latter. It is packed with a material similar to that of the analytical column. Its function is to collect any particulate matter or any strongly retained components of the sample and therefore to protect the expensive analytical column. A *precolumn* is positioned between the pump and the injection valve. It is always packed with silica, the purpose of which is to saturate the mobile phase with silicate and thus prevent dissolution of the packing material in the analytical column. This has reportedly allowed operation of silica columns at pHs of 10, far beyond the normal pH for dissolution of silica.

The analytical column has been described previously. The high efficiencies obtained with current HPLC columns result from the use of small (3, 5, or 10 μm), totally porous particles. To obtain efficient columns and reasonable operating pressures, the range between the largest and smallest particle must be as small as possible. Both spherical and irregularly shaped particles are available. Columns packed with spherical particles seem to give lower operating pressures and are more durable.

Microbore (1 mm ID) and small-bore (2 mm ID) columns are used because of the increase in sensitivity (as described previously) and because of the conservation of mobile phase in comparison to conventional HPLC columns, which is advantageous for cost, environmental, and detector compatibility reasons. Concerning detector compatibility, microbore columns are required for mass spectrometric detection. The reason is that mass spectrometers require the removal of as much mobile phase as possible, mandating the use of microbore columns, which introduce smaller amounts of mobile phase into the detector than conventional HPLC designs.

In addition to the columns, the connections made between system components are critical because the fittings should introduce as little peak spreading as possible. They should be of the zero dead volume or at least low dead volume type. An excellent article on the intricacies of HPLC plumbing is available.[27]

Detection systems

The final component in the chromatographic system is responsible for detecting the compounds as they elute from the column. Ideally a detector would respond to any compound, would detect picograms or less of the analytes, would be immune to any solvent-related phenomena, and would respond linearly to a wide range of concentrations. Unfortunately, liquid chromatography does not have such a detector. Three types of HPLC detectors routinely used in the clinical laboratory are absorbance, fluorescence, and electrochemical detectors. Mass spectrometric detection is important in clinical research. The selection of the appropriate detector will depend on the required selectivity and sensitivity. Several books giving a detailed description of various HPLC detection methods have been published.[28,29] Derivatization methods, though not covered below, are an important means of enhancing sensitivity or specificity of detection in HPLC analysis.[30] The performance characteristics of the common LC detectors are summarized in Table 6-7.

Absorbance detection. The most frequently used HPLC detection mode is absorbance spectrophotometry. The advantage of absorbance detectors over fluorescence or electrochemical detectors is that they can be used to detect a greater variety of compounds. However, absorbance detectors have poorer detection limit capabilities by factors of 10 and 100, in comparison to those of fluorescence and electrochemical detectors respectively. For absorbance detectors, wavelengths higher than 200 nm are required, since mobile-phase solvents absorb appreciably at the low ultraviolet wavelength region of the spectrum (<200 nm). In general, the number of compounds that can be detected increases as wavelength decreases. However, at lower wavelengths there is also an increased detection of interfering compounds and an increase in baseline shifts when gradient chromatography is used. It is thus desirable to use the highest wavelength at which a compound absorbs to increase the specificity of the technique.

There are three types of absorbance detectors that are used: fixed-wavelength, variable-wavelength, and multiple-wavelength absorbance detectors. These detectors, as described below, differ in the number of wavelengths available for monitoring and whether multiple wavelengths can be monitored simultaneously.

Fixed-wavelength detectors. This detector is popular because of its low cost. Fixed-wavelength detectors are limited in the choice of wavelengths that can be used. The

Table 6-7 Performance characteristics of commonly used detectors

Ideal detector characteristic	Fixed wavelength	Variable wavelength	Fluorescence	Electrochemical	
				Oxidation	Reduction
Selective?	No	No	Yes	Yes	Yes
Sensitivity to flow-rate changes?	Possibly	Possibly	No	Yes	Yes
Limit of detection?	10^{-10} g/L	10^{-9} g/L	10^{-11} g/L	10^{-12} g/L	10^{-9} g/L
Cell volume?	8-10 μL	8-10 μL	20 μL	$\leq$1 μL	
Compatible with gradient?	Yes	Yes	Yes	No	No

choice is determined by the specific light source that is used. Each kind of arc lamp emits specific spectral lines. The wavelengths of various lamps are given in Table 6-8. The low-pressure mercury vapor lamp is the most widely used lamp, with the 254 nm wavelength used most often. The cadmium and zinc lamps are used for shorter ultraviolet wavelengths. Phosphor-coated mercury lamps produce different wavelengths, increasing the number of wavelengths available for use.

Variable-wavelength detectors. These detectors are advantageous because a continuous-spectrum light source and a monochromator are used to allow unlimited choice of visible and ultraviolet wavelengths. However, these detectors are more complex and expensive than the fixed-wavelength detectors. Deuterium and tungsten lamps are used to provide ultraviolet and visible wavelengths respectively. Some detectors use a deuterium source for both the ultraviolet and the visible region; however, these detectors have decreased precision in the visible range in comparison with detectors with a tungsten light source.

Multiple-wavelength detectors. These detectors are variable-wavelength detectors that have the capability of monitoring multiple wavelengths simultaneously. This class of detectors includes detectors that differ greatly in complexity and sophistication from those detectors that have dual-channel capability, in which two wavelengths can be monitored simultaneously, to those detectors that can record an entire spectrum in fractions of a second. All multiple-wavelength detectors (dual channel, spectrum recording) are advantageous for several reasons. One reason is the optimization of analyte detection, since the detector allows the monitoring of each analyte at the particular wavelength at which there is a maximum analyte/interferent response ratio. Another reason is that the multiple-wavelength detector can be used for verification of peak purity. Multiple-wavelength detectors that are capable of ultrafast spectrum measurement can also be useful for compound identification and suppression of known interference peaks. The use of the photodiode array detector for the above-mentioned purposes has been described.[28]

There are two types of multiple-wavelength detectors that are capable of ultrafast spectral measurement: the photo-diode array detector (PDA) and an ultrafast scanning spectrophotometer known as a low-inertia scanning (LIS) detector. PDA detectors employ a reverse-optics scheme (meaning that the diffraction grating is placed after the sample cell instead of before it) in which the entire spectrum of light (usually a deuterium lamp source is used) is directed through the flow cell to a diffraction grating, which disperses the light into component wavelengths. The dispersed wavelengths are directed to an array consisting of 32 to 512 diodes (the higher-resolution PDAs have the larger number of diodes). When light strikes a diode, it produces a current proportional to the intensity of the light. Since the light hitting the array is spatially dispersed according to wavelength, each diode has a particular range of wavelengths that is striking it, and thus the detector records the entire spectrum simultaneously. The fastest PDAs can record a spectrum every 10 msec (specifications for one representative company are a spectrum acquisition rate of 12.5 msec for a wavelength range of 190 to 600 nm, with a 4 nm bandwidth, and a noise level during the scan of less than $\pm 2.5 \times 10^{-5}$ AU [at 254 nm]).

The LIS detector employs the usual forward-optics design. Modifications have been made in these detectors to allow rapid wavelength scanning. Deuterium and tungsten lamps are used for the ultraviolet and visible range, respectively. The LIS detector has a limited spectrum range, requiring one to select either the deuterium or the tungsten lamp in order to select wavelength ranges of either 190 to 365 nm or 366 to 800 nm. The LIS also has a slow scanning speed of 583 ms to scan 190 to 365 nm in 3 nm intervals, with a band pass of 2.7 nm. It should be noted, however, that the spectrum acquisition rate for the LIS detector is sufficient for most HPLC work. Only those HPLC techniques that yield extremely narrow peaks require faster scanning rates. An important advantage of the LIS detector is that is has less interferences from noise than the PDA detector ($< \pm 1 \times 10^{-5}$ AU [during a scan at 254 nm]). This results in better detection limits for the LIS by at least a factor of 2.5. It should be noted that the detection limit gains are much greater in the visible-wavelength region, since the LIS utilizes a tungsten lamp for the visible region, whereas the PDA commonly employs only a deuterium lamp.

Fluorescence detection. The technique of fluorescence is based on the ability of a molecule to emit light after it has been excited by light radiation. For a description of fluorescence spectroscopy, refer to Chapter 4. The main differences in fluorometer performance between manufacturers arise from differences in the lamp intensity and the detection efficiency. Commercially available instruments use emission from either deuterium or xenon arc lamps for exciting light. Because the fluorescent intensity is directly proportional to the excitation light intensity, there has been a great deal of interest recently in laser sources. Fluorescence is a highly sensitive detection method for those compounds that fluoresce, but because many mol-

Table 6-8 Wavelengths emitted by arc sources used in fixed-wavelength detectors[29]

Source	Mercury	Phosphor mercury	Cadmium	Zinc
Emission lines (nm)	254	280	229	214
	313	300	326	308
	365	320		
	405	340		
	436	470		
	546	510		
	578	610		
		660		

ecules do not fluoresce, numerous methods for derivatizing compounds have been developed. Epinephrine and other amine compounds can react with dimethylaminonaphthalenesulfonyl (dansyl) chloride or *o*-phthalaldehyde to produce highly fluorescent compounds.

Electrochemical detection.[31] For a select group of compounds electrochemical detection is the method of choice because of its superior detection limit capability (femtomole to picomole). The types of compounds that can be determined by liquid chromatography–electrochemical detection (LCEC detection) are compounds that undergo reversible electron transfer reactions. Characteristics of a small oxidation (or reduction) potential and fast kinetics are most desirable for sensitive and selective detection. The classes of organic compounds that have these characteristics are phenols (such as hydroquinones, catechols, and catecholamines), aromatic amines, thiols, nitro compounds, and quinones. Compounds such as aldehydes and ketones require too high a reduction potential, whereas alkyl amines and carboxylic acid functionalities require too high an oxidation potential for direct determination by LCEC. Highly conjugated compounds such as α,β-unsaturated ketones and imines may be determined by LCEC; however, UV detection techniques are better. The most common LCEC analyses done in the clinical laboratory, in which LCEC has a decided advantage because of its superior detection limit capabilities, are the determination of catecholamines, catecholamine metabolites, serotonin, and 5-hydroxyindoleacetic acid.

Amperometric and coulometric detection. In general, electrochemical detection of an analyte occurs through an electron transfer between the electrode surface and the analyte molecule, with subsequent measurement of the current. The oxidizing strength of the electrode surface (increasingly positive potential for stronger oxidizing capability), or reducing strength of the electrode surface (increasingly negative potential for stronger reducing capability), is determined by the potential applied. The potential thus establishes the selectivity of the detector. Operation at lower oxidative potentials (or less negative reductive potentials) provides greater selectivity. The name of the detection technique described above is *controlled potential amperometry.* In this technique, the detector cells consist of three electrodes: a working electrode (at which the redox reaction occurs), a reference electrode, and an auxiliary electrode. The potential is applied between the reference and working electrodes, and the current is passed between the auxiliary and working electrodes.

Detectors are classified as either *amperometric*, in which 1% to 10% of the analyte reacts at the electrode, or *coulometric*, in which 100% of the analyte reacts. Increasing the electrode surface area or slowing the flow rates to increase the percentage of electroconversion does not increase detection limits because there is a concomitant increase in background electrolysis and hence noise. Thus, coulomet-

ric detectors have no detection limit advantage over amperometric detectors. Factors such as variations in temperature, flow rate, and mobile-phase impurities, which are important contributors to noise, need to be controlled to achieve the lowest detection limits. For this reason gradients are not usually employed in LCEC. There are three amperometric detector designs used, which are diagrammed in Fig. 6-10: thin layer, wall jet, and tubular. The most common amperometric electrode is the thin-layer electrode, in which column effluent passes through a very small volume flat channel (<1 μL) in which the working electrode is contained on one side of the channel and the reference and counter electrodes are contained on the other side. The coulometric detector consists of porous material through which the mobile phase passes, providing the large surface area required for complete electroconversion of the analyte species. It should also be noted that a conductive mobile phase is required for electrochemical detection, with a concentration of electrolyte or buffer of 0.01 to 0.1 M normally employed.

The best choice of material for the active surface of the electrode depends on the compound to be measured and the conditions of analysis. The glassy carbon electrode is the most widely used material because of its wide potential range (+1.2 to −0.8 V versus Ag/AgCl), its mechanical stability with high flow rates, and its chemical stability with nonaqueous solvents. For substances requiring high reduction potentials, a mercury film on gold is used (+0.2 to −1.2 V versus Ag/AgCl). Mercury electrodes are used in the determination of thiols, since the association of thiol to mercury lowers the oxidation potential of complexed mercury to +0.1 V.

For cathodic reactions, several problems associated with oxygen reduction restrict the limit of detection to the nanogram range. To make the reductive mode more sensitive, all oxygen needs to be removed from the mobile phase.

Pulsed amperometric detection (PAD).[32] A significant development in electrochemical detectors that allowed sensitive detection of carbohydrates occurred in the early 1980s. Before this, derivatization of carbohydrates with fluorophoric or chromophoric reagents was needed for sensitive detection. Carbohydrate detection was accomplished by

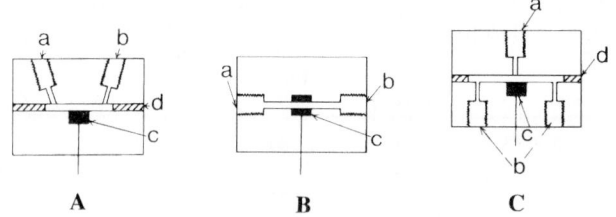

Fig. 6-10 Schematic diagram of thin layer of channel, **A;** tubular, **B;** and wall-jet, **C,** electrochemical flow cell designs. (From Weber SG: *I & EC Product Research and Development* 20:593, 1981.)

use of electrodes consisting of noble metals such as platinum or gold, which catalyze oxidation reactions of carbohydrate compounds, reactions that do not occur at reasonable potentials when other materials are used for the electrode. Electrodes made with noble metals, however, present unique problems that result from the formation of metal oxides at positive potentials and the irreversible absorption of compounds onto the surface. These problems were solved by the development of a triple-pulse waveform scheme. *Pulsed amperometric detection* (PAD) refers to the electrochemical detection technique that uses this triple-pulse waveform on platinum or gold electrodes. In this technique, a cycle of three potentials are applied over a 600 to 1000 msec period. These potentials, which are needed for the analytical process, are (1) a reducing potential, at which metal oxides on the electrode's surface are reduced and at which adsorption of the analyte occurs; (2) an oxidizing potential, at which the analyte is measured (the current resulting from the oxidation of hydrogen atoms that were removed catalytically by the metal surface); and (3) a yet higher oxidizing potential, at which desorption of molecules previously adsorbed to the electrode surface occurs. Besides carbohydrates, alcohols and amino acids have been determined by this technique.

Conductivity detection. Like the LCEC techniques described previously; measurement of conductivity is also considered to be an electrochemical detection method. The HPLC determination of inorganic anions uses anion-exchange chromatography with conductivity detection. Conductivity is a measure of conductance when a constant alternating potential is applied at a platinum electrode surface. The amount of current generated increases with increased solution conductance. Current in these electrodes is temperature dependent, and thus temperature must be strictly controlled.

Mass spectrometric detection.[31,33] The use of mass spectrometry in LC detection is increasing because of its unique ability to identify compounds through molecular weight and fragmentation information. Interfaces include thermospray, direct liquid injection, continuous-flow fast-atom bombardment, and atmospheric-pressure ionization methods (such as electrospray). The thermospray interface is the most widely used interface in the clinical setting, since it is useful for the determination of moderately polar compounds in the mass range of 200 to 1000 daltons. It does, however, require the compound to have some volatility. The continuous-flow fast-atom bombardment technique is useful for determining involatile compounds up to a molecular

Table 6-9   Clinically relevant compounds determined by HPLC

Compound		Most prevalent HPLC mode or modes used
Class	**Subclass**	
Amino acids		Reversed phase, ion exchange
Anions	Oxalate, citrate, sulfate, phosphate, iodide, bromide, chloride, thiocyanate, nitrate, nitrite	Ion exchange
Bile acids		Reversed phase
Bilirubins		Reversed phase
Bioamines	Catecholamines and catecholamine metabolites	Reversed phase, ion pair
	Serotonin and serotonin metabolites	Reversed phase, ion pair
Carbohydrates	Monosaccharides and oligosaccharides	Reversed phase, ion exchange, ion-moderated partition, normal phase
Drug and drug metabolites		Reversed phase
Fatty acids and organic acids	Fatty acids	Reversed phase
	Organic acids	Ion exchange, ion-moderated partition, reversed phase
Hemoglobins		
	Glycated hemoglobins	Ion exchange, affinity
	Hemoglobin variants	Ion exchange
Isomers, positional		Normal phase
Lipoproteins		Size exclusion
Nucleic acid compounds		
	Nucleic acid bases, nucleosides, nucleotides	Reversed phase, ion pair
	Oligonucleotides	Reversed phase, ion exchange
	DNA restriction fragments	Reversed phase, ion exchange
Phospholipids		Normal phase
Porphyrins		Reversed phase
Prostaglandins		Reversed phase
Steroids		Reversed phase
Vitamins	Biotins, folates, nicotinamides, pantothenic acids, retinoids (vitamin A), riboflavins, thiamines, tocopherols (vitamin E), vitamin B_6, vitamin B_{12}, vitamin C, vitamin D, vitamin K	Reversed phase

weight of 6000 daltons. Electrospray is useful for determining polar and ionic compounds and has the distinguishing feature of being able to analyze macromolecules with molecular weights up to 100,000 daltons. See Chapter 8 for a more detailed discussion of mass spectrometry.

APPLICATIONS

Several books on HPLC of clinical and biochemical analytes have been published.[34-41] Table 6-9 contains a comprehensive list of the classes of clinically relevant compounds in which HPLC plays a significant role in analysis. The HPLC modes given in Table 6-9 for each compound class are the modes most prevalently used (as determined by a survey of recent literature).

REFERENCES

1. Snyder LR, Kirkland JJ: *Introduction to modern liquid chromatography,* ed 2, New York, 1979, Wiley & Sons.
2. Scott RPW: *Liquid chromatography column theory,* Chichester, 1992, Wiley & Sons.
3. Karger BL, Snyder LR, Horvath C: *An introduction to separation science,* New York, 1973, Wiley & Sons.
4. Giddings JC: *Dynamics of chromatography,* New York, 1965, Marcel Dekker.
5. Guichon GG: In Horvath C, editor: *High performance liquid chromatography: advances and perspectives,* vol 2, New York, 1981, Academic Press.
6. van der Wal SJ, Snyder LR: Precision of 'high-performance' liquid-chromatographic assays with sample pretreatment: error analysis for the Technicon 'Fast-LC' system, *Clin Chem* 27:1233-1240, 1981.
7. Ghrist BFD, Cooperman BS, Snyder LR: Design of optimized high-performance liquid chromatographic gradients for the separation of either small or large molecules. I. Minimizing errors in computer simulations, *J Chromatogr* 459:1-23, 1988.
8. Ghrist BFD, Snyder LR: Design of optimized high-performance liquid chromatographic gradients for the separation of either small or large molecules. II. Background and theory, *J Chromatogr* 459:25-41, 1988.
9. Ghrist BFD, Snyder LR: Design of optimized high-performance liquid chromatographic gradients for the separation of either small or large molecules. III. An overall strategy and its application to several examples, *J Chromatogr* 459:43-63, 1988.
10. Snyder LR: *Principles of adsorption chromatography,* New York, 1963, Marcel Dekker.
11. Snyder LR, Glajch JL, Kirkland JJ: Theoretical basis for a systematic optimization of mobile phase selectivity in liquid-solid chromatography, *J Chromatogr* 218:299-326, 1981.
12. Majors RE: Trends in HPLC column usage, *LCGC* 9:686-693, 1991.
13. Dorsey JG, Dill KA: The molecular mechanism of retention in reversed-phase liquid chromatography, *Chem Rev* 89:331-346, 1989.
14. Szepesi G: *How to use reverse-phase HPLC,* New York, 1992, VCH.
15. Karger BL, LePage JN, Tanaka N: Secondary chemical equilibria in high-performance liquid chromatography. In Horvath C, editor: *High performance liquid chromatography: advances and perspectives,* vol 1, New York, 1980, Academic Press.
16. Turkova J: *Bioaffinity chromatography,* ed 2, Amsterdam, 1993, Elsevier.
17. Scouten WH: *Affinity chromatography: bioselective adsorption on inert matrices,* St. Louis, 1992, Sigma-Aldrich Co.
18. Allenmark S: *Chromatographic enantioseparation: methods and applications,* ed 2, New York, 1991, Ellis Horwood.
19. Krstulovic AM: *Chiral separations by HPLC,* Chichester, 1989, Ellis Horwood.
20. Unger KK, editor: *Packings and stationary phases in chromatographic analysis,* New York, 1990, Marcel Dekker.
21. Anderson DJ: High-performance liquid chromatography (advances in packing materials), *Anal Chem* 67:475R-486R, 1995.
22. Mikes O, Coupek J: Organic supports. In Gooding KM, Regnier FE, editors: *HPLC of biological macromolecules,* New York, 1990, Marcel Dekker, pp 25-46.
23. Tanaka N, Araki M: Polymer-based packing materials for reversed-phase chromatography, *Adv Chromatogr* 30:81-122, 1989.
24. Anderson DJ: High-performance liquid chromatography (direct injection techniques), *Anal Chem* 65:434R-443R, 1993.
25. Afeyan NB, Fulton SP, Regnier FE: Perfusion chromatography packing materials, *J Chromatogr* 544:267-279, 1991.
26. Dolan JW, Snyder LR: *Troubleshooting LC systems: a comprehensive approach to troubleshooting LC equipment and separations,* Clifton, N.J., 1989, Humana Press.
27. Dolan J, Upchurch P: *Interchangeability of HPLC fittings,* Oak Harbor, Wash., 1983, Upchurch Scientific; also *LC* 2:20-21, 1984, and 3:92-95, 1985.
28. Parriott D, editor: *A practical guide to HPLC detection,* San Diego, 1993, Academic Press.
29. Yeung ES, editor: *Detectors for liquid chromatography,* New York, 1986, Wiley & Sons.
30. Lingeman H, Underberg WJM, editors: *Detection-oriented derivatization techniques in liquid chromatography,* New York, 1990, Marcel Dekker.
31. Anderson DJ: High-performance liquid chromatography, *Anal Chem* 63:213R-219R, 262R-264R, 1991.
32. Johnson DC, LaCourse WR: Liquid chromatography with pulsed electrochemical detection at gold and platinum electrodes, *Anal Chem* 62:589A-597A, 1990.
33. Niessen WMA, van der Greef J: *Liquid chromatography–mass spectrometry: principles and applications,* New York, 1992, Marcel Dekker.
34. Heftmann E, editor: *Chromatography: fundamentals and applications of chromatography and related differential migration methods,* part B: *Applications,* ed 5, Amsterdam, 1992, Elsevier.
35. Hanai T, editor: *Liquid chromatography in biomedical analysis,* Amsterdam, 1991, Elsevier.
36. Papadoyannis IN: *HPLC in clinical chemistry,* New York, 1990, Marcel Dekker.
37. Hearn MTW, editor: *HPLC of proteins, peptides and polynucleotides, contemporary topics and applications,* New York, 1991, VCH.
38. Gooding KM, Regnier FE, editors: *HPLC of biological macromolecules,* New York, 1990, Marcel Dekker.
39. Fallon A, Booth RFG, Bell LD, editors: *Applications of HPLC in biochemistry,* Amsterdam, 1987, Elsevier.
40. Lim CK, editor: *HPLC of small molecules,* Oxford, U.K., 1986, IRL Press (Oxford University Press).
41. Henschen A, Hupe KP, Lottspeich F, Voelter W, editors: *High performance liquid chromatography in biochemistry,* Weinheim, Federal Republic of Germany, 1985, VCH.

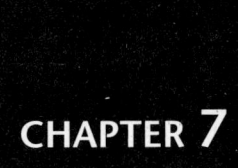

CHAPTER 7

Gas chromatography

Alphonse Poklis

Molecules that can be separated by gas chromatography

Theory of gas chromatographic separation
Partition coefficient (K_D)
Partitioning in GC systems
Temperature dependence
Column performance

Mobile-phase considerations

Stationary-phase considerations
Gas-solid stationary phases
Gas-liquid-solid supports for GLC
Liquid phases

Derivatization

Selection of a separation system
Choosing the mobile phase
Stationary-phase selection

Components of gas chromatograph
Carrier gas
Sample-injection port
Column tubing
Thermal compartment
Detectors

GC applications in clinical chemistry

OBJECTIVES

- Diagram the basic components of a gas chromatographic system, describe the function of each component, and outline the mechanisms of gas-liquid and gas-solid chromatography.

- Explain the significance of temperature dependence in gas chromatography and tell why temperature is the most important single parameter.

- Name four common carrier gases and state the function of a carrier gas, summarizing the criteria for selection of an appropriate carrier gas for chromatographic separation.

- Define derivatization and state why the process is used in gas chromatography.

- Describe the operation of the six types of detectors that may be used in gas chromatography.

KEY TERMS

active sites Places, usually on the stationary phase, that reversibly bind the compound to be separated.

capillary column An open tubular column with an inside diameter of 0.20 to 0.35 mm.

chemical ionization The component molecule to be analyzed is mixed with an ionized gas, such as methane or isobutane. A positive charge is transferred to the molecule, the $M + 1$ charged molecule and its fragments are separated by the mass spectrometer, and their size and relative abundance are measured. (M is 'mass'.)

corrected retention time The amount of time a compound is retained on a column minus the gas-holdup time.

derivative A molecule chemically altered from the original one. Usually in gas chromatography it refers to chemical groups added to increase the volatility of the initial compound.

diffusivity The ability of molecules to diffuse or spread because of the thermal energy inherent in the molecule.

effective plate (number of effective plates) The number of partitions that are practically available on a column.

electron-capture detector A device that releases beta particles into the carrier-gas stream, producing low-energy electrons, which are captured by eluted compounds and change in current measured. This type of detector is very sensitive and specific for compounds with chemical groups of high electronegativity, such as halogens.

electron impact Fragmentation of molecules into specific charged fragments by collision with high-energy electrons.

flame ionization detector A device in which eluted components are mixed with hydrogen and burned in the air to produce a flame, which ionizes these components. A pair of electrodes measures the number of ions.

flow regulator A system of valves that is set to yield a desired gas pressure and thus control the rate of gas movement (flow) through a gas chromatographic system.

Fourier-transform infrared spectrometer A device that may be considered as a gas chromatographic detector. The infrared spectral lines of compounds are obtained as the compounds elute from the chromatograph.

gas chromatography A physical technique that separates components based on their distribution between a gas and a stationary phase.

gas-holdup time The amount of time it takes for the carrier gas to move from the injection port to the detector, analogous to the void volume of liquid chromatography.

gas-liquid chromatography A separation technique in which the stationary phase is a liquid.

gas-solid chromatography A separation technique in which the stationary phase is a solid.

injection port A device usually having a septum and a heating block to volatilize the compounds to be separated. This is placed before the column.

Kovats index This index relates the logarithm of the retention time of a compound, regardless of its chemical nature, to those of the *n*-paraffins.

liquid phase The nonvolatile fluid that coats the immobile support medium. These fluids have the property of acting as solvents for the compounds to be separated.

mass fragment A degraded portion of a molecule containing one or more charges.

mass spectrometer A device that may be considered a gas chromatographic detector. Compounds are fragmented into specific groups of charged molecules, which are separated into their mass and charge components, and their relative abundance is measured.

mass transfer The movement of mass from one phase to another.

McReynolds constant A constant describing a system that classifies the stationary phase in terms of its ability to separate various compounds.

negative chemical ionizations Similar to chemical ionization except that the gas is oxygen or hydrogen, which produces primarily negative ions of the form $M - 1$. (*M* is 'mass'.)

nitrogen-phosphorus detector A device similar to a flame ionization detector but into which alkaline metals are introduced. When nitrogen- or phosphorus-containing compounds are burned, the rate of release of alkaline metal vapor and thus of current flow is increased.

nonvolatile liquid A fluid that does not vaporize or have a form that is readily gaseous in nature.

nonpolar Usually applied to molecules that have a hydrophobic affinity, that is, 'water hating'. Nonpolar substances tend to dissolve in nonpolar solvents.

open tubular column A gas chromatographic column in which the stationary phase coats the inside walls of the column.

overloading When too much of a compound is presented for adsorption by the stationary phase, nonequilibrium between the two phases occurs.

packed column A gas chromatographic column in which the stationary-phase support consists of particulate material filling the column.

phase ratio The ratio of mobile-phase (gas) volume to stationary-phase (column) volume. Usually indicated by the term "β."

plate A chromatographic term that refers to a single partitioning unit of the chromatographic system.

polar Usually applied to molecules that have a hydrophilic affinity, that is, 'water loving.' Polar substances tend to dissolve in polar solvents.

relative retention time The ratio of the corrected retention time of the reference compound to that of the sample compound.

retention index A system relating the retention time to a standard.

Rohrschneider constant Similar to the McReynolds constant.

selected-ion chromatogram A technique in which only mass fragments of a preselected size are recorded and quantified by the mass spectrometer.

separator A device that removes large portions of the carrier gas and concentrates the solutes before entrance to the mass spectrometer.

septum A device that separates the chromatographic column from the laboratory environment. Usually it is a small disk of silicone rubber through which the solution to be separated is injected into the column.

silanization The chemical process of converting the SiOH moiety of a stationary phase to the ester form.

sorbent A material that has the property of interacting with the compound of interest, usually to make it bind.

thermal compartment The temperature-regulated oven in which the chromatographic column is placed.

thermal-conductivity detector A device that measures the difference between the heat conductivities of the carrier gas and that of the sample-gas effluents. A sample carried in gas increases the heat conductivity.

van Deemter's equation Relates the HETP (height equivalent to the theoretical plate) to the linear velocity of the carrier gas.

wide-bore column An open tubular column with an inside diameter of 0.50 to 0.75 mm.

Chromatography is a physical technique that separates two or more compounds based on their distribution between two phases, a stationary and a mobile one. Review Chapter 5 for a description of the basic theory and practice of chromatographic separations. The stationary phase may be a liquid or a solid, and in gas chromatography (GC) the mobile phase is a gas that percolates over the stationary phase. When separation of sample components is accomplished by use of a mobile-gas phase and a stationary phase consisting of a thin layer of nonvolatile liquid held on a solid support, the technique is called gas-liquid chromatography (GLC). Gas-solid chromatography (GSC) employs a solid sorbent as the stationary phase. Both GLC and GSC may be further differentiated based upon the stationary-phase support. When the liquid phase in GLC is coated over the surface of small particles, or the solid sorbent in GSC consists of small particles, the column acts as a container for the stationary phase. This technique is known as "packed-column GC." When liquid-phase GLC or the solid sorbent coats the inner wall of the column, the column itself acts as a support for the stationary phase. This technique is known as "open-tubular GC," or "capillary GC." Regardless of the type of mobile or stationary phase, separation is achieved by the difference in partitioning of the various molecules of the sample between the two phases.

Gas chromatographic separation is illustrated by the following example: A sample containing the components to be separated is injected into a heated block in which they are immediately vaporized and swept by a stream of carrier gas through a column of stationary phase. The components are adsorbed onto the stationary phase at the head of the column and then are gradually desorbed by fresh carrier gas. The partitioning between the two phases occurs repeatedly as carrier gas sweeps the components toward the column outlet.

As the components are eluted, they enter a detector where

their presence is converted to an electric signal, which is then measured, usually by a strip chart recorder that produces a series of peaks charted versus time (Fig. 7-1). The appearance time, height, width, and area of these chromatogram peaks may be measured to yield valuable qualitative and quantitative data.

MOLECULES THAT CAN BE SEPARATED BY GAS CHROMATOGRAPHY

Theoretically any compound that can be vaporized or converted to a volatile derivative may be analyzed by gas chromatography. Compounds as small as carbon monoxide and methane and as large as 800 daltons have been successfully analyzed. Compounds larger than 800 daltons lack sufficient volatility. Generally a compound must be stable as a vapor to produce a single identifiable chromatographic peak. Unstable compounds may be converted to stable, volatile derivatives. However, if a compound degrades to known products or a consistent number of products, the resultant pattern of multiple compounds may be used as a means of tentative identification.

Inorganic compounds, or the inorganic salts of organic acids and bases, lack sufficient volatility for gas chromatographic analysis. Thus the technique is generally applied to analysis of organic molecules in their neutral nonionic forms. Before chromatographic analysis, compounds are generally isolated and concentrated by means of solvent extraction and evaporation to dryness. The residues containing the analytes are dissolved in small amounts of volatile organic solvents. The solvent-analyte solution is then chromatographed. The analyte vapor should not interact with the solvent. The solvent should have greater volatility and much less affinity for the stationary phase than the analyte compounds do, thereby eluting far ahead of the analyte and not interfering with the chromatogram.

THEORY OF GAS CHROMATOGRAPHIC SEPARATION

The following is a brief discussion of the basic chromatographic theory as it applies to gas-liquid chromatography. See Chapter 5 for a review of general chromatography theory. For a more complete treatment of the many complex variables that influence gas chromatographic separations, one should read references 1 and 2.

Partition coefficient (K_D)

The general concepts of sample *partitioning* and the *partition coefficient* (K_D) have been described in Chapter 5 (see equation 5-1 and pp. 109 and 121). Similarly, definitions of *retention* and *retention time* and *capacity factor* (or capacity rates) have been described in Chapter 5 on p. 113 and Fig. 7-1. These basic concepts apply to both liquid chromatography (LC) (Chapter 6) and gas chromatography (GC). The transit time required for the carrier gas to move from the point of injection to the end of the column is called the "gas-holdup time," or "dead time," t_M (Fig. 7-1). It arises from the internal volumes of the injector, column, and detector and is equivalent to the void volume in high performance liquid chromatography (HPLC). A compound that does not partition into the stationary phase ($K_D = 0$) will be eluted from the column at t_M.

Because the "dead time" is a characteristic of both the particular gas chromatograph used for analysis (injector and detector volumes) and the column volume, it is the same for all sample components and is of no significance in identification. The difference between the uncorrected retention time and the dead time is called the "corrected retention time," t'_R

$$t'_R = t_R - t_M \qquad \text{Eq. 7-1}$$

Partitioning in GC systems

The K_D, or corrected time, t'_R, of a solute in a specific system must be determined experimentally; it cannot be predicted easily. Both the partition coefficient and retention time of a solute are directly related and depend on the affinity of solute for the stationary phase. The old rule "like dissolves like" offers a simple guide to solute affinity. Polar solutes will have greater partition coefficients, K_D, hence longer retention times on hydrophilic (polar) phases than hydrophobic (nonpolar) stationary phases. Likewise, hydro-

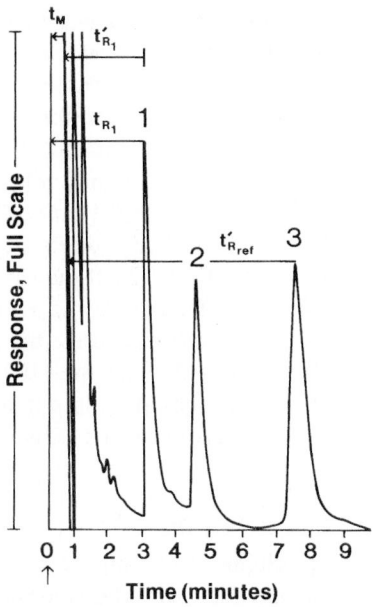

Fig. 7-1 Example of gas chromatogram showing detector response versus time. Vertical arrow (time = 0) indicates time of injection, and initial peak is "dead time," t_M. t_R designates uncorrected retention time, whereas t_R' is corrected retention time. t'_{Rref} is corrected retention time for internal standard or reference compound. Relative retention time for peak 1: $r = t'_{R1}/t'_{Rref}$. (Modified from Mackell MA, Poklis A: *J Chromatogr* 235(2):445, 1982.)

phobic solutes exhibit greater K_D's and longer retention times on the nonpolar rather than the polar stationary phase. If both a hydrophobic and a polar solute are chromatographed together on a polar stationary phase, the hydrophobic solute will have less affinity for the phase than the polar solute ($K_{D\ hydrophobic} < K_{D\ polar}$) and will be eluted before the polar solute ($t'_{R\ hydrophobic} < t'_{R\ polar}$).

The K_D of solute is expressed as a concentration (amount/volume) ratio and therefore may be written as

$$K_D = [W_s/V_s]/[W_m/V_m] = \frac{V_M}{V_S} \cdot \frac{W_S}{W_M}$$

W_S = Weight of the sample in the stationary phase
W_M = Weight of the sample in the mobile phase
V_S = Volume of the stationary phase
V_M = Volume of the mobile phase

The ratio of the mobile-phase (gas) and stationary-phase (column) volumes (V_M/V_S) is called the phase ratio (β). The ratio of sample weights (W_S/W_M) in each phase is equal to the capacity ratio, k. Therefore the partition coefficient can be expressed as

$$K_D = \beta k$$

The phase ratio and capacity ratio are characteristics for a particular column. However, their product, K_D, is independent of the particular column. Therefore the higher the phase ratio (and smaller the volume of stationary phase), the smaller is the capacity ratio (less time for elution, t_R). In general, the smaller the capacity ratio (shorter t_R), the more difficult it is to achieve a particular separation. The amount of solute analyzed on a column without overloading is dependent on the amount of stationary phase that influences β. The greater the amount of stationary phase, the smaller is the β and the larger the k (greater t_R).

Temperature dependence

Temperature is the most important single parameter in a gas chromatograph separation. This is attributable to the great dependence of the partition coefficient, K_D, on temperature. The inverse relationship between K_D and temperature is given by the equation

$$\log K_D = \frac{\Delta H}{2.3R \cdot T_c} + \text{Constant} \qquad \textit{Eq. 7-2}$$

ΔH is the partial molar heat of solution of the solute in the liquid state, R is the gas constant, and T_c is the column temperature.

This equation demonstrates that, in a given system, the higher the column temperature, the lower is the K_D, which means a lower capacity ratio, k (shorter retention time). Therefore the retention times of solute molecules may be readily altered when one changes the column temperatures. Roughly, a 30° C decrease in column temperature will approximately double the retention time. Conversely a 30° C increase in column temperature will approximately halve

the retention time. The influence of temperature on separation is discussed later.

Column performance

The ability of a column to produce optimum separations is measured by two quantities: *efficiency,* which is the ability to produce narrow peaks, and *resolution,* which is the ability to separate two adjacent peaks.

The general concepts of *resolution, theoretical plates,* and *height equivalent to a theoretical plate* (HETP), all used to describe the efficiency of a column, have been defined in Chapter 5 (pp. 110 to 113). HETP (or *H*) uses the uncorrected retention time, t_R. If the corrected retention time, t'_R, is employed instead, the expression *height equivalent to an effective plate,* or HEEP (*h*), is used. The term *HETP* defines not only the efficiency of the column, but also the overall efficiency of the system because of the gas-holdup times of the injector, column, and detector. Because the gas-holdup time varies in different instruments, the column efficiency is best expressed by the number of effective plates (HEEP, or *h*).

The relationship of the HETP to the linear gas velocity, μ, is complex. The factors affecting gas flow are expressed by the van Deemter equation:

$$\text{HETP} = A + B/\mu + C\mu$$

In packed column GC, *A* is the eddy diffusion term, which relates the effect of support-particle diameter and the column-packing procedure to the distance that a streamline of carrier gas persists before its velocity is drastically changed by the support. *B* is the longitudinal gas diffusion term, which relates peak broadening to the effect of diffusion in the flowing gas along the direction of flow. *C* is the resistance–to–mass transfer term, which relates the diffusion processes in the gas and liquid phases. The relationship of the HETP to linear velocity, when graphed, corresponds to a hyperbola (see Fig. 7-2). If the slope of the rising part of the curve is extended down, it intercepts the *y*-axis, yielding the value of the *A* term (the contribution of the obtrusion of the gas flow to the HETP). In open tubular columns where the gas path is not inhibited, the *A*-term intercept is zero and the van Deemter equation is reduced to

$$\text{HETP} = B/\mu + C\mu$$

Thus open tubular columns have much lower HETPs and much greater efficiency than packed columns[3] (Table 7-1). Eventually the van Deemter curve reaches a minimum, which is the optimum velocity (μ_{opt}) yielding the smallest HETP. For open tubular columns the minimum HETP is determined solely by flow rate and the resistance to mass transfer, $C\mu$. The descending part of the curve (from μ_{opt} to the *y*-axis) represents the longitudinal diffusion term *B*. Because there are no support or sorbent particles hindering diffusion along the column in open tubular columns, the

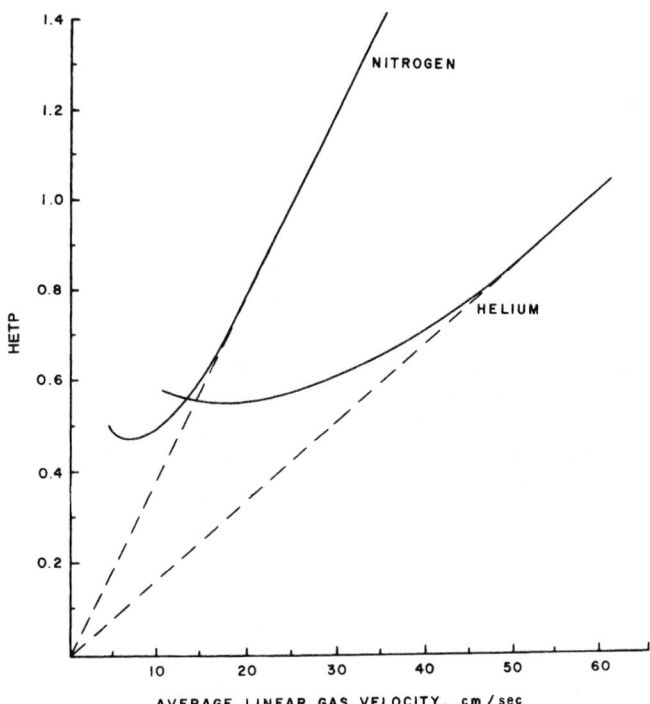

Fig. 7-2 Relationship between HETP (heat equivalent to a theoretical plate) and average linear gas velocity for two different carrier gases: nitrogen and helium. (From Ettre LS: *Practical gas chromatography*, Norwalk, Conn., 1973, Perkin-Elmer Corp.)

Table 7-1 Differences between packed and capillary columns

Parameter	Packed	Capillary
Length, meters	1.5 to 6.0	5 to 100
Inner diameter, millimeters	2 to 4	0.2 to 0.7
Specific permeability, (10^{-7}) cm^2	1 to 10	10 to 1000
Flow, mL/min	10 to 60	0.5 to 15.0
Pressure drop, psi	10 to 40	3 to 40
Total effective plates (2 meter, 50 meter)	5000	150,000
Effective plates per meter	2500 (ID 2 mm)	3000 (ID 0.25)
Capacity	10 μg/peak	<50 ng/peak
Liquid film thickness (μm)	1 to 10	0.05 to 0.5

carrier-gas velocity must be much greater than that in packed columns (Table 7-1). Thus the van Deemter plot is greatly shifted to the right (increased μ_{opt}) for open tubular columns.

The optimum velocity is ideal for only one compound; however, similar compounds have closely related optimum velocities, and a single flow rate is suitable for their separation. At higher flow rates, the gas sweeps the diffusing molecules from the liquid before all have emerged, thus broadening the peak.

MOBILE-PHASE CONSIDERATIONS

The most commonly used carrier gases are presented in Table 7-2. The carrier gas must be inert so as not to react with the sample components. Large quantities of relatively pure gas must be commercially available because appreciable amounts of carrier gas are used for analysis. Common impurities in carrier gases are moisture, oxygen, and hydrocarbons. Each of these contaminants may adversely affect various detectors, producing unstable recorder baseline or extraneous peaks. In certain situations, carrier-gas impurities may interact with sample components and prevent their analysis. For example, prepurified-grade nitrogen contains up to 20 ppm of oxygen. If high column temperatures are necessary to separate compounds that are readily oxidized, the oxygen impurity in nitrogen carrier gas may

degrade the compounds on the column and prevent their detection or may produce multiple extraneous peaks of the degradation products. In such a situation, helium, which contains less oxygen contamination, should replace nitrogen as the carrier gas.

The choice of carrier gas does influence column performance (efficiency and resolution) and time required for analysis (retention time). As presented by the van Deemter equation, the height equivalent to a theoretical plate (HETP) is related to the linear gas velocity (μ) of the carrier gas. This interaction is highly complex, but the following brief discussion presents the basic effects of carrier gas upon separation.

In a flowing system (column) where the gas is compressible, the density, pressure, and velocity of the gas are different at each point in the column. The carrier gas is compressible, and the value of the carrier-gas velocity must be corrected to average conditions. The average linear gas velocity (μ) is determined by two factors: (1) the time necessary for an unretained solute to pass through the column (dead time, t_M) (p. 153) and (2) the length of the column, L. These factors determine μ by the following equation:

$$\mu = L/t_M \qquad \textit{Eq. 7-3}$$

In a given column, the optimum linear gas velocity (μ_{opt}) is proportional to the diffusivity of the vapors of the substances being chromatographed. However, the kinetic theory of gases states that the diffusivity in gas is inversely proportional to the square root of the molecular weight or density of the gas (see Table 7-2). Therefore the μ_{opt} will be lower for high-density gases (low solute diffusivity), such as nitrogen and argon, and higher for low-density gases (high solute diffusivity), such as helium and hydrogen. Therefore in the same column different values of μ_{opt} will be obtained for different gases. Fig. 7-2 shows the relationship between the μ of two different carrier gases and the resultant HETP. Nitrogen has a minimum HETP of 0.465 at a μ_{opt} of 7 cm/sec, whereas helium has a minimum HETP of 0.55 at a μ_{opt} of 17.5 cm/sec. This demonstrates that in the same length of column, a high-density gas (nitrogen or argon) will produce better efficiency (more theoretical plates per unit length, lower HETP) than a low-density gas (helium or hydrogen). For a given system, the maximum resolution will be obtained at minimum h, which is determined at the μ_{opt} of the carrier gas. Also, for a given length of column, better resolution will be obtained by the carrier gas producing the lowest h value.

For a low-density gas, the diffusivity of the solute and the μ_{opt} in a given column are greater than those of a high-density gas. Therefore, shorter retention times (smaller t_R) are obtained with helium or hydrogen than with nitrogen or argon.

STATIONARY-PHASE CONSIDERATIONS
Gas-solid stationary phases

In gas-solid chromatography the column is packed or the inner wall is coated with an adsorptive solid material on which the sample components are partitioned by adsorption on the surface of the solid. This material should possess a large surface area per unit volume to ensure rapid equilibrium between the stationary and gas phases. It should possess uniform particle size and pore structure and be strong enough to resist breakdown during handling and column packing. Theoretically the smaller the particle size of support, the greater the efficiency of the column is. However, the smaller the particles, the greater the resistance to flow and the greater the necessary carrier-gas pressure.

The most common chromatographic solids for adsorption phases are made from diatomaceous earth (kieselguhr). The processed white kieselguhr is sold under many trade names: Chromosorb W, Celite, Gas Chrom, and Anakron. The diatomite may also be crushed, blended, pressed into brick, and processed such that mineral impurities form oxides and silicates, which give the material a pink color. It is marketed as crushed firebrick, or Chromosorb P. This material has greater density and is less fragile than the white material. The pore size of the pink material is only 2 mm compared to 9 mm for the white. Therefore greater efficiency is obtained with the pink material.

Each support possesses individual properties that may enhance or hinder its use for a particular application. The white material is slightly alkaline and will interact with acidic compounds. Its surface, however, is nonadsorptive, a property that favors its application for analysis of polar compounds. The pink material adsorbs polar compounds;

thus it is best suited for the separation of nonpolar molecules like hydrocarbons.

Another type of solid stationary phase consists of porous polymer beads, which allow the analyte molecules to go into partition directly from the gas phase into the amorphous polymer. Porapak, a polymer of ethylvinylbenzene cross-linked with vinylbenzene, is the most popular polymer phase. The material may be modified by copolymerization with various polar monomers to produce beads of varying polarity. Porapak columns are thermally stable up to 250° C. At temperatures above 250° C the column material will be degraded and eluted, a phenomenon called *column bleed*. These degradation products can be observed by the detector. Water and highly polar molecules are rapidly eluted from the polymer. Porapak is especially useful for baseline separation of aqueous samples containing low-molecular-weight alcohols, esters, halogens, hydrocarbons, ketones, and mercaptans (Table 7-3).

Gas-liquid-solid supports for GLC

The stationary phase in gas-liquid chromatography is a thin film of liquid held on an inert support. In capillary chromatography, the liquid is coated on the walls of the tubing. In packed columns, the liquid is held in a thin-layer film across the surface of an inert support (Fig. 7-3). Many materials that act as stationary phases for GSC are also supports for the liquid phase in GLC. Both the pink and white solid phases described earlier are popular liquid supports. Although the support should be inert and not influence separation, both pink and white materials have *active sites* because of metallic impurities and silanol (—SiOH) and siloxane (SiOSi—) groups, which form hydrogen bonds with polar compounds. This interaction gives rise to distorted (asymmetrical) peaks in the resultant GLC chromatogram. These *active sites* may be removed by acid washing of the mineral impurities from the support and by conversion of the silanol groups to silyl esters (silanization) of dimethyl-dichlorosilane or hexamethyldisilazone. Silanization reduces surface activity but also reduces the surface area of the support so that no more than 10% (v/w) of the liquid stationary phase to total column weight may be applied. In certain instances, special additives are mixed with the liquid phase to block the active sites of untreated support ma-

Table 7-2 Common carrier gases

Gas	Molecular weight	Density (g/L)	Impurities (ppm)
Argon	39.944	1.784	—
Helium	4.007	0.177	Hydrocarbons (1 to 100)
Hydrogen	2.018	0.089	—
Nitrogen	28.014	1.251	Oxygen (20)

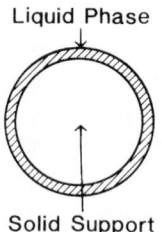

Liquid Phase

Solid Support

Fig. 7-3 Schema of solid support particle for gas chromatography with liquid stationary-phase coating.

Table 7-3 Examples of commonly used stationary phases and their applications

Stationary phase	Structures	Activity	Temperature (°C min/max)	Application	Specific compounds
Silicone OV-1 (100% methyl)	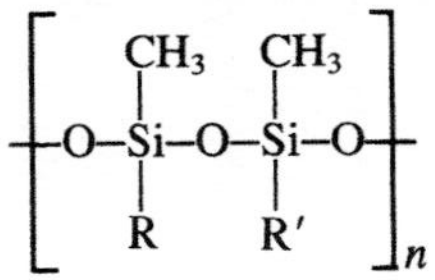 (structure)	Nonpolar	100/350	Bacteria, drugs	Fatty acid methyl esters, benzodiazepines
Silicone OV-17 (50% phenyl)	R and R' = CH_3 in above structure; R and R' = Phenyl in above structure	Intermediate polarity	20/350	Drugs, steroids	Tricyclic antidepressants, barbiturates, cholesterol
Silicone OV-210 (50%, 3,3,3-trifluoropropyl)	R and R' = $-CH_2-CH_2-CF_3$ in above structure	Polar	20/300	Drugs, pesticides	Basic drugs, lindane, aldrin, DDT
Silicone OV-225 (25% cyanopropyl, 25% phenyl)	R = Phenyl, R' = $-CH_2-CH_2-CH_2-CN$ in above structure	Polar	20/275	Steroids	TMS derivatives of 17-ketosteroids
10% Apiezon L 2% KOH NPGS (neopentyl glycol succinate)	Undefined mixture of high-boiling hydrocarbons; (structure)	Nonpolar	50/225, 50/240	Amines; Volatile fatty acids	Amphetamine; Acetic through caproic acids
Carbopack B/5%	(structure)	Polar		Alcohols, aldehydes, ketones	Methanol, ethanol, acetaldehyde acetone
DEGS (diethylene glycol succinate)	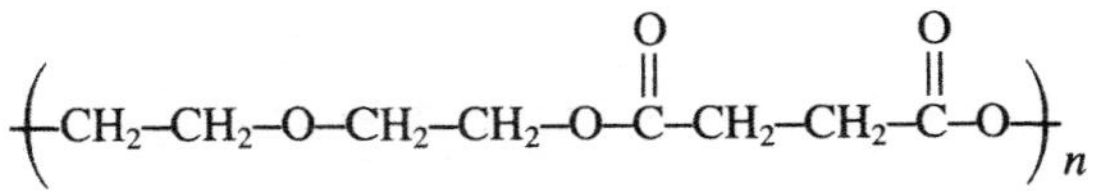 (structure)	Polar	20/200	Bacteria	Fatty acid methyl esters
EGA (ethylene glycol adipate)	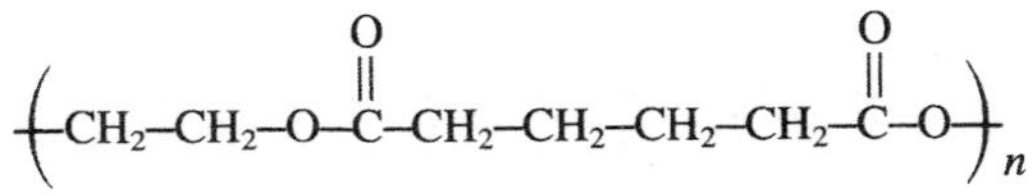 (structure)		100/210	Amino acids	NBTFA derivatives of amino acids
Chromosorb 102 (styrene divinyl benzene polymer)	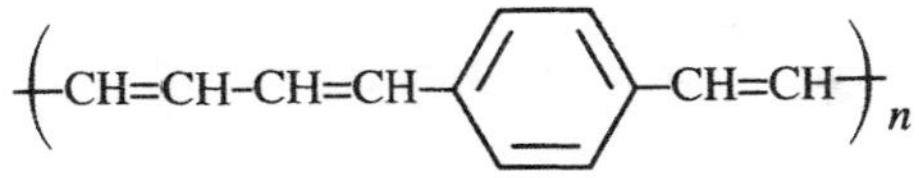 (structure)		<250° C	Alcohols, aldehydes	Methanol, ethanol, acetaldehyde
Porapak Q (ethylvinyl benzene + divinyl benzene polymer mixture)	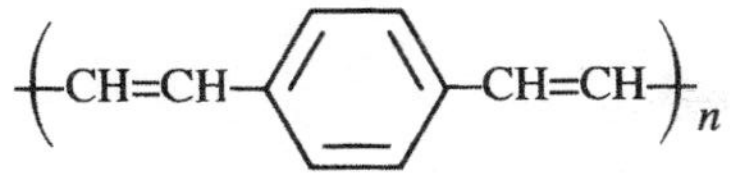 (structure)		<250° C	Low molecular weight	Chlorinated hydrocarbons

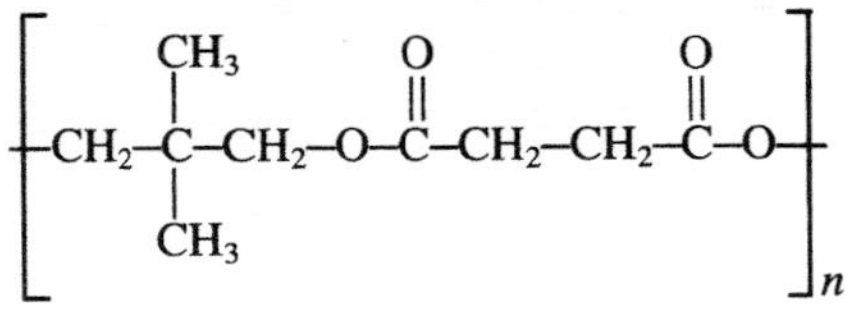

NBTFA, Nitroblue tetrazolium fatty acid.

terial. Two such examples are the incorporation of stearic acid in silicone oil used in separation of fatty acids and the addition of potassium hydroxide to polar liquid phases used to separate amines.

In open tubular chromatography, the liquid is coated on the walls of the tubing. The cohesive forces of most liquid phases are greater than the adhesive or wetting forces between the liquid and the glass surface of the column. Therefore, to create a uniform thin film the column is treated to produce an adhesive surface.[4] Several techniques are used: deposition of fumed silica, a microlayer of fine particles of salts such as barium carbonate or sodium chloride, quartz powder, or etching the glass with dry acid gas. These treatments increase the "roughness" of the surface, allowing the liquid to fill the holes and crevices and spread across the surface of the column. The character of the column surface may also be altered by treatment with wetting agents, such as Carbowax 20M, which are strongly attached to absorptive sites and deactivate the surface. After treatment, residual Carbowax 20M is washed from the column, and the liquid phase of choice is applied to the surface. Informative data describing preparation, applications, and limitations of support materials are readily available from commercial manufacturers and suppliers.

Liquid phases

The universal popularity of GLC as a separation method is attributable to the large variety of liquid phases with differing solution properties and therefore different affinities for various classes of analytes. The range of liquids used as stationary phases is limited only by their volatility, thermal stability, and ability to wet the support. No single stationary phase will achieve all desired separations. Commercial suppliers typically offer 100 to 200 liquid phases; however, many of these phases are duplicates sold under various trade names or are so similar in character as to have little difference in their separation abilities. In fact, few laboratories require the use of more than a half dozen different liquid phases. Eighty percent of a wide range of organic compounds may be successfully separated using only four to seven phases: OV-101, OV-17, Carbowax 20M, OV-225, DEGS, OV-275, and OV-210.[5,6] Examples of liquid phases, characteristics, and applications are presented in Table 7-3.

Liquid phases may be generally classified into five categories: (1) Nonpolar phases, which are hydrocarbon liquids such as squalane, silicone greases, Apiezon L, and silicone gum rubber. Generally, compounds are eluted from these phases in order of increasing boiling point. (2) Intermediate polarity phases that include polar or polarizable groups attached to a long nonpolar skeleton, such as esters of high molecular weight or alcohols such as diisodecylphthalate. Both polar and nonpolar compounds are separated by these phases, with the more polar ones eluted first. (3) Polar phases, which contain a high concentration of polar groups, such as carbowaxes. These phases differentiate

between polar and nonpolar compounds by interacting strongly only with polar compounds, separating these from the earlier eluting, less polar compounds. (4) Hydrogen-bonding phases, which contain many hydrogen atoms readily available for hydrogen bonding, such as glycol phases. Polar compounds have greater affinity for the stationary phase and are eluted more slowly. (5) Special-purpose phases that can be prepared to use a specific chemical interaction between the sample and the stationary phase. An example of a special-purpose phase is silver nitrate dissolved in glycol to enhance separation of unsaturated hydrocarbons by charge-transfer interactions.

Each liquid phase has a specific temperature range for efficient use (Table 7-3). The maximum temperature at which a phase may be used is determined by its volatility. Beyond this temperature the phase is lost because of decomposition or volatilization and is carried into the detector producing extensive background noise (column bleed). A column may be heated above the maximum temperature for brief periods of time as in temperature programming, but the maximum temperature must never be exceeded for isothermal (constant-temperature) analysis. Below the minimum temperature analysis of the increased viscosity or solidification of the liquid cannot be reproduced.

The amount of stationary phase in the column is expressed in percentage by weight of the liquid phase on the support. In general, packed columns contain 3% to 10% liquid phase. Deviations from these values may occur in specific applications: very low liquid loads for high-molecular-weight compounds and high loads for small, highly volatile compounds such as hydrocarbons containing one to four carbon atoms. The amount of stationary phase directly affects the sample capacity and efficiency of the column. The greater the amount of liquid phase, the larger the amount of sample that may be chromatographed.

The manufacturers of open tubular columns often use trade names for the liquid phases presented in Table 7-3. However, the name usually retains a numerical designation so that the chromatographer can recognize the composition of the liquid phase as given in the table. For example, a capillary column of HP-1 or DB-1 is a 100% dimethyl polysiloxane (simethicone) comparable to OV-1 (Table 7-3) produced by Hewlett-Packard and J&W Scientific, respectively.

Open tubular columns contain small amounts of stationary phase which significantly reduce the capacity of the column. Capillary columns with inside diameters (ID) of 0.2 mm have capacities of less than 100 ng of sample component. The sample capacity is increased by increasing the column ID. For example, columns with 0.32 mm will accept up to 500 ng of sample component, and columns with 0.53 mm up to 2000 ng of sample component. Columns with IDs of 0.75 mm approach the capacity of packed columns (15,000 ng). Such columns with increased IDs (0.50 to 0.75 mm) are referred to as "wide-bore" columns.

DERIVATIZATION

Often it is desirable to modify a molecule chemically so that a newly formed product has properties that are preferable to its precursors. One may need to derivatize a compound to make it volatile and stable as a gas and thus analyzable by GC. Derivatives are also prepared to achieve increased sensitivity, selectivity, or specificity for a given separation. Derivatives may be eluted from the column sooner, have less tailing, produce sharper peaks, provide stability to thermally labile compounds, and increase resolution. Derivatization involves a chemical reaction between some functional group on the sample molecule (usually a polar group, which reduces volatility or interacts with the stationary phase to increase retention time) and a smaller molecule (derivatizing agent), which forms a new product of increased volatility with a smaller partition coefficient (K_D). The derivatization may be carried out before sample injection or may occur in the injection port of the chromatograph ("on column" or "flash derivatization"). A few derivatization techniques are briefly presented, but for a more complete discussion consult the literature.[7,8]

A popular GC derivatization technique is the replacement of an active hydrogen by a trimethylsilyl (TMS) group. The resultant *silyl* derivatives are usually less polar and more volatile and display greater thermal stability than their parent compounds. Silylizing reagents react vigorously with water or alcohol-containing solvents; therefore the conversion reactions are carried out in anhydrous solvents such as acetonitrile or tetrahydrofuran. TMS reagents are flammable, and some are highly corrosive. They should be handled with care.

$$ROH \quad + \quad (CH_3)_3SiCl \rightarrow ROSi(CH_3)_3 + HCl$$
Alcohol   Trimethylchlorosilane

Esterification is often used for GC analysis of compounds containing a carboxylic acid group. Methyl esters possess the greatest volatility and hence are most popular. Alkylation reactions with quaternary alkylammonium hydroxides or dimethylformamide-dialkyl acetals have become popular as "flash-derivatizing" reagents. Fig. 7-4 presents the derivatization reaction of tetramethylammonium hydroxide and barbiturate drugs. To increase sensitivity, derivatizing reagents that produce halogen- or nitrogen-containing compounds are used with electron-capture detectors.

SELECTION OF A SEPARATION SYSTEM
Choosing the mobile phase

The mobile phase or carrier gas has one major function in gas chromatography: to carry the vaporized sample through the column and into the detector. As previously described, selection of the proper carrier gas is predicated upon three considerations: (1) the operating principles of the detector through which the gas will be continuously flowing, (2) the presence of impurities in the carrier gas, and (3) the desired speed of analysis and performance of the column. Compounds that are negligibly partitioned into a stationary phase cannot be separated from each other. Similarly, compounds with too great an affinity for the stationary phase will have unacceptably long retention times or may be irreversibly retarded.

Stationary-phase selection

Liquid phases with the same physical properties as the sample will retain the sample and generally effect a separation. However, this general rule does not aid in determining which specific stationary phase is potentially the best for a particular separation. Several approaches to the choice of liquid-phase selection for a desired separation are briefly presented.

Many sources of irreproducibility can affect GC analysis. These include variations in assay conditions and variations in stationary-phase packaging (lot to lot, company to company, and so on). To ensure reproducible identification of peaks of interest regardless of exact assay conditions, relative retention times are converted to indices or constants. These values can then be used to compare data between analyses, within a laboratory, or between laboratories.

Kovats index. If the components of the sample are known, the most likely stationary phase that will effect a separation may be selected by use of the Kovats retention index.[9,10] Retention indices relate the retention time of a compound, regardless of its chemical nature, to those of the *n*-paraffins (straight-chain hydrocarbons) eluted directly before and after it. Chromatographing the *n*-paraffins on a given column under set conditions yields a nearly linear relationship between the log of their retention time, t_R, and the number of carbon atoms in each paraffin, as shown in Fig. 7-5.

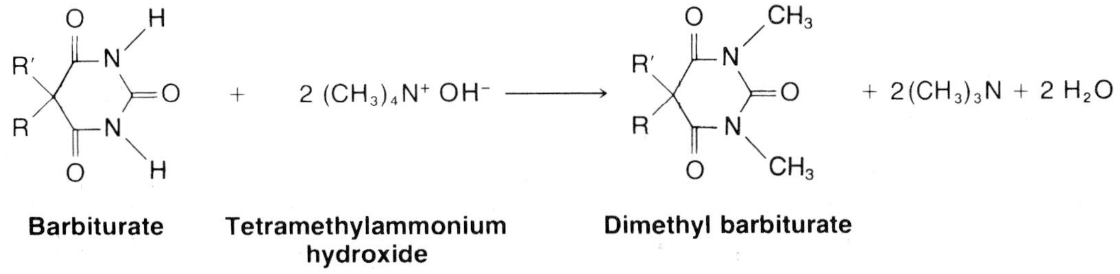

Barbiturate   **Tetramethylammonium hydroxide**   **Dimethyl barbiturate**

Fig. 7-4   Tetramethyl derivatization of barbiturate drugs.

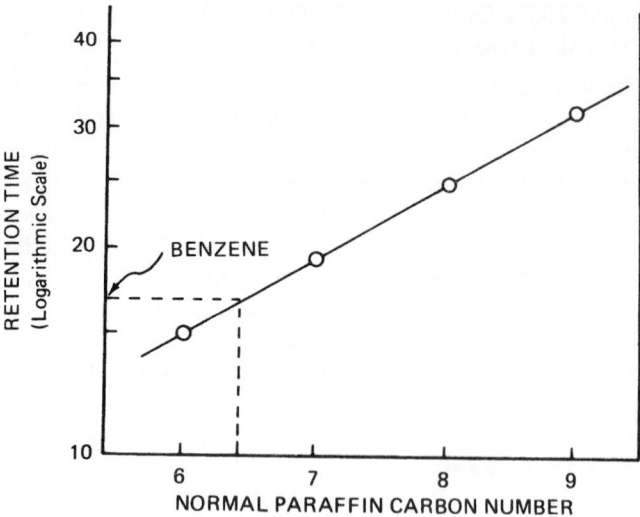

Fig. 7-5 Linear relationship between log of retention time and number of carbon atoms in a series of paraffin hydrocarbons. (From Rowland FW: *The practice of gas chromatography,* Palo Alto, Calif., 1974, Hewlett-Packard Co.)

Each *n*-paraffin is given a retention index, *I*, that equals 100 times the number of carbon atoms. The retention index of all other compounds is calculated from the following relationship:

$$I = 100z + 100 \left[(\log t_{Rx} - \log t_{Rz})/(\log t_{R(z+1)} - \log t_{Rz}) \right]$$

Eq. 7-4

z equals the number of carbon atoms in the unknown compound; t_{Rx} is the retention time of the unknown substance *x*; t_{Rz} is the retention time of the *n*-paraffin eluted immediately before *x*; and $t_{R(z+1)}$ is the retention time of the *n*-paraffin eluted immediately after *x*. For example, assume that the data presented in Table 7-4 and graphically represented in Fig. 7-5 were obtained by chromatography from a series of *n*-paraffins and benzene on a given liquid phase. The retention index, *I*, benzene ($z = 6$) on that liquid phase is calculated to be 650.

$$I = 100(6) + 100(0.052/0.104) = 600 + 50 = 650$$

The calculated *I* applies only to the particular stationary phase and temperature conditions. However, the effects of flow rate of the mobile phase and the percent loading (quantity of liquid phase) will change the retention time proportionally for all *n*-paraffins, and thus the calculated *I* values

are unchanged. Extensive lists of retention indices of numerous compounds on liquid phases are available in the *ASTM Gas Chromatography Data Compilation Catalog AMD 25A*[11] and a supplement catalog *AMD 25A S-1*.[12] If several compounds of a different chemical nature are to be separated simultaneously, the compounds of interest are located in the table and their respective *I* values for various stationary phases noted. A difference of at least 30 *I* units between the compounds will indicate that a particular phase will efficiently separate them. The *I* values are based on peak apex only and give no indication of peak width. Therefore *I* values do not indicate the resolution of the compounds. However, since the retention times increase with the retention index, *I*, the retention indices indicate the order in which compounds will be eluted from the column. A clinical application of *I* values has been the qualitative identification of drugs on standard liquid phases under both isothermal and temperature-programmed conditions.[13] Retention index data bases for packed columns may be used for preliminary identification of peaks eluting from open tubular columns.[14]

Rohrschneider and McReynolds constants. Rohrschneider and McReynolds constants are related systems that classify stationary phases in terms of their separating power.[15,16] The *I* values of a set of reference compounds of varying polarity are determined on the liquid phase being tested and compared against the *I* values for the same compounds obtained on a reference liquid phase. Squalane, a nonpolar liquid, is used as the reference phase. The constants are then calculated as indicated in the following equations:

Rohrschneider constant $(x) = 1/100 \, (I_{\text{test phase}} - I_{\text{squalene}})$ **Eq. 7-5**

McReynolds constant $(x') = I_{\text{test phase}} - I_{\text{squalene}}$ **Eq. 7-6**

Table 7-5 presents data related to five reference compounds used to determine the McReynolds constants. Both Rohrschneider and McReynolds constants may be used for two purposes: to select a liquid phase for a particular application and to classify liquid phases as to how similar or different they are in the ability to perform chromatographic separations.[17] An example of the use of McReynolds constants for selection of a liquid phase for a given application would be the separation of saturated and unsaturated fatty acid methyl esters. If one has available liquid phases 1 (DEGS) and 2 (Carbowax 20M), presented in Table 7-6, an

Table 7-4 Data used for calculation of retention index

Compound	Carbon atoms	Symbol	t_R (min)	log t_R (min)	Retention index (*I*)
Hexane	6	*z*	14.96	1.175	600 (by definition)
Benzene	6	*x*	16.86	1.227	650 (by experiment)
Heptane	7	*z* + 1	19.01	1.279	700 (by definition)
Octane	8	—	24.15	—	800 (by definition)
Nonane	9	—	30.76	—	900 (by definition)

Table 7-5   Reference compounds used to determine McReynolds constants

Reference compound	Abbreviation	I*	Organic compound expected to display similar behavior on liquid phase
Benzene	x'	650	Aromatics, olefins
Butanol	y'	590	Alcohols, phenols, weak acids
2-Pentanone	z'	627	Aldehydes, esters, ketones
Nitropropane	u'	652	Nitrogenous and nitrile compounds
Pyridine	s'	699	Nitrogenous aromatic heterocyclics, bases

*Absolute value of retention indices observed on squalane.

examination of their McReynolds constants permits one to choose the best phase for the separation. For the ability to separate saturated and unsaturated fatty acid esters, one considers the constants x' (olefinic compounds, unsaturated esters) and z' (esters) (Table 7-5). The McReynolds constants for x' and z' (in bold face in Table 7-5) are much higher for DEGS than for Carbowax 20M; therefore DEGS is better suited for the separation of the fatty acid esters.

The characterization of liquid phases as to their ability to perform separations by use of McReynolds constants is demonstrated by examination of phases 3 (Emulphor ON-870), 4 (Triton X-100), and 5 (XE-60) in Table 7-6. All liquid phases are commercially available, and one can determine differences or similarities in separating power as illustrated in Table 7-6. Liquid phases 3 and 4 are almost identical in their ability to separate the reference compounds. Therefore, if used as a liquid phase, they would yield very similar chromatograms. Liquid phase 5 is similar to phases 3 and 4 for constants x' and y'. Therefore separation of compounds characterized by these constants (Table 7-6) on phase 5 (XE-60) would be essentially the same on phases 3 (Emulphor EN-870) and 4 (Triton X-100). The constants z' and u' are higher for phase 5, and the separation of the compounds listed in Table 7-5 for these constants would be better on XE-60 than on the other two phases. However, although keto compounds (constant z') are better separated on phase 5, the separation of alcohols (constant y') would be practically identical on phases 3, 4, and 5. When using packed columns, one finds that differences in McReynolds constants of 20 or less are insignificant. Differences of 100 McReynolds units indicate significantly better separating ability of one phase compared to the other.

Table 7-6   McReynolds constant of various liquid phases

Liquid phase	McReynolds constant				
	x'	y'	z'	u'	s'
1. DEGS	**496**	746	**590**	837	835
2. Carbowax 20M	**322**	536	**368**	572	510
3. Emulphor ON-870	202	395	251	395	344
4. Triton X-100	203	399	268	402	362
5. XE-60	204	381	340	493	367

x', Benzene; y', butanol; z', 2-pentanone; u', nitropropane; s', pyridine. Numbers in bold-faced type are McReynolds constants that are much higher for DEGS than for Carbowax 20M.

COMPONENTS OF GAS CHROMATOGRAPH

Basically a gas chromatograph consists of six components (Fig. 7-6): (1) a pressurized carrier gas with ancillary pressure and flow regulators, (2) a sample-injection port, (3) a column, (4) a detector, (5) an electrometer and signal recorder, and (6) thermostated compartments encasing the column, detector, and injection port.

Carrier gas

The efficiency of a gas chromatograph depends on a constant flow of carrier gas. The carrier gas from a pressurized tank flows through a toggle valve, a flowmeter (range 1 to 1000 L/min), metal restrictors, and a pressure gauge (1 to 4 atmospheres). The flow is adjusted by a needle valve mounted at the base of the flowmeter. The gas moves more slowly at the head of the column than at the outlet because of a pressure drop in the column. Thus the flow rates are measured as the gas leaves the column. This is done with a soap-film flowmeter. A simple sidearm buret with a rubber bulb filled with soap solution is connected to the detector outlet. One determines the flow rate by noting the time required for a film (bubble) to pass between two calibrated volume marks on the buret.

Carrier gas should be inert, dry, and pure. The most common carrier gases are inert, but they may contain contaminants that affect column performance and the response of ionization detectors. Hydrocarbon gases and water are removed from the carrier gas by a molecular sieve trap between the gas cylinder and the chromatograph.

Sample-injection port

Most GC analyses are performed on nonaqueous, liquid samples that are injected by a glass microsyringe. A needle is inserted through a septum into a heated block where the sample is vaporized and swept by carrier gas into the column. The pressure inside the injection port is usually well above atmospheric pressure, and the stream of carrier gas sweeps away the sample and aids in vaporization. Thus a sample may be vaporized at temperatures below its atmospheric boiling point. However, the injection port temperature is usually set at 25° to 50° C higher than the boiling point of the highest boiling components in the sample. This assures that immediate vaporization will occur and that the components will not be diluted by carrier gas

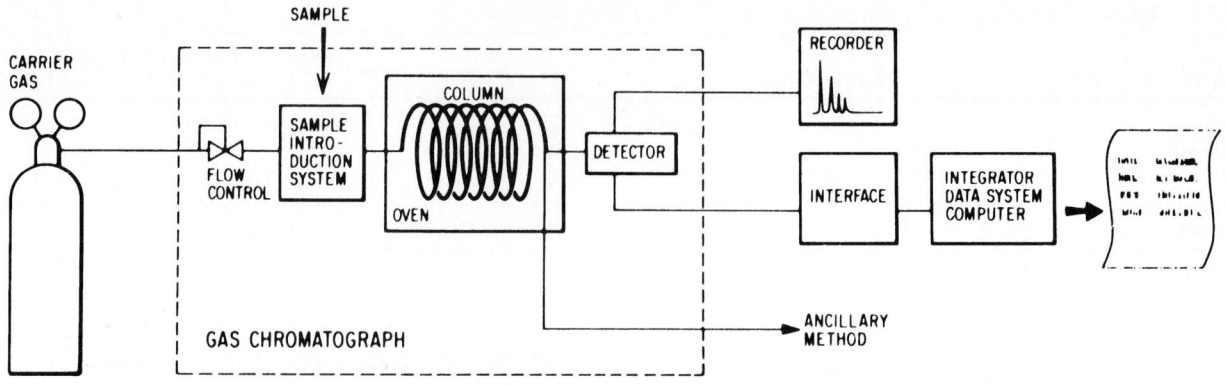

Fig. 7-6 Basic components of a gas chromatographic system. (From Ettre LS: *Practical gas chromatography,* Norwalk, Conn., 1973, Perkin-Elmer Corp.)

and will enter the head of the column as a single band. The time required for vaporization is dependent on the amount and volatility of the sample. Dilute samples vaporize faster than concentrated samples. High-boiling or temperature-sensitive compounds may be diluted with volatile solvents, which lower injection temperatures significantly.

Because heated metal may catalyze the degradation of many biological compounds, many injection ports are equipped with a glass liner or a glass column that extends through the injectors flush to the septum. The latter approach is called "on-column injection." For maximum efficiency it is imperative that the sample be the smallest possible volume (0.5 to 10 μL) consistent with detector sensitivity and be injected as a single, uniform band ("slug injection"). Insertion, injection, and withdrawal of the needle should be performed quickly and smoothly. Gaseous samples are injected by a gas-tight syringe or a calibrated bypass loop. The loop consists of a glass system of three stopcocks, between two of which a standard volume of gas is trapped and introduced into the carrier gas stream when the stopcocks are switched.

Because of the low capacity of capillary columns, injection of undiluted samples will often overload the column. This problem is avoided with capillary systems by splitting the carrier gas flow after vaporization. In the split-injection technique after vaporization of the sample, the carrier gas flow is divided into two parts with a variable ratio of flows. The smaller part of the gas/sample mixture enters the column while the larger flow bypasses the column inlet and leaves the system. The ratio of flow to the column and the outlet is controlled by a needle value. Splitting ratios may be adjusted over a wide range (1:5 to 1:250).

A septum separates the chromatographic column from the laboratory environment. Septums are small disks of silicone rubber, and numerous types are available, depending on analytic requirements. Silicone rubber septums may absorb certain types of samples. Special septums (such as Teflon R coated) will alleviate this problem. Low-molecular-weight solvents used in the manufacture of septums may

be released as the injection port is heated. This "bleed" of solvent may produce unwarranted peaks (ghost peaks) in chromatograms, and it increases the background level of the detector. Low-bleed septums from which the solvents have been extracted are available. Repeated injections through the septum will gradually destroy its mechanical strength, causing leakage. As a result, the retention time and sensitivity decrease as the carrier gas and part of the sample are released back through the septum into the atmosphere. This problem is easily avoided by regular insertion of new septums.

Various specialized injection systems are commercially available. If large numbers of similar analyses are to be performed, automatic sampling units are commonly used.

Column tubing

The column tubing is a container for the stationary phase (packing material) and directs the carrier gas flow. It should be inert and not affect the separation by reaction with the stationary phase or the sample. Depending on the gas chromatograph employed, the columns may be shaped as a U-tube or coiled in an open spiral or flat pancake shape.

Stainless steel and copper columns are often used for analyses requiring temperatures greater than 250° C. However, for the analysis of drugs, steroids, or other biological compounds, metal columns may absorb these analytes or catalyze their degradation. Therefore glass is the tubing of choice for the majority of clinical analyses. However, glass is fragile and inflexible, and if not properly handled, the columns are easily broken during transport or installation. Recently nickel has been recommended as a substitute for glass. Nickel tubing has been effectively used in the analysis of specific drugs, pesticides, and cholesterol, which previously required glass tubing.[18] However, the application of nickel tubing to the broad range of biological compounds has not yet been established. Until such time, glass tubing should remain the primary support when one is performing a clinical analysis.

The inside diameters of columns vary from capillary (0.2

Table 7-7 Detectors and appropriate gases

Detector	Carrier gas	Detector gas
Thermal conductivity (TCD)	Helium, hydrogen	—
Flame ionization (FID)	Helium, nitrogen	Air and hydrogen
Nitrogen-phosphorus (NPD)	Helium, nitrogen	1. Air and hydrogen
		2. Air and 8% hydrogen in helium
Electron capture	Nitrogen	5% methane in argon
	5% methane in argon	—

mm) to packed columns of 4 mm. Packed columns of 4 mm ID contain four times the stationary phase as 2 mm ID columns of the same length and therefore possess a greater sample capacity. However, the same separation will require higher temperatures and a longer analysis time on the wider column. In addition, columns should be only as long as necessary to effect the desired separation. A short column provides a short analysis time, low temperatures, long column life, and less background in the detector. Packed columns of 0.7 to 2 m (2 to 6 feet) or wide-bore columns of 15 m (45 feet) are sufficient for most chemical separations.

Thermal compartment

Precise control of column temperature is imperative in gas chromatography. The column oven is controlled by a system that is sensitive to changes of 0.01 Celsius degree and maintains the column temperature to ± 0.1 Celsius degree of the desired temperature. The column oven, injection block, and detectors should have separate heaters and controls. Analysis may be performed at a constant oven temperature (isothermal), or the temperature may be varied during the analysis (temperature programming). The temperature change during analysis can be programmed to vary with time according to predetermined, reproducible patterns, giving linear, convex, or concave curves when column temperature is plotted against time (Fig. 7-7). Temperature programming is often used in separating a complex mixture, the components of which have widely varying affinity for the stationary phase. Initially the column temperature is set low to permit separation and elution of the compounds with little affinity for the stationary phase. The temperature is then raised to elute compounds of higher stationary-phase affinity. Many chromatographs are equipped with specialized oven controls that uniformly raise the column temperature after each sample injection.

Detectors

As the carrier gas exits from the column, a detector senses the separated components of the sample and provides a corresponding electrical signal. Any physical device that accomplishes this may be used as a detector; however, only a few are commonly used. For proper operation or optimum response, each type of detector requires a specific carrier gas (Table 7-7). The most widely used detectors are discussed in the following section.[19,20]

Thermal-conductivity detector (TCD). A thermal-conductivity detector measures the difference in ability to conduct heat (thermal conductivity) between pure carrier gas and the carrier with sample mixture. A sample carried in the gas increases the thermal conductivity. Usually four heat-sensing elements, thermistors or wires, are mounted in a brass or stainless steel heat sink and connected to form the arms of a Wheatstone bridge (Fig. 7-8). An electric current is passed through the wires composing the bridge. Two filaments in opposite arms of the bridge are cooled by carrier gas (reference), and the other two by the column effluent (sample). The heat lost over both sets of wires is balanced by adjustment of the flow rate of the pure carrier gas. Emerging components from the column increase the rate of cooling of the sample wires because of the increased thermal conductivity of the gas mixture. This changes the electrical resistance of the sample wire pattern, making the Wheatstone bridge out of balance. This imbalance causes a response on the recorder. Important variables in optimum TCD response are carrier gas, flow rate, filament current, and detector temperature. TCDs lack selectivity because any compound cooling the wire will cause a response. They are not so sensitive as other detectors, with minimum detection ranging from 0.1 to 0.5 mg of analyte per microliter.

Flame-ionization detector (FID). In a flame-ionization detector, eluted components in the carrier gas are mixed with hydrogen and burned in air to produce a very hot flame to ionize organic compounds. A pair of electrodes, charged by a polarizing voltage, collects the ions and generates a current proportional to the number of ions collected. The resultant current is amplified by an electrometer, producing a response on the recorder. The response of an FID is directly proportional to the number of carbons in a molecule bound to hydrogen or other carbon atoms. It is insensitive to water, carbon monoxide, carbon dioxide, and most inorganic compounds. The FID is the most popular detector for the determination of organic compounds. Sensitivity depends on chemical structure; therefore, the detector response must be determined for each compound analyzed. At optimal conditions the minimal detectable quantity of organic compound is 1 ng. A cross section of an FID detector is shown in Fig. 7-9.

Nitrogen-phosphorus detector (NPD). A nitrogen-phosphorus detector is similar to an FID except that ions of an alkali metal (rubidium) are introduced into the hy-

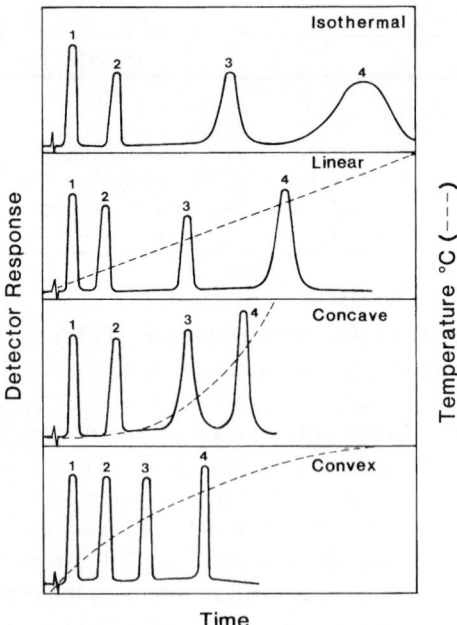

Fig. 7-7 Schema of theoretical separation of four compounds showing varying elution patterns with different temperature programming.

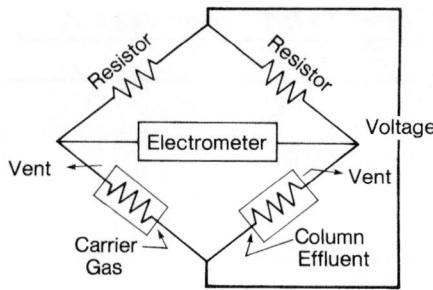

Fig. 7-8 Schema of thermal-conductivity detector. (From Werner M, Mohrbacher RJ, Riendeau CJ: In Baer DM, Dito WR: *Interpretation of therapeutic drug levels,* Chicago, 1981, American Society of Clinical Pathologists.)

drogen flame. When a compound containing nitrogen or phosphorus is burned in the flame, the rate of release of alkali metal vapor is increased. The alkali metal vapor readily ionizes in the flame and increases the current flow, which results in enhanced sensitivity for nitrogen and phosphorus. The optimum response is greatly dependent on the flow of hydrogen. The selective interaction of alkali metal ions with these compounds is complex and poorly understood. However, the sensitivity to organonitrogen compounds and lack of response to other organics make the NPD highly advantageous for the analysis of biological samples. At optimum conditions, the minimum detectable quantity of nitrogenous organic compounds is less than 1 ng. A cross section of an NPD detector is presented in Fig. 7-10.

Electron-capture detector (ECD). In an electron-capture detector, a radioactive isotope releases beta particles that collide with the carrier gas molecules, producing many low-energy electrons. The electrons are collected on electrodes and produce a small, measurable, *standing current.* As sample components that contain chemical groups with high electron affinity (electrophilic species), particularly halogen atoms, are eluted from the column, they capture the low-energy electrons generated by the isotope to form negatively charged ions. The detector measures the loss of cell current because of the recombination of the electrons. Three techniques are used for the collection of the electrons: (1) direct current (DC), (2) pulsed method, and (3) linear method. In the DC method, a constant voltage is applied to the cell electrodes, and the electrons are collected continu-

ously to produce a steady current. The sensitivity of the method is less than that of other ECD methods because both negative ions and free electrons are collected by the electrodes. The reduction in current is smaller than it would be if only free electrons were collected. In the pulsed method, a voltage is applied in continuous pulses of short duration; therefore the heavy negative ions do not have time to respond, and only free electrons are captured. Between pulses, the electron concentration in the detector builds up to levels exceeding those of the DC method. Thus the pulse method has greater sensitivity. The DC and pulsed methods inherently produce a nonlinear response over a wide range of sample concentrations. Such a response is attributable to the finite amount of beta radiation emitted by the detector source per unit time. Because a decrease in current is measured, once a concentration of eluting solute captures a majority of the available low-energy electrons, only small changes in current (detector response) will be observed with increasing concentrations of solute. The linear range is usually 400 to 500 times the detection limit of a solute for a tritium source and 100 times for a nickel-63 source. However, the linearized method uses electronic modifications that operate the detector in a pulsed mode such that constant cell current is produced. The linear range is thus expanded to ranges of 10,000:1 for a nickel-63 source. The sources of beta particles in an ECD are usually tritium or nickel-63. The ECD is the most sensitive detector available, since as little as 1 picogram of halogen-containing compound may be measured. Laboratories using electron-capture detectors must be licensed by the Nuclear Regulatory Commission and are subject to all regulations concerning employee safety and possible environmental contamination set forth by the commission.

Mass spectrometer (MS) as a detector. The mass spectrometer is a specialized chromatographic detector that provides extremely sensitive detection (picogram quantities) and specific analyte identification. GC and MS are presented in Chapter 8.

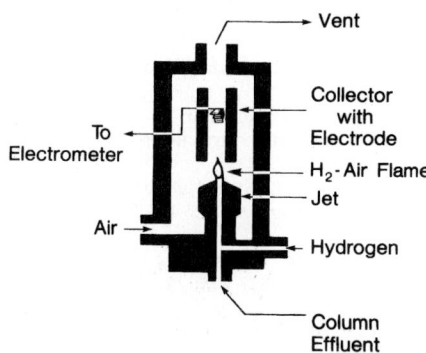

Fig. 7-9 Schema of flame-ionization detector. (From Werner M, Mohrbacher RJ, Riendeau CJ: In Baer DM, Dito WR: *Interpretation of therapeutic drug levels,* Chicago, 1981, American Society of Clinical Pathologists.)

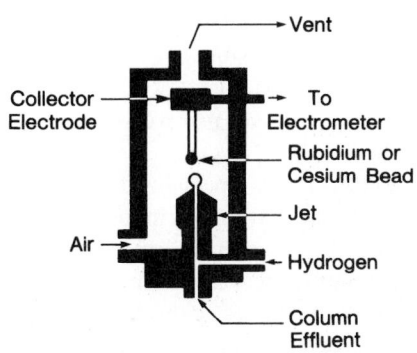

Fig. 7-10 Schema of alkali metal flame detector. (From Werner M, Mohrbacher RJ, Riendeau CJ: In Baer DM, Dito WR: *Interpretation of therapeutic drug levels,* Chicago, 1981, American Society of Clinical Pathologists.)

Fourier-transform infrared spectrometer (FTIR). The FTIR detector obtains the infrared spectra of a compound as it elutes from the GC column. The report format of FTIR detectors is similar to that of MS detectors (Chapter 8). A GC/FTIR produces chromatograms measured at specific IR bands similar to SIM mode GC/MS, or records the entire IR spectrum of the compound just as an MS records the mass spectrum of a compound. Recent developments in narrow-range IR photon detectors and photo sample cells now give GC/FTIR sensitivity and specificity that rivals that of GC/MS.[21] There are two types of interface for the GC to the FTIR detector: "vapor phase" and "cryogenic deposition." In vapor phase, a heated fused-silica line directs the GC effluent through a long narrow IR gas cell known as a "lightpipe." An IR beam transmits through the lightpipe, which is sealed at each end with IR-transparent windows. In cryogenic deposition, the column effluent is directed into a vacuum chamber (10^{-5} torr) that ends with a fused-silica restrictor positioned above a ZnSe IR-transparent plate. The effluent is deposited on the plate, which is held at liquid nitrogen temperatures. The plate with the frozen eluent is continuously exposed to the IR beam.

Both methods continuously collect the IR spectra of the eluted compounds. The detector does not destroy the compound, and the effluent for the FTIR may be directed into another detector system such as an MS(GC/FTIR/MS). GC/FTIR/MS is an extremely powerful identification technique. At present GC/FTIR is not routinely applied in the clinical chemistry laboratory; however, it is gaining popularity in forensic toxicology laboratories.[22]

Readout. Strip-chart recorders are the most common readout devices in gas chromatography. Recorder sensitivity is usually 1 to 10 mV, with a full-scale response of 1 second or less. Quantitative determinations of separate compounds are performed in two ways: peak-height or peak-area measurements. Both the peak height and peak area of the detector response to the effluent sample are proportional to its concentration. Peak-height measurements are useful in re-

petitive analyses that are performed by the same operator in a fixed system, that require extensive calibration, or that only partially resolve compounds, making peak-area determinations difficult. In general, peak-area measurements are more precise. Peak area can be determined by manual or automated methods. Electronic integration of the peak area produces both the most precise and the most accurate measurements. Today, detectors may be connected to microprocessor units or to a computerized data system that automatically records the response, identifies the sample components, integrates the signals, performs calculations, stores all data, and prints out the analytical results in final form.

GC APPLICATIONS IN CLINICAL CHEMISTRY

GC is an extremely versatile and powerful analytical methodology. Numerous sample components may be simultaneously separated, identified, and quantitated. By choosing the appropriate stationary phase, one can analyze any mixture of compounds that may be vaporized or converted to volatile derivatives. Selectivity and high sensitivity may be added by varying detectors. Yet, despite these advantages, application of GC in most clinical chemistry laboratories is limited to a few special areas of testing: therapeutic drug monitoring (TDM), toxicology, and testing for inborn errors of metabolism. Even in these areas, GC is applied to specific tests in only a relatively few laboratories because of the specialized training required for maintenance. GC is used to perform TDM analysis of psychoactive drugs, particularly those having active metabolites, which must be measured with the parent drug.

The determination of drugs or toxicants offers the widest potential arena for use of GC in the clinical laboratory because it provides a rapid, simple, reliable method for the simultaneous determination of volatile poisons such as methanol, ethanol, isopropanol, acetone, and acetaldehyde. GC coupled with mass spectrometry is required for drugs of abuse urine testing regulated by government agencies such as the Department of Defense, the Department of

Transportation, and the Nuclear Regulatory Agency. Laboratories performing such testing must be certified by the Department of Health and Human Services. Up to now about 80 laboratories, some associated with clinical laboratories, are so accredited.

GC is applied in highly specialized branches of clinical chemistry such as the testing for inborn errors of metabolism. Inherited defects in metabolism result in the accumulation in serum and excretion in urine of unusual or inappropriate amounts of organic acids and other byproducts of metabolism. The determination of organic acids and their concentrations in urine or serum is a valuable tool for these rare diseases.[23] Aciduria profiles are easily obtained with GC/FID, whereas serum profiles require more specific and sensitive GC/MS methods. At present, such testing is performed only in commercial reference laboratories or university medical centers.

REFERENCES

1. Willett J, Kealey D: *Gas chromatography,* New York, 1987, Wiley & Sons.
2. Grob RL: *Modern practice of gas chromatography,* ed 2, New York, 1985, Wiley & Sons.
3. Freeman RR: *High resolution gas chromatography,* ed 2, Palo Alto, Calif., 1981, Hewlett-Packard Co.
4. Schomburg F: *Gas chromatography, a practical course,* Weinheim, Germany, 1990, VCH Publishers.
5. Delley R, Friedrich K: System CG72 von bevorzugten Trennflüssigkeiten für die Gas-chromatographie, *Chromatographia* 10: 593-598, 1971.
6. Hawkes S, Grossman D, Hartkopf A, et al: Preferred stationary liquids for gas chromatography, *J Chromatogr Sci* 13:115-117, 1975.
7. Siggia S: *Instrumental methods of organic functional group analysis,* New York, 1972, Wiley & Sons.
8. Ahuja S: Derivatization in gas chromatography, *J Pharm Sci* 65:163, 1976.
9. Kovats E: The Kovats' retention index system, *Anal Chem* 36:31A, 1964.
10. Lorenz LJ, Roger LB: Specification of gas chromatographic behavior using Kovats' indices and Rohrschneider constants, *Anal Chem* 43:1593-1599, 1971.
11. American Society for Testing and Materials: *Gas chromatographic data compilation catalog AMD 25A,* Philadelphia, Penn., 1967, ASTM.
12. American Society for Testing and Materials: *Gas chromatographic data compilation catalog, suppl 25A S-1,* Philadelphia, Penn., 1971, ASTM.
13. Perrigo BJ, Peel HW: The use of retention indices and temperature-programmed gas chromatography in analytical toxicology, *J Chromatogr Sci* 19:219-226, 1981.
14. Japp M, Gill R, Osselton MD: Comparison of drug retention indices determined on packed, wide bore capillary and narrow bore capillary columns, *J Forensic Sci* 32:1574-1586, 1987.
15. Supina WR, Rose LP: The use of Rohrschneider constants for classification of GLC columns, *J Chromatogr Sci* 8:217-217, 1970.
16. McReynolds WO: Characterization of some liquid phases, *J Chromatogr Sci* 8:685-691, 1970.
17. Ettre LS: *Basic relationships of gas chromatography,* ed 2, Norwalk, Conn., 1979, Perkin-Elmer Corp.
18. Fenimore DC, Whitford JJ, Davis CM, Zlatkis A: Nickel gas chromatographic columns: an alternative to glass for biological samples, *J Chromatogr* 140:9-16, 1977.
19. David DJ: *Gas chromatographic detectors,* New York, 1974, Wiley & Sons.
20. Sevcik J: *Detectors in gas chromatography,* New York, 1975, Elsevier/North-Holland.
21. Bourne S, Hefner AM, Norton KL, Griffiths PR: Performance characteristics of a real-time direct deposition gas chromatography/Fourier transform infrared spectrometry system, *Anal Chem* 62:2448-2452, 1990.
22. Kalasinsky KS, Levine B, Smith ML: Feasibility of using GC/FTIR for drug analysis in the forensic toxicology laboratory, *J Anal Toxicol* 16:332-336, 1991.
23. Forman DT: Role of the laboratory in diagnosis of organic acidurias, *Ann Clin Lab Sci* 21:85-93, 1991.

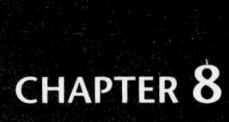

CHAPTER 8

Mass spectrometry

Michael Lehrer

Basic principles

Mass spectrometer
  Ion source
  Mass filter
  Detectors
  Computers

Creation of ion fragments
  Electron ionization (EI)
  Chemical ionization (CI)

Mass fragmentation

Comparison of electron ionization and chemical
  ionization

Use of the mass spectrometer
  Full-scan analysis
  Selected ion monitoring
  Quantitation

Separation techniques
  Gas chromatography/mass spectrometry
  Liquid chromatography/mass spectrometry
  Solids probe

Other mass spectrometers
  Ion trap detectors (ITD)
  Time-of-flight mass spectrometry
  Tandem mass spectrometry (MS/MS)

Forensic drug testing

OBJECTIVES

- Define the concepts of mass, charge, and mass fragmentation of molecules.
- Describe the basic components of a mass spectrometer.
- State how an ion source and mass filter are used to separate ions.
- Describe the key elements of a mass-fragmentation pattern.
- State the principles of how the mass-fragmentation pattern is used to identify molecules.

KEY TERMS

accelerating voltage A voltage potential in the ion source that helps propel charged ion fragments toward the detector.

base peak The most intense peak in the mass spectrum.

chemical ionization (CI) Low-energy ionization technique based on charge-transfer collision with an inert reagent gas.

daughter ions The ionic output of the second mass spectroscopy (MS) analyzer of an MS/MS system.

electron ionization (EI) High-energy electron bombardment transforming molecules into fragment ions.

fingerprint The unique fragmentation patterns of organic compounds.

fragmentation pattern A display of the intensity ion fragments formed versus mass-to-charge ratio.

full scan A mass spectrometric scanning sequence where all ions in the entire mass range of interest are detected.

GC/MS Gas chromatograph interfaced with a mass spectrometer.

ionization potential The amount of energy required to displace an electron from the outer shell of a compound.

ionization source Area within the mass spectrometer where molecules are ionized by an electron beam.

ion-molecule reaction The product of a collision between an ion fragment and an intact molecule within the ion source.

IonSpray A variation of thermospray technique used to introduce liquid chromatograph eluent into the ion source of the mass spectrometer at ambient temperature.

ion trap detector (ITD) Mass spectrometer that operates on the principle of ion accumulation over time.

isotope dilution Quantitation of chemicals different only in their isotope composition.

LC/MS Liquid chromatograph (LC) interfaced with a mass spectrometer (MS).

magnetic sector Mass spectrometer that separates ion fragments based on their passage through a magnetic field.

mass filter The electronic or magnetic device that separates ions based on their mass-to-charge ratio.

mass fragmentation The breakdown of a large unstable molecular ion, usually in a defined pattern unique to the test molecule.

mass spectrometer A device to separate ions based on their mass-to-charge ratio.

mass spectrum The output of a mass spectrometer displaying mass-to-charge (m/z) ratios versus intensity of the ion fragment.

mass-to-charge (m/z) A ratio of the mass of a given ion fragment divided by its ionic charge.

molecular ion (M⁺) The initial ion fragment corresponding to the molecular weight of the compound.

molecular weight The total molecular mass of a molecule.

National Institute of Drug Abuse (NIDA) A governmental agency charged with regulating and certifying forensic drugs of abuse testing laboratories.

negative-ion chemical ionization (NICI) Chemical ionization technique focusing on the generation of negatively charged ions.

parent ion The ionic output of the first mass spectrometer analyzer of an MS/MS system.

quadrupole Mass spectrometer that separates ion fragments based on their passage through an electronic field.

quasimolecular ion The ion fragment often formed by transfer of a proton in chemical ionization corresponding to the molecular weight plus one.

selected ion monitoring (SIM) Selective scanning of a few preselected ion fragments by the detector.

selected ion profile Selective scanning and area integration in the SIM mode of a significant ion fragment.

soft ionization A low-energy ionization technique such as chemical ionization.

solids probe A probe used to introduce crystalline material directly into the mass spectrometer.

tandem mass spectrometry (MS/MS) The coupling of 2 or more mass analyzers.

thermospray A technique utilized to introduce liquid chromatography eluent into the ion source of the mass spectrometer.

time-of-flight (TOF) mass spectrometer A spectrometer that separates ion fragments based on their transit time through a given path.

total ion current (TIC) Chromatographic integration and display of ion currents in GC/MS applications.

triple-stage quadrupole (TSQ) Instrumental configuration of a quadrupole MS/MS system.

unimolecular decomposition The high energy disintegration of an ion into smaller ion fragments.

BASIC PRINCIPLES

Mass spectrometry uses the creation and analysis of ions to analyze a wide variety of molecules. Mass spectrometers are devices that operate on the principle that charged particles moving through a magnetic or an electric field can be separated from other charged particles according to their mass-to-charge (m/z) ratios. Since molecules do not have a net charge, mass spectrometers induce them by an ionization process. Charged molecules are not stable and can break down into fragments and lose their charge by interacting with other molecules or surfaces. Implicit in the use of a mass spectrometer is the assumption that the ionized (including fragmented) products are formed in a reproducible manner if the ionization separation and detection systems are kept constant.

Each of the resulting ions has a specific molecular mass and charge, which the mass spectrometer separates and detects. Because the mass of each ion is discrete to greater than a thousandth of an atomic weight unit, the resulting separation of the ion masses is displayed as spectral lines of intensity versus the mass-to-charge ratio. The intensity of each ion is in proportion to the number of that ion reaching the detector.

Most ions have a single unit charge; consequently it is common practice to describe ions in terms of "mass" alone. However, doubly charged ions can occur and such ion fragments will have a mass value that is one half of its true mass spectrometric value. The m/z value for each ion is plotted on the *x*-axis, and the ion's intensity is plotted on the *y*-axis to yield a line graph output (Fig. 8-1). The most intense ion in the spectrum is termed the *base peak* and is

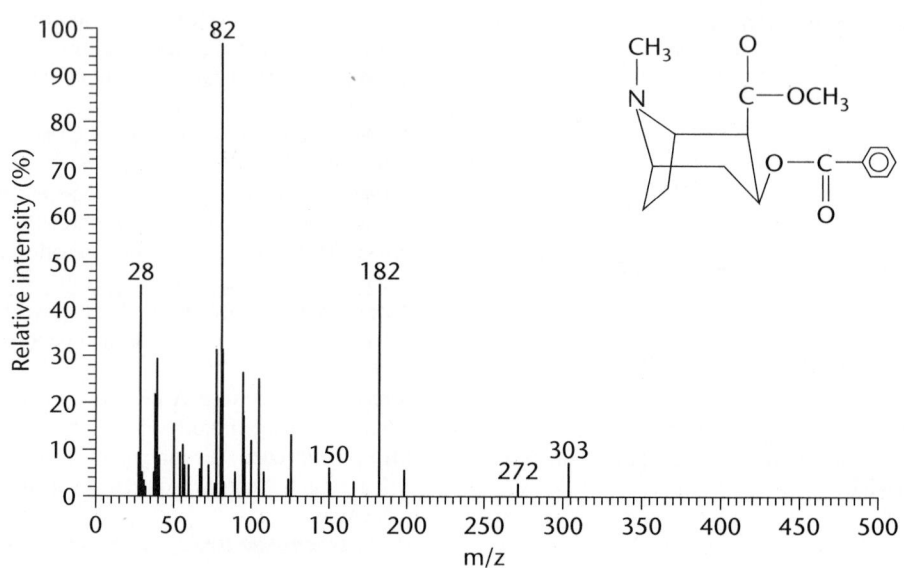

Fig. 8-1 Electron-impact mass spectrum of cocaine. (From Saferstein R: *Forensic science handbook*, Englewood Cliffs, N.J., 1982, Prentice Hall.)

arbitrarily assigned an abundance value of 100%. The intensity of other peaks is then normalized to the base peak intensity. The record of all ions formed and the relative abundance of each constitute the mass spectrum of that compound. This unique fragmentation pattern of the molecule is reproducible, and sample identification can be achieved when one compares an unknown compound's ion values and intensities against reference spectra. A match constitutes the chemical identification of the unknown compound.

MASS SPECTROMETER

All mass spectrometers include a system to create and maintain a vacuum; a device to introduce the samples (such as gas-liquid chromatography, GLC; liquid chromatography, LC; and solids probe); an ionization source, which serves to ionize the sample; a mass filter or analyzer where charged particles are separated according to their m/z ratios; and ion collection, amplification, and detection devices (Fig. 8-2). Contemporary mass spectrometers also incorporate computer systems for control of the instrument and for the acquisition, display, manipulation, and interpretation of data.

Ion source

The ion source is maintained in a high vacuum environment to enhance collision efficiency and ion formation. High-efficiency vacuum pumps maintain the ionization source pressure in the 10^{-5} to 10^{-7} torr range, which not only minimizes ion-molecule reactions (which would complicate the analysis), but also optimizes the detection, resolution, and transmission of the ions generated.

Ions are generated in the ion chamber or ion source of the mass spectrometer (Fig. 8-3). The source may be viewed as a small closed box containing several pinhole orifices that serve as inlets and outlets. Variable positive and negative electronic potentials are induced on specific metallic surfaces. An electron beam is directed into the source. Compounds undergoing analysis enter the ion source and are bombarded by the ionization beam operating at 70 eV (by convention). Some of the compounds are converted into positive and negative ions, and these ions are either attracted or repelled by the electronic potentials; that is, opposite charges attract, like charges repel. Electronic voltage programming optimizes the preservation of ions of a given polarity (either positive or negative ions). For example, the negative potential maintains the positive ions in motion within the volume defined by the source. If an ion comes into physical contact with the metallic surface, it is instantly grounded and eliminated. By manipulating the magnitude and polarity of the electronic potentials, the ions within the source can be stored, accelerated, and directed in space to the outlets that lead to the mass filter.

Mass filter

Electronic separation. The mass filter separates the ions of interest according to their m/z ratios and allows these ions ultimately to reach the detector. Separation of the ions by the mass filter can occur electronically as is the case in a quadrupole mass spectrometer. A quadrupole filter consists of a quadrant of four parallel hyperbolic or circular rods that provide a specific radio frequency field (Fig. 8-4). Opposite rods are electrically connected. The applied voltage consists of a constant direct current component U and a radio frequency component V_0 (cos wt). $W = 2\pi f$, where f is the radio frequency.[1] The potential difference between the two sets of rods is thus $U \pm V_0 \cos wt$. This creates a unique oscillating field where a positive ion injected into the quadrupole region will oscillate between the adjacent electrodes of opposite polarity. At specified radio frequency, ions of a given mass undergo stable oscillation between the electrodes. Ions of lower or higher mass undergo oscillation of increasing amplitude until they are grounded on the quadrupole electrodes. Within the quadrupole field, no force is exerted in the longitudinal direction, and so an ion with stable oscillation continues at its original velocity down the flight path to the detector. With 5 to 30 volts of ion acceleration potential, the ions undergo a sufficient number of oscillations during the flight period to provide reasonable mass separation.

Magnetic separation. Alternatively the mass filter can separate the ions magnetically, as is the case in magnetic sector mass spectrometers. Ions formed in the source are

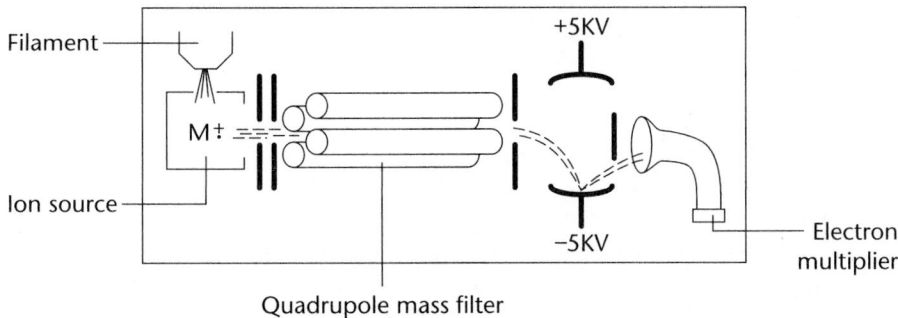

Fig. 8-2 A quadrupole mass spectrometer.

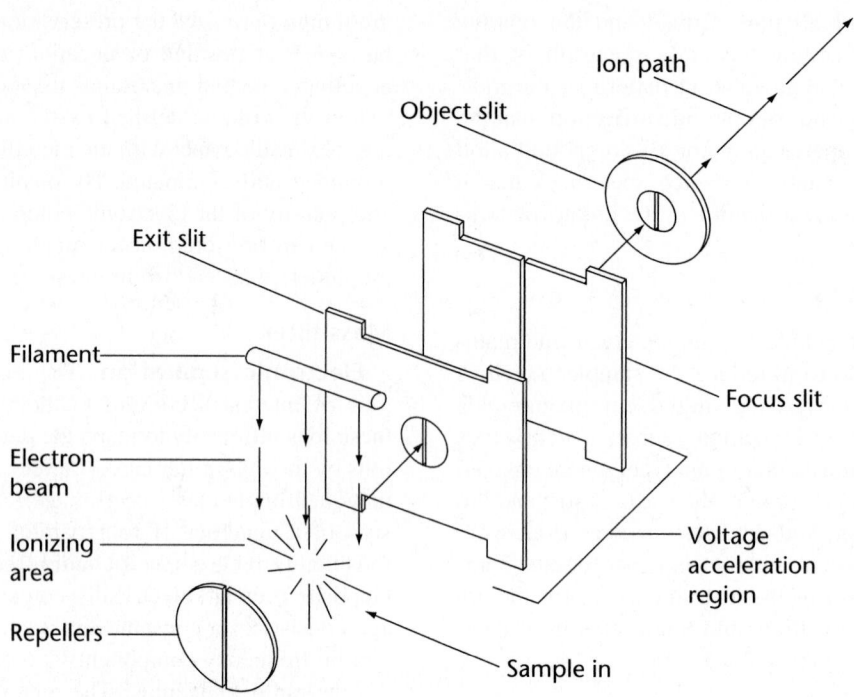

Fig. 8-3 Schema of an ion source. (From Saferstein R: *Forensic science handbook,* Englewood Cliffs, N.J., 1982, Prentice Hall.)

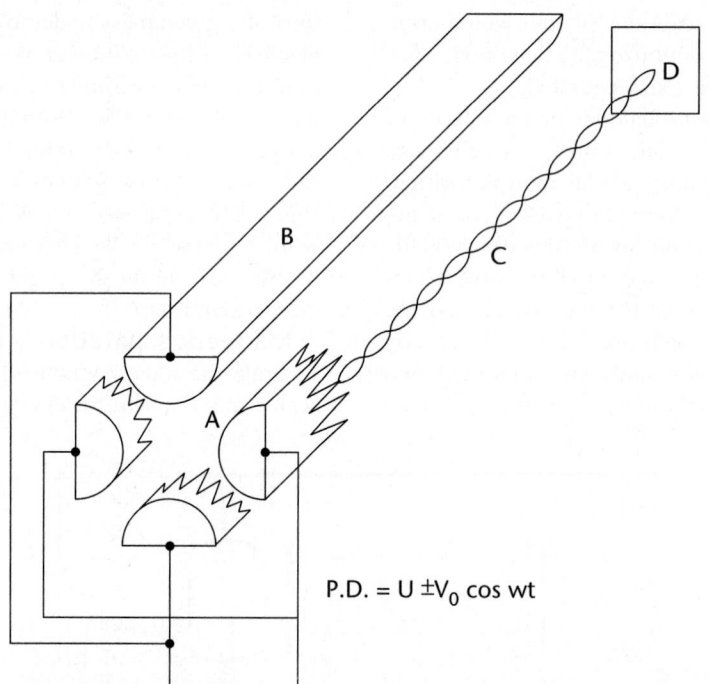

$$P.D. = U \pm V_0 \cos wt$$

Fig. 8-4 Schema of quadrupole mass filter. *A,* Ion injection; *B,* quadrupole rods; *C,* oscillating ion beams; *D,* collector. (From McFadden WH: *Techniques of combined gas chromatography/mass spectrometry,* New York, 1973, Wiley & Sons.)

accelerated toward a homogeneous magnetic field (Fig. 8-5). For ions with an electronic charge, z, and mass, m, the kinetic energy will be related to the accelerating voltage, V, by the equation

$$V_z = \tfrac{1}{2}\, mv^2$$

where v is the ion velocity. As the ions enter the magnetic field, H, they experience a force orthogonal to the field, which results in a curvature of the ion path. This accelerating force, Hev, is balanced by the centripetal force, so that

$$Hev = \frac{mv^2}{r}$$

where r is the radius of the curvature. Elimination of the velocity term gives the equation

$$m/z = H^2r^2/2V$$

Thus, at a fixed radius, r, and for a singly charged ion, the mass focused at S_2 and collected by the detector is proportional to the square of the magnetic field and inversely proportional to the accelerating voltage. By varying either of these two parameters, ions of different mass-to-charge ratio can be deflected to the detector, and in this fashion the mass spectrum is scanned.[1]

For most applications it is preferable to vary the magnetic field and maintain constant accelerating voltage. When the voltage is varied over a course of a mass scan (with constant magnetic field), the efficiency of transmitting ions of low mass is much greater than that for ions of high mass. This mass discrimination is attributable to the fact that an ion of mass 400 will have one tenth the accelerating voltage of an ion of mass 40. Since the higher mass region is the more important part of the spectrum, voltage scanning is used only for special cases where magnetic scanning is impractical.

Magnetic sector mass spectrometry. Magnetic sector instruments offer high resolution and consequently are more complex and expensive than either quadrupole or ion trap systems. Resolution requirement is an important consideration in choosing among systems. Resolution is defined by the following equation:

$$\text{Resolution} = M/\Delta M$$

M is the mass of the ion, and ΔM is the difference in mass between M and its adjacent ion. High-resolution systems have a resolution of 10,000 or greater. Such systems can separate an ion of mass 200.00 from an ion of mass 200.02. Systems with resolution of less than 1000 are considered low-resolution systems. An instrument with a resolution of 800 will separate an ion of mass 800 from 801. Most clinical, environmental, and forensic applications can readily be achieved with the less-expensive lower-resolution instruments.

Detectors

Almost all mass spectrometers detect ions by using electron multipliers. The impacting ion signal is amplified in the same manner as that described on p. 92 in Chapter 4.

Computers

Modern mass spectrometers use computer interfaces and data-handling capacity to operate, record, and analyze the data generated by the mass spectrometer.

CREATION OF ION FRAGMENTS
Electron ionization (EI)

Electron ionization (EI, electronic impact) is the most widely used method of ionization. For ionization to occur, the bombarding electrons must possess sufficient energy to displace an electron from the molecule's outer electron shell during the initial collision. The *ionization potential* of a molecule is the amount of energy required to displace that outer shell electron; most organic compounds have ionization potentials in the 7 to 13 electron volt (eV) range. Thus the energy of the incoming ionization beam must exceed the ionization potential of the molecule being analyzed to displace the molecule's valence electron successfully. Mass spectrometers are generally standardized on an ionization beam at 70 eV. At that setting, the electron beam always has sufficient energy to ionize incoming sample molecules efficiently. Additionally, bombardment at 70 eV results in collisions that impart excess energy to the ions generated, which enhances their decomposition to secondary fragments resulting in more structural information.

As gaseous sample molecules enter the ion source (Fig. 8-3), they are bombarded by the electron beam originating from a heated rhenium or tungsten filament. A small positive potential on the repeller plate focuses and repels the positive ions generated through the exit slit toward the mass analyzer. A much higher voltage potential is placed on one or more of the plates and is used to accelerate the velocity of the ions as they leave the exit slit. A focus slit is utilized

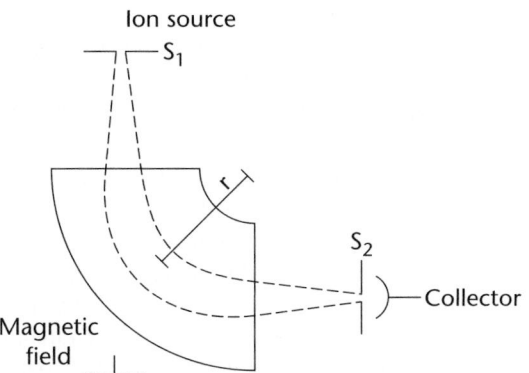

Fig. 8-5 Schema of 90-degree magnetic sector showing direction focusing of divergent ion beam. (From McFaddem WH: *Techniques of combined gas chromatography/mass spectrometry,* New York, 1973, Wiley & Sons.)

to direct the ion's trajectory toward the mass analyzer. Negative ions are also formed in the source. One can analyze such ions by reversing the voltage potentials of the repeller and accelerating plates. Compounds that can readily accommodate an extra electron such as halogen-containing drugs (or drugs derivatized with halogen-containing derivatives), polycyclic aromatics, and substituted phenols can generate significant negative ions, which allow sensitive detection by negative ion mass spectrometry. However, the resulting negative ion mass spectrum has fewer ion fragments, and they are usually at relatively low masses; consequently negative-ion EI provides less structural information than its positive-ion counterpart, and as a result most applications center on positive-ion mass spectrometry.

Chemical ionization (CI)

Chemical ionization (CI) is another ionization technique that has found great utility because it imparts the ability to exercise control over the site and degree of ion fragmentation. CI relies on an indirect approach to achieve sample molecule ion formation. A *reagent gas* is introduced into the source before the sample molecules enter. The reagent gas is ionized by the 70 eV ionization beam to generate *reagent gas ions*. When sample molecules enter the source, they collide with reagent gas ions, resulting in a charge transfer from the reagent gas ion to the sample molecule. This "gentle" ionization process results in ionized sample molecules that are relatively stable and hence long lived. The versatility of CI stems from the ability to select different reagent gases to influence the site and extent of sample ionization. This flexibility allows for the exercise of control over the complexity of the resulting spectrum and hence the degree of structural information derived. Methane, isobutane, water, and ammonia are some of the more commonly encountered CI reagent gases; fragments generated can differ depending on both the reagent gas utilized and on the chemical characteristics of the compound being analyzed. Choice of a particular reagent gas will influence the ionization process. Several different mechanisms for charge transfer, such as proton transfer, charge exchange, or negative ionization, can occur. Proton transfer reactions and, to a lesser extent, negative ionization have received the most attention and widespread application.

Methane reagent gas exemplifies the proton transfer process. High energy electron bombardment generates an abundance of CH_4^+ and CH_3^+ ions (equation 8-1) which quickly

$$M + e^- \rightarrow M^+ + 2e^-$$
$$M^+ \rightarrow F_1 + F_2 + F_3^+ \ldots$$

Fig. 8-6 Electron ionization. *F*, Fragment; *M*, molecule; *M*⁺, molecular ion.

react with excess methane gas to form stable CH_5^+ and $C_2H_5^+$ ions.[2]

$$2CH_4 + 2e^- \rightarrow CH_4^+ + CH_3^+ + H\bullet + 4e^- \qquad \textit{Eq. 8-1}$$
$$CH_4^+ + CH_4 \rightarrow CH_5^+ + CH_3\bullet \qquad \textit{Eq. 8-2}$$
$$CH_3^+ + CH_4 \rightarrow C_2H_5^+ + H_2 \qquad \textit{Eq. 8-3}$$

CH_5^+ and $C_2H_5^+$ are relatively stable adducts and constitute nearly 90% of the total methane ionization by the time the sample molecules enter the source. They react as Brönsted acids with most incoming sample molecules (M) protonating them to yield the *quasimolecular ion* $(MH)^+$ corresponding to their molecular weight plus one (equations 8-4 and 8-5).

$$M + CH_5^+ \rightarrow MH^+ + CH_4 \qquad \textit{Eq. 8-4}$$
$$M + C_2H_5^+ \rightarrow MH^+ + C_2H_4 \qquad \textit{Eq. 8-5}$$

In a similar fashion, isobutane reagent gas yields a predominant number of *tert*-butyl reagent gas ions that protonate the sample molecules as follows:

$$M + C_4H_9^+ \rightarrow MH^+ + C_4H_8 \qquad \textit{Eq. 8-6}$$

CI is considered a "soft ionization" technique because of its low-energy transfer ionization process when compared to EI. Consequently the quasimolecular ion produced is relatively stable and long lived when compared to the molecular ion produced in EI spectra. Because of this stability, the quasimolecular ion does not undergo as extensive fragmentation into secondary ion fragments as the molecular ion does in EI spectra. However, CI ionization does involve some energy transfer, since proton transfer reaction between the reagent gas ions and the sample molecule is an exothermic energy–producing process. The amount of energy transferred to the newly formed MH^+ ion is proportional to the exothermic reaction and will determine the stability and hence survival of MH^+ in the source. The higher the exothermicity of the reaction the more likely is MH^+ to decompose.

MASS FRAGMENTATION

During the collision, energy is transferred from the ionization beam to the sample molecule. This resulting moiety can dissipate some of its excess energy by freeing its outer shell electron to give rise to a positively charged *molecular ion* (M^+) corresponding to the molecular weight of the compound (Fig. 8-6). The molecular weight is one of the more important pieces of information obtained from a mass spectrum. The peak intensity of this molecular ion is directly proportional to the life-span of the ion. A stable molecular ion will last longer and hence generate an intense peak, whereas a short-lived ion will generate a small peak. Most molecular ions are short lived because of their high energy level. Often they are so unstable and short lived that they don't exist long enough to be detected. In such cases the mass spectrum will not exhibit the molecular ion at all. In general, ions that can easily dissipate their excess energy internally, such as extensively conjugated fragments, are more stable and hence longer lived.

EI ionization can be accomplished only when sample molecules exist in a gaseous state. Several suitable means for vaporizing and delivering the gaseous molecules into the ion source are available, as discussed later in this chapter.

In general, molecular ions are highly energized and thus inherently unstable. They dissipate their excess energy by breaking internal bonds and undergoing unimolecular decompositions that result in secondary ion fragments (F^+). Simultaneously, secondary fragments are also formed by means of ion-molecule and ion-ion collisions that are occurring randomly in the ion source. Secondary fragments have lower masses; such fragments continue the process of dissipating their energy by further decomposition as well as by random collisions with other molecules and ions. The resulting effect is the formation of a large number of fragment ions with m/z values ranging from the molecular weight of the compound at the high end of the spectrum down to the lowest m/z values scanned. These fragments are detected and plotted according to their m/z ratios versus intensity to generate the mass spectrum of the compound. Fragmentation patterns provide a wealth of structural information about the molecule of interest. They provide the "fingerprint" specificity to enable mass spectrometrists to make compound identification certain.

When one is conducting molecular structure elucidation of an unknown that cannot be identified by a spectral library match, the mass spectrum displaying the fragmentation patterns needs to be examined, since it can yield extensive structural information. The initial focus centers on identifying the molecular ion that arises by the loss of the first electron and corresponds to the molecular weight of the compound of interest. Knowledge of the compound's molecular weight is extremely helpful in identifying the unknown. Subsequent fragmentation attributable to unimolecular decomposition and ion-molecule reactions yield other characteristic fragments that can help identify the chemical moieties present in the compound. In general, the higher m/z ion fragments are more helpful in compound identification than the lower ones. The reason is that higher m/z fragments represent the fragmentation of the molecule of interest at the earlier stages of its breakdown in the ion source. Consequently these fragments are closer to the molecule's original structure and are thus more "unique" than the lower m/z fragments. The lower m/z fragments are smaller parts of the molecule, and, although they can provide structural information, this information is less specific information. Unfortunately the most abundant ions in the EI mass spectra generally occur at low mass and may not necessarily be unique to the compound of interest. Low m/z ion data are still useful, provided that the compound being

analyzed is pure. With either GC/MS or LC/MS this requires good chromatographic separation and the avoidance of co-eluting interfering components.

Fig. 8-7 shows the postulated EI fragmentation decomposition of cocaine.[3] The molecular ion is m/z 303, and, although weak, it is readily seen in the mass spectrum (see Fig. 8-1). The charge of the molecular ion is localized on the nitrogen atom and to a lesser extent on the two carbonyl oxygen atoms. Decomposition of the molecular ion occurs by several different pathways. Breakup of the molecular ion's six-membered ring with the loss of benzoic acid generates a relatively stable carbonium ion at m/z 182, which is seen as an intense fragment. The loss of the methoxyl moiety from the molecular ion generates the smaller fragment at m/z 272, and the aromatic carbonyl fragment at m/z 105 is also formed by cleavage from the molecular ion. The base peak is m/z 82 and represents the formation of a substituted pyrrole ring, which is very stable because of its highly resonant ring structure.

Certain elements that are often present in a wide variety of molecules, including drugs and their metabolites, have unique mass spectrometric behavior that imparts additional information. Nitrogen, for example, is the only commonly encountered element that has an even atomic mass and an odd valence. Thus, if the molecular ion has an even mass, it can be deduced that the compound of interest has either no nitrogen atom or an even number of nitrogen atoms. Additional structural information can be obtained from the mass spectrum when the compound of interest contains two or more abundant natural isotopes. Ion fragments containing halogen atoms have characteristic isotope clusters arising from the two different isotopes present. For example, chlorine's natural isotopes are ^{35}Cl and ^{37}Cl with a relative abundance of 75.8% and 24.2% respectively. Consequently, any fragments containing chlorine atoms will always generate a characteristic pattern consisting of a doublet peak two atomic mass units apart with a 3:1 ratio. Chlorine, bromine, and to a smaller degree silicon and sulfur are the only elements with sufficiently abundant natural isotopes to generate useful information with low-resolution mass spectrometers. Another useful fact to remember is that carbon-13 to carbon-12 abundance is approximately 1.1%. Increasing the number of carbon atoms in an ion increases the probability that one of these atoms will be a ^{13}C isotope. The $(M + 1)^+/M^+$ ratio for a 10-carbon ion will thus exhibit 10 times the probability for ^{13}C, or $10 \times 1.1\% = 11\%$. Although an approximation, this provides a means of determining the number of carbon atoms, which is paramount in interpreting the spectral lines of unknown organic compounds. To obtain more precise elemental composition, a high-resolution mass spectrometer is necessary.

Basic molecular structure and side chains of organic compounds can often be correlated to specific ion fragments in the mass spectrum. Metabolites frequently have similar

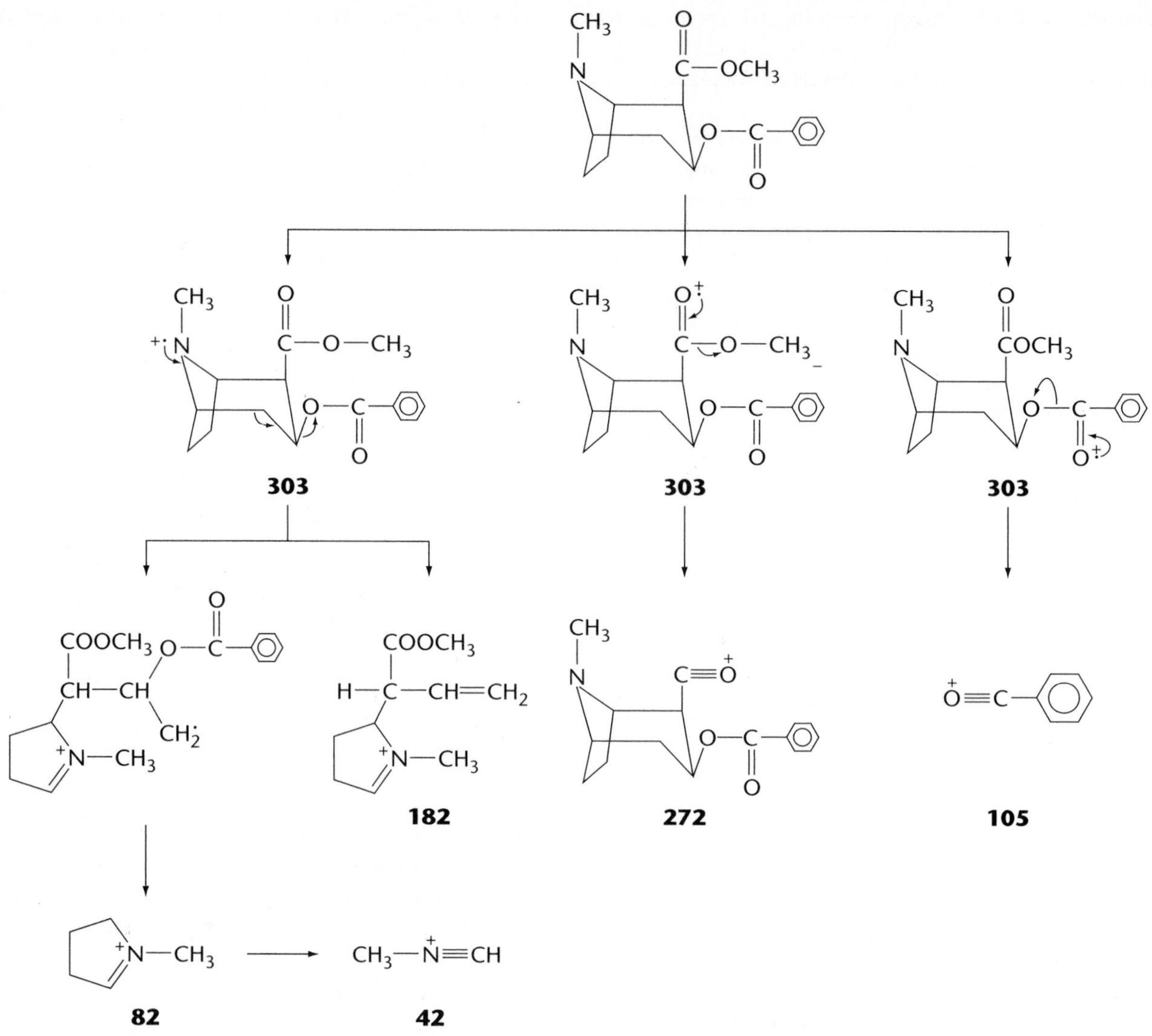

Fig. 8-7   Fragmentation pattern of cocaine.

structures and the same side chains as the parent compounds. Consequently, their mass spectra often contain similar or identical fragment ions. Chemically changing parent compounds either by metabolism or derivatization leads to anticipated fragment ions in the spectrum, making identification simpler. Such empirical observations are useful in the identification process. This pattern recognition is especially helpful in the identification of drug metabolites and known poisons. There are numerous molecular decomposition patterns of various chemical moieties that have been systematically applied to interpreting fragmentation patterns. A discussion of such interpretations is beyond the scope of this chapter, and one is referred to publications on this subject.[4-6]

A major advantage of CI spectra is their relative simplicity compared to the corresponding EI spectra. A comparison of CI isobutane spectrum of cocaine (Fig. 8-8) to that obtained by EI (see Fig. 8-1) demonstrates this. Compared with the complex EI fragmentation patterns the CI mass spectrum is simpler and contain only a few ions. The isobutane CI spectrum of cocaine is dominated by the quasimolecular ion that readily reveals the sample's molecular weight. As was discussed earlier, the molecular weight is one of the most important pieces of information that may be obtained from the mass spectrum. Hence, CI is useful in obtaining molecular weight information that may not be always readily available by EI techniques. Other major CI fragmentations arise from the loss of protonated acid-labile groups from the quasimolecular ion. For example, benzoate esters (such as cocaine) may show the loss of benzoic acid, acetate esters the loss of acetic acid, and aliphatic alcohols the loss of water.

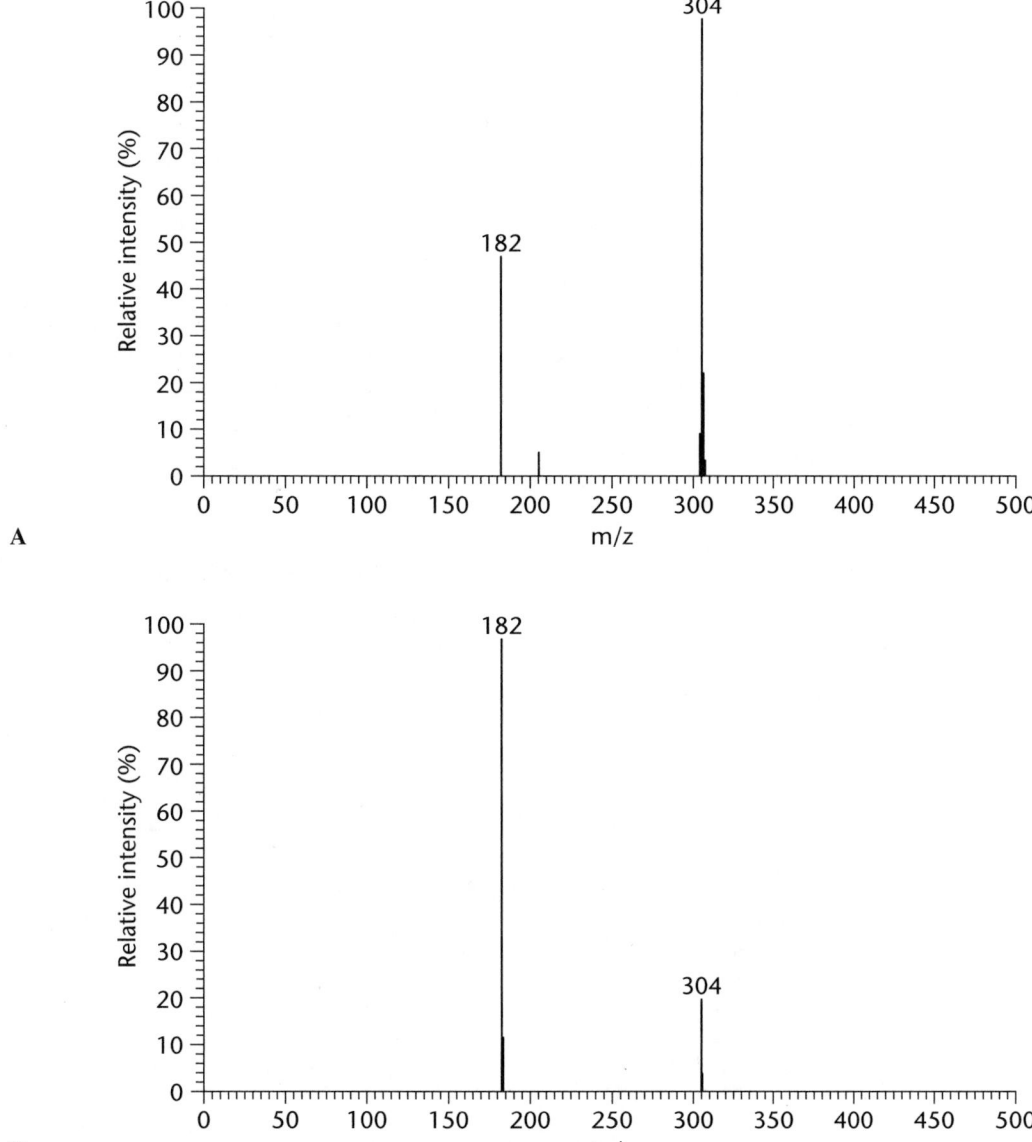

Fig. 8-8 **A,** Isobutane chemical ionization spectrum of cocaine. **B,** Methane chemical ionization spectrum of cocaine.

COMPARISON OF ELECTRON IONIZATION AND CHEMICAL IONIZATION

Sensitivity is another important factor that is affected by the ionization process. Typically, CI sensitivity can exceed that of EI by several orders of magnitude. This is attributable to CI's ability to concentrate total ion current into a small number of ions (because of the minimal fragmentation). Compare the cocaine CI fragmentation pattern with that obtained by EI. The CI spectrum (Fig. 8-8) demonstrates that m/z 304 and 182 account for almost all the CI fragments generated. This is in stark contrast to the EI fragmentation (see Fig. 8-1) where m/z 182 and 303 constitute only a small

portion of the total number of fragments generated. As can be readily seen, the prominent CI ions will typically have a higher response per unit weight of sample and hence greater sensitivity (compared to abundant EI ions). Additionally, such CI ions tend to have higher m/z values and hence are more unusual than the abundant EI ions, which tend to have a low m/z value. Notice that in the case of cocaine the base peak in EI is at a low mass (m/z 82), whereas it is at higher masses with CI (m/z 182 with methane CI and m/z 304 with isobutane CI). This example also serves to demonstrate that the selection of CI reagent gas will have a pronounced influence on the extent of fragmentation and the ultimate sensitivity of the analysis. Compounds that have different molecular weights generally give CI spectra with minimal overlap, enabling accurate identification of targeted compounds even when GLC fails to separate components of interest adequately.[7]

Chemical ionization data can supply significant mass spectral information that can be used by itself, or to supplement EI data. The additional CI data can provide greater specificity; it is valuable in enhancing the accuracy of results. Such a situation is demonstrated in Fig. 8-9, which illustrates the mass spectra of methamphetamine and phentermine in the EI and CI modes respectively. Although the two compounds are structural isomers, methamphetamine is an illicit drug, whereas phentermine is not. As can be seen

in Fig. 8-9, *A,* the EI mass spectra of these two compounds are virtually identical, and identification based on full-scan EI data or selected ion monitoring (SIM) is incapable of distinguishing the two compounds. Furthermore, the GC chromatographic retention times can be similar in many of the GC/MS protocols routinely used by drugs of abuse testing laboratories.[8] Consequently a false-positive methamphetamine result is quite possible when underivatized amphetamines are analyzed by the popular electron ionization SIM technique (see p. 178). In fact, some National Institute of Drug Abuse (NIDA) certified laboratories lost their certification to perform drug testing because of false-positive amphetamine results. All these laboratories were utilizing EI and were relying on three ion SIM techniques.

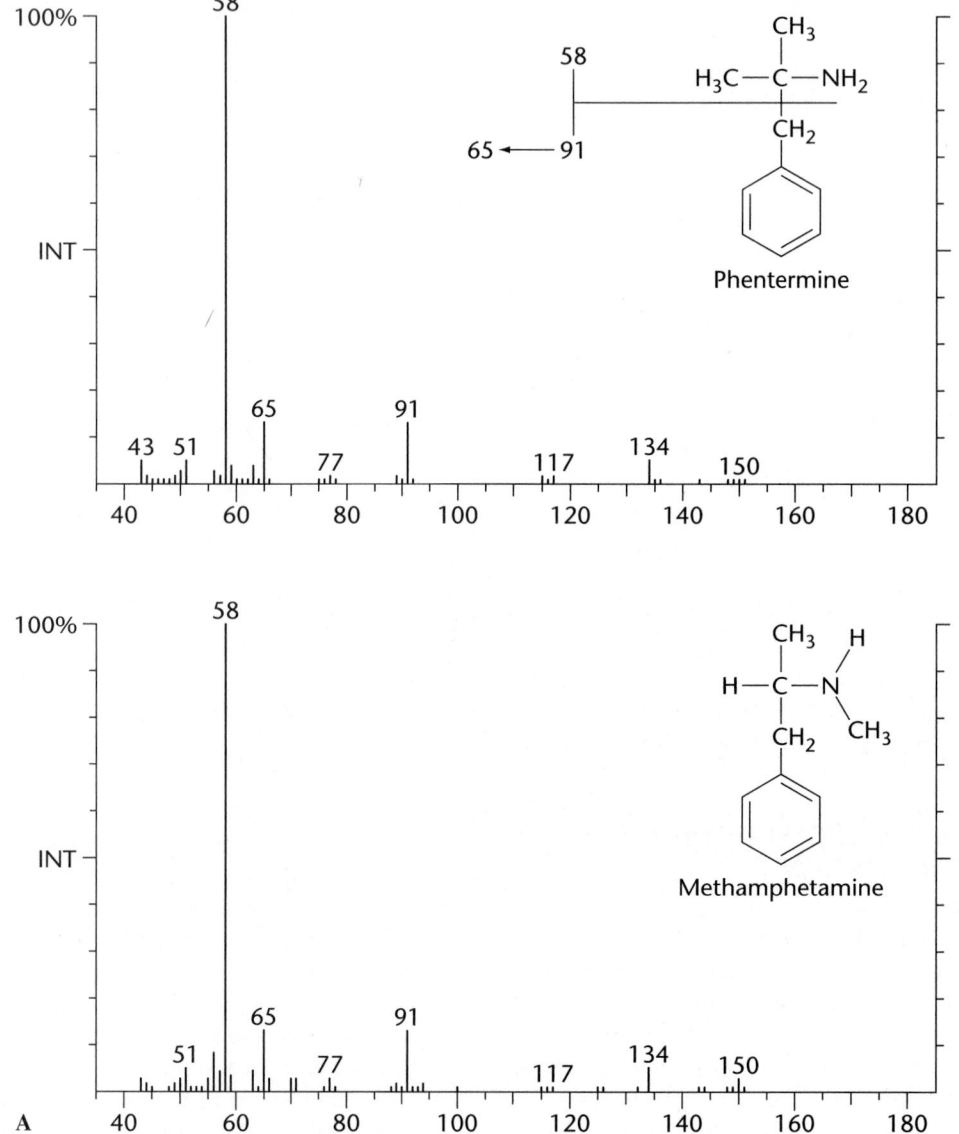

Fig. 8-9 **A,** Full-scan electronic ionization (EI) spectra of phentermine and methamphetamine. The two compounds have virtually identical EI mass spectra (performed on Finnigan-Mat ITS 40 GC/MS).

In contrast with the EI spectra, methamphetamine and phentermine are readily differentiated in CI by the presence of a significant ion at m/z 133 in phentermine that is nonexistent in the methamphetamine spectrum (Fig. 8-9, *B*). In this case, chemical ionization removes all ambiguities and totally eliminates the potential for false-positive results. CI techniques should be viewed as complimentary to EI, since they help minimize EI specificity gaps, which may be encountered. Because of these EI complimentary characteristics, it has been recommended that the International Olympics Committee require chemical ionization analysis for every positive sample.[9] Instrumental advances during the past few years have made CI practical and easy to use. Incorporation of CI analyses in drugs of abuse testing laboratories

can also be cost effective, since it can speed analytical analysis time by rapidly providing greater certainty of identification.

Negative ions produced under CI conditions are far more useful than under EI; significant negative-ion chemical ionization (NICI) applications exist. Whereas negative ions in EI tend to have low mass fragments that impart little structural information, negative ions in CI tend to have more useful high mass fragments. Information from NICI can also serve to complement information gained from positive-ion mass spectra generated under CI and EI conditions. The formation of negative sample ions under CI conditions occurs through three primary pathways: electron capture, proton abstraction, and association. Of the three primary pathways,

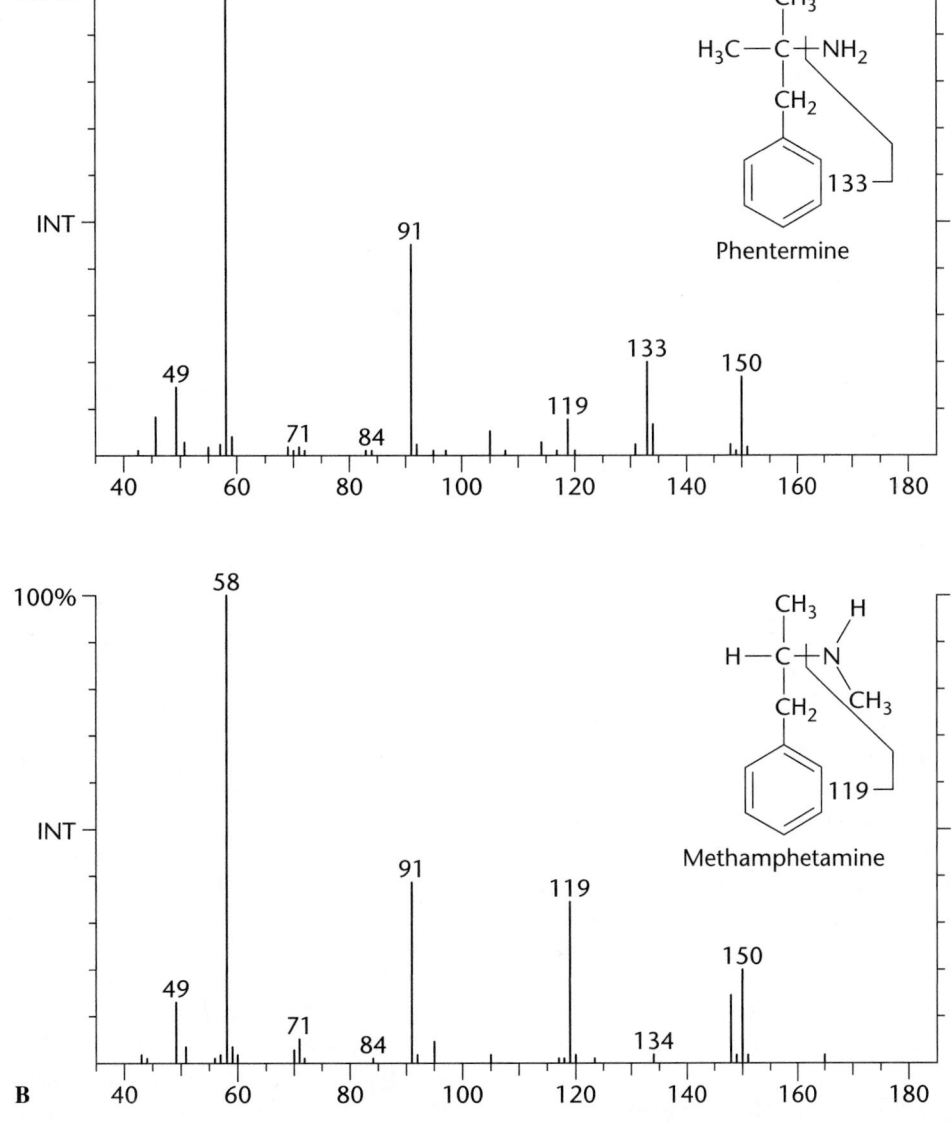

Fig. 8-9, cont'd. **B,** Full-scan methane chemical ionization (CI) spectra of phentermine and methamphetamine (performed on Finnigan-Mat ITS 40 GC/MS).

the electron capture (EC) process offers the most feasible approach for examining drugs and clinical samples. The EC ionization process takes place when the sample molecule captures a thermal or low-energy electron in the reagent gas plasma. For this to be the dominant process the reagent gas must be one that generates low-energy electrons upon electron bombardment. Additionally, the gas itself must not form negative ions capable of reacting with the sample molecule. Methane fulfills these criteria. Upon ionization, methane forms CH_4^+ and CH_3^+ (equation 8-1) as well as low-energy electrons. The capture of these electrons by sample molecules and the subsequent decomposition of the resultant negative ions produces the NICI fragmentation pattern. An intense $(M - 1)^-$ ion fragment is often generated. Very high sensitivity is characteristic of NICI. In many cases, the intensity of the base negative CI ion is 30 to 100 times greater than the base positive CI ion.[2] This can effectively extend routine detection levels to the femtogram level.

USE OF THE MASS SPECTROMETER
Full-scan analysis

Full-scan mass spectrometric analysis in the electron ionization mode is probably the best mass spectrometric technique for the unequivocal identification of a drug or its metabolite or metabolites. In the full-scan mode, the entire mass range of interest is repeatedly scanned. Scanning is programmed to start at the high m/z range and end at the low m/z value at the range of interest. In each scan every ion fragment generated is monitored and displayed. The scan rate must be slow enough so that the detector can register a given fragment but fast enough so that multiple scans can occur during a given analysis. Multiple scans are necessary for the resulting ion statistics to be meaningful. The resulting mass spectrum, consisting of all ion fragments generated, offers a very high degree of specificity. In combination with mass spectrometry's high sensitivity, this full-scan "fingerprint" is extremely effective in providing positive identification of organic compounds such as drugs and their metabolites.[10] Modern systems often rely on computer matching programs to identify unknown compounds. This is done by comparison of the acquired mass spectrum with an existing stored reference spectrum. A variety of different commercially available libraries exist. There are also many different library search algorithms to compare the unknown spectrum to existing stored reference spectra. Ten peak search, probability-based matching, forward or reverse search, purity search, and fit and reverse fit search algorithms are commonly utilized. Although a detailed description of the search algorithms and libraries is beyond the scope of this chapter, reference 11 offers a good discussion of the topic.

Full-scan techniques are more demanding in terms of sample cleanliness. Interfering or co-eluting compounds must be avoided. The presence of interfering compounds generates extraneous ions and complicates the resulting spectra. This can make identification difficult or even impossible. Consequently most samples are purified before analysis. Samples are purified by recrystallizing solids, performing organic cleanup extraction of samples utilizing biological fluids or particulate matter (such as organics in soil), and chromatographic separation by gas chromatography or liquid chromatography before mass spectrometric analysis.

A total ion current (TIC) chromatogram is commonly generated when chromatographic separation is utilized. The total ion current is integrated, and the resulting chromatographic output resembles the appearance of a conventional GLC chromatogram. The full-scan mass spectrum is typically generated at the top of the chromatographic peak to maximize sensitivity. However, multiple mass spectral lines can be generated from any part of the peak, which is helpful in assessing the purity and chromatographic resolution. Co-eluting components can be easily detected even in situations where TIC peak shape is fully symmetrical. Although full-scan analysis offers the highest specificity, its sensitivity is limited. Scanning each fragment in the spectrum means that the detector spends significant time in regions where fragments give low-intensity adducts. Consequently the same characteristics that make full-scan techniques highly specific are also responsible for limiting its sensitivity. Aspects greatly influencing sensitivity are discussed in greater detail later in this chapter.

Selected ion monitoring

Greater EI sensitivity can be obtained when the mass spectrometer is operated in the *selected ion monitoring* mode, in which it monitors ion currents at only a few preselected intense masses characteristic of the compound of interest. Use of few ion fragments for compound identification is less specific than use of a full scan, since all other ion fragments are discarded. This technique is frequently used for target compound identification applications such as forensic or clinical drugs of abuse analyses and is known by several names (such as SIM, selected, selective, or simultaneous ion monitoring; MID, multiple ion detection; and SMS, selective mass storage). Historically, the use of SIM techniques arose from sensitivity limitations of full-scan techniques in magnetic sector and quadrupole systems. In the full-scan mode, mass spectrometers do not always have sufficient sensitivity to detect low drug levels in complex matrices such as biological fluids. By focusing on just a few preselected intense ion fragments, one can enhance sensitivity because the detector can spend all its time on those few ions rather than dividing its time on the several hundred ions scanned in the typical full-scan mode. Consequently, SIM techniques tend to enhance sensitivity by 10 to 100 times. This enhanced sensitivity, however, is obtained at the expense of decreased specificity, since the vast amount of data from the mass spectrum is lost and unavailable. In summary, SIM affords higher sensitivity but provides a less specific identification.

Most SIM applications utilize only a few ions (generally three intense ions) from the mass spectrum to identify the drug. For example, SIM analysis of cocaine could utilize ion fragments m/z 303, 182, and 82 (see Fig. 8-1). Selection of these three ions is preferred because of their relatively high intensity or uniqueness. The molecular ion at m/z 303 has a high m/z value and is considered unique, which helps increase the analytical specificity. The pyrrole ring with m/z 82 is a likely choice because of its high intensity (base peak). Although its relatively low m/z value makes it less specific, its intensity helps the SIM analysis achieve sensitivity at lower levels. It should be stressed that in SIM mode all other ion fragments in the spectrum are lost, reducing the overall specificity of analysis. Consequently, other compounds may interfere if they generate ions with the same m/z value.

Often, SIM methods attempt to minimize specificity shortcomings by comparing to each other the relative ion intensities of major ions being monitored. This practice has been widely used in drugs of abuse testing and requires that the ratios of the ion intensities in the unknown match, within ±20%, the corresponding ratios in an extracted standard. One limitation of this approach is that ion intensities and therefore ratios can vary depending on the amount of drug or metabolite present in the ion source. Consequently the ion ratios of an unknown sample may not be consistent with that of the extracted standard, especially when the drug or metabolite concentrations are either much higher or lower than those in the standard.[12]

Although identification in SIM techniques is less specific than in full-scan mode, it is adequate for many applications. However, care must be used because it is possible to incorrectly identify compounds when conditions are not optimized. For example, some drugs of abuse testing laboratories analyze amphetamine by means of GC/MS using m/z 44 as a quantification ion and m/z 58 as a qualifying ion following a protocol published by Hewlett-Packard.[8] One problem with this method is the choice of ions. These ions have low m/z values and are subject to potential interference from a variety of other compounds and background ion currents that may be present in the sample. For example, in addition to amphetamine, many other sympathomimetic amine compounds exhibit a large peak at m/z 58, and carbon dioxide (a common background component) exhibits a peak at m/z 44. Consequently, significant problems can arise because commonly encountered legal drugs (such as ephedrine, phentermine, phenylpropanolamine, and other common over-the-counter [OTC] medications) have the same ion fragments as those selected to characterize illicit amphetamine. Such legal medications and OTC compounds are generally coextracted in the sample-preparation step and their chromatographic retention times can be close to those of the illicit drugs.

Under suboptimal conditions, SIM methods such as the described amphetamine procedure can essentially amount to identification based on incremental differences in chromatographic retention times. Since chromatographic retention times often shift, the possibility of a false-positive or a false-negative result exists. The probability of inaccurate drug confirmations may be further increased in laboratories where GC/MS operators, who sometimes have little knowledge of the principles of mass spectrometry, may be swamped under excessive work loads with demanding turn-around times. Some NIDA-certified forensic drugs of abuse testing laboratories have lost their testing accreditation because of false-positive amphetamine or methamphetamine results generated by such SIM analyses. In conclusion, it can be surmised that SIM techniques have specificity pitfalls and that these hold the potential for serious errors for the unsuspecting.

Employing mass spectrometric techniques offering greater specificity, such as full-scan EI or CI, or both, can help minimize analytical and interpretational errors. It is also possible to increase both mass spectral sensitivity and specificity by noninstrumental techniques. However, such a discussion is beyond the scope of this chapter, and this discussion primarily focuses on the instrumental MS means for enhancing sensitivity and specificity.

Quantitation

SIM techniques are well suited for quantitative analysis because several different ion fragments can be monitored simultaneously. This mass spectral output is frequently referred to as a *selected ion profile,* or a *selected ion chromatogram.* In mass spectrometry quantitative accuracy is best achieved by incorporating an internal standard, which is added at the beginning of the analytical process. The addition of a known quantity of internal standard compensates for material lost at any stage of the analysis including the extraction, derivatization, and analytical steps. Consequently, the internal standards selected should chemically resemble the compounds of interest as closely as possible so that their physical and chemical behavior matches those of the unknown. For this reason, deuterated compounds are widely used as internal standards. The technique of quantitation using chemicals different only in their isotope composition is termed *isotope dilution.* In the case of drug analysis one uses a deuterated internal standard that is identical to the drug being assayed except that one or more hydrogen atoms have been substituted by deuterium atoms. The number and position of the deuterated atoms are chosen by ease of synthesis and position in the fragmenting ion pattern. This results in an internal standard that has very close characteristics in terms of polarity, extraction partition coefficient, derivatization, and chromatography compared to the drug itself. In fact, the internal standard will have a chromatographic retention time that is almost identical to that of the drug itself because of its structural similarity (see Fig. 8-10). In conventional GLC, a deuterated internal standard cannot be utilized because it must be chromatographically resolved from the compound of interest. In mass spectrometry, this is not a problem because the atomic mass unit of a deuterium atom is 1 AMU greater than hydrogen. The deuterated internal standard has a different molecular weight and hence is differentiated from the drug by the difference in masses rather than by chromatographic retention time. Its fragmentation pattern will mimic that of the drug, but the fragments containing deuterium atoms will have a correspondingly higher m/z value.

The mass spectral SIM output displays only the ions exhibiting the m/z fragments being monitored. SIM quantitation simultaneously monitors the ion fragments of the compound and that of the internal standard. Fig. 8-10 shows selected ion profiles for two isotopes of silylated Δ^9-tetrahydrocannabinol analyzed by GC/MS. The internal standard contains the deuterated isotope (d_3), which is monitored at m/z 390. The ion profile of the compound of interest is the unlabeled analog, which is monitored at m/z 387. Chromatographic retention times of the two isotopes are essentially the same, and their detection is accomplished when one takes advantage of the difference in the molecular weights of the ion fragments. A quantitative value is obtained when one compares the peak area or intensity of the

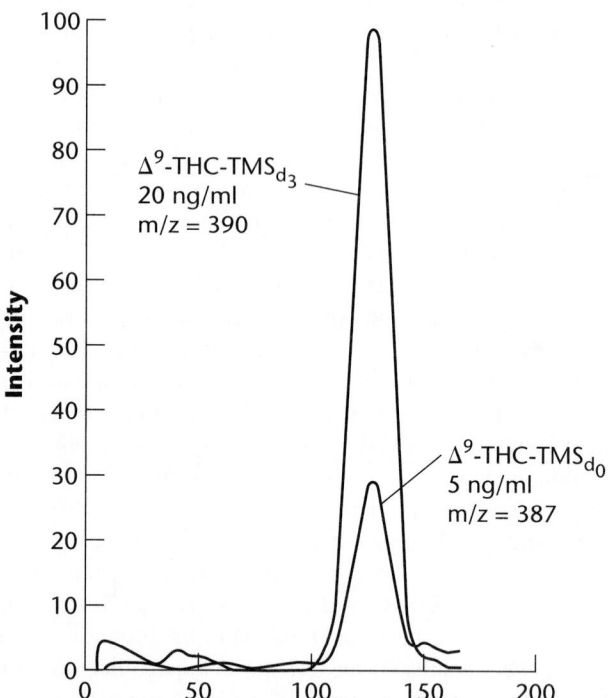

Fig. 8-10 Selected ion monitoring plot for quantitation of Δ^9-tetrahydrocannabinol in plasma. Undenterated (d_0) and denterated (d_3) drugs. (From Saferstein R: *Forensic science handbook,* Englewood Cliffs, N.J., 1982, Prentice Hall.)

compound of interest to that of the internal standard. This ratio is then utilized to generate a quantitative value from a previously established calibration curve.

SEPARATION TECHNIQUES

The mass spectrometer ionizes and separates all compounds entering the ion source. If there is more than one compound present, this results in a mass fragment pattern comprising all the components. For this reason, the clearest fragment patterns are those in which only one compound is analyzed at one time. Thus the mass spectrometer is usually coupled to a separation procedure such as gas or liquid chromatography.

Gas chromatography/mass spectrometry

Gas-liquid chromatography is one of the most versatile instrumental techniques for performing separation of complex mixtures because of its sensitivity, speed of analysis, and versatility. Capillary columns enable chromatographers to devise separation procedures for virtually every compound of interest in clinical chemistry. The combination of GLC separation versatility coupled with specificity and sensitivity of mass spectrometry makes GC/MS one of the most powerful techniques available for the identification of organic compounds. The same methods as described in Chapter 7 are used to prepare compounds for analysis by GC/MS.

The main technical issue in coupling these techniques arose from the incompatibility of pressure requirements. GLC requires a carrier gas flow at approximately atmospheric pressure to move the sample through the column. Mass spectrometers, on the other hand, require high vacuum (10^{-5} to 10^{-7} torr) to operate effectively. Molecular jet separators combined with differential vacuum pumps have been used to evacuate the carrier gas selectively just before the GLC effluent entry into the ion source of the mass spectrometer.[1] The more recent advent of capillary columns simplified the interface requirements because capillary columns function effectively at much lower carrier gas flow rates, which are within the pumping capacity of the mass spectrometer. Consequently, capillary column effluents can flow directly into the ion source.

Two different mass spectrometer data outputs are commonly obtained in GC/MS. The first, the TIC chromatogram, represents the integration of total ion current versus time of elution from the GLC column. That is, all the ions detected are summed together, and the total current is recorded. Its pattern resembles a conventional GLC chromatogram of detector response versus time. The full-scan mass spectrum is the second output. This analysis resolves the detected ions of the TIC into their mass fragment pattern. Mass spectral lines generated at different parts of the TIC peak can readily reveal whether the peak is pure or whether it contains multiple components. Additionally, the mass spectrum of a shoulder or minor peak can often reveal the identity of the component generating that ion current. The mass spectrum generated can either be a full scan or an SIM. In either case, sensitivity is maximized when the mass spectrum is generated at the apex of the TIC peak. TIC can also be monitored exclusively in the SIM mode, which generates a selective ion chromatogram. This is a common practice in target compound identification applications. The output is then composed of only the ions with the m/z value being monitored. SIM quantitations rely on this technique by simultaneously monitoring the ion fragments of the compound of interest and that of the internal standard.

Liquid chromatography/mass spectrometry

Another potentially useful combination is high-performance liquid chromatography (HPLC) and mass spectrometry. The barriers to interfacing LC are even greater than in the case of GC because the mobile phase used to propel the components through the HPLC column is less volatile and hence more difficult for selective removal (before mass spectrometric analysis) than the gaseous mobile phase used in GLC. Furthermore, LC is often used to separate components that are either not particularly volatile or are thermally labile. This further compounds the incompatibility because samples must first be volatilized into the gaseous state before they can be analyzed by mass spectrometry. The difficulty of converting relatively nonvolatile molecules solvated in a liquid into the gaseous form without inducing excessive decomposition has always been the basis for the incompatibility; it is the reason why the evolution of LC/MS has been slower than GC/MS.

Thermospray is one approach to LC analysis, and this process creates charged droplets. The tip of the capillary tube from which the HPLC eluate emerges is heated by application of a high voltage. By optimizing the temperature, small droplets can be made to be ejected (spray) from the end of the tube into the ion source.

Thermospray relies on an "ion-evaporation" process where ions are emitted from a liquid into the gas phase.[13] In theory, a charged droplet contains the solvent plus positive and negative ions, with ions of one polarity being domi-

nant. The difference is the net charge; it has been postulated that the excess charge resides at the surface of the droplet. As the solvent evaporates, the electric field at the surface of the droplet increases because of the decreasing radius. If the droplet evaporates far enough, a critical field is reached at which ions from the surface are emitted. Fig. 8-11 illustrates the ion-evaporation process. *IonSpray*[14] is a newer but related technique suited to the introduction of thermally labile compounds into the mass spectrometer. It differs from thermospray in that it does not utilize heat to produce the spray, and it can readily occur at atmospheric pressure. Thermospray is generally operated in high vacuum, though it can be used at pressures up to atmospheric. Elevated temperatures are required for thermospray. IonSpray allows the introduction of complex and polar compounds into the mass spectrometer. It also generates a quasimolecular ion and is especially suitable for polar and thermally labile compounds. In addition to HPLC, IonSpray can be interfaced with other separation techniques such as capillary zone electrophoresis to allow the analysis of complex biological samples.[15]

Solids probe

Direct mass spectrometry using solids probe sample introduction has been used by toxicologists for many years to rapidly identify targeted compounds.[16,17] This technique is advantageous for compounds of low volatility, which can be introduced directly into the ion source. Another advantage of solids probe MS is that it eliminates the chromatographic separation step; consequently, analysis can be completed very rapidly. MS analysis probing solids has been used extensively both in the EI and CI modes with pure compounds. For biological specimens CI is especially practical, since compound identification can be done based on molecular weight.

OTHER MASS SPECTROMETERS
Ion trap detector (ITD)

Mass spectrometers based on ion trap technology are different in design from other MS systems. All current com-

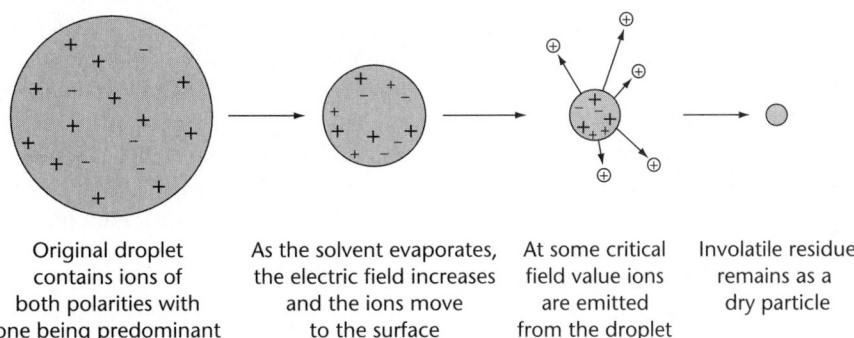

| Original droplet contains ions of both polarities with one being predominant | As the solvent evaporates, the electric field increases and the ions move to the surface | At some critical field value ions are emitted from the droplet | Involatile residue remains as a dry particle |

Fig. 8-11   Diagram of ion evaporation process. (From *The API book,* Eden Prairie, Minn., 1992, Perkin-Elmer Sciex.)

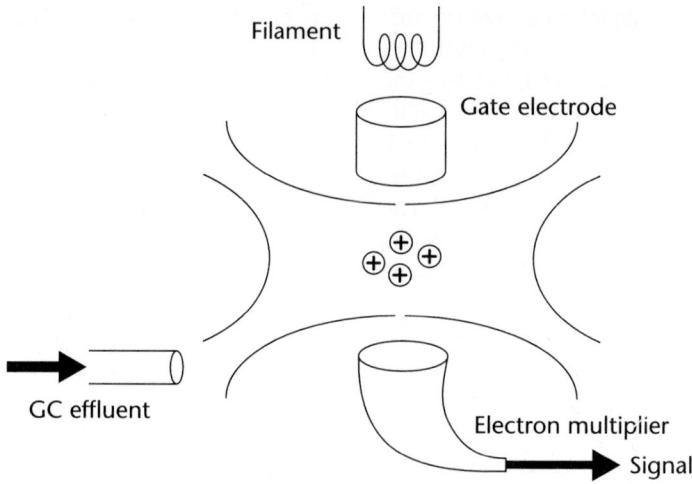

Fig. 8-12   The ion trap mass spectrometer.

mercial instruments are relatively inexpensive benchtop systems. Ion trap mass spectrometers combine the functions of an ion source and a mass analyzer. This is done in a simple three-electrode assembly consisting of a ring electrode and two end caps (Fig. 8-12). This simplicity is in sharp contrast to the complex mechanical assemblies commonly found in quadrupole and magnetic sector mass spectrometers. Electrons from a heated filament are pulsed into the central cavity by a gate electrode where they ionize the sample molecules, resulting in conventional EI fragmentation patterns characteristic of the compound. The unique feature of ion trap mass spectrometers is that they "trap" and "store" the ions generated over time within the ion source cavity. This is done by application of a radio frequency voltage to the central ring electrode, which causes ions of interest to be trapped and accumulated over time in the ion source. The trapped ions are then mass-selectively ejected from the cavity according to their m/z ratio onto the electron multiplier where they are detected. The effective trapping and accumulation of ions results in concentrating the ions of interest; consequently very high sensitivities are obtained with ITD. The ion trap's superior sensitivity allows the user to obtain full-scan mass spectra with limits of detection comparable to SIM analyses in conventional quadrupole detectors.

Time-of-flight mass spectrometry

The time-of-flight mass spectrometer is based on the requirement that ions generated in the source must travel a fixed distance to reach the detector. The accelerating voltage propels the ions into a "drift tube" that is typically 1 meter long. The velocity of ions is proportional to their mass. Consequently different mass ions travel at different speeds and reach the detector at different times. The m/z value of any given ion can be determined mathematically when one makes an accurate measurement of the time that an ion takes to traverse the distance and reach the detector.

Currently this type of mass spectrometer is used in research for the analysis of complex biopolymers at the picomole level. This type of instrument using laser desorption ionization is suited for the measurement of high mass molecules and can determine the molecular weights of peptides, intact proteins, and glycoproteins 300,000 daltons in size.

Tandem mass spectrometry (MS/MS)

In general, improving selectivity and detection limits of instrumental techniques can be achieved by extensive sample pretreatment (extraction, derivatization, chromatographic separation, and so on) before mass spectrometry. An alternative approach to improve detection limits and enhance selectivity is the coupling of two or more analytical techniques in tandem.[18] GC/MS, GC/MS/IR, MS/MS, and GC/MS/MS are examples (as compared to MS alone).

The acceptance of applications of tandem mass spectrometry (MS/MS) is attributable to the technique's ability to provide (1) increased speed of analysis; (2) decreased cost per sample; (3) improved limits of detection in complex mixtures; and (4) rapid, sensitive, and selective analysis of complex mixtures rapidly, often with minimal or no sample cleanup.[19-21] Solids probe MS/MS can be performed on drugs that are difficult to chromatograph and hence cannot be run on conventional GC/MS. In tandem MS/MS a mixture is introduced into the ion source of the first MS where ionization of the mixture produces ions characteristic of the individual drug components, termed *parent ions*. A characteristic parent ion of the targeted drug of interest is then selected and identified. This "separates" the analyte of interest from the other mixture components and can be thought of as analogous to the chromatographic separation step of GC/MS. The targeted parent ion is then subjected to second MS analysis where it is further fragmented into secondary ion fragments termed *daughter ions*. This step is analogous to the fragmentation occurring during the ionization step in GC/MS. Mass analysis of the daughter ions by

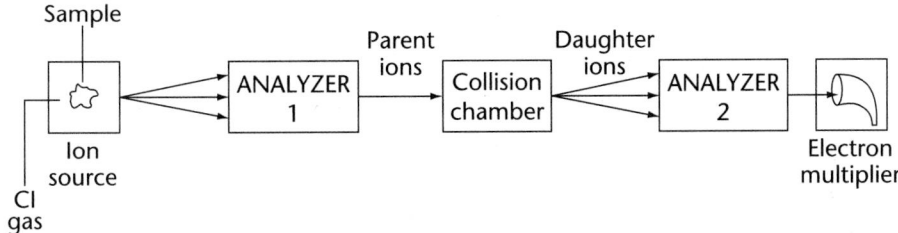

Fig. 8-13 Schema of a tandem mass spectrometer (MS/MS). CI, Chemical ionization. (From Yinon Y: *Forensic mass spectrometry,* Boca Raton, Fla., 1987, CRC Press.)

the second mass analyzer provides a unique and highly specific identification of the targeted parent ion.

Fig. 8-13 demonstrates the schema of a tandem mass spectrometer. It consists of two mass analyzers connected sequentially. A collision chamber for fragmentation of selected ions is situated between the two mass analyzers. Although different types of mass spectrometers can be combined, the triple-stage quadruple configuration is one of the more popular. Many applications utilize CI techniques for the initial ionization to generate an intense quasimolecular ion fragment. The ion selected should be as specific and as intense as possible. This ion is then subjected to collisions with inert gas in the collision chamber. The resulting daughter ions are then separated by the second mass analyzer. Daughter ions' spectral lines resemble conventional EI spectral lines and are used for the actual compound identification. MS/MS effectively generates highly characteristic fragmentation of a specific ion.

In summary, the first MS analysis is used to achieve separation of mixture into components, a process performed by the GC in conventional GC/MS. With MS/MS, however, this separation process is instantaneous, whereas with GC/MS it can take 5 to 15 minutes. This time advantage is the feature that gives MS/MS the potential for very rapid analysis. Whereas, the throughput of samples in conventional GC/MS may typically be 4 to 6 samples per hour, in MS/MS it can be 60 samples per hour. Additional time efficiency is gained, since sample extraction and derivatization can be drastically minimized and in some cases totally avoided.

FORENSIC DRUG TESTING

In 1987, the Department of Health and Human Services charged the NIDA to develop and implement a laboratory accreditation program for laboratories testing government workers for drugs of abuse. The need for regulation arose from the fact that different laboratories were utilizing different testing methodologies and different performance standards to designate a result as positive for drugs of abuse. The quality and reliability of results varied greatly. The NIDA regulations[22] were issued in 1988 and covered all aspects of the drugs of abuse testing. These included personnel requirements, security of facilities, chain-of-custody

(COC), specimen handling, record keeping, confidentiality of results, proficiency testing, quality control (QC), independent inspection of facilities, and analytical testing requirements. NIDA has successfully implemented a rigorous accreditation program propagating these standards. Certified laboratories that fail to meet the standards have been decertified from the program. The goal of the program is to ensure that labs do not generate false-positive results and that the results generated could stand up to legal challenges. Consequently, the term "forensic" drugs-of-abuse testing is used. The NIDA analytical protocols for the detection of drugs of abuse in urine are based upon the use of two independent analytical techniques of:

1. A sensitive initial screening procedure to identify negative specimens and to select presumptive positive specimens for further testing. Screening had to be done using an FDA-registered immunoassay technique.
2. A highly specific confirmatory technique that is at least as sensitive as the initial screen for confirmation of presumptive positive results. The confirmation method was limited to GC/MS.

Both screening and confirmation steps are incorporated into a forensic urine drug detection program where the consequences of such an analysis will be the basis of actions taken against the individual who supplied the sample.[23] Because of the potential negative effect on the individual, only rigorous and conclusive procedures are used. GC/MS is generally accepted as a rigorous confirmation technique, since it provides the best level of confidence in the result. A survey of experts, industrial arbitrators, and forensic toxicologists on the legal defensibility of laboratory analyses concluded "that most forensic experts believe that GC/MS is the gold standard and experts who must defend analytical data are of the opinion . . . that GC/MS confirmation is held to be the most defensible confirmation procedure by a considerable margin."[24] Other forensic drug workplace testing programs have also been instituted by various state and municipal localities (such as Florida, New York State, Commonwealth of Pennsylvania, and New York City). The College of American Pathologists together with the American Association of Clinical Chemists have also implemented a voluntary forensic urine drug testing accrediting program. Analytically, all follow the NIDA model requiring confirmation of an initial positive immunoassay screen.

It is worthy to remember that GC/MS is a technique combining GLC separation with mass spectrometric detection. This means that good GC/MS results are highly dependent on good chromatographic separations. Although it may seem self-evident, many users encounter GC/MS problems that could be readily avoided by optimizing chromatographic parameters. In fact, most GC/MS problems in the clinical and forensic toxicology laboratory are probably chromatographic in nature. Thus it is important to consider chromatographic as well as urine sample clean-up and derivatization issues in any discussion of the application of GC/MS to drug testing in biological fluids. For several of the NIDA-regulated drugs, derivatization is necessary to increase the compound's volatility and optimize the chromatographic process. Reactive groups such as hydroxyl, carboxylic acids, and amine moieties are converted to less reactive functional groups by means of derivatization. This enhances their volatility and minimizes their chromatographic reactivity resulting in better chromatographic performance as well as more rapid separation. Derivatization also increases the molecular weight of the compounds and hence increases specificity by generating more desirable higher m/z ion fragments. Several good in-depth discussions of derivatization techniques and related issues are readily available.[12,25-27] Deuterated internal standards should be utilized and should be added to the biological samples being assayed before the extraction process.

Two widespread misconceptions about mass spectrometry are (1) that GC/MS is a specific "method" and (2) that GC/MS is 100% accurate. GC/MS is in fact an instrumental analytical technique with many variations and a diverse variety of instrumental configurational possibilities. There are countless methods based on GC/MS techniques, each with its own set of advantages and disadvantages. Some GC/MS methods may be appropriate for a given analyte, whereas others may not be. Although forensics testing laboratories are required to utilize GC/MS, they have great flexibility and freedom in selecting instrumentation, mode of operation, as well as the actual analytical methodologies. When a correct method is performed correctly, it will result in the positive identification of a drug or metabolite. The result will be legally defensible if appropriate quality control is part of the laboratory's analysis. The QC program should include the analysis of threshold-cutoff standards, drug-free samples, blind controls, and known controls containing drugs below and above the threshold value with each batch of samples. In addition, forensic requirements call for strict COC and laboratory security. Such requirements are part of the forensic package and are necessary because of the implication of laboratory results for job applicants, employees, and companies and because of the potential legal challenges of the laboratory's results. When all these aspects of testing are incorporated, the lab results are legally defensible.

REFERENCES

1. McFadden WH: *Techniques of combined gas chromatography/mass spectrometry,* New York, 1973, Wiley & Sons.
2. Saferstein R: *Forensic science handbook,* Englewood Cliffs, N.J., 1982, Prentice-Hall, pp 92-182.
3. Jindal SP, Vestergaard P: Quantitation of cocaine and its principal metabolite, benzoylecgonine, by GLC/mass spectrometry using stable isotope labeled analogues as internal standards, *J Pharm Sci* 67:811-814, 1978.
4. McLafferty FW: *Interpretation of mass spectra,* ed 3, Mill Valley, Calif., 1980, University Science Book.
5. Silverstein RM, Bassler CG: *Spectrometrical identification of organic compounds,* New York, 1967, Wiley & Sons.
6. Budzikiewicz H, Djerassi C, Williams DH: *Mass spectrometry of organic compounds,* San Francisco, 1967, Holden-Day Inc.
7. Lehrer M: Application of gas chromatography/mass spectrometry instrument techniques to forensic urine drug testing, *Clin Lab Med* 10:271-288, 1990.
8. Hewlett-Packard technical application: *GC/MS confirmation of amphetamines,* publication #23-5954-8146, Waltham, Mass., Jan 1987, Hewlett-Packard Co.
9. deJong EG, Maes RA, van Rossum JM: *Why do doping control labs need MS/MS?* Presented at the International Symposium on Applied Mass Spectrometry in the Health Sciences, Barcelona, Spain, Sept 28, 1987.
10. Deutsch DG: *Analytical aspects of drug testing, chemical analysis series,* New York, 1989, Wiley & Sons, pp 87-128.
11. Pfleger K, Maurer H, Weber A: *Mass spectral and GC data of drugs, poisons, and their metabolites,* New York, 1985, VCH Publishers.
12. Peat MA: Analytical and technical aspects of testing for drug abuse: confirmatory procedures, *Clin Chem* 34(3):471-473, 1988.
13. Iribane JV, Thomson BA: On the evaporation of small ions from charged droplets, *J Chem Physiol* 64:2287, 1976.
14. Bruins AP, Covey TR, Henion JD: IonSpray interface for combined liquid chromatography/atmospheric pressure ionization mass spectrometry, *Anal Chem* 59:2642-2646, 1987.
15. *The API book,* Eden Prairie, Minn., 1992, Perkin-Elmer Sciex.
16. Lehrer M, Karmen A: Chemical ionization mass spectrometry for rapid assay of drugs in serum, *J Chromatogr* 126:615-624, 1976.
17. Saferstein R: Drug detection in urine by chemical ionization mass spectrometry, *J Forensic Sci* 23:29-39, 1978.
18. Yost RA, Johnson JV: Tandem mass spectrometry for trace analysis, *Anal Chem* 57(7):758A-768A, 1985.
19. Glish GL, Shaddock VM, Harmon K: Rapid analysis of complex mixtures by mass spectrometry, *Anal Chem* 52:165-167, 1980.
20. Lee MS, Yost RA: Rapid identification of drug metabolites with tandem mass spectrometry, *Biomed Environ Mass Spectrometry* 15:193-204, 1988.
21. Weiss MD: Chemistry is winning the war against crime, *Industrial Chemist* 15:28-34, Feb 1988.
22. Federal Register: Mandatory guidelines for federal workplace drug testing; final guidelines, April 11, 1988.
23. Lehrer M: Drug screening in the workplace, *Clin Lab Med* 7(2):389-400, 1987.
24. Hoyt DW, Finnigan RE, Nee T, et al: Drug testing in the workplace—are methods legally defensible? *JAMA* 258(4):504-509, 1987.
25. Blau K, King GS, editors: *Handbook of derivatives for chromatography,* Philadelphia, 1978, Heyden & Sons.
26. Foltz RL, Fentiman AF, Foltz RB: *GC/MS assays for abused drugs in body fluids,* National Institute of Drug Abuse monogr no 32, DHHS publ no (ADM) 80-1014, Washington, D.C., 1980.
27. Hawks RL, Chiang CN: *Urine testing for drugs of abuse,* National Institute of Drug Abuse monogr no 73, DHHS publ no (ADM) 87-1481, Washington, D.C., 1987.

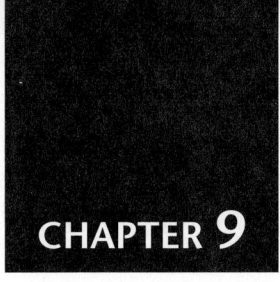

CHAPTER 9

Radioisotopes in clinical chemistry

I-Wen Chen

Basic structure of an atom
   Fundamental particles of an atom
   Atomic structure nomenclature
Principles of radiation and radioactivity
   Nuclear radiation
   Radiation energy
   Rate of radioactive decay
   Properties of radiation and interaction with matter
Measurement of nuclear radiation
   Gas-filled detectors
   Scintillation detectors
Radiation health safety
   Monitoring
   Contamination control
   Waste disposal

OBJECTIVES

- Describe the basic structure of the atom. Explain the significance of the atomic number and atomic mass number as they relate to the existence of isotopes.

- Describe the modes of radioactive decay associated with tritium, carbon-14, and iodine-125 and name the particles emitted.

- Define and explain the importance of decay constants, decay factors, half-life, and specific activity.

- Summarize the operation of scintillation detectors. Diagram and explain the use of the crystal and liquid scintillation counters and describe the operation of each component. Define quenching and outline correction methods.

- Describe the use of isotopes in the clinical laboratories and list radiation safety considerations for monitoring personnel and work areas, contamination control, and waste disposal.

KEY TERMS

becquerel (Bq) Système International d'Unités (SI) unit of radioactivity corresponding to a decay rate of 1/sec (1 Bq = 1 sec^{-1} = 2.7×10^{-11} Ci) (see *curie*).

chemiluminescence Production of light photons by an interaction of the sample material with the solute or solubilizer added to the scintillation solution in liquid scintillation counting.

circuit, anticoincident A circuit used in the pulse-height analyzer of a radioactive-particle counter for setting window width (see *window*). It transmits a pulse arriving at its input from the lower discriminator only if there is no pulse arriving from the upper discriminator at the same time (see *discriminator*).

circuit, coincident A circuit used in a liquid scintillation counter to eliminate the electronic noise. It determines if a pulse from one photomultiplier tube is accompanied by a corresponding pulse from the other within the allowed time interval (see *coincidence resolving time*).

coincidence resolving time A time interval within which the output pulses from each photomultiplier tube of a liquid scintillation counter have to arrive at the coincident circuit to be counted.

curie (Ci) Unit of radioactivity. One curie is defined as an activity of a sample decaying at a rate of 3.7×10^{10} disintegrations per second (dps).

decay constant A constant unique to each radioactive nuclide (see *nuclide*) representing the proportion of the atoms in a sample of that radionuclide undergoing decay in unit time.

decay factor The fraction of radionuclides remaining after a time, *t*.

discriminator(s) Device(s) used in the pulse-height analyzer of a radioactive-particle counter for setting upper (upper-level discriminator) and lower (lower-level discriminator) voltage limits for counting.

electron capture One mode of radioactive decay in which the neutron-poor nuclides decay by capturing electrons from orbits closest to the nucleus to transform a proton to a neutron. The orbital vacancy created by the electron capture is filled by the electron from a higher orbit, resulting in emission of characteristic x rays.

electron volt (eV) Basic unit of energy commonly used in radiation, defined as the amount of energy acquired by an electron when it is accelerated through an electrical potential of 1 volt.

half-life (t$_{1/2}$) Time required for a given number of radionuclides in the sample to decrease to one half its original value.

isobar Nuclides (see *nuclide*) with the same atomic mass number but different atomic number.

isotope Nuclides (see *nuclide*) with the same atomic number but different atomic mass number.

isotopic abundance Amounts of isotopes present for a given element.

nucleon A collective term for protons and neutrons in the nucleus.

nuclide A nucleus with a particular atomic number and atomic mass number.

radiation absorbed dose (rad) A measure of local energy deposition per unit mass of material irradiated. One rad is equal to 100 ergs of absorbed energy per gram of absorber. (No plural form.)

roentgen equivalent, man (rem) That dose of any ionizing radiation causing the same amount of biological injury to human tissue as 1 rad of x, gamma, or beta radiation. In the case of x, gamma, or beta radiation rem is equal to the absorbed dose in rad; in the case of alpha radiation, however, the dose in rem equals the dose in rad multiplied by 20, because only 0.05 rad of alpha radiation is needed to produce the same biological effect as 1 rad of x, gamma, or beta radiation. (No plural form.)

roentgen (R) A unit of x rays or gamma rays representing the quantity of ionization produced by photon radiation in a given sample of air. One roentgen equals that quantity of photon radiation capable of producing one electrostatic unit of ions of either sign in 0.001293 g of air.

specific activity Activity of the radionuclide per unit mass of the radioactive sample, expressed as curies (Ci) per μg, μCi per μmole, and so on.

specific ionization Number of ion pairs produced per unit path length of ionizing radiation.

summation circuit A circuit used in a liquid scintillation counter to sum all coincident pulses to improve counting efficiency for low-energy beta-particle emitters.

transmutation A radioactive decay process that results in a change in nuclear constitution, such as electron capture decay (see *electron capture*).

wavelength shifter The secondary scintillator added to scintillation liquid for shifting the wavelength of light emitted by the primary scintillator for more efficient detection by the photocathodes of photomultiplier tubes in liquid scintillation counting.

window The voltage limit set by the upper-level and lower-level discriminators (see *discriminator*) of the pulse-height analyzer of a radioactive-particle counter for differential counting.

The use of isotopes, both stable and radioactive, has provided a great body of information in the medical sciences, much of which could not have been obtained in any other way. The usefulness of isotopes depends on the fact that isotopes of an element have identical chemical properties but different isotopic properties, such as radioactivity and increased mass, and on the fact that the isotopic properties and chemical properties of an element are independent of each other. Therefore substitution of an atom in the molecule of a substance by other isotopes will not chemically alter that substance, and the isotopic properties of the isotopes incorporated into that substance will remain unchanged. The isotopic properties will make that substance more easily identifiable. For example, thyroxine is a thyroid hormone containing four atoms of iodine. One or all of these iodine atoms may be replaced by radioactive iodine without appreciable alteration of its chemical properties, and the radioiodine atoms incorporated into the thy-

roxine molecules will maintain their characteristic radioactivity. The radioiodine-labeled thyroxine molecules can be identified and quantified easily by virtue of their radioactivity. Radioiodine-labeled thyroxines are used in various thyroid-function tests.

The application of radioisotopically labeled compounds in clinical chemistry has greatly expanded since the advent of radioimmunoassays, in which the quantity of antigen bound to antibody is determined by measurement of radioactivity (see Chapters 12 and 13). The use of radioisotopes in clinical laboratories, however, has been decreasing in recent years because of the emergence of automated nonisotopic immunoassay technology, and radioimmunoassays will have more limited roles in the field of immunoassays for routine disease diagnosis. In this chapter, some basic principles involved in the measurement of isotopes are discussed.

BASIC STRUCTURE OF AN ATOM
Fundamental particles of an atom

An atom is the smallest unit of matter that still exhibits the chemical properties of an element. The primary building blocks of atoms, the electron, the proton, and the neutron, are termed *elementary particles*. According to the planetary model of the atom developed by Rutherford in 1911, the atom consists of a central, small, positively charged body (the nucleus, composed of protons and neutrons) around which the negatively charged electrons move in defined orbits. Although the Rutherford model is oversimplified, one can use it to explain many atomic phenomena satisfactorily. The planetary model of an atom of carbon is illustrated in Fig. 9-1.

The nucleus of carbon contains six protons and six neutrons. Since complete atoms are electrically neutral, six orbiting electrons are present in the carbon atom to match the six protons in the nucleus. They move around the nucleus in a series of orbits or shells, at varying distances from the nucleus, much as the planets of the solar system travel in different orbits at varying distances from the sun. The orbits, or shells, are called *K, L, M,* and so on, starting from

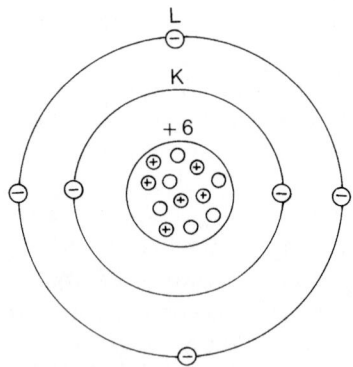

Fig. 9-1 Planetary model of carbon atom.

the inner one. Only two electrons can be accommodated in the K shell; the L shell of the carbon atom contains the remaining four.

The physical and chemical differences between the atoms of different elements depend on the number of protons and neutrons contained in an atomic nucleus, which determines both the mass and charge of the nucleus, and the number and arrangements of the electrons, which determine the chemical properties of elements.

Atomic structure nomenclature

There are several important terms that are helpful in understanding atomic structure:

nucleon A collective term for protons and neutrons in the nucleus.

atomic number, Z The number of protons in the nucleus.

atomic mass number, A The total number of nucleons in the nucleus.

neutron number, N The number of neutrons in the nucleus.

nuclide A nucleus with particular Z and A numbers.

element, E A nucleus with a given Z number.

isotope Nuclides with the same Z but different A numbers (various nuclear species of the same element).

isobar Nuclides with the same A but different Z numbers (different elements with the same atomic mass).

The atomic mass number is represented as a left superscript and the atomic number as a left subscript to the chemical symbol. Thus an element, E, is written as $^A_Z E$. The most abundant, naturally occurring, stable isotope of carbon has six protons and six neutrons in the nucleus. The atomic number, Z, is therefore 6; the atomic mass number, A, is 12 ($A = Z + N$); and the whole atom may be written as $^{12}_6 C$. The other naturally occurring but less abundant isotope of carbon is $^{13}_6 C$, which contains seven neutrons in the nucleus. $^{12}_6 C$ and $^{13}_6 C$ are both stable isotopes of carbon, and neither is radioactive. The best-known radioactive isotope of carbon is $^{14}_6 C$, which contains six protons and eight neutrons. Examples of other groups of isotopes of an element commonly used in clinical chemistry are $^1_1 H$, $^2_1 H$, and $^3_1 H$ and $^{125}_{53} I$, $^{127}_{53} I$, and $^{131}_{53} I$. $^1_1 H$ is the most abundant naturally occurring isotope of hydrogen and has one proton but no neutron in the nucleus. $^2_1 H$ is a stable isotope of hydrogen and is known as *deuterium* because its nucleus contains two nuclear particles, one proton and one neutron. $^3_1 H$, called *tritium*, is a radioactive isotope of hydrogen, the nucleus of which is formed by a combination of a proton and two neutrons. All isotopes of hydrogen have a single circling electron and therefore have identical chemical properties; however, their physical properties are different. For example, they will have different boiling and freezing points. The tritium nucleus is unstable and will undergo radioactive transitions to become a different and stable nucleus—the nucleus of helium. The naturally occurring stable isotope

of iodine is $^{127}_{53} I$. The other two isotopes of iodine mentioned here are radioactive isotopes with different numbers of neutrons in their nucleus, as indicated by their atomic mass numbers. In many cases the atomic number subscript is redundant because the atomic number and the chemical symbol both identify the chemical species. Therefore, except in some equations describing nuclear reactions, the subscript is normally omitted (such as $^{14} C$, $^3 H$, and $^{125} I$).

PRINCIPLES OF RADIATION AND RADIOACTIVITY
Nuclear radiation

The release of energy or matter during the transformation of an unstable atom to a more stable atom is termed *nuclear radiation*. The numbers and arrangement of protons and neutrons in the nucleus of an atom determine whether the nucleus is stable or unstable.

Nuclear stability. There are favored neutron-to-proton ratios among stable nuclides. The ratio is equal to or close to unity for the light nuclides. When the atomic mass number exceeds 40, no stable nuclides exist with equal numbers of neutrons and protons because, as the number of protons increases, the repulsive coulombic forces between the protons increase at a greater rate than the attractive nuclear force does. Therefore the addition of extra neutrons is necessary to increase the average distance between protons in the nucleus to reduce the coulombic force. For heavy nuclei the neutron-to-proton ratio is 1.5 or greater. For example, the heaviest stable isotope of lead, $^{208} Pb$, has a neutron-to-proton ratio of 1.53.

Fig. 9-2 illustrates the relationship between the neutron and proton numbers of the stable nuclides. An imaginary line, called the *line of stability*, represented by a dashed line in the graph, can be obtained from the neutron-proton plot; the stable nuclides are clustered around this line. Nuclides deficient in protons lie below the line of stability and are unstable. Nuclides deficient in neutrons lie above the line and are also unstable. The graph also illustrates the fact that, as nuclides become heavier, more neutrons are required to maintain stability.

In addition to the favored neutron-to-proton ratio, the stable nuclides tend to favor even numbers. For example, 168 out of approximately 280 known stable nuclides have even numbers of both protons and neutrons, reflecting the tendency of nuclides to achieve stable arrangements by pairing up nucleons in the nucleus.

Modes of radioactive decay. Unstable nuclides are generally transformed into stable nuclides by one of the radioactive-decay processes described in the text that follows.

Decay by alpha-particle emission. An alpha (α) particle consists of two neutrons and two protons and is essentially a helium nucleus. Heavy nuclides that must lose mass to achieve nuclear stability frequently decay by alpha-particle emission because alpha-particle emission is an effective way to reduce the mass number. The emission of

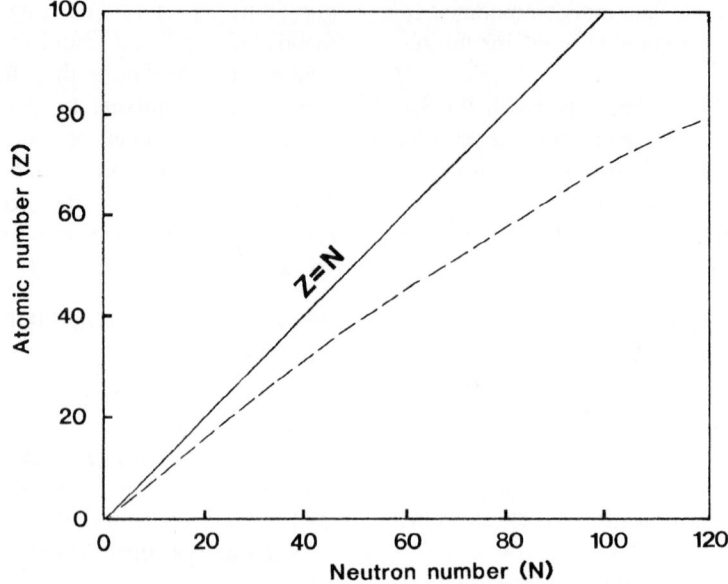

Fig. 9-2   Neutron-proton ratios for stable isotopes, *dashed line.*

one alpha particle removes two neutrons and two protons from the nucleus, resulting in the reduction of an atomic number by 2 and a mass number by 4. Very heavy radioactive nuclides that decay with alpha-particle emission are of little interest in clinical chemistry. An example of alpha-particle decay is as follows:

$$^{226}_{88}\text{Ra} \rightarrow ^{222}_{86}\text{Rn} + ^{4}_{2}\text{He (alpha particle)}$$

Decay by beta-particle emission. Beta (β) particles are either negatively charged electrons (negatrons, β^-) or positively charged electrons (positrons, β^+). Proton-deficient nuclides lying below the line of stability, shown in Fig. 9-2, usually decay by negatron emission, because this mode of decay transforms a neutron into a proton, moving the nucleus closer to the line of stability. Neutron-deficient nuclides lying above the line of stability usually decay by positron emission, since this mode transforms a proton into a neutron.

In beta-particle decay processes the mass number does not change because the total number of nucleons in the nucleus remains the same. Such decay processes are known as *isobaric* transitions. However, the atomic number increases by 1 in the negatron emission and decreases by 1 in the positron emission, resulting in a transmutation of elements (conversion of one element to another). Examples of decay by beta emission are as follows:

$$^{3}_{1}\text{H} \rightarrow ^{3}_{2}\text{He} + \beta^- + \nu \text{ (negatron emission)}$$

$$^{11}_{6}\text{C} \rightarrow ^{11}_{5}\text{B} + \beta^+ + \nu \text{ (positron emission)}$$

The neutrino *(ν)* is a particle with no mass or electrical charge and virtually does not interact with matter. The only practical consequence of its emission from the nucleus is

that it carries away some energy released in the decay process.

Decay by electron capture. In addition to the decay by positron emission, the neutron-deficient nuclides may decay by electron capture to transform a proton to a neutron. Thus the electron capture is sometimes called *inverse negatron decay.* It is also an isobaric transition leading to a transmutation of elements. In the electron-capture process the electron is captured from orbits closest to the nucleus, that is, the K and L shells (K and L capture; see Fig. 9-1). The orbital vacancy created by the electron capture is quickly filled by the electron from a higher orbit, resulting in emission of a characteristic x ray.

The daughter nucleus formed by this mode of decay is frequently in an excited or metastable state and may further undergo decay by gamma (γ)-ray emission, as described below.

Decay by gamma-ray emission. In some cases the isobaric transitions previously mentioned (negatron emission, positron emission, electron capture) result in a daughter nucleus in an excited, or metastable, state, which means that it possesses excess energy above its minimum possible ground-state energy. Such an excited, or metastable, nuclide decays promptly to a more stable nuclear arrangement by emitting gamma rays, electromagnetic radiation of very short wavelength:

$$^{125}_{53}\text{I} \xrightarrow[\text{capture}]{\text{Electron}} ^{125}_{52}\text{Te*} \rightarrow ^{125}_{52}\text{Te} + \gamma$$

*The nuclide is in an excited, or metastable, state.

Notice that gamma emission is not accompanied by any change in mass number, proton number, or neutron number. This is called an *isomeric transition.*

Radiation energy

In any of the radioactive decay processes mentioned previously, a fixed amount of energy is released with each disintegration. Most or all of the released energy will appear as the kinetic energy of the emitted particles or photons. The basic unit of energy commonly used in radiation is the electron volt (eV). One electron volt is defined as the amount of energy acquired by an electron when it is accelerated through an electrical potential of 1 V. Basic multiples are the kiloelectron volt (keV; 1 keV = 1000 eV) and the megaelectron volt (MeV; 1 MeV = 1000 keV = 1,000,000 eV). In general, the energy of beta particles emitted from radionuclides in clinical use ranges from 18 keV to 3.6 MeV, and that of gamma rays ranges from 27 keV to 2.8 MeV.

Rate of radioactive decay

Decay constant, decay factor, and half-life. Radioactive decay is a spontaneous process; that is, it is not possible to predict when a given radioactive atom will decay, and the probability of decay in a large number of atoms can be given only on a statistical basis. For a sample containing N radioactive nuclei, the number of nuclei decaying at any given moment (dN/dt) can be given by the following:

$$dN/dt = -\lambda N \qquad \textit{Eq. 9-1}$$

In this equation, λ is the decay constant of the radioactive nuclide, and the minus sign indicates that the number of radioactive nuclides is decreasing with time. Each radionuclide has a characteristic decay constant that represents the proportion of the atoms in a sample of that radionuclide undergoing decay per unit time. The decay constant, λ, is measured in units of (time)$^{-1}$. Therefore the equivalence $\lambda = 0.05$ sec^{-1} means that, on the average, 5% of the radionuclides are disintegrating per second. On integration of equation 9-1, we obtain

$$N = N_0 e^{-\lambda t} \qquad \textit{Eq. 9-2}$$

where N_0 is the number of radionuclides present at time $t = 0$, and e is the base of the natural logarithm. Therefore the number of radionuclides remaining after a time, $t(N)$, is equal to the number of radionuclides at a time, $t = 0$ (N_0), multiplied by the factor ($e^{-\lambda t}$). This factor is the fraction of radionuclides remaining after a time, t, and is termed the "decay factor." The decay factor, $e^{-\lambda t}$, is an exponential function of time, t; that is, a constant fraction of the number of radionuclides present in the sample disappears during a given time interval. A given time interval is customarily expressed as the time required for a given number of radionuclides in the sample to decrease to one half its original value. This time interval is termed the half-life ($t_{1/2}$). The half-life of a radionuclide is related to its decay constant as follows:

$$t_{1/2} = 0.693/\lambda \qquad \textit{Eq. 9-3}$$

Units of radioactivity. The average rate of decay of a sample (see equation 9-2), that is, the average number of nuclides disintegrating per second (dps) or per minute (dpm), is the activity of the sample and is used to determine the amount of radioactivity present in the sample.

Radioactivity is measured in curie (Ci) units. One curie is defined as the activity of a sample decaying at a rate of 3.7×10^{10} dps (2.22×10^{12} dpm), which is very close to the activity of 1 g of ^{226}Ra (3.656×10^{10} dps/g). In fact, the curie was originally defined as the activity of 1 g of ^{226}Ra. The basic multiples of the curie are as follows:

$$1 \text{ Ci} = 10^3 \text{ millicurie (mCi)} = 10^6 \text{ microcurie } (\mu\text{Ci}) = 10^9 \text{ nanocurie (nCi)} = 10^{12} \text{ picocurie (pCi)}$$

In clinical chemistry the amounts of radioactivity used are usually in the range of nanocuries to microcuries; occasionally, picocurie quantities are measured. The use of Système International d'Unités (SI) units in radioactivity measurements has been introduced. The basic unit of this system is the becquerel (Bq), in which 1 Bq = 1 dps. Thus

$$1 \text{ } \mu\text{Ci} = 3.7 \times 10^4 \text{ Bq}$$

This system has not gained widespread acceptance in the United States.

In equation 9-2, N_0 and N are the numbers of radionuclides present at times 0 and t, respectively. These quantities are extremely difficult to measure. However, the effects of the nuclear disintegrations can be measured more easily with use of one of the radioactive detectors described on pp. 192 to 197. In this way the total number of disintegrations per second occurring within the radioactive sample, or the radioactivity, at any given time can be estimated. Since the radioactivity, A, is proportional to the number of atoms, N, equation 9-2 can be written as

$$A = A_0 e^{-\lambda t} \qquad \textit{Eq. 9-4}$$

Therefore the decay constant, the decay factor, and the half-life are also applicable to activity versus time.

Decay factors of commonly used radionuclides can be obtained from decay-factor tables, which are available from most radiopharmaceutical companies and instrument manufacturers. An example of such a table for ^{125}I is Table 9-1. The decay factor can be used to calculate the amount of radioactivity remaining after a certain time. For example, the decay factor for ^{125}I 28 days after the manufacturer's calibration date is 0.724 according to Table 9-1. This num-

Table 9-1 Decay factors for ^{125}I

Days	Days				
	0	4	8	12	16
0	—	0.955	0.912	0.871	0.831
20	0.794	0.758	0.724	0.691	0.660
40	0.630	0.602	0.574	0.548	0.524
60	0.500	0.477	0.456	0.435	0.416

Table 9-2 Radiation characteristics of radionuclides commonly used in clinical chemistry

Nuclide	Half-life	Main radiation		Specific activity*	
		Type	Energy (keV)	mCi/μg	mCi/μmole
^{3}H	12.3 years	β⁻	18	9.7	29
^{14}C	5760 years	β⁻	158	0.0044	0.062
^{32}P	14.3 days	β⁻	1700	285	9120
^{35}S	87.1 days	β⁻	167	42.8	1500
^{51}Cr	27.8 days	EC†	γ320	92	4690
^{59}Fe	45 days	β⁻/γ	460/1099	49.1	2900
^{57}Co	270 days	EC†	γ122	8.5	480
^{125}I	60 days	EC†	γ35	17.3	2200
^{131}I	8.1 days	β⁻/γ	807/364	123	16,100

*Carrier free.
†Electron capture.

ber, multiplied by the initial amount of radioactivity, gives the level of radioactivity left at 28 days.

It is often necessary to know the specific activity of a radioactive sample. This is the activity of the radionuclide per unit mass of the radioactive sample and thus is measured in microcuries per microgram, microcuries per micromole, and so on or submultiples thereof. The specific activity of the nuclide is inversely proportional to the half-life of the radionuclide and is an important factor in determining the sensitivity of radioimmunoassay. A list of nuclides commonly used in clinical chemistry, and some of their radiation characteristics are presented in Table 9-2. The low decay rates of ^{3}H and ^{14}C with long half-lives give them low specific activity and make them less suitable for radioimmunoassay work. The specific activities of nuclides listed in Table 9-2 are calculated under the assumption that all nuclides present are radioactive (carrier free). This assumption does not always hold true. For example, the isotopic abundance of available ^{131}I preparations seldom exceeds 20%; that is, only about 20% of iodine atoms present in the ^{131}I preparation are ^{131}I—the rest are ^{127}I (stable iodine). Therefore the actual specific activity of ^{131}I preparations is only about one fourth of the theoretical specific activity shown in Table 9-2. Similarly, the specific activity of molecules depends on the isotopic abundance of the radionuclides present in the molecules. A thyroxine molecule contains four iodine atoms, and thus the specific radioactivity of radioiodine-labeled thyroxine preparations depends not only on the kind of radioactive iodine used for labeling but also on how many of the stable iodines are replaced by the radioactive iodine.

Properties of radiation and interaction with matter

An understanding of the properties of radiation and the mechanism of the energy loss of radiation as it passes through matter is important because the operation of every detecting device for any type of radiation depends on one or more of the particular properties of the radiation that is being measured and the interactions of radiation with mat-

ter. Further, the safe manipulation of radioactive substances requires a knowledge of the nature of radiation and its ability to penetrate matter. The harmful effects of radiation on tissues are highly dependent on the ability of the radiation to ionize matter and on the energy of the incident radiation.

The interactions of radiation with matter result in the transfer of energy from a radioactive nucleus to the surrounding material. This transfer is accomplished through processes of excitation and ionization; therefore radiation emitted from radionuclides is frequently termed *ionizing radiation.*

Excitation occurs when orbital electrons are perturbed from their normal arrangement by absorbing energy from the incident radiation. Ionization occurs when the energy absorbed is sufficient to cause an orbital electron to be ejected from its orbit, creating an ion pair (a free electron and a positively charged atom or molecule). This ionizing ability of radiation is best expressed by the number of ion pairs produced per unit path length, that is, the specific ionization. Properties of various forms of radiation are presented in Table 9-3.

Particulate radiation. Because of their relatively large mass and double charge, alpha particles produce a great deal of ionization, which causes them to lose their energy quickly in a short distance (high specific ionization; see Table 9-3). Therefore alpha particles are weakly penetrating and can be stopped completely by very thin layers of solid materials. For this reason, they are less hazardous externally. However, if they get into the body, they will irradiate the tissues around them intensely, causing a serious health hazard. Alpha-emitting nuclides are seldom used in medicine.

Beta particles may be negatively or positively charged. There is no known difference between the negatron particle and the electron except for their origin. Positrons are antiparticles of electrons. The energetic negatron and positron particles also lose their energy by excitation and ionization of molecules, but, because of their smaller mass and charge, their specific ionization is not so high as that of alpha par-

Table 9-3 Basic properties of radiation

| Radiation | Charge | Energy range | Approximate range of travel in | | Relative specific ionization* |
			Air	Water	
Particles					
α	+2	3-9 MeV	2-8 cm	20-40 μm	2500
β⁻	−1	0-3 MeV	0-10 m	0-1 mm	100
β⁺	+1	0-3 MeV	0-10 m	0-1 mm	100
Electromagnetic					
X rays	None	1 eV to 100 keV	1 mm to 10 m	1 μm to 1 cm	10
Gamma rays	None	10 keV to 10 MeV	1 cm to 100 m	1 mm to 10 cm	1

*The number of ion pairs produced per unit path length relative to that of gamma rays.

ticles (see Table 9-3). As described previously, the beta decay is always accompanied by the release of a neutrino and the energy released in the decay process is shared between the beta particle and the neutrino in the form of kinetic energy. Therefore, beta particles have a continuous energy ranging from zero to a maximum of E_{max} depending on the distribution of the decay energy between the beta particle and the neutrino and have an average energy approximately equivalent to one third of E_{max}. E_{max} is equivalent to the total energy available from the nuclear decay and is characteristic of each radionuclide. Fig. 9-3 shows the beta-particle energy spectrum of ^{14}C.

Electromagnetic radiation. Electromagnetic radiations usually encountered in the field of medicine include gamma-radiation and x radiation. Except for possible differences in energy, these photons are indistinguishable and engage in the same type of interactions with matter. Because photons have no mass, are uncharged, and travel with the velocity of light, they might travel through matter for a considerable distance without any interaction and then lose all or most of their energy in a single interaction. Photons can interact with matter in several different ways, depending on their energies and the properties of the material with which they interact.

Photoelectric effect is especially important for photons with low energy (below 0.5 MeV). The photon interacts directly with one of the orbital electrons in matter (a photon-electron interaction), and the entire photon energy is transferred to the electron. Some transferred energy is used to overcome the binding energy of the electron, and the remaining energy is carried by the electron as kinetic energy. The ejected electron (photoelectron) in turn transfers its kinetic energy to many other electrons in its path. The photoelectric effect is especially pronounced if the atomic number of the absorbing material is high.

Compton effect, or *Compton scattering,* occurs primarily with photons of medium energy (0.5 to 1 MeV). In this process a collision between a photon and an electron results in the transfer of only a portion of the photon energy to the electron. The scattered photon with reduced energy emerges from the site of interaction in a new direction. The ejected

electron (Compton electron) and the scattered photon lose more energy by subsequent interactions.

MEASUREMENT OF NUCLEAR RADIATION

Radioactivity measurements depend on the ability of radio-nuclides to produce ionized or excited atoms within the detector. Two basic types of radiation detectors are in common use: gas ionization and scintillation. The latter is capable of detecting both negatron and gamma radiation and providing information on the type and energy of the radiation and hence is currently the most commonly used detector in the field of medicine. Therefore the following discussion is devoted primarily to scintillation detectors; other detectors are described only briefly.

Gas-filled detectors

The Geiger-Müller counter and the ionization chamber are examples of gas ionization detectors. In the Geiger-Müller counter the radiation is detected through ionization produced within a suitable gas. Because the ions produced are accelerated by the relatively high voltage applied between the electrodes of the detector, considerable secondary ionization occurs, leading to a large output pulse (electron multiplication). The major advantage of this type of detector, as compared with ionization chambers, is its ability to detect low levels of radiation. The ionization chamber functions on a similar principle. However, because a lower voltage is used, electron multiplication does not occur in the ionization chamber, and the output signal is relatively small. Both detectors are widely used in survey meters for measuring exposure of personnel and locating a spilled radio-nuclide.

Scintillation detectors

Scintillation counting is based on the principle that a charged particle (alpha or beta) entering the detector, or an electron excited in the detector after an interaction with an incoming photon (gamma ray), will dissipate its energy within the scintillator contained in the detector by various processes of interaction mentioned previously. A portion of the energy absorbed by the scintillator is emitted as pho-

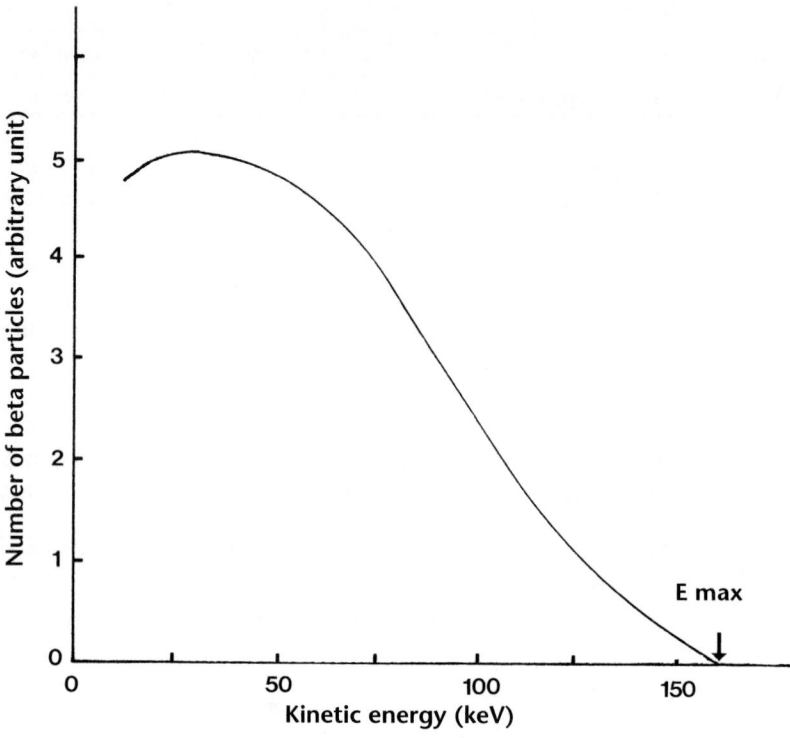

Fig. 9-3 Beta-particle spectrum for ^{14}C.

tons in the visible or near-ultraviolet region of the electromagnetic spectrum. Scintillators, or fluors, are substances capable of converting the kinetic energy of an incoming charged particle or photon into flashes of light (scintillation).

Crystal scintillation detectors. The most commonly used fluor for detecting gamma radiation by scintillation is a single crystal of sodium iodide containing small amounts of thallium (about 1%) as the activator. Fig. 9-4 is a block diagram of the common types of thallium-activated sodium iodide crystal scintillation detectors. The crystal is usually in the shape of a well, and the sample to be counted is allowed to sit in the well. The sodium iodide crystal is very hygroscopic. It is encapsulated in a metal (such as aluminum) can to prevent it from absorbing atmospheric moisture, except for one face (usually the bottom face) of the crystal well, which is covered by a transparent material such as Lucite and is optically coupled to the transparent face of a photomultiplier tube.

A gamma ray emitted from the sample placed in the crystal well is highly penetrating and therefore can pass through the glass or plastic wall of the test tube containing the radioactive sample and enter the crystal. As the gamma ray passes into the crystal, it produces excitation or ionization, and light photons are emitted. About 20 to 30 light photons are produced for each electron volt of energy absorbed. The photons pass through the transparent crystal and strike the photocathode of the photomultiplier tube, causing a release of electrons from the cathode. The energy required to re-

lease one photoelectron from the photocathode is about 300 to 2000 eV.

In addition to the conversion of the light photons emitted by the fluor into a pulse of detectable electrons, the photomultiplier also amplifies the minute amount of current produced from the photocathode to a level that can be effectively handled in conventional electronic amplifier circuits. This is achieved by a process of electron multiplication. As illustrated in Fig. 9-4, a series of metal plates, termed *dynodes,* are spaced along the length of the photomultiplier tube. The dynode surface is coated with a material capable of emitting secondary electrons when struck by an accelerated electron. Each dynode is maintained at a potential voltage higher than the preceding one. The initial photoelectrons are accelerated toward the first dynode and strike it to produce secondary electrons, which are then accelerated toward a second dynode. About three or four electrons are released from the dynode for each striking electron. This process is repeated until an amplification of about 10^8 is achieved.

The current output of the photomultiplier tube is amplified, and the resulting voltage pulse is shaped for optimal counting by conventional electronic circuitry such as that shown in Fig. 9-4. The preamplifier reduces the distortion of the electrical signal produced by the photomultiplier tube. The preamplifier output is further amplified by the amplifier to give a voltage of up to 10 V.

The function of the pulse-height analyzer is to sort out the pulses according to their pulse height and to allow those

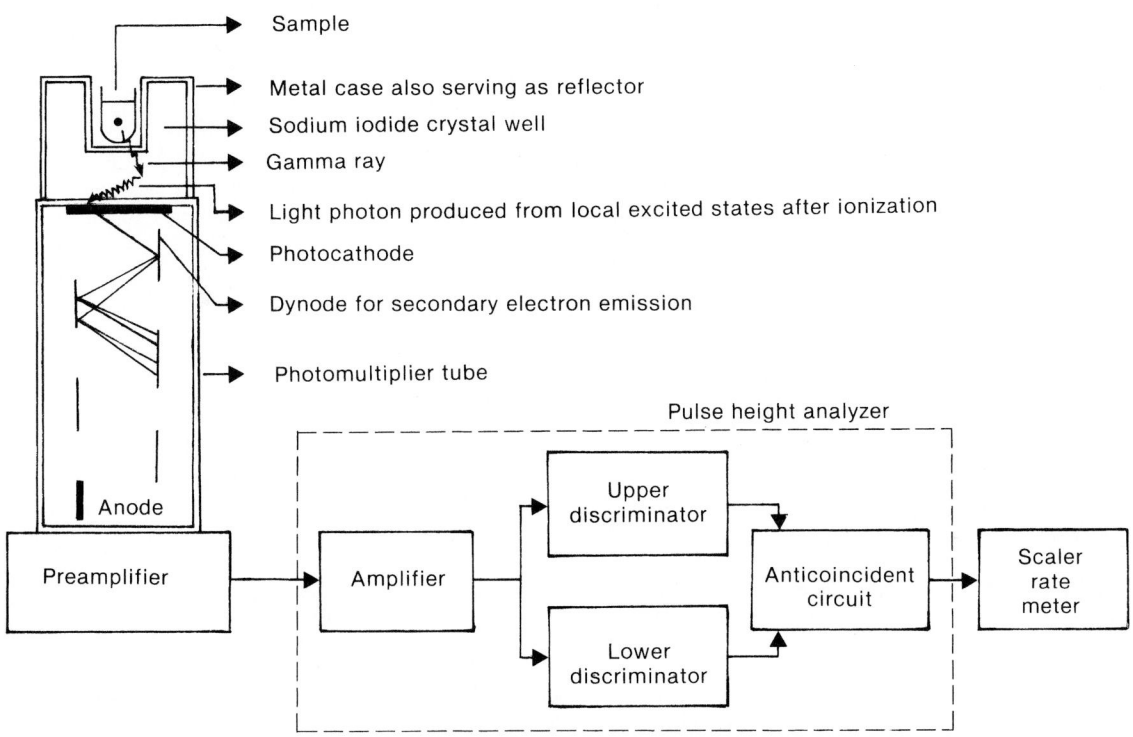

Sample

Metal case also serving as reflector

Sodium iodide crystal well

Gamma ray

Light photon produced from local excited states after ionization

Photocathode

Dynode for secondary electron emission

Photomultiplier tube

Anode

Pulse height analyzer

Upper discriminator

Lower discriminator

Anticoincident circuit

Scaler rate meter

Preamplifier

Amplifier

Fig. 9-4 Block diagram showing principal components of typical crystal scintillation counter.

pulses within a restricted range (the photopeak) to reach the rate meter for counting. This is accomplished by means of *discriminators*. A lower discriminator sets the lower limit, and an upper discriminator sets the upper limit of the energy range to be counted. The lower discriminator excludes all voltage pulses below the lower limit; the upper discriminator excludes voltage pulses above the upper limit. The energy interval represented by the difference between the two discrimination levels is called the *window width*. Only the pulses with energy in the preset discriminator window pass through the *anticoincident circuit* and are counted because the anticoincident circuit will transmit a pulse arriving at its input from the lower discriminator only if there is no pulse arriving from the upper discriminator at the same time.

It is important to note that the magnitude (height) of the output pulse of the photomultiplier tube is proportional to the intensity of light photons produced in the crystal by a gamma ray and hence to the gamma ray energy deposited in the crystal, whereas the number of voltage pulses per unit time is related to the activity of radioactive samples being analyzed. Each radionuclide has a characteristic spectrum of energies (pulse height), as noted earlier.

Unlike beta particles which give a continuous energy spectrum (see Fig. 9-3), photons produced by gamma decay have a discrete and specific energy value (see Table 9-2). This specific energy value would appear in the gamma ray energy spectrum as a single vertical line at that energy

level corresponding to the energy of the emitted gamma ray if the crystal scintillation detector used were perfect. In reality, however, the intensity of light produced in the crystal and transmitted to the photocathode, and the number of electrons collected at the anode for each total absorption interaction in the crystal detector are slightly different. These differences produce a bell-shaped curve (photopeak) instead of a single vertical line (Fig. 9-5).

All gamma ray–emitting nuclides have their own characteristic photopeaks in their energy spectra that are very useful in the identification of such radionuclides. Fig. 9-5 shows an energy spectrum of ^{125}I. As described previously, the nuclide ^{125}I decays into ^{125}Te by electron capture with the emission of 35 keV gamma rays by the ^{125}Te daughter nuclide in the excited state and 27 and 31 keV Te x rays. The photopeak at about 28.5 keV is attributable to the single-photon detection of the two x rays and the 35 keV gamma rays, whereas the photopeak at about 56.8 keV is attributable to the coincident summing of the two x rays or one x ray and the 35 keV gamma ray. The 56.8 keV photopeak is called the *coincident photopeak* and is the result of emission of a coincidence pair of photons during the ^{125}I decay process (that is, the emission of two photons within the resolving time of the detector). Both photons of the pair are detected by a high-efficiency sodium iodide crystal detector and are recorded as a single event with a pulse height equivalent to the sum of the energies of the two photons. This unique energy spectrum is used to determine the count-

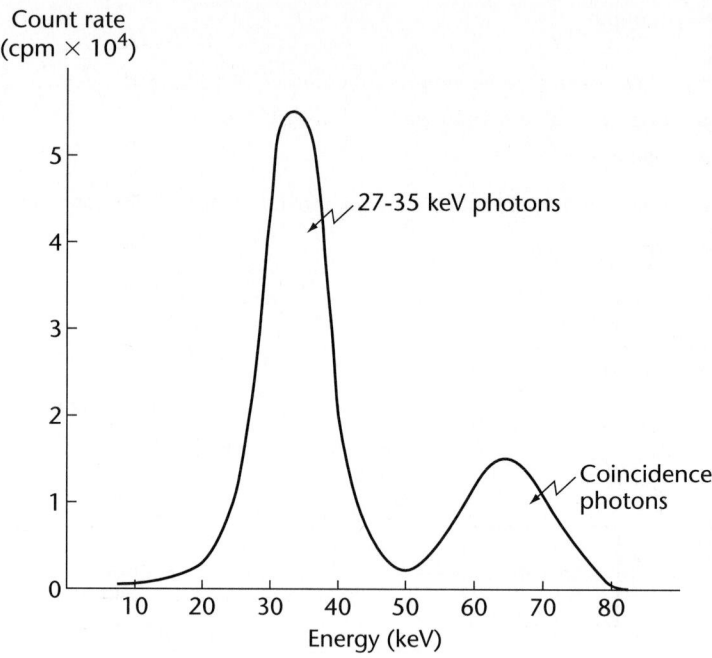

Fig. 9-5   Spectrum of ^{125}I showing the dominant peak of the x-ray photons (27 to 35 keV) and the apparent energy recorded in the detector when two photons happen to cause a scintillation simultaneously (coincidence photons). (From Thorell JI, Larson SM: *Radioimmunoassay and related techniques: methodology and clinical applications,* St. Louis, 1978, Mosby.)

ing efficiency for ^{125}I of some solid scintillation analyzers without the use of a standard of known disintegration rate.

A scintillation detector equipped with two or more pulse-height analyzers (multichannel analyzers) can be used to count two or more radionuclides simultaneously, either in the same sample or in different samples, provided that there is sufficient energy difference between them so that a certain portion of the energy of one radionuclide can be detected free from the second radionuclide. For example, the major photopeak of ^{125}I occurs at 27 keV and that of ^{131}I at 364 keV. In addition to the 364 keV photopeak, a minor ^{131}I photopeak occurs at 32 keV. For counting a mixture of these two isotopes, one analyzer channel (A) is centered at 27 keV and the other channel (B) at 364 keV, with the window width of about 20 to 40 keV. Channel B gives the true count for ^{131}I because ^{125}I does not contribute counts to channel B. Counts from channel A, however, represent the sum of the true counts for ^{125}I and the ^{131}I spillover. One can estimate the extent of the ^{131}I spillover by counting the pure ^{131}I standard in both channels.

In clinical laboratories performing radioimmunoassays, crystal scintillation counters equipped with multiple detectors are frequently used because these assays involve counting of a large number of radioactive samples. With the use of a multidetector instrument, the total counting time can be reduced considerably. However, it is absolutely necessary to make sure that all detectors in such counters perform in an equivalent fashion.

Liquid scintillation detectors.   Liquid scintillation detectors are primarily used for counting beta particle–emitting radionuclides such as ^{3}H, ^{14}C, and ^{32}P. Unlike that of gamma photons, the penetration of negatron particles is so short that they cannot penetrate the wall of the sample container for interaction with crystal scintillators. In liquid scintillation counting, the sample is dissolved or suspended in a solution, or "cocktail," consisting of a solvent such as toluene, a primary scintillator such as 2,5-diphenyloxazole (PPO), and a secondary scintillator such as 1,4-bis-2(5-phenyloxazolyl)benzene (POPOP) (Fig. 9-6). The beta particles from the radioactive sample dissolved in the scintillation cocktail ionize and excite the molecules of the solvent. The excitation energy is transferred to the primary scintillator, which emits light photons when the excited electrons return to the ground energy level. The wavelength of light emitted by the primary scintillator is frequently too short (about 350 to 400 nm) for efficient detection by the photocathodes of photomultiplier tubes. The secondary scintillator absorbs the photons emitted by the primary scintillator and reemits them at a longer wavelength (about 430 nm). Thus the secondary scintillator is also termed a *wavelength shifter.* However, the modern photomultiplier tubes are sensitive to the wavelength of the primary scintillator. The secondary scintillators are used today primarily for more effective transmission of the energy from the beta particle to produce light flashes especially when a large amount of color-quenched sample is placed in the scintillation so-

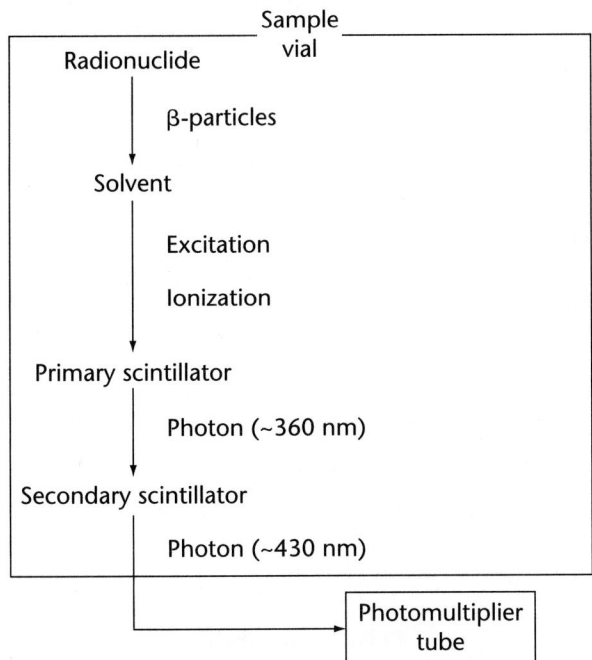

Fig. 9-6 Initial scintillation processes in a liquid scintillation analyzer. (From Thorell JI, Larson SM: *Radioimmunoassay and related techniques: methodology and clinical applications,* St. Louis, 1978, Mosby.)

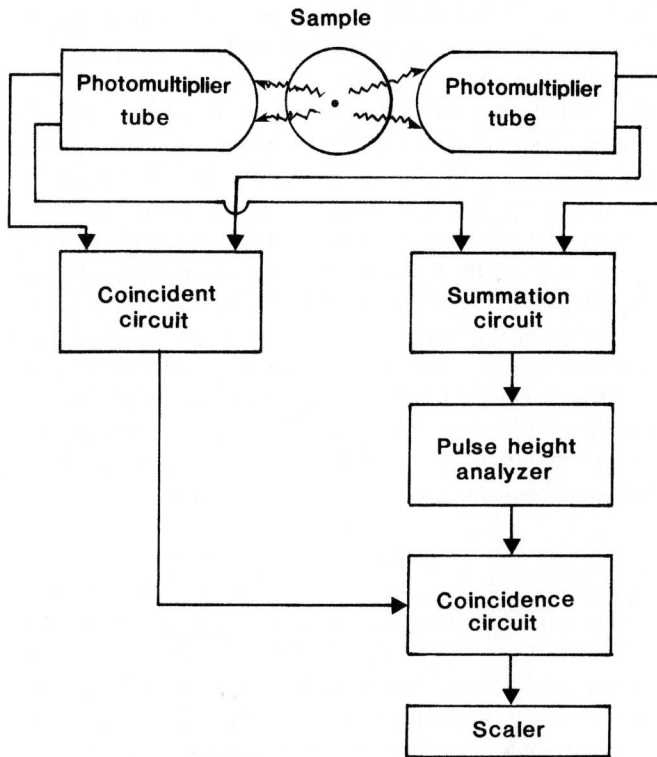

Fig. 9-7 Schema of liquid scintillation counter.

lution. Problems related to quenching are discussed later in this chapter.

The operating principles of solid crystal scintillation analyzers and liquid scintillation analyzers are basically the same except for the difference in scintillation detection. A typical arrangement of the principal components of a liquid scintillation counter is shown in Fig. 9-7. The light photons produced in the sample vial are detected and amplified by the photomultiplier tubes in the same manner as for the crystal scintillation counter. In the liquid scintillation detector, however, a second photomultiplier tube, a coincident circuit, and a summation circuit are incorporated to eliminate the electronic noise associated with the photomultiplier tube and to improve counting efficiency for low-energy beta-particle emitters.

Noise pulses are random events, and the probability of two photomultiplier tubes producing noise pulses simultaneously is relatively small. In contrast, the beta particle produces a burst of photons, and two photomultiplier tubes will receive photons almost simultaneously. The output pulses from each photomultiplier tube are fed into a coincident circuit to check if a pulse from one photomultiplier tube is accompanied by a corresponding pulse from the other within the allowed time interval (termed the *coincidence resolving time,* usually about 20×10^{-8} seconds). Pulses within the resolving time produce a coincident signal that is electrically sent to the coincident gate. Most noise pulses do not meet the requirement of the coincidence resolving

time and are excluded. The summation circuit is incorporated to sum all coincident pulses to obtain the true pulse height. The summed coincident pulses are amplified, sorted, and counted in a manner similar to that for the crystal scintillation counter.

In liquid scintillation counting, proper energy transfer cannot occur unless the sample is in contact with the scintillation solution to give a colorless, transparent, homogeneous solution. Some radioactive samples are not soluble in the scintillation solution, and so it may be necessary to add one or more substances to obtain a homogeneous scintillation mixture. Solubilizers such as methylbenzethonium chloride (Hyamine 10X) are used to facilitate dissolution of the sample in the scintillation solution, or jelling agents such as aluminum stearate are used to enhance the counting efficiency by stabilizing the sample suspension in liquid scintillators. Many commercial liquid scintillation cocktails of nonpolar mediums (toluene or xylene) contain some type of surfactant such as the Tritons (polyoxyethylene ethers and other surface-active compounds) to maintain aqueous samples in colloidal suspensions so that the aqueous samples can be counted at high efficiency. Nonvolatile, radioactive materials are also counted on solid supports such as filter paper disks or glass fibers immersed in a scintillation solution. The disadvantage of this counting method is the relatively low counting efficiency because of impurity quenching.

Quenching is basically a process that results in the reduction of the overall photon output of the sample. Impurities present in the radioactive sample may compete with the scintillators for energy transfer, that is, the energy is lost to a non–light producing process. This phenomenon is termed *impurity quenching*. Water in aqueous samples or a support medium such as a filter disk may cause impurity quenching. Colored substances such as hemoglobin may absorb the light photons produced by the scintillation process before they can be detected by the photomultiplier tubes or may change the wavelength of the light photons to a value not suitable for efficient detection by the photocathodes of photomultiplier tubes. Quenching in liquid scintillation counting is detected and corrected by efficiency determination. The efficiency of the measurement is defined as the ratio of the observed counts per minute (cpm) to the absolute units of disintegrations per minute (dpm):

$$\text{Efficiency} = \frac{\text{cpm}}{\text{dpm}}$$

Since the quenching characteristics of each sample are different, the efficiency must be determined for each sample. By knowing the counting rate (cpm) and the counting efficiency of a sample, one can calculate the absolute radioactivity (dpm) of the sample. Several methods for efficiency determination have been developed, but only those most frequently used are discussed.

Internal standardization. Internal standardization, one of the oldest methods, is the most accurate for efficiency determination when properly carried out. In this method the sample is counted before and after the introduction of a calibrated standard of the measured radionuclide. The difference between the count rates before and after the spike, divided by the calibrated activity of the spike in disintegrations per unit time, is termed the *counting efficiency*. The disadvantages of this method are the time-consuming manipulation of the sample and the loss of sample for recount after the introduction of the spike.

Sample-channels ratio. The sample-channels ratio method is based on a downward shift of the pulse-height spectrum of the photon as a result of the quenching-induced decrease in the pulse height of many energetic decays (Fig. 9-8). The degree of the shift is related to the extent of quenching or counting efficiency and is expressed by the change in the ratio of the sample counts obtained from two different discriminator window settings (channels). As shown in Fig. 9-8, one channel is usually set to measure the entire isotope spectrum (L_1 to L_3), and the second channel is restricted to only a portion of the spectrum (L_1 to L_2). In this method, channel ratios (L_1 to L_2) to (L_1 to L_3) of a set of artificially quenched standards of known efficiencies are determined and plotted against counting efficiency to obtain a quench curve. The efficiency of any unknown sample can be determined from its channel ratio and the quench curve. This method requires no additional sample manipulation, unlike internal standardization, and is

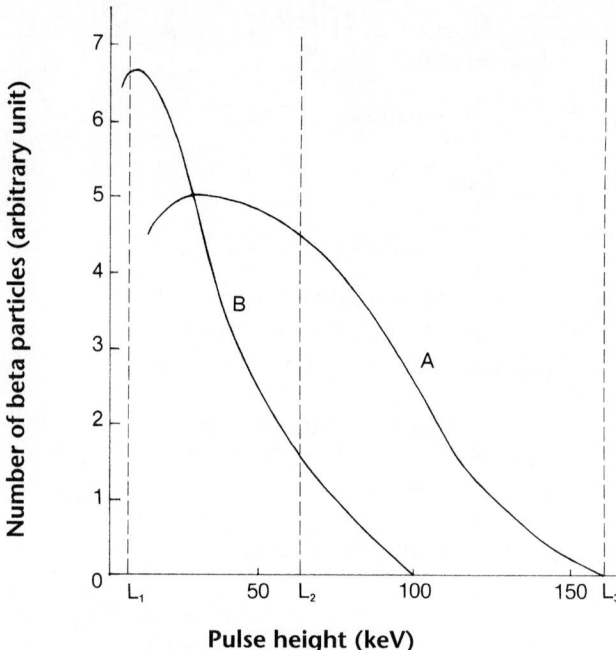

Fig. 9-8 Unquenched, *A*, and quenched, *B*, pulse-height spectra of ^{14}C. L_1 to L_3 denote discrimination levels.

suitable for handling a large number of samples through automation. This method, however, may result in large errors in highly quenched samples or samples with low count rates.

External standards. Unlike the internal standard method, the known activity in the external standard method is provided by an external source of gamma radiation, such as ^{226}Ra, placed at a fixed position adjacent to the sample vial. The external gamma-ray source generates electrons through the Compton collision process in the scintillation solution. The Compton electrons transfer energy to the solution and cause scintillation in the same way as beta particles do in the scintillation medium. The energy spectrum produced by Compton electrons is also affected by the presence of quenching materials, as in a typical beta-particle spectrum. The sample is counted twice, once in the absence of and once in the presence of an external standard. As in the sample-channels ratio method, a set of quenched standards of known efficiencies is used to obtain a correlation curve between the sample-counting efficiency and the count rate of the external standard. The counting efficiency of a sample can be determined from the count rate of the external standard counted with the sample and from the correlation curve. The external standard method has become an integral part of almost all modern liquid scintillation detectors.

Another problem encountered in liquid scintillation counting is *chemiluminescence*, the production of light photons by a chemical reaction between the sample material and the solute or solubilizer added to the scintillation solution. Chemiluminescence gives rise to single photons and can be excluded by the coincident circuit of the liquid scintillation counter. However, when chemiluminescence reactions are of sufficient intensity, non–beta particle coincident pulses may be generated that interfere with the beta-particle scintillation counting. The chemiluminescent effect will eventually disappear, but this may take several hours or longer, especially at low temperatures. Chemiluminescence can be monitored by repeated counting of the sample. Some modern instruments are capable of automatically monitoring and correcting for the chemiluminescent effects.

As with crystal scintillation counting, mixed-isotope counting is possible with a liquid scintillation counter with multichannel analyzers. A common example of dual-label counting involves a mixture of tritium, with a maximum beta-particle decay of 18.6 keV, and ^{14}C, with a maximum beta-particle decay of 156 keV.

Counting statistics. Since radioactive decay is essentially a random process, it is unlikely that successive measurements on a given sample will result in the same number of counts. However, radioactive decay obeys a *Poisson distribution*. The Poisson distribution density formula can be applied in the calculation of the precision of measurement at a given count rate. If a single measurement of total counts, *N,* is made, precision of this measurement in terms of the percent coefficient of variation (%CV) can be estimated to be as follows:

$$\%CV = \frac{\sqrt{N}}{N} \times 100\%$$

For example, at a total count of 100, CV = 10%; at 1000, CV = 3.2%; at 10,000, CV = 1%. This approximation is applicable only when the background count is negligible compared with the sample count. When significant background counts are present, the formula for the standard deviation of a difference must be used:

$$\%CV = \frac{\sqrt{N} + B}{S} \times 100\%$$

where *B* is the background count and *S* is the sample count (*N* − *B*). Thus a total count of 100 in the presence of a background count of 10 gives the following:

$$\%CV = \frac{\sqrt{100} + 10}{100 - 10} \times 100\% = 11.7\%$$

Precision can be increased if one prolongs the counting time, but a 1% CV (that is, 10,000 counts) is satisfactory in most applications.

RADIATION HEALTH SAFETY

Although the quantity of radioactivity handled in the clinical chemistry laboratory is usually very small, a basic knowledge of radiation safety is vital to every laboratory worker who has frequent contact with radioactive substances because the biological effects of long-term expo-

sure to very low doses of ionizing radiation are still largely unknown and may prove to be hazardous to health.

Radionuclides commonly used in the clinical laboratory are either beta-particle emitters, such as ^{14}C and ^{3}H, or gamma-ray emitters, such as ^{125}I and ^{57}Co. Both forms of radiation produce their biological effects by producing ionization and excitation along their paths in the tissue. However, beta radiation is less penetrating than gamma radiation; thus beta-particle emitters are considered to be more hazardous in terms of internal radiation and less hazardous in terms of external radiation than gamma-ray emitters. Therefore the primary concern with beta-particle emitters is to prevent the entry of radioactive materials into the body through inhalation, ingestion, or absorption by the skin; with gamma-ray emitters other factors, such as shielding, exposure time, and exposure distance, are also important when radiation safety is considered.

Monitoring

Regular monitoring of both personnel and work areas is an important radiation safety procedure. It is necessary to measure periodically the radiation exposure doses of personnel to ensure that radiation doses received are below the recommended limits. The following three basic units are used to measure radiation exposure and dose.

The roentgen (R) is a unit of x rays or gamma rays and measures the quantity of ionization produced by photon radiation in a given sample of air. One roentgen equals that quantity of photon radiation capable of producing one electrostatic unit of either sign in 0.001293 g of air.

The radiation absorbed dose (rad) is a measure of local energy deposition per unit mass of material irradiated by any ionizing radiation. One rad is equal to 100 ergs of absorbed energy per gram of absorber.

The roentgen equivalent, man (rem) is that dose of ionizing radiation causing the same amount of biological injury to human tissue as 1 rad of x, gamma, or beta radiation. In the case of alpha radiation, the dose in rem equals the dose in rad multiplied by 20 because only 0.05 rad of alpha radiation is needed to produce the same biological effect as 1 rad of x, gamma, or beta radiation. The recommended maximum permissible dose to the whole body is 0.5 rem per year for the general public and 5 rem per year for radiation workers.

Film badges are probably the most commonly used and cost-effective way of monitoring personnel. The photographic film becomes progressively optically dense when exposed to ionizing radiation and thus may be used to monitor the radiation dose received by the wearer. Since most clinical laboratory personnel working with radioimmunoassays routinely handle ^{125}I-labeled compounds, it is advisable to monitor possible accumulation of radioactive iodine in the thyroid glands. Arrangements should be made to have the radioactive content of each worker's thyroid measured at least twice each year or after each radioiodination experiment. It is necessary to keep all records of radiation exposure of all workers handling radioactive materials for at least 5 years. Each laboratory should have a portable radiation detector, such as a portable Geiger-Müller survey meter, to monitor radioactivity in an area in which radioactive materials are routinely handled. Monitoring of beta radiation usually requires taking samples of the work area with swabs and using a liquid scintillation counter to determine the presence of radioactivity.

Contamination control

Internal radiation exposure is controlled only by prevention of the entry of radioactive materials into the body. This requires strict adherence to the general rules for radiation safety. No smoking, eating, drinking, applying of cosmetics, or storing of food is allowed in work areas. Mouth pipetting of radioactive materials should never be done. All persons working in radioactive areas must wear the designated protective clothing (a standard laboratory coat is satisfactory in a clinical laboratory involved in radioimmunoassays) and disposable gloves. Such protective clothing should be removed when one is leaving the laboratory and should not be taken home for washing, and so on. Radioactive materials must be properly labeled, stored, and used only at specially designated areas. Work involving the possible generation of volatile, radioactive substances, such as radioiodination, should be performed in an exhaust hood. The working surface should be covered by a layer of disposable absorbent material. In addition to the proper operating technique, cleanliness and good housekeeping are essential to prevent and minimize the spread and buildup of contamination.

External radiation exposure is of minor concern in radioimmunoassay laboratories because the amount of radioactivity handled in any given time is very small (less than 1 μCi) and because the radiation energy of the most commonly used gamma ray–emitting radionuclide ^{125}I has weak energies ranging from 27 to 35 keV. Nevertheless, it is always a good practice to minimize the time spent in a radiation field, to maximize the distance from the source of radiation, and to utilize shielding between you and the source of radiation, especially for those involved in radioiodination.

Persons contaminated by radioactive materials should be quickly decontaminated to prevent the possible transfer of radioactivity to internal organs by absorption through the skin. Facilities for decontamination, such as a shower and an eyewash station, should be available in each laboratory. Absorbent materials should be used to remove spilled radioactive material. The contaminated area should then be scrubbed with soap and water. It is a good practice to cover the contaminated area immediately with a piece of paper to prevent spreading of the radioactivity to other parts of the laboratory.

Waste disposal

The radioactivity level of the radioactive waste materials generated in clinical laboratories involved in radioimmunoassays is usually very low, but such radioactive waste material should still be disposed of according to the guidelines established by the Nuclear Regulatory Commission (NRC) of the United States. Some states (NRC agreement states) are approved by the NRC to regulate the use, safety, and disposal of radioactive material in the state, provided that the regulations are more restrictive than the NRC regulations. Therefore it is important to be familiar with the state regulations on radioactive materials if the laboratory is located in an NRC agreement state.

BIBLIOGRAPHY

Bernier DR, Christian PE, Langan JK, Wells LD: *Nuclear medicine technology and techniques,* ed 2, St. Louis, 1989, Mosby.

Heal AV: Safety and disposal changes that affect regulations in radioassay labs, *Lab World,* pp 50-53, Dec 1981.

L'Annunziata MF: *Radionuclide tracers,* New York, 1987, Academic Press.

Radiation Protection for Medical and Allied Health Personnel, Recommendations of the National Council on Radiation Protection and Measurements, NCRP report no 105, Oct 1989.

CHAPTER 10

Electrophoresis

John M. Brewer

OBJECTIVES

- State the charge properties of amphoteric substances at acidic, isoelectric, and basic pH. Explain the significance of these properties in electrophoresis.

- Outline the principle of electrophoresis and summarize how electrophoretic separations of molecules are affected by the following:
    Enhanced resolution techniques
    Molecular size
    Molecular size and charge
    Thickness of support

- Describe the commonly encountered problems associated with electrophoresis and explain probable causes and corrective actions.

- List three common support media for electrophoresis and classify commonly used visualization stains according to the substance being separated. Describe the physical or chemical reactions that allow one to use a stain to visualize a specific substance.

- Describe the effect or effects on electrophoretic separations of the following parameters:
    Ionic strength of buffer
    pH of buffer
    Electro-osmosis
    Heating

KEY TERMS

ampholyte A trade name for a mixture of substances with a range of isoelectric points that have high buffering capacities at their isoelectric points.

amphoteric A substance that can have a positive, zero, or negative charge, depending on conditions.

anion Negatively charged particle or ion.

boundary Edge of a zone, as of a macromolecule solution next to the solvent.

buffer A mixture of proton-donating and proton-accepting substances the function of which is to keep the proton concentration (the pH) constant or nearly so. An example is a mixture of acetic acid and sodium acetate.

cation Positively charged particle or ion.

co-ion An ion of the same charge as the one under consideration; generally a much smaller ion.

conductivity The readiness of a substance to carry a current. In an ionic solution, the sum of the product of the charge concentrations and charge mobilities.

convection Mass or bulk movement of one part of a solution relative to the rest, usually because of density differences.

counterion An ion of charge opposite to the one under consideration; generally a smaller ion.

densitometry Measurement of the absorbance of analytes along the length of a support.

disk electrophoresis A stacking or isotachophoretic step followed by zone electrophoresis, usually on a polyacrylamide gel.

discontinuous solvent A solution consisting of at least two separate regions that have different ions in them.

effective mobility The actual mobility of a substance under certain conditions; generally less than the mobility because of a lower charge or resistance by a supporting medium.

electric field An influence measured in volts (or volts per centimeter) that is manifested by the behavior of a charged particle in it.

electrical neutrality A condition in which total positive charges equal total negative charges.

electroblot Substances separated on supporting medium by electrophoresis are transferred onto a facing sheet of material using an electric field perpendicular to the original separating field. The material on the facing sheet adsorbs and immobilizes the substances in the same pattern as the original separation.

electrodes Substances in contact with a conductor. The substances are connected to a source of an electric field.

electrolyte Ionic substances, usually of low molecular weight, added to provide as constant and uniform an ionic environment for electrophoresis as possible.

electro-osmosis Tendency of a solution to move relative to an adjacent stationary substance when an electric field is applied.

electrophoresis Movement of charged particles because of an external electric field.

frictional coefficient A measure of the resistance a particle offers to movement through a solvent.

gel A network of interacting fibers, or a polymer that is solid but traps large amounts of solvent in pores or channels inside.

ionic strength The sum of the concentrations of all ions in a solution, weighted by the squares of their charges.

isoelectric Condition of zero net charge on an amphoteric substance.

isoelectric focusing The ordering and concentration of substances according to their isoelectric points.

isoelectric point The pH at which a substance has a zero net charge.

isotachyphoresis The ordering and concentration of substances of intermediate effective mobilities between an ion of high effective mobility and one of much lower effective mobility, followed by their migration at a uniform velocity.

joule heating Heating of a conductor by the passage of an electrical current.

mobility The velocity a particle or ion attains for a given applied voltage. A relative measure of how quickly an ion moves in an electric field.

molecular sieving Separation of molecules on the basis of their effective sizes.

polyacrylamide Polymer of acrylamide and usually some cross-linking derivative.

polyelectrolyte Substance with many charged or potentially charged groups.

resolving power Ability to separate closely migrating substances.

sodium dodecyl sulfate (SDS) A detergent and an especially effective protein denaturant.

Southern blot A kind of *electroblot*, in which the substances separated and transferred are nucleic acids.

stacking Ordering or arranging and concentrating macromolecules according to their effective mobilities; cf. isotachophoresis.

Western blot A kind of *electroblot*, in which the substances separated and transferred are proteins.

zeta potential The potential produced by the effective charge of a macromolecule, usually taken at the boundary between

what is moving with the macromolecule and the rest of the solution.

zone A particular region or space within a larger one, generally distinguished by some property, such as its occupancy by a protein.

Movement of charged particles because of an *external* electrical field is called *electrophoresis*.[1] Since charged molecules can be made to move, different molecules can be separated if they have different velocities in an electric field. Therefore electrophoresis is a separation technique, just as chromatography and ultracentrifugation are, and there are similarities among these techniques.

The movement of a species in aqueous solution is affected by the species' interaction with water molecules, that is, hydration (Fig. 10-1). The more polar a molecule is, the greater is the cluster of water molecules about it.[2]

The electric field is applied to a solution through oppositely charged *electrodes* placed in the solution (Fig. 10-2). A particular ion then travels through the solution toward the electrode of opposite charge. Thus positively charged particles (cations) move to the negatively charged electrode (cathode), while negatively charged particles (anions) migrate to the positively charged electrode (anode).

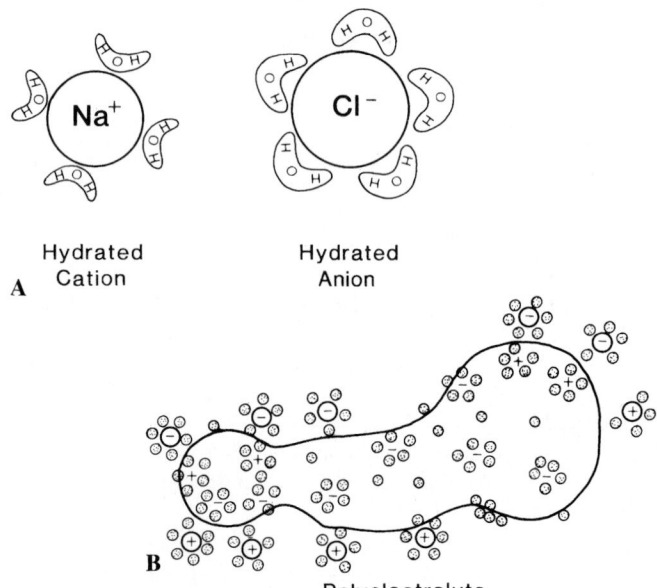

Fig. 10-1 State of charged particles in water solution. **A,** Small ions (Na^+ and Cl^-) with associated water molecules. **B,** Macromolecule with water molecules *(stippled smaller circles)* associated with charged and polar groups. Hydrated co-ions and counterions are also shown as larger circles around plus or minus signs.

APPLICATION OF ELECTRIC FIELD TO A SOLUTION CONTAINING A CHARGED PARTICLE

Forces on a particle

The force exerted on a charged particle depends on the electric field, V (in volts or volts per centimeter), and the charge on the particle, Q. The force on the charged particle is the product:

$$F_{elec} = QV \qquad \textit{Eq. 10-1}$$

This electrical force, F_{elec}, when exerted on the particle, will cause it to move. However, a particle moving in a solvent will experience resistance because of the viscosity of the solvent.[1,3] The resistance, which is itself a force, is proportional to the velocity[3]:

$$F_{resistance} = fv \qquad \textit{Eq. 10-2}$$

The proportionality constant, f, is called the *frictional coefficient*.

The frictional coefficient depends on the viscosity of the solvent and the size and shape of the particle. The greater the viscosity, the slower the movement is. The bigger or more asymmetrical the particle, the slower its movement through the solvent is. The frictional coefficient of a large particle such as a protein is a characteristic property of the particle.

Mobility of a particle

When an electric field is applied to a charged particle, the particle will begin to migrate. The electrophoretic and frictional forces oppose each other, and the particle's velocity increases until the forces are equal ($F_{resistance} = F_{elec}$). The velocity, v, a particle attains for a given electric field, V, is determined by two properties of the particle—its charge and its frictional coefficient. Consequently the value of v/V is also a characteristic property of the particle and is important enough to be given its own name. It is called the *mobility* of the particle.

Effect of pH on mobility

Each ion has a particular charge and mobility. However, when a solution contains a substance the pK of which is near the pH of the solution, that substance exists in both a charged and an uncharged form in the solution. The fraction of species with a charge will depend on the pK of the substance and the pH of the solution. When the pH is equal to the pK_a of a weak acid, only 50% of the particles will be charged. At 1 pH unit below the pK_a, 90% will be uncharged. At 1 pH unit above the pK_a, 90% will be in the charged state. Since the effective (average) charge of a substance varies with the pH, its *effective mobility* also varies with the pH.

This is particularly true for substances such as proteins. Proteins are clearly *amphoteric* substances; that is, they contain acidic and basic groups. Their overall (net) charge will be highly positive at low pH's, zero (isoelectric) at a particular higher pH, and negative at still more alkaline pH's. Since mobility is directly proportional to the magnitude of the charge, the effective mobility of a protein is very much a function of the pH.

The most important practical consequence of this is that electrophoretic solutions must be buffered to maintain a constant pH. The *buffer* pH is chosen to give an optimum net charge for maximum separation. For proteins, pH's in the 7 to 9 range are generally used. The buffer is used to maintain this pH and thus the net protein charge throughout the electrophoretic process. Buffers are ionic substances themselves and so take part in any electrophoretic process, a fact that must also be considered.

Electrolytes

In electrophoresis, a substance such as a protein is put in one limited region, or *zone*, of the system and is made to move into another region, or zone. Therefore much of the solution will not have protein in it at any particular time. If the protein and its associated counterions are not present to

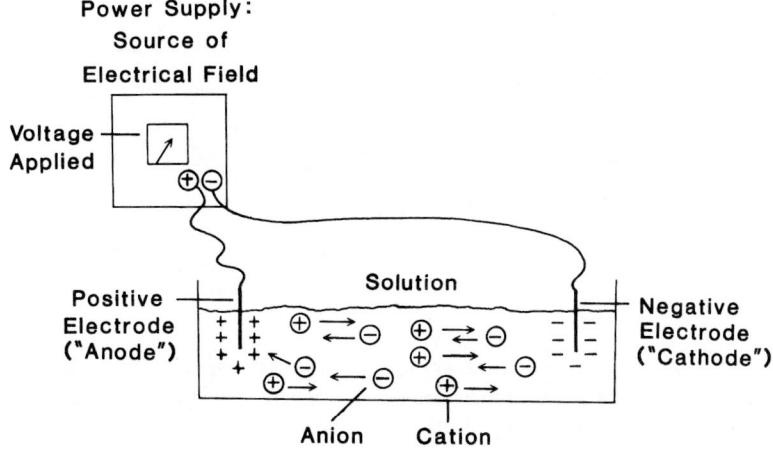

Fig. 10-2 Application of electric field to solution of ions makes ions move.

carry the current in a particular region, other ions must be present to carry the current. For this reason it is a common practice to add an excess, usually about 0.1 M, of low-molecular-weight buffer to the solution through which the protein must travel. The buffer and salt ions *(electrolytes)* provide a constant electrical environment so that the over-all movement of the protein will be as constant as possible and will be minimally influenced by other protein molecules.

Ion movement and conductivity

In any electrical system, the current produced is proportional to the voltage applied:

$$V = \text{Resistance} \times \text{Current} \qquad \textit{Eq. 10-3}$$

or

$$V = \frac{\text{Current}}{\text{Conductivity}} \qquad \textit{Eq. 10-4}$$

In electrophoresis, the current is the flow of ions (in both directions). The conductivity is the sum of the concentrations times the effective mobilities of all ions present. An ion with a higher effective mobility carries a larger fraction of the current.[2]

The voltage, conductivity, and current thus are all related (see equation 10-4). If the conductivity is increased by an increase in the salt concentration while the current is kept constant, the voltage must decrease. Such a decrease in voltage reduces the electrical force, F_{elec}, on charged particles, slowing the movement of the macromolecules. This increases the time needed for a given separation, and the resolution decreases because of increased diffusion. If the conductivity is increased at a fixed voltage, the current must increase, thus increasing the electric heat ("joule heating") generated by the system, since heating is proportional to the square of the current. Excessive heating produces convective disturbances in the solutions, which distort the electrophoretic patterns and may also denature macromolecules. Since increasing the conductivity at either a fixed voltage or current has deleterious effects, optimum results are achieved when one keeps the concentration of ions and therefore the conductivity at moderate values.

FACTORS AFFECTING MOBILITIES OF MACROMOLECULES
Charge and conformation

The clinical laboratory usually deals with polyelectrolytes, substances with many charged or potentially charged groups on them. The net charge of a polyelectrolyte is determined by the total number of charged groups within the polyelectrolyte and its conformation. The folding, or *conformation*, of a protein exposes sites for any small molecules that it may bind. In some cases electrolyte ions bind strongly and specifically to the macromolecule. For example, bovine serum albumin can bind several chloride ions. This changes the net charge of the macromolecule and therefore its mobility.

Ionic atmosphere and zeta potential

Counterions, ions of opposite charge, naturally tend to hover in the vicinity of the charged groups of macromolecules.[4] However, they do not actually neutralize the charges on the macromolecule but are instead located at a range of distances from the charged groups of the macromolecule, forming a double layer of charge about the macromolecule, called an *ionic atmosphere*.

The macromolecule moves with its entourage of hydration and hydrated counterions (Fig. 10-3). These reduce the effective charge of the macromolecule to a level given by the *zeta potential*. The zeta potential is the potential (volt-

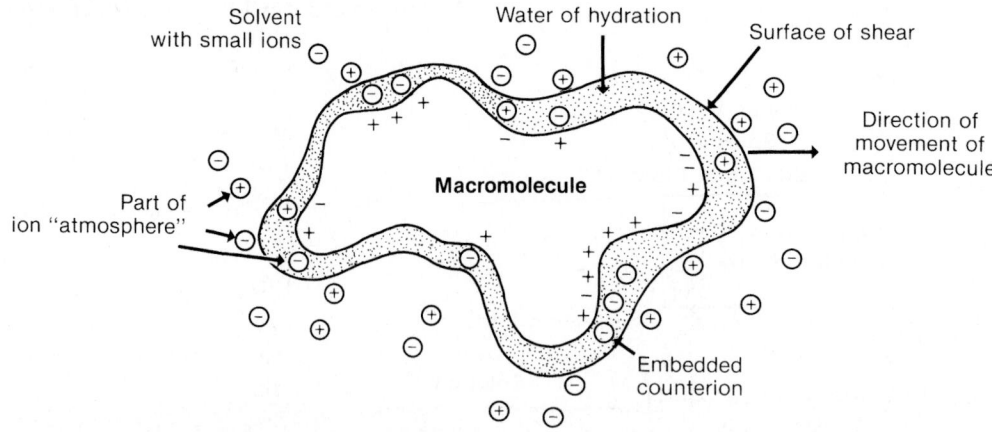

Fig. 10-3 Zeta potential of macromolecule is average effective electric field strength (potential) produced by charges on macromolecule and any charged particles embedded in solvent carried along (water of hydration) with macromolecule. *Stippled area,* Water of hydration. Zeta potential is measured at surface of shear: the boundary between water of hydration and rest of solvent.

age) produced by the effective charge of the macromolecule at the *surface of shear.* The surface of shear is the boundary between the entire macromolecular complex in solution (hydration layer and embedded counterions) and the material that is staying behind (the solvent).

Relaxation effect

Because of random thermal motion, electrophoresing macromolecules move irregularly, in jumps, rather than in a continuous straight line. At each jump, the counterion atmosphere is left somewhat behind. The counterions (or their replacements from other parts of the solution) then move to catch up or reposition themselves, but this takes a little time. This is called a *relaxation effect.* It also tends to lower the mobility of the macromolecule, since the retarded or misplaced counterions momentarily produce a field that acts in a direction opposite to that of the applied field.

Electrophoretic effect

Since ions in water solution are hydrated, the counterions of the electrolyte moving in the opposite direction carry solvent along with them. The macromolecule is thus moving against a *flow* of solvent, and its mobility is reduced.

SUPPORT MEDIUMS

The goal of electrophoresis is to separate a mixture of substances, such as macromolecules, into completely separate zones. The narrower (thinner) the original zone of a mixture of macromolecules is, the smaller the migration distance necessary to achieve separation will be. Use of narrower zones means that complete separation can be effected in less time. Blurring or remixing of the separated zones as a result of diffusion is also reduced.

The major technical difficulty in using narrow (thin) zones of relatively concentrated macromolecules is a mechanical one. Such zones will be considerably more dense than the solvent; thus the zones would "fall" through the solvent faster than the macromolecules would electrophorese. This is called *bulk flow,* or *convection.* The conventional solution to this problem is to use a supporting medium.

Functional basis

The supporting medium must allow as free a penetration of the material to be separated as possible and yet cut off bulk flow (convection). Most mediums do this by offering a restricted pore size for electrophoretic movement of the macromolecules. A capillary tube has the same effect. This is the basis of "capillary zone electrophoresis." The capillary tubes are as little as 25 to 50 μm (0.025-0.05 mm) across.

Electro-osmosis

The supporting medium should not interact with the molecules, since this will inhibit or stop migration. The usual interaction problem encountered is not the actual adsorp-

tion of the material. More commonly seen are the effects of charged groups attached to the medium that result in *electro-osmosis.* For example, agar, which is often used as a supporting medium in electrophoresis, is a mixture of agarose and agaropectin. The agaropectin has a relatively large number of carboxyl groups in it, which at neutral pH have counterions. If a voltage is applied, the counterions will move, but the carboxyl groups attached to the polysaccharide matrix will not. The counterions carry enough solvent with them to produce a *net* flow of solvent in *one* direction. This is the electro-osmosis effect, sometimes called *endosmosis.* However, electro-osmosis is a very general effect.[2] It is more pronounced when charged groups are present in the supporting medium, but it always occurs to some extent.

Electro-osmosis in glass capillary tubes occurs to such an extent that glass capillaries used in capillary zone electrophoresis are often coated with a cellulose or plastic to reduce the effect, which might otherwise seriously distort the separation pattern.

Types of supporting mediums

The supporting medium can be a solution such as a sucrose-density gradient, but, in general, insoluble materials are used. Some are self-supporting, whereas others are mechanically supported by the apparatus. Paper or sheets of plastic such as cellulose acetate have enough mechanical strength to allow electrophoresis on sheets hung or stretched over rods.

Support mediums can also be classified as particulate or continuous. Particulate support mediums include glass beads, Sephadex, and cellulose fibers. Continuous support mediums include polyacrylamide, starch, and agarose gels.

Gels are jellylike solids in which considerable solvent is included. Starch gels, for example, are made from starch suspensions that are heated and cooled. The starch fibers interact, tangling with each other but trapping the solvent so that large gaps or pores exist between the fibers. These gaps or pores are available for macromolecular movement. Similar gels can be made from agar, agarose, and some chemical polymers. Gels can also be made by polymerization of acrylamide with a small percentage of a bifunctional acrylamide derivative that cross-links the acrylamide polymers (Fig. 10-4).

Molecular sieving

The porosity, or average pore size, of some mediums is fixed, but the porosities of other mediums can be controlled. For example, by changing the gel concentrations of starch or agar, one can vary the pore size. If the average pore size is near the average diameter of the macromolecules that are being electrophoresed, the supporting medium will produce molecular sieving effects.

Sequencing of DNA is done by electrophoresis of a mixture of radiolabeled DNAs that vary in length from a few

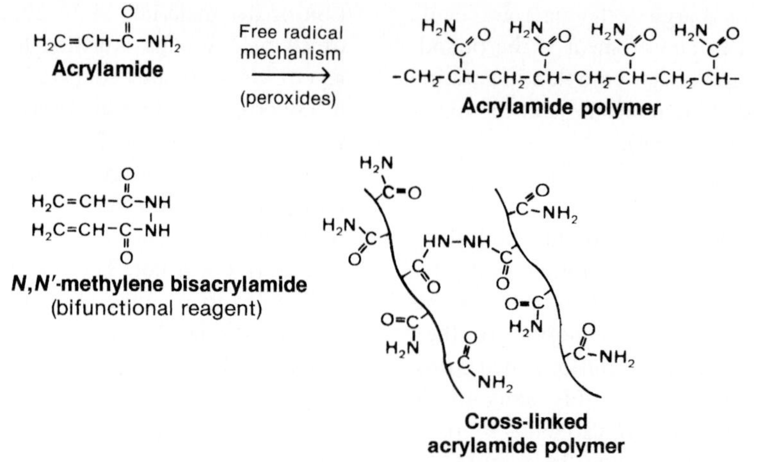

Fig. 10-4 Polyacrylamide gels are produced by polymerizing a mixture of acrylamide and a bifunctional (cross-linking) acrylamide derivative. Derivative shown is that in common use.

nucleotides to many hundreds of nucleotides. These are separated by electrophoresis on a 6% polyacrylamide gel containing 8 M urea and so efficiently that adjacent zones of separated polynucleotide differ in length by only one nucleotide. Up to several hundred base lengths can be separated (and "read") on one such gel. Note that oligonucleotides in general have one negative charge per nucleotide at neutral pH values, a constant "charge-to-mass ratio" in other words, and usually have the same shape and so are separated exclusively on the basis of their molecular weight.

The average pore size of polyacrylamide gels cast at 5% to 10% concentrations is also comparable to the effective diameters of many globular (relatively compact) proteins of 15,000 to 250,000 daltons. These gels will filter such solutions, separating proteins on the basis of *both* size and mobility (see Chapter 5, reference 6, and Chapter 6, reference 4). The molecular sieving effects can produce enhanced resolution, that is, narrower zones of macromolecules, as well.

ENHANCED-RESOLUTION TECHNIQUES
Discontinuous buffers

Several electrophoretic techniques employ a system in which different buffer cations or anions are placed along the electrophoretic path on either side of the protein zone. The mobilities are different for each ion. If the ionic species placed before and the species placed after a mixture of high-molecular-weight substances, proteins, for example, have suitable mobilities, the proteins become *stacked* between the two ions. If a series of proteins are electrophoresed in this discontinuous buffer system, they will arrange themselves according to their effective mobilities and become concentrated, resulting in a much greater (enhanced) resolution.

There are three major applications of the use of discontinuous systems to produce enhanced resolution: isotachy-

phoresis, isoelectric focusing, and disk electrophoresis. These techniques, briefly described in Table 10-1, are used frequently to analyze proteins.

Separations based on molecular size

By enabling separations on the basis of molecular size as well as molecular charge, the techniques briefly described in Table 10-2 provide enhanced separation ability. They usually employ polyacrylamide or agarose to prepare gels of known pore size. Molecules of smaller molecular size will electrophorese faster than larger molecules carrying similar charges.

Electrophoresis of such substances is sometimes used analytically to estimate molecular weights from how far a given substance moves, compared to how far substances of known molecular weight ("standards") move under the same conditions.

SELECTION OF METHODS AND CONDITIONS

Knowledge of the isoelectric point and the molecular weight of the compound to be examined can help determine the optimum conditions for an electrophoretic separation. A buffer should be chosen with a pH that will provide the maximum separation without destroying the properties of the sample. Very acidic or basic conditions pose problems for any system, since an increasing fraction of the current is carried by protons or hydroxyl ions, resulting in poorer separation. A summary of the effects of the various parameters on electrophoresis is provided in Table 10-3.

Support mediums

The choice of a supporting medium is based on many considerations. Slabs or sheets are useful when one is comparing different samples, and routine clinical electrophoresis is done using sheet supports. Gel cylinders are sometimes used in isoelectric focusing. Use of gel cylinders can pro-

Table 10-1 Enhanced-resolution techniques

Technique	Physical basis	Mechanism	Effect	Limitations	Advantages and uses
Isotachophoresis	Electrical neutrality; current in series circuit is constant.[7,8] Lower-conductivity solution after higher-conductivity solution must move at same velocity and carry same current, and so the two solutions experience different voltages and adjust in concentration.[4,7,8]	Solution of lower conductivity containing ion of lower mobility running behind solution of higher conductivity containing higher mobility ion (e.g., chloride); ion of intermediate mobility (e.g., protein) sandwiched between; concentration of protein increases to carry same current as lower and higher mobility ions.	Intermediate-mobility ions (e.g., proteins) stack in thin concentrated zones and move in discrete zones.	Ions not separated; resolution not so good as disk electrophoresis.	No widespread clinical applications currently.
Disk electrophoresis	Effective mobilities of some ions are pH dependent; it is often used with polyacrylamide gels.	As above; then stacked proteins overrun by following ion because of pH change; change in pH produced using counterion.	Proteins, now in thin zones, migrate independently.	Ion systems and pH's limited; technically more exacting than ordinary electrophoresis.	High sensitivity and resolving power; used extensively to separate proteins, mostly as research tool.
Isoelectric focusing[6,7,9,10]	Migration of ions must occur in both directions; amphoteric ions (with both basic and acid groups) have zero effective mobility and zero net charge at their isoelectric point.	Ion movement stops because of zero counterion concentration, leaving all ions stacked in pH gradient; leading and trailing ions are an acid and a base.	Proteins in zones at isoelectric (isoionic) points; pH gradient is buffered by carrier ampholytes.	More complicated and exacting than ordinary electrophoresis.	High capacity and resolution to 0.01 pH unit possible; primarily a research tool.

vide great sensitivity, whereas thin-layer methods provide even greater sensitivity.

Paper and cellulose acetate. Paper is especially favored for separation of low-molecular-weight substances in specialized biochemical laboratories. The main advantages of these materials are their thinness and mechanical strength. A thinner support means greater sensitivity because less material is needed to produce a detectable spot or zone. In a thicker support, the same amount of sample in a zone would be distributed in a greater volume and so would be more dilute and hence harder to detect. Otherwise, more sample must be applied to a thicker support for equal ease of detection. Use of thinner supports means smaller samples and less material is electrophoresed. This is advantageous if little sample is available though this is not usually the situation in clinical laboratories.

Cellulose acetate is prepared by treating cellulose with acetic anhydride. This puts acetyl groups on the sugar hydroxyl groups. The resulting material is pressed into sheets that are somewhat stronger than paper and a good deal more

chemically uniform. Adsorption of material to groups in the paper leads to losses of material and to *tailing* of zones. Cellulose acetate is more inert in this respect, and because of its uniformity and ease of preparation (the strips are merely soaked in electrophoretic buffer so that no air is trapped), it is very widely used in routine clinical work.

Gels. Gels can be cast with varying thicknesses to increase or decrease capacity (the amount of sample). Gels also offer the possibility of molecular sieving effects because their porosity can be controlled by changing their composition. On the other hand, their mechanical strength tends to be low.

Starch and agar. Starch gels are not so extensively used as agarose, acrylamide, or even Sephadex. The starch solution must be heated to 100° C, then degassed, an awkward process, and then cast. The starch gels tend to provide greater resolution than agar or agarose does. However, the inconvenience of preparing starch gels has limited their use.

Agar and agarose (agar without the agaropectin) are

Table 10-2 Use of supporting mediums in separation

Method	Principle	Effect	Limitations	Advantages and uses
Separation based on molecular size				
Gradient gels[11]	Gels cast with increasing gel concentrations going from origin to end of gel have gradient of pore sizes.	Larger macromolecules move more slowly as they encounter higher gel concentrations; can measure relative sizes and charges.	Difficult to reproduce gels.	Research tool.
Gels containing denaturants[12,13]	Gels cast with denaturants (e.g., urea or SDS) so that macromolecules migrate in denatured forms; SDS binds uniformly and in large amounts to most proteins.	Proteins in SDS and oligonucleotides migrate inversely to subunit molecular weights or number of nucleotides.	Exacting technique; disulfide bonds in proteins must be broken; not all proteins behave normally.	Research tool.
Separations based on molecular size and charge				
Gel electrophoresis[11]	Pore size is small enough to restrict diffusion.	Higher resolution.	Reproducibility.	Better resolution than cellulose acetate; agarose gels widely used; mostly research tool.
Immunoelectrophoretic methods (see Chapter 12)	Antigen and antibody are brought together using electrophoresis to form precipitate.	Can identify and quantitate specific antigen or antibody.	Sensitivity somewhat low.	Very widespread (e.g., *rocket immunoelectrophoresis*) clinical use.
Two-dimensional electrophoresis[14]	Separation occurs according to one parameter (e.g., isoelectric point) in one dimension (direction) and then according to a second parameter (e.g., size) at right angles.	Mixture of proteins spread over a surface; information proportional to square of length of side of surface.[14,15]	Exacting technique; difficult to reproduce patterns.	High information content; widely used in clinical research.

SDS, Sodium dodecyl sulfate.

easier to handle. Because agarose demonstrates a lower electro-osmotic effect and exhibits fewer problems with adsorption, it is preferred over agar. The pore size of agarose is much greater than that of polyacrylamide. This is the reason why agar or agarose is used in most immunoelectrophoretic techniques, since antigen and antibody must be able to migrate through the gel. Another advantage of agarose is that it may be poured after reheating to only about 50° C; thus some proteins, such as antibodies, can be mixed in without denaturing. Even so, the same disadvantages encountered when preparing starch gels are encountered when preparing agar and agarose gels. Precast agarose gels for a variety of separations are available commercially. These gels are used for separation of isoenzymes, hemoglobins, glycoproteins, and so on.

Polyacrylamide. Polyacrylamide gels are less frequently used in clinical laboratories but are a common research tool. They are clear, fairly easy to prepare, and exhibit reasonable mechanical strength over the acrylamide

concentration range normally employed for proteins. In addition, they show a low endosmosis effect and have a pore size well suited for the separation of the average proteins, ribonucleic acid (RNA) molecules, and smaller restriction fragments of DNA. A major clinical use of polyacrylamide gels is the separation of alkaline phosphatase isoenzymes. However, polyacrylamide gel preparation and casting are somewhat more exacting and time consuming, and reproducibility of gel preparation is difficult to achieve. It is now possible to buy commercially prepared polyacrylamide sheets from several firms.

Cellulose acetate sheets can be purchased in relatively uniform batches so that results of different electrophoresis experiments are more consistent. After electrophoresis, the strips can be sliced into bands containing stained or radioactive materials. These slices can be dissolved in a solvent such as acetone for easy quantitation.

On the other hand, resolution with cellulose acetate is not as good as with polyacrylamide. Eight or nine serum

Table 10-3 Common effects of electrophoretic parameters on separation

Parameter	Effect on electrophoresis
pH	Changes charge of analyte and hence effective mobility; can affect structure of analyte, such as denaturing or dissociating a protein.
Ionic strength	Changes voltage or current; increased ionic strength usually reduces migration velocity and increases heating.
Ions present	Can change migration velocity if interaction is strong; can cause tailing of bands.
Current	Too high a current causes overheating.
Voltage	Migration velocity is proportional to voltage.
Temperature	Temperature gradients in support mediums cause bowed bands. Overheating can denature (precipate) proteins. Lower temperatures reduce diffusion but also reduce migration velocity; there is no effect on resolution.
Time	Separation of bands (resolution) increases linearly with time, but dilution of bands (diffusion) increases with the square root of time.
Medium	Major factors are endosmosis and pore-size effects, which affect migration velocities.

protein fractions can be resolved using cellulose acetate, but up to 30 fractions can be detected using disk electrophoresis on polyacrylamide gels.[11] So cellulose acetate is used because it lends itself to fast, easy, reproducible measurements, though of comparatively low resolution.

Electroblotting. There is an exception to the requirement that a supporting medium not interact with the material being separated. In the *Western blot* technique,[15] a gel slab containing separated proteins is electrophoresed perpendicularly to the slab, with transferal of some or all of the separated proteins onto a facing sheet of material, often nitrocellulose, which adsorbs the proteins[16] (see Fig. 12-4). The sheet may be stained for protein or enzyme activity (see the text that follows). Usually, however, the sheet is washed with some neutral protein, such as milk protein or bovine serum albumin, to block unoccupied adsorption sites. Then the locations of specific transferred adsorbed proteins are determined, usually by immunochemical assays. The resulting pattern may be compared with the original slab that is stained or examined by autoradiography for all proteins or all labeled proteins.

A major virtue of Western blots is their sensitivity. (The adsorption *concentrates* the proteins.) Adsorption of antigens or antibodies takes place at concentrations of antigen and antibody that are far too low for a precipitate to form. As little as 10^{-10} g of protein can be detected and hence identified.[17] Consequently, antigens (and antibodies) in serum that are present at very low concentrations can be detected and even quantitated. This technique is used for detecting acquired immunodeficiency syndrome (AIDS) antigens and antibodies in patients.[15]

Conditions

Horizontal versus vertical position. Electrophoresis can be performed horizontally or vertically; there is no theoretical reason for preferring one or the other procedure. Horizontal electrophoresis places less mechanical stress on the support, whereas vertical electrophoresis supporting mediums are often supported between glass plates.

If horizontal electrophoresis is used and the surface of the medium is open to air, evaporation of the solvent can cause problems. As a result of evaporation, salt concentrations rise, usually unevenly along the support, leading to nonuniform current flow and heating. This can lead to problems of uneven migration, especially at the sides of a horizontal, flat electrophoresis bed. "Submarine" electrophoresis is horizontal electrophoresis in which the support is covered with buffer solution so that there is no evaporation from the support. The sample is inserted into slots or holes in the support and electrophoresed through the support. If one buffer reservoir is higher than the other, convective flow of the buffer through the supporting medium may occur. Therefore the electrophoresis apparatus should always be level.

Sample application. Sometimes samples are simply applied to the surface of the supporting medium and allowed to soak in. Sometimes special slots or holes are cast or cut in a gel. Occasionally, the sample may be polymerized into the gel or cast with the gel. Injection of the sample is rarely used, except with isotachophoresis. In capillary zone electrophoresis, a very small quantity (a few microliters) of the sample is electrophoresed into the capillary tube. Commercial sample applicators can simultaneously apply a desired number of 1 or 2 μL samples of, for example, blood serum to the support surfaces; such devices help ensure greater uniformity of the initial sample zone shapes and sizes, improving reproducibility of results in clinical laboratories. If electrophoresis takes place in stages (as in two-dimensional electrophoresis), the gel-containing part or all of the sample may be cut out and reattached, sometimes with an agarose "glue," to another gel for the next stage in the separation. Often the sample is layered onto the surface of a gel. The sample is then usually made denser than the solvent by the addition of sucrose or glycerol. All the above techniques are equally valid when combined with the appropriate type of assay.

Current and voltage considerations. Electrophoresis can be carried out at constant voltage, constant current, or constant power. Selection of any of these modes often depends on the power supply available. Since diffusion increases with the square root of time, it is best to complete the electrophoresis as quickly as possible. This requires use of the maximum voltage. However, the maximum voltage is always limited by the efficiency of cooling of the apparatus. Some workers claim that temperature gradients of more than 0.1° C across a gel or other support lead to noticeable distortions of macromolecule zones. For some current clinical applications, temperature control does not appear to be necessary, and separations are carried out at ambient temperatures.

Use of thinner supports (or capillaries) is now widespread because the temperature gradients that form are smaller because of the more efficient heat dissipation possible from thinner supports. This means higher voltages can be applied, producing faster separations and consequently less diffusion and clearer, sharper separation patterns. Also, more samples can be electrophoresed in a given time, an important consideration in routine clinical work. DNA-sequencing gels are about 1 mm thick. Such thin supports are very fragile and so require very careful handling. Commercial agarose or polyacrylamide supports are backed by plastic sheets to enable them to be used in routine clinical work.

One recently developed commercial electrophoresis system employs a very efficient cooling system and very thin, preformed agarose gels to perform high-voltage electrophoresis. By using 1000 to 2000 V instead of 100 V, the electrophoresis can be completed in 2 to 3 minutes instead of 20 minutes. This approach maximizes the efficiency of the electrophoretic system in time and resolution. Capillary zone electrophoresis employs voltages of 300 to 400 V/cm, resulting in electrophoresis times of often less than 10 minutes.

The conductivity of any electrophoretic system will change with time because the ionic composition will change as a result of movement (electrophoresis) of the sample along the system. Such changes are minimal in continuous systems, such as high-voltage paper electrophoresis, and application of constant voltage is satisfactory for these systems. For isotachophoresis, a constant velocity of zone migration is desired, and a constant current is used. For other electrophoretic systems, heating is usually the limiting factor (see above), and so constant power (wattage) should be used. Disk electrophoresis and isoelectric focusing fall into this category. Pulsed power supplies provide no advantage.[18]

Separation time. In the case of isotachophoresis, the electrophoresis is stopped when the trailing ion emerges. Isoelectric focusing is complete after the gradient is formed and the current has dropped to a stable value. The time to stop a disk or ordinary zone electrophoretic separation is usually indicated by the position of the *tracking dye,* usually when the dye band reaches a predetermined position in the stationary support (typically the end of the support). Dyes that have high mobilities, such as bromphenol blue, are employed. They are usually added to the sample. Since some proteins bind such dyes, their apparent mobilities may be changed.

LOCATING THE ANALYTE

Analysis involves determining where the substances to be identified or quantified are on the support. This can be accomplished by measurement of a physical property of a molecule, such as light absorption or refractive index, or by use of a chemical reaction such as staining. Measurements of physical properties may lack specificity, sensitivity, or resolution. For example, not all proteins absorb strongly at 280 nm.

Use of shorter wavelengths (such as 200 mm), where most things absorb more strongly, improves the sensitivity of direct measurement at the cost of possible interference from other absorbing substances. A commercial capillary zone electrophoresis apparatus uses microfocused optics to enable direct measurement of separated substances inside the capillary tube as they migrate past the light beam. One major problem with direct measurement is that with current instruments, the patterns of separated substances must be obtained one at a time.

Staining

Staining often achieves the desired goals of resolution, sensitivity, specificity, and speed (Table 10-4). Since the zones of material broaden by diffusion after electrophoresis is stopped, the first step in the analytical procedure is to eliminate diffusion. One can do this in paper electrophoresis by drying the paper or in autoradiography by drying or freezing the gels. In routine clinical electrophoresis, supports are usually dried in an oven before measurement.

Proteins

Protein in gels is often denatured (that is, precipitated in the gel matrix) by soaking the gels in dilute acetic acid or more effectively in trichloroacetic acid. Addition of sulfosalicylic acid further improves the denaturing ability of the staining solution. In the Western blot procedure, the proteins are immobilized by adsorption.

Sometimes heat must also be applied to make the proteins insoluble. However, some resist denaturation by all these conventional procedures and remain soluble in the stain. If detergents such as sodium dodecyl sulfate or other soluble agents are present, they will interfere with precipitation. Inclusion of methanol in the acid solutions helps remove such substances before staining.

Choice of stain

Many types of stains are employed, depending on the need. Sometimes it is desirable to stain everything, such as all proteins. A dye called *Stains-All* is suitable.[19] A *silver stain,* which reacts to both proteins and nucleic acids, is an alternative.[20] Proteins, after electrophoresis on cellulose acetate, are most often stained with Ponceau S.[21]

Stains and staining procedures are often specific for one chemical group. The Ninhydrin (triketohydrindene hydrate) stain for amino groups, often used after paper electrophore-

Table 10-4   Commonly used stains for various substances

Substance	Stain	Comments
Proteins	Ponceau S*	Less sensitive than amido black, but more specific for proteins; the most widely used stain
	Bromphenol blue†	
	Light green SF†	Low sensitivity, but can be used with ampholyte gels
	Coomassie brilliant blue R250*	Can detect less than 0.2 μg of protein; can be used with ampholyte gels
	Silver stain (silver reduced onto oxidized macromolecules)‡	10 to 50 times more sensitive than Coomassie; different proteins give different colors, for unknown reasons
	Stains-All (a cationic carbocyanine dye)§	General sensitivity, including phosphoproteins
	Amido black 10B ("buffalo black")‖	Very sensitive stain, but one-tenth as sensitive as Coomassie
	Colloidal Gold	About 100-fold more sensitive than Coomassie; most sensitive protein stain currently available; used with Western blots§§
Lipoproteins	Sudan black B¶	
	Oil red O#	
	Coomassie brilliant blue R250#	Used with SDS (sodium dodecyl sulfate) gels
Glycoproteins	PAS (periodic acid–Schiff)**	Best for neutral glycoproteins; 2 to 3 μg of carbohydrate detectable
	Stains-All§	Best for sialic acid–rich glycoproteins, and mucopolysaccharides
Nucleic acids	Stains-All§	Best for RNA, DNA
	Silver stain§	2 to 5 times more sensitive than ethidium bromide
	Ethidium bromide††	Fluorescent bands with DNA; less than 10 ng detectable
	TOTO-1‖‖	Fluorescent bands with DNA; 4 pg detectable
Enzymes		
Dehydrogenases	NADH (fluorescence)‡‡	
	Nitroblue tetrazolium chloride‡‡	
Esterases	Beta-naphthyl esters and tetrazotized *o*-dianisidine‡‡	
Cholinesterases		
Phosphatases	1-Naphthyl phosphate and fast blue B‡‡	

NOTE: The sensitivity factors given are averages; different proteins will stain with different intensities with any stain.
*Righetti PG, Drysdale JW: *Isoelectric focusing,* New York, 1976, Academic Press.
†Chapter 22, reference 7.
‡Merril CR, Goldman D, Sedman SA, Ebert MH: *Science* 211:1437, 1981.
§Green MR, Pastewka JV, Peacock AC: *Anal Biochem* 56:43, 1973.
‖Wilson CM: *Anal Biochem* 96:263, 1979.
¶Swahn B: *Scand J Clin Lab Invest* 4:98, 1952.
#Weller H: *Klin Wochenschr* 36:563, 1958.
**Matthieu JM, Quarles RH: *Anal Biochem* 55:313, 1973.
††Brunk CF, Simpson L: *Anal Biochem* 82:455, 1977.
‡‡Gabriel O: *Methods Enzymol* 22:578, 1971.
§§Gershoui J, Palade G: *Anal Biochem* B1:1, 1983.
‖‖Glazer AH, Rye HS, Quesada MA, Mathies RA: *Proc Nat Acad Sci USA* 8T:3851, 1990.

sis of peptides or amino acids, is an example of this. Glycoproteins can be treated with periodic acid (for oxidation) and color developed with a dye (fuchsin) in the presence of a reducing agent (sulfite). This periodic acid–Schiff stain treatment oxidizes carbohydrate groups to aldehydes, which react with the dye to form a Schiff base. The sulfite reduces the Schiff base, making the stain permanent. There is also a specific stain for phosphoproteins. A fairly complete list of stains is given by Righetti and Drysdale.[21] (See Table 10-4 for a list of commonly used stains.)

Once the stain has been introduced, usually by soaking the support in the stain solution, excess stain must be removed. This can be done electrophoretically or, most commonly, by diffusion. Electrophoretic removal is fast but can result in distortion of the stained zones. Diffusion involves changing the solvent or using a destainer to remove free stain.

Many enzymes are identified by the use of colored or fluorescent substrates or products (zymograms), even in gels or other support mediums. For example, alkaline phosphatase hydrolyzes *para*-nitrophenylphosphate to *para*-nitrophenol, which has a yellow color at pH 8. Soaking a gel in such assay solutions produces colored bands where the enzymes are. If the product of enzymatic activity is of low molecular weight, rapid diffusion of the product may broaden the zone, making location of the enzyme or identification of the isozyme difficult. Products that form polymers or insoluble substances are better, but if this is not possible, a contact print method may be used.[11] A sheet of paper or other material is impregnated with a chromophoric substrate and pressed against the support containing the separated enzyme or enzymes. Often the support is cut into slices, and the slices are incubated in assay solution. A list of such zymograms is given in the text by Righetti and Drysdale.[21]

Other localization techniques

A common technique for localization of proteins and nucleic acids employs radioactive labels, such as ^{125}I or ^{14}C, incorporated into the macromolecules. After electrophoresis, a piece of x-ray film is placed in contact with the stationary support in the dark for 12 to 24 hours. After the film is developed, a dark area corresponding to the position of the radioactively labeled macromolecule will be present. This technique, *autoradiography,* is commonly employed in the Western blot technique for proteins and also is used in the Southern blot technique for nucleic acids.

Some commonly encountered problems in electrophoresis, their most likely causes, and suggested corrective action are listed in Table 10-5.

CLINICAL APPLICATIONS

For clinical research, high sensitivity of detection of analyte, high resolution of adjacent zones of analyte, and high reproducibility of separations are required. For routine clinical work, some resolution and sensitivity of detection are sacrificed for speed or throughput; reproducibility remains important but is ensured by frequent use of comparison samples from healthy people.

The most common uses of electrophoretic techniques in the laboratory today are the following:

1. Specific protein electrophoresis
   a. Quantitative analysis of specific serum protein classes, such as gamma globulins and albumin (see Chapters 49 and 27, respectively)
   b. Identification and quantitation of hemoglobin and its subclasses (see Chapter 36)
   c. Identification of monoclonal proteins, such as Bence Jones gamma globulins in either serum or urine (see Chapter 49)
   d. Separation and quantitation of major lipoprotein classes (see Chapters 33 and 53)
2. Isoenzyme analysis: separation and quantitation of enzymes such as creatine kinase, lactate dehydrogenase, and alkaline phosphatase into their respective molecular subtypes (see Chapters 27 and 31)
3. Immunoelectrophoresis: most often used to determine qualitatively the elevation or deficiency of specific classes of immunoglobulins; also can be used to semi-quantitate serum proteins, such as transferrin and complement component C3 (see Chapter 12)
4. Western blot technique to identify a specific protein: used to confirm the presence of antibodies to human immunodeficiency virus (AIDS) (see Chapter 12)
5. Southern blot techniques to identify specific nucleic

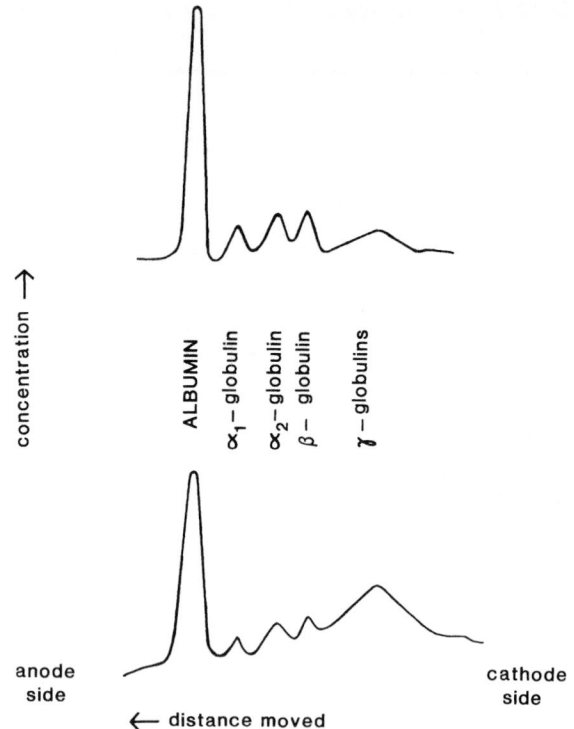

Fig. 10-5 Example of effect of disease, hepatic cirrhosis, on blood serum protein electrophoretic pattern. *Upper profile,* Distribution characteristic of healthy people.

acid sequences (DNA or RNA) (see Chapter 48): used for prenatal diagnosis of inborn errors, diagnosis of viral infections, and identification of risk factors for cancer (see Chapter 49)

The two-dimensional procedures will undoubtedly replace some or all of the preceding procedures, but at this time mostly exploratory work is being done. All the procedures involve measurement of alterations in an electrophoretic pattern compared with a normal control. One can often use these to diagnose specific diseases[14,22] (Fig. 10-5). Nephrotic syndrome, for example, may be accompanied by a decrease of more than 25% in alpha$_2$ globulin levels and a decrease of up to 25% in gamma globulin levels because of the loss of low-molecular-weight proteins in the urine. The pattern of decrease or increase in several disease conditions is fairly characteristic, and hence quantitation of stained cellulose acetate strips is useful in diagnosis.

The stained support may be either put through a strip scanner if the support is a strip or put through a modified spectrophotometer ("densitometer") if it is not. Cellulose acetate supports must sometimes be "cleared," made more transparent, before analysis by densitometry. This is done by soaking the support in a solvent. With due care, the dye absorbance on the support is a good measure of the amount of protein. With cellulose acetate electrophoresis, normal serum is electrophoresed next to the serum to be tested. The

Table 10-5   Commonly encountered problems in electrophoresis

Problem	Likely cause	Corrective action
No migration	Instrument not connected	Check electrical circuits.
	Wrong pH; electrodes connected backwards	Check isoelectric point of protein and pH of buffer; check electrode polarity.
Bowed electrophoretic pattern on edges of support	Overheating or drying out of support	Humidity chamber; check buffer ionic strength; reduce wattage.
Tailing of bands	Chemical reaction: subunit dissociation or adsorption to support	Use different support; try different pH.
	Salt in sample	Check sample for salt; dialyze sample against electrophoresis buffer.
	Buffer co-ion effect	Use different buffer co-ion.
Holes in staining pattern	Analyte present in too high a concentration	Apply less concentrated sample.
Very thin, sharp bands	Molecular weight of sample very high for support pore size	Use support with larger pore size.
	Sulfhydryl oxidation and aggregation	Run sample with sulfhydryl reducing compound or at lower pH.
Very slow migration	High molecular weight	Use support with larger pore size.
	Low charge	Change pH so that charge increases.
	Ionic strength too high	Check conductivity; dilute buffer.
	Voltage too low	Increase voltage.
Sample precipitates in support	pH too high or low	Run at different pH.
	Too much heating	Use lower wattage or external cooling.

Table 10-6   Compounds commonly separated by electrophoresis

Class of compound	Stain	Support medium
Amino acid	Ninhydrin	Paper, cellulose acetate
Serum protein	Ponceau S	Cellulose acetate
	Coomassie blue 250	Polyacrylamide (with or without isoelectric focusing)
Lipoproteins	Oil red O	Agarose
Glycoproteins	Periodic acid–Schiff	Agarose
Nucleic acids	Ethidium bromide (fluorescent)	Agarose
Hemoglobins	Silver stain	
	o-Dianisidine	Cellulose acetate, agar
	Ferricyanide	
	Peroxide	
Isoenzymes		
Lactate dehydrogenase	Fluorescent NADH or tetrazolium	Agarose
Creatine kinase	Fluorescent NADH or tetrazolium	Agarose
Alkaline phosphatase	1-Naphthylphosphate + fast blue B or 5-bromo-4-chloroindolyl phosphate	Polyacrylamide, cellulose acetate
Immunoglobulins	Coomassie blue 250	Agarose
Specific antigens by immunological electrophoretic techniques (such as Laurell rocket)	Amino black 10B	Agarose

plots of absorbance (color) versus distance obtained from a strip scanner (see Fig. 10-5) allow immediate comparison of relative amounts of each class of separated proteins. Routine clinical electrophoresis such as of blood serum samples can be done by use of highly automated instruments. Several companies sell such equipment, such as Beckman, Ciba-Corning, and Helena Laboratories.

Electrophoresis is sometimes used in assays of genetic defects. The two-dimensional techniques now being developed have tremendous potential in that area. Table 10-6 lists compounds normally separated by electrophoresis.

REFERENCES

1. Van Holde KE: *Physical biochemistry,* ed 2, Englewood Cliffs, N.J., 1985, Prentice-Hall.
2. Moore WJ: *Physical chemistry,* ed 4, Englewood Cliffs, N.J., 1970, Prentice-Hall.
3. Tanford C: *Physical chemistry of macromolecules,* New York, 1961, Academic Press.
4. Melvin M: *Electrophoresis,* New York, 1987, Wiley & Sons.
5. Righetti PG, Van Oss CJ, Vanderhoff JW: *Electrokinetic separation methods,* New York, 1979, Elsevier/North Holland.
6. Deyl Z, Everaerts FM, Prusik Z, Svendsen PJ: Electrophoresis: a survey of techniques and applications, *J Chromatogr* 18(series), 1979.
7. Ornstein L: Disc electrophoresis, *Ann NY Acad Sci* 121:321, 1964.

8. Brewer JM, Ashworth RB: Disc electrophoresis, *J Chem Educ* 46:41, 1969.
9. Jovin TM, Dante ML, Chrambach A: *Multiphasic buffer systems output PB 196085 to 196092 and 203016,* Springfield, Va., 1970, National Technical Information Service.
10. Fagerhol MK, Laurell CB: The Pi system–inherited variants of serum alpha-1-antitrypsin, *Prog Med Genet* 7:96, 1970.
11. Andrews AT: *Electrophoresis: theory, techniques, and biochemical and clinical applications,* ed 2, New York, 1986, Oxford University Press.
12. Laemmli UK: Cleavage of structural proteins during the assembly of the head of bacteriophage T4, *Nature* 227:680, 1970.
13. Wyckoff M, Rodbard D, Chrambach A: Polyacrylamide gel electrophoresis in sodium dodecyl sulfate–containing buffers using multiphasic buffer systems, *Anal Biochem* 78:459, 1977.
14. O'Farrell PH: High-resolution two-dimensional electrophoresis of proteins, *J Biol Chem* 250:4007, 1975.
15. Dunn MJ, editor: *Electrophoresis '86,* Deerfield Beach, Fla., 1986, VCH Verlagsgesellschaft.
16. Lemkin PF, Lipkin LE: GELLAB: a computer system for 2D gel electrophoresis analysis. II. Pairing spots, *Comput Biomed Res* 14:355, 1981.
17. Towbin H, Staehelin T, Gordon J: Electrophoretic transfer of proteins from polyacrylamide gels to nitrocellulose sheets, *Proc Nat Acad Sci USA* 76:4350, 1979.
18. Allington RW, Nelson JW, Aron GG: *ISCO Applications Research Bulletin,* no 18, Lincoln, Neb., 1975, Instrumentation Specialties Co. (ISCO, Inc.).
19. Green MR, Pastewka JV: Identification of sialic acid–rich glycoproteins on polyacrylamide gels, *Anal Biochem* 65:66, 1975.
20. Merril CR, Goldman D, Sedman SA, Ebert MH: Ultrasensitive stain for proteins in polyacrylamide gels shows regional variation in cerebrospinal fluid proteins, *Science* 211:1437, 1981.
21. Righetti PG, Drysdale JW: *Isoelectric focusing,* New York, 1976, Academic Press.
22. Annino JS, Giese RW: *Clinical chemistry, principles and procedures,* ed 4, Boston, 1976, Little, Brown & Co.
23. Righetti PG: *Isoelectric focusing: theory, methodology and applications,* ed 2, vol 5, *Laboratory techniques in biochemistry and molecular biology,* New York, 1983, Elsevier Biomedical Press.
24. Foret F, Bocek P: Capillary electrophoresis. In Chrambach A, Dunn MJ, Radola BJ, editors: *Advances in electrophoresis,* vol 3, New York, 1989, VCH Publishers.

CHAPTER 11

Immunological reactions

Susan Bassion

OBJECTIVES

- Define antigen and antibody.
- List and explain eight factors affecting antigenicity.
- Describe the composition and structural differences of antibodies. Name five human immunoglobulins and describe the physiological role of each.
- List and explain the forces involved in antigen-antibody reactions and the factors that influence the specificity of immunochemical reactions.
- Outline the mechanism of the following antigen-antibody gel-precipitation reactions and state the principle of each:
    Double immunodiffusion
    Radial immunodiffusion

KEY TERMS

affinity Measure of the binding strength of the antibody-antigen reaction.

antibodies Proteins that combine specifically with antigens.

antigenic determinant That portion of an antigen that reacts with antibody.

antigens Substances that induce an immune response.

avidity Measure of the binding strength of antibodies to multiple antigenic determinants on natural antigens.

B cells B lymphocytes that transform to plasma cells and produce antibodies.

constant region C-terminus of light and heavy chains, highly conserved. Not part of the antibody combining site.

cross-reactivity Binding of an antibody to an antigen other than the one initiating the immune response.

Fab fragment Portion of immunoglobulin molecule made by papain degradation and containing the antibody-combining site; composed of the light chain and a portion of the heavy chain.

Fc fragment Portion of immunoglobulin molecule produced by papain degradation that contains most of the heavy chain (including the complement-binding site).

flocculation Precipitation reaction producing large, loose precipitates.

haptens Low-molecular-weight substances that can induce an immune response only when coupled to high-molecular-weight immunogenic molecules.

heavy chain Portion of immunoglobulin molecule consisting of a polypeptide chain of about 50,000 daltons.

hypervariable regions Amino acid sequences in the variable region that have an increased likelihood of variation.

idiotype Portion of immunoglobulin molecule conferring unique character, most often including its binding site.

immunoglobulins (Ig) Proteins with antibody activity.

joining (J) chain Portion of IgM molecule possibly holding structure together.

lattice The cross-linked, three-dimensional structure formed by the reaction of multivalent antigens with antibody.

light chain Portion of an immunoglobulin molecule composed of a polypeptide chain of about 22,000 daltons.

plasma cells Immunoglobulin-producing cells that are the end stage of B-cell differentiation.

precipitin reaction, or precipitin line Refers to the precipitation of antigens and antibodies in gels. *Precipitin line* is an insoluble complex formed by proteins; for antigens and antibodies, it occurs when their relative concentrations are approximately equivalent or optimal for lattice formation.

secretory piece Polypeptide chain attached to IgA (may participate in secretion into mucosal spaces).

valency The effective number of antigenic determinants on an antigen molecule. Also sometimes used to describe the number of antibody-binding sites.

variable region N-terminal portion of immunoglobulin light and heavy chains whose amino acid sequence can change; this region includes the antigen-combining site.

zone of equivalence Region of antibody-antigen precipitin reaction in which concentrations of both reactants are equal.

Immunological reactions can occur between two types of substances, *antigens* and *antibodies*. This chapter examines these substances and the interactions between them.

ANTIGENS

Antigens, or *immunogens,* are defined as substances that induce an immune response. The immune response produced may be an antibody (humoral) response or the production of sensitized cells (cellular response). Usually both humoral and cellular responses are stimulated.

Factors affecting antigenicity

Many factors determine the antigenicity of a molecule. The nature and dosage of an antigen, the route of administration, the organism immunized, and the sensitivity of the detection method are important factors in the evaluation of antigenicity. Many other conditions must be satisfied for a molecule to be immunogenic. These conditions are discussed below.

Chemical nature. The first antigens investigated were bacteria and red blood cells that are complex macromolecular structures composed of many different proteins, carbohydrates, and lipids. Subsequent investigations have proved that immunogens are found in several chemical classes, including proteins, polysaccharides, glycolipids, nucleic acids, and polynucleotides.

Size. There is no absolute size requirement, but size is of considerable importance in determining the antigenicity of a molecule. The most potent immunogens are macromolecules with molecular weights greater than 100,000 daltons. The A and B polypeptide chains of insulin (2500 daltons) and of glucagon (3600 daltons) are immunogenic in guinea pigs. Nevertheless, most molecules with molecular weights less than 10,000 daltons are weakly immunogenic, if at all.

Haptens. Substances with low molecular weights can induce an immune response when coupled to higher-molecular-weight immunogenic *carrier* molecules. Such incomplete antigens, or *haptens,* do not elicit an immune response by themselves but do react with antibody. Many low-molecular-weight compounds have been shown to act as haptens, including monosaccharides, lipids, peptides, hormones such as adrenocorticotropic hormone and prostaglandins, toxins such as arsphenamide, and drugs such as barbiturates and sulfonamides.

Complexity. A molecule must exhibit a certain degree of chemical complexity to be antigenic. Synthetic amino acid homopolymers, composed of repeating units of a single amino acid, have been shown to be poor immunogens; copolymers of two or three amino acids are much better immunogens. Increasing immunogenicity follows increasing complexity. For example, the addition of aromatic amino acid residues such as tyrosine to synthetic amino acid copolymers increases their immunogenicity.

Antigenic determinants. The portion of an antigen involved in the reaction with an antibody is called an *antigenic determinant,* or *epitope.* An antigen may contain more than one type of antigenic determinant; the number of antigenic determinants per antigen varies with the size and complexity of the molecule (Fig. 11-1). The effective number of antigenic determinants on an antigen is its *valency.* This is the number of antibody molecules that can be bound to an antigen at the same time (see Fig. 11-1). Antibodies recognize the three-dimensional shape of an antigenic determinant (conformational antigenic determinant), as well as the basic amino acid structure (sequential antigenic determinant). An antigenic determinant sometimes comprises as few as four amino acid residues. The combining site of an antibody molecule reacts with an antigenic determinant in the complementary *lock-and-key* manner of protein-enzyme interactions. The affinity of an antibody for an antigenic determinant is directly proportional to the closeness of fit.

Conformation and accessibility. The tertiary structure or spatial folding of molecules is a significant factor in their immunogenicity. Antibodies to native proteins do not react with denatured molecules. Antibodies to native proteins are directed primarily to conformational rather than sequential antigenic determinants.

In addition, accessibility or exposure to the environment is an important factor in determining immunogenicity. The terminal side chains of polysaccharides, the portions of a polysaccharide molecule that stick out from the main part of the molecule, are the most immunopotent regions of polysaccharide antigens. Accessibility of an antigen to the environment is related to the solubility of an antigen in aqueous medium. The more soluble an antigen is, the greater the probability that it will interact with an antibody. The influence of charge on immunogenicity may be a manifestation of accessibility. Charged or hydrophilic residues are more in contact with the environment than hydrophobic residues, which tend to be sequestered in the interior of molecules.

Foreignness. The immune system is capable of distinguishing *self* from *nonself* in such a way that, under normal circumstances, a vigorous immune response is produced only to substances recognized as foreign. The more distant the evolutionary relationship between antigen and host, the more immunogenic the molecule. Thus, guinea pig albumin will not evoke an immune response when injected into another guinea pig. The same guinea pig albumin will evoke a strong immune response, however, when injected

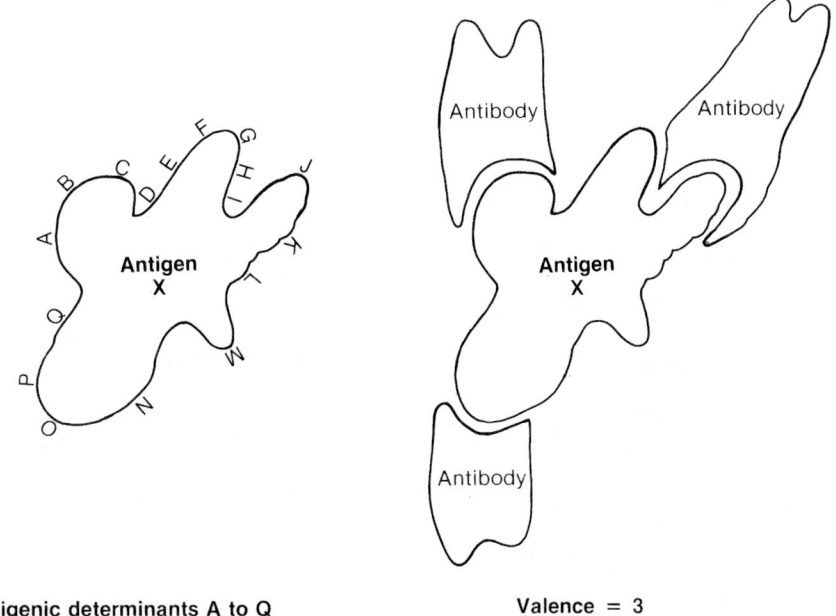

Antigenic determinants A to Q   Valence = 3

Fig. 11-1   Antigen X contains many different antigenic determinants, designated *A* to *Q* in this schematic representation. Antibody molecules when combined with antigen X bind to different sites. Maximum number of molecules of antibodies bound in this figure is 3; therefore, valence is 3.

into a different or more complex (higher) vertebrate, such as a rabbit or a monkey.

Genetics. It has recently been shown that the ability to recognize an antigen and the strength of the immune response produced may be under strict genetic control. Some strains of mice injected with synthetic polypeptides are capable of producing a vigorous immune response. Other mice, with closely related but nonidentical genetic backgrounds, may be poor responders or nonresponders.

. . .

In summary, many factors influence the immunogenicity of an antigen: chemical nature, size, molecular complexity, conformation, accessibility, foreignness, and genetics.

ANTIBODIES

The proteins that combine specifically with antigens are termed *antibodies*. Antibodies are produced by a subset of lymphocytes, called *B lymphocytes*, and by their progeny, *plasma cells*. B lymphocytes, through their production of antibodies, are responsible for the phenomenon of humoral immunity. Proteins with antibody activity are also called *immunoglobulins*. Immunoglobulins are an extremely heterogeneous group of molecules that constitute approximately 20% of the plasma proteins. Immunoglobulins are heterogeneous in their antigen specificity, amino acid sequence, migration within an electrical field, and functions. There may be as many as 10,000 different molecules circulating

in the human body that can be classified as immunoglobulins.

Structure

The discovery that electrophoretically homogeneous proteins found in the serum of patients with multiple myeloma were structurally homogeneous and very closely related to normal immunoglobulin was an important advance in the study of immunoglobulin structure. Such myeloma proteins could be isolated in large quantities and chemically characterized. These studies produced an understanding of the precise structure of the antibody molecule.

H and L chains. Antibodies are glycoproteins composed of 82% to 96% polypeptide and 4% to 18% carbohydrate. All immunoglobulin molecules have a common structure of four polypeptide chains. Two identical large, or *heavy*, chains (H chains) and two identical small, or *light*, chains (L chains) are held together by noncovalent forces and covalent interchain disulfide bonds (Fig. 11-2).

The carbohydrate portion of the immunoglobulin molecule is covalently bound to amino acids in the polypeptide chains. The carbohydrates are usually found bound to the C-terminal half (Fc) of the molecule. Their function is poorly understood. They may be involved in transporting the molecule or protecting it from metabolic degradation.

Fab and Fc fragments. Enzymatic digestion of immunoglobulin molecules has provided further evidence of their structure (see Fig. 11-2). Digestion with papain splits the

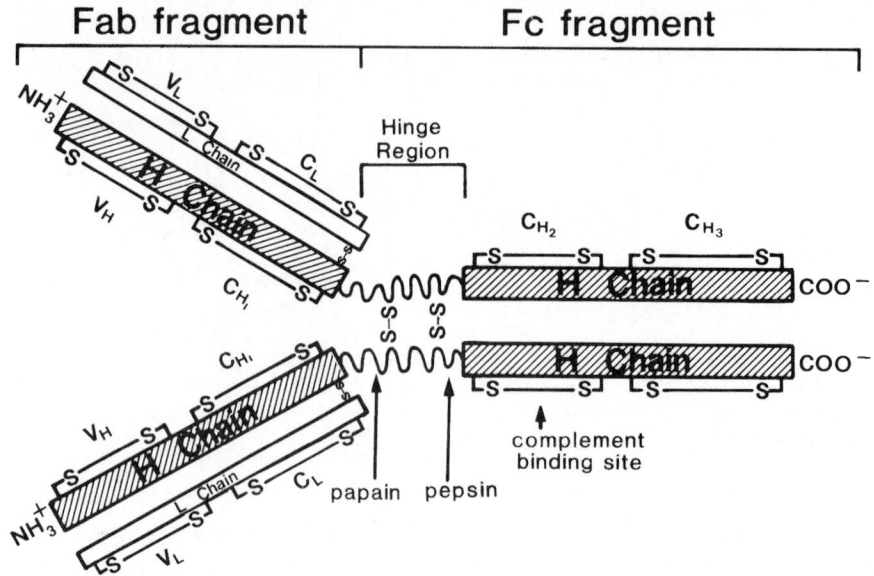

Fig. 11-2 Diagram of IgG molecule (immunoglobulin monomer). *H*, Heavy chain; *L*, light chain; *V*, variable region; *C*, constant region; *S—S*, disulfide bonds. *Arrows,* Papain and pepsin cleavage sites. *NH_3^+* indicates N-terminus, and *COO^-* indicates C-terminus of immunoglobulin.

molecule on the N-terminal side of the disulfide bonds, yielding three fragments of approximately equal size. Two of these fragments are identical and retain the antigen-binding capacity associated with an intact immunoglobulin molecule. The fragments with the antibody-combining site *(Fab fragments)* are each composed of an entire light chain and a portion of the heavy chain. The third fragment has no antigen-binding activity and is crystallizable *(Fc fragment)*. The Fc fragment retains the other biological activities associated with immunoglobulin molecules: interaction with the complement system and binding to tissue. The Fc fragment is composed of the C-terminal half of the heavy chain.

Digestion with pepsin cleaves the antibody molecule on the C-terminal side of the disulfide bonds. This digestion results in the $F(ab')_2$ fragment composed of the two Fab fragments linked by disulfide bonds. The remainder of the molecule undergoes extensive degradation.

V and C regions. Each polypeptide chain is composed of *domains,* or peptide sequences of uniform size (100 to 110 amino acid residues), that contain intrachain disulfide bonds. The domain of the N-terminal or antibody-combining site is more variable in its amino acid sequence than the rest of the polypeptide chain and is called the *variable region* (V region). The sequence and the spatial folding of the polypeptide chain are responsible for antibody specificity and affinity. The remainder of the polypeptide chain is composed of domains that are similar in immunoglobulin molecules of the same and other species. These domains are termed *constant regions* (C regions). Light chains

are composed of one variable and one constant region (V_L and C_L). Heavy chains are composed of one variable and three or four constant regions (V_H and C_{H1-4}) (see Fig. 11-2).

The specific amino acid sequences of the variable regions of the light and heavy chains of an antibody molecule confer a unique three-dimensional structure to the antigen-binding potential antibody. These sequences are termed the *idiotype* of the molecule. The idiotype is determined by the antigenic determinant to which the antibody is directed. The structure of the idiotype permits the complementary fit of the antigenic determinant to the antibody-combining site.

Light-chain types. There are two types of light chains found in immunoglobulin molecules, kappa (κ) and lambda (λ). Kappa and lambda light chains differ in the amino acid sequence of their constant regions. A given antibody molecule always has two identical kappa light chains or two identical lambda light chains. An antibody molecule can never have both a kappa and a lambda light chain together. In human serum the ratio of kappa to lambda antibody molecules is approximately 2:1.

Heavy-chain types. Five types of heavy chains are distinguished in humans, based on structural differences in the constant regions of the chains. These structural differences permit functional differences. The heavy-chain types are designated gamma (γ), alpha (α), mu (μ), delta (δ), and epsilon (ϵ). The heavy-chain types vary in molecular weight. The gamma, alpha, and delta heavy chains are composed of three constant regions. The mu and epsilon

Table 11-1   Properties of human immunoglobulin classes

Properties	IgG	IgA	IgM	IgD	IgE
Heavy chain	γ	α	μ	δ	ϵ
Subclasses	1 to 4	1 and 2	1 and 2	None	None
Light chain	κ and λ	κ and λ	κ and λ	κ and λ	κ and λ
Form	Monomer	Monomer and dimer	Pentamer (some monomer may circulate)	Monomer	Monomer
Formula	$\gamma_2\kappa_2$ or $\gamma_2\lambda_2$	$\alpha_2\kappa_2$ or $\alpha_2\lambda_2$	$\mu_{10}\kappa_{10}$ or $\mu_{10}\lambda_{10}$	$\delta_2\kappa_2$ or $\delta_2\lambda_2$	$\epsilon_2\kappa_2$ or $\epsilon_2\lambda_2$
J chain	No	On dimer	On pentamer	No	No
Molecular weight in daltons (approximate)	150,000	Monomer 160,000 Dimer 400,000	900,000	180,000	190,000
Complement fixation (classical pathway)	$G_3 > G_1 > G_2$	No	M_1 and M_2	No	No
Crosses placenta	Yes	No	No	No	No
Concentration in serum	8-16 mg/mL	1.4-3.5 mg/mL	0.5-2 mg/mL	Up to 0.14 mg/mL	$\leq$300 ng/mL

heavy chains have four constant regions. The heavy-chain type determines the class of immunoglobulin. In humans there are five immunoglobulin classes, corresponding to the five heavy-chain types: immunoglobulin G (IgG), immunoglobulin A (IgA), immunoglobulin M (IgM), immunoglobulin D (IgD), and immunoglobulin E (IgE) (Table 11-1).

In addition, some immunoglobulin classes have subclasses based on additional amino acid differences in their constant regions. IgG has four subclasses, and IgA and IgM have two subclasses each. The biological properties and concentrations of the subclasses may differ.

Immunoglobulin G

IgG molecules are monomers of the basic immunoglobulin subunit. They are composed of two kappa or two lambda light chains and two gamma heavy chains. IgG molecules may therefore be represented as $\gamma_2\lambda_2$ or $\gamma_2\kappa_2$. Approximately 75% of serum immunoglobulin is IgG. The frequency of IgG subclasses varies as follows: IgG$_1$, 60% to 70%; IgG$_2$, 14% to 20%; IgG$_3$, 4% to 8%; and IgG$_4$, 2% to 6%. There is evidence that antibodies to certain antigens may be restricted in their subclasses. Polysaccharide antigens tend to produce IgG$_2$ and IgG$_4$ antibodies. Antiviral and antinucleoprotein antibodies are found primarily in the IgG$_1$ and IgG$_3$ subclasses.

IgG molecules cross the placenta and are responsible for the immunological defense of the newborn. IgG molecules also fix to the surface of effector cells, which are then capable of antibody-mediated cytotoxic reactions important in protecting the host. IgG molecules bind or "fix" complement, a complex of serum proteins that assists in the lysis or elimination of foreign particles. Complement proteins are bound to the IgG molecule in the midpoint of the heavy chain, near the disulfide bond in the CH$_2$ domain. This area of increased flexibility is called the *hinge region.* After reaction with large antigens, this region undergoes spatial changes to expose the complement-binding site (see Fig. 11-

2). Molecules in the IgG subclasses differ in their ability to fix complement proteins. IgG$_3$ is most active, followed by IgG$_1$, IgG$_2$, and IgG$_4$.

Immunoglobulin M

IgM constitutes approximately 10% of serum immunoglobulins and exists primarily as a pentamer of the basic immunoglobulin structure. The five immunoglobulin monomers are held in a circle by disulfide bonds between H chains of the subunits. In addition, the IgM molecule contains a polypeptide chain, called the *joining* (or *J*) chain, that may help in maintaining its structure. The J chain is a small glycoprotein (15,000 daltons) that is covalently bound to the H chains of the molecule.

IgM is the predominant immunoglobulin in the initial immune response to an antigen. It is the most efficient immunoglobulin in a fixing complement. This efficiency is a result of its pentameric structure. The presence of 10 Fab units conveys on the IgM pentamer molecule a theoretical valency of 10. This means that an IgM molecule should be able to bind 10 antigen molecules simultaneously. Although this value has been computed in some experimental systems, it is not normally observed. Steric hindrance may be responsible for this disparity.

Immunoglobulin A

IgA constitutes approximately 15% of the serum immunoglobulin, but it is the predominant immunoglobulin in body secretions such as saliva, tears, sweat, human milk, and colostrum. In serum, IgA exists in both monomeric and polymeric forms. Polymeric serum IgA possesses the J chain. Secretory IgA exists as a dimer of the basic immunoglobulin unit combined with a J chain and an additional polypeptide chain called the *secretory piece.* The secretory piece is bound to dimeric secretory IgA by strong noncovalent linkages. It is important in secretory transport of the molecule and in its protection from proteolytic digestion in the gut. Secretory IgA provides the first line of defense against local infections and is important in the processing of food antigens in the gut.

Immunoglobulin D

IgD is a monomer of the basic immunoglobulin unit and is present in human serum in trace amounts. In addition, it is expressed on lymphocyte cell surface membranes. The main function of IgD is unknown. It may be involved in lymphocyte differentiation.

Immunoglobulin E

IgE is also a monomeric immunoglobulin. It is present in human serum in very low concentrations. IgE, which binds to cells by means of its Fc portion, is responsible for the physiological manifestations of allergy.

ANTIGEN-ANTIBODY REACTIONS

Antigen-antibody reactions were first recognized by bacteriologists who also surmised that such reactions exhibited specificity. Bacteriologists noted that the serum of patients recovering from infectious diseases could agglutinate the organism responsible for their disease but not unrelated organisms. Serum from persons not exposed to the disease or from patients before they contracted the disease could not agglutinate the same organisms. From such evidence, scientists proposed the existence of antibody molecules, the specificity of their interactions with antigens, and the importance of such interactions in host defense.

The following sections consider the forces involved in antigen-antibody binding, the specificity of the reaction, and the mechanism of the reaction.

Binding forces

The strength of the binding of an antigen to an antibody depends on the complementarity of fit of the antigenic determinant to the antibody idiotype and the resultant electrostatic attraction. It also depends on the sum of weak, noncovalent, intermolecular forces, such as hydrogen bonding, van der Waals forces, and hydrophobic interactions (see Table 53-2). Weak, short-range forces can operate between antigen and antibody if their closeness of fit brings them into proximity with one another.

In solution at physiological pH, charged polar groups on the amino acid residues of proteins can be strongly attracted to one another. These electrostatic forces are the strongest and most important contributors to noncovalent attraction between antigen and antibody.

Hydrogen bonding between the amino and carboxy groups of peptide bonds also contributes to the attractive forces. Hydrogen bonds are weaker than electrostatic forces, but their numbers make them an important factor.

Van der Waals forces are the weakest forces involved. They can function only within a very small radius because of their low power. The increasing approximation of anti-

genic determinant to idiotype induces charge fluctuations within the atoms of the molecules. At very close distances the nucleus of one atom can be attracted to the external orbit electrons of a second atom. These van der Waals forces contribute to binding strength.

The final component of the attractive forces involves hydrophobic bonding between apolar groups in solution. Hydrophobic bonding functions by the exclusion of polar water molecules to bring hydrophobic molecules together. Such interactions also serve to attract polar water molecules to hydrophilic amino acid residues on protein molecules. Antibody molecules have increased numbers of hydrophobic amino acid residues such as alanine, leucine, tyrosine, tryptophan, and methionine in their antibody-combining sites, where they enhance bonding to hydrophobic residues in antigenic determinants.

Antibody affinity

The strength of the binding of a single antigenic determinant to an antibody is a function of the closeness of fit and is called *antibody affinity.* Antibody affinity is an expression of the attraction between molecules of antibody and antigen. It is a function of the sum of the short-range, noncovalent, intermolecular forces.

Binding of antigen to antibody is a reversible reaction. The equilibrium of the reaction favors antigen-antibody association if the fit between molecules is good and the forces binding the molecules together are relatively strong and stable. The strength of the association between antigen and antibody is represented by the association constant, which may be derived as follows:

$$Ag + Ab \underset{k_2}{\overset{k_1}{\rightleftharpoons}} Ag \cdot Ab \qquad \textit{Eq. 11-1}$$

$$\frac{[Ag \cdot Ab]}{[Ag][Ab]} = K_a \text{ (Association constant)} \qquad \textit{Eq. 11-2}$$

To study these reactions, one places solutions of a small antigen, or hapten, on either side of a semipermeable membrane. As the hapten diffuses across the membrane, the reaction proceeds to the right of equation 11-1; that is, hapten and antibody associate to form complexes. Eventually, equilibrium is reached. At equilibrium, the rate of the forward reaction and the rate of the reverse reaction are constant. One rate constant, k_1, expresses the tendency of the reaction to move toward the right, or the tendency for association. The other rate constant, k_2, expresses the tendency of the reaction to move to the left, or the tendency for dissociation. These reaction-rate constants differ for each antigen and antibody pair. The concentrations of antigen, antibody, and complex at equilibrium are described by equation 11-2. The equilibrium constant, K_a, expresses the tendency of the reaction to favor association between antigen and antibody.

Heterogeneity of immune response

Analysis of the binding of a simple hapten containing a single antigenic determinant shows variation in binding strength of antibody molecules. Immunization with a single antigenic determinant produces a variety of antibodies with different antibody-combining sites and with a range of antibody affinities. This is termed the *heterogeneity* of the immune response. Because haptens are three dimensional, the immune system produces antibodies that have different areas of contact (Fig. 11-3). The antibody presents differing distributions of charged and hydrophobic residues, resulting in varying closeness of fit of hapten with each different antibody.

Antibody avidity

In natural situations *in vivo* a variety of antibody molecules are generated in response to a large number of multivalent antigenic stimuli. Thus there are two areas of complexity: (1) multiple antibodies generated to different conformations on a single antigenic determinant and (2) multiple antigenic determinants on a single natural antigen. Both of these generate the *diversity* of the immune response. The measure of binding strength of antibodies to multiple antigenic determinants on natural antigens is termed *avidity*. Avidity is a measure of the stability of the antigen-antibody complex. It is partially dependent on the affinity of each antibody for its complementary antigenic determinant. There is an enhanced effect, however, with multivalent antigens. The sum of the binding is greater than its individual parts because of the reversible nature of antigen-antibody bonds and because of the divalent nature of IgG molecules or the multivalent nature of IgM molecules. If the single bond between

antigen and antibody dissociates, the antigen escapes. If an antigen has two antigenic determinants, each of which is bound by antibody, the antigen is kept in place until the broken bond re-forms (Fig. 11-4). Thus avidity is a measure of the stability of the multivalent antigen–multivalent antibody complex.

Cross-reactivity

Cross-reactivity of antigen and antibody is a by-product of the heterogeneity of the immune response. As stated previously, immunization with a simple hapten produces a variety of antibodies of differing affinities. Some of these antibodies will combine with chemically related and structurally similar haptens. The reactivity of an antibody to a different antigen may also indicate that the two antigens in question share a previously unknown but common antigenic determinant. Thus cross-reactivity may result from similar or identical antigenic determinants in different antigens. Such cross-reactivity is often observed with antibodies produced to such drugs as penicillin. The reactivity of an antibody with penicillin may be very high, but metabolic derivatives containing the basic drug structure may also react with an antibody produced to the complete drug.

In cases of prolonged antigenic challenge, such as that occurring in natural infection, the initial response is with low-affinity, low-specificity molecules, which may react with other closely related antigens. With time, animals exhibit a natural selection for clones of plasma cells producing high-affinity antibodies. As the heterogeneity of the antibody response narrows, the specificity of antigen-antibody reactions increases. This adaptation of the immune re-

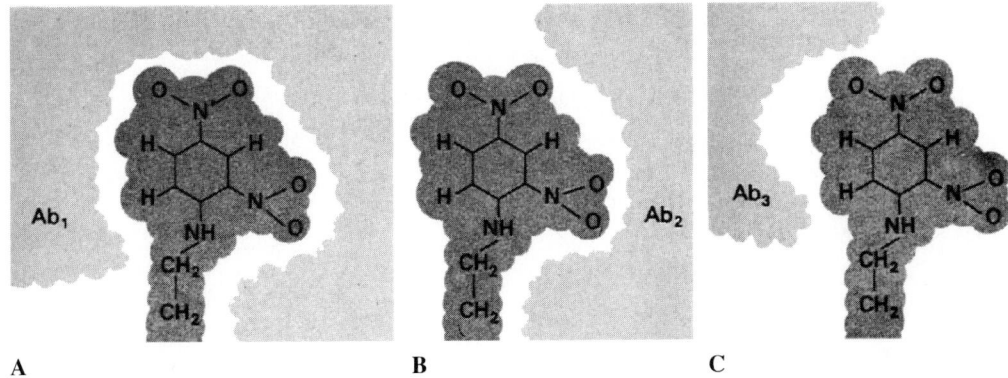

A   B   C

Fig. 11-3 Binding of antibodies present in the same antiserum with different affinities to same hapten (dinitrobenzene linked to amino group of lysine). **A,** Antibody₁ fits with nearly whole hapten and is thus of high affinity. **B,** Antibody₂ fits with less of molecule and not so closely and has a moderate binding affinity, whereas, **C,** low-affinity antibody₃, is complementary in shape to so little of hapten surface that its binding energy is very little above that occurring between completely unrelated proteins. Only a portion of antibody-combining site is shown. (From Roitt I: *Essential immunology,* ed 4, Oxford, England, 1980, Blackwell Scientific Publications.)

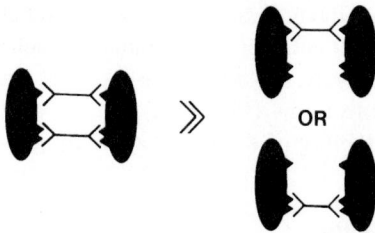

Fig. 11-4 Multivalent bonding of antigen-antibody increases bonding strength. A single bond created by divalent antibody molecules between a single antigenic determinant on two adjacent antigens is much weaker than binding created by two divalent antibodies bound simultaneously to two unique antigenic determinants on two adjacent antigens. Strength and complexity of this multivalent bonding are described by the term *avidity*.

sponse promotes effective protection of the host against infection.

Genetic basis of antibody diversity

The heterogeneity of the immune response or the variety of antibodies produced to a single antigen is known to be genetically determined. The variable (V) regions of light and heavy chains of the antibody molecule encode for antibody specificity. Some positions in the amino acid sequence of the V region have an even more increased likelihood of amino acid variation. These *hypervariable regions,* scattered throughout the amino acid sequence of the V region, are brought into proximity to each other by the natural folding (tertiary structure) of the antibody molecule. The amino acid sequence dictates possible attraction between polar amino acid residues, as well as the possibility of intrachain disulfide bonds. The approximation of hypervariable regions by the folding of the antibody mol-

ecule results in the formation of the antibody-combining site.

ANTIGEN-ANTIBODY PRECIPITATION REACTIONS

The primary reaction of antigen with antibody is usually detected by secondary manifestations of the reaction. The nature of the secondary manifestations depends on experimental conditions, the class of antibody involved in the reaction, the number of antigenic determinants on the antigen, and the size and solubility of the antigen. The reaction of antibody with soluble molecules possessing multiple antigenic determinants that permit cross-linking is detected by *precipitation* of the complex out of solution. The term *flocculation* may be used to describe a precipitation reaction that produces a large, loosely bound precipitate. The reaction of antibodies with large, particulate, multivalent antigens is detected by *agglutination* of the antigen. These reactions are considered separately.

Precipitation curve

When a known quantity of antibody is present in solution in a series of tubes to which increasing amounts of antigen are added, precipitation occurs in some of the test tubes. When the amount of precipitate is measured and correlated with the amount of antigen present, one obtains a curve similar to that shown in Fig. 11-5.

In the first phase of the reaction, called the *antibody-excess phase,* no free antigen (an antigen without bound antibody) can be detected in the fluid and essentially no precipitate can be found. Free (unbound) antibody can be detected, however. As increasing amounts of antigen are added, the amount of precipitate increases until a point of maximum precipitation is reached. At this point, no free antigen or free antibody can be detected in the fluid. This is called the *zone of equivalence.* As the amount of antigen

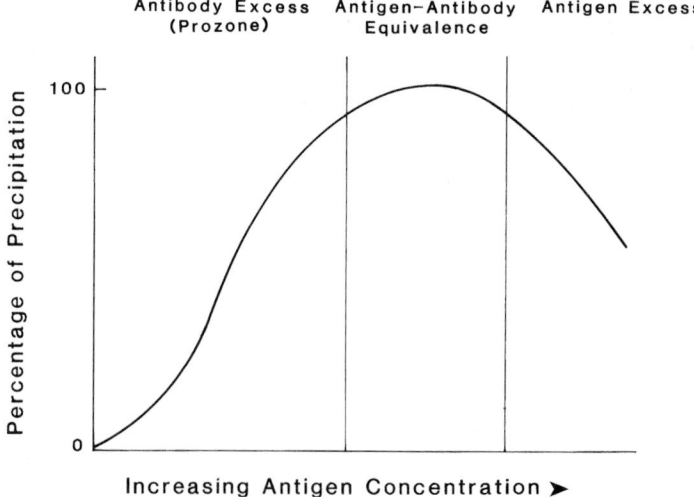

Fig. 11-5 Quantitative precipitin curve in which amount of antibody-antigen complex that precipitates is plotted as function of antigen concentration.

added continues to increase, the amount of precipitate detected diminishes. Examination of the fluid phase of the reaction at this time shows no free antibody but increasing amounts of free antigen. This area of the curve is called the *antigen-excess phase.*

Lattice theory

Antigen-antibody complexes precipitate out of solution because of the multivalent nature of both molecules. The reaction of antigens possessing multiple antigenic determinants and antibodies with two (as in IgG) or more (as in IgM) antibody-combining sites produces a lattice of interlocking molecules. Antibody molecules can cross-link antigenic sites on the same or different molecules of antigen. As the size and complexity of the lattice increase, the lattice becomes insoluble and precipitates out of solution (Fig. 11-6).

In the antibody-excess zone, a single molecule of antigen binds to each antibody molecule. The excess of antibody ensures that each molecule of antigen can encounter a free antibody molecule. The absence of cross-linking produces small soluble complexes.

As the antigen concentration increases and the zone of equivalence is entered, complexes of increasing size with increasing levels of cross-linking are formed. Such large, complex lattices precipitate out of solution.

As the antigen concentration continues to increase, the zone of antigen excess is reached. In this portion of the curve, smaller complexes are again seen. The size of the lattice decreases because there is sufficient antigen to permit binding of a free antigen molecule to each antibody-combining site. At high concentrations of antigen, lack of precipitation can result in false-negative results. Obviously, detection of antigen by antibody precipitation requires optimum concentration of both reactants. Formation of lattices best suited for precipitation occurs at an equal equivalent concentration of antigen and antibody or at a slight antigen excess.

Other factors affecting precipitation

The precipitation of antigen-antibody complexes out of solution can be affected by factors other than the ratio of antigen concentration to antibody concentration. Different antibody molecules can precipitate the same antigen to varying degrees. The efficiency of the antibody depends on its affinity and specificity. The charge and shape of the antigen-antibody complex are also important. Highly charged complexes are difficult to precipitate. The best precipitates are observed with protein antigens with molecular weights from 40,000 to 160,000 daltons. Proteins in this range are easily cross-linked by multivalent antibody molecules. Polysaccharide antigens, denatured proteins, and viruses produce broader precipitation curves. Their large size sterically hinders cross-linking. Precipitation can also be affected by temperature, pH, and ionic concentration. Such factors influence antigen-antibody interactions on a molecular level.

Precipitation reactions in gel

Precipitation reactions are frequently carried out in a gel-support matrix composed of agar or the more purified polysaccharide, agarose. The agar prevents convective mixing of antigen and antibody and thereby ensures establishment of concentration gradients of the two reactants. Precipitation in agar is only a moderately sensitive technique when compared with newer advances, such as radioimmunoassay, but it is widely employed because of its ease and versatility. In addition, precipitation reactions in gels can be modified to permit the study of antigenic relationships

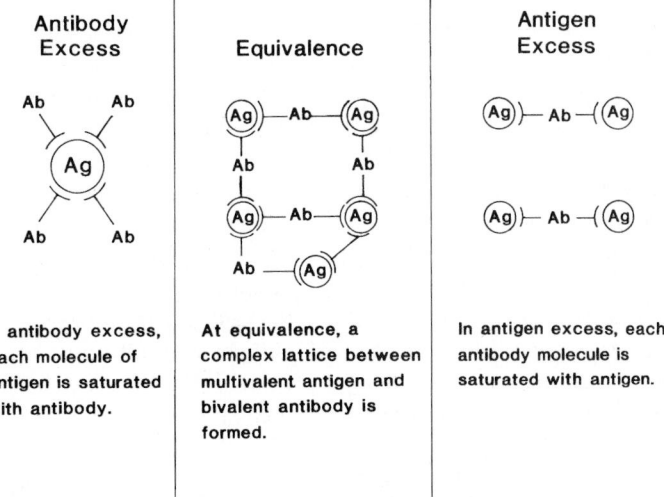

Fig. 11-6 Representation of sizes of molecular complexes formed at varying ratios of antigen and antibody.

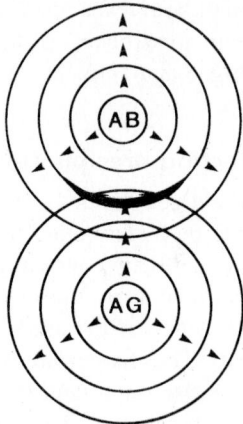

Fig. 11-7 Depiction of radial protein gradients in Ouchterlony immunodiffusion. Concentric circles represent decreasing protein concentrations. Both antigen *(AG)* and antibody *(AB)* diffuse radially from application wells. Precipitation, *heavy black arc,* occurs at point of antigen-antibody equivalence. Precipitin line is closer to well of lower concentration and concave toward reagent of higher molecular weight.

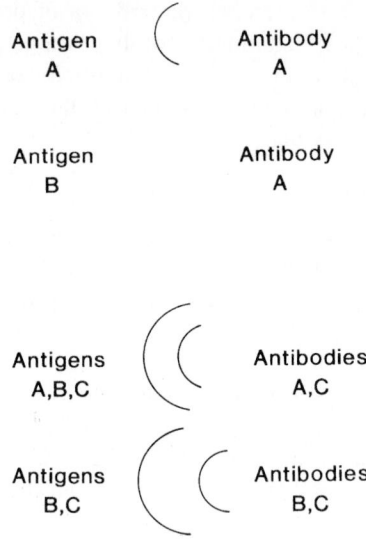

Fig. 11-8 Precipitation occurs at equivalence point of antigen with corresponding antibody. Multiple precipitation lines are seen with multiple antigens and corresponding multiple antibodies.

among different compounds. The following section discusses two gel-precipitation reactions, double immunodiffusion and radial immunodiffusion.

Double immunodiffusion. In double-immunodiffusion reactions, or *Ouchterlony technique,* agar or agarose is poured onto a solid support, such as a glass slide or petri dish. Wells are then cut into the agar. Antigen and antibody solutions are placed into separate wells. The solutions then diffuse toward one another in the gel in a radial fashion during room-temperature incubation (Fig. 11-7). With diffusion into the agar, the solutions establish concentration gradients that diminish with distance from the well. At the point of antigen-antibody equivalence at the interface of the diffusing fronts, a precipitation line is formed (see Fig. 11-7). The positioning and shape of the line are dictated by the concentration of the reactants and the size of the molecules. The line will be closer to the well with the reactant of lower concentration because the distance traveled is directly proportional to concentration. The rate of diffusion is also inversely proportional to molecular size. High-molecular-weight compounds, such as IgM, diffuse more slowly than lower-molecular-weight substances, such as IgG. The precipitation line that is formed at the interface of the two-concentration gradients will be concave to the higher-molecular-weight compound, whose diffusion rate is slower. Because precipitation occurs at a range of antigen-antibody equivalence to slight antigen excess, an inappropriate ratio of antigen to antibody will result in failure to form a precipitate.

The presence of different antigenic determinants on the same or different molecules can be detected by the production of more than one precipitation line if the antiserum used contains antibodies against the multiple antigens (Fig. 11-

8). Two antigens in the antigen solution will create two independent concentration gradients as they diffuse into the agar. Precipitation will occur at the point of equivalence of each antigen with its corresponding antibody. In this way the components of an antigen mixture can be studied.

Ouchterlony testing also permits analysis of the relationship between two antigenic mixtures. The antibody solution is placed in a center well, which is surrounded by several wells into which antigen solutions are placed. Unrelated antigens that have corresponding antibodies in the antibody solution will form separate precipitation lines corresponding to their distinct components. Radial diffusion from the adjacent wells causes superimposition of the two gradients, but because the concentration gradients of the antigens are independent, two separate and distinct lines are formed (Fig. 11-9). The double spurs formed at the two antigen interfaces are the hallmark of the *reaction of nonidentity.* The two antigens or antigen mixtures have nothing in common in relationship to the antibody solution used.

Two identical antigen solutions that are tested with their common antibody result in a *reaction of identity* (see Fig. 11-9). Precipitation lines form at their separate but adjacent points of equivalence against antibody. Because diffusion through the gel is radial, an area of shared and common antigen concentration between the two adjacent wells is formed. For this reason, there is fusion of the two separate precipitation lines. This fusion or reaction of identity indicates that the antigen solutions are identical with respect to the antibody employed or that the antigen solutions have one antigenic determinant in common. It does not imply molecular identity. If antigen concentrations in the adjacent wells differ, a common fused precipitation line is still

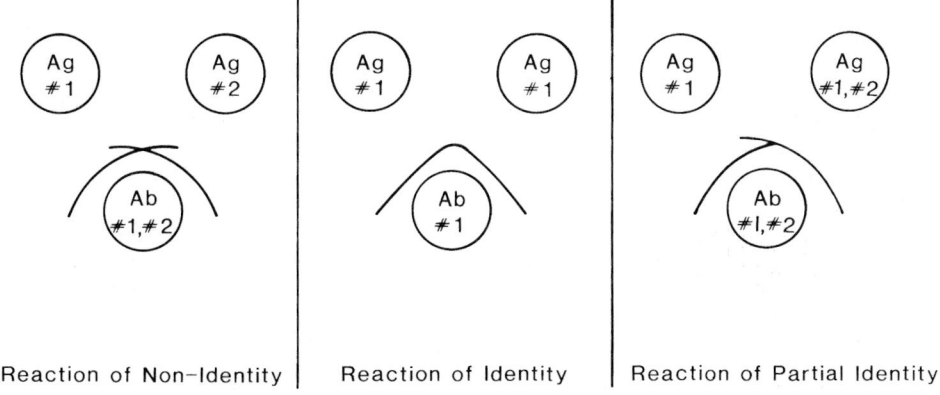

Fig. 11-9 Double-immunodiffusion patterns. *Ag,* Antigen; *Ab,* antibody; *heavy line,* pre-cipitin line; *circles,* application wells.

Well Content

1. Antigen A
2. Unknown
3. Unknown
4. Antigen B

Well Content

1. Antigen A
2. Unknown
3. Antigen B + Unknown
4. Unknown

Well Content

1. Unknown
2. Unknown
3. Antigen A + Unknown
4. Antigen B

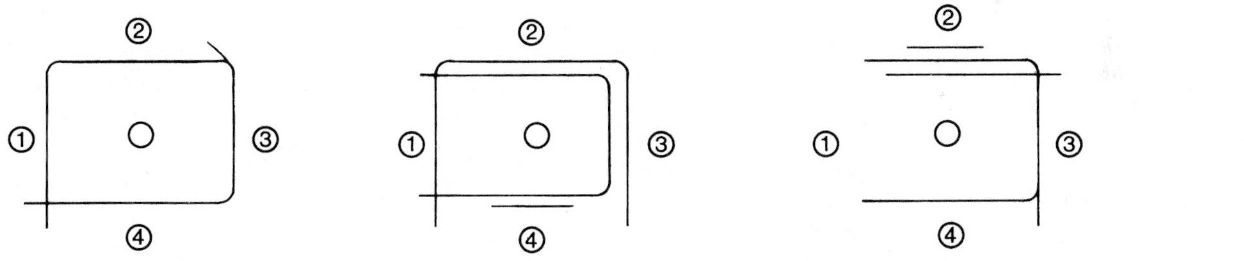

Conclusions:

  # 2 = Antigen A
  # 3 = Antigen A + Antigen B

Conclusions:

  #2 = Antigen A + Antigen B
  #3 = Antigen A + Antigen B
  #4 = Antigen B + Antigen C

Conclusions:

  # 1 = contains no antigens
      recognized by antisera
      or reagent concentrations
      are not correct
  Antigen A and B are the same
  #2 = contains antigen A plus
      antigens C and D
  #3 = contains A and E

Fig. 11-10 Interpretations of double-immunodiffusion patterns. Center well contains an antiserum to several possible antigens. Surrounding wells contain test antigens. *Heavy lines,* Precipitin reaction.

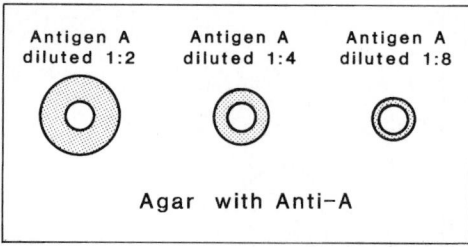

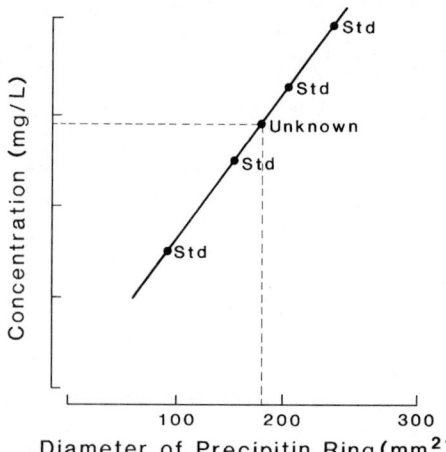

Fig. 11-11 Radial immunodiffusion patterns. Band of precipitation, *stippled area,* extends as a disk from center of each circular well. Area of precipitation is proportional to concentration.

Fig. 11-12 Graph of concentration of antigen expressed as milligrams per liter versus square of diameter of precipitin ring. *Std,* Standard.

formed at the point of average concentration of the two antigen fronts.

A *reaction of partial identity* is seen when adjacent wells share some but not all the antigens detected by the antibody solution. A reaction of partial identity is a reaction of nonidentity superimposed on a reaction of identity (see Fig. 11-9). A common fused line is formed by reaction of the shared antigen. A second identical equivalence point between the novel antibody and a common antigen creates a superimposed precipitation line that extends into the common area between the adjacent wells. The second antigen creates a concentration gradient that is not contributed to by the adjacent well. The spur indicates that the second antigen solution lacks an antigenic determinant present in the first antigen solution that is recognized by the antibody solution. The spur always points to the well of the antigen that is monospecific with respect to the antibody.

Two double-immunodiffusion patterns that show a complex relationship of antigen and antibody solutions are presented and discussed in Fig. 11-10.

Radial immunodiffusion. Radial immunodiffusion, the *Mancini technique,* is a precipitation reaction carried out by application of antigen solution to a gel that has been impregnated with a monospecific antibody solution. It is an adaptation of a gel-precipitation reaction that permits quantitation of antigen. The antibody-gel solution is applied to a solid support. Wells are then cut into the agar, and dilutions of antigen are placed in the wells. The antigen diffuses out radially into the agar. This diffusion produces a concentration gradient that is inversely proportional to the distance from the well. Antibody concentration within the gel is constant. At the point where antigen and antibody concentrations are equivalent, precipitation occurs. Because diffusion from the well is radial, the precipitation appears as a ring around the well. The precipitation reaction is not

a static but a dynamic one. The precipitation ring first forms close to the well at the initial point of antigen-antibody equivalence. As antigen continues to diffuse from the well, antigen excess causes conversion of the precipitate to soluble complexes that resolubilize and continue to diffuse outward. A new ring is formed at a new point of antigen-antibody equivalence. The square of the diameter of the ring (mm^2) is directly proportional to antigen concentration. The thickness of the ring is a function of the final concentration of antigen-antibody complexes at the equivalence point (Fig. 11-11).

With constant sample volume, temperature, pH, incubation time, and antibody concentration, an unknown antigen concentration can be determined. This is accomplished when one compares the square of the diameter of the precipitation ring of the unknown rings obtained by several dilutions of a standard antigen solution. When the concentrations of the diluted standard are plotted against ring area, the concentration of the unknown can be easily determined (Fig. 11-12).

BIBLIOGRAPHY

Gosling JP: A decade of development in immunoassay methodology, *Clin Chem* 36(8):1408-1427, 1990.

Roitt IM, Brostoff J, Male DK: *Immunology,* St. Louis, 1985, Mosby.

Butt WR, editor: *Practical immunoassay,* New York, 1984, Marcel Dekker.

Keren DF: *High resolution electrophoresis and immunofixation,* ed 2, Boston, 1994, Butterworth.

Weir DM et al, editors: *Immunochemistry,* ed 4, Oxford, England, 1986, Blackwell Scientific Publications.

CHAPTER 12

Immunochemical techniques

Carolyn S. Feldkamp

OBJECTIVES

- For each of the following techniques, state the principle of the immunoreaction, describe sample requirements and preparation, list common pitfalls, and explain the interpretation of results:
    Immunoelectrophoresis
    Counterimmunoelectrophoresis
    Two-dimensional immunoelectrophoresis
    Laurell rocket immunoelectrophoresis
    Immunonephelometry
    Western blot
- State the sample requirements and preparation and list common pitfalls for the Ouchterlony and radial immunodiffusion techniques.
- Define agglutination and differentiate between direct agglutination, indirect agglutination, and agglutination-inhibition reactions.
- Describe the principles of solid-phase, "sandwich" assays, distinguishing between those that measure antigen and those that measure antibody.
- List the labels used for "sandwich" assays, comparing their

sensitivity and their ability to be used in heterogeneous and homogeneous assays.

agglutination Clumping or aggregating together by specific antibody of particles, such as red blood cells or latex beads, to which the specific antigenic determinant is attached.

agglutinin Specific antibody that causes agglutination.

antiantibody An antibody with specificity for immunoglobulins.

antibody absorption The process of removing or tying up nonspecific undesired antibody in an antiserum reagent by allowing it to react with nonspecific antigens before using it as reagent.

antibody reagent A high-titer, high-affinity, IgG-class antibody prepared in animals for use in immunoassays.

antigen reagent A stabilized solution containing a known amount of an antigen that is used as a standard.

cold agglutinin An agglutinin that reacts better at temperatures less than body temperature; best reaction is usually at 4° C.

complement A group of serum proteins activated as a result of an antibody-antigen reaction. When the reaction is on the surface of a red blood cell, the activated complement can lyse the cell.

complement fixation A term applied to a set of assays in which complement is activated or "fixed" by a test reaction system.

Coombs' test A type of agglutination reaction. A direct Coombs' test measures the presence of antibody on cells; an indirect test measures its presence in serum.

counterimmunoelectrophoresis An assay in which antigen and antibody migrate toward each other under the influence of an electric field. The presence of antigen is observed by the formation of a precipitin line.

cryoglobulin Protein that precipitates at temperatures less than body temperature; precipitates maximally at 4° C.

fluoroimmunoassay Any immunoprocedure that uses a fluorescent molecule as the indicator label.

hemolysin Anti–sheep red blood cell antibody.

heterogeneous immunoassay Any technique that uses two phases, usually liquid and solid, to separate reacted from unreacted components.

immobilization The fixation of antigen or antibody onto a solid support such as a plastic tube or microtiter plate.

immunodiffusion Random, spreading movement of antibody or antigen or both in a support medium.

immunoelectrophoresis An immunoprecipitation technique in which antigens are separated from each other by migration in an electric field, followed by reaction with antibody by immunodiffusion.

indicator phase The portion of an immunochemical reaction that can be measured.

inhibition assay A term for those types of immunoassays in which an excess of antigens prevents or inhibits the completion of either the initial or indicator phase of the reaction.

monoclonal antibody A monospecific antibody that is produced by a single plasma cell or a single clone of plasma cells of a lymphocyte myeloma hybrid.

monospecific An antibody that will react with only one type of antigen molecule.

nephelometric assay Measurement of antigen or antibody by determination of the amount of light scattered as the result of the amount or rate of antibody-antigen aggregation.

nephelometric inhibition assay (NINIA) Measurement of haptens by inhibition of formation of an antibody-antigen lattice.

nephelometry Measurement of light-scattering properties of large particles (such as antigen-antibody complexes) in solution.

Ouchterlony double diffusion A version of the original gel diffusion technique invented by Oudin in which antigen and antibody in separate wells are allowed to spread (diffuse) toward each other.

polyclonal antibody Heterogeneous antibodies with diverse affinities produced by a large number of plasma cells.

prozone phenomenon Apparently lower reactivity or nonreactivity caused by a relative antigen excess. May be seen when antibody solution is used at low concentrations.

radial immunodiffusion (Mancini technique) Measurement of antigen concentration by allowing antigen to spread (by diffusion) into agarose containing the desired monospecific antibody. The area of the immunoprecipitin ring is proportional to antigen concentration.

rocket (Laurell) immunoelectrophoresis Assay system in which the antigen, under the influence of an electric field, migrates into agarose containing antibody, with a resultant immunoprecipitation reaction. The precipitin lines appear rocket shaped.

sandwich assay A term applied to a solid-phase immunoassay in which the first layer is immobilized antibody, the second is antigen, and the third is labeled antibody.

specificity Property of an antibody molecule that restricts its reactivity to a defined molecule or group of molecules.

titer Maximum dilution of a specific antibody that gives a measurable reaction with a specific antigen; usually expressed as the reciprocal of that dilution.

Chapter 11 describes the molecular nature of antigens and antibodies, as well as the general characteristics of the antigen-antibody reaction. This chapter deals with many techniques that use the antigen-antibody reaction as the basis to detect, characterize, or quantitate constituents in blood and other body fluids submitted to the laboratory for analysis. These constituents can range from small-molecular-weight drugs and their metabolites to large-molecular-weight proteins, such as IgM and alpha$_2$-macroglobulin. Most frequently, the patient's sample contains the antigen (analyte), and antibody is added as the reagent to detect or measure the antigen. In contrast, in cases of infectious disease, serological determinations, and autoimmune antibody testing, the patient's sample is the source of antibody, and it is the antibody measurement that is clinically important. For these determinations, antigen of known composition is used. The antigen may be soluble or tissue based. However, this latter form of testing is usually performed in the immunology section of the laboratory. Because this chapter is directed primarily at those techniques used in the clinical chemistry laboratory, it will concentrate on the procedures that detect antigen in the patient's sample.

REAGENTS
Antibody as reagent

Reagent antibodies are usually prepared in animals, such as rabbits or goats, by the repeated exposure of the animal to foreign substances. A group of cells are stimulated to respond by producing antibodies. Some of the groups of atoms of the immunizing material are the major determinants of the antigen molecule and cause the production of the largest amount of antibodies; minor determinants, however, also stimulate antibody production. Since there are many different antibodies that are attributable to the expansion of several clones of antibody-producing cells, the antiserum thus produced is a *polyclonal* reagent antiserum. For example, an antiserum against the protein human serum albumin (anti-HSA) is a reagent that has multiple antibodies to antigenic determinants or specific molecular configurations that are characteristic and specific for the surface of HSA.

It is important to demonstrate that this anti-HSA will not react with other serum proteins, such as IgG and transferrin. If this anti-HSA is to be used as a reagent in the clinical laboratory, its specificity (that is, its reactivity with only HSA) must be verified in the same immunological test system used to generate patient results. For every reagent antibody, the specificity of its immunochemical reactivity is the single most important factor in the success or failure of any immunological technique used in the clinical laboratory.

Monoclonal antibodies are formed by a technology that hybridizes a single antibody-producing cell (plasma cell) with an immortal cell line. After selecting one of many hundreds of these hybrids, the resulting cell line produces a unique antibody. These antibodies have a single homogeneous primary structure and are called *monoclonal antibodies*. These antibodies provide a reproducible reagent of known specificity and affinity. Monoclonal antibodies are used in competitive binding assays and in tissue assays to identify specific antigens. Fig. 12-1 is a schema of how monoclonal antibodies are produced.

Selection of antibody as a reagent in an immunological procedure requires information about its characteristics such as its strength (titer), affinity, and specificity. Because not all of the immunoglobulin in the antiserum is reactive, the amount of antibody that is available for reactivity in a specific immunological method is termed the "titer of the antibody." The titer is the reciprocal of the maximum dilution of the antibody that gives a detectable reaction for a specific method. The titer of the reagent antibody is often different for each kind of immunological procedure. For example, anti-HSA may react in an immunoprecipitation technique at a maximum dilution of 1:32, but the same antiserum may react at a maximum dilution of 1:6400 in a radioimmunoassay procedure. Occasionally the amount of reagent antibody present may be expressed in weight, that is, milligrams per milliliter. This expression of antibody amount is determined by precipitation techniques and is often helpful in determining the amount of reagent needed. For monoclonal antibodies that are virtually pure, the indicated amount describes the total reactive proteins.

Affinity. Reagent antibodies generally fall into two categories, those of high affinity and those of low affinity. The antibodies in the reagent may be a mixture of both, but one should use reagents where high-affinity antibodies are predominant. This will result in a strong union with the antigen that is not readily reversible and that will not be influenced greatly by alteration of the reaction conditions. Low-affinity antibodies do not bind well with the antigen and can be influenced by temperature, pH, and ionic strength with consequent changes in the reaction, resulting in dissociation of the antibody-antigen complex. Most commercial reagent antibodies are of the high-affinity type. However, if one is preparing reagents, they should be tested to be certain they are of the appropriate, preferably high, affinity.

Specificity. Specificity refers to the ability of the antibody to restrict its reaction to a defined group of molecules. Because these reagents are really a collection of antibodies, they are directed to multiple antigenic determinants on a single antigen and thus could have multiple reactivities. In some cases, other reagent antibodies may react with antigenic determinants that are common to several molecular forms of plasma proteins. For example, a reagent directed to the IgG molecule should recognize only the IgG molecule, but there may be antibody in the reagent that would also react with light chains of that IgG molecule. Because light chains are common to all the immunoglobulin classes (that is, IgA, IgM, and IgD) the reagent antibody would then react with all immunoglobulin molecules. It would not be appropriate to say that it was recognizing only the IgG molecule. The problem of cross-reactivity with other serum proteins can usually be controlled by a technique termed *antibody absorption,* which binds or removes from the reagent that population of antibody reacting inappropriately with other molecules of the test solution. Absorption is necessary for virtually all antibody reagents of the polyclonal type. It is often accomplished by addition of the undesired reacting antigen or by preparation of pure antibody by affinity columns.

Specificity of the reagent antibody is extremely important in the enzyme immunoassays and radioimmunoassays that are frequently used to measure the presence of small molecules such as drugs and hormones. However, often there is a residual reaction between the reagent antibody and a closely related compound. This reaction between antibody and the undesired antigen is termed *cross-reactivity.*

There are times, however, when the cross-reactivity with

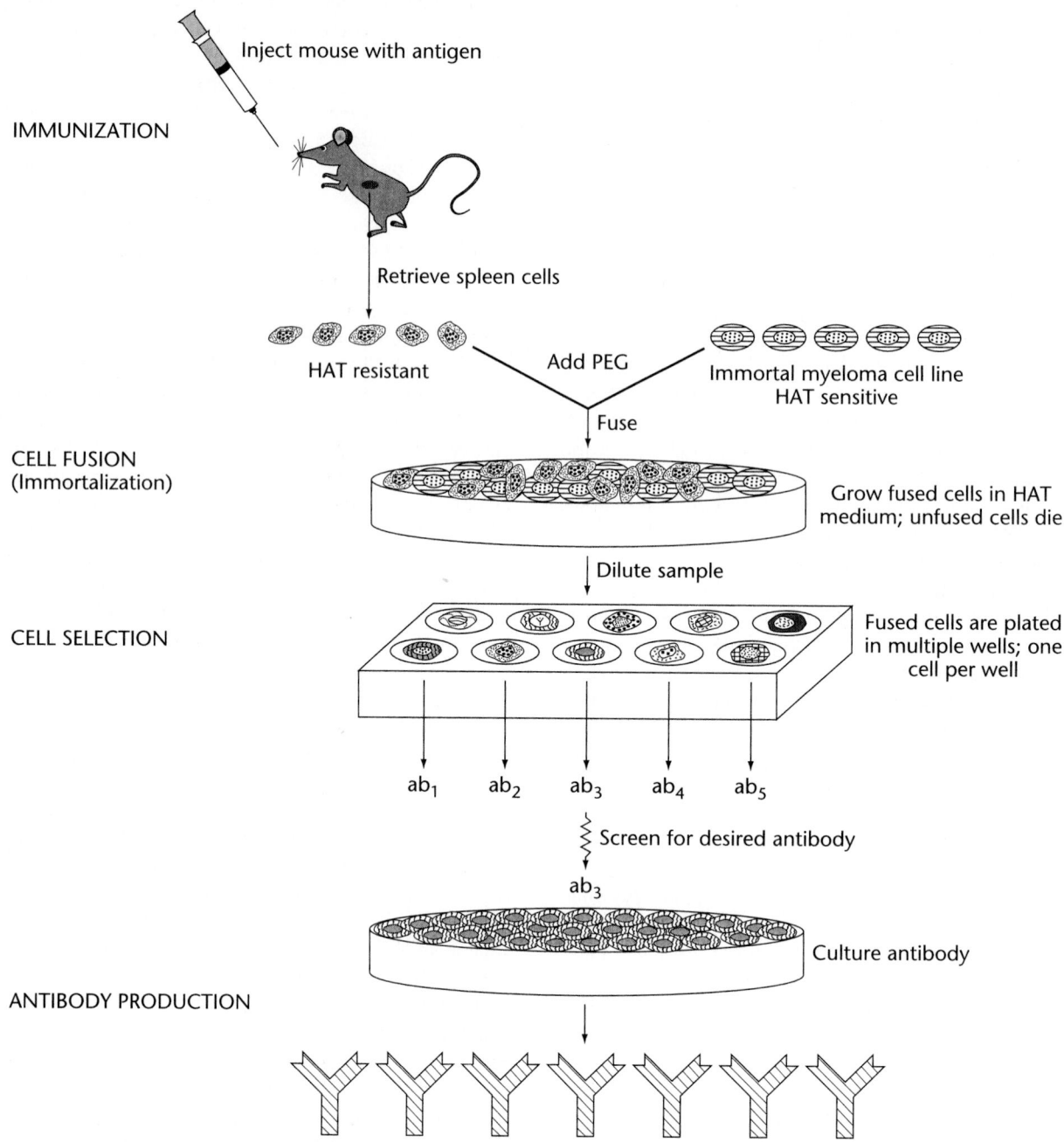

Fig. 12-1 Monoclonal antibody production. Antibody production is initiated by immunization of an animal with antigen. After the immune response, spleen cells are isolated, each of which produces a single, unique antibody. These cells are fused with an immortal myeloma cell line by exposure to polyethylene glycol (PEG). In the culture medium containing HAT (a mixture of hypoxanthine, aminopterin, and thymidine) unfused myeloma cells, which cannot bypass the metabolic block caused by aminopterin, die. Unfused spleen cells also die naturally after 1 to 2 weeks. Fused cells survive having the immortality of the myeloma cells and HAT resistance of the spleen cells. Fused cells are then cultured at high dilution and selected by screening for secretion of antibodies with the desired characteristics. Eventually a culture of antibody-secreting cells derived from a single spleen cell produces reagent amounts of monoclonal antibody.

very similar antigenic determinants cannot be avoided. For example, antibody directed to the small molecule trinitrophenol will cross-react with dinitrophenol. To the antibody, these small-molecular-weight entities look very similar. The only way to establish the specificity of the antibody is to determine the relative affinity of the reagent antibody to presumptive cross-reacting molecules at concentrations likely to occur in patients. Often, particularly in the case of antibody reagents used in therapeutic drug monitoring, the degree of cross-reactivity with the metabolites of the drug and with other drugs is given by the manufacturer.

Because reagent antibody is protein, all precautions to prevent denaturation and degradation should be taken. The reagent should be kept free of bacterial contamination and should be stored in the refrigerator (4° C) if it is to be used within several days. Long-term storage usually is adequate at −20° C.

Antigen as analyte

Numerous naturally occurring molecules or antigens that are protein, glycoprotein, or lipoprotein in nature can be detected and measured easily in biological fluids if specific reagent antibodies are available. In addition, many small molecules, such as drugs and hormones, can be measured. The following box lists examples of the large and small molecules that are frequently measured by immunological techniques. To ensure accurate detection and precise measurement of these molecules using immunological techniques, close attention by the technologist to the proper handling and storage of the biological fluid containing these antigens is necessary.

The biological fluids most commonly available to the laboratory for analysis are serum, urine, and cerebrospinal fluid. Antigens present in each of these fluids are subject to degradation depending on (1) the nature of the antigen, (2) its concentration, (3) its susceptibility to various enzymes in the body fluids, and (4) its relative stability at various storage temperatures (such as room temperature, 4° C, −20° C, and −70° C). Each specimen must be stored and handled properly to ensure that the antigen molecule is unaltered and

the reagent antibody can react with the appropriate antigenic determinants on the molecule. Stability of antigens must be established for each biological fluid. For example, the C4 component of complement of serum is stable and can be measured accurately up to a week after receipt of the serum if the specimen is stored at 4° C before analysis. However, the C4 component of cerebrospinal fluid is very labile and is usually present at very low concentrations. If this kind of sample is stored more than 8 hours at 4° C before analysis, the C4 will have been degraded and will be unmeasurable. Thus spinal fluid must be frozen and stored at −70° C to ensure that the C4 will not be degraded before measurement. Another example is that of antigen denaturation in urine specimens. Because most urine specimens are acidic, immunological measurement of various proteins is often suspect. Proteins are degraded in an acid pH, and many antigenic determinants on these proteins are lost. Beta$_2$-microglobulin is a protein found in both urine and plasma. In urine it is used to estimate renal tubular dysfunction. It is rapidly destroyed if the pH of urine is less than 6.0. Quantitation of specific proteins in urine samples requires immediate neutralization of the acid pH at the time of collection. In contrast, the protein is stable for a week in serum stored at 4° C. The problems associated with specific protein measurement and antigen degradation are not so acute when small molecules are measured, but it is always good laboratory practice to store biological fluids at 4° C if the analysis is to be performed on the same day and in a frozen state if the analysis is to be performed much later.

It should be emphasized that the immunological reactivity of a molecule may not be related to its biological activity. The importance of this distinction is illustrated by the immunological measurement of alpha$_1$-antitrypsin and C3, the third component of complement. Alpha$_1$-antitrypsin is a potent inhibitor of the proteolytic enzyme trypsin, and its production is under genetic control. In certain individuals there occur genetic variations in which the molecule is estimated to be present at normal levels when measured by immunochemical techniques, but the molecule's enzyme-

---

Examples of Molecules in Biological Fluids Frequently Measured by Immunological Techniques

Large molecules	Small molecules
Immunoglobulins (IgG, IgA, IgM, IgD, IgE)	Digoxin and digitonin
Complement components (C3, C4, factor B)	Antibiotics
Coagulation factors (factor VIII, fibrinogen)	Cytotoxic drugs
Lipoproteins	Prostaglandins
Protein hormones	Hormones (steroids, thyroid hormones)
Acute-phase proteins (α_1-antitrypsin, C-reactive protein)	Theophylline
Albumin	Anticonvulsant drugs
Selected urine and cerebrospinal fluid proteins	Antiarrhythmic drugs
Viral antigens	Drugs of abuse

inhibiting capability is greatly impaired. Immunochemically the genetic variants react as well as the normally functioning molecule does; however, there is a great biological difference. Another example, C3, is a reasonably stable molecule in serum, but in other body fluids, such as joint fluid and cerebrospinal fluid, the C3 molecule may not be present as an intact molecule. When levels of C3 are obtained by immunological methods, they can appear to be normal or increased when, in fact, there is a low level of the complete molecule. This discrepancy is attributable to the reaction of antibody with the breakdown products of C3, which retain the appropriate antigenic determinants. Examples of immunological reactivity without biological activity occur frequently and demonstrate that normal levels of molecules assayed by immunological methods do not necessarily predict normal functional activity.

Qualitative and quantitative measurements of antigen in biological fluids require the use of a highly specific reagent antibody and a known reference standard of antigen. The reactivity of the antibody with the antigen in the patient's biological fluid is compared to the reactivity of the antibody with the standard antigen. For the most part, standards are supplied in immunological test kits. If these test kits are approved by the Food and Drug Administration, the technologist is reasonably assured that the reagent antibody is detecting the antigen, as stated by the manufacturer. However, it is good practice when using immunological methods to evaluate the test system with reference antigen obtained from other sources. The World Health Organization supplies reference antigen for many of the serum proteins as primary standards. Secondary standards have been developed by the College of American Pathologists in collaboration with the Centers for Disease Control and Prevention (CDC) and are easily available. These reference materials provide the technologist with a level of confidence that the laboratory is providing valid measurements of antigens in biological fluids (Table 12-1). Federal regulations established in the Clinical Laboratories Improvement Act of 1988 (CLIA '88) define laboratory requirements to validate accuracy and precision of clinical assays. Manufacturers' data may be used for kits used with no modification. Otherwise, thorough documentation of accuracy, precision, linearity, sensitivity, and normal ranges must be maintained. Periodic calibration verification and quality control programs are also required by CLIA.

IMMUNODIFFUSION (OUCHTERLONY)

Immunodiffusion is commonly used to determine if antibody or antigen is present in a test solution. It can also be used to establish if there are changes in antigenic structure or to estimate the purity of either antigen or antibody.

Principles

The principles of this technique are discussed in Chapter 11.

Sample requirements and preparation

Samples must have a suitable concentration of the test antigen or antibody so that an observable reaction takes place. Usually, several dilutions of antibody and antigen must be tested before the desired result is observed. Serum or plasma is often suitable with appropriate dilution. Urine and cerebrospinal fluid often must be concentrated. After samples are concentrated, they must not contain too high a salt concentration or a pH that would prevent the reaction from occurring.

Reagents

If an antibody is to be tested for purity, it is desirable to have the pure antigen and a series of solutions containing possible cross-reacting antigens. In contrast, if an antigen is to be tested for purity, one should use antibodies that can react with possible antigen contaminants.

Common pitfall

Improper dilution of antigen or antibody may occur.

Interpretation of results

Interpretation of results is discussed in Chapter 11.

Limitations

The Ouchterlony technique requires a concentration of antigen greater than 45 μg/mL and thus is not so sensitive as other techniques. It is not so discriminatory as immunoelectrophoresis and resolves only a few antigens compared to other techniques. Large molecules do not diffuse readily into the gel, and the technique resolves these poorly.

IMMUNOELECTROPHORESIS

The immunological technique of immunoelectrophoresis (IEP) is used primarily as a qualitative procedure to evaluate the electrophoretic and immunological characteristics of proteins and glycoproteins in serum, urine, or cerebrospinal fluid. IEP is a technique more sophisticated than serum protein electrophoresis and is used routinely to characterize qualitative abnormalities of specific proteins or to analyze the composition of a complex mixture of proteins in biological fluids. Immunoelectrophoresis is not considered a screening method.

Principles

Immunoelectrophoresis is a two-stage procedure. The first stage involves the separation of the components of antigenic material in biological fluids by their differential migration in an electrical field. Generally, serum proteins can be separated into five discrete regions (albumin, α_1, α_2, β, and γ); this stage of the procedure is termed *zone electrophoresis*. The second stage of this technique is the immunological characterization of each of the separated proteins by immunodiffusion procedures. In this process, antibody diffuses into the gel, and the antigen-antibody reaction is visualized by precipitation.

Fig. 12-2 illustrates the technique of immunoelectrophoresis. The biological fluid to be analyzed is placed at the application point (antigen well). Because of the alkaline pH of the agarose buffer, most biological molecules assume a net negative charge and in an electrical field will migrate toward the anode. If serum samples are used, proteins are separated into five distinct regions when a potential difference of 3.3 V/cm is established across the agarose plate for 30 to 60 minutes. Albumin travels the farthest toward the anode. After the albumin are the α_1, α_2, β, and γ regions respectively. After the electrophoresis, antisera are placed in the parallel antibody trough and allowed to diffuse toward the electrophoretically separated proteins. The density, position, and shape of the resultant immunoprecipitin bands are then interpreted as a means of describing each of the precipitated proteins.

Permanent records of the immunoelectrophoretic patterns can be obtained when the precipitin bands are stained with protein stains, such as amido black or Coomassie blue. Some laboratories obtain permanent records by photographing the immunoprecipitin bands in indirect lighting in lieu of staining.

Sample requirements and preparation

Serum. Most immunoelectrophoretic procedures are established to characterize serum proteins that are present in concentrations greater than 500 μg/mL. The system can be used to detect albumin, the immunoglobulins, and about 30 other serum proteins present in at least these concentrations. No further preparation of the serum specimen is required. The sample should be stored in a frozen state to preserve antigens if the procedure is to be delayed more than a day after receipt of the specimen. Plasma is considered an inappropriate sample for immunoelectrophoresis because of the high concentrations of fibrinogen in an unclotted sample.

Urine. As mentioned earlier, immunoelectrophoretic techniques are used to characterize proteins that are present in concentrations greater than 500 μg/mL. Urine usually contains dilute concentrations of protein and must therefore be concentrated to bring the protein concentrations into the detectable range for the immunoelectrophoretic procedure. Concentration procedures usually involve the use of semipermeable membranes that allow water and salts, but not proteins, to pass through. Methods that concentrate the urinary salts, such as lyophilization, are not acceptable. Many of the urine proteins can be detected by immunoelectrophoretic procedures if the urine is concentrated 50 to 100 times. Urine specimens should be stored in a frozen state if any delay in immunoelectrophoretic analysis is anticipated.

Cerebrospinal fluid. Cerebrospinal fluid is also a dilute protein solution that requires concentration before immunoelectrophoresis can be performed. The original volume must be reduced 50 to 100 times so that albumin, transferrin, and immunoglobulins, the major proteins of clinical significance, can be detected. Again, storage of the sample in a frozen state is important if the analysis is to be delayed more than 1 day.

Reagents

In immunoelectrophoresis, three high-quality reagents are needed: agarose, buffered solution, and specific reagent an-

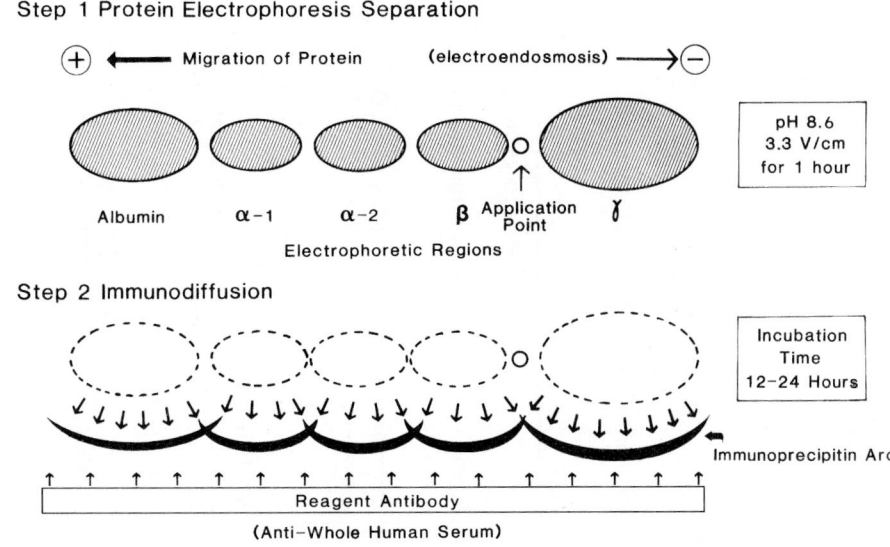

Step 1 Protein Electrophoresis Separation

Step 2 Immunodiffusion

Step 3 Interpretation of Immunoprecipitin Arcs

Fig. 12-2   Immunoelectrophoresis technique using normal human serum and anti–whole human serum. Usually many more than five immunoprecipitin arcs are seen.

Table 12-1 Summary of immunological techniques

Technique	Assay end point	Assay sensitivity	Time needed for assay results	Common analytes	Comments
Immunodiffusion (Ouchterlony)	Precipitation (qualitative)	45 µg/mL	8-72 hours	Bacterial, viral, or fungal antigens	Most frequently used to screen for presence of antigen
Immunoelectrophoresis	Precipitation (qualitative)	500 µg/mL	12-24 hours	Serum, urine, and cerebrospinal fluid protein	Used to assay complex mixture of analytes in biological fluids
Counterimmunoelectrophoresis	Precipitation (qualitative)	3 µg/mL	2-3 hours	Bacterial, viral, or fungal antigens	Commonly used to screen for antigens associated with infectious agents; more rapid than immunodiffusion
Two-dimensional immunoelectrophoresis	Precipitation (qualitative)	500 µg/mL	8-10 hours	Serum proteins	Research, used to examine subtle differences in proteins
Radial immunodiffusion (Mancini)	Precipitation (quantitative) CV, 10%-15%	50 µg/mL	12-24 hours	Serum and CSF proteins	Most commonly used immunological technique to measure serum and CSF proteins
Laurell (rocket) immunoelectrophoresis	Precipitation (quantitative) CV, 8%-12%	50 µg/mL	4-8 hours	Serum and CSF proteins	More rapid than radial immunodiffusion
Turbidimetry	Light-scattering of aggregates of antigen-antibody complexes (quantitative) CV, ~8%	50 µg/mL	15 minutes	Serum and CSF proteins	More rapid than radial immunodiffusion
Direct and indirect agglutination	Agglutination of bacteria or red blood cell-containing antigen (semiquantitative)	15 µg/mL	1-5 minutes	Antibodies to bacterial antigens (such as febrile agglutinins) and red blood cell antigens	Techniques commonly used by serology laboratory and blood bank; not often used in chemistry laboratory
Agglutination inhibition	Inhibition of agglutination (semiquantitative)	15 µg/mL	2-5 minutes	Detect antigens such as pregnancy hormones (hCG)	Rapid test procedure often used to screen urine of pregnant women for hCG

Technique	Principle	Sensitivity	Time	Uses	Comments
Immunofixation	Reaction of enzyme-labeled Ab with antigens fixed after electrophoresis	10 µg/mL	1-4 hours	Serum proteins including immunoglobulins	Used to study gammopathies and as western blot to find antibodies to HIV
Complement fixation	Lysis of red blood cells or inhibition of red blood cell lysis (semiquantitative)	10 µg/mL	24 hours	Detect complement-fixing antibodies to bacterial, viral, or fungal antigens	Worldwide, commonly used serological procedure; sensitivity of assay approaches radioimmunoassay; assay difficult to perform
Immunonephelometry	Light-scattering of aggregates of antigen-antibody complexes (quantitative) CV, 3%-8%	1 µg/mL	½-1 hour	*Direct mode:* Serum, urine, and CSF proteins. *Inhibition mode:* Drugs, such as theophylline and phenytoin	Popularly accepted technique to quantitate protein in many laboratories, this technique has replaced radial immunodiffusion
Enzyme immunoassay (ELISA, sandwich)	Color reaction between enzyme and substrate (quantitative) CV, 8%-15%	<1 ng/mL	1-24 hours	Serum proteins (such as IgE) Bacterial, viral, and fungal antigens Antibodies to infectious agents	Excellent assay for small amounts of antigen or antibody
Radioimmunoassay (competitive binding)	Measurement of radioactivity	<1 ng/mL	2-24 hours	Capable of measuring most molecules large and small	Traditional assay, less popular because of radioisotope concerns
Enzyme immunoassay (competitive binding)	Color reaction between enzyme and substrate (quantitative) CV, 8%-15%	<1 ng/mL	2-4 hours	Small amounts of antigen (such as hormones, drugs, viral antigens)	Excellent assay for measuring ligands
Immunoradiometric	Radioisotope decay emission	<1 ng/mL	1-24 hours	Same as ELISA above	Excellent assay for quantitative measurement of low levels of antigens or antibodies; problem with radioactive wastes
Immunofluorometric	Fluorescence of dye	<1 ng/mL	1-24 hours	Same as ELISA and RIA above	Same as for immunoradiometric but no waste problem
Chemiluminescent	Chemiluminescence of dye	<1 ng/mL	15-60 minutes	Same as ELISA and RIA above	Very sensitive for quantitative measurement of low levels of antigens

CSF, Cerebrospinal fluid; *CV,* coefficient of variation; *hCG,* human chorionic gonadotropin hormone.

tibody. Agarose, unlike agar, does not develop surface changes that can interfere with the migration of proteins during the electrophoresis. Electroendosmosis is less noticeable when agarose is used.

Immunoelectrophoresis is usually carried out in a buffered medium (pH 8.6). Barbital, or barbituric acid, is frequently added to the buffering solution, not only because it has good buffering properties, but also because it is an excellent bacteriostatic reagent. Close attention to the freshness of a buffer solution is necessary each time immunoelectrophoresis is performed.

The properties of the reagent antibody used to detect the various migrated proteins must be chosen carefully. This antibody should perform well in an immunoprecipitation reaction and should be titered to the dilution that will give the maximum precipitation band for those detectable proteins that are present in lowest concentration.

Instrumentation

Four specific pieces of equipment are needed for the performance of immunoelectrophoresis: power supply, buffer tanks, proper wicking material, and agar-cutting template. The power supply used in the electrophoretic stage of the procedure should be able to supply a constant voltage over a period of several hours at a rate of 3 to 5 V/cm. Buffer tanks should be able to hold enough buffer to prevent changes in pH during the electrophoresis stage of the technique. Electrodes should be made of platinum because of its high conductance and inertness to chemical degradation. The wicking material should be porous and inert and should allow free passage of buffer from the tank to the agarose-containing plate. The wicking material should have low electrical resistance. Material that has a high electrical resistance can cause the system to overheat, producing inaccurate results.

Common pitfalls

Immunoelectrophoresis is a multicomponent system that requires close attention to each of the major components. Following is a list of common pitfalls.

1. Spent buffer solution, causing improper migration of the proteins during electrophoretic separation. This can cause overheating in the agarose, which may result in some denaturation of the protein and destruction of antigenic determinants. A buffer solution becomes spent when it is used for too many electrophoretic runs.
2. Improper concentration of specimens, resulting in no precipitation, insoluble aggregated proteins, or a concentration too high to observe.
3. Inappropriate attachment of the wick to the agarose plate and buffer tanks, resulting in intermittent or nonuniform flow of electricity across the agarose plate during the electrophoretic procedure. Improper attachment of the wick to the agarose plate is a frequent source of errors in this technique.

4. Dull cutting blades in the template, causing ragged cutting of the agarose plate with consequent artifactual influence on the diffusion properties of the reagent antibody.
5. Improper dilution of the antiserum, usually with loss of precipitation reaction.
6. Improper ionic strength of the buffer. The ionic strength of the buffer solution used should be sufficiently low so that when migration of the antigenic material is induced, the electrical charge is conferred primarily to the antigens rather than to ions of the buffer.
7. Overheating, usually caused by improper wicking, spent buffer solutions, or too long an electrophoretic migration, with a resulting denaturation of the proteins.
8. Excessive time for the immunodiffusion step, resulting in immunoprecipitation lines in inappropriate positions, making interpretation questionable. Antisera and antigen concentrations should be titrated to a point where the maximum precipitation line can be observed between 14 and 24 hours.
9. Improper staining and photographic procedures.

Interpretation of results

Immunoelectrophoretic analysis of biological fluids requires a firm understanding of the processes of electrophoretic separation of proteins and immunodiffusion analysis. Fig. 12-3 illustrates the use of this technique in the interpretation of normal and abnormal serum. Analysis of these immunoprecipitin bands can provide much useful clinical information. The presence of monoclonal or oligoclonal immunoglobulins, the presence or absence of specific proteins, alpha$_1$-antitrypsin, and so on can be used for the diagnosis of disease processes.

COUNTERIMMUNOELECTROPHORESIS

Counterimmunoelectrophoresis is also called *double electroimmunodiffusion*. This technique was used for the detection of single antigens present in a patient sample. It has largely been replaced by immunofixation. Please refer to the second edition for details.

IMMUNOFIXATION (WESTERN BLOT)

The immunofixation technique, known as the western blot method, is often used in clinical applications to confirm the presence of antibody (such as Human Immunodeficiency Virus, HIV, antibody) to specific antigens. The technique is also used for the detection of specific proteins, such as apo E isoforms.

Principles

The method of immunofixation is a three-stage procedure that uses electrophoresis in the first two stages. An antigen mixture is first electrophoresed in an appropriate support medium, such as polyacrylamide, neutral agarose, or paper

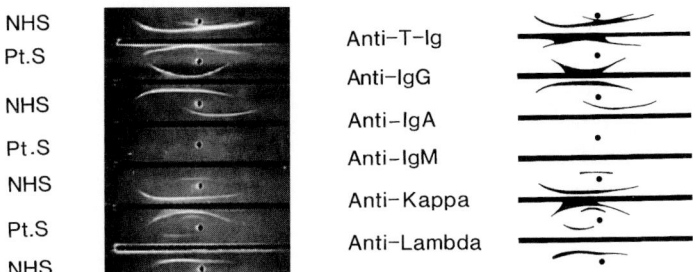

Fig. 12-3 Examples of immunoelectrophoresis patterns. *On left,* Actual gel. *On right,* Scheme drawn from photograph. *NHS,* Normal human serum; *Pt.S,* serum from a patient with IgG(K) myeloma; *Anti-T-Ig,* antiserum to all (total) human immunoglobulins; *Anti-IgG,* antiserum to human immunoglobulins.

strips to separate the components by charge-to-weight differences. After the first stage the agarose film is overlaid with a sheet of nitrocellulose-based filter paper. In a second electrophoretic step, the protein is transferred from the support to the nitrocellulose. The nitrocellulose has the property of effectively irreversibly binding the transferred protein. The nitrocellulose sheet is then treated with a protein solution, which reacts with all remaining binding sites, minimizing nonspecific binding in the next step. Next, an antibody solution, usually serum from a patient, is allowed to react with the nitrocellulose sheet. Excess antibody is then removed by washing. The nitrocellulose sheet is incubated with a second labeled antibody that has specificity for the first antibody. The label allows detection of the original antigen-antibody reaction. If the label is an enzyme, such as peroxidase, the reaction is detected by substrate precipitation of, for example, a benzidine dye. A diagram is presented in Fig. 12-4.

Reagents

The agarose film should contain an appropriate buffer so that adequate separation of the antigen mixture occurs. The nitrocellulose sheet should be able to absorb the proteins.

Reagent antibody. The reagent antibody label must have a high specificity and specific activity so that it can detect only the desired antibody or test protein and that the sensitivity of the assay will be great enough to determine the presence of the reaction.

Common pitfalls

The assays commonly use peroxidase dye reactions to detect the presence of antibody or antigen. The assays often require skilled individuals to read the patterns.

Test sensitivity and interpretation of results

This technique is nearly as sensitive as the enzyme immunoassay technique. However, whereas enzyme immunoassays are employed as quantitative assays, western blots and other immunofixation methods are used primarily as qualitative techniques; that is, they are used to determine the presence or absence of a particular protein or antibody. A widely used purpose of the technique is confirmation of the results of HIV screening. The sensitivity of the technique can be the detection of less than 1 ng/mL of test protein.

TWO-DIMENSIONAL IMMUNOELECTROPHORESIS

Two-dimensional immunoelectrophoresis is used as a research technique for the analytical separation of closely related antigens with similarly related electrophoretic properties. It is used in special situations to identify the heterogeneity of certain proteins such as factor VIII (antihemophilic factor) or to distinguish genetic variants of some proteins, such as alpha$_1$-antitrypsins. It is a difficult, time-consuming procedure that is not likely to be used in most laboratories.

Principles

This procedure is a two-stage technique that uses electrophoresis in both stages. The antigen mixture is first electrophoresed in a neutral agarose to separate components by charge. After this first stage, the agarose strip containing the separated protein is transferred to a larger plate and abutted to a gel-containing antibody. An electric current is applied in a direction perpendicular to the first electrophoretic separation so that the antigens migrate into the antibody-containing agarose, forming immunoprecipitation arcs. This second stage of electrophoresis may take as long as 20 hours. After the reaction, the plate is washed in saline solution to remove excess protein, excess fluid is pressed out with filter paper, and the plate is fixed and stained.

RADIAL IMMUNODIFFUSION

Because of its simplicity and accuracy, radial immunodiffusion is one of the most commonly used techniques for the quantification of antigens.

Principles

The principles of radial immunodiffusion are discussed in Chapter 11.

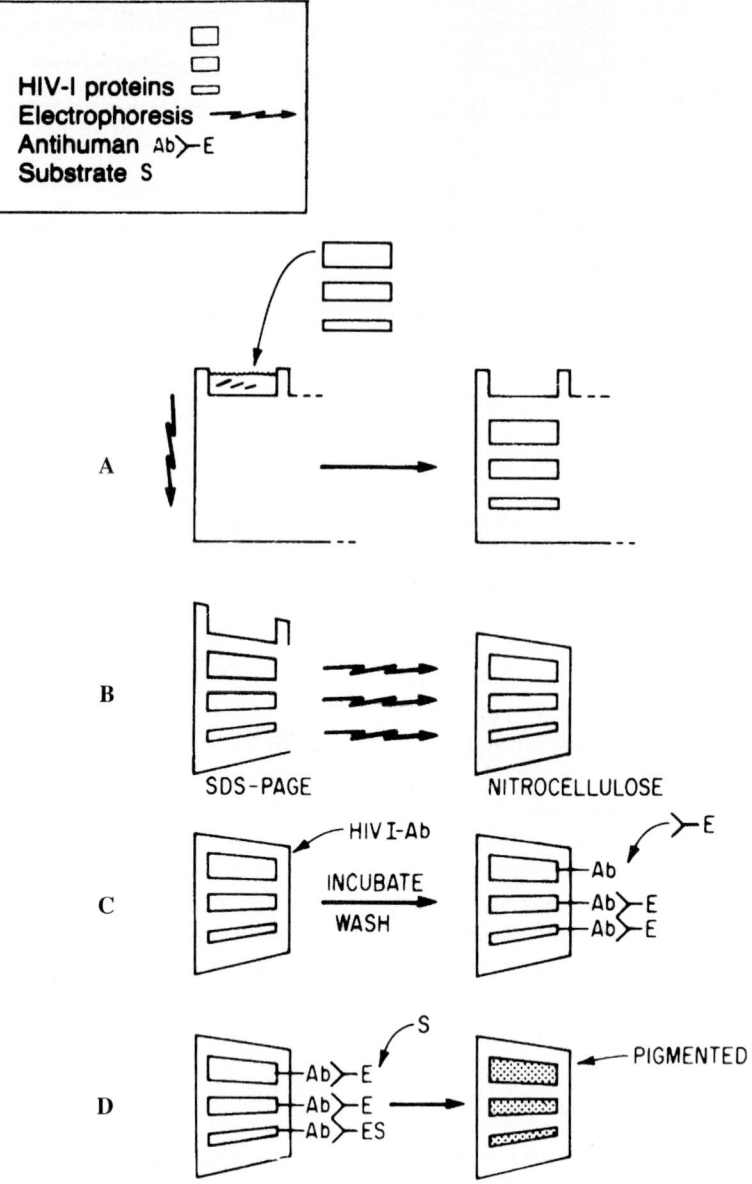

Fig. 12-4 Diagram of enzyme-linked immunoelectrotransfer blot technique (western blot). **A,** HIV-1 proteins are layered onto an SDS-PAGE, subjected to electrophoresis, and separated according to their molecular weight. **B,** The discrete proteins are then electrophoresed (blotted) to a nitrocellulose matrix and incubated, first with specimen containing HIV-1 antibody (Ab), which binds to the discrete HIV-1 Ag bands. **C,** Tagged anti-human Ab is then added. The excess is then washed away, and substrate is added. **D,** HIV-1 Ab directed toward the discrete HIV-1 antigen bands is present, the discrete bands can be visualized as pigmented bands. (From *American Clinical Products Review* 6(11):16, 1987, International Scientific Communications, Inc.)

Sample requirements and preparation

The assay is valid only over a rather narrow range of antigen concentrations. In part, this is dictated by the antibody concentration in the gel and by the ease of diffusion of the antigen into the gel. For some antigens, several dilutions are necessary to achieve the optimum concentration range. Urine and cerebrospinal fluid generally must be concen-

trated before they can be quantified by this technique. Excess salt must be removed from these specimens if they have been concentrated by lyophilization.

Reagents

Monospecific antibody to the desired antigen is the only crucial reagent.

Step 1 – Electrophoresis of
Antigen into Agarose
Containing Antibody

Step 2– Interpretation of Results

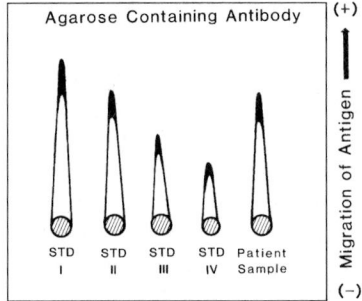

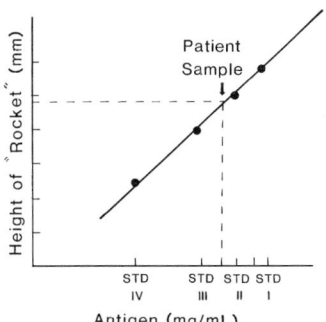

Fig. 12-5 "Rocket" immunoelectrophoresis. *STD,* Standard.

Common pitfalls

If the antiserum binds more than one antigen, a double ring may be seen. Temperature should be kept constant. If the antigen is too large or aggregated, the resulting diffusion pattern will not be quantitative.

Test sensitivity

Test sensitivity depends on antigen size; the greater the size, the poorer the diffusion. For most serum proteins, the assay is sensitive to 50 μg/mL.

LAURELL ("ROCKET") IMMUNOELECTROPHORESIS

Laurell immunoelectrophoresis is a quantitative method that is used to measure antigens in biological fluids. It provides data for individual antigens similar to those obtained by radial immunodiffusion. The advantage of this technique over radial immunodiffusion is that the time needed to produce results is 4 to 6 hours rather than 18 to 72 hours. This shortened time is attributable to the use of electrophoresis instead of passive diffusion. The "rocket" technique is usually more expensive to perform than radial immunodiffusion because of the need for electrophoretic equipment and the increased quantity of reagent antibody and agarose used. This technique is best used to measure antigens present in concentrations of 50 to 20,000 μg/mL. Antigens most frequently measured are the serum proteins.

Principles

In this technique the antigen combines with the antibody during electrophoresis of the antigen into an antibody-containing medium such as agarose. The pH of the agarose-antibody medium is usually 8.6, so that the antibody has little or no net negative charge and will not migrate when current is passed through the gel. The antigen to be measured must have a net negative charge so that it will migrate into the gel toward the anode in an electric current. Each sample is applied to a circular well cut at one end of the gel. Electrical current applied to the gel plate causes migration of the antigen toward the center of the plate. As the

antigen migrates and combines with the antibody in the gel, cones or rocket-shaped bands of precipitate are formed. As unbound antigen within the rocket-shaped band of precipitate migrates into the precipitate under the influence of the electrical current, precipitate dissolves in antigen excess. The leading edge of the rocket re-forms ahead of the antigen in the direction that the antigen is migrating. The amount of antigen within the leading edge is successively diminished until equivalence of the antigen-antibody complex is reached. At this point, a stable precipitate will form, and the antigen will no longer migrate. The length of the rocket in the test sample is proportional to the log concentration of the antigen in the reference standard run in the same gel (Fig. 12-5).

Sample requirements and preparation

As in the other immunological techniques, care must be taken to ensure that the antigen to be measured is not degraded or denatured. These precautions are especially important for complement components, such as C3 and C4, and the immunoglobulin IgM. Breakdown of the protein molecule can cause several peaks to form within the same rocket. In some disease states, breakdown of the proteins C3 and C4 occurs in vivo, and the formation of several peaks has clinical significance, but if the test sample has not been properly handled and stored before testing, the significance of the observation of several peaks would be difficult to interpret.

Common pitfalls

1. Improper antigen migration. For an accurate measurement of antigen concentration with this technique, the antigen must be able to assume a net negative charge at a pH of 8.6. If the antigen's isoelectric point is greater than 7.5, the antigen will not migrate adequately into the agarose-antibody medium to obtain peaks of high resolution.

2. Improper wicking. As in all electrophoretic procedures, proper placement of the wicks at the edge of the gel plate

such that all of the gel has a constant electrical current is necessary. If the contact point of the wick with the gel is improper, the antigen will not migrate consistently throughout the plate, and false peaks will result.

3. Overheating during electrophoresis. Since the electrophoresis time is prolonged in this technique, close attention to cooling of the gel plate during electrophoresis is essential. Overheating can cause the gel to dry, the antigen to denature, and the antigen to migrate improperly.

4. Improper measurement of peak height.

Test sensitivity and coefficient of variation

The Laurell (rocket) immunoelectrophoresis technique has a sensitivity of approximately 50 μg/mL for serum proteins found in biological fluids. The upper limits of detection are usually around 20,000 μg/mL for these antigens. Within-run variations are between 5% and 10%, whereas between-run variations, when the same antigen is measured, are 10% to 15%.

IMMUNONEPHELOMETRY (see Chapter 4, pp. 101-103)
Nephelometry

Principles. When an antibody and an antigen combine in solution, small aggregates that can scatter light form quickly, giving a turbid appearance to the solution. These aggregates then slowly associate to form a larger matrix, which eventually gives rise to the precipitate seen in immunoprecipitation assays such as double diffusion (Ouchterlony) or radial immunodiffusion (Mancini).

Development of a clinically useful assay was made possible by the observation that for some plasma proteins the intensity of scattered light was a measure of the amount of precipitate formed, *as long as the reaction was carried out in antibody excess.*

One successful nephelometer uses a laser as its light source and a fixed-time two-measurement protocol. A second instrument uses a tungsten light source and measures the rate of complex formation.

Fast (seconds to minutes) and precise methods for the specific measurement of plasma proteins, such as albumin, immunoglobulins, complement components, and acute-phase reactants, as well as hormones and therapeutic drugs, are now available.

In Chapter 11, the structure of the aggregates created by early lattice formation of immune complexes is shown. These aggregates from primary reactions occur within seconds to minutes, whereas the secondary interactions leading to precipitation occur over a period of hours.

Light-scattering assays measure this early second-order reaction, presumably between antigen and high-affinity antibody, in which there is formed a micelle of protein large enough to scatter light but not large enough to precipitate.

Although the initial reaction of antigen with antibody is fast, the buildup of small light-scattering complexes takes time. This reaction, aggregate formation, can be greatly enhanced with the addition of the water-soluble polymer polyethylene glycol (6000 daltons) at concentrations of 2% to 4%. The polymer causes a severalfold increase in light scatter while decreasing the reaction time tenfold.

Sample requirements and preparation. The most frequently measured biological fluids are serum and cerebrospinal fluids, though urine may also be measured.

Reagents. Reagent antibody must be of very high titer and affinity and must be specially clarified by microfiltration to minimize background light scatter.

Common pitfalls

1. Antibody is not in excess. In these circumstances the amount of precipitate formation will be recorded as a falsely low value.

2. Background scatter is too high. The rate-nephelometric determinations are preferred to end-point determinations because they minimize the contribution of background. For example, it is possible to detect a 5% increase in scattering over background using a rate measurement. In contrast, such a difference may not be measurable as an end-point change. Lipidemia will cause high background scatter.

3. Interference is caused by colored solution. End-point methods are most influenced by colored solutions. These absorb the scattered light, tending to yield lower values. However, even kinetic measurements are lower in highly colored solutions.

4. Mixing is insufficient. Because the rate method requires constant agitation to make uniform particles, the mixing efficacy must be constantly monitored.

5. Preformed immune complexes in the patient serum may cause false-high or false-low values, depending on whether the rate of reaction is measured and how the background correction is done.

Limitations. For most assays, quantitation is valid only when the reagent antibody is in excess. Although each instrument manufacturer has devised ways of recognizing antigen excess, the foolproof method requires the laboratorian to carry out the measurements at two different dilutions, or to have available a serum protein electrophoresis of the sample for comparison. The method is limited to measurements of antigens that form enough lattice to scatter light, such as proteins. Special steps are required for small molecules (see the following text).

Nephelometric inhibition immunoassay (NINIA)

Principles. If a small molecule, such as digoxin or a drug, is covalently linked to a large carrier protein such as bovine serum albumin, the resulting conjugate acts as a large light-scattering antigen when reacted with antibody to the small molecule. In this case the complex formation can be inhibited by the addition of the specific hapten. The in-

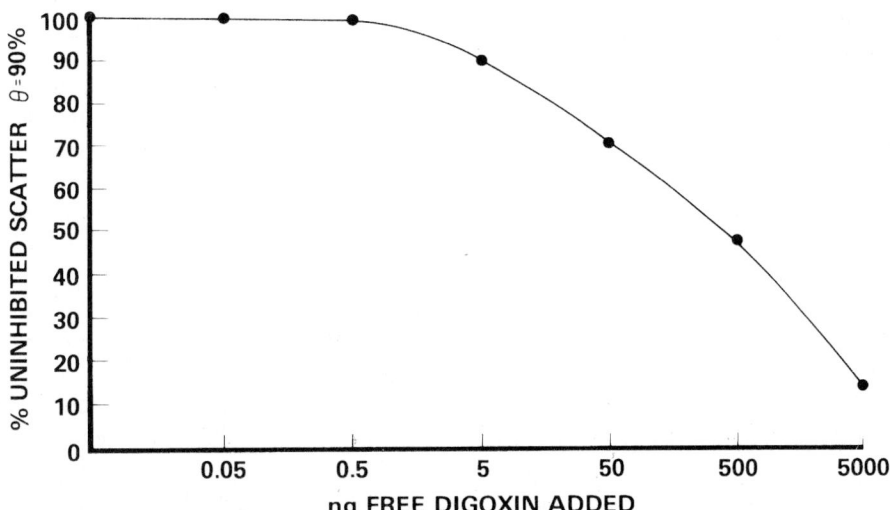

Fig. 12-6 Digoxin standard curve using nephelometric-inhibition immunoassay.

hibition is dose dependent, and a quantitative assay for the small molecule results. With appropriate manipulation of the parameters, one can adjust the number of haptenic groups for adequate precipitation while allowing maximum sensitivity for inhibition by free hapten.

Addition of sample containing free hapten to the reaction mixture decreases available antibody and causes a decrease in the signal generated by a standard hapten-conjugate preparation (Fig. 12-6).

Methods have been developed for rapid analysis of drugs occurring in milligram-per-liter amounts, such as phenytoin, phenobarbital, and theophylline.

Sample requirements and preparation. The most frequently measured biological fluid is serum. The most measured compounds are drugs such as theophylline and phenytoin.

Reagents. The requirements for reagent antibody are similar to those for any nephelometric technique. Reagent antigen is composed of the drug to be monitored covalently bound at several sites to a protein, usually albumin.

Instrumentation. Instrumentation is the same as that used for nephelometry.

Common pitfalls. Pitfalls are similar to those described for nephelometry, except that the reaction is titered to be always in antigen excess.

Additional assay modifications

Particle-enhanced light scattering. Because the amount of light scatter is dependent on the size, amount, and refractive index of the scattering species, an increase in any of these parameters should result in greater sensitivity. This potential is realized when either antigens or antibodies are coupled to various inert carrier particles, but, because of availability and better control of coupling conditions, polystyrene latex beads have become the particles of choice. This type of assay is essentially a type of aggluti-

nating procedure (see discussion of agglutination assays below). The method also offers faster signal generation and greater economy of reagents. The latex-fixation test for detection of rheumatoid factor is the classic example of this type of assay, though it depends on visual observation of agglutination and is thus only semiquantitative. More recently, several particle-enhanced methods have been developed for both direct and inhibition assays, and a wide variety of light-scatter detection techniques have been employed.

Monoclonal antibody reagents. The performance of light-scattering assays depends greatly on the quality of the antiserum used. With conventional polyclonal reagents there is a continual need to monitor and adjust antiserum titer, specificity, and affinity.

Such variability is often overcome with the use of a monoclonal antibody. However, unless the antigen has many identical antigenic sites, a single monoclonal antibody cannot cause matrix formation and will cause little or no light scatter. If an appropriate mixture of monoclonal antibodies can be made, complexes will form, causing measurable light scatter. This blending of monoclonal antibodies or the use of monoclonals in particle-enhanced light-scatter assays ensures constancy of reagent production and gives these assays further stability and specificity.

AGGLUTINATION ASSAYS

Agglutination is the clumping and sedimentation of antigen after reaction with antibody. It was first noted when the reaction of bacteria incubated with serum from an infected patient was observed. Observation of the agglutination of red blood cells after incubation with serum led to the discovery of ABO blood groups. Agglutination has been extensively used as a detection system because of its ease and versatility. It is, however, only semiquantitative, showing reproducibility only within fourfold dilutions. Agglutinating antibodies *(agglutinins)* may be directed against naturally occurring antigens on the surface of cells *(active or direct agglutination)* or against substances that have been applied to the surface of cells or inert particles *(passive or indirect agglutination).*

Principles

Agglutination reactions depend on the formation of antibody bridges by bivalent (IgG) or multivalent (IgM) antibody between antigen particles with multiple antigenic determinants. Large particles, such as red blood cells or bacteria, contain many different antigens, as well as antigens that appear hundreds of times on the cell or particle surface. Thus it is possible for antibody molecules to bind to more than one site on a single particle or to bind to equivalent sites on different particles. Such binding is called *cross-linking.* Antigens with a single antigenic determinant would not permit cross-linking and would therefore not agglutinate. Cross-linking may create a high-molecular-weight lattice that clumps together and precipitates. Because of its size and multivalency, IgM is said to be 750 times more efficient at agglutination than IgG. Agglutination reactions are generally used to detect antibody directed to particulate antigens; quantitation is by serial dilution of serum. *Reverse agglutination* can be used to detect soluble antigen by using antibody adsorbed onto cell or particle surfaces. Agglutination reactions are read by the naked eye or with the aid of magnification. The extent of agglutination is scored 1+ to 4+ by estimation. The titer of the serum is the reciprocal of the highest dilution giving visible (1+) agglutination.

Factors influencing agglutination reaction

Factors influencing agglutination include particle charge, antibody type, electrolyte concentration, viscosity of the medium, reactant concentrations, location and concentration of antigenic determinants, and time and temperature of incubation.

Particle charge. Red blood cells, bacteria, and inert particles such as latex have a net negative surface charge called the *zeta potential.* These charges must be overcome to permit the cross-linking that will result in agglutination.

Antibody type. IgM antibodies are more efficient at agglutination because of their multivalency and because their size permits more effective bridging of the gap between cells caused by charge repulsion.

Electrolyte concentration and viscosity. The ionic strength of the medium used for the agglutination reaction can assist in reducing the negative surface charge of particles. This can be accomplished by addition of charged molecules, such as albumin, to the medium. The pH of the medium should be near that present in physiological conditions. At neutral pH, high electrolyte concentrations act to neutralize the net negative charge of particles. Increasing the viscosity of the medium with polymerized mol-

ecules, such as dextran, also assists in bringing the charged particles together.

Antigenic determinants. As stated earlier, antigens with multiple antigenic determinants are necessary for agglutination. A monovalent antigen would not permit cross-linking. The placement of the antigenic determinants on the particle can also affect agglutinability. Antigenic determinants that are sparsely distributed will not be so easily cross-linked as antigenic determinants that are densely distributed. Antigenic determinants can also be inaccessible to antibody binding because they are buried within cell membranes.

Concentration, temperature, and time of incubation. At higher antigen concentrations, the reaction with antibody will be more rapid. Agitation of the antigen suspension with antibody solution will increase the reaction rate by increasing the surface area exposed to the antibody. At lower antigen concentrations, the reaction time can be shortened by centrifugation, which increases contact between the antigenic particles and the antibody. Concentration of reactants can therefore influence reaction time. The temperature of incubation is also an important variable. Some antigens are bound most readily by antibody at 37° C. These antigens include microbes. Some antigens react optimally with antibody at 4° C. These *cold agglutinins* include antibody to the *i* antigen of fetal and infant red blood cells. Optimum temperature for the agglutination reaction will vary with different antigen-antibody systems. Temperature also affects the behavior of antibodies in vitro.

Direct agglutination

Direct agglutination tests are frequently used in the immunological diagnosis of microbial infections. The titer of the serum reflects the concentration of the predominant antibody in the serum. Early detection of a high titer and documentation of a significant rise in titer are important tools in diagnosis. Antibodies to *Brucella* (brucellosis), *Salmonella* (typhoid fever), and *Proteus* (Rocky Mountain spotted fever) organisms are detected in this way. Direct agglutination tests are also used in the typing of human red blood cells in the blood bank.

Different bacterial antigens may give different patterns of agglutination. Antibodies to bacterial flagella cause cross-linking of the flagella themselves. These antibodies cause formation of a loose, rapidly formed agglutinate. Antibodies to antigens in the body of the bacterium cause cross-linking of the organisms themselves. This results in a granular, compact precipitate that develops more slowly.

Indirect agglutination

Indirect agglutination involves reaction of antibody with antigens that have been passively transferred onto the surface of particles (Fig. 12-7). Red blood cells, usually from humans, sheep, or turkey, are employed. Inert particles such as latex (0.81 μm in diameter) and bentonite (clay) are also

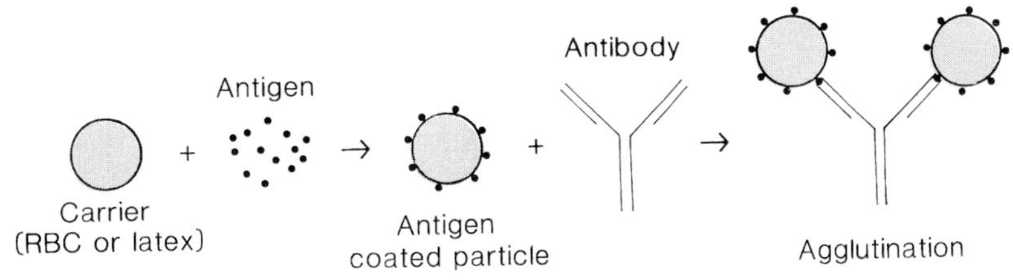

Fig. 12-7 Passive (indirect) agglutination reaction. Antigen is adsorbed onto surface of carrier particle, which is then agglutinated by antigen-specific antibody.

used. Polysaccharide and some protein antigens, such as albumin and purified protein derivative are easily adsorbed onto the particle surface. Other antigens require pretreatment of particles with tannic acid or chromium chloride, which modifies the cell surface. Antigen can be covalently bound to the cell surface by bifunctional molecules, such as bisdiazobenzidine or glutaraldehyde. Indirect agglutination is used in the diagnosis of syphilis. The Venereal Disease Research Laboratory test employs cholesterol crystals coated with cardiolipin antigen. Detection of rheumatoid factor, useful in the diagnosis of rheumatoidarthritis, uses agglutination of latex particles coated with human IgG.

Agglutination inhibition

Agglutination inhibition is an adaptation of the agglutination reaction that permits detection and quantitation of soluble antigen. The concentrations of antibody and particles are carefully controlled to prevent antibody excess. Antibody is incubated with the test antigen solution, and antigen is bound to available antibody-combining sites. The antibody is then added to particulate antigen suspensions. The failure to agglutinate indicates that enough antibody-combining sites have been saturated with a soluble form of the same antigen so that insufficient antibody-binding sites are available for binding and cross-linking of the particulate antigen. Quantitation of the soluble antigen can be accomplished by assessment of the degree of inhibition in serial dilutions of the antigen solution (Fig. 12-8).

Antiglobulin testing

Antiglobulin testing is a modification of the agglutination reaction to permit detection of an incomplete (IgG) antibody, which may not produce agglutination even after binding to the particle surface. IgG is less effective at agglutination than IgM because its smaller size is less effective at bridging antigen particles. If an anti-immunoglobulin, or *Coombs' reagent,* is added to the unagglutinated IgG-coated particles, the Coombs' reagent will bridge the gap between particles by bivalent binding (Fig. 12-9). This enables cross-linking to achieve agglutination. The *direct Coombs test* is used in blood banks to determine the presence of IgG antibodies to red blood cells.

The *indirect Coombs test* is a variation of the antiglobulin test and is used to detect free antibody to red blood cells in patient serum (Fig. 12-10). Serum is screened against a panel of red blood cells of known and varied antigenicity. Agglutination of cells to which patient serum and antiglobulin reagent have been added indicates the presence of antibody in patient serum to an antigen present on the agglutinated cells.

Sample requirements

Agglutination reactions can be used to measure components of plasma, serum, or cerebrospinal fluid. Urine must be buffered because of its usual acidity. Since serum complement may affect agglutination, inactivation or dilution to minimize complement may be necessary.

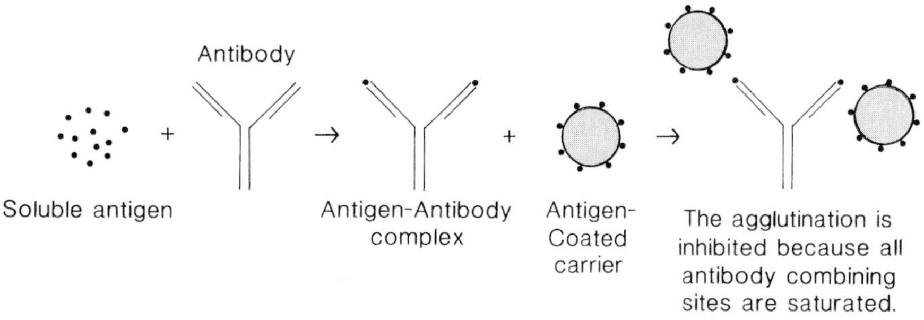

Fig. 12-8 Agglutination-inhibition reaction. Same reaction as that shown in Fig. 12-7 but inhibited by soluble antigen.

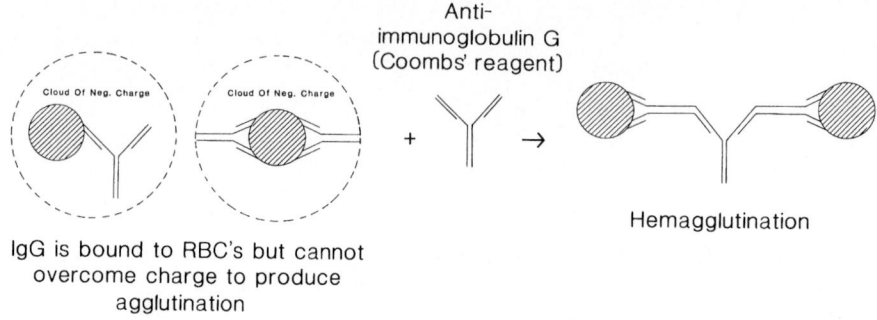

Fig. 12-9 Direct Coombs test for antibody to red blood cells (RBC).

Reagents

As for red blood cell agglutination techniques, the factors influencing the reactions are particle charge, type of antibody, electrolyte concentration, and viscosity. Red blood cells, when used fresh, have a shelf life of about 2 weeks. Therefore many manufacturers have developed fixed red blood cells (usually stabilized by tannic acid or glutaraldehyde) or latex beads to overcome the need to prepare the reagents every few weeks.

Instrumentation

The great advantage of this technique is the simplicity of instrumentation. Results can be detected by eye or with the aid of a mirror or magnifying glass.

Common pitfalls

Antigen excess often results in a prozone phenomenon with false-negative results. Use of expired red blood cells or other reagents can result in lack of agglutination.

Limitations

The technique is only semiquantitative and thus allows estimates of the true value within a dilution factor of two.

COMPLEMENT-FIXATION ASSAYS

The complement-fixation tests are probably the most sensitive of the immunological procedures that were developed early in the history of immunology. Tests more sensitive

than complement fixation, such as radioimmunoassay and enzyme immunoassay, have now been developed, but complement-fixation tests are still important, especially in the diagnosis of fungal, viral, and parasitic infections and in the quantitation of functional complement levels (total hemolytic complement) and complement components.

Complement proteins

The term *complement* is used to denote a series of plasma proteins that are activated in sequence after antigen-antibody reactions. Not all classes and subclasses of immunoglobulins are capable of activating complement or can activate it to the same degree (see Table 11-1, p. 217). The antigen-antibody complex used in complement-fixation tests therefore must involve an antibody that is capable of activating, or *fixing,* complement. As with agglutination reactions, pentameric IgM is 1000 times more efficient in fixing complement than IgG is.

The first protein in the complement sequence is bound to the second constant domain of the heavy chain (C_{H2}), which is inaccessible on an unreacted or unbound antibody. After interaction and binding with antigen, conformational changes in the immunoglobulin molecule cause the hinge region to open and the complement-binding site to be exposed. Subsequent complement proteins are then activated and can bind to the membrane of the cell to which the antigen-antibody complex is bound. Binding of the complete sequence of nine complement proteins results in small

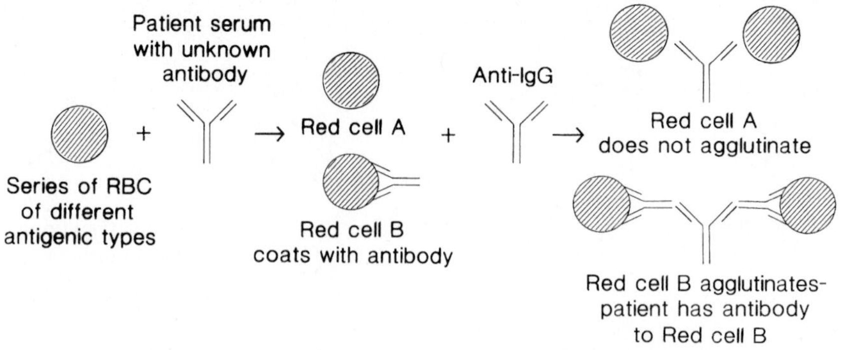

Fig. 12-10 Indirect Coombs test for antibody.

defects in the membranes of the cells. Cytoplasmic cell contents are lost through these holes, and extracellular fluid is admitted. This results in hypotonic swelling of the cell and ends in cell lysis. If the cells used in the test are red blood cells, cell lysis results in release of hemoglobin into the medium. The amount of hemoglobin is directly proportional to the amount of complement fixed to the surface of the cells.

One-stage testing

To assess total complement levels (complement activity that reflects all nine major complement proteins) or to assess individually the nine major complement proteins, a one-stage test system is used. A constant volume of red blood cells, usually sheep, is added to a constant amount of anti–sheep red blood cell antibody, or *hemolysin*. A source of complement is added. For total complement measurements, dilutions of the unknown serum are used. For measurement of complement components, serum with an added excess of every complement component but the component to be measured is used. The degree of hemolysis is measured in a spectrophotometer and is directly proportional to the amount of complement available for fixation in the test serum (Fig. 12-11).

Some immunologically mediated diseases cause a decrease in total serum complement levels or in the levels of individual complement components. In addition, hereditary deficiencies of certain components of the complement system have been described.

Two-stage testing

Two-stage complement-fixation testing is used to measure antigen or antibody. In the first reaction, antigen and antibody are incubated with a known amount of complement. In the second stage, the residual complement activity in the solution is determined by an indicator system, such as sheep red blood cells that are coated with hemolysin. The degree of hemolysis of the indicator cells is inversely proportional to the amount of complement fixed in the first reaction (Fig. 12-12).

To determine antigen levels, one uses a constant volume of antibody. To determine antibody levels, a constant amount of antigen is used.

Sample requirements and preparation

Ethylenediaminetetraacetic acid (EDTA) plasma, serum, and cerebrospinal fluid may be analyzed, but certain precautions are necessary. The samples cannot be hemolyzed. The endogenous complement of the sample must be inactivated, usually by heating of the specimen for 15 to 30 minutes at 56° C.

Reagents

Exogenous complement must be prepared daily and cannot be stored. The complement activity varies significantly from batch to batch and must be standardized daily.

Limitations

Complement-fixation tests are sensitive to many variables. They are inhibited by anticomplementary activity (factors that inactivate or interfere with any of the complement proteins) in serum, including factors such as circulating immune (antigen-antibody) complexes, lipemic sera, aggregated immunoglobulins, and heparin.

It is critical to keep all components in the test constant except the one that is to be measured. Red blood cell number, concentration of complement, and concentration of antigen should be rigorously defined for antibody determinations.

Tests are influenced by the instability of some complement proteins, variability in red blood cells, variation between lots of hemolysin, and the narrow range of optimum reactivity for many reagents. The need for fresh reagents and the great variability make this assay one of the most difficult performed by a laboratory.

The CDC evaluates complement-fixation reagents and has developed standardized procedures for complement-fixation tests.

INDICATOR-LABELED IMMUNOASSAYS

The immunoassays described above all used direct measurement of a physical property of the antigen-antibody complex or aggregates formed secondarily to the initial binding step (such as precipitation or light scatter). By introducing a labeled indicator antigen or antibody to trace the initial binding reaction, one can achieve an enhanced analytical

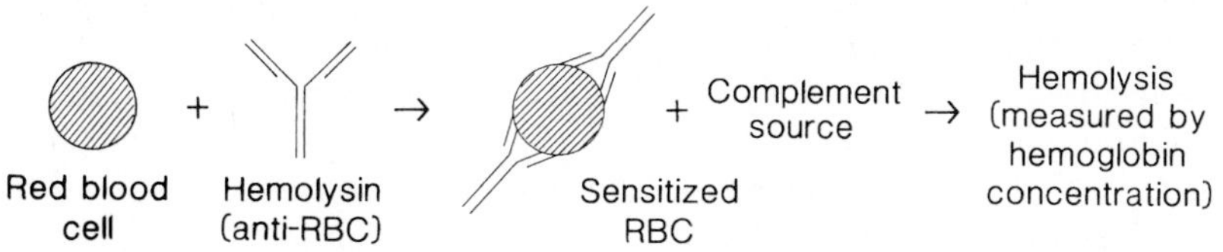

Fig. 12-11 Complement fixation one-stage testing. For measurement of total hemolytic complement, test serum is added as source of complement. For measurement of complement components as complement source, one uses test serums, to which purified complement components are added; for example, to measure complement component 3, one adds all components, except C3, in excess to test serum. Therefore reaction is limited only by concentration of C3 in test serum.

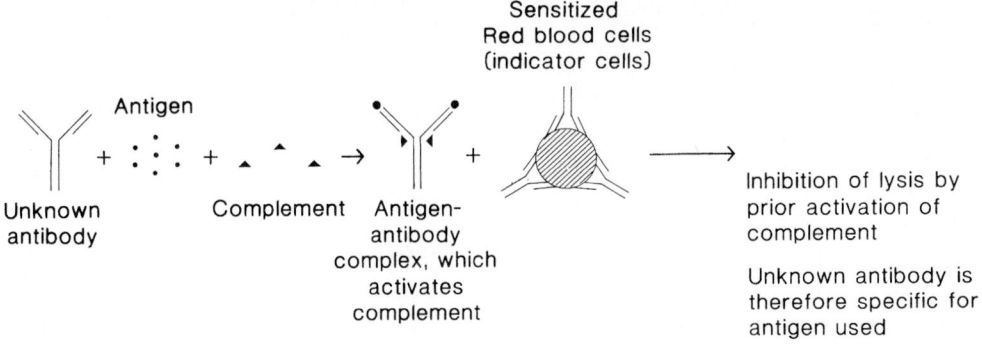

Fig. 12-12 Complement-fixation two-stage testing. One can measure antigen or antibody by holding constant all but the variable to be tested, in this case unknown antibody.

sensitivity. These *indicator-labeled* immunoassays use as a detection system the sensitive measurement of some property of the indicator molecule. The indicators, or labels, commonly used include enzymes, fluorescent or chemiluminescent molecules, and radioactive compounds.

Indicator-labeled assays are suitable for both qualitative and quantitative measurements. Their increasing popularity is due to the fact that they are sensitive, reproducible, use minimal reagents, and are suitable for automation. The nonisotopic immunoassays have the additional advantage over radioimmunoassays in that they do not require the special precautions and waste-disposal procedures necessary for handling radioisotopes.

Quantitative immunoassays of this type usually use IgG as the reagent antibody. Although they are quite specific by virtue of the antibody specificity, the binding reactions are sensitive to the usual variations in temperature, pH, ionic strength, and sample or standard matrix. Analytical sensitivity to nanograms-per-milliliter range or even lower allows this type of assay to be used for analytes that are present in low concentrations, such as hormones, vitamins, and drugs.

Qualitative indicator-labeled immunoassays frequently are less sensitive but are convenient and very popular in the serology laboratory for the detection of antibodies to infectious organisms and for the characterization of autoimmune antibodies such as antinuclear antibody and antithyroid antibodies.

Indicator-labeled immunoassays may be generally classified as competitive or noncompetitive and as heterogeneous or homogeneous. Competitive reactions usually use labeled antigen and are carried out in the presence of excess antigen. The analyte and labeled analyte compete for binding sites on the antibody. Radioimmunoassay (RIA) is the prototype of the heterogeneous type of competitive immunoassay, and enzyme-multiplied immunoassay technique (EMIT) (see next chapter) is an example of the homogeneous type. Noncompetitive assays usually employ a labeled antibody and are carried out in the presence of excess antibody. Frequently these assays are heterogeneous,

using a capture antibody bound to a solid phase such as a plastic bead or test tube and a second phase consisting of the labeled antibody in solution. This latter type of assay is synonymous with the terms *immunometric* or *sandwich* assay.

Labels. A label that is suitable for use as an immunochemical reagent must have certain qualities. The label must have high specific reactivity, that is, many detectable events per indicator molecule per unit of time. The specific activity must not be reduced, or quenched, by the conjugation of the indicator to the antigen or antibody. Enzyme labels should not be normally present in the sample in high enough concentrations to interfere with the measurement. This is crucial for homogeneous assays in which the sample matrix containing interfering substances remains in the reaction mixture during the measurement step. Several enzymes, metal chelates, radioisotopes, chemiluminescent dyes, and fluorophores fulfill most of these requirements and have been successfully used as labels in immunoassays. Examples of enzymes commonly used are horseradish peroxidase, alkaline phosphatase, glucose oxidase, and beta-galactosidase. Selection of the enzyme for use as a label for the immunochemical reagents is often empirical, and each enzyme has distinct advantages and disadvantages. (For the properties of enzymes, see Chapter 54.) Radioisotopes can be used to label either antigens or antibodies. The most commonly used radioisotope is ^{125}I, which has a high specific activity and a decay energy suitable for safe use in clinical laboratories (see Chapter 9).

In fluorometric immunoassays, either antigen or antibody can be conjugated, or covalently linked, with a fluorochrome molecule. The fluorochrome is a chemical that can absorb the electromagnetic energy of short-wavelength light (200 to 400 nm) and then emit light at a longer wavelength in the visible spectrum (400 to 700 nm) (p. 98). Intensity of the emitted light is the measurable indicator in fluorometric immunoassays. The most popular fluorochrome is fluorescein isothiocyanate, often abbreviated FITC, which can be easily conjugated to free amino groups; other fluorophores include rare-earth chelates. Chemiluminescent dyes are used in a similar manner. In this case, the conjugate is activated by a chemical reaction and subsequently emits light which can be measured. The chemiluminescent molecule may be directly conjugated to the label or a chemiluminescent substrate can be used with an enzyme label such as alkaline phosphatase.

IMMUNOMETRIC ASSAYS
Principles

Heterogeneous, noncompetitive, labeled antibody (immunometric technique). A popular format for this type of immunoassay is the heterogeneous immunoassay using a solid phase coated with antibody for the first step of the assay. The first antibody reacts with the antigen being tested. The extent of this reaction is assessed by subsequent reaction with a second labeled antibody. This forms the "sandwich" with the antigen between two different antibodies. The sandwich technique can be used to measure either antigens or antibodies (in which case the solid phase is coated with antigen). Antibodies have been immobilized to polystyrene (microtiter plates), latex, or ferromagnetic particles.

For the antigen-measuring system, two different molecules of antibody must bind to the antigen. Thus, only large antigens, such as proteins with multiple epitopes, can be measured by this type of immunoassay (Fig. 12-13). Antibody of the desired specificity is immobilized to a solid surface, which may be the wells in a microtiter plate or a plastic test tube. The solid surface is washed to remove all unreacted materials and may then be coated with other material (protein) to minimize nonspecific reactions, with subsequent possible false-positive results. In the second step, the fluid containing the antigen is reacted with the immobilized

antibody. All nonreacting material is then washed away. In the third step, the labeled antibody reacts with the antigen that has now been immobilized by the antibody onto the solid phase. All unreacted labeled antibody is then washed away. If enzyme is used as the label, substrate with appropriate cofactors is added. The amount of product is then measured by a color, fluorescence or light. Either end-point or kinetic measurements may be used. The intensity of the measured product is directly proportional to the amount of antigen bound to the solid phase. If a radioisotope was used as the label, the solid phase can be counted.

For an antibody-measuring system, the antigen of interest must be first immobilized on an insoluble matrix, such as a plastic surface or bead. Most often microtiter plates are used. Fig. 12-14 is a schema of this assay type. Immobilization with retention of antigenic reactivity is the first step of this procedure. In the second step, the biological fluid containing presumptive antibody toward the immobilized antigen is allowed to react. Any antibody present will be bound to the antigen immobilized on the solid phase. After separation of the unreacted components by washing of the support surface, the presence of antibody is detected and quantitated by addition of labeled anti-antibody that is directed toward the class specificity of the antibody being measured. Finally, the label is quantitated. This format is used to measure serum IgE that is specific for a particular allergen (the RAST test).

For both types of sandwich assays, the antibody or antigen coating the solid phase must be in excess over the analyte being measured. If the amount of antigen present exceeds the binding capacity of the capture molecule immobilized on the solid phase, the assay will not be quantita-

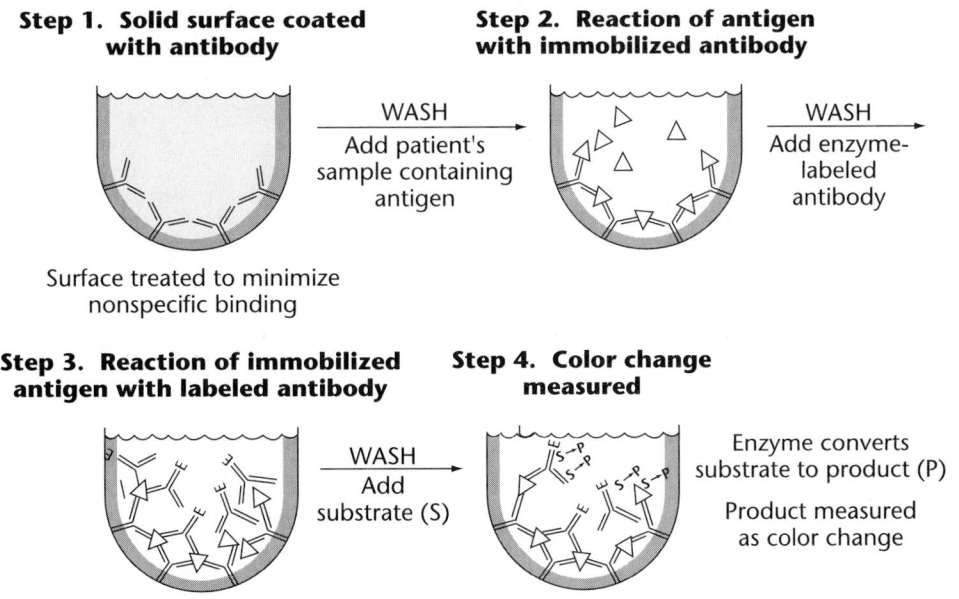

Step 1. Solid surface coated with antibody

WASH
Add patient's sample containing antigen

Surface treated to minimize nonspecific binding

Step 2. Reaction of antigen with immobilized antibody

WASH
Add enzyme-labeled antibody

Step 3. Reaction of immobilized antigen with labeled antibody

WASH
Add substrate (S)

Step 4. Color change measured

Enzyme converts substrate to product (P)

Product measured as color change

Fig. 12-13   Enzyme immunoassay. Sandwich technique with antibody label.

Step 1. Solid surface coated with test antigen

Step 2. Reaction of antibody with immobilized antigen

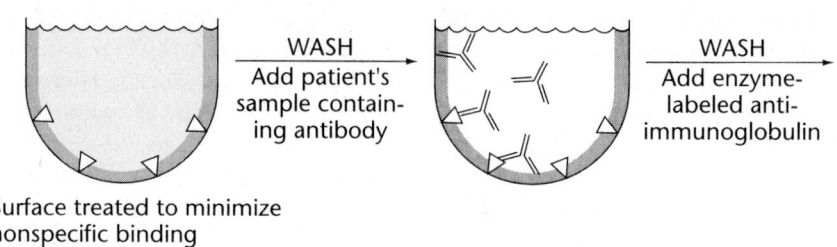

WASH
Add patient's sample contain- ing antibody

WASH
Add enzyme- labeled anti- immunoglobulin

Surface treated to minimize nonspecific binding

Step 3. Reaction of immobilized patient antibody with labeled antibody

Step 4. Color change measured

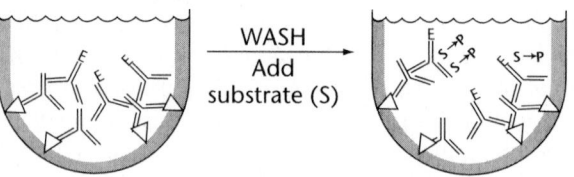

WASH
Add substrate (S)

Enzyme converts substrate to product (P)

Product measured as color change

Fig. 12-14   Enzyme immunoassay. Detection of IgE specific for an allergen.

tive, producing the so-called "high dose hook" effect. The labeled antibody must also be present in excess over the bound analyte in order to achieve a linear response and a quantitative assay.

Heterogeneous, competitive-binding assays. The simplest competitive-binding assay uses labeled antigen (Fig. 12-15) and a thorough treatment is given in Chapter 13. For the case of enzyme immunoassay, the enzyme-labeled antigen is mixed with the test solution, which contains an unknown amount of the antigen. The solution containing the labeled and unlabeled antigen is allowed to re-

act with a *limited* amount of antibody that is bound to a solid matrix. Unbound antigen (both labeled and unlabeled) is removed by washing, and the amount of labeled antigen is measured by determination of the amount of enzyme bound to the solid surface. This assay is always performed in antigen excess. The test solution contains the enzyme substrate and cofactors, and the enzymatic reaction, producing a colored product, proceeds continuously. The intensity of color is inversely proportional, but not linear, to the concentration of the antigen present in the test sample. This format of immunoassay can be used to detect small molecu-

Step 1. Solid surface coated with antibody

Step 2. Competitive binding of patient's antigen and enzyme-labeled antigen with immobilized antibody

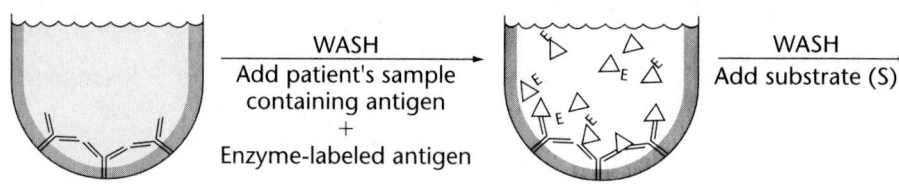

WASH
Add patient's sample containing antigen
+
Enzyme-labeled antigen

WASH
Add substrate (S)

Step 3. Color change measured

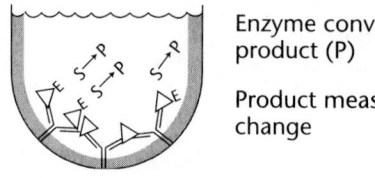

Enzyme converts substrate to product (P)

Product measured as color change

Fig. 12-15   Enzyme immunoassay. Competitive binding.

lar antigens or hapten groups, including drugs and hormones such as steroids and thyroid hormones, in biological fluids.

Sample requirements and preparation

All precautions required to preserve antibodies and antigen should be taken with indicator-labeled immunoassays. Many hormones, protein analytes, and antibodies are stable in serum for a short time at refrigerator temperatures. For long-term storage, freezing is preferable.

It is particularly important to establish and monitor that the antigen or antibody used in an assay does not bind nonspecifically to the support surface. Any component in the sample that can link the solid phase antibody with the label will be measured as analyte. Rheumatoid factor may interfere in this way. Also, systems using mouse monoclonal antibodies as reagents may show a positive interference with patients who have heterologous (antispecies) antibodies in their serum. This problem has been reported with patients who have been treated with mouse monoclonal antibodies for imaging or therapy and have subsequently developed human antimouse antibodies.

Reagents

Labeled reagents. The test reagents must be selected so that the conjugate has high specific activity, particularly when the concentration of the test analyte is low.

Solid phase. The plastic, latex, or magnetic bead should be chosen such that the bound ("capture") reagent is not removed by the wash solution under the assay conditions. Several manufacturers have developed plastic microtiter plates and test tubes specifically for enzyme immunoassays.

Substrate. In the case of enzyme labels, the appropriate pure substrate specific for the enzyme is selected to maximize the catalytic activity of the enzyme. As in any enzyme assay, care should be taken to add sufficient substrate so that it will not be depleted during the standard reaction time even if a large amount of enzyme label is bound to the solid phase.

Buffers. Pure buffers of appropriate ionic strength, pH, and composition are selected to optimize detection of enzyme and chemiluminescent labels.

Instrumentation

A spectrophotometer is usually used to measure the color changes that are a result of enzyme activity. With contemporary instruments, this process can be automated and kinetic measurements are possible. When the reaction occurs in microtiter plates with reaction volumes of 100 to 200 μL, special spectrophotometers called "microtiter readers," or "microELISA readers," are used. A drawback to the microtiter plate readers, however, is that they are frequently not as sensitive as a standard spectrophotometer. In addition, they are usually end-point readers. However, many have the ability to record the results of a standard 96-well microtiter plate in 1 to 2 minutes.

Instrumentation required for the measurement of radioisotopes is presented in Chapter 9. ^{125}I, the radioisotope most commonly used, requires a gamma counter. Specialized instrumentation is required for the measurement of fluorescent labels. If metal chelates are employed, techniques such as time-resolved fluorescence may be used (see Chapter 4). Both the indirect and direct fluoroimmunoassays require a fluorometer or spectrophotofluorometer to obtain accurate reading of the fluorochrome-labeled antibody. Luminometers, or photon counters, measure light flashes or the "glow" emitted in chemiluminescent assays.

Interfering substances

Substances in the sample matrix may interfere with the antigen-antibody binding reaction or the detection of the label, or they may simulate the specific binding by increasing nonspecific binding or by cross-linking the label with the solid phase. In addition, the sample may contain substances which have enzyme activity or that fluoresce under assay conditions. Care must be taken to avoid contact with compounds that interfere with the detection of the enzyme label, such as inhibitors or oxidizing reagents.

Common pitfalls

1. Improper storage of immunochemical reagents. Care should be taken to preserve the enzymatic or radioisotopic activity of the labeled reagents.
2. Inappropriate plastic used for the microtiter plates or test tubes. This is not a common problem when using kits but is a consideration when developing new assays. Lot changes, even from the same supplier, occasionally result in poor performance due to changes in the properties of the plastic support.
3. Improper pH and ionic strengths of buffer.
4. Nonspecific adsorption of reactants to plastic surface. This nonspecific adsorption can be minimized by incubation of the solid phase with proteinaceous material, such as gelatin or bovine serum albumin, after initial adsorption of the capture reagent to the solid phase.
5. Inadequate control of experimental conditions. Precision in enzyme immunoassays depends on strict control of temperature, pH, ionic strength of buffers, and concentrations of the various cofactors necessary for the enzymatic conversion of substrate into product. Finally, since enzymes are proteins and are subject to rapid denaturation under improper incubation conditions, close attention must be paid to preserve the enzyme activity during analysis.
6. Substrate depletion. If a large quantity of enzyme-labeled reagent is captured on the solid matrix, substrate can be depleted very rapidly. Sufficient substrate must be included in the reaction mixture so that a suitable

working range is available and the upper limits of linearity should be carefully defined.

Test sensitivity and precision

Numerous formats are described for the performance of indicator-labeled immunoassays. The sensitivity and precision of each of these immunoassays depend on the format selected and the instrumentations used to measure the label. Enzyme immunoassays and radioimmunoassays are generally considered to be sensitive in the nanogram-picogram/mL range. Most currently available enzyme immunoassays or radioimmunoassays have a coefficient of variation of less than 10% throughout the working range of the assay. Fluoroimmunoassays may have less sensitivity (about 100 to 200 µg/mL), but newer formats, including time-resolved fluoroimmunoassays, are as sensitive as most EIA or RIA. The variation observed within the same run is typically 3% to 6%. Immunoassay sensitivity depends on high specific activity labels, low nonspecific binding, and excellent precision.

SUMMARY

In this chapter, many immunological techniques are described and are summarized in Table 12-1. Each of these procedures was developed to meet a specific need to identify or quantitate an antigen present in a patient's sample. The immunoprecipitation techniques are the least sensitive but have high specificity in determining the presence of an antigen within the working range of the assay. Immunonephelometry is the most sensitive of the quantitative assays using precipitation as an end point and is fast becoming the most popular form of assay to quantitate many serum and cerebrospinal fluid proteins. Recent advances in instrumentation have made this technique the most precise of the direct immunological techniques, and it is preferred over radial immunodiffusion and rocket immunoelectrophoresis. Immunoelectrophoresis and western blot techniques are strictly qualitative tools. The former is commonly employed to assess the quality of an antigen present in a patient's sample, such as polyclonal IgG versus a monoclonal protein, or C3 breakdown versus C3 in native form. The western blot technique is commonly used for the verification of the presence of antibody to a specific antigen, such as HIV.

The agglutination and complement-fixation techniques are procedures used primarily in serology and blood bank laboratories.

Indicator-labeled immunoassays are becoming increasingly popular in the clinical laboratory as quantitative tools as they extend the sensitivity and specificity of antigen detection. Enzyme immunoassays are the most frequently used immunoassays for reasons previously cited. There are many assay formats, and numerous kits are commercially available to measure minute quantities of serum proteins, hormones, and drugs.

Selection of the appropriate immunological technique for detection of an antigen in the laboratory depends on many variables: technologist's skills, instrumentation, test volume and desired turnaround time, availability of test in kit form, quality control sample availability, ease of the technique, and cost to perform the assay. Whatever assay format is selected, the crucial factors that must be considered are the specificity of the reagent antibody, the antigen's structure, and sample preservation.

BIBLIOGRAPHY
General

Butt WR, editor: *Practical immunoassay: the state of the art,* New York, 1984, Marcel Dekker.

Chan D, Perlstein MT, editors: *Immunoassay: a practical guide,* Orlando, Fla., 1986, Academic Press.

Gosling JP: A decade of development in immunoassay methodology, *Clin Chem* 36(8):1408-1427, 1990.

Nakamura RM, Kasahara Y, Rechnitz GA, editors: *Immunochemical assays and biosensor technology for the 1990's,* Washington, D.C., 1992, American Society for Microbiology.

Roitt IM, Brostoff J, Male DK: *Immunology,* London, 1985, Gower Medical Publishing.

Roitt IM: *Essential immunology,* ed 6, Oxford, England, 1988, Blackwell Scientific Publications.

Rose NR, Friedman H, Fahey J, editors: *Manual of clinical immunology,* ed 3, New York, 1986, American Society of Microbiology.

Stites DP, Stobo JD, Wells JV, editors: *Basic and clinical immunology,* ed 6, Norwalk, Conn., 1987, Appleton & Lange.

Weir DM, editor: *Handbook of experimental immunology,* ed 4, Oxford, England, 1986, Blackwell Scientific Publications.

Immunodiffusion

Ouchterlony O: *Handbook of immunodiffusion and immunoelectrophoresis,* Ann Arbor, Mich., 1986, Ann Arbor Science Publishers.

Immunoelectrophoresis

Keren DF: *High resolution electrophoresis and immunofixation,* ed 2, Boston, 1994, Butterworth.

Two-dimensional immunoelectrophoresis

Dunbar BS: *Two-dimensional electrophoresis and immunological techniques,* New York, 1987, Plenum Publishing.

Radial immunodiffusion

Fahey JL, McKelney E: Quantitative determination of serum immunoglobulins in antibody-agar plates, *J Immunol* 94:84, 1965.

Mancini G, Vaerman JP, Carbonara AD, Heremans JF: A single radial immunodiffusion method for the immunological quantitation of proteins. In Peeters H, editor: *Protides of the biological fluid,* 11th colloquium, Amsterdam, 1964, Elsevier Publishing Co.

Ritzman SE, Fisher CL, Nakamura RM: Quantitative immunochemical procedures. In Ritzman SE, Daniels JC, editors: *Serum protein abnormalities: diagnostic and clinical aspects,* Boston, 1975, Little, Brown & Co.

Laurell rocket immunoelectrophoresis

Laurell CB: Quantitative estimation of proteins by electrophoresis in agarose gel containing antibodies, *Ann Biochem* 15:45, 1966.

Nephelometry

Ritchie RF: The maturation of light-scattering immunoassay. In Nakamura RM, Kasahara Y, Rechnitz GA, editors: Immunochemical assays and biosensor technology for the 1990s, Washington, D.C., 1992, American Society for Microbiology.

Whitcher JT, Perry DE: Nephelometric methods. In Nakamura RM, Kasahara Y, Rechnitz GA, editors: Immunochemical assays and biosensor technology for the 1990s, Washington, D.C., 1992, American Society for Microbiology.

Immunonephelometry

Price CP, Spencer K, Whitcher JT: Light scattering immunoassays of specific proteins: a review, *Ann Clin Biochem* 20:1-14, 1983.

Nishikawa T, Kubo H, Saito M: Competitive nephelometric immunoassay methods for antiepileptic drugs in patient blood, *J Immunol Methods* 29:85, 1979.

Agglutination

Bell CA, editor: *A seminar on antigen-antibody reaction revisited,* Washington, D.C., 1982, American Association of Blood Banks.

Kasahara Y: Principles and applications of particle immunoassay. In Nakamura RM, Kasahara Y, Rechnitz GA, editors: Immunochemical assays and biosensor technology for the 1990s, Washington, D.C., 1992, American Society for Microbiology.

Lennette EH, Valows A, Hausler WJ Jr, Truant JP, editors: *Manual of clinical microbiology,* ed 3, New York, 1980, American Society for Microbiology.

Williams CA, Chase MW: *Methods in immunology and immunochemistry;* vol 3, *Reactions of antibodies with soluble antigens;* vol 4, *Agglutination, complement, neutralization and inhibition,* New York, 1977, Academic Press.

Complement fixation

Stansfield WD: *Serology and immunology,* New York, 1981, McMillan.

Fluoroimmunoassays

Hemmilä L: Fluoroimmunoassays and immunofluorometric assays, *Clin Chem* 31:359-375, 1985.

Enzyme immunoassays

Avrameas S, Nakane PK, Papamichael M, Pesce AJ, editors: 25 years of enzyme immunoassay, *J Immunol Methods,* vol 150, no 1 and 2, 1992.

Engvall E, Perlmann P: Enzyme-linked immunosorbent assays (ELISA): quantitative assay of immunoglobin G, *Immunochemistry* 8:871, 1971.

Kemeny DM, Chaldacombe SJ: *ELISA and other solid phase immunoassays,* New York, 1988, Wiley & Sons.

CHAPTER 13

Principles for competitive-binding assays

Stephan G. Thompson

KEY TERMS

apoenzyme-reactivation immunoassay system (ARIS) A homogeneous immunoassay in which a ligand labeled with an enzyme prosthetic group combines with the apoenzyme for activity. This interaction is inhibited by a specific antiligand antibody, which in turn is competitively relieved with unlabeled ligand.

capture phase Ligand or specific binding protein attached to a solid surface or matrix to help separate bound from free label in a heterogeneous assay.

cloned-enzyme donor immunoassay (CEDIA) A homogeneous immunoassay in which a low-molecular-weight ligand is labeled with a genetically cloned fragment (enzyme donor) of β-galactosidase. The remaining portion of the molecule, complementary enzyme acceptor, is inactive unless the two components can combine to generate an active enzyme. In the assay, this combination is inhibited by antibody to the ligand-enzyme donor complex. The inhibition is relieved in a dose-response manner when the test ligand is present in the solution.

competitive-binding assay An analytical procedure based on the reversible binding of a ligand to a binding protein. The ligand competes in proportion to its concentration with a labeled derivative for binding to the limited number of binding sites.

conjugate Usually refers to the labeled reagent in which either the ligand (antigen) or antibody is covalently attached to the label.

cross-reactivity In competitive-binding assays this term is synonymous with specificity, that is, the specificity of the binding protein to bind only the ligand in contrast to other substances.

detection limit The smallest concentration of a ligand that can be statistically distinguished from a zero level in an assay. The detection limit is also referred to as the sensitivity of an assay.

enzyme-linked immunosorbent assay (ELISA) A heterogeneous immunoassay that in one configuration employs an enzyme-labeled ligand and antibody immobilized on a solid phase.

enzyme-multiplied immunoassay technique (EMIT) A homogeneous enzyme immunoassay in which a low-molecular-weight ligand is attached to an enzyme that is inhibited when the conjugate is bound by a specific antibody. Competitive binding of unlabeled ligand to the antibody relieves the inhibition in proportion to the ligand concentration.

fluorescence immunoassay (FIA) Competitive-binding assays that employ a fluorophore or fluorogen as the label.

fluorogen A nonfluorescent molecule that becomes fluorescent when modified by a chemical or enzymatic process.

heterogeneous assay A competitive-binding assay in which it is necessary to separate mechanically the protein-bound, labeled ligand from the unbound ligand before measurement of the signal generated by the label.

homogeneous assay Competitive-binding assay in which it is not necessary to separate protein-bound and free ligand fractions because the signal of the label is modulated by protein binding.

immunoassay Any binding assay in which the binding protein is an antibody.

immunogen A substance that stimulates an antibody response when administered to an appropriate animal. Immunogens include macromolecular antigens and otherwise nonantigenic haptens coupled to a macromolecular carrier.

immunometric assay Competitive and noncompetitive protein-binding assays in which the antibody rather than the ligand is labeled with a radioisotope or other suitable label.

label An atom or molecule attached to either the ligand or binding protein, capable of generating a signal for monitoring the binding reaction.

ligand A molecule or part of a molecule that is reversibly bound by the binding protein in a competitive-binding assay. It usually is the analyte but can also be a cross-reactant.

luminogenic substrates Enzyme substrates that emit light upon hydrolysis. Light emission is either a rapid (5- to 10-second) "flash" or a long-lived "glow" where the emission is measured up to 2 hours after the reaction is started.

prosthetic group Nonprotein components of enzymes and other functional proteins that are required for functional activity of the protein.

sensitivity The degree of response to a change in the ligand concentration in an assay. Sensitivity also refers to and is synonymous with the detection limit.

specificity The degree to which a binding protein binds its particular ligand while not binding structurally similar compounds.

time-resolved fluorescence Long-lasting fluorescence emitted from the chelates of lanthanide metals such as europium and terbium. Also characterized by its high quantum yield and enormous Stokes shift.

PROTEIN BINDING AND THE LAW OF MASS ACTION

Competitive-binding assays are based on the noncovalent, reversible binding of a ligand to a specific binding protein. The binding assay is most often described by the following reaction:

$$\text{Ligand} + \text{Binding protein} \rightleftharpoons \text{Binding protein:ligand} \quad \textbf{\textit{Eq. 13-1}}$$

where the binding protein has a measurable affinity for the ligand that interacts with it. In general, only one binding protein can bind a small molecule. This reaction can be considered simply as one molecule of ligand reacting with one protein binding site. The important molecular feature of binding proteins that enables them to be used in quantitative assays is their ability to bind compounds with a high specificity and affinity (see Chapters 11 and 12). Examples of specific binding proteins are listed in Table 13-1.

Nearly all competitive binding methods use antibodies as the binding protein for small molecules. These are usually

Table 13-1 Specific binding proteins present in blood or other tissues

Binding protein	Ligand
Antibodies	Varied antigens
Corticosteroid binding globulin (CBG)	Cortisol, corticosterone
Estrogen receptor	Estrogen
Intrinsic factor	Vitamin B_{12}
Thyroid binding globulin (TBG)	Thyroxine (T_4) Triiodothyronine (T_3)
Vitamin D receptor	1-α,25-Dihydroxyvitamin D_3

gamma immunoglobulins (IgG) directly produced in animals by a cellular response to immunization with the ligand or produced by monoclonal antibody hybridoma techniques with cells derived from an original antibody-secreting cell. These methods are discussed in great detail in Chapters 11 and 12 as well as other sources listed in the bibliography at the end of this chapter.

Small molecules by themselves normally do not provoke an immune response but do elicit antibodies when coupled with larger molecules; such small molecules are termed *haptens*. Because such small molecules participate in competitive-binding assays where the binding protein is an antibody, the ligand may be referred to as a "hapten."

The ligand in equation 13-1 is the analyte to be quantified. Often ligands are drugs (digoxin, theophylline), hormones (cortisol, T_4), or vitamins (B_{12}). For most competitive-binding reactions, the ligand refers to both the analyte and a labeled derivative of the analyte. Both must bind to the specific binding protein for the analyte to be measured. The final complex of binding protein and ligand is usually stable and dissociates only very slowly under favorable circumstances.

The binding reaction described in equation 13-1 is more complex for larger ligands such as proteins because macromolecules have many different binding sites (antigenic determinants) on their surface. A protein can therefore have more than one antibody simultaneously attached to it. Such binding determinants can be structurally quite different from one another, and so the population of antibodies generated in an immune response to large molecules is heterogeneous (polyclonal antiserum). The antigenic determinants of both high-molecular-weight immunogens and low-molecular-weight haptens are similar when one considers the behavior of antibody-binding reactions. Although macromolecules can be measured by competitive protein binding assays, noncompetitive methods are employed more often. These are discussed in Chapter 12.

The law of mass action describes some aspects of the phenomenon that occurs when molecules bind to one another. This is best illustrated when one examines the concentration of an antibody *(Ab)* and its ligand *(L)* or specific binding partner under equilibrium conditions. The bimolecular reaction

$$\text{Ab} + \text{L} \underset{k_{-1}}{\overset{k_1}{\rightleftharpoons}} \text{Ab:L} \qquad \textbf{\textit{Eq. 13-2}}$$

can be rearranged for calculation of the equilibrium association constant

$$K_a = \frac{k_1}{k_{-1}} = \frac{[\text{Ab:L}]}{[\text{Ab}][\text{L}]} \qquad \textbf{\textit{Eq. 13-3}}$$

where k_1 and k_{-1} are the respective rate constants for association and dissociation of the bound complex; *[Ab]* is the concentration of the unbound or free antibody at equilibrium; *[L]* is the equilibrium concentration of unbound ligand (a term denoting the antigen, *hapten,* or other substance); and *[Ab:L]* is the equilibrium concentration of the ligand-antibody complex. K_a, also referred to as the *affinity constant,* is defined in reciprocal molar concentrations (M^{-1}) or liters per mole (L/mol). This is the volume into which a mole of the binding protein can be diluted to yield 50% binding of the ligand. The larger the K_a, the greater the affinity of the antibody for the ligand. It follows that for a constant amount of antibody in the reaction, less ligand is required for a high-affinity antibody to bind 50% of the ligand than is required for 50% binding by a low-affinity antibody. Antiserum produced by an animal that has been immunized with a high-molecular-weight immunogen usually contains a mixture of different populations of antibody (polyclonal antisera) to that antigen. These different populations of antibody vary in their ability to bind the ligand (affinity) and in their ability to recognize different sites on the protein's surface.

There is only one uniform population of binding sites for a ligand when the binding protein or antibody is homogeneous, as in the case of monoclonal antibodies, which have a uniform binding affinity (K_a) and specificity for the antigen.

Low-affinity binding proteins and antibodies typically have association affinity constants in the order of 10^5 to 10^7 L/mol, whereas binders suitable for immunoassays and other competitive-binding assays have association constants between 10^8 and 10^{11} L/mol. A higher association constant enables one to design assays with sensitivities as low as 10^{-12} M, or lower, provided that the label itself is detectable at these low concentrations.

BEHAVIOR OF COMPETITIVE-BINDING ASSAYS

The competitive-binding assay can be imagined as the addition of increasing amounts of unlabeled ligand to reaction mixtures containing known, constant amounts of labeled ligand and a specific binding protein. In this case, labeled ligand, L*, and antibody, Ab, are added together in equimolar amounts. If one presumes that all the L* is bound, the reaction becomes

$$L^* + Ab \rightleftharpoons Ab:L^*$$

Two things happen with the addition of increasing amounts of unlabeled ligand (L): (1) unlabeled ligand competes with the labeled ligand for antibody-binding sites, and (2) there is an excess of the total ligand (L and L*) in solution compared to the number of binding sites. The concentration of antibody-binding sites is therefore limiting with respect to total ligand, thus modifying the preceding reaction as follows:

$$L + AbL^* \rightleftharpoons AbL + AbL^* + L^* + L$$

Less L* is antibody bound (as Ab:L*); thus, more L* is free as the amount of L increases. The amount or percent-

age of L* in the bound form can be calculated from the amount of L and L* present.

When the percentage of labeled ligand bound is plotted as a function of the concentration of the unlabeled ligand, it yields the dose-response curve shown in Fig. 13-1. The term *dose-response curve* applies to a plot of binding versus increasing amounts of ligand. The curvature of the dose-response plot in Fig. 13-1 is attributable to the logarithmic increase in the percentage of L that is bound when the concentration of L (dose) in the assay increases arithmetically. Thus the decrease in bound L* is also logarithmic. Conversion of the concentration of L to a logarithm makes the relationship become more linear.

COMPETITIVE-BINDING ASSAY FORMATS

Fig. 13-1 shows that to derive a dose-response curve one must know the amount of labeled ligand that is antibody bound as a function of the amount of unlabeled ligand added. A variety of techniques have been developed to measure either the bound or free forms of the labeled ligand in a competitive-binding format.

Some of these techniques require that the antibody-bound labeled ligand be physically separated from the free labeled ligand. These assays are called *heterogeneous assays.* Immunoassay approaches that do not require physical separation of bound and free labeled ligand are called *homogeneous assays.* The activity of the label in a homogeneous assay is altered when the labeled ligand is bound to the specific binding protein; thus the bound and free labeled ligands can be directly distinguished from one another.

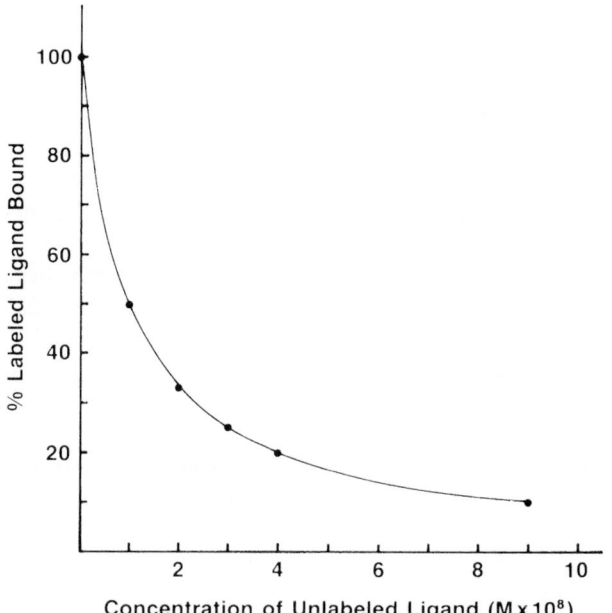

Fig. 13-1 Linear dose-response curve for a competitive protein-binding assay.

Heterogeneous assays

Table 13-2 lists some of the methods commonly used to separate the protein-bound from free-labeled ligand. In one example, the ligand or antibody is covalently attached or adsorbed to the hydrophobic plastic surfaces of microtiter plate reaction wells, providing a universally applied support for the *capture phases* of many different heterogeneous assays. The capture phase binds the labeled reactant in a competitive-binding heterogeneous assay, whether the latter is labeled ligand or labeled antibody. Another system, the microparticle-based capture phase, is widely used for two reasons: (1) suspended microparticle capture phases approach solution-like kinetics in that diffusion distances are very short compared to the surface of a microtiter plate well or a coated polystyrene tube, and (2) microparticles in comparison also provide a far greater surface area. For example, 1 mg of 1 μm diameter particles have 60 cm^2 of surface area for immobilization of antibody or ligand compared to the 1.0 to 1.5 cm^2 of surface area in a microtiter well. Both of these attributes shorten the assay time and potentially increase its sensitivity.

Latex and paramagnetic microparticles are used in similar heterogeneous assay formats; both can be used to readily separate the bound label from the unbound, one by filtration through a porous filter and the other by magnetic attraction.

Table 13-2 Techniques to separate protein-bound from free-labeled ligand

Technique	Principle
Adsorbents	
Nonspecific	Low-molecular-weight ligands are adsorbed by particles such as charcoal and removed by centrifugation.
Specific	Antibodies to the ligand or to the ligand-binding antibody are immobilized on the surface of a solid matrix such as glass fibers, latex microparticles, magnetic microparticles, membranes, or plastic. The immobilized antibody-ligand complex is separated from the unbound ligand by decantation, washing, filtration, diffusion, or centrifugation.
Chromatography	The protein-bound ligand moves at a rate through the chromatographic medium different from that of the free ligand. A similar behavior can occur with multilayer films.
Precipitation by ammonium sulfate	The antibody-bound ligand is precipitated by ammonium sulfate (Farr technique).
Double antibody	The antibody-bound ligand is precipitated by the addition of a second antibody specific for the antibody in the antibody-ligand or antibody-antigen complex.

Other methods for separating bound from free labeled ligand are listed in Table 13-2. Both the nonspecific adsorbent technique and the double antibody technique have been used with isotopic labels.

In some instances, competitive methods incorporate an indirect capture approach where an unrelated binding protein–ligand pair is used to bring the solid phase together with the capture antibody or ligand. In a classical example, immobilized streptavidin binds biotin that has been covalently attached to an antibody or to the ligand. Advantages to this approach are discussed below. Automation of some of the methods described in Table 13-2 has been accomplished, resulting in improved precision (see Chapter 16, pp. 304 to 309).

Homogeneous immunoassays

By definition, the activity of the label in a homogeneous assay is modulated when bound to the specific binding protein; an exception to this generalized definition for homogeneous immunoassays is based on the scattering of light by microparticles. Instead of an antibody modulating the signal per se, changes in light scattering are produced by the formation of antibody:ligand:particle complexes where either the antibody or ligand (or both) are multivalently attached to latex particles; the corresponding binding partner is also multivalent, thus enabling the components to form larger agglutinated complexes. An example is described later in this chapter.

LABELED LIGANDS
Types of labels

Common types of markers used to label ligands include radioisotopes, enzymes, and fluorophores. These can be used in both homogeneous and heterogeneous competitive-binding assays. The type of label, assay, and detection system are presented in Table 13-3.

Factors determining choice of label

Radioisotopes. Radioisotopic labels are used only with heterogeneous immunoassays because binding by antibody

Table 13-3 Some labels for competitive-binding assays

Label	Detector
Enzymes	
Chromogenic substrates	Spectrophotometer
Fluorogenic substrates	Fluorometer
Luminogenic substrates	Luminometer
Enzyme prosthetic groups	Spectrophotometer, fluorometer
Enzyme substrates	Spectrophotometer, fluorometer, luminometer
Fluorophores, fluorogens	Fluorometer
Microparticles	Spectrophotometer, nephelometer
Radioactive isotopes*	Radioactivity counter

*Usable only in heterogeneous assays.

Table 13-4 Radioisotopes used in competitive-binding assays

Isotope	Emission	Maximun specific activity* (Ci/g)	Half-life	Counter†
^3H	Beta	9.6×10^3	12.3 years	LS
^{14}C	Beta	4.5	5730 years	LS
^{32}P	Beta	2.85×10^5	14.2 days	LS
^{125}I	Gamma	1.74×10^4	60 days	Crystal
^{57}Co	Gamma	8.48×10^3	270 days	Crystal

*The curie (Ci) is a unit of radioactivity equal to 3.7×10^{10} disintegrations per second.
†Beta-particle emitters are counted in liquid scintillation (LS) counters by the release of photons from organic phosphors in solution. Gamma-ray emitters are counted in detectors with a sodium iodide crystal that contains fluor from which photons are released.

does not change the radioactive decay. In general, the desired sensitivity of the assay limits the choice of radioactive labels to certain specific isotopes that have high specific activity, high energy output, manageable half-lives, and ready availability. The radioisotope must be readily incorporated into or coupled to the ligand (or antibody) molecule, and its emission must be easily detected. Isotopes that meet these requirements are listed in Table 13-4. Consideration of all the factors, especially high specific activity, ease of incorporation, and reasonably short half-life, has made ^{125}I the label of choice for most radioassays.

Enzymes. Enzymes as labels differ from radioisotopes in that the binding reaction can modify their activity. Again, the enzymes must have high specific activity (that is, conversion of many moles of substrate to product per minute per mole of enzyme) and must also be easily attached to the ligand or antibody without losing significant activity. Enzymes that are commonly used include alkaline phosphatase, β-galactosidase, glucose oxidase, glucose-6-phosphate dehydrogenase, and peroxidase.

Some homogeneous enzyme immunoassays are based on the use of an inactive component of an enzyme molecule as the label. In the apoenzyme-reactivation immunoassay system (ARIS), the prosthetic group of glucose oxidase is a reactant label that recombines with inactive apoglucose oxidase to generate a fully active enzyme. Similarly, a polypeptide fragment of β-galactosidase is the reactant label for competitive protein-binding assays based on the cloned-enzyme donor immunoassay (CEDIA). Both technologies are discussed in greater detail later.

Substrates. Substrates for enzyme labels also help define the means for detection and in some cases the format for how the assay will be performed. Examples are shown in Table 13-3. Until recently, the most commonly used substrates were either chromogenic or fluorogenic, with the enzyme-catalyzed product being colored or fluorescent respectively. Luminogenic enzyme substrates that emit light upon enzyme catalysis have also been adopted for routine applications, particularly for the immunoassay of ligands that require greater sensitivity for detection and quantitation.

Although one can usually measure a thousandfold lower concentration of a fluorophore by fluorescence techniques than by colorimetric methods, the gain in assay sensitivity

with fluorogenic substrates for enzyme labels is at best only tenfold to a few hundredfold. Sensitivity greater than that seen with either fluorescence or colorimetry is generally achieved with luminogenic substrates. Since enzyme labels amplify the ligand or antibody molecules participating in the binding reaction, greater sensitivity can be achieved by longer incubation times for the conversion of substrate to product. This is an undesirable characteristic of some chromogenic substrates, particularly when more rapid assays are available that use either fluorogenic or luminogenic substrates. There are two types of luminogenic substrates. When a "flash" reaction occurs, the emitted light is measured within 5 to 10 seconds after the reaction is initiated, whereas the dioxetane substrates "glow" upon hydrolysis so that the light measurement can be made from 2 minutes up to 2 hours after the reaction is started.

Fluorophores. Fluorophores chosen as labels still fluoresce with a high degree of efficiency when attached to the ligand or antibody. The absorption (excitation) and emission wavelengths are well separated (Stokes shift) so that light scatter does not contribute to the fluorescence seen at the emission wavelength. Examples of fluorophores used as labels for competitive-binding assays and their properties are shown in Table 13-5. Of these, fluorescein and europium chelates are commonly used. Chelates of the rare-earth lanthanide metals europium and terbium strongly absorb light and fluoresce with properties that depend on the chelating ligand. The quantum yield (photon output/photon input) is very high, and the excitation and emission wavelengths are well separated. Europium and fluorescein have high extinction coefficients and quantum yields, but europium has the greatest separation between the excitation and emission wavelengths (273 nm).

Microparticles. When a microparticle multivalently coated with either antibody or ligand forms aggregated complexes upon binding to its specific binding partner, the increased particle size changes the amount and direction in which the light is scattered. To minimize background signal, the measured particle should be smaller in diameter than the detection wavelength; thus optimal unaggregated particles are less than 1 μm in diameter. Both turbidimetry and nephelometry are commonly used to measure the binding reactions for microparticle-based competitive light-scattering reactions. Turbidimetry measures the decrease of incident

Table 13-5 Fluorophores used as labels in competitive-binding assays

Fluorophore	Excitation wavelength (nm)	Emission wavelength (nm)	ε*	Fluorescence quantum yield†
Europium chelate‡	340	613	90,000	>0.95
Fluorescein	490	520	72,000	0.85
β-Phycoerythrin§	488	576	2,400,000	0.98
Rhodamine	550	585	50,000	0.70
Umbelliferone	380	450	20,000	0.50

*ε is the absorbance of a 1 M solution through a 1 cm light path.
†The fluorescence quantum yield is relative to the quantum yield of acridine, which is 1.0.
‡Europium:β-diketone chelate.
§β-Phycoerythrin is a 240,000 dalton phycobiliprotein.

light as a function of light scatter as the size of the aggregated particles increase. Thus these changes are detected as increases in absorbance at a particular wavelength. Nephelometry directly measures the scattered light at an angle greater than 90 degrees to the incident light (forward light scatter). Since turbidimetry can be performed with a spectrophotometer, it has greater applicability to different analytical or clinical systems. Nephelometry, like fluorescence and luminescence, requires special optical instrumentation.

Other labels

Two other labels that provide the basis for different homogeneous competitive protein-binding technologies are prosthetic group labels and substrate labels respectively. The ARIS employs the glucose oxidase prosthetic group FAD as its reactant label.

Fluorogenic β-galactosyl-umbelliferone, the reactant label for the competitive-binding substrate-labeled fluorescence immunoassay, is hydrolyzed by β-galactosidase to fluorescent umbelliferone when the labeled ligand is not bound by antibody.

DETECTION LIMITS (SENSITIVITY)

The sensitivity of a binding-reaction assay is a function of the affinity of the binding protein for its ligand. Consequently, for 50% binding to occur, a ligand present at a concentration of 1×10^{-7} M would require an antibody that had a K_a of 10^7 L/mol, whereas a ligand present at a concentration of 1×10^{-10} M would need an antibody that had a K_a of 1×10^{10} L/mol.

Ideally the binding protein in a competitive-binding assay would have the same affinity for both the labeled and unlabeled ligands. Usually this is not the case. In some instances the label or the labeling procedure will alter the immunochemical properties of the ligand to the extent that antibody does not bind it as well as it does the unlabeled compound, and in other instances, the converse is also true: antibodies made against haptens can include affinity for the chemical bridge used to couple the ligand to the protein carrier. Such antibodies may have a higher affinity for the labeled ligand with the chemical bridge than they do for the unmodified ligand.

The sensitivity of a competitive-binding assay is often improved if the ligand has sufficient time to bind to the antibody before the addition of the labeled ligand conjugate. This *sequentially* competitive-binding assay is particularly helpful when the antibody has greater affinity for the hapten conjugate than for the hapten alone compared to a *simultaneous* competitive format where the sample ligand and the ligand conjugate have equal access to the antibody. The response to the presence of sample ligand is usually greater in a sequential format, since the ligand has more opportunity to occupy the available antibody-binding sites than it would in a simultaneous format.

Besides the relationship to the affinity of the binding reaction, the detection limits or sensitivity of a competitive-binding assay is also dependent on the relative detectability of the labeled species. For example, a fluorophor should provide greater sensitivity than a chromophore; the fluorescent or luminescent product of enzyme-label catalysis will place the detection limit 1 to 2 orders of magnitude below that usually observed with chromogens as substrates; europium chelates can provide greater sensitivity than ^{125}I because of their greater label density compared to ^{125}I, which is limited (to avoid damage to the radioactivity-labeled reagent).

Detection limits can be defined as the lowest concentration of a ligand that can accurately and precisely be distinguished from zero (ligand). Therefore, by definition, any nonspecific interaction that contributes to the signal in the absence of ligand compromises the detection limit by lowering the signal-to-noise ratio (S/N), thus making it more difficult to distinguish the signal derived from the specific binding reaction from that attributable to nonspecific binding (NSB) and other nonspecific interferences. Although other types of interference are prevalent in both homogeneous and heterogeneous assays, NSB is a common problem in the latter where either a ligand-labeled conjugate or antibody-labeled conjugate nonspecifically adheres to the solid phase. This phenomenon can be attributable to sites on the solid phase available for hydrophobic or ionic adsorption because binding sites on the solid-phase surface are not saturated or there are surface changes after coating or chemical modification. Reduction of the NSB is often achieved by inclusion of blocking proteins or detergents in the reactions.

Table 13-6 Cross-reactant binding as a function of antibody affinity

Antibody	Bound species	K_a	Concentration (M) required for 50% binding*
1	Ligand₁	1×10^8	2×10^{-8}
	Cross-reactant_a	1×10^7	2×10^{-7}
	Cross-reactant_b	5×10^7	1×10^{-6}
2	Ligand₂	1×10^{10}	2×10^{-10}
	Cross-reactant_c	2×10^8	4×10^{-8}
	Cross-reactant_d	1×10^6	2×10^{-6}

*When 50% of the ligand or cross-reactant is bound, $B/F = 1$. Since

$$K_a = \frac{B}{F[Ab]}; \quad \text{when } B/F = 1, \text{ the } K_a = \frac{1}{[Ab]}$$

CROSS-REACTIVITY (SPECIFICITY)

The specificity of a binding protein for its ligand is measured by its ability to bind only the ligand in contrast to other substances. Cross-reacting molecules are structurally so similar to the ligand that they are also bound by the antibody. The greater the chemical difference between the ligand and a potential cross-reactant, the less likely it is that the cross-reactant will be bound. Examples of potential cross-reactants are drug analogs and metabolites for drug assays and low-molecular-weight hormones that are similar in structure, such as T_3 and T_4 for their respective assays. Differences in antibody binding of ligand and cross-reacting substances are a function of differences in affinity. These differences are reflected by responses to cross-reactants in competitive-binding assays. Table 13-6 gives two examples of the relationship between the K_a of the antibody for its li-

gand, two cross-reactants, and the concentration of each that is required in the assay to deliver the same binding response. The concentration of cross-reactant_a required for 50% binding to antibody₁ is 10 times the concentration necessary to bind 50% of ligand₁. Similarly, 10,000-fold less ligand₂ is required to achieve 50% binding to antibody₂ than is necessary to bind 50% of cross-reactant_d. Table 13-6 shows that with a lower K_a more antibody is required to bind 50% of the ligand or cross-reactant, further illustrating the relationship between sensitivity and K_a. The degree to which each cross-reactant in Table 13-6 interferes with the analysis of each ligand depends on the relative concentrations of ligand and cross-reactant in actual samples. For example, cross-reactants c and d would probably *not* interfere in the assay of ligand₂ *unless* they were present at concentrations 100 or 10,000 times higher, respectively, than that of ligand₂.

Ideally, antibodies or other binding proteins that participate in competitive-binding reactions are very specific for the ligand with essentially no cross-reactivity with closely related molecules. In reality, the antibodies present in a heterogeneous antiserum bind the ligand with different affinities and orientations and are therefore also likely to bind structurally similar molecules. One of the advantages of monoclonal antibodies is the potential for selecting very specific antibodies that have essentially no cross-reactivity with other compounds. Examples of the cross-reactivity of antiserums and a monoclonal antibody are shown in Figs. 13-2 and 13-3. The dose-response curves seen with antiserum, in Fig. 13-2, show that caffeine, which is structurally similar to the antiasthmatic drug theophylline, effectively competes only at much higher concentrations with the

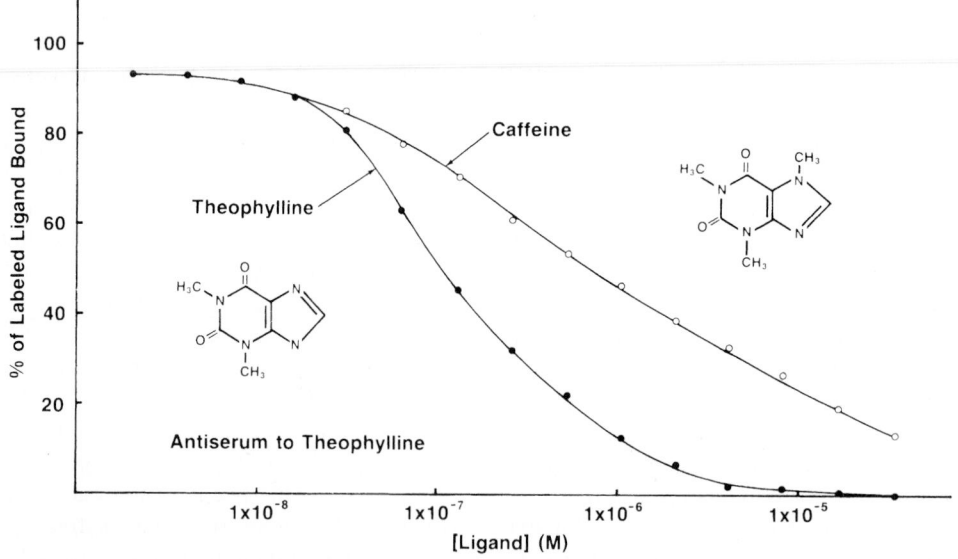

Fig. 13-2 Cross-reactivity of caffeine with a polyclonal antibody to theophylline in a homogeneous fluorescent immunoassay. Cross-reactivity is determined at concentrations of theophylline and caffeine required for 50% of the dose response. This is equivalent to 46.5% of the bound label. Refer to Table 13-7 for cross-reactivity data.

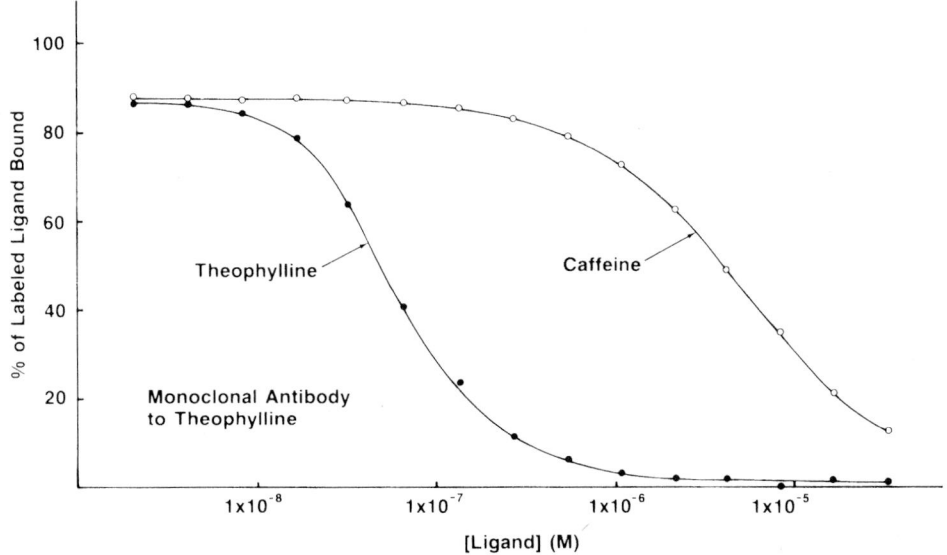

Fig. 13-3 Cross-reactivity of caffeine with a monoclonal antibody to theophylline in the same immunoassay. Cross-reactivity is determined at 43.2% of bound label.

Table 13-7 Caffeine cross-reactivity with polyclonal or monoclonal antibodies to theophylline

| | Concentration (M) when 50% of label is bound | | % Cross-reactivity |
	Theophylline	Caffeine	
Polyclonal	1.29×10^{-7}	1.05×10^{-6}	12.3
Monoclonal	6.15×10^{-8}	5.09×10^{-6}	1.2

label for theophylline-binding sites. The degree of caffeine cross-reactivity, determined by the "classical" approach, is calculated when one divides the concentration of ligand (in this case theophylline) at 50% of the maximum binding (indicated in Fig. 13-2) by the concentration of cross-reactant (caffeine), which also displaces 50% of the label according to the following equation:

$$\frac{[\text{Ligand}] \text{ at } 50\% \text{ binding}}{[\text{Cross-reactant}] \text{ at } 50\% \text{ binding}} (100) = \% \text{ cross-reactivity}$$

Eq. 13-4

There is 12.3% caffeine cross-reactivity for the antiserum shown in Fig. 13-2, but only 1.2% cross-reactivity with the

theophylline monoclonal antibody as shown in Fig. 13-3. Table 13-7 summarizes these results. A competitive-binding assay that uses the monoclonal antibody to theophylline is more specific than one that uses the antiserum; consequently based on this analysis, the former would be less prone to caffeine interference.

Although the classical approach to determining cross-reactivity is useful for evaluating the comparative assay response of ligand and cross-reactant, the *"functional"* approach is more meaningful. The latter determines the contribution of a potential cross-reactant to the competitive-binding assay response in the presence of the ligand. For example, both the ligand and the cross-reactant are com-

Table 13-8 Functional and classical cross-reactivity determinations for an antitheophylline monoclonal antibody

| | Classical* | | Functional† | |
Cross-reactant	µg/mL	%	µg/mL	%
1,3,7-trimethylxanthine (caffeine)	>10,000	<0.2	400	0.8
3,7-dimethylxanthine (theobromine)	760	2.8	390	0.8
1,3-dimethyluric acid	2,900	1.0	580	0.5
3-methylxanthine	760	2.8	280	1.1

*Classical cross-reactivity determined as described by Eq. 13-4. Theophylline concentration at 50% binding was 21.3 µg/mL.
†Functional cross-reactivity is defined by the concentration of cross-reactant that increases the observed concentration of 15 µg of theophylline/mL control by 20%. Therefore, functional cross-reactivity is calculated as follows:

$$\% \text{ Cross-reactivity} = (100) \frac{3 \text{ µg theophylline/mL}}{\text{µg cross-reactant/mL at } 20\% \text{ bias}}$$

peting with each other *and* with the ligand-label conjugate for antibody-binding sites. Consequently it is not surprising when a cross-reactant with cross-reactivity of 1% to 2% in the classical method increases the known concentration of a ligand by 10% to 20%. One approach to evaluate functional cross-reactivity is to determine the assay response to increasing concentrations of cross-reactant at different concentrations of ligand. Table 13-8 summarizes the cross-reactivity of caffeine, theobromine, and various theophylline metabolites at a midlevel theophylline concentration compared to that observed using the classical approach, whereas Fig. 13-4 illustrates the response of various cross-reactants in a functional assay.

Now that the monoclonal antibodies produced from immortal cell lines can be readily screened for very high affinity ($K_a = 10^{11} - 10^{12} \, M^{-1}$) with almost absolute specificity, these binding proteins are preferred to polyclonal antibodies, which are often inconsistent in quality and availability.

DATA REDUCTION

Earlier in this chapter the displacement reaction was described by the equation

$$L + AbL^* \rightleftharpoons AbL + AbL^* + L^* + L$$

where Ab is the antibody or another binding protein providing a limited number of ligand-binding sites. The concentration of the labeled ligand, L^*, is constant and in excess of the binding-site concentration. The ligand, L, will compete with L^* for the available binding sites. As shown in Fig. 13-1, the amount of L^* bound by the antibody is inversely proportional to the concentration of L in the assay. The dose response is a measure of either the bound L^* or the free L^* that has been displaced by L. Radioimmunoassay (RIA) will serve to illustrate the common methods for generating dose-response curves and quantifying concentrations of analytes.

The data shown in Table 13-9 were generated with a double-antibody RIA for the aminoglycoside antibiotic amikacin, where ^{125}I-amikacin was the labeled ligand. The primary antibody was rabbit antiserum to amikacin. Goat antiserum to rabbit antibodies is included in the assay to precipitate the antibody-bound labeled ligand. The precipitate is collected by centrifugation, and the pellet in the bottom of the tube is counted for radioactivity after the supernatant has been removed. The quantity *nonspecifically bound (NSB) counts per minute* refers to the radioactivity nonspecifically bound to the bottom of the tube in the absence of antibody to amikacin.

Table 13-9 shows how the amikacin RIA data are pro-

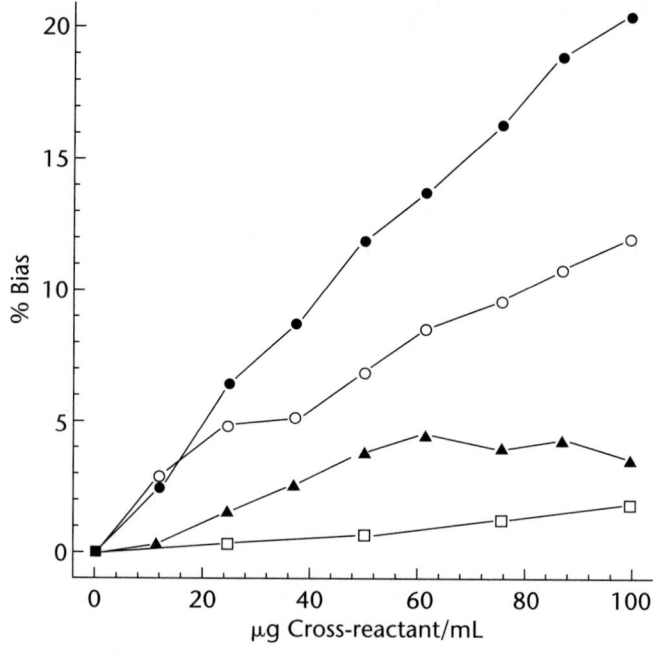

Fig. 13-4 Functional determination of cross-reactivity in a homogeneous turbidimetric inhibition assay. The observed increase in apparent concentration to a midrange control is measured in the presence of increasing concentrations of 1,3-dimethyluric acid, •; 1-methylxanthine, ▲; 3-methylxanthine, ○; and caffeine, □.

Table 13-9   Data for amikacin RIA radioactivity*

Dose of amikacin ($M \times 10^{-8}$)	Total bound cpm (TB)	Specifically bound cpm (B)†	%B‡	B/F§	B/B₀‖	Logit B/B₀
0	14019	13588(B_0)	64.0	1.78	1.00	—
1.07	10694	10264	48.4	0.94	0.76	1.13
2.14	9235	8805	41.5	0.71	0.65	0.61
4.28	7184	6754	31.8	0.47	0.50	−0.01
8.56	5360	4930	23.2	0.30	0.36	−0.56
17.12	3925	3495	16.5	0.20	0.26	−1.06
Unknown 1	8912	8482	40.0	0.67	0.62	0.51
Unknown 2	6910	6480	30.5	0.44	0.48	−0.09
Unknown 3	4340	3910	18.4	0.23	0.29	−0.91

*Total counts per minute (cpm), *T*, of ^{125}I-amikacin in each reaction are 21,225; nonspecifically bound (NSB) counts per minute are 430.
†Specifically bound cpm = *B* = Total bound cpm − NSB.
‡% bound = (*B/T*)100.
§$B/F = \dfrac{B}{TB - B}$
‖B_0 = *B* at zero dose of drug.

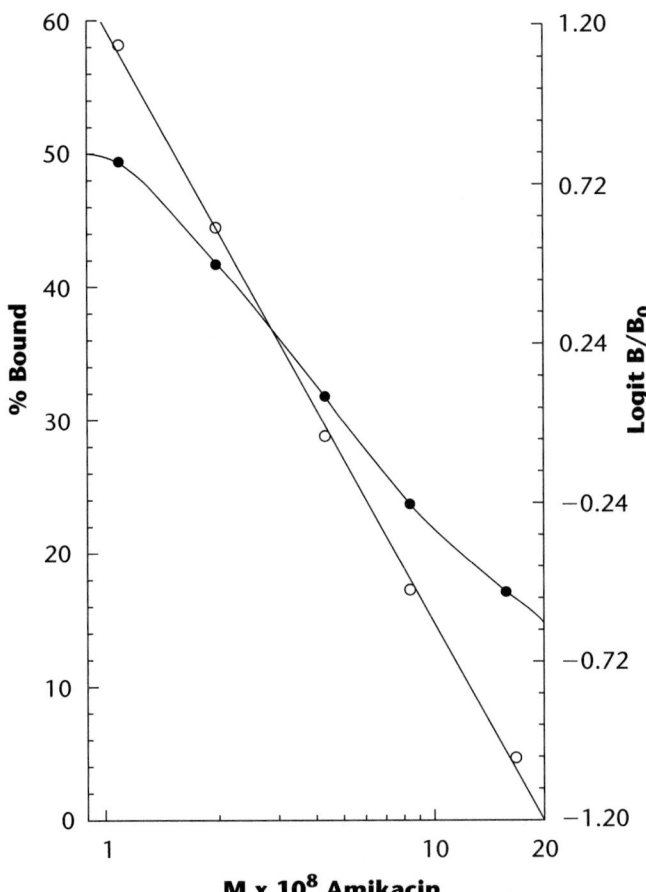

Fig. 13-5 Amikacin radioimmunoassay dose-response curves with the percentage of bound ^{125}I-amikacin, •, and logit (B/B_o), ○, plotted as a function of the log of the amikacin concentration.

cessed to generate two common dose-response curves. In addition to the total bound counts per minute (TB), the *y*-axis can be drawn as %B, or logit B/B_0. The logit transformation is the following:

$$\text{logit } (B/B_0) = \ln \frac{B/B_0}{1 - B/B_0} \qquad \textit{Eq. 13-5}$$

The bound counts per minute and %B can be plotted as a function of the arithmetic dose of the ligand concentration even though the resulting curves are nonlinear (see Fig. 13-1), or they can be plotted versus the log of the concentration to yield the slightly sigmoid dose-response curve seen in Fig. 13-5. The graph of log dose versus the logit B/B_0 (also shown in Fig. 13-5) has been the most accepted empirical method for linearizing competitive protein-binding dose-response curves, particularly for RIA. Automatic data reduction and processing of the log-logit transformation are easily performed with computerized instruments that offer various axis transforms with polynomial and four-parameter curve-fitting equations that are well suited for curvilinear calibration lines.

EXAMPLES OF COMPETITIVE-BINDING ASSAYS
Radioimmunoassay (RIA)

In radioimmunoassay, the ligand and a constant amount of radioactively labeled ligand compete for a limited number of antibody-binding sites. The concentration of antibody is usually sufficient to bind between 30% and 80% of the labeled material. In the above example, the antibody to amikacin bound 64% of the ^{125}I-amikacin in the absence of unlabeled ligand. Addition of unlabeled ligand to the reaction yields a net increase in the total ligand (labeled plus unlabeled), but because of competition for antibody-binding sites, there will be a decrease in the proportion of labeled ligand that will be bound by the antibody. If one counts the radioactivity bound to the antibody after the separation step, the dose-response curve will have a negative slope similar to that shown in Fig. 13-1. As the concentration of unlabeled ligand increases and the antibody-binding sites approach saturation, the slope levels off. When the unbound radioactively labeled ligand is monitored, the dose-response curve has a positive slope but with the same shape.

Radioimmunoassay is applicable to the measurement of both low- and high-molecular-weight ligands, provided that the labeling procedure or the labeled ligand conjugate itself does not adversely affect the immunoreactivity of the ligand. These problems are overcome by labeling the antibody rather than the ligand because the major structural differences between IgG molecules are substantially less than the differences between ligands. Losses in immunoreactivity are less likely to occur when the antibody is labeled.

Assays based on the use of a labeled antibody are called *immunometric* assays. One that uses a radiolabeled antibody is an immunoradiometric assay (IRMA). The ligand in the sample competes with the ligand attached to a solid surface for the binding sites of the labeled antibody (Fig. 13-6). The amount of labeled antibody bound to the solid surface is determined after excess label and sample have been removed. A representative dose-response curve is also shown in Fig. 13-6. The immunometric format is considered again in the discussion of ELISA techniques.

Enzyme-linked immunosorbent assay

The enzyme-linked immunosorbent assays (ELISA) are heterogeneous nonisotopic assays that usually have an antibody immobilized onto a solid support (see Table 13-2) whereas the ligand is labeled with an enzyme. Table 13-10 lists some enzymes used for ELISA (or other enzyme immunoassays). These enzymes are useful as labels because they satisfy the following criteria:

1. *High specific activity.* The signal amplification obtained with an enzyme label corresponds to the amount of substrate converted to product during the time of incubation. Enzymes with the highest specific activities yield the greatest amplification. Assays using such enzymes have excellent sensitivity and are able to measure very low concentrations of ligand.

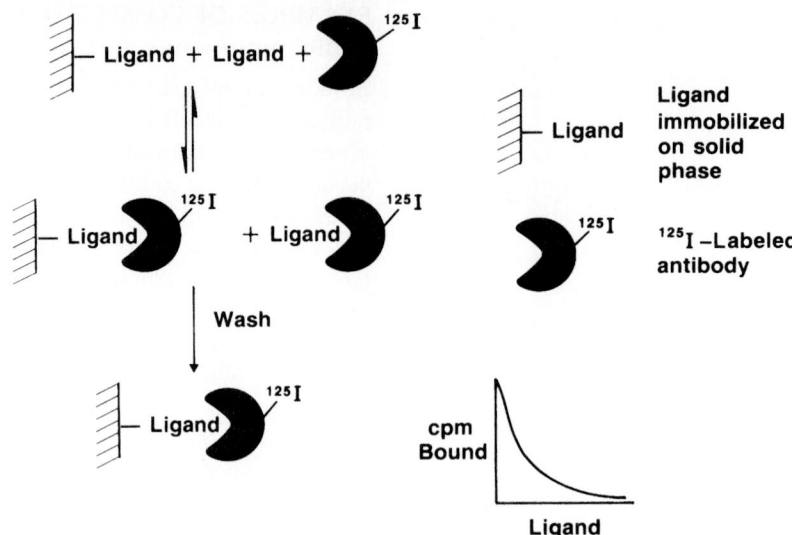

Fig. 13-6 Principle of the competitive immunoradiometric assay (IRMA) and a typical dose-response curve.

2. *Easily coupled to ligand.* The enzymes have sufficient acidic and basic amino acids, thiol groups, or carbohydrate to be easily coupled to the ligand without losing substantial enzymatic activity.

3. *Stability.* The enzyme labels are stable during the assay and under refrigerated storage conditions.

4. *Absent in fluid or tissue.* The enzymes are not usually present in the biological fluid or tissue sample that is to be analyzed.

5. *Retention of activity.* The enzymes retain most of their activity when attached to the ligand or antibody.

Alkaline phosphatase and horseradish peroxidase are inexpensively available in a highly purified form. For this and the reasons listed above, these two enzymes are most often used as labels for ELISA.

Some of the enzymes listed in Table 13-10 can use chromogens, fluorogens, or luminogens as substrates.

One advantage of a chromogenic substrate is that its product can be detected visually. Fluorescent and luminescent products can be detected at 100 to 1000 times lower concentrations than those of chromophores, and the incubation time can also be reduced.

Many configurations for ELISA have been devised. Some are based on competitive reactions, whereas others are di-

rect immunometric "sandwich" assays. The sandwich ELISA is discussed in Chapter 12. The two basic formats for the competitive assays and the shape of the respective typical dose-response curves that describe the signal remaining on the solid phase are shown in Figs. 13-7 and 13-8.

Of the two, the configuration in which the antibody has been immobilized onto the solid surface (Fig. 13-7) has been described more frequently. This is analogous to the configuration in an RIA because the ligand in the sample competes with the enzyme-labeled ligand for the limited amount of antibody-binding sites fixed to the solid phase. After the binding reaction has taken place, the solid phase is washed with buffer to remove the unbound labeled ligand so that it does not contribute to the signal. The amount of enzyme bound to the solid phase is proportional to the absorbance, fluorescence, or luminescence of the product formed after the addition of substrate, and it is inversely proportional to the concentration of unlabeled ligand. This method is applicable to both low- and high-molecular-weight analytes.

Instead of antibody, the ligand can be attached to the solid phase as shown in Fig. 13-8. Only those antibody-enzyme binding sites not occupied by the sample ligand will bind to the immobilized ligand. The solid-phase

Table 13-10 Enzyme labels for immunoassays

Enzyme	Source	Molecular weight	Activity	
			Turnover rate*	°C
Alkaline phosphatase	Calf intestine	140,000	420,000	37
β-Galactosidase	*Escherichia coli*	540,000	324,000	37
Glucose oxidase	*Aspergillus niger*	186,000	53,700	25
Glucose-6-phosphate dehydrogenase	*Leuconostoc mesenteroides*	130,000	93,600	30
Peroxidase	Horseradish	40,000	220,000	25
Urease	Jack bean	540,000	450,000	25

*The turnover rate is the number of moles of product released per minute per mole of enzyme at the designated temperature.

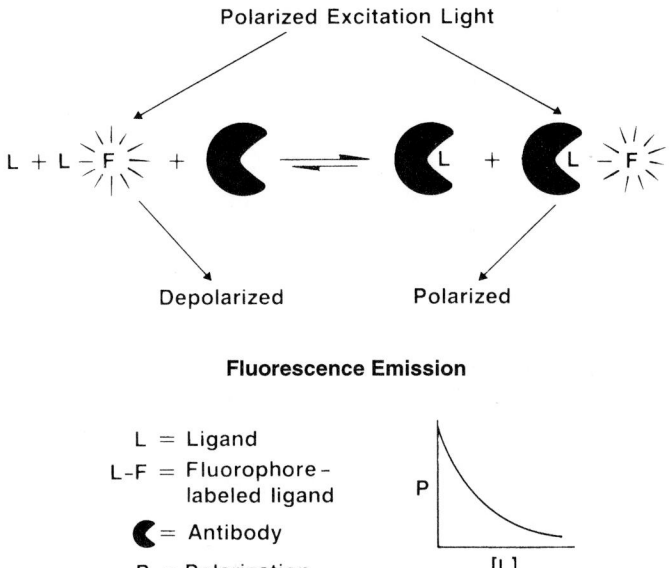

Fig. 13-15 Principle of the fluorescence polarization immunoassay (FPIA) and a typical dose-response curve.

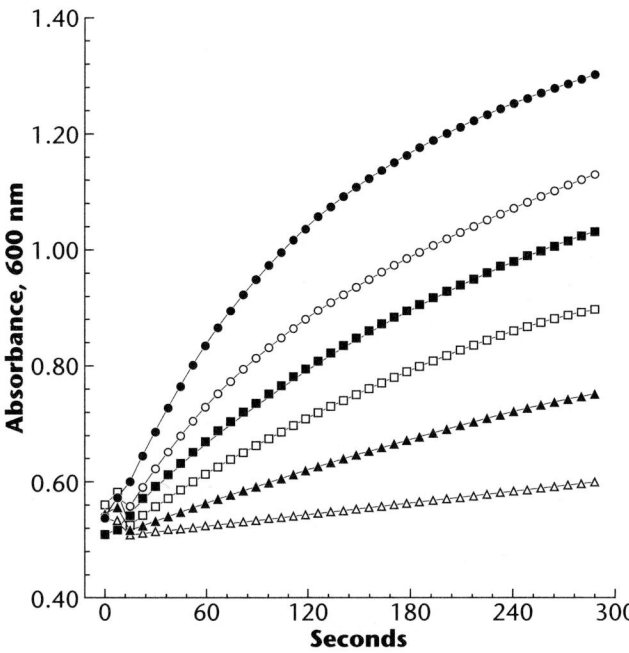

Fig. 13-16 Reaction time courses for a theophylline turbidimetric inhibition immunoassay in the absence, ● and presence of 2.5, ○; 5.0, ■; 10.0, □; 20.0, ▲; and 40.0, △, μg of theophylline per milliliter of sample.

taining a ligand-peroxidase conjugate and glucose oxidase. A dry paper chromatography strip that has ligand-specific antibody immobilized over its entire surface is then placed in the sample/enzyme reagent mixture so that the liquid reagents can migrate up the strip by capillary action. Since the enzyme conjugate competes with the ligand in the sample for binding to the immobilized antibody, conjugate migration is proportional to ligand concentration. During migration of the reagent mixture, the glucose oxidase is evenly dispersed throughout the strip. After reagent migration and chromatography are complete, the strip is placed in a developing solution containing glucose and a chromogenic indicator, which is oxidized by hydrogen peroxide (produced by glucose oxidase) by means of the peroxidase conjugate. Color will be produced in the strip to the height that the ligand peroxidase conjugate has migrated. Quantitation is performed by relating the height of color development to concentration using a conversion table. Enzyme immunochromatography tests have been developed for therapeutic drugs such as theophylline, phenytoin, and phenobarbital.

Microparticle-based light-scattering immunoassays

The competitive nephelometric and turbidimetric inhibition immunoassays differ only in how the scattered light is detected, as was discussed earlier. These methods consist of an *agglutinator,* usually a water-soluble polymeric carrier substance to which are coupled a multiple of haptenic ligands. Examples of carriers include dextran, polysucrose, and albumin. The antibody reagent is composed of antiligand antibodies adsorbed or covalently coupled to submicrometer-sized latex microparticles. For greater sensitivity, the ligand is also coupled to even smaller latex par-

ticles in a two-particle inhibition assay. The agglutination complex formed when the agglutinator and antibody reagent are combined can be measured kinetically or at a single time point. The presence of the ligand in the assay inhibits the rate of agglutination by competing for the antibody-binding sites. The course for agglutination at different ligand concentrations in a turbidimetric inhibition assay is presented in Fig. 13-16. The density of both ligand on the agglutinator and antibody on the latex microparticles is optimized to obtain maximum kinetics in the absence of ligand with appropriate inhibition in its presence. Measuring the rate of agglutination early in the reaction provides for the greatest sensitivity, whereas the rate or fixed time point can be taken at any time during the reaction for those assays that do not require low detection limits. Fig. 13-17 presents two dose-response curves derived from the reactions course shown in Fig. 13-16.

ATTRIBUTES AND LIMITATIONS OF DIFFERENT APPROACHES TO COMPETITIVE-BINDING ASSAYS

Before describing some advantages and limitations of the competitive-binding assays described earlier, I find it useful to discuss factors to be considered when one designs or chooses a particular assay format. Convenience, cost effectiveness, and performance for an assay must be addressed.

Convenience factors include:
1. Number of pipetting steps
2. Incubation time
3. Rate or end-point assay

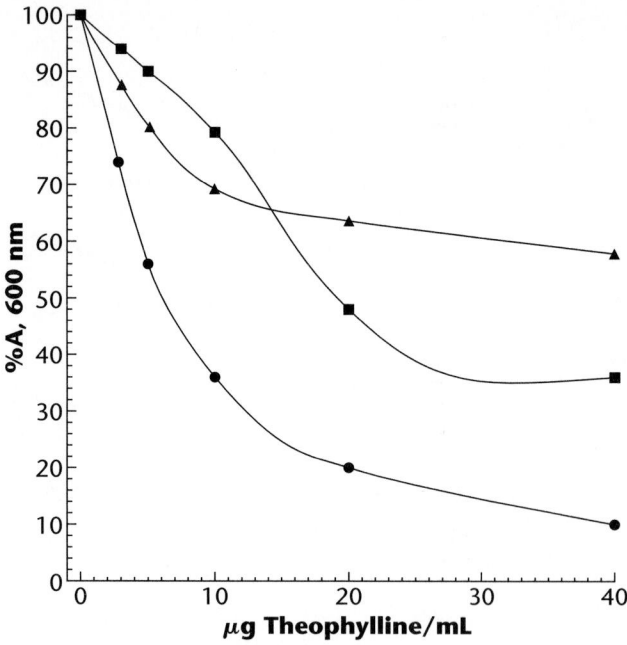

Fig. 13-17 Theophylline turbidimetric inhibition assay dose-response curves derived from the kinetic responses shown in Fig. 13-16. Rates were taken between 30 and 45 seconds, ●, and between 270 and 285 seconds, ■, and the dose response for a fixed time point at 285 seconds, ▲, is also shown. The respective responses were normalized to 100% for scaling purposes.

4. Need for additional equipment such as incubators, centrifuges, or specialized detectors
5. Automation and throughput
6. Sample volume requirement
7. Sample pretreatment (dilution, extraction, and so on)
8. Temperature-control requirements
9. Cost
10. Operator time
11. Radioactive-waste disposal
12. Applicability to a variety of analytes
13. Stability of reagents and storage temperatures

Obviously, the ideal assay would require very little sample with no pretreatment, a very short incubation time at ambient temperature, no pipetting steps, and no additional equipment other than the detector or an automated instrument. It would be able to be performed quickly, cheaply, with very little operator hands-on time, walk-away capability, and it would have a rapid data-reduction capability. The reagents would be stable for at least a year at room temperature or on board an automated system for at least 30 days.

Some of the most important performance factors are as follows:

1. Good assay response over the range of the standard curve.
2. A low background signal (that signal caused by either nonspecific interactions of the reagents in the assay or contributed by other substances in the standards or samples). The background must be kept to a minimum to maximize the S/N, detection limits, slope, and dynamic range.
3. High antibody affinity increases the slope of the dose-response curve and contributes to the sensitivity and detection limit of an assay. Sensitivity is related to the slope of the dose-response curve, to the experimental error (accuracy and precision of the assay), and to the activity and detectability of the label.
4. Good precision and accuracy depend on the accuracy of the values used for the concentrations of standards or calibrators and on the correct interpolation of the true shape of the dose-response curve between the standards.
5. Specificity is determined by the ability of the antibody to discriminate between the ligand and similarly structured substances. In most cases, the screening and selection process for suitable antiserums or monoclonal antibodies plays a very important part in determining antibody specificity. This is true for both native ligands (such as proteins) and the synthetic immunogens prepared to produce antibodies to low-molecular-weight substances.
6. Although some interferences are related to antibody specificity, others contributed by the patient sample can affect either homogeneous or heterogeneous competitive-binding assays, or both.

For example, homogeneous assays are influenced by endogenous enzyme activity that is the same as the enzyme label, or by substances that would interfere in the immunoreaction or signal measuring step. These may be removed by washing (heterogeneous method). Both types of immunoassay formats are subject to "heterophilic" antibody interferences from the patient sample. Heterophilic or endogenous antispecies antibodies can bind the assay antibody such that the signal is compromised. For example, human antimouse antibody (HAMA) will bind to the mouse immunoglobin coating the latex microparticle in a turbidimetric inhibition assay, with agglutination independent of the agglutinator resulting in a falsely elevated signal. HAMA is commonly neutralized by the inclusion of excessive mouse immunoglobulin in the assay.

Table 13-11 compares some characteristics of previously described competitive-binding assays, and Table 13-12 lists some of the interferences. The heterogeneous assays have the greatest potential for sensitivity, with picomolar or less detection limits. In addition to the high specific activities of the radiolabels or enzyme labels, fluorescent and luminescent labels are available. Interferences originating either from substances in the sample or from impurities in the reagents are removed by the separation or wash steps. By reducing the background signal, the heterogeneous procedure also allows one to increase the volume of sample to increase the sensitivity of the assay.

Table 13-11   Characteristics of some competitive-binding assays

Immunoassay	Homogeneous or heterogeneous	Detection limit (M)	Amplification	Low or high MW ligands
RIA	Heterogeneous	10^{-12} to 10^{-14}	No	Both
ELISA	Heterogeneous	10^{-11} to 10^{-15}	Yes	Both
EMIT	Homogeneous	5×10^{-10}	Yes	Low
CEDIA	Homogeneous	10^{-10}	Yes	Low
Light scattering	Homogeneous	10^{-10}	No	Low
FPIA	Homogeneous	5×10^{-9}	No	Low
Time-resolved fluorescence immunoassay	Heterogeneous	10^{-12}	No	Both
ARIS	Homogeneous	5×10^{-10}	Yes	Both

ARIS, Apoenzyme-reactivation immunoassay system; *CEDIA*, cloned-enzyme donor immunoassay; *ELISA*, enzyme-linked immunosorbent assay; *EMIT*, enzyme-multiplied immunoassay technique; *FPIA*, fluorescence polarization immunoassay; *MW*, molecular weight; *RIA*, radioimmunoassay.

The short half-life of the radioactive labels used in the clinical laboratory (such as ^{125}I) limits the use of RIA reagents to between 6 and 12 weeks after their receipt. This is a short period compared to reagents for the non–isotope labeled assays, which often are stable for a year or longer. In addition, radioisotopes are presumed to be hazardous and are subject to governmental regulation in their use and disposal.

ELISA and the other nonisotopic immunoassays have many advantages including the avoidance of radioisotope use. Because enzymes are biochemical amplifiers, the systems that employ enzyme labels are capable of producing a greatly amplified signal, depending on the specific activity of the enzyme and the incubation time for conversion of substrate to product. The use of fluorogenic or luminogenic substrates instead of chromogens can enhance the sensitivity of these assays 100 to 1000 times.

Disadvantages of ELISA include the inconvenience of required washing steps compared to homogeneous assays, though available instruments automated these washing steps. Other factors are listed in Table 13-12.

The homogeneous enzyme immunoassay (enzyme-multiplied immunoassay technique, EMIT), though limited by the absorbance of the product, is still sensitive to subnanomolar levels of ligand. Like ELISA, the sensitivity may be increased by use of a fluorogenic substrate. EMIT and other methods that use an absorbance readout

Table 13-12   Some potential immunoassay limitations and interferences

Assay type	Interferences/limitations	Effect on assay response
Heterogeneous	Antibody or antigen deformation or steric hindrance at solid phase	Loss of binding affinity and capacity; reduces sensitivity
	Nonspecific binding of labeled conjugate to solid surfaces	Reduces S/N, sensitivity, detection limit
	Desorption of adsorbed binder	Loss of binding capacity over time; enhanced competitive response
	Conjugation of ligand or antibody to enzyme lowers its activity	Reduced signal that is compensated for by longer incubation times
	Increased enzyme labeling increases NSB	Lower S/N, sensitivity, detection limit
	Europium contamination with time-resolved fluorescence-labeled chelates	Increased background, lower S/N
Homogeneous	Increased sample background because of endogenous:	Lower S/N alleviated by dilution (which also lowers
	•Fluorescence	sensitivity) or by kinetic measurements (if appropriate)
	•Enzyme activity	
	•Spectral interferences	
	•Label-like materials	
	•Antibodies to label	Reduction in signal, could interfere with ligand-conjugate antibody binding
	Imprecision	Overall noise increases, thereby lowering S/N
General	Exogenous substances	
	•Anticoagulants	Inhibit enzyme activity
	Endogenous substances	
	•Cross-reactants, metabolites	Increased signal response
	•Heterophilic antibodies, HAMA, rheumatoid factor	Bind antiligand antibody to simulate or interfere with normal response

HAMA, Human antimouse antibody; *NSB*, nonspecifically bound; *S/N*, signal-to-noise ratio.

are subject to possible interferences by hemolyzed, lipemic, and icteric samples. Because a rate measurement is used for EMIT, it is difficult to perform manually but is quickly and easily accomplished with automated equipment. However, the assay is not suitable for high-molecular-weight ligands because binding by antibody usually will not provide sufficient enzyme inhibition for unlabeled ligand to elicit a response.

Fluorescence assays are also sensitive to subpicomolar concentrations of ligand. The homogeneous fluorescence assays avoid errors that can be introduced by the separation steps of heterogeneous systems. With the possible exception of the time-resolved fluoroimmunoassay, which is a heterogeneous assay, these fluorescence assays are prone to interferences by hemolyzed, lipemic, and icteric samples. Possible sample interferences in homogeneous fluorescence immunoassays include light scattering from lipids and particulates, fluorescence quenching, and background fluorescence from the presence of endogenous fluorophores. The fluorescence polarization immunoassay is sensitive to the depolarized scattered light of particulates in the assay and requires sophisticated instrumentation. Some labeled ligands may be nonspecifically bound by endogenous proteins, resulting in an increased polarization background.

CEDIA and ARIS amplify the signal because an active enzyme is generated in each assay. Unlike other homogeneous enzyme immunoassays, antibody binds a ligand-label conjugate required to generate an active enzyme, rather than binding a ligand coupled to an enzyme that is already active. CEDIA, which has very high activity because of the generation of a high-turnover β-galactosidase label, would be more sensitive and require a shorter incubation time if the antiligand antibody complex was a more effective inhibitor of the donor-acceptor complementation for generating active enzymes. In addition, both fluorogenic and luminogenic substrates are available for β-galactosidase, making this method readily adaptable to most automatic instrumentation.

Although the nephelometric inhibition immunoassay requires a special instrument, the turbidimetric inhibition method is applicable to most immunoassay and clinical automatic instrumentation. Although perhaps not so potentially sensitive as CEDIA, in practice it is being used to quantitate lower-level analytes such as T_4 and digoxin.

BIBLIOGRAPHY

Ligand-binding and competitive-binding assays
Chan DW, Perlstein ET, editors: *Immunoassay, a practical guide,* New York, 1987, Academic Press.
Odell WD, Franchimont P, editors: *Principles of competitive protein binding assays,* ed 2, New York, 1983, Wiley & Sons.
Travis JC: *Fundamentals of RIA and other ligand assays,* Anaheim, Calif., 1977, Scientific Newsletter.
Voss EW Jr, editor: *Fluorescein haptens: an immunological probe,* Boca Raton, Fla., 1984, CRC Press.

Immunoassays (under a variety of formats)
Albertini A, Ekins R: *Monoclonal antibodies and developments in immunoassay,* Symposium of the Giovanni Lorenzini Foundation, vol 11, Amsterdam, 1981, Elsevier/North Holland Biomedical Press.
Diamandis EP: Detection techniques for immunoassay and DNA protein applications, *Clin Biochem* 23:437-443, 1990.
Gosling JP: A decade of development in immunoassay methodology, *Clin Chem* 36:1408-1427, 1990.
Nakamura RM, Dito WR, Tuckler ES III, editors: *Immunoassays: clinical laboratory techniques for the 1980's,* vol 4, *Laboratory and research methods in biology and medicine,* New York, 1980, Alan R Liss.

Radioimmunoassay
Chard T: *An introduction to radioimmunoassay and related techniques,* ed 3, New York, 1987, Elsevier Science Publishing.

Enzyme immunoassay
Maggio ET, editor: *Enzyme-immunoassay,* Boca Raton, Fla., 1980, CRC Press.
Porstmann T, Kiessig ST: Enzyme immunoassay techniques: an overview, *J Immunol Methods* 150:5-21, 1992.

Enzyme-linked immunosorbent assay (ELISA)
Avrameas S: Amplification systems in immunoenzymatic techniques, *J Immunol Methods* 150:23-32, 1992.
Butler JE, Peterman JH, Suter M, Dierks SE: The immunochemistry of solid phase sandwich enzyme linked immunosorbent assays, *Fed Proc* 46:2548-2556, 1987.
Pesce AJ, Michael JG: Artifacts and limitations of enzyme immunoassay, *J Immunol Methods* 150:111-119, 1992.

Homogeneous enzyme immunoassay
Henderson DR, Friedman SB, Harris JB, et al: CEDIA, a new homogeneous immunoassay system, *Clin Chem* 32:1637-1641, 1986.
Jenkins SG: Homogeneous enzyme immunoassay, *J Immunol Methods* 150:91-97, 1992.
Khanna PL, Dwarschock RT, Manning WB, Harris JD: A new homogeneous enzyme immunoassay using recombinant enzyme fragments, *Clin Chim Acta* 185:231-240, 1989.
Thompson SG, Boguslaski RC: Homogeneous dry reagent immunoassay strips for the determination of therapeutic drugs in human serum or plasma, *J Clin Lab Anal* 1:293-299, 1987.

Enzyme immunochromatography
Chen R, Li TM, Merrick H, et al: An internal clock reaction used in a one-step enzyme immunochromatographic assay of theophylline in whole blood, *Clin Chem* 33:1521-1525, 1987.
Zuk RF, Ginsburg VK, Houts T, et al: Enzyme immunochromatography—a quantitative immunoassay requiring no instrumentation, *Clin Chem* 31:1144-1150, 1985.

Immunoassay interference
Graves SW, Sharma K, Chandler AB: Methods for eliminating interferences in digoxin immunoassays caused by digoxin-like factors, *Clin Chem* 32:1506-1509, 1986.
Levinson SS: The nature of heterophilic antibodies and their role in immunoassay interference, *J Clin Immunoassay* 15:108-115, 1992.
Pesce AJ, Michael JG: Artifacts and limitations of enzyme immunoassay, *J Immunol Methods* 150:111-119, 1992.
Valdes R Jr, Miller TI: Increasing the specificity of immunoassays, *J Clin Immunoassay* 15:87-96, 1992.

Fluorescence immunoassay
Visor GC, Shulman SG: Fluorescence immunoassay, *J Pharm Sci* 70:469-475, 1981.

Fluorescence polarization immunoassay
Dandliker WB, Kelly RJ, Dandliker J, et al: Fluorescence polarization immunoassay: theory and experimental method, *Immunochemistry* 10:215-227, 1973.

Time-resolved fluorescence immunoassay

Diamandis EP: Multiple labeling and time-resolvable fluorophores, *Clin Chem* 37:1486-1491, 1991.

Soini E, Kojola H: Time-resolved fluorometer for lanthanide chelates—a new generation of nonisotopic immunoassays, *Clin Chem* 29:65-68, 1983.

Papanastasiou-Diamandis A, Christopoulos TK, Diamandis EP: Ultrasensitive thyrotropin immunoassay based on enzymatically amplified time-resolved fluorescence with a terbium chelate, *Clin Chem* 38:545-548, 1992.

Light-scattering assays

Newman DJ, Henneberry H, Price CP: Particle enhanced light scattering immunoassay, *Ann Clin Biochem* 29:22-42, 1992.

Luminescence immunoassays

Kricka LT: Chemiluminescent and bioluminescent techniques, *Clin Chem* 37:1472-1481, 1991.

Maeda M, Shimizu S, Tsuji A: Chemiluminescence assay of β-D-galactosidase and its application to competitive immunoassay for 17-hydroxyprogesterone and thyroxine, *Anal Chim Acta* 266:213-217, 1992.

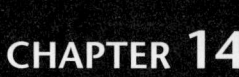

CHAPTER 14

Measurement of colligative properties

Lawrence A. Kaplan

Colligative properties
  Osmosis
  Osmolality
  Osmometry
  Osmolal gap
Clinical use of osmometry
  Plasma osmolality
  Urine osmolality
  Stool osmolality
  Serum or plasma osmolality
Principles of measurement
  Freezing-point depression
  Vapor-pressure depression
Colloid osmotic pressure
  Definitions
  Clinical use of colloid osmotic pressure
  Measurement of colloid osmotic pressure

OBJECTIVES

■ Identify the relationship between osmosis, osmotic pressure, osmolality, and osmometry.

■ List four measurements that depend on colligative properties and describe what happens to each property during sample concentration.

■ State the relationship between freezing-point depression and moles of particles dissolved per kilogram of water and calculate the osmolality from a given freezing point of a solution.

■ Describe the techniques of freezing-point depression and vapor-pressure depression for osmolality determinations.

■ State the clinical utility of performing plasma osmolality and urine osmolality determinations. State the clinical situations in which the measurement of the osmolal gap is useful.

KEY TERMS

"acetone" bodies The acetone and other ketones that are present in the serum of patients with diabetic ketoacidosis.

activity The effective concentration of the molecules of a solution.

boiling-point elevation A phenomenon in which addition of solute molecules raises the temperature at which the solution will boil. For water, this is 1.86 Celsius degrees per mole of solute per kilogram of solvent.

colligative property A characteristic to which all the molecules of a solution contribute, regardless of their individual composition or nature.

colloid A large molecule, usually in aqueous solution. Normally the term is applied to protein solutions.

colloid osmotic pressure (COP) The osmotic pressure generated by that portion of a solution with high molecular weight (greater than 30,000 daltons).

crystalloids The uncharged solute molecules of a solution.

dew point The temperature at which condensation of water from the vapor phase occurs.

diffusion Mixing or movement of molecules as a result of their random motion.

Donnan effect The distribution of ions caused by having a high-molecular-weight ion on one side of a semipermeable membrane.

freezing-point depression A phenomenon in which the addition of solute molecules to a solution lowers the temperature at which the solution will freeze.

molality The number of moles of solute per kilogram of water or solvent.

oncotic pressure Another term for colloid osmotic pressure.

osmolal gap The difference between the observed and calculated serum osmolalities. The calculated osmolar values include sodium concentration multiplied by 2, plus glucose and blood urea nitrogen.

osmolality The measurement of the number of moles of particles per kilogram of water.

osmometry The measurement of a colligative property of a solution in which the number of moles of a solute per unit volume (concentration) are determined.

osmosis Water flow across a semipermeable membrane.

osmotic pressure The hydrostatic pressure required to prevent a change in volume when two solutions of different concentrations are placed on opposite sides of a semipermeable membrane.

plasma expander Usually a high-molecular-weight dextran that is administered intravenously to increase the oncotic pressure of a patient.

Seebeck effect Voltage difference seen when two ends of a specially made wire are at two different temperatures.

semipermeable membrane A barrier that allows one type of molecule, such as water, to pass but does not allow another type of molecule, such as protein, to pass.

thermistor A temperature measuring device in which the

changes of resistance is temperature dependent. It is derived from the words *thermal resistor.*

thermocouple A device that generates a voltage (Seebeck effect) when the two ends of a wire are at different temperatures.

ultrafiltrate The solution remaining after passage through a semipermeable membrane. Usually it contains only low-molecular-weight solutes.

vapor-pressure depression The phenomenon in which the addition of a solute molecule to a solvent will decrease the amount of solvent in equilibrium between the vapor phase and the liquid phase.

COLLIGATIVE PROPERTIES
Osmosis

Osmosis is neither simply a mixing of two fluids nor simply a diffusion. Diffusion is the mixing of molecules as a result of random motion caused by thermal kinetic energy (brownian motion). For example, if an albumin solution were carefully overlaid with water, the albumin molecules would randomly move back and forth across the original interface boundary. Because there are more albumin molecules in the albumin solution, the odds are great that an albumin molecule will cross into the water side. Thus albumin will diffuse into the water layer until the solutions become homogeneous, that is, until the odds are equal that an albumin molecule will diffuse one way or the other across the original boundary because the concentration is equal on both sides.

The term *osmosis* specifically applies to water flow across a semipermeable membrane such as a cell wall. Although osmosis can occur with any fluid, water is the most important fluid for this discussion. A semipermeable membrane allows some particles (molecules, ions, or aggregates of molecules) to pass through it, but it inhibits the passage of others; hence it is *semi*permeable. The simplest example of a semipermeable membrane is a dialysis membrane, which is usually made of cellophane. It has very small pores through which water and some small molecules and ions pass. However, large molecules, such as proteins, cannot pass through the membrane. To demonstrate, place an albumin solution in a section of dialysis tubing and tie the ends of the tubing. If the tubing is placed in a beaker of water, the albumin molecules cannot move out of the membrane, but water molecules will move in and affect dilution of the albumin. As a result, the tubing will swell as water flows into the albumin solution inside the tubing, increasing the pressure inside the membrane. If the tubing does not burst from this pressure, an equilibrium will be maintained between the water flowing in and the water being forced out by the internal pressure. The hydrostatic pressure built up and maintained by this process is called *osmotic pressure.*

Perhaps the most graphic example of osmosis is lysis of red blood cells by water. So much water flows into the more concentrated intracellular fluid that the cell swells and bursts. Cells can also shrink if exposed to a fluid of high osmolality. In this case the water in the cell flows out of the cell into the concentrated solution outside. In the laboratory the measurement of mean corpuscular volume (MCV) is affected by this process. If the diluent is not isotonic, that is, of equal osmotic pressure, the cells will swell or shrink, giving an erroneous mean corpuscular volume and hematocrit value because the latter is calculated from the MCV.

Osmolality

The term *molarity* is used to characterize concentration, that is, the number of moles of solute per liter of water. *Molality* is the number of moles of solute per kilogram of water. Because a liter of water has a mass of 1 kg, the difference between these two expressions of concentration is usually small. Only for concentrated solutions is the difference appreciable. In practice it is the difference between adding material to a liter of water (molality) and adding water to material to make a liter of solution (molarity).

Molality is the term best suited to osmometry because it gives a simpler theoretical formula for osmotic pressure than molarity does. The term *osmolality* is used to identify the number of moles of particles per kilogram of water.

Because the osmolality of a solution does not depend on the kind of particles but only on the number of particles, it is called a *colligative* property. A solution that is 1 millimolal in sodium chloride is 2 milliosmolal because sodium chloride separates into sodium and chloride ions. Each kind of ion represents a particle that contributes to the osmolality. Furthermore, a 1 millimolal calcium chloride solution is 3 milliosmolal because each molecule ionizes to give one calcium ion and two chloride ions.

Osmometry

Osmometry is the measurement of the concentration, not of a particular molecule, but of molecules and ions in general. In this chapter the clinical importance and use of osmometry are discussed, the techniques for measuring osmolality are reviewed, and examples of instrumentation are provided.

Osmolal gap

There are just a few substances in plasma that contribute significantly to the osmolality, and they are mostly small molecules and ions. For example, plasma usually contains 40 g of albumin per liter, but the number of moles of albumin is very small (only about 50 mmol). In contrast, plasma contains about 150 mmol of sodium ion and 100 mmol of a corresponding anion such as chloride. This is only 5.8 g of sodium chloride per liter. Thus sodium chloride contrib-

Table 14-1 Toxic substances affecting plasma osmolality

Substances	Toxic or lethal concentrations		Corresponding increase in osmolality (mOsm/kg)
	Historical units (mg/dL)	SI units (mmol/L)	
Ethanol	350	80	80
Isopropanol	340	60	60
Methanol	80	24	24
Ethyl ether	180	24	24
Trichloroethane	100	9	9
Acetone (including other ketones or ketone metabolites)	55	10	10

utes 3000 times more to osmolality than a similar mass of albumin does.

Many formulas have been used to calculate the approximate osmolality of serum or plasma. Most formulas attempt to combine accuracy with simplicity in calculation. A formula that requires measurement of many substances is not very useful clinically. The calculated osmolality can be compared with the measured osmolality; the difference is called the *osmolal gap*. An abnormal osmolal gap is an important indication of abnormal concentrations of unmeasured substances in the blood. Because the formula predicts the plasma osmolality so well, there is little new information to be gained from *routine* measurements of the osmolality. However, in certain special situations described in the next section, the measurement is informative and worthwhile.

The formulas shown below for the calculation of serum osmolality are approximations because they include only the most important contributors to osmolality:

Historical units

$$\text{Calculated osmolality (mOsm/kg)} = 2 \cdot Na^+ \text{ (mEq/L)} +$$

$$\frac{\text{Glucose (mg/dL)}}{18} + \frac{\text{BUN (mg/dL)}}{2.8} \qquad \textit{Eq. 14-1}$$

SI* units

$$\text{Calculated osmolality (mOsm/kg)} =$$
$$2 \cdot Na^+ \text{ (mmol/L)} + \text{Glucose (mmol/L)} + \text{BUN (mmol/L)}$$
$$\textit{Eq. 14-2}$$

The SI units formula is very straightforward. The factor 2 in both equations counts the cation (sodium) once and the corresponding anion once. Glucose and blood urea nitrogen (BUN) are undissociated molecules and are counted once each. All other components are ignored. In the historical-units formula the dividing factors represent the respective molecular weights and conversion from deciliters to liters. The calculated osmolality is not corrected for the actual water content of plasma (lipids and protein take up some of the volume) because this correction does not improve the clinical utility of the osmolal gap or of osmolality in general.

*Système International d'Unités, or simply "metric" units.

Notice that these formulas use molarity rather than molality. This approximation fortuitously compensates for some of the serum components and theoretical corrections that were ignored.

The osmolal gap is defined as:

$$\text{Osmolal gap, Osm/kg} =$$
$$\text{Measured Osm/kg} - \text{Calculated Osm/kg} \qquad \textit{Eq. 14-3}$$

The average osmolal gap is near zero.

CLINICAL USE OF OSMOMETRY

There are several clinical uses of osmometry. Serum osmolality can be used to screen for the ingestion of toxic substances and to monitor mannitol therapy. In addition, osmolality measurements of urine are used to assess renal concentrating ability. Measurements of stool osmolality can be useful in differentiating various causes of diarrheic stools.

Plasma osmolality

Screening for toxin ingestion. Only a few exogenous substances can be ingested in amounts sufficient to affect the plasma osmolality. Table 14-1 lists the substances and the concentrations necessary to increase the osmolal gap to 10 or more milliosmoles per kilogram. The most common substances are alcohols. If the measured concentration of ethanol (mmol/L) does not correspond within 10 mOsm to the calculated osmolal gap, an *excess osmolal gap* is present. An excess osmolal gap would be suggestive that another of the substances listed in Table 14-1 is also present. When calculating the osmolal gap, one needs to be confident that methodological and calculation errors have been avoided.[1] Table 14-1 shows that trichloroethane can be at near-lethal levels in the blood without being readily detected by osmometry.

Although osmometry has long been recommended as a means to detect alcohol, it should be noted that vapor-pressure osmometers are not useful for the detection of alcohol because dissolved alcohol is also volatile and thus contributes to the solution's vapor pressure.

An increase in the osmolal gap will also reflect an increase in the anion gap in patients with metabolic imbalance. These changes are caused by the presence of ketone "bodies" (see Chapter 32).

Screening for mannitol toxicity. Mannitol is often used as an osmotic diuretic to treat cases of edema, especially cerebral edema, by reducing the amount of intracellular water. Although mannitol is a relatively nontoxic substance, it can cause renal damage at levels greater than 50 mmol/L. Measurement of the osmolality gap for patients undergoing mannitol therapy can be useful in estimating the serum levels of mannitol. If the osmolal gap is greater than 10 mOsm/L but less than 50 mOsm/L, it is likely that mannitol is present at a therapeutic, nontoxic level.

Urine osmolality

Renal concentrating ability is a sensitive measure of kidney function. The urine that is delivered to the bladder is typically one to three times more concentrated than the plasma. A random urine specimen is sufficient to demonstrate the kidney's ability to concentrate urine if the osmolality of the random urine specimen is greater than 600 mOsm/kg. However, if the random urine specimen is dilute, no conclusion about concentrating ability can be made. A definitive follow-up test involves overnight water restriction. After the morning void, at least one urine specimen should exceed 850 mOsm/kg. Patients who are compulsive water drinkers may need continuous observation to assure that no water has been ingested.

The specific gravity as estimated by the refractive index can also be used to measure urine concentration. However, osmometry is less affected by the presence of protein or radiocontrast dyes.

Stool osmolality

The measurement of the osmolality of watery (diarrheic) stools can be used to diagnose the cause of chronic diarrhea. Diarrheic stools can be caused by maldigestion of foods; the undigested nutrients cause an osmotic diuresis in the intestines, producing a stool with a high osmolality (see Chapter 30). Watery stools can also result from excessive intestinal excretion of fluids and electrolytes; this produces a stool with a low osmolality.

These two types of chronic diarrheic disorders can often be differentiated by the calculation of the *stool osmolal gap*. The stool osmolal gap is the difference between the measured stool osmolality and twice the sum of the measured stool sodium and potassium.

Stool osmolal gap =
$$\text{Measured osmolality}_{stool} - 2([Na^+] + [K^+])_{stool}$$

If the stool osmolal gap is less than 50 mOsm/L, the patient most likely has a secretional diarrhea.[2] A stool osmolal gap greater than 50 mOsm/L would be suggestive of the presence of unabsorbed, osmotic materials such as food. A large gap may also be seen in cases of excessive use of laxatives, some of which, such as the magnesium-containing laxatives, can be detected in stool water by the measurement of magnesium.

Table 14-2 Estimated effect of anticoagulants on osmolality (compared to serum)

Anticoagulant	Full tube (mOsm/kg)	Half-full tube (mOsm/kg)
Heparin	+0	+0
EDTA (disodium salt)	+15	+30
Fluoride-oxalate (sodium fluoride–potassium oxalate)*	+150	+300
Iodoacetic acid (lithium salt)	+5	+10

*This hyperosmolal state accounts for the hemolysis usually observed in the plasma of these samples.

The osmolality of fresh liquid stool is approximately equal to that of serum. A hypo-osmolar watery stool (approximately less than 280 mOsm/L) might be suggestive of a factitious diarrhea, that is, one created by the patient himor herself, such as by adding water to the stool (Munchausen syndrome).[3]

Intestinal bacteria present in the stool can very rapidly convert stool carbohydrates into osmotically active fragments, raising the stool water osmolality. Thus stool osmolality measurements should be performed within 30 minutes of the collection of the stool sample.

Serum or plasma osmolality

Sample-collection technique is important to obtain a valid specimen for measurement of osmolality. For example, stasis during phlebotomy should be avoided. In addition, the patient's position, supine or upright, will affect the osmolality. Thus a sample from a fasting, hospitalized patient will give the most uniform results, not because lipemia or other effects are avoided but because it is more likely that the patient was supine at the time of the morning phlebotomy rounds.

Serum and heparinized plasma have similar osmolality values. The contribution to the osmolality by fibrinogen in plasma is small, and it is important only in the measurement of colloid osmotic pressure. Freezing-point depression techniques can use whole blood and are not affected by lipemia or hemolysis. Anticoagulants other than heparin increase the measured osmolality. Table 14-2 shows the estimated effect of four anticoagulants. On occasion, the kind of anticoagulant used can be verified by measurement of the osmolality of the plasma.

PRINCIPLES OF MEASUREMENT

Osmolality is a colligative property; thus any of four measurements that depend on colligative properties may be used to measure osmolality. The measurements are (1) osmotic pressure, (2) boiling-point elevation, (3) freezing-point depression, and (4) vapor-pressure depression. Osmotic-pressure measurement has been used only in a special form of osmometry called "colloid osmotic pressure" and is discussed separately in a later section of this chapter. Boiling-point elevation is not useful for clinical samples because proteins will coagulate, causing gross changes in the sample composition. Of the remaining two, freezing-point depression is the most frequently used technique. Vapor-pressure depression as measured by the dew point is more commonly used in pediatric laboratories.

Freezing-point depression

The use of salt to melt ice and snow is a well-known practice. This is an example of freezing-point depression; that is, dissolved salt increases the osmolality, thereby lowering the freezing point of the solution compared to that of the pure solvent (ice or snow). The temperature at which ice and the water solution are in equilibrium is a function of the salt concentration. More precisely, the temperature at equilibrium is a function of the number of particles in solution. The freezing-point temperature is depressed 1.86 Celsius degrees for each mole of particles dissolved per kilogram of water. Because the osmolality of blood is about 0.285 Osm/kg (285 mOsm/kg), the freezing point is $-0.53°$ C. Precise measurement of this temperature requires a sensitive thermometer. A thermistor (thermal resistor) is made from a mixture of transition metal oxides such as manganese, cobalt, and nickel. These materials are semiconductors, and the number of electrons in the conduction band (valence electrons of the metal lattice capable of conducting a current) depends on the temperature. They become better conductors as the temperature rises. The conductance or resistance of the metals can be related to the temperature and hence to the osmolality.

Freezing-point depression is measured as follows:

1. The sample is either cooled by a bath containing an antifreeze solution that is maintained at about $-5°$ C by a conventional refrigerator or by a thermoelectric cooler.
2. The sample is supercooled; that is, its temperature falls below the equilibrium freezing point. This occurs because pure ice crystals are slow to form.
3. The crystallization process is induced by vigorous stirring. Once ice crystals begin to form, additional water molecules are rapidly added to the ice crystals. However, heat is released in the freezing process just as it is absorbed in the melting process. The heat that is released from the formation of the ice crystals raises the temperature of the sample until the rapid freezing stops and an equilibrium temperature is established.
4. The temperature is measured at the plateau, that is, at the temperature at which the heat removed by the cooling bath is matched by the heat released by the freezing process. The temperature at this equilibrium is the freezing point of the solution and is inversely related to osmolality. The plateau's temperature is measured electronically by the thermistor, and the temperature reading is converted to milliosmoles per

kilogram and displayed. At this time, before complete freezing can cause mechanical damage to the thermistor probe, the thermistor is removed from the sample.

Because 1 osmole of solute lowers the freezing point by 1.86° C, osmolality can be calculated directly by the formula:

$$\text{Osmolality (mOsmol/kg)} = \frac{\text{Freezing-point depression}}{1.86°\text{ C}} \times \text{mOsmol/kg}$$

Eq. 14-4

However, it is more practical to calibrate the osmometer using saline solutions. Calibration also corrects for systematic or procedural effects, such as the increase in concentration of the sample because of the removal of pure water (as ice) before measurement of the temperature.

Several factors must be controlled to achieve high precision in freezing-point depression osmometry. These include the bath temperature, fluid composition, and amount of fluid. The fluid composition and volume change as moisture condenses from the room air. The thickness of the sample container and the amount of sample must be standardized. The probe must be rinsed and wiped to minimize carryover from one sample to the next. This is especially important between samples of widely differing osmolality, such as standards and urine samples. Samples can be remeasured, but great care must be taken to warm the sample (for example, by holding the sample cup in one's hand) until *all* the ice is melted; otherwise the sample will freeze prematurely. Any sample droplets on the side of the cup should be joined with the sample by tipping the cup to coalesce the droplets.

The most common freezing-point osmometers are listed in Table 14-3, along with several key characteristics.

Vapor-pressure depression

Solvent molecules on the surface of a liquid are in constant thermal motion; some of these molecules escape from the surface into the atmosphere above the surface, forming a gaseous vapor phase in equilibrium with the liquid phase. This process is called *evaporation*. If the liquid contains dissolved solute, some of these solute molecules will occupy the surface layer of the liquid. Generally a solute molecule will not evaporate but will, by its presence, prevent a solvent molecule from evaporating. As the number of solute molecules increases, the chance that a solvent molecule will evaporate decreases, reducing the vapor phase in equilibrium above the liquid. Thus there is an inverse relationship between the concentration of dissolved solute particles (osmolality) and the vapor pressure above a solution. In vapor-pressure osmometry, the vapor-pressure depression of a solution is compared with that of a standard to determine the osmolality of a solution.

The temperature at which the atmosphere is saturated

Table 14-3   Characteristics of clinical osmometers

Manufacturer	Model*	Technique†	Routine sample size (μL)	Precision (%)‡	Measurement time (sec)
Advanced Instrument, Inc.	3D3	FP	200	1.4	120-180
(Needham Heights, Mass.)	3M0 Plus	FP§	20		60
Fiske Associates, Inc.	One-Ten	FP§	15	1.6	60
(Needham Heights, Mass.)					
Precision Systems, Inc.	5002	FP	200	1.6	180
(Natick, Mass.)	μOsmette	FP§	50		
Wescor, Inc. (Logan, Utah)	5500	VP	10	2.8	60-90
	4420	COP	450	6.7	90-120

*All models are manually loaded with sample and have automated measurement and reporting. Variations in sample size, automated sampling, and printing are available.
†*COP*, Colloid osmotic pressure; *FP*, freezing-point depression; *VP*, vapor pressure.
‡From College of American Pathologists' survey for osmolalities in normal range.
§Does not use liquid cooling bath; uses electronic cooling.

with solvent can be measured by a thermocouple. A thermocouple generates a voltage (Seebeck effect) between the ends of a wire. The voltage difference between the ends depends on the difference in temperature of the ends.

Thermocouples also exhibit the Peltier effect, which is the opposite of the Seebeck effect. An electrical current through the thermocouple transfers heat from one junction to the other. One junction cools, whereas the other heats. The vapor-pressure osmometer passes an electrical current through the thermocouple in the measurement chamber, causing it to cool. When its temperature falls low enough, water (solvent) begins to condense on it. The electrical current is discontinued, and the thermocouple comes to an equilibrium temperature at which the water condensing on it is matched by the water evaporating from it. This equilibrium temperature is measured by the Seebeck voltage, which is linearly related to the osmolality.

Vapor-pressure depression is measured as follows:
1. The sample is sealed in a chamber. The air quickly changes humidity until its humidity is in equilibrium with the sample.
2. The thermocouple cools until its temperature is below the dew point. The electrical current is turned off, and the junction temperature rises as vapor condenses on it.
3. The plateau temperature (the temperature at which an equilibrium exists between condensation and evaporation) is measured.

The vapor pressure of the sample is directly proportional to the thermocouple voltage. Again, it is more practical to calibrate this type of osmometer than to apply theoretical factors. Systematic or procedural effects that must be controlled include the sample volume, the size and composition of the sample absorbent disk, the time delay between sample application and sealing of the chamber, cleanliness of the chamber, and changes in room temperature.

Table 14-3 provides information on the only available clinical vapor pressure osmometer.

COLLOID OSMOTIC PRESSURE
Definitions

Osmotic pressure is a colligative property and hence reflects osmolality. This is strictly true for a semipermeable membrane that is permeable to water only. The difficulty in finding such a membrane has kept the measurement of osmotic pressure from being used as a technique in the assessment of osmolality in clinical samples. However, measurement of the osmolal contribution of a group of molecules responsible for the colloid osmotic pressure (COP) is practical and useful. This property is measured by use of membranes that are permeable to small molecules. Small molecules, less than 30,000 daltons molecular weight, are called *crystalloids* if they are uncharged and *ions* if they are charged. Large molecules are called *colloids*. Hence colloid osmotic pressure measures only the contribution made to osmolality by large, essentially only protein, molecules. An alternative term is the *oncotic* pressure.

Clinical use of colloid osmotic pressure

The major use for the measurement of the COP is detection of conditions leading to pulmonary edema.

In this condition, there is an accumulation of water in the lungs, which interferes with oxygen and carbon dioxide exchange. The actual diagnosis can be obtained from x-ray measurements. Two measurements are needed to predict pulmonary edema: left ventricular heart pressure and COP. As long as the COP is greater than the pulmonary blood pressure (as measured by the "pulmonary artery wedge pressure"), pulmonary edema is unlikely. If heart failure is not present, that is, if the pulmonary blood pressure is normal, COP measurements *alone* will allow one to predict the probability of pulmonary edema.

Knowledge of the albumin or total protein content of the plasma permits the calculation of the COP. However, the formula is inaccurate when used for acutely ill patients (especially patients with heart failure) and for patients who have received dextrans, or "plasma expanders." For these groups of patients, measurement of COP is very useful.

Measurement of colloid osmotic pressure

The COP is measured with a microporous filter or membrane that contains pores or channels whose diameters are carefully controlled to be impermeable to large molecules (proteins). Physiological saline is placed in a sealed chamber on one side of the membrane, and the sample is placed on the other. Saline flows into the sample until the backpressure stops further flow. This backpressure, or negative pressure, is sensed by a pressure gauge. In addition to the osmotic pressure, an additional pressure is created by the Donnan effect. This effect arises because at physiological pH most proteins are negatively charged. Because the sample is electrically neutral, there are positive charges equal in number to the negative charges on the proteins. These positive charges are mostly in the form of sodium ions. Charged sodium ions diffuse through the membrane, whereas the corresponding negatively charged proteins do not. This leads to a separation of electrical charges. Because of the charge separation, additional small, negatively charged molecules will be attracted across the membrane. As a result, the number of particles that diffuse will be larger than that resulting from simple osmosis, and the pressure across the membrane will be larger. Because the net charge on proteins changes with pH, the measured COP will also change with pH.

Customarily, COP is reported in millimeters of mercury (mm Hg). In practice a maximum pressure occurs 30 to 90 seconds after the sample is placed into the instrument. This value is chosen because the pressure decays with time as a result of imperfections in the membrane that slowly allow large molecules to diffuse to the saline side, thus reducing the true pressure. Characteristics of a commercially available colloid osmometer are listed in Table 14-3.

BIBLIOGRAPHY

Dorman HR, Sondheimer JH, Cadnapaphornchai P: Mannitol-induced acute renal failure, *Medicine* 69:153-159, 1990.

Dorwart VW, Chalmers L: Comparison of methods for calculating serum osmolality from chemical concentrations and the prognostic value of such calculations, *Clin Chem* 21:190-194, 1975.

Epstein FB: Osmolality, *Emerg Med Clin North Am* 4:253-261, 1986.

Eskew L, Speicher CE: Using anion and osmolar gaps to diagnose the cause of intoxification, *Diagn Med,* p 6, Feb 1985.

Geheb MA: Clinical approach to the hyperosmolar patient, *Crit Care Clin* 3:797-815, 1987.

REFERENCES

1. Demedts P, Theunis L, Wauters A, et al: Excess serum osmolality gap after ingestion of methanol: a methodology associated phenomenon? *Clin Chem* 40:1587-1590, 1994.
2. Binder HJ: The gastroenterologist's osmotic gap: fact or fiction? *Gastroenterology* 103:702-704, 1992.
3. Topazian M, Binder HJ: Brief report: factitious diarrhea detected by measurement of stool osmolality, *N Engl J Med* 330:1418-1419, 1994.

Electrochemistry: principles and measurements

Jon R. Kirchhoff
John F. Wheeler
Craig E. Lunte
Sarah H. Jenkins
William R. Heineman

Potentiometric methods
  Reference electrodes
  Indicator electrodes
  Care and methodology
  Experimental considerations and interferences
Voltammetric methods
  Voltammetry electrodes
  Oxygen electrode
  Glucose electrode
  Liquid chromatography with electrochemical
    detection
  Anodic stripping voltammetry
Coulometric methods
  Titration of chloride

OBJECTIVES

■ Understand the fundamental differences between potentiometric and voltammetric techniques and understand how each technique is used for clinical measurements.

■ Understand the process by which ion-selective electrodes respond to the presence of an analyte.

■ Develop a knowledge of the methodology and possible interferences associated with using electrochemistry in the clinical laboratory.

■ Understand how various voltammetric and coulometric techniques are used for clinical measurements.

KEY TERMS

activity The effective concentration of a solution species that accounts for interactions with other solution species.
activity coefficient Effective concentration (activity) divided by molar concentration. A measure of the degree with which a species interacts with other solution species.
amperometry A controlled-potential technique in which current is measured at a fixed applied potential.

anode The electrode (positive) at which oxidation occurs.
auxiliary electrode The electrode in the three-electrode electrochemical cell that carries the current to maintain electrolysis at the working electrode.
cathode The electrode (negative) at which reduction occurs.
cell potential The quantitative measure of the energy of an electrochemical cell; the difference in electron energy between two electrodes.
charge A quantity of electricity that reflects the total current during a given time: $Q = it$.
conductivity A measure of the relative ability of materials to carry an electrical current.
coulometry A technique in which the charge required to electrolyze a sample completely is measured.
current The rate of charge flow (1 ampere = 1 coulomb/second).
electrolysis A nonspontaneous electrochemical reaction that results from the application of potential to an electrochemical cell.
electrolyte solution A solution of ions that provides a conducting medium for electrochemistry.
half-cell potential The quantitative measure of the energy of a half-cell reaction relative to a reference electrode.
half-cell reaction An electrochemical reaction that represents either an oxidation or reduction at one of the electrodes in an electrochemical cell.
hydrodynamic voltammogram A graphical representation of current versus applied potential for a particular electrochemical reaction that occurs in a stirred or flowing solution.
indicator electrode An electrode whose potential varies as the concentration of reactants and products change in solution. This potential is governed by the Nernst equation.
ionic strength (μ) One-half the sum of the concentration (C_i) multiplied by the square of the charge (Z_i) for each ionic species in solution: $\mu = \frac{1}{2}\Sigma_i C_i Z_i^2$
ionophore A neutral carrier molecule incorporated into an ion-selective electrode to detect a specific ion.
ion-selective electrode An indicator electrode used in potentiometry to respond to specific ions in solution.
limiting current The portion of a hydrodynamic voltammogram where electrolysis is occurring and the current remains constant as a function of increased applied potential.
liquid junction potential A potential that develops at the interface between two nonidentical solutions.
Nernst equation The expression that relates the cell potential

to the standard cell potential and the activities of reactants and products in the electrochemical cell.

oxidation The process whereby a chemical species loses one or more electrons.

polarography Voltammetry performed at a dropping mercury working electrode.

potentiometry The technique in which the potential difference between two electrodes is measured under equilibrium conditions.

potentiostat An instrument designed to control the potential of an electrochemical cell.

reduction The process whereby a chemical species gains one or more electrons.

reference electrode An electrode with a stable half-cell potential that is used to measure and control the relative potential of the working electrode.

salt bridge A device that allows ionic movement between compartments of an electrochemical cell to maintain electrical contact and at the same time prevent mixing of the separate solutions.

standard cell potential The electrochemical cell potential measured under standard state conditions.

standard state The condition in which each species is present with unit activity.

stripping voltammetry A voltammetric technique that allows sample preconcentration at the electrode before voltammetric analysis.

voltammetry A technique whereby current is measured as a function of applied potential.

Electrochemistry involves the measurement of electrical signals associated with chemical systems that are incorporated into an electrochemical cell. The cell consists of two or more electrodes that interface a chemical system and an electrical system. The electrical system measures or controls the electrical parameters of voltage and current, which are characteristic of a particular chemical system.

Electroanalytical chemistry makes use of electrochemistry for the purpose of analysis. In this application the magnitude of a voltage or current signal originating from an electrochemical cell is related to the activity or concentration of a particular chemical species in the cell. Excellent detection limits coupled with a wide dynamic range are exhibited by many electroanalytical techniques, with an operating range of 10^{-8} to 10^{-3} M. Measurements can generally be made on very small volumes of sample, that is, in the microliter range. The combination of low detection limits and microliter volume samples allows picomole amounts of analyte to be measured routinely in some instances. Furthermore, electroanalysis lends itself to measurements made in vivo. For example, miniature electrochemical sensors are used to measure pH and Po_2 in the bloodstream of patients with indwelling catheters.

In the clinical laboratory, electroanalysis is routinely used for the determination of many ions, drugs, hormones, metals, and gases. Methods are available for the rapid determination of analytes present at relatively high concentrations, such as blood electrolytes (Na^+, Cl^-, HCO_3^-), and analytes present at very low concentrations, such as heavy metals and drug metabolites in blood and urine samples.

The purpose of this chapter is to provide a fundamental background for understanding the electroanalytical techniques found in the clinical laboratory and to illustrate some of the practical applications of electroanalysis. These fundamental electrochemical techniques are divided into three basic categories: potentiometric, voltammetric, and coulometric. Potentiometry is the most widely used clinical application of electrochemistry and involves the measurement of a cell potential under equilibrium conditions. Voltammetry and coulometry are considered dynamic techniques and are based on measurements made on a cell in which electrolysis is occurring. Many common definitions, symbols, and electrochemical nomenclature used in potentiometry, voltammetry, and coulometry are listed in Table 15-1.

POTENTIOMETRIC METHODS

Potentiometric methods are based on the measurement of a potential (voltage) difference between two electrodes immersed in solution under the condition of zero current. The electrodes and the solution constitute an *electrochemical cell*. Each electrode in the electrochemical cell is characterized by a *half-cell reaction* with a corresponding *half-cell potential*. Since no current passes through the cell while the potential is measured, no net electrochemical reaction is occurring; thus a potentiometric technique is an equilibrium method. Potentiometric techniques are important because they can provide accurate measurements of activities, concentrations, or activity coefficients of many solution species. In general, a solution of ions or molecules is characterized by its molar concentration. However, these species can interact with other ions, molecules, or solvent. Depending on the type of interactions that occur, the *effective concentration* of the species may be less than, equal to, or greater than the actual molar concentration of species. The effective concentration is referred to as the *activity* of the species and is related to the molar concentration by an activity coefficient as shown in the equation

$$a_i = \gamma C_i,$$

where a_i is the activity of an ionic species, γ is the activity coefficient, and C_i is the molar concentration of that species.

A typical apparatus for potentiometry is shown in Fig. 15-1. The potential difference between the two electrodes is usually measured with a pH-millivolt meter. One electrode, the *indicator electrode*, is chosen so that its half-cell potential responds to changes in the activity or concentration of the particular species in solution to be measured. The other electrode is a *reference electrode* whose half-cell

Table 15-1   Electrochemical terms, units, constants, symbols, and conversions

Term	Symbol	Unit or constant	Symbol	Conversion or value
Potential	E	Volt	V	$V = J/C$
Standard potential	(E^0)			$E = i \cdot R$
Formal potential	$(E^{0'})$			
Current	i	Ampere	A	$A = C/s$
				$1A = 1.05 \times 10^{-5}$ mol of electrons per second
Charge	Q	Coulomb	C	$C = A \cdot s$
				$1C = 1.05 \times 10^{-5}$ mol of electrons
Energy	H	Joule	J	
Resistance	R	Ohm	Ω	
Time	t	Second	s	
Temperature	T	Kelvin	K	
Activity	a	Moles per liter	mol/L	
Concentration	C	Moles per liter (or moles per cubic centimeter)	mol/L (mol/cm^3)	
Area	A	Square centimeters	cm^2	
Diffusion coefficient	D	Square centimeters per second	cm^2/s	
		Gas constant	R	8.31441 J/mol·K
		Faraday constant	F	9.64846×10^4 C/mol
		Number of electrons in electrode or redox reaction	n	

potential does not change. It is important to understand that one does *not* measure an individual half-cell potential, but only the potential *difference* between one half-cell and a reference electrode. The most commonly used reference electrodes for potentiometry are the saturated calomel electrode and the silver/silver chloride electrode. The potential of the potentiometric electrochemical cell, E_{cell}, is given by:

$$E_{cell} = E_{ind} - E_{ref} + E_{lj} \qquad \textit{Eq. 15-1}$$

where E_{ind} is the half-cell potential of the indicator electrode, E_{ref} is the half-cell potential of the reference electrode, and E_{lj} is the *liquid junction potential*. The liquid junction potential is the electrical potential that develops at the interface between two liquids as a result of differences in the rates with which ions move from one liquid to the other. For example, the liquid junction potential arises in Fig. 15-1 at the point where the tip of the reference electrode meets the solution. Thus, E_{lj} is a potential that results from differences in charge rather than from an electrochemical reaction at an electrode.

Reference electrodes

Since every electrochemical measurement must be made with respect to a reference potential, further discussion is needed with regard to the properties and types of reference electrodes. A reference electrode is an electrochemical half-cell that is used as a fixed reference for the measurement of cell potentials. Ideally, a reference electrode should possess the following characteristics: a stable, easily reproducible half-cell potential; a reversible half-cell reaction; chemical stability of its components; and ease of fabrica-

tion and use. Three reference electrodes are discussed below; one is of fundamental significance, and two are of practical importance.

The *standard hydrogen electrode (SHE)* has been chosen as the reference half-cell electrode on which tables of standard electrode potentials are based. In this half-cell, hydrogen gas at a pressure of 1 atmosphere is bubbled over a platinum electrode immersed in acid solution for which the activity of H^+ is unity. The potential of the SHE is defined as 0.0 V at all temperatures, and the potentials of other half-cell couples are referenced to this value. The potentials of other half-cells are either negative or positive of 0.0 V. Since other reference electrodes are easier to construct and use, the SHE is rarely used in practical applications of electrochemistry.

A commonly used reference electrode is the *saturated calomel electrode* (SCE). A schema of a common type of SCE, its half-cell reaction, and standard half-cell potential are shown in Fig. 15-2, *A*. The electrode consists of elemental mercury covered with a thin coating of calomel (Hg_2Cl_2) that is in contact with an aqueous solution saturated with KCl. The potential of the half-cell will be constant so long as the activity of Cl^- does not change. The easiest way to set the activity of Cl^- to a fixed value that is easily verifiable is to saturate the solution with a chloride salt such as KCl. So long as crystals of KCl are present, the experimenter knows that the solution is saturated and that the activity of Cl^- is constant. Notice that the other participants in the electrochemical reaction (Hg_2Cl_2 and Hg) are solid and liquid components and consequently exhibit unit activity regardless of the amounts present in the cell. Thus, the SCE offers the extraordinary convenience of being easily

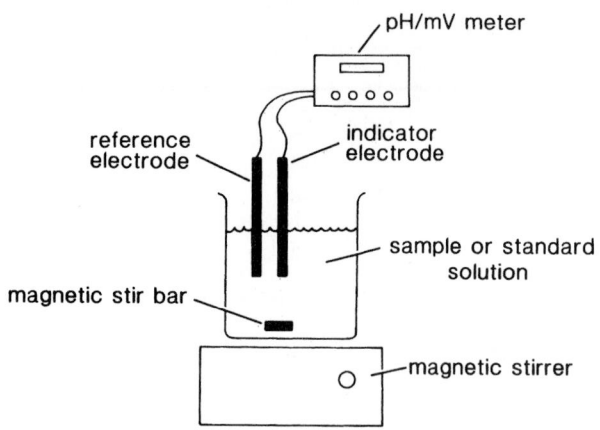

Fig. 15-1 Schema of apparatus for potentiometry.

fabricated without the need for accurate preparation of the activities of any of the components.

Another commonly used reference electrode is the *silver/ silver chloride electrode (Ag/AgCl)*. A representative Ag/AgCl reference electrode is shown in Fig. 15-2, *B*. The electrode is prepared by coating a silver wire with a thin film of AgCl and immersing it in a solution of constant chloride concentration, which fixes the half-cell potential. The Ag/AgCl reference electrode is used routinely, especially as the inner reference electrode in potentiometric membrane electrodes. The SCE and Ag/AgCl electrodes are commercially available or conveniently constructed.

Indicator electrodes

The indicator electrode is the essence of potentiometric analysis. This electrode should interact with the analyte of interest so that the E_{ind} reflects the activity of this species in solution and not of other compounds in the sample that might interfere. The relative response of an electrode to one species and not to another species is defined as the *selectivity* of the electrode. The importance of having indicator electrodes that selectively respond to species of analytical significance has stimulated the development of many types of these electrodes.

Ion-selective electrodes. The most common indicator electrode used in clinical chemistry is the *ion-selective electrode* (ISE). The ISE is based on the measurement of a potential that develops across a selective membrane. The response of the electrochemical cell is therefore based on an interaction between the membrane and the analyte that alters the potential across the membrane. The selectivity of the potential response to an analyte depends on the specificity of the membrane interaction for the analyte.

A representative ISE is shown schematically in Fig. 15-3. The electrode consists of a membrane, an internal reference electrolyte of fixed activity, $(a_i)_{internal}$, and an internal reference electrode. The ISE is immersed in a sample solution that contains analyte of some activity, $(a_i)_{sample}$. An external reference electrode is also immersed in this solution. The internal and external reference electrodes constitute the two half-cells of the electrochemical cell. The potential measured by the pH/mV meter (E_{cell}) is equal to the differ-

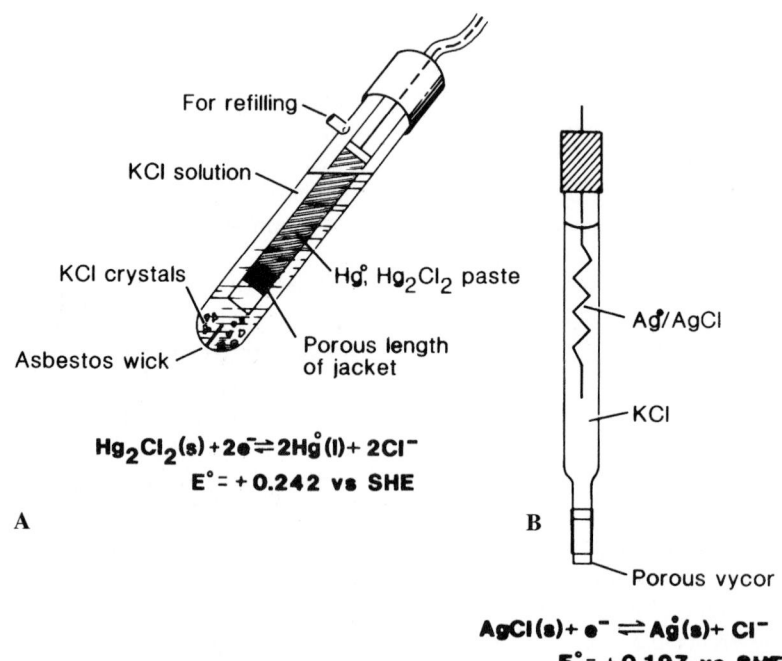

Fig. 15-2 Reference electrodes. **A,** Saturated calomel electrode, *SCE,* with asbestos wick for salt bridge junction. **B,** Silver/silver chloride electrode, Ag/AgCl.

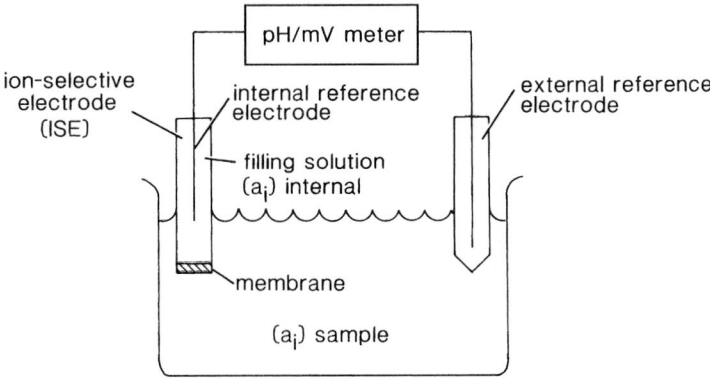

Fig. 15-3 Schema of an ion-selective electrode (ISE).

ence in potential between the external ($E_{ref,ext}$) and the internal ($E_{ref,int}$) reference electrodes, plus the membrane potential (E_{memb}), plus the liquid junction potential (E_{lj}) that exists at the junction between the external reference electrode and the sample solution.

$$E_{cell} = E_{ref,ext} - E_{ref,int} + E_{memb} + E_{lj} \qquad \textit{Eq. 15-2}$$

If the membrane is permeable to a particular ion [i], a potential develops across the membrane that depends on the ratio of activities of the ion on either side of the membrane. The half-cell potentials of the two reference electrodes are constant, sample solution conditions can be controlled so that E_{lj} is effectively constant, and the composition of the internal solution can be maintained so that $(a_i)_{internal}$ is fixed. Consequently, E_{cell} is described by the Nernst equation:

$$E_{cell} = K + 2.3 \frac{RT}{zF} \log (a_i)_{sample} \qquad \textit{Eq. 15-3}$$

where K represents the constant terms and z is the charge on the analyte ion (cations: $+1$, $+2$, $+3$, and so on; anions: -1, -2, -3, and so on). This logarithmic relationship between cell potential and analyte activity is the basis of the ISE as an analytical device. A plot of E_{cell} versus log a_i for a series of standard solutions should be linear over the working range of the electrode and have a slope of 2.3 RT/zF or $0.0591/z$ for measurements made at 25° C. Since membranes respond to a certain degree to ions other than the analyte (that is, interferents), a more general expression than equation 15-3 is needed:

$$E_{cell} = K + 2.3 \frac{RT}{zF} \log [(a_i)_{sample} + k_{ij}a^{z/x}_j] \qquad \textit{Eq. 15-4}$$

where a_j is the activity of the interferent ion [j], x is the charge of the interferent ion, and k_{ij} is the selectivity constant. Small values of k_{ij} are characteristic of electrodes with good selectivity for the analyte, i.

The development of successful ISEs has hinged on the search for membranes that exhibit both sensitivity and selectivity for the analyte of interest. Of the two properties,

selectivity is by far the more difficult to achieve. ISEs with selectivity for cations and anions have been developed with three basic types of membranes: liquid and polymer, solid state, and glass. All of these membranes function by selectively incorporating the analyte ion into the membrane and thereby establishing a membrane potential. An ISE membrane must exhibit low solubility in the analyte medium to provide a durable electrode with a stable response. This requirement imposes a severe restriction on the material that can be used for membranes. Also, the membrane must exhibit some electrical conductivity to function in an electrochemical cell. The scope of ISEs has been expanded to include the measurement of gases and neutral organic compounds by combining ISEs with gas-permeable membranes and layers of enzymes, bacteria, and tissues. These general categories of electrodes and specific ISEs are considered in the following sections.

Liquid and polymer membrane electrodes. A selective liquid membrane is the basis for many excellent ISEs. The liquid consists of a water-insoluble, viscous solvent in which is dissolved an *ionophore,* a hydrophobic organic ion-exchanger or a neutral carrier molecule that reacts selectively with the ion of interest. The liquid is typically soaked into a thin, porous solid membrane such as cellulose acetate, which is then incorporated into the ISE.

Fig. 15-4 shows the schema of the membrane portion of a liquid membrane ISE and the mechanism whereby an electrode responds to M^+ activity. The liquid membrane is in contact with internal and sample aqueous solutions of analyte M^+. The neutral carrier ionophore (R) reacts with M^+ at each membrane-solution interface and extracts M^+ into the membrane as MR^+. The extraction of M^+ into the membrane generates a positive membrane potential at each interface as a result of the charge difference that occurs when M^+ is extracted into the membrane in the form of MR^+ and the counter anion X^- that remains in the aqueous solution. As the activity of M^+ in solution is increased, the activity of MR^+ in the membrane increases, and the membrane potential increases. This reaction exists at both the outer membrane surface, which is exposed to the sample,

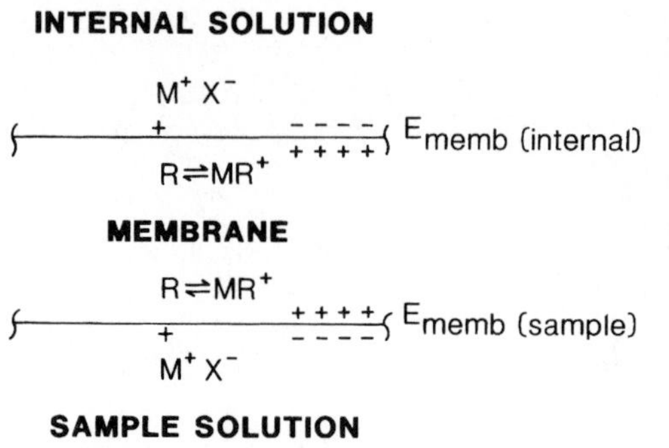

INTERNAL SOLUTION

$$M^+ X^-$$

$$+$$

$$\{\underline{\hspace{3cm}}\}_{++++}^{----} E_{memb} \text{ (internal)}$$

$$R \rightleftharpoons MR^+$$

MEMBRANE

$$R \rightleftharpoons MR^+$$

$$\{\underline{\hspace{3cm}}\}_{----}^{++++} E_{memb} \text{ (sample)}$$

$$+$$

$$M^+ X^-$$

SAMPLE SOLUTION

Fig. 15-4   Schema of liquid membrane ISE, where M^+ represents analyte cation, and R represents neutral carrier ionophore.

and the inner membrane surface, which contacts the inner filling solution of the ISE. The potential of the inner surface of the membrane, $E_{memb(internal)}$, is kept constant by maintenance of a constant activity of M^+ in the internal solution. Thus the only potential change measured in the circuit is the potential of the membrane surface contacting the sample, $E_{memb(sample)}$.

The availability of liquid and polymer membrane electrodes for a variety of ions is the result of the development of different neutral carrier ionophores and liquid ion exchangers that react selectively with particular ions. In the surface equilibria shown in Fig. 15-4, any ionic species other than M^+ that react to an appreciable degree with R will also generate a membrane potential and thereby cause an interference. The selectivity of the electrode for M^+ is therefore determined by the relative affinity between R and M^+ and R and the various interferent ions in the sample.

Several ionophores that selectively bind cations to nonaqueous membranes have been found. When it reacts with an ionophore, a cation is essentially inserted in a hydrophobic cavity within the ionophore that allows the cation to exist within a nonaqueous membrane medium. Selectivity for a particular cationic species is controlled by provision of an optimum environment in terms of number and position of binding atoms. An excellent example is the antibiotic, valinomycin, which exhibits selectivity for K^+. Fig. 15-5 illustrates the K^+ complex of valinomycin. The K^+ cation fits into a snug cavity surrounded by oxygen atoms. The electrode exhibits excellent selectivity for K^+ against Na^+ because the smaller Na^+ ion is bound less tightly in the valinomycin cavity. This feature is of considerable practical importance in the clinical determination of K^+ in serum, which contains higher concentrations of Na^+ than of K^+. Ionophores for the selective determination of NH_4^+, Ca^{2+}, Na^+, Li^+, and Mg^{2+} have also been incorporated into ISEs. The selective incorporation of these cations occurs by the same principle described for the K^+ electrode. The development of liquid and polymer membrane ISEs has allowed the measurement of ions in samples of diverse origin. The electrodes have been especially successful in clinical laboratories and are now used routinely for measuring

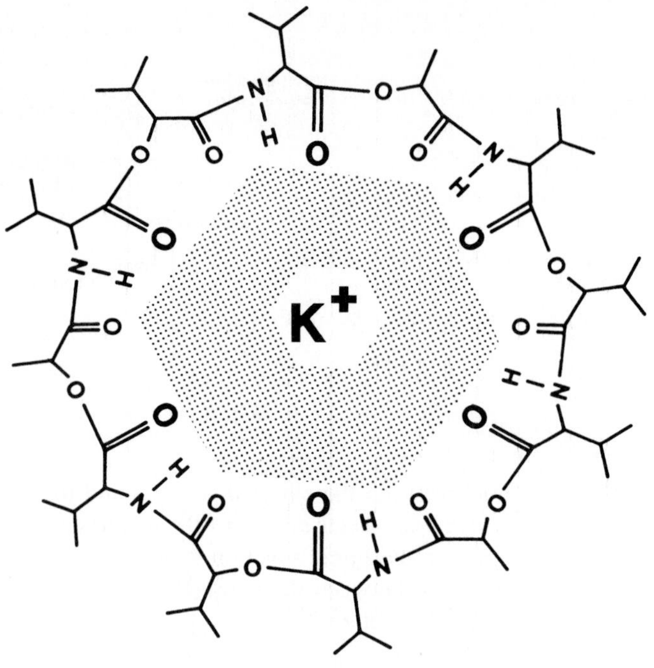

Fig. 15-5   Model of K^+ complex of valinomycin. Stippled region represents K^+ ion. Bold oxygens are binding atoms.

Ca^{2+}, K^+, Na^+, and Cl^- in biological fluids. The response characteristics for liquid and polymer membrane ISE systems commonly used in biomedical investigations are shown in Table 15-2.

Electrodes based on ion-pairing reactions have been developed for numerous organic compounds. These electrodes are based on insoluble ion pairs between an ionic form of the organic compound and an ion-pairing reagent. An example is an electrode for the antiepileptic drug phenytoin (5,5-diphenylhydantoin) based on the ion-pair complex between the 5,5-diphenylhydantoinate anion and the quaternary ammonium cation, tricaprylmethyl ammonium, which is immobilized in poly(vinyl chloride).

The electrode measures phenytoin over the range of 10^{-1} to 10^{-4} mol/L and has a detection limit of 1.5×10^{-5} mol/L. This electrode can be used to determine phenytoin in tablets and capsules. New ion exchangers and neutral carriers are continually being evaluated in an effort to improve selectivity of existing electrodes and to develop electrodes for other ions and molecules.

Solid-state membrane electrodes. Solid-state membranes consist of single crystals or pressed pellets of salts of the ions of interest. The crystal or pellet must have some degree of electrical conductivity and exhibit very low solubility in the solvent in which the electrode is to be used—usually water. An excellent ISE for F^- uses LaF_3 that is doped with Eu^{2+} to provide electrical conductivity. The membrane potential is generated by a selective surface reaction between LaF_3 and F^- in which solution F^- is incorporated into vacancies in the crystal lattice. The selectivity is very good because other anions do not fit well into the

Table 15-2   Ion-selective electrodes (ISEs) used in clinical chemistry

	Analyte	Membrane composition	Linear response range (mol/L)	Possible interferences
Glass	H^+	72.17% SiO_2, 6.44% CaO, 21.39% Na_2O (mol %)	10^{-12} to 10^{-2}	Na^+
	Na^+	11% Na_2O, 18% Al_2O_3, 71% SiO_2	10^{-6} to 10^{-1}	K^+, Ag^+
Solid state	F^-	LaF_3 crystal	10^{-6} to sat'd	OH^-
	Cl^-	$Ag_2S/AgCl$	$5 \times 10^{-5} - 1$	Br^-, CN^-, S^{2-}
Liquid or polymer membrane	Na^+	Na^+ ionophore (ETH 227) 2-nitrophenyloctyl ether, sodium tetraphenylborate	10^{-3} to 10^{-1}	Li^+, K^+, Ca^{++}
	Cl^-	Tri-*n*-octylpropylammonium chloride, decanol	10^{-3} to 10^{-1}	OH^-, Br^-, F^-
	K^+	Valinomycin, dioctyladipate, PVC	3×10^{-5} to 1	NH_4^+
	Li^+	Li^+ ionophores, such as crown ethers	$10^{-4} - 10^{-2}$	Ca^{++}, Na^+
	Ca^{++}	Ca^{++} ionophore (ETH 1001), 2-nitrophenyloctyl ether, sodium tetraphenylborate	10^{-7} to 10^{-2}	—
	Ca^{++}	Calcium di(*n*-decyl)phosphate, di(*n*-octylphenyl)phosphonate, PVC	3×10^{-5} to 1	Mg^{++}
Gas sensors	CO_2	Combination glass pH electrode, 0.01-0.1 M $NaHCO_3$-NaCl filling solution; behind silicone rubber membrane	10^{-4} to 10^{-1}	Organic acids
	NH_3	Combination glass pH electrode, 0.1 M NH_4Cl filling solution; behind porous Teflon gas-permeable membrane	10^{-5} to 5×10^{-2}	Volatile amines

Modified from Meyerhoff ME, Opdycke WN: *Adv Clin Chem* 25:1-47, 1986.

crystal structure. The properties of the F^- ISE are shown in Table 15-2. Another clinically important solid-state membrane electrode for determination of Cl^- is based on pressed-pellet membranes of the ionic conductor, Ag_2S, and AgCl. Similar electrodes have also been developed for the detection of Br^-, CN^-, I^-, SCN^-, S^{2-}, Ag^+, Cu^{2+}, Pb^{2+}, and Cd^{2+}.

Glass membrane electrodes. The first and most widely used ISE is the glass membrane electrode for pH measurements. Glasses of certain compositions respond to pH when a membrane potential develops as a result of an ion-exchange mechanism with H^+ that occurs in the thin, hydrated outer layer of the glass membrane that has been soaked in solution. The outstanding properties of the glass pH electrode are attributable to the remarkable selectivity of this surface reaction for H^+.

The basic design of the glass electrode for pH is shown in Fig. 15-6. The electrode consists of a glass or plastic tube with a thin, pH-sensitive glass membrane sealed in the tip. Ordinarily the membrane is only about 50 μm thick and hence is very fragile. The bulb at the end contains an internal solution composed of 0.1 M HCl into which is dipped a silver wire coated with AgCl, which provides an internal Ag/AgCl reference electrode. This solution also maintains a fixed activity of H^+ to which the internal surface of the membrane is exposed. A shielded cable makes electrical contact between the internal Ag wire and the external pH meter.

The pH response of the glass membrane is determined by the composition of the glass. The glass consists of Na_2O, CaO, and SiO_2. Pure SiO_2 is essentially an insulator that is unresponsive to pH. The addition of Na_2O to the glass for-

mulation disrupts the SiO_2 structure so that negatively charged oxide sites (SiO^-) are paired with Na^+. The mobility of Na^+ in the glass renders the glass membrane slightly conductive to electrical charge. The negative oxide sites serve as ion-exchange sites in aqueous solution and provide the basis for pH response. The potential response to pH is extraordinarily accurate over a pH range of 0 to 14. At pH values above about 9 to 10 the electrode exhibits significant response to other monovalent cations such as Na^+ and K^+. This response to alkali cations at high pH is termed the *alkaline error*. It can be minimized by replacement of Na_2O and CaO to a certain extent in the glass with Li_2O and BaO.

The membrane response to H^+ is attributed to an ion-exchange process that occurs in the vicinity of the membrane solution interface. On immersion of a dry glass membrane in an aqueous solution, the membrane surface becomes hydrated during the course of a few hours. This uptake of water leads to a gradual dissolving of the glass; this process generally determines the useful lifetime of an electrode. However, surface hydration is essential for electrode function; new electrodes immersed in solution respond poorly until adequately soaked. Soaking establishes a hydrated layer that is only 10^{-4} mm or less in thickness. This hydrated layer then functions as a cation-exchange layer in which negatively charged oxygen sites are linked to the glass matrix but in which Na^+ is mobile. Soaking the electrode in acid, for example, results in the replacement of Na^+ with H^+. The membrane response to H^+ can be understood in terms of a surface potential that results from the ion exchange of Na^+ with H^+ in the hydrated gel. Immersion of the electrode membrane in alkaline solution results in ex-

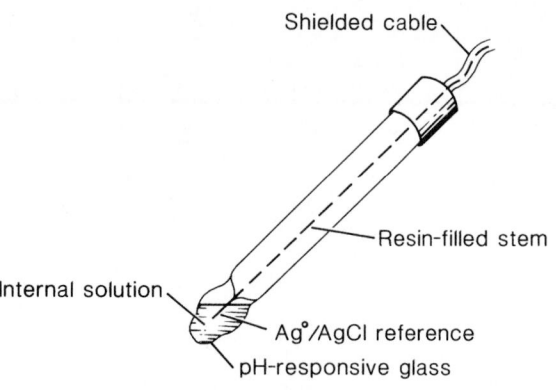

Fig. 15-6 Representative pH electrode. Usually only membrane at tip of electrode bulb is of H^+ ion-selective glass.

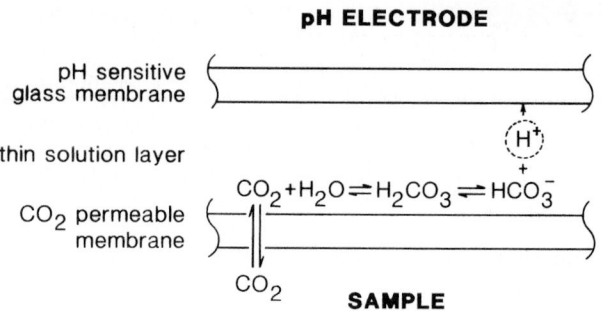

Fig. 15-7 Schema of gas-sensing electrode for CO_2.

change of H^+ in the membrane with Na^+ as membrane H^+ moves into solution. The inner membrane potential is held constant by exposure to a fixed activity of H^+ in the internal solution. Glass electrodes for Na^+, Ag^+, and NH_4^+ have been developed by varying the composition of the glass.

Gas-sensing electrodes. Gas-sensing electrodes consist of an ISE in contact with a thin layer of aqueous electrolyte that is confined to the electrode surface by an outer membrane, as shown schematically for a CO_2 electrode in Fig. 15-7. The outer membrane is very thin and is chosen so that it is permeable to the gas of interest; for CO_2, the membrane is made of silicone rubber. This membrane allows CO_2 gas in the sample to pass through the membrane. Dissolution of the CO_2 in the thin layer of electrolyte causes a change in pH because of a shift in the equilibrium position of the chemical reaction shown in Fig. 15-7. The change in pH sensed by the internal ion-selective pH electrode is in proportion to the P_{CO_2} of the sample. One of the most important applications of the CO_2 electrode is the measurement of blood P_{CO_2}.

The NH_3 electrode in principle is identical to the CO_2 electrode; here the filling solution is aqueous ammonium chloride. The internal pH electrode senses the change in pH from the ammonium/ammonia (NH_4^+/NH_3) acid-base equilibrium. The pH change is thus proportional to P_{NH_3} of the sample.

Gas electrodes have been used for other bioanalytical applications such as the measurement of CO_2 in general assays of decarboxylating enzyme activities and the measurement of NH_3 in tissue and serum. Characteristics of the CO_2 and NH_3 electrodes are shown in Table 15-2.

Care and methodology

The care of ISEs is essentially similar for every ion type. Since the sensing tip of the electrodes is made from extremely fragile and sensitive materials, care must be taken to prevent breakage and maintain the tip in a moist environment. Most commercially available electrodes are supplied with protective coverings to help prevent careless

damage to the electrodes while they are not in use. Each electrode is also accompanied by manufacturer's recommendations for specific cleaning and storage requirements. Storage conditions depend on the frequency of use, the type of electrode, and the application. For example, cleaning procedures are different for a pH electrode used in a protein solution and for one used in a solution of inorganic ions. Protein layers are removed by rinsing the electrode with pepsin, bleach, or 0.1 M HCl, whereas an inorganic deposit can be removed with ethylenediaminetetraacetic acid (EDTA) or acids. After each cleaning procedure, the electrode tip is thoroughly rinsed with distilled water, and the electrode is returned to the storage container.

pH measurements are easily made in the clinical laboratory with a two-point calibration procedure. Standard buffer solutions, which are commercially available, are chosen to bracket the pH of the sample solution. Electrode calibration is always initiated with a pH 7 standard buffer. The meter is adjusted to read 7.00 after the temperature control has been set to the temperature of the buffer. Subsequently, either an acidic or alkaline buffer is used to complete the calibration, depending on the sample to be measured. Samples can then be measured. Multiple calibrations may be necessary for a large number of samples.

For non–H^+ sensing electrodes a calibration curve that relates the potential difference in millivolts to concentration is needed. Although ISEs measure analyte activity, the concentration can be related to millivolts as long as the ionic strength is constant between standards and samples. This is accomplished by addition of a small amount of a solution of high ionic strength to the calibrating standards. This solution must not contain any interfering ions. A potential reading is determined for each standard solution, beginning with the lowest concentration. A plot of log $(C_i)_{standard}$ versus potential is linear for a properly responding ISE. Ion concentrations in samples are then obtained by measurement of the response in millivolts of the sample and use of the calibration curve. The sample ion concentrations are valid as long as the matrix of the standard solutions is made to closely mimic the samples. Most laboratory electrodes and instruments routinely use a two-point standardization procedure to ensure similar response from analysis to analysis. Other standardization and analysis methods have been developed for various electrodes and applications.

In the clinical laboratory, the analysis of large numbers of samples is a necessity. Thus many ISEs are incorporated into automatic analyzers in a flow-through configuration. This arrangement takes advantage of the rapid response of ISEs by placing them into multi-ion analyzers with large sample throughput capabilities. Calibrants, samples, and rinsing solutions are pumped across the electrode surfaces of the ISEs, which are placed in series. A single reference electrode is used for all ISEs in a system with the exception of the CO_2 sensor, which has its own reference electrode behind the gas-permeable membrane. Calibrants have constant ionic strength that closely matches that of physiological samples to minimize errors that result from differences in liquid junction potentials between samples and standards. It cannot be emphasized enough that the proper care and use of the ISEs in these instruments are essential to ensure accurate and reproducible analyses. This requires a constant monitoring of the performance of both the individual electrodes and the instrument as a whole. The following section is a discussion of some of the common errors and interferences that can occur with ISE measurements.

Experimental considerations and interferences

Errors in ISE measurement can result for any ion determination if standards and samples are not run at approximately the same temperature, since the Nernst equation is temperature dependent. Perhaps the most important source of error is the response of an ISE to a nonanalyte or interferent ion in the sample. It is therefore important to know the selectivity properties of the electrode being used and to ensure that nonanalyte ions to which the electrode responds are not present in high enough concentrations to constitute an interference. Components in certain samples can also change the sensitivity of an electrode by adsorbing on its surface and thereby blocking access of the analyte to the surface. Such contamination is a problem in samples containing surface-adsorbing species such as proteins. For single electrode determinations in whole blood or serum, techniques that isolate the ISE from direct contact with the sample are available. However, the demand for multiple sample and ion analyses has made single electrode measurements impractical. Modern multi-ion analyzers incorporate a small size–exclusion membrane that protects the ion-selective membrane from the high-molecular-weight components of biological fluids but allows analyte molecules access to the electrodes.

Although many ISEs are very selective, under certain conditions some ions may interfere and yield erroneous results. Specific examples are listed in Table 15-2 and are briefly discussed below. Detailed descriptions of clinical analyses for many ions can also be found in Chapters 24, 25, and 28.

pH measurements have few specific interferences associated with them. The linear response range is from pH 2 to 12. Sensitivity of the glass pH electrode may be reduced at pH values above 10 because of the interference of monovalent cations, especially Na^+. Although monovalent cations can enter and slowly move through the hydrated layer, multivalent cations of $2+$ or $3+$ charge do not interfere. In solutions of pH less than 1, low water activities also give rise to measurement error.

Na^+ ions are determined by either a glass electrode or a polymer type of liquid membrane electrode. Interferences are minimal because of the high concentration of sodium in biological fluids, especially in blood. The glass electrode exhibits excellent selectivity over K^+ and H^+ because of this fact. Highly acidic urine samples are an exception. The polymer-based ISE, however, can be subject to an interference from Li^+ if a patient is being treated with a lithium compound.

K^+ is usually measured by the valinomycin/polymer electrode described above. Good results are obtained for measurements in blood; however, in undiluted urine samples a negative error may result because of the partitioning of a negatively charged lipophilic component of the urine that is permeable to the polymer. This component can be excluded by use of an ISE with a silicone-rubber membrane instead of the polymer. Alternatively, accurate measurements can be obtained by sample dilution.

Determination of Na^+ and K^+ levels in undiluted blood and urine samples requires special attention. Measurements made by the nondilutional ISE method may differ from results obtained by flame atomic emission spectroscopy (FAES), which determines the concentration of ions in the total sample volume. In contrast, the ISE method measures the activity of the ions in the sample. Since the activity can be influenced by the sample environment (such as protein and water content), deviations may occur between these methods. Agreement between these methods is usually realized by sample dilution. Methodological differences may be greater in the case of Na^+ determinations because of the higher relative concentration of Na^+ in biological fluids. The influence of physiological effects on Na^+ and K^+ determinations in biological fluids is discussed in further detail elsewhere.

Much care must be taken in the determination of *Ca^{++}*. Ca^{++} exists in both the bound form (with proteins or other biological molecules) and the unbound, ionized Ca^{++} form. The Ca^{++} ISE is one of the easiest ways to measure ionized Ca^{++}, since it responds to only the ionized form, which is believed to be the physiologically important form.

The determination of *Cl^-* in biological fluids by an ISE suffers from frequent fouling of the surface by proteins present in the sample. This problem can be minimized when one uses the semipermeable membrane described above to exclude the large molecules from the electrode surface. Recently a liquid membrane electrode made of polymer that exhibits selectivity for chloride has been developed and used in electrolyte analyzers for biomedical use. The chloride ISE is subject to interference from Br^-, I^-, F^-, CN^-, OH^-, and S^{--}, but, except for Br^-, these ions are usually not present in physiological samples at a level high enough to interfere.

The F^- ISE exhibits excellent selectivity and suffers only from interference of OH^- at high pH.

ISEs for the measurement of CO_2 are relatively easy to use and are interference free. Undiluted blood can be used directly as the sample, and calibration is typically accomplished with 5% and 10% mixtures of CO_2 in an inert gas. Total CO_2 measurements require acidification to convert CO_3^{--} and HCO_3^- to CO_2. In this case, calibration is performed with standard $NaHCO_3$ solutions. Response times for total CO_2 measurements are generally longer because of the necessity of establishing equilibrium conditions. CO_3^{--}-selective membranes are available in some instruments for total CO_2 measurements. Interferents are mainly organic acids to which the gas membrane is also permeable. The carbonate-selective membranes are subject to interferences from anions such as salicylate, but placement of the ISE behind the silicone-rubber membrane alleviates this problem.

The NH_3 ISE responds selectively and rapidly to the ammonia concentration in solution. The major drawback is the questionable stability of the membrane and the electrode. Interference can result from nonpolar volatile amines present in the sample. With both the CO_2 and NH_3 electrodes it is important to have a rapidly responding electrode. A decrease in the response time signifies a loss in electrode performance and may require the replacement of the membrane.

VOLTAMMETRIC METHODS

Electrochemical techniques in which a potential is applied to an electrochemical cell and the resulting current from an electrochemical reaction is measured are generally categorized as *voltammetric* methods. Electrochemical cells for voltammetry use a three-electrode configuration. The cell consists of a *working electrode*, a *reference electrode*, and an *auxiliary electrode*. The potential is applied between the working and reference electrode by a *potentiostat;* this applied potential can force changes to occur to any electroactive species at the working electrode surface by *electrolysis*. Electrolysis can occur by a *reduction*, a gain of one or more electrons, or an *oxidation*, a loss of one or more electrons. The current required to sustain the electrolysis at the working electrode and maintain electroneutrality in the cell is provided by the auxiliary electrode. This arrangement prevents the reference electrode from being subjected to large currents that could change its potential. Some voltammetry instrumentation is based on the two-electrode system. Here the auxiliary electrode is absent, and the reference electrode is subjected to the entire cell current.

The basic concept of applying a potential to an electrochemical cell and measuring the current that results from electrolysis can be implemented in numerous ways. Several different techniques have been developed by variations in how the potential is applied or how the current is measured. Although the resultant output and the practical applications of these techniques are varied, they all share the common basis of applying a potential, E, and measuring a current, i, or charge, Q. In addition, the solution may be moving or stationary with respect to the working electrode. Voltammetry in an unstirred solution is referred to as *stationary* solution voltammetry. *Hydrodynamic* voltammetry involves the forced movement of solution either through stirring the solution or flowing the solution over the electrode as in *liquid chromatography with electrochemical detection* (LCEC).

The result of a voltammetric technique is called a *voltammogram* (that is, a current-potential curve). Voltammograms give useful quantitative and qualitative information about the electrochemical reaction. A typical hydrodynamic voltammogram is shown in Fig. 15-8 for the reduction of species *Ox* by one electron to species *Red*. As the potential is scanned in the negative direction, the voltammogram can be described by three distinct regions. In region A, the potential applied at the working electrode is insufficient to cause electrolysis to occur; therefore no current is observed. The onset of electrolysis is signaled by the rise in current in region B. The current continues to rise until a maximum value is reached. This is region C, where electrolysis is occurring at the maximum rate possible. The maximum current in region C is defined as the *limiting current* (i_l), and is defined by equation 15-5:

$$i_l = \frac{nFAD_0C_0}{\delta} \qquad \textit{Eq. 15-5}$$

where A is the electrode area, D_0 is the diffusion coefficient of *Ox*, C_0 is the concentration of *Ox*, and δ is the diffusion distance. As is illustrated by equation 15-5, the magnitude of i_l is directly proportional to the concentration of the electrochemically active analyte. Thus voltammetry can be used to quantitatively measure analyte concentration. The practical unit for current is the ampere (A), which is the transfer of one coulomb of charge per second. This corresponds to the passage of 1.05×10^{-5} moles of electrons per second. Since the current involved in most electroanalytical techniques is very small, milliamperes (mA), microamperes (μA), and nanoamperes (nA) are commonly used units.

The *half-wave potential* ($E_{1/2}$) is defined as the potential at one half the limiting current. $E_{1/2}$ is uniquely characteristic of the species undergoing electrolysis just as the half-cell potential is for the reference electrode, and it can be used for qualitative identification. By convention a reduction is described by a positive, or *cathodic*, current, whereas

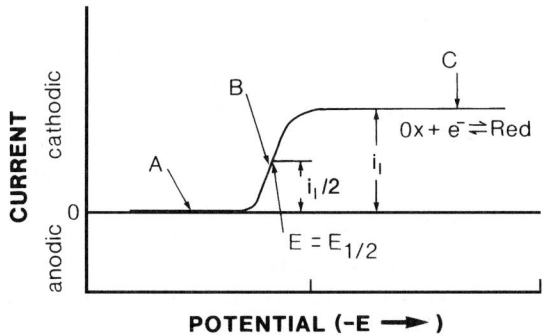

Fig. 15-8 Generalized hydrodynamic voltammogram for reduction of *Ox* to *Red*. Potential scanned negatively left to right. i_l is limiting current, and $E_{1/2}$ is half-wave potential.

an oxidation is described by a negative, or *anodic,* current. The principles for an oxidation are similar and can be applied for a positive potential scan.

One specific type of voltammetry that is clinically useful is amperometry. Amperometric sensors are devices that measure the current generated at a fixed potential by an electroactive analyte in solution. The potential is set to a value of *E* where i_l occurs (Fig. 15-8, region C), and i_l is then measured for each sample. The current measured is directly proportional to the concentration of species present. Three clinically important amperometric sensors discussed below are the oxygen electrode, the glucose electrode, and LCEC.

Voltammetry electrodes

Working electrodes. Working electrodes have certain properties in common. Good electrical conductance is of foremost importance. Consequently, working electrodes are generally metals or semiconductors. Chemical and electrochemical inertness is important in applications for which the electrode should function simply to transfer electrons to and from species dissolved in solution. This inertness gives a

wide potential region with minimum background contributions from electrode and solvent redox properties in which the electrochemistry of the analyte or analytes can be easily monitored.

Platinum, gold, mercury, and glassy carbon are commonly used materials for voltammetric electrodes. When used for voltammetry, mercury can be used in the form of a *hanging mercury drop electrode.* To provide the working electrode surface, one can extrude a reproducible mercury drop through a narrow glass capillary by means of a commercially available micrometer syringe. One can form a new drop by simply dislodging the old one and extruding more mercury. The *dropping mercury electrode* is the working electrode for *polarography.* In this technique, mercury is forced by gravity through a very fine capillary to provide a continuous stream of identical droplets. Each droplet expands, becomes too heavy to be suspended, and breaks loose from the capillary.

Auxiliary electrodes. Auxiliary electrodes are made from any conductive material, typically a piece of platinum wire.

Reference electrodes. The commonly used reference electrodes for voltammetry are the SCE and Ag/AgCl electrodes, which have been previously described in detail.

Oxygen electrode

The oxygen electrode is designed as a complete electrochemical cell. The basic design, which is shown in Fig. 15-9, incorporates a platinum disk as the cathode and a Ag/AgCl electrode as the anode in a buffered electrolyte solution. The electrochemical cell is isolated from the sample by an oxygen-permeable membrane. Oxygen diffuses through the membrane and is reduced electrochemically at the platinum electrode, which is held at a potential that quantitatively reduces oxygen (-0.5 to -0.6 V versus Ag/AgCl).

$$O_2 + 2H^+ + 2e^- \rightarrow H_2O_2 \qquad \textit{Eq. 15-6}$$

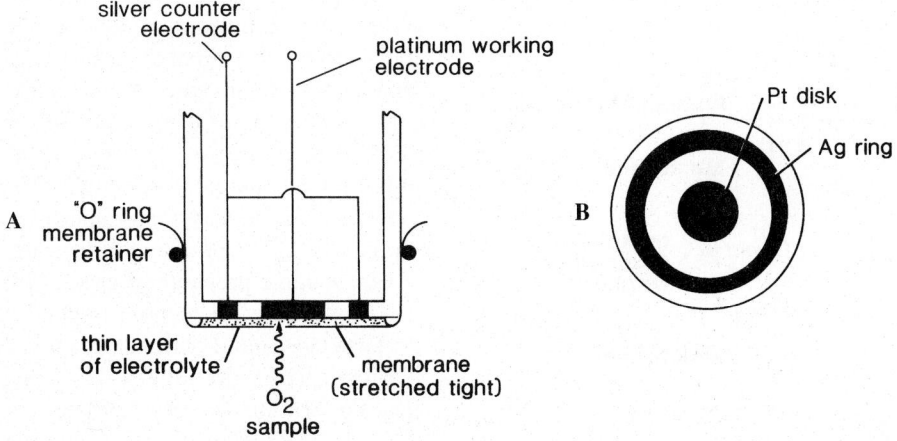

Fig. 15-9 Schema of oxygen electrode. **A,** Cross-sectional view showing diffusion of O_2 sample through membrane. **B,** View of electrode assembly from bottom.

The current generated at the platinum electrode is directly proportional to the concentration (partial pressure) of oxygen dissolved in the sample. As with potentiometric indicator electrodes, the membrane inhibits electrode fouling from serum proteins in blood and also prevents other electroactive substances from being reduced at the electrode. Calibration of the electrode system is done with standard solutions or gases containing known concentrations of oxygen.

Few interferences are associated with the use of the oxygen electrode. Poor response times and variable results may indicate that degradation of the membrane or a change in pH of the buffer solution has occurred. Silver metal may deposit on the platinum cathode and also affect the electrode response. Polishing the electrode with electrode polishing compound will regenerate the platinum surface.

The oxygen electrode is usually incorporated into a blood gas analyzer, which routinely measures oxygen, CO_2, and pH on samples of less than 250 μL of whole blood. Miniaturized O_2 electrodes have been developed, and they can be used for transcutaneous measurements, eliminating the need for drawing blood samples. However, the accuracy and response time of these electrodes depend on the physical characteristics of the patient's skin tissue. The oxygen electrode has been used to monitor many reactions that involve consumption of O_2 to measure glucose (glucose oxidase), cholesterol (cholesterol oxidase), and uric acid (uricase).

Glucose electrode

Glucose is another important constituent of serum and plasma that can be measured by an amperometric sensor. A diagram of a typical glucose electrode is shown in Fig. 15-10. The basic design of this electrode uses the enzyme glucose oxidase, immobilized between two membranes. Glucose oxidase reacts with the glucose in the sample to generate hydrogen peroxide (H_2O_2) and gluconic acid. The inner membrane is permeable to H_2O_2, which is determined amperometrically by the underlying platinum electrode held at a positive potential sufficient to oxidize H_2O_2 to O_2 (the reverse of the reaction shown in equation 15-6). The cur-

rent measured from the H_2O_2 oxidation is directly proportional to the glucose concentration; glucose concentrations have been reported to be quantified in the range of 10^{-7} to 10^{-3} M. Few interferences are noted for this electrode. The inner membrane is impermeable to ascorbic acid, uric acid, and acetaminophen, which are electroactive at positive potentials and may be present in clinical samples. The glucose electrode may be limited by the depletion of O_2 in the internal buffer solution. Current research is involved in constructing future generations of glucose electrodes to overcome this problem. The design for this glucose electrode has been developed by the Yellow Springs Instrument Company (Yellow Springs, Ohio).

Liquid chromatography with electrochemical detection

LCEC is a hybrid technique that combines chromatography with electrochemistry. As discussed in Chapters 5 and 6, high-performance liquid chromatography provides a means of separating various components of solutions by making use of their chemical affinities to column-packing materials. In LCEC, electroactive materials are detected sequentially as they elute from a chromatographic column and flow across or through the working electrode. Very low detection limits (approximately 1.0 pmol) may be obtained with relatively simple instrumentation. As a result of these features, LCEC has become recognized as a powerful tool for the trace determinations of many clinically important biomolecules. These include several metabolites of the central nervous system that are easily oxidized or reduced at an electrode surface.

To optimize an LCEC determination, it is necessary to consider both chromatographic and electrochemical requirements simultaneously. A primary requirement for electrochemical detection is that the mobile phase has a relatively high conductivity. To this end, buffered mobile phases of moderate ionic strength (0.01 to 0.1 M) are typically used. Most LCEC applications use reverse-phase, ion-exchange, or ion-pair chromatographic columns for separation (see Chapter 6). Significant amounts (up to 90% v/v) of organic modifiers, such as methanol, acetonitrile, and propanol, can be added to the aqueous mobile phase to shorten chromatographic retention. Of great advantage in LCEC is the inherent specificity of electrochemical detection, in which only compounds electroactive at the applied potential are detected. In this way many interferences that have similar chromatographic retention times are eliminated. For this reason, sample preparation may be quite facile in comparison with other detection methods available for high-performance liquid chromatography.

Most LCEC applications use a single working electrode in a conventional three-electrode system (see Chapter 6). The choice of working electrode material is an important consideration for LCEC. Carbon paste, a mixture of graphite powder and a coagulant such as paraffin oil, exhibits low

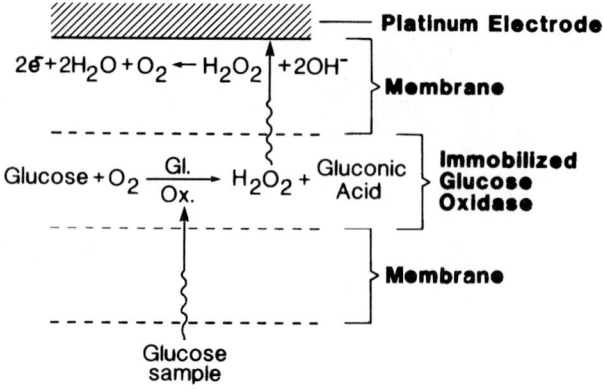

Fig. 15-10   Schema of glucose electrode.

background currents at positive potentials and is well suited to oxidative applications. Unfortunately, carbon paste electrodes are incompatible with mobile phases containing significant amounts of organic modifier. Glassy carbon electrodes are compatible with modifiers and may be used at negative potentials. Mercury or mercury-gold amalgam electrodes have the best characteristics when operated at negative potentials, and they are used principally for reductive LCEC. Any of these types of electrode surfaces can become fouled and inefficient when one is detecting high concentrations of some compounds. Additionally, high concentrations of proteins or other large biomolecules can lead to electrode fouling. This will result in irreproducible data. To alleviate the permanent loss of electrode performance, both physical and chemical cleaning procedures have been developed.

To obtain the best detector sensitivity and detection limits, it is important to know the minimum potential that need be applied to the working electrode for the desired electrochemical reaction to occur. This is most often accomplished by obtaining a hydrodynamic voltammogram (Fig. 15-8) of each component being detected. To generate such a voltammogram, multiple injections are made using various applied detector potentials, and the resulting current is plotted as a function of potential. To achieve maximum sensitivity, the applied potential should be selected so that the observed oxidations or reductions are at the limiting current for all compounds to be detected.

LCEC has become a widely used analytical technique for biomedical analysis. Although space does not permit a complete review of all biochemical applications, it is important to consider many general classes of compounds detectable by both oxidative and reductive techniques. Table 15-3 lists several compounds of pharmaceutical origin that may be determined using LCEC. Table 15-4 provides the approximate oxidation potentials obtained from hydrodynamic voltammograms that are used to detect some neurochemically important compounds by LCEC.

Oxidative applications. Most phenols are readily oxidized at carbon electrodes. The first and still most common LCEC application is the determination of catecholamines in biological samples. A second major use of LCEC is in the determination of the hydroxyindole metabolites of tryptophan. More recently, there has been developed an electrochemical enzyme immunoassay in which phenols are detected as the electroactive product of the enzyme reaction. Aromatic amines are likewise easily oxidized at carbon electrodes and may be studied by LCEC.

Many compounds of biomedical interest are heterocyclic in structure, and electroactive at potentials easily attained using LCEC. Methods for the determination of such heterocycles as ascorbic acid, uric acid, reduced nicotinamide adenine dinucleotide (NADH), biotin, and the folates have been developed. Although most amino acids are not electroactive at analytically usable potentials with reduced carbon electrodes, derivatization methods have been developed to produce electroactive products. These methods provide excellent determination of amino acids. Thiols may also be determined at a gold-mercury amalgam electrode.

Reductive applications. Wide-scale reductive LCEC applications have not been well established in the clinical laboratory because of the difficulties presented by oxygen and trace metal–ion interferences at negative potentials. These problems can be overcome with established mobile-phase deoxygenation procedures and the use of high-purity salts, leading to more clinical applications of reductive LCEC.

Aromatic nitro and nitroso compounds are easily reduced at carbon or mercury electrodes. Other nitro compounds such as nitrate esters, nitroamines, and nitrosamines are also easily reduced. Additionally, several heterocycles of clinical interest may be detected by reductive LCEC, including the K vitamins, the pterins, and several pharmaceuticals.

Anodic stripping voltammetry

Anodic stripping voltammetry is a voltammetric technique that is useful in clinical chemistry for the determination of heavy metals. The determination of Pb^{2+} in biological flu-

Table 15-3   Application of LCEC to drug analysis

Class	Compound
Analgesic	Acetaminophen, codeine, naproxen, phenacetin, salicylic acid, ketobemidone, morphine
Tranquilizer	Diazepam
Anticonvulsant	Nitrazepam
Antibacterial	Amoxicillin
Adrenergic blockers	Labetalol, mepindolol
Antineoplastic	Methotrexate, procarbazine hydrochloride
Muscle relaxant	Theophylline
Antihypertensive	Sulfinalol hydrochloride
Antitubercular	Rifampin
Antipsychotic	Chlorpromazine
Antiarthritic	Penicillamine

Modified from Lunte CE, Heineman WR: *Top Curr Chem* 143:1-48, 1988.

Table 15-4   Approximate oxidation potentials of neurochemically important compounds

Compound	Oxidation potential
Dopamine	0.3 V
Epinephrine	0.3 V
5-Hydroxyindoleacetic acid (5-HIAA)	0.3 V
Norepinephrine	0.3 V
Ascorbic acid	0.3 V
Vanillylmandelic acid (VMA)	0.6 V
Metanephrine	0.6 V
Normetanephrine	0.6 V
3-Methoxy-4-hydroxyphenylglycol (MHPG)	0.7 V
Homovanillic acid (HVA)	0.7 V

Modified from Lunte CE, Heineman WR: *Top Curr Chem* 143:1-48, 1988.

ids of patients suspected of having lead poisoning is an example of its use. Stripping voltammetry has the lowest detection limit of the commonly used electroanalytical techniques. Analyte concentrations as low as 10^{-10} M have been determined. The technique consists of two steps. In the first step, analyte is deposited at a mercury electrode by the application of a potential that is sufficient to reduce the species of interest at the working electrode. This step serves to preconcentrate the analyte by electrochemically extracting it into a mercury electrode. It is this preconcentration feature that enables such low concentrations to be reached by stripping voltammetry. In the second step, the deposited analyte is removed, or "stripped," from the electrode by application of increasingly positive potentials, and the resulting current signal is a measure of the concentration of analyte in solution. Since the stripping step gives anodic current (that is, the species is oxidized), the technique is termed "anodic stripping voltammetry."

In anodic stripping voltammetry only a fraction of the total analyte is deposited into the mercury electrode by electrolysis during the preconcentration step. Complete deposition of all of the analyte into the electrode is time consuming and generally unnecessary, since adequate concentrations can usually be deposited into the electrode to give a satisfactory stripping signal in much shorter times. Since the deposition is not exhaustive, it is important to deposit the same fraction of analyte for each stripping voltammogram. The parameters of electrode surface area, deposition time, and stirring must be carefully duplicated for all standards and samples. Deposition times vary from 60 seconds to 30 minutes, depending on the analyte concentration, the type of working electrode, and the stripping technique.

Anodic stripping voltammetry has become a useful method in the clinical laboratory for the determination of Pb^{++} in blood and urine since the development of automated instrumentation by Environmental Science Associates (ESA). ESA also markets a digestion reagent, Metexchange, which frees bound Pb^{++} from biological components of blood and urine. Detailed procedures for Pb^{++} determination in blood and urine by anodic stripping voltammetry can be found in the literature.

COULOMETRIC METHODS

Coulometry is a very useful electrochemical method for quantitative analysis. Clinical applications use one form of coulometry that involves the application of a constant current to generate a titrating agent. In principle, the time required to titrate a sample at constant current is measured and is related to the amount of analyte in a sample by Faraday's law (equation 15-7):

$$Q = it = nFN \qquad \textit{Eq. 15-7}$$

where Q is the charge passed for a finite time, t, at constant current, i; n is the number of electrons involved in the electrochemical reaction; F is Faraday's constant; and N is the number of moles of analyte in the sample. Charge is a quantity of electricity. The unit for charge is the coulomb (C) and corresponds to 1.05×10^{-5} moles of electrons. Since N is measured directly without the need for standards, coulometry is an absolute method and can be used for very precise determinations of analyte.

Titration of chloride

Although not in wide use currently, coulometric determination of chloride is of historical importance and has been used for the determination of Cl^- in serum, plasma, urine, and other body fluids. The analysis of Cl^- takes advantage of the quantitative formation and low solubility of AgCl. Ag^+ ions (the titrating agent) are electrochemically generated at the Ag anode by application of a constant current. Cl^- ions in the sample are rapidly consumed as they react with Ag^+ to form insoluble AgCl. At any point in the titration, the Ag^+ concentration is very low.

$$\textit{Anode reaction:}\ \ Ag \rightarrow Ag+ + e-$$
$$\textit{Solution reaction:}\ \ Ag+ + Cl- \rightarrow AgCl\ (s)$$

However, the end point is signaled by a sudden increase in Ag^+ concentration that follows the consumption of all of the Cl^-. A second pair of Ag^+-specific electrodes detects the rise in concentration of silver ions in solution and immediately stops the titration. The amount of Cl^- in the sample is proportional to the amount of Ag^+ ions generated at the anode.

Coulometric determination of chloride is very precise; however, other anions that form insoluble complexes with silver ion can result in Cl^- determinations that are falsely elevated. Poor reproducibility can be a problem at high chloride concentrations because of the large amount of precipitate.

BIBLIOGRAPHY
General

Koryta J, Dvorak J, Kavan L: *Principles of electrochemistry,* ed 2, New York, 1993, Wiley & Sons.

Wang J: *Electroanalytical techniques in clinical chemistry and laboratory medicine,* New York, 1988, VCH Publishers.

Potentiometric methods

Bates RG: *Determination of pH: theory and practice,* New York, 1964, Wiley & Sons.

Freiser H, editor: *Ion-selective electrodes in analytical chemistry,* vols I and II, New York, 1978, 1980, Plenum Publishing.

Koryta J, editor: *Medical and biological applications of electrochemical devices,* New York, 1980, Wiley & Sons.

Meyerhoff ME, Opdyke WN: Ion-selective electrodes, *Adv Clin Chem* 25:1, 1986.

Morf WR: *The principles of ion-selective electrodes and of membrane transport,* New York, 1981, Elsevier Science.

Simon W, Ammann D, Bussmann W, Meier PC: Ion-selective electrodes in biology and medicine. In Laidler KJ, editor: *Frontiers of chemistry,* New York, 1982, Pergamon Press.

Solsky RL: Ion-selective electrodes in biomedical analysis, *CRC Crit Rev Anal Chem* 14:1, 1982.

Voltammetric methods

Bard AJ, Faulkner LR: *Electrochemical methods,* New York, 1980, Wiley & Sons.

Kissinger PT, Heineman WR, editors: *Laboratory techniques in electro-analytical chemistry,* New York, 1984, Marcel Dekker.

Lunte CE, Heineman WR: Electrochemical techniques in bioanalysis, *Top Curr Chem* 143:1-48, 1988.

Enzyme electrodes

Kessler M, Clark LC Jr, Lubbers DW, et al, editors: *Ion and enzyme electrodes in biology and medicine,* Baltimore, 1976, University Park Press.

Phenytoin electrode

Cosofret VV, Buck RP: A poly(vinyl chloride) membrane electrode for determination of phenytoin in pharmaceutical formulations, *J Pharm Biomed Anal* 4:45, 1986.

Biosensors

Blum LJ, Coulet PR, editors: *Biosensor principles and applications,* New York, 1991, Marcel Dekker.

Turner APF: *Advances in biosensors,* vol 1, Greenwich, Conn., 1991, JAI Press Ltd.

Automation

Michael A. Pesce

OBJECTIVES

- Outline the steps in sample processing. Outline the steps in analysis and describe how they may be adapted to automation.

- Describe the proportioning of samples to reagents as accomplished by the following analytical systems:
  1. Dry-film reagent systems
  2. Discrete test analyzers

- Define sample carryover, identifying systems where it is commonly seen and suggest at least two ways by which it can be minimized.

- Outline the processes of mixing, incubation, and sensing, and describe how they are handled in dry-film reagent systems, continuous-flow systems, and discrete test analyzers.

- List and interpret the eight basic concepts of automation, explaining how the concepts are applied to commonly used automated instruments.

KEY TERMS

analog A measurement derived directly from an instrument's continuous signal (such as voltage) and usually presented in graphic form.

automation Use of a machine designed to follow repeatedly and automatically a predetermined sequence of individual operations.

bar-coding A computer-driven sample-recognition system that identifies both the specimen and the analyses to be performed and relays this information to the automated analyzer.

bulk reagents Those that must be measured before being added to a reaction mixture to attain the desired proportion. Usually a reservoir contains the reagents for more than one analysis.

carryover Contamination of a specimen by the previous one.

centrifugal analyzer Uses centrifugal force to mix the sample aliquot with reagent and to pass the reaction cuvette past a detector.

computation Calculation of a desired result from the signal or readout of an instrument; it can be electronically automated by use of either digital or analog conversion.

continuous flow Process in instruments that constantly pump reagent and sample through tubing and coils, forming a continuous stream.

dead volume The volume in a sampling container that must be present for proper sample aliquoting but is not consumed.

digital Relating to data available in the form of discrete units or the calculations using such data.

discrete Term applied to instruments that compartmentalize each sample reaction.

dwell time The minimum time required for an instrument to obtain a result, calculated from the initial sampling of the specimen.

flow injection Placement of a sample into the stream of a continuous-flow analyzer.

incubation time The time allowed for a chemical reaction or process to proceed to completion.

mixing Process by which individual components of a chemical assay are formed into a homogeneous solution.

proportioning Addition of individual components of a chemical assay in proper ratios or amounts.

readout Written or computer display of the result of an analysis performed on an instrument.

selective instrument An instrument capable of performing multiple tests on a sample. Instead of performing all possible tests on each sample, these instruments are capable of performing only those tests programmed.

sensor A system or device that monitors changes in the reaction mixture that are related to analyte concentration.

test menu The number of different tests available at one time without changing reagents or components.

test repertoire All the different tests that are available on an instrument, including those that can be made available by changing reagents or instrument components.

throughput The maximum number of individual samples or test analyses that can be practically performed per hour by an assay system, with the required dwell time being taken into account.

unit reagents Premeasured reaction chemicals packaged so that only one package (unit) is used per sample test.

DEFINITIONS

In this chapter the reasons for laboratory automation and the ways to achieve it are considered. Examples of the major automated instrument categories are examined.

In this section the concept of automation is examined from a historical perspective. It is a fact that more laboratory tests are being performed per patient every year. This has come about for several reasons: the repertoire of available tests has increased; more patients survive acute illnesses and trauma, thus continuing to need additional tests; and results are able to be generated more rapidly and be reported in time to affect medical decisions. The perceived need for results to be returned to physicians in the shortest possible time has, in turn, affected the types of instrumentation available for test analyses, including testing devices that are intended to be used at the patient's bedside.

Increases in test work load have been fueled and sustained by improvements in productivity, some of which derive from automation. A major result of automation has been the almost unlimited access to laboratory analyses by physicians. The salutary effect of this phenomenon on patient care and the cost to the health system is still to be determined.

Automation in a hospital must be viewed as a global, industrial process, encompassing the entire sequence that begins when a physician orders a test and ends when that result is delivered to the physician. Laboratorians must be aware of each step in that process and what can cause a breakdown in the step, resulting in a longer turnaround time or a misplaced sample. The overall process can be broken down into the following components: test ordering, sample acquisition (phlebotomy), sample transport, sample processing, sample analysis, result acquisition, and result reporting.

A discussion of the automation of the first three steps can be found in Chapter 3 and the use of a laboratory information system (LIS) to automate the last three steps can be found in Chapter 18. This chapter reviews the automation in the sample processing and sample analysis steps of this process.

Automation, as applied to the clinical chemistry laboratory, can be defined as the self-moving or mechanical transfer of a specimen within a complex industrial assembly to a succession of self-acting machines, each of which completes a specified stage in the total analytical process from crude sample to analytical result. A second definition is the application of fully automated procedures in the efficient performance and control of operations involving a sequence of complex standardized or repetitive processes. Automation in the laboratory may be considered in the broader context of the need to transfer information about a patient within a hospital or outpatient setting.

One way to visualize how information is transferred is shown in the block diagram of Fig. 16-1. The patient is examined by a physician, and there is a decision to obtain specific laboratory information. A specimen is collected, transferred to the laboratory, received and processed by the laboratory, and analyzed to obtain the desired results, which are then transferred back to the requesting physician. In general, laboratory automation has focused on those steps from the receipt of the sample in the laboratory to the transfer of information back to the requesting physician. There is, however, increasing interest in automating the process of transferring the sample to the laboratory.

Automating the transfer of samples to the laboratory can reduce some of the preanalytical errors associated with this step (see Chapter 3) and reduce the overall time required to produce a test result. Automation of sample transfer is usually accomplished by means of a vacuum tube system. Phlebotomy tubes are placed in a cushioned holder that is introduced into a sending station. The sending station can be programmed to send the holder to a specific receiving station. Vacuum tube systems can rapidly (in less than 5 minutes) transport samples with insignificant physiological changes to the samples, that is, hemolysis and gas cavita-

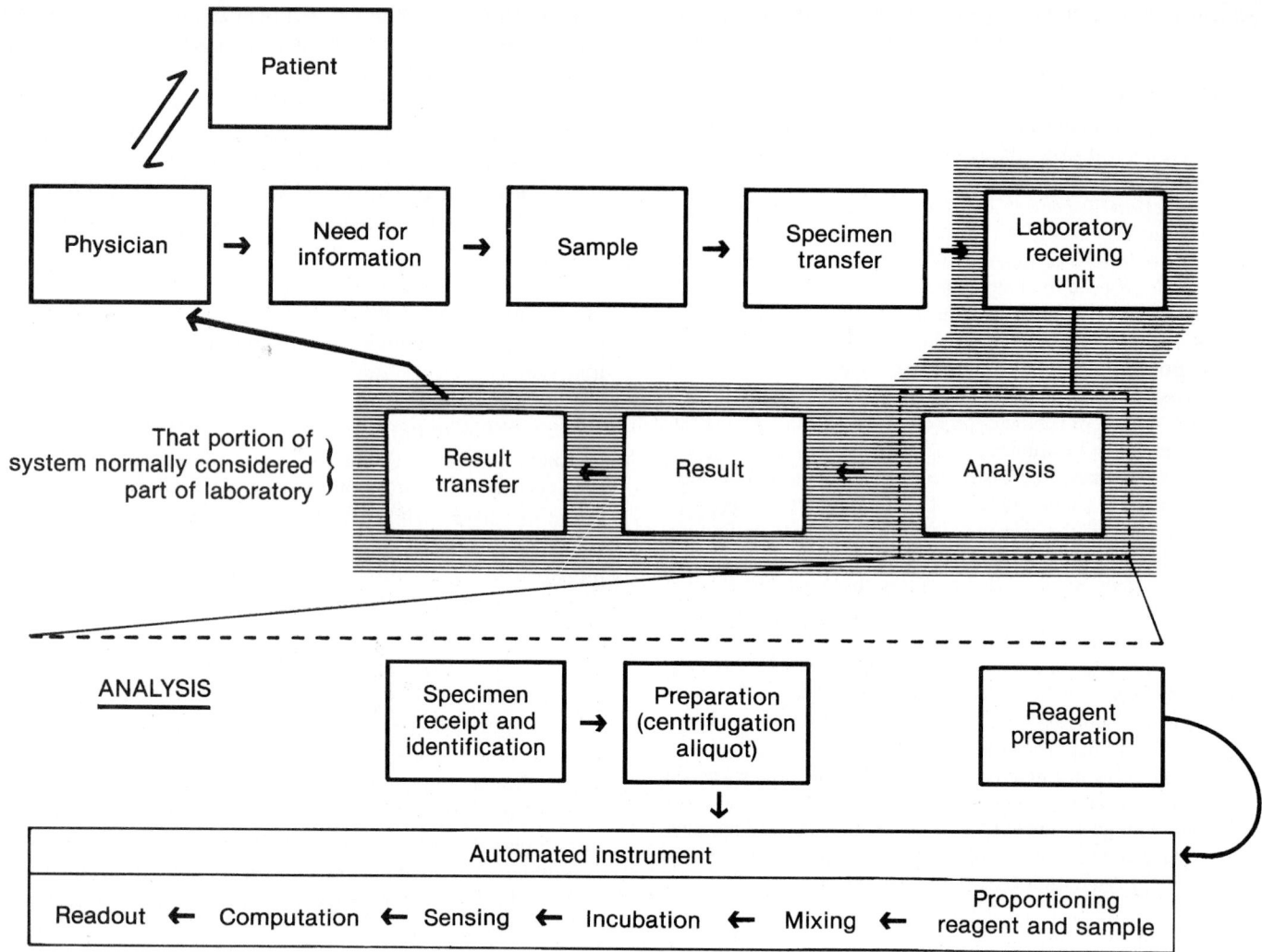

Fig. 16-1 Diagram illustrating specimen and information flow between physician and laboratory. Lower portion outlines steps in sample processing and analysis.

tion in blood-gas samples, obviating the need for slower, less reliable human transporters.

Most laboratories have concentrated on purchasing instruments that will automate the steps of analysis that are outlined in the lower part of Fig. 16-1 and discussed in detail below. Although the term "automation" implies the processing of large numbers of samples, the principles inherent in automation can be applied to the analysis of single samples as well. For example, a blood-gas analyzer is a single-sample analyzer but is commonly highly automated.

The goals of automation in the clinical laboratory are (1) to increase flexibility—ability of the laboratory to expand the test menu; (2) to consolidate work stations; (3) to make more efficient use of laboratory space and personnel; (4) to improve turnaround time for reporting of test results; (5) to improve analytical precision of test results and minimize laboratory errors; (6) to decrease overall cost, including the costs of reagents, supplies, and personnel; and (7) to im-

prove transfer of laboratory results to the requesting physician. With proper planning, there is no reason why these goals cannot be achieved.

AUTOMATION OF CHEMICAL ANALYSIS

To understand how patient samples are processed by automated procedures, one needs to divide the process of analysis, as might be performed in a manual assay, into a series of stages or steps. Commonly the following series of steps is performed during the course of an analysis: (1) obtaining a patient sample in the proper form, (2) mixing an aliquot of the sample with a series of reagents in an ordered sequence with defined amounts, (3) incubating the reaction mixture at a specified temperature for a specified amount of time, (4) monitoring or sensing the result of the reaction, (5) quantitating the extent of the reaction, and (6) providing an appropriate readout of the permanent record. Automation may be applied to any or all of these steps. The automation of each one of these steps is now discussed in some detail.

Sample preparation and identification

Until recently, little automation was applied to the sample processing steps that occur before sample analysis. By and large, specimens were manually labeled, centrifuged, and divided into aliquots if tests for more than one work station had been requested for a specimen. The manual performance of these procedures can often lead to errors, which result in the generation of inaccurate patient results. Mislabeling patient samples leads to laboratory information being erroneously transferred. Similarly, the necessity of dividing the sample into aliquots for separate work stations also can lead to improper patient identification.

Various approaches are now being employed to avoid or to minimize these manual processing steps. Coulter, Olympus, Lab Interlink, and others have introduced systems to automate the initial sample processing steps of the laboratory. These systems employ robotic techniques that have been used in Japan for the past decade to develop highly automated laboratories.

The Coulter system includes modular sample preparation stations with tracks that move samples between work stations. This system automates the centrifugation step, sample aliquoting (with bar-coding), and uncapping and recapping of specimens. Bar-code labels are used to identify samples and tests requested. After preparation the samples are automatically transported to the appropriate analyzers for chemical analysis, hematological and urinalysis testing, or coagulation procedures. The software for running the Coulter system must be linked with the laboratory information system.

The Olympus system is designed to perform triage on specimens, which are then automatically moved to the Olympus AU-5000 system. The carrier is a 10-position sample rack that uses 16 mm tubes. Five secondary tubes can be filled from a primary tube and sent to the laboratory. The system is driven by bar codes and requires a laboratory information system with a computer for control of the system.

The Lab Interlink system is used to automate sample transport within a hospital. Conveyer rails transport specimens from a collection station to analytical work stations by a series of tracks, which can be installed overhead or in between locations. Bar-code readers direct samples to different locations. The Lab Interlink system lacks a centrifuge and aliquot splitting stations.

Adequate laboratory space must be available to install these systems, and highly skilled technologists and bioengineers are needed to support the operation of these systems.

Reagent preparation

Although bulk reagents can be manually prepared, almost all laboratories use concentrates or lyophilates. Thus simple dilution or reconstitution of the reagent with water is all that is required. This simple step, however, can lead to analytical errors because of improper dilution or processing. These errors can be avoided by purchasing reagent in a form suitable for instrument use without any processing. *Unit test-reagent* preparation, where sufficient reagent is present for the performance of a single test, has been automated in two ways. The first is the dry-film or impregnated-paper technique. The dry-chemical techniques use either paper or a series of thin films impregnated with the desired reagent. The analytical reactions take place when the sample is placed on the dry reagent (see Johnson and Johnson Ektachem, Table 16-1 and p. 302). In this type of reagent, preparation consists in wetting the reagent with water, buffer, or sample. The second kind of unit test reagent is a container or test tube containing premeasured liquids or powders to which water, buffer, or sample is added. Because reagent preparation errors are avoided, unit test reagents tend to be more consistent on a long-term, within-lot basis. However, unit test reagents also tend to be more expensive than bulk reagents, a consideration that can be important for many laboratories.

Proportioning of samples and reagents

Most chemical reactions require the combining of reagent and sample in exact amounts to yield specific, final concentrations of analyte and reagents. Since the reagents, as just described, are prepared in predetermined amounts, the ratio, or proportion, of reagent to sample must be kept constant to achieve reproducible and accurate final reagent concentrations. Thus the addition of sample to reagent is termed *proportioning*. The case of unit test reagents is considered first. In these systems the reagents are already proportioned in the required amounts; therefore only the sample must be proportioned. The dry-film reagent may have the sample added volumetrically or by saturation addition. The latter technique requires some explanation. The film is exposed to an excess of the sample, and the pores of the film allow only a fixed amount of the sample to be absorbed. This fixed amount of sample required to wet the film represents the proportioning mechanism. In some cases of saturation addition, the rate of diffusion of the sample into the film may also affect the proportioning step.

In the case of bulk reagents, proportioning is always accomplished by volumetric addition. There are three automated volumetric dispensing methods in common use. Syringes or volumetric overflow devices are used in discrete test analyzers where sample and reagents are volumetrically added to a test tube or container. The second mechanism is the continuous-flow technique used where sample and reagents are proportioned by their relative flow rates. Typically, peristaltic pumps are used to move the reagents through tubing, and the flow rate is controlled by the cross-sectional area (diameter) of the pump tubing. Usually the sample and reagent streams are allowed to flow continu-

Table 16-1   Comparison of operational features for several automated clinical chemistry analyzers

	ACA V	Dimension AR	Hitachi 747-200	Hitachi 911	CX7	Ektachem 750 XRC	RA-2000	Chem-1	DAX	Paramax 720ZX
Type	D, SL, B	D, SL, B	D, SL, B	D, SL, B	D, SL, B	D, SL, B	D, SL, B	C, SL, B	D, SL, B	D, SL, B
Sample volume (μL)*	10-540	2-80	1-20	3-31	3-69	10-11	2-30	1-11	180-250	2-151
Minimum volume (μL)†	20-660	52-112	150	73	53-210	50	52	51	300	12-161
Sample ID‡	Bar code, keyboard	Keyboard	Bar code, keyboard	Bar code, keyboard	Bar code, keyboard	Keyboard	Bar code, keyboard	Bar code, keyboard	Bar code, keyboard	Bar code
Reagent	Unit, M	Bulk, M	Bulk, A	Bulk, A	Bulk, A, M	Unit, M	Bulk, A	Bulk, M	Bulk, A	Bulk, M, A
Proportioning§	Prepackaged, vol add	Vol add	Vol add	Vol add	Vol add	Prepackaged, saturation	Vol add	Ready to use	Premeasured diluent	Vol add
Minimization of matrix (protein) interferences	Dilution	Dilution	Dilution	Dilution	Dilution	Filtration	Autodilution	Dilution	Autodilution	Dilution
Mixing	Vibration (mechanical)	Ultrasonic	Mechanical stirring	Mechanical stirring	Vibration (rotational)	Diffusion	Lateral movement	Coils	Mechanical	Ultrasonic mixer, air mixer
Sensing‖	Spec, electrode	Spec, electrode	Spec, electrode	Spec, electrode	Spec, electrode	Reflectance, electrodes	Spec, electrode	Spec, electrode	Spec, electrode	Spec, electrode
Optical characteristics Lamp	Tungsten-halogen	Tungsten-halogen	Tungsten-halogen	Tungsten-halogen	Xenon Arc	Tungsten-halogen	Tungsten-halogen	Tungsten-halogen	Tungsten-halogen	Tungsten-halogen

Wavelength, nm	340-600	293-700	340-800	340-800	340-700	340-670	340-600	340-600	340-804	340-630
Test menu	Gen chem TDM Coag Ltd hormones	Gen chem TDM Ltd hormones	Gen chem Ltd hormones	Gen chem DAU Ltd hormones TDM	Gen chem TDM Ltd hormones Specific proteins	Gen chem Ltd TDM	Gen chem TDM Specific proteins Ltd hormones	Gen chem DAU TDM	Gen chem	Gen chem Ltd TDM
Test repertoire¶	88	45	32	32	32	46	26	32	26-34	48
Total repertoire#	98	48	70	88	63	46	55	43	32	45
Stat. capability	Yes	Yes	Yes	Yes	Yes	Yes	Yes	Yes	Yes	Yes
Dwell time (min)**	7	1-12	10	0.5-15	1-5	3-5	0.5-5	17	14	3.5-10
Throughput (samples/hr)††	50	60	150-600	360	69-225	60	100	518	100-300	240
Throughput (tests/hr)‡‡	50	540	6600	720	825	750	240-720	720-1800	2600-10200	720
Readout	Digital	Digital	Digital	Digital	Digital	Digital	Printer, CRT	Printer, CRT	Printer, CRT	Digital

A, Available from alternative sources; *B*, batch analyzer; *C*, continuous flow; *Coag*, coagulation analysis; *CRT*, cathode-ray tube; *D*, discrete analyzer; *DAU*, drugs of abuse; *ID*, identification; *Ltd*, limited; *M*, available from manufacturer only; *SL*, selective; *Spec*, that is, photometric; *TDM*, therapeutic drug monitoring; *vol add*, volumetric addition.

*Sample volume needed to perform a test (discrete analyzer) or simultaneous profile.

†Sample volume plus dead space in sample cup.

‡Means of identifying sample for final printout.

§Manner of adding reagent, diluent, and sample.

‖Spec, photometric; electrodes, ion-selective electrodes.

¶The number of tests available at one time, without a change of reagents or instrument module.

#Total number of analytes for which reagents are commercially available.

**Approximate time between sampling and availability of test.

††Number of samples capable of being processed per hour. Data listed are for one simultaneous profile or a single test per sample.

‡‡Calculated by multiplication of maximum number of tests per sample available times number of samples capable of being processed per hour.

ously through the tubing where mixing and incubation are also accomplished. The third type uses electrical valves to control the time reagents can flow. The flow rate is controlled by the air pressure applied to the reagent container and the flow resistance in the tubing that is connected to the reaction vessel.

In almost all systems the sample is introduced into the analyzer with a thin, stainless steel probe. This probe passes into a sample either by direct penetration of a stopper or after the stopper is removed from the Vacutainer tube, aspirates a defined quantity of sample, and moves from the sample to dispense the aliquot into an appropriate vessel. A potential problem with these probes is the risk of clots; this risk is directly related to sample size. As the amount of sample pipetted decreases, the diameter of the probe decreases and the risk of clots increases. Some sample probes are designed to detect clots specifically and to reject clotted samples. Many sample probes have an associated level-sensing device that permits the tip of the probe to go a specified distance below the level of the sample to detect short samples. Since the same probe is used repeatedly for sequential samples, there is the potential for contamination of a specimen by a preceding one. This is called *sample carryover*. Various techniques have been used to minimize the interaction between samples. These include (1) aspiration of a wash liquid (such as saline solution or water) between sample aspirations, and (2) a backflush of the probe. In the latter technique, the wash liquid flows through the probe in a direction opposite to that of the aspiration into a waste container. This procedure has the advantage of minimizing the risk of pulling a small clot further into the system.

One can determine the degree of sample carryover by assaying four identical high-level samples immediately followed by four identical low-level samples. Carryover is calculated by use of the following equation:

$$\text{Percent carryover} = \frac{L1 - (L3 + L4)/2 \times 100}{\dfrac{(H3 + H2)}{2} - \dfrac{(L3 + L4)}{2}}$$

where *L1*, *L2*, *L3*, and *L4* are the consecutive low samples and *H1*, *H2*, *H3*, and *H4* are the consecutive high samples.

Carryover affects the test results by contaminating the current sample with a proportional part of the previous sample. The amount of contamination attributable to carryover that is permitted affects the instrument's throughput. If less carryover is permitted, a longer time must be allowed for the previous sample to be flushed out, reducing the number of samples that are processed per hour.

Mixing

Those instruments using the dry-film technique mix sample and reagents by the diffusion of sample into the reagents. Most dry-film reagents are premixed during manufacturing, though some are mixed by diffusion, which becomes possible only when the film is wet. The discrete test analyzers

can mix the reagent and sample by (1) motion of a test tube or container, (2) stirring by paddle or stick, (3) agitation by air bubbles or ultrasonic waves, or (4) convection resulting from forceful addition of sample into the container.

Incubation

Automated incubation is merely a delay station where the test mixture is allowed to react. This is performed, in most cases, under conditions of a specified, constant temperature, which is most frequently achieved by the use of heating blocks or air or water baths. These constant temperature devices are monitored electronically by thermocouples. Discrete analyzers accomplish incubation by allowing the reaction mixture to dwell in a chamber (test tube or cuvette) for a specified time. A similar approach is used for the dry-film analyzers. It should be noted that many test methods require an addition of a second reagent, possibly followed by an additional incubation period. The automated means for doing this are not different from those just discussed.

Sensing

The techniques of automation do not depend on the method of sensing, whether optical, thermal, or electrical. There are two major approaches to automated sensing: in situ and external. The term "in situ" refers to measurement in the vessel where the reaction has taken place, for example, in the reaction cuvette. The term "external" is applied to systems of measurement where the sample is transferred from its original incubation position in the reaction vessel to the sensing device. The dry-film tests are measured in situ by reflectance photometry (see Chapter 4) or by means of integral electrodes (electrometric, see Chapter 15). Discrete test instruments use both in situ and external sensing mechanisms. External sensing generally exposes the sensing chamber to many samples, and so care must be taken to eliminate carryover from one sample to the next. Optical or electrode surfaces may also be contaminated by components from the samples. On the other hand, in situ sensing makes special demands on the test chamber or requires an elaborate, automated washing procedure. If the test container is disposable, it is impractical to calibrate it for optical or electrical characteristics. Such containers, therefore, must be manufactured with very good reproducibility. However, disposable containers are meant to eliminate the mechanical complexity required to wash and recertify the sensing chamber. Most sensing is done in situ because this approach decreases the mechanical complexity of the instrument.

Chemical reactions can be monitored either at one time point or at many. Commonly, single-point monitoring is used for end-point analyses in which the reaction has gone to completion. Multiple-point monitoring is used for kinetic analyses. Discrete analyzers are easily adapted for multiple time-point monitoring.

Spectrophotometric instruments often have the capability of automatically sensing the presence of common interferents, such as icterus, hemolysis, and lipemia. A rough "index" of the presence of these interferents is printed with test results. This helps to automate the technologist's review of results and to alert the technologist that a result may not be accurate (see below).

Computation

Automated computation has taken two forms: *analog* and *digital.* Analog computations use the electrical signal such as a voltage or current from a sensor (such as a phototube) and quantify the signal by comparing it to a reference signal. For example, a "blank" reaction mixture will give a 100% T (blank transmittance), resulting in a certain electronic signal. A test standard will give a lower percentage of T and thus a decreased electronic signal. The analog computer compares the two signals and takes the logarithm of the result. The final result is related to the quantitation of the reaction.

Some reaction signals by their very nature are in the form of discrete numbers. Two examples are individual photon-counting events and counting of radioactive decay. These signals, consisting of a number of individual events, can be monitored by a digital computer that can process the signal. Digital processing is restricted to certain arithmetical functions (such as subtraction or addition) unless the computer is programmable.

For a digital computer to process signals from many types of sensing devices in automated instruments (such as the spectrophotometer and ion-selective electrodes), an analog-to-digital converter is necessary. This converts the voltage or current signal into a digital form, which can be processed by the digital computer.

There are no straightforward rules as to which is the best form of computation. The decision is usually based on economics. However, if any part of the signal processing is done digitally, virtually all the processing is done digitally. Perhaps the major exception is the analog conversion of transmittance to absorbance, which is performed to improve analytical performance.

Readouts and result reporting

The simplest method that can be used to visualize an instrument readout is the use of light-emitting diodes (LED) or a television monitor (cathode-ray tube) to report the data in a numerical form. These devices allow the technologist to review the data before accepting the results. Some LISs and instruments have the capability of "automatic data review." In this process, criteria are established for patient results; if the results fall within the accepted criteria, the results are automatically validated and entered into patients' files. Criteria for automatic data validation can include results falling within a specified range (typically, the reference range), the absence of common interferents (see above), and delta checks. This process speeds up the result-

validation process for routine results and permits the technologist to perform a more careful review of results with potential problems.

The instrument readout is usually converted to a hard copy, such as a paper printout. The data must then be transferred to laboratory slips or other permanent records. If this step is performed manually, transcription errors may occur. More sophisticated, automated computer systems are usually used to collate all the test results for each patient and print the results directly on the report form. When the results are transferred into a laboratory computer, the instrument readout can be directly interfaced, or connected, to the computer. Although analog connections are possible, most connections are digital. Chapter 18 discusses the use of computer interfaces for the automation of the process of reporting results.

There is usually a delay between the time when a result is entered into the LIS and becomes available to a physician and the time when a physician actually sees the result. This delay occurs because a physician never knows exactly when a result will be available and must either waste time looking for a result that is not yet in the LIS or delay looking for that result. This delay is often a very large component of the overall turnaround time for a sample result. There are available improved hospital paging systems that permit the laboratory, using the LIS, to send a result directly to a physician's pager. As soon as a technologist verifies the result in the LIS, the result is transmitted to the pager. Patient identification and the test result, as well as small amounts of text, can be displayed on the pager's screen. Automated data transfer directly to physicians will decrease turnaround time, especially for critical values.

Troubleshooting and training

Medical technologists intervene to correct problems encountered when an instrument fails (see p. 394). This process, called *troubleshooting,* is limited by a technologist's training and the availability of in-laboratory resources, such as instrument manuals. These resources have been greatly expanded by the application of electronic technology, such as on-line modems and CD-ROMs.

Modems allow electronic information to be rapidly transferred over normal telephone lines. Sophisticated computers that are part of new laboratory instruments can detect an instrument problem, often before a technologist has become aware of it, and automatically transmit data about that problem to the instrument manufacturer. The manufacturer's technicians can provide the laboratory technologist with detailed instructions for resolving the problem.

On-board CD-ROMs can provide the same service within the laboratory. Multimedia CD-ROMs can contain sophisticated electronic troubleshooting manuals. Once a problem has been detected by the computer, the computer will alert the technologist and inform the technologist where the information to correct the problem can be found. If additional help is needed, video tapes of how to repair a problem may be available within the CD-ROM database.

The electronic troubleshooting guide and its accompanying video guides can also be used to train technologists to use instruments.

CONCEPTS OF AUTOMATION: DEFINITIONS
Test repertoire

Economic priorities require that instruments perform more than one kind of test. Once an investment has been made in an automated instrument, increasing the number of tests performed on each sample reduces the cost and labor required to produce each result. Following this logic to an extreme would require that an instrument be capable of performing every conceivable kind of test. This has not been possible. However, six chemistry tests account for 50% of the work load in the average chemistry laboratory, and 14 tests account for another 40% of the total work load. Thus automated instruments have been designed to perform the most frequently ordered tests. Automation, though usually not essential, is desirable for rarely ordered tests as well.

The automation of tests may also be done on the basis of type of analysis rather than test volume (number of samples); that is, an automated immunoassay instrument will perform immunoassays for many different analytes, regardless of the numbers of specimens per analysis.

The *immediate test repertoire* of an instrument can therefore be defined as the number of tests that can be performed by that instrument at any one time, whereas the *total test repertoire* includes the total number of different tests that can possibly be performed on the instrument (that is, by the changing of reagents and a few components). Improvements in techniques and changes in economic priorities have led to a new phenomenon called *work-site consolidation*. This phenomenon involves increasing the immediate test repertoire of random-access analyzers (see below) and having many high-volume tests on the least number of instruments. The possibility of performing automated immunoassays on traditional, automated chemistry analyzers has further stimulated this movement.

Selective

Instruments that are capable of performing multiple tests are selective if the particular tests to be performed on an individual sample can be specified and if no sample and no reagent are consumed by tests that are not requested. For example, the SMAC was a nonselective instrument because all tests in the immediate repertoire were performed on each sample, regardless of the exact tests requested. A discrete analyzer, such as the ACA, performs only the tests requested.

Selective analyzers have also been termed *random-access* analyzers for their ability to process different test combinations for individual specimens.

Discrete

Instruments that compartmentalize each sample reaction are discrete analyzers. Typically the sample aliquot and reagent are contained in a single cuvette that is physically separated from all other cuvettes. Most current instruments are discrete analyzers.

Continuous flow

Instruments that continuously pump reagent through tubing and coils to form a flowing stream and continuously pump sample into that stream are called *continuous-flow analyzers*. The proportioning of sample and reagents is accomplished by control of the respective volumetric flow rates.

Batch analyzer

Instruments that perform the same test simultaneously on all samples presented to it are termed *batch analyzers*. The type of test can vary widely, but usually only a limited number of samples are processed per analysis.

Dwell time

The dwell time is the minimum time required to obtain a result after the initial sampling of the specimen. Some instruments can give results in as little as 15 seconds for single tests such as glucose. Commonly, instruments that perform multiple tests on a single sample have longer dwell times, ranging from 60 seconds to 15 minutes. Certain test procedures, such as kinetic analyses for enzyme activity or radioimmunoassays, that require long incubations will, of course, have longer dwell times. Dwell time is extremely important when significant or life-threatening physiological changes can take place rapidly. Thus blood-gas determinations (pH, P_{CO_2}, and P_{O_2}) need instruments with dwell times on the order of seconds. On the other hand, a "dwell time" of several days for a vitamin assay would be clinically acceptable.

Throughput

The throughput is the maximum number of samples or tests that can be processed in an hour. For similar analyzers one can calculate the total test throughput by multiplying the number of samples processed per hour by the number of tests performed on each specimen. For discrete analyzers, the sample throughput will obviously depend on the number of different tests requested on each sample. In addition, the time required per test can vary widely (that is, from less than 30 seconds to more than 10 minutes). In general, the more tests ordered per sample, the slower is the sample throughput on a discrete analyzer. Thus it is more difficult to give a simple, accurate value for the sample throughput for a discrete analyzer. The calculation for throughput does take into account the dwell time; that is, the fact that no results are produced until the dwell time has elapsed. The desired throughput of an instrument is usually matched to the number of samples that need to be processed in a given time period. For example, a higher throughput (and more costly) instrument may be required to process samples from a clinic so that results can be made available before the patient's return home. In general, an automated analyzer is chosen on the basis of its ability to process the bulk of the routine work load in time for routine clinical decision making.

Stat. testing

The word *stat.* is an abbreviation of the Latin word *statim* meaning "immediately." Stat. tests account for a large portion (up to 30% to 50% in many laboratories) of the laboratory work load. Stat. tests must be analyzed before the non–stat. test samples, resulting in the interruption of the normal work flow of the laboratory. Unfortunately, many stat. requests are not ordered because of a medical emergency.

The acceptable within-laboratory turnaround time (TAT, beginning from when the sample is received in the laboratory) must be defined for each stat. test, usually after consultation with the appropriate clinical staff. The Clinical Laboratory Improvement Amendments of 1988 require that the laboratory's ability to achieve the target TATs be routinely monitored. TATs are usually kept well within 60 minutes for most stat. tests but may be greater for tests that are needed quickly but not immediately (see p. 61). Instruments are also available for the performance of stat. tests by the patient's bedside. These devices may be used to improve TAT in critical areas of the hospital (see below and Chapter 2). A "superstat." test, which has a turnaround time of less than 10 minutes, can be obtained by use of whole blood samples for measurement of blood gases, glucose, urea nitrogen, lactate, hematocrit, and electrolytes.

Instruments that are to be used for stat. testing need not necessarily have a high throughput but should have a short dwell time. Many stat. instruments are dedicated instruments that analyze no more than a half dozen high-frequency tests simultaneously.

Cost

The resources consumed in producing a patient's test result represent the cost of that test. The cost consists of a labor cost (which is the monetary value of the time spent by technologists processing and analyzing the sample and reporting the result) and the cost associated with the use of the instrument, including the costs of instrument maintenance, service contracts, reagents (which are calculated from the cost of the chemicals used for the test and a proportionate part of those required for instrument start-up), calibration and quality control, consumables (constituting the cost of sample containers and paper), and capital cost (which is the proportionate amount of the life of the instrument consumed and hospital overhead including the cost of items such as laboratory slips and maintenance). See p. 59, for a more in-depth discussion of calculating costs.

AUTOMATED CLINICAL CHEMISTRY INSTRUMENTS

This section describes a number of instruments that are used for routine chemistry testing in the hospital laboratory or that illustrate a category of instrument type. A comparison of operational parameters for some automated instruments is shown in Table 16-1. Obviously this table is not meant to be all inclusive but rather to demonstrate the features available for common types of instruments.

Du Pont ACA V, ACA Star, Dimension AR

ACA V, ACA Star. The ACA V (Du Pont, Wilmington, Delaware) can serve as a general chemistry analyzer in small-sized hospitals and a specialty analyzer in medium and large-sized hospitals. Samples for the ACA can be serum, plasma, urine, or cerebrospinal fluid. Reagents are prepackaged in plastic packs, which also serve as the reaction cuvettes.

The probe aspirates sample and buffer and dispenses it into the header of the test pack. For some assays the analyte is partially purified when the sample is passed through a column before it reaches the test pack. The reagents, isolated in separate compartments of the pack, are released and mixed with the sample and buffer. Photometric measurements are taken when the plastic pack is formed into a 1 cm path-length cuvette. End-point methods are measured bichromatically, except for several methods that use two packs to permit blank absorbance measurement at the desired wavelength. Rate ("kinetic") and enzyme methods are measured at a single wavelength over a 17-second interval. The ACA requires little operator interaction and is suited for off-hour shifts.

The ACA Star contains several features that are not available with the ACA V. The throughput of the ACA Star is significantly increased to 90 tests per hour. Primary tube sampling, bar-code sample identification, liquid level sensing capability, storage of a calibration curve for two different reagent lots, bidirectional LIS interface, and a comprehensive quality control and patient management system are available. The ACA Star uses the same methodology as the ACA V.

Dimension. The Dimension is a stand-alone analyzer that can be used for routine and profile testing or for stat. tests. The Dimension has two sample wheels, each of which can hold up to 60 samples. Specimens are aspirated either from bar-coded sample cups or primary sample tubes. Stat. samples can be introduced at any time and are processed ahead of the routine samples.

Reagents are lyophilized and packaged in multiwell Flex cartridges that are placed into the refrigerated compartment of the analyzer. Forty-five cartridges can be placed in the analyzer. Each Flex cartridge is bar coded, and such coding allows the Dimension to monitor reagent inventory and track expiration dates. A unique feature of the Dimension is that the reagents in each well are hydrated as needed.

For example, if a cartridge holds 240 tests with 40 tests in each of 6 wells, the analyzer will reconstitute only as much reagent as needed to perform the requested assays. This feature extends the stability of the calibration curve and decreases reagent waste. Du Pont provides empty Flex cartridges for user-defined chemical analyses.

The chemical reaction takes place in small, clear, disposable plastic cuvettes that are manufactured on board by the analyzer from Surlyn Resin film. The Dimension can hold enough film for over 12,000 cuvettes. Samples will be automatically diluted and rerun if the linearity of the method is exceeded.

Boehringer-Mannheim Hitachi 747-200 and 911 systems

Hitachi 747-200. The Hitachi 747-200 is a high throughput analyzer that is used for routine profile and panel chemistry testing. The 747 achieves its high throughput by aspirating sample for 4 different assays simultaneously during a 6-second period. The samples are pipetted from bar-coded primary sample tubes or cups by positive displacement pipettors. The probes dip deep enough into the sample to ensure bubble-free aspiration and at the same time act as sensors for liquid level detection. Stat. samples are placed in red-colored racks that are loaded in a special area. The analyzer detects the stat. rack and gives it priority. The first stat. result is usually available in 12 to 20 minutes, depending on the number of tests being run on the racks ahead of it.

Two reagents are available for 32 tests and are stored in the refrigerated compartment of the analyzer. After the sample has been injected into the reaction cell, the first reagent is added. The cell then moves to a position where mixing panels are lowered into the liquid to mix the solution. After the second reagent is added and incubated, the color intensity is determined by the photometer. Samples are automatically rerun when the linearity of the assay is exceeded or when laboratory defined criteria are not met. The instrument prints "serum indices," which can be used by the technologist to assess the degree of interference from lipemia, hemolysis, or icterus.

Hitachi 911. The 911 is a floor model analyzer that consists of a sample carousel, two reagent carousels each holding 32 reagent containers, and a reaction disk with 120 reusable cuvettes. Samples can be pipetted every 10 seconds from cups or primary collection tubes. Insufficient sample volume is detected by a liquid level sensor. Samples are bar coded to ensure positive patient identification, and stat. results for most chemistries are available in less than 5 minutes. Reagents are bar coded and placed in the refrigerated compartment of the analyzer. A unique feature of the 911 is the ability to add multiple reagents per method. Empty reagent containers can be obtained from BMC for user-defined applications. The 911 has autodilution capabilities for serum and urine samples, autorerun, and autocalibration features.

Beckman CX7 Synchron analyzer

The CX7 is a combination of the CX3 module and the CX4 CE module. The CX3 module is usually dedicated for stat. samples. The CX4CE is a photometric module that uses bichromatic or polychromatic spectrophotometric readings for kinetic, end-point, or turbidimetric reactions. Bar-coded samples are placed in sectors that can accommodate primary blood tubes or sample cups. Each sector can hold 7 samples. Six sectors can be transferred to the sample carousel and three sectors placed into the autoloader allowing for 63 samples to be processed at any one time. A unique feature of the CX7 system is that primary sample tubes can be placed in sectors, centrifuged in the Beckman centrifuge, and subsequently placed into the CX7 analyzer. This minimizes handling of the specimens and provides for more efficient laboratory work flow.

The reagent compartment of the analyzer is refrigerated and provides storage for 24 bar-coded reagent cartridges. A reagent inventory check is performed after loading of the reagents. Most reagents are ready to use and each cartridge contains wells for 3 reagents. Because more than one cartridge of the same chemistry can be placed in the reagent carousel, the instrument will automatically use the second cartridge after the first is depleted. The CX7 is an open system and Beckman provides empty cartridges for user-defined chemistries. Stat. samples are automatically processed before routine samples, and results are usually available in less than 5 minutes.

Johnson and Johnson Ektachem 750 XRC

The Ektachem 750 XRC uses the multilayer, dry-film slide technology. The slide is composed of layers, some of which serve to ultrafilter the sample (remove protein), whereas others serve to provide reactive reagents. The addition of serum sample provides the solvent (water) necessary to rehydrate the dry reagents. The colored reaction products are measured by reflectance on the side opposite that used for sample addition. The reflected light is converted into concentration units (of the reaction products) by the Williams-Clapper formula (analogous to Beer's law) for converting light transmission into absorbance units (see Chapter 4, p. 94).

Samples can be pipetted from either bar-coded primary tubes or sample cups. The slides are automatically dispensed from analyte-specific test cartridges. Sixty bar-coded cartridges, each containing 50 slides for a capacity of 3000 tests, can be stored in the analyzer. The slides are incubated at 37° C for colorimetric and 25° C for the potentiometric assays. After completion of the assay the slides are dropped into disposable containers.

Bayer (Technicon) RA-2000, Chem-1, DAX

RA-2000. For dispensing sample and reagent the RA-2000 uses separate probes, the internal and external sides of which are coated with a fluorocarbon. This prevents contact of the sample with the walls of the probe. Sample is aspirated into the probe together with an air bubble and a fluorocarbon solution that completely covers the probe tip. Sample, together with the fluorocarbon, is dispensed into a disposable cuvette. Because fluorocarbon is very dense, it will settle to the bottom of the cuvette and will not affect photometric measurements. The fluorocarbon material provides an inert surface that prevents sample-to-sample and reagent-to-reagent carryover. The reactions in the cuvettes (at 30° or 37° C) are monitored photometrically. The RA-2000 can determine general chemistry tests by endpoint, fixed-time, or kinetic assays. Ion-selective electrodes are available for measurement of electrolytes.

Chem-1. The Chem-1 analyzer is a continuous-flow system in which a capsule is generated for the performance of each test and the reaction occurs in a Teflon tube. A capsule consists of one reagent and sample separated from another reagent by a small air bubble. The capsule is transported through a Teflon tube, samples and reagents are mixed together, and the absorbance measured at a series of optical stations. Introduction of an inert fluorocarbon into the Teflon tube provides an interface between the sample and the air bubble and allows the air bubble to move over the fluorocarbon film preventing sample and reagent from touching the walls of the tube thus eliminating carryover. With the Chem-1 there are no disposable or reusable cuvettes.

Reagents in bar-coded cassettes are placed in a refrigerated compartment of the analyzer that holds 32 reagent cassettes. Reagents are automatically activated and have a 30 day on-line stability. Multiple cassettes of the same reagent can be loaded in the analyzer.

The Chem-1 holds 272 samples, which can be aspirated from a primary collection tube or sample cup. A novel feature of the Chem-1 is the small sample and reagent volume that is used for each assay. Photometric assays require 1 µL of sample and 14 µL of reagents, whereas ion-selective assays require 10 µL of sample and 140 µL of buffer.

DAX. A unique feature of the DAX is that a fixed number of samples are processed per hour, regardless of the number of tests ordered on these samples. For example, with the DAX 48, 150 samples are processed per hour.

Samples are loaded into a turntable that holds 60 racks of samples. Each rack has 5 wells for sample tubes. Samples are bar coded and aspirated from primary collection tubes or from sample cups. A liquid level sensor detects inadequate sample volumes and bubbles. Stat. samples are processed ahead of the routine samples.

The reagent compartment holds 12 reagents at ambient temperature and 36 reagents at 2° to 8° C. Depending on the assay, reagents are either ready to use or are lyophilized. Samples and reagents are dispensed into reusable cuvettes at the reaction turntable, which contains 96 sets of 4 cuvettes for a total of 384 cuvettes. Printed serum indices allow the technologist to assess the degree of lipemia, hemolysis, and icterus for each sample. A test result that exceeds linearity is automatically rerun with a preset dilution factor.

Baxter Paramax 720ZX

A unique feature of the Paramax 720ZX is the dry reagent technology. Reagents are packaged in dispensers of 100 or 300 tablets and placed in a 48-position carousel. Reagent tablets are automatically reconstituted as needed, which enhances calibration curve stability to 90 days for most assays. For each test a calibration curve can be stored for 5 different reagent lots. The instrument uses disposable reaction cuvettes packaged in reels of 2100 cuvettes. Since the cuvettes are used only once, there is no cross-contamination of reaction mixtures, and the need for complex washing systems to clean the cuvettes is eliminated.

Samples are bar coded and placed in a loading carousel that can hold up to 96 samples. Uncapped and closed phlebotomy tube sampling is possible. With closed-tube sampling laboratory personnel do not have to uncap the tube, eliminating the possibility of splashing biological fluids and the problem of resealing the tubes after they have been processed.

When a test is ordered, a reagent tablet is dispensed into the cuvette. Diluent is added, and the cuvette is immersed in a water bath at 37° C. The tablet is dissolved in 45 seconds by a high-efficiency ultrasound device, reagent blank is measured, and sample is added. Stat. samples can be loaded at any time. Because the sample must wait for five preceding samples to be processed, turnaround time for a stat. result can vary from 5 to more than 20 minutes. When the analysis is complete, the tops of the cuvettes are heat sealed and the cuvettes are dropped into a disposable bin.

Centrifugal analyzers

The key element in a centrifugal analyzer is the rotor. Sample and reagent are pipetted into discrete compartments and mixed together first by the action of centrifugal force when the rotor is accelerated and then by braking and accelerating, which mixes the solution by agitation. The cuvettes rotate past a stationary light source to permit absorbance readings at a preselected wavelength. These analyzers are useful for rate ("kinetic") measurements and for endpoint analyses.

The flexibility of these instruments allows for easy adaptation of "in-house" reagents and the use of bulk reagents available from a wide variety of commercial suppliers. Reagent consumption is small, a feature that makes them economical to operate. Some instruments use disposable rotor cuvettes, whereas others wash the rotor for reuse. Centrifugal analyzers can perform spectrophotometric, turbidimetric, nephelometric, and fluorometric analysis.

Although the theoretical test throughput can be high, in practice it is considerably lower because subsequent runs are often required for reanalysis of samples that give unsatisfactory results, such as that for excess enzymatic activity.

AUTOMATED IMMUNOCHEMISTRY INSTRUMENTS

During the past several years the number of immunochemistry systems available for use in the clinical laboratory has increased greatly, and the laboratory director is now in the enviable position of being able to select the optimal system for the laboratory. The immunochemistry system that best fits into a laboratory depends on the size and work flow of the laboratory. Requirements for test menu, turnaround time, throughput, degree of automation, data management system, and cost must all be considered when one is choosing an immunochemistry system. A comparison of the operational features for some immunochemistry systems is shown in Tables 16-2 and 16-3.

Abbott TDx/FLx, IMx, AXSYM

TDx. The TDx system was primarily designed for use in the measurement of therapeutic drugs by fluorescent polarization immunoassay (FPIA; see Chapter 4, p. 100). The TDx system can also perform some nondrug chemical analyses (such as glucose, lactate, and creatinine) by a radiation attenuation procedure and can measure specific proteins by nephelometric analysis with a specially designed carousel that contains the light source. The TDx system has unit dose reagents for measuring specific proteins and some drug assays. The TDx is also available as the FLx, which has some random-access capabilities.

IMx. The IMx is a benchtop analyzer that uses latex-microparticle enzyme immunoassay (MEIA) technology to measure high-molecular-weight analytes and FPIA technology to measure therapeutic drugs. The IMx consists of a reaction chamber, reagent compartment, and a control pad. A 24-position carousel is placed in the reagent chamber. Reaction cells that contain a glass-fiber matrix and sample and incubation wells are placed in the carousel. Sample is manually dispensed by the operator into the sample well. Latex-coated antibody and sample are pipetted into the reaction well and incubated at 34° C to form an immunocomplex. An aliquot of the immunocomplex is transferred to the glass-fiber matrix where it is irreversibly bound to the matrix. After the glass fiber is washed, an alkaline phosphatase conjugate and substrate are added, and the reaction is allowed to proceed. The fluorescence of the product is measured and related to the concentration of the analyte. Although the IMx system is essentially a batch analyzer, there is a select reaction carousel that allows the operator to run 3 chemical analyses per sample.

AXSYM. The AXSYM is a random-access analyzer that combines the FPIA and MEIA technologies into a single automated system. The analyzer is divided into sampling and processing centers. The sampling center contains three concentric carousels, one for samples, another for reagent, and a third for reaction vessels. The specimens can be pipetted either from primary sample tubes or sample cups. Sixty bar-coded primary tubes or 90 sample cups are placed in the sample ring. Twenty 100-test bar-coded reagent cartridges can be placed in the reagent compartment. The reagents are mixed by being shaken for 3 minutes every 8 hours or when new reagents are placed on board. Reaction vessels, in strips of 10, are placed in the sample wheel. Each reaction vessel contains a plastic cuvette and several wells for reagents. Sample and reagents are pipetted into separate wells of the reaction vessels every 30 seconds. A stat. sample is processed as soon as the pipetting sequence for the routine assay is completed.

After samples and reagents are pipetted, the reaction vessel is transferred into the processing center of the AXSYM. The processing center is temperature controlled at 34° C and contains a tungsten-halogen lamp for the FPIA assays and a low-pressure mercury lamp for the MEIA assays. For the FPIA assay, sample and reagents are pipetted into a plastic cuvette, and after incubation the fluorescence is measured. For the MEIA assay, sample and latex-coated antibody reagent are pipetted into an incubation well of the reaction vessel. A glass-fiber matrix cell is automatically dispensed into the processing center, and an aliquot of the immunocomplex is transferred to the glass-fiber matrix. The matrix cell is washed, conjugate and substrate are added, and the fluorescence is measured. The reaction vessel is then emptied into a disposable waste bin.

Baxter Stratus II Intellect

The Stratus II Intellect is a benchtop, batch analyzer consisting of a sample carousel, a reagent-tab transport system, and a fluorometer. The sample carousel holds up to 30 sample holders. Each sample holder contains 3 cups. Sample is placed into the first cup. The 2 remaining cups are used for dilution of samples that are outside the linear range of the assay. Below the sample carousel is the tab transport system, which is maintained at 38° C. Thirty tabs can be loaded for one run. The key to the Stratus is a one and a half–inch wide by two-inch deep tab that contains a glass-fiber filter impregnated with antibody. At the start of the assay the tab is removed from the top of the stack and placed on the transport pad. The tab moves along the transport pad, and sample and alkaline phosphatase–labeled conjugate is pipetted in the center of the tab where the entire

Table 16-2 Comparison of operational features for several immunochemistry analyzers

	TDx/FLx	IMx	AXSYM	Stratus Intellect	ALA 1200	Opus Plus	ES300
Type	B, D	B, D	SL, B, D	D, B	SL, B, D,	SL, B, D	B, SL
Sample volume (μL)*	10-25	50-150	10-200	20-200	10-100	10-40	10-200
Minimum volume (μL)†	60-75	150	60-250	70-250	110-200	70-100	260
Sample ID‡	Bar-code wand, keyboard	Keyboard, bar code	Keyboard, bar code	Keyboard	Keyboard, bar code	Keypad, bar code	Bar code, keyboard
Reagent	Unit dose, bulk, M	Bulk, M	Bulk, M	Unit dose, M	Unit dose bulk, M	Unit dose, M	Bulk, M
Proportioning§	Vol add	Aspiration	Aspiration	Saturation	Vol add	Saturation, vol add	Vol add
Minimization of matrix (protein) interferences‖	Dilution, vol add	Dilution, vol add	Dilution	Filtration	Dilution	NA	Multistep washing
Mixing	Forced turbulence	Forced turbulence	Automated vibration/forced turbulence	Diffusion	Mechanical movement of magnetic beads	Diffusion, forced turbulence	Mechanical stirring
Test menu	TDM, Ltd chemistry, DAU	TDM, AM, Hormones, Tumor markers, Cardiac markers	TDM, AM, Hormones, Tumor markers, Cardiac markers	TDM, AM, Hormones, Cardiac markers	Hormones, Tumor markers, Cardiac markers	TDM, Hormones, Tumor markers, Cardiac markers	Hormones, Tumor markers
Sensing¶	Fluorescence	Fluorescence	Fluorescence	Fluorescence	Fluorescence	Fluorescence	Spec
Test repertoire#	1	1	20	1	21	29	12
Total repertoire**	73	32	N/A	30	22	29	19
Stat. capability	Yes	Yes	Yes	Yes	Yes	Yes	N/A
Dwell time (min)††	5-20	15-45	8-30	8	60	6-18	55-170
Throughput (samples/hr)‡‡	60	30-40	100	49	120	20-80	100
Throughput (tests/hr)§§	60	30-40	80-120	49	120	20-80	100
Readout	Digital	Digital	Digital	Digital	Digital	Digital	Digital

AM, Anemia profile (vitamins B_{12}, folate, and ferritin); B, batch analyzer; D, discrete analyzer; DAU, drugs of abuse; ID, identification; Ltd, limited; M, available only from manufacturer; N/A, not available; SL, selective; Spec, that is, photometric; TDM, therapeutic drug monitoring; vol add, volumetric addition.
*Sample volume plus dead space in sample cup.
†Sample volume needed to perform a test (discrete analyzer) or simultaneous profile.
‡Means of identifying sample for final printout.
§Manner of adding reagent, diluent, and sample.
‖Means of minimizing protein interference.
¶Spec, photometric.
#The number of tests available at one time, without a change of reagents or instrument module.
**Total number of analytes for which reagents are commercially available.
††Approximate time between sampling and availability of test.
‡‡Number of samples capable of being processed per hour. Data listed are for one simultaneous profile or a single test per sample.
§§Calculate by multiplication of maximum number of tests per sample available times number of samples capable of being processed per hour.

Table 16-3 Comparison of operational features for several immunochemistry analyzers

	Access	Immulite	ACS-180	Vista	Vidas	Array 360 CE
Type	B, SL, D	B, SL, D	B, SL, D	B, SL, D	B, SL	B, D, SL
Sample volume (µL)*	5-200	10-75	25-200	10-150	100-350	20-350
Minimum volume (µL)†	105-300	110-175	225	110-250	100-350	40-525
Sample ID‡	Keyboard, bar code	Keyboard, bar code	Keyboard, bar code	Keyboard	Keyboard, bar code	Keyboard, bar code
Reagent	Bulk, M	Bulk, M	Bulk, M	Bulk, M	Unit dose	Bulk, M
Proportioning§	Autopipet, vol add	Vol add	Vol add	Vol add	Prepackaged, vol add	Vol add
Minimization of matrix interferences‖	Vol add	NA	NA	NA	Prepackaged	Vol add, autodilution
Mixing	Ultrasonic, spin	Shaking	Rotation	Vibration, turbulence	Kinetic action	Dilution/magnetic stirring
Sensing	Chemiluminescence	Chemiluminescence	Chemiluminescence	Fluorescence	Fluorescence	Nephelometry
Test menu	TDM, AM Hormones	Hormones Tumor markers	Hormones, AM Cardiac markers Tumor markers	Hormones	Hormones Infectious disease panel	TDM Specific proteins
Test repertoire¶	24	12	13	15	16	18
Total repertoire**	22	18	17	9	26	40
Stat. capability	Yes	Yes	Yes	N/A	Yes	Yes
Dwell time (min)††	12-75	40-70	20	78-114	20-150	1-2
Throughput (samples/hr)‡‡	100	120	Up to 180	19	15-90	40
Throughput (tests/hr)§§	100	120	Up to 180	38	15-90	40-80
Readout	Digital	Digital	Digital, CRT	Digital	Printer	Digital

AM, Anemia profile (vitamins B$_{12}$, folate, and ferritin); *B*, batch analyzer; *CRT*, cathode-ray tube; *D*, discrete analyzer; *ID*, identification; *M*, available only from manufacturer; *NA*, not applicable; *N/A*, not available; *SL*, selective; *TDM*, therapeutic drug monitoring; *vol add*, volumetric addition.

*Sample volume needed to perform a test (discrete analyzer) or simultaneous profile.

†Sample volume plus dead space in sample cup.

‡Means of identifying sample for final printout.

§Manner of adding reagent, diluent, and sample.

‖Means of minimizing protein interference.

¶The number of tests available at one time, without a change of reagents or instrument module.

**Total number of analytes for which reagents are commercially available.

††Approximate time between sampling and availability of test.

‡‡Number of samples capable of being processed per hour. Data listed are for one simultaneous profile or a single test per sample.

§§Calculated by multiplication of maximum number of tests per sample available times number of samples capable of being processed per hour.

immunoreaction takes place. The antibody-bound fraction remains at the center of the tab, while the unbound fraction diffuses toward the periphery. The tab is washed, substrate is added, and fluorescence is determined.

The Stratus can be programmed for preset serial dilutions, which is useful for tests like that for human chorionic gonadotrophin. Stat. samples can be placed in the next available position in the carousel, and the results are usually available in less than 10 minutes. The Stratus II Intellect uses Microsoft Windows software, which allows the user to store multiple calibration curves for a single analyte and to collect a substantial patient data base.

Tosoh ALA 1200

The ALA 1200 consists of a sample and reagent processing center, pipettor, and photometer. A novel feature of the ALA 1200 is the test pack, which contains capture antibody immobilized on magnetic beads. Depending on the assay, either alkaline phosphatase–labeled antigen or antibody is lyophilized in the pack. All immunochemistry reactions, incubations, washings, and fluorescent measurements are performed in this ready-to-use test pack.

The test packs are loaded on a reagent tray located beneath the sample-processing area. When loading is complete, the tray containing the packs is lifted to the sample-processing area by an air-activated elevator. The packs are punctured, sample and diluent are added, and the reaction mixture is incubated at 37° C. After each sample is pipetted, the pipet tips are automatically changed so as to eliminate sample-to-sample carryover. Vibration of the tray agitates the magnetic beads to ensure mixing. The cups are washed to remove the unbound fraction, substrate is added, and the fluorescence is measured. After the reaction is complete, the cups are automatically emptied into a waste bin.

Stat. specimens can be placed in the instrument at any time and are given priority. There is an autodilution feature available for assays exceeding the linearity of the method, and calibration curves can be stored for two different lot numbers of the same analyte. With the ALA 1200, samples cannot be pipetted from primary collection tubes. This feature is available only with the ALA 1200DX.

Behring Opus Plus

The Opus Plus is a benchtop system that features single-use, disposable test modules. The Opus can operate in either a random-access or a batch mode, with continuous sample addition during a run. Depending on the analyte measured, two different methodologies are used, a multilayer dry-film test module that uses the competitive-binding technique for measuring low-molecular-weight analytes and an enzyme-linked immunoabsorbent (ELISA) assay for measuring high-molecular-weight analytes.

The multilayer film module contains a spreading layer, top coat, optical screen, and signal layer on a polyester film base. Sample is added to the spreading layer and travels through the top layer and optical screen to the signal layer. The top layer blocks the passage of proteins and large molecules. The signal layer contains fluorescent-labeled hapten bound to the antibody. Analyte from the sample displaces the labeled hapten from the binding sites on the antibody. The unbound labeled hapten diffuses into the screen layer, which contains iron oxide, and prevents excitation of the unbound hapten. The fluorescent intensity of the bound complex in the signal layer is measured and is related to the analyte concentration.

The ELISA module consists of a fiberglass matrix and two wells containing conjugate and substrate. Sample is added to the glass-fiber matrix, which contains the antibody. After incubation an enzyme-labeled conjugate and substrate are added. The unbound antigen is washed onto absorbent strips, and the bound fluorescent antibody complex is measured and related to the analyte concentration.

The operation of the Opus involves the manual loading of bar-coded test modules, sample trays, which hold 20 cups, and pipet tips. Each pipetting step involves the use of a new pipet tip, which eliminates carryover. The Opus Plus offers liquid-level sensing and on-line dilution. The Opus Plus cannot sample directly from primary collection tubes, and there is no on-board reagent storage for the test module. These features are available with the Opus Magnum.

Boehringer-Mannheim ES300

The ES300 is a benchtop analyzer that consists of sample, reagent, and incubator rotors; a multifunctional arm; and a photomultiplier. The sample rotor holds 150 cups that can be used for samples, calibrators, or controls. Reagents are placed in a 12-position reagent rotor. Streptavidin-coated tubes are placed in the incubator rotor. A multifunctional arm contains four needles that are used for sample pipetting, separating the bound and unbound fractions, mixing, and aspiration. Sample and either peroxidase-labeled antibody or peroxidase-labeled antigen are pipetted into the coated tubes. Mixing is accomplished by rapid movement of the needle in the tube. After incubation at 25° C, the unbound fraction is removed. After substrate addition and color development, the solution is aspirated into a 3 mm flowthrough cuvette where absorbance readings are taken at 420 nm.

Sample and reagent bar-coding and automatic sample dilution are not available with the ES300. A stat. result is not possible with the ES300 because once the assay is initiated it must go to completion before the next series of tests can be determined.

Sanofi Access

The Access is a benchtop instrument that employs heterogeneous immunochemiluminescent assays. The Access consists of a sample- and reagent-processing station, a wash/separation station, and a luminometer. The sample rotor can hold up to 60 samples. Pipetting is possible from bar-coded sample cups or primary collection tubes. After 10 samples are pipetted, they can be removed and an additional set of samples placed in the rotor. Twenty-four bar-coded, ready-to-use reagent packs can be placed in the refrigerator rotor. Fifty tests can be determined with each reagent pack. Two hundred eighty-five disposable cuvettes are placed in the analyzer, which corresponds to about 3 hours of continuous sample processing.

The technology used with the Access requires the addition of samples to paramagnetic particles that are coated with antibody or antigen, followed by the addition of an alkaline phosphatase conjugate. The cuvettes are incubated at 37° C and transferred to the separation wash station where magnets force the particles to the side of the tube. After washing and aspiration of the fluids, a dioxetane-based chemiluminescent substrate is added and the cuvettes are moved to the luminometer where the emitted light is quantitated. After the reaction is complete, the cuvettes are dispensed into a waste bin.

Diagnostic Products Corporation Immulite

The Immulite is a benchtop immunoassay system that employs chemiluminescent heterogeneous assays. The Immulite consists of a loading platform, reagent and incubator carousels, and a photometer. Sample is manually transferred by the operator to a clear plastic cup and placed in bar-coded carriers that are loaded onto a continuous chain. An assay tube is placed behind the sample cup. A unique feature of this system is that all the immunochemical reaction, separation, washing, and measurement steps occur in the assay tube, which contains antibody bound to a bead.

Sample and alkaline phosphatase–labeled conjugate are added to the tube, which is then incubated at 37° C for 30 or 60 minutes with intermittent shaking. The tubes are transferred to the spin/wash station where the unbound fraction is removed by spinning the tube at high speed on its vertical axis. Fluids are transferred to a chamber within the unit, and the bead is washed several times to ensure that separation of the bound from free label is complete. Dioxetane substrate is added, and the intensity of the light produced is measured by the photometer.

Although the Immulite does not have direct tube sampling, once the sample is placed on the instrument the assay is entirely automated. Five tests can be performed for each specimen. Stat. samples can be loaded at any time and placed at the head of the queue.

Ciba-Corning ACS-180

The ACS-180 is a benchtop system that employs heterogeneous immunochemiluminometric assays. The ACS-180 consists of a cuvette loader, a sample and reagent handling system, fluid separation and wash stations, and a luminometer. The cuvettes are single-well, disposable, polypropylene vessels that are loaded by the operator in quantities of 200. The cuvettes are sequentially dispensed onto a linear track

at 20-second intervals. Sample trays hold up to 60 bar-coded tubes on two rings and can accept either sample cups or primary blood-drawing tubes. The reagent tray holds reagent cartridges for 13 tests. Each reagent cartridge contains enough reagent for 50 analyses. Each test requires two reagent bottles, one containing magnetic particles with bound antibody or antigen, and the other containing the acridinium ester–labeled antibody. After the reagents and cuvettes are preheated to 37° C, samples and reagents are added to the cuvette and incubated at 37° C. The cuvettes then move along a track to the separation/wash station containing two magnets where the paramagnetic particles are forced onto the walls of the cuvettes. Liquid containing the unbound fraction is aspirated from the cuvette, and the cuvette is washed with distilled water. The paramagnetic particles are then resuspended in a hydrogen peroxide solution, and the cuvettes are transported to the luminometer. A sodium hydroxide solution is dispensed into the cuvette, which oxidizes the acridinium ester tracer resulting in the emission of a chemiluminescent signal at a wavelength of 430 nm. The intensity of the emission is measured over a 5-second interval. The signal collected at the photomultiplier tube is converted to relative light units and related to the concentration of the analyte. The contents of the cuvette are aspirated into a liquid waste compartment, and the cuvette falls into a waste bin.

A master dose-response calibration curve is generated for each lot of reagents by the manufacturer. Calibration can be performed by use of two calibrators that are used to adjust the master curve.

Syva Vista

The Vista is a benchtop system that employs heterogeneous enzyme fluorescent immunoassays. The Vista uses chromium dioxide magnetic particles as a solid support and alkaline phosphatase as the enzyme label. In competitive-binding assays, streptavidin is coupled with chromium dioxide. Enzyme-labeled analyte competes with analyte in the sample for binding sites on biotinylated antibodies. Biotinylated antibodies are captured by the streptavidin-coated magnetic particles. A magnetic field separates the bound particles, and after several washing steps, substrate is added and the fluorescence is measured. In the sandwich format the chromium dioxide particles are bound to an antibody. Sample is added, and analyte binds to the antibody. The enzyme-labeled conjugate is added, and after separation, washing, and substrate addition, fluorescence is determined.

The Vista consists of a sample, reagent, and incubator carousel, a fluorometer, and a computer. Fifty samples can be placed in the sample rotor, and 20 bar-coded reagent cartridges can be put in the refrigerated reagent compartment. Each reagent cartridge is ready to use and can perform up to 32 tests. One hundred cuvettes are placed in the incubator tray. Each cuvette contains a plastic-coated ball bearing to ensure complete mixing of sample and reagent. The user enters the sample number through the computer and can order a single test or profiles on each patient's sample. Stat. assays are not practical with the Vista because once the run is initiated it must go to completion. With the Vista there is no direct tube sampling.

BioMérieux Vitek Vidas

The Vidas is a benchtop system that employs enzyme-linked, heterogeneous fluorescent assays. The key to the Vidas is the disposable reagent strip and solid-phase receptor (SPR). Each reagent strip is bar coded and has 10 wells, 1 for sample and 8 for diluent, wash solutions, conjugate, and substrate. The last well is the optical cuvette. The SPR, a long tube coated with antigen or antibody, also serves as a pipettor for accurate sampling and transfer of reagents during the assay. Sample must be manually placed in the first well of the reagent strip. An exact volume is not required. After the strip is placed into the analyzer, the test process is entirely automated. A precise volume of sample is drawn into the SPR tube. Analyte is captured on the solid phase followed by addition of an alkaline phosphatase conjugate solution. After incubation and washing, substrate is added, and fluorescence is measured at an excitation wavelength of 370 nm and an emission wavelength of 450 nm.

The operator requests the test and enters a patient identification through the keyboard function of the computer. There is no capability for bar coding of samples, direct tube sampling, or automatic dilution. Because each assay uses a discrete set of reagents and cuvettes, there is no sample carryover or cross contamination of reagents.

Beckman Array 360 CE

The Array 360 CE is a benchtop nephelometric system. The analyzer contains a 20-position reagent wheel and a 40-position sample wheel. Sample segments containing three wells are placed in the sample wheel. Samples can be pipetted from bar-coded primary collection tubes into the sample well of the segment. Depending on the assay, sample dilutions are automatically performed, and diluted sample and antibody are added to the flow cell, which is maintained at 26.7° C.

For protein assays the rate of formation of the antigen-antibody complex increases with increasing protein concentrations. To determine whether an antigen excess exists, one adds more antigen during the reaction. If further reaction takes place, the antigen is not in excess, and the results are valid. If more antigen is added and an increase in complex formation is not observed, the value is flagged and the assay is repeated at a higher dilution. Therapeutic drugs are measured by their ability to inhibit the precipitation of an immunodrug complex. A drug-protein complex and drug in the sample compete for binding sites on an antibody. The rate of formation of the precipitate decreases with increasing drug concentration in the sample and is determined nephelometrically. Samples that are outside the linear range

of the assay are automatically diluted. Stat. samples can be added at any time. Reagents are bar coded, prepackaged, and ready to use.

INSTRUMENTS FOR USE OUTSIDE OF THE HOSPITAL LABORATORY

Automated and semiautomated analyzers have been introduced for use outside of the traditional hospital laboratory. These instruments have been targeted for near-patient testing and the physician's office. The criteria used to choose the ideal instrument can include many factors: ability to generate single test results or perform chemistry profiling, adequacy of turnaround time, cost of the analyzer and reagents, labor cost, ease of operation, availability of quality control programs, and a simple maintenance schedule. The ideal instrument would use whole blood as the specimen, and pipetting of sample and reagent would be automated, requiring little interaction from the operator. Calibration curves would be stable for at least 1 month, and a quality control program and 24-hour service would be available from the instrument manufacturer. The instrument would be interfaced with a computer to provide documentation of laboratory results and a printout of quality control charts. The system should be extremely easy to operate because it will be used by personnel with little or no laboratory background. The reagents, dry or wet, should be bar coded, prepackaged, and stable for at least 6 months. Dry chemistry reagents can usually be stored in a small area, which is a significant advantage in a physician's office laboratory. Some of the instruments available are shown in Table 16-4. They have been categorized as having either dry or wet chemistry reagent systems.

Dry reagent systems

The Seralyzer system uses test strips consisting of cellulose fibers impregnated with reagents. The reagent strips are stored in vials and are stable for 1 to 4 months after the container is opened. The reaction parameters for each assay are programmed by a dedicated module that is inserted into the analyzer. The sample, which usually requires predilution, is pipetted onto the strip, and the strip is moved into the analyzer. Light from a xenon lamp strikes the strip, and the vertically reflected light is passed through a collimator to the interference filter and is sensed by the sample photodetector. Reflected light is also sensed by the reference photodetector. The ratio of the sample-to-reference reflectance is used to compensate for the drift in electronics and variations in the intensity of the lamp. Profile testing is difficult because each test requires a separate plug-in module.

The Kodak DT systems use multilayered film technology similar to that of the Ektachem 750 analyzer. Each test slide is bar-coded to identify the assay and the lot number of the reagent. The reagents are stable for about 1 year. With a specially designed battery-driven pipet, sample is placed on the slide and incubated for 5 minutes at 37° C. Light

Table 16-4 Clinical chemistry systems for use outside of the hospital clinical laboratory

Instrument	Manufacturer	Sample type	Sample volume (µL)	Chemistry	Reagents	Reagents bar coded	Reagent choice	Available assays	Assay time (min)	Maximum throughput per hour	Output
Seralyzer	Bayer	S, P	Prediluted sample, 30	Dry	Strip	No	No	General chemistries, enzymes, TDM	0.5-4.0	60	Digital display
DT-60 System DT-SC DT-E	Johnson and Johnson	S, P	10	Dry	Slide	Yes	No	Enzymes, electrolytes, TDM, general chemistries	5 3 4	65 20 15	Printer
Analyst	Du Pont	S, P	Prediluted sample, 90	Dry	Unitized in rotors	Yes	No	General chemistries, enzymes	10	72	Digital display/ printer
Reflotron	Boehringer-Mannheim	B, S, P	30	Dry	Tab/strips	Yes	No	General chemistries, enzymes	1.5-3.0	20	Digital display/ printer
i-STAT	i-STAT	B	~65	Dry	Individual reagent	No	No	Electrolytes, HCT, glucose, BUN	<2.0	90	Digital display
Vision	Abbott	B, S, P	2 drops or 1 capillary tube	Wet	Individual reagent packs	Yes	No	General chemistries, enzymes, TDM limited	8	60	Printer

B, Whole blood; *BUN,* blood urea nitrogen; *HCT,* hematocrit; *P,* plasma; *S,* serum; *TDM,* therapeutic drug monitoring.

illuminates the slide, and the amount of reflected light is related to the concentration of analyte in the sample. The incubator can hold up to five slides, thus allowing for batch or profile testing of up to five assays. The DT-60 can perform only colorimetric assays. The DT-SC Analyzer, which uses a xenon lamp as a light source with ultraviolet or visible wavelength detection, is available to perform enzyme assays and some therapeutic drug testing. The DT-SC analyzer uses the same pipet and basic technology as the DT-60. The DT-E module can be obtained for measuring electrolytes.

The Reflotron system uses solid-phase reagent tabs containing a magnetic code to identify the tests, reaction parameters, and the calibration curve for each assay. The calibration curve is established by the manufacturer for each reagent lot. The shelf life of each test tab is from 1.5 to 2 years. Blood is placed on a glass-fiber pad, and the plasma is separated from the erythrocytes. Plasma is transported away from the erythrocytes by capillary action, and the required sample volume is added to the reagent at a temperature of 37° C. Excess plasma is removed from the reaction area. The analyte concentration is determined by reflectance photometry. With this system, blood obtained by finger or heel stick can be used for analysis. Since this is a single test system, profile testing is not practical.

The Analyst is a benchtop system that consists of specially designed disposable plastic rotors. The rotors contain bar-coded lyophilized reagents, which are stable for 1 year when stored in a refrigerator. Rotors are available for profile or discrete analysis. Sample, which must be prediluted tenfold or sixtyfold with pipets supplied by Du Pont, is automatically pipetted into the rotor. The diluted sample is transferred by centrifugal force through capillaries into the cuvettes along the rotor's perimeter that contain the reagent tablets. The chemical reactions are monitored at a temperature of 37° C using bichromatic spectrophotometry. After each test profile, the rotor must be discarded whether a complete or partial chemistry profile is performed. With the Analyst, rotors are available for performing a 7- or 12-test general chemistry profile, a lipid profile, or a discrete analysis of a single analyte. An ion-selective electrode system for measuring sodium and potassium is also available from Du Pont.

The i-STAT is a hand-held clinical analyzer that can measure sodium, potassium, chloride, glucose, urea (BUN), and hematocrit in whole blood using biosensor technology. The biosensors are microfabricated thin-film electrodes. Sodium, potassium, and chloride are determined by direct-measuring potentiometric ion-selective electrodes, urea is determined by an ammonium ion–selective electrode, glucose is determined by amperometric electrochemical detection of hydrogen peroxide as a result of the glucose oxidase reaction, and hematocrit is measured by conductivity. The operator introduces about 65 μL of whole blood into a disposable cartridge that contains a biosensor and cali-

brant and inserts the cartridge into the analyzer. The calibrant solution is transported over the biosensors, and the data are stored. Sample is then moved to the sensors where the concentration of each analyte is determined by comparison of each sensor result of the sample with that of the calibrant. The analytical results are available in less than 2 minutes. When the analysis is complete, the results are viewed on a liquid crystal display on the analyzer. Data can also be transmitted to a printer or to a personal computer and then to the laboratory information system.

Wet chemistry systems

The Vision system uses two-dimensional centrifugation with specially designed disposable reagent packs for analysis. The reagent pack is a self-contained unit with a cuvette, liquid reagents, and bar codes to identify the assay. Two drops of sample, either blood, serum, or plasma, are placed into the multichambered reagent pack, and the packs are placed into a 10-position rotor in the analyzer. The plasma is separated from the erythrocytes by centrifugal force. The packs are rotated at a 90-degree angle, which results in a premeasured amount of sample and reagent being transferred into the cuvette. The reaction is monitored at 37° C, and the absorbances are measured bichromatically. Blood can be obtained by finger or heel stick in a special tube provided by Abbott. The tube is then inserted directly into the reagent pack, so as to eliminate the pipetting of blood from the capillary tube into the analyzer. The reagents are stable for several months, and with this system one to 10 analytes can be measured.

TRENDS IN AUTOMATION

The ideal scenario for the clinical laboratory is the automation of all the steps that are involved in obtaining and analyzing the specimen and reporting of laboratory results. Order entry is performed at the nurses' station and bar-coded labels with patient demographics and tests requested are printed and placed on the Vacutainer tube. After the phlebotomist draws the blood, the specimens are put in a pneumatic tube, which transfers the specimens to the laboratory or to a central processing area, significantly decreasing the amount of time it takes for specimens to reach the laboratory. The samples' arrival in the laboratory is monitored, by means of the bar codes, by the specimen-processing person.

Once the specimen arrives in the laboratory or in the central processing area the steps that are required for processing the sample should be automated. For example, centrifugation and aliquoting specimens for the appropriate work stations in the laboratory are a manual, time-consuming task that needs to be automated.

Whole blood would be the ideal specimen for analysis because it would eliminate the problems associated with centrifugation of blood. Whether blood, serum, or plasma is used in obtaining the test results, the specimen should be pipetted directly from the primary collection tube. This would avoid specimen mixup that can occur when samples are transferred from the tube to the sample cups. Closed-tube sampling, which eliminates splashing of biological fluids when the tube is uncapped, should be used for tests that require a single work station for analysis.

The reagents must be bar coded, prepackaged, and ready for use without the necessity of any interaction by laboratory personnel. The sample size required for each assay should be small, less than 15 μL, so that a chemistry profile, a drug analysis, and hormone testing can be determined from a 10 mL sample of blood.

Work-station consolidation and continuous analysis of samples as they come into the laboratory are essential for the efficient operation of the clinical laboratory. A single immunochemistry analyzer should be able to measure a thyroid panel, fertility hormones, cardiac and tumor markers, and drugs. In addition, a single general chemistry system should be used for both chemistry profiles and stat. assays. Any instrument used must be able to generate quality control charts for each assay and should be able to be interfaced to the main laboratory computer to receive ordering information for each sample and to directly transfer laboratory results to the requesting physician.

BIBLIOGRAPHY

Alpert N, editor: *Chemical Instrument Systems Newsletter,* Stamford, CT 06906.

Lifshitz MS, DeCresce RP: *The Instrument Report,* Applied Technology Associates, Inc., Chicago, IL 60614.

Pesce MA: Instrument systems for the physician's office laboratory, *J Med Technol* 2:566-569, 1985.

CHAPTER 17

Point-of-care (near-patient) testing

Ellis Jacobs

Use of near-patient testing
  Driving forces and potential benefits
  Immediate medical management benefits
  Contraindications
Implementation and monitoring of POCT
  Regulations
  Training
  Coordination of central laboratory and POCT
Cost assessment of POCT
Technology used in POCT
  Non–instrument-based systems
  Instrument-based systems
  Quality control of single-use devices

OBJECTIVES

- Describe what is meant by near-patient testing.
- Describe the perceived medical management benefits of point-of-care testing, distinguishing between true and perceived management benefits.
- Be able to list the regulations and describe the interdepartmental coordination required for point-of-care testing.
- List the tests most frequently measured by point-of-care testing.
- Describe some of the technology used in point-of-care testing devices, including reagents and instruments.
- Describe the philosophical differences in approach to quality control between point-of-care testing and the testing performed in a central laboratory.

KEY WORDS

alternative site testing Laboratory testing that is performed under hospital jurisdiction but outside the central laboratory environment.

CLIA '88 (Clinical Laboratory Improvement Amendments of 1988) Set of federal regulations that govern the operations of clinical laboratories and the performance of diagnostic testing.

ex vivo A diagnostic test that is performed on a specimen that is temporarily removed 'from a living organism' for analysis and then returned to the organism.

in vitro Literally 'in glass'; a diagnostic test that is performed on a specimen that is permanently removed from the organism.

in vivo Literally 'within the living body'; a diagnostic test in which an analyte is measured within a living organism.

point-of-care testing (POCT) Diagnostic testing that is performed near or at the site of patient care. If performed within a hospital, it can also be called alternate site testing.

total quality management (TQM) A management philosophy that encompasses an expansion of continuous quality management. TQM emphasizes team or institutional performance rather than individual or departmental performance.

waived tests A CLIA test complexity category that includes tests that have an insignificant risk of an erroneous result. Tests that have been approved for home use by the Food and Drug Administration are in this category.

There are many names for the style of testing that involves laboratory procedures performed near the patient's bed or room (Table 17-1). The College of American Pathologists (CAP) recently changed the title of its inspection checklist (Section 30) from *ancillary testing* to *point-of-care testing* (POCT). The Joint Commission on Accreditation of Healthcare Organizations (JCAHO) has replaced the term *decentralized testing* with *waived tests* in their accreditation requirements for diagnostic testing that is not performed within a "traditional" laboratory setting. Regardless of the name, it is a form of diagnostic testing that will be predominantly performed by nonlaboratorians. Currently, in vivo and externally attached patient-dedicated monitoring devices, such as intra-arterial blood gas catheters and pulse oximeters respectively, are not subject to federal, CAP, or JCAHO regulations even though they are forms of diagnostic testing because, with these techniques, a specimen is not withdrawn from the body.

Before the decision is made to proceed with POC testing, the true costs and benefits of this modality of testing must be carefully analyzed in each clinical setting. Is there a significant improvement in patient care or outcome? What is the *total* financial effect, not just the cost of equipment and supplies, of the various options for the provision of ex-

Table 17-1 Names for POCT

Alternative site testing
Ancillary testing
Bedside testing
Decentralized testing
Distributed testing
Near-patient testing
Patient-focused testing
Value-added testing
Waived testing

Table 17-2 Potential benefits of POCT

To physicians:	Improved therapeutic turnaround time
	Better and more immediate care
To patients:	Patient-focused system
	Less traumatic (for fingerstick systems)
	Improved convenience
	Less blood withdrawn
To lab:	Decreased preanalytical errors
	Improved visibility
	Decreased manpower needs
	Collaboration with clinicians
	Direct patient involvement
	Team management system
To administration:	Shorter intensive care unit stays
	Decreased overall length of stays
	Financial savings
	Total quality management (TQM) program

pedient diagnostic services? Additional considerations include integration of the data into the medical record and proper control and supervision of the testing, as mandated by professional standards and regulatory agencies.

USE OF NEAR-PATIENT TESTING
Driving forces and potential benefits

There are distinctly different driving forces behind point-of-care testing dependent on the clinical setting. In the ambulatory care setting, the ability to obtain test results *during* the patient's visit is important for both patient and physician and is a strong economic motivator for POCT. However, in the in-patient setting, other than for diabetic patients, the desire for POCT is based upon other factors. POCT can meet the demands of critical care medicine in the intensive care unit (ICU), operating room (OR), or emergency department (ED) for the faster delivery of results. In addition, certain point-of-care (POC) tests, such as fecal occult blood and urine dipsticks, can be used conveniently and easily in the nursing units. Finally, because intensive insulin therapy of diabetic patients requires that preprandial glucose determinations be performed four times a day, bedside glucose testing programs have been established in most hospitals. For both inpatients and outpatients, there is the assumption that more rapid testing will improve immediate medical management.

For hospitalized patients, economic forces within the health care industry are demanding improved patient medical management to reduce the length of stay (LOS) of the patient in either an ICU or the hospital in general. The costs associated with a hospital stay are one of the largest components of the overall costs of the health care system. Within a hospital, the costs associated with ICUs, such as cardiac (CICU), neonatal (NICU), and surgical (SICU), are much greater than the costs of regular nursing units. If more rapid testing could decrease the LOS of patients in the ICU and the hospital in general, the added costs of the rapid testing could be justified. As of now, this has *not* been demonstrated (see below). In hospitals, the rise of POCT is the result, in part, of the "failure" of the traditional, central laboratory to meet some of the current clinical needs. However, with proper modernization of facilities and services the central laboratory is able to compete with bedside testing on

both cost and turnaround time bases (refer to the work by Winkelman et al., 1994, in the Bibliography).

The potential benefits of POCT in the hospital setting are shown in Table 17-2. Most of the benefits for the physicians, nurses, patients, and administration are based on the belief that "faster is better" and that more rapid testing by POCT would improve medical care and decrease utilization of hospital resources (supplies, room, and personnel). Other possible benefits include minimizing sample size because of the ability to use fingersticks rather than tubes of blood and increasing the patient's sense of involvement in his or her medical care. For the laboratory, the benefits are based on possible improvements in the preanalytical and postanalytical phases of the test cycle. Improvements in the preanalytical phase include fewer problems with sample identification and lost specimens. In addition, changes in concentration caused by time delays between sampling and testing would be minimized, as would the time needed for calling the results back to the physician or caregiver. With a decrease in both the amount of specimen handling and time-dependent specimen degradation, POCT should reduce preanalytical variance.

Immediate medical management benefits

The most significant use of POCT in the hospital setting is for the immediate assessment and management of critically ill patients. Even though over 40 different analytes have been evaluated as potential POC tests, based on the criteria of immediate medical need, only blood gases, electrolytes (Na^+, K^+, Ca^{++}), prothrombin time (PT), partial thromboplastin time (PTT) or activated clotting time (ACT), hematocrit or hemoglobin, and glucose should be considered for analysis at the point of care.

Other tests may be performed at the point of care for reasons of convenience or as parts of critical-care diagnostic profiles. It still must be demonstrated that utilization of these diagnostic tests by POCT will improve patient care. However, intraoperative monitoring of potassium during cardiac surgery has been associated with a 50% reduction in arrhythmias and a decreased use of antiarrhythmic pharmacological agents. Studies have also indicated that faster coagulation testing may improve management of anticoagulation therapy after thrombolytic therapy or decrease microvascular bleeding after cardiopulmonary bypass surgery.

Contraindications

The most important consideration for the use of POCT is whether it is the most appropriate testing mechanism in a particular setting. There are several ways of providing critical test results, of which POCT is one. Testing can be performed in a stat. section of the main laboratory or in a stat. laboratory that is separate and distinct from the main laboratory. A variant on the latter would be the development and use of dedicated satellite laboratories at the point of need, such as an operating unit's blood-gas laboratory. It is necessary to look at all aspects of a service delivery model, as well as the unique characteristics of each clinical setting, to determine which testing system best services both the financial (see p. 318) and the clinical needs of the institution. To make this decision, outcome data on the efficacy of POCT under different clinical conditions are needed. The major negative aspect of POCT is its cost. POCT analyzers have higher disposable and reagent costs than traditional laboratory systems, and thus POCT systems are more costly to operate. Other areas of concern are (1) performance and documentation of quality control and quality assurance, (2) control of diagnostic testing, and (3) proper data integration and flow. Despite a projected reduction in preanalytical variance because of the decrease in specimen handling and in time delay between sampling and analysis, other preanalytical causes of variance arise in POCT. When obtaining microliter samples by fingerstick, if the site is not properly prepared, significant specimen contamination with alcohol or other disinfectant can occur. The physiological status of the patient influences the results obtained with fingerstick and noninvasive testing more significantly than it does the analysis of arterial or venous specimens. In a patient with poor peripheral circulation, fingerstick samples are difficult to obtain and are often contaminated with interstitial fluids (see Chapter 3). Additionally, POCT results may not correlate with results from the main laboratory because of biochemical differences between specimen source (arterial, venous, or capillary) or type (whole blood, plasma, serum).

The rapid availability of results with POCT creates a quality assurance dilemma. Data can be seen and acted upon before any quality control checks or other external mechanisms of assuring test result reliability can be applied to the systems. Therefore it is critical that POCT devices have built-in quality control/quality assurance (QC/QA) systems. These automatic functions prevent erroneous data from being seen by the health care provider.

Table 17-3   CLIA '88 waived tests

Dipstick or tablet reagent urinalysis (nonautomated) for bilirubin, glucose, hemoglobin, ketones, leukocytes, nitrites, pH, protein, specific gravity, and urobilinogen
Fecal occult blood
Ovulation tests (visual comparison of color)
Urine pregnancy tests (visual comparison of color)
Erythrocyte sedimentation rate
Hemoglobin (copper sulfate)
Blood glucose (FDA approved for home use)
Spun hematocrit
Automated hemoglobin using single-analyte instruments with a self-contained specimen-reagent interaction and direct measurement and readout

IMPLEMENTATION AND MONITORING OF POCT
Regulations

Despite its relative simplicity, the implementation and use of POCT is subject to the various regulations associated with clinical laboratory testing. The Clinical Laboratory Improvement Amendment of 1988 (CLIA '88) subjects virtually all clinical laboratory testing to federal regulation and inspection. These regulations are considered "site neutral," which means that all laboratory testing must meet the same quality standards regardless of where it is performed. State and city governments and nongovernmental agencies (such as CAP and JCAHO) may enact regulations that are more, but not less, stringent than federal regulations.

Test procedures are grouped into one of four categories: waived, moderate complexity, high complexity, or physician-performed microscopy (see also Chapter 2). Test complexity is determined by seven criteria that assess knowledge, training, reagent and material preparation, operational technique, QC/QA characteristics, maintenance and troubleshooting, and interpretation and judgment. There are nine tests in the waived category (Table 17-3), and the federal regulations and inspections of laboratories that perform only these tests are minimal. However, if these tests are performed in a JCAHO- or a CAP-accredited institution, they are regulated in essentially the same way as laboratory-based testing. Also, six physician-performed microscopy tests have been waived from accreditation requirements: wet mounts, potassium hydroxide preps, pinworm preps, fern tests, urine sedimentation exams, and postcoital exams. All POCT falls within either the waived or moderate-complexity categories. Laboratories that either perform or are in charge of moderate-complexity POC tests may also perform or be responsible for waived tests and must fulfill all the requirements for personnel credentials, proficiency testing, QC, patient test management, QA, and inspections.

Personnel standards for the performance of waived tests are minimal. However, in 10 states (such as California, Florida, and New York) medical technologist training or licensure is required even for performance of tests in the waived category. When one is reviewing personnel requirements for diagnostic testing, regardless of testing category and location, the following are necessary:

- Those responsible for testing, direction, and supervision are identified.
- There is an adequate number of trained individuals to perform the test.
- Testing personnel receive regular in-service training.
- Competency to perform test is checked triannually.

As for any laboratory test, written policies and procedures must be established to encompass every aspect of POCT. There should be policies and procedures for patient preparation, specimen collection and preservation, instrument calibration, QC and remedial actions, equipment performance evaluations, test performance, and result reporting and recording. State regulations in several states, including New York, New Jersey, and Pennsylvania, require that the central laboratory must supervise POCT and that the laboratory director is responsible for the standards of performance in all areas, such as QC, QA, and cost-effective test utilization.

Each laboratory, or testing site, performing nonwaived tests must establish written policies regarding quality assurance. There must be an ongoing system to monitor and evaluate QC and proficiency testing data. Quality control specimens at two or three different analyte concentrations must be analyzed on a daily basis. Records of actions taken to correct out-of-range QC results must be maintained. Linearity studies, for assessment of the analytical range of the system, are performed before devices are initially placed into use and then every 6 months. Split-sample correlation studies with a primary testing system are performed before each POCT device is initially placed into use and then every 6 months. Some states may require more frequent evaluations. Triannual proficiency testing is required only for the primary method of patient testing by federal standards but may be required on all testing systems by state and CAP regulations.

Finally, regulations require adequate record keeping. An integral component of both patient test management and a laboratory QA system is proper record keeping. The following information must be recorded in various logs and records:

- Time, date, test result, and operator ID for each analysis
- Quality control data (result, time, date, and operator ID)
- Maintenance and revalidation of POC device
- Actions taken to correct out-of-range QC results
- Initial training and recertification of personnel

Training

Point-of-care testing may or may not be performed by laboratory personnel. Nurses, anesthesiologists, respiratory therapists, operating room technologists, and physician assistants are among those who may be involved in the performance of POCT. Qualifications for personnel perform-

Table 17-4   Point-of-care training program agenda

Theory of instrument/device
Specimen collection/preservation
Instrument maintenance
Quality control procedures
Testing procedure
Sources and degree of preanalytical errors
Clinical significance

ing bedside testing are set as a minimum by state, local, and federal requirements. The laboratory director, who is responsible for the testing, will often set additional requirements. The minimum educational and experience requirements for personnel performing POC laboratory tests range from the requirement for a high school diploma with no experience to a Bachelor of Science degree with 2 years of experience. In specific cases, other health care professionals may be qualified by state-defined scopes of practice to perform select testing, such as respiratory therapists performing blood-gas analysis.

The degree of training required to allow an individual to perform POCT depends on both the background of the individual involved and on the analytical system being employed, that is, the amount of technique dependency of the POCT device. There are seven main subjects that should be included in the training program (Table 17-4). The amount of time required for each item varies depending on the personnel and system being used. In addition to teaching the specific steps involved in performing the test, it is very important that quality control and quality assurance issues be addressed. The greatest source of error in POCT, as well as testing in general, is preanalytical error, and it is essential that it be adequately addressed in the training program. Sources of preanalytical error are fully discussed in Chapter 3. The training program should include pretraining and posttraining written tests and practical tests that demonstrate acceptable performance for obtaining patient specimens and for performing the analysis. All individuals should participate in an annual recertification course, which should also include a written test and demonstration of test performance. There must be a mechanism for the withdrawal of authorization for the performance of POCT for either an individual or a testing site when there is failure to follow policy or poor technical performance. Authorization will then be reinstituted after retraining and demonstration of competency.

Coordination of central laboratory and POCT

Decentralization of testing away from the traditional laboratory increases the direct involvement of the laboratory with other members of the health care team. Because POCT can be used to provide cost-effective improvement of medical care, the implementation of POCT is a total quality management (TQM) project (Table 17-5). The quality improve-

Table 17-5   Point-of-care testing as a total quality management project

Multidisciplinary team approach
Looking at entire system rather than individual performance
Ongoing evaluation and refinement (CQI)
Improvement in delivery of critical-care laboratory services
Cost savings

ment issues are complex, and their effect is compounded by the fact that POCT is an interdisciplinary concept that crosses many boundaries within a hospital. Therefore, proper implementation of point-of-care testing requires an interdepartmental approach to the establishment, compliance review, and setting of the future direction of the program or programs.

Interdisciplinary committee. In order for a POCT program to work efficiently, a multidisciplinary team approach must be employed. An interdisciplinary POCT committee must be established with representation from all involved disciplines, such as medicine, nursing, laboratory, respiratory therapy, and administration. The committee should be chaired by the laboratory director or designee. The function of the committee is to determine institutional policies, define levels of service provided, evaluate and select the equipment that will be utilized, and assign work assignments to meet the various regulatory requirements. The committee should review all requests for additional POC programs, and if a request is approved, the committee should provide guidelines, that is, which analytical system, who will operate it, and so forth. It is the clinical laboratory staff who are in the best position to assess new technology, design training programs, and help identify potential pitfalls in the use of new systems.

Ancillary testing personnel. Ultimate responsibility and control of POCT must reside within a CLIA-certified laboratory, and a minimum of one laboratorian should be assigned by that laboratory to the POCT program. The duties of this POC technologist are outlined in the box below.

Duties of Laboratory Technologist Assigned to POCT Program

Evaluate and test devices

Help choose final testing instrument

Perform validation studies before devices are placed into service, including linearity and correlation studies

Assist in training and retraining

Coordinate proficiency testing

Ensure compliance with documentation of procedural requirements

Provide preliminary review of QC data

Provide technical guidance and troubleshooting

If there is more than one POCT program, a laboratorian should be appointed as an ancillary testing coordinator to overview and coordinate the entire POC system. The duties of this individual are reviewed in the following box.

Quality assurance monitoring. As previously mentioned, even waived tests are associated with specific standards. For example, some state regulations, such as those of New York, New Jersey, and Pennsylvania, require that the laboratory director be responsible for the standards of performance in all areas of POCT, including QA. As for the testing within the central laboratory, QA monitoring entails much more than a simple review of QC data. All POCT systems will have problems with noncompliance with the different QA requirements, especially record keeping and QC performance. The degree of noncompliance will be directly related to the size and complexity of the program. Some of these problems are caused by a lack of understanding of the regulatory requirements regarding record keeping, of what QC testing really means, and of the causes of erroneous results. Additionally, external pressures, like being overworked in a busy ICU or emergency department, may also lead to noncompliance. Once a POCT system has been established, the monitoring of the compliance by POC personnel with all policies and procedures requires more attention than is needed for the monitoring of the analytical systems.

Motivation of personnel is critical for a successful QA program, especially with large POCT programs like bedside glucose testing, which may have several hundred operators. These systems are so complicated and are so sensitive to various factors outside the control of the laboratory that continuous monitoring is required so that changes can be made to maintain, if not improve, the overall quality of service.

The QA monitoring and control of POCT is performed on many levels, with overall responsibility residing in the laboratory (Table 17-6). Nursing or unit supervisors observe work performance and compliance with policies and procedures on a daily basis. Weekly and monthly reviews of system operations by ancillary testing personnel and supervisors are important to ensure a high degree of continuous compliance with existing policies and procedures. Once a

---

Duties of Ancillary Testing Coordinator

Train and supervise POC technologist(s) (see previous box)

Ensure that all aspects of POCT are in compliance with regulatory requirements

Review QC data on a regular basis

Submit monthly and quarterly QC reports, reviewing individual units' activities

Provide yearly overview report on hospital-wide ancillary testing program

Develop and coordinate training programs for POC individuals

---

month the ancillary testing personnel generates a QC report that includes a report on each unit's degree of compliance with policies and procedures, focusing on record keeping and instrument maintenance. The QC report should also include both a statistical and a narrative analysis of QC testing and should summarize test volumes for individual units and the entire system. Monthly QA audit rounds should be performed by the individual in charge of the program, either the lab director or ancillary testing coordinator, with a representative from nursing management. In addition to being a second level of review, one of the main focus items on these rounds is to ensure that there is the proper entry of patient data in both the medical record or laboratory computer system as well as in the workstation logs. Furthermore, these rounds open up another feedback channel for the program and send a clear signal to the system operators of the program's importance and the institution's commitment to quality. For each QC/QA monitor, limits of acceptable criteria need to be established. For example, more than 95% of all results generated by glucose meters *must* be properly charted. A proper response when criteria are not met must also be defined. This TQM approach will help to improve the overall POCT system. Either the interdisciplinary or the end-users committee can define these criteria and responses.

A critical component of a POCT program is an end-user committee, which is different from the interdisciplinary committee that establishes and overviews all POCT programs. Such a committee, which should be established for each POCT program, should meet bimonthly to discuss the various compliance reports, as well as ongoing issues and problems with the program. Recommendations for change should be forwarded to the interdisciplinary committee for consideration. The interdisciplinary committee should meet on a biannual basis, or sooner if circumstances demand it, to consider any recommendations from the user committees, to review and discuss the overall program, and to set future directions.

COST ASSESSMENT OF POCT

A cost/benefit evaluation of the true efficacy of point-of-care testing is extremely difficult to perform at this time because sufficient patient outcome data for POCT systems are not available. The costs associated with POCT depend on the services that have usually been provided and on the new services that are planned.

When one is assessing the financial effect of POCT, it is necessary to look at the entire picture, not just the specific direct costs of test performance (see Chapter 2). There are often cost savings associated with an improved level or quality of work, such as reduced repeat testing, decreased preanalytical variables, and improved management of patient service. Bedside testing systems will tend to have greater variable expenses, reflecting the costs of reagents, disposables, and flexible staffing, rather than traditional laboratory methodologies. However, fixed expenses are significantly lower, such as equipment costs, instrument maintenance and QC, stepped-down space-allocation costs, and minimal staffing required to maintain needed levels of service.

Either a cost-centered (microeconomic) or defect-rate inclusive (macroeconomic) approach can be used to determine the costs of any laboratory testing, whether by the central laboratory or by POCT. The cost center–based approach takes into account all the fixed and variable expenses related to testing within the affected cost center, that is, laboratory, nursing unit, or operating room expenses. However, should every minute of labor time associated with testing be accounted for in a cost analysis, or is it correct to assume the capture of "free," structurally idle time? It is very important that all labor associated with testing be taken into account and that none is assumed to be free. Even though POCT takes only a couple of minutes per test, that time adds up. At The Mount Sinai Medical Center over 15,000 fingerstick glucose tests per month are performed by the nursing staff. At approximately 9 minutes per test for sample collection, analysis, and paperwork (Winkelman et al., 1994) this translates into over 27,000 nursing hours per annum, not including time for quality control testing and other functions such as training and supervision. Currently that time may be thought of as being recaptured and thus "free"; however, as institutions go through restructuring and work-function reassignments, that time has to be taken into account.

The defect-rate inclusive approach is a subset of total cost management. Total cost management is a means by which all the costs, including preventive, appraisal, and internal and external failure costs, associated with the quality of a system are assessed. *Preventive costs* are costs associated with the mechanisms used to protect against process errors. These include QC testing, personnel training and continuing education, and preventive maintenance. The costs of ascertaining the degree to which a system meets its service requirements are *appraisal costs*. Appraisal costs include the costs of proficiency testing, inspections and accreditation, and internal QA audits. *Internal failure costs* are costs within the actual testing cycle that result from poor laboratory performance. Specimen re-collections, results considered useless because of the lack of timely reporting

Table 17-6 Quality assurance monitoring of POCT

Frequency	Task
Daily	Work performance and compliance are observed
Monthly	Quality control/quality assurance reports are generated and distributed
	Individual in charge of program makes quality assurance round of test sites
Bimonthly	End-users committee meets
Semiannually	Interdisciplinary committee meeting is held

Table 17-7 "Ideal" POCT system characteristics

Is self-contained and portable
Has a flexible test menu
Requires minimal training; simple to operate
Uses small volumes of whole blood
Has an accuracy and precision comparable to main laboratory
    systems
Performs automatic, periodic calibrations
Requires minimal routine and preventive maintenance
Has bar codes for test packs, controls, and bar-code reader for
    specimens
Reagents stable at ambient temperature storage
Generates result printouts
Can be interfaced with a laboratory information system
Provides QA software, system lockouts, and data management

(test wastage), and repeat testing or confirmation by a second methodology because of questionable first-time results are examples of internal failure costs. *External failure costs* are the costs of poor performance that are outside the testing cycle and are incurred by the receiver of testing results. They include inappropriate clinical decisions based on inaccurate or untimely results, excessive duplicate testing, and excessive use of expensive stat. testing.

Again, however calculated, testing costs must be judged worthwhile based on the value added to patient care (does the additional cost yield better patient outcomes?) and the economic effect on the overall system (does testing reduce the length of stays?; see Table 17-2).

TECHNOLOGY USED IN POCT

The environment in which POCT is performed is different from that of the traditional laboratory setting because of different work-flow and work-load characteristics. Furthermore, the personnel involved with POCT are more oriented to obtaining results rapidly for their immediate use for patient care and are not, like laboratorians, necessarily committed to all the procedures associated with laboratory medicine, such as QC, analytical procedures, record keeping, and regulatory requirements. Therefore the desirable characteristics of POC diagnostic systems (Table 17-7) are similar but distinct from laboratory-based diagnostic systems. Significant differences include the desire for POC systems that are easy and convenient to use, that is, no venipuncture or precise pipetting is required, that are as technique independent as possible, and that have automated record keeping that fulfills regulatory requirements.

Non–instrument-based systems

The predominant forms of POCT are non–instrument-based systems that utilize competitive and noncompetitive immunoassays, enzymatic assays, or chemical reactions with a visually read end point (Table 17-8). A variety of specimen types, such as whole blood, serum or plasma, urine, amniotic fluid, saliva, and feces, can be analyzed with non–instrument-based POCT systems. Qualitative assays with a visually read positive or negative indicator are the predominant form of non–instrument-based POCT. Systems based on either competitive or noncompetitive immunoassays are used for detecting a variety of analytes including human chorionic gonadotropin, drugs of abuse, fetal lung maturity, cardiac markers, and markers for infectious diseases. Other major qualitative assays are occult fecal blood testing, which employs chemically impregnated paper and a color developer, and visually read blood glucose reagent strips,

Table 17-8 Non–instrument-based technology employed in POCT

Type of assay	Assay principle	Format	Specimen	Analytes
Qualitative	Chemical reactions	Impregnated paper strips	Feces	Occult blood
	Immunoconcentration	Dry reagent cartridges—single use	Urine and serum	hCG; streptomycin A
	Competitive immunoassay	Dry reagent cartridges—single use	Urine	Drugs of abuse
		Latex agglutination slides	Amniotic fluid	Fetal lung maturity
	Immunochromatographic	Dry reagent cartridges—single use	Blood	CK-MB; troponin I and T; myoglobin
		Dry reagent cartridges—single use	Urine	hCG
		Dry reagent cartridges—single use	Swabs	*Chlamydia;* streptomycin A; herpes
Semiquantitative	Chemical/enzymatic reactions	Impregnated paper strips	Urine	Urinalysis
		Impregnated paper strips	Blood	Glucose
		Dry reagent cartridges—single use	Saliva	Ethanol
Quantitative	Chemical/enzymatic reactions	Dry reagent cartridges—single use	Blood	Lipids
	Immunochromatographic	Dry reagent cartridges—single use	Blood	Therapeutic drugs

CK-MB, Creatine kinase–MB; *hCG,* human chorionic gonadotropin.

which utilize coupled enzyme reactions to form a colored product. The glucose concentration can be semiquantified by visual comparison of the color development on the glucose reagent strips to a color chart, or by reflectance colorimetry. Urine dipstick systems are also semiquantitative and utilize both chemical and enzymatic reactions to generate a colored product. There are a few non–instrument-based quantitative POC test systems that employ chemical or enzymatic reactions and immunochromatographic techniques to determine lipid and therapeutic drug concentrations.

Instrument-based systems

Instrument-based POCT systems are becoming very sophisticated. They are highly automated, using a small sample size, requiring minimal routine and preventive maintenance, and eliminating or automating calibration functions. These improvements in functionality have been facilitated by advances in reagent stabilization, in the development and miniaturization of electrodes and biosensors, in the ability to produce relatively inexpensive, precise, disposable devices, and in the development of microcomputers and microelectronics. These advances in engineering and technology have allowed reformulation of currently used reagents into different testing formats, the incorporation of real-time process control and monitoring of the analytical process, and the encoding (through microchips and bar codes) of information (such as calibration data, lot number, and test name) into the system. Through the application of these technologies and processes the responsibility for the quality of the analytical result moves significantly toward the manufacturer.

Most but not all of the characteristics of the "ideal" POCT device listed in Table 17-7 are found in the various instruments on the market today. Automatic record keeping of patient result logs, QC/QA logs, and maintenance logs with attached comments and operator ID are part of several systems. Quality assurance software that allows for automatic lockouts of users who are either not authorized or who do not adhere to QC/QA procedures is available in some analyzers. System lockouts can occur if QC has not been performed or is out of range, if a valid operator ID is not entered, or if patient ID is not entered. However, not all the systems on the market today have the capability of interfacing with a laboratory information system. Integration of the data generated with POCT into the medical record is important.

Most POC instruments require only a few microliters of whole blood, and either the analytes are tested for directly in the whole blood sample or the system internally separates the red blood cells and analyzes the plasma obtained. Where necessary, size filtration or centrifugation is used to retain the erythrocytes. Table 17-9 identifies the current technologies that are utilized in instrument-based POCT systems. The most common instrument systems used today are those based on reflectance photometry. Representative

devices of the various technology and format combinations are given along with some of the other characteristics of these testing systems. Some of these systems employ new analytical concepts, such as biosensors, paramagnetism, and optical immunoassays. Other POC instruments, taking advantage of the process improvements discussed earlier, are miniaturized versions of traditional laboratory analyzers utilizing the same chemistries (see Chapter 16, p. 309).

The ability to perform analytical processes on only a few microliters of whole blood, minimizing iatrogenic blood loss, is one of the significant benefits of POCT. Noninvasive POCT, such as the use of pulse oximeters for the measurement of O_2 saturation, end-tidal CO_2 measurements for PCO_2, and transcutaneous and conjunctival PO_2/PCO_2 measurements, eliminates the need for blood withdrawal. However, since these systems do not provide measurements with the highest accuracy, they are used as trend indicators, allowing for a continuous monitoring of information and the ability to recognize a change in physiological status. Other advantages of noninvasive systems include less infection control problems and better compliance rates with self-monitoring because of the elimination of the inconvenience and discomfort of multiple fingersticks. Noninvasive systems now being developed employ infrared spectroscopy, near-infrared spectroscopy with signature analysis, and photoacoustic technology.

Quality control of single-use devices

Quality control has been traditionally accomplished by running multiple levels of stabilized, matrix-matched specimens (QC material) within each analytical run (see Chapter 21). After applying various statistical rules (for example, 2SD) to the results, the technologist determines whether the run is "in control," and the patient results can be released. As defined by the National Committee for Clinical Laboratory Standards (NCCLS) and incorporated into the CLIA '88 regulations, an analytical run for the purpose of QC "is an interval (that is, a period of time or series of measurements) within which the accuracy and precision of the measuring system are expected to be stable." Maximum run length has been set at 24 hours. The concept of run length does not exist with single-use diagnostic testing devices where, strictly speaking, each test is a run unto itself. With instrument-based systems, every time a new cartridge, pack, or strip is inserted into the base instrument, a new test system is created. Therefore, QC must take a different form in POCT devices from that used in traditional testing systems.

How can POC systems be evaluated to assure the continued quality of the results generated? In certain non-instrument devices, QC has been integrated directly into the device by the use of visual indicators that test for positive and negative reaction zones as well as for the adequacy of specimen flow. With these devices, external QC material should be analyzed only upon initial receipt of a shipment and then, depending on the system, on a periodic basis.

Table 17-9   Current technology employed in instrument-based POCT

Technology	Format	Sample type	Precise pipetting	Sample volume (μL)	Representative systems	Testing
Photometry, reflectance	Dry reagent strip, single test	Whole blood	No	10-45	Glucose meters	Glucose
		Serum/plasma	No	30	Reflotron (Boehringer)	Chemistry and TDM
			Yes	10	Ektachem (J & J)	Chemistry
Photometry, transmittance	Wet reagent cartridges, single test	Whole blood	No	(~20)	Vision (Abbott)	Chemistry
		Serum/plasma	No	2 drops	Biotrack (Boehringer)	Drugs
	Dry reagent cartridges, single test	Whole blood	No	10	HemoCue (Hemocue)	Glucose and hemoglobin
	Dry reagent rotors, multiple tests	Whole blood	No	~90	Picolo (Abaxis)	Chemistry
		Serum/plasma	No	90	Analyst (DuPont)	Chemistry
Fluorometry	Dry reagent cartridges, multiple tests	Serum	No	20	IOS (Biocircuits)	Hormones
Potentiometry/ electrochemistry	Biosensor strips, single test	Whole blood	No	10	Satellite G (Medisence)	Glucose
			No	10	AccuChek (Boehringer)	
	Biosensor chips, multiple tests	Whole blood	No	~70	PCA (i-Stat)	Chemistry/blood gases
			No	500	IRMA (Diametrics)	
	Miniature electrodes, multiple tests, multiple use	Whole blood	No	200	Gem Stat/Premier (Mallinckrodt Sensor Systems)	
Turbidimetry	Dry, coated latex particle cartridges, single use	Whole blood	No	10	DCA 2000 (Bayer)	Hemoglobin A1c
Optical motion detection	Dry, paramagnetic particle motion reagent card, single use	Whole blood	No	1 large drop	TAS (Cardiovascular Diagnostics)	Coagulation
	Dry, sample motion cartridges, single use	Whole blood	No	1 large drop	Biotrack (Boehringer)	Coagulation
			No		Hemochron Jr. (International Technidyne)	Coagulation
Luminescence/fiber optic	Intra-arterial catheter	Not applicable	Not applicable	Not applicable	PB3300 (Puritan Bennett)	Blood gases

TDM, Therapeutic drug monitoring.

Quality control has been integrated into various POCT instruments by incorporating the following:

- Automation of calibration function
- Encoding (via bar code or microchip) crucial quality control and quality assurance information on unit dose packages
- Real-time process monitoring
- Inclusion of calibration solution in units using electrode-based systems.

Through these means the company ensures the reliability of the test results as long as the disposable test devices have been stored properly and are used before a stated expiration date. Thus, with these POCT systems, part of the laboratory QC is dependent on the ability of the company to manufacture reliably and reproducibly its consumable product.

An analytical instrument can be divided into three sections: mechanical/electronic, analytical, and reagent/calibrants. The mechanical/electronic component consists of various parts, such as pumps, levers, gears, chains, memory chips, logic circuits, and software. The analytical components are those parts of the system that come into contact with the sample being analyzed or produce the signal for the electronics to convert into results, such as ion-selective electrodes, pH electrodes, biosensors, reaction cups, and optics. However, with instrument-based POCT systems, the mechanical/electronic and analytical components have been completely separated from the reagent/calibrant components. In some systems, the analytical components are individually packaged with the reagents and calibrants. With these devices, the only consistent part from test to test is the mechanical/electronic component. All biosensors, electrodes, reagents, and calibrants are replaced with every analysis.

Traditional QC testing programs validate the entire system, not its components. However, with modern electronics and software, it is possible to isolate and test some of the subsystems independent of the others. In this manner it may be possible to devise a QC program for instrument-based POCT systems that is more cost effective than that used for traditional testing systems. The functionality of the mechanical/electronic component of each analytical device in operation should be tested on a daily basis, that is, once every 24 hours. Reflectance standard strips with established ranges for acceptable values are used with some of the reflectance photometry systems to validate optical performance. Electronic test modules are available for some POCT systems. The electronic test module is inserted into the analyzer and simulates the analytical output of a test cartridge at one or more specimen concentrations. Additionally, the electronic test module may perform a series of mechanical and electronic tests on the base unit. Comparison of the various results to predefined limits allows the analyst to determine if the base system is working properly. Furthermore, with some systems the electronic test module is not a passive testing system but requires operator intervention to further stimulate sample analysis; this provides additional validation of operator technique.

One can verify the analytical reliability of the test cartridges, that is, the analytical/reagent/calibrant component, by analyzing matrix-matched QC material with the test cartridges. Because the operational characteristics of all the base units are verified with the electronic test module, it is necessary only to verify the analytical performance of a test cartridge lot with one base unit. By using the electronic test module and liquid QC material in this manner, one can be properly assured that all test cartridges are in control, with a minimal utilization of test cartridges. Because the stability and reliability of the test cartridges are contingent upon proper storage conditions, such as temperature, humidity, and light, it is necessary that every testing site that stores its own stock of reagents perform QC testing on each lot in storage.

Process control features of some POCT systems allow detection of deteriorating reactivity and inappropriate biosensor response. In the PCA device, the controlling software monitors the rehydration, calibration, and analytical response curves from the individual biosensors. If any of the biosensor parameters monitored fall outside acceptable ranges, the output of that sensor is automatically suppressed. The Picolo analyzer has an enzyme reagent in the rotor that is sensitive to temperature, humidity, and light. If the enzyme activity is not great enough, one can assume that the rotor has been affected by the environment and the run is aborted. With the expansion of the application of real time process controls in POCT devices, the need for external QC testing will continue to diminish. Furthermore, the definition of a run for quality control purposes may either be changed to allow for time periods greater than 24 hours

or eliminated completely for systems that incorporate on-board process control.

BIBLIOGRAPHY

Chernow B: The bedside laboratory: a critical step forward in ICU care, *Chest* 97:183S-184S, 1990.

Claremont DJ: Biosensors: clinical requirements and scientific promise, *J Med Engl Technol* 11:51-56, 1987.

Department of Health and Human Services, Health Care Financing Administration: Clinical Laboratory Improvement Amendments of 1988; final rule, *Fed Register* 7:7002-7186, 1992.

Despotis GJ, Gresalfi NJ, Enney-O'Mara LA, et al: Prospective evaluation and clinical utility of on-site coagulation monitoring in cardiac surgical patients, *J Thorac Cardiovasc Surg* 107:271-279, 1994.

Fleisher M, Schwartz MK: Strategies of organization and service for the critical-care laboratory, *Clin Chem* 36:1557B-1561B, 1990.

Friedman BA, Mitchell W: Integrating information from decentralized laboratory testing sites, *Am J Clin Pathol* 99:637-642, 1993.

Handorf CR: Quality control and quality management of alternate-site testing, *Clin Lab Med* 14:539-558, 1994.

Handorf CR: POC testing: must quality cost more?, *Med Lab Observer* 25(9S):28-33, 1993.

Jacobs E, Sarkozi L, Coleman N: A centralized critical care (stat) laboratory: the Mount Sinai experience, *Crit Care Rep* 2:397-405, 1991.

Jacobs E, Vadasdi E, Sarkozi L, Coleman N: Analytical evaluation of i-Stat portable clinical analyzer and use by non-laboratory health-care professionals, *Clin Chem* 39:1069-1074, 1993.

Jacobs E: Total quality management and point-of-care testing, *Med Lab Observer* 25(9S):2-6, 1993.

Jacobs E: Bedside glucose testing: sources of variation, *ASCP Check Sample-Core Analytes* 10:1-11, 1994 (American Society of Clinical Pathologists).

Kost JG, Jammal MA, Ward RE, Safwat AM: Monitoring of ionized calcium during human hepatic transplantation: critical values and their relevance to cardiac and hemodynamic management, *Am J Clin Pathol* 86:61-70, 1986.

Kost JG: The hybrid laboratory: shifting the focus to the point of care, *Med Lab Observer* 24(9S):17-28, 1992.

Korpman RA: Health care information systems—patient centered integration is the key, *Clin Lab Med* 11:203-220, 1991.

Lee-Lewandowski E, Laposata M, Eschenbach K, et al: Utilization and cost analysis of bedside capillary glucose testing: implications for managing point of care testing, *Am J Med* 97:222-230, 1994.

Marks V: Advantages and disadvantages of performing clinical biochemistry nearer the patient. In Zinder O, editor: *Optimal use of the laboratory,* New York, 1986, Karger.

Nanji AA, Poon R, Hinberg I: Near-patient testing: quality of laboratory test results obtained by non-technical personnel in a decentralized setting, *Am J Clin Pathol* 89:797-801, 1988.

NCCLS Approved Guideline C30-A: *Ancillary (bedside) testing in acute and chronic care facilities,* Villanova, Penn., June 1994, National Committee for Clinical Laboratory Standards.

Rock RC: Why testing is being moved to the site of patient care, *Med Lab Observer* 23(9S):2-5, 1991.

Robinson MR, Eaton RP, Haaland DM, et al: Noninvasive glucose monitoring in diabetic patients: a preliminary evaluation, *Clin Chem* 38:1618-1622, 1992.

Salem M, Chernow B, Burke R, et al: Bedside diagnostic testing: its accuracy, rapidity, and utility in blood conservation, *JAMA* 266:382-389, 1991.

Suver JD, Neumann BR, Boles EE: Accounting for the costs of quality, *Health Finance Management* 9:29-37, 1992.

Winkelman JW, Wybenga DR, Tanasijevic MJ: The fiscal consequences of central vs. distributed testing of glucose, *Clin Chem* 40:1628-1630, 1994.

Laboratory information systems

David Chou

OBJECTIVES

■ Describe the functions, operational characteristics, and work flow of a laboratory information system (LIS) in a clinical laboratory.

■ Describe the problems, importance, and needs for instrument interfaces, computer interfaces, and data information interchange between computers.

■ Describe the basic computer terminology and the technology associated with laboratory information systems.

■ Describe the type of information generated by the LIS, which can track the quality of health care in the hospital setting.

KEY TERMS

ADT (admissions/discharge/transfer) Administrative and demographic patient information that is provided by a central computer system. In particular, this information concerns patient admissions, transfers, and discharges.

applications programs Programs written to support specific end-user functions, such as ADT (above). The computer interactions visible to most users are those with applications programs.

archived data Patient data that are removed from immediate access on the LIS system, placed in a form not immediately accessible by the user, and that require intervention on the part of a computer operator.

backup A procedure, usually performed daily, where operational data on disks are transferred to a secondary medium, usually magnetic tape. Normally data on these tapes will be restored to disk only in the event that the disk fails.

bar code A series of parallel lines of varying thicknesses, printed in a fashion to represent numbers or numbers and letters and that can be read by automated equipment.

bidirectional interface A program that allows electronic communications between an instrument and an LIS, permitting the interchange of information in both directions.

central processing unit (CPU) The part of the computer responsible for the execution of programs and making decisions (that is, the brains of the computer).

client/server A system design where two or more computers share in the processing of data. Information stored on the "server" computer is downloaded to the "client" computer for independent processing. This process is then reversed when data are uploaded.

cumulative report A report designed to display results over a period of time for a single patient in a tabular fashion.

data structure The organization of the data as it is stored in the computer.

database manager A program designed to manage the storage and retrieval of data to and from computer storage media such as disks or tapes.

delta check A method of quality control where the current patient result is compared to a previous patient result.

downtime Any period of time when a computer system is unavailable for use.

duplicate order The same test ordered within a short time frame that may or may not be necessary for patient care.

file maintenance A program that is executed on a regular basis for managing and reorganizing data, usually on disk, for optimal storage and retrieval.

hardware The physical parts of a computer. Hardware remains largely unchanged after manufacturing.

hierarchical database A database design that treats data as a hierarchical or treelike relationship.

incomplete list A report printed by the LIS listing specimens and tests that have not yet been processed. Different incomplete lists may be printed for each task performed in the laboratory.

interface A program or programs that allow two computers to interchange data electronically.

interpretive reports Reports generated providing information to the clinician that differ depending on the results and describe possible treatment or diagnostic possibilities for the given set of results.

laboratory information system (LIS) One or more applications software packages and the associated operating system software and the hardware needed to run computer programs that support the operational and management needs of a clinical laboratory.

local area network (LAN) A digital computer network that services a localized area, usually limited to under several miles in distance.

mainframe computer A computer characterized by costs exceeding $500,000 and supported interdepartmentally. Mainframes usually require special electrical power and air conditioning.

minicomputer A computer characterized by costs in the $25,000 to $500,000 range most often supported at the departmental level.

network or digital computer network The use of cable television, microwave, or fiber-optic technology to permit high-speed communications between a group of computers.

network database A database design that attempts to keep only a single copy of data through the use of complex indices or pointers to the data.

on-line Data that are kept in a computer in a manner that allows immediate access.

operating system Software designed to supervise the orderly execution of programs and provide support for basic functions utilized by most programs.

order entry The action of entering test orders into a computer system. This order process may occur on the LIS or a remote computer linked to the LIS.

patient demographics Pertinent clinical and administrative patient information collected at the time of patient admission. These include the patient number, name, sex, age, birth date, and other information relating to the patient. This information defines and identifies the patient in the system.

personal computer A small desktop computer designed to be used by a single user in the office or home environment and costing between $1000 and $5000.

program A series of instructions directing computer hardware to perform specified actions.

programming languages A structured set of instructions designed to be translated into detailed instructions for the computer hardware. Most languages are English-like and are designed to make writing instructions for the computer easier.

relational database A database design defined by E.F. Codd based on set theory. The operations allowable in a relational database are similar to that for sets. This database allows information to be retrieved as it is related (in sets), not as a file where only the information in the file can be retrieved.

run As defined by the Clinical Laboratory Improvement Amendments of 1988 (CLIA' 88), a run is an interval within which the accuracy and precision of a testing system are expected to be stable but cannot be greater than 24 hours.

software Collectively, the programs that operate the computer.

software maintenance Changes in software intended to fix problems, to improve functionality, or to provide new capabilities.

specimen number A number, usually 4 to 10 digits in length, assigned by the LIS to a sample for identification purposes. The number may be reused periodically and must not duplicate any specimen still being processed.

unidirectional interface A program that permits electronic communication between an LIS and instrument, permitting the instrument to send or upload information to the LIS.

validation The process whereby a technologist reviews one or more analyses and releases the results to the patient file for reporting.

virus A software program, often destructive in nature, designed to embed itself into the operating system or other commonly available software.

wide area network (WAN) A digital computer network that services an area larger than 1 to 2 miles in distance. WANs are usually networks that provide intercity services.

worklist A list of specimen numbers generated by a technologist before performing a specified task, such as an analytical run or a specimen collection.

The function of the laboratory is to provide information to physicians. This information is usually in the form of data derived from the analysis of patient samples. This information transfer requires that the data be integrated with the patient's entire database. To perform the information transfer rapidly and efficiently, a computer-based information system, called a laboratory information system, is needed.

The *laboratory information system,* or *LIS,* can be defined as one or more applications software packages along with the associated operating system software and the hardware needed to run computer programs that support the operational and management needs of a clinical laboratory. Because the spectrum of services required by an LIS can significantly differ from one laboratory to another, both the software and the hardware can significantly vary. Most successful information systems structure routine tasks and assist in the integration of diversified processes. As a secondary benefit, the LIS provides management data and imposes management controls. An LIS, therefore, must be closely tuned to the operating needs of each laboratory and its organization. The computer can be a powerful tool for improving both productivity and quality, and, unlike an automated instrument, which primarily affects the technologists operating it, the LIS directly influences almost everyone within the laboratory and many users outside the laboratory.

Most LIS's depend on the joining of technologies provided by two or more vendors. Each vendor in the technology chain builds upon products and systems developed by other vendors. At the highest level in this chain are software called *applications programs.* This is the end product that is recognized as the LIS by most users. The vendor developing a modern LIS will write applications programs utilizing the second layer of the technology chain. These consist of software development tools such as the *database manager,* the *programming language* or *languages,* and the *operating system.* Such tools are typically provided by one or more vendors unrelated to the LIS applications software vendor. Finally, a vendor provides the *hardware,* or the physical computer that executes the software. Because of the close relationship between the hardware and the operating system, these are frequently provided by a single vendor. A single vendor minimizes the likelihood that a problem with an LIS program may be related to a defect in the operating system developed by another vendor. The use of more than one vendor allows the user to dissociate applications software changes from changes in the hardware.

LIS CHARACTERISTICS
Overall functions

Over the last several years, LIS's available in the marketplace have become increasingly standardized. Most systems contain modules supporting many tasks such as specimen collection, order entry, manual results entry, results reporting, and interfaces to automated instrumentation and computers (see box). Additional modules usually included are those providing management reports and other ad hoc reports. LIS's for hospitals support phlebotomy by providing blood drawing lists, the ability to print labels, and other essential organizing duties; systems for independent laboratories usually include specimen tracking and financial and billing functions. Separation of the LIS into discrete modules is done for marketing and functional reasons. Typically one such module supports general laboratory functions for high-volume testing areas that provide numeric answers, as in hematology and chemistry. Other modules support microbiology, blood banking, and anatomic pathology. Larger institutions may use two or more LIS vendors to meet their needs. In such cases, one vendor may provide a system to meet the needs of general laboratory functions, whereas another vendor provides supports for one or more additional areas such as blood bank, anatomic pathology, or customer billing. Many LIS vendors interface to third-party blood bank software to minimize Food and Drug Administration regulatory requirements. The following sections cover features of an LIS that supports the sample analysis process in the general laboratory areas.

Patient demographics

Before any test requesting can occur, the patient must first be identified and defined in the system. Most hospitals as-

---

LIS Functions

Preanalytical
Test ordering
Phlebotomy draw lists
Phlebotomy (labels, collection times)
Specimen accessioning and aliquoting
Specimen tracking

Analytical
Manual worklist
Instrument worklist
Manual results entry
Automated results entry through interfaces
Patient delta check
Quality control
Results validation

Postanalytical
Noncumulative patient chart reports
Patient cumulative chart reports
Immediate remote report printing
Electronic results inquiry
Historical patient archiving
Work-load recording
Results correction
Billing

---

sign a permanent, unique patient identification number for this purpose. This combined with other related information is called *patient demographics.* Systems servicing reference laboratories or outreach programs may define patients under the auspices of the client sending the test. A clerk can manually enter the demographic information into the LIS. Alternatively, an interface between an LIS and an ADT (for admissions, discharge, and transfer) administrative computer system allows the information to be transmitted to the LIS when needed during test request processing or transmitted automatically upon admission of the patient elsewhere in the hospital. Automated ADT interfaces can significantly reduce the errors and entry time associated with manual data entry. Demographic information entered at this time include (1) the patient number (which may be the social security number), (2) patient name, (3) sex, (4) age or birth date, (5) race, (6) referring or attending physician who will receive reports by default, and (7) admitting diagnosis. Most systems also capture some patient information such as height and weight as well as billing and accounting information. If a patient number cannot be determined, as when one is handling an unconscious accident patient treated in an emergency room, the laboratory may assign a temporary number and pseudonym. The temporary patient information must be changed later and merged into a record with the proper patient information.

Order entry

After the admission of the patient, the next LIS interaction is usually the processing of a test request, also known as *order entry*. Orders may be received by the LIS through a computer-to-computer interface, for example, with a hospital information system (HIS), from which nursing personnel or physicians[1] can directly order the test. Alternatively, the laboratory receives a paper requisition from a clinical area, and laboratory personnel enter the test request into the LIS. Typically, order entry requires the entry of the information listed in the following box. This process is known as *data acquisition*.

Numerous checks are performed by the LIS as a part of the data entry process. Most systems maintain internal tables that contain lists of valid test entry personnel, physicians, patient locations, available laboratory tests, and even reasonable dates. These tables prevent the entry of erroneous information but also require updates, also referred to as *table maintenance*. Most institutions also incorporate a *check digit* with patient numbers or any other long number that requires some form of self-validation. This is usually a single digit included as a part of the patient number that is computed during data entry from digits in the patient number. If the computed number does not match the check digit, the datum entry is rejected. For example, if the patient number is 12345676 and the last digit is the check digit, one way to generate a check-digit calculation is to use the formula:

check digit

$$= [2*C_1 + 3*C_2 + 4*C_3 + 5*C_4 + 6*C_5 + 7*C_6 + 2*C_7] \text{ module } 10$$

where the *module* function is the remainder after dividing the result by 10. Therefore the calculated result is:

check digit

$$= [2*(1) + 3*(2) + 4*(3) + 5*(4) + 6*(5) + 7*(6) + 2*(7)]$$
$$= 126 \text{ module } 10$$
$$= 6$$

If the clerk types 22345676, the check-digit calculation will

result in a 7. Since 6 is expected, the patient number is rejected by the computer. Check digits do not guarantee accuracy but if properly designed help reduce errors. In this example, the odds of matching the check digit by a random process are 1 in 10.

During the order-entry step, the LIS may also check for duplicate orders. A *duplicate order* occurs when the same test or test panel is ordered more than once within a defined sequence of time. Duplicate-order checks are complicated, since any check for a single test must investigate that test ordered by itself as well as a component of any ordering groups, such as a test panel. The allowable interval between duplicate test orders depends on the preferences of the ordering physician, the patient location, the test, economics, and a multitude of other factors. For example, the interval for a duplicate electrolyte panel in an intensive care unit might be less than an hour, whereas the time for a duplicate testosterone level in an outpatient setting might be several days. For most tests, knowledge of the clinical situation is required before it is possible to determine whether it has been inappropriately ordered. Unless ordering is performed by the physician caring for the patient, such information is rarely available at the time tests are ordered. Determination of the appropriate duplicate-test interval through the consensus of all ordering clinicians or a detailed review of their practices is a formidable task, and physicians generally resist performing their own test ordering because of the time required with current technology. Most laboratories check for duplicate orders only to resolve operational problems and to control situations when the same test is accidentally ordered twice. Duplicate-order checking by itself is rarely effective in changing ordering behavior or for reducing test utilization.

Sample identification

If the specimen has already been collected, laboratory personnel log it into the LIS as received. Otherwise the computer places the test requisition onto a collection list for future collection. In either case, a specimen label will usually be generated by the LIS, which contains patient demographics, patient location, tests ordered, and collection tube type (Fig. 18-1). Most specimen labels also include a *specimen*

Data Acquired During Order-Entry Process

1. A patient identifier, such as a patient number and a patient name
2. One or more ordering physicians
3. One or more physicians receiving reports with their reporting locations
4. Test request time and date
5. Time the specimen was collected or will be collected
6. Person entering the request
7. Tests to be performed
8. Priority of the test request (such as stat., now, routine)
9. Any special comments or instructions pertaining to the request

---

VALIDATION PATIENT
9-999-999-3

PLC   02/28/94 11:05

DIGOXIN

398291

AUPS

Fig. 18-1 An example of a bar-coded specimen label. The six-digit specimen number (398291) is bar coded. The patient number, patient demographics, time/date, and test are written in human readable form.

number, or *accession number,* an identification number that allows the computer to reference that sample back to a specific test request and patient. Specimen numbers may be assigned for each phlebotomy transaction or, less commonly, for each orderable test. Another approach utilized by larger laboratories requires separate specimen number sequences for different processing areas. For example, numbers from 100,000 to 199,999 are reserved for chemistry, from 200,000 to 299,999 for hematology, and so on. To keep numbers short, most systems will recycle specimen numbers. Systems that reuse specimen numbers must check to see if a number is being used on an active specimen before reassigning it. Some systems assign a permanent specimen number by combining a date code with a short sequence number. Although this offers advantages of a permanent specimen number, the larger number complicates manual data entry. In most cases the LIS produces an assignation of a specimen number at the time of test requisition, but for tests ordered far into the future this assignment may occur later. Some systems allow users to reserve specimen numbers for manual assignment. Although this is convenient under conditions such as computer failure, manual assignment of specimen numbers greatly increases errors, especially if users accidentally assign the same specimen number to unrelated samples.

The sample identification number is usually printed on the sample label as an arabic number and is often duplicated in a bar-code format. *Bar codes* consist of a series of small parallel lines of varying widths that are used to represent numbers or letters and numbers and that are readable by automated equipment. A number of bar-code formats exist, but the most commonly used format in hospitals is Code 39. The older Codabar format has been used for labeling blood bank products. Codabar is limited to representing numbers, whereas Code 39 can represent both numeric and upper-case alphabetic characters. Code 128 is recommended for new applications, since it can represent lower case and other characters not available in Code 39. Most current bar-code readers and printers automatically read and print several formats. Bar-code labels are typically printed using thermally sensitive paper or with a thermally sensitive ribbon that transfers images to the label. Bar-code readers may be self-scanning, such as laser-based units found in grocery stores, or user scanned with a penlike device. Self-scanning bar-code readers are more expensive than pens but are easier to use.

Bar coding the specimen label greatly decreases errors in specimen handling as well as increases productivity.[2] For maximum benefit, specimen bar-coding must be coordinated with automated instrumentation, preferably those that directly sample from the venipuncture tube and automatically read bar codes. Mechanical limitations of instruments and venipuncture tubes limit the bar-code size. Larger bar codes read more reliably, but consume label space and may prevent printing of valuable human-readable information.

Since the patient number is both larger and not unique to a given test request, only the specimen number or a part of the specimen number is typically bar coded.

Phlebotomy

For samples to be collected on some future scheduled phlebotomy runs, the computer prints up a collection list and specimen-collection labels. The specimen labels can also serve as the collection list for the phlebotomist. The LIS may also be able to print the collection list in an order that will optimize the phlebotomist's rounds. After specimen collection, the phlebotomist or a clerk verifies collected samples and deletes or reschedules uncollected requests in the LIS. Hand-held computers with built-in bar-code readers also allow phlebotomists to verify collection at the bedside and download the status of each collection to the host computer upon return to the laboratory, thus reducing time for phlebotomy verification and increasing the accuracy of the draw time. To further increase phlebotomy accuracy, bar coding of the patient identification band allows a phlebotomist with a hand-held unit to match specimen requests to the proper patient.

Sample transport and tracking

After collection, the specimen must be prepared for transport or analysis. The LIS often prints additional labels for aliquoting or other purposes, either as part of the initial test request or on demand. If processing occurs at a satellite location, the LIS can track the sample for transportation time and specimen location to help determine transportation time and for locating lost specimens, but because of the additional effort, tracking is not commonly used. Specimen tracking may be useful in larger laboratories with long transport times where clinicians frequently request additional tests on a sample that is presumed to be already in the laboratory. In such cases, tracking assists the technologist in locating an acceptable sample, after which he or she enters the new "add-on" test into the LIS and prints a new specimen label. If an acceptable specimen cannot be found, the test request must be entered into the LIS to allow a phlebotomist or nurse to recollect it. The complexity of the process for handling add-on testing frequently results in errors.

Analytical instrument interfaces

Automated instruments perform most testing in clinical laboratories. Interfacing between an instrument and the LIS requires compatibility of software and hardware but once accomplished greatly improves productivity and decreases errors. The LIS and the instrument must be linked by a compatible physical connection. Most clinical laboratory instruments expect the physical data interface to adhere to the Electronic Industries Association RS-232C standard.[3] To reduce variations in this specification, the American Society for Testing and Materials (ASTM) issued the E1381 standard, which more closely specifies the physical requirements and electrical interactions.[4] Interface software must be available on the LIS to allow it to receive data from and transmit data to the instrument. Although the physical connection between instruments and the LIS requires minimal adaptation, considerable software differences exist among automated instruments even with software standards such as ASTM E1394.[5] Since current standards are not satisfactory, most instrument manufacturers provide LIS vendors with instrument-interface specifications before they are introduced into the marketplace to allow time for interface software development. This usually requires separate software programs (and expense) for each instrument. For some instruments, several software-interface programs are needed to handle different versions of the same instrument.

An interfaced instrument must link each specimen to its specific test request. Many modern instruments link the specimen through its bar-coded specimen number on the specimen label. Typically the instrument reads the bar-coded specimen label and transmits the number to the LIS along with the analytical results. An interface is *unidirectional* if the instrument only transmits, or *uploads,* results to the LIS computer; the interface is *bidirectional* if the LIS can transmit, or *download,* information to the instrument while it receives uploaded information from the instrument. The most common information downloaded to an instrument from the LIS are the tests that have been requested for the specimen. In a bidirectionally interfaced instrument, the instrument first transmits the specimen number to the LIS, the LIS then returns the information of which tests have been ordered, the instrument automatically performs the requested tests, and finally the instrument sends the results to the LIS. The communications and interactions between the host LIS computer and the instrument can be complex. Adding to this complexity is the requirement of some instruments for an immediate response from the LIS upon reading the bar-coded specimen number. The software required for a unidirectional interface, therefore, is considerably simpler than that for a bidirectional interface.

If the instrument does not have the ability to identify the specimen automatically through the interface, the operator must manually link the sample at the instrument to the specimen number in the computer. The order in which the LIS processes specimens for a specified instrument is called a *worklist,* or a *loadlist.* At least three ways are used to create the worklist. One method is to have the instrument operator manually create ("build") a worklist on the LIS by entering specimen numbers and the instrument position. For example, position 1 on the instrument contains specimen A, position 2 contains specimen B, and so on. Alternatively, only the specimen number can be entered, and the instrument position order is implicitly provided without a physical cup or tray position. This method requires that results are released from the instrument in the order that specimens are processed. Using a hand-held bar-code scanner, the technologist can use the LIS to build the worklist rapidly in a more automated fashion that is less prone to error. The third approach is to have the computer automatically build a worklist, typically in the order that specimens are received or in sample number order, and to have the operator load the instrument in that order. This frees the operator from entering the information needed for the worklist but requires him or her to locate specimens and load them in the specified order. For the smaller laboratory, the computer-generated worklist is usually more efficient, since the receiving area can often place the specimens in the computer specified order. In the larger laboratory, multiple receiving areas complicate the specimen receipt order, making it easier for the operator to specify explicitly the worklist with one of the first two approaches rather than searching for a specific specimen.

Problems arise when two or more bar-coded instruments are used to perform the same test and each instrument has a different bar-code label requirement. This problem is further complicated by the limited space available on the small venipuncture tubes, preventing the application of multiple bar codes. If the different requirements do not allow for a common label format, the user must decide on a default format or, if the LIS allows, set up criteria to select the most likely format. Misapplication of the specimen label also causes instruments to misread bar codes. If a correct bar-code label is required, the user must reprint it before running the sample at the instrument. The ASTM has published a standard for placement of bar codes on specimens. Because of mechanical limitations of some existing instrument designs, actual adaptation of the bar-code standard[6] may be delayed until older designs are replaced.

Data verification

With any interfaced instrument, the operator reviews and approves, or *validates,* test results before they are released for patient reporting. Usually validation is performed by a worklist. This validation process starts with the LIS printing a *validation report,* followed by the technologist excluding results and then batch validating the entire worklist on a terminal. An alternative procedure is a paperless one, validating one specimen at a time on an LIS terminal without a validation report. Batch validation may be more efficient for the instrument operator but delays reporting. For most systems, the validation review occurs in the specimen order the worksheet was created or in the numeric order of specimen numbers. If results exceed predetermined parameters, the instrument operator must perform specified activities, such as a dilution or a repeat analysis. Frequently, the LIS displays both the initial and reanalyzed results and allows the operator to validate one of the results, or reject both.

Some instruments, particularly those for blood-gas analyses, process samples on a one-at-a-time basis. Test ordering frequently occurs at the time of analysis rather than in advance. For such instruments, the interaction between the analyzer, the LIS, and the operator will be greater and more labor intensive than that for other instruments. The test request, result entry, and validation processes are similar to instruments mentioned earlier but occur serially and manually for each sample. Some older hematology analyzers also operate in this fashion.

Results entry

Automated. The interaction between a technologist and automated instrumentation has been partially discussed previously. For a bidirectionally interfaced instrument, the results entry process proceeds automatically. Most LIS's place the results in a pending area, waiting for the technologist to manually review and validate the entered results (see previous section). This holding area limits results access only to those in the laboratory. Upon validation, results are released for reporting to external users. Several features may be available through the LIS to help the technologist during the review process. Typically these include the display of flags signifying results outside reference ranges, life-threatening results (critical, or "panic," values), results outside technical ranges, or those failing delta checks (*"delta check"*; see Chapter 3). Most LIS can also display previous results for the same tests, allowing the operator to do a check for sample misidentification. Calculations, such as the anion gap, may also be performed during the validation process. All the specifications of these features must be built into the LIS by laboratory personnel.

Manual. The laboratory must perform manual results entry for specimens analyzed manually or for tests performed on instruments that are not interfaced. Low-volume instruments may not be interfaced because of the economic restraints of an interface or because of the complexity of building worklists and validating them. Manual results entry may also be used when interfaces have failed or under special conditions such as abnormal tests being repeated on a different instrument. For batched tests, the operator first generates a manual worklist, similar to that described for an instrument, and prints a worksheet. The printed worksheet will usually contain a list of specimen numbers with patient demographics and blank spaces for a user to write in results. This worksheet is a guide for the specimen-processing order and provides a place for manual transcription of results so that they can be later entered with a terminal.

As the technologist manually enters results into the computer terminal, most systems will check the data for technical credibility, life-threatening conditions, delta checks, abnormal limits, previous results, and other conditions that may have been specified by the site, similar to that for automated systems. To assist in the data entry process, software can perform automatic calculations, and terminals can be set up so that keyboards perform special functions. For example, programs can convert the numeric pad on a data entry terminal to a differential counter. To support the uri-

nalysis area the computer can translate the single keystroke *m* into the word *many.* After results are entered, a validation report similar to that for an automated instrument is printed. This report is similar to the initial worklist with test results replacing blank lines. Normally, the technologist performing the test will also validate the worklist in a manner similar to that for automated instruments. In some areas, a second technologist may be required to validate critical results in addition to, or in lieu of, the first technologist. Even with computer assistance, manual data entry can be tedious and error prone, particularly if worklists are much longer than 100 to 150 tests. For efficiency, manual data entry occurs at the end of the work day or at the end of a run. This may also delay results reporting if completed results are held for data entry.

Results reporting

The end product of any clinical laboratory is its results, usually in the form of paper reports. Paper reports continue to be required as a legal entry of results into the patient's chart, and they remain an important method for communication of laboratory results. Electronic transmittal of results by the LIS to printers, computer terminals, or hand-held pager terminals provides a more rapid alternative for making results available to physicians at any time, without user intervention. Remote terminals allow users to retrieve both current and historical data at any time. Depending on location and user expertise, any combination of these LIS options may be installed to reduce the delays associated with test-result availability to seconds, even though physical charting of reports continues to take hours to days. In many institutions, electronic reporting and retrieval of results have replaced all paper reports except those required for the patient chart. Terminals and remote pagers can greatly reduce the use of the telephone for results queries, saving personnel time and reducing associated transcription errors.

Accreditation agencies and medical practice continue to require paper reports for the medical chart. Paper reports continue to be important for accessing test results not required immediately. For outpatients, the LIS prints a report nightly with all test results that have been completed. In addition to the report needed for the patient's chart, duplicate copies are sent to ordering physicians or other clinical personnel. Most outpatient reports record the result in a straightforward manner containing (1) patient demographics, (2) time of report generation, (3) name of laboratory reporting and performing the test, if all the results are not from the same laboratory, (4) test name or names, (5) collection date and time for a test or tests, (6) result with abnormal flags as needed, (7) reference range, (8) result and order comments, and (9) ordering physician or physicians. With electronic reporting, location reports serve little or no purpose, since they are less timely and more difficult to use. Federal regulations (Clinical Laboratory Improvement Amendment of 1988, CLIA '88) and common sense dictate

THE CLEVELAND CLINIC FOUNDATION
Division of Pathology and Laboratory Medicine
Department of Clinical Pathology
9500 Euclid Avenue, Cleveland, Ohio 44195
LABORATORY REPORT

Page 2
1/29/93
21:42

PATIENT LOCATION	NUMBER	NAME	AGE	SEX	CATEGORY
G110-06		Gladys M	78Y	F	O
F15					

PRIMARY PHYSICIAN;   04019   MILLER, PAUL

ADMIT DATE: 01/25/93   DISCHARGED: 01/29/93

* * * * * * * * * * * * * * * * * HEMATOLOGY BLOOD COUNTS * * * * * * * * * * * * * * * * * *

		WBC	RBC	HGB	HCT	PLTCT	MCV	MCH	MCHC
Ref. Range:		4.0	4.2	12	37	150.0	80	27	32
		11.0	5.4	16	47	400.0	100	34	36
UNIT:		K/UL	M/UL	G/DL	%	K/UL	FL	PG	G/DL
DATE	TIME								
0126	0800	8.30	4.18*	9.9*	32.6	275	77.9*	23.6*	30.2*
0126	1825	9.53	3.83*	8.7*	30.2*	264	78.8*	22.8*	28.9
0127	0900			10.0*	33.8*				
0127	1600			10.7*	33.3*				
0128	0400	7.71	4.01*	9.9*	32.3*	236	78.0*	24.7*	31.7*
0128	1605			9.7*	32.6*				
0129	0500	8.43	4.20	9.6*	32.7*	225	77.9*	22.8*	29.3*
0129	1430			11.3*	35.7*				

Fig. 18-2   A cumulative patient report.

that LISs have the capability to reprint reports easily on demand. Printer jams and, more commonly, lost reports occur frequently in most institutions using location reports.

For inpatients, chart reports are usually printed in a *cumulative* format (Fig. 18-2), in which current and past results are printed in a tabular format. Most commonly, tests appear as a column on the page with test-result dates displayed in rows horizontally. An alternative format is to have the dates appear in columns and tests in rows. With this tabular format, a very high density of results can appear on a page. Upon admission, any results reported within the last 3 to 5 days may be included in the cumulative report. Typically, the report will accumulate results for an entire inpatient stay or some other predetermined interval. Temporary reports are printed until the end of this interval (as on patient discharge), at which time a final permanent report is

printed. The cumulative format is almost always used for inpatients but rarely for outpatients. For these patients, reports typically contain one or more lines for a single test result (Fig. 18-3). The main reason for not using cumulative reports on outpatients is the difficulty in charting reports and difficulty in determining the next time tests will be ordered.

Printer technology continues to change, resulting in changing appearances in patient reports. With conventional impact printers, the uniformity of the typefaces in reports makes them difficult to read and prohibits graphics. With laser printers, varying sizes and typefaces help emphasize significant findings and make reports more readable but at higher costs for printer consumables. Many LIS's allow the inclusion of *interpretive reports* to assist clinicians. These reports contain comments to explain one or more result patterns. Such reports, though welcomed by primary care prac-

THE CLEVELAND CLINIC FOUNDATION
Division of Pathology and Laboratory Medicine
Department of Clinical Pathology
9500 Euclid Avenue, Cleveland, Ohio 44195
LABORATORY REPORT

Page 1
9/15/93
03:56

PATIENT LOCATION	NUMBER	NAME	AGE	SEX	CATEGORY
F25		Catherine	62Y	F	O

REQUESTING PHYSICIAN: 00300 HEUPLER, FREDERICK A

SPC-#/COLL	TEST	RESULT	UNIT	REF. RANGE	N COMMENTS
259024 A	SMA-16 PROFILE				
9/13 09:21					
	TP	8.8*	G/DL	6.0-8.0	
	ALB	4.9	G/DL	3.5-5.0	
	CA	9.5	MG/DL	8.5-10.5	
	PHOS	3.6	MG/DL	2.5-4.5	
	GLUCOSE	88	MG/DL	65-110	
	URIC A	6.8	MG/DL	2.0-7.0	
	T BILI	0.3	MG/DL	0-1.5	
	ALK P	167*	U/L	20-120	
	LD	164	U/L	100-220	
	AST	17	U/L	7-40	
	NA	138	MMOL/L	134-145	
	K	4.2	MMOL/L	3.5-5.0	
	CL	106	MMOL/L	98-108	
	CO2	21*	MMOL/L	24-32	
	BUN	53*	MG/DL	8-25	
	CREAT	1.9*	MG/DL	0.7-1.4	

Fig. 18-3 A noncumulative patient report.

titioners, are likely to be ignored by specialists, and the laboratory must use them selectively. Most systems still do not allow inclusion of graphical images in reports.

Quality control

(See also Chapter 21.)

The LIS can also contribute greatly to improve the efficiency of benchside technologists and laboratory managers by supporting quality control (QC) procedures. The daily QC activities that maintain the precision and accuracy of results tend to be fairly consistent among most laboratories, particularly with respect to the regulatory requirements that require strict adherence to specified guidelines. These regulations (CLIA '88; DHHS, 1990) require that laboratories retain quality control information associated with any re-

leased test result, and most LIS's automatically or manually capture these data.

CLIA '88 defines a *run* as an interval for which the accuracy and precision of a testing system are expected to be stable but cannot be greater than 24 hours (CLIA '88, 1992). Most LIS's allow users to define a run that matches a physical sample tray or to perform continuous analyses between controls. These runs, however, may not meet CLIA requirements if they do not have proper control samples. Some LIS's treat controls as if they were patient samples and perform statistical analyses later; others treat controls in a manner that provides the user with immediate feedback. Most instruments have built-in computers, and it is uncommon for an LIS to support the derivation of standard curves from calibration samples. Although the LIS can restrict release of results for runs by producing a review of the results for controls, of status instrument, and patient demographics, most systems leave such decisions to the operator.

Numerous quality control calculations and checks are easily and commonly performed by an LIS, allowing the technologists to review and interpret QC data conveniently. These include routine checking for controls that deviate more than a specified number of standard deviations from an expected mean or values that deviate from expected limits according to more complex rules.[7] In larger laboratories interinstrument, intermethod, and test-level comparisons of controls and calibrations help assure result consistency. Most LIS systems can typically provide such quality control information both in summary format and as the analysis is performed. The Levy-Jennings plot is a popular tool for following and displaying such information. Typically the LIS will stratify quality control statistics by instrument, by methodology, and by analyte and allow comparisons of controls at all three levels. Delta checking a patient value with his or her own previous result can also assist in identifying a specimen identification problem.[8,9]

Quality assurance

(See also Chapters 2, 3, and 21.)

The LIS can collect and provide information useful for quality assurance (QA) activities. The ability of the LIS to perform 100% sampling with little effort encourages a level of laboratory monitoring not possible with a manual system. QA activities are used by management to uncover and correct problems related to the laboratory's ability to provide the required level of service. Several examples of how the LIS can assist in QA activities follow.

First, turnaround time has become an important indicator of the overall average quality of service for high-accuracy areas of the hospital. Coupled with specimen tracking, such information assists the laboratory manager in identifying operational bottlenecks by looking at samples that exceed predetermined parameters. This helps to staff areas properly and identify peak work periods.

Second, reports on error corrections can assist in identifying sources of error. Errors can occur during the preanalytical processing, during test analysis, or after analysis. The most frequent error in the preanalytical process is misidentification of the patient or the specimen. Preanalytically and postanalytically, manual data entry can have as much as a 1% to 3% error rate, most of which is unlikely to be detected even with sophisticated tools such as delta checking, or supervisor validation. One way of evaluating errors is to compare the data entered into the computer automatically with the data expected to be entered manually. Although this comparison can be tedious, it can identify systematic problems associated with data entry of results or requisitions. The computer can also provide information regarding the test results that have been corrected. Most systems provide a way to change results after they have been validated. De-

pending on the laboratory, the function to correct results may be limited to a few individuals. Possibly the most difficult aspect about changing results lies in the effect on patient reports. Although reports may be reprinted, older reports remain in the chart and are potentially confusing. Most federal and other regulatory agencies require that corrected results be indicated as such on patient reports.

Third, the laboratory can monitor the quality of patient care by combining data available in other hospital computer systems of the hospital, such as a pharmacy system. Adverse effects associated with gentamicin, for example, can be reduced by coupling drug dispensation records with drug levels, renal function tests, and antimicrobial sensitivity patterns. This information can then be used to warn a clinician of either toxic or ineffective dosing.

Fourth, a simple report of patients with grossly abnormal results provides interesting laboratory teaching cases as well as detecting possible problems.

Most LISs perform significant QA reporting through epidemiology and cytology subsystems to meet Joint Committee on Accreditation of Health Organizations and CLIA regulations. Although these activities can be performed on other computers, the level of detail contained in most LISs in these areas allows more accurate reporting. Most information systems are capable of generating far more data than can be reviewed. Such customized reports require human resources and computer time and must be justified by their usefulness in meeting QA goals.

The following box provides some examples of management reports available through an LIS. See Chapter 2 for additional examples.

Management reporting

Management reports and QA reports differ only in their intended purpose. In theory, management reports provide information that can be used to improve efficiency of operations through reallocation of people and resources.

Examples of LIS Reports*

Quality assurance
Turnaround time
Correction of results after release
Correlation of lab results with drug administration
Correlation of antimicrobial sensitivities with antibiotic administration

Management report
Test volume by laboratory area
Work-load statistics
Utilization patterns
Revenue and cost/revenue patterns

---

*A more complete list is in Chapter 2.

QA reports are used to improve the overall quality of service.

Although some view the management reports as a by-product of implementing a computer system, others view them as a principal benefit of a computer. However, the management information provided by information systems may not prove useful until trends have been established after several years. Much of the information collected for QC and QA mentioned earlier may also be used as management reports. One of the more commonly used reports from any LIS is a list of tests and their ordering frequency. This information may be utilized from an operational perspective for projecting the need for instrumentation, personnel, and other resources. Using computer statistics, standard methods for monitoring work load provide information regarding appropriate personnel staffing and can help to reschedule employees as test-ordering patterns change.[10] Work-load information also helps to identify inefficient work areas or individuals. Another common report is a list of billing transactions, usually generated nightly.

All laboratory computer systems can provide data on physician test-ordering patterns. Unfortunately, these data are frequently difficult to interpret, since requisitions may not allow one to identify the ordering physician, or the test was requested by a medical student using an attending physician's name. The politics of managing test ordering are also difficult. With the advent of cost containment in healthcare, however, such data are being utilized more frequently to focus on and to eliminate unnecessary testing.

LIS TECHNOLOGY

Hardware refers to the physical parts of a computer, which largely remain unchanged after manufacturing. Most hardware is mass produced in factories. *Software* collectively refers to a series of instructions, called *programs,* that direct the actions of a computer. In contrast to hardware, software is frequently updated after its delivery. Programming, the intellectual process of creating programs, requires large amounts of time and effort. As a consequence, software costs have risen dramatically even as hardware costs drop. In 1970, software contributed to approximately 10% of the total cost of a computer system, and by 1980 that contribution increased to more than 60%. Today an LIS includes applications software, database managers, interpreters, and operating systems, and this software contributes more than 75% of the total cost of a system. Rapidly dropping hardware costs, increasing demands for more information, and interfacing between systems will further increase the software-to-hardware cost ratio. Since software represents such a major investment in a purchased system and hardware vendors change products rapidly and may not be able to support their products for long-term periods, most software companies try to design their products to be somewhat hardware independent.

Hardware

Computer hardware continues to change dramatically even after more than 30 years of continuous evolution. Traditionally, LIS vendors have used *minicomputers,* a class of computers loosely characterized by costs in the $50,000 to $500,000 range and supported at the departmental level. LIS vendors, particularly those supporting the smaller laboratories, have also produced products using personal computers that cost less than $1500 each to take advantage of the lower hardware costs. Less commonly, vendors distribute LIS software for *mainframes,* a class of computers that often cost more than $500,000. Economics dictate that an LIS operating on a mainframe can be cost effective only if it is shared with other software, such as a financial system. LIS application software operating on one class of computers will usually require significant reprogramming if it is to be used on other classes of computers.

At the heart of any computer hardware design lies the *central processing unit,* or *CPU.* A CPU is responsible for making logical decisions, performing computations, and translating program instructions into actions. Typically, the CPU consists of one (or more) silicon chip along with some associated circuitry. The terms *RISC,* for *reduced instruction set computer,* or *CISC,* for *complex instruction set computer,* have been used to describe the various classifications of CPU designs. Compared to a CISC design, an RISC design is simpler but requires more instructions to be executed for a given task. An RISC computer typically runs faster than a CISC design but requires more memory and disk resources. As memory and disk prices drop, RISC designs are becoming more common. A CPU also requires *RAM,* for *random-access memory,* which is used by the CPU to store data temporarily and reaccess it rapidly. It is analogous to short-term memory in humans.

Data requiring longer term storage are moved to *disks* and *tapes.* Disks are devices that store data in either magnetic or optical form on a rotating medium. Optical media possess the advantage of having a higher density, that is, being able to store more data in a given area, but retrieval from and storage to magnetic media are faster. The optical medium is frequently used for historical data where access speed is unimportant. Optical disks in a CD-ROM format can be used for distribution of mass-produced information. Old information may also be transferred to magnetic tape, but the linear format of tape makes data retrieval slower than optical disk. Since writing to magnetic tape is rapid, this medium is often utilized to back up disks. Disk backups are performed periodically to prevent the loss of data resulting from failures, often called *disk crashes.* Tape media are also a convenient way to transfer information between electronically separate computers.

Operating systems

An *operating system* is software that supervises the orderly execution of programs and provides support for basic functions commonly utilized by all programs. Some of these functions include management of disks and disk files, supporting the operation of computer terminals (cathode-ray tubes) and printers, and support for computer networking (see following section). *MS-DOS* is an example of an operating system for the IBM-PC. *Unix* is an example of a minicomputer operating system. Operating systems may be designated as being single-user/single-tasking where a single user can run a single program at a time, single-user/multitasking where a single user can run more than one program at the same time, or multiuser where several users can run many programs at the same time. Most LIS's operate under multiuser operating systems. For applications such as the laboratory, a *real-time* capability is also necessary. Real time refers to the need to capture and process input data immediately within specified time limits. For example, some high-volume analyzers can tolerate only a 5-second delay between inputting a specimen number and obtaining the test requests that have been made on the sample.

Programming languages

Early computers were programmed in a primitive and native *machine language* consisting of numbers entered through switches or punched cards. Because of the difficulty of associating binary numbers with instructions, there was developed a symbolic *assembly language* that performed some of these tasks. LIS's designed up to the late 1970s were often programmed with assembly language because it efficiently utilized expensive hardware. This approach, however, was still too slow for developing software.[12] Because of these limitations, computer scientist designers developed *higher level languages* to further improve productivity. In one approach, a *compiler* translates higher level language, or *source code*, into machine language, or *object code*. Once produced, data in object code can be stored and used without the compiler or source code. Frequently, vendors maintain LIS proprietary by not making source codes available to the user. If source codes are lost, as after bankruptcy, the user may not be able to make any programming changes. Examples of compiled high-level languages include C, COBOL, Fortran, and Pascal. In a second approach, high-level languages are processed by an *interpreter*. Interpreters produce no object code but examine each instruction in the source code and execute commands as they are understood. A popular interpreted language in the laboratory is MUMPS (Massachusetts General Updating and Multi-Programming Systems), or M. The trade-offs between compilers and interpreters depend on specific application and preferences.

Database managers

Most LIS's developed since 1984 utilize specialized software systems known as *database management systems*, or *DBMSs*, for the physical storage and retrieval of data, freeing the vendor of direct interaction with hardware and op-

erating systems software. A DBMS may be viewed as a very high level programming language. Their use has greatly speeded up programming of new systems and has added versatility to database expansion and alterations. Some database systems may be designed so that end users without programming experience can also perform inquiries into the database.

Computers are synonymous with data management and data processing. Programs generally operate on *data* that may be included within the program itself or on data acquired from sources external to the program, such as patient data. In either case, such data and their organization are called the *data structure*. Data stored on disks, tapes, and other devices external to the main memory, or the CPU, are organized and grouped into *files*. Although files and data structures may contain some explicit information about the purpose and type of information that is stored, additional information needed for meaningful interpretation of the data may be implicit. For example, an accounting system will almost always omit the dollar sign ($) and often omits the decimal point. In other words, $15.25 will appear as 1525 in a disk file. Such implicit information makes the use of data in files nearly impossible without prior knowledge of other information. Since the number of possibilities for data structures is limitless, implicit information holds significant importance.

The purpose of any database design is to store data in such a fashion as to permit their retrieval in a sufficiently fast manner. Although it is possible to store data unorganized and attempt their retrieval sequentially, computers will reach practical limits despite their speed. To make retrieval practical, data are usually stored in a manner reflecting the way they will be used. Four models have been developed for describing common organization of databases. These include the *hierarchical, network,* and *relational* database models. Although most databases do not utilize any single model in a pure fashion, the various models provide insights to some of the complications and trade-offs associated with implementing real systems.

The simplest and most often used model in laboratory systems is the hierarchical model. In this model, all data are treated as an inverted treelike structure with all data elements descending from a root. In an LIS, the root element is usually a unique patient identifier such as the patient name or a patient number (Fig. 18-4). For routine retrievals of patient care data, this data model usually works very well and can efficiently utilize computer resources. For retrieving abnormal laboratory results, however, this model fails, since it forces the computer to search all results on all patients. If such cases are frequently encountered, another tree must be built for storing the data again to gain satisfactory performance. Multiple copies of data introduce other problems, particularly if data are changed. Despite the performance of modern hardware, efficiency is still important when one is working with very large data sets, such as

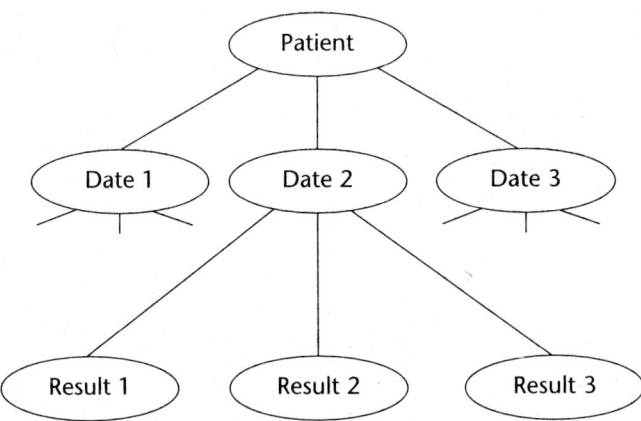

Fig. 18-4 A database with a hierarchical data relationship. These data are organized so that they are retrieved by the patient as the main starting index.

those with 2 to 3 years of historical data from a large institution. The M programming language is an example of a system that directly supports a hierarchical database manager.

Network databases allow users to retrieve data in multiple ways and resolve the problems associated with having multiple copies of the same data by setting up multiple access pointers to a single data element (Fig. 18-5). This data model very efficiently utilizes computer resources and can be very effective in many situations. Unfortunately, the relationships between the various data elements can become very complex and difficult to understand. Such complexities can become particularly problematic should data relationships change; that is, systems built using network model database managers are easily created but are difficult to maintain. Most common database managers are based on the network model.

The *relational database management system* has become popular because of its ease of use. The data appear as tables, and database operations become operations on tables that can be performed by users with ease (Fig. 18-6). This flexibility has earned relational databases a strong role in situations where data are manipulated frequently, as in a research setting. A side effect of this flexibility is that relational databases less efficiently utilize computer resources than simpler models do, and this may present problems with very large datasets. Some examples of relational databases are IBM's DB2, Oracle, and Sybase. Many other databases often claim to be relational but are based on the network model. Few LIS's use relational databases for high-volume data transactions because of performance and cost issues, though some systems transfer data from a nonrelational production database manager to a relational database manager for ad hoc queries. These hybrid approaches may completely move to a relational database manager as hardware resources become cheaper.

Data structures are critical to the design of programs. First, stored patient data in an LIS consume most of the disk and memory storage. In an LIS, the amount of laboratory data easily exceeds the programs needed to run a system by several orders of magnitude. The design of the data structure may impose limitations on the stored information. One system might be limited to storing data on 2000 patients, whereas a second system might be limited to 64,000 patients. The vendor of the smaller system may have made this restriction so that their LIS runs faster and more efficiently and requires less disk storage, thus producing a less expensive system than the larger system. But this efficiency is irrelevant if the user's needs exceed 2000 active patient files.

Computer networks

A *computer network,* or *network,* is a separate concept from the network database model. A network is any interconnection between computer systems or between a computer terminal and a computer system that supports the interchange

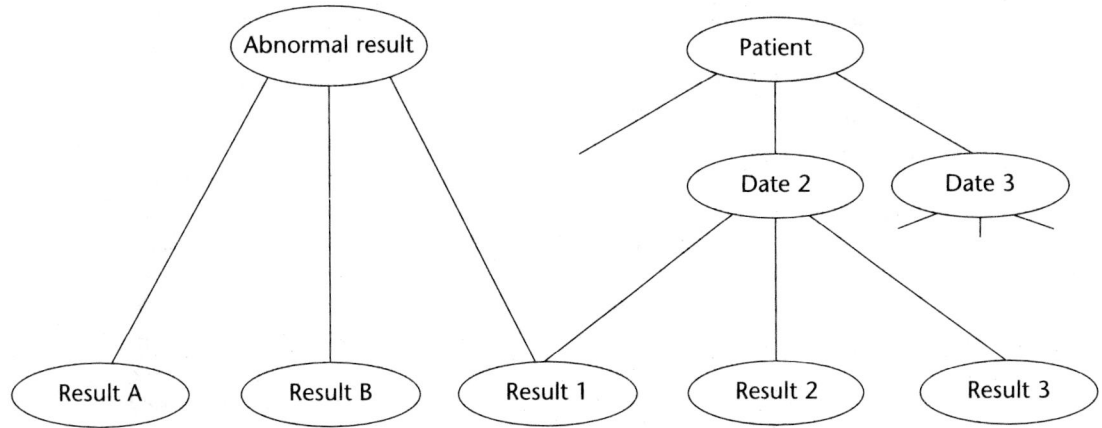

Fig. 18-5 A database with a networked data relationship. The data are organized so that they can be retrieved either by the patient or by abnormal results.

For a data relationship which follows the structure:

{patient–1, date–1, sodium–1, potassium–1, calcium–1, TSH–1}

{patient–2, date–2, sodium–2, potassium–2, calcium–2, TSH–2}

{patient–3, date–3, sodium–3, potassium–3, calcium–3, TSH–3}

⋮
⋮

The data appear as a table:

PATIENT	DATE	SODIUM	POTASSIUM	CALCIUM	TSH
James Smith	10/3/87	144mEq/L	4.5 mEq/L	10.1mg/dL	none
James Smith	10/20/87	138mEq/L	none	none	3.4μU/mL
John Jones	11/30/87	154mEq/L	none	none	none

Fig. 18-6 Structure and data elements in a relational database. Data can be retrieved either by any single or combination of columns and rows.

of data. If the network is physically located within a limited locale, such as 1 to 2 miles, it is called a *local area network,* or *LAN.* If the network spans a larger area, it is called a *wide-area network,* or *WAN.* High-speed LAN technology is inexpensive and is often user installed. Most computers found in businesses include *Ethernet* as an integral part of the hardware, and such systems require networks to communicate with other computers, such as the network for ADT and billing functions. Interchanging data between different computers requires software to support a common protocol, or an agreed-upon way to interchange data. Unfortunately, incompatibilities between software vendors, hardware vendors, and applications software often make this interchange highly complex.

As networks advance in speed and capability, computer systems implementing a *client/server* architecture have emerged. This term describes a specific interaction between two networked computers. The server computer holds the database from which the client retrieves and processes data for its use. If the client updates the data, it will generally update the data on the server. The client/server approach has become popular with LIS systems in two areas. With smaller systems, some vendors have implemented LISs with inexpensive personal computers and client/server software, replacing more expensive minicomputer-based systems. Larger systems have implemented a server architecture to allow users with personal computers to download data so that they can process it independently.

Microwave, satellite, cellular telephone, and other radio frequency systems are supporting mobile information-gathering activities. For example, some vendors are providing hand-held portable units for phlebotomists to increase the accuracy of collection times and for better patient identification. Advanced paging devices linked to the LIS allow physicians to have immediate access to patient data as soon as it has been verified. These systems may also be used to interconnect computer systems where cables cannot be used or are inconvenient. Most of these mobile technologies are substantially more expensive than cable-based systems. The effect of all these network technologies has been to allow the integration of information from physically diverse locations. In many institutions, networks are critical in supporting satellite laboratory facilities, allowing the satellites to have access to patient data, and in many cases allowing the creation of structures that support a decentralized physical and organizational operation.[12] Such satellite operations are becoming increasingly important as laboratories grow to meet expanding health care alliances.

MISCELLANEOUS
Maintenance

After the installation of a computer system, the user must perform numerous routine activities, often referred to as maintenance. *System maintenance* refers to housekeeping activities that must be performed to allow the LIS to operate optimally and to allow for data recovery in case of failures. *Backup,* the process of making a copy of files, is one maintenance activity mentioned previously. Most computers also require regular *file maintenance* activities during which the computer physically reorganizes its data on disk in a manner that maximizes performance. Most operating systems and database managers allow backup and file maintenance activities to occur with the system still available to any potential users of the LIS. Since the disk space on computers is frequently limited, inactive patient files must be *archived,* transferred to storage tapes or optical disks periodically, and *purged* from the active disk. Such archived data require either arranged or special permission to be accessed. Data purged to magnetic media are not permanent and do not meet the legal definitions for archival data, since they may "fade" in about 5 to 10 years. It is likely that optical disk media will satisfy future legal definitions for archival data.

Software maintenance refers to the periodic updating of

programs after their installation. These updates include both applications and systems software, usually for the purposes of fixing software defects or design problems, providing enhancements or new functionality, and providing support for new hardware or operating systems that have been updated by other vendors. These periodic updates may occur as often as several times a year. For many modern systems, the software-updating process will cause more computer downtime than unanticipated failures.

Software-maintenance charges remain a significant source of revenue for most software vendors, often amounting to 1% to 1.5% per year of the purchase price. However, these maintenance charges are a significant expense for users. Unskilled users often treat software support as a service contract. Skilled users may terminate software support to save expenses, especially when they perceive that they are getting little benefit. Vendors will often entice users to continue software support by offering enhancements. In addition to vendor-supplied updates, software maintenance must also address changes mandated by intrainstitutional events. In the laboratory, these might include changes in automated instrumentation. Changes external to the laboratory might result from replacement of interdependent systems, such as a computerized financial system. Locally mandated changes during a period of high activity can easily add another 25% to maintenance costs as well as require additional capital expenses. Often, for their own administrative requirements, some vendors require users to perform updates whether or not they are useful to the users. This often serves to cause problems in otherwise stable systems.

Maintenance activities can result in computer system *downtime* or periods of time when the system is unavailable to users. Downtime may be *scheduled* or *unscheduled*. Daily scheduled maintenance should be minimal, typically less than 15 minutes. Additional hardware and software may be needed to achieve this short a time, however. Hardware and software updates are more difficult to perform without longer periods of downtime and may be needed 2 to 4 times a year. Unscheduled downtimes are usually a result of hardware failures or software crashes. Total downtimes under 1% or 87.6 hours a year should be possible with most LIS's. High-availability systems can easily reach downtimes under 0.1% or 8.76 hours a year. Considering that a single scheduled downtime can take 4 hours or more, this is a significant achievement. A laboratory should decide on an acceptable level of downtime for an LIS.

Data security and privacy

Balancing the needs for confidentiality of patient information, data security, and access to medical information challenges computer systems, especially as the use of computerized databases increases. The LIS creates a database that can be directly accessed throughout the hospital or indirectly accessed through a secondary computer, such as a hospital information system. As the technology for the electronic medical record improves, the availability of prepaid medical care (Health Maintenance Organization) increases, and national health care progresses, these concerns come into even greater conflict by creating greater demands for information. Computers can both provide ready access to information and control ordering but can achieve this only at the risk of reducing privacy.

Early LISs using minicomputers were designed only for intralaboratory use and provided only minimal data security functions. Access codes identified the technologist and the functions that were allowed to the user. Since external access at low cost benefitted both laboratories and clinicians, LIS terminals were added to nursing stations. Even then, security was unimportant, since most of the data being accessed were not very sensitive and the number of users was limited. However, newer systems store data for longer periods of time, adding to the likelihood of exposing sensitive information. Many of these systems have not been designed to prevent systematic and determined attempts at gaining access to sensitive information.

To control access into the LIS, most current systems require the use of a user name, followed by a password. Security system design should allow users to select only passwords that are of sufficient length and complexity to prevent access by guessing. Even long passwords based on common dictionary words can be guessed by computers programmed to gain access illegally to an LIS. Security systems or laboratory procedures should force the changing of passwords at regular intervals. Most security systems of the LIS limit access to system functions and test results by user codes. For example, physicians might have access only for test results inquiry, laboratory technologists might have access to ordering, resulting, and inquiry functions, and order entry clerks might have access only to test-ordering functions. A special access privilege might be needed for accessing sensitive confidential data such as human immunodeficiency virus (HIV) results. LIS security systems should automatically disconnect inactive terminals to prevent inappropriate access.[13] Managing access rights in a large institution can be an extraordinarily difficult problem, since residents, interns, and students change services frequently and information regarding their role can be difficult to obtain. Personal information implied by data, such as home address, patient location, appointments, and billing transactions, also affect privacy but are difficult to block because of the large number of people requiring access to such data.

New technologies have introduced several additional challenges. First, data networks have become ubiquitous, with most newer computers requiring networking. Many institutional networks are connected to the Internet, a network with international access. Networks allow the less scrupulous to access confidential information electronically from physically remote sites in other parts of the world. In infrequent cases, malicious intruders even destroy or alter data. Technical complexity has prevented vendors and users from responding. For example, data encryption on networks is seldom utilized, making interception of data easy.[13]

Second, national health care and health care costs have resulted in increased use of databases. For example, Medicare is collecting data regarding appropriate patient care profiles and resource utilization. Private insurance carriers also routinely collect and store patient information. Interchange and dissemination of such information, both for patient and provider benefits, will further compromise privacy and security. Lastly, the common use of networks and microcomputers in LIS products have exposed many systems to destructive *computer viruses,* computer programs that embed themselves into the operating system programs. Many viruses remain dormant for periods of time and are not destructive. Some, however, perform destructive actions when triggered by a predefined event.

LIS vendors can and must enhance system security, but this is difficult because of (1) conflicting laws, (2) diversified medical practices, and (3) the fact that adding security inhibits the convenience of the systems. Gostin and associates reviewed the legal implications of privacy and security in a national health care system.[14] Several voluntary groups are also exploring privacy issues associated with computerization, but with little progress. Even with existing technologies, users must be educated and encouraged to take steps to guard privacy. For example, networks and computers must be designed with data security considerations as a forethought rather than an afterthought. Patient care computers should be isolated from outside network access, either physically or by use of electronic barriers.

Regulatory requirements

The Clinical Laboratory Improvement Amendment of 1988 has already led to major changes in clinical laboratories.[15] Information systems are the most appropriate tool for managing record keeping and work-load provisions required by this law. In addition to the capture of quality control data, technologist work-load, and proficiency records, specific provisions are included for the proper operation of information systems. LIS vendors prefer to implement software only after legal details are clear, and this often leads to significant delays in meeting regulations. The major effect of CLIA '88 on the LIS lies in data-retention requirements. Records of test requests and results must be retained in a conveniently retrievable manner for 10 years for anatomic pathology and cytology results, for 5 years for blood bank and tissue typing results, and for 2 years for all other results. Although it may be possible to retain data on-line in computer systems for this period of time, most laboratories archive the data to microfiche or optical disks for greater permanence.

The Health and Human Services detailing of CLIA '88 provides general guidelines for the proper operation of an LIS.[15] Before this, the FDA made specific rulings in 1988 classifying a blood bank's information system software as a medical device,[16] thus making requirements for the testing and documentation of such software to be similar to the requirements for devices such as patient monitors.[17] This ruling is based on the assumption that software errors result in the erroneous dispensation of blood products without physician review.[18] LISs servicing other laboratory areas are not currently subject to similar testing and validation guidelines, but some vendors have adopted them in anticipation of additional regulatory changes. Although these procedures may reduce errors, they are certain to increase the cost of and delay changes to information systems available to the consumer. Most voluntary accreditation agencies, such as the College of American Pathologists, are requiring documentation of software development and computer system operations similar to but less stringent than those found in CLIA '88.[19]

Role of the LIS in hospital computing

As previously mentioned, LIS's often interact with other computers for receiving or transmitting critical information. In a hospital setting, an administrative computer typically maintains patient information through interactions with other systems. These interactions include verifying patient identification numbers and patient accounting information and updating patient locations through an ADT system, receiving patients' test requests through an order entry system, and sending test results to a hospital information system. After storing the test results, the LIS may send an account of the laboratory transactions to a financial system to inform it of services that have been performed by the laboratory. The financial system then performs any needed billing and accounting, usually translating the LIS transactions into charges, CPT codes, and other information required by most insurance carriers. If the LIS performs its own billing and accounting, it must send similar information to an insurance carrier either through EDI (electronic data interchange) or by filling out an HCFA 1500 form. Unfortunately, these complex interchanges between computers remain a problem and require constant maintenance, since regulations constantly change. Updates of test definitions in the laboratory require coordination with financial computer systems. Patient locations, test definitions, and other information must be coordinated with HIS and other clinical systems.

In most institutions, LISs participate as one member in a complex quilt of unrelated and interconnected computerized information systems (Fig. 18-7). Pressure to integrate hospital information will increase as economic pressures to reduce costs increase.

The importance of sharing information has been mentioned previously in the section on quality assurance. The simple interchange of information between pharmacy and the laboratory helps detect adverse drug reactions, inappropriate dosing, inappropriate specimen drawing time, and drug toxicity, all of which negatively influence the costs of

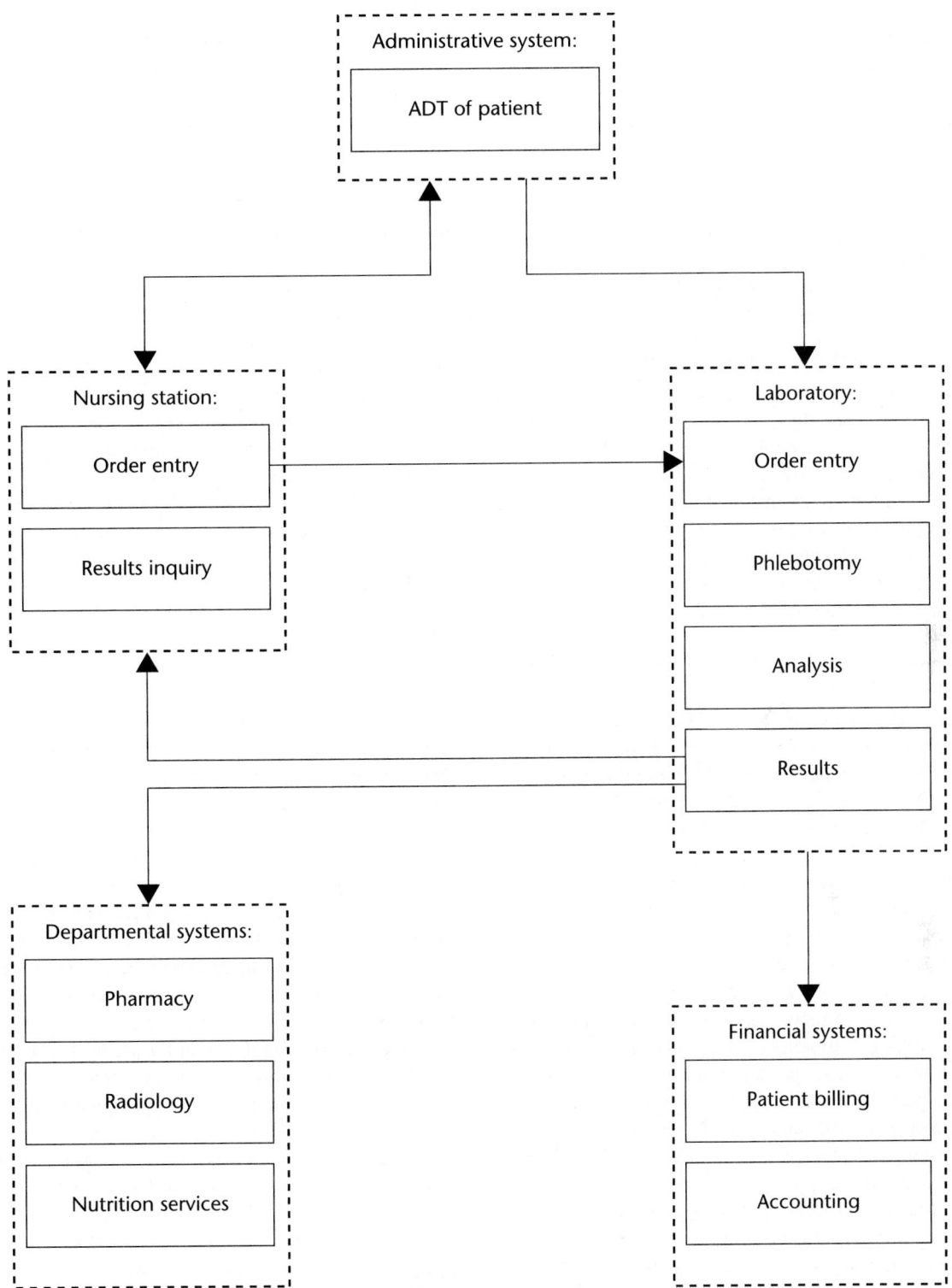

Fig. 18-7 The interchange of information between computer systems in a hospital environment. Most laboratory computer systems today are expected to interact with hospital administrative, financial, nursing, and other departmental systems.

patient care. A surgical pathologist benefits when he or she can review liver biopsy specimens along with the results of liver function tests. The blood bank benefits when it has access to the operating room schedule. The integration of ancillary and nursing data allows the hospital to determine the cost of providing care for a patient classified by a specific DRG (diagnosis-related group). The LIS is an essential component in a large matrix of information systems designed to support the delivery of patient care and cannot be considered to operate as an isolated stand-alone system. Coordinating the information in these various systems has received considerable attention recently and has been identified as being a problem in a survey of LIS installations.[20]

Standards development and data interchange

To address the high cost of software development and the lack of coordination between the various information systems, the health care computer industry, LIS and HIS users, and the federal government have created voluntary groups to set standards, particularly for the interconnection between information systems and between an information system and computerized equipment. For the clinical laboratory, standards address the interchange of data (1) with bedside monitoring systems, (2) with administrative systems, including those associated with payers and government agencies, and (3) between laboratory systems. Of particular importance are those functions covering the interchange of laboratory test requests and results. Three voluntary groups that have created standards in the laboratory arena include ASTM, already mentioned earlier with regard to automated instrumentation, the Institute of Electrical and Electronics Engineers, and the HL7 committee.

The HL7 committee was specifically formed to develop standards for supporting the interchange of information between computers in the hospital environment. Areas covered by the HL7 committee have included ADT, billing, patient demographics, orders, and results.

The ASTM E1238 protocol has become the basis for systems interchanging laboratory data between different systems.[21-23] Many reference laboratory systems exchange data with hospital laboratory systems using this standard. Interfaces between an HIS and an LIS often use the E1238 standard or a similar subset as defined by HL7. These hospital standards for information interchange carry profound implications for LIS's, for they offer large systemwide benefits at low additional LIS cost. For example, significant savings result when physicians directly perform order entry and retrieve results electronically, a task that requires integration of the HIS and the LIS. The ultimate goal of integrating interfaces is the migration toward a reduction in paper use and toward the electronic patient chart. This will be difficult until medical terminology becomes more consistent.[24,25]

Future directions

Rapid changes in laboratory technology, health care economics, and computer technology will force the continued evolution of laboratory systems. For example, point-of-care testing (POCT) has emerged in settings requiring rapid turnaround times. However, many POCT devices are currently limited in their ability to interact with the LIS, leading to conflicts with regulations that require proper documentation of the result and other parameters associated with the testing. POCT results are infrequently documented in the patient chart, if at all. More often, results are utilized by clinical personnel without documentation because of time and labor constraints. In comparison, results that are entered into an LIS or HIS are available for use by all clinical personnel.

The Institute of Medicine[26] and the Government Accounting Office,[27] along with users and computer vendors,[28] have proposed the computerized medical chart as an effective way to decrease costs. The successes of computerizing the clinical laboratory and the availability of large numbers of patient documents in an electronic format through the wide use of word processors have all contributed to this proposal. The electronic medical record, according to its proponents, would more readily transfer information between users of the chart in a more cost-effective fashion.[29] Coupled with order entry and medical practice guidelines, it can structure patient care for maximum benefits. Unfortunately, the lack of a common medical terminology, the politics associated with any large project, the difficulty of entering critical data such as those associated with nursing care, and the high cost and technical challenge of developing complex software make this goal formidable.[30,31]

Possibly the greatest potential for changing the human-computer interaction comes from new computer technology being introduced today. This technology includes voice-recognition devices, voice-response units, and portable handwriting tablets. These technologies have the advantage of being potentially easier to use than the keyboard, but reliability of these devices must increase before they are acceptable for use in most areas of the clinical laboratory.

The use of the computer in the clinical laboratory is still in the development stage. The potential of LIS systems to help manage the automation flow required for good patient care and to help effectively manage the resources required (costs) has barely been used. We can imagine a future where informatics is as important as the analytical result.

REFERENCES

1. Sittig DF, Stead WW: Computer-based physician order entry: the state of the art, *JAMA* 1(2):108-123, 1994.
2. Weilert M, Tilzer LL: Putting bar codes to work for improved patient care, *Clin Lab Med* 11:227-238, 1991.
3. EIA standard RS-232-C, Washington, D.C., 1969, Electronic Industries Association.
4. ASTM designation E1381-91, specification for low-level protocol to transfer messages between clinical laboratory instruments and computer systems, *1994 Annual book of ASTM standards,*

vol 14.01, Philadelphia, 1994, American Society for Testing and Materials, pp 311-317.

5. ASTM designation E1394-91, standard specification for transferring information between clinical instruments and computer systems, *1994 Annual book of ASTM standards,* vol 14.01, Philadelphia, 1994, American Society for Testing and Materials, pp 335-349.

6. ASTM designation E1466-92, standard specification for use of bar codes on specimen tubes in the clinical laboratory, *1994 Annual book of ASTM standards,* vol 14.01, Philadelphia, 1994, American Society for Testing and Materials, pp 407-409.

7. Westgard JO, Barry PL, Hunt MR, et al: A multi-rule Shewhart chart for quality control in clinical chemistry, *Clin Chem* 27:493-501, 1981.

8. Ladensen JH: Patients as their own controls: use of the computer to identify "laboratory error," *Clin Chem* 21:1648-1653, 1975.

9. Lezotte D, Grams RR: Determining clinical significance in repeated laboratory measurements—the "clinical delta range," *J Med Systems* 3:175-191, 1979.

10. Koss W, Sodeman T: The workload recording method: a laboratory management tool, *Clin Lab Med* 12:337-350, 1991.

11. Carlton J, Hays L: New computer chip hits desktop market with Intel in its sights, *Wall Street Journal* 75(102):A1, A4, 1994.

12. Friedman B, Mitchell W: Horizontal and vertical integration in hospital laboratories and the laboratory information system, *Clin Lab Med* 10:627-641, 1990.

13. Bakker AR: Security in medical information systems. In Bemmel JH, McCray AT, editors: *1993 Yearbook of medical informatics, sharing knowledge and information,* Stuttgart, Germany, 1993, Schattauer, pp 52-60.

14. Gostin LO, Turek-Brezina J, Powers M, et al: Privacy and security of personal information in a new health care system, *JAMA* 270 (20):2487-2493, 1993.

15. Department of Health and Human Services, Health Care Financing Organization, Department of Health and Human Services, 42 CFR part 405 et al: Clinical Laboratory Improvement Amendments of 1988, Final Rule, *Fed Register* 57(40):7001-7288, 1992.

16. Parkman PD: FDA letter to registered blood banks on recommendations for implementation of computerization in blood establishments, April 6, 1988.

17. Application of the medical device GMPS to computerized devices and manufacturing processes: medical device GMP guidance for FDA investigators, first draft, Office of Compliance and Surveillance, Division of Compliance Programs, Food and Drug Administration, Public Health Service, Department of Health and Human Services, Rockville, Md., Nov 1990.

18. Butch SH: Computer software quality assurance, *Lab Med* 22:18-22, 1991.

19. Commission on Laboratory Accreditation: *Inspection Checklist,* Section 1, Laboratory general—computer services, College of American Pathologists, Northfield, Ill., 1993.

20. Elevitch F, Treling C, Spackman K, et al: A clinical laboratory information systems survey: a challenge for the decade, *Arch Pathol Lab Med* 117:12-21, 1993.

21. ASTM designation E1238-94, standard specification for transferring clinical laboratory data messages between independent computer systems, *1994 Annual book of ASTM standards,* vol 14.01, Philadelphia, 1994, American Society for Testing and Materials, pp 132-210.

22. McDonald CJ, Hammond WE: Standards formats for electronic transfer of data, *Ann Intern Med* 110:333-335, 1989.

23. McDonald CJ: *Standards for the electronic transfer of clinical data: progress, promises, and the conductor's wand,* Proceedings of the 14th Annual Symposium on Computer Applications in Medical Care, Los Alamitos, Calif., 1990, IEEE Computer Society Press, pp 9-14.

24. *GAO/IMTEC-93-17, Automated medical records—leadership needed to expedite standards development,* Washington, D.C., 1993, General Accounting Office.

25. deMoor GJE: Standardization in medical informatics. In Bemmel JH, McCray AT, editors: *1993 Yearbook of medical informatics, sharing knowledge and information,* Stuttgart, Germany, 1993, Schattauer, pp 61-66.

26. Dick RS, Steen EB, editors: *The computer-based patient record, an essential technology for health care,* Washington, D.C., 1991, National Academy Press.

27. *GAO/IMTEC-91-5, Medical ADP systems—automated medical records hold promise to improve patient care,* Washington, D.C., 1991, General Accounting Office.

28. Korpman R: Health care information systems: patient-centered integration is the key, *Clin Lab Med* 11:203-220, 1991.

29. Barnett GO, Jenders RA, Cheuh HC: The computer-based clinical record—where do we stand? *Ann Intern Med* 119:1046-1048, 1993.

30. Brooks F: *The mythical man month: essays on software engineering,* Reading, Mass., 1979, Addison-Wesley.

31. Brooks F: No silver bullet: essence and accidents of software engineering, *IEEE Computer* 20:10-19, 1987.

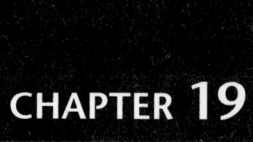

CHAPTER 19

Laboratory statistics

Stephen E. Kahn
Mark A. Jandreski

Population distributions
  Populations and samples
  Frequency distributions
Basic distribution statistics
  Measures of central tendencies
  Measures of variation
  Confidence intervals
  Measures of accuracy and precision
Parametric comparisons of populations
  The null hypothesis and statistical significance
  Comparison of random variation (precision)—the
    F-test
  Comparison of means (accuracy or bias)—the
    t-test
  One-way analysis of variance (ANOVA)
  Testing a sample for outliers using the gap test
Nonparametric comparisons of populations
  Nonparametric distribution statistics
  Sign test
  Mann-Whitney rank sum test
  χ^2 (chi-square) analysis
Linear regression and correlation
  Basic statistics of simple linear regression and
    correlation
  Testing for outliers using residual analysis
  Limitations of simple linear-regression analysis

OBJECTIVES

■ Given the appropriate data, construct a frequency and a relative frequency histogram.

■ List three measures of central tendency and describe their utility when applied to normal and nonnormal distributions.

■ List three measures of variation, calculate values for each given appropriate data, and describe their utility when applied to normal and nonnormal distributions.

■ State the percentage of the values falling within the $\pm 1s$, $\pm 2s$, and $\pm 3s$ confidence intervals in a normally distributed population.

■ Describe three parametric techniques for comparison of populations and their utility when applied to normal distributions.

■ Describe three nonparametric techniques for comparisons of populations and their utility when applied to normal and nonnormal distributions.

■ Explain the use of ANOVA.

■ Describe the uses and limitations of regression analysis for comparing sets of data.

KEY TERMS

accuracy Estimate of nonrandom, systematic bias between samples of data or between a sample of data and the true population value.

ANOVA Statistical method for comparison of three or more means.

central tendency The value about which a population is centered. The mean, the median, and the mode are all used to describe the central tendency of a population.

chi-square (χ^2) A test statistic that measures the difference between the observed and expected frequencies of occurrences in two or more populations.

coefficient of variation (CV) A relative standard deviation in which the standard deviation is divided by the mean and multiplied by 100%.

confidence interval A range around an experimentally determined statistic that has a known probability of including the true parameter.

correlation coefficient A statistic that measures the distribution of data about the estimated linear-regression line.

degrees of freedom (df) The number of independent observations in a data set. It is the number of observations minus the number of restrictions for a set of data.

F-test A statistical test used to determine whether there are differences between two variances.

gaussian distribution See *normal distribution.*

histogram A graphic display of data in which the frequency of a certain value (or range of values) is plotted against a scale of all values.

Mann-Whitney test A nonparametric statistical test based on the ranks of data and used to test the null hypothesis that the central tendencies of two independent populations are identical.

mean Arithmetic average of a set of data.

median A value or interval of a population occurring in the middle of a population, half of which falls above and half below the median.

mode The value or interval of a population occurring with the greatest frequency.

nonparametric statistics Statistics employed when the assumption of a normal or symmetrical (that is, gaussian) distribution of data is not valid.

normal distribution A population of data that has a tendency to cluster symmetrically around a central value such that the mean, median, and mode of the data are the same; also known as a gaussian distribution.

null hypothesis The working hypothesis of a statistical test stating that there is no difference between the statistics of two different populations.

outlier A result or data point that lies far outside the range of all other results or data points. The outlier is not considered to be from the population that has been sampled.

parametric statistics Statistics employed when the assumption that a population has a symmetrical distribution (such as gaussian or log-normal) of data is valid.

precision A descriptor of the random variation in a population of data.

random error Error that affects reproducibility of a method (precision).

range The difference between the highest and lowest values in a population.

sign test A nonparametric statistical test used to assess differences between population medians.

standard deviation Square root of a variance.

standard error A descriptor of the variability that results from sampling data from a population.

statistic A number that describes a property of a set of data or other numbers.

statistics The plural of statistic; also the science that deals with the use and classification of numbers or data.

systematic error Nonrandom error that affects the mean of a population of data and defines the bias between the means of two populations (see *accuracy*).

t-test A statistical test used to determine whether there are differences between two means or between a target value and a calculated mean in populations having a normal distribution.

variance A statistic used to describe the distribution or spread of data in a population.

Generating test results, using effective quality control procedures, monitoring the performance of existing methods, and assessing the utility of new test methods are routine analytical activities performed in the clinical laboratory. All analytical techniques and methods are subject to several types of errors, or variation, that create a degree of uncertainty in the quantitative test results that a laboratory produces. The clinical laboratorian must be able to apply basic statistical techniques in order to evaluate the validity of test results. Statistics, therefore, are an important laboratory tool.

Webster[1] defines statistics as "(1) a branch of mathematics dealing with the collection, analysis, interpretation, and presentation of masses of numerical data, and (2) a collection of quantitative data."

A statistic (singular) is a number that describes some property of a set of other numbers. In the clinical laboratory, statistical descriptions of data sets can be useful in many ways:

1. To identify how a population of data is distributed
2. To assess random variation in a population of data
3. To compare the amounts of random variation within populations of data
4. To analyze which parameters are significant components of variance
5. To test for a systematic difference between populations of data
6. To assess the degree of correlation between populations of data

This chapter describes each of these uses of statistics and illustrates how each can be effectively applied in laboratory situations.

A basic and theoretical knowledge of appropriate statistical methods is critically important in the clinical chemistry laboratory. Equally important, however, is the correct application of statistical methods to relevant laboratory problems. You are encouraged to refer to basic statistics textbooks, such as references 2 to 8, for an understanding of statistics beyond that presented in this chapter.

POPULATION DISTRIBUTIONS
Populations and samples

The term *population* usually refers to a number of animate creatures or people such as the inhabitants of the United States. However, in statistics, population may also refer to a collection of objects, events, procedures, or observations. For example, all the serum glucose values for all the people living in Chicago on a given day could be considered a population of glucose values. As a second example, if the glucose concentration of a single blood specimen were measured 10,000 times, a population of slightly different glucose results would be obtained, since no chemical measurement is exact because of the random variation inherent in all laboratory measurements.

The number of observations in these glucose examples is too large to study conveniently; therefore, a representative sample must be drawn from the population for an investigation. Before the sample is drawn, the population from which it comes must be carefully described. Once the attributes of the population are known, sample criteria for such variables as age, sex, occupation, family history, disease state, or any other parameter that might be relevant to the study can be applied. For example, if a serum glucose reference range analysis were carried out, serum samples from diabetic patients could not be used. The number of individual data points needed must be defined as well. If the number is too large, the study may be too difficult to carry out. If the number is too small, the sample may not be a statistically significant representation of the population. The sample must be chosen such that true inferences can be made about the population under study from results obtained from the sample. Most of the concepts and applications discussed in this chapter focus on statistical evaluations of samples of data obtained from a population.

Frequency distributions

Conceptually, perhaps the simplest way to describe a population of data is to construct a *histogram,* also called a *frequency distribution diagram.* A histogram shows the frequency, or the number of times, a particular value or range of values is obtained versus the scale of all values. Fig. 19-1, *A,* is a histogram of 20 glucose results obtained by the repeated measurement of an individual blood specimen. The horizontal axis is glucose concentration divided into small convenient ranges, or *bins.* The vertical axis is the frequency (or relative frequency) with which results from each bin are obtained, such as the number of patients having a given range of glucose values. When relative frequencies are used, each bin frequency is presented as a percentage of the total number of samples. The histogram's horizontal axis can also represent cumulative percentiles (cumulative percentage of the population up to and including each bin) as well as concentration units. When the number of observations, *N,* is small and the bins are relatively wide, the histogram has a choppy appearance (Fig. 19-1, *A*). As *N* increases and the bins are made narrower, the shape of the histogram becomes smoother and the histogram becomes more truly representative of the population (Fig. 19-1, *B*). As *N* increases further, the histogram takes on the appearance of a continuous function (Fig. 19-1, *C*). In the histogram of hypothetical glucose data in Fig. 19-1, *C,* one can see that the population is centered around 1000 mg/L with few observations less than 920 mg/L and few greater than 1080 mg/L. The general spread of the data can also be assessed.

If enough data are represented in the histogram and the data are truly random (that is, each result was affected by random processes alone), the histogram can be used to predict the probability of obtaining future results above or below a certain value. Fig. 19-1, *C,* shows that there is about a 2.3% chance that a future glucose result from this population will be less than 920 mg/L, and a 2.3% chance that a future glucose result will be greater than 1080 mg/L.

The curve approximated by the glucose histogram in Fig. 19-1, *C,* is a smooth "bell-shaped" curve called a *gaussian,* or *normal,* distribution, which is depicted in Fig. 19-2. This symmetrical curve was first described by the French mathematician Abraham de Moivre in 1733 and further developed by the astronomer-mathematician Karl Friedrich Gauss during the 1800s. The portion of the curve on the right is usually referred to as the *upper tail* and the portion on the left is called the *lower tail.* Many random variables of interest in medicine and health care, such as

reference ranges, have distributions similar to normal distributions.

The *parametric* statistical tests that are discussed in this chapter are used under the assumption that the population being tested is distributed in a gaussian fashion. Before we proceed with parametric statistical comparisons, it is important to establish whether the population is normally distributed. A graphical analysis utilizing *normal probability paper* can be used to test for a normal distribution. However, this method requires a visual evaluation of the sample data for deviation from a straight line and can therefore be very subjective. One constructs the graph by plotting the bin values, such as glucose concentration, along a linear *x*-axis and the cumulative frequency of the distribution on a nonlinear *y*-axis, the mathematical function of which is based on a normal distribution. Fig. 19-1, *D,* shows a normal probability plot for 600 glucose values drawn from a group of normal healthy volunteers.

The *Kolmogorov-Smirnov test* can be used to test for normally distributed data. This analysis measures the vertical distances between the cumulative distribution and the straight line on normal probability paper. Critical values for the statistically significant difference are obtained from a statistical table.

Another way to measure how well data fit a normal distribution is to calculate *skewness* and *kurtosis coefficients.* Skewness measures the asymmetry of the data distribution. Values greater than zero indicate that the upper tail of the curve is longer than the lower tail. Negative values indicate that the lower tail is longer. Kurtosis measures how steep or flat the distribution is with respect to a true normal distribution. Kurtosis coefficients greater than zero indicate that the curve is steep in the center and that the tails are relatively long. Values less than zero indicate that the curve is flat in the center and that the tails are short. For data that follow a reasonably gaussian distribution, the skewness and kurtosis coefficients should be between 1 and −1. Different types of coefficients called *standard skewness* and *kurtosis coefficients* test for significant deviations from the normal distribution and, analogous to standard deviation, should be between 2 and −2 for normally distributed data.[6] These calculations are usually done with computer software.

When a nonsymmetrical or nongaussian distribution is observed, one option is to *transform* the nongaussian distribution into one that is more normally distributed. This can be accomplished by conversion of the population values into another form. Transformation techniques include taking the logarithm (base 10, or natural) of the data, taking the reciprocal of the data, and raising the numbers exponentially. After using one of these methods, the resulting data set is often distributed in a gaussian fashion. If the data are still not normally distributed, *nonparametric* statistical tests are used to analyze the data. In the medical and healthcare fields, nonparametric distributions are usually either *skewed*

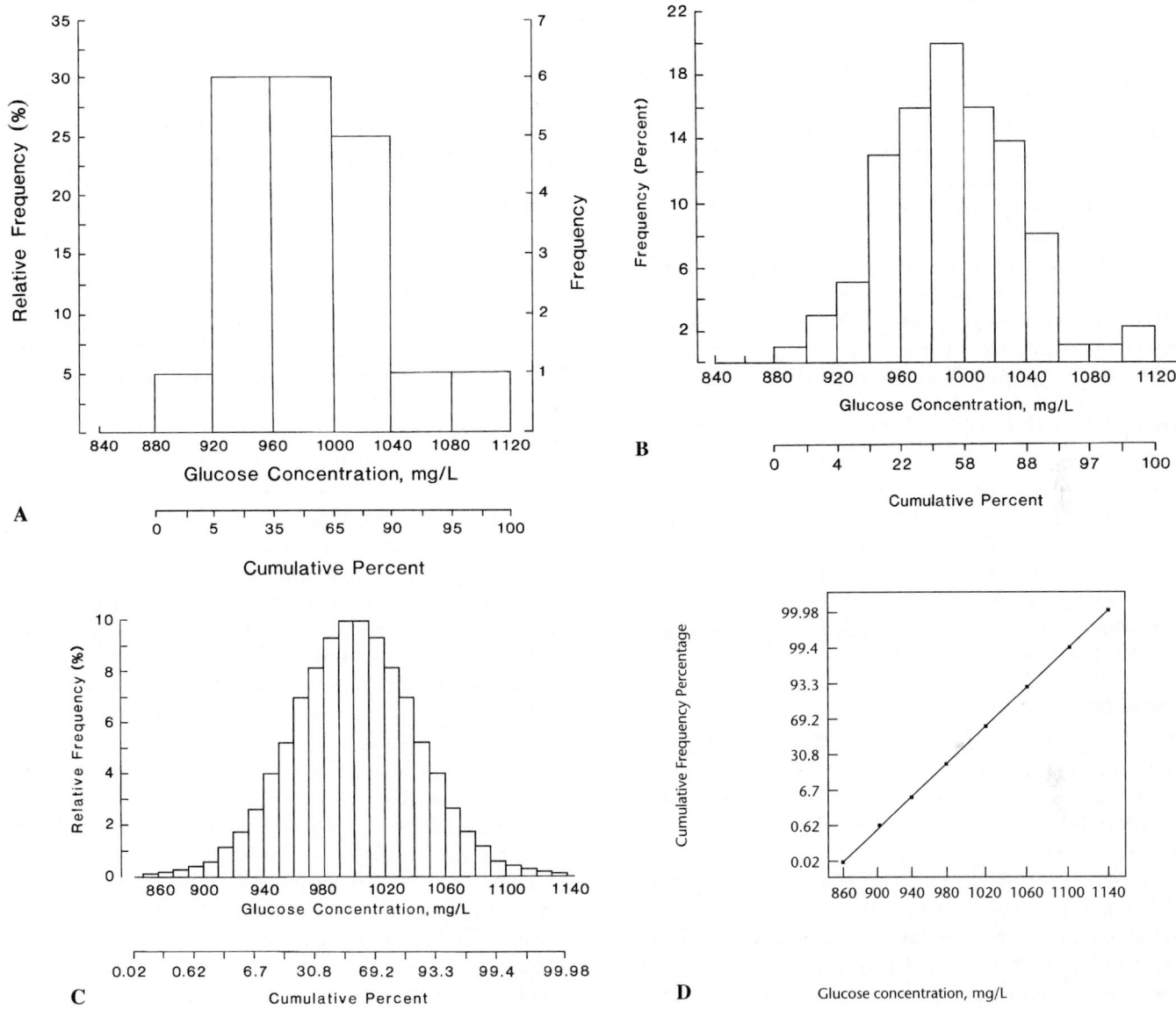

Fig. 19-1 **A,** Histogram (frequency distribution) of glucose results obtained from 20 repetitive measurements of the same specimen using bin width 40 mg/L. **B,** With $N = 100$ and bin width = 20 mg/L. **C,** With infinite N and bin width = 10 mg/L. **D,** Normal probability plot of glucose results obtained as described in **C.**

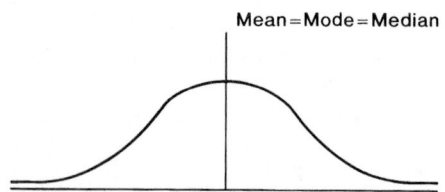

Fig. 19-2 Normal (gaussian) distribution, symmetric about mean.

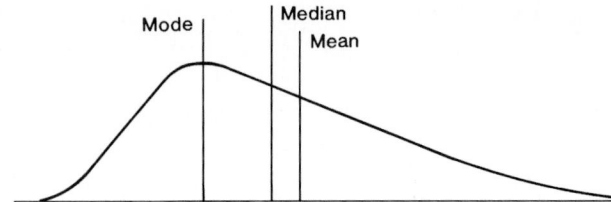

Fig. 19-3 Nonnormal distribution.

or *bimodal*. As alluded to previously, a skewed distribution is one where either the upper or lower tail of the distribution is longer than the other (Fig. 19-3). Serum gamma-glutamyl transferase reference interval data obtained from healthy individuals are usually skewed to the right. A bimodal distribution is seen when data are composed of two related populations (Fig. 19-4). Combined serum uric acid reference interval data obtained from healthy males and females typically demonstrate the appearance of a bimodal distribution when plotted appropriately. This type of distribution often indicates that separate, sex-based reference ranges should be established for the analyte under study.

BASIC DISTRIBUTION STATISTICS

In the previous section, plotting a histogram or frequency distribution was identified as a simple method for visually describing a population of data to assess, at least initially, whether the data set is distributed in a gaussian or a nongaussian fashion. There are two general categories of statistics that can also be used to describe the distribution of data. These two categories are measures of central tendencies and measures of variation.

Measures of central tendencies

Measures of central tendencies are statistics that represent some central value around which the data are distributed. Three measures of central tendencies that are often calculated for clinical laboratory applications are the mean, the median, and the mode.

The *mean* is probably the most widely used statistic and is a simple *arithmetic average*. One calculates the mean by adding up all the observations and dividing by the number of observations, *N*. For a sample of data, calculation of the mean, designated as $\bar{x}$, is illustrated by equation 19-1, where x_i is an individual observation:

$$\bar{x} = \frac{\Sigma\, x_i}{N} \qquad \textbf{\textit{Eq. 19-1}}$$

If the entire population of data is used to calculate the mean, the calculated mean is the actual mean of the population, indicated by the symbol "μ." For clinical laboratory applications, it is usually impossible to have collected the entire population of data (that is, one can always make another measurement unless the population is restrictively defined). For these applications, use of the symbol for the

sample mean, $\bar{x}$, is appropriate. This convention indicates that a subset of data from the population was used to calculate $\bar{x}$, which is an estimate of the true population mean.

If the sample data are distributed symmetrically about the mean, the arithmetic mean is actually representative of the central tendency of the sample. This feature is illustrated in Fig. 19-1, *D*, which depicts a *normal*, or *gaussian*, distribution. But any sample of data from a population would have a mean value whether the distribution was gaussian or nongaussian.

A second measure of central tendency is the *mode*. The mode of a sample of data is that value that is most frequently observed in the sample. It is the value at the peak of the frequency distribution (Fig. 19-3). If a frequency distribution of data has two peaks, the distribution is *bimodal*. An example of a bimodal distribution is illustrated in Fig. 19-4. For practical applications in the laboratory, every frequency distribution has a minimum of one mode (that is, the distribution is at least unimodal).

A third measure of the central tendency is the *median*. The median is the middle value in a sample of data when all the values in the distribution are ranked individually from lowest to highest (or vice versa). Unlike the mean and mode, the median value describes a true central tendency for all types of distributions, since half of the observations are greater than the median and half of the observations are less than the median.

One characteristic of a perfect normal distribution is that the arithmetic average is the value that is observed most frequently and is also the middle value observed in the sample when values are ranked from lowest to highest. As illustrated in Fig. 19-1, *D*, this results in the mean, median, and mode all being the same value. All three of these statistics are true measures of central tendency in a true gaussian, or normal, distribution.

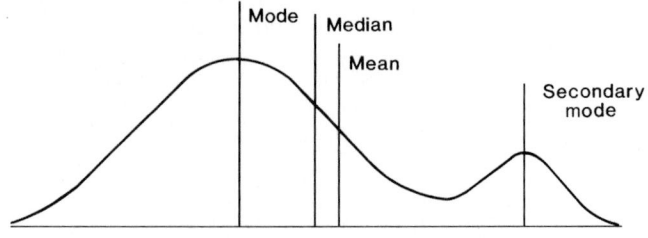

Fig. 19-4 Bimodal distribution.

In contrast, in a nonnormal distribution, such as that depicted in Fig. 19-3, the mean, median, and mode are all different values. The mean does not accurately describe the center of the distribution (though it is still an arithmetic average of the data). It is also apparent that the mode of this distribution does not describe a true central tendency of the sample of data. The median is the only value that can be considered a true measure of this distribution's central tendency. For those nonnormal distributions where the mean and median might be considerably different, it may be more appropriate to use both values, or the median alone, to describe central tendencies of the distribution.

There is a significant and often overlooked limitation to using mean values to describe samples of data, even those samples that are normally distributed. Means can be strongly influenced by values in the data that lie at the extremes of the data range. This feature indicates that when calculating a mean value for a sample of data one should be critical in evaluating which values may not be representative of the data set, that is, which values are outliers that should be excluded by the use of appropriate techniques (see below). The median is less affected than the mean by extreme values in the data set.

Measures of variation

In addition to measures of central tendencies, other kinds of statistical data are required to characterize effectively a sample of data or a distribution. Measures of central tendencies do not provide sufficient information on how close together or far apart the values in a sample of data are. Statistics that indicate the degree to which observed values vary, or the spread of the distribution, are measures of variation. Three measures of variation that are often calculated for clinical laboratory applications are range, variance, and standard deviation.

The *range* is simply the difference between the largest and smallest values in the sample of data. The range is useful for indicating the spread of data when N is small, but when one is using the range, no assumptions can be made concerning the shape of the distribution. But a limitation of the range as a measure of variation is that it is based on only two values in the sample of data.

More useful measures of variation are the *variance* and *standard deviation*. One calculates the variance by first determining the mean of the sample of data and then subtracting the mean from each value to get N differences. The squares of the differences between the individual values (x_i) and the mean are added. The sum of the squared differences is divided by $N - 1$, which yields the variance (equation 19-2,A):

$$\text{Variance} = s^2 = \frac{\Sigma(x_i - \bar{x})^2}{N - 1} \qquad \textbf{\textit{Eq. 19-2,A}}$$

The *standard deviation (s)* is the square root of the variance and is often represented as *SD*. The denominator of

equation 19-2,A is $N - 1$ rather than N because there are only $N - 1$ degrees of freedom for the variance once $\bar{x}$ has been used to calculate the variance. The concept of degrees of freedom is explained more fully later in this chapter.

Although s is normally calculated by use of the results of single analyses, one frequently needs to know the imprecision of replicate analyses. To calculate this estimate of variation, the following equation can be employed:

$$s_{\text{rep}} = \left(\frac{\Sigma d^2}{N}\right)^{1/2} \qquad \textbf{\textit{Eq. 19-2,B}}$$

where d is the difference between the replicate measurements. This calculation can be useful for determining if duplicate analyses can help to achieve a desired level of within-run imprecision for an assay.

Another statistic that is often calculated in laboratory applications is the *coefficient of variation,* or *CV*. The CV indicates what percentage of the mean is represented by the standard deviation, as illustrated in equation 19-3:

$$\%\text{CV} = \frac{100\% \, s}{\bar{x}} \qquad \textbf{\textit{Eq. 19-3}}$$

One advantage in using the CV to express the variation of analytical methods is that the variation is reported in units that are independent of the particular analytical method. One must keep in mind, however, that the magnitude of the CV of an analytical method is not completely independent of concentration. In certain instances, routine statistics on two levels of quality control materials may indicate a larger CV at the lower level simply because the numerator of the CV calculation, the mean, is a smaller number than the mean of the higher level of control material.

Example 1 depicts the calculation of basic measures of central tendencies and basic measures of variation using data from a single level of quality control material.

Example 1. Calculation of basic statistics using a sample of data from repeated cholesterol measurements on one level of quality control material.

Calculate the mean, mode, median, variance, standard deviation, and coefficient of variation.

Sample x_i (mg/L)	$x_i - \bar{x}$	$(x_i - \bar{x})^2$
2080	−1.4	1.96
2090	8.6	73.96
2110	28.6	817.96
2100	18.6	345.96
2010	−71.4	5097.96
2090	8.6	73.96
2040	−41.4	1713.96
2140	58.6	3433.96
2070	−11.4	129.96
2070	−11.4	129.96
2100	18.6	345.96
2110	28.6	817.96
2030	−51.4	2641.96

Continued.

Sample—cont'd

x_i (mg/L)	$x_i - \bar{x}$	$(x_i - \bar{x})^2$
2090	8.6	73.96
2080	−1.4	1.96
2060	−21.4	457.96
2170	88.6	7849.96
2060	−21.4	457.96
2130	48.6	2361.96
2090	8.6	73.96
2080	−1.4	1.96
2100	18.6	345.96
2000	−81.4	6625.96
2090	8.6	73.96
2040	−41.4	1713.96
2070	−11.4	129.96
2100	18.6	345.96
2080	−1.4	1.96

$\Sigma = 58280$ $(x_i - \bar{x})^2 = (x_i - \bar{x})^2 = 36142.88$

Mean

$$= \bar{x} = \frac{\Sigma x_i}{N} = 2081.4 \text{ mg/L}$$

Median*
= 2085 mg/L

Mode
= 2090 mg/L

Measures of Variance

$$s^2 = \frac{\Sigma(x_i - \bar{x})^2}{N - 1}$$

$$= 36142.88/27 = 1338.6 \text{ mg/L}$$

$$s = 36.5 \text{ mg/L}$$

$$\%CV = 100\% \ s/x$$

$$= \frac{36.5 \text{ mg/L } (100\%)}{2081.4 \text{ mg/L}}$$

$$= 1.75\%$$

Confidence intervals

Use of the mean and standard deviation values for the purposes of assessing quality control results and the determination of reference ranges are important laboratory applications. To use these statistics for these applications, the data in the sample must be normally distributed. In a normal distribution, the standard deviation and mean (which are in the same units) can be used to describe the proportion of the values falling in a given area under the normal curve.

The total area under the normal curve theoretically represents all the values in the given population. As illustrated in Fig. 19-5, the area under the perfect normal distribution from $+1s$ to $-1s$ represents 68.3% of the values, from $+2s$ to $-2s$ represents 95.4% of the values, and from $+3s$ to $-3s$ represents 99.7% of the values. These intervals that

contain a stated percentage of the data are called *confidence intervals*. For samples of data that are normally distributed, confidence intervals calculated using the mean and standard deviation can be used as the basis of statistical quality control rules for acceptance and rejection decisions concerning specific analytical runs (see Chapter 21).

If the results from analyzing the quality control material discussed in Example 1 were perfectly distributed, it would be expected that the range between the mean plus $2s$ and the mean minus $2s$ (2008.4 to 2154.4 mg/L) would exclude 4.6% of the data. In reality, this range excludes 7.1% of the data (2 of 28 values, 2000 mg/L and 2170 mg/L, are outside of the $2s$ range). For this sample of data, the $2s$ range should not be expected to include exactly 95.4% of the values. It was known that the distribution was not perfectly normal once different results for the mean, median, and mode were obtained.

The measurement of cholesterol levels in Example 1 is characterized by a certain degree of imprecision (the %CV is 1.75%). Since the error of the measurement of the mean of the set of values is smaller than that of a single measurement, the more times a measurement is made, the more certain one can be of its true value. If several means are calculated from different groups of measurements of this quality control specimen, the individual means are distributed about the actual population mean. The random variation in this group of means is described by the *standard error of the mean*, $s_{\bar{x}}$, in equation 19-4:

$$s_{\bar{x}} = \frac{s}{\sqrt{N}} \qquad \textit{Eq. 19-4}$$

Suppose that for the cholesterol QC measurements discussed in Example 1 one wished to determine the $s_{\bar{x}}$ and the likelihood that the population mean is within a certain range. Putting the appropriate values into equation 19-4:

$$s_{\bar{x}} = \frac{36.5 \text{ mg/L}}{\sqrt{28}} = 6.9 \text{ mg/L}$$

It would then be expected that 68.3% of the various sample means (with N's of 28) would be within 1×6.9 mg/L of the population mean (2074.5 to 2088.3 mg/L), 95.4% of the means would be within 2×6.9 mg/L of the population mean (2067.6 to 2095.2 mg/L), and 99.7% of the means would be within 3×6.9 mg/L of the true population mean (2060.7 to 2102.1 mg/L). Therefore it can be assumed with a 95% confidence that the *true* population mean lies within the range of 2067.6 to 2095.2 mg/L. This is termed the *95% confidence interval*.

The true mean cholesterol concentration of the quality control material in Example 1 cannot be exactly determined unless an infinite number of measurements are made. In practice, the population is sampled when one obtains groups of quality control values such as those shown in Example 1. The mean obtained is therefore not the true mean but an

---

*When even-numbered samples of data are collected, the two middle values are averaged to obtain the median.[6] For an N of 28, the two middle values are the 14th and 15th values, 2090 mg/L and 2080 mg/L, respectively.

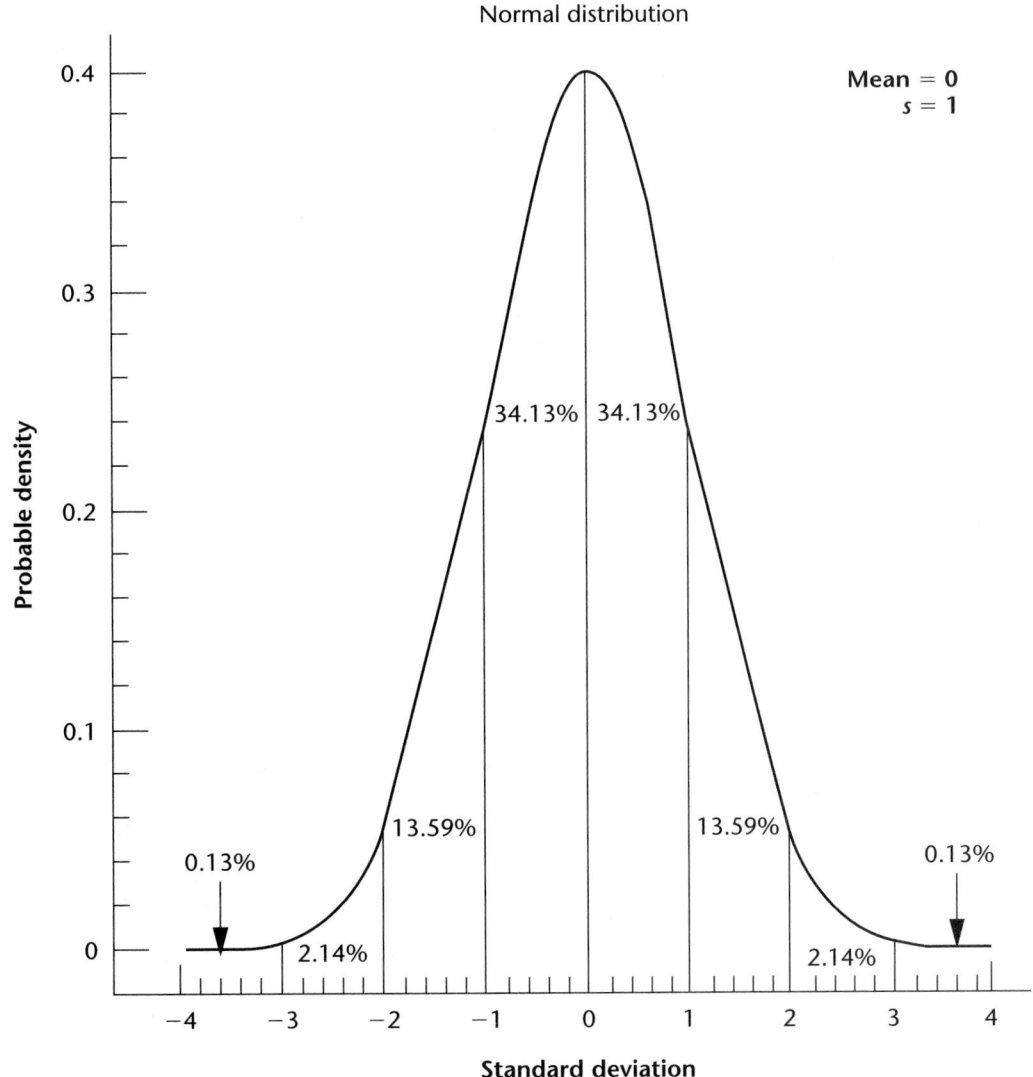

Fig. 19-5 Perfect normal distribution, with a mean = 0, indicating the percentage of results that are in each standard deviation interval between −4 and +4 standard deviations.

estimate of the true mean. The standard error of the experimentally derived mean, $\bar{x}$, can be used to develop a more exact *confidence interval* that has a known probability of including the true population mean, μ. This interval is described in equation 19-5:

$$\mu = \bar{x} \pm t \cdot s_{\bar{x}} \qquad \textit{Eq. 19-5}$$

The t value is obtained from a t table (Table 19-1). The t value depends on the number of degrees of freedom ($N - 1$) and the desired probability, p, that the true mean is outside the confidence interval because of chance alone. A probability of $p = 0.05$ implies a 95% confidence [$100 \times (1 - p)\%$] that the interval includes the true mean.

The t values describe the same probability distribution depicted in Fig. 19-5, but use of the distribution in Fig. 19-5 should be made under the assumption that the true popula-

tion mean and standard deviation are known. Use of the t table makes allowances for decreasing confidence in the estimated values of specific parameters as N decreases. Therefore an appropriate use of t values is to calculate more accurate confidence intervals for statistics obtained from small samples. An illustration of this is given in Example 2. To construct a confidence interval that includes a true mean, one should be sure that the 0.05 probability that the true mean is beyond the calculated limits is spread over both ends or tails of the distribution, as shown in Fig. 19-6. For these purposes, a two-sided, $p = 0.05$, t value is used. To state that the true mean is greater than some single limit, a one-sided t value should be used. Notice that the t value for a two-sided interval for a $p = 0.05$ is the same as the t value for a one-sided limit of $p = 0.025$. The practical application of confidence limits is demonstrated on pp. 416-418.

Table 19-1 Critical values of *t* for selected probabilities, *p,* and degrees of freedom, *df*

df	Two-sided intervals or tests		
	p = 0.10	**p = 0.05**	**p = 0.01**
	One-sided limits or tests		
	p = 0.05	**p = 0.025**	**p = 0.005**
1	6.31	12.70	63.70
2	2.92	4.30	9.92
3	2.35	3.18	5.84
4	2.13	2.78	4.60
5	2.01	2.57	4.03
6	1.94	2.45	3.71
7	1.89	2.36	3.50
8	1.86	2.31	3.36
9	1.83	2.26	3.25
10	1.81	2.23	3.17
12	1.78	2.18	3.05
14	1.76	2.14	2.98
16	1.75	2.12	2.92
18	1.73	2.10	2.88
20	1.72	2.09	2.85
30	1.70	2.04	2.75
40	1.68	2.02	2.70
60	1.67	2.00	2.66
120	1.66	1.98	2.62
∞	1.64	1.96	2.58

Condensed from Davies OL, Goldsmith PL: *Statistical methods in research and production,* ed 4, New York, 1972, Longman.

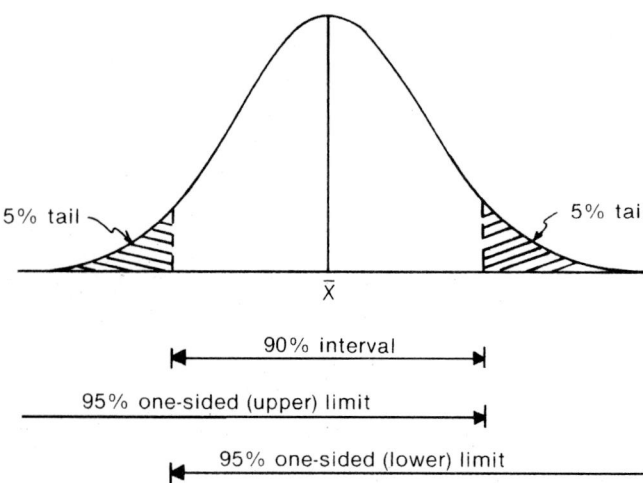

Fig. 19-6 One-sided versus two-sided *t* values. *t* values to calculate 90% interval and 95% one-sided limits are the same.

Example 2. Calculating 95% confidence intervals for the mean of a small sample.

Calculate the 95% confidence interval for the mean value of the lactate dehydrogenase (LD) activity of a stable control material after performing only 15 daily determinations.

Sample: All LD values are in IU/L: 324, 337, 350, 295, 284, 322, 339, 350, 309, 322, 348, 320, 298, 345, 335.

The calculated mean and standard deviation of the sample are 325 and 21 IU/L, respectively.

The standard error of the mean (SEM) is calculated:

$$s_{\bar{x}} = s/\sqrt{N} = 21/\sqrt{15} = 5.42 \text{ IU/L}$$

Using the *t* table in Table 19-1, find the two-sided *t* value for $p = 0.05$ and $N - 1$ degrees of freedom ($df = 14$). The *t* value of 2.14 is the factor that is used to adjust the SEM so that the correct lower and upper limits of the 95% confidence interval for the mean can be determined for this small sample. Using equation 19-5:

$$\mu = \bar{x} \pm t \cdot s_{\bar{x}}$$

Lower limit of confidence interval: 325 − (2.14) (5.42) = 313.4 IU/L

Upper limit of confidence interval: 325 + (2.14) (5.42) = 336.6 IU/L

There is a 95% probability that the mean LD activity of this sample of quality control measurements is between 313.4 and 336.6 IU/L.

Measures of accuracy and precision

In previous sections, the mean and standard deviations of a normally distributed population were described. When a new analytical method is evaluated by the laboratory, these parameters are used to describe the accuracy and precision of the method (see Chapter 22). *Accuracy* describes the ability of an analytical method to obtain the "true" or correct result after a number of replicate analyses. The closer the mean of *N* replicate analyses of a sample comes to the "true" or known value of that sample, the more accurate the method. *Precision* describes the reproducibility of a method. The narrower the distribution of results, that is, the smaller the standard deviation, after a number of replicate analyses, the better the precision of a method.

Fig. 19-7 shows the results of replicate analyses of the same sample by three different methods. All three methods have a similar mean and thus similar accuracy. However, the distributions or standard deviations of the results by each method are different. Method A has the narrowest distribution or smallest standard deviation and hence has the best precision of the three methods. Method C has the widest distribution or largest standard deviation and has the poorest precision.

Fig. 19-8 shows the results of replicate analyses of the same sample by two different methods. The two methods have a similar distribution of data or similar standard deviations; therefore their precision is about the same. The means, however, are not equal, and the relative accuracies for the two methods are not the same, which indicates a nonrandom bias between the methods. Which method has the better accuracy will depend on which mean is closer to the "true" value of the analyte examined in the sample.

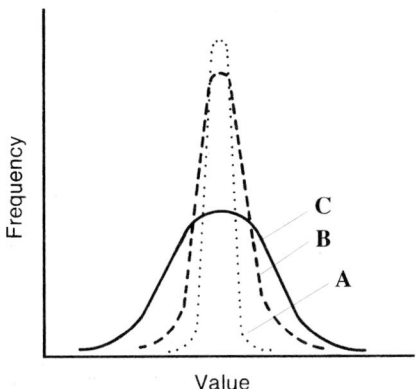

Fig. 19-7 Frequency distributions for three methods having same means, but different distributions, σ. A (•••) has narrowest distribution, whereas distribution of C (—) is wider than that of B (---).

Although the terms are sometimes used interchangeably, accuracy and precision are two distinctly different concepts and must never be interchanged with one another. This is shown in Fig. 19-9. Repeated attempts to hit the middle of the target, the true value, are indicated by dots. A method can be accurate but not very precise, as shown in Fig. 19-9, *A*. Inaccuracy but good precision is shown in Fig. 19-9, *B*, where the values fall close together but are grouped far from the middle, or "true," value. Fig. 19-9, *C*, shows the goal of all good analytical methods—excellent accuracy and precision.

PARAMETRIC COMPARISONS OF POPULATIONS
The null hypothesis and statistical significance

When a comparison is made between two samples from two populations, invariably a difference between the means *(x̄)* and standard deviations *(s)* is observed. These observed differences may or may not reflect a true difference between the populations. Therefore, it is necessary to test the *null hypothesis*, which states that there is no difference between the true means *(μ)* or the true standard deviations *(σ)* of the two populations. The corresponding calculated values, *x̄* or *s*, are used for this purpose.

Two hypotheses

$$s_1^2 = s_2^2 \quad \text{or} \quad \bar{x}_1 = \bar{x}_2 \quad \text{Null hypothesis}$$
$$s_1^2 \neq s_2^2 \quad \text{or} \quad \bar{x}_1 \neq \bar{x}_2 \quad \text{Alternative hypothesis}$$

There are many different statistical tests that can be used to generate a test *statistic* that indicates whether to accept or reject the null hypothesis. If the statistical test result indicates that the null hypothesis should be accepted, there is a chance that the calculated test statistic that forms the basis for the test results does not reflect the truth and the null

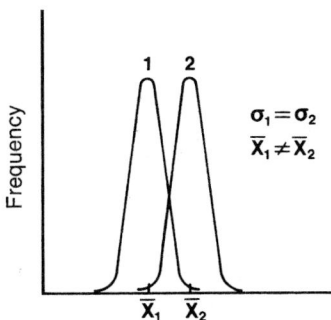

Fig. 19-8 Frequency distribution for replicate analysis by two different methods, *1* and *2*. Both methods are equally precise ($\sigma_1 = \sigma_2$) but are biased in relationship to each other ($\bar{x}_1$ does not equal $\bar{x}_2$).

hypothesis may be incorrectly accepted. The level of significance or chance of this occurring is defined by the value *p*, where $100\% \, (1 - p)$ is the percent confidence that the test results are statistically significant. A minimum value of $p = 0.05$ is customarily used to test for significance. This would mean that there is a 95% chance that the results of a statistical test are significant or conversely that there is a 5% chance that accepting the statistical test result is wrong.

For many applications in clinical chemistry, a difference that is only statistically different may still be acceptable for routine applications. It is of course important to identify differences that *are* medically significant or that do not meet regulatory requirements (see Chapters 21 and 22).

Degrees of freedom. The term *degrees of freedom* is usually defined as the number of ways in which a group of numbers can vary independently. This is often a difficult idea to explain or define. It is calculated by subtraction of the number of estimated parameters from the sample size. For example, consider 20 bilirubin measurements; the sample size is 20, and for this series the number of degrees of freedom is 20. Any one of these 20 values can be altered, and the change will not affect the value of any of the other measurements in the series. However, if the mean of the 20 values is calculated, the mean has only 19, or $n - 1$, degrees of freedom. It is possible to change 19 values with-

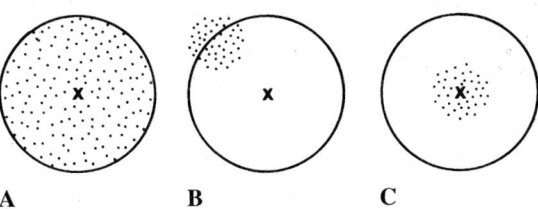

Fig. 19-9 x's of these targets each denote the true value for a sample. The dots shown on each of the circles **A** to **C** denote the results of three replicate analyses by three different methods: **A**, imprecise but accurate; **B**, precise but inaccurate; **C**, accurate and precise.

out changing the mean, but the 20th value will need to be a specific number so that the mean remains the same. Therefore, for the calculation of the mean, the degrees of freedom are calculated as $n - 1$. The number of degrees of freedom is an important parameter that is used in the calculation of many statistical tests, such as the *t*-test.

Comparison of random variation (precision)—the *F*-test

The *t*-test is often used to compare the means $(\bar{x})$ of two groups of observations in order for one to test whether there is a significant difference between the two group means (see p. 353). Two assumptions are made with the *t*-test: that the groups are *normally* distributed and that there is no significant difference between the group variances. It is not possible to tell simply by observation of the data how different the variances in the two groups must be before the *t*-test cannot be used. However, the null hypothesis that there is no significant difference between the variances can be tested by use of the *F*-test.

The *F*-test, or *variance ratio test*, is used to determine whether an observed difference between the standard deviations (s) of two sets of data is statistically significant. One calculates the *F*-test statistic by dividing the larger variance (s_1^2) by the smaller variance (s_2^2), as shown in equation 19-6:

$$F = \frac{s_1^2}{s_2^2} \qquad \textit{Eq. 19-6}$$

The calculated *F* value is compared with a critical *F* value obtained from an *F* table (Table 19-2) by using the numbers of degrees of freedom from each group at a specified level of *p*, such as $p = 0.05$. If the calculated *F* value is less than the critical value, the null hypothesis is accepted as true. If the calculated *F* value is greater than the critical value, the alternative hypothesis is accepted as true.

Example 3. *F*-test

A comparison between folate levels in two groups is needed, but the standard deviations look considerably different. The data below show folate levels from 21 laboratory workers and 16 individuals suspected of having dietary anemia.

Serum folate (μg/L)	
Workers (*n* = 21)	Patients (*n* = 16)
13	5
18	15
14	2
16	21
19	6
15	7
12	16
17	4
13	3
16	5
15	18
17	2
18	6
20	1
17	4
13	16
21	
15	
16	
19	
16	
Average 16.2	8.2
Standard deviation 2.44	6.59

$$F = \frac{(6.59)^2}{(2.44)^2} = \frac{43.43}{5.95} = 7.30$$

Table 19-2 Critical values of *F* for $p = 0.05$ and selected degrees of freedom, *df*

df for denominator	Degrees of freedom for numerator						
	5	10	15	20	30	60	∞
1	230.00	242.00	246.00	248.00	250.00	252.00	254.00
2	19.30	19.40	19.40	19.40	19.50	19.50	19.50
3	9.01	8.79	8.70	8.66	8.62	8.57	8.53
4	6.26	5.96	5.86	5.80	5.75	5.69	5.63
5	5.05	4.74	4.62	4.56	4.50	4.43	4.36
6	4.39	4.06	3.94	3.87	3.81	3.74	3.67
7	3.97	3.64	3.51	3.44	3.38	3.30	3.23
8	3.69	3.35	3.22	3.15	3.08	3.01	2.93
9	3.48	3.14	3.01	2.94	2.86	2.79	2.71
10	3.33	2.98	2.85	2.77	2.70	2.62	2.54
15	2.90	2.54	2.40	2.33	2.25	2.16	2.07
20	2.71	2.35	2.20	2.12	2.04	1.95	1.84
30	2.53	2.16	2.01	1.93	1.84	1.74	1.62
60	2.37	1.99	1.84	1.75	1.65	1.53	1.39
∞	2.21	1.83	1.67	1.57	1.46	1.32	1.00

Modified from Barnett RN: *Clinical laboratory statistics*, ed 2, Boston, 1979, Little, Brown & Co.

Use the *F*-table (Table 19-2) to find a critical *F*-value. Scan across the *F*-table to the column that corresponds to $n - 1$ degrees of freedom in the numerator (15) and down to the row that corresponds to $n - 1$ degrees of freedom in the denominator (20) and note a critical value of 2.20. Since the calculated value exceeds this value, the difference in precision is significant with $p < 0.05$.

The results of this test indicate that the *t*-test should *not* be used to compare the two means. The Mann-Whitney test may be a better alternative and is discussed later in this chapter.

Comparison of means (accuracy or bias)— the *t*-test

The *t*-test is used to check for statistically significant differences between two experimental means or between an experimental mean and a stated value.

Hypothesis testing. Testing the difference between an experimental mean and a stated or known value involves testing to see if the stated value is included in the confidence interval around the experimental mean. If it is not, the null hypothesis is rejected, and there appears to be a difference between the stated value and the experimental mean value. In this case, equations 19-7 and 19-8 are used to calculate the paired *t* statistic, which is used to determine if the null hypothesis will be accepted or rejected.

$$t = \frac{\text{Sample mean} - \text{Hypothesized mean}}{\text{Standard error of sample mean}} \qquad \textit{Eq. 19-7}$$

$$t = \frac{\bar{x} - \mu}{s/\sqrt{n}} \qquad \textit{Eq. 19-8}$$

For example, assume that the glucose concentration in a quality control specimen obtained from the National Institute of Standards and Technology is stated to be 1120 mg/L. This material is used as a quality control sample for 30 consecutive days.

For these data, the mean is 1110 mg/L and the s_d is 25 mg/L. Is the mean of the data significantly different from the stated value?

$$t = \frac{1110 - 1120}{\dfrac{25}{\sqrt{30}}} = -2.19$$

The critical *t* value for $p = 0.05$ and 29 *df* (rounded to 30 in Table 19-1) is 2.04. Thus this month's mean of 1110 mg/L is significantly different from the assigned glucose concentration of 1120 mg/L. See also p. 413 for an application of the *t*-test to assess bias in a methods-comparison experiment.

Testing the statistical significance between two measured means using the *t*-test actually involves testing the degree of overlap of their respective probability distributions. If there is little or no overlap, the populations are considered to be different. If there is significant overlap, one cannot be sure that there is any difference. A *t* value is calculated from the data and compared to a critical *t* value. Table 19-1

gives many of the critical values from the *t* distributions. If the absolute value of the calculated *t* value does not exceed the critical *t* value, the null hypothesis is accepted, and such acceptance indicates that a statistically significant difference between the two distributions does not exist; that is, the means are the same.

When one is comparing the means of different sample populations, two different *t*-tests are available, the *unpaired t-test* and the *paired t-test*.

Unpaired *t*-test. The unpaired *t*-test is used when the difference between the means of two independent populations is being analyzed. One example is the comparison of the means of patients' glucose values from two different hospitals. When the unpaired *t*-test is used, it is assumed that the variances of the two populations are equal, and this must first be verified with the *F*-test. If there is no statistically significant difference between the variances, it is proper to proceed with the *t*-test. The *pooled sample variance* $(s_p{}^2)$ is first calculated as shown in equation 19-9:

$$s_p{}^2 = \frac{(n_1 - 1)s_1{}^2 + (n_2 - 1)s_2{}^2}{n_1 + n_2 - 2} \qquad \textit{Eq. 19-9}$$

where s_1 and s_2 are the standard deviations of the two groups of sizes n_1 and n_2. Using $\bar{x}_1$ and $\bar{x}_2$ for the means of the two groups the *unpaired t-statistic* is calculated as shown in equation 19-10:

$$t = \frac{\bar{x}_1 - \bar{x}_2}{s_p \sqrt{1/n_1 + 1/n_2}} \qquad \textit{Eq. 19-10}$$

where s_p is the pooled standard deviation. Each group contributes to the degrees of freedom associated with s_p, so that the calculated unpaired *t* statistic has $(n_1 - 1) + (n_2 - 1)$ or $n_1 + n_2 - 2$ degrees of freedom. The critical *t* value is found from a *t*-table using the calculated degrees of freedom and compared to the calculated *t* value.

Example 4. Equal variance unpaired *t*-test

A reference laboratory begins using a new method for serum immunoglobulin A. Samples are received from two regions of the country. Random samples from healthy patients from each region are tested to find out if the reference range for these two regions is the same.

	Region A	Region B
Mean $(\bar{x})$ (mg/L)	2260	2650
Standard deviation (s) (mg/L)	584	473
Number of samples (n)	33	29

The unpaired *t*-test is used to determine whether the observed differences between the two means are significant. The *F*-test is first performed so that one can make sure that the variances are statistically the same.

$$F = \frac{(584)^2}{(473)^2} = \frac{341056}{223729} = 1.52$$

Use the *F*-table (Table 19-2) to find a critical *F*-value. Scan across the *F*-table to the column that corresponds to $n - 1$ degrees of freedom in the numerator (32) and down to the row that corresponds to $n - 1$ degrees of freedom in the denominator (28) and note a critical value of 1.84. (One can interpolate the table to obtain the exact value for $n_1 = 32$ and $n_2 = 28$, or one can round off to 30, as shown in this example.) Since the calculated value is less than the critical value, the difference in precision is insignificant with $p < 0.05$. The result of this test indicates that the t-test can be used to compare the two mean values.

To calculate the t statistic, s_p must first be calculated.

$$s_p^2 = \frac{(33 - 1)(584)^2 + (29 - 1)(473)^2}{33 + 29 - 2}$$

$$s_p^2 = 286303$$

$$s_p = \sqrt{286303} = 535$$

The t statistic is then calculated:

$$t = \frac{2260 - 2650}{535 \times \sqrt{1/33 + 1/29}} = -2.86$$

Use the t-table (Table 19-1) to find a critical t-value. Scan down the t-table to the column that corresponds to $n_A + n_B - 2$, or 60 degrees of freedom, and note a critical value of 2.00. Since the absolute value of the calculated t value, $|-2.86| = 2.86$ and this is greater than 2.00, the difference in the means is significant with $p < 0.05$. Thus the sample distributions for the two regions do not overlap enough to declare them the same. The laboratory would need separate regional reference ranges for the samples it is testing.

Suppose that $s_1 \neq s_2$, but it is reasonably certain that the two populations are normally distributed. In this case, the pooled estimate of the variance, s_p^2, cannot be used. However, another form of the unpaired t-test sometimes called the *separate-variance t-test* can be utilized. The formula in equation 19-11 approximates a student's t distribution for normally distributed response variables and does not require that the population variances be equal:

$$t = \frac{\bar{x}_1 - \bar{x}_2}{(s_1^2/n_1 + s_2^2/n_2)^{1/2}} \qquad \textit{Eq. 19-11}$$

The number of degrees of freedom can be found by use of the formula shown in equation 19-12. The answer is rounded down to the next lowest integer. For example, 7.6 becomes 7 degrees of freedom.

$$df = \frac{(w_1 + w_2)^2}{w_1^2/(n_1 - 1) + w_2^2/(n_2 - 1)} \qquad \textit{Eq. 19-12}$$

where df = degrees of freedom and $w_1 = s_1^2/n_1$ and $w_2 = s_2^2/n_2$.

Example 5. Separate variance unpaired t-test

In a study of chronic hepatitis, serum alkaline phosphatase levels were reported for 9 patients with inactive disease and 25 patients with active disease. Use the unpaired t-test to test the hypothesis that there is a difference between the alkaline phosphatase means for the active-disease and the inactive-disease populations.

Serum alkaline phosphatase (IU/L)	
Inactive	Active
65	103
72	210
84	92
68	225
89	110
110	286
77	96
95	216
81	94
	150
	195
	208
	95
	163
	184
	89
	238
	99
	116
	224
	124
	135
	201
	92
	176
$\bar{x}$ 82	157
s 14.2	58.5
n 9	25

The F statistic for the sample variances is $(58.5)^2/(14.2)^2 = 16.74$, which is much greater than the critical value of 3.12 (Table 19-2). Since the variances are very different, the separate-variance t-test is used.

$$t = \frac{82 - 157}{[(14.2)^2/9 + (58.5)^2/25]^{1/2}}$$

$$t = -75/12.6 = -5.95$$

The degrees of freedom are:

$$w_1 = (14.2)^2/9 = 22.4$$

$$w_2 = (58.5)^2/25 = 136.9$$

$$df = \frac{(w_1 + w_2)^2}{w_1^2/(n_1 - 1) + w_2^2/(n_2 - 1)}$$

$$df = \frac{(22.4 + 136.9)^2}{(22.4)^2/(9 - 1) + (136.9)^2/(25 - 1)}$$

$$df = 25376/843 = 30.1 \approx 30.$$

For 30 degrees of freedom from Table 19-1, the critical t value at $p = 0.05$ is 2.04.

Since the absolute value of the calculated t value $|-5.95| = 5.95$, and this is greater than 2.04, the difference in the means is significant with $p < 0.05$. Thus the sample distributions for the two disease groups do not overlap enough to declare them the same.

Paired *t*-test. A special case of comparison of means is the paired-sample *t*-test. Paired sample testing (also called "split" sample testing) is used to minimize the effects of sample variations, which can lead to ambiguous results. For example, if the blood gas Po_2 method *x* were being compared to the blood gas Po_2 method *y* and specimens were drawn from different random patient populations for each method, extraneous variations in the populations could mask true methodological differences. To eliminate this variance, the same specimens are analyzed by both methods (see Example 6). The equation used to calculate the paired *t* statistic is shown in equation 19-13:

$$t = \frac{\bar{x}_1 - \bar{x}_2}{s_d/\sqrt{n}} \qquad \textbf{\textit{Eq. 19-13}}$$

where $\bar{x}_1$ and $\bar{x}_2$ are the means of the two paired populations, s_d is the standard deviation of the *difference* between the populations, and *n* is the number of samples. There are $n - 1$ degrees of freedom. One calculates s_d by finding the standard deviation of the differences between each pair of results or between each result and a known or stated value. Example 6 shows the calculation of a paired *t*-test between two groups of data.

Example 6. Paired *t*-test

A laboratory examines a new method for Po_2 by running 40 samples in a paired fashion on the old and new instruments. Using a paired *t*-test, compare the data to determine if there is any bias between the methods.

Po₂ (mm Hg)		
Old	**New**	**Difference**
88	88	0
118	121	−3
115	119	−4
189	198	−9
36	36	0
123	123	0
123	118	5
200	203	−3
60	62	−2
86	86	0
61	62	−1
81	87	−6
33	31	2
223	232	−9
47	48	−1
38	36	2
140	142	−2
67	67	0
87	90	−3
218	225	−7
79	80	−1
56	56	0
228	224	4
65	67	−2
86	88	−2
327	334	−7

59	62	−3
36	36	0
100	101	−1
146	140	6
112	106	6
218	212	6
95	94	1
67	68	−1
71	72	−1
102	100	2
92	91	1
106	105	1
64	60	4
105	114	−9
Avg 108.7	109.6	−0.93
s 64.1	65.3	3.86

First the variances must be checked by use of the *F*-test to see that there is no significant difference between them. The *F* statistic for the sample variances is: $(65.3)^2/(64.1)^2 = 1.04$, which is less than the critical *F* value of 1.69 (Table 19-2) for $p = 0.05$ at 39 degrees of freedom. Since the variances are not significantly different, the *t*-test can be used.

$$t = \frac{\bar{x}_1 - \bar{x}_2}{s/\sqrt{n}}$$

$$t = \frac{-0.93}{3.86/\sqrt{40}}$$

$$t = -1.52$$

The critical *t* value for $p = 0.05$ at 39 degrees of freedom is 2.02. Since the absolute calculated *t* value $|-1.52| = 1.52$, which according to Table 19-1 is less than the critical value, 2.02, the means are not significantly different. The methods are yielding results that are not statistically biased from one another.

One-way analysis of variance (ANOVA)

ANOVA is a method for testing the hypothesis that several different groups (three or more), the distributions of which are normal, all have the same mean. A logical approach to this problem might be to perform a *t*-test on each difference, beginning with the largest until the null hypothesis is rejected for one test. For example, if three population means were compared by testing of the hypothesis that all three population means are equal, it would be necessary to carry out three *t*-tests: a test of the hypothesis that $\bar{x}_1 = \bar{x}_2$, a test of the hypothesis that $\bar{x}_1 = \bar{x}_3$, and a test of the hypothesis that $\bar{x}_2 = \bar{x}_3$. However, this approach would become increasingly inefficient as the number of populations increased. Also, when many comparisons are being performed, some may fail because of chance alone.

In ANOVA, *k* means (where $k \geq 3$) are compared by testing with the null hypothesis that: $\bar{x}_1 = \bar{x}_2 = \bar{x}_3 = \ldots = \bar{x}_k$. An *F* statistic is calculated, and if this statistic is less than a specified value, the null hypothesis is accepted and the means for all groups are not significantly different from one another. The alternative hypothesis is always that at least one sample mean does not equal another sample mean. If the null hypothesis is rejected, it cannot be stated that all the sample means are different. It can only be concluded that one of the sample means does not equal one other sample mean. Since ANOVA analysis cannot tell which of the means is significantly different from the others, other methods, such as the Bonferroni method for multiple comparisons,[6] are used to determine which of the means are different.

A major advantage of ANOVA compared with the use of individual *t*-tests is that ANOVA deals with the larger overall sample population. By using as many data as possible, ANOVA is essentially calculating the best estimate of the true population variance. Differences among the group means are then tested with reference to this best estimate of the population variance. This decreases the possibility that random differences in the variances within individual groups will obscure true findings. In the clinical chemistry laboratory, ANOVA can be a useful statistical tool.

Testing a sample for outliers using the gap test (See also p. 371)

When results or data points are distributed in gaussian fashion, graphing a frequency plot of the data allows the data to be visually assessed. It is possible that during this assessment the investigator may identify an *outlier,* which is a result or data point that is so far outside the range of all other results or data points that it is not considered likely that the result is from the population that has been sampled. Unfortunately, although the experienced investigator might feel comfortable with this assessment, a visual inspection of a frequency distribution or histogram is subjective in nature.

Certain samples of data can be evaluated for the presence of outliers using a more rigorous criterion established by the investigator, for example, exclusion of data points that exceed a given percentage of the mean or median value. A statistical technique that allows the investigator to test a sample for outliers is the *gap test.*[9]

Use of the gap test provides valid statistical evidence that justifies the exclusion of an outlier from a particular sample. In order to use the gap test on a sample, the series of results must be arranged, in order, from the lowest to the highest value. The results are then assigned particular values of *x* in one of the following two ways:

$$x_1 < x_2 < \ldots < x_n \text{ when testing an extreme high value}$$

$$x_n < x_{n-1} < \ldots < x_1 \text{ when testing an extreme low value}$$

In the first case, the smallest value is designated as x_1; whereas in the second, the largest value is x_1. Particular sample test quotients are then selected from standard statistical tables comparing different values of *n* and varying levels of significance.[9] A sample test quotient is a ratio of

two different equations that describe the relationship of *x* to the overall range of data. Once the sample test quotient is calculated, it is possible to determine if there is a statistically unacceptable "gap" between this *x* and the rest of the data. If so, one can justifiably discard the *x* from the data set as an outlier. Since there are different levels of significance and different values of *n*, there are different sample test quotients that can be used. Texts that provide these tables indicate which sample test quotient should be used given the value of *n*, the level of significance selected, and the value (extreme high or extreme low value) that is to be tested. Tests of an extreme high value require the use of a table different from that used for the test of extreme low values.

Use of the sample test quotient allows for calculation of a gap using specific data points in the ordered list. As an example, the sample test quotient used for an *n* of 15 when one is testing an extremely high value would require a gap calculation based on the ordered results designated as:

$$\frac{x_n - x_{n-2}}{x_n - x_3}$$

The recommended gap is then calculated based on the *n* of the sample and compared to the value listed in the statistical table in the significance column of choice (for example, $p < 0.05$). If the calculated gap is greater than the value listed in the table (at the desired probability level and *n* value), the investigator is justified in discarding this value as an outlier with the significance limit selected in the table.

NONPARAMETRIC COMPARISONS OF POPULATIONS
Nonparametric distribution statistics

The statistical tests described above are termed parametric statistics because they assume a gaussian, or normal, distribution of the data. Many populations do not meet this criterion, and the analyst needs techniques for describing and comparing these populations statistically. Nonparametric statistics require no assumptions about the distribution and thus can be considered more general than parametric statistics.

The simplest nonparametric procedure is to rank the data in order from the lowest (value = 1) to the highest (value = *n*). The range of the data set is the difference between the lowest and highest value, and the median value indicates the central tendency of the data set. The ranked data can be used, for example, to determine the limits of reference intervals for those analytes whose distributions are not gaussian. The lower 2.5 percentile and upper 97.5 percentile of the ranked data are usually selected as the lower and upper limits of a reference interval. The central 95% of the data are within the reference interval limits (see p. 348).

Sign test

One of the simplest nonparametric tests for the comparison of two nongaussian populations is the *sign test,* which is analogous to the *t*-test. This test essentially uses the median rather than the mean of a data set. In one application, all the data in a single data set can be compared to some stated (critical) value. Data points higher than the stated value are assigned a plus value (+), lower points are assigned a minus value (−), and zeros are assigned to those values equal to the critical value. The sign test can also be used to compare the results of two methods (A to B) using paired samples. If the B value is higher than A for a given sample, the sample is assigned a plus value. If the B value is less than A, it is assigned a minus value, and zeros are assigned to those samples in which A = B. A hypothesis is assumed that there is no difference between the median of the sample data set and the critical value or between the two samples in each pair, depending on how the test is used. If this hypothesis is correct, the median difference (A − B) should be zero and there should be approximately equal numbers of positive and negative differences.

One performs the test by designating the difference between each data pair as negative, positive, or zero, with the actual numerical difference being unimportant, and then tabulating the results. One then compares the number of negative results to a critical range from a table of "exact" confidence limits for *Np* (Table 19-3) entering the table at the level of the number of nonzero differences observed between the two populations. *Np* is a short-term designation for the sample size, *N,* and the significance level of probability, *p.* So, Table 19-3 can be said to describe exact confidence limits for a given sample size at a given probability. If the negative difference value (the number of negative results) is outside the critical range, the difference between the median values of the two populations is considered significant. Example 7 demonstrates the use of the sign test.

Example 7. Sign test

In order to determine whether there is a significant difference between plasma and serum potassium concentrations (mmol/L),

both types of samples are obtained from 18 volunteers for analysis.

Plasma	Serum	Difference
4.0	4.2	−
3.8	3.8	0
3.6	3.7	−
3.9	3.8	+
4.4	4.5	−
4.6	4.4	+
4.8	4.9	−
4.5	4.7	−
4.3	4.5	−
4.0	3.9	+
4.1	4.1	0
4.0	4.1	−
3.5	3.6	−
3.7	3.7	0
3.6	3.7	−
4.2	4.2	0
4.1	4.0	+
4.5	4.5	0

The null hypothesis assumes that there is no difference between the medians of the two samples, and if this hypothesis is correct, the difference between the median of the plasma samples and the median of the serum samples should be zero. There should be approximately equal numbers of positive and negative differences.

Negatives 9

Positives 4

Zeros 5

Take the number of negative differences to a table of "exact" confidence limits for *Np.* Enter the table at N = (total number of data pairs) − (number of zero differences) (see Table 19-3).

$$N = 18 - 5 = 13$$

The critical range for an adjusted sample size of 13 is 2 − 11. Since the observed number of negative differences, 9, does not fall outside this range, the median difference between the paired-plasma and serum samples is not significantly different from zero at the 5% level.

Table 19-3   Exact confidence limits for *Np* (binomial distribution), *p* = 0.05; *N* = 0 to 99

N	0	1	2	3	4	5	6	7	8	9
0	—	—	—	—	—	—	0-6	0-7	0-8	1-8
10	1-9	1-10	2-10	2-11	2-12	3-12	3-13	4-13	4-14	4-15
20	5-15	5-16	5-17	6-17	6-18	7-18	7-19	7-20	8-20	8-21
30	9-21	9-22	9-23	10-23	10-24	11-24	11-25	12-25	12-26	12-27
40	13-28	13-28	14-28	14-29	15-29	15-30	15-31	16-31	16-32	17-32
50	17-33	18-33	18-34	18-35	19-35	19-36	20-36	20-37	21-37	21-38
60	21-39	22-39	22-40	23-40	23-41	24-41	21-42	25-42	25-43	25-44
70	26-44	26-45	27-45	27-46	28-46	28-47	28-48	29-48	29-49	30-49
80	30-50	31-50	31-51	32-51	32-52	32-53	33-53	33-54	34-54	34-55
90	35-55	35-56	36-56	36-57	37-57	37-58	37-59	38-59	38-60	39-60

Condensed from Lenter C: *Geigy scientific tables,* vol 2, *Introduction to statistics, statistical tables, mathematical formulae,* ed 8, Allschwil, Switzerland, 1982, Ciba-Geigy.

Mann-Whitney rank sum test (see Example 8)

Another alternative to the *t*-test is the *rank sum test*. There are two forms of this test, one by Wilcoxon, the other by Mann and Whitney. The test is usually called the Mann-Whitney test in order to avoid confusion with the paired test also developed by Wilcoxon.

To perform the test, one ranks the sample data from the two populations being compared as if they belonged to one population and then calculates the sum of the ranks of each group. The sum of the smaller N is designated T and is used in a table of *Acceptance regions for the rank sum T* (Table 19-4); the larger N is designated in the table as N_2. If the T *value* is outside the acceptance range for the number of values in each sample, the difference in the median values of the two populations is taken to be significant at a chosen p value.

If the populations were identical, an even distribution among the ranks of the two samples would be expected. An extremely large or extremely small rank sum in one of the samples should not be observed when the populations are the same. The rank sum table gives the limits for these extremes, and if these limits are exceeded, it makes sense to reject the null hypothesis of equality between the two populations.

Example 8. Mann-Whitney rank sum test

A comparison is carried out to determine if there is any difference between the blood urea nitrogen (BUN) concentrations in renal transplant recipients with stable graft function and a group of patients with urinary tract infections (UTI). The following results in milligrams per liter are observed in the two groups:

UTI ($n_1 = 14$)		Transplant ($n_2 = 12$)	
Rank	BUN	Rank	BUN
1	150		
2	170		
3	180		
*4.5	190		
		*4.5	190
**7	200		
**7	200		
		**7	200
9.5	210		
		9.5	210
12	220		
		12	220
		12	220
14	230		
16.5	240		
16.5	240		
		16.5	240
		16.5	240
		19	250
20.5	260		
		20.5	260
		22	270
23	280		
24	290		
		25	310
		26	320
Sum =	160.5	Sum =	190.5

The smaller of the two sums ($T = 160.5$) is taken to a table of acceptance ranges for the rank sum T (Table 19-4) at a level of $p = 0.05$ for $n_1 = 14$, $n_2 = 12$. The range of acceptance is 150 to 228. The calculated T value falls within this range, and the difference in the median values of BUN between these two populations is not considered significant at the 5% level.

$$*4.5 = \frac{4 + 5}{2}$$

$$**7 = \frac{6 + 7 + 8}{3}$$

χ^2 (chi-square) analysis

When populations contain a continuum of numbers, regression analysis and correlation coefficients can usually be used to measure their association. However, when the values of two populations are discrete, with few possible values such as yes/no, or positive/negative, *chi-square analysis* is used to test whether the populations are related. The analysis is based on the difference between the observed frequency of the values in a population and the expected frequency of the values of a population.

Often, the results obtained with real samples do not agree exactly with the theoretical results expected according to the rules of probability. For example, if a fair coin is tossed 100 times, 50 heads and 50 tails would be the expected result. However, these exact results are rarely obtained. A statistical method would be needed to determine whether the observed frequencies, say 47 heads and 53 tails, differ significantly from the expected frequencies (50 heads and 50 tails). The χ^2 statistical method provides a measure of the chance discrepancy that may exist between the observed and expected frequencies of the results of an analysis. The formula for the calculation of χ^2 is shown in equation 19-14:

$$\chi^2 = \frac{(o_1 - e_1)^2}{e_1} + \frac{(o_2 - e_2)^2}{e_2} + \ldots \frac{(o_k - e_k)^2}{e_k} \quad \textbf{\textit{Eq. 19-14}}$$

where o = the observed frequency result and e = the expected frequency result. If $\chi^2 = 0$, the observed and expected frequencies agree, whereas if $\chi^2 > 0$, they do not agree exactly. The larger the value for χ^2, the greater is the discrepancy between the observed and the expected frequencies.

In medical and healthcare research, chi-square analysis is often used to answer questions about the relationship between sex, age, race, or hormonal status, and some laboratory test result or physical condition of a patient (such as diabetes or hypertension).

Example 9. χ^2 (chi-square analysis)

In a study designed to determine whether there was a significant difference in estrogen receptor positivity between breast tumors resected from premenopausal and postmenopausal women, the following frequency of positive results were observed:

Premenopausal women:	ER+	308/581
Postmenopausal women:	ER+	648/1079

Table 19-4 Acceptance region for the rank sum *T* (Mann-Whitney-Wilcoxon 2 sample test), *p* = 0.05

N_1	1	2	3	4	5	6	7	8	9	10	11	12	13	14	15
N_2															
1	—	—	—	—	—	—	—	—	—	—	—	—	—	—	—
2	—	—	—	—	—	—	—	36-52	45-63	55-75	66-88	79-101	92-116	106-132	121-149
3	—	—	—	—	15-30	22-38	29-48	38-58	47-70	58-82	69-96	82-110	95-126	110-142	125-160
4	—	—	—	10-26	16-34	23-43	31-53	40-64	49-77	60-90	72-104	85-119	99-135	114-152	130-170
5	—	—	6-21	11-29	17-38	24-48	33-58	42-70	52-83	63-97	75-112	89-127	103-144	118-162	134-181
6	—	—	7-23	12-32	18-42	26-52	34-64	44-76	55-89	64-104	79-119	92-136	107-153	122-172	139-191
7	—	—	7-26	13-35	20-45	27-57	36-69	46-82	57-96	69-111	82-127	96-144	111-162	127-181	144-201
8	—	3-19	8-28	14-38	21-49	29-61	38-74	49-87	60-102	72-118	85-135	100-152	115-171	131-191	149-211
9	—	3-21	8-31	14-42	22-53	31-65	40-79	51-93	62-109	75-125	89-142	104-160	119-180	136-200	154-221
10	—	3-23	9-33	15-45	23-57	32-70	42-84	53-99	65-115	78-132	92-150	107-169	124-188	141-209	159-231
11	—	3-25	9-36	16-48	24-61	34-74	44-89	55-105	68-121	81-139	96-157	111-177	128-197	145-219	164-241
12	—	4-26	10-38	17-51	26-64	35-79	46-94	58-110	71-127	84-146	99-165	115-185	132-206	150-228	169-251
13	—	4-28	10-41	18-54	27-68	37-83	48-99	60-116	73-134	88-152	103-172	119-193	136-215	155-237	174-261
14	—	4-30	11-43	19-57	28-72	38-88	50-104	62-122	76-140	91-159	106-180	123-201	141-223	160-246	179-271
15	—	4-32	11-46	20-60	29-76	40-92	52-109	65-127	79-146	94-166	110-187	127-209	145-232	164-256	184-281

Condensed from Lenter C: *Geigy scientific tables*, vol 2, *Introduction to statistics, statistical tables, mathematical formulae*, ed 8, Allschwil, Switzerland, 1982, Ciba-Geigy.

Is the observed difference in ER (estrogen receptor) positivity among the two groups significant?

	Pos	Neg	Total
Observed			
Pre	308	273	581
Post	648	431	1079
Total	956	704	1660
Expected			
Pre	335	246	581
Post	621	458	1079
Total	956	704	1660

$$\chi^2 = \frac{(308 - 335)^2}{335} + \frac{(648 - 621)^2}{621} +$$

$$\frac{(273 - 246)^2}{246} + \frac{(431 - 458)^2}{458}$$

$$\chi^2 = 7.90$$

The critical value $\chi^2_{0.05}$ for 1 degree of freedom is 3.84 (see Table 19-5). Since 7.90 > 3.84, the hypothesis that there is no difference between the groups is rejected, and the hypothesis that there is a significantly higher estrogen receptor rate of positivity in breast tumors resected from postmenopausal women is accepted.

When a comparison is made between one sample and another, as in this estrogen receptor sample, an easy rule for the degrees of freedom is that they equal:

(Number of variables in columns − 1) ×
  (Number of variables in rows − 1)

Sample: (Pos + Neg −1) × (Pre + Post − 1) = 1

Example 10. A continuation of χ^2 (chi-square analysis)

The numbers in the previous chi-square table are represented by variables in the chart at right. The expected values are calculated under the assumption that the percent distribution between the positive and negative values should be equal for both the premenopausal and postmenopausal populations. This is true with any 2 × 2 chi-square table.

Table 19-5 Critical values for chi-square

Level	0.10	0.05	0.01
df			
1	2.706	3.841	6.635
2	4.605	5.991	9.210
3	6.251	7.815	11.345
4	7.779	9.488	13.277
5	9.236	11.070	15.086
6	10.654	12.592	16.812
7	12.017	14.067	18.475
8	13.362	15.507	20.090
9	14.684	16.919	21.666
10	15.987	18.307	23.209

Condensed from Lenter C: *Geigy scientific tables*, vol 2, *Introduction to statistics, statistical tables, mathematical formulae*, 1982, Ciba-Geigy.

	Pos	Neg	Total
Observed			
Pre	a_1	a_2	N_a
Post	b_1	b_2	N_b
Total	N_1	N_2	N_T
Expected			
Pre	$N_1 (N_a/N_T)$	$N_2 (N_a/N_T)$	N_a
Post	$N_1(N_b/N_T)$	$N_2(N_b/N_T)$	N_b
Total	N_1	N_2	N_T

There are simple formulas for computing χ^2 that use only the observed frequencies. The following give results for the 2 × 2 contingency table used in the estrogen receptor example above.

$$\chi^2 = \frac{N(a_1b_2 - a_2b_1)^2}{(a_1 + b_1)(a_2 + b_2)(a_1 + a_2)(b_1 + b_2)} = \frac{N\Delta^2}{N_1 N_2 N_a N_b}$$

$$\chi^2 = \frac{1660(132{,}748 - 176{,}904)^2}{956 \times 704 \times 581 \times 1079} = 7.67$$

LINEAR REGRESSION AND CORRELATION

For a wide variety of clinical laboratory applications it is useful to determine the relationship between two variables, *x* and *y*. If *x* can be considered a "fixed," or an *independent,* variable and *y* can be considered to be a "not fixed," or a *dependent,* variable, then it is mathematically valid to describe *y* as a *function* of *x*. A widely used and sometimes misused statistical procedure for assessing this relationship, or describing this function, is regression analysis.

Simple "linear"-regression analysis can be used when the relationship between the independent *x* and dependent *y* variables is a linear one. This type of regression analysis is termed "simple" because there is one independent variable. The simplest model for a relationship between two variables would be a straight line. Linear-regression analysis can be graphed on a rectilinear *x,y* plot where each pair of values is a point on the graph. Once all the *x,y* pairs are plotted, a straight line of "best fit" can be manually drawn through the points. If the straight-line model appears to be a valid depiction of the relationship between *x* and *y*, the line is termed the *regression line,* and its calculation is termed "regressing *y* on *x*."

Simple linear-regression analysis is used to answer the question: If we know what one variable *(x)* is, can we calculate what the other variable *(y)* would be under certain conditions? There is another way to ask this question. Can changes in *x* be used to predict changes in *y?* In consideration of this question, the *x* variable can also be termed the "predictor" variable and the *y* variable can also be termed the "response" variable.

In simple linear-regression analysis, the equation that de-scribes the linear relationship between *x* and *y* also can be said to describe *y* as a function of *x*, that is, $y = f(x)$. This function is described in equation 19-15:

$$y = \alpha + \beta x + \epsilon \qquad \textit{Eq. 19-15}$$

where α is the true value of the intercept of the regression line and β is the true value of the slope of the regression line. Using this function, *x* can be used to make a prediction of *y*.

In practice, the values of α and β in equation 19-15 are unknown and must be estimated as *a* and *b* respectively. It is also expected that the majority of the data points will not fall precisely on the regression line. The term ϵ is included in equation 19-15 to describe the distance between any observed value of *y* and the corresponding value of *y* that would be predicted or expected for *y*, which is denoted as $\hat{y}$. This value of ϵ is also termed the *residual* and exists because there is variability expected in *y* for any fixed, accurately known value of *x*. This basic assumption for using simple regression analysis is that for every known value of *x*, there is a corresponding normal distribution of *y* values. This assumption is graphically illustrated in Fig. 19-10, *A*. Notice that the regression line passes through the means of the distributions.

Use of the simple linear-regression model for appropriate applications requires that the two variables *x* and *y*, in fact, satisfy several conditions.

1. The *x* values are considered fixed, and any random error in the measurement of *x* can be considered "negligible."
2. For every value of *x*, there is a normal distribution of *y* values as illustrated in Fig. 19-10, *A*.

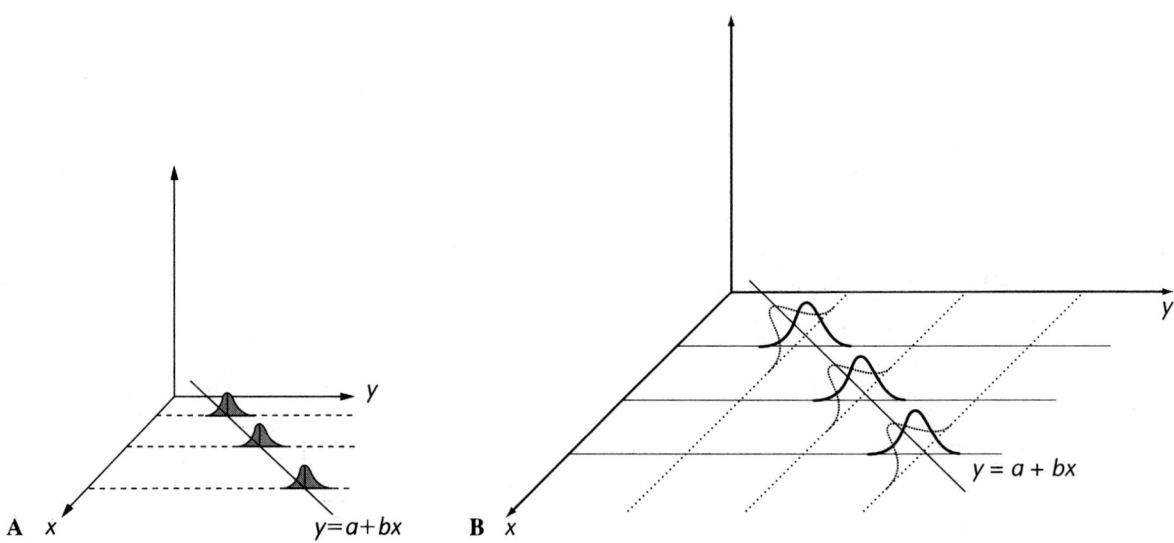

Fig. 19-10 **A,** Gaussian distributions of *y* values around simple linear-regression line. **B,** Gaussian distribution around Deming regression.

3. The distribution of y values for every value of x has the same variance; that is, the variance around the line is independent of the value of x.
4. The expected values of y for each x generally fit the straight-line model.
5. The straight-line model that is estimated is not horizontal (that is, β does not equal 0). If the straight line were horizontal, the values of y on the regression line would not be a better predictor of y than the mean y value, or $\bar{y}$.

If these conditions are met, use of the simple linear-regression model will allow the correct estimates of expected y values for each fixed value of x to be inferred.

The above conditions for simple linear regression should be satisfied for the majority of clinical laboratory applications. But in certain instances, the x values cannot be considered "fixed" or "invariable" as defined in condition 1. The most common misuse of simple linear-regression analysis involves the false assumption that values of x are fixed or that x is an independent variable when, in fact, it is not. For example, in a typical comparison of two methods, the results of one method will be considered to be the "x," independent variable (see p. 415). Although this may be the current method, each "x" result cannot be considered "fixed" but is reported with a certain error. In this instance, it is appropriate to consider using a different type of regression analysis. Although there are several types of regression techniques described in the literature, the technique that may be most appropriate to apply when there is variability in the values of x and in the values of y is the *Deming regression* technique (Fig. 19-10, *B*).[10,11]

In a simple linear-regression analysis, one could attempt to determine values for a and b using the manual plot of the data and the "best-fit" regression line (see p. 360). Conventionally, however, the method used to determine the correct regression parameters is the *method of least squares.* Using this method, the sum of the squares of the residuals of all the y values is minimized mathematically. Predicting expected y values based on the actual x,y data points using this method and calculating the subsequent regression statistics, for either the simple or Deming's model, are most easily done with the use of a calculator or software program that can generate the appropriate statistics automatically.

The method of least squares is valid if the residuals are random (that is, independent of values of x and y) and have a gaussian distribution with a mean of 0 and a standard deviation, $S_{y,x}$.[11] The standard deviation of the residuals, or *standard error of the estimate,* should be constant at every x value (see p. 362). It has been reported that within the range of measurement commonly encountered in most clinical laboratory applications, the method of least squares also correctly calculates a regression line when $S_{y,x}$ is proportional to x.[11]

Appropriate clinical laboratory applications for simple linear-regression analysis, when x can legitimately be considered a fixed or independent variable, are as follows:

1. Comparison of results from a new procedure to results from an established procedure.
2. Comparison of a technique to a reference method (see Chapter 22 for these two applications).
3. Comparison of paired results for the same test or analyte collected from two different analytical systems in current use. This application could be used to validate test systems secondarily with a test system that has been validated by external proficiency testing. This application would satisfy the Clinical Laboratory Improvement Amendments of 1988 regulations for proficiency testing.
4. Comparison of results from the same analytical system collected during two different analytical runs.

In either simple linear or Deming regression analysis, a relationship exists between the x and y variables, though the mathematical description of this relationship would be somewhat different for each type of regression technique. When a linear relationship exists between two variables, these variables can be considered to have a *correlation* with each other. If increasing values of x are related in a linear fashion to increasing values of y, there is a *positive correlation* between these variables. If increasing values of x are related in a linear fashion to decreasing values of y, there is a *negative correlation* between these variables (see p. 362).

It is, of course, possible that the relationship between two variables is a nonlinear relationship. If this is the case, the computation of basic linear-regression parameters may reflect this relationship. For example, determination of the correlation coefficient, r, may indicate a value much closer to 0 than either 1 or -1. It is also likely that a nonlinear relationship would be reflected in an increased value $s_{y,x}$. If this were the case, the application of either simple linear regression or Deming regression analysis would be inappropriate and other regression techniques should be utilized.[4-8] Of course, it is also true that a nonlinear relationship or an increased amount of scatter may be apparent upon visual inspection of the regression plot.

Basic statistics of simple linear regression and correlation

With the two methods of linear regression described above, the line of best fit would be determined by either the method of least squares or the method of Deming. In either case, once the correct line to fit the appropriate model is identified, this line can then be described by equation 19-16:

$$y = bx + a \qquad\qquad \textit{Eq. 19-16}$$

where b is the estimated slope of the regression line and a is the estimated intercept of the regression line on the y-axis.

Although the "best fit" of the regression line may appear

obvious by visual examination of the graphed scatterplot, this method is not recommended. More appropriately, calculation of the regression parameters, *a* and *b,* with the use of a calculator or software program allows for an exact prediction of any additional value of *y* once the *x* value is known. Automatic calculation of the regression parameters and the subsequent determination of two predicted *y* values from two different *x* values would then allow for the correct graphical placement of the regression line, since two points determine the location of a straight line.

In simple linear regression, the statistical parameters, *a* and *b,* the *y*-intercept, and the slope of the regression line respectively can be calculated by use of equations 19-17 and 19-18:

$$a = \bar{y} - b\bar{x} \qquad \qquad \textit{Eq. 19-17}$$

$$b = \frac{\Sigma(x - \bar{x})(y - \bar{y})}{\Sigma(x - \bar{x})^2} \qquad \qquad \textit{Eq. 19-18}$$

To measure the variability of the data points about the regression line, one needs to determine the standard deviation about the regression line of the differences between the observed and the predicted values of *y* (that is, the residuals). This variability, termed the *standard error of the estimate,* is calculated by use of equation 19-19:

$$S_{y,x} = \left(\frac{\Sigma(y - \bar{y})^2}{N - 2} \right)^{1/2} \qquad \qquad \textit{Eq. 19-19}$$

Use of $(N - 2)$ degrees of freedom in the denominator is appropriate because two regression coefficients, *a* and *b,* had to be determined from the data in order to calculate the predicted values of *y.* That is, two restrictions are placed on the *N* observations.

One determines the variability of the estimated slope, *b,* of the simple linear-regression line by first calculating the standard deviation of the slope, s_b, using equation 19-20:

$$s_b = s_{y,x} / [\Sigma(x_i - \bar{x})^2]^{1/2} \qquad \qquad \textit{Eq. 19-20}$$

and then determining a $100(1 - p)\%$ confidence interval for the true slope, β, using equation 19-21:

$$\beta = b \pm t \cdot s_b \qquad \qquad \textit{Eq. 19-21}$$

where *t* is obtained from a two-sided *t*-table for $N - 2$ degrees of freedom and the desired level of significance.

The variability of the estimated intercept, *a,* of the simple linear-regression line is determined in a similar manner. The estimated standard deviation of *a,* s_a, is calculated by use of equation 19-22:

$$s_a = s_{y,x} [\Sigma x_i^2 / N \Sigma (x_i - \bar{x})^2]^{1/2} \qquad \qquad \textit{Eq. 19-22}$$

and then by determination of a $100(1 - p)\%$ confidence interval for the true intercept, α, by use of equation 19-23:

$$\alpha = a \pm t \cdot s_a \qquad \qquad \textit{Eq. 19-23}$$

where *t* is, again, obtained from a two-sided *t*-table for $N - 2$ degrees of freedom and the desired level of significance.

The statistic that provides a measure of how closely the data points lie to the regression line is *r,* or the Pearson correlation coefficient. This correlation coefficient, *r,* is a measure of the degree that two variables are linearly related. The calculation of *r* is illustrated in equation 19-24:

$$r = \frac{\Sigma (x_i - \bar{x}) (y_i - \bar{y})}{\{\Sigma [(x_i - \bar{x})^2] [\Sigma(y_i - \bar{y})^2]\}^{1/2}} \qquad \textit{Eq. 19-24}$$

Essentially, *r* describes how strong a correlation there is between the *x* and *y* variables.

The correlation coefficient, *r,* can range in value from -1 to 1. If *r* is equal to 1, there is a perfect positive correlation between the variables. If *r* is equal to -1, there is a perfect negative correlation between the variables. The further the correlation coefficient is from 0, the stronger the correlation is, positive or negative, between the variables. If the correlation coefficient is equal to 0, there is no *linear* relationship between the variables. This should not be interpreted to mean that there is no relationship between the two variables. It is possible that these two uncorrelated variables are strongly related in nonlinear fashion (this would be apparent from a visual inspection of the *x,y* scatterplot).

At what value of *r* can one assume there is not a linear relationship between the *x* and *y* variables? From an empirical perspective, an *r* value between -0.7 and 0.7 would indicate that the probability of the relationship between *x* and *y* being linear is less than 50%. As *r* approaches zero, this probability also approaches zero. If the data collected for analysis by linear regression is from routine laboratory methods, a practical consideration is that a low *r* value can be caused by very poor precision in the method used to obtain *x* values, *y* values, or both variables.

An example of the use of equations 19-17 to 19-24 for calculation of basic statistics of simple linear-regression analysis is illustrated in Example 11. This example illustrates the use of simple linear-regression analysis and Deming regression analysis for the comparison of two potassium methods. Equations for the calculated Deming regression statistics are given elsewhere.[10]

Example 11. Linear-regression analysis

In an initial method comparison study, 42 pairs of potassium measurements are obtained from an established method (old) and an experimental method (new). Calculate regression statistics, first assuming that there is negligible variability in the old method (use simple linear-regression analysis) and then assuming that there is variability in the established method (using Deming regression equations, as cited in references 10 and 11).

Assuming there is negligible variability in the established method, calculate the standard error of the estimate, variability of the estimated slope and intercept, and the 95% confidence intervals for the actual slope and intercept for the population.

All *x,y* (old,new) potassium results are in millimoles per liter:

3.9, 3.9	3.9, 3.9	3.4, 3.4	5.4, 5.2	4.0, 4.0
4.6, 4.5	4.2, 4.2	4.3, 4.1	4.3, 4.3	4.8, 4.7
3.7, 3.6	4.4, 4.3	4.4, 4.4	4.5, 4.4	3.9, 3.9
4.3, 4.3	3.8, 3.7	3.8, 3.7	3.9, 3.8	4.0, 3.9
4.6, 4.5	3.4, 3.4	4.2, 4.1	3.8, 3.8	3.6, 3.6
4.3, 4.3	4.1, 4.0	3.5, 3.4	4.6, 4.8	4.1, 4.2
3.7, 3.1	4.1, 4.1	4.8, 4.7	3.3, 3.2	5.4, 5.4
4.0, 3.9	4.5, 4.4	3.5, 3.6	3.7, 3.7	4.1, 4.1
3.6, 3.5	3.0, 3.1			

	Simple linear-regression analysis	Deming regression
Slope *(b)*	0.99	0.98
Intercept *(a)*	−0.03	0.22
$S_{y,x}$	0.12	0.09
r	0.97	0.98

For 95% confidence intervals and $N - 2$ degrees of freedom (40), *t* value from a two-sided table = 2.021.

Variability of estimated slope:

Standard deviation of estimated slope $(b) =$
$$s_b = s_x \Big/ [\Sigma(x_i - \bar{x})^2]^{1/2} = 0.12/3.24 = 0.04$$

Confidence interval for the true slope $(\beta) =$
$$\beta = b \pm t \cdot s_b = 0.99 \pm 2.021\,(0.04) = 0.99 \pm 0.07$$

Variability of estimated intercept:

Standard deviation of estimated intercept $(a) =$
$$s_a = s_{y,x}[\Sigma x_i^2 \big/ N\Sigma\,(x_i - \bar{x})^2]^{1/2} = 0.12(1.28) = 0.15$$

Confidence interval for the true intercept $(\alpha) =$
$$\alpha = a \pm t \cdot s_a = -0.03 \pm 2.021(0.15) = -0.03 \pm 0.30$$

Testing for outliers using residual analysis

Simple linear-regression analysis can be used to identify outliers, or extreme paired values, in the *x,y* data points. This procedure involves the plotting of the residuals, or ϵ, against the independent variable *x*.[8] It may then be appropriate to exclude any data points that generate residuals greater than 4 $s_{y,x}$. The plot of residuals can be evaluated against the independent variable *x* for assessment of the equality of variances. If the variances are equal, the plotted residuals will be seen as a horizontal band of points that are independent of *x* (one of the conditions necessary to apply simple linear regression to a pair of variables).

One can obtain additional information by plotting the residuals against the predicted values of *y*. If there is truly a linear relationship between the *x* and *y* variables, the residuals would be randomly scattered, in horizontal fashion, around zero.

Limitations of simple linear-regression analysis

When paired data spanning a limited range are analyzed by the simple linear-regression method, an acceptable level of random error can still result in inaccurate estimates of the slope and intercept of the regression line. This problem is magnified if the *x* variable should really not be considered fixed or independent. In this instance, an unacceptably large standard error of the slope and intercept as well as an unacceptably low correlation coefficient may also be calculated, and it is appropriate to use Deming regression analysis instead of simple linear-regression analysis.

There are other considerations that may suggest that Deming regression should be utilized instead of simple linear-regression analysis. One can make an initial assessment of this question by plotting one variable on the *x*-axis in a first *x,y* plot and generating regression statistics. Then the procedure is repeated with the second variable plotted on the *x*-axis. If the two least-squares regression lines are substantially different from one another, the Deming regression should be used. The Deming method will yield one regression line between *x* and *y* that takes into account the error in measuring both variables. A characteristic of the Deming regression technique is that switching the variables and recalculating regression statistics will give identical statistics to the initial calculation.

Finally, it must be noted that the value of *r* in simple linear-regression analysis is sensitive to both the scatter of the data points and the range of data points. The scatter of the data points is a characteristic of the dependent method being evaluated. But it is possible to increase the value of *r* by simply extending the range of data. Extension of the range of data by one single point farther away from the majority of data points where this single point coincidentally happens to demonstrate close agreement between *x* and *y* will dramatically increase the value of *r*. This characteristic is described in equation 19-25:

$$r = (1/s_x)\,(s_x^2 + s_{y,x}^2)^{1/2} \qquad \textbf{\textit{Eq. 19-25}}$$

where s_x is the standard deviation of the *x* population, an indication of the spread in the *x* data. As s_x becomes very large relative to $s_{y,x}$, *r* approaches 1.0. Because of this characteristic, it is always wise to evaluate an *x,y* plot, visually examining the simple linear-regression line generated from the data. It may be obvious that a point lying far above or below the regression line is an outlier. But a more insidious outlier might be the point that lies exactly on the regression line but is considerably removed from the range of the remaining data points used to generate the regression statistics.

REFERENCES

1. Barnett RN: *Clinical laboratory statistics,* ed 2, Boston, 1979, Little, Brown & Co.
2. Lenter C: *Geigy scientific tables,* vol 2, *Introduction to statistics, statistical tables, mathematical formulae,* ed 8, Allschwil, Switzerland, 1982, Ciba-Geigy.
3. Spiegel MR: *Schaum's outline series theory and problems of statistics,* ed 2, New York, 1988, McGraw-Hill.
4. Mason RL, Gunst RF, Hess JL: *Statistical design and analysis of experiments with applications to engineering and science,* New York, 1989, Wiley & Sons.

5. Snedecor GW, Cochran WG: *Statistical methods,* ed 8, Ames, Iowa, 1989, Iowa State University Press.
6. Shott S: *Statistics for health professionals,* Philadelphia, 1990, Saunders.
7. Altman DG: *Practical statistics for medical research,* New York, 1991, Chapman & Hall.
8. Dowdy S, Wearden S: *Statistics for research,* ed 2, New York, 1991, Wiley & Sons.
9. Lenter C: *Geigy scientific tables,* vol 2, *Introduction to statistics, statistical tables, mathematical formulae,* ed 8, Allschwil, Switzerland, 1982, Ciba-Geigy.
   Significance limits for testing extreme values of a sample, p. 60.
10. Wallers PJM, Hellendoorn HBA, Op de Weegh GJ, Heerspink W: Applications of statistics in clinical chemistry—a critical evaluation of regression lines, *Clin Chim Acta* 64:173-184, 1975.
11. Cornbleet PJ, Gochman N: Incorrect least-squares regression coefficients in method-comparison analysis, *Clin Chem* 25(3):432-438, 1979.

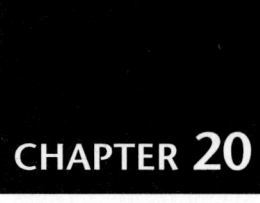

CHAPTER 20

Reference intervals and clinical decision limits

Edward A. Sasse

OBJECTIVES

- State the purpose of reference intervals and identify primary considerations of the sampling process when one is establishing a reference interval.

- Suggest a statistical approach for establishing the reference interval for nongaussian distributions.

KEY TERMS

abnormal Test results outside of reference intervals observed in people with disease or in less than good health.

cutoff values Those limits above or below which the patient is abnormal or positive for a condition such as substance abuse.

decision analysis Strategy comparing risks and benefits of predicting the true diagnosis or outcome.

gaussian A particular symmetrical statistical distribution; also called the *normal distribution.*

healthy A relative term that must be defined for each reference population.

log normal A symmetrical gaussian population distribution obtained by a plot of the logarithm of the data.

log-normal distribution A sample of values with a long tail to the right can often be made to act as a gaussian distribution when one uses the logarithms of values.

medical decision limits The values or changes in values that result in immediate medical intervention or change in medical management.

negative predictive value The probability that a laboratory result falling within the reference interval reflects the true absence of disease; defined as true negatives divided by the sum of true negatives and false negatives.

normal A term with many meanings, including those persons in the nondiseased population and an equivalent term for a gaussian distribution (see this chapter for a discussion).

observed value The quantitative value (test result) obtained for a test subject (such as a patient) to be compared with reference values, reference distributions, reference limits, or reference intervals.

outlier An observation that arises from a population different from the reference population. The outlier can be an erroneous result or an observation on a subject that does not conform to the characteristics of a reference individual.

partitioning of reference values The process of separating reference intervals of subjects based on criteria of age, sex, and race, as well as statistical analysis showing significant differences between the populations.

positive predictive value The probability that a laboratory result outside the reference interval actually reflects the presence of disease; defined as true positives divided by the sum of true positives and false positives.

predictive value Probability that a laboratory result accurately reflects the true presence or absence of disease. It is dependent on the actual prevalence of the disease.

prevalence The number of persons who have a disease in a given population at any one point in time, or more often the rate of such disease, which is also called the *disease frequency.*

receiver-operating characteristic curve (ROC) A graphical presentation of discrimination of disease from nondisease by plotting sensitivity.

reference distribution The distribution of reference values. Hypotheses regarding the distribution of reference values of a reference population may be tested statistically.

reference individual An individual selected on the basis of well-defined criteria. It is usually important to define the individual's state of health, age, sex, and race.

reference interval (Listed in the Clinical Laboratory Improvement Amendments of 1988, CLIA '88, as reference range.) The interval between and including two reference limits. It is designed as the central interval of values bounded by the lower reference limit and upper reference limit at certain designated percentiles. For example, for fasting glucose the central 95th percentile reference interval is 65 to 110 mg/dL (3.6 to 6.1 mmol/L), that is, 95% of the apparently healthy reference population will have a fasting glucose value of 65 to 110 mg/dL.

reference limit A numeric value or values derived from the reference distribution and used for descriptive purposes. It is common practice to define a reference limit so that a stated fraction of the reference values will be less than or equal to, or more than or equal to, the respective upper or lower limit.

reference population A group consisting of all the reference individuals. The reference population usually has an unknown number of members and therefore is a hypothetical entity.

reference range The entire range (actual minimal to maximal measured values) of laboratory values of people without disease.

reference sample group An adequate number of reference individuals selected to represent the reference population.

reference value The value (test result) obtained by the observation or measurement of a particular analyte for a reference individual. Reference values are obtained from a reference sample group.

sensitivity A term used to describe the probability that a laboratory test is positive (that is, outside of the reference interval) in the presence of disease; defined as true positives divided by the sum of true positives and false negatives.

specificity Used to describe the probability that a laboratory test will be negative (that is, within the reference interval) in the absence of disease; defined as true negatives divided by the sum of true negatives and false positives.

standard deviation A measure of variability. In the gaussian distribution, two standard deviations above and below the mean encompass the central 95% of the population data, and one standard deviation above and below encompasses 68.3% of the data.

DEFINITION OF REFERENCE INTERVAL

The medical interpretation of clinical laboratory data is a comparative decision-making process in which a laboratory test result for an individual is compared with a reference interval derived from reference values. Therefore, reliable reference values are required for all tests in the clinical laboratory and must be provided by clinical laboratories and diagnostic test manufacturers. The reference intervals most commonly used (often known as "normal values" and sometimes "expected values") are often poorly defined.

Reference intervals should be determined in a systematic

and scientific manner that provides an acceptable degree of confidence for the clinical decision-making process, which includes a consideration of the significant factors and variables introduced by the specific individual's reference sample or by the analytical process itself. Understanding the process used to establish a reference interval yields a better understanding of the limitations of the defined reference interval.

To facilitate the generation of reliable reference intervals, the National Committee for Clinical Laboratory Standards (NCCLS) has recently published a document entitled *How to define and determine reference intervals in the clinical laboratory; approved guideline* (NCCLS Document C28-A),[1] which establishes guidelines and procedures for determining valid reference values and reference intervals for quantitative clinical laboratory tests. The NCCLS document catalogs the significant factors and variables that may affect the reference interval and is based on the recommendations of the Expert Panel on Theory of Reference Values (EPTRV) of the International Federation of Clinical Chemistry (IFCC).[2-7] The recommendations given in the NCCLS guideline are intended to compose a standard protocol for determining reference intervals that meet the minimum, mandatory requirements for reliability.

Consequently, reference interval determination should follow the guidelines of the NCCLS protocol. However, there are instances, particularly for geriatric and pediatric populations, when it is difficult to collect data from the recommended number of reference individuals. In these instances, the proper and well-defined selection of reference individuals becomes preeminent. These reference values, with their limitations, are still useful to the practice of medicine in these particular patient categories.

Reference values may be associated with good health or with specific physiological or pathological conditions and may be used for different reasons. For example, to establish the sensitivity and specificity of a laboratory test, the laboratory must carefully define the population. In all cases, the reference values allow comparison of observed data to reference data for a defined population of subjects. This comparison then becomes part of the decision-making process.

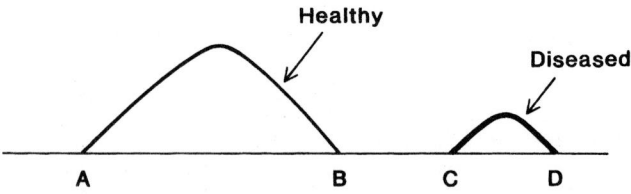

Fig. 20-1 Perfectly separated test result distributions of healthy and diseased populations. This clear separation rarely occurs in reality.

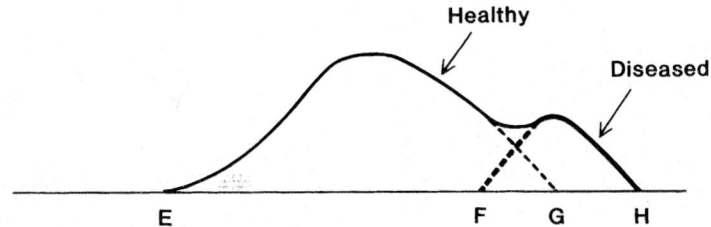

Fig. 20-2   Usual test result distributions of healthy and diseased populations in which an overlap between the two occur.

TERMINOLOGY

Specific definitions for terms permit relatively unambiguous description and discussion of the subject of reference values. The definitions listed in the key terms have been proposed by the EPTRV of the IFCC[2] and International Council for Standardization in Hematology and have been endorsed by the World Health Organization and other organizations worldwide.

The following scheme[2] demonstrates the relationship between the defined terms.

(1) REFERENCE INDIVIDUALS
compose a
↓
(2) REFERENCE POPULATION
from which is selected a
↓
(3) REFERENCE SAMPLE GROUP
on which are determined
↓
(4) REFERENCE VALUES
on which is observed a
↓
(8) OBSERVED VALUE in an individual may be compared with (5) (5) REFERENCE DISTRIBUTION
from which are calculated
↓
(6) REFERENCE LIMITS
which may define
↓
(7) REFERENCE INTERVALS

The reference limits and associated reference interval are usually estimated by a statistical method. Reference limits serve only to describe the reference sample group or reference population and are strictly a function of the characteristics of the designated population.

The term *reference range* has commonly been used as a substitute for "reference interval"; however, such a term

should be avoided. "Range" should be reserved for describing a set of values defined by the actual minimal and maximal measured values, that is, the entire range of values of the measured set.

The reference intervals most commonly used to describe healthy individuals have been known as "normal values," referring to reference values that have been observed in "normal," or healthy, people. Test results outside of these reference intervals may, therefore, be observed in people with disease or in states of less than good health and have consequently been termed as "abnormal." However, there is often an overlap of "normal" and "abnormal" values in disease because most disease processes and associated biological analytes change in a continuing fashion. Consequently "normal" values do not always indicate a lack of disease (Figs. 20-1 to 20-3), nor does a value exceeding a defined limit always indicate disease. The use of the term "normal" in this context is now considered to be an ambiguous term.

The word "normal" has several different connotations in laboratory medicine that can cause confusion. Values are often described as normal if their observed distribution seems to follow the theoretical gaussian ("normal") distribution. However, biological data from a reference sample group is often not gaussian, and the use of "normal" may be misleading by inferring that the data are symmetrical or bell-shaped in distribution. Other meanings of "normal" are "common," "frequent," "usual," and "typical," which also may be used in statements referring to biological or clinical values. Therefore it is more precise and less confusing to avoid the terminology "normal values" and replace it with "reference values (or reference interval) obtained from healthy individuals," "health-associated reference values (or reference intervals)," or colloquially, "healthy reference val-

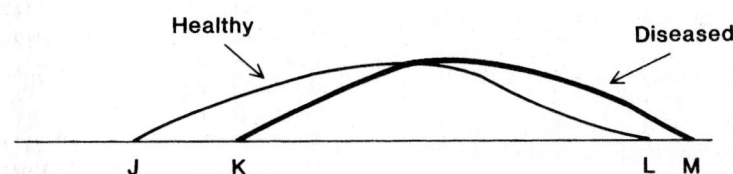

Fig. 20-3   Degree of test result overlap does not permit differentiation between healthy and diseased populations.

ues (intervals)." As previously mentioned, reference intervals can also be established for physiological conditions other than good health.

PROTOCOL OUTLINE FOR OBTAINING REFERENCE VALUES AND ESTABLISHING HEALTH-ASSOCIATED REFERENCE INTERVALS[1]

The collection or verification of reference values from healthy subjects and the subsequent estimation of the reference interval for a given analyte is a requirement of CLIA '88 regulations (§493.1213), *Federal Register* 57(40) Feb 28, 1992, and must be carried out in accordance with a well-defined protocol. This involves following the sequence of operations listed in the following box.

It is sometimes acceptable to transfer a previously established reference interval that is based on a valid reference value study from a donor laboratory or manufacturer to a receiving laboratory without performing a new, full-scale study. Such a transfer is acceptable only if the test subject population and the entire methodology, from preparation of the test individual to the analytical measurement in the receiving laboratory, is the same as or appropriately compa-

rable to that of the donor laboratory (see proceeding text). The comparability of the analytical measuring system can be validated using the techniques discussed in NCCLS Document EP9-P, *User Comparisons of Quantitative Clinical Laboratory Methods Using Patient Samples: Proposed Guideline.*[8] It may be necessary to carry out an abbreviated reference value study, as described later, to validate the transferred reference interval.

SELECTION OF REFERENCE INDIVIDUALS

Health is a relative condition lacking a universal definition. Defining what is to be considered healthy becomes the initial problem in any study, and establishing the criteria used to exclude nonhealthy subjects from the reference sample is the first step in selecting reference individuals. Frequently, one can only determine that a particular individual is apparently "disease free," that is, does not have a specific medical condition that might affect the reference interval study. In some cases, individuals with minor illnesses or "unrelated" conditions may be used as reference individuals. However, it is often difficult to estimate the potential physiological and pharmacological influences in these subjects, and appropriate caution is required.

The selection of reference individuals for a reference value study is important and should be systematic.[1,3,9] Each institution or investigator may have different criteria for health; these criteria should be defined *before* one proceeds. As a minimum it is recommended that the investigator establish lists of selection, exclusion, and potential partition criteria (examples are shown in Tables 20-1 and 20-2) and utilize a questionnaire to evaluate these criteria in the potential reference individuals. The use of designed questionnaires is one of the best ways to consistently implement the exclusion and partitioning criteria. Forms should be simple and nonintimidating, requiring only *yes* or *no* responses to questions. The questionnaire may be used with simple measurements, such as blood pressure, height, and weight, and with an interview during which it is appropriate to ask individuals if they consider themselves to be in good health. Name, address, and phone number and any additional information, such as a patient identification number, should

---

Protocol Outline for Obtaining Reference Values and Reference Intervals

1. Consult the medical and scientific literature and list possible biological variations and analytical interferences. (In the case of a totally new analyte, a laboratory may need to perform its own studies.)
2. Establish selection (or exclusion) and partition criteria and an appropriate questionnaire designed to reveal these criteria in the potential reference individuals.
3. Categorize the potential reference individuals based on the questionnaire findings and the results of other appropriate health assessments.
4. Exclude individuals from the reference sample group, based on the exclusion criteria or other assessments indicating a lack of good health.
5. Select the appropriate reference individuals.
6. Prepare the reference individuals properly and consistently for specimen collection following the specific requirements for the analyte and consistent with routine practice for patients.
7. Collect and process the biological specimens properly and uniformly and consistent with the routine practice for patient specimens.
8. Determine the reference values by analyzing the specimens according to the respective analytical methodology under well-defined conditions.
9. Inspect the reference value data and prepare a histogram.
10. Identify data errors and values that are outliers.
11. Analyze the reference values, that is, select a statistical method of estimation and estimate reference limits and the reference interval (include partitioning into subclasses for separate reference intervals, if appropriate).
12. Document all the above steps and procedures.

Table 20-1   Examples of possible exclusion criteria

Alcohol consumption	Recent illness
Abnormal blood pressure	Lactation
Blood donor, frequent	Obesity
Drug abuse	Occupation
Prescription drugs	Oral contraceptives
Over-the-counter drugs	Pregnancy
Environment	Recent surgery
Fasting or nonfasting	Tobacco use
Genetic factors	Recent transfusion
Current/recent hospitalization	Vitamin abuse

From National Committee for Clinical Laboratory Standards: *How to define, determine and utilize reference intervals in the clinical laboratory: proposed guideline,* NCCLS Document C28-A, Villanova, Penn., 1995, NCCLS.

be included to facilitate contacting the reference individual when abnormal results are obtained. Certainly there is an obligation to notify the individual or the individual's physician in such cases. In some situations anonymous questionnaires may be a better vehicle for obtaining the required information. In these instances a numbering system can be used. (The reference individual would then be responsible for contacting the laboratory to determine if the testing showed any problems that require follow-up study.) In all cases, the usual policy for patient confidentiality must be enforced.

Informed consent should be obtained from reference individuals for specimen collection and testing. In some cases, protocol review and approval by an institutional research committee (human use committee) may be necessary. A sample questionnaire is provided in the NCCLS C28-A document.[1] Determination of the health status of the individuals by medical examinations and laboratory testing is not considered to be essential. However, if these assessments are performed, they will, of course, strengthen the reliability of the reference interval determination. All criteria and assessments used should be documented so that others can evaluate the health status of the reference sample group.

Reference individuals used for the determination of a health-associated reference interval do not have to be young healthy adults but should closely resemble the patient population in the specific hospital or practice that will be using the results. However, for some particular analytes a "standard" population of young healthy adults may be appropriate. For others, age-related sets of reference intervals may be more appropriate. In the elderly population, it may be particularly important to rule out disease by use of additional diagnostic assessments. Patient populations should not be used as disease-free reference individuals unless it is absolutely essential, as in certain instances for pediatric or geriatric populations.

It is necessary to determine for each analyte whether there are age-related differences, whether these differences are clinically important, and whether the use of age subgroups for reference intervals will be clinically appropriate. For certain biological constituents, age-related differences are consistent with good health and are part of a nor-

mal process of growth or maturation, such as alkaline phosphatase levels in children versus those in adults. However, for levels of other substances, such as cholesterol or possibly growth hormone in the elderly, the use of different levels to reflect age differences may not be medically suitable when developing health-associated reference intervals. Consequently, determination of the need for separate reference intervals for age subgroups at specified age-group intervals is a rather complex medical decision. Review of the literature can be very helpful in making this evaluation.

The terms *a priori* and *a posteriori* are used to describe two general methods of selecting reference individuals from the reference population. *A priori* sampling is a method that is best used for well-studied, established laboratory procedures. Well-defined exclusion and partitioning criteria are established before the selection of the reference individuals. For established methods, a thorough search of the literature should allow one to identify known sources of biological variation, enabling the researchers to establish exclusion and partitioning criteria and to develop an appropriate questionnaire. Reference individuals are then selected and partitioned into subclasses, if necessary. This process should take place *before* any blood samples are collected. The number of reference individuals selected for analysis must closely match the number required to be statistically valid.

The *a posteriori* approach is especially appropriate for new or poorly studied laboratory procedures for which the literature contains little information. In *a posteriori* sampling the process of exclusion and partitioning takes place after sampling and analyte testing rather than before. Since the factors defining a subclass are not usually known, the questionnaire for this approach should be more detailed than the one designed for the *a priori* sampling process. Generally the *a posteriori* approach requires large numbers of subjects and substantial computing power to be implemented effectively.

PREANALYTICAL AND ANALYTICAL VARIABLES

Analytical results from reference populations are affected by preanalytical and analytical variables. Therefore, all these variables must be considered and controlled consistently when one is determining reference intervals.[10-15] In addition, it is important that reference subjects and samples be handled in an approved manner[16-22] and in exactly the same manner as patients and patient samples will be handled in the actual clinical analysis situation. All the preanalytical variables discussed in detail in Chapter 3 and reviewed in Table 20-3 must be carefully considered, controlled if necessary, and documented.

ANALYTICAL METHOD CHARACTERISTICS

The validity of information provided by the laboratory is critical; thus one must describe in detail the methods chosen for specimen analysis, clearly stating accuracy, preci-

Table 20-2   Examples of possible partitioning factors

Age	Posture when sampled
Blood group	Race
Circadian variation	Sex
Diet	Stage of menstrual cycle
Ethnic background	Stage of pregnancy
Exercise	Time of day when sampled
Fasting or nonfasting	Tobacco use
Geographic location	

From National Committee for Clinical Laboratory Standards: *How to define, determine, and utilize reference intervals in the clinical laboratory: proposed guideline,* NCCLS Document C28-A, Villanova, Penn., 1995, NCCLS.

Table 20-3 Examples of preanalytical variables

Subject preparation	Specimen collection	Specimen handling
Prior diet	Environmental conditions during collection	Transport
Fasting versus nonfasting	Time	Clotting
Abstinence from pharmacologic agents	Body posture	Separation of serum/plasma
Drug regimen	Specimen type	Storage
Synchronization in analysis	Collection site analysis	Preparation for analysis
Relation to biological rhythms	Site preparation	
Physical activity	Blood flow promotion	
Rest period before collection	Equipment	
Stress	Technique	

From National Committee for Clinical Laboratory Standards: *How to define and determine reference intervals in the clinical laboratory: approved guideline*, NCCLS Document C28-A, Villanova, Penn., 1995, NCCLS.

sion, minimum detection limit, linearity, recovery, and interference characteristics.[10-12] Other factors that affect analytical performance also require control and documentation. These include equipment or instrumentation, reagents (including water), calibration standards, and calculation methods.

Reagent lot-to-lot and technologist variability, as well as instrument-to-instrument variability (if the test will be performed on more than one instrument), must be determined. Thus the use of more than one technologist and more than one lot of reagent should be incorporated in the study protocol.

It is important to document the validity of the data generated during the reference interval study. Therefore, during the determination of reference intervals, quality control materials are routinely analyzed in the same format used for patient samples. This not only monitors the analytical protocol used during the process, but also ensures equivalence of results over the long term.[13] Ideally, one will gather data by analyzing specimens over several days, resulting in values that reflect average run-to-run variation (see Chapter 21). In addition, an assessment of the interference from naturally occurring constituents is essential.

ANALYSIS OF REFERENCE VALUES[1]
Statistical methods

The reference interval is defined here as the interval between and including two numbers, an upper and lower reference limit. These two numbers are estimated to enclose a specified percentage (usually 95%) of the values for a population from which the reference subjects have been drawn. For most analytes, the lower and upper reference limits are assumed to demarcate the estimated 2.5th and 97.5th percentiles, respectively, of the underlying distribution of values. In some cases, only one reference limit is of medical importance, usually an upper limit, say, the 97.5th percentile.

Two general statistical methods for determining such limits are the nonparametric and the parametric procedures (see also Chapter 19). Detailed presentations of these procedures have been published by Solberg.[6,9] The nonparametric method of estimation makes no specific assumption concerning the mathematical form of the probability distribution represented by the observed reference values. The parametric method, as applied in practice, is used under the assumption that the observed values, or some mathematical transformation of those values, follow a gaussian (that is, "normal") probability curve. Since the reference values of many analytes do not follow the gaussian form, use of the parametric method requires that they be transformed to some other measurement scale that will "normalize" them. This requires selecting the most suitable transform (such as log, power, or some other function of the original scale) and then testing whether, on this new scale, the reference values do indeed appear to conform to a gaussian distribution. The chi-squared goodness-of-fit test and the Kolmogorov-Smitnov nonparametric test of the cumulative distribution may be used to determine if the reference values have a gaussian distribution. This may involve some moderately complex statistical theory and corresponding computer programs.

The NCCLS Guideline document[1] recommends that the reference interval be estimated by the nonparametric method and that a minimum of 120 reference values be used for the reference interval determination. The nonparametric method is simple, depending only on the ranks of reference data arrayed in order of increasing values. As an example, the frequency distribution for calcium reference values is shown in Table 20-4. The rank of the percentile observation is the percentile time $(n + 1)$ the number of degrees of freedom thus for 120 values, the rank of the 2.5th percentile observation is 3, that is, $0.025 \times 121 = 3.025$; and the rank for the 97.5th percentile observation is 118, that is, $0.975 \times 121 = 117.975$. These are indicated in Table 20-4 by ● and ◆ respectively. Using these rank values to estimate upper and lower reference limits, we obtain the following 95% reference intervals: 89 to 102 mg/L for females and 92 to 103 mg/L for males, or 91 to 103 mg/L for the combined population.

Using the nonparametric method, it is impossible to distinguish between two percentiles of a distribution unless the number of observations, n, equals $(100/P) - 1$, where P is the difference between the two percentiles. Consequently, the nonparametric method requires an absolute minimum of

Table 20-4 Frequency distributions of calcium levels in 240 medical students, by sex

| Analyte (mg/L) | Frequency | | |
	Women	Men	Combined
Calcium			
88	1	0	1
89	2•	0	2
91	1	0	1
91	3	2	5•
92	11	1•	12
93	11	8	19
94	8	6	14
95	16	11	27
96	16	12	28
97	26	13	29
98	8	16	24
99	7	14	21
100	3	7	10
101	2	10	12
102	3◆	11	14
103	2	7◆	9◆
104	0	1	1
106	0	1	1
TOTAL	120	120	240

From National Committee for Clinical Laboratory Standards: *How to define and determine reference intervals in the clinical laboratory: approved guideline,* NCCLS Document C28-A, Villanova, Penn., 1995, NCCLS.
•Indicates the 2.5th percentile.
◆Indicates the 97.5th percentile.

39 measurements to distinguish the 2.5th percentile from the 5th percentile or the 95th percentile from the 97.5th percentile, $n = (100/2.5) - 1 = 39$. Reed and associates[23] have suggested that a minimum of 120 observations be secured, one from each reference group, allowing 90% confidence limits to be computed nonparametrically for each reference limit at the 2.5th and 97.5th percentiles. To estimate the reference limits for these same percentiles with 95% confidence, 153 reference values are needed; for 99% confidence, 198 reference values are needed. Recently Lott and associates,[24] using a Monte Carlo simulation technique and large numbers of samplings of a medical student population, found that increasing the size of the sample had a stabilizing effect on the 2.5th and 97.5th percentiles. At about 200 individuals, the lower and upper reference limits for seven tests (Na, K, Cl, glucose, hemoglobin, erythrocytes, hematocrit), as determined by the nonparametric method, became stable. This experimental finding agrees with the 198 subjects required by strictly statistical criteria to define the same limits with a 99% confidence level. Linnet[25] has proposed that up to 700 observations should be obtained for highly skewed distributions. Clearly, a greater number of observations will improve the statistical accuracy of the estimation.

The minimum number of 120 samples is made under the assumption that no observations have been deleted from the reference set. If aberrant or outlying observations have been deleted, additional subjects should be selected until at least

Table 20-5 90% confidence intervals for lower and upper 95% reference limits

Analyte	Lower reference limit	Upper reference limit
Calcium (mg/L)		
Women (*n* = 120)	88-91	101-103
Men (*n* = 120)	91-93	103-106
Combined (*n* = 240)	88-91	103-106

From National Committee for Clinical Laboratory Standards: *How to define and determine reference intervals in the clinical laboratory: approved guideline,* NCCLS Document C28-A, Villanova, Penn., 1995, NCCLS.

120 acceptable reference values have been obtained for each determination of a reference interval. Moreover, if separate intervals are needed for different subclasses (for sex or age class, for example), one should determine each such interval using the recommended number (at least 120) of reference observations.

Confidence intervals

The reference limits computed from a sample of selected subjects are estimates of the corresponding percentiles in the population of individuals studied. Confidence intervals are useful for two reasons. First, they remind the investigator of the variability of estimates and provide a quantitative measure of this variability. Second, confidence intervals narrow as the size of the sampling increases. Therefore the investigator can get an idea of the improved precision in an estimated 95% reference interval that would be obtained from a larger sampling of reference individuals.

Table 20-5 demonstrates the 90% confidence intervals for the lower and upper 95% reference limits for calcium.

TREATMENT OF OUTLYING OBSERVATIONS

An important implicit assumption in the estimation of reference limits is that the set of measured reference values represents a "homogeneous" collection of observations. This means that all values come from the same underlying probability distribution.

It may be that this condition is satisfied by almost all the reference values but that one or two arise from a probability distribution different from that of their fellows. When such values fall within the expected distribution, they are practically impossible to identify unless the individual performing the biochemical analysis happens to know that these observations represent atypical analytical conditions or are the result of some arithmetic or procedural mistake. Often, however, such "aberrant" values lie outside the range of the remaining measurements and often can be identified as "outliers" requiring special attention.

Unless outliers are known to be aberrant observations, that is, the result of a mistake in the analysis or a lapse in the preanalytic controls applied to the remaining subjects, the emphasis should be on retaining rather than deleting them. Nonparametrically estimated reference limits based on at least 120 observations would be only slightly changed, or not changed at all, if an extreme value were deleted. There are many statistical techniques available for testing the atypicality of outlying observations (see Barnett and Lewis).[26] A test proposed by Dixon[27] uses the ratio D/R, where D is the absolute difference between an extreme observation (large or small) and the next largest (or smallest) observation, and R is the range of all observations including extremes to evaluate outlying observations. Reed and associates[23] have suggested the use of $1/3$ as a cutoff value for the ratio D/R; that is, if the observed value of D were equal to or greater than one third of the range R, the extreme observation would be deleted. For sample sizes as large as 120, this criterion is rather conservative[23]; that is, it would often fail to reject outliers that are really not part of the distribution. However, in the absence of evidence that an outlier is indeed an aberrant observation and given that the underlying distribution will often not be exactly gaussian in form, the one third rule for the ratio D/R seems appropriate, especially when reference intervals are determined by the nonparametric method. Therefore the NCCLS guideline supports the use of this test and the cutoff value of one third suggested by Reed and associates when one is looking for statistically significant outliers in a set of observed reference values.

When two or three outliers are present on the same side of the distribution (that is, all are extremely large or extremely small), the one third rule (or any similar D/R rule) can fail to label the most extreme outlier as statistically significant and thereby mask the presence of the other outliers just slightly less extreme. Common sense indicates that, in such a case, the one third rule should be applied to the least extreme outlier as if it were the only outlier. If the rule leads to rejection of this outlier, the more extreme observations should naturally be rejected as well. If the rule does not reject the least extreme value, one should either accept all the extreme values or, alternatively, apply a test that considers all the outliers together. Such a test is called a *block procedure*; examples are given in Barnett and Lewis.[26] When any outlier is rejected, it is appropriate to test the remaining data for an additional outlier or outliers.

PARTITIONING OF REFERENCE VALUES

The possibility that separate reference intervals will be required for subclasses of subjects should be considered before one begins the process of securing and analyzing subject specimens. However, the use of separate reference intervals for men and women or for different age groups, for example, may not be justified unless these separate intervals will be clinically useful or are well grounded physiologically. When necessary, at least 120 subjects of each sex or age or other subclass should be sampled. The information necessary to decide whether partitioning is needed may not be available in advance for a new analyte.

It has been generally assumed that when the difference between the observed means of two subclass populations is statistically significant (at the 5% or 1% probability level), each subclass warrants its own reference interval. However, any observed difference, no matter how unimportant clinically, will become statistically significant if the sample sizes are large enough. It is important to consult with an appropriate clinician in order to define what a *clinically* significant difference is. If the difference between subgroups is *not clinically significant,* the reference values should not be partitioned, even if there is a statistically significant difference between the means (as determined by a *t*-test).

Recent research by Harris and Boyd[28] has shown that differences between subclass means or differences in the standard deviations (SD) of the subclasses, even when the means are identical, can lead to deviations in the sensitivity and specificity for disease detection. They found that at times there is a statistical need for separate reference intervals, which, if ignored, could potentially hamper the interpretation of laboratory results as part of the diagnostic process. An approach suggested by Harris and Boyd[1,28] tests the *statistical* significance of the difference between subclass means by the standard normal deviate test (z-test), beginning with a pilot sample of 60 subjects in each subclass. If the calculated statistic z exceeds a "critical" z value (see Chapter 19), separate reference intervals should be calculated for each subclass. In addition, if the larger SD of the two subclasses exceeds 1.5 times the smaller SD regardless of the z value, separate reference intervals should be calculated.

For two subclasses, such as men and women or two age groups, the statistical significance of the difference between subclass means should be tested by the standard normal deviate test:

$$z = \frac{|\bar{x}_1 - \bar{x}_2|}{[(s_1^2/n_1) + (s_2^2/n_2)]^{1/2}} \qquad \text{Eq. 20-1}$$

where $\bar{x}_1$ and $\bar{x}_2$ are the observed means of the two subgroups, s_1^2 and s_2^2 are the observed variances, and n_1 and n_2 are the number of reference values in each subclass, respectively. If one assumes at least 60 subjects in each subclass, the z-test is essentially a nonparametric test and may be applied to the original data whether or not the values represent a gaussian distribution. The calculated statistic z should be compared with a "critical" value z^*:

$$z^* = 3 \, (n_{\text{average}}/120)^{1/2} = 3[(n_1 + n_2)/240]^{1/2} \quad \text{Eq. 20-2}$$

In addition, the larger standard deviation, for example s_2, should be checked to see whether it exceeds $1.5s_1$, or, equivalently, whether $s_2/(s_2 - s_1)$ is less than 3. (See box on the following page.)

For example, suppose that at the end of the first stage of sampling the average number of reference values in each subclass is 60. Then, if the calculated z exceeds a z^* that is $3(60/120)^{1/2} = 2.12$, or if the larger standard deviation exceeds 1.5 times the smaller standard deviation, sampling should be continued to obtain at least 120 subjects in each subclass. The *z*-test and standard deviation comparisons should be repeated. If the average number of subjects in each subclass is now 120, $z^* = 3$.

At this point, if the calculated *z* value exceeds z^*, or if the larger standard deviation exceeds 1.5 times the smaller, regardless of the *z* value, separate reference intervals should be calculated for each subclass, under the assumption that the difference between the two reference intervals is likely to be of importance in medical practice. If these conditions do not hold, a single reference interval for the combined group of reference subjects should be calculated for general use. The box at right gives an example of this calculation.

When more than two subclasses are being compared, the problem is more complicated. A statistically significant difference found when the means of all subclasses are compared may, in fact, be attributable only to a difference between two means, such as the mean of one subclass versus the mean of the other subgroups combined. For three or more subclasses, the common statistical analysis of results would be the analysis of variance, if one assumes that all subclasses have equal standard deviations. In this case, a critical *F*-statistic comparable to the z^* value defined above (and therefore dependent on the sample sizes in each subclass) would have to be defined. It is suggested that in this situation the aid of a statistical consultant should be sought.

The statistical tests and criteria recommended above may also be applied to the question of whether reference intervals determined in one laboratory should be transferred without change for use in another laboratory (see the proceeding discussion of transference).

In the preceding examples, the differences in calcium values between men and women, although statistically significant, are small and may not be clinically significant. The *z*-test in this case is certainly sensitive. Considering the imprecision of the assay and the 90% confidence intervals calculated previously for calcium, a laboratory may choose to provide only a single reference range of 91 to 103 g/L for both men and women in this age group. The final decision may be made based on the clinical relevance of the statistically significant difference.

TRANSFERENCE

Because the determination of reliable reference intervals can be a major and costly task, it is cost-effective to transfer a reference interval from one laboratory to another by a convenient process of validation. As new tests and methods are introduced in laboratories, it is unrealistic to expect each laboratory, large or small, to develop its own reference intervals. Consequently, clinical laboratories will rely on other laboratories or on manufacturers of diagnostic tests to provide adequate reference value data that can be transferred. To transfer reference values properly, certain conditions must be fulfilled. For example, the original reference

---

Calculation of a *z* Statistic to Test for Subclass Difference

Example: To test for subclass difference between the calcium reference values for men and women, one needs the means and standard deviations of each group:

Calcium (mg/L), $n_1 = n_2$

$\bar{x}$, *men*	$\bar{x}$, *women*	*SD, men*	*SD, women*
98.0	95.7	3.1	2.9

Inserting these statistics into the formula previously given on p. 372 for *z*, the results are:

Calcium: $$z = \frac{|98.0 - 95.7|}{\left[\dfrac{(3.1)^2}{120} + \dfrac{(2.9)^2}{120}\right]^{1/2}} = 5.94$$

The *z* value exceeds the critical value $z^* = 3$ for $n = 120$, indicating that separate reference intervals for men and women should be considered. The SD of the male population is not greater than 1.5× the SD of the female group and thus does not indicate a subclass difference on this basis.

---

value study must meet the minimum requirements of a valid study as outlined by NCCLS C28-A. The preanalytical and the analytical procedural details, analytical performance, the complete set of reference values, and the method of estimating the reference interval must be stated.

If one assumes that the original reference value study was properly performed, the transference of a reference interval from one testing agency to another involves two problems: the comparability of the two analytical systems and the comparability of the two test subject populations. If both testing agencies do not use the same closed analytical system, the comparability of the two systems can be assessed as outlined by the NCCLS Proposed Guideline EP9-P.[8] In addition, all preanalytical procedures used during the reference value study, such as preparation of the test subjects and specimen collection and handling procedures, must also be the same as those used by the receiving laboratory. The factors that must be considered before one transfers a reference interval are reviewed in the box on the following page. If, in the judgment of the laboratorian, these factors are consistent with the receiving laboratory's operation and test subject population, the reference interval may be transferred.

The NCCLS approved guideline[1] has two alternative procedures for the transference protocol that uses either $n = 20$ or $n = 60$. Both shorter protocols require the same considerations as the larger protocol does (see the following box).

PRESENTATION OF REFERENCE INTERVALS

Every quantitative clinical result should be accompanied by an appropriately presented *reference interval*. The reference intervals should reflect the subclass partitions that have

---

Factors to Consider for Transference of Reference Intervals:

1. Appropriateness of donor laboratory reference interval (that is, selection of reference individuals, exclusions and partitions, number of reference values, method of estimation, and valid reference interval determination according to NCCLS C28-A requirements).
2. Comparability of preanalytical factors (that is, subject preparation and specimen collection and handling and other items listed in Table 20-3).
3. Comparability of analytical method (that is, same [closed method] or different [use NCCLS EP9-P] method).
4. Comparability of test subjects in terms of factors listed in Table 20-2.
5. Validation study, if necessary.

---

been determined to be significant for that laboratory's particular reference population. Reports that include the results of many tests should clearly highlight those results that are not within the reference interval. It is helpful to indicate the relationship of a patient's results to those of the reference interval. Printing "high" or "low" adjacent to a result is an acceptable option.

When forms with preprinted reference intervals are used, reference intervals for all appropriate subclasses should be included. This can result in a confusing report. A better approach is for the computer or instrument to print the reference interval appropriate for the particular patient. In most cases, the subclass reference intervals will be determined by the age and sex of the patient. Any report that uses subclass reference intervals should have the patient's partitioning factors included in the heading or in the demographics portion of the report.

Ideally, detailed information describing the reference population and the details of the reference interval study should be available to all users of a laboratory service. This information should be updated any time a change is made in the laboratory that affects the reference intervals in use. A memo addressing changes in a reference interval should be sent to all users of the laboratory.

INTRAINDIVIDUAL REFERENCE INTERVALS

The National Institutes of Health (NIH) has shown that even healthy individuals studied over several weeks under standardized conditions exhibited a range of values for numerous analytes.[30,31] (See Table 3-1, Chapter 3, for examples of intraindividual variations.) For the same analyte, some individuals had analyte values that fell within a narrow range, whereas for others the variability was quite large. The larger component of variability in some analytes was the preanalytical and analytical variation, whereas in others it was biological variability. In the NIH study, the spread of results obtained in any one individual was consistently less

than the population-based reference interval. Thus an intraindividual abnormal result for a particular individual could fall within the so-called healthy population–based reference interval. The variability of results also means that a healthy individual might occasionally have test results that fall outside a reference interval derived from a central 95% population–based interval and therefore be falsely categorized as having abnormal test results, whereas another individual might have a result that was abnormal for his or her specific range but fall within the population-based reference interval and therefore have a falsely normal result.

These studies showed that it is clearly impossible to develop a reference interval from 120 healthy individuals that would be appropriate for every individual. They also showed that it was impractical to develop a series of reference intervals that would consider each and every possible variable that might affect the concentration of an analyte. Consequently, we are left with the compromise of the population-based reference interval developed under those conditions that can be controlled and that are reasonably consistent with the patient testing conditions. This is discussed in detail by D.S. Young.[32]

Many clinicians are unaware of the preanalytical and analytical factors that may affect the interpretation of test results. It is important for all clinicians to understand that all results within the reference interval are not always considered healthy, nor are all results outside the reference interval considered abnormal. Thus it is essential that clinical laboratories interact with the clinicians who use their services to ensure the proper interpretation of test values in patients.

CLINICAL DECISION LIMITS
Predictive value theory

Clinical decision limits are different from reference intervals because they are based on medical information related to a specific medical condition. They may be "critical values," describing limits of analyte concentrations that demand immediate medical intervention or change in management, they may be diagnostic cutoff values with a high association for a disease or clinical condition, or they may be therapeutic window limits for pharmaceutical agents (see Table 20-6).

Decision analysis is a practical strategy for considering the risks and benefits of decision-making based on the quantitative probability of predicting the true diagnosis or outcome. The respective quantitative approaches used by the laboratorian or clinician in evaluating clinical laboratory measurements and data have been well described[33,34] and have been generally accepted. The concepts of sensitivity, specificity, and predictive values of test results are fundamentally important to these probabilistic approaches. These concepts are now being applied more frequently in the clinical laboratory, not only to establish clinical decision limits

Table 20-6 Purposes for which laboratory tests are ordered and importance of reference intervals in interpretation of their results

Purpose	Reference interval
Diagnosis of disease	++
Screening for disease	+++
Determination of severity of disease	+
Monitoring progress of disease	+
Monitoring response to therapy	+
Monitoring therapy	+++
Monitoring drug toxicity	++
Predicting response to treatment	+
Predicting prognosis	+
Reassurance of patient	++

From Young DS: *Arch Pathol Lab Med* 116:704-709, 1992.
+, Minor importance; ++, moderate importance; +++, great importance.

but also to assist in determining the relative clinical merits of a given test (see Fig. 20-4).[32]

The *diagnostic sensitivity* of a test is the probability of obtaining a positive result for a patient with a given disease, that is, the percentage of individuals with the disease who test positive. In contrast, the *diagnostic specificity* of a test is the probability of obtaining a negative result for a patient without the disease, that is, the percentage of individuals without the disease who test negative. The true positives (TP) are the individuals with the disease who are correctly classified by the test, that is, individuals with the disease who have positive test results. The false positives (FP) are the individuals without the disease who are incorrectly classified by the test, that is, healthy individuals who have positive test results. The false negatives (FN) are the individuals with the disease who are incorrectly classified by a negative test result. The true negatives (TN) are the individuals without the disease that correctly test negative. Since sensitivity is the true-positive rate, the complement, 100% minus sensitivity, is the false-negative rate. For example, if the sensitivity is 75%, the false-negative rate will be 25%. Accordingly, since specificity is the true-negative rate, 100% minus specificity is the false-positive rate.

The *predictive value of a positive test* is the probability that the patient with a positive test result has the given disease, that is, the fraction obtained when one divides the

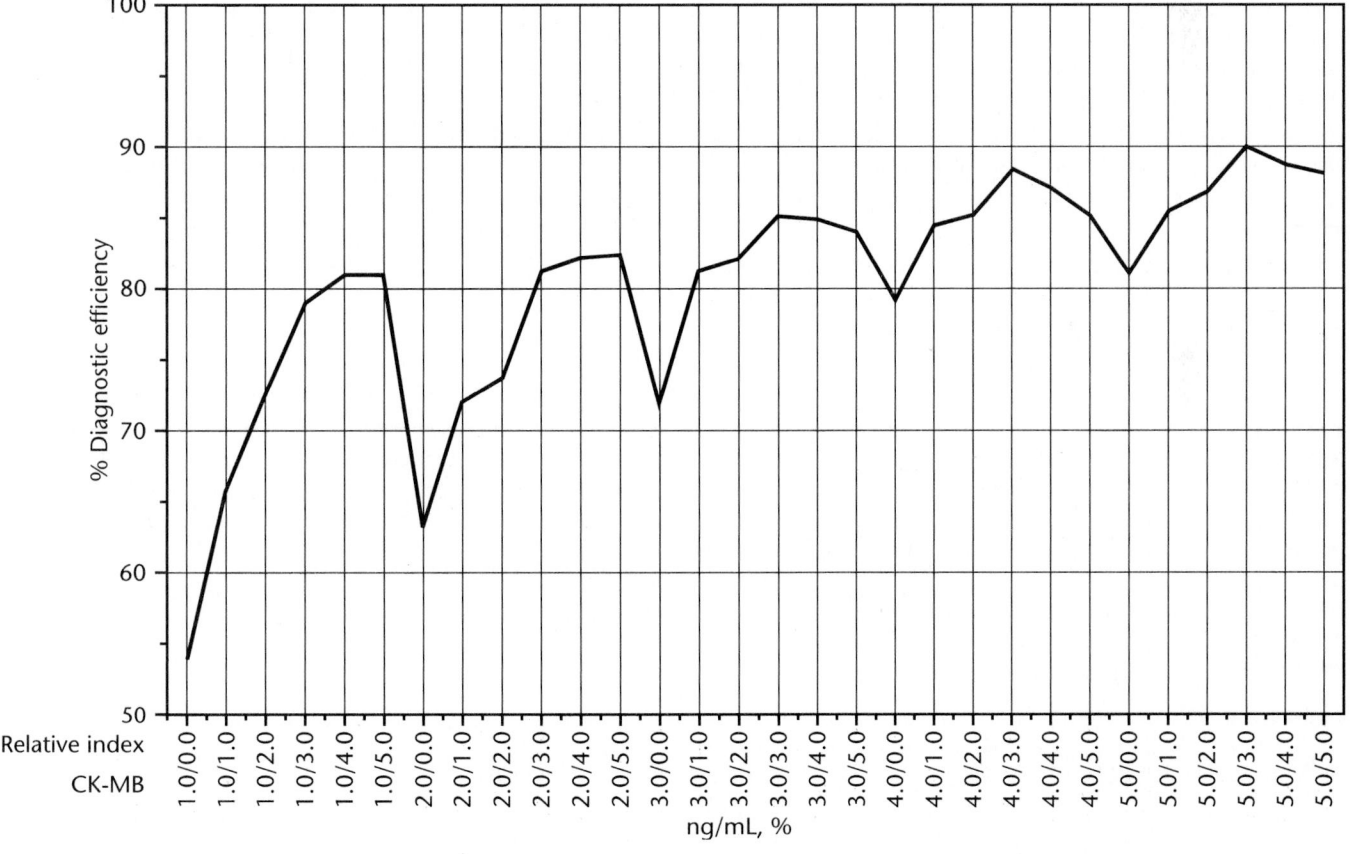

Fig. 20-4 Percent diagnostic efficiency versus combined cutoff levels of CK-MB in nanograms per milliliter (lower set of values on *x*-axis) and percent relative index, expressed as (CK-MB/total CK) × 100. Combining these two tests at different respective cutoff levels produced the highest diagnostic efficiency, 90%, at a cutoff of 5 ng/mL for CK-MB and 3% for the relative index. (Courtesy D. Obzansky, Du Pont Co., Wilmington, Del.)

number of true-positive results by the total number of positive test results. The *predictive value of a negative result* is the probability that the patient with a negative result does not have the disease, that is, the fraction obtained when one divides the number of true-negative results by the total number of negative test results. The *efficiency* of the test is the fraction of all the tested individuals who were correctly classified as either having or not having the disease. These probabilities are often converted to and discussed as percentages.

Predictive values and diagnostic efficiency are greatly influenced by the false-positive and false-negative rates and the prevalence of the disease in the population being tested (see Table 20-7). The importance of prevalence in determining the predictive value (expressed as a percentage) can be seen by rearrangement and substitution of the terms for the predictive value of a positive result (PV+) to give the following equivalent equation:

$$PV+ = \frac{[\text{Prevalence} \cdot \text{Sensitivity}] \times 100\%}{[\text{Prevalence} \cdot \text{Sensitivity}] + [(1 - \text{Prevalence}) \cdot (1 - \text{Specificity})]} \quad \textit{Eq. 20-3}$$

Thus, for a test with a diagnostic sensitivity of 95% and a diagnostic specificity of 95%, the predictive value for a positive result in a population with a prevalence of the disease of 50% is 95%. However, if the prevalence is 5%, the PV+ is 50%, or for a prevalence of 1%, the PV+ is only 16.1%. When the PV+ is 50%, the predictive value of the test is no better than chance; thus one may toss a coin to decide if a patient with a positive test result actually has the disease.

It is clear that even though a test has high sensitivity and specificity and is a good diagnostic test in a defined population of patients, it will perform less well in another population where the prevalence is very low. For example, a positive creatine kinase-MB (CK-MB) result is more significant (has a higher PV+) in a population of patients in a cardiac care unit (with prevalence at 30% to 50%) than in an emergency unit (with prevalence of myocardial infarction at ~5%).

The sensitivity of a specific laboratory test can vary as the disease progresses through various stages in the continuum of disease development over a relatively long term. This variability is seen, for example, with atherosclerosis, cancer, and diabetes. Thus a tumor marker test may have low sensitivity for very early cancer, but a much higher sensitivity for detecting advanced stages of the same cancer. On the other hand, certain tests can be so sensitive as to detect or predict disease before there are symptoms. The predictive value of the test in a population will then also be, in part, dependent on the relative proportion of patients with disease that has advanced to a detectable level.

As a general rule, tests that are used for the screening of occult disease in the general population (low disease prevalence) should have as high a diagnostic sensitivity as possible, consistent with an acceptable level of false-positive results (specificity). Generally, one wants to maximize both sensitivity and specificity. In the example above of a test with 95% sensitivity and specificity, if the test is used to screen for a disease present in a population with a 1% prevalence, 83.9% of the people who have a positive test result will *not* have the disease. If this rate of false-positive values is unacceptable, the specificity of the test will have to

Table 20-7 Sensitivity, specificity, predictive value*

	Number of subjects with positive test result	Number of subjects with negative test result	Total
Number of subjects with disease	TP	FN	TP + FN
Number of subjects without disease	FP	TN	FP + TN
TOTALS	TP + FP	FN + TN	TP + FP + TN + FN

TP, True positives, or number of diseased patients correctly classified by the test.
FP, False positives, or number of patients without the disease misclassified by the test.
FN, False negatives, or number of diseased patients misclassified by the test.
TN, True negatives, or number of patients without the disease correctly classified by the test.

Diagnostic sensitivity $= \dfrac{TP}{TP + FN}$

Diagnostic specificity $= \dfrac{TN}{FP + TN}$

Predictive value of positive test, $PV+ = \dfrac{TP}{TP + FP}$

Predictive value of negative test, $PV- = \dfrac{TN}{TN + FN}$

Efficiency of the test (number fraction of patients correctly classified), that is, $\dfrac{TP + TN}{TP + FP + TN + FN}$

Prevalence $= \dfrac{TP + FN}{TP + FP + TN + FN}$

*From Statland BE, Winkel P, Burke DM, Galen RS: Quantitative approaches used in evaluating laboratory measurements and other clinical data. In Henry JB, editor: *Clinical diagnosis and management by laboratory methods,* Philadelphia, 1979, Saunders.

be increased at the expense of the sensitivity. Alternatively, if the diagnostic sensitivity and positive predictive value are not mutually acceptable, the test should not be used for screening but should be applied only to populations with a higher prevalence of the disease.

Galen and Gambino[34] have suggested the following guidelines for deciding whether a test should have the highest sensitivity, the highest specificity, the highest positive predictive value, or the highest efficiency. Please note that it is *not* possible to have all these attributes at the same time.

The highest sensitivity (preferably 100%) is desired in the following diagnostic situations:

- The disease is serious and should not be missed and
- The disease is treatable and
- False-positive results do not lead to serious physical, psychological, or economic trauma to the patient.

Example. Pheochromocytoma. This disease can be fatal if missed, but if diagnosed, it is nearly 100% curable. Other examples include phenylketonuria, venereal disease, and other treatable infections.

The highest specificity (preferably 100%) is desired in the following diagnostic situations:
- The disease is serious but is not treatable or curable and
- The knowledge that the disease is absent has psychological or public health value and
- False-positive results can lead to serious psychological or economic trauma to the patient.

Example. Multiple sclerosis and most occult cancers. These diseases are serious but not generally treatable or curable.

A high predictive value for a positive result is essential in the following diagnostic situation:
- Treatment of a false-positive individual might have serious consequences.

Example. Occult cancer of the lung where the treatment of lobectomy or radiation has significant morbidity.

The highest efficiency is desired in the following diagnostic situations:
- The disease is serious but treatable and
- False-positive results and false-negative results are essentially equally serious or damaging.

Example. Myocardial infarction. The disease may be fatal but is treatable. Other examples include lupus erythematosus, some forms of leukemia and lymphoma, and diabetes mellitus.

It is apparent that the predictive value or efficiency estimation for a given test is highly dependent on the popula-tion of patients tested. Comparisons of the predictive value or efficiency of different tests or different methodologies are valid only if the populations studied are the same. Unless the patient populations studied are carefully defined, sufficiently large, and very similar, predictive values from different studies may be misleading if one is to judge the relative merits of the tests. For example, as suggested above, a study of the predictive value or efficiency of a CK-MB assay for diagnosing myocardial injury will most certainly give different results when the patient population consists of patients in the cardiac intensive care unit from the results it would give for a population of patients with chest pain in the emergency room. One even has to use caution in comparing predictive values between different studies of critical care unit patients from different institutions because the institutions may treat different patient populations and may use different specific criteria for admission to the unit or for making a final diagnosis.

Medical decision limits

Another important use of the concepts of sensitivity, specificity, and predictive value is in the determination of an optimal cutoff value or *medical decision limit* for a clinical laboratory test. The diagnostic sensitivity and specificity are dependent on the cutoff value selected. When a relatively low medical decision limit is used for CK-MB, the diagnostic sensitivity of the test may approach 100% for the diagnosis of myocardial injury (few or no false-negative results); however, the diagnostic specificity may decrease to a range of 50% to 60% (a large number of false-positive results). When a higher cutoff value is used, the specificity will improve but the sensitivity will decrease. Whenever a medical decision limit is changed, there is a tradeoff between the diagnostic sensitivity and the specificity of the test. The perfect test, if it were to exist, at a perfect cutoff value would have both a sensitivity and a specificity of 100% and a diagnostic efficiency of 100%.

Certainly, laboratories and clinicians have to collaborate and agree on the balance of false positives versus false negatives for each diagnostic situation. Some knowledge of the distributions of test results for diseased versus nondiseased populations can be very helpful when medical decision limits (Figs. 20-1, 20-2, and 20-3) are chosen. As illustrated in Figs. 20-2 and 20-3, test result distributions of healthy and diseased populations will commonly overlap. For some diseases and certain tests, not all individuals with a particular disease will ever have a test result for a particular test outside the healthy reference interval. Also the test results may be affected by more than one disease. In addition, the test results distribution can reflect the continuum from good health to the diseased condition or the stage of a given disease. For example, knowledge of the distribution of prostate-specific antigen (PSA) levels in men with BPH (benign prostate hypertrophy), in men with prostate cancer, and in men with normal prostates has led to the adoption of four decision limits: 0 to 4 ng/mL associated with normal prostates; 4 to 10 ng/mL normally associated with BPH but rarely with prostate cancer; 10 to 20 ng/mL often associated with prostate cancer; and >20 ng/mL associated almost always with prostate cancer. Thus, as the concentration of PSA increases, the likelihood of disease increases, and the specificity of the assay increases. Most experienced clinicians have a practical feel for such medical decision limits, using a relative high (or low) analyte level as an inclusion level to include confidently that a patient is in the population with the disease, or vice versa, to exclude the patient from the population with the disease. The medical decision limit helps the clinician make choices regarding diagnosis, follow-up care, or the need for adjunct diagnostic testing.

The intended clinical use of a test will also be a factor in selecting the best cutoff value. In a given clinical setting the consequences of a false-negative result may be far more serious than those of a false-positive result. False negatives are entirely unacceptable when one is testing for human immunodeficiency virus (HIV) infection among blood donors and organ transplant donors. Alternatively, less harm may be caused by classifying a patient as having myocardial injury by a CK-MB test when the patient in fact did not have a myocardial infarction (MI) (a false positive) than by classifying a patient with an MI as negative (a false negative). Clearly, discharging a patient with an MI from the emer-

gency department or clinic could be catastrophic for that patient. On the other hand, needlessly subjecting a patient with a falsely positive test result to other diagnostic procedures or interventions associated with a certain amount of risk is also not desirable. In addition, it could be prohibitively expensive to admit too many patients who have not had an MI to the cardiac intensive care unit. Galen and Gambino[34] have suggested that the best cutoff value to use for classifying a patient as having had an MI is the value that produces the highest diagnostic efficiency.

There is no simple way to select the optimum combination of sensitivity and specificity. The choice, as discussed earlier, depends on the nature of the disease, the clinical population, and the relative cost of a false-positive or false-negative result. Additional sequential, supplemental, or confirmation testing can often compensate for a test with a high rate of false-positive results and minimize the associated undesirable consequences.

Receiver-operating characteristic curve

The ability of a test, using a specific analyte concentration, to discriminate disease from nondisease can be graphically portrayed by use of receiver-operating characteristic (ROC) curve analysis. Plotting several ROC curves on the same graph, the laboratory staff can compare the merits of two different tests or the performance of one test under different conditions such as different cutoff values or different

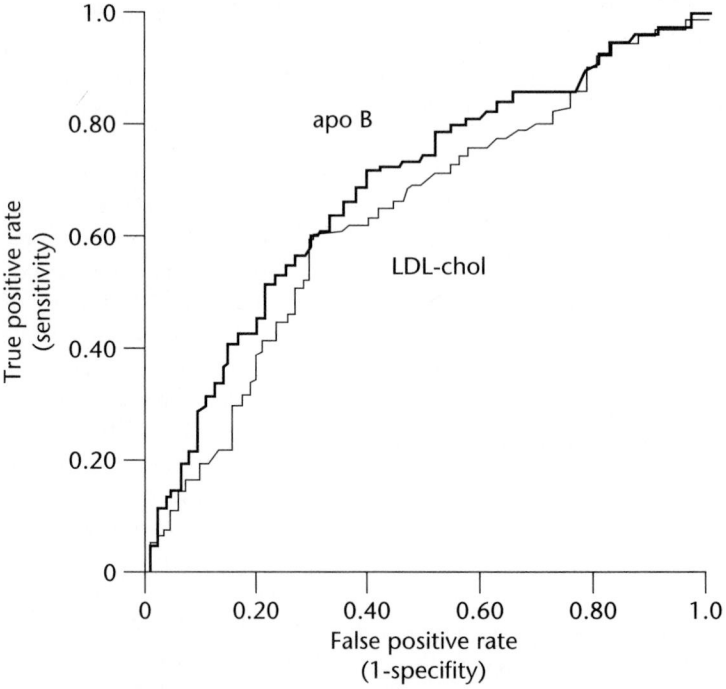

Fig. 20-5 Receiver-operating characteristic (ROC) curves showing discrimination between subjects with and without any coronary artery disease as measured by cardiac catheterization for two different biochemical indicators. (From Zweig MH, Broste SK, Reinhart RA: *Clin Chem* 38:1425-1428, 1992.)

patient populations. An example of such curves is shown in Fig. 20-5 (from Zweig and associates[35]) showing the discrimination between subjects with and without coronary artery disease at different decision levels for apolipoprotein B, low-density lipoprotein (LDL) cholesterol, the ratio of apolipoprotein A-1 to apolipoprotein B, and the ratio of high-density lipoprotein (HDL) cholesterol to total cholesterol. Refer to the article by Zweig and associates[35] and the

review by Zweig and Campbell[36] for a good discussion of the use of ROC curves.

One derives an ROC curve by plotting the sensitivity (the true-positive rate) of the test versus 1.0 minus specificity (the false-positive rate). The multiple points on a curve represent the true-positive rate and false-positive rate using different cutoff values for the diagnosis or differentiation of illness versus nonillness. The point on the curve that is the

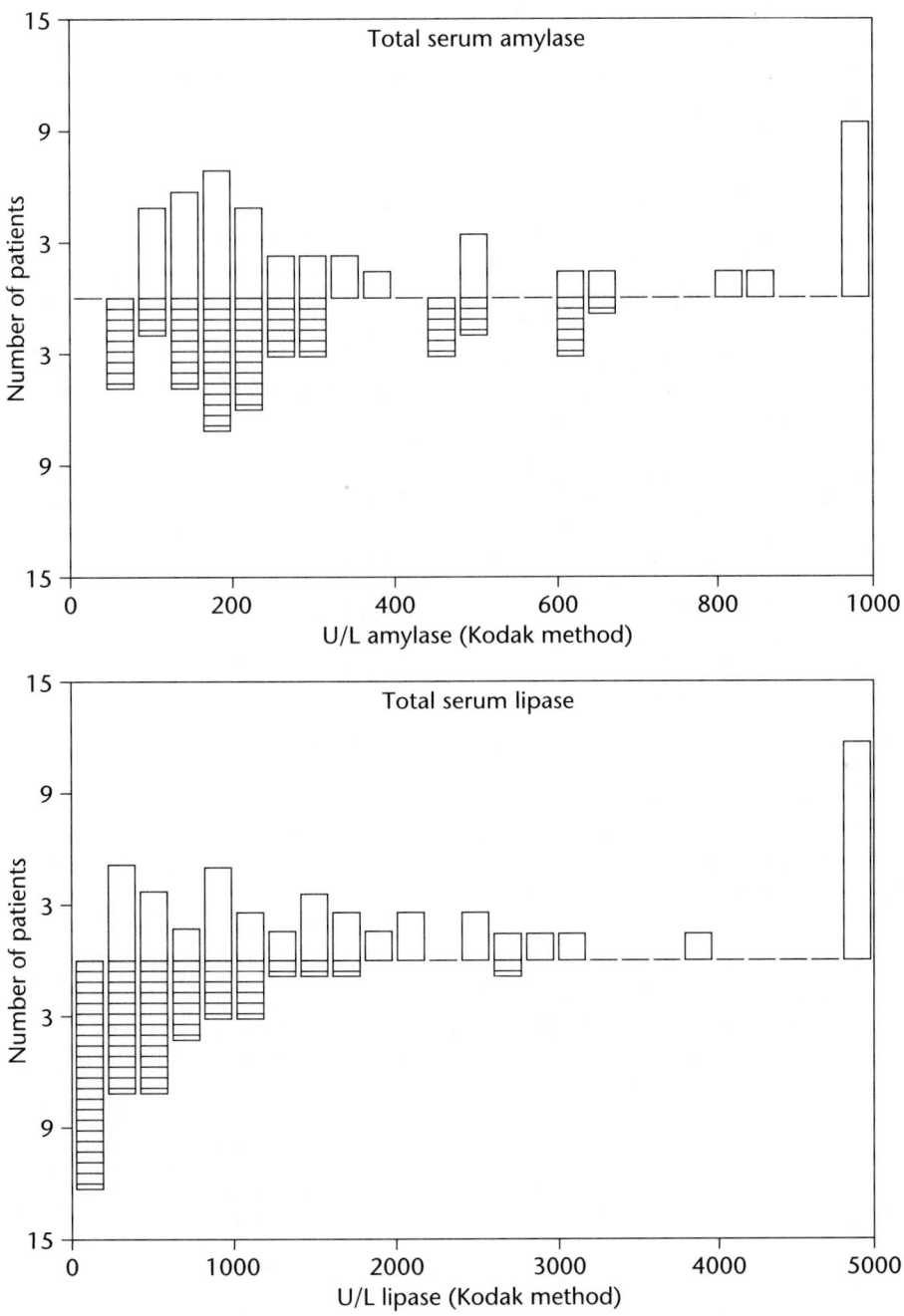

Fig. 20-6   Modified Gerhardt plots for serum amylase, lipase, and in the diagnosis of acute pancreatitis. (From Gerhardt W: The Bayes approach: systematic graphic evaluation of diagnostic tests. *In Keller H, Trendelenburg CH, editors: Data presentation, interpretation,* New York, 1989, Walter de Gruyter.)

closest to the upper left-hand corner of the plot represents the cutoff value or decision limit that provides the greatest diagnostic accuracy, that is, the efficiency of the test. The area under the curve represents the overall accuracy of the test.

There are other useful ways of representing and examining the relative diagnostic value of different cutoff values. One example is the modified Gerhardt plot,[37] as utilized in a study of the relative utility of serum total amylase, total lipase, pancreatic amylase isoenzyme, and a lipase isoform in the diagnosis of acute pancreatitis.[38] These four tests were used on the same population of 81 patients with suspected acute pancreatitis. In this population, 41 of the patients did have pancreatitis and 40 did not. In Fig. 20-6, the open bars in the plots above the zero line represent patients with pancreatitis, and the striped bars, below the line, represent patients without pancreatitis. Using these graphs, the investigators could judge the best discrimination or cutoff point to maximize the sensitivity or specificity of each test. They also concluded that, at least in this set of patients studied, total amylase was a poor test for evaluating patients with an "acute abdomen," and better test choice would be total lipase.

Other representations of cutoff values are also useful, such as those shown in Figs. 20-4 and 20-7, for a hypothetical immunochemical CK-MB assay for use in the diagnosis of myocardial injury.[39] When diagnostic efficiency is the goal, a simple plot of the percent efficiency versus the diagnostic cutoff values is helpful. The highest efficiency at the lowest cutoff is the most appropriate, since increasing the cutoff value will produce more false-negative results. Fig. 20-4 is interesting in that the diagnostic efficiency is plotted as a function of the combination of two cutoff values, the CK-MB in nanograms per milliliter and the percent relative index of CK-MB to total CK. The maximum diagnostic efficiency for this studied and defined patient population for these specific CK-MB and CK assays appears to be 90% at a CK-MB cutoff of 5 ng/mL and a relative index of 3%.

The decision analysis involving multiple testing or combination testing may be similar to the concepts presented here for the measurement of a single variant value and is discussed in Galen and Gambino's text.[34] It can also be quite complex regarding the sequential or simultaneous assessment of multiple variate values according to the Bayes theorem as discussed by Statland and associates.[33]

ACKNOWLEDGMENT

We wish to acknowledge the efforts of the members of the NCCLS Subcommittee on Reference Intervals who prepared the C28-P Guideline: Edward A. Sasse (Chairman), Kaiser J. Aziz, Eugene K. Harris, Sandy Krishnamurthy, Henry T. Lee, Jr., Andy Ruland, and Bette Seamonds. The C28-P was revised to C28-A, 1995.

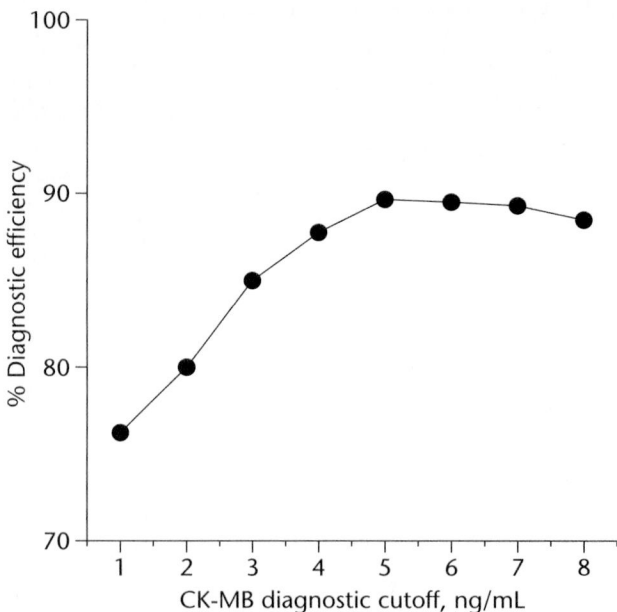

Fig. 20-7 Percent diagnostic efficiency plotted versus different diagnostic cutoff levels in nanograms per milliliter for a hypothetical immunochemical serum CK-MB assay. The highest diagnostic efficiency, 90%, at the lowest cutoff, 5 ng/mL, for CK-MB is the optimal decision level. (Courtesy D. Obzansky, Du Pont Co., Wilmington, Del.)

REFERENCES

1. National Committee for Clinical Laboratory Standards: *How to define and determine reference intervals in the clinical laboratory: approved guideline,* NCCLS document C28-A (ISBN 1-56238-269-1), Villanova, Penn., 1995, NCCLS. Copies of the current edition may be obtained from NCCLS, 771 E. Lancaster Avenue, Villanova, PA 19085.
2. Solberg HE: Approved recommendation (1986) on the theory of reference values. Part 1. The concept of reference values, *Clin Chim Acta* 167:111-118, 1987; *J Clin Chem Clin Biochem* 25:337-342, 1987; *Ann Biol Clin* 45:237-241, 1987; *Labmedica* 4:27-31, 1987.
3. PetitClerc C, Solberg HEL: Approved recommendation (1987) on the theory of reference values. Part 2. Selection of individuals for the production of reference values, *J Clin Chem Clin Biochem* 25:639-644, 1987; *Clin Chim Acta* 170:S1-S12, 1987.
4. Solberg HE, PetitClerc C: Approved recommendation (1988) on the theory of reference values. Part 3. Preparation of individuals and collection of specimens for the production of reference values, *Clin Chim Acta* 177:S1-S12, 1988.
5. Solberg HE, Stamm, D: Approved recommendation on the theory of reference values. Part 4. Control of analytical variation in the production, transfer and application of reference values, *Eur J Clin Chem Clin Biochem* 29:531-535, 1991.
6. Solberg HE: Approved recommendations (1987) on the theory of reference values. Part 5. Statistical treatment of collected reference values: determination of reference limits, *J Clin Chem Clin Biochem* 25:645-656, 1987; *Clin Chim Acta* 170:S13-S32, 1987.
7. Dybkaer R, Solberg HE: Approved recommendations (1987) on the theory of reference values. Part 6. Presentation of observed values related to reference values, *J Clin Chem Clin Biochem* 25:657-662, 1987; *Clin Chim Acta* 170:S33-S42, 1987; *Labmedica* 5:27-30, 1988.

8. National Committee for Clinical Laboratory Standards: *User comparison of quantitative clinical laboratory methods using patient samples: proposed guideline.* NCCLS document EP9-P (ISBN 1-56238-021-4), Villanova, Penn., 1985, NCCLS.

9. Solberg HE: Establishment and use of reference values. In Tietz *Textbook of clinical chemistry, 2nd ed.,* Burtis CA, Ashwood ER, editors, Philadelphia, 1994, Saunders.

10. Schultz EK: Analytical goals and clinical relevance of laboratory procedures. In Tietz NW, editor: *Textbook of clinical chemistry,* Philadelphia, 1986, Saunders.

11. Koch DD, Peters T Jr: Selection and evaluation of methods. In Tietz *Textbook of Clinical Chemistry, 2nd ed.,* Burtis CA, Ashwood ER, editors, Philadelphia, 1994, Saunders.

12. Stamm D: Control of analytical variation in the production of reference values. In Grasbeck R, Alstrom T, editors: *Reference values in laboratory medicine,* New York, 1981, Wiley & Sons.

13. National Committee for Clinical Laboratory Standards: *Internal quality control testing: principles and definitions: approved guideline,* NCCLS document C24-A (ISBN 1-56338-112-1), Villanova, Penn., 1990, NCCLS.

14. Statland BE, Winkel P: Selected preanalytical sources of variation in reference values. In Grasbeck R, Alstrom T, editors: *Reference values in laboratory medicine,* New York, 1981, Wiley & Sons.

15. Hjelm M: Preparing reference individuals for blood collection. In Grasbeck R, Alstrom T, editors: *Reference values in laboratory medicine,* New York, 1981, Wiley & Sons.

16. National Committee for Clinical Laboratory Standards: *Procedures for the collection of diagnostic blood specimens by venipuncture: approved standard,* ed 3, NCCLS document H3-A3 (ISBN 1-56238-108-3), Villanova, Penn., 1991, NCCLS.

17. National Committee for Clinical Laboratory Standards: *Procedures for the collection of diagnostic blood specimens by skin puncture: approved standard,* ed 3, NCCLS document H4-A3 (ISBN 1-56238-035-2), Villanova, Penn., 1991, NCCLS.

18. National Committee for Clinical Laboratory Standards: *Percutaneous collection of arterial blood for laboratory analysis: approved standard,* NCCLS document H11-A (ISBN 1-56238-041-9), Villanova, Penn., 1985, NCCLS.

19. National Committee for Clinical Laboratory Standards: *Collection, transport, and preparation of blood specimens for coagulation testing and performance of coagulation assays: approved guideline,* ed 2, NCCLS document H21-A2 (ISBN 1-56238-050-8), Villanova, Penn., 1986, NCCLS.

20. National Committee for Clinical Laboratory Standards: *Collection and transportation of single-collection urine specimens: proposed guideline,* NCCLS document GP8-P (ISBN 1-56238-027-3), Villanova, Penn., 1985, NCCLS.

21. National Committee for Clinical Laboratory Standards: *Collection and preservation of timed urine specimens: proposed guideline,* NCCLS document GP13-P (ISBN 1-56238-030-3), Villanova, Penn., 1987, NCCLS.

22. National Committee for Clinical Laboratory Standards: *Procedures for the handling and processing of blood specimens: approved guideline,* NCCLS document H18-A (ISBN 1-56238-110-5), Villanova, Penn., 1990, NCCLS.

23. Reed AH, Henry RJ, Mason WB: Influence of statistical method used on the resulting estimate of normal range, *Clin Chem* 17:275-284, 1971.

24. Lott JA, Mitchell LC, Moeschberger ML, Sutherland DE: Estimation of reference ranges: how many subjects are needed, *Clin Chem* 38:648-650, 1992.

25. Linnet K: Two-stage transformation systems for normalization of reference distributions evaluated, *Clin Chem* 33:381-386, 1987.

26. Barnett V, Lewis T: *Outliers in statistical data,* New York, 1978, Wiley & Sons, pp 68-73.

27. Dixon WJ: Processing data for outliers, *Biometrics* 9:74-89, 1953.

28. Harris EK, Boyd JC: On dividing reference data into subgroups to produce separate reference ranges, *Clin Chem* 36:265-270, 1990.

29. Harris EK: Personal communication.

30. Cotlove E, Harris EK, Williams GZ: Biological and analytical components of variation in long-term studies of serum constituents in normal subjects, III: physiological and medical implications, *Clin Chem* 16:1028-1032, 1970.

31. Young DS, Harris EK, Cotlove E: Biological and analytical components of variation in long-term studies of serum constituents in normal subjects, IV: results of a study designed to eliminate long-term analytic deviations, *Clin Chem* 17:403-410, 1971.

32. Young DS: Determination and validation of reference intervals, *Arch Pathol Lab Med* 116:704-709, 1992.

33. Statland BE, Winkel P, Burke DM, Galen RS: Quantitative approaches used in evaluating laboratory measurements and other clinical data. In *Clinical diagnosis and management by laboratory methods,* Henry JB, editor: Philadelphia, 1979, Saunders.

34. Galen RS, Gambino SR: *Beyond normality: the predictive value and efficacy of medical diagnoses,* New York, 1975, Wiley & Sons.

35. Zweig MH, Broste SK, Reinhart RA: ROC curve analysis: an example showing the relationships among serum lipid and apolipoprotein concentrations in identifying patients with coronary artery disease, *Clin Chem* 38:1425-1428, 1992.

36. Zweig MH, Campbell G: Receiver-operating characteristic (ROC) plots: a fundamental evaluation tool in clinical medicine, *Clin Chem* 39:561-577, 1993.

37. Gerhardt W: The Bayes approach: systematic graphic evaluation of diagnostic tests. In Keller H, Trendelenburg CH, editors: *Data presentation, interpretation,* New York, 1989, Walter de Gruyter.

38. Lott JA, Lu CJ: Lipase isoforms and amylase isoenzymes: assays and application in the diagnosis of acute pancreatitis, *Clin Chem* 37:361-368, 1991.

39. Obzansky D: Personal communication, Wilmington, Del.

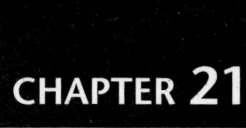

CHAPTER 21

Quality control for the clinical chemistry laboratory

Richard B. Passey

(Special thanks to **Bradley E. Copeland, M.D.**, *for his previous authorship of this chapter, much of which is retained.)*

Goals for a quality control program
    Setting goals
    Total allowable error
    Performance required for proficiency testing
    Medical decision limits
    Meeting medical usefulness criteria by calculating the significant change limit
Control of quality (process control) and error detection
    Levels of activity in the process control
    Testing quality control specimens—daily decision making
    Quality control mechanics
    Preliminary considerations for estimating limits for quality control pools
    A simple method for establishing average temporary target values for quality control pools
    Calculation of the usual standard deviation
    Setting the action control limits for each level of control pool
    Setting quality control limits by power curves
Detection and resolution of quality problems
    The out-of-control decision
    Detection of quality problems
    Using patients' data in decision making
    Actions to bring a testing system back into control
    Actions to be taken when a method is out of control
    Procedures to follow during a testing system failure
Calibration and quality control
    Use of calibrators
    A practical system for a new calibrator verification
    Quality control of reagent changes and instrument maintenance
External quality control programs and other tools for accuracy control
    Accuracy control is required by CLIA '88
    Definitive and reference methods
    Reference materials
    Selection of a reference laboratory for assistance in accuracy control
    Manufacturer's responsibility in the control of testing systems

---

OBJECTIVES

- Provide a practical approach to quality control.
- Establish a method to evaluate performance specifications during the process of controlling quality.
- Furnish practical methods for carrying out quality control.

- Develop criteria for judging the out-of-control condition.
- Provide a practical approach to solving an out-of-control condition.

KEY TERMS

action limits Ranges set for quality control pools that, if exceeded, signal a possible deterioration of the quality of the testing system and requires an investigation by a technologist. (See *out of control*.)

certified reference material (CRM) "A reference material that has one or more property values certified by a technically valid procedure and is accompanied by, or traceable to, a certificate or another document issued by a certifying body."[28] The material has high purity for the specified compound. Certified reference materials are used in preparing calibrators or specimens of known concentration.

CLIA, or CLIA '88 The Clinical Laboratory Improvement Amendment (CLIA) of 1988 regulates clinical laboratory operation in the United States. This law is interpreted by administrative regulations developed by certifying organizations.

control limits Numerical limits (expressed in the test units) within which the assay values of control samples must fall for the assay to be considered valid or in control.

definitive method An analytical method that has been subjected to thorough investigation and evaluation for sources of inaccuracy, including nonspecificity. The magnitude of the definitive method's final imprecision and bias, expressed in the uncertainty statement, is compatible with the definitive method's stated end purpose. The value obtained by a definitive method is taken as the true value.[26]

error budget A testing system's total allowable error. The total allowable error is determined by each laboratory on the basis of medical or regulatory requirements. The error expenditure comprises all sources of error including imprecision, bias, interferences, and other errors.

external quality control A program in which an external agency provides unknown samples for analysis. (See *survey or proficiency testing specimen*.) The results are returned to the participant with an evaluation of "acceptable" or "not acceptable" performance. Under CLIA '88 this process is called *proficiency testing*.

false rejection Rejection of an analytical run because quality control results indicate analytical problems that are not really present.

inherent variability Repeated measurements on the same material vary around an average value. The standard deviation measures the magnitude of this variability.

internal quality control An analysis program, using quality control samples, that is used to verify the acceptability and stability of laboratory results.

method The methodological principle used in the performance of a test; the chemical or physical basis of the test.

monthly average Daily quality control values averaged over the period of 1 month.

monthly standard deviation Standard deviation calculated using the daily quality control values over the period of 1 month.

out of control A circumstance when a testing system has been shown, by quality control results or other indicators, to be unusable for patient care. This circumstance must be formally declared by the laboratory director or technical supervisor, since this decision implies that specified actions need to be taken under CLIA '88 regulations (see §493.1219, Remedial Actions, and §493.1705, Quality Assurance of Quality Control). Routine responses to quality control results that exceed set limits should be documented; see *action limits*.

peer group When used in proficiency testing programs, it indicates a group of laboratories that use the same or similar methods.

performance specifications Numerical limits established by each laboratory for each analyte and each testing system, which delineate acceptable performance. Performance specifications often include accuracy, precision, analytical sensitivity (minimum reportable amount), analytical specificity (interfering substances) if applicable, the reportable range of patient test results, and the reference range or normal values.

power curves Plots of the magnitude of the error detected by a control system versus the probability of detecting that size error under various control rules.

primary standard Chemicals of the highest known purity that can be used to produce calibrators for analytical systems.

procedure A set of instructions for using a particular method that, when followed, will produce an analytical test value.

proficiency testing See *external quality control*.

quality control pool A quantity of stable material (such as serum, plasma, or urine) that is used in an internal quality control program to evaluate the acceptability and stability of a testing system.

reference method "A thoroughly investigated method, in which exact and clear descriptions of the necessary conditions and procedures are given for the accurate determination of one or more property values; the documented accuracy and precision of the method are commensurate with the method's use for assessing the accuracy of other methods, for measuring the same property values, or for assigning reference method values to reference materials."[27]

regional quality control A group of laboratories that jointly purchase a large amount of quality control material so that target values can be established.

run "A run is an interval within which the accuracy and precision of a testing system are expected to be stable but cannot be greater than 24 hours." (CLIA '88 §493.1218[b])

shift A shift is an abrupt and sustained change (in one direction) in control values. A shift usually indicates a problem with the analytical system or the control material.

significant difference A difference that is statistically shown to be outside the expected variability limit; *medically* it is a difference that is large enough to influence a medical decision; *operationally* it is a statistically significant difference that testing personnel and supervisors believe to be large enough to require investigation.

standard deviation (SD) A descriptor of the extent of dispersion of a population of test values (set of measurement data).

survey or proficiency testing specimen A sample that is prepared by an independent agency and submitted to a laboratory that is participating in an external quality control program.

systemic bias Systemic bias can be constant or proportional. *Constant systemic bias* denotes a constant difference between the true value and the observed value regardless of the concentration level. *Proportional systemic bias* denotes a difference between the true value and the observed value, which changes proportionally as the concentration level changes.

target value The established mean value for an analyte in a quality control pool.

testing system The combination of an analytical method; a procedure for using the method; reagents, calibrators, and supplies; and an instrument.

trend A gradual change in the test results obtained from control material that is suggestive of a problem with the testing system or control material, also termed *drift*.

true rejection The rejection of an analytical run because the control specimens indicate that a problem truly exists.

usual standard deviation (USD) The average of 3- to 6-monthly average standard deviation values based on consecutive quality control values. This estimates the usual precision that a laboratory's testing system is capable of achieving.

This discussion of quality control, as practiced in clinical laboratories, is designed to provide a practical guide for establishing and maintaining quality in laboratory practice. Breitenberg[4] identified 10 quality ensuring items from the International Organization for Standardization series 9000 standards that are common to all quality control systems. They are (1) effective quality system; (2) ensuring valid measurements; (3) using calibrated measuring and testing equipment; (4) using appropriate statistical techniques; (5) developing a product identification and traceability system; (6) maintaining adequate record-keeping systems; (7) ensuring adequate product handling, storage, packaging, and delivery systems; (8) maintaining an adequate inspection and testing system; (9) establishing processes for dealing with nonconforming items; and (10) ensuring adequate personnel training and experience. It should be the goal of quality control procedures to meet all 10 of these standards. Careful examination of the rules delineated by Clinical Laboratory Improvement Amendment of 1988 (CLIA '88) shows that all these items must be included in a laboratory's quality control system.

The primary analytical goals of a clinical laboratory's quality control program should be:

1. Establishing and maintaining accurate methods.
2. Determining the level of precision needed by the laboratory, and maintaining that level of reproducibility.
3. Ensuring that analytical systems are stable and operating according to performance specifications. This increases the reliability of both short- and long-term medical decisions.

To achieve its analytical goals a laboratory must meet the 10 quality-assuring goals listed above, institute policies that govern patient preparation, reduce preanalytical errors (see Chapter 3), and maximize the effective use of the laboratory's personnel and physical facilities. A laboratory's quality control program is designed to evaluate how well these analytical goals are being met.

GOALS FOR A QUALITY CONTROL PROGRAM
Setting goals

When you are establishing a laboratory quality control program, the first step is to establish criteria for acceptable laboratory performance. How accurate and precise *should* your laboratory be? How precise and accurate *must* it be? These considerations include the determination of what constitutes acceptable analytical error based on the test result's use.[8,18] Control beyond that required for medical purposes can be wasteful of time and materials, and it is therefore important to evaluate whether error reduction improves medical diagnosis, treatment, or prognosis.

There are several bases upon which performance criteria can be formulated. The first is the body of regulatory standards; for example, the precision and accuracy demanded by CLIA '88 regulations. The second is the precision and accuracy that appear to be attainable performance by most laboratories. This information can be obtained by communication with other laboratory professionals or from data derived from proficiency surveys, such as that of the College of American Pathology (CAP). Third and probably most important, it is essential to determine the precision and accuracy required by the clinical staff, the users of data produced by the laboratory. A testing system's analytical error should be much smaller than the allowable error in the regulatory requirements. If this is not so, the laboratory cannot meet its regulatory and perhaps medical requirements. The following section will review the medical criteria that are used to set up and evaluate performance.

Total allowable error

The total allowable error of a testing system is composed of individual components. In general each component of a testing system can be a source of imprecision or bias. If the total error can be likened to an error budget, the individual components of the total allowable error make up the total error expenditure of that budget. When the error budget is exceeded, more error than can be tolerated exists in the testing system. The more completely one can identify the components of error, the better one can adjust the test-

ing system to reduce these errors. Medical and CLIA '88 requirements don't depend on whether the error is introduced by imprecision or bias; it is the combination that determines the effect of the total error. The laboratory staff, however, must know what parts imprecision and bias play in the error expenditure because the resolution processes for these errors are often different.

Total error[20] is estimated from imprecision and bias by:

$$\text{Total error} = \text{Sum of bias errors} + 1.96 \times \text{SD (standard deviation)} \qquad \textit{Eq. 21-1}$$

Notice that 1.96 is the 95% confidence limit (often rounded to 2.0 for convenience) for a normally distributed set of results.

Example. If your medical requirements for glucose require that the total error be less than 60 mg/L at a concentration of 1200 mg/L and you know that your imprecision is 20 mg/L, the maximum bias that your method can have is calculated as follows:

$$60 \text{ mg/L} = x \text{ mg/L} + 1.96 \times 20 \text{ mg/L}$$

$$\text{Maximum bias} = x = 60 - (1.96 \times 20) = 20.8 \text{ mg/L}$$

If the bias of the assay is too large, it can often be reduced by more accurate calibration procedures and materials. Imprecision is often increased by poor mechanical and electronic components. The state of instrument maintenance can affect both bias and imprecision. An accuracy-based quality control system can provide information on both accuracy and precision.

Table 21-1 contains analytical data from the Oklahoma Medical Center showing the total error for each listed test. The total errors are large because they include error contributions from all the instruments used to report the test values. Accurate error budgeting must include the bias introduced by the use of multiple testing systems. The problem of bias between different testing systems is one that can affect the medical use of test results because a test is often performed by more than one testing system.

Performance required for proficiency testing

The federal government has set allowable error criteria for 154 tests in 13 laboratory disciplines plus cytology (proficiency testing rules of CLIA '88 *Federal Register* February 28, 1990, pp. 7152-7162). The CLIA criteria for chemistry tests are listed in Table 21-2. These allowable error criteria define the total amounts of error a proficiency testing value can have. The target value that is used to determine bias is defined by the proficiency testing service using either the overall mean, a peer group mean, or the value established by a definitive or reference method. CLIA '88 error windows (budgets) are too large for routine quality control limits because imprecision errors this large will cause frequent proficiency testing failure.[11]

Compare the total errors listed in Table 21-1 to the sug-

Table 21-1   Performance specifications for total error (%)*

Test	Analytical†	Medical‡	CLIA '88§
Albumin	13-15	—	10
Alkaline phosphatase	10-15	—	30
AST (aspartate aminotransferase)	5-20	14-26	20
Bilirubin, total	12-16	5-28	20% or 4 mg/L
BUN (blood urea nitrogen)	18-33	12-25	9% or 20 mg/L
Calcium	5.5-6.4	5-7	10 mg/L
Chloride	5	—	5
Cholesterol	11-14	9‖	10
Cholesterol, high-density lipoprotein	5	—	30
Creatine kinase (CK)	8-10	—	30
Creatinine	15-47	10-20	15% or 3 mg/L
Glucose	5-11	11-16	10% or 60 mg/L
Iron	—	17	20
Lactate dehydrogenase (LD)	7-8	—	20
Phosphorus	4-10	14-17	NA
Potassium	10-12	5-10	0.5 mmol/L
Protein, total	7-8	8	10
Sodium	5-6	2-3	4 mmol/L
Triglycerides	10-16	16	25

NA, Not applicable.
*Total analytical error calculated by: T.E. = Bias + 1.96 × standard deviation.
†Data from Oklahoma Medical Center, University of Oklahoma. Tested systems include Beckman CX3 and Kodak 700XRC; bias differences between these two systems are important sources of the high total error. The difference between the systems is part of the error for a patient's results when different systems are used interchangeably.
‡Rounded to the nearest whole percentage. (From Skendzel LP, Barnett RN, Platt R: *Am J Clin Pathol* 83:200-205, 1985.)
§Tests and acceptable performance are from the *Federal Register,* p 7158, Feb. 28, 1990.
‖Cholesterol medical goals are now set at 3% bias and 3% imprecision. (From NCEP: NIH Pub. no. 90-2964, 1990[25]).

gested allowable medical errors and the maximum error windows specified by CLIA '88. Notice that several tests in Table 21-2 show potential problems with proficiency testing because of unacceptably high total errors when the analysis is performed by more than one testing system. This would be the case if proficiency testing truly mimicked laboratory practice. However, as currently practiced, proficiency testing usually compares testing systems only to their instrument peer grouping.

Medical decision limits

For true control of quality, it is necessary to evaluate, from the customer's perspective, the performance required for each aspect of the clinical laboratory's operation.[1,10,11,36] The elements of a good quality control program include establishment of analytical accuracy and precision performance criteria based on medical usefulness requirements.[2,9,14,20,32,35,37]

In Table 21-1, the total analytical error for several analytical instruments is compared to the allowable error suggested by medical requirements and to the CLIA '88 mandated allowable error. An example of medically defined criteria for precision and accuracy are the guidelines formulated by the National Institutes of Health (NIH) for cholesterol analysis.[25,29] To minimize the errors in diagnosing hyperlipidemias, the NIH established a target of 3% for the limits of imprecision and 3% for an acceptable degree of bias (inaccuracy). Each laboratory should consult the ap-

propriate users or clinicians to obtain their estimate of allowable error based on their medical practice.[7,12,24,34] If their suggestions are reasonable and would not place the laboratory in conflict with regulatory requirements, the laboratory should try to attain these limits of error. If no information is available about the precision and accuracy needed for medical decision making, one can estimate a theoretical error based on the degree of intraindividual and interindividual variation for each analyte.[13,44] Page 405 lists the equations relating total analytical imprecision with these biological variabilities. Table 3-1 lists some examples of the intrapersonnel variability of certain analytes. Once the allowable total error based on medical requirements has been decided, the methods and testing systems chosen must be capable of producing values that meet those requirements. In addition, the quality control program must be designed to ensure that the testing system maintains these limits.

Reference ranges for tests describe the expected values for carefully selected groups of individuals determined by testing systems that are assumed to be performing appropriately (see Chapter 20). Increased bias will cause a shift in test values and will thus invalidate the medical usefulness of the established reference ranges.

Meeting medical usefulness criteria by calculating the significant change limit

The day-to-day medical usefulness of clinical laboratory tests depends on maintaining the accuracy and precision of

Table 21-2   CLIA required performance on proficiency testing (*Federal Register,* Feb. 28, 1992)

Analyte or test	Criteria for acceptable performance
Immunology tests	
Alpha$_1$-antitrypsin	Target value ±3 SD
Alpha-fetoprotein (tumor marker)	Target value ±3 SD
Antinuclear antibody	Target value ±2 dilutions or positive or negative
Antistreptolysin 0	Target value ±2 dilutions or positive or negative
Antihuman immunodeficiency virus	Reactive or nonreactive
Complement C3	Target value ±3 SD
Complement C4	Target value ±3 SD
Hepatitis (HBsAg, anti-HBc, HBeAg)	Reactive (positive) or nonreactive (negative)
IgA	Target value ±3 SD
IgE	Target value ±3 SD
IgG	Target value ±25%
IgM	Target value ±3 SD
Infectious mononucleosis	Target value ±2 dilutions or positive or negative
Rheumatoid factor	Target value ±2 dilutions or positive or negative
Rubella	Target value ±2 dilutions or immune or nonimmune or positive or negative
Chemistry tests	
Alanine aminotransferase (ALT/SGPT)	Target value ±20%
Albumin	Target value ±10%
Alkaline phosphatase	Target value ±30%
Amylase	Target value ±30%
Aspartate aminotransferase (AST/SGOT)	Target value ±20%
Bilirubin, total	Target value ±4 mg/L or ±20% (greater)
Blood gas P$_{O_2}$	Target value ±3 SD
P$_{CO_2}$	Target value ±5 mm Hg or ±8% (greater)
pH	Target value ±0.04
Calcium, total	Target value ±10 mg/L
Chloride	Target value ±5%
Cholesterol, total	Target value ±10%
Cholesterol, high density lipoprotein	Target value ±30%
Creatine kinase	Target value ±30%
Creatine kinase isoenzymes	MB elevated (presence or absence) or target value ±3 SD
Creatinine	Target value ±3 mg/L or ±15% (greater)
Glucose (excluding glucose performed on monitoring devices cleared by FDA for home use)	Target value ±60 mg/L or ±10% (greater)
Iron, total	Target value ±20%
Lactate dehydrogenase (LD)	Target value ±20%
LD isoenzymes	LD$_1$/LD$_2$ (+ or −), or target value ±30%
Magnesium	Target value ±25%
Potassium	Target value ±0.5 mmol/L
Sodium	Target value ±4 mmol/L
Total protein	Target value ±10%
Triglycerides	Target value ±25%
Urea nitrogen	Target value ±20 mg/L or ±9% (greater)
Uric acid	Target value ±17%
Endocrinology	
Cortisol	Target value ±25%
Free thyroxine	Target value ±3 SD
Human chorionic gonadotropin	Target value ±3 SD positive or negative
Triiodothyronine uptake	Target value ±3 SD
Triiodothyronine	Target value ±3 SD
Thyroid-stimulating hormone	Target value ±3 SD
Thyroxine	Target value ±20% or 10 μg/L (greater)
Toxicology	
Alcohol, blood	Target value ±25%
Blood lead	Target value ±10% or 40 μg/L (greater)
Carbamazepine	Target value ±25%
Digoxin	Target value ±20% or ±0.2 ng/mL (greater)
Ethosuximide	Target value ±20%

Table 21-2   CLIA required performance on proficiency testing (*Federal Register,* Feb. 28, 1992)—cont'd

Analyte or test	Criteria for acceptable performance
Toxicology	
Gentamicin	Target value ±25%
Lithium	Target value ±0.3 mmol/L or ±20% (greater)
Phenobarbital	Target value ±20%
Phenytoin	Target value ±25%
Primidone	Target value ±25%
Procainamide (and metabolite)	Target value ±25%
Quinidine	Target value ±25%
Tobramycin	Target value ±25%
Theophylline	Target value ±25%
Valproic acid	Target value ±25%
Hematology	
Cell identification	90% or greater consensus on identification
White blood cell differential	Target ±3 SD based on the percentage of different types of white blood cells in the samples
Erythrocyte count	Target ±6%
Hematocrit (excluding spun hematocrits)	Target ±6%
Hemoglobin	Target ±7%
Leukocyte count	Target ±15%
Platelet count	Target ±25%
Fibrinogen	Target ±20%
Partial thromboplastin time	Target ±15%
Prothrombin time	Target ±15%

the testing system. Physicians make many clinical decisions on the basis of the day-to-day differences in patient test values, assuming that the day-to-day accuracy and precision are maintained at the same level from month to month and year to year. Thus the actual accuracy and precision of the measurement procedure directly influence the medical interpretation of these day-to-day changes in test values. One key element in interpreting the medical usefulness of a test result is an estimate of the magnitude of an analytically significant change in concentration. This estimate is called the *significant change limit* (SCL).

The significant change limit is a decision-making tool that helps physicians distinguish day-to-day changes in results that are caused by the inherent variability of the analytical procedure from changes that are caused by modifications in the patient's physiology and pathology. The significant change limit is based on the assumption that the usual standard deviation represents day-to-day method variability. The theoretical standard deviation of the difference (SD_{diff}) between two separate analyses of the same material on different days is related to the usual standard deviation (USD) of the procedure by the following formula:

$$SD_{diff} = \sqrt{2(USD)^2} = 1.4\ USD \qquad \textit{Eq. 21-2}$$

The SCL is then the 95% confidence limits (or $\pm 2\ SD_{diff}$) that define the extent of the inherent method variability:

$$SCL = \text{Mean value} \pm 2\ SD_{diff} = \text{Mean value} \pm 2.8\ USD$$

$$\textit{Eq. 21-3}$$

As an approximation, the significant change limit is three times the usual standard deviation (Table 21-3). Changes

greater than the significant change limit are likely to represent a real change in the patient. For example, if the usual standard deviation for cholesterol is 50 mg/L, the significant change limit is 2.8 times 50, or 140 mg/L. A change from 2000 to 2200 mg/L would exceed the significant change limit and would represent a real change in the patient. A change from 2000 to 1900 mg/L would not exceed the SCL and could be the result of the method's imprecision. To facilitate consistent decision making by the attending physician, it is important to maintain a consistent level of precision from month to month and year to year.

CONTROL OF QUALITY (PROCESS CONTROL) AND ERROR DETECTION

Once a laboratory's performance criteria have been established, a process control system must be put into place. This system will allow continuous monitoring of the entire testing (including preanalytical and postanalytical) process to ensure that either the performance goals are met or that sufficient steps are taken to achieve the goals. It is important to recognize the role of laboratory personnel as the core of the quality process.

Levels of activity in the process control

The control process that we call quality control (QC) is designed to detect error in the measurement system. There are at least three levels in this process, each the responsibility of different individuals. For the control process to be most effective, active communication between the individuals within each level of responsibility is crucial.

Table 21-3 Calculation of quality control parameters

Test/method: Potassium by ABC flame photometer
Analyst: RBP **Start/finish date:** 3/15/93—3/26/93
Control source and level: Superior control—elevated
Manufacturer's target value: 6.02 mEq/L
How determined: By NRSCL Definitive Method
Manufacturer's typical standard deviation for users: 0.15 mEq/L

Day	Vial 1		Vial 2	
	Sample A	Sample B	Sample A	Sample B
1	6.1	6.1	6.2	5.9
2	6.2	6.2	6.0	6.0
3	5.7	5.8	6.0	6.0
4	5.9	5.8	5.9	5.8
5	6.0	6.0	6.0	6.0
6	5.9	6.0	6.0	6.0
7	5.9	6.0	6.0	6.0
8	5.9	5.8	6.0	5.9
9	6.0	6.1	6.1	6.2
10	6.0	6.1	6.1	6.1

Grand total (sum of all observations) = 239.7; n = 40 observations.
Average initial target value = 239.7/40 = 5.99 mEq/L.
Temporary standard deviation = 0.12 mEq/L.

Calculation of average final target and usual standard deviation (USD) values

Initial target value	Average target value	Standard deviation
Data	5.99	0.12 mEq/L
1 April	6.07	0.13 mEq/L
2 May	6.02	0.11 mEq/L
3 June	6.01	0.13 mEq/L

Average final target = 6.02 (average of 5.99, 6.07, 6.02, and 6.01)
Usual standard deviation (USD) = 0.12 mEq/L (average of 0.12, 0.13, 0.11, and 0.13)
Medically allowable error = 0.3 mEq/L (set by the medical staff Jan. 14, 1993)
Number of USDs in the medically allowable error = 0.3/0.12 = 2.5
Significant change value = 2.8 × USD = 2.8 × 0.12 = 0.34 mEq/L
Chosen control range is the average final target value ±2.5 USD, or 6.02 ±2.5(0.12) = 6.02 ±0.3 mEq/L, or 5.72 to 6.32 mEq/L.

If the chosen control range is the average final target value ±3 USD, range = 6.02 ±3(0.12) = 6.02 ±0.36, or 5.66 to 6.38 mEq/L (larger than the medical requirements).

Also be careful when less than 2.5 SD are contained in the medically allowable error because the imprecision may be too large to show medically required changes in test results.

The first level is the responsibility of the bench medical technologist and the supervisors. The control process at this level includes the daily analysis of quality control specimens, which is discussed in this section, and the review of patient results and reports. The technologist is responsible for performing quality control analyses at the appropriate intervals and for determining that, during any given run, there is no apparent systematic error in that run. Both the technologists and the supervisor are responsible for reviewing patient data to ensure that there is no random error.

The second level of control ensures that minimal systematic bias enters into the system over a relatively short period of weeks to months. The responsibility for this level of error control is usually shared by supervisors and the laboratory director, though technologists often contribute greatly. The control process at this level requires review of the quality control data and proficiency testing that have accumulated over that period of time.

The third level of the control process ensures that the analytical systems are as precise and accurate as possible. The responsibility for this falls to the laboratory director or technical consultant. The control process at this level requires review of proficiency testing results, knowledge of the levels of precision and accuracy achievable by other laboratories, and, when applicable, the use of accuracy-based standards to verify or correct errors. This level of quality control review occurs over a longer period of time, from months to years. Discussion of proficiency testing is found in a later section.

Quality control of the entire testing system, from phlebotomy to generating a patient report, requires additional process control measures. Many of these measures include regulatory-mandated monitors of individual steps in the process and are reviewed in Chapter 2. One important factor that is rarely formally recognized is the complaints of physicians about perceived problems. Physicians' complaints are very often based on real deficiencies in one part of the testing system. These errors may not be known to the laboratory until revealed by the laboratory staff's investigation of a complaint. Monitoring physicians' complaints and their resolutions is thus an important monitor to help control the overall quality of the testing system.

Testing quality control specimens—daily decision making

The daily preparation and analysis of quality control samples is a regular responsibility of the analyst. The quality control pools are analyzed as "known" controls during analysis of patient samples. The values are "known" because some attempt has been made to determine the actual levels of each constituent. The laboratory can estimate the target values of the control samples by repeated analysis, use the manufacturer's estimates of the values, or, ideally, determine the values by definitive or reference methods (see below, p. 399). The frequency of analysis of the QC material is established by each laboratory for each method. CLIA '88 requires the analysis of at least two controls of different values for each run (defined as up to 24 hours of stable operation).

Most laboratories use two different pools, one normal and one abnormal. A normal pool contains constituents at concentrations within the nondiseased reference interval whereas an abnormal pool contains the analytes at concentrations outside the reference interval. Some laboratories may employ three pools—low abnormal, normal, and high abnormal, especially when medically significant decisions are made at each level. CLIA allows each laboratory to set its own protocols for chemistry testing assay control samples as long as at least two control samples of different concentrations are assayed every 24 hours. Some states mandate three pools for some tests. CLIA mandates special rules for blood gases requiring, as a minimum, the analysis of one QC sample every 8 hours of testing and the use of a combination of QC samples and calibrators that includes samples with both high and low concentrations each day of testing. The Clinical Laboratory Improvement Amendment also requires the use of one calibrator or control each time a patient sample is analyzed, unless the blood-gas instrument is calibrated at least every 30 minutes (§493.1243). The manufacturer of a testing system generally recommends the testing frequency that should be used as a basis for a laboratory's quality control policy.

Testing personnel must use the data from each quality control analysis to make a decision about the validity of patients' test data. Generally, if the results for a quality control sample are within the accepted target range, technologists will assume that the patients' results obtained during the same run are equally valid and can "accept" the run. On the other hand, if the results for the quality control pool are unacceptable, the run is not acceptable (see p. 391). The decision to accept or reject an analytical run should be documented with the decision "accept" or "reject," the analyst's name (or code number), and the date on a work sheet, in a separate log book, on a data sheet, or in the laboratory information system (LIS) (see Chapter 18). Usually, the process of data verification in the LIS is recognized as a decision by the technologist to accept the data.

Daily bench-level quality control testing is most useful for detecting systematic errors. It can also be used to detect increases in imprecision. However, random errors, which occur unpredictably, are not usually detectable by a quality control system. Random errors can be detected only by review of reported problems and patients' results (see pp. 394-396).

Quality control mechanics

How to choose a quality control pool. Quality control material should have a matrix that closely matches that of the specimens in the analytical run. This means that if the run includes cerebrospinal fluid, serum, and urine then controls composed of cerebrospinal fluid (CSF), serum, and urine should be included in the analytical run.

Because the quality control material is analyzed in every run along with patients' specimens, large amounts of control material are needed each year. There are currently several sources from which a laboratory can obtain sufficient quantities of quality control material. These are (1) commercial lyophilized pool material; (2) commercial stabilized liquid pools; and (3) frozen, pooled, patient specimens. Patient serum is more frequently used than plasma because it is more readily available and is less likely to include precipitated material. Frozen liquid or clarified (with materials that reduce turbidity) pools show smaller standard deviations than lyophilized pools do.[17] The smaller imprecision errors of the liquid pools derive, in part, from the absence of the errors involved with the lyophilization process. However, the liquid pools may experience greater instability errors associated with shipping batches of a lot to the customer. Some characteristics of three sources of quality control material are listed in Table 21-4. It is important to select a pool that has a matrix that interacts least with the methods employed in the laboratory. Certain characteristics of a pool, whether its turbidity or chemical constituents, can render it unusable.

Notice that control pools prepared in the laboratory from pooled patient samples (serum, plasma, urine, and CSF) can be contaminated with dangerous viruses, and it is essential to test each specimen or group of specimens and the final pool for harmful viruses.

The following statements apply to all specimen pools used for quality control. First, all pooled human material should be monitored for the presence of the human immunodeficiency virus and the hepatitis B virus. No pools should be used if there is evidence of the presence of either virus. Second, all control material requires refrigerator or freezer space for storage of a 1- to 2-year supply. Alternatively, commercial distributors may supply quantities from a single lot number of stored material on a monthly or quarterly basis so that the laboratory can use the same lot number over 1 to 2 years. This helps bring long-term stability to the quality control process, though the possibility of shipment-to-shipment variations within the same lot must still be considered.

Some professional groups and manufacturers offer participation in regional quality control programs in which

Table 21-4 Comparison of quality control materials

Criteria	Frozen	Lyophilized	Low-temperature liquid
Cost	Low, if not manipulated* Medium, if manipulated	High	Highest
Clarity	Clear, if carefully collected	Turbid	Clear
Stability	12 months	18 to 24 months	18 to 24 months
Validation	Compare with accurately measured materials (NIST and CAP†)	Regional and manufacturer's peer group analysis available, or by NIST and CAP	Regional and manufacturer's peer group analysis available
Lyophilization error	Absent	Present	Absent

*That is, if additional analyte is added.
†*NIST*, National Institute of Standards and Technology; *CAP*, College of American Pathologists.

laboratories use the same batch of pooled serum. This offers both cost and scientific advantages. The comparison between laboratories can help predict how the testing system will perform in proficiency testing. This comparison becomes more valuable when the accuracy of the quality control pool is established by reference or definitive methods.[3,6,22,26-28]

Preliminary considerations for estimating limits for quality control pools

Unless the true value of a pool is established by definitive or reference methods, the target values are only averages of repeated measurements of the pool. The average temporary or the average final target values of the quality control pool are the estimated concentrations of each analyte within the pool. Each laboratory usually establishes its own average target values for the analytes by performing the laboratory's procedures on each pool. CLIA '88 allows the pool's manufacturer to establish target values, with the laboratory confirming that each target value is applicable to its testing system.

Laboratories must resolve a dilemma regarding target limits that result from CLIA's new rules. On one hand there is the need to optimize a testing system's calibration according to the manufacturer's instructions, but on the other hand there is the need to meet proficiency testing requirements. The Health Care Financing Administration allows each proficiency testing provider to determine how the program will establish the target values that will be used to judge acceptable performance. If the target value is calculated from peer group means for each testing system, it is better to establish the laboratory's QC system target values by use of the manufacturer's recommendations for both calibration and QC. However, if the target values for proficiency testing are set by the mean of all participants or by the true target values established by definitive methods, optimizing assays to the manufacturer's specifications may result in problems with the proficiency testing results if a bias is present as a result of those specifications.

Part of the problem with establishing a quality control program using manufacturers' recommendations is the effect of lyophilization (which causes matrix changes) on various constituents, causing method-specific interferences or bias (for example, as a result of the turbidity of these specimens). The dilemma, therefore, is that if a laboratory follows the requirement of CLIA '88 to follow the manufacturer's instructions, failure in proficiency testing may result. However, a laboratory can, by the rules of CLIA '88, modify the manufacturer's instructions if the laboratory has data validating any changes.

When new target values are established for a new lot of quality control material, it is important to be sure that, during the data-collection period, the analytical systems are performing according to normal performance specifications. The new lot of quality control material should be tested in parallel with the current lot of quality control material. If the analytical data from the current quality control material indicate satisfactory performance of the methods, the data for the new lot can be assumed to be valid. When setting up a quality control system for the first time, the current methodology is accepted as valid if the method meets its performance specifications. The choice of the laboratory's testing method (or testing system) is based on experience with medical usefulness, significant change limits, external quality control and accuracy comparisons, and quality control performance.

There are basically three approaches that can be used to establish the limits of acceptable values for a control pool. One approach is to use the medically allowable error for choosing the range. The other, more usual approach is to estimate the target value and usual standard deviation (SD) for the method and use some number of SDs to establish the range. The third technique is to employ the more statistically accurate method of power curves. On the following pages these alternatives are described.

A simple method for establishing average temporary target values for quality control pools

1. Procure a minimum of a 1-year supply of quality control test material.

2. It is preferable to plan a 6-week lead time before changing control pools to allow for (a) comparative analy-

ses of old and new lots of control materials (3 weeks), (b) data reduction and calculation and evaluation of control limits (1 week), and (c) 2 weeks for safety because not all planning is perfect. It is also advisable to retain 20 or 30 vials of each expiring pool for evaluating problems resulting from system changes. Clearly identify the expiring pool to ensure that it is not used beyond its expiration date and that it is not mistaken for the current lot of control materials. CLIA prohibits a laboratory from using out-of-date reagents, solutions, controls, calibrators, or culture media (§493.1205[e][1]). Any exception must be specifically granted by the Food and Drug Administration (FDA).

3. Always reconstitute the lyophilized material carefully, following the label's directions. Mixing too quickly or too vigorously may interfere with the solubilization of the lyophilized material or denature its protein constituents. Denatured enzymes have reduced activity. The date, time, and technologist's initials should be recorded on each vial of control material after reconstitution. If a frozen liquid pool is used, after thawing, mix the sample six times by inversion because the protein and other compounds become concentrated at the bottom of the vial during freezing.

4. Test duplicate samples from two separate vials (20 vials, 40 measurements) each day for 10 days. An alternative procedure is to reconstitute one vial per day and perform the tests in duplicate on each of 20 consecutive days (20 vials, 40 measurements). See Table 21-3 for an example of these calculations.

5. Determine temporary target values for each constituent by calculating the mean of these 40 analytical values ($n = 40$). This temporary target value is replaced after 2 months with a final average target value (see following text).

6. Calculate the standard deviation of the 40 values. Note that this calculated standard deviation is a hybrid between within-run and total imprecision because the tests are done both in single runs and over several days. Set the range of allowable control values around the average temporary target by using the newly calculated standard deviation multiplied by the laboratory's control limit, expressed as the number of standard deviations (such as 2.5 or 3.0). The number of standard deviations for the control range can also be set according to the size of the USD and the test's allowable error (see following text and Table 21-3). If the allowable error for glucose at 1200 mg/L is ±60 mg/L, the control range should fit within these boundaries. In other words, the testing system's full control range (such as ±3 standard deviations) should fit within the allowable ±60 mg/L. For this example, a single standard deviation can be as large as 20 mg/L. Alternatively, if the usual standard deviation is 15 mg/L, then ±4 standard deviations can fit within the allowable window.

The temporary average target and range of allowable control values are now used for routine quality control in the laboratory for the next 2 months.

7. After the second month there are three values to use in calculating the average final target value: the temporary target value and two monthly averages (Table 21-3). If the control material is slightly unstable over time (for example, alkaline phosphatase activity often changes over time), the process used to change the target value must include evidence that the test value of the control material changed while the testing system remained constant. Such evidence can be provided by the use of additional stable materials with known values (such as a different control, excess proficiency testing material, or additional calibrator materials). The decision process for changing the target value must be well documented. It is best to avoid unstable control material.

Calculation of the usual standard deviation

Every method has a characteristic inherent variability termed the *usual standard deviation*. The USD is calculated from a series of three to six consecutive monthly standard deviations that are obtained during a time when the testing instrument is assumed to be stable. The USD is a valid estimate of the usual day-to-day variability of individual measurements. The USD can eventually be used instead of the temporary SD to establish the daily control limits around the average final target value. Table 21-3 shows how the USD can be used to calculate the allowable number of standard deviations for control values that will still maintain the medical usefulness of the testing system. The medically allowable error is divided by the USD to calculate the number of USDs in the medically allowable error. This calculation assumes no significant bias. If significant bias is present, first subtract the bias from the total medically allowable error and then divide the result by the USD. This calculated number of standard deviations should be equal to or more than the number of standard deviations used for the laboratory's control range. Otherwise the test will either be persistently out of control or its medical usefulness will be compromised.

The USD can also be used to establish the statistical significance of the difference between two values from the same patient. The latter is often referred to as the significant change limit (see p. 387).

Setting the action control limits for each level of control pool

The limits of acceptable results are used to determine the action limits of the control range. Historically, a QC result that exceeded the set limits was known as an *out-of-control* value. However, CLIA regulations now specifically define the term *out of control* as a situation in which a testing system cannot be used for reporting patients' results. Thus the term *exceeding action limits* is now used to designate the less serious condition in which the result of a routine QC analysis exceeds the set limits. The documented response of a medical technologist to a QC result that exceeds action limits (see following text) does not include shutting the procedure down. This occurs only when the laboratory director formally declares that a testing system is *out of control* and the laboratory begins a formal remedial process to correct this more serious situation (see following text). A laboratory will be best served by designating in their laboratory manual the conditions that will define these two situations.

Historically the ranges were ±2 standard deviations and covered 95% of expected control values. However, this means that 5% of results for control pools are expected to exceed action limits even when the method is working perfectly. A false rejection of a run will result in excessive re-running of samples and will necessitate performing the documentation that is required under CLIA regulations. Therefore, limits other than ±2 SDs have been suggested for establishing control limits. Currently many laboratories use 2.5 or 3 standard deviations for the acceptable limits in an attempt to reduce false-run rejection time and unnecessary retesting.

However, the use of 2.5 or 3 standard deviations to set error limits may not result in error detection that is sufficient for medical and CLIA requirements.[10,11,32] Thus a second approach is to establish daily quality control ranges based on the considerations discussed earlier. The target range must be equal to or less than the total allowable error (see p. 384), which in turn is equal to or less than the allowable medical and legal (CLIA) error. The target control limits will therefore be some multiples of the USD or temporary SD that will fulfill these requirements. The number of multiples chosen will be based on the need to detect true cases of inaccurate measurements and yet minimize false rejections of acceptable runs (see following text).

Another approach is to set the allowable range based only on medical usefulness criteria. The range is expressed as plus or minus the medically allowable error window around the target value. This process does not require that the laboratory use ±2 or more standard deviations. The control window is as wide as medical use will allow. An "action limit" situation is demonstrated when the test value of the control material exceeds the error limits. One should determine that this approach will not place the laboratory at risk for failure of proficiency testing.

For all these approaches, the final control range must not be so large that the testing system will fail to detect true instances of failure of the method.

Setting quality control limits by power curves

Among the main questions in quality control are: "How much quality control testing is enough?" "Am I sure that I am detecting appropriately small errors?" and "Is my error detection sensitive enough to show if the testing system is appropriate for its medical needs?" If a laboratory has adequately set allowable errors for medical needs, the second question is of academic interest only because the pursuit of the smallest errors is costly and time consuming.

A more scientific approach to answering these questions uses power curves to determine how many controls should be run, how frequently controls should be run, and what control rules should be used. Power curves are plots of the size of the error detected by a control system versus the probability of detecting that size error by various control rules. The power curve rules can calculate the probability of falsely rejecting a valid test run, the probability of true rejection (the detection of a significant error in the run), the probability of error detection, and the average number of control observations required to identify a given error.[5,16,20,30,31,40,41,43] The design of specific control rules for a laboratory requires a five-step process[41] that includes (1) defining total allowable analytical error, (2) estimating the method's actual standard deviation and bias at the medical decision concentrations, (3) determining the systematic and random error that must be detected by the control system, (4) determining the probability level used for error detection (that is, do you want to detect 90%, 95%, or 99% of errors?), and (5) plotting and inspecting the power curves to determine the number of control specimens that should be tested per run. The most difficult part of these evaluations is determining how much error is allowable.

Westgard used these power curves to develop a series of specific control guidelines, popularly called the "Westgard rules." The rules, which are used to determine whether an analytical run is out of control, are written in shorthand as follows: (1) 1_{2s}, $1_{2.5s}$, and 1_{3s} mean one control value exceeding two, two and one half, or three standard deviations, (2) 2_{2s} means two control values exceeding two standard deviations, and (3) R_{4s} means the range of two control specimens exceeds four standard deviations. For many testing situations the sequential application of the $1_{3s}/2_{2s}/R_{4s}$ set of control rules allows two control specimens to give sufficient error detection for a single run.[42] These rules mean that the run is rejected (action limits are exceeded) if *any* of the following happen: (1) 1_{3s}, if one control value differs by more than three standard deviations from the mean value, (2) 2_{2s}, if two control values differ by more than two standard deviations from the mean value, and (3) R_{4s}, if the range between two controls in the same run exceeds a combination of four standard deviations (that is, one control ≥1.5 SD from mean and the other >−2.5 SD from mean). The first two rules will detect excessive bias, whereas the last rejects the run because of excessive imprecision. With use of these rules, the data in Fig. 21-1 for one control show values that exceed the action limits on days 10 (1_{3s}) and 20 (1_{3s}). Notice that, for rejection, the control value should exceed the control limit, not just be equal to that value. For many chemistry tests, power curves allow cost-effective detection of significant total errors (based on clinical usefulness) when two controls are used and the limits are set somewhere between 2.5 to 3.5 standard deviations.[20] For this reason, many use 3.0 usual standard deviations as a generalized control limit.

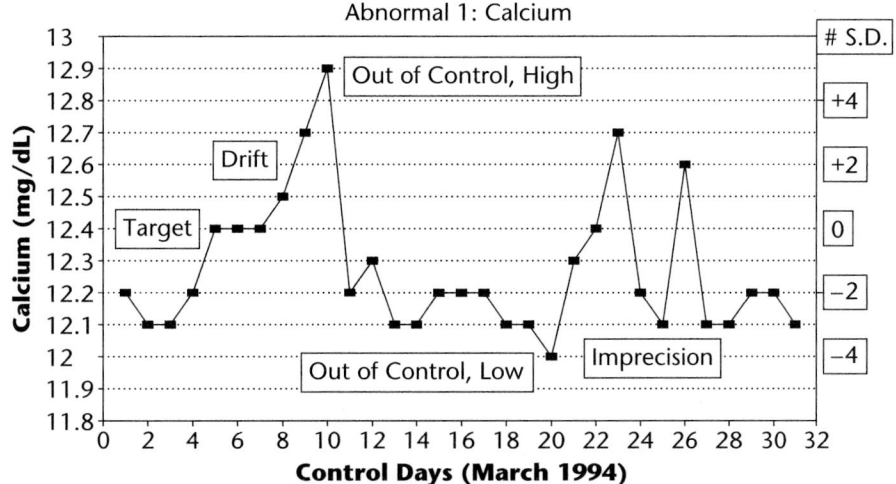

Fig. 21-1   Levey-Jennings plot of quality control values. *quality control actions (testing personnel documentation of how all out-of-control values were resolved):* Days 5-7 represent a shift from the target value (monitor carefully). Days 6-10 demonstrate a gradual trend toward higher values. Day 10 patients' results were not reported, an unresolved problem (one control > 3 SD), probably need new bottle of calibrator. On day 11 recalibrated using new bottle of calibrator. Control values are now in control range; the patients' specimens from day 9 were retested. Day 13 begins a shift to lower values. This shift was investigated on day 20 when one control was low by more than 3 SD. Recalibration on day 21 resolved the problem because values were nearer to the target value (RBP). Days 23 through 26 show increased imprecision. On day 27 cleaning the flow cell resolved the problem, however, the low bias is still present. *General note:* When this method shows acceptable imprecision, the values are below the target. It was subsequently determined that the manufacturer's target value for this QC pool was inaccurate. Proficiency results from testing performed on March 16 were within 0.01 mg/dL from the all participants' target value. After this documentation, the laboratory director approved a new target value for this QC pool.

DETECTION AND RESOLUTION OF QUALITY PROBLEMS
The out-of-control decision

A testing system is designated as "out of control" when the validity of the results is not considered to be appropriate. Grossly out-of-control testing systems are usually unsuitable for medical purposes. This determination is made by the director or technical supervisor.

The conditions for an out-of-control determination should be set by each laboratory; as a minimum, the criteria for an out-of-control decision include the following elements:

1. Control values exceed predetermined out-of-control limits within a specified period. Technologists must be directed to document their response to *every* control value that exceeds the established limits.
2. A method is determined to have an inappropriate reference interval; if the range is not immediately correctable, the method is "out of control."
3. A method demonstrates unacceptable imprecision, nonlinearity, or interferences. Interferences usually are limited to specific specimen types or substances.

4. A pattern of inappropriate patient results with large numbers of abnormals is observed.
5. The laboratory director, section director, or technical supervisor declares the method out of control for other reasons.

Techniques for detecting and resolving "out-of-control" situations are discussed in the following text.

Detection of quality problems

Computer assistance. The target values and limits for acceptable results that are established for each control pool areused in daily practice to detect analytical problems. There are several ways that a control result can be reviewed by a technologist to evaluate its acceptability. The technologist can simply compare the result to the posted range. This limits the technologist's ability to employ the Westgard rules or to evaluate the trend of previous results. More complex selection rules are now available as part of some computer programs, either on the instrument or as part of the laboratory's information system (LIS, see Chapter 18). Computer assistance allows real-time review of control results, early detection of QC problems, and better documentation of the quality control process.

Levey-Jennings plots. [23,33] The data obtained from daily analysis of quality control pools can be plotted to give a visual presentation of the data. The most common visual analysis is the Levey-Jennings plot. The expected analyte concentrations, the established target value, and the desired number of standard deviations are drawn on the *y*-axis and the days of the month (typically 31) are indicated on the *x*-axis (Fig. 21-1). A large piece of graph paper can be used to show the data for several months. Thus cumulative information from quality control results can be observed at one time. Levey-Jennings plots are usually available from the LIS (see Chapter 18).

Fig. 21-1 shows an example of a Levey-Jennings plot. The sudden change in control values (days 1-4 versus 5-7) from one average to a new average is called a *shift*. The increasing deviation from the target value, seen from day 8 to day 10, is called a *trend*. Changes in the precision of the testing system are shown on days 21 to 26, that is, a greater dispersion of data points than that shown for days 13 to 19. This system was judged as unacceptable for the reasons documented at the bottom of Fig. 21-1. On day 32, the laboratory director reevaluated the target value and concluded that it had been set too high. A lower value was set, and QC results for the next month were closely monitored to assess this change.

Either positive or negative trends (or drifts) or shifts from the target value represent biases that should be evaluated. Levey-Jennings plots should be routinely evaluated by technologists and supervisory personnel looking for trends or shifts in the data that could indicate problems in the testing system. Normally a trend or a shift is noticed within 6 to 10 days after it begins. A shift or trend that exists over this period is usually a nonrandom, permanent change.

Using patients' data in decision making

Pattern of patients' results. The results of most patients' sample analyses fall within reference (healthy) intervals established for each analyte.[21] Thus, for an analytical run of patients' samples, the results fall into a familiar pattern; that is, most results are within the nondiseased patient reference interval and a few results are abnormal. The distribution of abnormal results, that is, the percentage of high or low results, will vary from test to test and even from hospital to hospital. Deviations from the usual pattern of results should alert the testing personnel that a shift in the system's performance may be occurring and that the patient analyses may be invalid. For example, a series of patient results for potassium greater than 5 should alert a technologist to a possible bias problem (Table 21-5). The example in Table 21-5 shows a typical set of potassium values (patient set A) and a clearly abnormal series (patient set B). The technologist should, of course, evaluate special circumstances. For example, a work load that includes a larger number than usual of patients' specimens from renal dialy-

Table 21-5   Use of patient data in daily quality control

Sample number	Patient set A	Patient set B
Control I	4.4—in control	4.4—in control
Control II	6.9—in control	6.8—in control
1	3.8	4.1
2	4.6	3.9
3	5.0	5.7
4	4.3	6.1
5	4.2	6.5
6	3.6	5.8
7	4.7	6.4
8	4.0	6.2
9	4.6	5.1
10	3.9	4.7
Control I	4.3—in control	4.6—in control (at +2 SD)
Control II	6.8—in control	7.0—in control (at +2 SD)

Would you wait until the quality control samples after the tenth sample to make a judgment about the system? No. After about the third or fourth patient sample with an extremely high or low value, quality control could be moved ahead and trouble detection should begin. Keep in mind that occasionally, by chance, a series of specimens from very ill patients may fall in consecutive order. Repeated testing will usually solve the problem.

sis or cancer chemotherapy clinics will abnormally skew the otherwise typical pattern of test results.

The delta check. Another important quality control check is the pattern of consecutive results for an individual patient. For most analyses, it is unlikely that a consecutive series of two or three test values from one patient will show large differences unless a major medical change has occurred. Unexpected changes from a single patient's serial specimens are called *delta changes,* meaning that a value for a single patient changed from the previous results more than the laboratory's delta limit allows. Delta limits are set to detect mixed-up specimens or other errors (see p. 80). When these types of changes are noted, one must determine if the change is real or if problems exist that are not identified by analysis of quality control specimens.

Actions to bring a testing system back into control

When analytic problems are found, it is best to have a plan of action that is executed sequentially until the problem is resolved. For CLIA '88 it is necessary to document the problem, the investigation, the problem resolution, and any data that indicate that the problem is resolved. Typically, this documentation is kept in a separate "action limits" or "out-of-control" log book. A list of actions follows that are among the sequential actions that might be taken to identify a problem. After each step is taken, the routine QC pools are analyzed; if the results are now within limits, it is assumed that the problem has been resolved, and patient results can be released. If the QC results are still not satisfactory, the next step is taken.

1. Repeat assays on control specimens using fresh aliquots of QC pools.

2. Repeat assays on control specimens using a separate or newly reconstituted set of controls. A set of controls can

be mishandled, resulting in changed analyte concentrations because of either enzyme deterioration or evaporation.

3. Look for obvious problems: clots, reagent levels, mechanical fault.

4. Recalibrate the instrument for the "out-of-control" analyte, then reassay all the controls.

5. Install a new bottle or new lot number for one or all of the reagents, recalibrate, and reassay all the controls.

6. Perform periodic maintenance, recalibrate, and reassay all the controls.

If these responses now result in acceptable QC data, results for patients' results can be released if and *only* if at least three (or the entire run, whichever is less) patients' specimens taken from the last run are reassayed and the differences between previous and new results are within the performance specification for precision (see p. 391). This requirement is established by CLIA, which states (§493.1219[b]) that "all patient test results obtained in the unacceptable test run or since the last acceptable test run must be evaluated to determine if patient test results have been adversely affected and the laboratory must take the remedial action necessary to ensure the reporting of accurate and reliable patient test results."

Technologists should be encouraged to perform all the above steps by themselves before requesting help from a supervisor. However, in a critical testing area time limits for instrument downtime should be set. For an instrument in a stat. area, probably no more than 15 to 20 minutes should be spent in problem solving before supervisors are notified.

Example. At the start of the day, the laboratory's method for potassium produced results for controls that were elevated by over 5 standard deviations. The change coincided with a reagent change. New reagents were installed, the instrument was recalibrated, and the controls were retested; they were then back in control. Three patient samples from the last run were retested to see if the problem affected the reported values. The potassium results reported for the previous runs were 3.9, 4.6, and 5.3 mmol/L and, when repeated, the results were 4.1, 4.5, and 5.3 mmol/L. The method's performance specification for potassium precision is 1 SD = 0.11 mmol/L. The patients' potassium results each changed by <0.22 mmol/L. This is less than a 2 SD change; therefore, the old report does not have to be changed. This reevaluation of a patient's results should continue until either a significant difference is seen or the previously accepted quality control sample is reached.

When reevaluation of previous patients' results shows unacceptable differences, *all* the patients' specimens that were tested after the last in-control QC sample must be reassayed. If problems persist, the test may need to be performed on an alternative system or sent to a reference laboratory. If there is insufficient quantity (or quantity not sufficient) of a patient's specimen to reevaluate, the labora-

tory should request another specimen. It is inappropriate to report a result when the assay quality is in question.

7. Assay a different control of similar known concentration (to determine if the original control material is at fault). It is good policy to have some control materials different from the QC materials routinely used, with reliable assay values, which are saved for use in these situations. The determination of a shift in the control material's assay value (which requires resetting the target value) is to be made only by the director or technical supervisor. If the values for a routine QC pool have changed slightly, assuming a new, stable pattern, but the test system appears stable (as judged by values from separate QC materials), then the target values of the routine QC pool may be changed. Such changes must be authorized by the laboratory director, and the decision process is documented. If only one of the controls is showing the slight shift while a material of similar concentration continues to give a stable value and the test system shows stable performance, the initial estimation of the control material's target value was probably incorrectly set. In this case the target value should be modified. If both controls and additional controls show similar shifts or trends, the problem is probably in the testing system.

8. Call the manufacturer to help determine the cause of the problem. Follow the manufacturer's instructions and then reassay all the controls.

9. Have the instrument serviced by the manufacturer, recalibrate, and reassay all the controls.

10. Use commercial accuracy–based materials to evaluate the quality of the analytical system, checking linearity (reportable range), accuracy, bias, precision, analytical sensitivity, and minimal detectable change (smallest concentration change that is significant). Evaluate these data to see if they reveal the cause of the control problem. Performing parallel testing on patient samples on a second instrument can be very helpful at this point.

11. Determine if the testing system has changed by reevaluating the reference interval. You can do this by obtaining data on the last 100 patients who have near-normal chemistry profiles with 2 or fewer slight abnormalities (acceptable patients are determined by the director or technical supervisor). Estimate the reference interval by excluding the 2.5% of the values from the tails of the distribution. This interval should agree (within ±1 SD) with the laboratory's established reference interval. This procedure will only demonstrate gross changes in the system. The director or technical supervisor should determine if there has been a significant shift in the reference interval.

12. Reestablish the method's linearity using either the National Committee for Clinical Laboratory Standards (NCCLS) protocols EP-6 or EP-10. If the method is linear over the reporting range and the reference interval has not changed, the method is probably usable with adjustments to the appropriate target values for the control specimens.

13. Consult with the director or technical supervisor to declare the method out of control if the above steps fail.

14. A final action is replacement of the method or instrument with one that will allow the laboratory to meet its medical and proficiency testing goals.

Every quality control decision should be recorded in a permanent record. To meet CLIA '88's requirements, the quality control records should state acceptable limits and include a place where the actions taken in response to out-of-range values are noted. These responses must include date, analyte, complete testing system (that is, source of reagents, instrument, calibrators, and controls), description of the problem, its resolution, and names of the persons performing the test and approving the final actions. It may be convenient to prepare check-off forms or graphs for each control and analyte (Fig. 21-2). These records are also useful for predicting the need for maintenance, repair, or replacement of deteriorating reagents as indicated by the circled check marks in Fig. 21-2. Computerized records can greatly simplify and speed the documentation process.

Actions to be taken when a method is out of control

1. The decision that a testing system is out of control and must be suspended is communicated to all laboratory personnel including the director, technical consultant, technical supervisor, clinical consultant, general supervisor, and all appropriate testing personnel. As stated above, the time frame for making this problem known will vary from section to section and should be stated in the laboratory's manual.

2. Suspension of a testing system means that no further patient test results are to be released until the out-of-control condition is corrected and the director or technical supervisor approves resumption of the testing.

3. Steps must be taken to have the test performed either by an alternative method or by a reference laboratory. The alternative procedure must be listed in the laboratory manual. Notify the appropriate clinicians if the alternative method will have any adverse influence on test results or turnaround times.

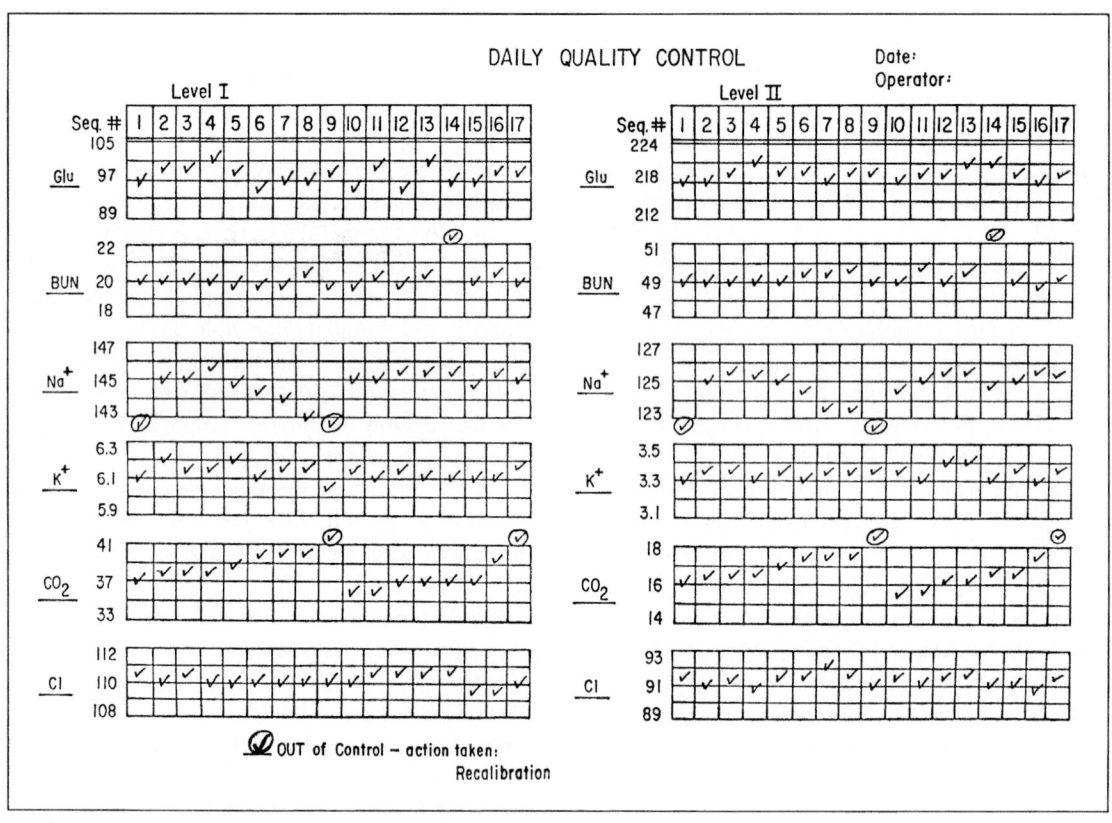

Fig. 21-2 Multiple analyte daily quality control check-off record. As each control is reported, it is quickly logged in on a data sheet. Notes of out-of-control values and action taken are included. A daily value for quality control calculation is selected by use of a random-number table basis. (Form developed by Rosvoll RV: In Copeland BE, Rosvoll RV, Casella JM: *Quality control workshop manual,* Chicago, 1978, American Society of Clinical Pathologists Commission on Continuing Education.)

4. An out-of-control condition that cannot be dealt with by use of alternative methods or testing systems must be communicated within a reasonable time to the medical staff and any other authorized persons (such as senior administrative staff).

5. Supervisory personnel may define, for medical or analytical reasons, out-of-control conditions that differ from those stated in the general policy. These special conditions must be documented in the procedure as well as in the method's file.

6. Bringing a suspended test back into production requires the following actions as a minimum. The method must be recalibrated, or a calibration verification must be performed. Two levels of controls and at least one other material, such as proficiency testing materials of known or established value, must be used. The method can be used when the results of the known specimens are within the expected mean ± 2 times the appropriate usual standard deviation (established at a concentration close to the control value that was out of control). The method's reuse must be authorized by the technical supervisor or director. This authorization must be entered into the laboratory's problem log and formally signed and dated.

Procedures to follow during a testing system failure

An out-of-control condition that is not immediately repairable can constitute a laboratory emergency. These emergencies can be managed by using a backup method, sending the test to a reference laboratory, or temporarily discontinuing the test. A laboratory must list an alternative or backup method of analysis in the procedure manual. Laboratory policy should define how much time the technologist can spend troubleshooting a method before using the alternative system. Other factors that affect the decision include the medical requirements of the test (stat. versus routine), laboratory staffing, and the laboratory's work load. For example, a stat. potassium analysis would be treated very differently from a 72-hour fecal fat determination. In the case of a potassium test, a delay of more than 30 minutes in providing a backup stat. analysis may affect the medical decision; whereas several days' delay in the fecal fat analysis may not be crucial to patient care. Decisions about processing patient samples during a testing system failure should be made in consultation with the laboratory technical supervisor/consultant and the laboratory director, as specified by laboratory policy.

CALIBRATION AND QUALITY CONTROL
Use of calibrators

Controls may not be used as calibrators. Controls and calibrators must be different because each has a separate and important function. Calibrators set the reported values accurately, whereas controls check on the stability and accu-

racy of the calibration and the testing system. However, for those tests that do not have suitable controls available, CLIA '88 allows calibration materials to be used as controls. For evaluation of the system's stability, in these cases it is best to find calibrator materials other than those used for calibration of the testing system.

A commercially available calibrator has an assigned value that the manufacturer establishes by using a definitive or reference method or by using reference materials (traceable to primary standards). The calibrator is then used to set the value reported by the laboratory's method or instrument. This process establishes correspondence of the instrument output with known concentrations. Differences between an aqueous and serum matrix can affect the transfer of known concentrations to a reported result. These matrix differences include turbidity, surface tension, which can affect sample pipetting, interactions between analytes and proteins, and the effect of the volume fraction occupied by protein or other large molecules (especially lipoproteins) on the actual concentration of the analytes.

Calibrators are usually purchased in lots large enough to last 12 or more months. It is recommended that a new lot of calibrator material be tested 6 weeks before it is used. This time delay allows the laboratory to detect any systematic bias between the values of the current and the new calibrator. Bias in a new lot of calibrator is detected when changes are seen in the mean value of quality control pools or patients' test results. Some testing systems do not allow calibrators (especially calibrators from other systems) to be run as an unknown because of matrix mismatch. Often a calibrator will have assigned values that don't represent actual analyte values. These assigned-value calibrators are designed to calibrate testing systems to produce accurate test values when patients' samples are used. Although the FDA requires manufacturers to use reference methods to assign calibrator values, there are frequently significant differences between calibrator lots. Because of matrix effects, errors can be introduced into the calibration process when calibrators are used that are not specifically designed for the analytic system. Under CLIA '88 any modification of the manufacturer's instructions for the analytical portion of an FDA-cleared procedure requires documentation of the validity of the change. A laboratory that wishes to change a manufacturer's calibration set point must document that the change does not adversely affect the method's performance specifications.

A practical system for new calibrator verification

1. Use a 10-day verification period.

2. If the manufacturer allows the assay of calibrators as unknowns, each day insert 2 aliquots from one vial of new calibrator as an unknown into the regular daily run ($n = 10$ vials; 20 values). Calculate the average for each analyte. Compare each average with the value assigned by the

manufacturer. Any difference between the assigned and measured values will allow one to predict the average change expected in the quality control pool's target value (and also in patients' test values) when the new calibrator is introduced. A change in the quality control pool's target value greater than 1.0 usual standard deviation is statistically significant, and a decision must be made as to which calibrator value is truly accurate. This decision must include consideration of CLIA's requirements (especially those that concern proficiency testing) and consultation with the manufacturer.

CLIA '88 requires that, when control values demonstrate significant changes (defined by each laboratory), the laboratory must establish, through calibration verification, that calibration has not been changed. Calibration verification requires that three specimens with high, low, and normal analyte concentrations be run to verify the quality of the test results. These specimens can be controls, calibrators, or other specimens with known values. If the manufacturer has specified a calibration verification protocol, you may follow it (§493.1217). The CLIA rules do not set the quantity of allowable error except as judged by proficiency testing. By setting an allowable error that is too large, however, a laboratory increases the danger of failing proficiency testing and may compromise patients' test values. Performance specifications can be used to judge excessive change (see Table 21-3).

Quality control of reagent changes and instrument maintenance

Each lot of reagent or separate shipment must be evaluated for quality before it is put into use. The laboratory can show that new lots or shipments of reagents (including calibrators and quality control pools) are acceptable if, after their use, the control values do not change significantly. It is also a good practice, after any maintenance is performed, to test a set of controls and run several patient samples from a previous batch before testing is resumed. Maintenance problems can lead to an "action-limits" situation because operating parameters may be changed. A chronological record of all reagent changes, instrument repairs, and maintenance procedures along with any calibration-verification tests must be kept.

EXTERNAL QUALITY CONTROL PROGRAMS AND OTHER TOOLS FOR ACCURACY CONTROL
Accuracy control is required by CLIA '88

CLIA '88 requires that all laboratories holding a certificate that allows testing of moderately or highly complex tests must participate successfully in proficiency testing. Proficiency testing (PT) specimens are used to evaluate the adequacy of laboratory performance in all laboratory specialties. The analyst must test these specimens in the same manner as patients' specimens. Historically, PT has been an educational process. Proficiency testing is now regulatory, and

failure has serious penalties. However, the value of proficiency testing is the provision of independent validation of the internal quality control programs. Some of the providers of proficiency testing programs approved by the Health Care Financing Administration (as of March 1993) are listed in Table 21-6. Because the analyst does not know the target value of the PT sample, it is difficult for the operator to influence the results. These programs, if properly used, can give an estimation of the inherent accuracy of a system, at least as compared to a peer group or to the overall mean.[19] Continued or significant deviations from the PT target levels, even if there is no failure, should alert the laboratory to a possible accuracy problem. If a method's USD is not significantly smaller than the comparative group's SD, that method is at increased risk for PT failure.

An *estimation* of a system's bias can also be made from proficiency testing performance. To do this, evaluate the specific test method's observed values against a comparison value, which is either the mean value reported for all similar methods (peer group mean), the mean value for all methods, or the definitive method value. Bias is calculated by subtracting the comparison value from your method's value. The algebraic sign shows whether your method's value is higher or lower than the group mean. Notice that comparison to a peer group mean or even to the mean of all participants doesn't establish accuracy. These comparisons show bias only from the comparison value. Accuracy is determined only when the comparison value is the true value. Certainly repeated bias on proficiency tests must raise the suspicion of a true

Table 21-6 Partial list of HCFA-approved providers of proficiency testing programs for CLIA '88

Provider	Telephone number
Accutest	800-356-6788
American Academy of Family Physicians	800-274-2237
American Association for Bioanalysts	800-234-5315
American Association of Pediatrics	800-433-9016
American Osteopathic Association	800-621-1773
American Proficiency Institute	800-333-0958
American Society of Internal Medicine	800-338-2746
American Thoracic Society	212-315-8789
California Thoracic Society	714-730-1944
College of American Pathologists/Excel	800-323-4040
College of American Pathologists/Surveys	800-323-4040
Commonwealth of Pennsylvania	215-363-8500
Commonwealth of Puerto Rico	809-764-6945
Pacific Biometrics Research Foundation	206-233-9151
State of Idaho	208-334-2235
State of New Jersey	609-530-6172
State of New York	518-474-8739
State of Ohio	614-466-2278
Solomon Park Research Institute	206-821-7005
Wisconsin State Laboratory of Hygiene	800-462-5261

HCFA, Health Care Financing Administration.
From the American Association for Clinical Chemistry, Clinical Laboratories Improvement Act, Fax no. 800-254-2329.

bias and will require additional steps to be taken to either prove or disprove a real bias.

Definitive and reference methods

Definitive and reference methods are established by the National Reference System for the Clinical Laboratory (NRSCL) through applications by groups of interested persons representing different disciplines and organizations from professional societies or practitioners, industrial companies, and governmental agencies. The NRSCL is a part of the NCCLS. Definitive and reference methods are used to establish accuracy-based reference materials (see below).

A *definitive method*[15,26,39] is the most accurate way to measure a particular chemical substance. Analysis by definitive methods usually involves instrumentation of the most sophisticated type and a separation procedure to purify the analyte before its concentration is measured. These methods are available in institutions such as the National Institute of Standards and Technology (NIST), the Centers for Disease Control and Prevention, and large reference laboratories. Table 21-7 lists the seven definitive and 18 reference methods defined by the NRSCL.

A *reference method*[27] is less rigorously proved than a definitive method, but it is well accepted because there is considerable evidence of its analytical ability. Thus the refer-

ence method has a demonstrated record of transferability of accuracy. The equipment and methodology are such that these methods are usually available in a university hospital–level laboratory. If a definitive method is not available for comparison, the reference method is established by consensus among authorities in the field. Reference methods credentialed by the NRSCL are listed in Table 21-7. There are other reference methods that will become NRSCL-credentialed in the near future. The NRSCL is currently designing specifications for designated comparison methods that could be readily used by many laboratories.

A *field method* is one that is in common use. It is not classified as a reference or definitive method. It has been compared to a reference method and has been shown to give comparable results acceptable to the user. Information on these method comparisons and evaluations is available in the medical literature and often from the manufacturer of a testing system.

Reference materials

There are now commercially available aqueous and protein-based materials that may be used as calibrators or controls to determine or monitor the accuracy of assays. Each of these reference materials is useful for investigating the accuracy of a method. True target concentrations are assigned by use of definitive or reference methods. Alternatively the reference material is prepared with a specific concentration by use of known amounts of high-purity analytes. These true target values are the most accurate values obtainable by state-of-the-art technology and thus are preferable when they are available. An example of such a reference material is the lyophilized human serum product, SRM909, produced by the NIST. A number of constituents in this material have levels measured by reference and definitive methods.

There are other materials (similar to quality control materials) that have consensus values established by thousands of laboratories. These values are reported as overall average values or average values of methods performed by a specific testing system. The College of American Pathologists produces survey-validated sera that have values established by thousands of individual assays from laboratories participating in proficiency testing.[19] Some systems will show matrix effects caused by the lyophilization process or the presence of interfering compounds, and so one must be careful when using these materials as the sole judge of a testing system's bias.

Primary standards are always required for definitive and reference methods. The NIST provides a number of reference materials that may be used to prepare primary liquid standards. These include albumin, angiotensin, anticonvulsant drugs, aspartate aminotransferase, bilirubin, blood gases, calcium, chloride, cholesterol, cortisol, creatinine, electrolytes for ion-selective electrodes, fat-soluble vitamins, glucose, hydrogen ion, inorganic ions in bovine serum, iron, lead, lithium, magnesium, potassium, phospho-

Table 21-7 NRSCL definitive and reference methods

Document number	Analyte
Definitive methods	
NCCLS RS1-A	Glucose
NCCLS RS3-A	Cholesterol
NCCLS RS7-P	Sodium
NCCLS RS8-P	Potassium
NCCLS RS9-P	Calcium
NCCLS RS10-P	Chloride
NCCLS RS11-P	Urea
Reference methods	
NCCLS RS1-A	Glucose
NCCLS RS2-A	Aspartate aminotransferase (AST)
NCCLS RS3-A	Cholesterol
NCCLS RS4-A	Alanine aminotransferase (ALT)
NCCLS RS5-A	Total protein
NCCLS RS6-A	Total bilirubin
NCCLS RS7-P	Sodium
NCCLS RS8-P	Potassium
NCCLS RS9-P	Calcium
NCCLS RS10-P	Chloride
NCCLS RS11-P	Urea
NCCLS RS12-P	Creatinine*
NCCLS RS13-P	Rubella antibody
NCCLS RS14-P	Creatine kinase
NCCLS RS15-P	Hemoglobin*
NCCLS RS16	Antimicrobial susceptibility testing
NCCLS RS17	Gamma-glutamyl transferase
NCCLS RS18	Uric acid*

NRSCL, National Reference System for the Clinical Laboratory.
A, Approved; *P,* proposed.
*In development.

rus, sodium, trace metals in serum, tripalmate, urea, and uric acid. Aqueous materials in sealed vials prepared from these NIST primary standards are available from CAP. When NIST reference materials are used for calibration, a method's accuracy may be said to be "traceable to NIST reference materials." It is essential that the matrix of the prepared calibrator is consistent with the requirements of the testing system. Some testing systems require protein or other constituents in the calibrator before it will behave appropriately in the testing system. A catalog of reference materials (NIST Special Publication 260) can be obtained from NIST at 1-301-975-6776.

Selection of a reference laboratory for assistance in accuracy control

One procedure that a laboratory can use to confirm the accuracy of a method is to send aliquots of patients' samples to a reliable reference laboratory. It is important, however, to be completely confident of the quality of the reference laboratory's analytical work. Always obtain information on the accuracy and precision of their analytical methods. The laboratory should request a list of the exact methods and performance specifications used by the reference laboratory as well as the results of their proficiency testing. The laboratory should evaluate all data carefully to determine whether the methods are appropriate for its needs. The laboratory's method is considered accurate if its results are not significantly different from those of the reference laboratory.

Manufacturer's responsibility in the control of testing systems

The responsibility for solving systematic and random bias problems does not belong solely to the user but should also be shared by the manufacturer of equipment and reagents. Manufacturers should provide performance specifications so that the laboratory can determine whether the system can be used appropriately to meet its medical and CLIA requirements. After the laboratory chooses a testing system, the technical supervisor must determine (often with the manufacturer) that the performance specifications are met by laboratory operation. Careful perusal of national proficiency surveys quickly reveals instrument systems and reagent systems that show the presence of significant systematic bias in the analysis of proficiency testing specimens. Proficiency testing specimens are the same or very similar to the specimens used for quality control evaluation. However, some bias may be shown only because of the difference in the matrix of the control materials.[38] These matrix-specific biases are not seen when fresh patients' specimens are tested. The presence of matrix bias is shown by testing of fresh human specimens and control materials by the laboratory's test method and a different method that doesn't show the matrix bias. Any differences found between the methods may be the result of the matrix effect.

Analytical problems that cannot be resolved after consultation with the manufacturer should be reported through the FDA's reporting system, administered by the U.S. Pharmacopeia, at 1-800-638-6725.

BIBLIOGRAPHY

Internal quality control testing: principles and definitions, approved guideline (1991), C24-A', NCCLS, 771 East Lancaster Avenue, Villanova, PA 19085.

Method comparisons and bias estimation using patient samples, tentative guideline (1993), EP9-T, NCCLS, 771 East Lancaster Avenue, Villanova, PA 19085.

Precision performance of clinical chemistry devices, ed 2, *tentative guidelines (1992)*, EP5-T2, NCCLS, 771 East Lancaster Avenue, Villanova, PA 19085.

Preliminary evaluation of clinical laboratory methods, ed 2, *tentative guidelines (1993)*, EP10-T2, NCCLS, 771 East Lancaster Avenue, Villanova, PA 19085.

REFERENCES

1. Barnett RN: Analytic goals in clinical chemistry: the pathologist's viewpoint. In *Analytical goals in clinical chemistry,* Northfield, Ill., June 1977, College of American Pathologists, pp 319-322.
2. Barnett RN: *Clinical laboratory statistics,* ed 2, Boston, 1979, Little, Brown & Co.
3. Bowers GN Jr: Clinical chemistry analyte reference systems based on true value, *Clin Chem* 37:1665-1666, 1991.
4. Breitenberg M: *Questions and answers on quality, the ISO 9000 standard series, quality systems registration, and related issues,* US Department of Commerce, National Institute of Standards and Technology Publication NISTIR 4721, Gaithersburg, Md., 1991, USDC.
5. Carey RN: Implementation of multi-rule quality control procedures, *Lab Med,* pp 393-399, June 1989.
6. Castañeda-Méndez K, Chemometrics: measurement reliability, *Clin Chem* 34:2494-2498, 1988.
7. Cotlove E, Harris EK, Williams GZ: Biological and analytic components of variation in long-term studies of serum constituents in normal subjects: III. Physiological and medical implications, *Clin Chem* 16:1028-1032, 1970.
8. Dorsey DB: Evolving concepts of quality in laboratory practice: a historical overview of quality assurance in clinical laboratories, *Arch Pathol Lab Med* 113:1329-1334, 1989.
9. Douville P, Cembrowski, GS: An approach to the use of clinical limits for quality control, *Lab Med,* pp 406-409, June 1989.
10. Ehrmeyer SS, Laessig RH: The relationship of intralaboratory bias and imprecision on laboratories' ability to meet medical usefulness limits, *Am J Clin Pathol* 89:14-18, 1988.
11. Ehrmeyer SS, Laessig RH, Leinweber JE, Oryall JJ: 1990 Medicare/CLIA final rules for proficiency testing: minimum intralaboratory performance characteristics (CV and bias) needed to pass, *Clin Chem* 36:1736-1740, 1990.
12. Elion-Gerritzen WE: Analytic precision in clinical chemistry and medical decisions, *Am J Clin Pathol* 73:183-195, 1980.
13. Fraser CG: The application of theoretical goals based on biological variation data in proficiency testing, *Arch Pathol Lab Med* 112:404-415, 1988.
14. Gilbert RK: Progress and analytic goals in clinical chemistry, *Am J Clin Pathol* 63:960-973, 1975.
15. Gilbert RK: Accuracy of clinical laboratories studied by comparison with definitive methods, *Am J Clin Pathol* 70:450-470, 1978.
16. Groth T, Falk H, Westgard JO: An interactive computer simulation program for the design of statistical control procedures in clinical chemistry, *Comput Programs Biomed* 13:73-86, 1981.
17. Hardin E, Passey R, Gillum RL, et al: The use of "clear" enzyme control materials, *Am J Med Technol* 45:183-185, 1979.
18. Harris EK: Statistical principles underlying analytic goal-setting in clinical chemistry, *Am J Clin Pathol* 72:374-382, 1979.
19. Hartmann AE, Naito HK, Burnett RW, Welch MJ: Accuracy of participant results utilized as target values in the CAP

Chemistry Survey Program, *Arch Pathol Lab Med* 109:894-903, 1985.

20. Koch DD, Oryall JJ, Quam EF, et al: Selection of medically useful quality-control procedures for individual tests done in a multi-test analytical system, *Clin Chem* 36:230-233, 1990.

21. Ladenson JH: Patients as their own controls: use of the computer to identify "laboratory error," *Clin Chem* 21:1648-1653, 1975.

22. Lasky FD: Proficiency testing linked to the National Reference System for the Clinical Laboratory: a proposal for achieving accuracy, *Clin Chem* 38:1260-1267, 1992.

23. Levey S, Jennings ER: The use of control charts in the clinical laboratory, *Am J Clin Pathol* 20:1059-1066, 1950.

24. Linnet K: Choosing quality-control systems to detect maximum clinically allowable analytical errors, *Clin Chem* 35:284-288, 1989.

25. National Cholesterol Education Program: *Recommendations for improving cholesterol measurements,* NIH Publication No. 90-2964, Bethesda, Md., Feb. 1990, US Department of Health and Human Services, National Institutes of Health.

26. National Committee for Clinical Laboratory Standards: *Development of definitive methods for the National Reference System for the Clinical Laboratory, approved guideline,* NCCLS publication NRSCL1-A (ISBN 1-56238-104-0), Villanova, Penn., 1991, NCCLS.

27. National Committee for Clinical Laboratory Standards: *Development of Reference Methods for the National Reference System for the Clinical Laboratory, approved guideline,* NCCLS publication NRSCL2-A (ISBN 1-56238-105-9), Villanova, Penn., 1991, NCCLS.

28. National Committee for Clinical Laboratory Standards: *Development of certified reference materials for the National Reference System for the Clinical Laboratory, approved guideline,* NCCLS publication NRSCL3-A (ISBN 1-56238-106-7), Villanova, Penn., 1991, NCCLS.

29. Oxley DK: Cholesterol measurements: quality assurance and medical usefulness interrelationships, *Arch Pathol Lab Med* 112:387-391, 1988.

30. Parvin CA: Comparing the power of quality-control rules to detect persistent systematic error, *Clin Chem* 38:358-363, 1992.

31. Parvin CA: Comparing the power of quality-control rules to detect persistent increases in random error, *Clin Chem* 38:364-369, 1992.

32. Ross JW, et al: Goals for allowable analytical error better based on medical usefulness criteria, *Am J Clin Pathol* 85:391-392, 1986.

33. Shewhart WA: *Economic control of quality of the manufactured product,* New York, 1931, Van Nostrand Co.

34. Skendzel LP: How physicians use laboratory tests, *JAMA* 239:1077-1080, 1978.

35. Skendzel LP, Barnett RN, Platt R: Medically useful criteria for analytic performance of laboratory tests, *Am J Clin Pathol* 83:200-205, 1985.

36. Tonks DB: A study of the accuracy and precision of clinical chemistry determination in 170 Canadian laboratories, *Clin Chem* 9:217-233, 1963.

37. Turcotte G, Bourget C, Talbot J, et al: Analytic clinical chemistry precision and medical needs: the Canadian interlab program (CID), *Am J Clin Pathol* 74:336-339, 1980.

38. Uldall A: Quality assurance within clinical chemistry—a brief review emphasizing "good laboratory practice," *Scand J Clin Lab Invest* 47(suppl 187):507-518, 1987.

39. Velapoldi RA, Paule RC, Schaffer R, et al: *A reference method for the determination of potassium in serum,* NBS spec pub no 260-63, Washington, D.C., 1979, National Measurement Laboratory, National Bureau of Standards.

40. Westgard JO, Groth T, Aronsson T, et al: Performance characteristics of rules for internal quality control: probabilities for false rejection and error detection, *Clin Chem* 23:1857-1867, 1977.

41. Westgard JO, Groth T: Power functions for statistical control rules, *Clin Chem* 25:863-869, 1979.

42. Westgard JO, Barry PL, Hunt MR, Groth T: A multi-rule Shewhart chart for quality control in clinical chemistry, *Clin Chem* 27:493-501, 1981.

43. Westgard JO, Oryall JJ, Koch DD: Predicting effects of quality-control practices on the cost-effective operation of a stable multitest analytical system, *Clin Chem* 36:1760-1764, 1990.

44. Young DS, Harris EK, Cotlove E: Biological and analytic components of variation in long-term studies of serum constituents in normal subjects. IV. Results of a study designed to eliminate long-term analytic deviations, *Clin Chem* 17:403-410, 1971.

CHAPTER 22

Evaluation of methods

Carl C. Garber
R. Neill Carey

OBJECTIVES

- List three purposes of a method evaluation.
- List aspects to consider when selecting a method to evaluate for use in a clinical chemistry laboratory.
- Differentiate between random, constant, proportional, and total error.

KEY TERMS

accuracy The agreement between the mean estimate of a quantity and its true value.[29]

allowable error (E_A) The amount of error that can be tolerated without invalidating the medical usefulness of the analytical result, or the maximum amount of error defined for successful performance in proficiency testing.[1]

assigned value The value assigned either arbitrarily (as by convention) or from preliminary evidence (as in the absence of a recognized reference method).[29]

bias A systematic component of analytical error, estimated from a comparison-of-methods experiment.[7] Also known as the difference between two quantities. A measure of inaccuracy.

comparative method The analytical method to which the test method is compared in the comparison-of-methods experiment. This term makes no inference about the quality of the comparative method.[3]

comparison-of-methods experiment An evaluation experiment in which a series of patient samples are analyzed by both the test method and comparative method. The results are assessed to determine whether differences exist between the two methods.[3,7]

confidence interval The numerical interval that contains the population parameter with a specified probability.

constant systematic error (CE) An error that is always in the same direction and of the same magnitude, even as the concentration of analytes changes.[3]

error The difference between a single estimate of a quantity and its true value. If a good estimate of the true value is not available, the difference may have to be expressed as the deviation from an assigned value.[29]

ideal value The value of a parameter under conditions of zero error.

imprecision The standard deviation or coefficient of variation of the results in a set of replicate measurements. The mean value and number of replicates must be stated as well as the particular type of imprecision, such as between-laboratory, within-day, or between-day imprecision.[29]

inaccuracy The systematic error estimated by the difference between the mean of a set of data and the true value known or estimated from other approaches.

interference The effect of any component of the sample on the accuracy of measurement of the desired analyte.[29]

interference experiment An evaluation experiment that is used to estimate the systematic error in a method, resulting from interference or lack of specificity.[3,6]

linear regression An approach that is used to choose a single line through a data set that "best" describes the relation between two subsets or two methods. One uses this approach assuming there are no errors in the data by the X method. (Also see Chapter 19, Laboratory Statistics.)

medical decision level (X_c) A concentration of analyte at which some medical action is indicated for proper patient care. There may be several medical decision levels for a given analyte.

parameter A number that describes a feature of a population. This is in contrast to a statistic, which is an estimate of a parameter derived from a sample of the population.

precision The agreement among replicate measurements.[29]

proficiency testing A program in which specimens are periodically sent to laboratories for analysis for the purpose of assessing overall analytical performance relative to defined target values as defined by reference methods or by peer groups as appropriate. Participation in proficiency testing is required under CLIA '88.[1]

proportional systematic error (PE) An error that is always in one direction and the magnitude of which is a percentage of the concentration of the analyte being measured.[3]

random analytical error (RE) An error, either positive or negative, the direction and exact magnitude of which cannot be predicted; imprecision.[3]

recovery experiment An evaluation experiment that estimates proportional systematic error.[3] The amount of analyte recovered is divided by the amount of analyte added to a sample, and the ratio is expressed as the percentage of recovery. The deviation of the percentage of recovery from 100% is the proportional error.

replication experiment An evaluation experiment that estimates random analytical error.[3,4] Measurements are made on aliquots of a stable sample over specified periods of time, as within a run, within a day, or over a period of days.

reportable range The concentration range of a method over which the analytical performance (that is, imprecision and inaccuracy) has been determined and judged to meet medical application requirements.

sample The appropriately representative part of a specimen used in the analysis. This sample should be called a *test sample* when it is necessary to avoid confusion with the statistical term *random sample from a population.*[29]

standard error of the estimate The standard deviation of the differences, $s_{y,x}$, between the observed y values and the y values predicted by the regression line for a given x. This statistic measures the dispersion or spread of the data around the regression line.

systematic analytical error (SE) An error that is always in one direction; inaccuracy.[3]

test method In this chapter, the method that is chosen for experimental testing or study by means of method evaluation.[3]

total error (TE) A combination of the random and systematic analytical errors; an estimate of the magnitude of error that might occur in a single measurement.

true value A term considered to have self-evident meaning requiring no definition. In practice the true value is closely approximated by the definitive (method) value and somewhat less closely by the reference (method) value.[29]

variance The square of the standard deviation.

Over the past several decades the quantitative analytical methods used in clinical laboratories have become more reliable and more standardized. Most analytical procedures are supplied by commercial manufacturers. The emphasis of the hospital clinical chemist has shifted away from methods development to the selection and evaluation of those commercially available methods that suit a particular laboratory situation best. Since implementation of the Clinical Laboratory Improvement Amendment of 1988[1] (CLIA '88), this selection and evaluation process has taken on more serious significance because these regulations require, among other things, successful performance in proficiency testing for any laboratory to continue to perform tests in that specialty, subspecialty, or test procedure.

The process of method evaluation has been evolving.[2] It is critical to recognize that a method's performance can be objectively judged as acceptable only if its errors are small enough to be acceptable for medical use. The protocols developed by Westgard and associates[3] and the National Committee for Clinical Laboratory Standards (NCCLS)[4-8] measure error in terms of analyte concentration units, but present different criteria for assessment of error. Westgard and associates take a quality management approach and include an error budget for the operation of the quality control procedure when they compare derived estimates of error to medically allowable error. NCCLS protocols provide procedures for comparing observed errors either to manufacturers' claims or to an allowable error specified in terms of a statistical parameter (such as allowable standard deviation or allowable bias). Yet another source of performance requirements are those stated in CLIA '88 for proficiency testing. We discuss each of these three approaches: acceptance from a medical need, a statistical significance, and a proficiency testing point of view.

PURPOSE OF METHOD EVALUATION
Laboratory requirements

New analytical methods are usually developed to improve accuracy or precision over existing methods, to allow automation, to reduce reagent or labor cost, or to measure a new analyte. In any case the method's analytical performance in a clinical laboratory setting must be verified experimentally, even if the new method is believed to be an improvement over all previous methods. The extent of the experiments and the interpretation of the data vary, depending on the purpose of the evaluation and who performs the evaluation, but the basic approach and basic experimental design are similar for all evaluations. Beyond the scientific and medical reasons for performing an evaluation, the federal regulations in CLIA '88[1] provide specific requirements in Subpart K, Section 493.1213 for performing a method evaluation before using the method to report patient results. However, in Section 493.1202, a phase-in provision was defined, extending from September 1, 1992 (the effective date for CLIA '88) to September 1, 1994, during which time if the laboratory follows manufacturer instructions exactly, some tests may be used based on manufacturer-derived performance data. This phase-in period has been extended for two additional years. State or local regulations with more specific requirements supersede the federal CLIA '88 regulations.

The process of evaluating a method is different from the process of routine quality control of a method after it has been introduced into daily use. Routine (daily) quality control (see Chapter 21) is a process established to detect increases in the analytical errors of a method in order to avoid the release of incorrect patient data. Routine quality control detects errors only when they exceed the error that was present in the method when the control ranges were established. The use of routine quality control does not enable the investigator to determine the magnitude of the inherent errors of the method or to decide whether they are acceptable. Method-evaluation experiments are required to assess the inherent analytical errors of the method and relate them to medical or regulatory requirements.

Manufacturer requirements

When a manufacturer develops a new method and prepares to market it, the manufacturer is required by the Food and Drug Administration (FDA) to make claims about the analytical performance of the method, specifically about its precision and accuracy.[9] In addition, the final rule of CLIA '88 requires that the FDA assess whether the manufacturer's claims meet the CLIA '88 requirements for general quality control.[10] All claims must be supported by experimental method-evaluation data. It is essential that these claims be realistic and conservative. The level of performance of the method in most laboratories must be at least as good as that claimed by the manufacturer. However, potential customers often compare claims made by different manufacturers as they select methods, and thus the claims must be competitive. Extensive experimental data will be required for the manufacturer to develop defensible claims. The protocols proposed by NCCLS have been modified for manufacturers to enable them to produce defensible performance claims that can be verified by the laboratory.

Most method evaluations are performed by laboratory personnel in hospital and commercial laboratories. These evaluations are performed to determine whether the performance of a method meets, primarily, the requirements for the medical applications intended by the user and, secondly, the quality goals specified by CLIA '88 for successful performance in proficiency testing. The method may be a commercial method, a "home-grown" method, or a method the user has seen in the literature and is setting up in his or her own laboratory. The user needs to perform the evaluation as efficiently as possible and to determine with a minimum of experimental work whether the method's performance is unacceptable. If this is the case, the user can reject the method without performing all the time-consuming studies that would be required for acceptance.

Medical requirements (see also Chapter 21)

The decision to accept or reject a candidate laboratory method should be based on the ability of the method to meet the requirements of the final user, the physician who is using the results of a laboratory test for patient care. The error of the test result is excessive if it causes a misdiagnosis. The greatest chance for misdiagnosis caused by an analytical error in a test result occurs at the concentration at which a medical diagnosis is made; this concentration is termed the *medical decision-level concentration*. For example, a fasting glucose concentration below 500 mg/L may be diagnostic of hypoglycemia.[11] For each decision-level concentration, a performance standard consisting of the decision-level concentration, X_C, and the allowable error, E_A, may be formulated. Allowable error is stated in concentration units so that errors of the test method may be judged by comparison with clinically allowable error. One interprets the method-evaluation data by using the data to estimate the error of the method at the medical decision level of concentration and then comparing this estimate with the allowable error. If the method's error exceeds allowable error, performance is not acceptable. If the error is less than the allowable error, performance is acceptable.

The amount of error present in the single measurement of an analyte is different each time the analyte is measured because a portion of the error is purely random. Thus the magnitude of error for a measurement on a given patient specimen cannot be known exactly, and one cannot predict the absolute maximum error a method could ever make on the analysis of a single patient specimen. However, one can calculate an estimate of the upper limit of the error such that there is only a 5% or 1% chance that the actual error would exceed the upper limit. Thus, one can define allowable error as a 95% or 99% upper limit of error. There will be only a 5% or 1% chance that the error will be larger than this defined amount and thus could cause a misdiagnosis.

Exact performance standards for allowable error based on medical criteria have not been defined for most analytes. Performance standards have been proposed for those analytes that are measured most often, but generally one must use one's own professional judgment and input from clinicians to establish the performance standard for a particular analyte. Barnett[12,13] presented a summary of medically allowable standard deviations. Tonks[14] proposed that allowable error be either one fourth of the reference range or 10%, whichever is less. For enzymes, the limit is expanded to 20%.[15] Other sources include Gilbert's[16] recommendations for allowable bias and allowable standard deviation and Cotlove's et al.[17] recommendations for "tolerable analytical variation" based on one half the individual and group biological variation.

The 1976 Aspen Conference[18] sponsored by the College of American Pathologists (CAP) also recommended the use of intraindividual and interindividual biological variations for determining the goals for the precision of a method used for group testing. The analytical coefficient of variation is denoted as CV_A,

$$CV_A = \frac{1}{2}\sqrt{CV_{Intra}^2 + CV_{Inter}^2} \qquad \textit{Eq. 22-1}$$

where CV_{Intra} is the biological variation observed within an individual and CV_{Inter} is the biological variation observed between individuals.[18] To enable the physician to monitor intraindividual changes, the method must be even more precise:

$$CV_A = \frac{1}{2}CV_{Intra} \qquad \textit{Eq. 22-2}$$

Fraser et al.[21-23] reviewed various approaches that have been used to establish quality goals, concluding that biological variation should be a key consideration for establishing allowable error for most analytes, whereas for therapeutic drugs, quality goals were based on pharmacokinetic theory.

Other factors, such as turnaround time, may affect the medically allowable error. Clinicians may sometimes accept increased error if turnaround time is small.

Performance standards based on proficiency testing

Another source of performance standards is the CLIA '88 specification for proficiency testing.[1] Not only must a laboratory consider medical requirements, but it is now necessary to select, evaluate, and then monitor (by statistical quality control, see Chapters 19 and 21) the test method so that when it is in routine use the laboratory will have confidence that the method will meet proficiency testing requirements. These requirements are given as (1) fixed limits, such as an absolute limit of the amount of variability or a limit expressed in terms of a fixed percentage of concentration or activity, or as (2) three–standard deviation limits based on the overall or peer-groups standard deviation, or as (3) within ± two dilutions of the target number of dilutions (titers) for assays reported in terms of the number of dilutions needed to titrate a positive sample to a negative reading (that is, titer). It has been shown[24] that if the internal laboratory precision is one third the fixed-limit criteria and the assay's bias is "small," the likelihood for passing proficiency testing is greater than 99%. Another analysis of this issue[25] indicates that the assay's bias +4 SD should be less than the specified limit. In practice, this indicates that the internal SD should be less than 25% of the fixed limit, or less than one fourth of a 3 SD limit (that is, less than three fourths of the peer-group SD). To say that the internal laboratory SD should be three fourths of the group SD is not at all unrealistic. Table 22-1 lists the CLIA '88 proficiency testing requirements. The fifth column shows the maximum allowable within-laboratory SD

(using the 4 SD criteria and zero bias). For comparison, the recommendations by Fraser et al.[21-23] for maximum internal SD are listed. Note that in some cases the SDs are quite similar whereas in others they are different. A laboratory method must be able to pass proficiency testing *and* also provide medically useful test results. For a further comparison of medical, testing, and proficiency errors, see p. 385.

SELECTION OF METHODS
Evaluation of need

The quality of service achievable by a laboratory is determined by selection of personnel, equipment, and analytical methods. The many considerations involved in the process of method selection are shown in Fig. 22-1 on p. 408. Unless this process is well organized, method selection can be a traumatic and costly experience. The left box on p. 407 provides a logical sequence to follow in method selection.

Often the decision to set up a new method or instrument is based on a medical or economic requirement for the laboratory to provide a new test on site. A change in the methodology of a presently offered test may also be dictated by advances in laboratory practice. For example, in recent years many laboratories have converted their immunoassays from radiolabeled to nonisotopically labeled reagents to reduce or eliminate the special procedures required for managing radioactive materials and to take advantage of the longer shelf lives of newer reagents. The need for a new method or device may also be dictated by the age and lack of operational reliability of the present method.

Application characteristics

After the need for a new method or analyzer has been determined, all the practical features required of the method are defined. These are termed *application characteristics* (see right box on p. 407). Emphasis will be placed on sample size for pediatric applications, on turnaround time and interrupt features for stat. applications, and on the sample throughput rate for high-volume screening applications. It is essential that a candidate method meet these fundamental requirements before one considers it any further.

Cost per test has been defined as an application characteristic. This item can also be considered separately in light of the present emphasis on reducing medical costs. The factors that affect direct cost should be considered when one compares candidate methods. These include the depreciated capital cost, reagent (including water for many analyzers) and supplies cost, service and repair cost, computer interface cost, and labor cost. Much of this information is available from the manufacturer including initial equipment cost, estimated reagent and supplies consumption and cost, estimated productivity, and service cost (by contract or per visit). Other information, such as the expected work load and anticipated modifications in the productivity based on the internal quality control procedures, is available from within the laboratory. One can use CAP work-load record-

Table 22-1   Considerations in the process of method selection

Analyte	Acceptable performance criteria, CLIA '88	Decision level (X_c*)	Allowable error (CLIA '88†)	Maximum SD (CLIA '88‡)	Medically based maximum SD (Fraser§)
Routine chemistry					
Albumin	±10%	3.5 g/dL	0.35	0.09	0.05
Bilirubin	±0.4 mg/dL or ±20%	1.0 mg/dL	0.40	0.10	0.11
		20 mg/dL	4.0	1.0	2.2
Calcium	±1.0 mg/dL	7.0 mg/dL	1.0	0.25	0.08
		10.8 mg/dL	1.0	0.25	0.10
		13.0 mg/dL	1.0	0.25	0.12
Chloride	±5%	90 mmol/L	4.5	1.1	0.63
		110 mmol/L	5.5	1.4	0.77
Cholesterol	±10%	200 mg/dL	20	5.0	5.4
Creatinine	±0.3 mg/dL or ±15%	1.0 mg/dL	0.30	0.08	0.02
		3.0 mg/dL	0.45	0.11	0.07
Glucose	±6 mg/dL or ±10%	50 mg/dL	6.0	1.5	1.1
		120 mg/dL	12	3.0	2.6
		200 mg/dL	20	5.0	4.4
Iron	±20%	150 mg/dL	30	7.5	24
Magnesium	±25%	2.0 mg/dL	0.50	0.12	0.02
pH	±0.04	7.35	0.04	0.01	0.01
P_{CO_2}	±5 mm Hg or ±8%	35 mm Hg	5.0	1.2	0.84
		50 mm Hg	5.0	1.2	1.2
P_{O_2}	±3 SD	30 mm Hg	3 SD	0.75 SD	
		80 mm Hg	3 SD	0.75 SD	
Potassium	±0.5 mmol/L	3.0 mmol/L	0.50	0.12	0.07
		6.0 mmol/L	0.50	0.12	0.14
Protein, total	±10%	7.0 g/dL	0.70	0.18	0.10
Sodium	±4 mmol/L	130 mmol/L	4.0	1.0	0.38
		150 mmol/L	4.0	1.0	0.44
Triglycerides	±25%	160 mg/dL	40	10	18
Urea nitrogen	±2 mg/dL or ±9%	27.0 mg/dL	2.4	0.6	1.7
Uric acid	±17%	6.0 mg/dL	1.0	0.25	0.25
Enzymes					
Alkaline phosphatase	±30%	150 U/L	45	11	5.1
ALT	±20%	50 U/L	10	2.5	6.8
Amylase	±30%	100 U/L	30	7.5	3.7
AST	±20%	30 U/L	6.0	1.5	2.2
		70 U/L	14	3.5	5.0
CK	±30%	200 U/L	60	15	40
LD	±20%	300 U/L	60	15	12
Endocrinology					
Cortisol	±25%	5 μg/dL	1.25	0.3	
		30 μg/dL	7.5	1.8	
Free thyroxine	±3 SD	2.3 ng/dL	3 SD	0.75 SD	0.1
HCG	±3 SD or positive/negative	25 IU/L	3 SD	0.75 SD	
T_3 uptake	±3 SD	25%	3 SD	0.75 SD	
Triiodothyronine	±3 SD	100 ng/dL	3 SD	0.75 SD	4.0
		200 ng/dL	3 SD	0.75 SD	8.0
TSH	±3 SD	0.1 mIU/L	3 SD	0.75 SD	0.025
		5.0 mIU/L	3 SD	0.75 SD	0.4
Thyroxine	±1.0 μg/dL or ±20%	3 μg/dL	1.0	0.25	0.1
		13 μg/dL	2.6	0.65	0.45
Toxicology					
Alcohol, blood	±25%	0.10 g/dL	0.025	0.006	
Blood lead	±4 μg/dL or ±10%	10 μg/dL	4.0	1.0	
		40 μg/dL	4.0	1.0	
Carbamazepine	±25%	8 mg/L	2.0	0.5	0.8
		12 mg/L	3.0	0.8	1.2

Table 22-1　Considerations in the process of method selection—cont'd

Analyte	Acceptable performance criteria, CLIA '88	Decision level (X_C*)	Allowable error (CLIA '88†)	Maximum SD (CLIA '88‡)	Medically based maximum SD (Fraser§)
Toxicology					
Digoxin	±0.2 μg/L or ±20%	0.8 μg/L	0.2	0.05	0.04
		2.0 μg/L	0.4	0.10	0.10
Ethosuximide	±20%	40 mg/L	8.0	2.0	2.0
		100 mg/L	20.0	5.0	4.9
Gentamicin	±25%	10 mg/L	2.5	0.6	
Lithium	±0.3 mmol/L or ±20%	0.5 mmol/L	0.3	0.08	0.06
		1.5 mmol/L	0.3	0.08	0.18
Phenobarbital	±20%	15 mg/L	3.0	0.75	1.3
		40 mg/L	8.0	2.0	3.6
Phenytoin	±25%	10 mg/L	2.5	0.6	0.7
		20 mg/L	5.0	1.2	1.3
Primidone	±25%	5 mg/L	1.2	0.3	0.56
		12 mg/L	3.0	0.75	1.36
Procainamide	±25%	4 mg/L	1.0	0.25	
		20 mg/L	5.0	1.25	
Quinidine	±25%	7 mg/L	1.8	0.45	
Theophylline	±25%	10 mg/L	2.5	0.6	0.7
		20 mg/L	5.0	1.2	1.4
Valproic acid	±25%	50 mg/L	12	3.0	3.3
		100 mg/L	25	6.2	6.7

ALT, Alanine aminotransferase; *AST,* aspartate aminotransferase; *CK,* creatine kinase; *CLIA,* Clinical Laboratories Improvement Amendment; *HCG,* human chorionic gonadotropin; *IU,* international units; *LD,* lactate dehydrogenase; *SD,* standard deviation; T_3, triiodothyronine; *TSH,* thyroid-stimulating hormone; *U,* units; X_C, concentration of x analyte to indicate medical intervention.
*Medical decision levels, most of which are based on Barnett.[12,13]
†Allowable error based on CLIA '88 performance requirements at the respective medical decision level.[1] SD limits are based on peer group data.
‡Maximum internal SD based on criteria that 4 SD is less than the allowable error[24,25] (see column 3 for units).
§Maximum internal SD based on biovariability criteria (Fraser et al[21-23]) (see column 3 for units).

ing units to make an initial estimate of the direct labor cost. Users must adjust this information to their own laboratory situations. The example in the box on p. 409 illustrates how this information may be combined to arrive at a total direct cost per test. By far the largest cost component is labor at 84% of the total. If the laboratory wishes to add new tests in a way that minimizes added overall cost, the new tests that will have the smallest labor component should be selected.

Method characteristics

The next step in the selection process is the definition of ideal methodological characteristics that will enable the selected method to have a good chance for success in the us-

er's laboratory. These characteristics include preferred methodology, which will potentially have the necessary chemical specificity (freedom from interferences) and chemical sensitivity (ability to detect small quantities or changes in the analyte's concentration). The ability to use primary aqueous standards for calibration (freedom from matrix effects) is also important. The reagents, temperature, reaction time, measurement time, and measurement approach (such as end-point, two-point, or multipoint

---

Steps in the Selection Process

Determine need
Define requirements
　Application
　Methodological
　Performance
Review literature
Select candidate methods

Application Characteristics

Sample size
Turnaround time
Sample throughput rate
Specimen type
Automated calibration
On-line quality control review
Self-diagnostics
Laboratory space required
Reagent storage facilities required
Availability and skill of laboratory staff
Time available for training
Cost per test
Safety and environmental hazards

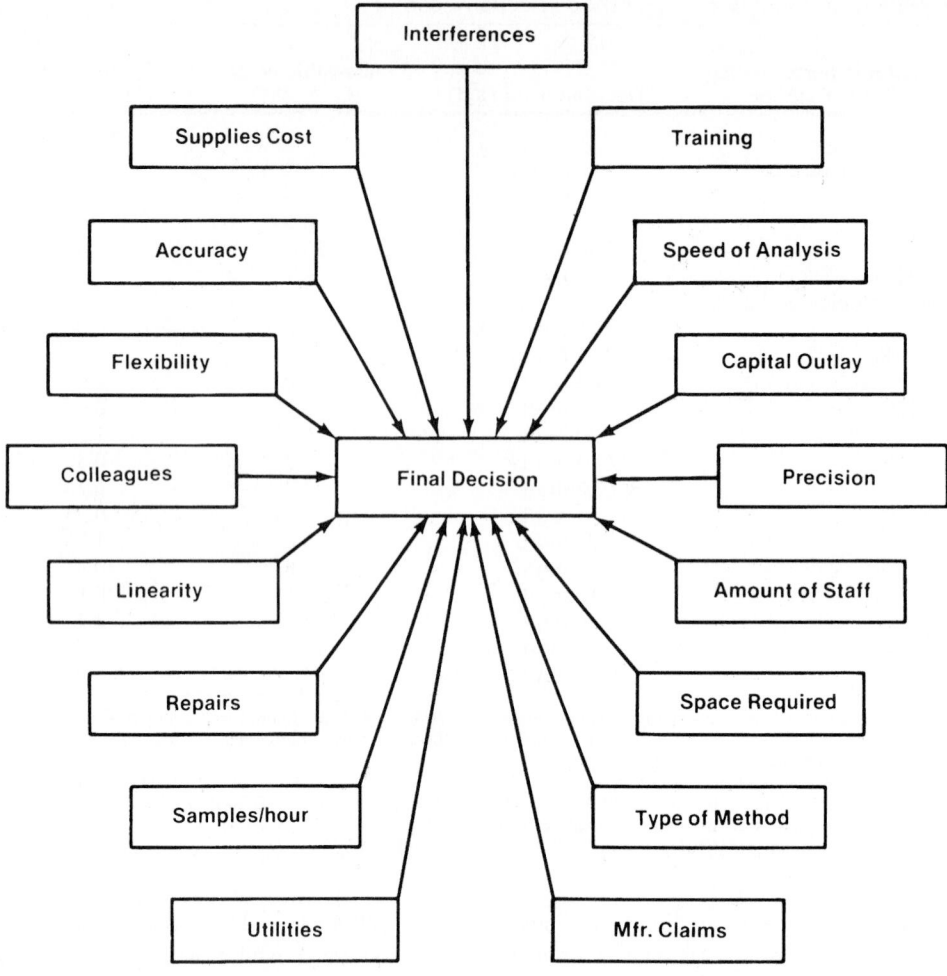

Fig. 22-1 Factors in method selection.

kinetic methods) are all characteristics of a method and should be defined. A source of recommended principles for clinical chemistry methods has been developed by the National Reference System for the Clinical Laboratory (NRSCL).[26]

Analytical performance characteristics

The method should also be defined in terms of its analytical performance capabilities. Overall goals for analytical performance have been discussed in terms of allowable error based on the medical application of the test and on proficiency testing requirements. Other aspects of performance that must be defined are working range of the method (*reportable range,* which may or may not be the same as the linear range), stability of the reagents and calibration materials, ability of the analyzer to detect reagent depletion in the case of enzyme substrates, expected reference range, amount of error caused by interfering substances, precision (within-run, between-run, between-day, and total), and accuracy of the method (determined by comparison of results to those obtained by a reference or standard method). The

manufacturer is now required to provide information about precision and accuracy. The selected method must be evaluated experimentally to determine if the method's actual performance in the user's laboratory is good enough to meet the medical application needs in the user's institution. The manufacturer's claimed performance should be considered only as a starting point for determining the actual performance in the user's laboratory setting.

Next, one should review the technical and professional literature and proficiency testing data to determine what methods are available and to obtain some information about their application and methodological and performance characteristics. It is also very useful to confer with colleagues about their experience and recommendations.

The final step in the selection process involves putting all the information together to arrive at a final choice. The use of a rating scheme enables one to arrive at a more objective overall ranking of the candidate methods.[27,28] The rating scheme can be customized by use of appropriate weighting factors for the characteristics that are more important. The final choice may include several candidate

---

Estimation of Direct Costs

Laboratory information
    8000 patient tests (samples) per year
    50% estimated test yield (samples, quality control, repeats, dilutions, troubleshooting)
    16,000 total number of assays
    4 CAP units per sample = 64,000 total units
    Five-year depreciation of capital
    $750 setup costs (change laboratory bench)
Manufacturer information
    $11,000: cost of equipment
    $1200: cost of reagents and supplies (for 16,000 assays)
    $1100: service contract (two visits)
    $500: replacement parts
Calculate equipment costs
    Capital and setup: $11,750 ÷ 5 yr = $2350/yr ÷ 8000 = $0.294/sample
    Service and repair: $1100 + $500 = $1600/yr ÷ 8000 = $0.20/sample
    Subtotal = $0.494/sample
Calculate labor costs (assume $25.00/hour including benefits)
    [(64,000 CAP units ÷ 60 units/hour) × $25.00/hour] ÷ 8000 samples = $3.333/sample
Calculate reagent costs
    $1200.00 ÷ 8000 samples = $0.15/sample
Total direct costs = $3.977/sample

---

methods that meet the desired criteria. These methods can then be subjected to the evaluation process described below to choose the method with the best analytical performance characteristics.

LABORATORY EVALUATION OF A METHOD

Usually a method-evaluation study is not performed to test all methods to determine the method with the smallest error but to determine whether the selected method has acceptably small analytical errors. The process of method evaluation involves estimation of the magnitude of analytical error for a single patient specimen. The laboratory experiments performed to obtain data for estimating the errors are chosen because they give quantitative estimates of random and systematic errors with a minimum of experimental work. The error estimates obtained may be invalid, however, if certain underlying assumptions are not true. These assumptions include operator familiarity with the method's procedure; stability of calibrators, controls, and reagents; and linearity of response throughout the working range.

Familiarization

It is essential that the operators of the method become thoroughly familiar with the details of the method and instrument operation before the collection of any data that will be used to characterize the method's performance. This familiarization period has been addressed by NCCLS[4-8] and

may include training by the manufacturer. It should be of sufficient duration so that, at its completion, one can perform all aspects of the method or instrument operation comfortably. Obviously the length of time for device familiarization varies with the complexity of the method or analyzer.

Stability

Verification of the stability of reagents, calibrators, and control materials, especially those prepared in house, can be a lengthy procedure. The matter is simplified considerably for commercially prepared materials. One can use the manufacturer's expiration date during the method evaluation because serious stability problems will be detectable through unacceptable analytical performance of the method. For in-house preparations it is necessary to document these characteristics. One should perform preliminary studies with crossover analyses comparing the results of patient samples analyzed using both fresh calibrators and old calibrators and fresh reagents to test the stability of calibrators. This should be done several times, and the differences for each specific age of calibrator should be averaged to reduce the effects of different preparations. Similarly, one can test the stability of reagents by periodically (daily, weekly, or monthly, depending on the anticipated decay rate) preparing new reagents and testing them against the older reagents by analyzing patient samples under both configurations of reagents. The older reagents should be stored under specified conditions for the subsequent measurements. One can test the observed differences between the old and new reagents by use of a *t*-test (see p. 413).

Linearity

The International Federation of Clinical Chemistry has defined the analytical range in a qualitative sense, stating that it is "the range of concentration or other quantity in the specimen over which the method is applicable without modification."[29] CLIA '88 regulations do not explicitly require that a "linearity" experiment be performed but instead discuss "verification" of the *reportable range* (see Section 493.1217), which is the range defined by a minimum (or zero) value and a maximum-value calibration material. When the limits of linearity are studied experimentally, the range of concentrations included should at least encompass the limits claimed by the manufacturer. The absolute minimum number of different concentrations that must be measured for linearity verification is three. Duplicate measurements should be made on each concentration sample.

An initial linearity study could use aqueous standards to identify the capabilities of the method in an ideal specimen matrix. This should be followed by the analysis of an analyte dilution series of samples containing the biological matrix,[5] such as serum or urine, that will be used for patient tests. The aqueous and matrix samples will provide important information about the influence of the biological matrix on the method. It may be difficult to prepare specimens in a biological matrix with a range of analyte concentrations from zero to the limit of linearity. For analytes not normally present in the matrix, such as drugs, the analyte is simply added to an analyte-free specimen to obtain the desired maximum concentration, and a dilution series is prepared using analyte-free serum or urine. One can also approximate serum matrices by diluting stock aqueous pools of analyte with human serum albumin, enzyme-inactivated serum, or Plasmonate (Miles, Inc., Elkhart, Indiana). One can also use a patient specimen containing the analyte at a concentration known to exceed the linearity of the method and then construct a dilution series using analyte-free materials. The accuracy of the volumetric dilutions is very important, and serial dilutions are not recommended because errors are propagated through the subsequent samples. Rather, each sample should be prepared by direct dilution from the original high sample or pool.

Finally, all the data points should be plotted for visual inspection of linear performance. The actual result of the analysis of each dilution is plotted against the percentage of high pool present in each dilution (or against known concentrations). The straight portion of the resulting curve represents the linear portion of the assay. In the case of methods with curvilinear response, such as radioimmunoassay procedures, the results obtained from the recommended curve-straightening algorithms should be plotted to show linearity of final results.

Random and systematic error

In general, errors that affect the performance of analytical procedures are classified as either random or systematic. Factors contributing to random error are those that affect the reproducibility of the measurement. These include (1) instability of the instrument, (2) variations in the temperature, (3) variations in the reagents and calibrators (and calibration-curve stability), (4) variability in handling techniques such as pipetting, mixing, and timing, and (5) variability in operators. These factors superimpose their effects on each other at different times. Some cause rapid fluctuations, and others occur over a longer time. Thus random error (RE) has different components of variation that are related to the actual laboratory setting. The *within-run* component of variation (σ_{wr}) is caused by specific steps in the procedure, such as pipetting precision, and short-term variations in the temperature and stability of the instrument. Within-day, *between-run* variation (σ_{br}) is caused by instability of the calibration curve or by differences in recalibration that occur throughout the day, longer-term variations in the instrument, small changes in the condition of the calibrator and reagents, changes in the condition of the laboratory during the day, and fatigue of the laboratory staff. The *between-day* component of variation (σ_{bd}) is caused by variations in the instrument that occur over days, changes

in calibrators and reagents (especially if new vials are opened each day), and changes in staff from day to day. Although not a true random component of variation, any drift in the stability of the calibration curve over time will greatly affect the between-day component of variation as well. One can combine these components in such a way as to produce an estimate of the total variance of a method (σ_t^2).

$$\sigma_t^2 = \sigma_{wr}^2 + \sigma_{br}^2 + \sigma_{bd}^2 \qquad \textit{Eq. 22-3}$$

Terms used to indicate random error include *precision, imprecision, reproducibility,* and *repeatability.* In each case they refer to the random dispersion of results or measurements around some point of central tendency.

Systematic error (SE) describes error that is consistently low or high. If the error is consistently low or high by the same amount, regardless of the concentration, it is called *constant* systematic error (Fig. 22-2). If the error is consistently low or high by an amount proportional to the concentration of the analyte, it is called *proportional* systematic error.

Factors that contribute to constant systematic error are independent of the analyte concentration, and the magnitude of this error is constant throughout the concentration range of the analyte. Constant systematic error is caused by an interfering substance in all samples or in reagents that gives rise to a false signal. The error can be positive or negative. A reaction between an interfering substance and the reagents, caused by a lack of specificity, is an example of a constant systematic error.

Another cause of systematic error is an interfering substance that interferes in the reaction between the analyte and the reagents. This type of error is seen in enzymatic methods using oxidase-peroxidase–coupled reactions in which the hydrogen peroxide intermediate is destroyed by endogenous reducing agents, such as ascorbic acid. An interfer-

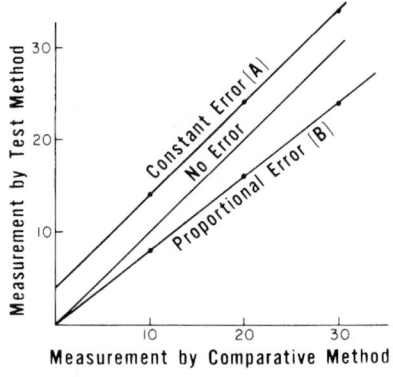

Fig. 22-2 Constant and proportional errors. (From Westgard JO, de Vos DJ, Hunt MR, et al: *Am J Med Technol* 44:290, 1978.)

ing substance may also inhibit or destroy the reagent, and so it remains in suboptimum amounts for the reaction with the analyte. A nonchemical source of constant systematic error is the error caused by improper blanking of the sample or the reagents.

Proportional error is most often caused by incorrect assignment of the amount of substance in the calibrator. If the calibrator has more analyte than is labeled, all the unknown determinations will be low; less analyte than is labeled will result in a positive error. The error will be proportional to the original calibration error. Proportional error may also be caused by a side reaction of the analyte. The percentage of analyte that undergoes a side reaction will be the percentage of error in the method.

EXPERIMENTS TO ESTIMATE MAGNITUDE OF SPECIFIC ERRORS

In designing experiments that will be used to determine the analytical errors of a method, it is imperative that the experiments be carefully conceived to avoid ambiguous conclusions. The aim of this section is to describe specific experiments that will enable one to estimate the magnitude of a specific error. One can then compare the size of the error to the allowable error to determine the acceptability of the method. This approach is used for all the types of errors described previously. Each type of error is considered individually before combinations of errors are considered. Fig. 22-3 presents an organization of experiments to be performed for specific error determinations, arranged in such a way that the easy experiments can be done first. The more extensive (and expensive) final studies are performed only if the errors estimated by these preliminary experiments are acceptable.

Random error estimated from replication studies

The within-run replication experiment is the simplest type of study and should be one of the first performed to assess the performance of a new method. Because it allows assessment of precision over a very short time, the results cannot be extrapolated to indicate long-term performance. The short-term performance must be judged acceptable before one goes on to study the long-term performance of the method.

The replication study should first be performed with an aqueous solution of calibrator or standard and then repeated with samples whose matrix is as similar as possible to that of the intended patient samples. The concentrations to be studied should be at or near the medical-decision concentrations for the analyte. This is where the laboratory data will be interpreted most critically; thus one must be certain of the method's performance at these concentrations.

An estimate of random error is developed by consideration of repeated analyses of the same specimen. Sixty-eight percent of the results are within ± 1.0 standard deviation of the test mean, and 95% of the results are within 1.96 SD of the mean (see p. 348). Based on recommendations that will yield a high likelihood of passing proficiency testing,[24,25] we define the random error as four times the standard deviation. If the estimate of random error is less than the allowable error, random error is acceptable. An example of the calculation of random error is shown on p. 420.

Constant error estimated from interference studies

The interference study measures the constant error caused by the presence of a substance suspected of interfering with the test method. To perform the study, one takes a sample that is spiked with the interferent. The volume of this addition should be small, less than 10% of the sample volume, so that the disruption of the matrix is minimal. To compensate for the dilution of the spiked sample, a baseline sample should be prepared by addition of an equal amount of the solvent that was used for the interferent to another aliquot of the sample. The two samples should then be analyzed, at least in duplicate. The difference between the results in the two samples is attributable to an interference caused by the added substance.

A scheme for studying the effects of hemolysis involves taking two blood samples. One is centrifuged and analyzed directly (baseline sample), and the red blood cells in the other blood tube are physically traumatized to rupture the cell membranes to yield an elevated amount of serum hemoglobin. After centrifugation, this hemolyzed sample is analyzed. The difference between the two samples is attributable to the effects of hemolysis. Mild, moderate, or severe hemolysis may be simulated, depending on the volume of red blood cells traumatized. This approach is more consistent with the actual problems encountered in the laboratory than the approach in which pure hemoglobin is added

TYPE OF ANALYTIC ERROR	EVALUATION EXPERIMENTS	
	PRELIMINARY	FINAL
RANDOM ERROR	REPLICATION WITHIN RUN PURE MATERIALS REAL SAMPLES	REPLICATION RUN TO RUN REAL SAMPLES
CONSTANT ERROR	INTERFERENCE	COMPARISON WITH COMPARATIVE METHOD
PROPORTIONAL ERROR	RECOVERY	

Fig. 22-3 Specific evaluation experiments for estimating specific types of analytical error. (From Westgard JO, de Vos, DJ, Hunt MR, et al: *Am J Med Technol* 44:290, 1978.)

to a sample. However, this procedure is not valid if red blood cells contain the analyte.

One may study the effects of lipemia by dividing a lipemic sample into two portions and analyzing one directly while centrifuging the other with an ultrahigh-speed centrifuge to remove the lipoproteins before analysis. The difference in results is attributable to the effects of lipemia. Alternatively, one may also prepare turbid specimens for each decision-level concentration by adding small amounts of IntraLipid (Cutter Laboratories, Inc., Berkeley, California) to nonlipemic specimens of appropriate analyte concentrations to obtain slightly, moderately, and grossly lipemic samples. Baseline concentrations are prepared by addition of equal volumes of water to the original specimens.

Pools with increased amounts of unconjugated bilirubin are produced from a stock solution of bilirubin prepared by dissolving pure bilirubin in dimethylsulfoxide to 2500 mg/L. Clear, nonicteric patient sera are spiked to the desired bilirubin concentration. Baseline specimens are prepared as already described. This technique does not test the effect of the more water-soluble conjugated bilirubin on the analysis.

The choice of substances to be tested is almost infinite. For all spectrophotometric methods, the effects of hemolysis, icterus, and lipemia should be determined. Other substances that have been reported to affect methods similar to the one under review should be tested (see NCCLS guideline EP-7[6]). Pipetting should be (1) precise so that the baseline and spiked samples reflect the same extent of dilution and (2) accurate so that a known amount of interfering substance is added. Again, it is important that the concentration of the analyte in the sample be near the medical-decision levels. A substance that is a possible interferent should be added so that its final concentration is at the maximum, physiologically expected concentration. If no errors are caused at this high concentration, one can assume that lower concentrations will not adversely affect the performance of the method. If an error is too large at the maximum concentration of interfering substance, it is appropriate to test the interference at lower concentrations. A slightly icteric sample may be acceptable, but a grossly icteric one may not. It is recommended that these interference studies be conducted on the comparative method (see later discussion) at the same time, as a check on the experimental technique.

An example of the calculation of constant error from data obtained from an interference experiment is shown on p. 420. The overall average difference (bias) is called a *constant error (CE)* because it is independent of the analyte concentration. This constant error is compared directly to the allowable error for the appropriate decision level. If the constant error is less than allowable error, the constant error caused by the interference is judged acceptable. This decision is based on clinical limits instead of a statistical test of significance (see pp. 406 and 407). The standard deviation of the interference values is a measure of the uncertainty of the estimated constant error.

Proportional error estimated from a recovery experiment

Another preliminary study is the recovery experiment. This procedure involves the addition of a known amount of analyte to an aliquot of sample. As in the interference experiment, the sample is divided into two aliquots. One aliquot is spiked with a stock solution that contains the analyte. An equal volume of diluent is added to the second; this is the baseline sample. The two samples are then analyzed. The baseline sample provides the original amount of analyte. The difference between the results of the analyses of the spiked sample and the baseline sample indicates the amount of added analyte "recovered." The amount of analyte "added" to the sample is calculated from the concentration of the stock solution of the analyte and the volume added. The volume of analyte added to the sample should be less than 10% to avoid major disruption of the sample matrix. Pipetting accuracy is critical because the amount of added analyte is calculated from the volume. The concentration of the sample and the amount added should be such that they test the performance of the method near the medical-decision levels of the analyte. In some instances a very small amount of analyte is added to the sample, and the amount recovered is lost in the randomness of the method. Thus it is advisable to make two to four measurements on each sample to reduce the effects of the imprecision of the method. Analysis of these samples with the comparison method is recommended as a check on the experimental technique.

The calculation of recovery is illustrated with an example on p. 421. *Recovery* is defined as the ratio of the amount of analyte recovered to the amount added and is given as a percentage. The difference between the calculated percentage of recovery and 100% recovery is the percentage of proportional error. The standard deviation of the percentage of recovery is a measure of the uncertainty of the percentage of proportional error. One cannot compare percentage of proportional error directly to allowable error to decide acceptability because the percentage of proportional error is not in concentration units. One can convert proportional error to concentration units at the medical-decision level, as shown on pp. 406-407. If the proportional error is less than the allowable error, the proportional error is acceptable. Again, the decision is based on medical requirements rather than statistical tests of significance.

If within-run random error, constant error, and proportional error are acceptable, the day-to-day replication and comparison-of-methods experiments are performed.

FINAL-EVALUATION EXPERIMENTS

The final-evaluation experiments take the most time to perform and potentially yield the most definitive information about the test method's day-to-day performance on real patient specimens.

Between-day replication experiment

The between-day replication experiment is an expansion of the within-run experiment over many days, usually 20. This period must be long enough to allow the random effects occurring over several days to influence the long-term estimate of random error. This experiment and the comparison-of-methods experiment described next are usually combined for better efficiency in the study.

A material known to be stable for the time of the experiment is used, usually a frozen serum or plasma pool or a lyophilized control product. Aliquot-to-aliquot variation of the material must be minimal because it will appear to be day-to-day variance of the test method.

Random error is estimated as four times the total standard deviation and compared to allowable error, as described previously for the within-run study.

Comparison-of-methods experiment

The comparison-of-methods experiment determines the systematic error of the test method, using real patient specimens. A group of patient specimens are analyzed by both the test method and a comparative method, a method known to be accurate and precise. Systematic differences between the two methods are interpreted as errors of the test method if the results of the comparison method are known to have little or no error (negligible random and systematic errors). Thus the comparative method should be of the highest quality possible so that errors will not be erroneously assigned to the test method. Methods may be classified in terms of the quality of their performance as definitive, reference, or routine methods. See Chapter 20 for a description of definitive and reference methods.

In practice the comparative method is often the method in routine use in the laboratory and not a method of reference quality. It is useful to see how results from the test method compare with those of the routine method, but differences between the two methods should be interpreted cautiously unless the quality of the comparative method is known to be high.

At least 40 and preferably 100 or more patient specimens should be analyzed. They should include the variety of disease states that will be encountered by the test in routine use. Analyte concentrations of the specimens should be evenly distributed throughout the analytical range; otherwise regression analysis of the comparison data will be inaccurate. However, even distributions are not always practical. The NCCLS guideline for comparison of methods[7] has suggested some alternative distributions. Hemolyzed, lipemic, and icteric specimens should be included if they are not proscribed by the manufacturer of the test method and if they do not cause errors by the comparative method. If included in the study, they should be identified.

Specimens must be carefully selected from the routine work load to be an efficient representation of the patient mix; preanalysis by the routine method is usually necessary.

Specimens are analyzed in duplicate by each method. Results should be examined carefully and plotted daily. Any specimen whose duplicates do not agree closely by either method (that is, differences greater than 5.5 SD[4]) should be reanalyzed in duplicate by both methods in the next run. Any specimen with large differences between results by the two methods (that is, differences exceeding the allowable error) should also be reanalyzed immediately. If the large difference is confirmed, one should investigate the patient for disease or diseases present and the specimen for other analytes (possible interferents) to determine the cause of the large difference. An immediate follow-up examination is essential to avoid unanswerable questions about outliers later.

The test and comparative methods should be run at the same time, or as close in time to each other as possible. If this is not possible, specimens must be stored in a manner that guarantees analyte stability.

The comparison-of-methods experiment is usually combined with the between-day replication experiment. Patient specimens should be evenly spread over at least five runs and preferably all 20 runs, to ensure that day-to-day effects have a chance to influence the data and to ensure that day-to-day effects are "fully confounded" (in statistical parlance). Both methods must be maintained in acceptable quality control during the period.

***t*-Test statistics: bias, s_d.** The systematic differences between the test and comparative methods are most easily estimated from the comparison-of-methods data by the bias. The bias is the difference between the average result by the test method and the average result by the comparative method. Bias can indicate the magnitude of the systematic error between the two methods. (Each patient specimen must be analyzed by both methods for bias to be valid.) Bias is given by equation 22-4, in which y_i and x_i are the analyte concentrations of the individual specimens by the test method and comparative method respectively and N is the number of paired results compared.

$$\text{Bias} = \frac{\Sigma(y_i - x_i)}{N} \qquad \textit{Eq. 22-4}$$

The standard deviation about the bias, called the *standard deviation of the differences*, s_d, is calculated in a manner analogous to that used to calculate the standard deviation in the replication experiment. One may view s_d as an indicator of the random error between the two methods.

$$s_d = \sqrt{\frac{\Sigma(y_i - x_i - \text{Bias})^2}{(N-1)}} \qquad \textit{Eq. 22-5}$$

The statistical significance of the bias, that is, whether it really differs from zero, or no bias, is determined by use of the *t*-test. A *t* value is calculated according to the formula

$$t = \frac{\text{Bias} \cdot \sqrt{N}}{s_d}$$ *Eq. 22-6*

This is the same *t* statistic described in equation 19-13. The *t* value is the ratio of a systematic-error term (bias) to a random-error term (s_d). If the bias increases relative to the standard deviation of differences, there is less of a probability that the observed bias is caused by random variations and more of a probability that there really is a systematic difference between the test and comparative-method mean values. For example, in a comparison of glucose methods there were 101 specimens, the bias was 30 mg/L, and the *t* value was 2.11. The critical *t* value for $p = 0.05$ and for 100 degrees of freedom (obtainable from a statistics textbook) is 1.99. (The two-sided critical *t* value is used because the bias could be either positive or negative.) The calculated *t* value exceeds the critical *t* value; therefore a statistically real bias exists between the two methods (see also p. 353).

The acceptability of the systematic error, as estimated by the bias, is judged by comparison with allowable error. If bias is less than allowable error, the systematic error is acceptable. If bias exceeds allowable error, the systematic error is not acceptable. Decisions about acceptability should never be based on the *t* value alone. A large bias and large s_d may combine to give an insignificant *t* value, even though the bias is unacceptably large. Also from this equation, it can be seen that if *N* is very large, the value of *t* can become statistically significant for some ratio of bias to s_d, indicating a statistically significant bias even though that bias may be medically unimportant.

Westgard and Hunt[30] have shown that bias can give inaccurate estimates of systematic error if a proportional error is present, since both proportional and constant errors are combined in the bias. Proportional error also increases s_d. Bias should not be used as an estimator of systematic error unless proportional error is absent, or unless the mean analyte concentration as measured by the comparative method is very near the decision-level concentration (X_C) and the data are well distributed around X_C. Otherwise the bias will be weighted toward the side of X_C that has the most samples with large individual biases.

Correlation coefficient. The statistic most frequently cited in reports of comparison-of-methods experiments is the correlation coefficient *(r)*. An *r* value of zero indicates that there is no correlation between the methods. A value of +1 indicates perfect positive correlation. See Chapter 19 for a more extensive discussion of the calculation of linear-regression statistics and their interpretation.

The correlation coefficient is frequently misused in method evaluation reports. Westgard and Hunt[30] demonstrated that the correlation coefficient is extremely sensitive to the range of analyte concentrations of the patient specimens in the comparison-of-methods experiment. In a comparison of bilirubin methods over a range of 0 to 45 mg/L, a correlation coefficient of 0.950 was obtained. When data pairs with bilirubin concentrations above 15 mg/L were eliminated, the correlation coefficient dropped to 0.773. This is shown in Fig. 22-4.

The correlation coefficient is simply a means to look for a correlation, not agreement, between pairs. Thus, if the values for one population were twice that of the other, as one population's value doubled, the other population's value would be doubled as well. The correlation between the two

Statistic	Range of Concentrations Studied		
	0-1.5 mg/dL	0-2.5 mg/dL	0-4.5 mg/dL
r	0.773	0.878	0.950
bias	0.17	0.17	0.17
s_d	0.30	0.29	0.31
$s_{y/x}$	0.29	0.29	0.31
a	0.17	0.17	0.20
b	1.025	1.007	0.966

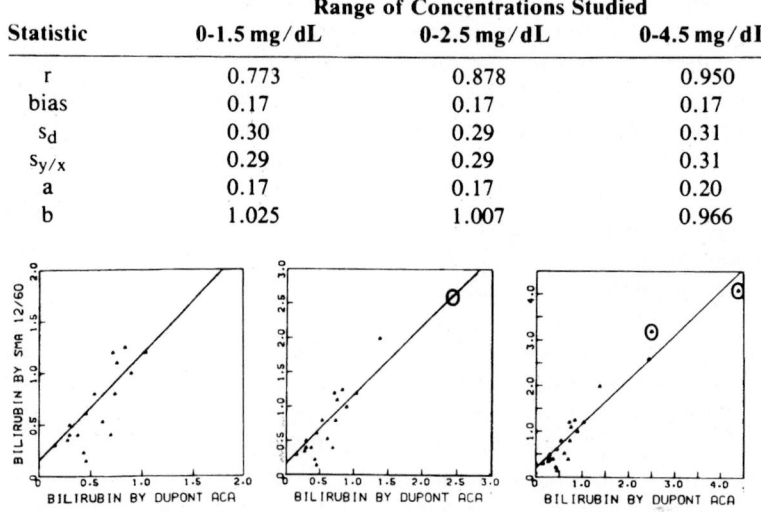

Fig. 22-4   Effect of range of data on correlation coefficient, *r*. (From Westgard JO, de Vos DJ, Hunt MR, et al: *Am J Med Technol* 44:552, 1978.)

methods would be excellent (high *r*). Thus decisions about the acceptability of the analytical performance of a method should never be based on the value of the correlation coefficient alone.

Linear-regression statistics. If the test method and comparative method do correlate with each other, an $x:y$ plot of results resembles a straight line, which can be described by the linear-regression expression

$$Y_i = a + bx_i \qquad \textit{Eq. 22-7}$$

where Y_i is the calculated value on the straight line corresponding to the actual comparative method result, x_i. The proportionality between the methods is given by the slope, b, the ideal value of which (no proportional error) is 1. Constant error is indicated by the y intercept, a. Random error between the methods is indicated by the standard error of the regression, $s_{y,x}$, also called the "standard error of the estimate," or the "standard deviation of the residuals."

An estimate of systematic error at X_C, the decision-level concentration, may be obtained from the linear-regression statistics by substitution of X_C for x_i in equation 22-7, to calculate Y_C, the concentration the test method would measure for a specimen whose true analyte concentration is designated as X_C. The systematic error, SE, is calculated by subtraction of X_C from this Y_C:

$$\text{SE} = |Y_C - X_C| = |a + bX_C - X_C| \qquad \textit{Eq. 22-8}$$

This estimate of error will be valid only if the following limitations of linear regression are observed.

The data used to calculate the regression equation (equation 22-7) must first be plotted and carefully examined for nonlinearity, and the data used for the final calculation must be limited to the data in the linear range. Nonlinearity at higher concentrations will lower the slope, increase the y intercept, and increase $s_{y,x}$.

The data must be carefully examined for outliers. The importance of daily examination and plotting of comparison-of-methods data cannot be overemphasized. Outlier specimens (for example, for which $|y_i - Y_i| > 3.5\, s_{y,x}$) must be detected immediately and reanalyzed by both methods so that the data can correct or confirm the outlier. The linear-regression line is "pulled" toward the outlier, with the greatest effects caused by outliers at the extreme ranges of the data. Confirmed outliers should be investigated for their causes. A confirmed outlier really is representative of the true analytical performance of the method. The systematic error of the test method should be calculated both with the outlier included in the data set and with it excluded. If errors are acceptable with the outlier excluded and excessive with it included, extreme caution should be exercised. There are statistical tests for removal of an outlier[31] (see pp. 363), but no more than one outlier should be excluded in a set of 40 patient comparisons. If the outlier discrepancy is less than the allowable error, do not exclude it

even though it may be a statistically significant outlier. If more than one clinically significant outlier is present per 40 patient comparison samples, the test method should be rejected until a cause for the outliers can be found and corrected.

The range of analytical concentrations must be wide. The effects of a narrow range of data on the least-squares statistics are seen in Fig. 22-5. Methods-comparison data often fail to meet one additional assumption of linear-regression calculations. This assumption requires that the x data (comparison) be known without error. Actually, in a methods-comparison experiment, random errors do affect the results of the comparison method. When the range of the data is sufficiently large, the effect of the failure to know the x values without error becomes negligible.[32,33]

Waakers and associates[32] have suggested that the correlation coefficient be used to decide whether the range of data is sufficient for using traditional least-squares calculation. If the correlation coefficient is greater than 0.99, the traditional least-squares approach by calculation will produce a slope whose mathematical error will be less than 1%. If the correlation coefficient is less than 0.99, the slope will be falsely low and the y intercept will be too high. Cornbleet and Gochman[33] have suggested another decision limit. If the ratio of the analytic standard deviation of the comparative method, S_{CM}, to the standard deviation of the x-method population, S_x, is less than 0.2, the least-squares calculation will be appropriate. If these tests on the data fail, one should use another regression approach, such as those discussed by Cornbleet and Gochman[33] (see also Chapter 19).

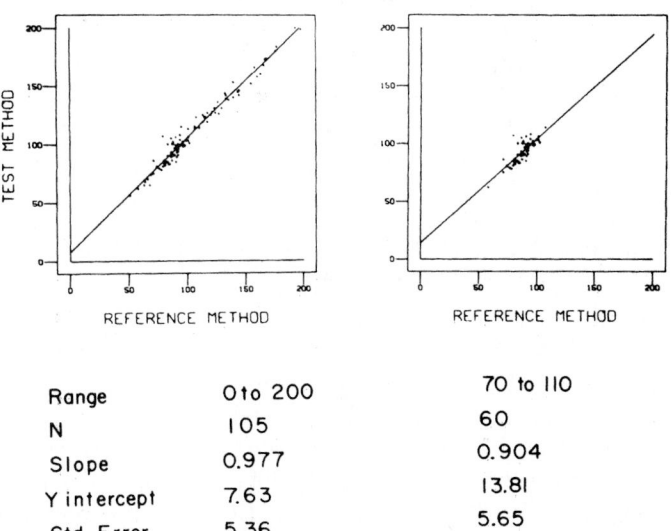

Range	0 to 200	70 to 110
N	105	60
Slope	0.977	0.904
Y intercept	7.63	13.81
Std Error	5.36	5.65

Fig. 22-5 Effect of range of data on linear-regression statistics. (From Westgard JO, Hunt MR: *Clin Chem* 19:49, 1973.)

Calculation of systematic error by use of linear-regression statistics is demonstrated on p. 422.

ESTIMATION OF TOTAL ERROR

Estimates of random error and systematic error are combined to estimate the total error of the test method. This is the most severe criterion for the test method to meet. The rationale for the total error concept is shown in Fig. 22-6. The horizontal line is error in concentration units, and the vertical line is located at the true-value concentration, the medical decision-level concentration, or zero error. The vertical distance from the horizontal line represents the probability of obtaining a test-method result at any given amount of error (difference from X_C). The bell-shaped curve shows the distribution of test-method data obtained from repeated analyses of a patient specimen whose true analyte concentration is designated as X_C. The distance from the mean of that curve to the true value is the systematic error. The dispersion around the mean of the data is the random error, which is defined as four times the standard deviation. There will be (1) instances in which the combined error will be exactly equal to the systematic error, (2) other times when the combined error for a given result will be less than the average systematic error by some amount because of the random error of the method, and (3) other times when the combined error will be greater than the systematic error, again by some amount caused by the random error of the method. The physician has no way of knowing what the various components of error are or when they will cause a larger error. Therefore it is essential to consider the worst-case combination and to define this as total error, TE:

$$TE = RE + SE \qquad \textit{Eq. 22-9}$$

If total error is less than allowable error, the method's overall performance is acceptable. Calculation of total error is demonstrated on p. 422.

Equations for estimating the magnitudes of the various errors and the criteria for judging their acceptability are summarized in Table 22-2.

CONFIDENCE-INTERVAL CRITERIA FOR JUDGING ANALYTICAL PERFORMANCE

To this point it has been assumed that the error estimated by each of the previous equations is absolutely accurate. However, if the same experiment were to be repeated in as identical a manner as possible, a slightly different estimate of error would probably be obtained. Exact measurements of random and systematic error cannot be obtained from the limited numbers of specimens analyzed in the procedures recommended above.

In the approach developed by Westgard, Carey, and Wold,[34] 95% upper and lower limits of error are calculated. If the 95% upper limit of an error is smaller than the allowable error, one can be at least 95% sure that the meth-

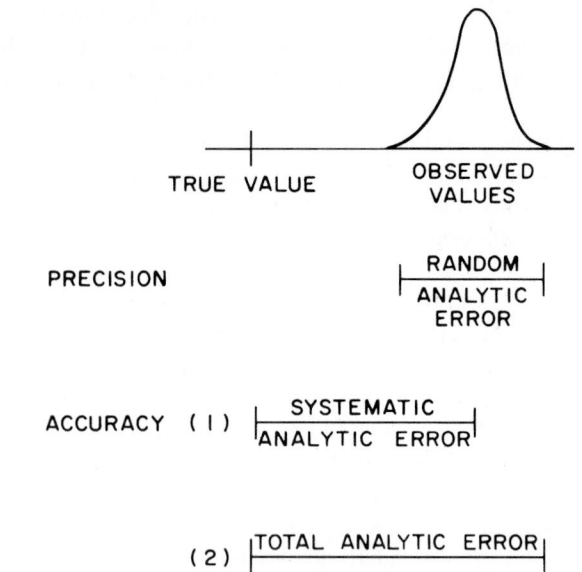

Fig. 22-6 Total analytical error. (From Westgard JO, Carey RN, Wold S: *Clin Chem* 20:825, 1974.)

od's performance is acceptable. If the 95% lower limit is greater than the allowable error, one can be at least 95% sure the method's performance is not acceptable, and no further testing is indicated. The method should be rejected or modified to improve its analytical performance. When the lower 95% limit is less than allowable error and the 95% upper limit of error exceeds allowable error, one cannot decide whether the method is unacceptable or acceptable, and more data are required to make a definitive decision.

Calculations of confidence-interval estimates of each type of error are demonstrated on pp. 420-422. For additional discussion of confidence limits, see pp. 348-350.

Confidence-interval criterion for random error

In the calculation of random error, the true value of the standard deviation is not known. One can estimate upper and lower confidence limits of the standard deviation by multiplying the observed standard deviation by the appropriate one-sided 95% factors. These factors

Table 22-2 Point-estimate criteria for acceptable performance

Type of error	Criteria
Random (RE)	$4 \cdot s_{TM} < E_A$
Constant (CE)	Bias $< E_A$
Proportional (PE)	$\dfrac{|R - 100|}{100} \cdot X_C < E_A$
Systematic (SE)	If $X = X_C$, $|\bar{Y} - \bar{X}| < E_A$
	or $|Y_C - X_C| = |a + bX_C - X_C| < E_C$
Total (TE)	$RE + SE = 4 \cdot s_{TM} + |a + bX_C - X_C| < E_A$

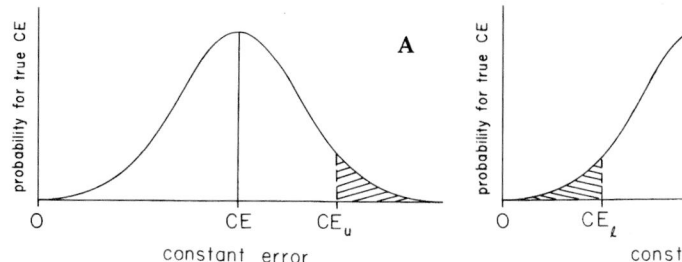

Fig. 22-7 **A,** One-sided 95% upper limit of constant error, CE_u. **B,** One-sided 95% lower limit of constant error, CE_l.

(see Table 22-3) are referenced to $N - 1$ degrees of freedom.

$$s_{TM_u} = s_{TM} \cdot A_u \qquad \textit{Eq. 22-10, a}$$

and

$$s_{TM_l} = s_{TM} \cdot A_l \qquad \textit{Eq. 22-10, b}$$

where A_u and A_l are the factors for computing the upper and lower one-sided limits of the standard deviation.[35]

The upper confidence limit of random error is four times the upper confidence limit of the standard deviation, and the lower confidence limit of random error is four times the lower confidence limit of the standard deviation.

$$RE_u = 4 \cdot s_{TM_u} \qquad \textit{Eq. 22-11, a}$$

and

$$RE_l = 4 \cdot s_{TM_l} \qquad \textit{Eq. 22-11, b}$$

Confidence-interval criterion for constant error

Upper and lower limits for constant error are estimated from the interference study data. Again, an upper limit is derived

Table 22-3 Factors for computing one-sided confidence limits for standard deviation

Degrees of freedom ($N - 1$)	$A_{.05}$	$A_{.95}$
1	.5103	15.947
5	.6721	2.089
10	.7391	1.593
15	.7747	1.437
20	.7979	1.358
25	.8149	1.308
30	.8279	1.274
40	.8470	1.228
50	.8606	1.199
60	.8710	1.179
70	.8793	1.163
80	.8861	1.151
90	.8919	1.141
100	.8968	1.133

From Natrella MG: *Experimental statistics,* National Bureau of Standards Handbook 91, Washington, D.C., 1963, US Government Printing Office.

such that there is a 95% probability that the true error is less than that limit.

$$CE_u = CE + \frac{t \cdot s}{\sqrt{N}} \qquad \textit{Eq. 22-12, a}$$

and

$$CE_l = CE - \frac{t \cdot s}{\sqrt{N}} \qquad \textit{Eq. 22-12, b}$$

The t value is a one-sided 95% t. Fig. 22-7, *A*, shows the upper 95% limit of constant error, leaving only a 5% chance that the error exceeds this upper limit, CE_u. Similarly, Fig. 22-7, *B*, shows the lower 95% limit of constant error, CE_l. A one-sided t is used only when one is concerned with an upper limit on the constant error without regard for how small the constant error is and vice versa for a lower limit. (A two-sided t is used to answer the question, "Is there a difference?" without regard to whether the difference is positive or negative, as in the t-test used in the interpretation of the comparison-of-methods experiment.)

Confidence-interval criterion for proportional error

A similar approach is used to estimate the upper and lower limits for recovery. A one-sided t value is used in the following equation for $N - 1$ degrees of freedom and a 95% limit.

$$\bar{R}_u = \bar{R} + \frac{t \cdot s}{\sqrt{N}} \qquad \textit{Eq. 22-13, a}$$

and

$$\bar{R}_l = \bar{R} - \frac{t \cdot s}{\sqrt{N}} \qquad \textit{Eq. 22-13, b}$$

where $\bar{R}$ is the percent mean recovery and s is the standard deviation of the recovery (see p. 412). The upper confidence limit of the percentage of proportional error is the confidence limit that is the greater distance from the ideal value of 100%. The lower confidence limit of the percentage of proportional error is the confidence limit that is closer to 100%. These percentages are converted to concentration units at the critical concentration or concentrations to make the comparison with allowable error.

$$PE_u = X_C \left| \frac{\bar{R}_u \text{ or } (\bar{R}_l - 100)}{100} \right|_u \qquad \textit{Eq. 22-14, a}$$

and

$$PE_l = X_C \left| \frac{\bar{R}_l \text{ or } (\bar{R}_u - 100)}{100} \right|_l \qquad \textit{Eq. 22-14, b}$$

Confidence-interval criterion for systematic error

Fig. 22-8 shows the profile of a confidence interval around a least-squares regression line. The expression for the limits, w, of this interval is given as

$$w = t \cdot s_{y,x} \sqrt{\frac{1}{N} + \frac{(X_C - \bar{X})^2}{\Sigma(x_i - \bar{X})^2}} \qquad \textit{Eq. 22-15}$$

This equation is similar to those used to calculate the limits for constant and proportional error in terms of the component $t \cdot s_{y,x}$. The component under the square-root sign becomes $1/N$ if X_C equals the mean of the patient data by the comparative method. As X_C moves away from the mean, the right term begins to contribute to the widening of the limits. One can calculate the denominator of this second term from the standard deviation of the patient population by the comparative method (s_x) as follows:

$$\Sigma(x_i - \bar{X})^2 = s_x^2 (N - 1) \qquad \textit{Eq. 22-16}$$

In this situation, one cannot know exactly what the regression line is, and for a given X_C, the corresponding Y_C could be as large as $(Y_C + w)$ or as small as $(Y_C - w)$. The limit that is farther from the ideal value is used to estimate the upper limit of systematic error, and the limit closer to the ideal value is used to estimate the lower limit of systematic error:

$$SE_u = |(Y_c \pm w) - X_c|_u \qquad \textit{Eq. 22-17, a}$$

and

$$SE_l = |(Y_c \pm w) - X_c|_l \qquad \textit{Eq. 22-17, b}$$

Equation 22-15 may not provide a valid estimate of the confidence limits of the linear-regression line if the precision of the test method is not reasonably constant throughout the concentration range of the patient specimens included in the comparison-of-methods experiment.

Confidence-interval criterion for total error

As described before, total error is the worst-case combination of the random and systematic errors. Since both the random and systematic errors have variances included in the equations used to calculate them, they must be combined vectorially. Their variances are combined as shown:

$$TE_u = \sqrt{RE_u^2 + w^2} + SE \qquad \textit{Eq. 22-18, a}$$

and

$$TE_l = \sqrt{RE_l^2 + w^2} + SE \qquad \textit{Eq. 22-18, b}$$

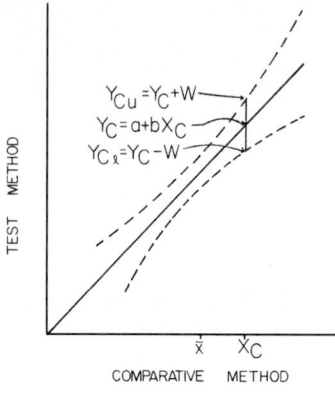

Fig. 22-8 Confidence interval around regression line. (From Westgard JO, de Vos DJ, Hunt MR, et al: *Am J Med Technol* 44:727, 1978.)

If the upper 95% limit of the total error is less than the allowable error, one can be 95% sure that the method performs acceptably. If the lower 95% limit of the total error exceeds allowable error, one can be 95% sure the method does not perform acceptably and should be modified or rejected.

One should note that whenever the ideal value (zero error condition) is between the upper and lower limits of the estimated error there is a chance that the true error might be zero. Thus in these situations the lower limit of error is simply zero. The upper limit of error remains as just calculated. This situation can arise for the constant, proportional, or systematic error estimates but not of course for random error. If the lower limit of systematic error is zero, the lower limit of the estimate of total error is equal to the lower limit of the estimate of random error because there may not be a systematic error present.

Equations for calculating confidence intervals of the various errors and criteria for judging their acceptabilities are summarized in Table 22-4.

OTHER EVALUATION PROTOCOLS AND APPROACHES FOR DATA ANALYSIS

The NCCLS has proposed a series of evaluation protocols. The first, EP5-P, is for evaluation of precision and verification of manufacturer's precision claims.[4] It requires duplicate measurements on sample pools that contain at least two different levels of the analyte in a run, two runs per day, for 20 days. An analysis of variance calculation is used to determine within-run, within-day, and day-to-day components of variance. These are combined to estimate the total standard deviation.

Guideline EP6-P addresses both experimental procedure and data analysis for evaluating the linearity of an assay.[5] Statistical procedures are presented for determining the limit of linearity and for estimating errors caused by nonlinearity at a particular concentration.

Another NCCLS guideline, EP7-P, presents two approaches for interference testing in the clinical chemistry

Table 22-4 Point-estimate criteria for acceptable performance

Error	Acceptable performance	Unacceptable performance
Random (RE)	$4 \times s_{TM_u} < E_A$	$4 \times s_{TM_l} > E_A$
Constant (CE)	$\left|\text{Bias}\right| + \dfrac{t \cdot s}{\sqrt{N}} < E_A$	$\left|\text{Bias}\right| - \dfrac{t \cdot s}{\sqrt{N}} > E_A{}^*$
Proportional (PE)	$\dfrac{\left|\bar{R}_u \text{ or } \bar{R}_l - 100\right|_u}{100} \cdot X_C < E_A$	$\dfrac{\left|\bar{R}_l \text{ or } \bar{R}_u - 100\right|_l}{100} \cdot X_c > E_A{}^*$
Systematic (SE)	$\left|(a + bX_c \pm w) - X_c\right|_u < E_A$	$\left|(a + bX_c \pm w) - X_c\right|_l > E_A{}^*$
Total error (TE)	$\sqrt{RE_u{}^2 + w^2} + SE < E_A$	$\sqrt{RE_l{}^2 + w^2} + SE > E_A{}^*$

*If the ideal value is between the two limits, it is possible that there is no error, and thus the lower limit of error might be zero. In these cases, therefore, CE_l is defined as zero, or PE_l is redefined as zero, or SE_l is redefined as zero, whatever the case might be. If $SE_l = 0$, TE_l becomes RE_l.

laboratory.[6] The first approach is similar to that already discussed on pp. 411-412. The second approach describes the determination of interferences with increasing concentrations of interferent (dose-response method). This guideline also presents extensive lists of exogenous and endogenous interferents and recommended testing concentrations.

The NCCLS guideline EP9-P[7] addresses key issues in method-comparison studies. The protocol requires that duplicate results be obtained for each procedure to facilitate tests for outliers. A minimum of 40 specimens distributed over the reportable range are to be tested. Various approaches to estimate the bias between the two methods and its confidence interval are described for use, depending on the nature of the data as determined in the preliminary review.

Multifactor experimental designs have been proposed to look at several method characteristics at one time.[36] A special example of this approach is the NCCLS guideline EP-10, which is entitled *Preliminary Evaluation of Quantitative Clinical Laboratory Methods.*[8] This protocol enables the estimation of imprecision, inaccuracy, nonlinearity, carryover, and drift in one series of studies over 5 days, using three levels of analyte. Samples must be measured in a specific sequence for a total of three readings each day as well as two "primer" samples of the midlevel sample, for a total of 11 analyses per day, or 55 for the whole study. It should be noted that if unusual effects are observed, each effect should be investigated more thoroughly with a specific study performed for each factor separately, as we have described in this chapter.

Another statistical approach that has been used to summarize the comparison between two methods is the multivariate approach in which both the *x* value and the *y* value vary with imprecision. The traditional linear least-squares regression analysis is made under the assumption that the *x* value is known without error. The Deming approach[32,33] determines the best slope as the one that minimizes the sum of squares of residuals determined perpendicularly from the line (as opposed to only in the *y* direction by the traditional least-squares method). The Deming approach is much more robust and provides a good estimate of the slope, even when the data are not precise, or when the data are limited to a narrow range (see also p. 363). The method of Passing-

Bablock[37] involves drawing straight lines between each pair of data points and then ranking the slopes and selecting the median slope as the best nonparametric estimate of the slope. This approach makes no assumption about the distribution of the data. A disadvantage of this approach is that the number of computations increases dramatically with increasing numbers of data points, thus placing a practical limit on the size of the study that can be analyzed.

DISCUSSION

There are situations, as in the study of different enzyme methods, in which suitably close agreement is not expected or possible because of different reaction conditions or different definitions of enzyme units. In these cases, rather than conclude that the method is unacceptable, a new clinical baseline of information is necessary, and a new reference interval is needed (see Chapter 20). Specific disease-related data should be obtained to provide new clinical information for interpretation of test-method results.

Evaluation of a method for a "new" analyte previously not measured in the user's laboratory is an analogous situation. Since there is no comparative method on site, accurate estimates of systematic error are harder to obtain. Reliance on published evaluation reports increases. The conclusions of these reports must be reviewed cautiously after the analysis of one's own experimental data is completed. If an analyte is not usually measured, the emphasis of the laboratory should shift to experiments to estimate specific errors. Accurate recovery studies are essential. The interference studies are expanded to include a broader range of chemicals that could interfere with the measurement reactions. Patient specimens that have been analyzed in another laboratory may be analyzed for comparison purposes, but the reliability of the systematic-error estimate may be decreased by specimen instability and lack of user control of the other laboratory's procedure. However, if the other laboratory is the reference laboratory to which the user has previously referred specimens for measurement of this analyte, the comparison is really being made to present practice.

Smaller laboratories often do not have the resources for exhaustive method-evaluation studies, but fortunately these are usually not among the first to evaluate a new method. Usually some evaluation reports have been published. Even when a method's performance is well documented by published evaluation studies, the user should still evaluate random error and perform the comparison-of-methods experiment to verify acceptable performance in his or her own laboratory. A reference interval study should be performed (see Chapter 20).

Using the decision-making approaches and tools that have been described in this chapter, it is possible to perform evaluations of methods efficiently and objectively. Conducting a method evaluation enables the laboratorian to understand the capabilities and quality of an assay before its routine use for patient testing, regardless of whether an evaluation is required by government regulation.

EXAMPLE CALCULATIONS AND DECISION MAKING FOR A PERFORMANCE EVALUATION STUDY FOR GLUCOSE

1. Estimation of random error from replication data

a. Statistics calculations. (y_i = Results from the method being tested)

Mean:

$$\bar{y} = \frac{\Sigma\, y_i}{N}$$

Standard deviation:

$$s_{TM} = \sqrt{\frac{\Sigma\,(y_i - \bar{y})^2}{N - 1}}$$

or

$$s_{TM} = \sqrt{\frac{\Sigma\, y_i^2 - (\Sigma\, y_i)^2/N}{N - 1}}$$

Coefficient of variation:

$$CV = \frac{s_{TM}}{\bar{y}} \cdot 100\%$$

Example. For glucose

$$N = 20,\ \Sigma\, y_i = 23{,}840,\ \text{and}\ \Sigma\, y_i^2 = 284{,}180{,}470$$

$$\bar{y} = 1192\ \text{mg/L}$$

$$s_{TM} = 20.1\ \text{mg/L}$$

$$CV = 1.7\%$$

b. Point estimate of random error (RE)

$$RE = 4 \cdot s_{TM}$$

If $RE < E_A$, performance is acceptable.
Example. For glucose, $E_A = 120$ mg/L at $Y_C = 1200$ mg/L

$$\bar{y} = 1192\ \text{mg/L}$$

$$s_{TM} = 20.1\ \text{mg/L}$$

$RE = 4 \cdot 20.1 = 80.4$ mg/L; RE is acceptable.

c. Confidence-interval estimate of random error (RE_u, RE_l)

$$s_{TM_u} = s_{TM} \times (A_{.95})\ \ldots \text{(see Table 22-3)}$$

$$= 20.1 \times 1.358 = 27.3\ \text{mg/L}$$

$$s_{TM_l} = s_{TM} \times (A_{.05})$$

$$= 20.1 \times 0.7979 = 16.0\ \text{mg/L}$$

$$RE_u = 4 \cdot s_{TMu} = 4 \cdot 27.3 = 109\ \text{mg/L}$$

$$RE_l = 4 \cdot s_{TMl} = 4 \cdot 16 = 64\ \text{mg/L}$$

Since $RE_u < E_A$, we are 95% certain that random error is acceptable.

2. Estimation of constant error from an interference study for a glucose method

a. Sample preparation
(1) 1.00 mL of serum A + 0.10 mL of water
(2) 1.00 mL of serum A + 0.10 mL of 1000 mg/L of creatinine standard
(3) 1.00 mL of serum A + 0.10 mL of 3000 mg/L of creatinine standard

b. Results

	Creatinine added (mg/L)	Glucose measured (mg/L)	Interference (mg/L)	Average interference (CE) (mg/L)
(1)	—	1200, 1220, 1190	—	—
(2)	91	1240, 1240, 1230	+40, +20, +40	+33
(3)	273	1310, 1340, 1290	+110, +120, +100	+110

c. Formulas for calculations

Concentration added =

$$\text{Concentration of standard} \times \frac{\text{Volume standard}}{\text{Total volume}}$$

Interference = Concentration (test) − Concentration (baseline)

d. Point estimate of constant error (CE)

$$CE = \text{Interference}$$

If $CE < E_A$, performance is acceptable.
Example. For glucose, $E_A = 120$ mg/L at $X_C = 1200$ mg/L

In the presence of 91 mg/L of creatinine, CE = 33 mg/L; CE is acceptable.

In the presence of 273 mg/L of creatinine, CE = 110 mg/L; CE is just barely acceptable but doesn't allow for much imprecision.

e. Confidence-interval estimate of constant error (CE_u, CE_l)

(1) In the presence of 91 mg/L of creatinine, CE = 33 mg/L, $s = 11.5$ mg/L, $N = 3$, and t for $(N - 1)$, or 2 degrees of freedom; 95% one-sided limit is 2.92 (see p. 350).

$$CE_u = CE + \frac{t \cdot s}{\sqrt{N}}$$

$$CE_u = 33 + \frac{2.92 \cdot 11.5}{\sqrt{3}} = 52 \text{ mg/L}$$

$$CE_l = CE - \frac{t \cdot s}{\sqrt{N}}$$

$$CE_l = 33 - \frac{2.92 \cdot 11.5}{\sqrt{3}} = 14 \text{ mg/L}$$

Since $CE_u < E_A$ (52 < 120 mg/L), the constant error caused by creatinine of 91 mg/L is acceptably small.

(2) In the presence of 273 mg/L of creatinine, CE = 110, s = 10 mg/L, N = 3.

$$CE_u = 110 + \frac{2.92 \cdot 10}{\sqrt{3}} = 127 \text{ mg/L}$$

$$CE_l = 110 - 2.92 \cdot 103 = 93 \text{ mg/L}$$

Since $CE_l < E_A < CE_u$, we cannot be 95% sure the method is acceptable or 95% sure the method is not acceptable for glucose analysis in the presence of 273 mg/L of creatinine. More data should be obtained to narrow the confidence limits to one side of E_A or the other.

3. Estimation of proportional error from a recovery study for a glucose method

a. Sample preparation

(1) 2.0 mL of serum A + 0.1 mL of water
(2) 2.0 mL of serum A + 0.1 mL of 10,000 mg/L of glucose standard
(3) 2.0 mL of serum B + 0.1 mL of water
(4) 2.0 mL of serum B + 0.1 mL of 10,000 mg/L of glucose standard

b. Results (mg/L): see table at the bottom of this page.

c. Formulas for calculations

$$\text{Concentration added} = \text{Concentration of standard} \times \frac{\text{Volume standard}}{\text{Total volume}}$$

$$\text{Concentration recovered} = \text{Concentration (test)} - \text{Concentration (baseline)}$$

$$\% \text{ Recovery} = \frac{\text{Concentration recovered}}{\text{Concentration added}} \cdot 100$$

d. Point estimate of proportional error (PE)

$$PE(\%) = |\bar{R} - 100|$$

$$PE \text{ (concentration units)} = \left| \frac{\bar{R} - 100}{100} \right| \cdot X_C$$

If PE $< E_A$, performance is acceptable.

Example: For glucose, E_A = 120 mg/L at X_C = 1200 mg/L

$$\bar{R} = 94.8\%$$

$$PE(\%) = |94.8 - 100| = 5.2\%$$

or

$$PE = \left| \frac{94.8 - 100}{100} \right| \cdot 1200 \text{ mg/L} = 62 \text{ mg/L}$$

PE is acceptable.

e. Confidence-interval estimate of proportional error (PE_u, PE_l)

$\bar{R}$ = 94.8%, s = 3.09%, N = 6, and t for ($N - 1$), or 5 degrees of freedom, and the 95% one-sided limit is 2.02.

$$\bar{R}_u = \bar{R} + \frac{t \cdot s}{\sqrt{N}}$$

$$\bar{R}_u = 94.8 + \frac{2.02 \cdot 3.09}{\sqrt{6}} = 97.4\%$$

$$\bar{R}_l = \bar{R} - \frac{t \cdot s}{\sqrt{N}}$$

$$\bar{R}_l = 94.8 - \frac{2.02 \cdot 3.09}{\sqrt{6}} = 92.3\%$$

The limit that deviates more from the ideal recovery of 100% is used to estimate the upper limit of proportional error, $PE_u\%$.

$$PE_u\% = |92.3 - 100| = 7.7\%$$

and for the lower limit

$$PE_l\% = |97.3 - 100| = 2.7\%$$

To relate $PE_u\%$ or $PE_l\%$ to E_A, convert them to concentration units at X_C.

b. Results (mg/L)

	Sample	Glucose added	Glucose measured	Glucose recovered (Test − Baseline)	Percentage of recovery*
(1)	Baseline	—	510, 530, 540	—	—
(2)	Spike	476	970, 1000, 980	460, 470, 440	96.6%, 98.7%, 92.4%
(3)	Baseline	—	1240, 1200, 1210	—	—
(4)	Spike	476	1690, 1660, 1640	450, 460, 430	94.5%, 96.6%, 90.3%

*Average recovery ($\bar{R}$) = 94.8%; SD of recovery (s_R) = 3.09%; SD of average recovery = 1.26%.

$$PE_u = \frac{PE_u\%}{100} \cdot X_C$$

$$= \frac{7.7\%}{100} \cdot 1200 = 92 \text{ mg/L}$$

$$PE_l = \frac{PE_l\%}{100} \cdot X_C$$

$$= \frac{2.7\%}{100} \cdot 1200 = 32 \text{ mg/L}$$

Since $PE_u < E_A$, one can be 95% sure proportional error is acceptably small for this glucose method.

4. Estimation of systematic error from a comparison-of-methods study for glucose

a. In the comparison of an automated glucose oxidase method (y) versus the manual glucose national reference method (x), the following statistics were obtained by linear-regression analysis: $y = 0.973 \cdot x - 57$ mg/L, $s_{y,x} = 37$ mg/L, $N = 82$, $\bar{x} = 1723$, $\bar{y} = 1619$, $s_x = 571$ mg/L (where s_x is the standard deviation of the x values for the 82 samples), and $r = 0.9941$.

b. Point estimate of systematic error (SE)

Consider bias:

$$\text{Bias} = |\bar{y} - \bar{x}| = 104 \text{ mg/L}$$

The bias provides an estimate of systematic error at the mean of the data. However, if x is not equal to the X_C of interest, there must be no proportional error between methods for the bias to provide an accurate estimate of systematic error at these other concentrations. If proportional error is present, use linear-regression statistics or calculate the bias using only those samples close to X_C.

Consider linear regression:

$$\text{SE} = |Y_C - X_C|$$

where $Y_C = a + b \cdot X_C$

For

$$X_C = 1200 \text{ mg/L of glucose,}$$

Then

$$Y_C = 0.973 \times 1200 - 57 \text{ mg/L}$$

$$= 1111 \text{ mg/L}$$

$$\text{and SE} = |1111 - 1200| = 89 \text{ mg/L}$$

Since $SE < E_A$, the systematic error is acceptable.

c. Confidence-interval estimate of systematic error (SE$_u$, SE$_l$)

$$Y_{C_u} = Y_C + w$$

and

$$Y_{C_l} = Y_C - w$$

where

$$w = t \cdot s_{y,x} \sqrt{\frac{1}{N} + \frac{(X_C - \bar{X})^2}{\Sigma (x_i - \bar{X})^2}}$$

where

$$\Sigma(x_i - \bar{X})^2 = s_x^2 (N - 1)$$

where w is the width of the confidence interval around the regression line (see Fig. 22-8). The value for t, obtained from a 95% one-sided t table and $N - 2$ degrees of freedom, has the value of 1.66.

$$w = 1.66 \cdot 37 \sqrt{\frac{1}{82} + \frac{(1200 - 1723)^2}{571^2 \cdot 81}} = 9 \text{ mg/L}$$

thus

$$Y_{C_u} = 1111 + 9 = 1120 \text{ mg/L}$$

$$Y_{C_l} = 1111 - 9 = 1102 \text{ mg/L}$$

The limit that deviates more from the ideal value for Y_C (ideally, $Y_C = X_C$) will be used to estimate the upper limit of systematic error.

$$SE_u = |(Y_{C_u} \pm w) - X_C|_u$$

$$= |1102 - 1200| = 98 \text{ mg/L}$$

and

$$SE_l = |(Y_{C_l} \pm w) - X_C|_l$$

$$= |1120 - 1200| = 80 \text{ mg/L}$$

Since $SE_u < E_A$, we can be 95% sure that the systematic error is acceptable between these methods.

5. Estimation of total error

a. Point estimate of total error (TE)

$$\text{TE} = \text{RE} + \text{SE} \quad (\text{See Fig. 22-6})$$

$$= 4 \cdot s_{TM} + |Y_C - X_C|$$

$$\text{TE} = 80 + 89 \text{ mg/L} = 169 \text{ mg/L}$$

Since $TE > E_A$, the total error of the new glucose method is not acceptable.

b. Confidence-interval estimate of total error (TE$_u$, TE$_l$)

$$TE_u = \sqrt{RE_u^2 + w^2} + SE$$

and

$$TE_l = \sqrt{RE_l^2 + w^2} + SE$$

Notice that the variances of the uncertainty in repetitive measurements and the uncertainty in the regression line are added, and the square root of the sum is taken to estimate the overall uncertainty, which is then combined with the point estimate of systematic error to yield the appropriate limit for total error. Thus

$$TE_u = \sqrt{109^2 + 9^2} + 89 = 198 \text{ mg/L}$$

and

$$TE_l = \sqrt{64^2 + 9^2} + 89 = 154 \text{ mg/L}$$

Because $TE_l > E_A$, we are at least 95% sure that the total error is not acceptable. Although both components of error—random and systematic—are fairly large, the errors that are easiest to reduce or eliminate are systematic errors. However, in this example, both RE_u and SE_u are individually almost as large as E_A (120 mg/L). Steps should be taken to reduce both types of error before the automated method is acceptable.

REFERENCES

1. Health Care Financing Administration (42 CFR Part 405, et al.), the Public Health Service, U.S. Department of Health and Human Services: Clinical Laboratory Improvement Amendments of 1988, Final Rule; *Fed Reg* 57:7003-7288, Feb 28, 1992.
2. Westgard JO: Precision and accuracy: concepts and assessment by method evaluation testing, *CRC Crit Rev Clin Lab Sci,* pp 283-330, Boca Raton, Fla., 1981, CRC Press.
3. Westgard JO, de Vos DJ, Hunt MR, et al: Concepts and practices in the selection and evaluation of methods, *Am J Med Technol:* Part I, Background and approach, 44:290-300, 1978; Part II, Experimental procedures, 44:420-430, 1978; Part III, Statistics, 44:552-571, 1978; Part IV, Decision on acceptability, 44:727-742, 1978; Part V, Applications, 44:803-813, 1978.
4. National Committee for Clinical Laboratory Standards: *NCCLS proposed guideline EP5-T2, Proposed guidelines for user evaluation of precision performance of clinical chemistry devices,* Subcommittee for User Evaluation of Precision of the Evaluation Protocols Area Committee, Villanova, Penn., 1992, NCCLS.
5. National Committee for Clinical Laboratory Standards: *NCCLS proposed guideline EP6-P, Evaluation of the linearity of quantitative analytical methods,* Subcommittee on Linearity Performance of the Evaluation Protocols Area Committee, Villanova, Penn., 1986, NCCLS.
6. National Committee for Clinical Laboratory Standards: *NCCLS proposed guideline EP7-P, Interference testing in clinical chemistry,* Subcommittee on Interference Testing of the Evaluation Protocols Area Committee, Villanova, Penn., 1986, NCCLS.
7. National Committee for Clinical Laboratory Standards: *NCCLS proposed guideline EP9-T, User comparison of quantitative clinical laboratory methods using patient samples,* Subcommittee on User Comparison of Methods of the Evaluation Protocols Area Committee, Villanova, Penn., 1993, NCCLS.
8. National Committee for Clinical Laboratory Standards: *NCCLS tentative guideline EP10-T, preliminary evaluation of quantitative clinical methods,* ed 2, *tentative guideline,* Evaluation Protocols Area Committee, Villanova, Penn., 1993, NCCLS.
9. Labeling requirements and standards development for in-vitro diagnostic products, *Fed Reg* 21 CFR:809-810, 1974.
10. Draft guidance to manufacturers of in vitro analytical test systems for preparation of premarket submissions implementing CLIA '88, *Fed Reg,* pp 3592ff, Jan 12, 1993.
11. Berkow R, editor: *The Merck manual of diagnosis and therapy,* ed 16, Rahway, N.J., 1992, Merck Sharp & Dohme Research Laboratories, p 1129.
12. Barnett RN: Medical significance of laboratory results, *Am J Clin Pathol* 50:671-676, 1968.
13. Barnett RN: Analytic goals in clinical chemistry: the pathologist's viewpoint. In Elevitch FR, editor: *Proceedings of the 1976 Aspen conference on analytic goals in clinical chemistry,* Skokie, Ill., 1977, College of American Pathologists, pp 20-24.
14. Tonks D: A study of the accuracy and precision of clinical chemistry determinations in 170 Canadian laboratories, *Clin Chem* 9:217-233, 1963.
15. Tonks D: A quality control program for quantitative clinical chemistry estimations, *Can J Med Technol* 30:38-54, 1968.
16. Gilbert R: Progress and analytic goals in clinical chemistry, *Am J Clin Pathol* 63:960-973, 1975.
17. Cotlove E, Harris E, Williams G: Biological and analytic components of variation in long-term studies of serum constituents in normal subjects. III. Physiological and medical implications, *Clin Chem* 16:1028-1032, 1970.
18. Elevitch FR, editor: *CAP Aspen Conference 1976: analytical goals in clinical chemistry,* Skokie, Ill., 1977, College of American Pathologists.
19. Elion-Gerritzen WE: Analytic precision in clinical chemistry and medical decisions, *Am J Clin Pathol* 73:183-195, 1980.
20. Ross JW: Blood gas internal quality control, *Pathologist* 34:377-379, 1980.
21. Fraser CG: The application of theoretical goals based upon biological variation in proficiency testing, *Arch Pathol Lab Med* 112:404-415, 1988.
22. Fraser CG: Desirable standards of performance for therapeutic drug monitoring, *Clin Chem* 33:387-389, 1987.
23. Fraser CG, Petersen PH, Ricos C, Haeckel R: Quality specifications. In Haeckel R, editor: *Evaluation methods in laboratory medicine,* New York, 1993, VCH Publishers.
24. Ehrmeyer SS, Laessig RH, Leinweber JE, Oryall JJ: 1990 Medicare/CLIA final rules for proficiency testing: minimum intralaboratory performance characteristics (CV and bias) needed to pass, *Clin Chem* 36:1736-1740, 1990.
25. Westgard JO, Burnett RW: Precision requirements for cost-effective operation of analytical processes, *Clin Chem* 36:1629-1632, 1990.
26. National Reference System for the Clinical Laboratory, *NRSCL6-T, Development of methodological principles documents for analytes in the clinical laboratory: tentative guideline,* National Committee for Clinical Laboratory Standards, Villanova, Penn., 1989, NRSCL.
27. Tremblay MM: Evaluation of instruments in biochemistry, *Can J Med Technol* 41:65-76, 1979.
28. Shaikh AH: A systematic procedure for selection of automated instruments in the clinical laboratory, *Am J Med Technol* 45:710-714, 1979.
29. Büttner R, Borth R, Boutwell JH, et al: Approved recommendation (1978) on quality control in clinical chemistry. Part 1. General principles and terminology, *Clin Chim Acta* 98:129F-143F, 1979.
30. Westgard JO, Hunt MR: Use and interpretation of common statistical tests in method-comparison studies, *Clin Chem* 19:49-57, 1973.
31. American Society for Testing and Materials: *ASTM Standard E178-68: standard recommended practice for dealing with outlying observations,* Philadelphia, 1968, ASTM.
32. Waakers PJM, Hellendoorn HBA, Op De Weegh GJ, Heerspink W: Applications of statistics in clinical chemistry: a critical evaluation of regression lines, *Clin Chim Acta* 64:173-184, 1975.
33. Cornbleet PJ, Gochman N: Incorrect least-squares regression coefficients in method-comparison analysis, *Clin Chem* 25:432-438, 1979.
34. Westgard JO, Carey RN, Wold S: Criteria for judging precision and accuracy in method development and evaluation, *Clin Chem* 20:825-833, 1974.
35. Natrella MG: *Experimental statistics,* National Bureau of Standards Handbook 91, Washington, D.C., 1963, US Government Printing Office.
36. Krouwer J: A multifactor experimental design for evaluating random access analyzers, *Clin Chem* 34:1984-1986, 1988.
37. Passing H, Bablock W: Comparison of several regression procedures for method comparison studies and determination of sample sizes, *J Clin Chem Clin Biochem* 22:431-445, 1984.

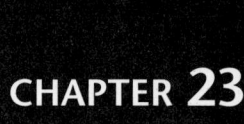

CHAPTER 23

Interferences in chemical analysis

Lawrence A. Kaplan
Amadeo J. Pesce

OBJECTIVES

- To understand how the accuracy of analytical results are minimized by reducing errors from interferents in instrumentation, methodology, and sample.
- To be aware of limitations to analytical accuracy.
- To be able to discuss the levels of inaccuracy of laboratory data that can be tolerated.

KEY TERMS

Allen correction Multichromatic analysis of a reaction to correct for background absorbance. Two wavelengths, in addition to the A_{max} (maximum absorption) of the chromophore, are monitored to subtract average background absorbance.

bichromatic analysis Spectrophotometric monitoring of a reaction at two wavelengths. Used to correct for background color.

chemical interferent A compound that either produces an endogenous color or interferes directly in the reaction or process being monitored.

DLIF Digoxin-like immunoreactive factor. An endogenous substance that cross reacts with antibody to digoxin.

end-point analysis Monitoring of a reaction after the reaction has been essentially completed.

HAMA Human antimouse antibody found in serum of individuals.

hemolysis Breakage of red blood cells, either in vitro or in vivo. Hemolysis will give a plasma specimen a red color.

icteria Pertaining to the orange color imparted to a sample because of the presence of bilirubin.

interferent Any chemical or physical phenomenon that can interfere in or disrupt a reaction or process.

in vitro interferent An interferent that is not caused by any in situ physiological process. Also called exogenous interferent.

in vivo interferent An interfering process resulting from physiological processes within the body. Also called endogenous interferent.

kinetic analysis Analysis in which the *change* of the monitored parameter with time is related to concentration, such as change of absorbance per minute. Measurements are made very early in the reaction period.

lipemia Presence of lipid particles (usually very-low-density lipoprotein) in a sample, which gives the sample a turbid appearance.

reagent blank Reaction mixture *minus* the sample; used to subtract endogenous reagent color from the absorbance of the complete reaction (plus sample).

sample blank Sample plus diluent; used to correct absorbance of complete reaction mixture for endogenous sample color.

turbidity Scatter of light in a liquid containing suspended particles.

window Term used to denote a specific time during which reactions are monitored, a phenomenon can be observed, or a procedure can be initiated.

A chemistry laboratory uses many techniques for measuring the concentration of specific biochemicals. All these techniques are subject to interferences from a variety of sources. Specific interferences that affect one technique may not be important for another. There are, however, general concepts that, when understood, help to control and minimize the effects of interferences on method accuracy and precision.

There are four basic types of interferences in laboratory analysis: (1) those that arise from limitations of detectors; (2) chemical substances in the sample that directly interfere with the analytical method; (3) disease states or exogenous agents that modify certain physiological processes, thus changing the concentrations of an analyte in vivo; and (4) those that occur as a result of sample (blood) processing.

LIMITATIONS OF DETECTORS

Methods yielding quantitative answers usually employ a detector, such as a spectrophotometer. It is then possible to obtain a relationship between the detector response and the concentrations of analytes in various samples. In the case of absorption spectrophotometry, there is a complex logarithmic relationship between concentration and detector response (see Chapter 4). When fluorescence is used, there is a linear relationship between concentration and the fluorescence signal. Similarly, when other optical properties, such as refractive index, or electrochemical properties, such as ion current from oxidation, are used by detectors, the response is also linear. Knowledge of the type of relationship that exists between concentration and detector response is important.

The first section describes errors in absorption spectrophotometry. Because the clinical chemistry laboratory quantifies most of its analytes by this technique, it is most important to understand the interference problems associated with this mode of measurement. As the nature and sophistication of the laboratory change, other types of interferences will become important to consider when one is performing a laboratory analysis.

Absorption spectrophotometer

There are two interrelated types of error in spectrophotometric measurement. The first is caused by the nature of the mathematical relationship between absorbancy and percentage of transmittance, and the second is related to limitations of the instrument.

Absorbance variance. As discussed in Chapter 4, there is a logarithmic relationship between the percentage of transmittance (%T), which is the quantity actually measured, and the absorbance (A), which is calculated. Fig. 23-1 shows the relationship between the linear percentage of transmittance and the log absorbance scales. At very low percentages of transmittances, small changes in the percentage of transmittance result in large changes in absorbance. For example, a change in percentage of transmittance of 60% to 50% T produces only a small absorbance change of approximately 0.08 A. A change in percent transmittance from 15% to 5%, however, results in a change of absorbance of 0.65 A. Thus, small changes of

Table 23-1 Absorbance error as a function of percentage of transmittance

%T and error	Absorbance	Variation in absorbance	Percent error of absorbance measurement
4 ±1	1.398	0.22	15.8
10 ±1	1.000	0.041	8.60
25 ±1	0.602	0.035	5.79
35 ±1	0.456	0.025	5.44
50 ±1	0.301	0.017	5.78
70 ±1	0.155	0.012	8.03
90 ±1	0.046	0.0097	21.2

percent T at very low transmittances will result in disproportionately large changes in the calculated absorbance at this part of the scale and will lead to an increased error of analysis.

One can consider the error of a spectrophotometric measurement as a function of the total or full-scale deflection of the detection meter or its electronics. When the absorbance scale is set at 0.000 or the transmittance scale is adjusted to 100%, the maximum electronic signal is obtained. For error analysis, the variation in this measurement is presumed to be constant throughout all readings on the scale. Because percent T directly reflects the electrical signal, some simple calculations using percent T can be done. At full-scale deflection (100% T), a 1% variation in percent T means an error of ±1% T. At half scale, a 1% variation of the 50% T value means a 2% absolute error ($\frac{1}{50}$), and at 10% T, this becomes a 10% error ($\frac{1}{10}$). However, it is not percent T that is directly proportional to concentration; it is absorbance. One can convert these percent T values into absorbance and calculate the error (Table 23-1).

Because the conversion of percent T to absorbance is a logarithmic function, both ends of the scale, 0.000 absorbance and high absorbance (more than 1.0), have the greatest error. In simple terms, when the solution has little color, it is difficult to tell the difference between no color and some color. The relative error can be huge because this difference is so small. At high absorbances, it is not easy to record accurately a small amount of light passing through the solution. Thus, differences between the two values are minute compared to the total incident light used to calibrate 100% T, and it is difficult to measure these small changes.

The relative error of spectrophotometric measurements versus percentage of transmittance and absorbance is shown in Fig. 23-2. One should make most spectrophotometric measurements at absorbances between 0.1 and 1.1 to minimize this type of error.

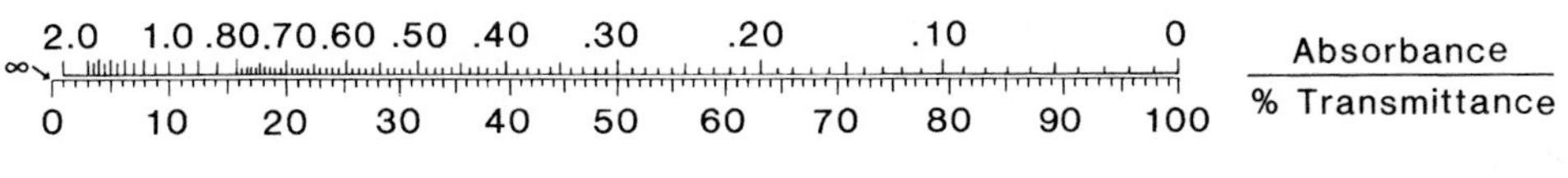

Fig. 23-1 Absorbance and percentage of transmittance scales juxtaposed.

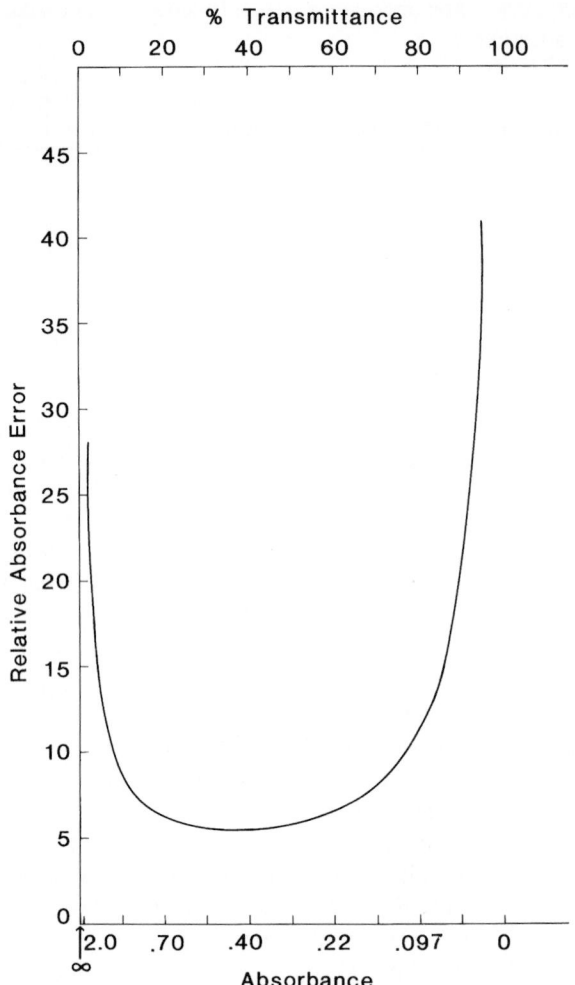

% Transmittance

Relative Absorbance Error

Absorbance

Fig. 23-2 Relative absorbance error versus absorbance *(A)* and percentage transmittance *(%T)* for a ±1% error in measurement of transmitted light. Relative error is minimum at 36.8% *T,* and *A* is 0.434.

Instrument limitations. Consider how a spectrophotometer functions. At 100% T, or zero absorbance, all the light signal is converted to an electronic signal. Assume that this signal measures 1000 nanoamps (nA). If the absorbance changes by 0.010, there is a decrease to 990 nA, and the instrument must measure accurately $^{10}/_{1000}$ nA, or a 1% change in signal. To do this accurately (1%), it must measure the signal to ±0.10 nA (1% of 10). Thus, at zero absorbance there is the difficulty of accurate measurement of one part in 10^4 of signal. In contrast, if the absorbance is 2.0, the signal to the photomultiplier is only 10 nA because only 1% of the light reaches the photodetector. To achieve the same degree of accuracy between a value of absorbance of 2.00 and 2.02, the instrument must measure the difference between 10 and 9.9 nA, or 0.1 nA. To do this accurately, it must measure to within 0.001 nA (1% of 0.1). Thus, at high absorbances the limitations are caused by the

inability of the detection system to measure small differences between high levels of absorbance accurately.

Thus, in analyses with relatively high levels of absorbing compound or interferent there will be a large spectrophotometric error. An initial dilution to lower total absorption *in addition to* a sample blank may be needed to eliminate this problem (see the discussion of turbidity on pp. 427-428 for an example).

Fluorescence spectrophotometer

Fluorescence measurements are different from those of transmission spectrophotometry in that the intensity of the fluorescence signal is linearly related to concentration. A doubling of the fluorescence signal is indicative of a two-fold increase in concentration. This is true only if there is very little light absorbed by the sample. If a significant portion of the light passing through a fluorescence sample is absorbed, the relationship is no longer linear; it becomes a more complex mathematical function. Thus, to minimize error, fluorescence analysis should be performed with relatively dilute solutions, the absorbance of which is less than 0.1.

Scattering of light or the presence of stray light has pronounced effects on fluorescence measurements. If the sample scatters light, some may be observed by the detector as fluorescence. Similarly, if there is *stray light* (a term meaning that the light used to excite the sample was not pure, that is, not of a very narrow color band), this also may be recorded by the detector. Because only a small fraction of the incident light (less than 1% and often less than one part in a million of the total light input into the instrument) is detected as fluorescence, these extraneous signals have a disproportionate effect on the reading and thus on the error.

Fluorescence measurements, like absorption measurements, can be inaccurate or invalid because of high signals. Unlike absorption spectrophotometry, this usually occurs because of the blanking system. If the fluorometer is adjusted to read zero for the blank, the entire detector sensitivity is adjusted for this zero reading. Assume that there is a blank solution that the instrument records as 10 units on its most sensitive scale. The instrument is now set to read zero fluorescence units. If the instrument can record accurately this zero unit to ±1 unit and if it can also measure a full scale of 100 units in the same way, it can accurately measure a signal of 100 ±1 units. If a different blank solution is used and this is recorded as 100 units, this value can be set at zero by use of an electronic manipulation (subtraction of the signal). At this new full-scale deflection of 100, the detector is really recording 200, of which 100 is subtracted as the blank. Because the instrument is accurate to 1%, it is now accurate to 1% of the new full scale of 200 units. The inaccuracy of measurement is now ±2 units. The accuracy is therefore twice as poor as that for the first example. Similarly, if a blank records as 1000, the accuracy is one tenth as great. Therefore the blank limits the accuracy of fluorescence measurements.

This same line of argument also applies to other linear measurements as in electrochemical analysis. The background can be blanked, but this must be considered in relation to the total signal.

IN VITRO INTERFERENCES

In vitro interferences arise from the fact that biochemical analyses are performed in the complex matrices that make up biological fluids (serum, plasma, urine, cerebrospinal fluid, and so on). These fluids contain hundreds of compounds that either have chemical groups that can react to some extent with the test reagents or can mimic the physical, chromatographic, or spectral properties of the desired analyte. This situation is further complicated because the chemical composition of body fluids can vary with the nature and extent of disease processes. This variability is increased by the possible presence of a large number of drugs. Each of these factors, alone or in combination, can result in a possible interference.

The in vitro interferences can be subclassified into those of a spectral nature and those caused by competing chemical reactions. The most commonly observed interferences are hemolysis, icteria, and lipemia. From one fourth to one third of samples obtained from clinic patients[1] or hospitalized patients[2] are lipemic, icteric, or hemolyzed. A compendium listing the degree of interference by hemolysis, icterus, and lipemia on the analysis of 21 analytes on 22 different instruments is available.[3]

Spectral interferences

Absorbance. Spectral interferences are observed when a compound causes a response in the spectrophotometer similar to that of the analyte of interest, though the interferents themselves do not necessarily undergo any chemical change during the analytical reaction. The simplest and most common example is the effect of hemoglobin (Hb) on many analytical procedures. A partial spectrum of HbO_2 (Fig. 23-3) shows significant absorption in the 500 to 600 nm portion of the visible spectrum. If one were monitoring the reaction of a colorimetric procedure in this region of the visible spectrum, there would be significant positive interference whenever Hb was contaminating the specimen. Other molecules, such as bilirubin, cause a similar interference.

An example of hemoglobin interference can be seen when a serum total protein (TP) concentration is determined by monitoring the biuret reaction at 540 nm. A standard curve for this reaction is depicted in Fig. 23-4. If a significant concentration of hemoglobin is added to a sample, the absorption at 540 nm is increased, thus giving a falsely high total protein reading. In this example, the A_{540} of a 50 g/L standard is 0.550. If small amounts of hemoglobin are added to this standard, the A_{540} is 0.650. When this solution is

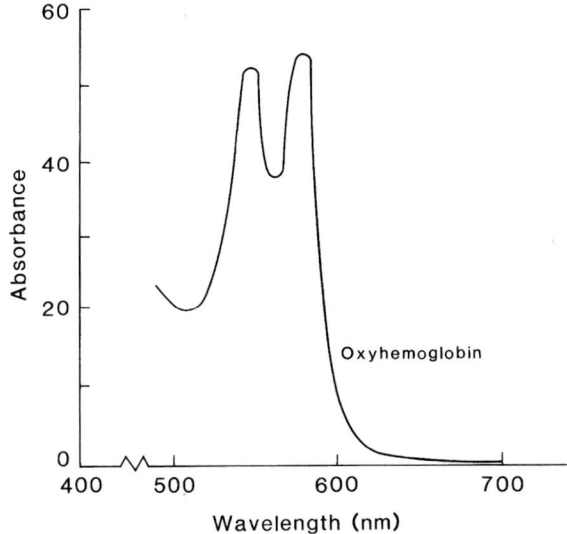

Fig. 23-3 Partial spectrum of oxyhemoglobin (HbO_2).

read from the standard curve, a higher apparent concentration of protein is calculated *(dotted line)*. Most spectral interferences give falsely elevated results in this manner.

Turbidity. A common type of spectral interference is caused by the turbidity of the sample. Turbidity is caused by large lipoprotein molecules called very-low-density lipoproteins (VLDL), which are suspended in serum. When a turbid specimen is analyzed in a colorimetric reaction, the lipoproteins cause the incident light to scatter, much as in nephelometry (see Chapter 4).

Because spectrophotometric analysis normally measures transmitted light at 180 degrees to the incident light, any light scattering tends to decrease the transmitted light and therefore to increase the apparent absorbance of the specimen. This, of course, results in falsely elevated results.

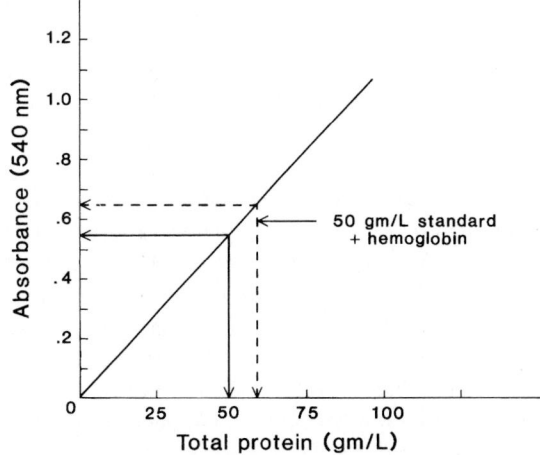

Fig. 23-4 Standard curve for measurement of total protein by the biuret reaction: A_{540} versus concentrations: *Solid arrow*, A_{540} for 50 g/L standard; *dotted arrow*, A_{540} for same standard containing hemoglobin.

Table 23-2   Effect of turbidity on measurement of LD activity (U/L)

Dilution (with saline)	LD Activity (U/L)			
	Nonturbid sample		Turbid sample	
	Uncorrected	Corrected	Uncorrected	Corrected
Undiluted	440	—	28	—
1:2	245	450	32	64
1:4	136	444	30	120
1:8	62	496	26	208
1:16	30	480	25	400
1:32	14	450	13	416

Sample blanks normally work poorly here, just as two-point kinetic analysis does (see below), because of the error resulting from the very high absorbances often encountered. The best method for eliminating the interference caused by turbidity is dilution of the specimen. The extent that the sample can be diluted to minimize turbidimetric interference is limited by the ability of the analytic procedure to measure the diluted analyte. If possible, several dilutions should be analyzed simultaneously to determine the best response. An example of the effect and elimination of turbidometric interference is presented in the analysis of equal amounts of lactate dehydrogenase (LD) activity in a turbid and a nonturbid specimen (Table 23-2). When the nonturbid specimen is diluted, all the corrected LD activities calculate out to the same approximate value. This indicates linearity of dilution. In contrast, when the turbid specimen is diluted, the calculated LD activity changes with dilution. Only at higher dilutions containing minimum turbidity do the calculated LD activities converge with the true values of the nonturbid specimen.

Fluorescence. Turbidity affects fluorescence measurements in a similar fashion. Here, some scattered light will reach the detector set at 90 degrees to the incident light, thus giving an apparent increase in fluorescence and falsely elevated concentrations. Reducing problems of turbidity in fluorescence measurements is more difficult than for absorption spectroscopy. The best approach is the elimination of the source of light scattering by filtration or centrifugation.

Correction of spectral interferences

Sample blank. One can minimize spectral interferences by measuring the absorbance of the assay against a sample blank. The simplest sample blank is obtained by a mixture of the sample and diluent (instead of reagent). The correction for spectral interference is made by subtracting the absorbance value of the blank from the absorbance of the complete reaction mixture. Any significant color inherent to the sample is eliminated by this calculation. In the example of the biuret reaction discussed previously, the absorbance of the sample and the hemoglobin diluted with saline is 0.100. If this is subtracted from the absorbance of the complete reaction mixture (0.650), the true absorbance of the stan-

dard (0.550) is obtained. Such a sample blank can usually work unless there are gross amounts of the interferent present. In these cases, the very large total absorption ($A_{interferent} + A_{reaction}$) results in large spectrophotometric and calculation errors. Random access analyses (see Chapter 16) easily permit the measurement of sample blank absorbances before the addition of reagent.

Reagent blanks (reagent plus diluent) are used in a similar fashion to correct for high absorbance of the reagent.

In the case of fluorescence, the sample blank allows for the correction of nonspecific fluorescence; however, the fluorescence of this blank cannot be a great portion of the total fluorescence signal (see preceding text).

Kinetic measurements. One frequently used method for the correction of spectral interference is the measurement of a typical end-point reaction as a two-point kinetic reaction. If the absorbance of a noninstantaneous, colorimetric reaction is monitored versus time, a reaction curve as shown in Fig. 23-5 will be observed. An *end-point* reaction is monitored at a single time point when the reaction is mostly completed (Fig. 23-5, arrow 3). If no spectral interferences are present, the reaction curve should pass through the origin. If such interferences are present, the curve will be *parallel* to the original curve but biased high because of the endogenous color in the sample. If a sample blank was used to subtract endogenous color, a line identical to the sample containing no interferences would be obtained.

In a *two-point kinetic* assay, the absorbance is measured at *two* different time points (Fig. 23-5, arrows 1 and 2) when (1) the final color development has not occurred and in fact may be small and (2) the response of absorbance versus time response is still linear.

The initial absorbance reading (Fig. 23-5, arrow 1) is actually taken when almost no color formation has occurred. Thus any absorbance at this time is primarily caused by endogenous spectral interferents. A second reading is taken a short time later when only a small amount of color has formed and the response of absorbance versus time is still linear (Fig. 23-5, arrow 2). This absorbance therefore includes both the original endogenous color and the color formed because of the specific analytical reaction. By subtraction of the first reading from the second, the calculated

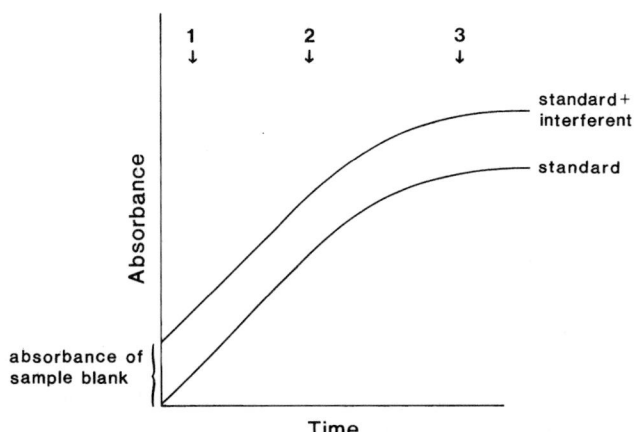

Fig. 23-5 Absorbance changes versus time for colorimetric reaction, with and without interferent present. *Arrows 1 and 2,* Time frame for kinetic analysis; *arrow 3,* end-point reading.

delta absorbance (ΔA) is caused only by the specific color formed by the analytical reaction. Standard curves based on kinetic analysis have the change in absorbance (ΔA) plotted versus concentration (Fig. 23-6). In this standard curve the presence of a *nonreacting,* endogenous, colored interferent has no effect. Thus no separate sample blank measurement needs to be made; a two-point kinetic reaction is self-blanking when there is no change in the nature of the interferent during the reaction. This is an important technique when one is performing automated chemical analysis on large numbers of specimens.

Biochromatic analysis.[4] Many instruments in current use employ a different technique for correction of spectral interferences. This technique involves measurement of the absorbance of the reaction mixture simultaneously at two different wavelengths. These are the primary wavelength (λ_1) and one other wavelength (λ_2) close by. As shown in Fig. 23-7, λ_1 is the wavelength at which the chromogen

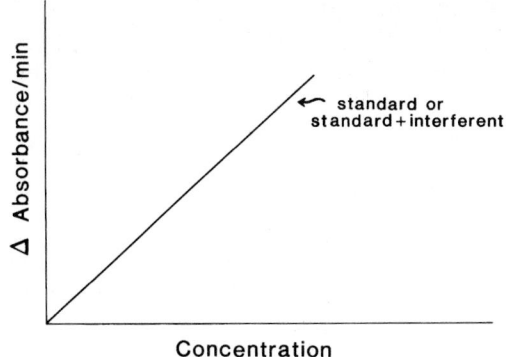

Fig. 23-6 Kinetic analysis of both reactions shown in Fig. 23-5. Change in absorbance (ΔA) per minute versus concentration during linear portion of curve of absorbance versus time between arrows 1 and 2 in Fig. 23-5.

maximally absorbs. At λ_2 there is minimum absorbance of the chromogen. Because the reaction is monitored simultaneously at two wavelengths, this is known as *bichromatic analysis.* This technique is based on the premise that although a compound may give a spectral interference, the absorbance maxima of the interferent will differ from that of the actual analytical reaction. In addition, this procedure is made under the assumption that the absorption caused by the interfering compound is approximately the same at λ_1 as at λ_2. Although the measured absorbance at λ_1 will be caused by both the analytical reaction and the interferent, the absorbance at the second wavelength (λ_2) will be caused by only the interferent. This technique can also correct for instrument problems such as dirt on the cell, which causes light scattering or reflectance. Standard curves are then based on either $A_1 - A_2$ or the ratio of the two absorbances (A_1/A_2). Use of this procedure also allows each sample to serve as its own blank for endogenous color.

Another similar method for the correction of background interference is the measurement of absorbance at the primary wavelength A_{max} and at two additional wavelengths, usually equidistant from the peak, A_1 and A_2. The absorbance readings at these last two wavelengths are averaged to give the average background absorbance in the specimen. This technique for the correction of background absorbance from interfering substances is known as the *Allen correction.*[5]

The Allen correction is valid only if the background absorbance is approximately linear with wavelength over the region in which the measurements are being taken. Thus the shape of the absorption curve for both the analyte and the interferent *(solid line)* and the interferent or interferents *(dotted line)* must be obtained as shown in Fig. 23-8. Use of the Allen correction in this example, when the wavelengths used to correct for background are equidistant from the absorbance maxima, would give the following equation:

$$A_{300}\ \text{corrected} = A_{300} - \frac{A_{320} + A_{280}}{2} \qquad \textit{Eq. 23-1}$$

The "A_{300} corrected" has the average background absorbance subtracted from the absorbance maximum to give the actual absorbance above base-line value. The Allen correction is widely used, but improper use of the Allen correction, that is, with nonlinear background interference, can lead to even larger errors. Because the final corrected absorbance is based on three measurements, there is a decrease in the precision of the assay.

Dilution. As discussed for turbidity, dilution of a sample containing a spectral interferent can sometimes reduce the problem. One must be careful not to overdilute the desired analyte or chromogen to a concentration below the minimum detectable level for a given assay. Several dilutions should be assayed simultaneously to determine the most effective dilution.

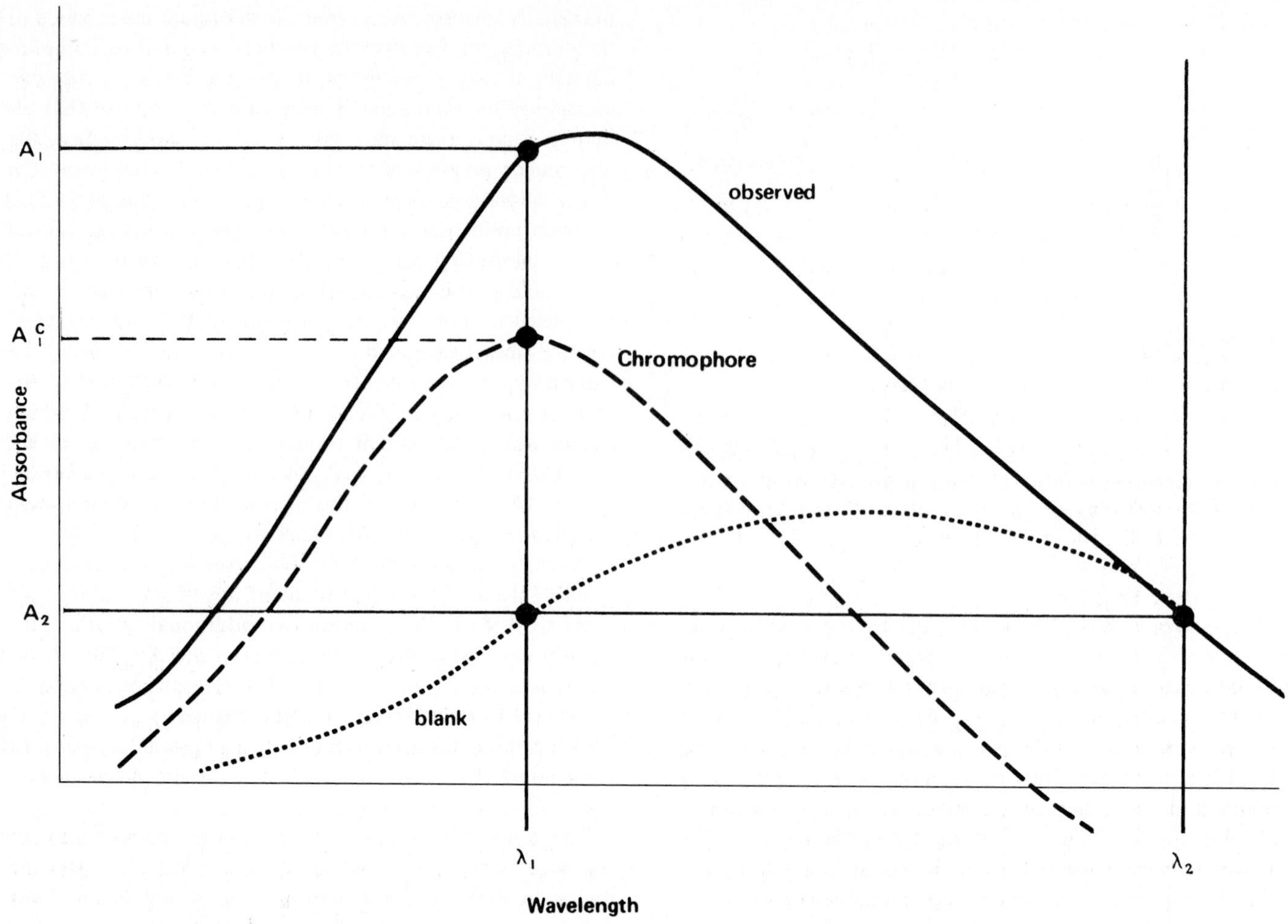

Fig. 23-7 Spectral curves for chromophore and nonreactive blank, where blank absorbance is equal at λ_1 and λ_2.

Chemical interferences

All the interferences discussed so far have been spectral interferences caused by compounds that do not react in the analytical chemical reaction. However, many interferents do react with the chemicals of the analytical reaction. The re-

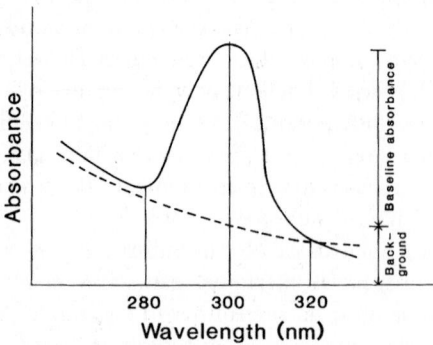

Fig. 23-8 Spectral curves of chromophore and interferent, *solid line,* and background interferents, *dotted line.* Average of A_{280} and A_{320} represents background absorbance at A_{max} for chromophore (300 nm).

action products of these interferences usually result in positive interferences, though negative interferences are observed.

The types of nonspecific, chemically reacting interferents can vary greatly, as seen in the examples in Table 23-3. Uric acid produces a positive interference, and bilirubin and ascorbic acid yield negative interferences in the glucose oxidase methods used for glucose measurement. The alkaline picrate reaction for the measurement of creatinine is known to have both positive (ketones, protein) and negative (bilirubin) interferences.

Correction of chemical interferences

Elimination of many nonspecific chemical interferents is often achieved by one or more of the following techniques:
1. Diluting the interferent
2. Increasing the specificity of the reaction
3. Removing the interferent
4. Monitoring an assay by kinetic measurement
5. Monitoring an assay by bichromatic measurement

Dilution of the sample is an effective method in the case of interferents that do not react at the same rate or produce

Table 23-3 Examples of chemically interfering biochemicals

Analyte	Method	Interferences
Glucose	Reducing sugar	Uric acid (+), creatinine (+), protein (+), glutathione (+)
	Glucose oxidase–horseradish peroxidase	Uric acid (+), ascorbic acid (−), bilirubin (−)
	Glucose oxidase—O_2 consumption	Hemoglobin (−), ascorbic acid (+)
	Hexokinase	Fructose
Creatinine	Alkaline picrate	Ascorbic acid (+), glucose (+), protein (+), ketones (+)
Vanillylmandelic acid	Pisano	Certain foods (such as bananas), vanilla, aspirin (+)
	High-performance liquid chromatography	Certain drugs and their metabolites (+)

+, positive interference; −, negative interference.

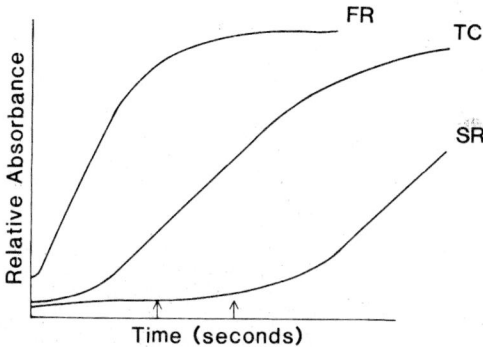

Fig. 23-9 Relative absorbance versus time curves for alkaline picrate reaction, for creatinine *(TC)*, slow-reacting interferents *(SR)*, and fast-reacting interferents *(FR)*. *Arrows,* Time during which absorbance, over time, primarily reflects change attributable to the TC reaction.

the same color intensity as the analyte. Interference by protein is minimized in many automated analyzers by a large specimen dilution.

Increased specificity of an analytic reaction is often achieved by use of specific enzymes as reagents. Examples of this approach include the measurement of glucose by hexokinase or glucose oxidase, uric acid by uricase, and urea by urease. Immunochemical-based reactions are also used to increase the specificity of the analysis. An example would be the measurement of theophylline by enzyme immunoassay versus the older methods, which employed ultraviolet absorbance.

Separation of an interferent from the analyte may be achieved by the use of (1) a protein-free sample, (2) liquid-liquid extraction, or (3) adsorption or partition chromatography. Protein-free samples were originally prepared by precipitation of serum proteins and separation of the protein-free sample by filtration or centrifugation. Agents used to precipitate proteins include tungstic acid (Folin-Wu procedure) and heavy-metal salts (such as barium and zinc; Somogyi-Nelson procedure). protein-free specimens obtained by the dialysis technique were the basis of many Technicon Auto-Analyzer procedures.

Liquid-liquid extractions are used when the analyte and interferent or interferents can be separated into different liquid phases. Similarly, in adsorption and partition chromatography, the analyte and interferent are separated by their differential affinity for the stationary phase (see Chapters 5 to 7).

The basis for the elimination of nonspecific chemical reactants by use of a two-point kinetic reaction is that many interferents react at a different *rate* from the one at which the specific analyte of interest does. This is ob-

served in the example of the Jaffé reaction with creatinine.[6]

Creatinine reacts with alkaline picrate at a finite rate (curve TC, true creatinine) (Fig. 23-9). Many of the nonspecific interferents (such as acetone) react at a faster kinetic rate (FR), whereas some (such as protein) react at a slower rate (SR), giving a complex change of absorbance with time for the reaction of a mixture of all three species (Fig. 23-10). Therefore, by properly choosing an optimal window of time for the two absorbance readings for the kinetic analysis (*arrows,* Fig. 23-9), one can minimize the effect of the fast-reacting and slow-reacting nonspecific interferents and isolate the absorbance change caused primarily by creatinine. During the window of time, the reaction of the FR interferents is essentially complete, whereas that of the SR interferents is not yet occurring (Fig. 23-10). The ΔA during this time is caused by the analyte, that is, creatinine. This concept has also been used for the glucose oxidase reaction and is, in fact, a popular technique for increasing the specificity of reactions in many instruments.

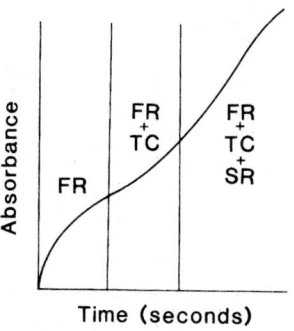

Fig. 23-10 Complex reaction of mixture containing fast-reacting *(FR)* and slow-reacting *(SR)* interferents plus creatinine *(TC)*. Only by measurement of the change in absorbance over time can TC reaction be isolated and SR and FR interferences minimized.

Chromatographic interferences

The third type of common in vitro, or methodological, interference is chromatographic interference. This often occurs when an interfering compound cochromatographs with the compound of interest to give falsely elevated results.

Currently, many analytical procedures use chromatography to separate the analyte to be measured from interfering compounds. A chromatographic method is made under the assumption that the desired analyte is completely isolated from other compounds that may be recorded by the detection system. However, no single set of chromatography conditions can possibly prevent interferences from cochromatographing or closely chromatographing compounds, especially when the patient may be receiving several potentially interfering drugs.

An example of this type of interference and its correction can be seen in the high-performance liquid chromatographic (HPLC) separation of catecholamines and the drug methyldopa (Aldomet), which is used in the treatment of hypertension. In some HPLC assays, methyldopa is eluted from the column just before norepinephrine. Because the pharmacological dose of Aldomet is much greater than the physiological concentrations of norepinephrine, it will obliterate or be confused with the norepinephrine peak. The only way to eliminate this type of interference is to remove the source of exogenous interferent. In the case of methyldopa, removal of the drug from the patient for 2 to 10 days is required. Drug or diet restrictions before biochemical analysis are often a necessity for many compounds.

There are two primary modes of minimizing chromatographic interferents: (1) increasing the specificity of the detector and (2) removing the interferent from the analyte. Detectors can measure compounds based on a variety of different principles. If the interferent has physical or chemical properties different from those of the analyte, it is possible to select a detector that will not respond significantly to a potential interferent. In liquid chromatography, refractive index detectors can detect almost any compound in the eluant; thus, they are very nonspecific. Fluorescence detectors have much higher specificities because not all compounds fluoresce. By appropriate setting of excitation and emission wavelengths, the detector can be made even more specific. Electrochemical detectors also have high specificities because not all compounds are electrochemically active. The specificity can be further increased by selection of an electrode voltage at which the interferent will not react.

As discussed earlier, separation of the analytes from potentially interfering compounds is achieved by several techniques. These techniques are based on differences in solubility or chromatographic behavior between the analyte and interferents. The techniques commonly used are single liquid-liquid extractions, multiple extractions including back-extractions, and adsorption and ion-exchange chromatography. The complexity of the procedure used depends on the nature of the interference and required sensitivity. HPLC methods for serum theophylline, present in relatively large amounts, usually employ only a simple liquid-liquid extraction. In contrast, the HPLC analysis of the tricyclic antidepressants present in nanogram quantities requires several extraction steps, including back-extractions. Chapter 5 discusses these types of procedures in more detail.

A technique for detecting contaminating or cochromatographing compounds is dual-detection analysis. This technique uses two different types of detectors or parameters, such as multiple wavelengths, to monitor the column eluate. The response of the two different detectors (D_1 and D_2) is determined for a standard, and the ratio of the responses is calculated (D_1 standard/D_2 standard). The probability that another compound would have a similar characteristic ratio is quite small. Thus, significant deviations of the ratio found in patient analyses would be strongly suggestive that the analyte peak contains a contaminating, coeluting compound.

Often the presence of a cochromatographing interferent is recognized because of the abnormal shape of the peak. The presence of a contaminant often causes a normally symmetric peak to be skewed. In these cases, rerunning the chromatogram at lower flow rates will sometimes separate or partially separate the analyte from the interfering compound, allowing quantitation.

Immunochemical interferences

Immunochemical methods are subject to the usual causes of exogenous interference (see box below).[7] In addition, however, they are subject to matrix effects of the reaction solution and, in some cases, the surface where the reaction is occurring. Hyperlipidemia can greatly affect immunochem-

---

Interferences Common to Immunoassays*

Exogenous interference
  Sample collection and preparation, including anticoagulants, sample storage, drugs, and serum-separating gels
  Calibration matrix
  Changes in solid-phase surface binding caused by coating molecule
  Incomplete saturation of solid-phase binding sites for antigen or antibody
Endogenous interference
  Hyperlipidemia—turbidity
  Heterophilic anti-immunoglobulin antibodies (HAMAs)
  Iatrogenic antibodies, such as Digabind [see p. 433]
  Rheumatoid factor
  Autoantibodies against analyte
  Complement
  Cross-reacting substance, such as DLIF
  Competing immunospecific antibodies to analyte

DLIF, Digoxinlike immunoreactive factor; *HAMAs*, human antimouse antibodies.
*Modified from Pesce AJ, Michael JG: *J Immunol Methods* 150:111-119,1992.

ical reactions that use turbiditometric or nephelometric measurements because of the increased sample turbidity. The most difficult interference to detect is that in which the patient has antibodies to the test reagent antibodies (heterophile antibodies), or to the actual test antigen. The most frequently encountered heterophile antibodies, those against mouse antibodies (HAMAs), can cause interference in assays employing mouse monoclonal antibodies. Methods for reducing these interferents include adding specific animal sera, such as mouse serum, to the test reagent to combine with the heterophile antibodies and neutralize them. Often the only indication that the patient has antibodies to the test analyte is the patient history, which can indicate that the test results are not consistent with the clinical findings. An interesting example of the problem of endogenous antibodies can be seen in the measurement of digoxin. In acute digoxin overdoses, the patient may be treated with Digabind, an Fc fragment of IgG antibodies to digoxin that binds digoxin, minimizes toxicity, and increases clearance. Digabind will also react with labeled digoxin in an immunoassay and cause apparently highly elevated digoxin levels.

For enzyme immunoassays, some of the interferences are the same as those observed in ordinary enzyme assays, as shown in the following box.

IN VIVO INTERFERENCES

Factors such as age and sex, time of day, diet, pregnancy and menses, as well as sample-processing errors can affect the test result. These are discussed in Chapter 3. The presence of drugs in the patient is a common source of interference.

Drugs

Virtually every drug affects some laboratory procedure, and any laboratory procedure may be affected by one or more drugs. The interference may be either in vivo or in vitro.

Interferences for Enzyme Immunoassays*

Exogenous interference
  Enzyme inhibitor
Endogenous interference
  Endogenous enzyme
  Endogenous substrate
  Spectral: lipids, hemoglobin
  Drugs that inhibit enzyme activity
Measurement of enzyme activity
  Temperature
  Substrate reaction on solid phase
  Non-linear kinetics
  Limited sensitivity
  Substrate depletion

---

*Modified from Pesce AJ, Michael JG: *J Immunol Methods* 150:111-119, 1992.

An example of a commonly encountered drug is alcohol, whose ingestion may affect glucose, lactate, urate, bicarbonate, γ-glutaryltransferase, and creatine phosphokinase levels.[8] Smoking may alter catecholamine, cortisol, and blood-gas results. Reference to source material is needed to determine the effect of any one of the huge number of drugs on a specific test.

SOURCE-REFERENCE MATERIAL

This chapter provides only a brief description of the wide variety and types of interferences in chemistry laboratory testing. Many common interfering substances are well documented, and an alert laboratory staff can often eliminate these as a source of interference. For example, the development of the interferogram[2] allows the laboratory to estimate the effect of hemolysis, icterus, and lipemia on the analyses performed on frequently used instruments. Newer automated chemistry analyzers can be calibrated to detect increased levels of hemolysis, lipemia, and icterus.

However, as the number of drugs produced by pharmaceutical companies and consumed by the public increases, the laboratory must determine both the in vivo and in vitro effects exerted by each of these drugs on clinical laboratory analysis.

A list of the known effects of drugs and other interferences on chemical analysis was developed by Donald Young and published as an issue of *Clinical Chemistry* in April of 1975[9] and published in a third edition in 1990 with a supplement in 1991.[10,11] Although it was outdated when published, it remains the best and only single listing of drug effects on laboratory tests. In one of the two major sections, possible interferents (not only drugs) are listed in alphabetical order. Listed under each interferent are those laboratory tests that may be affected by that interferent.

One section of Young's study is shown in Fig. 23-11. Barbiturates are the tested interferent. The initial capital letter indicates the type of body fluid in which the laboratory test was analyzed (U = urine, S = serum, and so on); the laboratory tests are then given in alphabetical order. After each test is the indication of how the tested interferent affects the laboratory test (*inc* = increases, *dec* = decreases, and z = no effect). The next capital letter indicates the type of interference (V = in vivo; M = methodological). A comment and a reference completes the test listing.

The section listing interferents is cross-indexed by another section that lists, in alphabetical order, laboratory tests. Each laboratory test is listed by subsections according to decreased *(dec)*, increased *(inc)*, or no effects *(z)* of the listed interferents on that test. The laboratory test is also listed as either a urinary *(U)* or serum *(S)* analyte. Under each laboratory test is listed the interferent for which the effect *(inc, dec,* or *z)* has been shown.

The complexity and extent of Young's work highlight the

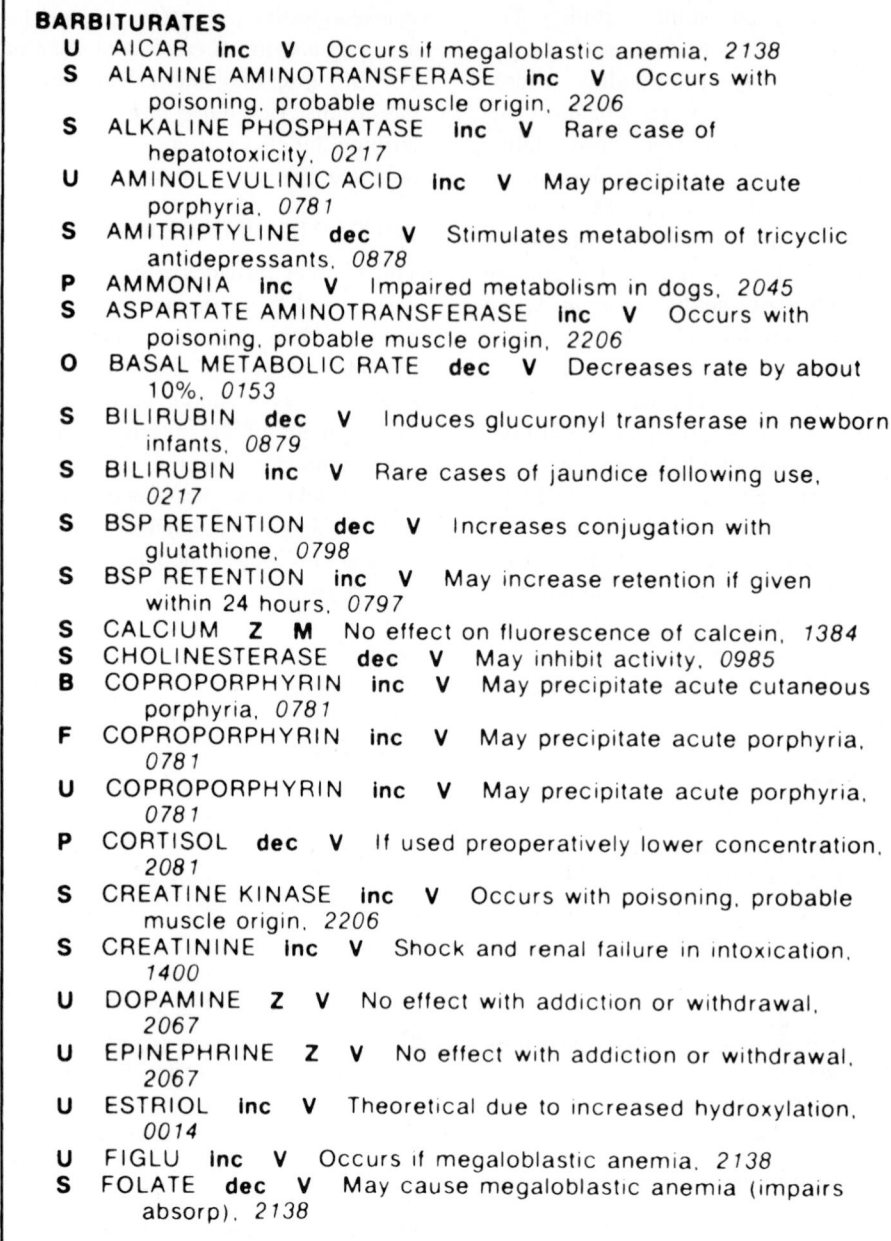

BARBITURATES

U	AICAR	inc	V	Occurs if megaloblastic anemia, *2138*
S	ALANINE AMINOTRANSFERASE	inc	V	Occurs with poisoning, probable muscle origin, *2206*
S	ALKALINE PHOSPHATASE	inc	V	Rare case of hepatotoxicity, *0217*
U	AMINOLEVULINIC ACID	inc	V	May precipitate acute porphyria, *0781*
S	AMITRIPTYLINE	dec	V	Stimulates metabolism of tricyclic antidepressants, *0878*
P	AMMONIA	inc	V	Impaired metabolism in dogs, *2045*
S	ASPARTATE AMINOTRANSFERASE	inc	V	Occurs with poisoning, probable muscle origin, *2206*
O	BASAL METABOLIC RATE	dec	V	Decreases rate by about 10%, *0153*
S	BILIRUBIN	dec	V	Induces glucuronyl transferase in newborn infants, *0879*
S	BILIRUBIN	inc	V	Rare cases of jaundice following use, *0217*
S	BSP RETENTION	dec	V	Increases conjugation with glutathione, *0798*
S	BSP RETENTION	inc	V	May increase retention if given within 24 hours, *0797*
S	CALCIUM	Z	M	No effect on fluorescence of calcein, *1384*
S	CHOLINESTERASE	dec	V	May inhibit activity, *0985*
B	COPROPORPHYRIN	inc	V	May precipitate acute cutaneous porphyria, *0781*
F	COPROPORPHYRIN	inc	V	May precipitate acute porphyria, *0781*
U	COPROPORPHYRIN	inc	V	May precipitate acute porphyria, *0781*
P	CORTISOL	dec	V	If used preoperatively lower concentration, *2081*
S	CREATINE KINASE	inc	V	Occurs with poisoning, probable muscle origin, *2206*
S	CREATININE	inc	V	Shock and renal failure in intoxication, *1400*
U	DOPAMINE	Z	V	No effect with addiction or withdrawal, *2067*
U	EPINEPHRINE	Z	V	No effect with addiction or withdrawal, *2067*
U	ESTRIOL	inc	V	Theoretical due to increased hydroxylation, *0014*
U	FIGLU	inc	V	Occurs if megaloblastic anemia, *2138*
S	FOLATE	dec	V	May cause megaloblastic anemia (impairs absorp), *2138*

Fig. 23-11 Example of format used in special issue of *Clinical Chemistry:* "Effects of drugs on clinical laboratory tests." (From O'Kell RT, Elliott JR: *Clin Chem* 16:161-165, 1970.)

awareness laboratory personnel must have concerning interferences with clinical laboratory tests. A complementary issue to the 1975 listing was published in 1980[12] and updated in 1989.[13] This volume lists the effects of disease on clinical laboratory tests. The format for this volume is similar to the one just described. The first section lists each analyte and those disease states in which changes in the concentration of that analyte have been noted. The second section lists diseases and those analytes that change during the course of the disease.

Evaluation of analytical interference

Because virtually all clinical chemistry analytical procedures can be interfered with by the factors of preanalytical variation and the patient specimen itself (see Chapter 3), many protocols for evaluating the extent of the potential interference have been proposed.[14-17]

Often the testing of spectral interference involves the addition of a lipid substance Intralipid (Kabi Vitrum, Alameda, California), a hemolysate, or bilirubin.[3] In some cases the test method is compared to a reference or definitive method that is not subject to the interference being evaluated. These techniques include isotope dilution mass spectroscopy, neutron activation, atomic absorption, and other specialized techniques. The most extensive proposal for interference testing can be found in reference 16.

Allowable interference

Because some interference is potentially present for every assay, clinical chemists must determine how much interference is allowable. A statistically significant interferent may not be a clinically significant one. One approach is to use the medical decision limit.[18] The concept of clinically important errors is reviewed in Chapter 21, and examples of its application are found in Chapter 22. The size of allowable error is determined from consultations with the clinicians who are using the results of the testing and from discussions of allowable error in the literature.

The total analytical error, E_A, of a method is the sum of its imprecision, which equals the sum of twice the standard deviation (2SD), its analytical bias (E_B), and the error resulting from interferents (E_I):

$$E_A = 2SD + E_B + E_I \qquad \textit{Eq. 23-2}$$

For an assay to be clinically useful, the total analytical error, E_A, *must* be less than the total allowable error at the medical decision level, E_{MDL}, for each analyte. If the laboratory knows the errors SD + E_B and can estimate E_{MDL}, the allowable contribution from an interferent, E_I, can be calculated:

$$E_I = E_{MDL} - 2SD - E_B \qquad \textit{Eq. 23-3}$$

This discussion is made under the assumption that the total allowable error based on medical decision making needs is greater than the total allowable error permitted for CLIA '88–regulated analytes. These calculations can be used to determine the analytical errors permissible under these regulations (see Chapter 21).

Thus, for precise assays with small standard deviations and large changes before the medical decision value is reached, larger errors caused by interferences can be tolerated. In contrast, some measurements, such as creatinine in transplant patients, have a small allowable error (often less than 20%), which must include bias, method variability, and

interference. Thus, in these methods there is less tolerance to interference.

REFERENCES

1. Glick MR: Ohio Valley Section Meeting on "Interferences," Cincinnati, Ohio, Feb 27, 1988.
2. Kaplan LA: Ohio Valley Section Meeting on "Interferences," Cincinnati, Ohio, Feb 27, 1988.
3. Glick MR, Ryder KW: *Interferographs: user's guide to interferences in clinical chemistry instruments,* Indianapolis, 1987, Science Enterprises, Inc.
4. Hahn B, Vlastelica DL, Snyder LR, et al: Polychromatic analysis: new applications of an old technique, *Clin Chem* 25:951-959, 1979.
5. Allen E, Rieman W: Determining only one compound in a mixture, short spectrophotometric method, *Anal Chem* 25:1325-1331, 1953.
6. Soldin SJ, Henderson L, Hill JG: The effect of bilirubin and ketones on reaction rate methods for the measurement of creatinine, *Clin Biochem* 11:82-86, 1978.
7. Pesce AJ, Michael JG: Artifacts and limitations of enzyme immunoassay, *J Immunol Methods* 150:111-119, 1992.
8. Freer DE, Statland BE: The effect of ethanol (0.75 g/kg body weight) on the activities of selected enzymes in sera of healthy young adults. I. Intermediate-term effect, *Clin Chem* 23:830-834, 1977.
9. Young DS, Pestaner LC, Gibberman V: Effects of drugs on clinical laboratory tests, *Clin Chem* 21:1D-432D, 1975.
10. Young DS: *Effects of drugs on clinical laboratory tests,* ed 3, Washington, D.C., 1990, American Association for Clinical Chemistry.
11. Young DS: *1991 supplement* to the *effects of drugs on clinical laboratory tests,* Washington, D.C., 1991, American Association for Clinical Chemistry.
12. Friedman RB, Anderson RE, Entine SM, Hirshberg SB: Effect of diseases on clinical laboratory tests, *Clin Chem* 26:1D-476D, 1980.
13. Friedman KB, Young DS, *Effect of diseases on clinical laboratory tests,* ed 2, Washington, D.C., 1989, American Association for Clinical Chemistry.
14. Buttner R, Dorth R, Boutwell JH, et al: International Federation of Clinical Chemistry expert panel on nomenclature and principles of quality control in clinical chemistry. Approved recommendation (1978). Part 2: Assessment of analytical methods for routine use, *Clin Chim Acta* 98:129F-143F, 1979.
15. Galteaux MM, Siest G: IFCC. Drug effects in clinical chemistry. Part 2: Guidelines for evaluation of an analytical interference, *J Clin Chem Clin Biochem* 22:275-279, 1984.
16. Interference testing in clinical chemistry; proposed guideline, NCCLS Publication EP7-P, Villanova, Penn., 1986, National Committee on Clinical Laboratory Standards.
17. Glick MR, Ryder KW, Jackson SA: Graphical comparison of interferences in clinical chemistry instrumentation, *Clin Chem* 32:470-475, 1986.
18. Castano-Vidriales JL: Interferences in clinical chemistry, *J Int Fed Clin Chem* 6:7-9, 1994.

SECTION TWO

Pathophysiology

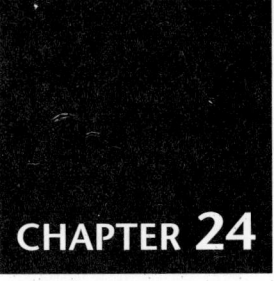

CHAPTER 24

Physiology and pathophysiology of body water and electrolytes

Leonard I. Kleinman
John M. Lorenz

Body water compartments
  Definitions
  Volume of body water compartments
  Maturational changes in body water compartment
    volumes
  Composition of body water compartments
  Osmotic pressure and osmolarity of body fluids
Regulation of body fluid compartment osmolarity and
    volume
  Extracellular compartment
  Sodium metabolism and natriuretic factors
  Plasma and interstitial fluid compartments
  Intracellular compartment
Water metabolism
  Water balance
  Disorders of water imbalance
  Dehydration
  Overhydration
Sodium metabolism
  Sodium balance
  Disorders of sodium balance
  Abnormalities of plasma sodium concentration
Potassium metabolism
  Potassium balance
  Disorders of potassium balance
  Abnormalities of plasma potassium concentration
Chloride metabolism
  Chloride balance
  Disorders of chloride balance
  Abnormalities of plasma chloride concentration
Methods of analysis
  Anion gap
  Chloride
  Osmolality
  Sodium and potassium

OBJECTIVES

- List the electrolyte composition of the two main
  compartments of total body water.
- Define anion gap and state its clinical significance; calculate
  and interpret anion gap results from given data.
- Outline the homeostatic regulation of sodium, potassium,
  chloride, and body water.

- Define the various states of decreased or increased plasma
  electrolyte concentrations in terms of an excess or deficit of
  water or electrolyte.
- List and briefly describe the symptoms and at least two
  causes or clinical conditions associated with increased and
  decreased amounts of electrolytes and body water.

KEY TERMS

acidosis Abnormally low body fluid pH. *Respiratory*—caused by
an abnormally high Pco_2; *metabolic*—caused by an abnormally
low bicarbonate concentration.

active transport The passage of ions or molecules across a cell
membrane by an energy-consuming process. This energy is generated by cellular metabolism.

adipsia Absence of thirst.

aldosterone A mineralocorticoid hormone secreted by the adrenal cortex that influences sodium and potassium metabolism.

alkalosis Abnormally high body fluid pH. *Respiratory*—caused
by an abnormally low Pco_2; *metabolic*—caused by an abnormally high bicarbonate concentration.

anabolism The process of assimilation of nutritive matter and
its conversion into living substance.

angiotensin A vasoconstrictive polypeptide produced by the enzymatic action of renin on angiotensinogen. A converting enzyme from the lung removes two C-terminal amino acids from
the inactive decapeptide angiotensin I to form the biologically
active octapeptide angiotensin II.

angiotensinogen A serum globulin produced in the liver that
is the precursor of angiotensin.

anion An ion that carries a negative charge.

anorexia Diminished appetite for food.

antidiuretic hormone A peptide hormone of the neurohypophysis that acts on the collecting tubule of the kidneys to allow increased water reabsorption and therefore decreased free
water excretion by the kidney. Also known as *vasopressin*.

arrhythmia Irregularity of the heartbeat.

ascites The accumulation of fluid in the peritoneal cavity.

asphyxia Interference with oxygen delivery to and carbon dioxide removal from the tissue.

atrial natriuretic peptides (ANP) A number of peptides released from the atria of the heart that increase sodium excretion by the kidney. Some peptides are also released by the brain
(BNP) and by the kidney (urodilatin).

baroreceptor A nerve ending that responds to change in pressure.

catabolism The breaking down of complex chemical compounds in the body into simpler ones, often with the production of energy.

cation An ion that carries a positive charge.

cirrhosis Progressive disease of the liver characterized by damage to hepatic parenchymal cells.

colloid As used in this chapter, this term applies to the large molecules in the body to which the capillary endothelium and cell membrane are impermeable.

colloid osmotic pressure The effective osmotic pressure of plasma and interstitial fluid across the capillary endothelium, largely the result of the presence of protein.

dehydration Abnormal decrease in total body water (see Table 24-4). *Hypernatremic*—net loss of sodium and water from the body, with net water loss exceeding net sodium loss; *hyponatremic*—net loss of sodium and water from the body, with net sodium loss exceeding net water loss; *normonatremic*—net loss of sodium and water from the body in equal extracellular proportions; *simple*—net loss of body water alone with no net sodium loss.

diabetes insipidus The chronic excretion of very large amounts of hyposmotic urine caused by inability to concentrate urine because of the lack of antidiuretic hormone (ADH) production, secretion, or effect. *Pituitary*—caused by inadequate ADH synthesis or secretion; *nephrogenic*—caused by unresponsiveness of the renal tubules to ADH.

distension receptor A nerve ending that responds to stretch.

edema An increase in the interstitial fluid volume.

extracellular water (ECW) Water external to cell membranes. *Anatomical*—all body water external to cell membranes; *physiological*—plasma and body water into which small solutes can freely diffuse; excludes the transcellular portion of the anatomical extracellular water; includes the plasma and interstitial fluid (see Fig. 24-1).

free water Water containing no solute.

Gibbs-Donnan equilibrium The steady-state distribution of permeable ions and transmembrane potential that results across a semipermeable membrane when an impermeant ion exists in unequal amounts on either side of the membrane and solvent movement across the semipermeable membrane is exactly opposed (Fig. 24-7).

hyperaldosteronism A disorder caused by excessive secretion of aldosterone and characterized by hypokalemic alkalosis, muscular weakness, hypertension, polyuria, polydipsia, and normal or elevated plasma sodium concentration.

hyperchloremia An abnormally high plasma chloride concentration.

hyperkalemia An abnormally high plasma potassium concentration.

hypernatremia An abnormally high plasma sodium concentration.

hyperosmotic Denoting an effective osmotic pressure higher than that of plasma.

hypertonic Denoting a theoretical osmotic pressure higher than that of plasma.

hypochloremia An abnormally low plasma chloride concentration.

hypokalemia An abnormally low plasma potassium concentration.

hyponatremia An abnormally low plasma sodium concentration. *Dilutional*—hyponatremia caused by an excess of water (relative to sodium) in the extracellular compartment.

hyposmotic Denoting an effective osmotic pressure lower than that of plasma.

hypothalamus Portion of brain beneath the thalamus and connected to the pituitary gland (see Chapter 43).

hypotonic Denoting a theoretical osmotic pressure lower than that of plasma.

hypovolemia An abnormally low blood volume.

insensible water loss Evaporation of water through the skin or from the respiratory tract.

interstitial fluid (ISF) Extravascular, extracellular water (see Fig. 24-2).

intracellular water (ICW) Water inside the cells of the body; water within cell membranes.

ischemia A decrease in arterial blood flow below the minimum level necessary to meet the metabolic demands of the tissue or organ in question.

juxtaglomerular cells Smooth muscle cells that synthesize and store renin and release it in response to decreased renal perfusion pressure, increased sympathetic nerve stimulation of the kidneys, or decreased sodium concentration in fluid in the distal tubule.

macromolecule A molecule of colloidal size, notably proteins, nucleic acids, and polysaccharides.

nephrotoxin A substance that causes dysfunction or death of renal parenchymal cells with some degree of specificity.

obligatory water requirements The minimum volume of water necessary to replace insensible water loss and to excrete the existing renal solute load when the urine is maximally concentrated.

oliguria Abnormally low urine output, that is, less than 400 mL/day in an adult.

osmolarity Osmotic concentration expressed as osmoles or milliosmoles of solute per liter of solvent (see Chapter 14).

osmole The total number of moles of a solute in solution after dissociation.

osmosis The movement of water across a semipermeable membrane from a solution with low solute particle concentration to a solution with high solute particle concentration.

osmotic pressure The force necessary to exactly oppose osmosis into a solution across a semipermeable membrane.

paresthesia An abnormal spontaneous sensation, such as burning, pricking, numbness, and so on.

passive diffusion Movement of ions or solute across a membrane, down electrical or chemical gradients without energy consumption or a carrier process.

plasma The extracellular, intravascular fluid of the body (see Fig. 24-2).

polyanionic Possessing multiple negative charges.

polydipsia Excessive fluid intake secondary to extreme thirst. *Psychogenic polydipsia* secondary to a psychiatric disorder, without a demonstrable organic lesion.

polyuria Excessive urine output, that is, more than 1 to 2 L/day in the adult.

pseudohyperkalemia Abnormally high plasma potassium concentration in a sample obtained from a patient in the absence of true elevation of plasma potassium concentration in that patient.

renin An enzyme produced, stored, and secreted by the juxtaglomerular cells of the kidney, which acts on circulating angiotensinogen to form angiotensin I.

semipermeable Permeable to certain molecules but not to others; usually permeable to water.

syndrome of inappropriate antidiuretic hormone secretion (SIADH) A grouping of findings, including hypotonicity of the plasma, hyponatremia, and hypertonicity of the urine with continued sodium excretion, that is produced by excessive ADH secretion and that improves with water restriction.

total body water (TBW) All water within the body, both inside and outside the cells, including that contained in the gastrointestinal and genitourinary systems.

transcellular water That portion of extracellular water that is enclosed by an epithelial membrane, the volume and composition of which are determined by the cellular activity of that membrane.

transudation The passage of a fluid through a membrane with nearly all the solutes the fluid contains remaining in solution or suspension.

urodilatin A peptide similar in structure to atrial natriuretic peptide (ANP) but released by the kidney. Urodilatin increases renal sodium excretion.

water intoxication An increase in free water in the body; results in dilutional hyponatremia.

Water is the most abundant constituent of the human body, accounting for approximately 60% of the body mass in a normal adult. Water is important not only because of its abundance but also because it is the medium in which body solutes, both organic and inorganic, are dissolved and metabolic reactions take place. The discussion in this chapter focuses on (1) description of the dynamic steady-state compartmentalization of body fluid and its inorganic solutes, (2) physiological mechanisms involved in the maintenance of this compartmentalization, and (3) pathophysiological events that occur during certain clinical states that alter the composition of body fluids.

BODY WATER COMPARTMENTS
Definitions (Figs. 24-1 and 24-2)

Total body water (TBW) includes water both inside and outside of cells and water normally present in the gastrointestinal and genitourinary systems. TBW can be theoretically divided into two main compartments. The *anatomical extracellular water (ECW)* includes all water external to cell membranes and constitutes the medium through which all metabolic exchange occurs. *Intracellular water (ICW)* includes all water within cell membranes and constitutes the medium in which chemical reactions of cell metabolism occur. This compartment is heterogeneous and discontinuous; the interior of each cell is separated from the extracellular water and from the interior of every other cell by the semipermeable cell membrane.

The anatomical ECW is functionally subdivided into *physiological extracellular water* and *transcellular water.* The physiological ECW is the portion of the anatomical ECW whose volume is accessible to direct measurement; it includes *plasma* (intravascular water) and *interstitial fluid* (ISF). The ISF, which includes extravascular, extracellular water into which ions and small molecules diffuse freely from plasma, is the fluid that directly bathes the cells of the body. In addition, there are potential spaces in the body (pericardial, pleural, peritoneal, and synovial) that are normally empty except for a few milliliters of viscous lubricating fluid and are considered to be part of the ISF compartment. Transcellular water includes water in extracellular compartments enclosed by an epithelial membrane, the volume and composition of which are determined by the cellular activity of that membrane. These heterogeneous compartments include the aqueous humor in the eye, the cerebrospinal fluid, and water within the gastrointestinal, genitourinary, and nasorespiratory systems. The volume of the transcellular water portion of the anatomical ECW is

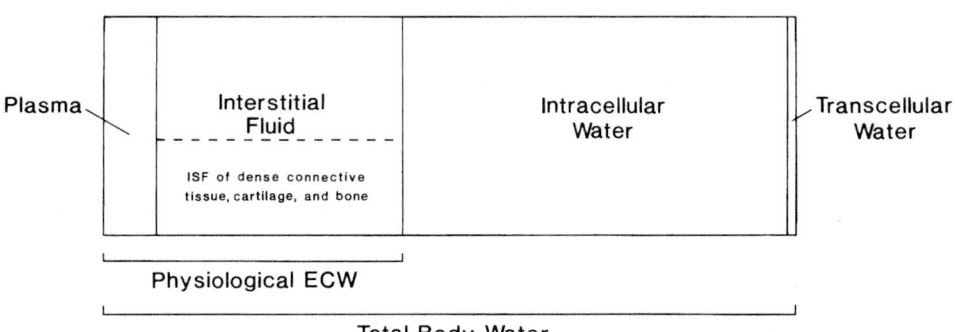

Fig. 24-1 Body water compartments. Keep in mind that anatomical extracellular water (*ECW*) includes physiological extracellular water and transcellular water. *ISF,* Interstitial fluid.

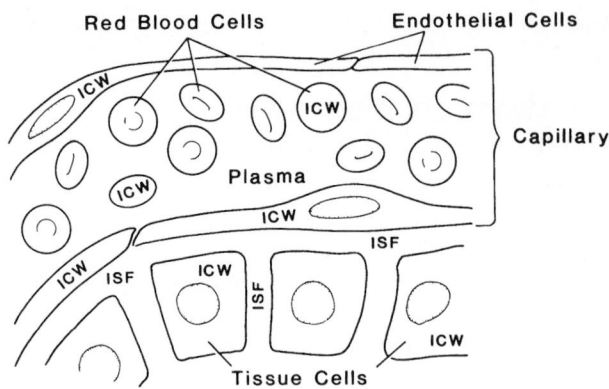

Fig. 24-2 Diagram of plasma, interstitial fluid, *ISF,* and intracellular water, *ICW,* in tissue at microscopic level.

not included in conventional measurements of extracellular water (see Chapter 41).

Volume of body water compartments (Table 24-1)

TBW is 65% of body weight in average adult men and 55% of body weight in women. This difference between men and women is largely the result of differences in body fat. As a percentage of total body weight, TBW varies inversely with body fat content, from approximately 70% in very thin persons to 50% in very obese persons.

Physiological ECW volume is approximately 20% of body weight and one third of TBW in the average adult. Unlike TBW, neither physiological nor anatomical ECW volumes can be accurately measured. Plasma volume can be accurately measured and is approximately 5% of body weight. Interstitial fluid volume is calculated as the difference between the ECW and plasma volumes. It is approximately 15% of body weight and one fourth of TBW. Intracellular water is calculated as the difference between the TBW and ECW volumes. It is equal to 40% of body weight and two thirds of TBW in the average adult. Intracellular water volume calculated in this manner includes transcellular water, which has been estimated to be 1% to 3% of body weight.

Maturational changes in body water compartment volumes (Fig. 24-3)

The fraction of body weight that is water and the proportion of TBW that is ECW and ICW do not remain constant during growth. When expressed as a percentage of body weight, TBW gradually decreases during intrauterine gestation and early childhood, reaching a value approximating that in the adult by about 3 years of age. During this time ECW (expressed as a percentage of body weight) decreases and ICW (expressed as a percentage of body weight) increases. Thus, ECW becomes a lesser and ICW a greater proportion of TBW. Plasma volume remains constant at 4% to 5% of body weight throughout life. Of course, the abso-

Table 24-1 Compartment volumes

	Percentage of body weight	Percentage of total body water	Volume in 70 kg man
Total body water	60		42 L
Extracellular water	20	33	14 L
Plasma	5	8	3.5 L
Interstitial fluid	15	25	10.5 L
Intracellular water	40	67	28 L

lute volumes of TBW, ECW, ICW, and plasma all increase with growth.

Composition of body water compartments (Table 24-2)

Plasma compartment. The plasma compartment is the only compartment the composition of which is directly measurable. Notice that the concentration of ions in the plasma is lower than that in *plasma water*. The reason is that plasma is composed of water, ions, and macromolecules. Ions are present only in the water phase. The term *plasma water* is used to indicate this aqueous fraction in distinction to the remainder, which is composed of protein, lipid, and other macromolecules. The concentration of ions in plasma is lower than that in plasma water because plasma contains both the plasma water (in which plasma ions are dissolved) and the macromolecule fraction (in which no ions are dissolved). Plasma water represents only 93% of total plasma volume. Consequently the concentration of ions in plasma is 93% of that in plasma water (see p. 461). It should be emphasized that although the concentration of ions in plasma is that portion conventionally measured and reported, it is the concentration of ions in plasma water that affects the distribution of ions across the capillary endothe-

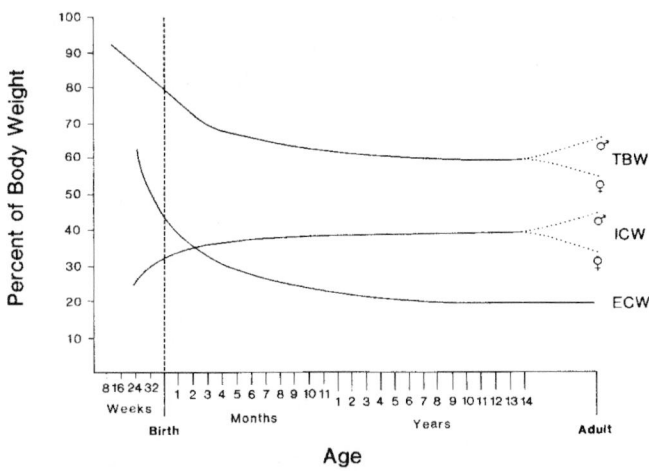

Fig. 24-3 Changes in body water compartments (expressed as a percentage of body weight) with age. *TBW,* Total body water; *ICW,* intracellular water; *ECW,* extracellular water. (Adapted from data of Friis-Hansen B: *Acta Paediatr Scand* 46[suppl 110]:1, 1957.)

Table 24-2   Composition of body compartments

	Plasma (mEq/L)	Plasma water (mEq/L)	Interstitial fluid (mEq/L H₂O)	Intracellular water (mEq/L H₂O)
Cations	153	164.6	153	195
Na⁺	142	152.7	145	10
K⁺	4	4.3	4	156
Ca⁺⁺	5	5.4	(2-3)	3.2
Mg⁺⁺	2	2.2	(1-2)	26
Anions	153	164.6	153	195
Cl⁻	103	110.8	116	2
HCO₃⁻	28	30.1	31	8
Protein	17	18.3	—	55
Others	5	5.4	(6)	130
Osmolarity (mOsm/L)		296	294.6	294.6
Theoretical osmotic pressure (mm Hg)		5712.8	5685.8	5685.8

lium. If there is an abnormally increased amount of macromolecules in the plasma (such as lipids), the measured plasma concentration of ions will be low even though the concentration of ions in plasma water and the resultant chemical activities of these ions may be normal. In addition to protein, plasma contains high concentrations of sodium and chloride, moderate concentrations of bicarbonate, and low concentrations of calcium, magnesium, phosphate, sulfate, and organic acids.

The sum of all the charges of positively charged ions (cations) must be equal to the sum of all the charges of negatively charged ions (anions) to maintain electrical neutrality in the plasma. Most often in clinical medicine, however, the plasma concentrations only of sodium, potassium, chloride, and bicarbonate are measured. The sum of these *measured* cations exceeds that of the *measured* anions. Therefore the sum of unmeasured plasma anions must be greater than that of the unmeasured cations. The difference between the sum of measured cations and the sum of measured anions is known as the *anion gap* and is calculated either as $[Na^+] + [K^+] - [Cl^-] - [HCO_3^-]$ or as $[Na^+] - [Cl^-] - [HCO_3^-]$ (see p. 457). The latter is frequently used because the plasma potassium concentration is relatively constant and may be spuriously elevated because of hemolysis (see p. 463). Because total plasma cation concentration must equal total plasma anion concentration and decreases in unmeasured cations have little effect in the calculation, an increased anion gap is usually indicative of an increase in the concentration of one or more of the unmeasured anions (Fig. 24-4). A decrease in the anion gap is suggestive of the opposite possibility. The most frequent use of the anion gap clinically is in the differential diagnosis of metabolic acidosis (see Chapter 25).

Interstitial fluid compartment. The interstitial fluid cannot normally be sampled in amounts sufficient for chemical analysis. The major difference between the ISF and plasma is the presence of protein in the plasma and its relative absence in the ISF. Although the concentrations of freely diffusible solute in ISF might be expected to be equal to those in plasma water, this is true only for uncharged solutes. The presence of polyanionic protein molecules in plasma, which cannot cross semipermeable membranes, leads to the Gibbs-Donnan equilibrium (see p. 448). This equilibrium results in plasma water cation concentrations slightly greater than those in ISF and plasma water anion concentrations slightly less than those in ISF. Values for ISF ion concentrations given in Table 24-2 are theoretical approximations based on Gibbs-Donnan equilibrium calculations.

Intracellular water compartment. Solute concentrations in cell water cannot be directly determined. The ICW compartment is heterogeneous; important differences exist in intracellular solute concentrations between different cell types. However, certain features of most cell fluids are quantitatively similar and distinguish ICW from ECW. The major cations of ICW are potassium and magnesium, and the concentration of sodium is always low; the major anions of cell fluids are protein, organic phosphates, and sulfates, whereas chloride and bicarbonate concentrations are low. The profile presented in Table 24-2 is for muscle cells.

Osmotic pressure and osmolarity of body fluids

Osmotic pressure is an important factor determining the distribution of water among the body water compartments. (See Chapter 14 for a description of colligative properties that determine osmotic pressure.) The *theoretical* osmotic pressure (and water attractability) of a solution is proportional to its osmolarity. The theoretical osmotic pressure of a solution at body temperature is calculated as follows:

Theoretical osmotic pressure (mm Hg) =
    19.3 (mm Hg/mOsm/L) × Osmolarity (mOsm/L)   *Eq. 24-1*

Notice that the solute permeability of specific biological membranes is not considered in this calculation. The osmolarity and theoretical osmotic pressure of each of the body water compartments are listed in Table 24-2.

Osmotic pressure can be simply seen as the force that

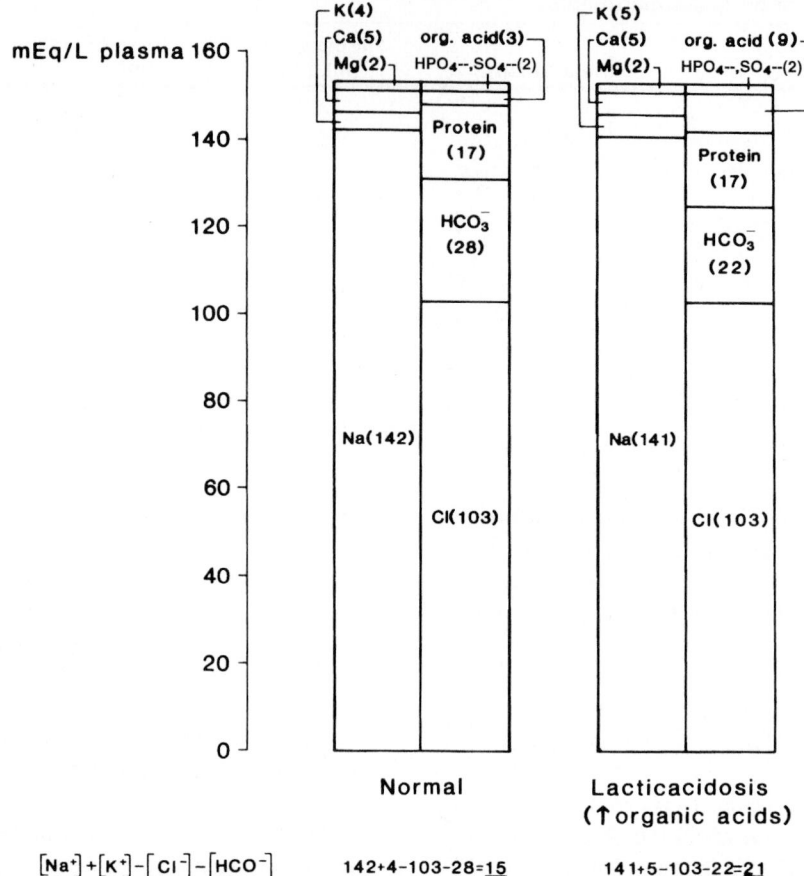

mEq/L plasma

Fig. 24-4 Increased anion gap because of an increase in unmeasured anions. *Numbers in parentheses,* concentration of ions in units of mEq/L plasma. Notice that the sum of cations (left-hand side of each bar graph) is always equal to the sum of anions (right-hand side of each bar graph), both under normal conditions and in the presence of lactic acidosis. The sum of concentrations of unmeasured anions (organic acids, HPO_4^{--}, SO_4^{--}, and proteins) is larger than the sum of concentrations of unmeasured cations (Ca^{++} and Mg^{++}). During lactic acidosis, the difference between unmeasured anions and cations becomes greater because production of lactic acid increases the concentration of organic acids.

tends to move water from dilute solutions to concentrated solutions. When a membrane is permeable to a solute, the solute exerts no osmotic pressure across the membrane—it does not contribute to the *effective* osmotic pressure of the solution. The effective osmotic pressure of a solution thus depends on the total number of solute particles in solution *and* the permeability characteristics of the particular membrane in question. The higher the permeability of a membrane to a solute, the lower is the effective osmotic pressure of a solution of that solute at any given osmolarity. For example, cell membranes are much more permeable to urea than to sodium and chloride. Therefore the effective osmotic pressure of a solution of urea across the cell membrane would be much less than that of a solution of NaCl of the same osmolarity. Measurement of the osmolarity of body compartment water is a measure only of its *theoretical,* not effective, osmotic pressure.

A solution with an *effective* osmotic pressure greater than that of plasma is said to be *hyperosmotic* with respect to plasma. A solution with a *theoretical* osmotic pressure greater than plasma is said to be *hypertonic. Hyposmotic* and *hypotonic* solutions are those with effective and theoretical osmotic pressures, respectively, less than those of plasma.

The effective osmotic pressure of plasma and ISF across the capillary endothelium by which they are separated is referred to as their *colloid* osmotic pressure. The capillary endothelium is freely permeable to most solutes in plasma and ISF. Therefore these solutes contribute to theoretical but not to effective osmotic pressure. The capillary endothelium is impermeable to large protein molecules (colloids) under usual circumstances. It is these colloids that are responsible for the effective osmotic pressure of plasma and ISF.

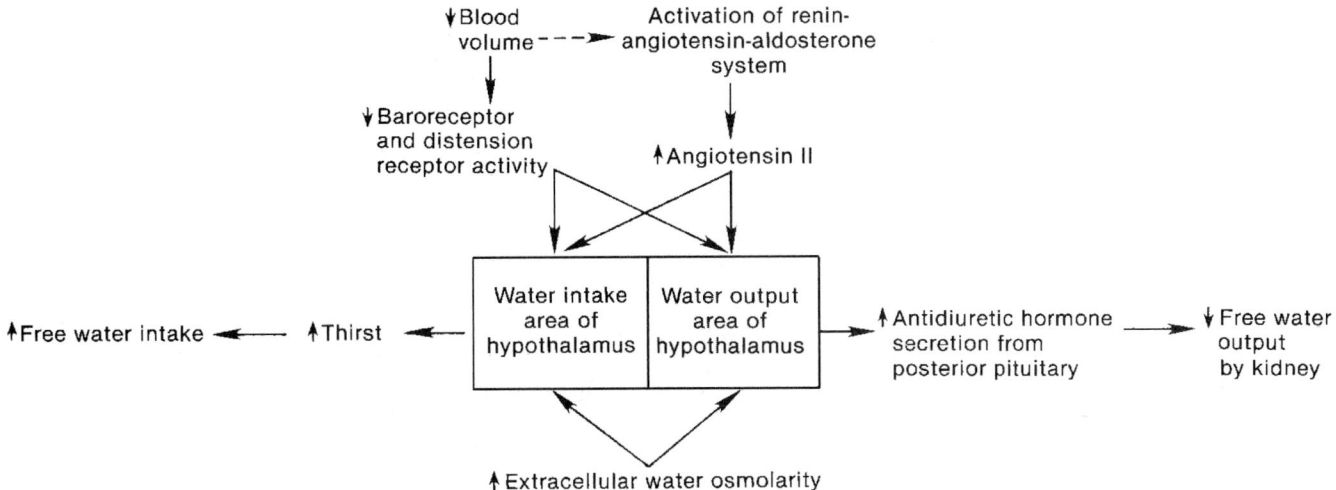

Fig. 24-5   Hypothalamic regulation of water balance.

REGULATION OF BODY FLUID COMPARTMENT OSMOLARITY AND VOLUME
Extracellular compartment

Regulation of the ECW osmolarity and volume depends on the independent control of each of these variables by the hypothalamus, the renin-angiotensin-aldosterone system, atrial natriuretic factor, and the kidney.

Water metabolism and hypothalamus (Fig. 24-5). The regulatory centers for water intake and water output are located in separate areas of the hypothalamus in the brain. Neurons in each of these areas respond to increases in ECW osmolarity, to decreases in intravascular volume, and to angiotensin II. Increased ECW osmolarity stimulates these neurons directly by causing them to shrink (increased osmolarity of ISF bathing any cell will cause water to move out of the cell into the ISF; see p. 447). A decrease in intravascular volume causes a reduction in activity of distension receptors located in the atria of the heart, the inferior vena cava, and the pulmonary veins and a reduction in activity of blood pressure receptors in the aorta and the carotid arteries. Relay of this information to the central nervous system stimulates neurons in the water-intake and water-output areas of the hypothalamus. Circulating angiotensin II seems to act directly to stimulate neurons located in these water-control areas of the hypothalamus. Stimulation of neurons located in the water-intake area produces the conscious sensation of thirst and thereby stimulates water intake. Stimulation of neurons located in the water-output area results in the release of antidiuretic hormone (ADH) from the posterior pituitary gland. Antidiuretic hormone stimulates water reabsorption in the collecting ducts of the kidney, which results in the formation of hypertonic urine and decreased output of free water (water without solute). The integration of all these control mechanisms governing water intake and output ensures maintenance of appropriate water balance.

Water and sodium metabolism and renin-angiotensin-aldosterone system (Fig. 24-6). The renin-angiotensin-aldosterone system functions as a neurohormonal regulating mechanism for body sodium and water content, arterial blood pressure, and potassium balance. Renin is a proteolytic enzyme synthesized, stored, and secreted by cells in the juxtaglomerular bodies of the kidney. Renin secretion is increased by decreased renal perfusion pressure, stimulation of sympathetic nerves to the kidneys, and decreased sodium concentration in the fluid of the distal tubule. Renin converts angiotensinogen (a polypeptide synthesized in the liver) to angiotensin I. Angiotensin I is converted to angiotensin II in the lung and kidney. Angiotensin II is a potent vasoconstrictor. In addition, angiotensin II stimulates aldosterone secretion by the adrenal cortex, thirsting behavior, and ADH secretion. Aldosterone stimulates sodium reabsorption in the distal nephron. As a consequence of this sodium reabsorption, water is retained by the body.

Sodium metabolism and natriuretic factors

There are humoral substances other than those of the renin-angiotensin-aldosterone system that play a role in regulation of sodium balance. The most widely studied is a natriuretic substance produced by cells in the cardiac atria called *atrial natriuretic peptide* (ANP), or atriopeptin. Atrial natriuretic peptide consists of at least three forms; the A-form (ANP), the B-form (BNP, also called "brain natriuretic peptide" because it is found in the brain as well as the heart), and the C-form peptide (CNP). Early studies suggested that ANP may play a major role in sodium regulation by increasing renal sodium excretion. However, more recent studies indicate that ANP's effects are modest under normal conditions but may be more important under certain clinical conditions such as congestive heart failure. Although there

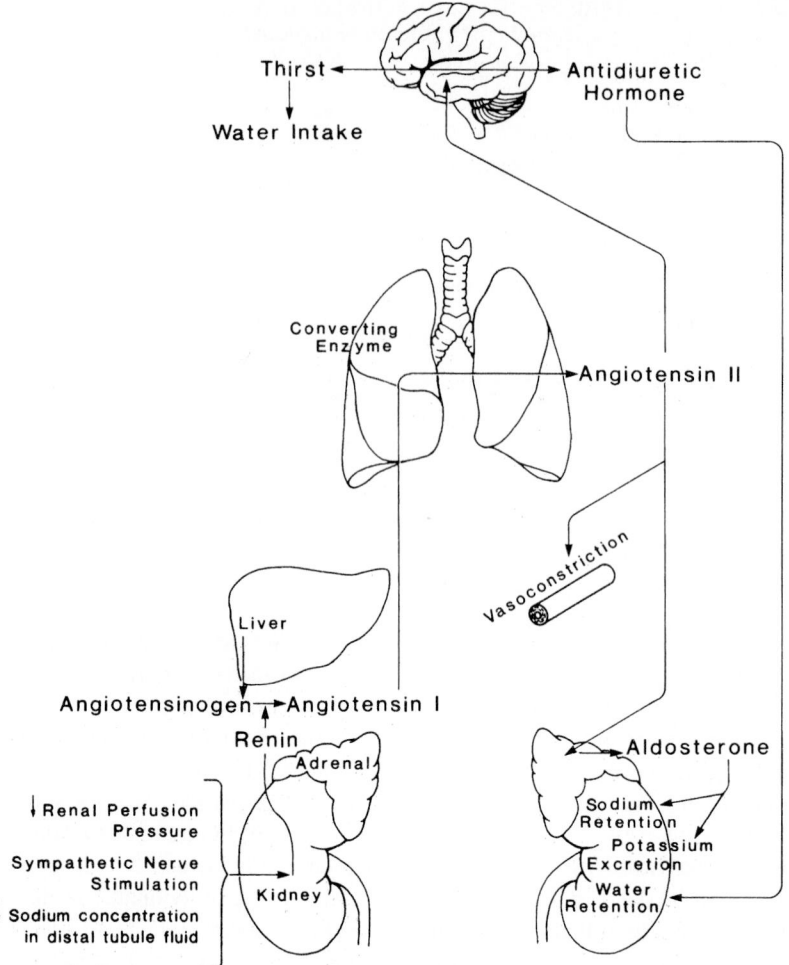

Fig. 24-6   Renin-angiotensin-aldosterone system.

is a direct effect of ANP on the kidney, much of its actions are secondary to inhibition of the renin-angiotensin-aldosterone system. *Urodilatin,* a peptide similar in chemical structure to ANP but formed directly in the kidney, may be more important in the renal regulation of sodium balance than ANP itself.

Another humoral substance that may be important in sodium regulation is the Na$^+$,K$^+$-ATPase inhibitory substance (also called "digitalis-like substance"), which inhibits the sodium pump responsible for sodium reabsorption by the renal tubules.

Factors and mechanisms involved in the control of water and sodium excretion by the kidney are discussed in Chapter 26.

Control of extracellular water osmolarity. ECW *osmolarity* is regulated by the hypothalamic control of water intake (regulatory thirst) and renal excretion of free water (see Fig. 24-5). Increased ECW osmolarity stimulates water intake and ADH secretion. Antidiuretic hormone secretion decreases renal water excretion. Increased water intake and decreased renal water excretion results in a positive wa-

ter balance, that is, water gain in excess of water loss. Positive water balance decreases ECW osmolarity to normal. The opposite occurs with decreased ECW osmolarity: thirst and ADH secretion are inhibited. Negative water balance (water loss in excess of water gain) results, and ECW osmolarity is restored to normal.

Control of extracellular water volume. Control of ECW *volume* depends on the integrated control of *water and sodium balance* by the water intake and output areas of the hypothalamus, the renin-angiotensin-aldosterone system, atrial natriuretic factor, and the kidney.

When water and sodium output exceed intake (water and sodium balance are negative), the ECW volume contracts. The associated decrease in plasma volume results in decrease in venous blood return to the heart and decrease in cardiac output. These cardiovascular changes produce the following effects:

1. Stimulation of the water-intake area of the hypothalamus and thirst center (see Fig. 24-5)
2. Stimulation of the water-output area of the hypothalamus and ADH secretion (see Fig. 24-5)

3. Stimulation of the renin-angiotensin-aldosterone system and increase in angiotensin II (see Fig. 24-6)
4. Inhibition of release of atrial natriuretic factor
5. Retention of sodium and water by the kidney

The net result of these effects is that water and sodium balance become positive, and ECW volume is restored to normal.

Expansion of the ECW volume results in the opposite sequence of events, with net loss of water and sodium and restoration of ECW balance to normal.

Plasma and interstitial fluid compartments

Water and solute distribution between the plasma and ISF compartments depends on an intact capillary endothelial surface and is controlled passively by the interaction of hydrostatic, osmotic, and electrochemical forces. The capillary endothelium functions as a continuous tube, with numerous 4 to 5 nm–diameter intercellular channels. It is freely permeable to water and small solutes and relatively impermeable to protein.

Water distribution. Water distribution across the capillary endothelial surface is controlled by the balance of forces that tend to move water from the plasma to the ISF (filtration forces) and forces that tend to move water from the ISF into the plasma (reabsorption forces). The major filtration force is plasma hydrostatic pressure in the capillary. A much weaker filtration force is the ISF colloid osmotic pressure. Since the protein concentration in ISF is negligible, colloid osmotic pressure is low. Another weak filtration force is a small *negative* ISF hydrostatic pressure. The major reabsorption force is the colloid osmotic pressure exerted across the capillary endothelium by plasma proteins. As a broad generalization, plasma hydrostatic pressure (which tends to drive water out of the capillary) exceeds plasma colloid osmotic pressure (which tends to draw water into the capillary) at the arteriolar end of the capillary so that net filtration occurs. As plasma moves along the capillary and filtration occurs, plasma hydrostatic pressure decreases and plasma protein concentration (and therefore plasma colloid osmotic pressure) increases along the course of the capillary so that net reabsorption occurs toward the venous end of the capillary. This is depicted schematically in Fig. 24-7. Overall, filtration exceeds reabsorption; therefore water must be returned to the plasma from the ISF compartment by way of the lymphatic system to prevent edema (defined as an abnormal increase in ISF volume).

Solute distribution. The small differences in the concentrations of the various extracellular solutes across the capillary endothelium are the result of the presence of polyanionic protein molecules (that is, having multiple negative charges) in plasma to which the capillary endothelium is relatively impermeable. This results in the Gibbs-Donnan equilibrium (Fig. 24-8): the presence of impermeant polyanionic macromolecules restricted to one side of a membrane permeable to solvent and small ions establishes

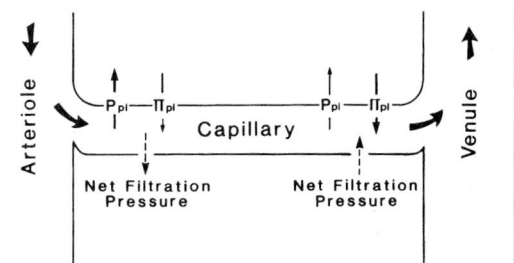

Fig. 24-7 Starling's hypothesis of water distribution between plasma and interstitial fluid compartments. Thickness of arrows representing plasma hydrostatic pressure, P_{p1}, and plasma oncotic pressure, Π_{p1}, indicate their relative magnitudes. *Dashed arrows,* Direction of net filtration pressure.

a characteristic distribution of the permeable ions. At electrochemical equilibrium, the concentrations of *diffusible cations* are slightly *higher* and the concentrations of *diffusible anions* slightly *lower* in the compartment containing the impermeant polyanionic macromolecule.

In the cases of calcium and magnesium, the larger differences between plasma water and ISF concentrations result from the fact that approximately 45% of plasma calcium and 25% of plasma magnesium is protein bound and therefore is nondiffusible.

Intracellular compartment

Water and solute distribution across the cell membrane between the ISF and ICW depends on the integrity of the cell membrane and on osmotic and electrochemical forces; all these factors are sustained by cell metabolism. The cell membrane behaves as though it were an oil film with numerous 0.7 nm–diameter pores. This membrane is highly permeable to water but differentially permeable to solutes. The permeability of the cell membrane to a solute is directly related to the lipid solubility of the solute and inversely related to its hydrophilicity (water attractability) and molecular size. Other factors being constant, membrane permeability is greater to anions than to cations.

Cell volume. Cell volume is controlled by ISF osmolarity. Osmolarity inside the cell must equal osmolarity outside the cell because the cell membrane is highly permeable to water and no hydrostatic pressure gradient can be maintained across animal cell membranes. The osmotic content of the intracellular compartment is maintained relatively constant by cell metabolism. Therefore osmotic equilibrium across the cell membrane can be maintained in the face of changes in ISF osmolarity only by the movement of water between the intracellular compartment and interstitial space. A decrease in ISF osmolarity causes movement of water into cells and an increase in intracellular volume. Conversely, an increase in ISF osmolarity causes movement of water out of cells and a decrease in intracellular volume.

Cell solute content. The ionic composition of the intracellular fluid is shown in Table 24-2. This composition

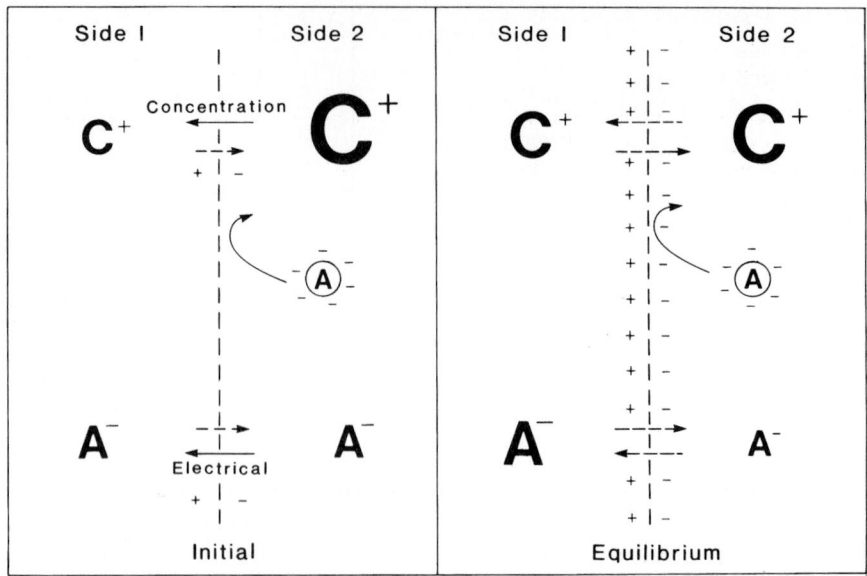

Fig. 24-8 Gibbs-Donnan equilibrium. Distribution of diffusible and nondiffusible ions and development of an electrical potential gradient across a membrane when a nondiffusible, polyvalent anion ($\overline{\underline{A}}$) with a diffusible cation (C^+) is added to one side of membrane in solution of diffusible cation (C^+) and anion (A^-). Initially, a diffusible cation moves down its concentration gradient from side 2 to side 1. This movement generates an electrical potential gradient across the membrane (side 2 negative with respect to side 1). The diffusible anion moves down this electrical potential gradient from side 2 to side 1. At equilibrium, the concentration of diffusible cation will be greater on side 2 than side 1 (as indicated by size of symbols), whereas the concentration of diffusible anion will be greater on side 1 than on side 2. No *net* movement of diffusible ions occurs across the membrane because no net electrochemical gradients exist. The concentration gradient for each ion is balanced by an equal but oppositely directed electrical gradient.

is largely the result of an energy-dependent ion-transport pump (Na^+,K^+-ATPase) found in the cell membrane that extrudes sodium from the cell in exchange for potassium. In addition, the intracellular solute composition depends on the intracellular production of nonpermeable polyanionic macromolecules. The cellular content of the other, permeable ions results from (1) electrochemical gradients produced by Na-K exchange and nonpermeable intracellular polyanionic macromolecules (Gibbs-Donnan effect), (2) the specific permeability characteristics of the cell membrane to the various ions, and (3) other energy-dependent ion-specific transport pumps. The latter two factors vary from cell type to cell type and are responsible for the differences in ionic content among various cell types.

All factors influencing cell solute content depend on normal cellular metabolism. When cellular metabolism is disrupted, as during asphyxia, solute and water enter the cell, causing it to swell.

WATER METABOLISM
Water balance

Extracellular water osmolarity is maintained constant at 285 to 298 mOsm/L as a consequence of the dynamic balance between water intake and water excretion, which is controlled by the mechanisms discussed previously. Average daily water turnover in the adult is approximately 2500 mL; however, the range of water turnover possible is great and depends on intake, environment, and activity (Table 24-3).

Under normal conditions approximately one half to two thirds of water intake is in the form of oral fluid intake, and approximately one half to one third is in the form of oral intake of water in food. In addition, a small amount of water (150 to 350 mL/day) is produced by oxidative metabolism. Oral fluid intake is the only source of water that is regulated in response to changes in ECW volume and osmolarity.

Routes of water excretion include urinary water loss, insensible water loss, sensible perspiration (sweating), and gastrointestinal water loss. The kidney is the principal organ regulating the volume and composition of the body fluids. Urine volume varies over a wide range in response to changes in ECW volume and osmolarity. Solute excretion is regulated independently.

Loss of water by diffusion through the skin and through the respiratory tract is known as *insensible water loss* be-

Table 24-3   Water balance in average adult under various conditions

	Intake (mL/day)				Output (mL/day)		
	Normal	Hot environment	Strenuous work		Normal	Hot environment	Strenuous work
Drinking water	1200	2200	3400	Urine	1400	1200	500
Water from food	1000	1000	1150	Insensible water			
Water of oxidation	300	300	450	Skin	400	400	400
				Lungs	400	300	600
				Sweat	100	1400	3300
				Stool	200	200	200
Total	2500	3500	5000		2500	3500	5000

cause it is not apparent. It is the only route by which water is lost without solute. Normally, half of insensible water loss occurs through the skin and half through the respiratory tract. The magnitude of cutaneous insensible water loss is a function of body surface area; therefore it is disproportionately greater in infants and children for weight. Insensible water loss varies directly with ambient temperature, body temperature, and activity and inversely with ambient humidity.

Sensible perspiration is negligible in a cool environment but may be quite large with increases in ambient temperature, body temperature, or physical activity. Sodium and chloride are the major ionic components of sweat, but sweat is almost invariably hypotonic to plasma. An increase in ECW osmolarity causes a decrease in the rate of sensible perspiration.

Net water loss from the gastrointestinal tract is normally small, approximately 150 mL/day. However, the *flux* of water and electrolytes between the gastrointestinal tract and ECW compartment is quite large. Therefore, if reabsorption is impaired, water and electrolyte losses from the gastrointestinal tract can be great, as with diarrhea. Except for saliva, which is hypotonic, the total solute concentration of most gastrointestinal secretions is similar to ISF.

Disorders of water imbalance

Disorders of water balance (dehydration and overhydration) result from an imbalance of water intake and output or sodium intake and output (Table 24-4).

Dehydration

Deficit of water. *Simple dehydration,* defined as a decrease in total body water with relatively normal total body sodium, may result from failure to replace obligatory water losses or failure of the regulatory or effector mechanisms that promote conservation of water by the kidney (see left box, p. 450). Simple dehydration is by definition associated with hypernatremia and hyperosmolarity because water balance is negative and sodium balance is normal. The increase in ECW osmolarity as water is lost from the body results in movement of water out of the ICW compartment. Therefore simple dehydration results in contraction of both the ECW and ICW compartments (Table 24-4).

Deficit of water and sodium. More often dehydration results from a net negative balance of both water and sodium. In this case water balance may be more negative than, equal to, or less negative than sodium balance (see Table 24-4). If water balance is more negative than sodium balance, the result is *hypernatremic* or *hyperosmolar* dehydration; if it is equally negative, *normonatremic* or *isomolar*

Table 24-4   Changes in total body water volume and distribution, total body sodium content, and plasma sodium concentration with dehydration and overhydration

	Total body water	Extracellular water	Intracellular water	Total body sodium	Plasma sodium concentration
Dehydration					
Hypernatremic	↓	sl ↓	↓	nl or sl ↓	↑
Normonatremic	↓	↓	nl	↓	nl
Hyponatremic	↓	↓↓	↑	↓↓	↓
Overhydration					
Water intoxication	↑	↑	↑	nl	↓
Extracellular water volume expansion					
Normonatremic	↑	↑	nl	↑	nl
Hyponatremic	↑	↑	↑	sl ↑	↓

nl, Normal; *sl,* slightly.

Causes of Dehydration (Water and Sodium Deficits)

Hypernatremic dehydration
  Water and food deprivation
  Excessive sweating*
  Osmotic diuresis (with glucosuria)
  Diuretic therapy*

Normonatremic dehydration
  Vomiting, diarrhea
  Replacement of losses in the above conditions with low-
    sodium liquids

Hyponatremic dehydration
  Diuretic therapy†
  Excessive sweating
  Salt-wasting renal disease
  Adrenocortical insufficiency

*If free water intake is inadequate.
†If free water intake is excessive.

Causes of Water Intoxication

Polydipsia
Psychogenic—secondary to a psychiatric disturbance
Organic—secondary to an anterior thalamic lesion

SIADH
Increased secretion of ADH by hypothalamus secondary to de-
  creased venous return to heart with no decrease in total blood
  volume
  Asthma
  Pneumothorax
  Bacterial or viral pneumonia
  Positive pressure ventilation
  Chronic obstructive pulmonary disease
  Right-sided heart failure
  Disease of spinal cord or peripheral nerves (Guillain-Barré syn-
    drome, poliomyelitis)
Increased secretion of ADH by hypothalamus in absence of ap-
  propriate osmolar or volume stimuli
  Central nervous system disorders (intracranial hemorrhage,
    hydrocephalus, skull fracture, severe asphyxia, brain tumors,
    cerebrovascular thrombosis, meningitis, encephalitis, sei-
    zures, acute psychoses, and cerebral atrophy)
  Hypothyroidism
  Pain, fear
  Anesthesia or surgical stress
  Drugs such as morphine, barbiturates, cyclophosphamide, vin-
    cristine, and carbamazepine

Ectopic, autonomous secretion of ADH
Bronchogenic carcinoma
Adenosarcoma of pancreas
Lymphosarcoma
Duodenal adenocarcinoma
Pulmonary tuberculosis
Pulmonary abscess

---

dehydration results; and if it is less negative, *hyponatremic* or *hyposmolar* dehydration results. Hypernatremic dehydration is most common. Some causes of water and sodium deficits are listed in the box above.

The degree of extracellular volume contraction for a given sodium deficit and the associated change in intracellular volume is different for each of these types of dehydration (see Table 24-4). The degree of extracellular volume contraction is least with hypernatremic dehydration because the increase in ECW osmolarity causes water to move out of the cell; contraction of ICW volume occurs. Thus the total body water deficit is "shared" by the extracellular and intracellular compartments. The degree of extracellular volume contraction is intermediate with normonatremic dehydration, since no water moves out of or into cells because there is no change in ECW osmolarity. There is also no change in ICW volume. The degree of ECW volume depletion is largest with hyponatremic dehydration because the decrease in ECW osmolarity causes water to move into cells. Intracellular water volume is actually increased.

Symptoms of dehydration. The signs and symptoms of dehydration include thirst, dry mucous membranes, decreased skin turgor, decreased urine output, and increased urine osmolarity (except when caused by failure of the kidney to conserve free water), increased blood urea nitrogen, and increased hematocrit. With increasing severity, weakness, lethargy, hypotension, and shock may occur.

Overhydration

Excessive water. Water intoxication is defined as an increase in total body water with normal total body sodium. It rarely results from excessive water consumption (polydipsia). More often water intoxication results from impaired renal free water excretion as the result of ADH secretion in excess of that required to maintain normal ECW osmolar-

ity (syndrome of inappropriate ADH secretion, SIADH; see the right-hand box above).

With water intoxication the *dilutional* hyponatremia and hyposmolarity of the ECW results in water movement into the cells. Therefore water intoxication produces expansion of the ECW and ICW compartments (see Table 24-4).

The symptoms of water intoxication are related to the degree and rate of fall in sodium. With an acute fall in serum sodium to 120 to 125 mmol/L, nausea, vomiting, seizures, and coma can occur.

Excessive water and sodium. Expansion of the extracellular compartment usually results from retention of sodium and water. This occurs with oliguric renal failure, nephrotic syndrome, congestive heart failure, cirrhosis, and primary hyperaldosteronism. In these conditions total body water excess is associated with normal or low serum sodium and osmolarity (see Table 24-4). Hypernatremia is rare with water excess. If the serum sodium is normal, the increase in TBW will be limited to the ECW.

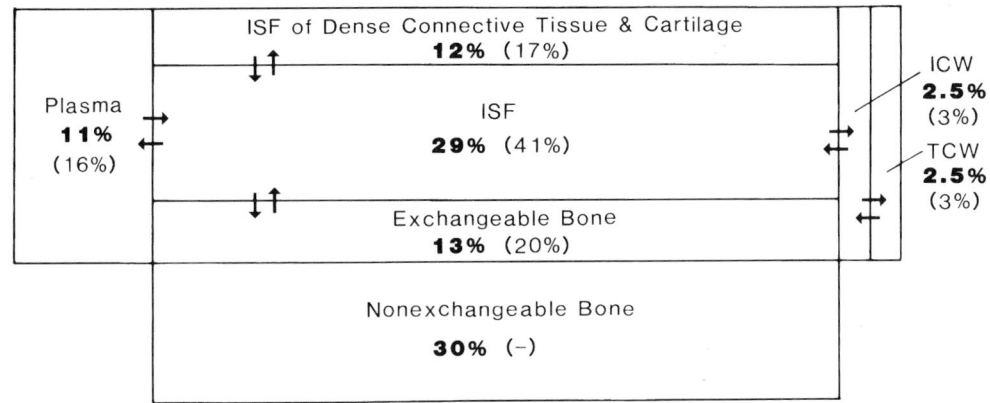

Fig. 24-9   Distribution of sodium among body compartments. *Bold numbers,* Percentages of *total body* sodium in various compartments; *numbers in parentheses,* percentages of *exchangeable* sodium in various compartments; *ICW,* intracellular water; *ISF,* interstitial fluid; *TCW,* transcellular water.

With hyponatremia the increase of TBW will be shared by the ECW and ICW compartments.

SODIUM METABOLISM
Sodium balance

In a normal adult the total body sodium is about 55 mmol/kg of body weight; about 30% is tightly bound in the crystalline structure of bone and thus is nonexchangeable. Thus, only 40 mEq/kg is exchangeable among the various compartments and accessible to measurement. The exchangeable sodium is distributed primarily in the extracellular space (Fig. 24-9). About 97% to 98% of the exchangeable sodium is found in the ECW space and only 2% to 3% in the ICW space. Approximately 16% of exchangeable sodium is in plasma, 41% is in ISF that is readily accessible to the plasma compartment, 17% is in ISF of dense connective tissue and cartilage, 20% is in ISF of bone, and 3% to 4% in the transcellular water compartment. Total bone sodium (exchangeable and nonexchangeable) accounts for 40% to 45% of the total body sodium. The concentrations of sodium in the various fluid compartments are displayed in Table 24-2. As discussed previously, the difference in sodium concentration between plasma and ISF is the result of the Gibbs-Donnan equilibrium. The difference in sodium concentration between ISF and ICW is the result of the active transport of sodium out of the cell in exchange for potassium.

The amount of sodium in the body is a reflection of the balance between sodium intake and output. Sodium intake depends on the quantity and type of food intake. Under normal conditions the average adult takes in about 50 to 200 mmol of sodium/day. Sodium output occurs through three primary routes: the gastrointestinal tract, the skin, and the urine.

Under normal circumstances loss of sodium through the gastrointestinal tract is very small. Fecal water excretion is only 100 to 200 mL/day for a normal adult, and fecal sodium excretion only 1 to 2 mmol/day. However, one should bear in mind that although fecal losses of water and electrolytes are normally small, the total volume of gastrointestinal fluid secreted is large, averaging about 8 L/day. Almost all this volume is normally reabsorbed. However, with impaired gastrointestinal reabsorption, losses of water and electrolytes are large. The volume and electrolyte content of various gastrointestinal secretions are shown in Table 24-5. Notice that most of the secretions have sodium contents much higher than that of the feces. Thus, with severe diarrhea or with gastric or intestinal drainage tubes, sodium losses through the gastrointestinal tract may exceed 100 mmol/day.

The sodium content of sweat averages about 50 mmol/L but is somewhat variable. The sweat sodium concentration is decreased by aldosterone and increased in cystic fibrosis. The rate of sweat production is highly variable, increasing in hot environments, during exercise, and with fever. Under extreme conditions sweat production can exceed 5 L/day, accounting for a loss of more than 250 mmol of sodium. Under normal conditions, in a cool environment, sodium losses from the skin are small. With extensive burns or exudative skin lesions there is great loss of sodium and water.

The major route of sodium excretion is through the kidney. Furthermore, the urinary excretion of sodium is carefully regulated to maintain body sodium homeostasis, which in turn is critical to control of extracellular volume. The details of the mechanisms and regulation of renal sodium excretion are discussed in Chapter 26.

Sodium is freely filtered by the glomerulus. Approximately 70% of the filtered sodium is reabsorbed by the proximal tubule, about 15% by the loop of Henle, about 5% by the distal convoluted tubule, 5% by the cortical collecting tubule, and another 5% by the med-

Table 24-5   Electrolyte composition and volume of various gastrointestinal secretions in a normal adult

Fluid	Volume secreted (mL/day)	Electrolyte concentration (mmol/L)			
		Na$^+$	K$^+$	Cl$^-$	HCO$_3^-$
Gastric juice*	2500	8-120	1-30	8-100	0-20
Bile	700-1000	134-156	4-6	83-110	38
Pancreatic juice	>1000	113-153	2-7	54-95	110
Small bowel	3000	72-120	3.5-7	69-127	30
Ileostomy	100-4000	112-142	4.5-14	43-122	30
Cecostomy	100-300	480-116	11-28	35-70	15
Feces	100	<10	<10	<15	<15

*Electrolyte composition of gastric juice varies, depending on acidity. The higher the acidity, the lower the sodium concentration, the higher the chloride concentration, and the lower the bicarbonate concentration. The average sodium concentration is approximately 100 mmol/L. (From Lockwood JS, Randall HT: *Bull NY Acad Med* 25:228-243, April 1949.)

Clinical Conditions Resulting in Excess Body Sodium

Cardiac failure
Liver disease
Renal disease—nephrotic syndrome
Hyperaldosteronism
Pregnancy

Clinical Conditions that Can Result in Deficits of Body Sodium

Gastrointestinal losses—vomiting, diarrhea, fistulas, drainage tubes
Excessive sweating—exercise, fever, hot environment
Renal disease
Adrenal insufficiency—hypoaldosteronism
Diuretic therapy
Osmotic diuresis—diabetes mellitus
Burns
SIADH

---

ullary collecting duct; thus normally less than 1% of the filtered sodium is excreted.

Disorders of sodium balance

Sodium excess. Sodium accumulates in the body when sodium intake exceeds sodium output because of some abnormality of sodium homeostatic mechanisms. Some major clinical causes of sodium retention appear in the box above.

Since sodium is distributed in the extracellular space, an increase in total body sodium is usually accompanied by an increase in ECW volume. An abnormal increase in ECW volume, particularly an increase in the interstitial space, produces tissue swelling known as *edema*. Thus those clinical conditions associated with sodium retention are frequently characterized by the presence of edema. Clinically, edema is characterized by swelling and puffiness of the body.

Congestive heart failure. When the heart begins to fail as a pump, a series of pathophysiological mechanisms occur leading to retention of sodium. The failing heart does not pump as much blood to the kidney, resulting in less sodium filtration, greater reabsorption, and consequently less excretion. The greater venous backpressure generated from the failing heart causes fluid to move from the vascular space to the interstitial space, decreasing the effective plasma volume and cardiac output. These factors stimulate the secretion of angiotensin II, aldosterone, and ADH and decrease release of atrial natriuretic factor. These hormone responses further enhance salt and water retention.

Liver disease. In some liver diseases there is venous obstruction, which results in increased sinusoidal and portal venous pressure. These in turn lead to leakage of fluid out of the vascular space into the peritoneal space (ascites), which lowers the effective plasma volume. The lowered plasma volume leads to salt and water retention by mechanisms similar to those described for heart failure.

Renal disease. If the kidneys are damaged to such a degree that the glomerular filtration rate is greatly reduced and sodium excretion is thereby compromised, sodium retention will occur (see Chapter 26). Sodium retention occurs by another mechanism in the nephrotic syndrome. This syndrome is characterized by proteinuria and decreased serum albumin levels, which result in low plasma colloid osmotic pressure and therefore a shift of fluid from the vascular space to the ISF space. This in turn results in hypovolemia with consequent salt and water retention, as previously discussed.

Pregnancy. The reasons for sodium accumulation during pregnancy are still unclear, but there is no question that most women accumulate between 500 and 800 mmol of sodium during a normal pregnancy. Some suggest that the sodium accumulation may be a resetting of the normal homeostatic mechanism regulating body sodium and water.

Sodium depletion. Sodium depletion occurs when the output of sodium exceeds the intake (see the preceding box). As discussed previously, only small amounts of sodium are lost in the feces under normal conditions. However, under conditions of severe diarrhea or drainage of gastrointestinal secretions, gastrointestinal sodium excretion can be quite large. If this is not replaced by increased intake, sodium depletion will result. Moreover, since the gastrointestinal route may not be available, the intravenous replacement of water and electrolytes may be necessary. Similarly, losses of sodium through the skin are normally relatively small. However, when the volume of sweat becomes large, when the concentration of sodium in sweat is abnormally high (as with cystic fibrosis), or when there is abnormal exudation of fluid and electrolytes from the surface of the body (as occurs with extensive burns), the amount of sodium lost from the skin may be substantial and sodium depletion may occur.

When the tubules of the kidney are unable to reabsorb sodium because of disease or hormonal abnormalities, sodium loss can be excessive. For example, aldosterone deficiency, caused by disease of the adrenal gland or abnormalities in the aldosterone-regulating system, leads to decreased reabsorption of sodium in the distal nephron and total body sodium depletion. Inhibition of tubular sodium reabsorption by a diuretic also may lead to body sodium depletion.

In SIADH (see p. 450) there is water retention and hypotonic expansion of the ECW and ICW spaces. This in turn inhibits sodium reabsorption in the proximal nephron and also perhaps the distal nephron, leading to body salt depletion.

Abnormalities of plasma sodium concentration

Changes in total body sodium are not necessarily associated with similar changes in plasma sodium concentration. That is, with salt retention, plasma sodium concentration is not necessarily increased. In fact, plasma sodium is frequently decreased in sodium-retentive states. Similarly, salt depletion is not necessarily associated with decreased plasma sodium concentrations. Plasma sodium concentration reflects the relative balances of extracellular sodium and water.

Hyponatremia (low serum sodium) occurs when there is a greater excess of extracellular water than of sodium or a greater deficit of sodium than of water. Some causes of hyponatremia are listed in the upper box at the right. Notice that in many cases there is an excess of total body sodium.

The symptoms of hyponatremia depend on the cause, magnitude, and rate of fall in serum sodium. With acute, pronounced hyponatremia caused by water intoxication, nausea, vomiting, seizures, and coma occur. Symptoms are less fulminant with chronic hyponatremia caused by salt depletion in excess of water depletion. With progressively severe degrees of chronic hyponatremia, constant thirst, muscle cramps, nausea, vomiting, abdominal cramps, weakness, lethargy, and finally delirium and impaired consciousness occur.

Hypernatremia (high plasma sodium) occurs when there

Clinical Conditions Associated with Hyponatremia

Water excess greater than sodium excess
   Heart failure*
   Liver disease*
   Nephrotic syndrome*
   Renal failure*
   Inappropriate ADH secretion
   Psychogenic polydipsia (excessive fluid intake)
   Essential hyponatremia (reset "osmostat")
Sodium deficit greater than water deficit
   Certain gastrointestinal abnormalities—vomiting, diarrhea, fistulas, and intestinal obstruction
   Burns
   Diuretic therapy
   Adrenal insufficiency—hypoaldosteronism
Movement of sodium from extracellular to intracellular water space
   Adrenal insufficiency—hypoaldosteronism
   Sick cell syndrome—shock
Pseudohyponatremia—hyperglycemia, hyperlipidemia, hyperglobulinemia

*Hyponatremia is dilutional, that is, secondary to excessive water retention. Total body sodium may even increase.

Clinical Conditions Associated with Hypernatremia

Sodium excess greater than water excess
   Ingestions of large amounts of sodium
   Administration of hypertonic $NaCl$ or $NaHCO_3$
   Primary hyperaldosteronism
Water deficiency greater than sodium deficiency
   Excessive sweating*—exercise, fever, hot environment
   Burns*
   Hyperventilation
   Diabetes insipidus
      ADH deficiency
      Nephrogenic—kidney unresponsive to ADH
   Osmotic diuresis*—diabetes, mannitol infusion
   Diminished fluid input—diminished thirst
   Essential hypernatremia—reset "osmostat"
   Certain diarrheal states and vomiting*

*Total body sodium is decreased. Serum sodium concentration is increased because the magnitude of water loss exceeds the magnitude of sodium loss.

---

is greater deficit of extracellular water than of sodium. Greater excess of sodium than of water rarely occurs. Causes of hypernatremia are listed in the box just above. Notice that in many cases there is actually a deficit of total body sodium.

Hypernatremia usually occurs as a chronic process secondary to loss of water in excess of sodium. Symptoms are therefore those of dehydration (see Methods, Sodium and potassium, p. 461).

POTASSIUM METABOLISM
Potassium balance

Approximately 98% of the total body potassium is found in the ICW space, reaching a concentration there of about 150 to 160 mmol/L. In the ECW space, the concentration of potassium is only 3.5 to 5 mmol/L. Total body potassium in an adult male is about 50 mmol/kg of body weight and is influenced by age, sex, and, very importantly, muscle mass, since most of the body's potassium is contained in muscle.

The concentrations of potassium in the various fluid compartments are listed in Table 24-2. The difference in potassium concentration between plasma and interstitial fluid (ISF) is attributable to the Gibbs-Donnan equilibrium. The difference in potassium concentration in ISF and intracellular fluid is the result of the active transport of potassium into the cell in exchange for sodium. Factors that enhance potassium transport into the cell and thereby increase the ratio of intracellular to extracellular potassium are insulin, aldosterone, alkalosis, and β-adrenergic stimulation. Factors that decrease potassium transport into the cell or enhance leakage out of the cell include acidosis, α-adrenergic stimulation, and tissue hypoxia.

The amount of potassium in the body is a reflection of the balance between potassium intake and output. Potassium intake depends on the quantity and type of food intake. Under normal conditions the average adult takes in about 50 to 100 mmol of potassium/day, about the same amount as sodium. Potassium output occurs through three primary routes: the gastrointestinal tract, the skin, and the urine.

Under normal conditions loss of potassium through the gastrointestinal tract is very small, amounting to less than 5 mmol/day for an adult. The concentration of potassium in the sweat is less than that of sodium, and so potassium losses through the skin are usually quite small.

The major means of potassium excretion is by the kidney. The kidney is capable of regulating the excretion of potassium to maintain body potassium homeostasis. The details of the mechanisms of renal potassium excretion are discussed in Chapter 26.

Disorders of potassium balance

Potassium excess. Potassium accumulates in the body when the intake of potassium exceeds output because of some abnormality of the potassium homeostatic mechanisms. Some major conditions causing potassium retention are presented in the upper box. It should be noted that under most conditions the normal kidney is capable of excreting a great deal of potassium, and a high-potassium intake leads to potassium retention only when kidney function is compromised.

Potassium depletion. Potassium depletion occurs when potassium output exceeds intake. As discussed previously, only small amounts of potassium are lost in the fe-

ces under normal conditions. As is the case for water and sodium, however, gastrointestinal potassium loss during diarrhea or drainage of gastrointestinal secretions can be quite large (see Table 24-5). Some major clinical conditions causing potassium depletion are presented in the lower box.

Note that alkalosis results in total body potassium depletion. With alkalosis, potassium moves from the extracellular to the intracellular space. In the cells of the distal nephron of the kidney, this increase in intracellular potassium stimulates potassium secretion and therefore increases renal excretion of potassium.

Causes of Potassium Retention

Increased potassium intake
  High-potassium diet
  Oral potassium supplementation
  Intravenous potassium administration
  Potassium penicillin in high doses
  Transfusion of aged blood
Decreased potassium excretion
  Renal failure
  Hypoaldosteronism—adrenal failure
  Diuretics that block distal tubular potassium secretion:
    triamterene, amiloride, spironolactone
  Primary defects in renal tubular potassium secretion

Causes of Potassium Depletion

Decreased potassium intake
  Low-potassium diet
  Alcoholism
  Anorexia nervosa
Increased gastrointestinal losses
  Vomiting
  Diarrhea
  Fistulas
  Gastrointestinal drainage tube
  Malabsorption
  Laxative or enema abuse
Increased urinary losses
  Increased aldosterone
    Primary aldosteronism
    Adrenal hyperplasia
    Bartter's syndrome
  Adrenogenital syndrome
  Renal disease
    Renal tubular acidosis
    Fanconi syndrome
Diuretics
  Thiazides
  Loop diuretics—ethacrynic acid, furosemide
  Carbonic anhydrase inhibitors—acetazolamide
Alkalosis

Abnormalities of plasma potassium concentration

Abnormalities in plasma potassium concentration can occur, not only because of abnormalities in total body potassium, but also because of shifts of potassium between the extracellular and intracellular compartments. Although similar shifts may occur with sodium, the effect of intracellular to extracellular shifting on plasma concentration is more pronounced for potassium, since 98% of the total potassium is intracellular. For example, if only 2% of the intracellular potassium were to shift to the extracellular space, plasma potassium concentration would double. Fortunately the plasma potassium concentration is held fairly constant despite large fluctuations in potassium intake. This homeostatic mechanism is depicted in Fig. 24-10 for increased potassium intake. The opposite effect occurs with decreased potassium intake.

Hyperkalemia. Clinical conditions associated with elevated plasma potassium are listed in the following box. Actual plasma potassium may be normal, but measured plasma potassium may be elevated (pseudohyperkalemia) if the blood sample is hemolyzed or if there is leakage of potassium from white blood cells where there is leukocytosis (elevated white blood cell number). In addition, vigorous arm exercise, tight application of the tourniquet, or squeezing of the area around the venipuncture site may result in cellular potassium release and spurious elevation of plasma potassium concentration.

True hyperkalemia can result from movement of potassium out of the cell into the extracellular water space, increased intake, or decreased output. Hyperkalemia caused by potassium shifts may in fact be associated with total body potassium depletion. This is the case in diabetic ketoacidosis. Hyperkalemia caused by increased intake or de-creased output is associated with total body potassium excess.

The clinical signs and symptoms of hyperkalemia include changes in the electrocardiogram, cardiac arrhythmia, muscular weakness, and paresthesias. The greatest danger of hyperkalemia is life-threatening cardiac arrhythmia or arrest.

Hypokalemia. Low plasma potassium concentration (hypokalemia) can be caused by movement of potassium into the cell from the extracellular water space, increased output, or decreased intake (see box on p. 456). Hypokalemia caused by potassium shifts may in fact be associated with increased total body potassium. Hypokalemia caused by increased excretion or decreased intake is associated with total body potassium depletion.

Signs and symptoms of hypokalemia are numerous and include anorexia, nausea, vomiting, abdominal distension,

---

Causes of Hyperkalemia
Pseudohyperkalemia
Hemolysis
Leukocytosis
Intracellular to extracellular shift
Acidosis*
Crush injuries
Tissue hypoxia*
Insulin deficiency*
Digitalis overdose*
High potassium intake (see upper box, p. 454)
Decreased potassium excretion (see upper box, p. 454)

*May be associated with total body potassium depletion.

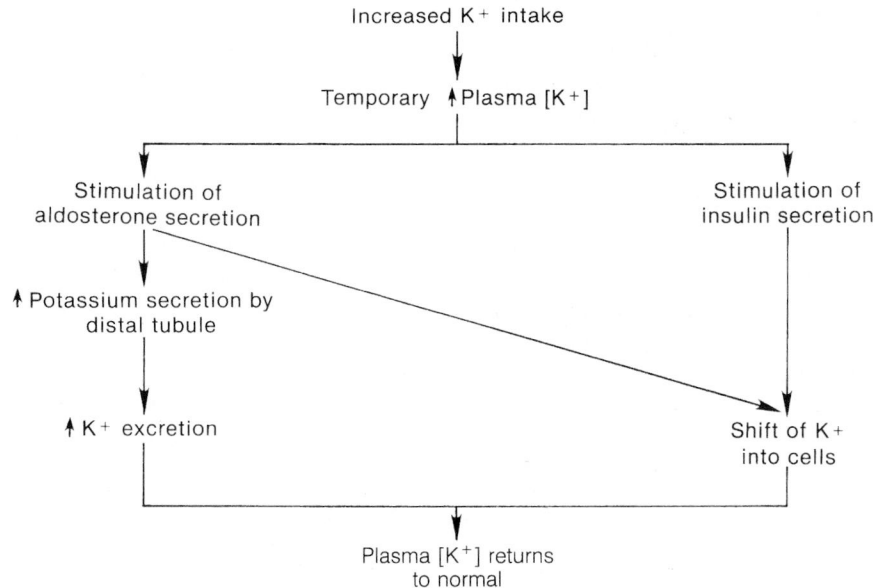

Fig. 24-10 Control of plasma potassium concentration.

Causes of Hypokalemia

Extracellular to intracellular potassium shift
  Alkalosis
  Increased plasma insulin*
  Diuretic administration
Decreased potassium intake ⎫
Increased gastrointestinal losses ⎬ See lower box, p. 454
Increased urinary losses ⎭

---

*May be associated with total body potassium excess.

muscle cramps or tenderness, paresthesias, electrocardiographic changes, arrhythmias, inability to concentrate the urine with resultant polyuria and polydipsia, lethargy, and confusion. For methods of analysis see sodium and potassium described previously and p. 461.

CHLORIDE METABOLISM
Chloride balance

Chloride is the major anion in the ECW space. In a normal adult the total body chloride is about 30 mmol/kg of body weight. Approximately 88% of chloride is found in the ECW space and 12% in the ICW space. Approximately 14% of total body chloride is in the plasma, 27% in ISF that is readily accessible to plasma, 17% in ISF of dense connective tissue and cartilage, 15% in ISF of bone, and 5% in the transcellular space. The concentrations of chloride in the various fluid compartments are listed in Table 24-2. Notice that the concentration of chloride in ISF is greater than that in plasma water, whereas the concentrations of sodium and potassium in ISF are less than that in plasma water. These differences between plasma and ISF are caused by the Gibbs-Donnan equilibrium. Chloride is passively distributed across the cell membrane. The difference in chloride concentration between ISF and ICW is caused by the electrical potential difference across the cell membrane. Because the inside of the cell is negative compared to the outside, the concentration of chloride outside the cell will be higher than that inside.

The amount of chloride in the body is a reflection of the balance between chloride intake and output. Chloride intake depends on the quantity and type of food intake. The chloride content of most foods parallels that of sodium. Under normal conditions the average adult takes in about 50 to 200 mmol of chloride/day. Chloride output occurs by way of three primary routes: the gastrointestinal tract, the skin, and the urinary tract.

Under normal circumstances loss of chloride through the gastrointestinal tract is very small. Fecal chloride excretion for a normal adult is only 1 to 2 mmol/day. The concentrations of chloride in gastrointestinal secretions are shown in Table 24-5. With severe diarrhea or with gastric or intestinal drainage tubes, chloride loss through the gastrointestinal tract may exceed 100 mmol/day.

The chloride composition of sweat averages about 40 mEq/L but is somewhat variable. As in the case of sodium, the concentration of chloride in sweat is decreased by aldosterone and increased in cystic fibrosis. Under conditions of excessive sweating, chloride losses through the skin can exceed 200 mmol/day. However, under normal conditions chloride losses through the skin are small.

The major route of chloride excretion is through the kidney. Details of the mechanisms of renal chloride excretion are discussed in Chapter 26.

Disorders of chloride balance

Chloride excess. Chloride accumulates in the body when the intake of chloride exceeds output because of some abnormality of chloride homeostasis mechanism. For the most part, the causes of chloride retention mainly are the same as those of sodium retention. Therefore the pathophysiology of chloride excess is in most cases similar to that of sodium excess (see left box, p. 452). However, there is one clinical condition in which chloride excess may not be associated with sodium excess: certain types of metabolic acidosis. The two major extracellular anions are chloride and bicarbonate. Extracellular bicarbonate is consumed by the reaction with hydrogen ions produced in metabolic acidosis. If no organic anions are produced with the H^+, chloride ions are needed to replace the consumed bicarbonate ions to maintain electrical neutrality. The increase in chloride concentration is caused by the reabsorption of a relatively greater proportion of sodium with chloride than with bicarbonate by the tubules of the kidney.

Chloride depletion. Chloride depletion occurs when the output of chloride exceeds intake. For the most part, the causes of chloride depletion are the same as those of sodium depletion (see right box, p. 452). However, in one clinical condition, hypochloremic metabolic alkalosis, there may be chloride depletion without sodium depletion. Hypochloremic metabolic alkalosis may result from loss of chloride in excess of sodium loss, usually from abnormal loss of gastric fluid. Bicarbonate must be retained to maintain electrical neutrality. Hypochloremia may also be associated with other disorders that involve bicarbonate retention, such as renal compensation for chronic respiratory acidosis (see Chapter 25).

Abnormalities of plasma chloride concentration

As for sodium, changes in total body chloride are not necessarily associated with similar changes in plasma chloride concentration. That is, with body chloride retention the plasma chloride concentration will remain normal if there is a proportional increase in ECW and will decrease if there is a relatively greater increase in ECW. Similarly, plasma chloride concentration may remain normal or even increase with chloride depletion, depending on the concomitant change in ECW.

In most cases the causes of hypochloremia and hyperchloremia are the same as those of hyponatremia and hy-

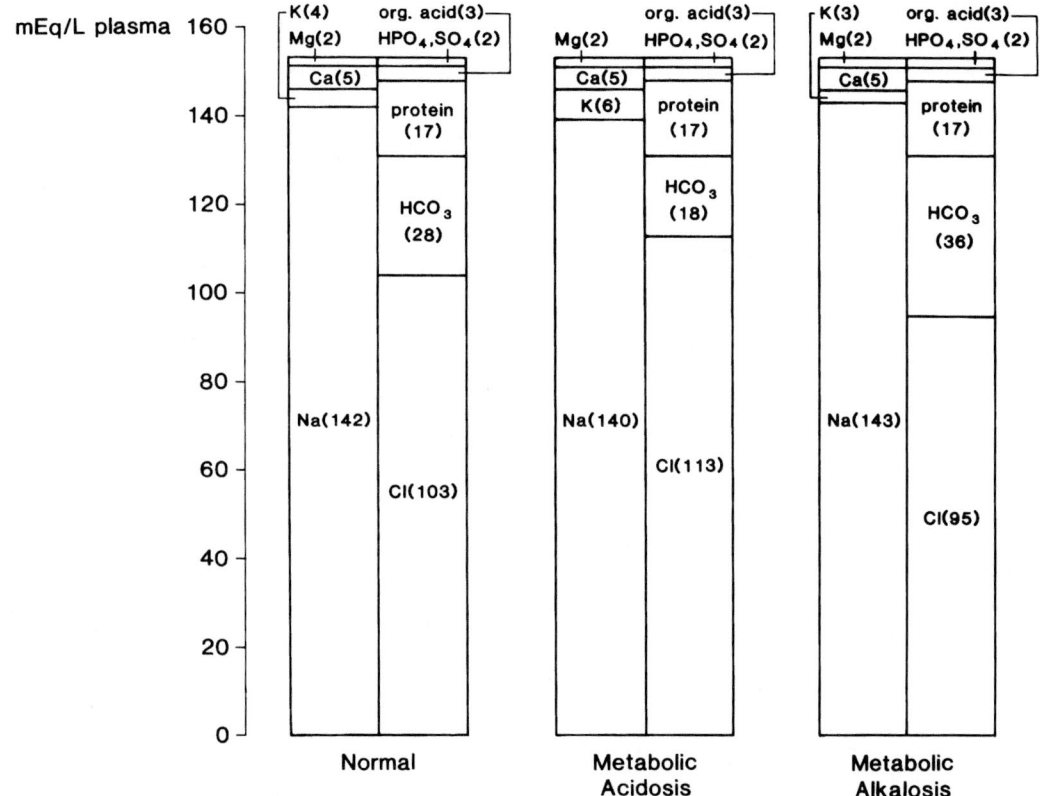

Fig. 24-11 Concentration of electrolytes in plasma (mEq/L) with metabolic acidosis and metabolic alkalosis compared to normal. In the example of metabolic acidosis shown, there is no increase in organic acids, only loss of bicarbonate. Metabolic acidosis may be attributable to an increase in organic acids (see Fig. 24-4). In these cases chloride may not be increased. Notice that the extracellular potassium concentration is elevated in metabolic acidosis and lowered in metabolic alkalosis. Under all conditions the concentration of anions equals concentration of cations.

pernatremia (see p. 453). The major clinical exceptions to the usual parallel changes in plasma sodium and chloride concentrations occur during chronic metabolic acidosis and alkalosis. With metabolic acidosis, hyperchloremia may not be associated with hypernatremia; with metabolic alkalosis, hypochloremia may not be associated with hyponatremia. The reasons for this are those previously discussed for chloride excess and depletion.

Symptoms are not directly attributable to hypochloremia or hyperchloremia. Rather, symptoms that occur in patients with an abnormal serum chloride concentration are caused by the associated abnormality in serum sodium or pH.

A summary of the plasma electrolyte changes in metabolic acidosis and alkalosis is presented in Fig. 24-11 (see the chloride method on the next page).

METHODS OF ANALYSIS

Anion gap

F. PHILLIP ANDERSON
W. GREGORY MILLER

Principles of analysis and current usage The anion gap, commonly calculated as $Na^+ - (Cl^- + CO_2)$ is an estimate

of the concentration of those anions not normally measured in serum. Because the sum of all cations must equal the sum of all anions to maintain electrical neutrality within the blood, there is no true anion gap. The anion gap is the difference between the usually unmeasured cations and the usually unmeasured anions, as follows[1]:

Unmeasured cations	mEq/L
Calcium	5
Magnesium	2
Potassium	4
TOTAL	11

Unmeasured anions	mEq/L
Protein	15
Phosphate	2
Sulfate	1
Organic acids	5
TOTAL	23
ANION GAP	12

The anion gap is used clinically to detect the potential presence of metabolic disorders affecting electrolyte balance. Table 24-6 lists disease states associated with increased and decreased anion gaps. It should be noted, however, that the use of anion gap suffers from poor diagnostic accuracy, and reliance on the anion gap value can result in misinterpretation of the patient's actual condition. The anion gap is no substitute for measurement of electrolytes, blood pH, lactate, and other data pertinent to the management of the patient.[2]

Reference interval The original studies that established the usual anion gap range measured sodium by flame photometry, chloride by the mercuric-nitrate-thiocyanate colorimetric assay, and total CO_2 by colorimetric acidification titration. Currently most laboratories measure sodium, potassium, and chloride using ion-selective electrodes. When this technology is used, chloride concentrations tend to be overestimated systematically and the sodium concentration underestimated when compared to the older methods used for quantitating these analytes.[3-6] Because the anion gap is calculated as Na^+, or $(Na^+ + K^+)$, $- (Cl^- + HCO_3^-)$, this results in a consistently smaller anion gap than that presented previously. With the newer methods for measuring electrolytes, the estimated anion gap is often ≤ 6 mEq/L and almost always ≤ 11 mEq/L.[6] These values contrast sharply to the "traditional" anion gap reference interval of 8 to 16 mEq/L.[7,8] Ideally, to be useful clinically, each laboratory should establish the anion gap based on methodologies currently used for measuring sodium, chloride, and bicarbonate.

Table 24-6 Causes of increased and decreased anion gaps

Causes of increased anion gap

Decreased unmeasured cations
   Hypocalcemia
   Hypomagnesemia
Increased unmeasured anions
   Associated with metabolic acidosis
   Uremia (renal failure)
   Ketoacidosis
   Salicylate poisoning
Not necessarily associated with metabolic acidosis
   Hyperphosphatemia
   Hypersulfatemia
   Large doses of antibiotics (such as penicillin and carbenicillin)
   Treatment with lactate, citrate, or acetate
   Increase in net protein charge as in alkalosis

Causes of decreased anion gap

Decreased unmeasured anions
   Hypoalbuminemia
   Hypophosphatemia
Increased unmeasured cations
   Hypercalcemia
   Hypermagnesemia
   Paraproteins
   Polyclonal gamma globulins
   Drugs such as polymyxin B or lithium
Underestimation of serum sodium
   Hyperproteinemia
   Hypertriglyceridemia (turbidity)
Overestimation of serum chloride
   Bromism
   Turbidity (for ferric thiocyanate method)

Chloride

W. GREGORY MILLER
F. PHILLIP ANDERSON

Principles of analysis Early methods to quantitate chloride made use of the very low solubility of chloride when combined with silver or mercury to form silver chloride or mercury chloride salts.[9]

Currently available chloride assays for routine clinical laboratory use fall into three categories: colorimetry, coulometric titration, and ion-selective electrodes. One common colorimetric method for chloride measurement utilizes the ability of chloride to displace thiocyanate from mercuric thiocyanate (Table 24-7, method 1).[10] The displaced thiocyanate reacts with ferric iron, also present in the reaction mixture, to form a red-colored ferric thiocyanate complex that can be measured colorimetrically at 525 nm. This technique is adversely affected by temperature fluctuations, necessitating that constant temperature be maintained for accurate results. Bilirubin, hemoglobin, and lipemia can also interfere in the analysis. However, the effects of these interfering compounds can be significantly reduced if a small ratio of sample to reagent volume is used (such as 0.01 mL of serum to 1 mL of reagent).

Another common method used to quantitate chloride concentrations is coulometric titration (Table 24-7, method 2).[11] The principles underlying coulometric titrations have much in common with classic titrations except that coulometry makes use of an electrochemically generated titrant. The sample is placed into a solution containing a supporting electrolyte, and a voltage is applied to electrodes immersed in the solution. The voltage causes an electrolytic reaction to occur at each of the electrodes. One of the electrode reactions results in the generation of silver ions, which then react with chloride in the sample to produce insoluble silver chloride. The end point of the titration is detected amperometrically by a second pair of electrodes as the sudden increase in free silver ions, which occurs when all the chloride ions are consumed. The number of equivalents of silver ions required to titrate the chloride ions in solution can be calculated from the number of coulombs (current × time) produced and Faraday's constant (96,487 coulombs/equivalent). In practice however, the time required to titrate a chloride standard solution or unknown sample is measured. The concentration of chloride in the unknown solution is then calculated by direct proportion of the time required to titrate a standard chloride solution. Coulometric titration is accepted as the reference method for chloride.

The precision of coulometric titration is limited by the rate of mass transfer of silver ions from the generating electrode into the sample mixture. The time needed to detect the end point once all the chloride is consumed is called the "blank time" and depends on the rate of mixing in the vessel and the rate of silver formation. The blank time should be a small fraction of the total titration time for maximum precision. Dirty electrodes will cause poor reproducibility of results; cleaning with ammonium hydroxide and nitric acid solutions between each titration has been recommended.[12] The addition of gelatin, used in the original procedure, or polyvinyl alcohol, which is more stable, in current procedures prevents reduction of silver chloride at the indicating electrodes and promotes uniform deposition of excess silver ions on the indicator cathode. This results in a smooth amperometric current and a reproducible detection of the end point. It is necessary for the titration mixture to have an acid pH to prevent the formation of poorly soluble basic silver salts. An acidic pH of the reagent mixture provides ionic conductivity and sharpens the end point by reducing the slight solubility of silver chloride.[13]

The most common method us use today for measurement of chloride concentrations is ion-selective based methods (Table 24-7, method 3). Limitations of this technology are essentially the same as those described for sodium and potassium. The ion-selective sensing element is usually silver/silver chloride or silver sulfide. Chloride measurements using ion-selective electrodes may be performed using either diluted or undiluted specimens.

Another technique for chloride analysis that has recently been described is based upon the determination of chloride-dependent α-amylase activity (Table 24-7, method 4).[12] α-Amylase, which requires calcium ion for activity, is deactivated by removal of a calcium ion with a chelating agent (that is, ethylenediaminetetraacetic acid, or EDTA) in the absence of chloride ion. The deactivated α-amylase is reactivated by the addition of a specimen containing chloride. The chloride ion in the sample allows the calcium to reassociate with α-amylase causing reactivation of the enzyme. The amount of enzyme that is reactivated is proportional to the chloride concentration of the sample. The reactivated α-amylase is allowed to act on a synthetic substrate liberating 2-chloro-4-nitrophenol, which can be detected at 405 nm with a spectrophotometer. This enzyme-based assay for serum chloride, though generally applicable to a wide range of automated chemistry analyzers, is not in current use.

All methods of chloride analysis show positive interference from other halides. The only clinically important interfering halide is bromide, which is administered in some drug preparations. Although bromide interferes with all chloride assays, ion-selective electrodes are reportedly the most vulnerable to bromide interference.[13] Although erroneously high chloride values may be obtained when specimens containing bromide are analyzed, the laboratory may have the opportunity to improve patient care by identifying bromide toxicity.

Specimen Chloride measurements may be performed on serum, heparinized plasma, urine, and other body fluids. Some nonselective analyzers can measure chloride concentrations in whole blood. Serum should be separated promptly from red blood cells because changes in the pH of the specimen will alter the distribution of chloride between cells and sera. Chloride in venous samples is approximately 3 to 4 mmol/L less than in arterial samples.

Reference interval The reference interval for chloride in serum or plasma is 98 to 107 mmol/L. Chloride in urine of healthy adults is 110 to 250 mmol/L; however, values can vary greatly depending on the chloride intake.

Osmolality

STEVEN C. KAZMIERCZAK
LAWRENCE A. KAPLAN

Principles of analysis and current usage Osmolality is a colligative property of solutions that depends on the number of molecules of solutes present in a given volume of solution. Physical characteristics of the solute, such as particle size, molecular weight, or chemical composition, do not exert an effect on the colligative properties of a solution; only the number of particles present in the solution is responsible for colligative effects (see Chapter 14 for a further discussion). As the number of dissolved particles in a solution increases, the colligative changes that occur to a solution include a *decrease* in the freezing point and vapor pressure and an *increase* in the osmotic pressure and boiling point.[14] The three types of solutes most often encountered in biological fluids are electrolytes, organic molecules, and colloids. It is important to realize that it is not the mass concentration but the molar concentration, that is, moles per kilogram of solvent, that is the basis of colligative properties. For example, the concentration of salts and low-molecular-weight organic compounds in biological fluids, such as glucose and urea, affect osmolality much more than albumin, which is present

Table 24-7 Methods of chloride measurement

Method	Type of analysis	Principle	Usage	Comments
1. Mercuric/ferric thiocyanate	Quantitative, end point	$2\ Cl^- + Hg(SCN)_2 \longrightarrow HgCl_2 + 2(SCN)^-$ $3\ (SCN)^- + Fe^{+++} \longrightarrow A_{max}Fe(SCN)_3\ (red)$	Serum, plasma, urine; manual, automated	Relatively uncommon, good accuracy and precision
2. Coulometric titration	Quantitative titration, end point	$Ag^+ + Cl^- \longrightarrow AgCl(\downarrow)$	Serum, plasma, urine, fluids, highly accurate manual; automated	Reference method
3. Ion-selective	Quantitative, potentiometric end point, or kinetic	$Ag^+/AgCl(s)$, and $Cl^- + AgCl/Ag(s)$ **Test solution Reference electrode**	Serum, plasma, urine, fluids, sweat; manual, automated	Most common method, good accuracy and precision
4. Enzymatic	Quantitative, kinetic	$EDTA\text{-}Ca^{++} + \alpha\text{-Amylase}\ (inactive) \xrightarrow{Cl^-} EDT$ $EDTA + \alpha\text{-Amylase-}Ca^{++}\ (active)$ $\alpha\text{-Amylase-}Ca^{++}\ (active) + CNP\text{-}G7$ $\xrightarrow{\alpha\text{-} \&\ \beta\text{-glucosidase}} 2\text{-Chloro-4-nitrophenol}$ $(\lambda_{max} = 405\ nm)$	Adaptable to wide variety of instruments	Under investigation

CNP-G7, 2-Chloro-4-nitrophenol–β-ᴅ-maltoheptaoside.

in a large mass amounts but is present at low molar concentrations. Thus, the molar concentration of serum NaCl, present at approximately 9 g/L, is approximately 150 mmol/L. The molar concentration of serum albumin, present at approximately 40 g/L, is approximately 0.58 mmol/L.

Osmolality determinations in the clinical laboratory are usually performed on serum or urine specimens. These fluids typically have an osmolality between 200 and 1200 mmol/kg (mOsm). The relationship between serum or urine osmolality and the molality of the substances present in these fluids are nearly linear over this range. Thus, a measured change in the osmolality of these fluids will be proportional to the change in molal concentration of one or more components present in the solution.

In principle, the measurement of any of the colligative properties could be used to calculate the osmolality of a solution. In practice, the colligative properties used to quantitate fluid osmolality are freezing-point depression and vapor-pressure depression. The most frequently measured colligative property used to measure fluid osmolality is freezing-point depression. When 1 mol of a nondissociating solute is added to 1 kg of water, the freezing point is depressed by 1.858° C. Adding 1 mol of a dissociating compound, such as NaCl, to 1 kg of water would depress the freezing point by 3.716° C (1.858° C/mol × 2) because 1 mol of NaCl would dissolve to form 1 mol of Na^+ and 1 mol of Cl^-.

One can measure the freezing point of the specimen by rapidly cooling the solution below its freezing point. Actual freezing of the solution is initiated by mechanical motion or vibration. The temperature of the solution is monitored throughout this whole process by use of a sensitive heat thermistor. As the solution begins to freeze, energy in the form of heat is released from the fusion of the ice crystals. As the solution warms, the temperature reaches a plateau where frozen solution (ice) is in equilibrium with solution that is still unfrozen. This temperature recorded at this plateau is the freezing point of the solution. The temperature value is converted to solution osmolality by comparison to calibration factors that are derived from freezing-point measurements performed on solutions of known osmolality.

A less common measured colligative property used to quantitate fluid osmolality is vapor-pressure depression. The vapor-pressure osmometer does not actually measure vapor pressure but instead measures the dew-point temperature of the vapor. The dew-point is the temperature at which air is saturated with solvent vapor that is at equilibrium with solvent in the liquid phase.[14] The greater the amount of dissolved particles present in solution (increased osmolality), the lower is the vapor pressure of the aqueous component of the solution. An important exception to this rule occurs when the solute itself is a volatile substance. Examples of commonly encountered volatile compounds include ethanol, methanol, isopropanol, and ethylene glycol. A major disadvantage of vapor-pressure osmometers is that they do not detect these volatile solutes. Volatile solutes contribute to the total vapor pressure present above the solution, though they decrease the vapor pressure of the water portion of the solution. Thus, the decreased vapor pressure of water is counterbalanced by the increase in vapor pressure caused by the presence of a volatile substance. However, as the concentration of the volatile substance increases in aqueous solu-

tions, the vapor pressure above the solution actually increases, resulting in falsely low osmolality values.

A quick procedure frequently used to estimate the osmolality of serum or plasma is performed by summation of the molar concentrations of the principle active osmolar solutes present in these fluids.[15] Several formulas for calculating serum osmolality have been proposed; the simplest and most frequently used is the following:

$$\text{Calculated mOsm/L } H_2O = $$
$$1.86\,[Na^+] + \frac{\text{Glucose (mg/L)}}{180 \text{ mg/mmol}} + \frac{\text{BUN (mg/L)}}{28 \text{ mg/mmol}} \qquad \textit{Eq. 24-2}^{16}$$

where sodium concentrations are expressed in millimoles per liter (mmol/L), and the concentrations of glucose and blood urea nitrogen (BUN) are divided by their respective formula equivalent weights, 180 and 28, to convert these mass concentrations into millimoles per liter (mmol/L).[3] Other formulas that have been proposed include the following two:

$$\text{Calculated mOsm/L } H_2O = $$
$$1.86\,[Na^+] + \frac{\text{Glucose (mg/L)}}{180 \text{ mg/mmol}} + \frac{\text{BUN (mg/L)}}{28 \text{ mg/mmol}} + 9 \quad \textit{Eq. 24-3}^{17}$$

$$\text{Calculated mOsm/L } H_2O = $$
$$2\,[NA^+] + \frac{\text{Glucose (mg/L)}}{200} + \frac{\text{BUN (mg/L)}}{30} \qquad \textit{Eq. 24-4}^{15}$$

These formulas are designed to balance simplicity and ease of calculation with the goal of obtaining results that closely compare to a measured osmolality. It is important to note that although osmolality should be expressed as milliosmoles per kilogram (mOsm/kg) of water, it is most frequently calculated and reported as milliosmoles per liter (mOsm/L) of water. The slight error introduced has little clinical significance.[17] The difference between the measured and calculated serum osmolality, the "osmolality gap," has been suggested as a rapid test for the detection of ingested volatile substances, especially alcohols.[18] There is very good correlation between the alcohol concentration measured enzymatically and that determined by calculation.[19]

Specimen Blood collected without the use of any anticoagulant is the preferred specimen. The serum should be removed from the clotted blood cells as rapidly as possible. Urine or other body fluids are also acceptable provided they have been well centrifuged to remove cellular debris. Random urine samples can vary considerably in the concentration of analytes and thus are rarely useful clinically. The preferred specimen for the measurement of urine osmolality is an aliquot of a 24-hour urine collection.

Any fluid that is left uncovered will have an increased osmolality because of evaporation and concentration of sample solutes. Serum osmolality is stable for 3 hours at room temperature and for up to 3 days at 4° C.[20] Urine osmolality may be stable at 4° C for up to 24 hours[20] and for several weeks if frozen.

Reference interval

SERUM. Reported reference intervals for serum osmolality typically range between 282 and 300 mOsm/kg. No sex- or age-related differences for serum osmolality have been reported.

URINE. Urine osmolality will vary considerably with diet. Twenty-four-hour osmolalities will vary between 50 and 1200 mOsm/24 hours.

CEREBROSPINAL FLUID. Cerebrospinal fluid and other normal body fluids will have an osmolality that is essentially equal to that of serum drawn at the same time.

Sodium and potassium

WILLIAM J. KORZUN
W. GREGORY MILLER

Principles of analysis and current usage The most common method in use today for quantitation of sodium and potassium is ion-selective electrode potentiometry (ISE). Only a small percentage of laboratories utilize flame atomic emission spectroscopy (FAES). Spectrophotometric methods for sodium and potassium based upon the interaction of sodium or potassium with chromogenic macrocyclic ionophores that are capable of selectively complexing the analyte of interest have also been described.

The FAES method (Table 24-8, method 1) has a broad range of clinical applications for quantitation of alkali metals, including sodium, potassium, and lithium. Chapter 4 describes the principles of FAES. Briefly, when a sample containing sodium or chloride is aspirated into a propane flame, fine droplets of solution are formed. The heat of the propane flame (about 1925° C) evaporates the solvent leaving sodium and potassium salt particles dispersed in the flame. The heat breaks down the salt particles into gaseous ions of sodium and potassium. These ions gain electrons from reducing gases present in the flame to form the ground-state atoms, Na^0 and K^0. A small percentage of these ground-state atoms absorb enough heat energy to attain the more highly energetic, or excited, states of Na* and K*. After about 10^{-13} seconds, the excited atoms reemit this gained energy as a photon of light. Sodium emission is usually monitored at 589 nm, potassium at 766 nm, lithium at 671 nm, and cesium (used as an internal standard) at 852 nm. The amount of emitted light is directly proportional to the concentration of these metals. Although only 1% to 5% of the atoms in the flame are excited to emission, this is sufficient for accurate and precise quantitation of these elements.

FAES methods typically employ a 1:100 or 1:200 dilution of sample with a diluent containing lithium or cesium as an internal standard. Thus the FAES method for sodium and potassium is an indirect method (see proceeding text) because predilution of the sample occurs before analysis. The use of internal standards minimizes measurement errors (see Chapter 23).

Measurement of sodium and potassium with ion-selective electrode (ISE) methods use glass ion-exchange membranes for sodium and liquid ion-exchange membranes incorporating valinomycin for potassium. Figs. 24-12 and 24-13 are schemas of sodium-selective and potassium-selective electrodes. Typical sodium electrodes have a thousandfold greater selectivity for Na^+ than for K^+ and are insensitive to pH above 1. Although the Na^+/K^+ ratio in serum is approximately 30, the potassium electrode has adequate selectivity, and so sodium does not interfere.

There are two general types of ISE measurements made on clinical samples, "direct" and "indirect." Direct potentiometric systems measure the ion activity in an undiluted sample, whereas indirect ISE systems measure the ion activity in a prediluted sample. There are significant differences in sodium concentrations when measured by either the direct or the indirect methods, especially for certain pathophysiological conditions. Artifactually low values of sodium may be measured in samples that have elevated lipid or protein concentrations when indirect ISE methods are used.[21] The reasons for the low values obtained in these conditions is the decrease in the percentage of water (water content) in plasma; sodium is dissolved only in the water portion of serum. A decrease in the percentage of the sample that is water results in there being less sodium present in a given volume of sample; the rest of the sample may be protein or lipid, even though the concentration of sodium present in the water phase may be unaltered.

When the interference is caused by lipemia, one can use an ultracentrifuge to remove the excess lipid volume from the sample to get a physiologically meaningful result. If the interference is caused by protein, indirect ISE methods are inappropriate and a "direct" ISE method must be used to obtain a clinically reliable result. In patients with hyperproteinemia resulting from conditions such as multiple myeloma, low sodium values may also be caused by the cationic nature of some of the paraproteins or to sampling errors caused by high serum viscosity.[21]

Table 24-8 Methods of sodium and potassium analysis

Method	Type of analysis	Principle	Usage	Comments
1. Flame atomic emission spectroscopy (FAES)	Quantitation of mass concentration	Excited atom emits photon	Serum, urine CSF, other body fluids	Reference method; dilution error possible
2. Ion-selective electrode potentiometry (ISE)	Quantitation of chemical activity	Ion-selective electrode measures potentiometric change as function of ion concentration	Serum, urine CSF	Dilution error possible by indirect procedure; urine analysis may have limited linear range
3. Chromogenic ionophore	Quantitative ionic complexation	K^+ + Ionophore $\longrightarrow$ *Colored complex*	Serum	Physician's office instruments; dilution error possible
4. Enzymatic	Quantitation of Na^+- or K^+-dependent enzyme activity	Na^+ or K^+ in sample modifies activity of Na^+- or K^+-dependent enzyme	Serum	Currently under investigation

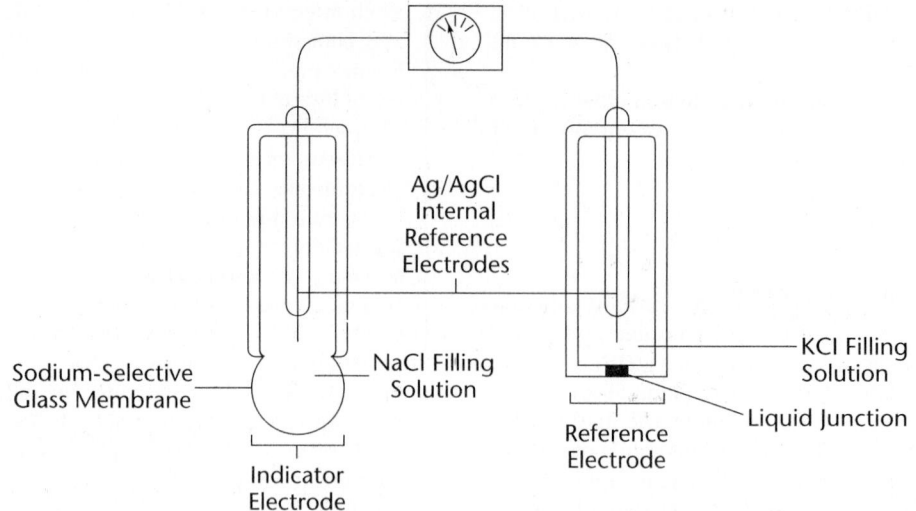

Fig. 24-12 Schema of a sodium-selective glass electrode. Glass membrane is made selective for sodium by molar ratios of Na_2O and Al_2O_3 in the SiO_2 matrix.

The effect of hyperlipidemia or hyperproteinemia does not usually create a problem of clinical interpretation for potassium because the reference interval for potassium is fairly large with respect to the magnitude of concentration of potassium in serum. For potassium, the size of the reference interval (3.6 to 5.0 mmol/L) represents a 33% change in concentration, whereas for sodium the reference interval (135 to 145 mmol/L) extends over only a 7% change in concentration.

Spectrophotometric methods for sodium and potassium have recently been developed based on the use of chromogenic macrocyclic ionophores. Chromogenic ionophores are novel molecular structures capable of selectively complexing alkali metal cations, a property previously attributable only to certain naturally occurring compounds such as the potassium-selective valinomycin molecule. The specificity and selectivity of ion binding is strongly dependent on the size and stability of the three-dimensional structure of the cyclic organic ionophore molecule. One type of complexation reaction specifically extracts K^+ into an organic phase containing the ionophore. The charged K^+-ionophore complex then mediates protonation of an organic-phase dye molecule with a subsequent spectral change that is proportional to K^+ concentration.[22] A similar organic extraction phase using valinomycin and a pH indicator is used to measure potassium in a dry film format. A third approach for K^+ and Na^+ employs a water-soluble ionophore that is covalently attached to an acid-base indicator dye. Complexation at constant pH pro-

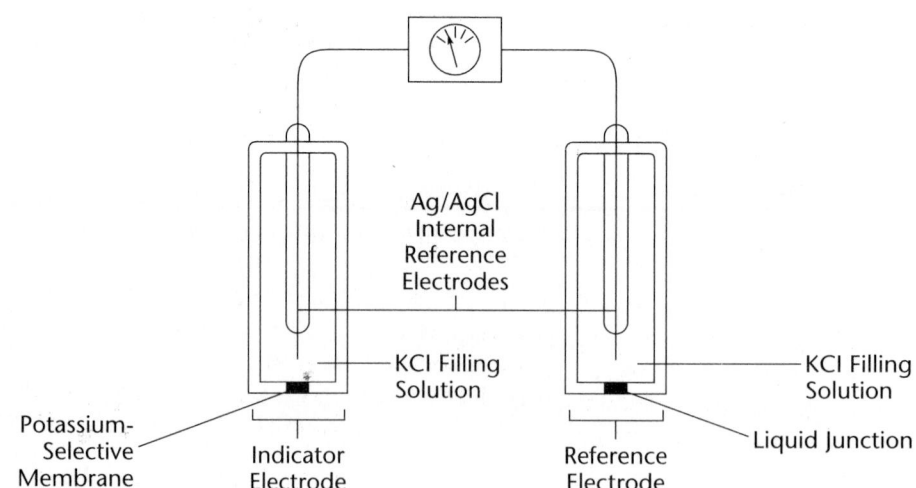

Fig. 24-13 Schema of potassium-selective electrode. The potassium-selective membrane is typically composed of a polyvinyl chloride film in which molecules of valinomycin are dissolved.

duces a change in the dye pK_a that results in an absorbance spectral shift proportional to the concentration of ion.[23]

Enzymatic methods for sodium and potassium that are adaptable to routine laboratory analyzers have been reported. A kinetic assay for sodium based on the measurement of sodium-dependent β-galactosidase (EC 3.2.1.23) activity has been described,[24] whereas measurement of potassium based on the activation of pyruvate kinase (EC 2.7.1.40) has also been reported.[25]

Specimen Serum, heparinized plasma or whole blood, urine, and other body fluids are acceptable specimens. Potassium concentrations in plasma may be 0.1 to 0.2 mmol/L lower than those in serum because of the release of potassium from platelets during the coagulation process. Heparinized plasma in which the heparin is present as the sodium salt is unacceptable for sodium analysis unless the tube is completely filled with blood. Ammonium heparin is unacceptable when ion-selective electrodes or chromogenic methods are used because ammonium ions in high concentrations give falsely high values.

Hemolysis must be strictly avoided when one is measuring potassium because even minimal red blood cell lysis can significantly increase the potassium concentration of the sample. Erythrocytes contain minimal amounts of sodium, as compared to sodium found in plasma; thus hemolysis does not affect the measured sodium concentration unless the hemolysis is severe, whereby a dilutional effect will cause a decrease in measured sodium concentrations. Serum, plasma, and other fluids should be separated from cells within 3 hours. Plasma and serum sodium and potassium are stable for at least 1 week at room or refrigerator temperatures and for at least 1 year frozen.

Reference interval

Sodium	135-145 mmol/L
Potassium	3.6-5.0 mmol/L

These intervals were obtained by use of indirect FAES or ISE methods. When measured by direct FAES and ISE, these intervals will be approximately higher than when measured by indirect techniques. As previously stated, plasma potassium values may be 0.1 to 0.2 mmol/L lower than serum values.

REFERENCES

1. Goldstein RJ, Lichtenstein NS, Souder S: The myth of the low anion gap, *JAMA* 243:1737-1738, 1980.
2. Natelson S: On the significance of the expression "anion gap," *Clin Chem* 29:282-283, 1983.
3. Berger R: Anion gap: low sensitivity or erroneous reference range? *Crit Care Med* 19:129-130, 1991.
4. Cembrowski GS, Westgard JO, Kurtycz DFI: Use of anion gap for the quality control of electrolyte analyzers, *Am J Clin Pathol* 79:688, 1983.
5. Bockelman HW, Cembrowski GS, Kurtcyz DFI, et al: Quality control of electrolyte analyzers: evaluation of the anion gap average, *Am J Clin Pathol* 81:219, 1984.
6. Winter SD, Pearson JR, Gabow PA, et al: The fall of the serum anion gap, *Arch Intern Med* 150:311, 1990.
7. Emmett ME, Narins RG: Clinical use of the anion gap, *Medicine* 56:38-54, 1977.
8. Oh MS, Carroll WJ: Current concepts: anion gap, *N Engl J Med* 297:814-817, 1977.
9. Mather A: Chloride, direct mercurimetric titration (provisional). In Faulkner WR, Meites S, editors: *Selected methods of clinical chemistry,* Washington, D.C., 1982, American Association for Clinical Chemistry, vol 9, pp 153-155.
10. Levinson SS: Chloride, colorimetric method. In Faulkner WR, Meites S, editors: *Selected methods of clinical chemistry,* Washington, D.C., 1982, American Association for Clinical Chemistry, vol 9, pp 143-148.
11. Dietz AA, Bond EE: Chloride, coulometric-amperometric methods. In Faulkner WR, Meites S, editors: *Selected methods of clinical chemistry,* Washington, D.C., 1982, American Association for Clinical Chemistry, vol 9, pp 149-52.
12. Ono T, Taniguchi J, Mitsumaki H, et al: A new enzymatic assay of chloride in serum, *Clin Chem* 34:552-553, 1988.
13. Emancipator K, Kroll MH: Bromide interference: Is less really better? *Clin Chem* 36:1470-1473, 1990.
14. Kayne FJ: *Osmolality: review of methods,* American Society of Clinical Pathologists, Check Sample, vol 9, no 7, Chicago, 1993; PTS 93-7 (PTS-73).
15. Weisberg HF: Osmolality—calculated "delta" and more formulas, *Clin Chem* 21:1182-1184, 1975.
16. Holmes JH: Measurement of osmolality in serum urine and other biologic fluids by the freezing point determination. In preworkshop manual on *Urinalysis of renal function studies,* Chicago, 1962, American Society of Clinical Pathologists, Commission on Continuing Education.
17. Dorwart WV, Chalmers L: Comparison of methods for calculating serum osmolality from chemical concentrations, and the prognostic value of such calculations, *Clin Chem* 21:190-194, 1975.
18. Bhagat CI, Garcia-Webb P, Fletcher E, Beilby JP: Calculated vs. measured plasma osmolalities revisited, *Clin Chem* 30:1703-1705, 1985.
19. Loeb JN: The hyperosmolar state, *N Engl J Med* 290:1184-1187, 1974.
20. Weissman N, Pilegg VJ: Inorganic ions. In Henry RJ, Cannon DC, Winkleman JW, editors: *Clinical chemistry principles and techniques,* New York, 1974, Harper & Row.
21. Ladenson JH, Apple FS, Aguanno JJ, Koch DD. Sodium measurements in multiple myeloma: two techniques compared, *Clin Chem* 28:2383-2386, 1982.
22. Sumiyoshih H, Nakahara K, Ueno K: New convenient colorimetric determination of potassium in blood serum, *Talanta* 24:763-765, 1977.
23. Kumar A, Chapoteau E, Czech BP, et al: Chromogenic ionophore–based methods for spectrophotometric assay of sodium and potassium in serum and plasma, *Clin Chem* 34:1709-1712, 1988.
24. Berry MN, Mazzachi RD, Pejakovic M, Peake MJ: Enzymatic determination of sodium in serum, *Clin Chem* 34:2295-2298, 1988.
25. Berry MN, Mazzachi RD, Pejakovic M, Peake MJ: Enzymatic determination of potassium in serum, *Clin Chem* 35:817-820, 1989.

BIBLIOGRAPHY

Atlas SA: Atrial natriuretic factor: renal and systemic effects, *Hosp Pract* 21(7):67, 1986.
Badrick T, Hickman PE: The anion gap—a reappraisal, *Am J Clin Pathol* 98:249-252, 1992.
Cohen JJ: Disorders of potassium balance, *Hosp Pract* 14(1):119, 1979.
Collins RD: *Illustrated manual of fluid and electrolyte disorders,* Philadelphia, 1983, Lippincott.
Hays RM: Antidiuretic hormone, *N Engl J Med* 295:659, 1976.
Inagami T: Atrial natriuretic factor as a volume regulator, *J Clin Pharmacol* 34:424, 1994.
Kokko JP, Tannen RL: *Fluids and electrolytes,* Philadelphia, 1986, Saunders.
Levey M: The pathophysiology of sodium balance, *Hosp Pract* 13:95, 1978.
Lolekha PH, Lolekha S: Value of the anion gap in clinical diagnosis and laboratory evaluation, *Clin Chem* 29:279-283, 1983.
Narins RG, editor: *Maxwell and Kleeman's clinical disorders of fluid and electrolyte metabolism,* ed 5, New York, 1994, McGraw-Hill.
Oh MS, Carroll HJ: The anion gap, *N Engl J Med* 297:814, 1977.

CHAPTER 25

Acid-base control and acid-base disorders

John E. Sherwin

OBJECTIVES

- Outline the blood-buffering mechanism of the bicarbonate and hemoglobin buffering systems.
- Explain acid-base balance regulation by the kidney with respect to the following:
  Hydrogen ion excretion
  Bicarbonate ion reaction
  Sodium-hydrogen exchange
  Ammonium secretion
- State the Henderson-Hasselbalch equation, identifying the respiratory and metabolic components; relate the equation to acid-base disorders; and calculate the pH given appropriate data.
- For each of the following pathological states, identify the expected pH, P_{O_2}, and P_{CO_2} values as normal, increased, or decreased, and state the physiological response to the disease states.
  Drug-induced hyperventilation
  Acute hyperglycemic ketoacidosis
  Hypochloremia resulting from persistent vomiting
  Chronic emphysema
- Define oxygen saturation and P_{50}, and describe the effect of the following on dissociation of oxygen from hemoglobin:
  2,3-DPG
  pH
  P_{CO_2}

KEY TERMS

acidemia A condition of decreased pH of the blood.

acidosis A pathological condition resulting from accumulation of acid in the blood or loss of base from the blood.

alkalemia A condition of increased pH of the blood.

alkalosis A pathological condition resulting from accumulation of base or loss of acid from the body.

alveoli Small outpouchings of walls of alveolar space through which gas exchange takes place between alveolar air and pulmonary capillary blood.

anion gap The concentration of undetermined anions, calculated as the difference between the measured cations and the measured anions.

apnea Cessation of breathing.

base excess or deficit The difference between the titratable acids and bases of a blood sample and a normal blood sample at a pH of 7.4, a P_{CO_2} of 40 mm Hg, and a temperature of 37° C.

bradycardia Slowing of the heartbeat to less than 60 beats per minute.

buffer A solution consisting of a weak acid and its conjugate base, which resists change in pH on addition of strong acid or base.

carbamino reaction A covalent chemical reaction between CO_2 and the primary amino group (—NH_2) of a protein to form a stable, bound form of CO_2.

carbonic anhydrase An enzyme that catalyzes the reaction between CO_2 and water to form carbonic acid (H_2CO_3).

chloride shift Exchange of Cl^- in serum for HCO_3^- in red blood cells in peripheral tissues in response to the P_{CO_2} of the blood. The shift reverses in the lungs.

conjugate base Unprotonated anionic form of a corresponding weak acid.

Henderson-Hasselbalch equation Describes the relationship between pH, the pK_a of a buffer system, and the ratio of the conjugate base to a weak acid.

hypercapnia A condition of excess carbon dioxide in the blood.

hypochloremic alkalosis A metabolic alkalosis resulting from increased blood bicarbonate secondary to loss of chloride from the body.

hypoxia A condition of low oxygen content in tissues.

isohydric shift The series of reactions in red blood cells in which CO_2 is taken up and oxygen is released without the production of excess hydrogen ions.

metabolic acidosis Pathological loss of base in the body.

metabolic alkalosis Pathological accumulation of base in the body.

metabolic component The bicarbonate concentration of plasma.

oxygen saturation A term that defines the fraction of total hemoglobin (Hb) in the form of HbO_2 at a defined Po_2. Percentage of saturation = $100(HbO_2)/(HbO_2 + Hb)$.

P_{50} The partial pressure of oxygen at which hemoglobin is half-saturated with bound oxygen.

partial pressure The pressure exerted by a gas, whether it is alone or mixed with other gases. The partial pressure of a gas is denoted by the letter P preceding the symbol for that gas (usually in small capital letters); for example, the partial pressure of CO_2 is Pco_2.

pH The negative logarithm of the hydrogen-ion concentration.

pK_a The negative logarithm of the dissociation constant of a weak acid; also, the pH of a buffer at which the concentration of a weak acid and its conjugate base are equal. Maximum overall buffering capacity occurs when pK_a = pH.

relative base deficit A term that describes the lowered HCO_3^-/H_2CO_3 ratio caused by an increase in Pco_2. The HCO_3^- (base) is low relative to the Pco_2.

relative base excess Name for the elevated HCO_3^-/H_2CO_3 ratio caused by a decrease in Pco_2. The HCO_3^- (base) is elevated relative to the Pco_2.

respiratory acidosis Pathological retention of CO_2 in the body caused by respiratory change.

respiratory alkalosis Pathological decrease in CO_2 caused by respiratory change.

respiratory component The "αPco_2," or acid component, which is immediately modified by respiratory status. "α" is the solubility (or Bunsen) coefficient of CO_2.

surfactant An agent that decreases surface tension. Applies to agents that coat pulmonary alveolar surfaces.

ventilation The exchange of gases between the lungs and ambient air.

ACID-BASE CONTROL
Acids and bases (see also p. 39)

Definitions. Using the simplest definition, an acid is defined as a substance that releases protons or hydrogen ions (H^+), whereas a base is simply defined as a substance that accepts protons or H^+. Both acids and bases are further defined by their degree of affinity for H^+. A strong acid has little affinity for H^+ and so readily dissociates H^+, whereas a weak acid has some affinity for H^+ and thus less readily dissociates H^+. A strong base has a high affinity for H^+; a weak base has low affinity for H^+. If one molecule differs from another by only a proton, the two are called a conjugate acid-base pair. Physiological examples of a weak acid and its conjugate base are carbonic acid (H_2CO_3) and bicarbonate (HCO_3^-). The equilibrium reaction is as follows in equation 25-1:

$$H_2CO_3 \rightleftharpoons H^+ + HCO_3^- \qquad \textit{Eq. 25-1}$$

This equilibrium lies to the right at physiological pH because bicarbonate, the conjugate base, has a weak affinity for hydrogen ion.

Dietary and metabolic sources of acids and bases.

Two types of acids are dealt with in physiological states: fixed acids and volatile acids. Fixed acids are nongaseous acids such as phosphate (HPO_4^{2-}) and sulfate (HSO_4^-) ions or organic acids such as lactic acid, acetoacetic acid, and beta-hydroxybutyric acid. The physiologically important volatile acid is carbonic acid (H_2CO_3). The volatility of carbonic acid arises from its ability to dissociate into water and carbon dioxide (CO_2), which can be released as a gas. The reaction scheme for carbonic acid is as follows:

$$CO_2 \text{ (gas)} \rightleftharpoons CO_2 \text{ (dissolved)} \underset{-H_2O}{\overset{+H_2O}{\rightleftharpoons}} H_2CO_3 \rightleftharpoons H^+ + HCO_3^-$$
$$\textit{Eq. 25-2}$$

At one end of the equilibrium is carbon dioxide, which can be considered the anhydrous form of H_2CO_3, and at the other end is HCO_3^-, the conjugate base of H_2CO_3. Although the reaction of CO_2 and water to form H_2CO_3 will occur spontaneously, the enzyme carbonic anhydrase facilitates this reaction in vivo.

Carbohydrates, lipids, and proteins are metabolized by oxidation reactions that generate acids that must be neutralized in order to maintain constant cellular pH. Under anaerobic conditions such as those produced by respiratory distress or strenuous exercise, carbohydrates are metabolized to lactic and pyruvic acids, which accumulate until normal oxygenation is achieved. These acids can be further metabolized to the ultimate oxidation product, carbon dioxide, when aerobic metabolism is resumed. Triglycerides are metabolized to fatty acids, which can be further metabolized to ketone bodies (acetoacetic acid and β-hydroxybutyric acid) under anaerobic conditions. Ultimately these lipid metabolites are further oxidized to carbon dioxide. Proteins are hydrolyzed to amino acids, which are then converted to carbon dioxide. Those proteins composed of sulfur-containing amino acids are catabolized in part to the salt of sulfuric acid. Nucleic acids and some lipids contain phosphorus and are metabolized to salts of phosphoric acid.

pH, hydrogen ion, and buffers. Please review the discussion of pH and buffer calculations in Chapter 1. Remember, rather than describing the concentration of H^+ in moles per liter (M), the accepted convention is the use of pH, which is defined as the negative logarithm of the concentration of H^+.

Physiological buffers. Normal human whole blood is buffered at a slightly alkaline pH in a range of 7.35 to 7.45, which corresponds to an H^+ concentration of 4.5×10^{-8} M to 3.5 to 10^{-8} M. Buffering capacity depends on the concentration of the buffer and the relationship between the pK_a of the buffer and the desired pH. A buffer is considered most effective within ± 2 pH units of its pK_a. It has maximum buffering capacity when its pK_a equals the pH. For maximum blood buffering the pK_a of the buffers should therefore be near physiological pH, that is, pH 7.4. The physi-

Table 25-1 Physiologically important buffers and their concentration, pK_a, and buffering capacity

Buffer	pK_a	Concentration (mmol/L)	Relative buffering capacity (mEq/L)
Bicarbonate	6.33	25	1
Hemoglobin	7.2	53	40
Phosphate	6.8	1.2	0.3
Protein	—	—	8

ologically important buffers that maintain this narrow pH range observed in the body are hemoglobin, bicarbonate, phosphate, and proteins. Table 25-1 lists the pK_a and concentrations of these buffer systems and their relative buffering capacities.

Bicarbonate buffer system. The Henderson-Hasselbalch equation for the bicarbonate-carbonic acid buffer system (equation 25-3) is as follows:

$$pH = pK_a + \log \frac{[HCO_3^-]}{[H_2CO_3]} \qquad Eq.\ 25\text{-}3$$

The measured pK_a is 6.33 at 37° C. Instead of being at the maximum buffer capacity with a 1:1 ratio of HCO_3^- to H_2CO_3, the bicarbonate-carbonic acid buffer system at the blood pH of 7.4 is at a ratio of 20:1.

$$pH = pK_a + \log \frac{[HCO_3^-]}{[H_2CO_3]} = 6.33 + \log 20 = 7.4 \qquad Eq.\ 25\text{-}4$$

This 20:1 ratio is maintained primarily by the lungs, which expel CO_2 produced during the metabolism of nutrients.

In equation 25-3 there are three unknowns: pH, $[HCO_3^-]$, and $[H_2CO_3]$. Although pH is measurable, there is no direct measure of $[HCO_3^-]$ or $[H_2CO_3]$. To use this equation, the term H_2CO_3 is replaced by an analyte that is measurable. The concentration of H_2CO_3 is proportional to the amount of dissolved CO_2 (equation 25-2). Thus, one can replace $[H_2CO_3]$ with the term αP_{CO_2} where α (the Bunson coefficient) is the solubility coefficient of CO_2. The pK_a term in the Henderson-Hasselbalch equation is modified to reflect the equilibrium between CO_2 (dissolved) and HCO_3^-. The modified Henderson-Hasselbalch equation describing the equilibrium in equation 25-2 is as follows:

$$pH = pK'_a + \log \frac{[HCO_3^-]}{\alpha P_{CO_2}} \qquad Eq.\ 25\text{-}5$$

The apparent pK'_a in human plasma is 6.1 at 37° C. The solubility coefficient for CO_2 in plasma at 37° C is 0.031 mmol $\times$ L^{-1} $\times$ mm Hg^{-1}. The concentration of base greatly exceeds that of acid in this plasma buffer system, reflecting the demands put on the body by metabolism, which primarily produces acids. This buffer system is designed to process the primary metabolic waste product, CO_2. The CO_2 component of the buffer system is eliminated by the lungs.

The total CO_2 content (T_{CO_2}) of plasma is described as

$$T_{CO_2} = CO_2 \text{ (dissolved)} + [HCO_3^-] + [H_2CO_3] \qquad Eq.\ 25\text{-}6,\ a$$

One can disregard the $[H_2CO_3]$ term because it is so small (one twentieth the $[HCO_3^-]$) and can replace CO_2 (dissolved) with the term αCO_2. Thus the equation can be reduced to

$$T_{CO_2} = \alpha P_{CO_2} + [HCO_3^-] \qquad Eq.\ 25\text{-}6,\ b$$

Two of the three unknowns are readily determined, allowing calculation of the third (see pp. 474 and 480).

Hemoglobin. The major buffer of blood is hemoglobin, which is localized in the red blood cells. Hemoglobin (Hb) takes up free H^+ so that the following reaction proceeds to the right:

$$CO_2 + H_2O \rightleftharpoons H_2CO_3 \rightleftharpoons HCO_3^- + H^+$$

$$\searrow HHb^+ + O_2$$

$$HbO_2 \qquad Eq.\ 25\text{-}7$$

Hemoglobin and serum proteins have high concentrations of histidine residues. The imidazole group of histidine (Fig. 25-1) has a pK_a of approximately 7.3. It is this combination of high concentration and appropriate pK_a that makes hemoglobin the dominant buffering agent of blood at physiological pH. The bulk of the CO_2 formed in peripheral tissues is transported in the plasma portion of blood as HCO_3^- with the H^+ bound to hemoglobin within the erythrocyte (Fig. 25-2). The CO_2 of carbonic acid accounts for about 2 mmol/L of CO_2 in venous blood but accounts for only about 1 mmol/L in arterial blood.

Significant amounts of CO_2 are transported as a protein-bound moiety. CO_2 reacts nonenzymatically with the accessible amino groups of proteins to form a *carbamino group:*

$$\begin{array}{ccc} O\ O & H & O \\ \backslash\!/ & | & \| \\ C & + \ N\text{-Protein} \rightarrow \ ^-O\text{-}C\text{-}N\text{-Protein} + H^+ \\ | & & \textbf{Carbamino} \\ H & & \textbf{group} \qquad Eq.\ 25\text{-}8 \end{array}$$

Approximately 0.5 mmol/L of CO_2 is transported in this fashion.

The observed arteriovenous difference in total CO_2 con-

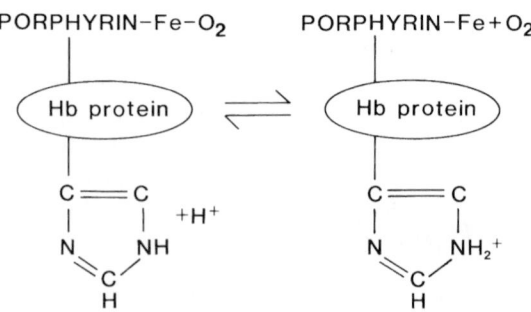

Fig. 25-1 Effect of hemoglobin oxygenation on buffering action of imidazole group of histidine. Binding affects the pK_a of the imidazole ring, making the ring more acidic with release of an H^+.

tent is almost entirely the result of formation of bicarbonate in the red blood cell. In the lungs, as deoxygenated hemoglobin becomes oxygenated and the CO_2 is expelled, the H^+ is released from hemoglobin because oxygenated hemoglobin (HbO_2) is a stronger acid than deoxyhemoglobin (HbH). In the lungs then, the reaction in equation 25-7 proceeds to the left. H^+ is released and reacts with the transported HCO_3^- to form CO_2 that the lungs can now release (Fig. 25-2). The overall equation linking the oxygenation process to buffering is

$$H^+ + HbO_2 \rightleftharpoons HbH^+ + O_2 \qquad Eq.\ 25\text{-}9$$

The forward reaction occurs in tissues in which there is a relatively high H^+ and a relatively low O_2 concentration, whereas the reverse reaction occurs in the lungs, where the O_2 concentration is relatively high.

Phosphate and proteins. Phosphate is a minor buffering component of the blood, with the following equilibrium reaction occurring:

$$H_2PO_4^- \rightleftharpoons H^+ + HPO_4^{2-} \qquad Eq.\ 25\text{-}10$$

The pK_a of this reaction is 6.8. Phosphate buffer is an important buffer in urine, which has relatively little protein, hemoglobin, or bicarbonate. The phosphate buffers in the blood are inorganic phosphates, but both inorganic and organic phosphates act as intracellular buffers.

Plasma proteins also act as buffers in the blood. This buffering effect is minor compared to the bicarbonate system or hemoglobin system (Table 25-1).

Oxygen and carbon dioxide homeostasis

Partial pressure. Blood gas analysis is performed to determine the partial pressures of oxygen and carbon dioxide (Po_2 and Pco_2 respectively). Historically, the units of Po_2 and Pco_2 have been millimeters of mercury (mm Hg), or torr, and these are still used by a majority of laboratories in

Table 25-2 Comparison of air (partial pressure expressed in mm Hg)

Air	N_2	O_2	CO_2	H_2O	Total pressure
Atmospheric air	598.0	158.0	0.3	3.7	760
Alveolar air	573.0	100.0	40.0	47.0	760
Expired air	566.0	115.0	32.0	47.0	760

the United States. The international unit for partial pressure is the *pascal,* or Pa (1 mm Hg = 133.3224 Pa).

Table 25-2 shows the composition of atmospheric air, alveolar air (air inside the lung), and expired air. Humidity makes a substantial contribution to the composition of air in the lungs, thus altering the partial pressures of the other gases. A correction for the gas-volume contributed by water vapor is therefore essential; at 37° C, the P_{H_2O} of blood is approximately 47 mm Hg.

Two terms used in discussing the oxygen content of blood are *oxygen saturation* and P_{50}. Oxygen saturation is the percentage of the total hemoglobin present as oxygenated hemoglobin. The term P_{50} denotes that partial pressure of oxygen at which the hemoglobin is 50% saturated with oxygen.

Ventilation. Ventilation is differentiated from respiration in that *ventilation* is the mechanical process of moving air in and out of the lungs, and *respiration* is the exchange of gases between the atmosphere and the body. The exchange of gases between air and the capillaries of the pulmonary circulation occurs in the *alveoli.* The normal respiration rate is 13 to 16 times per minute.

The walls of the lung contain elastic connective tissues that would collapse the lung were it not for the surface tension between the surface of the lung and the wall of the thoracic cavity. The surface tension of the inner walls of the alveoli, in contrast, has a tendency to collapse the

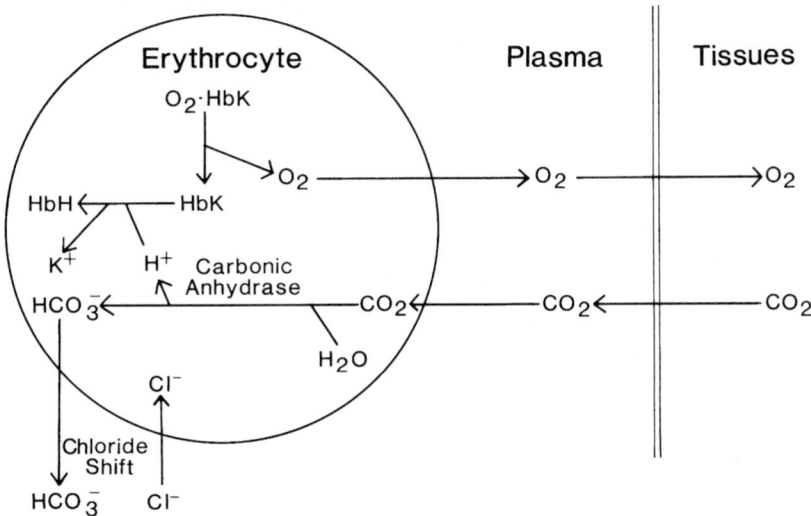

Fig. 25-2 Hemoglobin buffering action in peripheral tissues. HbK is a potassium salt of hemoglobin. HbH is the protonated form of hemoglobin.

alveoli after expiration, when the alveoli are deflated. This surface tension is reduced by the presence of a phospholipid-lipoprotein complex, a *surfactant,* that lines the alveolar walls in a thin film and allows the alveolar walls to be easily reinflated. Premature babies without sufficient surfactant lining the alveolar walls can have respiratory difficulties because of the tendency of alveoli to collapse. It is for this reason that the lecithin/sphingomyelin ratio in amniotic fluid is determined to assess fetal lung development (see Chapter 40).

Gas exchange. Gas transfer in the alveoli is a concentration-dependent phenomenon. Inspired (room) air has a relatively high Po_2 (158 mm Hg) and a low Pco_2 (0.3 mm Hg). Pressures of oxygen and carbon dioxide in capillary blood in the lungs are 50 and 40 mm Hg respectively. Because the Po_2 of blood is lower than that of inspired air and the Pco_2 of blood is higher than the Pco_2 of room air, the gases diffuse from higher to lower concentration areas. That is, CO_2 gas moves from the capillaries to the alveolar air space, while O_2 moves from the alveoli to the capillaries. Reference values for adult blood-gas parameters in arterial and venous blood are summarized in Table 25-3. Because of its greater water solubility, CO_2 exchanges more rapidly and more efficiently than O_2 does. In respiratory acidosis, this phenomenon of differential gas diffusibility can result in low blood Po_2 but relatively normal Pco_2.

Control of ventilation. Ventilatory control regulates the carbohydrate-bicarbonate buffer system but is in turn regulated by the resulting pH of cerebrospinal fluid and plasma. Control of ventilation is localized in a respiratory center of the brain where chemoreceptors are influenced by the pH of the cerebrospinal fluid. Other chemoreceptors influenced by the changes in pH of arterial blood are located in the carotid and aortic vessels. A rise in Pco_2 of arterial blood will result in a fall in pH. This will in turn stimulate the chemoreceptors, initiating a rise in the respiration rate that will result in the release of more CO_2 from the blood in the lungs.

Acid-base balance

The maintenance of a constant pH is important because changes in pH will alter the functioning of enzymes, the cellular uptake and use of metabolites and minerals, the con-

formation of biological structural components, and the uptake and release of oxygen.

In the body, physiological buffers act to maintain a constant pH in the following manner. Fixed acids enter into the blood and are immediately neutralized by the bicarbonate buffering system.

$$H^+A^- \text{ (fixed acid)} + HCO_3^- \rightleftharpoons H_2CO_3 + A^- \text{ (unmeasured anions)}$$
$$\Updownarrow$$
$$H_2O + CO_2 \qquad \textit{Eq. 25-11}$$

However, the volatile acid, CO_2, is neutralized by the hemoglobin buffering system, because all the buffering systems are at equilibrium with each other. It is this overall equilibrium that gives the blood the relative buffering capacities described in Table 25-1.

Thus one of the important buffer systems required to maintain the pH of the blood is the carbonic acid–bicarbonate buffer system. Although this system has relatively low buffering capacity (see Table 25-1), it plays a large role in maintaining blood pH because it acts as the immediate buffer when fixed acids enter the blood.

Changes in respiration rate will alter the bicarbonate-carbonic acid ratio and pH. To understand this process, one must reconsider equations 25-2 and 25-5. A decrease in the ventilation rate will cause a decrease in release of CO_2 from the blood in the lungs. The increased blood CO_2 will result in the formation of more bicarbonate (shifting equation 25-2 to the right), though the increase in bicarbonate will be less than the increase in Pco_2. Thus, there will be a decrease in the bicarbonate-carbonate ratio and a decrease in the pH (see equation 25-5). If the ventilation rate were to stay constant and the metabolic release of fixed acid were to increase, the same effect would be observed. In this case H^+ reacts with HCO_3^- to form CO_2, which is released in the lungs. There is an immediate decrease in the concentration of bicarbonate with essentially no change in Pco_2, resulting in a decreased bicarbonate/αPco_2 ratio and a decreased pH. If the ventilation rate increases, more CO_2 is released from the blood at the lungs and the bicarbonate–carbonic acid ratio and pH increase. The ventilation rate can range from zero to 15 times the normal, allowing a significant degree of regulation of the bicarbonate–carbonic acid ratio. Thus, when the rate of ventilation is increased, excess acid in the form of CO_2 is quickly removed. Similarly, when the rate of ventilation is decreased, acid (CO_2) is added to neutralize excess alkali (HCO_3^-).

The other important blood buffer, hemoglobin, which is vital for the regulation of blood pH, buffers the CO_2 from the tissues. The major function of hemoglobin is the transport of oxygen through the blood to the cells of the body. There is a complex relationship between the degree of oxygenation of hemoglobin and the pH, Pco_2, and total CO_2 (Tco_2) of blood. Oxygenated hemoglobin is a stronger acid than deoxygenated hemoglobin, and therefore in the lungs hemoglobin will release H^+ as it becomes oxygenated

Table 25-3 Reference values for adult blood-gas parameters in arterial and venous blood

Parameters	Arterial	Venous
pH	7.35-7.45	7.33-7.43
Pco_2	35-45 mm Hg	38-50 mm Hg
Po_2	80-100 mm Hg	30-50 mm Hg
HCO_3^-	22-26 mmol/L	23-27 mmol/L
Total CO_2	23-27 mmol/L	24-28 mmol/L
O_2 saturation	94%-100%	60%-85%
Venous anion gap	5-14 mmol/L	5-14 mmol/L
Base excess	−2 to +2 mEq/L	−2 to +2 mEq/L

(equations 25-7 and 25-12), decreasing the bicarbonate level and increasing the levels of carbonic acid and its anhydrous form CO_2, and thus increasing the P_{CO_2} of the blood. The rate at which this reaction proceeds is enormously increased by the presence in the red blood cells of the enzyme *carbonic anhydrase*. It is the action of this enzyme that allows the rapid transfer of CO_2 into and out of red blood cells, with consequent buffering by hemoglobin. This process is summarized by the following series of reactions and Fig. 25-3.

$$\text{Gas exchange in the lungs } \underset{\text{(gas)}}{CO_2} \rightleftharpoons \underset{\text{(dissolved)}}{\overset{\overset{\text{Carbonic}}{\underset{\downarrow}{\text{anhydrase}}}}{dCO_2}} \rightleftharpoons$$

$$H_2CO_3 \rightleftharpoons H^+ + HCO_3^-$$

$$T_{CO_2} = dCO_2 + HCO_3^- \text{ or } T_{CO_2} = \alpha P_{CO_2} + HCO_3^- \quad \textit{Eq. 25-12}$$

In the lungs ventilation will eliminate this increased P_{CO_2} by releasing the CO_2 from the blood and thereby return the ratio of bicarbonate to carbonic acid to 20.

Oxygenated hemoglobin is transported in the blood to cells that have relatively low P_{O_2} tension and are releasing metabolic products, such as CO_2 and organic acids, into the blood, thus raising the P_{CO_2} and T_{CO_2} and lowering the pH. The relatively low P_{O_2} causes the dissociation of O_2 from HbO_2 and the consequent delivery of O_2 to the cells. The high CO_2 pressure in the cells drives the CO_2 along a concentration gradient into the red blood cells. Carbonic anhydrase rapidly converts the CO_2 into H^+ and HCO_3^- (see Fig. 25-2). Deoxygenated hemoglobin is a weaker acid than oxygenated hemoglobin. It neutralizes the H^+ to raise the pH and causes the dissociation reaction of carbonic acid to proceed to the right to increase the level of bicarbonate and decrease the P_{CO_2}.

The dissociation of oxygen from hemoglobin as a function of the P_{CO_2} is shown in Fig. 25-4, which is a graph of the percentage of O_2 saturation of hemoglobin versus P_{O_2}. The sigmoidal shape of the curve indicates that at critical levels of P_{O_2} near the P_{50} there is a strong increase or decrease in the percentage of O_2 saturation, with a minimal shift in P_{O_2}. In an area of the body in which there is a drop in P_{O_2} below that of P_{50} on the sigmoid curve, the hemoglobin will release a larger portion of O_2 than at a P_{O_2} level above the P_{50}. Similarly, in areas of high O_2, such as the lungs, the hemoglobin will be essentially saturated with O_2.

Another factor that has an effect on the position of the oxygen dissociation curve is 2,3-diphosphoglycerate (2,3-DPG), an intermediate in glycolysis. By interacting with the N-terminal amino groups of the hemoglobin molecule itself, 2,3-DPG induces the release of oxygen from hemoglobin. This is reflected in the shift to the right of the O_2 dissociation curve (Fig. 25-4). With a shift to the right, the critical P_{O_2} level that causes 50% saturation of hemoglobin by oxygen is increased so that areas of active metabolism, which contain increased 2,3-DPG levels, do not require P_{O_2} levels as low as those required in areas without increased 2,3-DPG for significant O_2 release from hemoglobin. See Chapter 36 for additional details on factors affecting oxygen binding by hemoglobin.

As more oxygen is released in response to increased levels of P_{CO_2} and H^+, more deoxyhemoglobin, which acts as a buffer, is formed. Increased P_{CO_2} leads to formation of bicarbonate (HCO_3^-). Most H^+ ions are bound by the deoxygenated hemoglobin, and the rest are buffered by the proteins and phosphate buffer in the plasma. Because all the H^+ formed is buffered, there is essentially no change in the pH. This buffering phenomenon is referred to as the *isohydric shift*. The HCO_3^- formed in the red blood cells as a result of uptake of H^+ by the hemoglobin diffuses out

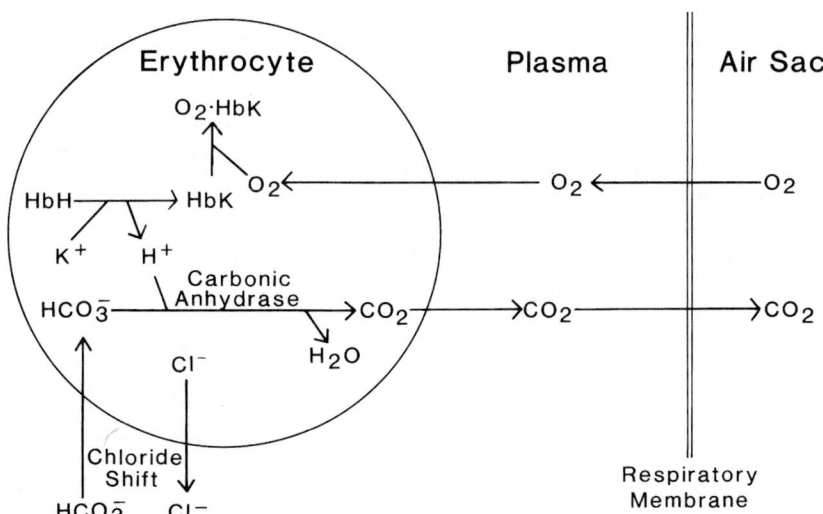

Fig. 25-3 Transfer of CO_2 in lungs from erythrocytes to air sacks. *HbK*, Potassium salt of hemoglobin; *HbH*, protonated form of hemoglobin.

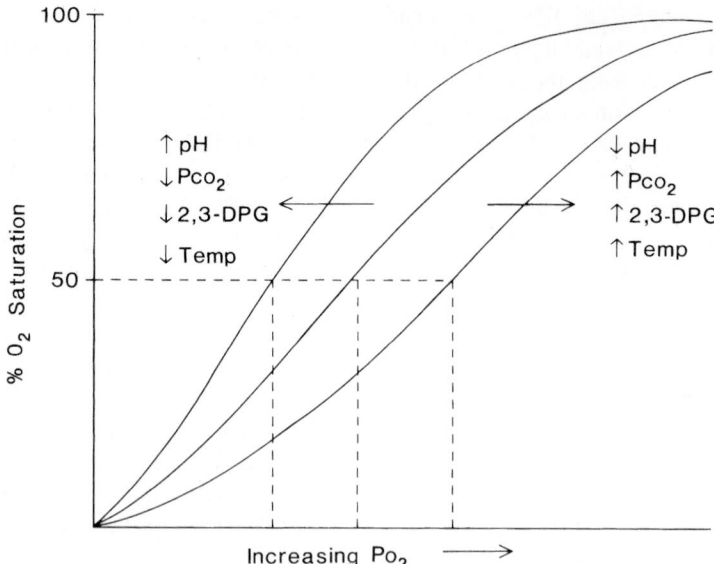

Fig. 25-4 Hemoglobin-oxygen dissociation curves and factors that shift the curve right and left. A shift of curve right or left changes the level of Po_2 at which hemoglobin is 50% saturated (P_{50}).

of the cells into the plasma. To preserve the electrical neutrality of the red blood cell, as HCO_3^- diffuses out of the cell, Cl^- diffuses into the erythrocytes from the plasma. This increase in the erythrocyte Cl^- is termed the *chloride shift*. Thus, the plasma chloride concentration of venous blood (where HCO_3^- is formed in red blood cells) is *lower* than that of arterial blood. When CO_2 is expelled from the lungs, Cl^- again shifts out of red blood cells into plasma (see Figs. 25-2 and 25-3). As the polyvalent hemoglobin anions are replaced by the diffusing monovalent chloride anions, the osmolality of the erythrocyte increases, leading to diffusion of water into the erythrocyte, slightly increasing the mean volume of venous red blood cells over the mean cell volume (MCV) in arterial blood.

Although the intact respiratory system acts as an imme-

diate regulator of the $HCO_3^-/\alpha Pco_2$ system, long-term control is exerted by renal mechanisms (see Chapter 26 for details). The kidneys excrete nonvolatile acids such as sulfuric, hydrochloric, phosphoric, and some of the organic acids into the urine. Hydrogen ions are excreted by the kidneys into the urine and are buffered by HPO_4^{2-} and ammonia, which is derived from deamidation of the amino acid glutamine. Sodium is the cation exchanged for excreted hydrogen ions by the kidney. The kidney also affects the bicarbonate–carbonic acid buffer system by regulating the excretion of bicarbonate (Fig. 25-5). The kidney reabsorbs almost all filtered bicarbonate at plasma bicarbonate concentrations below 25 mEq/L. Only when bicarbonate levels become elevated above 25 mEq/L will bicarbonate be excreted into the urine. The reabsorbed bicarbonate is neu-

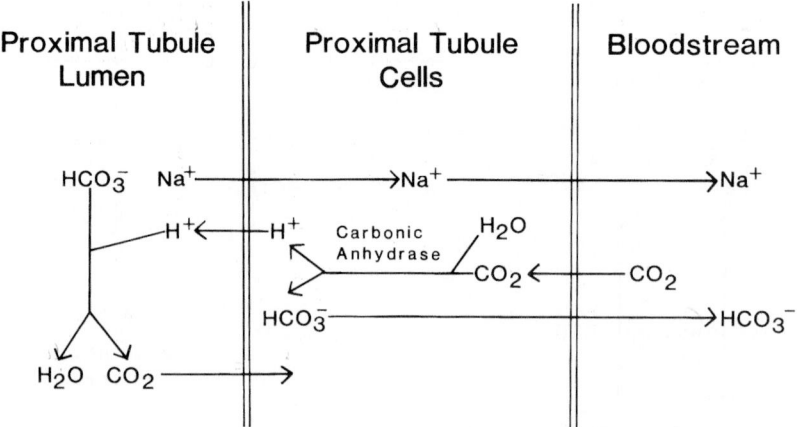

Fig. 25-5 Kidney reabsorption of bicarbonate with excretion of H^+.

tralized by the reabsorbed sodium ions, which have been exchanged for the hydrogen ions excreted in the urine (Fig. 25-5).

ACID-BASE DISORDERS
Definitions

Acid-base disorders are most readily classified in terms of their immediate cause. Thus acidoses and alkaloses are described as of either respiratory or metabolic origin.

These classifications should always be considered in terms of the modified Henderson-Hasselbalch equation:

$$pH = pK'_a + \log \frac{[HCO_3^-]}{\alpha P_{CO_2}} \qquad \textit{Eq. 25-13}$$

The term αP_{CO_2} represents the acid component that is directly and immediately modified by respiratory status. Thus, the term αP_{CO_2} is called the *respiratory component*. The concentration of bicarbonate is most immediately affected by changes in the hydrogen-ion concentration caused by production of metabolic acids other than CO_2 (that is, fixed acids) and by physiological processes that directly change the concentration of serum bicarbonate. Thus, the bicarbonate concentration of plasma is called the *metabolic component* of acid-base status. Acid-base homeostasis is accomplished when one controls one or both of these components. Keep in mind that the pH of plasma depends on the *ratio* of the concentration of bicarbonate to αP_{CO_2} rather than on the absolute concentration of these components (see equation 25-13).

Base excess. *Base excess* is a calculated parameter that is used to assess the metabolic component of the patient's acid-base disturbance. The term *base excess* is used to describe clinical situations in which there is an excess of bicarbonate (positive base excess) or a deficit of bicarbonate (negative base excess). We use the term *base deficit* for a negative base excess because this term is a more accurate description of the physiological condition. Base excess in the blood at a pH of 7.40, P_{CO_2} of 40 mm Hg, a hemoglobin concentration of 150 g/L, and a temperature of 37° C is zero. The hemoglobin concentration is important because the blood-buffering capacity is greatly dependent on this quantity. The addition of a base, such as bicarbonate, raises the buffer content of the blood and results in a positive base excess. The loss of base, as occurs in diarrhea or with the addition of acids, lowers the blood buffer content and results in a base deficit. The calculation of the base excess or deficit is useful in the management of patients with acid-base disturbances because it permits estimation of the number of milliequivalents of sodium bicarbonate or ammonium chloride that should be administered to correct the patient's pH to normal. In practice the base excess is only a crude estimate because as the patient's condition improves, changes in respiration and metabolism will invalidate the original calculation. It is for this reason that blood-gas status is closely monitored by the analysis of sequential blood specimens.

$$\text{Base excess} = (1.0 - 0.0143\ \text{Hgb})(HCO_3^-) - $$
$$(9.5 + 1.63\ \text{Hgb})(7.4\ \text{pH}) - 24 \qquad \textit{Eq. 25-14}$$

where Hgb is the hemoglobin concentration in g/dL.

Oxygen saturation. *Oxygen saturation* indicates the amount of oxygen bound to hemoglobin and is used to determine the effectiveness of respiration or oxygen therapy. Oxygen saturation is calculated by use of the measured parameters of pH and P_{O_2} and the equation for a normal oxygen dissociation curve. A nomogram to derive O_2 saturation from pH and P_{O_2} values is presented in Fig. 25-6. Oxygen saturation is also measured directly by use of the difference in the wavelengths of maximum absorbance for oxyhemoglobin and deoxyhemoglobin. This measurement is performed with a co-oximeter. Table 25-3 contains reference values for the calculated blood-gas parameters.

Anion gap. If the total measured cations are subtracted from the total measured anions as shown below, the difference is the anion gap, or the amount of unmeasured anions present. Or more simply:

$$\text{Anion gap} = [Na^+] + [K^+] - [Cl^-] - [HCO_3^-] \qquad \textit{Eq. 25-15}$$

Usually the only electrolytes measured are sodium, potassium, chloride, and bicarbonate (as total CO_2). However, other anions exist in blood, such as phosphates, ketones, lactic acid, proteins, and sulfates. Because these other anions are not measured whereas their counterions are, there is an apparent excess, or gap, of measured cations over measured anions. Increases in the amounts of these unmeasured anions and of the accompanying Na^+ ions will increase the apparent gap. Usually the anion gap averages 12 mEq/L. The anion gap increases with production of organic acids. Diabetic ketoacidosis is the most common cause of an elevated anion gap. If diabetes is ruled out, other causes of the acidosis must be sought, such as lactic acidosis, dehydration, renal tubular acidosis, sepsis, and toxic acidosis.

Base-deficient disorders

Any condition associated with a lower-than-normal blood pH (acidemia) is referred to as *acidosis*.

Metabolic acidosis. In base-deficient disorders the pH is below the reference interval. Such disorders occur if metabolic processes result in the accumulation of abnormal amounts of organic acids other than carbonic acid. Examples of acids that accumulate are lactic acid, β-hydroxybutyric acid, and acetoacetic acid. Metabolic organic acids entering plasma react with plasma bicarbonate to form H_2CO_3, which is immediately converted to CO_2 gas, which is in turn rapidly eliminated from the body by the lungs. The net result is an immediate decrease in bicarbonate concentration with essentially no loss of P_{CO_2}. This leads to a lowered bicarbonate/αP_{CO_2} ratio and a lowered pH, or metabolic acidosis.

In contrast to this accumulation of acids is the pathological loss of base from the body. In severe diarrhea, bicar-

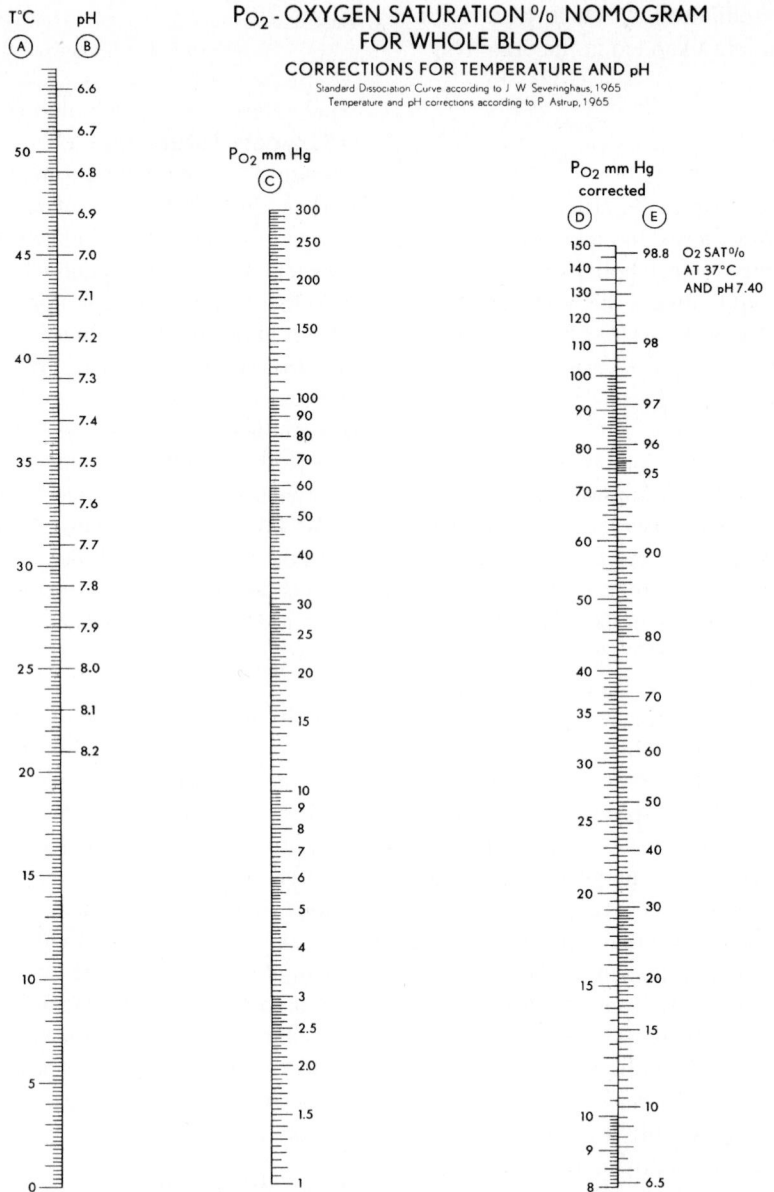

Fig. 25-6 Nomogram of relationship between pH, P_{O_2}, and O_2 saturation. A straight line through a value of pH and of P_{O_2} will connect with a calculated value of O_2 saturation at 37° C. (Courtesy Radiometer Corp., Copenhagen, Denmark.)

bonate ion is lost as part of the watery stool, resulting in a base deficit ($\downarrow$ [HCO_3^-], $\downarrow$ bicarbonate/αP_{CO_2} ratio). These types of disorders are termed *metabolic acidoses*.

Respiratory acidosis. A relative base-deficient disorder can result from a decrease in the bicarbonate-carbonic acid ratio as a result of an increase in carbonic acid. This occurs if the lungs are not able to expel CO_2 from the blood. This disorder is termed *respiratory acidosis*. The increase in P_{CO_2} results in an increase in the concentration of bicarbonate as the CO_2 is buffered by hemoglobin. However, the rise in bicarbonate is less than the increase in P_{CO_2}, resulting in a relative base deficit and a decrease in the bicarbonate/αP_{CO_2} ratio, which results in a below-normal serum pH below the reference interval.

Base-excess disorders

Any condition associated with a blood pH above the reference interval (alkalemia) is an *alkalosis*.

Metabolic alkalosis. In base-excess disorders, the pH is above the reference interval. If the disorder is caused by an increase in bicarbonate, with little or no change in carbonic acid, the disorder is termed *metabolic alkalosis*. Such a disorder occurs when excess amounts of bicarbonate of soda are ingested or administered or when there is an increased renal reabsorption of bicarbonate, as in *hypochloremic alkalosis*.

Respiratory alkalosis. If the disorder is caused by a decrease in carbonic acid, as when respiration is overly stimulated, the disorder is termed *respiratory alkalosis*. In this condition, rapid ventilation greatly decreases the P_{CO_2} of blood, with minimal change in bicarbonate concentration. This results in a relative excess of bicarbonate so that the bicarbonate/αP_{CO_2} ratio increases. This increased ratio yields a higher plasma pH.

Instrumentation (see also pp. 320 and 477-480

The traditional laboratory blood-gas analyzer includes a pH electrode, a P_{O_2} electrode, and a P_{CO_2} electrode. As point-of-care testing has gained acceptance, the use of noninvasive electrodes has expanded. Current technology permits reliable assessment of both P_{O_2} and P_{CO_2} using noninvasive techniques but *not* blood pH. The noninvasive devices use essentially the same electrodes as the traditional blood-gas analyzer. They are widely used in neonatal intensive care units because they do not require blood collection from these small infants. It is common practice to verify the performance of these noninvasive instruments by performing a traditional blood-gas analysis periodically.

With the development of disposable microelectrodes and fully automated analyzers that are reliable, blood-gas analysis is now being done in the surgery suite and other nonlaboratory settings, resulting in shortened turnaround times for results and permitting more rapid medical intervention.

The central laboratory is usually responsible for maintaining the devices, whereas the operator, physician, or respiratory therapist is responsible for performing quality control. Documentation of operator training is required.

Calculated parameters. The remainder of the blood acid-base parameters are not measured but are instead calculated using equations 25-6 and 25-13. One of the parameters is bicarbonate, which is calculated by use of the measured parameters pH and P_{CO_2} in the Henderson-Hasselbalch equation:

$$HCO_3^- = [\alpha P_{CO_2}] \text{ antilog } [pH - pK'_a] \qquad \textit{Eq. 25-16}$$

Nomograms have also been developed to derive bicarbonate levels from pH and P_{CO_2} measurements (Fig. 25-7). Bicarbonate levels are useful in the assessment of the degree to which metabolic and renal control are involved in the acid-base status of the patient.

ACIDOSIS
Metabolic acidosis
Etiology. Increased organic acid production resulting in metabolic acidosis can have many causes. Uncontrolled diabetes results in accumulation of acetoacetic and hydroxybutyric acids, which are produced by the excessive oxidation of fatty acids (see Chapter 33). Fasting or fad diets also lead to increased levels of these acids.

Lactic acid increases as a result of increases in anaerobic metabolism caused by strenuous muscular exercise or systemic infections. Lactic acidosis also results from local tissue hypoxia (low tissue P_{O_2}), which is caused by dehy-

dration, poor perfusion as a result of circulatory collapse, or cardiac failure.

Renal tubular acidosis results from a failure of the kidney to acidify the urine by exchanging H^+ for Na^+. This renal insufficiency is acquired as a result of infection or is congenital, as in cases of severe de Toni-Fanconi syndrome. Liver disease that impairs the formation of urea and ammonia will also result in a metabolic acidosis because of retention of H^+.

Salicylate intoxication initially induces respiratory alkalosis because of hyperventilation, which is a result of a stimulatory effect of the drug on the respiratory center. The ingested drug is converted to an acid before excretion, and the large quantities of acid formed ultimately result in metabolic acidosis. Other poisons that are ingested as acids or as compounds that will lead to acid metabolites are methanol (converted to formic acid), ethylene glycol (converted to oxalic acid), paraldehyde, and ammonium chloride. These compounds initially cause respiratory alkalosis, followed by metabolic acidosis. Infusion of large quantities of isotonic sodium chloride results in a metabolic acidosis because the high sodium load competes with hydrogen ions for renal excretion. Metabolic acidosis is also caused by the ingestion of carbonic anhydrase inhibitors, such as acetazolamide or sulfonamides, which interfere with the formation of bicarbonate in the erythrocyte and the renal tubule cells (see Figs. 25-2, 25-3, and 25-5).

A metabolic acidosis may also be caused by a decreased bicarbonate concentration. Diarrhea and colitis lead to losses of intestinal fluids, which contain high concentrations of bicarbonate. The resultant reduction of the HCO_3^-/H_2CO_3 ratio causes acidemia.

Physiological response. The acidoses just described usually result from the presentation to the body of an acid load that is compensated for at least in part by retention of bicarbonate. When acidemia occurs as a result of acute metabolic acidosis, the body attempts to correct this acidemia by hyperventilation. Hyperventilation lowers the P_{CO_2}, and to a smaller extent the HCO_3^-, and at least partially increases the ratio of HCO_3^-/H_2CO_3, thereby returning the pH toward normal. This mechanism of correcting the pH during acidosis is known as *compensatory respiratory alkalosis*. The result is a decrease in the P_{CO_2} and HCO_3^- concentration and a pH value closer to the reference interval.

In a metabolic acidosis that does not involve renal dysfunction, the kidney will excrete organic acids and exchange H^+ for Na^+ in the distal region of the tubule, resulting in a more acid urine. This renal compensatory mechanism becomes effective over a period of time and will eventually correct both the blood pH and the bicarbonate toward the reference interval. This correction can take place only when the underlying cause of the acidosis has been eliminated. Part of the renal response to chronic acidosis is the excretion of ammonia by the renal tubular cells. This excretion of ammonia into the presumptive

SIGGAARD-ANDERSEN ALIGNMENT NOMOGRAM

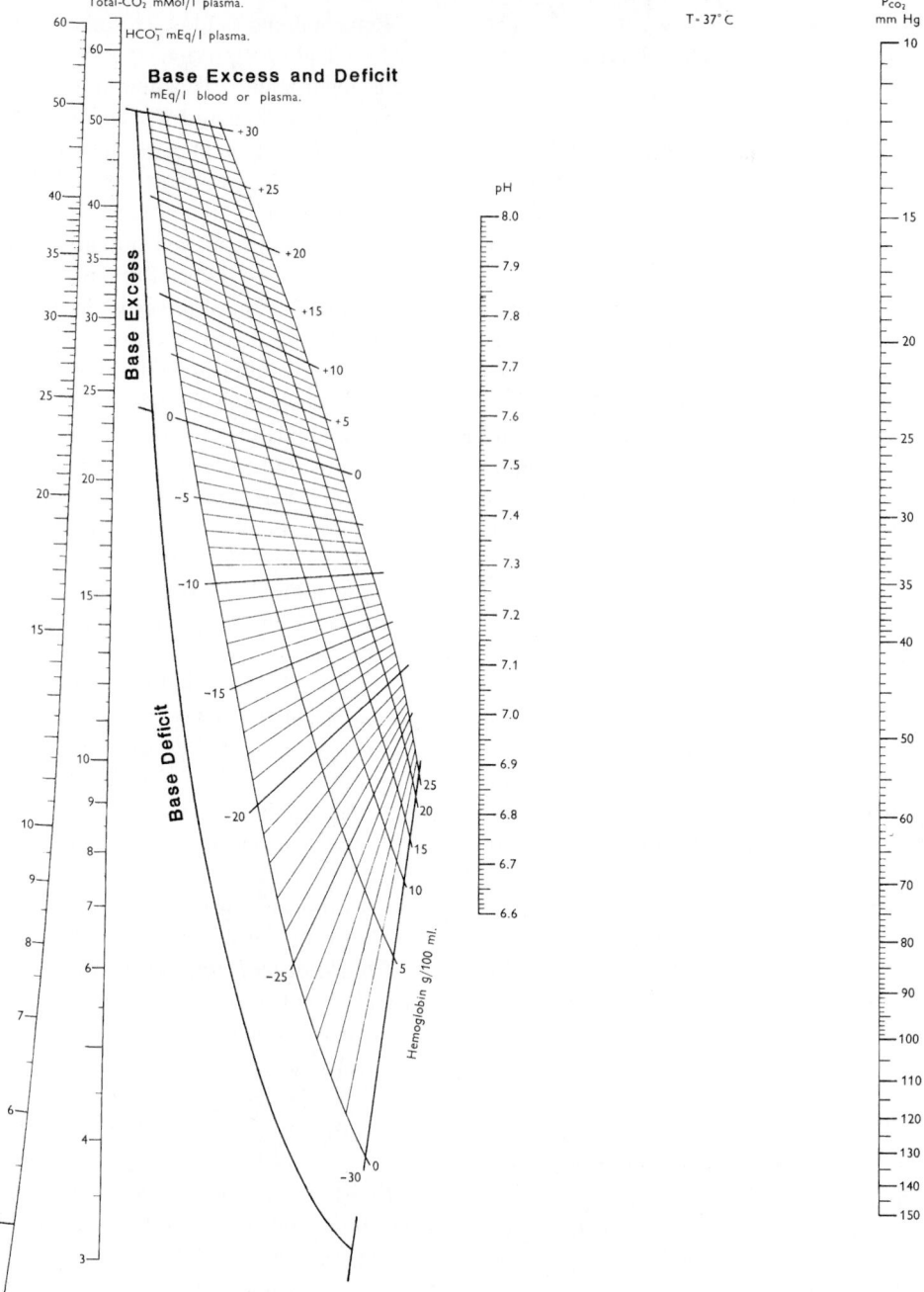

Fig. 25-7 Nomogram of relationship between P_{CO_2}, pH, base excess, hemoglobin, bicarbonate, and total CO_2. A straight line through a value of pH and of P_{CO_2} will connect with a calculated value of HCO_3^- and total CO_2. Base excess or deficit can be derived from that straight line if the hemoglobin level is known. (Modified from Radiometer Corp., Copenhagen, Denmark.)

urine allows additional H^+ to be excreted and thus reduces the H^+ load in blood.

Laboratory findings. The findings seen in metabolic acidosis, summarized in Table 25-4, include a decrease in both pH and HCO_3^-. Initially the P_{CO_2} may be within the reference interval but it will decrease as a result of the respiratory response to the acidemia. A base deficit (negative base excess) will also be present.

The laboratory findings in lactic acidosis are those of a metabolic acidosis with a decreased pH, an initially normal

Table 25-4 Classes of acid-base disorders with corresponding effects on selected blood-gas parameters

Disorder	pH	P_{CO_2}	HCO_3^-	Base excess
Metabolic acidosis	↓	↓ N	↓	↓
Respiratory acidosis	↓	↑	↑ N	↑ N
Metabolic alkalosis	↑	↑ N	↑	↑
Respiratory alkalosis	↑	↓	↓ N	↓N

N, Initially normal (within the reference interval).

P_{CO_2} and P_{O_2}, a decreased O_2 saturation (the hemoglobin saturation curve is shifted to the right), a decreased bicarbonate and total CO_2, an increased anion gap, a negative base excess, and increased potassium and lactic acid concentrations. As the body attempts to correct the metabolic acidosis, the P_{CO_2} decreases.

In cases of toxic drug ingestion, such as methanol, ethylene glycol, or paraldehyde poisoning, the patient develops a metabolic acidosis. Laboratory findings include a decreased pH, an initially normal P_{CO_2} and P_{O_2}, a decreased O_2 saturation, bicarbonate, and total CO_2, an increased anion gap (caused by the ingested poisons or their metabolites), and a negative base excess. As the body attempts to compensate for the acidosis, the P_{CO_2} decreases initially and the bicarbonate slowly increases toward normal as the kidney reabsorbs increasing amounts of bicarbonate.

Treatment. Initially the cause of the acidemia is corrected if possible, for example, by insulin treatment of diabetes. If the pH falls below 7.2, there is sometimes a deleterious effect on the cardiovascular system, and the base deficit may have to be corrected immediately. This is frequently accomplished by administration of bicarbonate, which corrects the base deficit by raising the HCO_3^-/H_2CO_3 ratio. In all cases the cause of the metabolic acidosis must ultimately be corrected.

Respiratory acidosis
Etiology. Respiratory acidoses are caused by disorders that interfere with the usual ability of the lungs to expel CO_2. These disorders include pulmonary edema, bronchoconstriction, pneumonia, emphysema, apnea, and bradycardia. Morphine injection and barbiturate poisoning cause an immediate respiratory depression, resulting in respiratory acidosis.

Respiratory distress syndrome (RDS), which is common in premature infants, results in a respiratory acidosis because the infants lack sufficient levels of surfactant in their lungs to allow the alveoli to expand in their usual manner. Gas exchange is thus inhibited. Respiratory distress is also seen in some adults who experience systemic shock or oxygen toxicity. Initially, the observed blood-gas parameters are decreased pH, increased P_{CO_2}, decreased P_{O_2}, and decreased oxygen saturation. Base excess, bicarbonate, and anion gap are initially within normal limits.

Physiological response. The physiological response to respiratory acidosis includes the increased renal excretion of acids, the retention of sodium and bicarbonate, and, if possible, hyperventilation. If a response compensates for the respiratory acidosis and results in its correction, the acidosis is referred to as *compensated respiratory acidosis.* This response may be viewed as the development of a metabolic alkalosis that compensates for the respiratory acidosis. In chronic respiratory acidosis, the pH becomes essentially normal but a base excess remains. When the respiratory disorder is corrected, the usual respiratory response to the acidosis removes the excess CO_2, and a transient metabolic alkalosis may result. Generally this alkalosis does not require treatment.

Laboratory findings. Respiratory disorders frequently lead to an increase in plasma CO_2 concentration with a smaller increase in HCO_3^- and a concurrent decrease in the ratio of HCO_3^-/H_2CO_3, which results in respiratory acidosis. However, as a result of the low oxygen levels in the tissue, a coexisting metabolic lactic acidosis can develop. This metabolic acidosis results in an increased anion gap, and the decrease in bicarbonate results in a negative base excess. Table 25-4 is a review of these findings.

As a result of the renal compensatory response, very elevated concentrations of HCO_3^- with almost normal pH are often seen. In chronic respiratory disease the concentration of HCO_3^- and pH are near normal, though the P_{O_2} may be rather depressed.

Medical treatment. Medical treatment is primarily aimed at correction of the respiratory disorder and ventilation of the patient with gases containing higher P_{O_2} and lower P_{CO_2} by use of mechanical respirators. However, initial correction of the acidemia may be achieved by injection of sodium bicarbonate.

ALKALOSIS
Metabolic alkalosis
Etiology. Occasionally, excessive, chronic ingestion of bicarbonate of soda for gastrointestinal distress results in an increased concentration of blood bicarbonate and a resultant metabolic alkalosis. Similarly, treatment of peptic ulcers with ingestion of large quantities of alkali antacids will also produce metabolic alkalosis. More commonly, metabolic alkalosis arises from the loss of chloride. Prolonged vomiting or aspiration of gastric fluids leads to loss of gastric hydrochloric acid. This in turn raises the pH of the blood because the loss of the chloride anion results in increased renal retention of bicarbonate to counter the sodium reabsorbed by the proximal tubule. This condition is known as *hypochloremic alkalosis.* Corticosteroid administration and diseases such as hyperaldosteronism and Cushing's syndrome, which affect the ability of the kidney to regulate electrolyte balance, will also raise the blood pH. In the distal tubule, Na^+ is retained at the expense of K^+ and H^+. The resultant hypokalemia causes a release of K^+ by cells

into the blood and a concurrent balanced movement of H^+ from blood into the cells, thereby leading to a rise in the pH of the blood.

Physiological response. To compensate for the increase in the HCO_3^-/H_2CO_3 ratio during metabolic alkalosis, the respiratory system slows, raising the Pco_2 and the bicarbonate concentration of the blood. The Pco_2 rises more rapidly than the HCO_3^-, thereby decreasing the pH. This mechanism of readjusting the pH during metabolic alkalosis is termed *compensatory respiratory acidosis.* The result is a pH closer to the reference interval in the presence of an elevated concentration of HCO_3^-.

If the alkalosis persists, the body will attempt to correct the alkalosis by increasing the renal excretion of the excess bicarbonate unless the proximal tubule of the kidney actually increases the reabsorption of bicarbonate, as in hypokalemia, dehydration, or hypochloremia.

Laboratory findings. During metabolic alkalosis, the ratio of HCO_3^-/H_2CO_3 increases as a result of a rise in the concentration of blood bicarbonate. Because of the physiological response to the alkalemia, additional laboratory findings are an increased Pco_2 and an alkaline urine containing titratable bicarbonate (Table 25-4).

Treatment. Treatment of metabolic alkalosis involves administration of NaCl or KCl, depending on the degree of hypokalemia, and perhaps also administration of NH_4Cl if the alkalosis is severe and persistent. The Cl^- anion of NH_4Cl compensates for the chloride deficit, which may have led to excessive retention of bicarbonate initially. This permits the kidney to begin to excrete the excess bicarbonate and correct the alkalosis.

Respiratory alkalosis

Etiology. Hyperventilation causes respiratory alkalosis. The conditions resulting in hyperventilation include hysteria, excessive crying, pregnancy, salicylate intoxication, impairment of the central nervous system's control of the respiratory system, asthma, fever, pulmonary embolism, and excessive use of a mechanical respirator.

Physiological response. The kidneys respond to the alkalosis by excreting increased amounts of bicarbonate under the conditions of lower Pco_2 that occur during respiratory alkalosis. In response to the alkalosis, the proximal tubules of the kidney decrease the reabsorption of bicarbon-

ate. This renal response to respiratory alkalosis is termed *compensatory metabolic acidosis.*

Laboratory findings. Hyperventilation leads to increased loss of CO_2 from the blood at the alveolar surface, which causes the HCO_3^-/H_2CO_3 ratio to increase as carbonic acid is lost. Because of the physiological response to the alkalemia, additional laboratory findings include decreased Pco_2 and an alkaline urine containing titratable bicarbonate (Table 25-3).

Treatment. One corrects respiratory alkalosis by lowering the respiration rate with drugs, such as sedatives, or by having the patient breathe air with a higher CO_2 content. One easily accomplishes this by having the patient breathe in a restricted environment, as into a paper bag, which raises the Pco_2 of the air and the blood. The increased Pco_2 returns the HCO_3^-/H_2CO_3 ratio to within the reference interval and corrects the respiratory alkalosis. Table 25-4 summarizes the changes in blood-gas parameters seen in several diseases.

CHANGE OF ANALYTE IN DISEASE (Table 25-5)

Diabetic ketoacidosis in patients with uncontrolled diabetes is an example of metabolic acidosis. Laboratory findings include a decreased pH, acidemia, a decreased Pco_2, a normal Po_2, a decreased O_2 saturation (see p. 477 for blood-gas methods), a decreased bicarbonate and total CO_2 (see p. 480, Tco_2), an increased anion gap, a negative base excess, and increased serum potassium, ketones (see p. 632), and lactic and pyruvic acids (see pp. 481-482) caused by the disturbed carbohydrate and fat metabolism.

Emphysema is a disease of impaired respiration that frequently results in respiratory acidosis. Laboratory findings include a decreased pH and Po_2, an increased Pco_2 and potassium, and a decreased oxygen saturation. Initially the anion gap, base excess, bicarbonate, and Tco_2 are within the reference interval. As the body compensates for the acidosis, the bicarbonate and Tco_2 rise. As in RDS, the low Po_2 may result in a metabolic acidosis caused by a rise in blood lactate because of increased anaerobic metabolism.

Hemoglobinopathies, such as sickle cell anemia, can lead to unusual oxygen-saturation kinetics caused by the abnormal hemoglobin molecule. Some laboratory findings associated with hemoglobinopathies are decreased oxygen saturation and Po_2 levels, which result in increased anaerobic metabolism and thereby metabolic acidosis. Persistence of

Table 25-5 Common disorders of acid-base balance and effects on selected blood-gas parameters

Disorder	pH	Pco_2	Po_2	HCO_3^-	Base excess	Anion gap	O_2 saturation
Respiratory distress syndrome	↓	↑	↓	N	N	N	↓
Lactic acidosis	↓	N*	N	↓	↓	↑	↓
Diabetic ketosis	↓	N*	N	↓	↓	↑	↓
Emphysema	↓	↑	↓	N*	N	N	↓
Methanol poisoning	↓	N*	N	↓	↓	↑	↓
Renal failure	↓	N*	N	↓	↓	↑	↓

N*, initially normal; *N,* always normal (within the reference interval).

the hypoxemia results in decreased bicarbonate and total CO_2, an increased anion gap (see p. 457) and blood lactate, and a negative base excess. The respiratory response to this acidosis is hyperventilation, which decreases the Pco_2. The renal response to this acidosis is an increase in the reabsorption of bicarbonate, which tends to return the HCO_3^-/H_2CO_3 ratio to normal.

Renal failure leads to metabolic acidosis with the associated laboratory findings of a decreased pH, initially normal Pco_2 and Po_2, decreased oxygen saturation, increased potassium level, and decreased bicarbonate level and Tco_2. As the anion gap increases because of organic acid production and retention, the base excess becomes negative. The respiratory compensation for the metabolic acidosis will lead eventually to a decrease in Pco_2.

METHODS OF ANALYSIS
Blood-gas analysis and oxygen saturation
JOHN E. SHERWIN

Principles of analysis and current usage Assessment of an individual's acid-base status is aided by measurement of the

blood pH, Pco_2, and Po_2. Measurement of these parameters also allows for the calculation of a variety of other indices, including oxygen content, oxygen saturation, total CO_2, bicarbonate, and base excess, which reflect an individual's metabolic and oxygenation status.

Modern pH electrode measuring systems comprise a glass electrode, a reference electrode, and a liquid junction between the two electrodes (Fig. 25-8). The reference electrode serves as a reference potential source that is in contact with the unknown solution. Reference electrodes commonly used are the silver/silver chloride electrode and the calomel electrode. The saturated calomel electrode is probably the most common. The calomel electrode comprises a glass tube containing a calomel paste (mercurous chloride, Hg_2Cl_2 and mercury, Hg) and a saturated solution of potassium chloride (KCl). The KCl solution is saturated or kept at a high enough concentration so that the ionic composition of blood that is in contact with the electrode does not alter the constant electrical potential of the reference electrode. A platinum wire extends into the calomel solution.

The potential of the glass electrode varies with changes in the pH. Hydrogen ions in the blood sample will exchange with metallic ions in the glass membrane of the glass electrode. The glass layer of the electrode must be hydrated for the electrode to function properly. The hydrated glass layer

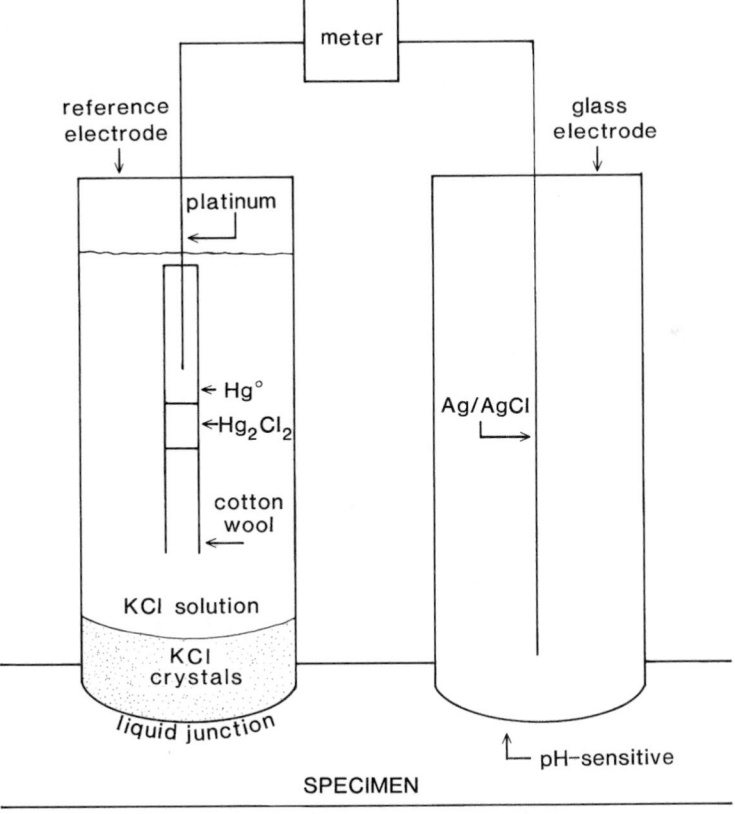

Fig. 25-8   Schema of a pH electrode and calomel reference electrode. A potential develops across pH-sensitive glass membrane of pH electrode because of the difference in pH of outer sample and inner electrode buffer solution. Calomel electrode is in electrical contact with sample and pH electrode through a KCl salt bridge and acts as a reference against the potential developed at the pH electrode.

continuously dissolves from the surface as the dry glass becomes hydrated. The interior of the glass electrode is filled with a solution of a constant pH that is in contact with the glass membrane. A silver/silver chloride wire in contact with the solution of constant pH is connected to a voltmeter. Hydrogen ions present in blood that comes in contact with the glass electrode change the potential of this electrode with respect to the reference electrode. This change in electrical potential is recorded by the voltmeter and related to the pH of the blood specimen.

The pH electrode can be modified and used to measure the P_{CO_2} of blood. The modifications include placing the glass electrode in a weak bicarbonate buffer solution and physically preventing this buffer from coming into direct contact with the blood specimen by use of a gas-permeable membrane. Carbon dioxide present in the blood will diffuse through the gas-permeable membrane into the bicarbonate buffer solution where it can react with water in the following sequence of reactions:

$$CO_2 + H_2O \rightleftharpoons H_2CO_3 \rightleftharpoons H^+ + HCO_3^- \qquad Eq.\ 25\text{-}17$$

The change in the concentration of hydrogen ion is measured by the same system used for measuring the pH of a blood specimen, as illustrated in Fig. 25-9. Hydrogen ions present in the blood sample do not affect the pH inside the bicarbonate buffer system because hydrogen ions do not penetrate the gas-permeable membrane.

Measurement of the partial pressure of oxygen, or P_{O_2}, in a blood specimen is achieved with use of a Clark polarographic electrode (Fig. 25-10). The Clark electrode comprises a silver anode and a platinum cathode immersed in an electrolyte buffer. The buffer solution consists of potassium chloride and phosphate buffer, or buffered potassium hydroxide, in water. The electrical potential of the cathode is held constant with respect to that of the anode. Oxygen present in the blood sample diffuses across a gas-permeable membrane into the electrolyte buffer where it is reduced at the platinum cathode as follows:

$$O_2 + 2H^+ + 4e^- \rightarrow H_2O_2 + 2e^- \rightarrow 2OH^- \qquad Eq.\ 25\text{-}18$$

The reduction of oxygen at the cathode results in the flow of current between the cathode and anode. The amount of current flow is measured and related to the amount of oxygen present in the sample.

Calibration of a P_{O_2} and P_{CO_2} electrode can be achieved either with a flowing gas or a liquid sample that has been equilibrated with gas. The gases used for instrument calibra-

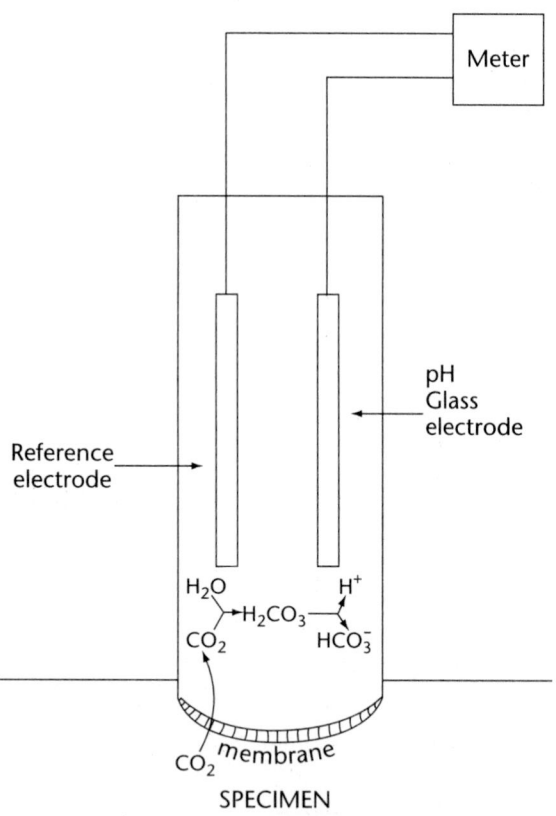

Fig. 25-9 Schema of P_{CO_2} electrode. CO_2 diffuses across the outer membrane, which is not permeable to HCO_3^- or H^+, into a layer of bicarbonate solution. Reaction of diffused CO_2 and H_2O to form carbonic acid changes the pH of bicarbonate solution, which is detected by inner pH electrode.

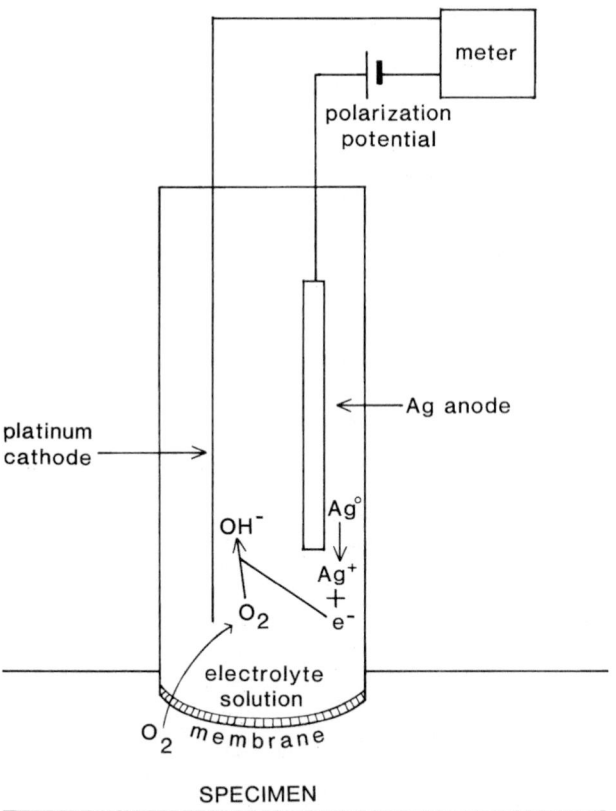

Fig. 25-10 Schema of Clark polarographic electrode. A constant voltage is generated between the platinum cathode and silver anode. Oxygen molecules that diffuse past the outer membrane into a layer of electrolyte solution in contact with the platinum cathode are reduced at the cathode, producing a current that can be measured and related to the amount of diffusing oxygen.

tion are usually bubbled through humidifiers at 37° C to saturate the gases with water vapor. Saturating the gases with water vapor is necessary to eliminate the problem of trying to maintain totally "dry" gas for instrument calibration. Any residual moisture that is present in the measuring chamber will contaminate a "dry" gas by introducing water vapor into the gas. Water vapor exerts its own partial pressure and will therefore reduce the partial pressures of the other gases in the mixture by a proportional amount. For example, a gas that is saturated with water at 37° C will have a partial pressure of 47 mm Hg contributed by water vapor. Therefore, to produce consistently a gas mixture with known partial pressures of O_2 and CO_2 and to eliminate the possible error associated with maintaining a "dry" calibrating gas, the gas is saturated with water before instrument calibration.

The use of a flowing gas for instrument calibration does have some drawbacks however. The gas flow rate through the measuring chamber must be strictly controlled because variations in flow rate can affect electrode cooling and result in incomplete saturation of the gas with water vapor. Both these factors can adversely affect instrument calibration. Another drawback of using this type of calibration concerns the difference in matrices between the gas calibrator and the patient sample, which is a liquid.

Another calibration scheme for blood gas analyzers makes use of a gas-tonometered, buffered liquid for calibration. Use of liquid calibrators offers the advantage that they have similar matrices to the sample being analyzed, calibration is independent of the flow rate of the gas, and saturation of the gas with water vapor is not a consideration. When a liquid-calibration technique is used, a positive bias of approximately 5% to 8% for both P_{CO_2} and P_{O_2} may be observed, as compared to the use of a gas calibrator.

In addition to the analysis of blood specimens for analysis of P_{CO_2} and P_{O_2}, noninvasive transcutaneous techniques for measurement of these parameters have also been developed. Transcutaneous measurements of P_{CO_2} and P_{O_2} make use of the same technologies as those used for blood specimens, though with minor modifications. Transcutaneous measurement of P_{CO_2} and P_{O_2} makes use of the small amount of diffusion of gases from the capillary bed in the skin to the skin surface. This diffusion of gas from the capillary bed can be increased by heating the skin to 42° or 43° C to increase local blood flow. With maximal blood flow, the P_{O_2} measured at the skin surface correlates very well with the arterial P_{O_2}. For P_{CO_2} measured transcutaneously, the increased temperature necessary for maximizing blood flow also increases metabolism within the tissue being heated, and such an increase results in an increase in the P_{CO_2}. In addition, in contrast to the P_{O_2} electrode, which consumes oxygen in the process of its reduction to peroxide and hydroxide ion, the P_{CO_2} electrode does not consume or eliminate the P_{CO_2} that diffuses through the skin surface. Thus, the P_{CO_2} is higher at the electrode surface than at the area of the capillary closest to the skin surface. The adverse effects of temperature and electrode arrangement make it necessary for use of a correction factor to compensate for these factors on P_{CO_2} measurements.

Measurement of pH and P_{O_2} allows for the calculation of the percentage of hemoglobin that is saturated with oxygen.[2] The percentage of oxygen saturation is the percentage of total hemoglobin that has oxygen bound to it (see p. 471). The percentage of oxygen saturation can also be quantitated by direct measurement of the difference between the absorption spectral profiles of oxygenated hemoglobin and deoxygenated hemoglobin. For the direct measurement of percent saturation, hemoglobin is measured at two wavelengths. The first wavelength chosen is one at which a large difference in absorbance occurs between the oxygenated and deoxygenated forms of hemoglobin (such as 600 or 577 nm). The second wavelength chosen is the isosbestic point. The isosbestic point is the wavelength (such as 506 or 548 nm) at which the absorbance for the oxygenated and deoxygenated forms of hemoglobin are identical. The absorbance at the isosbestic point indicates the total amount of hemoglobin present, whereas the absorbance at the other wavelength indicates the difference in the concentration of the oxygenated and deoxygenated forms of hemoglobin. The formula used for calculating the percentage of oxygen saturation is the following:

$$\text{Percent } O_2 \text{ saturation} = \left[K_1 \times \frac{\text{Absorbance at first wavelength}}{\text{Absorbance at isosbestic point}} - K_2 \right] \times 100\%$$

Eq. 25-19

where K_1 and K_2 are constants derived from the light path and molar extinction coefficients for oxygenated and deoxygenated hemoglobin.

Specimen Three different types of blood specimens—arterial, venous, and capillary—may be used for blood-gas determinations. Blood may be collected either in syringes or in capillary tubes. Both glass and plastic material are used. Glass syringes and glass capillary tubes are more suitable for sampling, storage, and transport of specimens as compared to devices made of plastic. A well-stopped glass syringe or glass capillary tube is gastight for at least 2 hours.[3,4] Plastic containers are permeable to gases and thus are not perfectly gastight.[5,6] The gas permeability of the plastic containers may cause a shift in the values of P_{O_2} and P_{CO_2} toward the corresponding values of the surrounding atmosphere.[6,7] The magnitude of this change is dependent on the thickness of the syringe wall, the surface-to-volume relationship, and the tightness of fit between the plunger and stopper. Plastic syringes are entirely suitable for collection of specimens for blood-gas analysis if the storage interval is not longer than 30 minutes.[3]

Regardless of the type of collection container used, several key requirements must be met for accurate measurement of blood gases. Samples must be collected and handled without contact with air (anaerobically) to prevent equilibration of blood-gas parameters with the atmosphere. Also, the sample must be properly anticoagulated. Insufficient coagulant or sample mixing will allow the formation of fibrin clots, which may interfere with instrument function, whereas an excessive amount of anticoagulant can yield incorrect data, an increased P_{CO_2}, and a decreased pH. If there is a delay of more than 5 minutes between sample collection and analysis, the blood-gas sample should be preserved in an ice-water mixture.

Reference intervals The reference intervals for pH, P_{O_2}, P_{CO_2}, and percent oxygen saturation at 37° C for arterial and venous blood are as follows:

	ARTERIAL	VENOUS
pH	7.35-7.45	7.33-7.43
P_{CO_2}	35-45 mm Hg	38-50 mm Hg
P_{O_2}	80-100 mm Hg	30-50 mm Hg
O_2 saturation (%)	95%-100%	60%-85%

Carbon dioxide

W. GREGORY MILLER
WILLIAM J. KORZUN

Principles of analysis Total carbon dioxide in serum or plasma consists of dissolved CO_2, CO_2 loosely bound to amine groups of plasma proteins, and bicarbonate (HCO_3^-) anion. Other quantitatively minor forms include carbonic acid (H_2CO_3) and carbonate ions (CO_3^{2-}). Since bicarbonate alone constitutes the majority of total carbon dioxide present in plasma, the measurement of total carbon dioxide is useful primarily to indicate bicarbonate concentration.

Procedures to quantitate total carbon dioxide content in serum or plasma may be of two types. In the first, acidification of the sample converts all the different carbon dioxide forms to CO_2 gas; measurement of the amount of gas formed is proportional to total CO_2 content. Another approach for measurement of total CO_2 involves the enzymatic reaction of bicarbonate with phosphoenolpyruvate carboxylase coupled to an indicator reaction that is monitored spectrophotometrically.

The historical reference method for CO_2 is the manometric method using the Natelson microgasometer (Table 25-6, method 1).[8,9] Sample is placed in a closed system and CO_2 and other gases present are released after acidification. The pressure exerted by the gases in the closed system is measured. The CO_2 gas is then absorbed by alkali and the residual pressure caused by the gases other than CO_2 is measured. The difference in pressures after acidification and after absorption of CO_2 by alkali is attributable to the CO_2 content of the sample.

Another older, infrequently used method for carbon dioxide determination is continuous-flow analysis (Table 25-6, method 2).[10] CO_2 gas is released from the sample by acidification of the sample stream. The gaseous CO_2 diffuses across a silicon-rubber membrane, dissolving in an alkaline bicarbonate buffer containing a pH-indicating dye (phenolphthalein or cresol red). The dissolved CO_2 gas is converted to bicarbonate and hydrogen ions producing a pH change that results in a change in the color intensity of the indicator. The increase in color is determined spectrophotometrically and is proportional to the CO_2 content of the sample. Because other gases dissolved in the serum do not produce a pH change, they do not interfere.

One commonly used method for CO_2 determinations employs a CO_2 electrode to quantitate the CO_2 gas produced after acidification of the sample (Table 25-6, method 3). This method, similar to continuous-flow analysis, has the CO_2 gas diffuse across a silicon-rubber membrane and dissolving in a buffer. This results in a change of the pH of a bicarbonate electrode buffer. However, the pH is not detected by a pH-indicating dye, but, instead, the pH change is detected by a glass pH electrode within the CO_2 electrode assembly (see p. 478).

Another common method used to measure total carbon dioxide is based on an enzymatic and spectrophotometric assay. This method has been adapted to many automated analyzers. All CO_2 forms are converted to HCO_3^- after the addition of alkali to the serum. The HCO_3^- is then enzymatically converted to oxaloacetic acid, which in turn is reduced to malate by NADH. The decrease in NADH concentration, monitored at 340 nm, is directly related to the bicarbonate concentration in the specimen (Table 25-6, method 4).

Table 25-6 Methods of total CO_2 analysis

Method	Analysis	Principle	Usage	Comment
1. Gas release	Manometric or thermometric	CO_2 is released from samples after addition of acid, and the gas pressure is measured manometrically or by thermal conductivity.	Rare	The reference method, used for calibration purposes
2. pH indicator	Spectrophotometric	CO_2 + Acid → CO_2 gas CO_2 gas $\xrightarrow{\text{Silicone membrane}}$ CO_2 dissolved, ↓ pH H^+ + pH indicator → *Color change*	Rare	Used in continuous-flow analyzers
3. CO_2 electrode	Ion-selective (pH) electrode	After acidification of sample, CO_2 diffuses across a silicone membrane into dilute bicarbonate buffer. The resulting pH change, as measured by a pH electrode, is related to total CO_2 content.	Common	Same electrode by which P_{CO_2} is measured in blood-gas analyzers
4. Enzymatic	Spectrophotometric	$HCO_3^- + PEP \xrightarrow{\text{PEPC}} OX + P_i$ $OX + NADH + H^+ \xrightarrow{\text{MDH}} MAL + NAD^+$ (↓ A, 340 nm)	Common	Used on discrete analyzers
5. Calculation	Ion-selective (pH and P_{CO_2}) electrode	Total CO_2 calculated from data obtained in blood-gas analysis $$\text{Total } CO_2 = \alpha P_{CO_2} + [HCO_3^-]$$	Common	Although only an estimate, it compares well with measured values

MAL, Malate; *MDH*, malate dehydrogenase; *NADH*, dihydronicotinamide adenine dinucleotide; *OX*, oxaloacetate; P_i, inorganic phosphate; *PEP*, phosphoenolpyruvate; *PEPC*, phosphoenolpyruvate carboxylase.

$$HCO_3^- + \text{Phospho}enol\text{pyruvate} \xrightarrow{\text{PEPC}} \text{Oxaloacetate} + P_i$$
$$\text{Oxaloacetate} + NADH + H^+ \xrightarrow{\text{MDH}} \text{Malate} + NAD^+$$

$$Eq.\ 25\text{-}20$$

PEPC is phospho*enol*pyruvate carboxylase, P_i is inorganic phosphate, and *MDH* is malate dehydrogenase.

Total CO_2 can also be calculated from measured pH and P_{CO_2} obtained during a blood-gas analysis (Table 25-6, method 5). Although this calculation can provide only an indirect, unmeasured estimate of total CO_2, it is frequently performed by many blood-gas analyzers. Agreement between calculated and measured total CO_2 is generally good.[11]

Specimen Serum or heparinized plasma are acceptable specimens for total CO_2 analysis. Venous blood drawn into an evacuated tube is the usual specimen, though capillary blood may also be used. Other anticoagulants cannot be used because they disturb the equilibrium between erythrocyte and plasma CO_2. They also lower the pH of the sample and accelerate the loss of CO_2 to ambient air. Whole blood cannot be used because the heme-bound CO_2 and carbamino-bound CO_2 vary with the hematocrit and oxygen saturation and produce variable results.

Reference intervals The reference intervals listed are based on the manometric procedure. The values obtained by many automated methods range from 22 to 32 mmol/L, according to various manufacturers' product information.

Children, 18-27 mmol/L
Adults, 21-31 mmol/L

Lactic acid

STEVEN C. KAZMIERCZAK

Principles of analysis and current usage Early methods for measurement of lactic acid were based on the oxidation of lactate by permanganate or manganese dioxide to form ac-etaldehyde and CO_2 or CO. The amount of lactate in the sample is proportional to the amount of products formed, which can be determined by a variety of techniques. Acetaldehyde can be measured colorimetrically,[12,13] by titration,[14] or by gas chromatography.[15] The CO formed (Table 25-7, method 1b) can be determined by titration[16] or gasometric analysis.[17] The CO_2 formed (Table 25-7, method 1c) can be quantified gasometrically by a Van Slyke manometer.[18]

Enzymatic methods for lactate employ lactate dehydrogenase or lactate oxidase. Lactate dehydrogenase (LD)-based methods monitor the oxidation of lactate to pyruvate with concomitant formation of NADH (Table 25-7, method 2).

$$\text{L-Lactate} + NAD^+ \xrightarrow{\text{LD}} \text{Pyruvate} + NADH + H^+ \quad Eq.\ 25\text{-}21$$

Because the equilibrium for this reaction lies far to the left, modifications are required to reverse this equilibrium in favor of formation of pyruvate. The use of an alkaline (pH 9.0) reaction medium, presence of excess NAD^+, and the use of trapping agents such as hydrazine, to remove pyruvate as it is formed, helps to shift the equilibrium of this reaction to the right. The formation of NADH may be monitored by spectrophotometric (340 nm) or fluorometric methods.

Lactate oxidase (LO) has also been used in several enzymatic lactate methods including colorimetric methods and the development of a reagent dipstick. Lactate oxidase catalyzes the following reaction:

$$\text{L-Lactate} + O_2 \xrightarrow{\text{LO}} \text{Pyruvate} + H_2O_2 \quad Eq.\ 25\text{-}22$$

The hydrogen peroxide generated in this reaction can oxidize various indicator compounds to produce a color change that is detected spectrophotometrically or usually using a visual dipstick technique.

Lactate oxidase has also been used in the production of lactate-specific electrodes (Table 25-7, method 3). Lactate

Table 25-7 Methods of lactate analysis

Method	Type of analysis	Principle	Usage	Comments
1. Chemical oxidation with formation of:		Permanganate (MnO_4) or MnO_2 oxidizes lactate to one of several products in one of the following reactions:	Historical	Accurate, precise, and sensitive, but time consuming
a. Acetaldehyde (CH_3CHO)	Quantitative, EP	Lactate $\xrightarrow[\text{Heat}]{H_2SO_4}$ Acetaldehyde + H_2O + CO		
b. CO (carbon monoxide)	Quantitative, EP	As above		
c. CO_2 (carbon dioxide)	Quantitative	2 lactate + $O_2 \rightarrow$ 2 acetaldehyde + $2CO_2$ + H_2O		
2. Enzymatic	Quantitative, EP or K	Lactate + NAD $\xrightarrow{\text{LD}}$ Pyruvate + NADH + H^+	Automated	Accurate and precise; automatable and rapid
3. Enzyme electrode senser	Quantitative, EP	Lactate + $O_2 \xrightarrow{\text{LO}} H_2O_2$ + Pyruvate $H_2O_2 \rightleftharpoons 2H^+ + O_2 + 2e^-$ Current measured is proportional to hydrogen peroxide (H_2O_2) concentration	Semiautomated	Incorporated in blood-gas analyzers
4. Electrochemical	Quantitative, EP	Lactate + $2Fe(CN)_6^{3-} \rightarrow$ Pyruvate + $2H^+ + 2Fe(CN)_6^{4-}$ $2Fe(CN)_6^{4-} \xrightarrow{\text{Pt electrode}} 2Fe(CN)_6^{3-} + 2e^-$	Automated	Accurate, precise, sensitive, and rapid analysis, but equipment not readily available

EP, End point; *K*, kinetic; *LD*, lactate dehydrogenase; *LO*, lactate oxidase.

Table 25-8 Methods of pyruvic acid analysis

Method	Principle	Usage	Comments
1. Enzymatic	Pyruvate converted to lactate with concomitant oxidation of NADH to NAD by lactate dehydrogenase. NADH monitored spectrophotometrically at 340 nm. Pyruvate + NADH + H $\overset{LD}{\rightleftharpoons}$ Lactate + NAD	Plasma, serum	Specific, most commonly used method, easily automated
2. Amperometric	Pyruvate reacts with pyruvate oxidase that has been immobilized on an artificial membrane. H_2O_2 produced is measured amperometrically. Pyruvate + HPO_4^{2-} + O_2 + H_2O $\xrightarrow[\text{oxidase}]{\text{Pyruvate}}$ Acetylphosphate + CO_2 + H_2O_2	Plasma, serum, whole blood	Experimental; correlates well with enzymatic pyruvate method

oxidase is immobilized in the membrane of an electrode. Hydrogen peroxide produced during the oxidation of lactate to pyruvate is detected by oxidation at a platinum anode:

$$Lactate + O_2 \xrightarrow{LO} H_2O_2 + Pyruvate$$

$$H_2O_2 \overset{\text{Platinum}}{\underset{\text{electrode}}{\rightleftharpoons}} 2H^+ + O_2 + 2e^- \qquad Eq.\ 25\text{-}23$$

This method has the advantage of being able to use whole blood samples.

A method to quantitate lactate by use of electrochemical detection has also been developed. The principle of this technique relies on the oxidation of lactate by ferricyanide, which is catalyzed by lactate dehydrogenase (Table 25-7, method 4). The hexacyanoferrate II that is produced by this reaction is then oxidized at a platinum electrode. The amount of current generated at the platinum electrode is proportional to the amount of hexacyanoferrate formed and thus the concentration of lactic acid initially present in the sample.

Specimen Accurate lactic acid measurements require special attention to sample processing. Venous stasis will increase blood lactate; tourniquet restriction time should be minimized, or, if a tourniquet is used, 1 to 2 minutes should elapse after release of the tourniquet before blood is collected. In specimens containing metabolically active cells, glucose is converted to lactate by cellular glycolytic pathways. Blood can be kept at 4° C for up to 2 hours with no significant change in lactate concentrations. However, the recommended sample for lactic acid analysis is a serum sample drawn in a sodium iodoacetate phlebotomy tube. Lactic acid concentrations in samples collected with sodium iodoacetate are suitable for up to 2 hours at room temperature.[19] Fluoride can also be used as an inhibitor of the glycolytic pathway.[20] Oxaloacetate cannot be used as an anticoagulant, since it will inhibit lactate dehydrogenase used in some enzymatic lactate assays. Certain drugs, including epinephrine, isoniazid, oral contraceptives, morphine, aspirin, valproic acid, phenytoin, and phenobarbital can change lactate concentrations by altering lactate metabolism.[21]

Reference intervals

SPECIMEN TYPE	LACTATE, mmol/L
Venous blood	0.5-2.2
Arterial blood	0.5-1.6
Cerebrospinal fluid	
<16 years	1.1-2.2
Adult	<2.8

These lactate concentrations in blood are for a patient at rest; higher values may be seen otherwise. Lactate concentrations may increase 20% to 50% over baseline values after a meal.[22] Lactic acid concentrations in cerebrospinal fluid are independent of serum levels but are usually close to those seen in blood.[23]

Pyruvic acid
STEVEN C. KAZMIERCZAK

Principles of analysis and current usage Measurement of pyruvate in blood is valuable in critical care medicine and exercise physiology.[24] The most common method in use for the analysis of pyruvic acid utilizes the enzyme lactate dehydrogenase (LD) to catalyze the following reaction (Table 25-8, method 1)[25]:

$$Pyruvate + NADH + H^+ \overset{LD}{\underset{\text{pH 7.4}}{\rightleftharpoons}} Lactate + NAD^+$$

$$Eq.\ 25\text{-}24$$

The consumption of NADH is monitored at 340 nm and is related to pyruvate concentrations in the sample. The reaction can be followed kinetically, by measuring the rate of disappearance of NADH, or it can be performed in an end-point mode. The reaction is performed at pH 7.4 with an excess of NADH, which favors the conversion of pyruvate to lactate. This is the same reaction that is used to measure lactate except that the analysis for lactic acid is performed at pH 9.8, and an excess of NAD^+ is present, which strongly favors the oxidation of lactate to pyruvate.

A biosensor has also been developed for measurement of pyruvate in whole blood or serum (Table 25-8, method 2).[26] The pyruvate sensor comprises a hydrogen peroxide sensor covered with a membrane containing immobilized pyruvate oxidase and protected with a cellulose acetate membrane. The reaction of pyruvate in the presence of pyruvate oxidase is as follows:

$$Pyruvate + HPO_3^{2-} + O_2 + H_2O \xrightarrow{\text{Pyruvate oxidase}}$$
$$Acetylphosphate + CO_2 + H_2O_2 \qquad Eq.\ 25\text{-}25$$

The H_2O_2 produced is measured amperometrically and related to the pyruvate concentration present in the sample. Several cofactors, including thiamine pyrophosphate (TPP), phosphate, and calcium chloride, are required for the reaction catalyzed by pyruvate oxidase.[27]

Specimen Blood should be drawn from a fasting patient. To prevent the metabolism of glucose by red blood cells, blood should be drawn in a tube containing iodoacetate (with a gray top). Mild exercise will increase the blood pyruvate concentration. Pyruvic acid is very unstable at room temperature. The serum should be separated immediately and kept at 4° to 8° C until analysis. Preservation of the sample by preparation of a protein-free supernatant of serum or plasma is recommended. Delays of 1 hour or more before deproteinization have been found unacceptable.[28] The use of metaphosphoric acid (MPA) for preparation of the protein-free supernatant is recommended over other precipitating agents because NADH is much more stable when MPA is used.[29] The protein-free supernatant is stable for 6 days at room temperature, 8 days if kept refrigerated, and for up to 42 days if stored frozen.[30]

Reference interval The concentration of pyruvate in healthy adults is <0.10 mmol/L.

REFERENCES

1. Clark LC: Monitor and control of blood and tissue oxygen tensions, *Trans Am Soc Artif Intern Organs* 2:41-48, 1956.
2. Rem J, Siggard-Andersen O, Norgard-Pedersen B, Sørensen S: Hemoglobin pigments: photometer for oxygen saturation, carboxyhemoglobin, and methemoglobin in capillary blood, *Clin Chim Acta* 42:101, 1972.
3. Burnett RW, Covington AK, Fogh-Andersen N, et al: Recommendations on whole blood sampling, transport, and storage for simultaneous determination of pH, blood gases, and electrolytes. *J Int Fed Clin Chem* 6:115-120, 1994.
4. Siggard-Andersen O: In *The acid-base status of the blood,* ed 4, Copenhagen, 1974, Munksgaard, p 152.
5. Rosenberg E, Price N: Diffusion of CO_2 and O_2 through the walls of plastic syringes, *Clin Chem* 37:1244-1248, 1991.
6. Mahoney JJ, Harvey JA, Wong RJ, Van Kessel AL: Changes in oxygen measurements when whole blood is stored in iced plastic or glass syringes, *Clin Chem* 37:1244-1248, 1991.
7. Hilty H, Karendal B: Effect of syringe material on oxygen tension in stored blood, *Acta Soc Upsal* 193-205, 1969.
8. Natelson S: Routine use of ultramicro methods in the clinical laboratory, *Am J Clin Pathol* 21:1153-1172, 1951.
9. Meites S, Faulkner WR: *Manual of practical micro and general procedures in clinical chemistry,* Springfield, Ill., 1961, Charles C Thomas.
10. Skeggs LT Jr: An automatic method for the determination of carbon dioxide in blood plasma, *Am J Clin Pathol* 33:181-185, 1960.
11. Ungerer JP, Ungerer MJ, Vermaak JH: Discordance between measured and calculated total carbon dioxide, *Clin Chem* 36:2093-2096, 1990.
12. Hochella NJ, Weinhouse S: Automated lactic acid determination in serum and tissue extracts, *Anal Biochem* 10:304, 1965.
13. Barker SB: Lactic acid. In Seligson D, editor: *Standard methods of clinical chemistry,* New York, 1961, Academic Press, vol 3.
14. Long C: The stabilization and estimation of lactic acid in blood samples, *Biochem J* 40:27, 1946.
15. Savory J, Kaplan A: A gas chromatographic method for the determination of lactic acid in blood, *Clin Chem* 12:559-569, 1966.
16. Ronzoni E, Wallen-Lawrence Z: Determination of lactic acid in blood, *J Biol Chem* 74:363-377, 1927.
17. Schneyer J: Eine methode zur quantitativen Milchsäurebestimmung im Harne, *Biochem Z* 70:294, 1915.
18. Avery BF, Hastings AB: A gasometric method for the determination of lactic acid in the blood, *J Biol Chem* 94:273-280, 1931.
19. Kaplan LA, Gau N, Stein EA: Collection and storage of serum lactic acid samples at room temperature without deproteinization, *Clin Chem* 26:175-176, 1980.
20. Astles R, Williams CP, Sedor F: Stability of plasma lactate in vitro in the presence of antiglycolytic agents, *Clin Chem* 40:1327-1330, 1994.
21. Kiechle FL: *Lactate: review of methods,* ASCP check sample volume 8, no 7, PTS 92-7 (PTS-65), American Society of Clinical Pathologists.
22. Friedmann TE, Haugen GE, Kmieciak TC: Pyruvic acid III, *J Biol Chem* 157:673-689, 1945.
23. Glasser L: Body fluids III: tapping the wealth of information in CSF, *Diagn Med,* pp 23-33, Jan-Feb 1981.
24. Bonora R, Pagani F, Panteghini M: Pyruvate measured in whole blood with the Cobas Bio analyzer, *Clin Chem* 35:325, 1989.
25. Hansen JL, Freier EF: Direct assays of lactate, pyruvate, β-hydroxybutyrate and acetoacetate with a centrifugal analyzer, *Clin Chem* 24:475-479, 1978.
26. Chariot P, Ratiney R, Ammi-Said M, et al: Optimal handling of blood samples for routine measurement of lactate and pyruvate, *Arch Pathol Lab Med* 118:695-697, 1994.
27. Mascini M, Mazzei F, Moscone D, et al: Lactate and pyruvate electrochemical biosensors for whole blood in extracorporeal experiments with an endocrine artificial pancreas, *Clin Chem* 33:591-593, 1987.

BIBLIOGRAPHY

Arieff AI, DeFronzo RA: *Fluid, electrolyte and acid-base disorders,* ed 2, New York, 1995, Churchill Livingstone.
Cohen JJ, Kassirer JP: *Acid-base,* Boston, 1982, Little, Brown & Co.
Davenport HW: *The ABC of acid-base chemistry,* ed 6, Chicago, 1974, University of Chicago Press.
Haber RJ: A practical approach to acid-base disorders, *West J Med* 155(2):146-151, 1991.
Soloway HB: How the body maintains acid-base balance, *Diagn Med,* pp 32-41, Feb 1979.
Scanlon CL, Spearman CD, Sheldon R: *Egan's fundamentals of respiratory care,* ed 6, St. Louis, 1995, Mosby.

Renal function

M. Roy First

OBJECTIVES

- List the five main functions of the kidney and outline the formation of urine, including the function of the following:
  Glomerulus
  Proximal tubule
  Loop of Henle
  Distal convoluted tubule
  Collecting duct

- Outline the mechanism by which the kidney conserves protein and describe the metabolic production and renal control of blood urea nitrogen, serum creatinine, and uric acid.

- Given pathological conditions associated with the kidney, state the expected abnormal laboratory results.

- State the purpose of performing a renal clearance test and the reasons why creatinine is most frequently used for renal clearance testing. State the advantages and disadvantages of using inulin or urea for clearance testing.

- Outline two types of studies used to evaluate renal tubular function.

KEY TERMS

albuminuria The presence of albumin in urine.

absorption (active and passive) The process of uptake of substance into tissues or cells. Active absorption requires the expenditure of energy to move substances against a concentration gradient, whereas, in the case of passive absorption, substances move from higher to lower concentrations.

aldosterone A steroid hormone produced in the adrenal cortex that acts on the distal tubules to stimulate sodium reabsorption and potassium and hydrogen excretion.

antidiuretic hormone (ADH) Also called *vasopressin;* a pituitary hormone that acts at the collecting duct to increase absorption of water, resulting in the formation of a more concentrated urine.

anuria A condition in which no urine is formed.

ascending limb The straight portion of the loop of Henle in which the presumptive urine flows up toward the convoluted distal tubule. Osmolality of urine decreases because of loss of chloride (plus Na^+).

Bence Jones protein The light-chain portion of a monoclonal immunoglobulin produced in excess and excreted into urine by patients with multiple myeloma.

bladder A sac used to collect formed urine before voiding.

Bowman's capsule A structure consisting of glomeruli and extended opening of the proximal tubule.

carbonic anhydrase The enzyme at the brush border of the proximal tubule that catalyzes the reaction $H_2O + CO_2 \rightarrow H_2CO_3$.

casts Protein aggregates, outlined in the shape of renal tubules, secreted into the urine.

clearance A theoretical concept expressing that volume of plasma filtered at the glomeruli per unit of time from which an analyte would be completely removed and placed in final urine. It is usually expressed as milliliters of plasma per minute.

collecting tubule The last portion of the nephron, connecting the distal convoluted tubule and the larger collecting ducts, which in turn empty into the ureter. The final concentrating processes under the influence of antidiuretic hormone occur here.

countercurrent mechanism The process by which two streams flowing in opposite directions exchange material. In the kidney, urine and blood form opposing flows, and this mechanism allows reabsorption of substances.

creatinine clearance An estimate of the glomerular filtration rate obtained by measurement of the amount of creatinine in the plasma and its rate of excretion into the urine.

descending limb The straight portion of the loop of Henle in which forming urine flows down from the convoluted proximal tubule. This portion of the loop of Henle is freely permeable to water, which leaves the presumptive urine.

distal convoluted tubule The convoluted tubule connecting the ascending loop of Henle with the collecting tubule. It has secretory and reabsorptive functions as part of the final urine formation and acidification process.

diuretic A drug the action of which promotes the increased excretion of salt and water, thus increasing the flow of urine.

filtered load The amount of a substance presented to the tubules for reabsorption.

glomerular filtration rate (GFR) The rate in milliliters per minute at which plasma substances are filtered through the glomeruli into the proximal tubule.

glomerulus Cluster of small blood vessels in the kidney that projects into the expanded end (capsule) of the proximal tubule and functions as a filtering mechanism of the nephron.

hematuria The presence of blood or red blood cells in the urine.

loop of Henle A U-shaped tubule connecting the proximal and distal convoluted tubules. It reduces the volume of tubule fluid.

microalbuminuria Low-grade, dipstick-negative increase in urine albumin excretion.

micturition Urination.

nephron The functional unit of the kidney containing Bowman's capsule, the proximal and convoluted tubules, the ascending and descending limbs of the loop of Henle, and the collecting tubules.

oliguria The formation of small amounts of urine.

proteinuria The presence of protein in urine.

proximal tubule The convoluted tubule beginning at the glomeruli and connecting to the descending loop of Henle. It has secretory and reabsorptive functions as part of the mechanism for urine formation.

pyuria The presence of pus (an inflammation fluid with leukocytes and dead cells) in the urine.

renal cortex The outer part of the kidney that contains mostly glomeruli and convoluted tubules.

renal medulla The inner part of the kidney that contains mostly collecting ducts and the loop of Henle.

renal threshold The plasma concentration of a substance above which it will be present in urine.

renin An enzyme formed by the juxtaglomerular apparatus in the kidney. It converts plasma angiotensinogen to angiotensin I.

specific gravity The ratio of the weight in grams per milliliter of a body fluid compared with water.

titratable acid The combination of hydrogen ion with phosphate present in final urine.

urethra A membranous tube through which urine passes from the bladder to the exterior of the body.

urine The aqueous liquid and dissolved substances excreted by the kidney.

ANATOMY OF KIDNEY
Gross anatomy

The kidneys are paired organs located in the posterior part of the abdomen on either side of the vertebral column. Underneath the capsule of fibrous tissue that encloses the kidney lies the cortex, which contains the glomeruli. The inner portion of the kidney, the medulla, contains the collecting ducts. A vertical section through the kidney is shown on the left-hand side of Fig. 26-1.

The urinary system is illustrated on the right-hand side of Fig. 26-1. The renal pelvis rapidly diminishes in caliber and merges into the ureter. Each ureter descends in the abdomen alongside the vertebral column to join the bladder. The bladder provides temporary storage for urine, which is eventually voided through the urethra to the exterior.

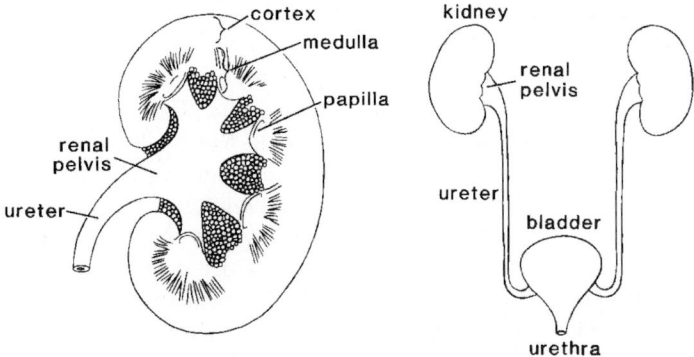

Fig. 26-1   Gross anatomy of kidney and urinary system.

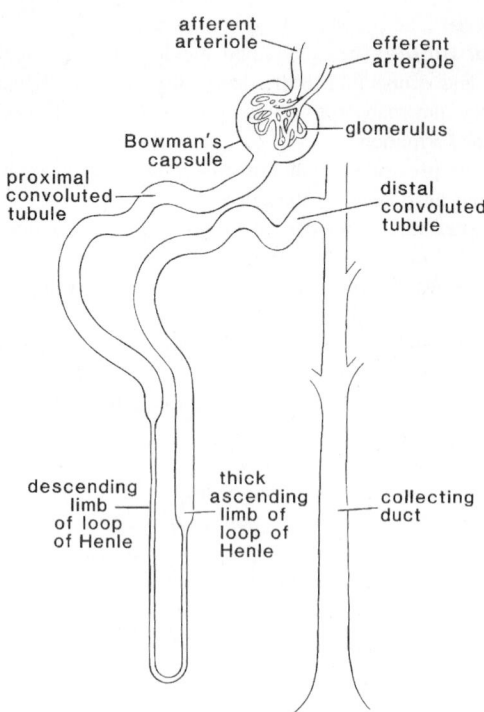

Fig. 26-2 Components of the nephron.

Microscopic anatomy

Each kidney is made up of approximately 1 million functional units, or *nephrons*. The component parts of the nephron are illustrated in Fig. 26-2. The nephron begins with the glomerulus, which is a tuft of capillaries that is formed from the afferent (incoming) arteriole and drained by a smaller efferent (outgoing) arteriole. The glomerulus is surrounded by Bowman's capsule, which is formed by the blind, dilated end of the renal tubule. The proximal convoluted tubule runs a tortuous course through the cortex, entering the medulla and forming first the descending limb of the loop of Henle and then the ascending limb of the loop of Henle. The thick section of the ascending limb of the loop of Henle reenters the cortex, forming the distal convoluted tubule. The merging of two or more distal tubules marks the beginning of a collecting duct. As the collecting duct descends through the cortex and medulla, it receives the effluent from a dozen or more distal tubules. The collecting ducts join and increase in size as they pass down the medulla. The ducts of each pyramid coalesce to form a central duct, which empties through the papilla into a minor calyx, eventually draining into the renal pelvis.

RENAL PHYSIOLOGY

The kidney is the chief regulator of all body fluids and is primarily responsible for maintaining homeostasis, or equilibrium of fluid and electrolytes in the body. The kidney has six main functions:

1. Urine formation
2. Regulation of fluid and electrolyte balance
3. Regulation of acid-base balance
4. Excretion of waste products of protein metabolism
5. Hormonal function
6. Protein conservation

The kidney is able to carry out these complex functions because approximately 25% of the volume of blood pumped by the heart into the systemic circulation is circulated through the kidneys; therefore the kidneys, which constitute about 0.5% of total body weight, receive one fourth of the cardiac output.

Urine formation

The removal of potentially toxic waste products is a major function of the kidneys and is accomplished through the formation of urine. The basic processes involved in the formation of urine are *filtration, reabsorption,* and *secretion.* The kidneys filter large volumes of plasma, reabsorb most of what is filtered, and leave behind for elimination from the body a concentrated solution of metabolic wastes called *urine.* In healthy individuals the kidneys, highly sensitive to fluctuations in diet and fluid and electrolyte intake, compensate for any changes by varying the volume and consistency of the urine.

Glomerular filtration. Each minute 1000 to 1500 mL of blood pass through the kidneys. The glomerulus has a semipermeable basement membrane that allows free passage of water and electrolytes but is relatively impermeable to larger molecules. The architecture of the human glomerular capillary wall is illustrated in Fig. 26-3. In the process of transfer from capillary lumen (CL) to Bowman's space, or urinary space (US), water, solutes, and macromolecules must traverse three layers: (1) The endothelial wall cytoplasm (En), containing numerous fenestra with a mean diameter of 70 nm; (2) the basement membranes (B) with a mean thickness of 320 nm; and (3) the layer of foot process (F), which are separated 25 to 60 nm from each other by slit pores. The cytoplasm (EpCy) and nucleus (EpN) of an epithelial cell are also shown. In glomerular capillaries the hydrostatic pressure is approximately three times greater than the pressure in other capillaries. As a result of this high pressure, substances are filtered through the semipermeable membrane into Bowman's capsule at a rate of approximately 130 mL/min; this is known as the *glomerular filtration rate* (GFR). Cells and the large-molecular-size plasma proteins are unable to pass through the semipermeable membrane. Therefore the glomerular filtrate is essentially plasma without the proteins. The GFR is an extremely important parameter in both the study of kidney physiology and the clinical assessment of renal function. In the average healthy person, more than 187,000 mL of filtrate are formed per day. Normal urine output is around 1500 mL per day, which is only about 1% of the amount of filtrate formed; therefore the other 99% must be reabsorbed.

Proximal tubule. The proximal tubular cells perform a variety of physiological tasks. Approximately 80% of salt and water are reabsorbed from the glomerular filtrate in the

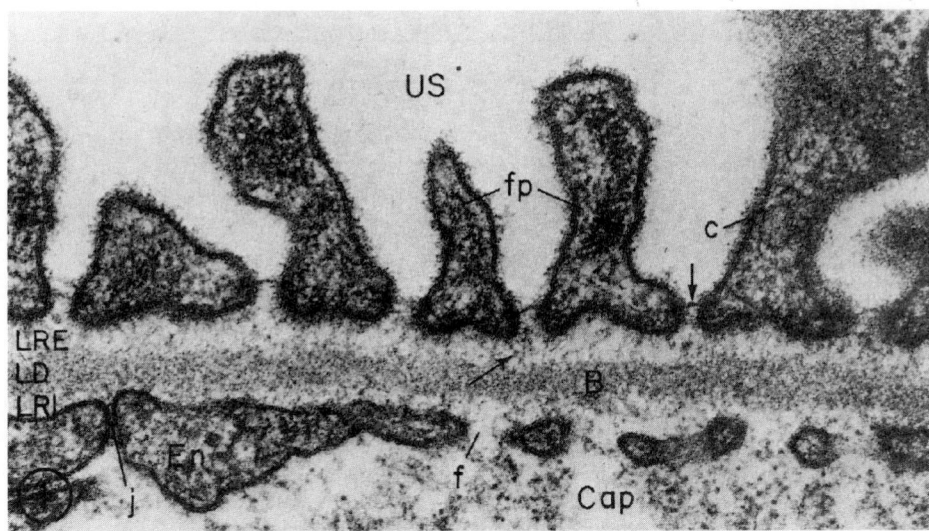

Fig. 26-3 Portion of a glomerulus showing a peripheral region of a capillary loop cut into a healthy section. The filtration surface consists of the endothelium *(En)* with its open fenestrae *(f)* lacking diaphragms, the glomerular basement membrane *(B)*, and the epithelial foot processes *(fp)* between which are the filtration slits, bridged at their base by slit membranes *(short arrow)*. Notice that the GBM consists of three layers—a central dense layer, the lamina densa *(LD)*, and two adjoining layers of lower density, the lamina rara interna *(LRI)* and externa *(LRE)*. A thick cell coat *(c)* is visible on the membrane of the foot processes. The lamina densa is composed of a fine (~3 nm) filamentous meshwork, and wispy filaments are seen extending from the lamina densa to the endothelial and epithelial *(long arrow)* membranes on either side. *Cap,* Capillary lumen; *J,* junction between two endothelial cells; *US,* urinary spaces; 80,000 ×. (From Farquhar MG, Kanwan YS: In Cummings NB, Michael AF, Wilson CB, editors: *Immune mechanisms in renal disease,* New York, 1983, Plenum Medical Books.)

proximal tubule. All the filtered glucose and most of the filtered amino acids are normally reabsorbed here. Low-molecular-weight proteins, urea, uric acid, bicarbonate, phosphate, chloride, potassium, magnesium, and calcium are reabsorbed to varying extents. A variety of organic acids and bases, as well as hydrogen ions and ammonia, are secreted into the tubular fluid by tubular cells. Under normal conditions, no glucose is excreted in the urine; all that is filtered is reabsorbed. As the plasma concentration of glucose is increased above some critical level, termed the *renal plasma threshold,* the tubular maximum for glucose is exceeded, and glucose appears in the urine. The higher the plasma concentration of glucose, the greater is the quantity excreted in the urine. Renal plasma thresholds also exist for phosphate and bicarbonate ions.

Most of the metabolic energy consumed by the kidney is used to promote *active reabsorption.* Active reabsorption can produce net movement of a substance against a concentration or electrical gradient and therefore requires energy expenditure by the transporting cells. Active reabsorption of glucose, amino acids, low-molecular-weight proteins, uric acid, sodium, potassium, magnesium, calcium, chloride, and bicarbonate is regulated by the kidney according to the levels of these substances in the blood and the body's needs. *Passive reabsorption* occurs when a substance moves by simple diffusion as the result of an electrical or chemical concentration gradient, and no cellular energy is involved in the process. Water, urea, and chloride are reabsorbed in this way.

Tubular secretion, which transports substances into the tubular lumen (that is, in the direction opposite to tubular reabsorption), may also be an active or passive process. Substances that are transported from the blood to the tubules and excreted in the urine include potassium, hydrogen ions, ammonia, uric acid, and certain drugs, such as penicillin. Table 26-1 gives an idea of the magnitude and importance of these reabsorptive mechanisms.

Loop of Henle. The descending limb of the loop of Henle is highly permeable to water. In the medulla, the loop of Henle descends into an environment that is increasingly hypertonic as the papilla is approached. Passive reabsorption of water occurs in response to this osmotic gradient, leaving the presumptive urine highly concentrated at the bottom of the loop. The ascending limb is relatively impermeable to the passage of water but actively reabsorbs sodium and chloride. This segment of the nephron is often called the *diluting segment* because the removal of salt with little water from the tubular contents lowers the salt and osmotic concentration, in effect diluting the tubular fluid. The ascending thick limb of the loop of Henle transfers sodium

Table 26-1 Filtration, reabsorption, and excretion by kidney

Component	Amount filtered per day	Amount excreted per day	Percentage reabsorbed
Water	180 L	1.5 L	99.2
Sodium	24,000 mEq	100 mEq	99.6
Chloride	20,000 mEq	100 mEq	99.5
Bicarbonate	5,000 mEq	2 mEq	99.9
Potassium	700 mEq	50 mEq	92.9
Glucose	180 g	0	100
Albumin	360 mg	18 mg	95.0

chloride actively from its lumen into the interstitial fluid. The tubular fluid in its lumen becomes hypotonic, and the interstitial fluid becomes hypertonic. This phenomenon is known as the *countercurrent mechanism*. A series of successive steps results in sodium chloride being trapped in the interstitial fluid of the medulla. As the isotonic fluid in the descending limb reaches the area into which the ascending limb is pumping out sodium, it becomes slightly hypertonic because of the movement of water into the hypertonic interstitium. The first step repeats itself, and again, as more sodium and chloride are added to the interstitium by the ascending limb, more water is drawn out of the descending limb.

Distal convoluted tubule. A small fraction of the filtered sodium, chloride, and water is reabsorbed in the distal tubule. The distal tubule responds to the antidiuretic hormone (ADH), and so its water permeability is high in the presence of the hormone and low in its absence. Potassium can be reabsorbed or secreted in the distal tubule. Aldosterone stimulates both sodium reabsorption and potassium secretion in the distal tubule. Hydrogen, ammonia, and uric acid secretion and bicarbonate reabsorption occur, but there is little transport of organic substances. This segment of the nephron has a low permeability to urea.

Collecting duct. ADH controls the water permeability of the collecting tubule throughout its length. In the presence of the hormone, the hypotonic tubular fluid entering the duct loses water. Sodium and chloride are reabsorbed by the collecting tubule, with the transport of sodium stimulated by aldosterone. Potassium, hydrogen, and ammonia are also reabsorbed by the collecting duct. When ADH is present, the rate of water reabsorption exceeds the rate of solute reabsorption, and the concentration of sodium and chloride in the presumptive urine rises. The collecting duct is relatively impermeable to urea.

Regulation of fluid and electrolyte balance

Water. Water is the most abundant component of the human body, constituting approximately 60% of body weight. Body water, and therefore body weight, remains fairly constant from day to day in normal persons, despite wide fluctuations in fluid and salt intake.[1,2] One of the most remarkable properties of the human kidney is its ability to elaborate urine that is either more concentrated or more dilute

than the plasma from which it is derived. When the human body needs to conserve water, as in dehydration, the concentrating mechanism operates maximally, and urine osmolality increases to about 1200 mOsm/kg. Conversely, when there is excess water in the body, urine flow increases, and the diluting mechanism reduces urine osmolality to as low as 50 mOsm/kg. The capacity of the kidney to form urine of greatly varying osmolality enables it to regulate the solute concentration and hence the osmolality of body fluids within narrow physiological limits, despite wide fluctuations in intake of salt and water.[1,2] Water balance is controlled primarily through voluntary intake (which is regulated through the thirst center in the hypothalamus) and urinary loss of water. The control of urinary water loss is the major automatic mechanism by which body water is regulated. In dehydrated states the urine is concentrated when the kidney reabsorbs water without solute. Conversely, urine is diluted when the kidney reabsorbs solute without water.

Sodium. Sodium is the main cation found in extracellular fluid. Sodium is freely filtered through the glomerulus and actively reabsorbed by the tubules. Sodium reabsorption is very important because it affects the regulation of several other electrolytes. Active reabsorption of the sodium ion in the proximal tubule results in passive transport of chloride and bicarbonate as counterions and in passive reabsorption of water. In normal persons, daily urinary sodium excretion fluctuates widely according to the dietary intake, thereby keeping the body sodium content remarkably constant. In the normal person, more than 99% of the filtered load of sodium is reabsorbed by the kidneys. The sodium reabsorption by the nephron is controlled by the renin-angiotensin-aldosterone system (see Chapters 24 and 31).[3,4]

Chloride. The concentration of chloride in the extracellular fluid parallels that of sodium and is influenced by the same factors. However, chloride reabsorption is passive in the proximal tubule and probably active in the distal tubule and collecting duct.

Potassium. Potassium is the chief cation of the intracellular fluid. Maintenance of a normal potassium level is essential to the life of the cells. The distribution of potassium is such that 90% of total body potassium is intracellular and only 2% is extracellular. The high intracellular-to-extracellular potassium ratio is maintained by the

Na^+,K^+-ATPase pump.[5] The normal person maintains potassium balance by excreting daily an amount of potassium equal to the amount ingested minus the small amount eliminated in the feces and sweat. Renal function is the major mechanism by which the body potassium is regulated. Potassium is freely filtered at the glomerulus, and active tubular reabsorption occurs throughout the nephron, except in the descending loop of Henle. Only about 10% of the filtered potassium enters the distal tubule. The distal tubule and collecting ducts are able to both secrete and reabsorb potassium, thus regulating potassium excretion.[6] The hormone aldosterone, which stimulates tubular sodium reabsorption, simultaneously enhances potassium secretion in the distal tubule.[6,7]

Calcium. Calcium reabsorption in the proximal tubule parallels that of sodium and water. The maintenance of calcium homeostasis depends on the balance between calcium intake and calcium loss. The body loses calcium in the urine, through the gastrointestinal tract, and in sweat. Calcium balance is achieved largely by the control of calcium absorption rather than by the regulation of calcium excretion. The percentage of ingested calcium absorbed decreases as the dietary calcium content increases, and so the amount absorbed can remain relatively constant. The slight increase in absorption that occurs on a high-calcium diet is reflected in an increased renal excretion.[8]

Phosphorus. Over a wide range of dietary intakes, roughly two thirds of ingested phosphorus is absorbed into the bloodstream. The maintenance of the phosphorus balance is achieved largely through renal excretion.[8,9] Proximal tubular reabsorption of inorganic phosphate is normally about 90% of the filtered load. Parathyroid hormone depresses the renal tubular reabsorption of inorganic phosphate. In progressive chronic renal failure, there is a progressive increase in the serum phosphorus level.[10]

Magnesium. The filtration of magnesium at the glomerulus and its reabsorption from the proximal tubules parallels that of calcium and is also under the influence of parathyroid hormone. A moderate elevation of the plasma magnesium concentration occurs in patients with advanced chronic renal failure.[11]

Acid-base balance

Each day acid waste products are produced in the body. If they were not disposed of efficiently, they would accumulate and cause cellular damage. Body pH is controlled by three systems: acid-base buffers, the lungs, and the kidneys. (See Chapter 25.)

Excretion of hydrogen ions. In subjects on a normal diet, about 50 to 100 mEq of hydrogen ions are generated each day.[12] To prevent a progressive metabolic acidosis, these hydrogen ions are excreted in the urine. Hydrogen ions are generated in the cells of the proximal and distal tubule and the collecting duct as a result of the formation of carbonic acid by the enzyme carbonic anhydrase (CA).

These hydrogen ions are secreted by the cells into the lumen[13]:

$$H_2O + CO_2 \xrightleftharpoons{CA} H_2CO_3 \rightleftharpoons H^+ + HCO_3^- \qquad \textit{Eq. 26-1}$$

The kidneys' role in the maintenance of the acid-base balance centers on the generation of bicarbonate. The hydrogen ions are excreted into the urine while newly generated bicarbonate ions pass from the tubular cells into the blood at the same rate as bicarbonate is consumed by the metabolic processes.[13] Four mechanisms exist to handle the hydrogen ions that have been secreted into the tubular fluid.

Reaction with filtered bicarbonate ions. Bicarbonate is completely filterable at the glomerulus. In the tubular lumen, the excreted hydrogen ion combines with the filtered bicarbonate to form carbonic acid, which decomposes to water and carbon dioxide, the latter then diffusing into the cell, where it can be converted by CA to carbonic acid to generate another hydrogen ion. One bicarbonate ion is regenerated for every hydrogen ion that is secreted into the tubular lumen. The bicarbonate ion is reabsorbed into the blood as sodium bicarbonate, thus conserving most of the filtered bicarbonate. The renal threshold for bicarbonate is 28 mM; at a plasma level below this, all filtered bicarbonate is reabsorbed.

Reaction with filtered buffers to form titratable acids. Inorganic monohydrogen phosphate is present in the tubular lumen as the disodium salt. The secreted hydrogen ions react with the filtered phosphate, releasing sodium that combines with the bicarbonate; the sodium bicarbonate is reabsorbed, and dihydrogen phosphate is excreted:

$$Na_2HPO_4 + H^+ \rightarrow NaH_2PO_4 + Na^+$$
$$Na^+ + HCO_3^- \rightarrow NaHCO_3 \text{ (reabsorbed)} \qquad \textit{Eq. 26-2}$$

Hydrogen ions combine with phosphate to form titratable acid. The rate of excretion of titratable acid is limited by the filtered load of buffer and cannot increase greatly in acidosis. The lowest possible pH of urine is 4.4.

Reaction with secreted ammonia to form ammonium ion. The glomerular filtrate does not contain ammonia. This compound is synthesized in renal tubular cells by deamination of glutamine in the presence of glutaminase.[13] The ammonia diffuses into the tubular fluid, where it reacts with a secreted hydrogen ion to form an ammonium ion. Once again this results in the addition of new bicarbonate to the blood. The most important renal adaptation to acidosis is the increased excretion of ammonium ions[13]:

$$\text{Glutamine} \xrightarrow{\text{Glutaminase}} \text{Glutamic acid} + NH_3$$
$$NH_3 + H^+ \rightarrow NH_4^+ \qquad \textit{Eq. 26-3}$$

Excretion as free hydrogen ions. Only negligible quantities of hydrogen ions are handled in this way by the kidneys.

Nitrogenous waste excretion

One of the major functions of the kidney is the elimination of nitrogenous products of protein catabolism. The enormous reserves of the kidney for excretion of the products of protein catabolism are indicated by the fact that the blood concentrations of these products are not elevated in renal failure until renal function is reduced to less than one half of normal.[14]

Urea. As amino acids are deaminated, ammonia is produced. The development of toxic levels of ammonia in the blood is prevented by the conversion of ammonia to urea. This takes place in the liver. Urea in the blood is reported as the blood urea nitrogen (BUN). Urea production and the BUN are increased when more amino acids are metabolized in the liver. This can occur with a high-protein diet, tissue breakdown, or decreased protein synthesis. In contrast, urea production and the BUN are reduced in the presence of a low-protein intake and severe liver disease. Urea production exceeds renal urea excretion in normal persons. The remaining urea is degraded to ammonium ions by intestinal bacteria. Urea is readily filtered, but approximately 40% to 50% of the filtered urea is normally reabsorbed by the proximal tubules. Since many factors may influence the BUN level while the GFR remains constant, BUN is a less specific indicator of renal function and should not be relied on for that purpose.

Creatinine. Serum creatinine levels and urinary creatinine excretion are a function of muscle mass in normal persons and shows little response to dietary changes.[16] Creatinine is derived from the nonenzymatic dehydration of creatine in skeletal muscle. The amount of creatine per unit of muscle mass is constant, and thus the rate of spontaneous breakdown of creatine is also constant. As a result, the plasma creatinine concentration is very stable, varying less than 10% per day in serial observations in normal subjects. Since the serum creatinine concentration is a direct reflection of muscle mass, the serum level is higher in males than in females. Creatinine is freely filtered at the glomerulus and is not reabsorbed by the tubules. A small amount of the creatinine in the final urine is derived from tubular secretion. Because of these properties of creatinine, the creatinine clearance can be used to estimate the GFR (see tests of glomerular function, p. 493):

$$CH_3-NCH_2-COOH \qquad CH_3-N-CH_2$$
$$| \qquad\qquad\qquad \backslash$$
$$C=NH \quad \longrightarrow \quad | \qquad C=O + H_2O$$
$$| \qquad\qquad\qquad /$$
$$NH_2 \qquad\qquad HN=C-NH$$

Creatine **Creatinine** *Eq. 26-4*

Uric acid. Uric acid is derived from the oxidation of purine bases. Plasma levels of uric acid are quite variable and are higher in males than in females. Plasma urates are completely filterable, and both proximal tubular resorption and distal tubular secretion occur. With advanced chronic renal failure there is a progressive increase in the plasma uric acid level.

Hormonal function

The kidneys have important metabolic and endocrine functions. The kidney as an endocrine organ is discussed in this section.[17]

Vitamin D metabolism. In vitamin D metabolism the kidney produces the major biologically active hormone 1,25-dihydroxycholecalciferol.[18] The enzyme responsible for the production of 1,25-dihydroxycholecalciferol is present only in the mitochondria of the renal cortex. (See Chapter 28.)

Renin. The kidney releases renin in response to a decrease in extracellular fluid volume. This results in stimulation of the renin-angiotensin-aldosterone axis, with subsequent sodium and water conservation. (See Chapters 24 and 31.)

Erythropoietin. The kidneys play a major role in the production and release of erythropoietin, a hormone that stimulates red blood cell production. The central role of the kidneys in erythropoietin production explains the anemia associated with chronic renal failure.[19]

Protein conservation

Under normal physiological conditions, the kidney helps to maintain the homeostasis of the body's proteins. In humans 180 L of plasma, each liter containing 70 g of protein, are filtered each day by the glomerulus.[20] Without an efficient conservation mechanism, body protein stores would be depleted very rapidly. Yet normal urine contains less than 200 mg of protein per day, with only a minute percentage of the 12,600 g passing through the glomerulus daily.[20] Most of the filtered proteins are absorbed by the proximal tubules and returned to the circulation. Most plasma proteins, except those of very high molecular weight, have been found in the urine. Albumin excretion is less than 20 mg/day.[20] Many proteins of nonserum origin are also found in the urine. One of these, uromucoid or Tamm-Horsfall mucoprotein, is the predominant protein in normal urine, with about 40 mg excreted daily.[21] This high-molecular-weight mucoprotein is excreted by the cells of the distal tubule and collecting ducts. Commercially available dipsticks (Albustix) are in widespread use and are accurate for rapid assessments of urinary protein concentration.

PATHOLOGICAL CONDITIONS OF KIDNEY

There are many syndromes that singly or in combination indicate possible renal disease. These have been elegantly described by Coe.[22]

Acute glomerulonephritis

Acute glomerulonephritis is an acute inflammation of the glomeruli, resulting in oliguria, hematuria, increased BUN and serum creatinine levels, decreased GFR, edema formation, and hypertension. The presence of red blood cells in the urine (hematuria) alone is insufficient evidence of acute glomerulonephritis, for blood can originate from elsewhere in the kidney or from the urinary tract. The presence of red blood cell casts in the urine indicates glomerular inflammation and is a finding of great importance. Other abnormalities present in acute nephritis include proteinuria and anemia.

Nephrotic syndrome

The nephrotic syndrome has been classically defined as a clinical entity characterized by massive proteinuria, edema, hypoalbuminemia, hyperlipidemia, and lipiduria.[20] This syndrome, which can have many causes, is characterized by increased glomerular membrane permeability that results in massive proteinuria and excretion of fat bodies. Protein excretion rates are usually greater than 2 to 3 g/day in the absence of a depressed GFR. Hematuria and oliguria may be present. The causes of the nephrotic syndrome are illustrated in the following box. As a result of the massive loss of serum proteins, primarily albumin, into urine, the plasma protein concentration is decreased, with a concomitant reduction in plasma oncotic pressure. This results in fluid movement from the vascular to interstitial space with consequent edema formation.

Tubular disease

In some disorders of renal tubular function, the depressed renal function cannot be explained by the reduction in the GFR. Defects of tubular function may result in depressed

---

Causes of Nephrotic Syndrome

Associated with various forms of glomerulonephritis
Associated with generalized disease processes
    Amyloidosis
    Carcinoma
    Systemic lupus erythematosus
    Diabetic glomerulosclerosis
    Polyarteritis nodosa
Associated with mechanical or circulating disorders
    Renal vein thrombosis
    Constrictive pericarditis
Associated with infection
    Syphilis
    Malaria
    Subacute bacterial endocarditis
Associated with toxins and allergens
    Penicillamine
    Gold salts
    Bee sting
    Serum sickness
Miscellaneous
    Severe preeclampsia
    Transplant rejection

---

secretion or reabsorption of specific biochemicals or impairment of urine concentration and dilution mechanisms. Renal tubular acidosis (RTA) is the most important clinical disorder of tubular function.[23] There are two main types of RTA: (1) proximal RTA, which is a result of reduced proximal tubular bicarbonate reabsorption and causes *hyperchloremic acidosis,* and (2) distal RTA, in which there is an inability of the tubular cells to create and maintain the usual pH difference between tubular fluid and blood. Failure of either the proximal or distal secretory mechanisms occurs in several disease states. Failure of the proximal tubule to reabsorb bicarbonate causes acidosis because more bicarbonate is passed on to the low-capacity distal mechanism than it can reabsorb. The loss of alkali in the urine causes the blood to become acidotic. Defects in potassium and uric acid secretion may result in elevations of the serum potassium and uric acid levels that cannot be explained by the reduction in the GFR. Reabsorptive disorders of the proximal tubules may result in hypouricemia, hypophosphatemia, aminoaciduria, and renal glucosuria. The Fanconi syndrome is a group of renal defects resulting in glucosuria, aminoaciduria, hypophosphatemia, and renal tubular acidosis. Tubular proteinuria may occur as a result of a tubular defect in the handling of proteins. In tubular proteinuria, less than 2 g/day of protein are excreted. Disorders of urine concentration and dilution occur in all renal disease as the GFR falls appreciably, but occasionally these disorders become extreme and dominate the clinical presentation.[22]

Urinary tract infection

Infection of the urinary tract may occur in the bladder *(cystitis)* or may involve the kidneys *(pyelonephritis)*. The presence of a urine bacterial concentration of more than 100,000 colonies/mL is diagnostic of urinary tract infections. In a urinary tract infection there is an increased number of white blood cells in the urine. The presence of white blood cell casts indicates pyelonephritis. An increased number of red blood cells may also be present in the urine.

Vascular diseases

Hypertension. Long-standing and severe hypertension can result in progressive renal damage and chronic renal insufficiency (hypertensive nephrosclerosis). In contrast, hypertension can be caused by the sodium and water retention that occurs in chronic renal failure, acute glomerulonephritis, and the nephrotic syndrome (volume-dependent hypertension), or it can occur as a result of increased renin release from chronically damaged kidneys (renin-dependent hypertension).

Arteriolar disease. Disease of the small arteries of the kidneys (arteritis) may occur in association with generalized disease processes affecting the kidney, such as systemic lupus erythematosus, polyarteritis nodosa, and progressive systemic sclerosis (scleroderma). These diseases may result in the clinical and biochemical abnormalities seen in acute glomerulonephritis, the nephrotic syndrome, or chronic renal insufficiency.

Renal vein thrombosis. Thrombosis of the renal veins results in massive proteinuria and the nephrotic syndrome. Hypertension, edema, hematuria, and impaired renal function may accompany the proteinuria.

Diabetes mellitus

Diabetes mellitus results in a wide variety of abnormalities in kidney function. The early phases of the disease are manifested by the presence of pronounced glucosuria, polyuria, and nocturia as a result of the osmotic diuresis caused by the glucose load. In insulin-dependent diabetes (type I diabetes mellitus), kidney disease is the leading cause of death. In the juvenile diabetic, overt proteinuria develops approximately 17 years after the diagnosis has been made, hypertension develops 1 to 2 years later, and chronic renal insufficiency is seen after another year.[24] Early in the course of this disease, protein excretion, particularly albumin and IgG, is increased. A urinary albumin excretion in the range of 50 to 200 mg/24 hr is usually predictive of diabetic nephropathy.[25] The level of albumin excretion rate has been shown to be increased with age and disease duration after 10 years in patients with type I diabetes mellitus.[26] A significant link also occurred with a declining renal function and elevation of blood pressure. In recent years, attention has been focused on dipstick-negative, low-grade increase in albumin excretion, or microalbuminuria. This latent phase has been shown to be predictive of clinical nephropathy and eventual renal failure in patients with type I diabetes mellitus.[27,28]

Urinary tract obstruction

Lower urinary tract obstruction is characterized by residual urine in the bladder after micturition or urinary retention, whereas the presence of upper tract obstruction is established by the demonstration of a dilated collecting system above a constricting lesion.[14] Lower urinary tract obstruction is characterized by a slow urinary stream, difficulty in emptying the bladder, hesitancy in initiating micturition, and dribbling. Chronic renal damage may result from obstruction and incomplete bladder emptying, and symptoms of chronic renal insufficiency may develop. With complete obstruction, oliguria or anuria will occur. Symptoms of urinary tract infection may also be seen. Urinary tract obstruction may occur as a result of congenital disorders of the lower urinary tract, neoplastic lesions (benign prostatic hypertrophy, carcinoma of the prostate or bladder, or lymph nodes compressing the ureters), or acquired disorders (retroperitoneal fibrosis, renal calculi, or urethral strictures).

Renal calculi

Renal calculi, or stones, are seen in combination with renal colic, hematuria, and symptoms of urinary tract infection or obstruction. Kidney stones may form after recurrent urinary tract infections by urease-producing organisms or when the urine is supersaturated by large quantities of calcium, uric acid, cystine, or xanthine.

Acute renal failure

In acute renal failure there is an abrupt deterioration in renal function. Acute renal failure can be classified as follows:

1. Prerenal (occurring before blood reaches the kidney) because of hypovolemia or poor perfusion as a result of cardiovascular failure
2. Renal (occurring in the kidney) because of acute tubular necrosis, which is the most frequently observed cause of acute renal failure, or because of other renal diseases, causing rapid deterioration in renal function, including arterial or venous obstruction
3. Postrenal (occurring after urine leaves the kidney) because of obstruction

The causes of acute renal failure are listed in the following box. Acute renal failure is usually accompanied by oliguria or anuria; in addition, nonoliguric acute tubular necrosis can occur. Acute renal failure is associated with varying degrees of proteinuria, hematuria, and the presence of red blood cell casts and other casts in the urine. Serum urea nitrogen and creatinine levels increase rapidly, and metabolic acidosis becomes evident. Depending on the cause, acute renal failure can progress to chronic renal insufficiency or failure, or can be followed by recovery of renal function. Most patients with acute tubular necrosis recover once the offending cause has been treated or removed.

Chronic renal failure

Chronic renal failure is a clinical syndrome resulting from the progressive loss of renal function. The symptoms of

---

Causes of Acute Renal Failure

Prerenal
Hypovolemia
Cardiovascular failure

Renal
Acute tubular necrosis
Glomerulonephritis
Vasculitis
Malignant nephrosclerosis
Vascular obstruction
Arterial
Venous

Postrenal
Obstruction of lower urinary tract
Rupture of bladder

chronic renal failure result not only from simple excretory failure but also from the onset of regulatory failure, the kidney's failure to regulate certain substances, such as sodium and water; from biosynthetic failure, such as the kidney's inadequate production of erythropoietin, resulting in anemia; and from the excessive production of certain normal substances in response to the chemical derangements that occur in chronic renal failure, such as the excessive production of parathyroid hormone.[14] There are four stages in chronic, progressive renal disease. In the first stage renal function is diminished, but plasma urea and creatinine levels remain normal. At least 50% of normal function must be lost before the concentrations of these chemicals rise above the normal range. The second stage is characterized by mild renal insufficiency. The third stage is the development of frank renal failure with advancing anemia, acidosis, and other clinical and biochemical manifestations. The fourth and final stage is that of uremia, when all the consequences of renal failure become overt.[14] A classification of the causes of chronic renal failure is shown in the following box.

RENAL FUNCTION TESTS

The kidney performs many physiological and excretory functions. By performing a relatively small number of tests, a physician can deduce accurately the functional state of

---

Classification of Causes of Chronic Renal Failure

Primary glomerular diseases
    Chronic glomerulonephritis of various types
    Systemic lupus erythematosus
    Polyarteritis nodosa
Renal vascular disease
    Malignant hypertension
    Renal vein thrombosis
Inflammatory disease
    Chronic pyelonephritis
    Tuberculosis
Metabolic disease with renal involvement
    Diabetes mellitus
    Gout
    Amyloidosis
Nephrotoxins
    Aminoglycosides
    Analgesic nephropathy
    Chronic heavy metal poisoning
Obstructive hypertrophy
    Calculi
    Prostatic hypertrophy
    Congenital anomalies of lower urinary tract
Congenital anomalies of kidneys
    Hypoplastic kidneys
    Polycystic kidney disease
Miscellaneous
    Chronic radiation nephritis
    Balkan nephropathy

---

the kidney.[29] The clinician first determines whether any significant impairment of renal function exists and then assesses a particular renal function to make a specific diagnosis. In this section evaluation of glomerular and tubular function and urinalysis is discussed.

Tests of glomerular function

Glomerular function is most conveniently measured by the creatinine clearance test. Clearance is defined as that volume of plasma from which a measured amount of substance can be completely eliminated into the urine per unit of time. This depends on the plasma concentration of the substance and its excretory rate, which in turn depends on the GFR and renal plasma flow. The creatinine clearance is a renal function test based on the rate of excretion by the kidneys of metabolically produced creatinine. The amount of creatinine produced by endogenous creatine metabolism is relatively constant and directly proportional to the body surface area. The amount of creatinine present in the urine depends on renal excretion. Creatinine is freely filtered at the glomerulus and is not reabsorbed by the tubules. The creatinine clearance can therefore be used to estimate the GFR. Generally, a 24-hour urine collection is performed. However, shorter collection periods are acceptable. Precise timing is critical to this test. The bladder is emptied at the beginning of the test period and the urine discarded; all urine passed subsequently during the timed collection is kept in a single container. A sample of blood is drawn during the urine collection period. The creatinine clearance is calculated from the following formula:

$$\text{Creatinine clearance (mL/min)} = UV/P \qquad \textit{Eq. 26-5}$$

where U is urinary creatinine (mg/L), V is volume of urine excreted per time (mL/min), and P is plasma creatinine (mg/L). The healthy reference interval for creatinine clearance corrected to a surface area of 1.73 m^2 is 90 to 120 mL/min (see p. 499). The creatinine clearance usually parallels true GFR. However, at low filtration rates, creatinine clearance becomes increasingly inaccurate.[16] The creatinine clearance is lower in women, the elderly, and smaller persons. Measurement of creatinine clearance by collection of a timed (24-hour) urine specimen is burdensome to the patient and frequently difficult to perform. Inaccurate results caused by incomplete bladder emptying, failure to collect the entire specimen, and wide intraindividual variation impair the usefulness of this procedure.[16] Numerous formulas and nomograms have been developed for estimating creatinine clearance from the serum creatinine concentration, thereby bypassing the need for urine collection. The simplest and most widely used is the formula described by Cockcroft and Gault.[30]

$$C_{cr} \text{ (males)} = \frac{[140 - \text{Age (years)} \times \text{Weight (kg)}]}{[7.2 \times \text{Serum creatinine (mg/L)}]}$$

C_{cr} (females) = Above equation result $\times$ 0.85 (based on 15% lower muscle mass on average)   *Eq. 26-6*

Inulin clearance is the method of choice when precise determination of the GFR is required.[16] The glomerular capillary wall is freely permeable to inulin, and inulin is not reabsorbed, secreted, or metabolically altered by the renal tubule. The clearance of endogenous creatinine may exceed that of inulin by up to 30% in healthy individuals. The main disadvantages in the measurement of inulin clearance are the need for its intravenous administration and the technical difficulty of the analysis.

Urea clearance may also be employed as a measure of the GFR. Urea is freely filtered at the glomerulus, and approximately 40% is reabsorbed in the tubules. Thus, urea clearance values will parallel the true GFR.

From a practical point of view, creatinine clearance is used in clinical medicine as an assessment of the GFR. It is important to understand that there is a large margin of reserve in renal function; more than two thirds of the GFR may be lost in the course of chronic renal disease with few clinical symptoms and biochemical abnormalities.[29] For a person whose usual serum creatinine is 7 mg/L, an increase to 14 mg/L, which is still defined as within the reference interval for healthy individuals for serum creatinine, is indicative of a fall in the GFR to 50% of normal.

Tests of tubular function

Concentration-dilution studies. Assessment of the concentrating and diluting ability of the kidney can provide the most sensitive means of detecting early impairment in renal function, since the ability to concentrate urine and conserve water requires an adequate GFR, renal plasma flow, and tubular mass and healthy tubular cells that are able to pump salt against a sizable electrochemical gradient.[29] The urinary *specific gravity* and *osmolality* are used as measures of the concentrating and diluting ability of the tubules. As long as the urine does not contain appreciable amounts of protein, sugar, or exogenous material such as contrast dye, specific gravity is proportional to osmolality, and a specific gravity of 1.032 will correspond to an osmolality of 1200 mOsm/kg.[29]

Impairment of renal concentrating ability is a relatively early manifestation of chronic renal disease and becomes evident before changes in other function tests appear. However, it is a nonspecific test for reduced renal function, and any disease resulting in chronic renal failure, diabetes insipidus, or the use of diuretics may impair renal concentrating ability. The test is performed after 15 hours of fluid deprivation, and urine is then collected on the hour for 3 hours. Dehydration maximally stimulates endogenous ADH secretion. Under these conditions the urine osmolality should be at least three times that of plasma (286 mOsm/kg). A specific gravity of 1.025 or more or an osmolality of 850 mOsm/kg or above in one of the specimens is accepted as evidence of concentrating ability within the healthy reference interval. A patient within the healthy reference interval of concentrating ability is unlikely to have a serious kidney malfunction of any type.[29] As chronic renal disease progresses, tubular ability to concentrate urine slowly decreases until the urine has the same specific gravity as the plasma ultrafiltrate—1.010. Clinically the loss of concentrating ability is manifested by nocturia and polyuria.

To test the urinary diluting capacity, one uses the following procedure. The patient empties the bladder and is given 1000 to 1200 mL of water. Urine specimens are then collected every hour for the next 4 hours. Under these circumstances, the urinary specific gravity should fall to 1.005 or less or an osmolality of less than 100 mOsm/kg. In the patient with chronic renal disease who is unable to dilute the urine, there is a danger of fluid overload with this test.

In diabetes insipidus, which can arise from inadequate ADH production or from insensitivity of the renal tubules to ADH, the distal tubular walls are impervious to water. As sodium is reabsorbed, the fluid left behind may be very dilute. In this disease the baseline urine might have a specific gravity of less than 1.005 and an osmolality of 50 mOsm/kg.

Urinalysis

Urinalysis is an indispensable tool for assessing renal disease. It may reveal disease anywhere in the urinary tract. Observations that can be made in the standard urinalysis include the appearance of the specimen, pH, specific gravity, protein semiquantitation, presence or absence of glucose and ketones, and a microscopic examination of the centrifuged urinary sediment. The importance of the urinalysis is indicated in Table 26-2. Microscopic examination of the centrifuged urinary sediment for cells, crystals, and casts should be done on a freshly voided specimen.

Casts are protein conglomerates outlining the shape of the renal tubules in which they were formed. Hyaline casts are composed almost exclusively of protein. Cellular elements may be trapped within hyaline casts, resulting in the formation of granular casts. When there is heavy proteinuria, accumulation of protein within tubular cells leads to fatty degeneration of the cells and desquamation of cells into the urine; these appear in the urine as oval fat bodies. In acute pyelonephritis, white blood cells may aggregate in the tubules to form pus casts. Red blood cell casts are important markers of glomerular inflammation and should be diligently searched for when any form of glomerular nephritis is suspected.

Microscopic examination of the urinary sediment is completed by a search for bacteria and crystals. The presence of crystals in the urine may be a clue to the diagnosis of a specific type of renal calculus. The characteristic urine microscopic findings in healthy individuals and in renal disease are indicated in Table 26-3. (See Chapter 57.)

CHANGE OF ANALYTE IN DISEASE

The changes that occur in analytes are discussed in the section on pathological conditions of the kidney and summa-

Table 26-2   Association of pathological conditions affecting the kidney and clinical and biochemical abnormalities

	AGN	NS	TD	UTI	HT	RVT	DM	UTO	RC	ARF	CRF
Hypertension	++	+	0	0	++	±	±	0	0	+	+
Edema	+	++	0	0	0	+	+	0	0	+	+
Oliguria or anuria	+	±	0	0	0	±	0	+	0	+	+
Polyuria	0	0	+	0	0	0	+	0	0	0	0
Nocturia	0	±	+	±	0	0	+	±	0	0	0
Frequency	0	0	0	+	0	0	0	±	±	0	0
Loin pain	0	0	0	+	0	+	0	+	+	0	0
Anemia	+	0	0	0	0	0	0	0	0	0	++
↑Blood urea nitrogen	+	0	0	0	±	±	±	±	0	+	+
↑Serum creatinine	+	−	−	−	±	±	±	±	0	+	+
↓GFR	+	0	0	0	±	±	±	±	0	+	+
↑Serum potassium	±	±	0	0	0	0	0	0	0	+	+
↑Serum phosphorus	±	0	0	0	0	0	0	0	0	+	+
↓Serum calcium	0	+	0	0	0	0	0	0	0	+	+
↑Serum uric acid	0	0	+	0	±	0	±	0	±	+	+
Acidosis	0	0	+	0	0	0	0	0	0	+	+
Proteinuria	+	++++	+	±	±	++	+	0	0	±	±
Hematuria	++	+	±	+	0	+	0	0	++	+	±
RBC casts	+	0	0	0	0	0	0	0	0	±	0
Pyuria	±	0	0	++	0	0	0	±	±	0	0
WBC casts	0	0	0	+	0	0	0	+	0	0	0
Glucosuria	0	0	+	0	0	0	++	0	0	0	0

AGN, Acute glomerulonephritis; *ARF,* acute renal failure; *CRF,* chronic renal failure; *DM,* diabetes mellitus; *GFR,* glomerular filtration rate; *HT,* hypertension; *NS,* nephrotic syndrome; *RBC,* red blood cells; *RC,* renal calculi; *RVT,* renal vein thrombosis; *TD,* tubular disease; *UTI,* urinary tract infection; *UTO,* urinary tract obstruction; *WBC,* white blood cells. 0, Absent; ±, variable; +, present.

rized in Table 26-2. In this section the following question is examined from a different perspective: What does the finding of a biochemical abnormality or group of abnormalities mean in the diagnosis of the pathological condition in the kidney?

Serum electrolytes (see also pp. 451-457)

Sodium. Sodium is the major cation in the extracellular fluid and usually has a serum concentration of 136 to 145 mmol/L. Sodium and its attendant anions are the major contributors to serum osmolality.[31]

Hyponatremia. Hyponatremia with hyposmolality can occur in renal disease because of an increased extracellular fluid volume resulting from the kidney's inability to excrete water. This state occurs in chronic renal insufficiency and the nephrotic syndrome. Hyponatremia, with decreased extracellular fluid, can be associated with the use of diuretic agents and the syndrome of inappropriate ADH secretion.

Hypernatremia. Hypernatremia, by definition a relative water deficit, can occur in patients with hypotonic fluid loss. Hypernatremia also occurs in diabetes insipidus whenever the oral fluid intake cannot keep pace with urinary losses.

Chloride. The concentration of chloride in extracellular fluid parallels that of sodium and is influenced by the same factors. Chloride imbalances occur concurrently with sodium imbalances. Hyperchloremia occurs in association with renal tubular acidosis.

Potassium. Potassium is the major cation of intracellular fluid.

Hypokalemia. Hypokalemia is usually associated with overt potassium depletion as a result of excessive losses of potassium-rich fluids. Potassium loss may be renal or extrarenal. Increased renal excretion of potassium occurs with diuretic agents, prolonged use of corticosteroids, primary or secondary aldosteronism, and Cushing's syndrome. Hypokalemia from extrarenal potassium losses usually occurs in the gastrointestinal tract and is seen with prolonged vomit

Table 26-3   Characteristic urine microscopic findings in renal disease

Condition	Protein	Red blood cells (per high-power field)	White blood cells (per high-power field)	Bacteria	Casts (per low-power field)
Normal	0-Trace	0-3	0-5	0	Hyaline, occasionally
Glomerulonephritis	1-2+	>20	0-10	0	Granular red blood cells
Nephrotic syndrome	4+	0-10	0-5	0	Oval fat bodies; hyaline
Pyelonephritis	0-1+	0-10	>30	++	Granular white blood cells

ing, diarrhea, fistulas of the intestinal tract, and villous adenomas of the colon.

Hyperkalemia. Hyperkalemia, an acute medical emergency, is usually caused by either increased cellular breakdown exceeding the normal renal excretory capacity or impaired renal excretion.[31] Hyperkalemia may result from (1) increased intake of potassium, as occurs with dietary excess or intravenous potassium administration in the patient with compromised renal function; (2) cellular breakdown, as occurs with extensive burns or rhabdomyolysis (acute muscle necrosis); (3) decreased potassium excretion, as occurs in acute or chronic renal failure, secondary to potassium-sparing diuretics, in adrenal insufficiency, and in hypoaldosteronism; or (4) transcellular redistribution of potassium, as occurs with acute acidosis, diabetic ketoacidosis, familial hyperkalemic periodic paralysis, and certain drugs (see Chapter 24 for specific methods).

Urinary electrolytes

Sodium. Urinary sodium determinations are diagnostically useful in three clinical settings. First, in volume depletion, the measurement of urinary sodium excretion is helpful in determining the route of sodium loss. A low urinary sodium concentration (less than 10 mEq/L) indicates an extrarenal sodium loss, whereas the presence of a high concentration of sodium in the urine indicates renal salt wasting or adrenal insufficiency. Second, in the differential diagnosis of acute renal failure, the urinary sodium excretion will be less than 10 mEq/L in patients with volume depletion who have no intrinsic renal disease and usually more than 30 mEq/L in patients with acute tubular necrosis.[32] In volume depletion a urine-to-plasma osmolality ratio of more than 1.1 and a urine-to-plasma urea ratio of more than 10 is observed, compared with values of less than 1.05 and less than 10, respectively, in acute tubular necrosis.[32] Third, in hyponatremia a low urinary sodium concentration (less than 10 mEq/L) indicates avid renal sodium retention, which may be attributable to either severe volume depletion or sodium-retaining states seen in cirrhosis, the nephrotic syndrome, and congestive heart failure. When hyponatremia is associated with urinary sodium excretion that equals or exceeds the dietary sodium intake, it is likely that the syndrome of inappropriate ADH secretion is present.[31] In these three situations a random urinary sodium concentration can rapidly supply valuable diagnostic information (see Chapter 24 for specific methods).

Chloride. The measurement of urinary chloride is of clinical value only in patients with persistent metabolic alkalosis who are not receiving diuretics (see Chapter 24 for specific methods).[31]

Potassium. Urinary potassium levels are helpful in the evaluation of patients with unexplained hypokalemia.[31] The finding of a urinary potassium concentration of more than 10 mEq/L indicates that the kidney is responsible for the potassium loss, whereas a urinary potassium concentration of less than 10 mEq/L in the presence of hypokalemia is strongly suggestive that the gastrointestinal tract is the route of potassium loss (see Chapter 24 for specific methods).

Anion gap

An increased anion gap occurs in renal failure because of the retention of sulfate, phosphate, and organic acid anions. (See Chapters 24 and 25.)

Creatinine, urea, and uric acid (see text below for methods)

With progressive renal insufficiency there is retention in the blood of urea, creatinine, and uric acid. Normally the ratio of serum urea nitrogen to serum creatinine is between 10:1 and 20:1. In the usual case of renal failure, a similar ratio is seen. Ratios higher than 20:1 occur in disease states of extrarenal origin, such as prerenal azotemia, gastrointestinal bleeding, or excessive protein intake with marginally adequate renal function. In contrast, urea production and the BUN are reduced in the presence of a low protein intake and in severe liver disease. Uric acid concentration in the blood rises in advanced chronic renal failure, but this rarely results in classical gout.

Calcium and phosphorus

In chronic renal failure there is impaired excretion of phosphate, and progressive hyperphosphatemia occurs. This results in a fall in the plasma calcium concentration (hypocalcemia), giving rise to secondary hyperparathyroidism. The elevated parathyroid hormone level causes calcium resorption from bone, and normocalcemia or hypercalcemia may result. However, hypocalcemia is more prevalent in uremia, both as a result of the reciprocal fall in the plasma calcium concentration as the plasma phosphate level rises and because of reduced calcium absorption in the gut as a result of impaired 1,25-dihydroxycholecalciferol production.[10,18] Hypocalcemia is also present in the nephrotic syndrome, as a result of the hypoalbuminemia. However, the ionized serum calcium level remains normal in this condition.

Proteinuria (see p. 502 for methods)

Proteinuria may be of two types. In *glomerular proteinuria* large quantities of high-molecular-weight proteins enter the glomerular filtrate and ultimately appear in the urine. Heavy proteinuria (more than 2 g/day) results from increased glomerular permeability, and the protein loss may be great enough to result in the nephrotic syndrome.[20] In *tubular proteinuria* the amount of protein filtered by the glomeruli is not increased, but the low-molecular-weight proteins, which are normally filtered, appear in larger quantities in the final urine because tubular reabsorption is incomplete. Impaired tubular reabsorption of filtered proteins results in modest increases (1 to 3 g/day) in the urinary excretion of low-molecular-weight proteins and albumin.[20] Physiological increases in protein excretion occur during the maintenance of an upright posture, after strenuous exercise, and in normal pregnancy.[20]

Enzymes in urine

Enzymes may appear in urine because of filtration, secretion, or tissue damage.[20] Enzymes of low molecular weight, such as lysozyme and amylase, appear because they are filtered and not completely reabsorbed. High-molecular-weight enzymes, such as lactic dehydrogenase, can be excreted because of parenchymal renal damage.

Hemoglobin and hematocrit

Anemia is a common feature of chronic renal failure, and its severity reflects the extent of renal impairment.[19] Progressive anemia usually occurs when the GFR falls below 25 mL/min. The anemia of chronic renal failure is attributable to (1) reduced erythropoietin production as renal mass decreases, (2) inhibitors of erythropoiesis present in the serum of the uremic patient, (3) reduced red blood cell survival in advanced renal failure, and (4) iron deficiency caused by blood loss as a result of the hemostatic defect characteristic of renal failure.[19]

METHODS OF ANALYSIS

Creatinine

STEVEN C. KAZMIERCZAK

Principles of analysis and current usage The Jaffé method for creatinine analysis (Table 26-4, method 1), has the distinction of being the oldest clinical chemistry method still in common use.[33] In 1886, Jaffé described the reaction of creatinine with alkaline picrate, and in 1904, Folin demonstrated the utility of this assay for measurement of creatinine in urine and blood.[34] In the Jaffé reaction, creatinine reacts directly with picrate ion under alkaline conditions to form a red-orange compound, called a Janovski complex, with an absorbance peak at 520 nm.

The advantages of the Jaffé reaction are its simplicity and wide clinical acceptance gained over years of use.[35] However, a major disadvantage of this reaction is the significant interference that occurs from substances other than creatinine. Substances reported to cause a positive interference when the original Jaffé reaction (without fuller's earth) is used include ascorbic acid, pyruvate, acetone, acetoacetic acid, levulose, glucose, aminohippurate, uric acid, protein, cephalosporin antibiotics, and nitromethane.[39,40] By their oxidation in strong base to colorless compounds, bilirubin or other hemoglobin degradation products cause a negative bias. The re-

Table 26-4   Methods of creatinine analysis

Method	Type of analysis	Principle	Usage	Comments
1. Jaffé	Spectrophotometric (520 nm) end point, quantitative	Creatinine + Picrate $\xrightarrow{OH^-}$ Janovski complex *(red)*	Serum, plasma, diluted urine	Described by Jaffé, 1886
2. Jaffé/fuller's earth	Same as 1. Creatinine isolated before analysis. Can be removed with buffer or picrate reagent added directly to creatinine adsorbent suspension	As above	Serum, plasma, diluted urine	Reference method; alternatively one can use cation exchangers as adsorbent
3. Jaffé, kinetic automated	Spectrophotometric, quantitative, kinetic analysis during early color formation	As above	Serum, plasma, diluted urine	Requires equipment for accurate, precise absorbance measurements, commonly used
4. Creatinine amidohydrolase	Enzymatic hydrolysis to creatine, which reacts in indicator reactions	Creatinine + H_2O $\xrightarrow[\text{amidohydrolase}]{\text{Creatinine}}$ Creatine Creatine measured via indicator reactions	Serum	Commonly used
5. Creatinine iminohydrolase	Enzymatic hydrolysis of creatinine with formation of ammonia, which can be quantitated spectrophotometrically or electrometrically	Creatinine $\xrightarrow[\text{iminohydrolase}]{\text{Creatinine}}$ *N*-methylhydantoin + NH_3 NH_3 measured by GLDH reaction, ammonia electrode, or colorimetrically	Serum	Least common of enzymatic methods
6. High-performance liquid chromatography (HPLC)	Cation-exchange or reversed-phase chromatographic separation of creatinine from other compounds	Creatinine quantitated by method 1 or absorption at 200 nm	Serum, plasma, specific, not urine	Highly useful for analysis, possible reference method

*GLDH, Glutamate dehydrogenase.

sulting decrease in background color decreases the measured absorbance and is interpreted as a lower creatinine concentration. This negative bias is also seen in kinetic analyses for creatinine.[39]

Substances such as glucose, ascorbate, and uric acid interfere by slowly reducing alkaline picrate, whereas other compounds, such as ketoacids, pyruvate, proteins, and cephalosporin drugs react with alkaline picrate to form colored complexes.[35,36] The presence of these noncreatinine chromogen compounds may cause overestimation of the actual creatinine concentrations in serum by as much as 20%. However, noncreatinine chromogens do not interfere significantly with creatinine measurements made in urine.

Bacterial contamination, which can occur in samples stored for long periods of time, has also been found falsely to lower creatinine values measured using the Jaffé reaction.[37] The mechanism of this interference appears to be bacterial production of a substance that retards the rate of the Jaffé reaction. In cases where the concentration of interferant is low, prolonging the reaction time can overcome the effect of the interferent. For plasma that is to be stored for long periods of time, the addition of 1 gram of sodium azide per liter or freezing of the specimen can reduce the likelihood of bacterial interference.

Various modifications of the original Jaffé reaction have been developed to increase the specificity of the assay. The use of a protein-free sample instead of serum was shown to increase specificity greatly. Also the addition of porus aluminum silicate clay (fuller's earth, Lloyd's reagent) to the filtrates, to absorb the creatinine present in the protein-free filtrate, further removed most potential interferents (Table 26-4, method 2). Creatinine is adsorbed by these compounds with approximately 92% efficiency and after centrifugation and decanting of the interferent-containing supernatant, one can add the alkaline picrate directly to the creatinine-absorbent pellet. Most potential interferents are not adsorbed. However, pyruvate in excess of 0.9 mmol/L and 2-oxoglutarate in excess of 0.5 mmol/L are adsorbed and can thus cause interference.[38] The use of adsorption methods for measurement of creatinine are infrequently used because of their laborious nature.

Alternative methods now used in clinical practice include kinetic alkaline picrate methods and enzymatic creatinine methods. The kinetic method for determination of creatinine (Table 26-4, method 3) makes use of the differential rate of color development for noncreatinine chromogens versus that for creatinine. Although the kinetic method significantly reduces the interference caused by most noncreatine chromogens, compounds such as bilirubin still interfere and can substantially reduce the measured creatinine concentration.[39]

Enzymatic methods for measurement of creatinine have been developed. Creatinine amidohydrolase (E.C. 3.5.3.10), also referred to as "creatinase," or "creatinine hydrolase," is commonly used in enzymatic methods for creatinine. This enzyme is used to convert creatinine to creatine, coupled to an indicator reaction (Table 26-4, method 4). Different types of indicator reactions have been developed as described as follows:

I.

$$Creatinine + H_2O \xrightarrow{Creatinine\ amidohydrolase} Creatine$$

$$Creatine + ATP \xrightarrow{Creatine\ kinase} Creatine\ phosphate + ADP$$

$$ADP + PEP \xrightarrow{Pyruvate\ kinase} ATP + Pyruvate$$

$$Pyruvate + NADH + H^+ \xrightarrow{Lactate\ dehydrogenase}$$
$$Lactate + NAD^+ \qquad Eq.\ 26\text{-}7,\ a$$

II.

$$Creatinine + H_2O \xrightarrow{Creatinine\ amidohydrolase} Creatine$$

$$Creatine \xrightarrow{Creatine\ amidohydrolase} Urea + Sarcosine$$

$$Sarcosine \xrightarrow{Sarcosine\ oxidase} Formaldehyde$$
$$+ Glycine + Hydrogen\ peroxide \qquad Eq.\ 26\text{-}7,\ b$$

The indicator reaction described above in reaction I allows continuous monitoring of NADH disappearance at 340 nm.[41] In reaction II, the hydrogen peroxide can be quantified by its reaction with a suitable indicator dye.[42]

Another enzyme system less frequently used for creatinine quantitation is creatinine deaminase (E.C. 3.5.4.21), also known as "creatinine iminohydrolase" (Table 26-4, method 5).

$$Creatinine + H_2O \xrightarrow[iminohydrolase]{Creatinine} N\text{-}Methylhydantoin + NH_3$$

$$NADPH + NH_4^+ + \alpha\text{-}Ketoglutarate \xrightarrow{GLDH}$$
$$L\text{-}Glutamate + NADP^+ \qquad Eq.\ 26\text{-}8$$

With this method, ammonia can be quantitated directly by monitoring of the reaction of NADPH with α-ketoglutarate in the presence of glutamate dehydrogenase[43] or by use of an ammonia electrode.[44] The reaction mixture must be free of ammonia-producing and ammonia-consuming materials. In addition, a correction for endogenous ammonia must be made.

Separation and quantitation of creatinine using high-performance liquid chromatography (HPLC) (Table 26-4, method 6) has been proposed as a reference method, and several HPLC applications have been reported.[45,46] Measurement of creatinine by HPLC has been found to be accurate, precise, and specific.

Specimen Serum, plasma, and urine are acceptable specimens for analysis. No differences in creatinine concentrations between serum and plasma have been noted. Urine should be diluted to a final creatinine concentration of approximately 300 to 600 μmol/L (34 to 68 mg/L); a 1:100 dilution will usually accomplish this. The common preservatives and anticoagulants (fluoride and heparin) do not cause interference, though heparin, which can be formulated as the ammonium salt, must be avoided in enzymatic methods that measure ammonia production. This type of enzymatic assay also requires prompt removal of serum from red blood cells and prompt analysis to minimize in vitro ammonia production; both of these precautions are necessary because of the imprecision that results from an elevated ammonia background. If analyzed by the Jaffé reaction, specimens are stable for at least 7 days at 4° C.

Table 26-5   Reference intervals for creatinine and creatinine clearance*

Age	Serum creatinine mg/L (µmol/L)	Urine creatinine g/day (mmol/day)	Creatinine clearance (mL/min)
<12 years	2.5-8.5 (22-75)	0.057 g (0.5 mmol/kg) of muscle	50-90
Adult male	6.4-10.4 (57-92)	1.0-2.0 (8.8-17.7)	97-137
Adult female	5.7-9.2 (50-81)	0.8-1.8 (7.1-15.9)	88-128

*From Meites S, editor: *Pediatric clinical chemistry,* Washington, D.C., 1981, American Association for Clinical Chemistry, pp 171-177; and from Newkirk RE, Rawnsley HM: *Creatinine clearance, ASCP check sample clinical chemistry no. CC-110,* Chicago, 1978, American Society of Clinical Pathologists.

Reference ranges (Table 26-5)   An individual's serum creatinine level is dependent on two factors: the rate of creatinine production and the rate of creatinine excretion. Because the source of serum creatinine is muscle creatine and creatine phosphate, a greater amount of muscle mass results in a higher serum creatinine. The second and much more significant determinant of serum creatinine levels is the rate of renal excretion. As a measure of renal function, however, the creatinine clearance determination is more sensitive than the serum creatinine level. Infants and children have lower clearance rates, and the clearance gradually rises to adult rates by the onset of puberty. Creatinine clearance rates are relatively constant from puberty to midlife, generally decreasing from the fifth decade on. Urine determinations of creatinine output are of value only with creatinine clearance determinations or as a check of the completeness of a 24-hour collection. Urinary excretion is directly proportional to muscle mass; approximately 0.5 mmol of creatinine is excreted per kilogram of muscle mass. Diet, urine volume, and exercise have little effect on serum creatinine levels. Urinary creatinine concentrations are slightly increased by exercise and are slightly decreased in individuals on a protein-deficient diet.[47]

The reference ranges given in Table 26-5 were determined with the fuller's earth modification of the Jaffé reaction. A less specific method would be expected to result in slightly increased serum levels but would have little effect on the urine levels. Because of this nonuniform effect, a less specific method would result in a lower calculated creatinine-clearance rate.

Urea
STEVEN C. KAZMIERCZAK

Principles of analysis and current usage   The results of blood urea measurements were originally reported in terms of the amounts of released nitrogen, with urea concentration being expressed in terms of milligrams of blood urea nitrogen (BUN) per volume (usually in deciliters). This terminology still continues despite the fact that serum and plasma, not whole blood, are the preferred specimens for analysis, and urea is measured directly. Values for BUN can be converted to urea concentrations as follows:

1. Atomic weight of nitrogen = 14.0 g/mol; molecular weight of urea = 60.1 g/mol.
2. One urea molecule contains two nitrogen atoms.
3. Urea nitrogen (urea-N) makes up 46.6% of the weight of urea (28.0 divided by 60.1).
4. Therefore

   100 mg/L of BUN divided by 0.466 = 214.6 mg/L of urea

or

$$\text{mg of urea-N/L} \times 2.146 = \text{mg of urea/L}$$

$$\text{mg of urea-N/L} \times 0.036 = \text{mmol of urea/L}$$

Measurement of urea may be performed by use of *indirect* methods whereby urea is hydrolyzed by the enzyme urease to form ammonia, which can then be quantitated, or *directly* by reaction of urea with compounds to form a chromogenic product. Historical methods for urea determinations were based on the chemical quantitation of ammonia released from urea after heating at 125° C or by enzymatic breakdown of urea by urease. These methods are rarely used today; additional information can be found in the second edition of this text.

The most common method in use today for determining urea concentrations is based on the enzymatic measurement of the NH_3 formed by the action of urease on urea. An indicator reaction, employing glutamate dehydrogenase (GLDH) to oxidize NADH to NAD^+, is used to measure the NH_3 that is formed (Table 26-6, method 1).[48] Endogenous enzymes, such as GLDH, that may be present in the sera of some patients can interfere with the assay.[49] In addition, ammonia, which may be present in the reagent or the specimen (such as urine) being analyzed can interfere with the assay. This interference can be eliminated if the reaction is performed using a kinetic analysis mode. When a kinetic analysis mode is used, endogenous ammonia is rapidly consumed during the initial seconds of the reaction, and the subsequent changes in absorbance are essentially caused by ammonia generated by the reaction of urease with urea. Also, if the reaction is run in the kinetic mode with large dilutions of the sample, no significant interferences by bilirubin, hemoglobin, or lipemia are seen.

A very common method for urea analysis employs the reaction between NH_3 (produced by the action of urease) and a pH indicator dye to produce a color change (Table 26-6, method 2).[50,51] This approach is utilized with dry reagent technology, either thin-film[50] or reagent strips.[51] Urease immobilized in an initial spreading layer reacts with urea to produce NH_4^+. Under alkaline conditions, NH_3 passes through a semipermeable layer and reacts with a pH indicator dye. The color change that occurs is monitored by reflectance photometry. These methods show excellent accuracy, and there appears to be little significant interference from commonly encountered biochemicals.

Another common assay for quantitating urea is based upon the change in conductivity of a sample that occurs after the action of urease on urea (Table 26-6, method 3).[52] The CO_2 and ammonia that are produced by the urease re-

Table 26-6 Methods of urea analysis

Method	Type of analysis	Principle	Usage	Comments
1. Coupled enzymatic (urease/glutamate dehydrogenase [GLDH])	Quantitative, end-point, kinetic, spectrophotometric	Urea + H_2O $\xrightarrow{\text{Urease}}$ $(NH_4)_2CO_3$ NH_4^+ + α-Ketoglutaric acid + NADH $\xrightarrow{\text{GLDH}}$ ADP + H^+ + NAD^+ + Glutamic acid	Most frequently used procedure	Very specific, rapid
2. Indicator dye	Quantitative, endpoint	Urea $\xrightarrow{\text{Urease}}$ $(NH_4)_2CO_3$ → $2NH_4^+$ + CO_3^{2-} NH_3 + pH indicator dye → Change in absorbance spectrum of dye	Very commonly used	Very specific, used with dry chemistry technology
3. Conductimetric	Quantitative, kinetic	Urea $\xrightarrow{\text{Urease}}$ $(NH_4)_2CO_3$ → $2NH_4^+$ + CO_3^{2-} Increased ions change conductivity	Frequently used	Very specific, rapid
4. Ion-selective electrode	Quantitative, enzymatic, potentiametric	Urea $\xrightarrow{\text{Urease}}$ $(NH_4)_2CO_3$ NH_3 measured by electrode	Rarely used	Very specific; may see increased use in future
5. o-Phthalaldehyde	Colorimetric, quantitative, endpoint	Urea + o-Phthalaldehyde $\xrightarrow{H^+}$ Isoindoline Isoindoline + 8-(4-amino-1-methylamino)-6-methoxyquinoline $\xrightarrow{H^+}$ Chromophore (510 nm)	Rarely used	Interferences, often primary amines
6. Diacetyl monoxime	Colorimetric, quantitative, endpoint	Diacetyl monoxime $\xrightarrow[H^+]{H_2O}$ Diacetyl + Hydroxlamine Urea + Diacetyl $\xrightarrow{H^+}$ Diazine + $2H_2O$	Rarely used	Some nonspecificity of reaction; uses noxious, dangerous reagents

action form ammonium carbonate ($[NH_4]_2CO_3$), which increases the conductivity of the reaction mixture. When performed in a kinetic analysis mode to correct for the endogenous conductivity of the sample, both serum and urine samples can be measured using this method.

Urea determinations can be performed using an ammonia ion-selective electrode to monitor the urease reaction (Table 26-6, method 4). Although this technology has been available for some time, it has not been widely used in the clinical laboratory. This method employs urease, bonded to a membrane affixed to the electrode, to convert urea to ammonia and CO_2; an ammonium electrode is used to detect ammonia formed by the reaction. Use of this technology has been found to be very specific for urea, and results for urea obtained by this method closely agree with those obtained using other methods.[53]

Other infrequently used urea methods include the reaction of o-phthalaldehyde with primary amines, such as urea (Table 26-6, method 5), and the diacetyl monoxime reaction (Table 26-6, method 6) (see second edition). The isoindoline product of the o-phthalaldehyde reaction is coupled to a complex quinoline to form a chromogen that is monitored at 510 nm. Other primary amines can interfere in this assay. The diacetyl monoxime does not directly react with urea but is first hydrolyzed to form diacetyl and hydroxylamine. The diacetyl condenses with urea in an acid solution to form a yellow diazine product. One disadvantage of this method is the photosensitivity and rapid fading of the colored products.

Specimen Serum and heparinized plasma can be used for the urea methods that have been described. Fluoride will inhibit the urease reaction; therefore methods employing urease cannot use serum preserved with fluoride. Ammonium heparin also cannot be used as an anticoagulant for urease-based methods. Urea in urine can be analyzed after one performs a dilution (typically 1:20 to 1:50) of the sample. Because of the susceptibility of urea to bacterial degradation, serum and urine samples should be kept at 4° to 8° C until analysis. Urine samples can also be preserved by maintenance of pH less than 4.

Reference ranges The reference range for serum BUN will vary depending on the method used for its measurement (Table 26-7). Young children have slightly lower serum urea values than older children and adults have. Individual varia-

Table 26-7

Method	Adult reference range (serum)	Urine urea output (average diet)
1. Urease/GLDH	50 to 170 mg BUN/L (107 to 365 mg of urea/L, 1.8 to 6.1 mmol/L)	7 to 16 g of BUN/24 hours (0.25 to 0.57 mol of urea/24 hours)
2. Urease conductivity	60 to 200 mg BUN/L (129 to 429 mg of urea/L, 2.2 to 7.2 mmol/L)	
3. Diacetyl monoxime	80 to 260 mg BUN/L (172 to 558 mg of urea/L, 2.9 to 9.4 mmol/L)	

Table 26-8   Methods of uric acid measurement

Method	Type of analysis	Principle	Usage	Comments
1. Phosphotungstic acid	Spectrophotometric	Oxidation of uric acid to allantoin and carbon dioxide with reduction of phosphotungstic acid to tungsten blue (A_{max}, 700 nm)	Serum, urine	Nonspecific infrequently used
2. Uricase	Enzymatic	Oxidation of uric acid to allantoin, hydrogen peroxide, and carbon dioxide	Serum, urine	
	a. Differential absorption	Uric acid absorbs in the 290 to 293 nm (at pH ≥7) and 283 nm (at pH <7) region of the ultraviolet spectrum, but allantoin does not		Basis for a candidate reference method, increased specificity
	b. Colorimetric	Quantitation of the hydrogen peroxide produced, especially when coupled to a NAD^+/NADH indicator reaction		Specificity varies from method to method, NADH reaction widely used
	c. Polarographic	Rate of oxygen consumption measured		Not widely used, some interferences
3. High-performance liquid chromatography	Chromatographic			
	a. Spectrophotometric	Reversed-phase chromatography	Serum, urine	Increased specificity and sensitivity
	b. Electrochemical	Ion-exchange separation	Serum, urine	Proposed selected method

tions in BUN concentrations also depend on the dietary habits of the person: those consuming less protein will have lower serum urea concentrations. Similarly, urine output of urea will vary with diet.

Uric acid

ARNOLD L. SCHULTZ

Principles of analysis and current usage   The earliest methods for uric acid utilized the ability of an alkaline solution of uric acid to reduce phosphotungstic acid to tungsten blue.[54] The original method used protein precipitation and subsequent isolation of uric acid from the filtrate before reaction with phosphotungstic acid (Table 26-8, method 1). Few laboratories currently measure uric acid using the phosphotungstate method. Drawbacks of this method include its lack of specificity for uric acid because of interference from compounds that can also reduce phosphotungstic acid.

The use of the enzyme uricase has led to the development of more specific assays for uric acid (Table 26-8, method 2). The oxidation of uric acid to allantoin and hydrogen peroxide by the enzyme uricase allows uric acid to be quantitated by a variety of techniques. One method for quantitating uric acid makes use of the differential absorption spectra of allantoin and uric acid (Table 26-8, method 2a). Allantoin, unlike uric acid, does not have an absorption peak in the 290 to 293 nm region of the ultraviolet spectrum. Absorption measurements at these wavelengths before and after incubation of uric acid with uricase have been used to quantitate uric acid in serum, plasma, and urine.[55]

Alternatively, the hydrogen peroxide that is produced after the oxidation of uric acid by uricase can be quantified by measurement of the chromogenic product that is formed when dye, such as *o*-dianisidine, is oxidized by hydrogen peroxide (Table 26-8, method 2b).[56] Other compounds that can react with hydrogen peroxide to produce colored chromophores include 3-methyl-2-benzothiazolinone and *N,N*-dimethylalinine to produce a blue indamine dye[57] and 3,5-dichloro-2-hydroxybenzenesulfonic acid and 4-aminophenazone to form a red quinoneimine dye.[58]

Hydrogen peroxide production can also be monitored by its ability to oxidize ethanol to acetaldehyde. This reaction is coupled to the enzymatic oxidation of acetaldehyde and NADH to acetate and NAD^+ by aldehyde dehydrogenase. The change in absorbance at 340 nm is related to uric acid concentration.[59]

The oxidation of uric acid by uricase can also be monitored when the rate of oxygen consumption during the reaction is followed (Table 26-8, method 2c).[60] The rate of oxygen consumption is proportional to uric acid concentrations and can be measured with a polarographic oxygen sensor.

High-performance liquid chromatography (HPLC) for the quantitation of uric acid in serum[61] and urine[62] have been developed (Table 26-8, method 3). Although HPLC is not used routinely, the sensitivity and specificity of HPLC for uric acid determinations has led to this method being proposed as the selected method for uric acid.[61]

Specimen   Serum or plasma may be used for uric acid determinations. Collection of specimens in tubes containing EDTA or fluoride should be avoided because they can contribute a positive interference in uricase-based methods. Uric acid is stable at 2° to 6° C for 3 to 5 days and for at least 6 months at −20° C.

Determination of uric acid concentrations in urine may also be performed provided that the specimen is properly preserved. To prevent precipitation of salts of uric acid, 10 mL of sodium hydroxide (500 g/L) should be added to the collection bottle before collection of a 24-hour specimen. Uric acid in urine that has been properly preserved is stable for approximately 3 days at room temperature, provided that no bacterial growth is present to degrade it.

Reference ranges

SERUM OR PLASMA

36 to 77 mg/L (214 to 458 μmol/L) for males
25 to 68 mg/L (149 to 405 μmol/L) for females

URINE

250 to 750 mg (1.49 to 4.46 mmol) per 24 hours for average diet
Up to 450 mg (2.68 mmol) per 24 hours for low-purine diet
Up to 1 g (5.95 mmol) per 24 hours for high-purine diet

Urine protein, total

STEVEN C. KAZMIERCZAK

Principles of analysis
Total urine protein is measured by turbidimetry, colorimetry, and dye-binding methods. In turbidimetry, a protein precipitant is added to the sample, and the denatured protein precipitates in a fine suspension that is quantitated turbidimetrically (Table 26-9, method 1). Reagents that are used to precipitate protein include trichloroacetic acid (TCA), sulfosalicylic acid (SSA), and benzethonium chloride (BZC) in alkali; BZC is the most commonly used precipitant. The turbidity varies appreciably with the chemical nature of the precipitant. For example, SSA produces four times more turbidity with albumin than it does with γ-globulin and also precipitates significant quantities of polypeptides from urine.[63] Methods that use SSA as the precipitant generally suffer from poor precision, different responses to different proteins, and lack of agreement with other protein methods. The turbidity that is produced by TCA is not affected by changes in the albumin/globulin ratio when the temperature is kept between 20° to 25° C. Above 25° C however, much more turbidity is produced with albumin than with globulin.[63] Another drawback associated with use of TCA is that total urine protein concentrations are underestimated when α_1-acid glycoprotein concentrations are increased; a common finding in patients with an acute phase reaction.[64] Some drugs have also been shown to interfere with the TCA procedure.[63,65]

The BZC protein-denaturing agent is the most sensitive of the turbidimetric methods in use. However, even this procedure is not without its drawbacks. γ-globulin has been found to produce 11% to 31% less turbidity than albumin, depending on the total protein concentration of the sample.[63] In addition, fluorescein, a pharmacologic agent frequently used for the evaluation of diabetic retinopathies and retinal vas-

Table 26-9   Methods for total urine protein analysis

Method	Sensitivity (mg/L)	Principle	Usage	Comments
1. Turbidimetric		A protein-denaturing agent precipitates proteins; resulting turbidity is measured photometrically at either 450 or 620 nm.	Most frequently used method	Technically simple, rapid, fairly accurate
a. Sulfosalicylic acid (SSA)	10 to 25		Commonly used method	Overestimates albumin, which produces 4 times greater turbidity than for γ-globulins
b. Trichloroacetic acid (TCA)	20		Infrequently used	Estimates albumin and γ-globulin equally
c. Benzethonium chloride (BZC)	10		Most frequently used method	Most sensitive of turbidimetric techniques
2. Coomassie Brilliant Blue	2.5	Dye binds to NH_3^+ residues of proteins with resulting absorption at 595 nm.	Frequently used	Rapid, highly sensitive; overestimation of albumin
3. Pyrogallol red	35	Dye binds basic amino groups forming a blue complex measured photometrically at 600 nm.	Frequently used	Reacts with albumin and γ-globulins equally
4. Biuret (modified)	5 to 17	Proteins are concentrated by precipitation with TCA or ethanolic-HCl-phosphotungstic acid (Tsuchiya's reagent) and redissolved in biuret reagent (alkaline-Cu^{++}); the Cu^{++} reagent forms a colored complex with peptide bonds, which is measured at 540 nm.	Used by small percentage of laboratories	With Tsuchiya's reagent this method is very sensitive with a good linear range
5. pH indicator	100	Protein (principally albumin) binds to pH indicator dye causing color change.	Semiquantitative method; most frequently used	Reacts primarily with albumin; false positive if urine pH >8

culopathies, has been found to interfere with this method.[66]

Dye-binding techniques for measurement of protein are based on the shift in the absorbance maximum of the dye when it is bound to a protein. The change in the absorbance maximum of the dye allows the resulting color to be measured in the presence of excess dye. One frequently used dye-binding method utilizes Coomassie Brilliant Blue (G-250) (CBB, Table 26-9, method 2). The method is sensitive and precise, the binding is complete within 2 minutes, and the color is stable for an hour. Unfortunately, the dye produces more color per gram of protein with albumin than with globulins.[63] Thymol, often used as a urine preservative, and salicylates have been shown to interfere in the CBB procedure[63]; others have found tolbutamide and urea, at concentrations of 2 to 4 g/L and 90 to 180 g/L respectively, to give positive interference. In addition, the Coomassie Blue reagent can stick to the wall of cuvettes, limiting its application.

Another frequently used dye-binding method utilizes pyrogallol red–molybdate (Table 26-9, method 3).[67] This procedure measures the blue color formed when the pyrogallol red–molybdate complex binds to basic amino groups.[68] The resulting blue color is measured photometrically at 600 nm. Like other dye-binding methods, the sensitivity of the procedure depends on the type of protein being measured. However, the addition of a surfactant such as sodium dodecyl sulfate (25 mg/L) to the reagent mixture equalizes the color produced when the reagent reacts with either albumin or γ-globulin.[68] Like the Coomassie Blue dye-binding method, the one potential drawback to the procedure is that the blue product that is formed can absorb onto the wall of the cuvette causing a drift in the baseline absorbance readings. Automation of this method should probably be limited to instruments with single-use cuvettes.[69]

The reaction of biuret reagent (Cu^{++} ions) with the peptide bonds in proteins is still used by some laboratories for quantitation of protein in urine (Table 26-9, method 4). Since the biuret reaction is relatively insensitive, the protein must be concentrated before analysis. Concentration is accomplished by precipitation of the protein with TCA or ethanolic hydrochloride-phosphotungstic acid. The precipitated protein is isolated by centrifugation, redissolved, and then reacted with biuret reagent. The biuret reaction suffers from interferences from colored metabolites (such as bilirubin) and ammonium ion.[70]

A semiquantitative technique for estimating urinary protein concentrations uses a dye binding-pH indicator technique (Table 26-9, method 5). This technique, usually incorporated into urine dipsticks, employs a pH indicator dye, such as tetrabromo blue, embedded in a pad. When protein binds to the dye, there is a change in the pH environment of the dye, resulting in a change in the color of the dye. This methodology is most sensitive to albumin and relatively insensitive to γ-globulin. The presence of large amounts of bilirubin or other highly colored compounds in the urine can also discolor the reagent pad and make interpretation of the dipstick color change difficult. False-positive results are not an infrequent finding when this method is used; therefore, the reagent-strip test is best used as a screening procedure. Positive test results obtained by this method should be verified by use of another method.

Specimen   A 24-hour or 12-hour urine specimen with no preservatives is preferred. However, because of the inconvenience and difficulty in collecting accurate and complete 12- or 24-hour urine samples, determination of the urinary protein/creatinine concentration ratio in random (untimed) urine samples can be used to estimate the more exact determinations of a 12- or 24-hour urine protein excretion.[71,72] The sample should be well mixed and an aliquot frozen if the sample cannot be analyzed within 48 hours after collection. Frozen specimens are stable for at least 1 year.

Reference ranges   In healthy adults, urinary protein excretion averages approximately 40 mg/day, with the upper limit of protein excretion being less than 150 mg/day.[70,73] Of the protein that is normally excreted, approximately one third is albumin and two thirds are globulins.

For random or untimed urine samples collected from healthy adults with urinary protein excretion rates of <150 mg/day, the ratio of protein to creatinine is <100 mg protein per gram of creatinine. Protein/creatinine concentration ratios >2000 mg/g are comparable with daily urinary protein excretion rates of >3 to 4 g/day.[73]

REFERENCES

1. Kokko JP: Renal concentrating and diluting mechanism, *Hosp Pract* 14:110-116, 1979.
2. Schrier RW: *Renal and electrolyte disorders,* ed 3, Boston, 1986, Little, Brown & Co.
3. Peart WS: Renin-angiotensin system, *N Engl J Med* 292:302-306, 1975.
4. Rose BD: *Pathophysiology of renal disease,* New York, 1981, McGraw-Hill, pp 579-585.
5. MacKnight ADC: Epithelial transport of potassium, *Kidney Int* 11:391-414, 1977.
6. Suki WN: Disposition and regulation of body potassium: an overview, *Am J Med Sci* 272:31-41, 1976.
7. Giebisch G, Malnic G, Berliner RW: Renal transport and control of potassium excretion. In Brenner BM, Rector FC, editors: *The kidney,* Philadelphia, 1991, Saunders.
8. Massry SG, Friedler RM, Coburn JW: Excretion of phosphate and calcium, *Arch Intern Med* 131:828-859, 1973.
9. Agus ZS, Gardner LB, Beck LH, Goldberg M: Effects of parathyroid hormone on renal tubular reabsorption of calcium, sodium, and phosphate, *Am J Physiol* 224:1143-1148, 1973.
10. Slatopolsky E, Robson AM, Elkan I, Bricker NS: Control of phosphate excretion in uremic man, *J Clin Invest* 47:1865-1874, 1968.
11. Contiguglia SR, Alfrey AC, Miller N, Butkus D: Total-body magnesium excess in chronic renal failure, *Lancet* 1:1300-1302, 1972.
12. Richardson RMA, Goldstein MB, Stinebaugh BJ, Halperin ML: Influence of diet and metabolism on urinary acid secretion in the rat and the rabbit, *J Lab Clin Med* 94:510-518, 1979.
13. Flessner MF, Knepper MA: Renal acid-base transport. In Schrier RW, Gottchalk CW, editors: *Diseases of the kidney,* Boston, 1993, Little, Brown & Co.
14. First MR: *Chronic renal failure,* Garden City, N.Y., 1982, Medical Examining Publishing Co, pp 1-5, 15-18.
15. Walser M: Urea metabolism in chronic renal failure, *J Clin Invest* 53:1385-1392, 1974.
16. Perrone RD, Madias NE, Levey AS: Serum creatinine as an index of renal function: new insights into old concepts, *Clin Chem* 38:1933-1953, 1992.
17. Stein JH: Hormones and the kidney, *Hosp Pract* 14:91-105, 1979.
18. Haussler MR, McCain TA: Basic and clinical concepts related to vitamin D metabolism and action, *N Engl J Med* 297:974-983, 1041-1050, 1977.
19. Eschbach JW, Adamson JW, Cook JB: Disorders of red blood cell production in uremia, *Arch Intern Med* 26:812-815, 1970.

20. Pesce AJ, First MR: *Proteinuria: an integrated review,* New York, 1979, Marcel Dekker, pp 80-99, 100-143.

21. Perlmann GE, Tamm I, Horsfall FL: An electrophoretic examination of a urinary mucoprotein which reacts with various viruses, *J Exp Med* 95:99-104, 1952.

22. Coe FL: Clinical and laboratory assessment of the patient with renal disease. In Brenner BM, Rector FC, editors: *The kidney,* vol 1, Philadelphia, 1986, Saunders.

23. Madias NE, Perrone RD: Acid-base disorders in association with renal disease. In Schrier RW, Gottschalk CW, editors: *Disease of the kidney,* Boston, 1993, Little, Brown & Co.

24. First MR, Pollak VE: Renal insufficiency in the diabetic patient with heart disease. In Scott RC, editor: *Clinical cardiology and diabetes,* vol 3, part 2, Mount Kisco, N.Y., 1981, Futura Publishing.

25. Viberti GC, Keen H: The patterns of proteinuria in diabetes mellitus: relevance to pathogenesis and prevention of diabetic nephropathy, *Diabetes* 33:686-692, 1984.

26. Wiegmann TB, Chonko AM, McDougall ML, Moore WV: The role of disease duration and hypertension in albumin excretion of type I diabetes mellitus, *J Am Soc Nephrol* 2:1587-1592, 1992.

27. Mogensen CE, Christensen CK: Predicting diabetic nephropathy in insulin-dependent patients, *N Engl J Med* 311:356-360, 1984.

28. Mathiesen ER, Ronn B, Jensen T, et al: Relationship between blood pressure and urinary albumin excretion in development of microalbuminuria, *Diabetes* 39:245-249, 1990.

29. Ware F: Renal function tests: a guide to interpretation, *Hosp Med* 9:77-92, 1981.

30. Cockcroft DW, Gault MH: Prediction of creatinine clearance from serum creatinine, *Nephron* 16:31-41, 1976.

31. Harrington JT: Evaluation of serum and urinary electrolytes, *Hosp Pract* 17:28-39, 1982.

32. Oken DE: On the differential diagnosis of acute renal failure, *Am J Med* 71:916-920, 1981.

33. Jaffé M. Ueber den Niederschlag welchen Pikrinsäure in normalen Harn erzeugt und über eine neue Reaction des Kreatinins, *Z Physiol Chem* 10:391-400, 1886.

34. Folin O: On the determination of creatinine and creatine in blood, milk and tissues, *J Biol Chem* 17:475-481, 1914.

35. Perrone RD, Madias NE, Levey AS: Serum creatinine as an index of renal function: new insights into old concepts, *Clin Chem* 38:1933-1953, 1992.

36. Rajs G, Mayer M: Oxidation markedly reduces bilirubin interference in the Jaffé creatinine assay, *Clin Chem* 38:2411-2413, 1992.

37. Dilena BA: Bacterial interference with measurement of creatinine in stored plasma, *Clin Chem* 34:1007-1008, 1988.

38. Haeckel R: Assay of creatinine in serum with use of fuller's earth to remove interferents, *Clin Chem* 27:179-183, 1981.

39. Weber JA, van Zanten AP: Interferences in current methods for measurement of creatinine, *Clin Chem* 37:965-700, 1991.

40. Swain RR, Briggs SL: Positive interference with the Jaffé reaction by cephalosporin antibiotics, *Clin Chem* 23:1340-1342, 1977.

41. Moss GA, Bondar RJL, Buzzelli DM: Kinetic enzymatic method for determining serum creatinine, *Clin Chem* 21:1422-1426, 1975.

42. *Kodak Ektachem clinical chemistry slides (CREA), test methodology sheet,* pub no MP2-49 (revision 1992), Rochester, N.Y., 1992, Eastman Kodak Co.

43. Tanganelli E, Prencipe L, Bassi D, et al: Enzymic assay of creatinine in serum and urine with creatinine iminohydrolase and glutamate dehydrogenase, *Clin Chem* 28:1461-1464, 1982.

44. Thompson H, Rechnitz GA: Ion electrode-based enzymatic analysis of creatinine, *Anal Chem* 46:246-249, 1974.

45. Zhiri A, Houot O, Wellman-Bednawska M, Siest G: Simultaneous determination of uric acid and creatinine in plasma by reversed-phase liquid chromatography, *Clin Chem* 31:109-112, 1985.

46. Rosano TG, Ambrose RT, Wu AHB, et al: Candidate reference method for determining creatinine in serum: method development and interlaboratory validation, *Clin Chem* 36:1951-1955, 1990.

47. Delanghe J, Slypere JPD, Buyzere MD, et al: Normal reference values for creatine, creatinine, and carnitine are lower in vegetarians, *Clin Chem* 35:1802-1803, 1989.

48. Tiffany TO, Jansen JM, Burtis CA, et al: Enzymatic kinetic rate and endpoint analysis of substrate, by use of a GeMSAEC fast analyzer, *Clin Chem* 18:829-840, 1972.

49. Harrison SP: Interference in coupled-enzyme assay of urea nitrogen by excess endogenous enzyme, *Clin Chem* 39:911, 1993.

50. Ohkubo A, Kamei S, Yamanaka M, et al: Multilayer-film analysis for urea nitrogen in blood, serum, or plasma, *Clin Chem* 30:1222-1225, 1984.

51. Hammond BR, Lester E: Evaluation of a reflectance photometric method for determination of urea in blood, plasma, or serum, *Clin Chem* 30:596-597, 1984.

52. Chin WT, Kroontje W: Conductivity method for determination of urea, *Anal Chem* 33:1757-1760, 1961.

53. Gourmelin Y, Gouget B, Truchaud A: Electrode measurement of glucose and urea in undiluted samples, *Clin Chem* 36:1646-1649, 1990.

54. Folin O: An improved method for the determination of uric acid in blood, *J Biol Chem* 86:179-187, 1930.

55. Feichtmeier TV, Wrenn HT: Direct determination of uric acid using uricase, *Am J Clin Pathol* 25:833-839, 1955.

56. Marymount JH, London M: Analyses performed with heat-coagulated blood and serum. VI. Direct determination of urates by means of o-dianisidine oxidation, *Am J Clin Pathol* 42:630-633, 1964.

57. Gochman N, Schmitz JM: Automated determination of uric acid, with use of a uricase-peroxidase system, *Clin Chem* 17:1154-1159, 1971.

58. Fossati P, Prencipe L, Berti G: Use of 3,5-dichloro-2-hydroxy-benzenesulfonic acid/4-aminophenazone chromogenic system in direct enzymatic assay of uric acid in serum and urine, *Clin Chem* 26:227-231, 1980.

59. Haeckel R: The use of aldehyde dehydrogenase to determine H_2O_2-producing reactions. I. The determination of the uric acid concentration, *J Clin Chem Clin Biochem* 14:101-107, 1976.

60. Bell R, Ray RA: A rate-sensing approach to the measurement of uric acid in serum and urine, *Clin Chem* 17:644, 1971.

61. Pachla LA, Kissinger PT: Measurement of serum uric acid by liquid chromatography, *Clin Chem* 25:1847-1852, 1979.

62. Hausen A, Fuchs D, König K, Wachter H: Quantitation of urinary uric acid by reversed-phase liquid chromatography, *Clin Chem* 27:1455-1456, 1981.

63. Hohnadel DC, Koller A: Urine protein, total. In Pesce AJ, Kaplan LA, editors: *Methods in clinical chemistry,* St. Louis, 1987, Mosby.

64. Beilby JP, O'Leary BA: α_1-Acid glycoprotein decreases recovery of total protein in urine when trichloroacetic acid is used to precipitate the proteins, *Clin Chem* 36:565-567, 1990.

65. Lievens MM, Celis PJ: Drug interference in turbidimetry and colorimetry of proteins in urine, *Clin Chem* 28:2328, 1982 (Letter).

66. Koumantakis G, Wyndham L: Fluorescein interference with urinary creatinine and protein measurements, *Clin Chem* 37:1799, 1991.

67. Fujita Y, Mori I, Kitano S: Color reaction between pyrogallol red–molybdenum (IV) complex and protein, *Bunseki Kagaku* 32:E379-386, 1983.

68. Orsonneau JL, Douet P, Massoubre C, et al: An improved pyrogallol red–molybdate method for determining total urinary protein, *Clin Chem* 35:2233-2236, 1989.

69. van Ingen HE: Automated analysis for urinary protein by pyrogallol red–molybdate method, *Clin Chem* 36:702, 1990.

70. Waller KV, Ward KM, Mahan JD, Wismatt DK: Current concepts in proteinuria. *Clin Chem* 35:755-765, 1989.

71. Lemann J Jr, Doumas BT: Proteinuria in health and disease assessed by measuring the urinary protein/creatinine ratio, *Clin Chem* 33:297-299, 1987.

72. Ginsberg JM, Chang BS, Matarese RA, Garella S: Use of single voided urine samples to estimate quantitative proteinuria, *N Engl J Med* 309:1543-1546, 1983.

73. Cohen EP, Lemann J Jr: The role of the laboratory in evaluation of kidney function, *Clin Chem* 37:785-796, 1991.

CHAPTER 27   *Liver function*

John E. Sherwin
Juan R. Sobenes

OBJECTIVES

- Explain the role of the liver in carbohydrate metabolism, nitrogen metabolism, bile pigment formation, and metabolic end-product excretion and detoxification.

- Describe pathological liver conditions and the serum biochemical alterations associated with these diseases.

- Describe the processing of bilirubin by the liver, define jaundice, and describe the various pathological states associated with jaundice.

- List the serum proteins derived from the liver and describe their functions.

KEY TERMS

biliary canaliculi Fine channels running between liver cells.

cirrhosis A liver disorder characterized by loss of normal micro-

scopic architecture with fibrosis. Cirrhosis has a variety of causes but is most commonly secondary to chronic alcohol abuse. Obstructive biliary cirrhosis may also be caused by obstruction of major intrahepatic or extrahepatic bile ducts.

Crigler-Najjar syndrome A familial form of nonhemolytic jaundice caused by the absence of glucuronide transferase activity from the liver. Associated with increased serum unconjugated bilirubin and nervous system disorders.

cytochrome P-450 A series of cellular proteins, whose active centers are heme groups, that are one-electron carriers. These are involved in hydroxylation reactions of drugs and other xenobiotics. The 450 refers to the nanometer position of the *Soret* absorption band.

detoxification The process of changing the chemical structure of a foreign substance or poison to make it less poisonous or more readily eliminated.

Dubin-Johnson syndrome A familial form of chronic, nonhemolytic jaundice caused by a defect in the hepatic excretion of conjugated bilirubin.

focal necrosis The death of cells in a small area of tissue.

Gilbert's disease A benign, hereditary form of hyperbilirubinemia and jaundice caused by a defect in the hepatic uptake of unconjugated bilirubin from serum.

gluconeogenesis The formation of glucose from lactate or amino acids by means of the Cori cycle.

glycogenesis The biochemical formation of glycogen from glucose.

glycogenolysis The biochemical degradation of glycogen to form glucose.

hepatitis Inflammation of liver produced by a variety of infections, toxins, and other causes, such as obstruction of the biliary tract in obstructive hepatitis.

hepatobiliary Relating to liver and biliary ducts.

hepatocellular disease Diseases in which the liver cells are destroyed.

hepatocyte A parenchymal liver cell that performs all the functions ascribed to the liver.

jaundice A syndrome characterized by hyperbilirubinemia and deposition of bilirubin pigment in skin and mucosal membranes, giving a yellow appearance to the skin (also called *icterus*).

kernicterus Literally 'nuclear jaundice,' resulting from deposition of unconjugated bilirubin in nuclei of brain and nerve cells, which causes cell destruction and encephalopathy.

ketone bodies Compounds with carbonyl groups, usually referring to acetoacetic acid, acetone, and beta-hydroxybutyric acid (though the latter compound is chemically not a ketone).

LCAT Lecithin-cholesterol acyltransferase; esterifies cholesterol with fatty acids.

505

mRNA   Messenger ribonucleic acid; is translated into specific proteins.

MSH   Melanocyte-stimulating hormone.

neonatal jaundice (physiological jaundice)   A disorder of newborns characterized by increased serum levels of unconjugated bilirubin and caused by transient immaturity of liver.

oncofetal proteins   Any protein, such as alpha-fetoprotein, produced by embryological tumors.

parenchymal cells   A general term indicating the functional elements of an organ (see hepatocyte).

periportal fibrosis   The deposition of fibers or fibrous material in the cells lining the portal blood vessels of the liver.

porphyrias   A group of disorders caused by disturbances of porphyrin metabolism characterized by increased formation and excretion of porphyrins and their precursors.

Reye's syndrome   Acute, often fatal encephalopathy and fatty degeneration of the liver, seen primarily in children.

Wilson's disease   Hepatocellular degeneration, also associated with a change in the iris and lens of the eye and caused by a defect in copper metabolism.

xenobiotics   Any organic compound that is foreign to the body, such as drugs and organic poisons.

ANATOMY AND NORMAL FUNCTION OF LIVER

The liver is the largest organ of the body and is responsible for producing most of the endogenous energy sources used by the body. The liver is divided into two primary lobes and is located in the abdominal cavity just below the diaphragm. The two primary cells of the liver are the *hepatocytes* and the *Kupffer cells* (Fig. 27-1). The parenchymal hepatocytes secrete metabolites into veins or the biliary

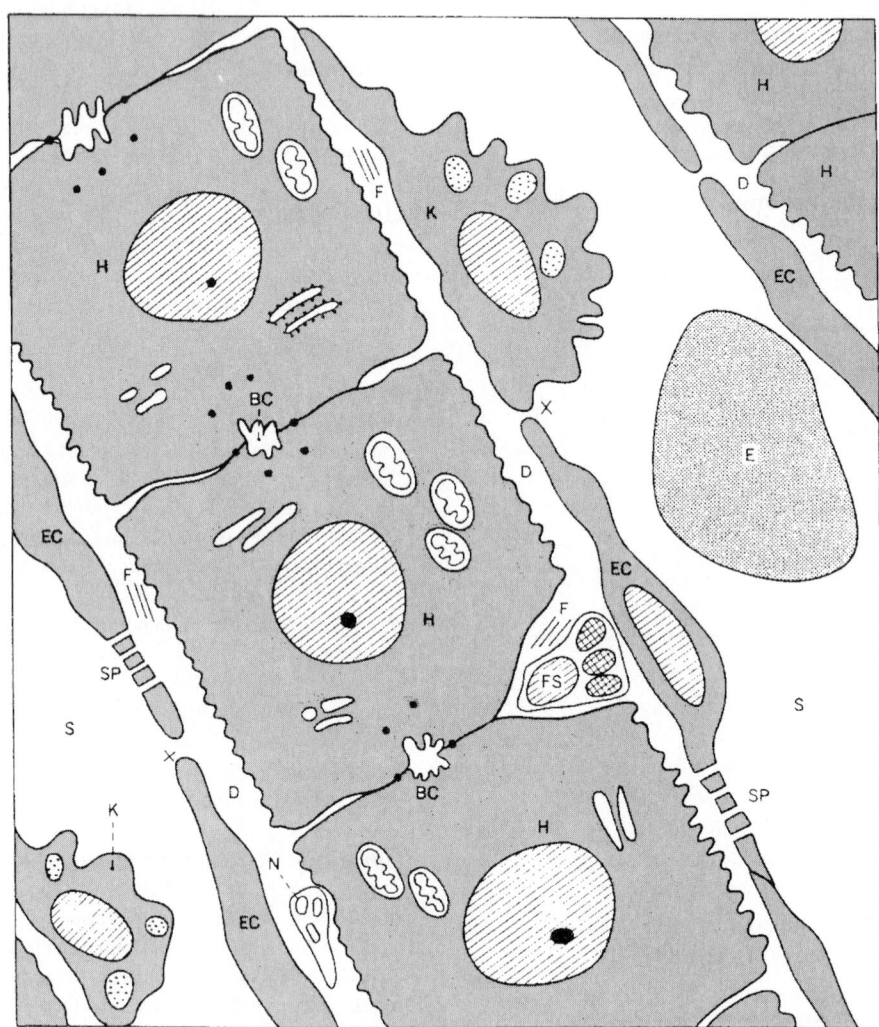

Fig. 27-1   Schema of structures within the lobule. *BC*, Bile canaliculus; *D*, space of Disse; *E*, erythrocyte; *EC*, endothelial cell; *F*, reticulum fibers; *FS*, fat-storing cell; *H*, hepatocyte; *K*, Kupffer cell; *N*, nerve fiber; *S*, sinusoid; *SP*, fenestrae of endothelial cell forming a sieve plate; ×, intercellular gap. (From Tanikawa K, editor: *Ultrastructural aspects of the liver and its disorders*, ed 2, Tokyo, New York, 1979, Igaku-Shoin.

canaliculi; the canaliculi eventually dispense wastes into the bile duct and gallbladder. The hepatocytes are responsible for the metabolic functions of the liver.[1]

The liver is the principal organ for the metabolism of carbohydrates, proteins, lipids, porphyrins, and bile acids. It is capable of synthesizing most body proteins except the immunoglobulins, which are produced by the lymphocytic plasma cell system. The liver is also the major site for storage of iron, glycogen, lipids, and vitamins. The liver plays an important role in the detoxification of xenobiotics and excretion of metabolic end products such as bilirubin, ammonia, and urea.

Carbohydrate metabolism and liver function

Polysaccharides are a form of energy storage. The liver is capable of producing glycogen, the principal storage polysaccharide, by glycogenesis and degrading glycogen by glycogenolysis. Whether the glycogen synthetic reaction or the glycogen degradation reaction predominates depends on an individual's metabolic status. Only liver glycogen is available for maintenance of a constant blood glucose, since only the liver and kidneys contain the enzyme glucose-6-phosphatase, which converts glucose-6-phosphate to glucose. As a result of the highly branched structure of glycogen, approximately 10% of the glucose of glycogen is available for immediate enzymatic release (see Chapter 32 for details on glucose metabolism). Liver glycogen in the normal adult is not a static storage pool; instead it functions as a source of glucose for the rest of the body, except for muscle. Under conditions of stress, increased body energy requirements must be met by increased glucose use, that is, glycogenolysis and glycolysis. Additional glucose required for the body is provided by increased secretion of glucose by the liver. This is accomplished when the rate of glycogen degradation and the rate of *gluconeogenesis* are increased. Gluconeogenesis is not simply a reversal of glycolysis, since several of the glycolytic enzymes, such as pyruvate kinase, phosphofructokinase, and hexokinase, are not reversible. Lactate and amino acids serve as the precursors for the gluconeogenic pathway. The use of blood lactic acid (of muscle origin) by the liver is an important factor in the clearance of this analyte from serum. Gluconeogenesis is an important source of blood glucose when liver glycogen has been depleted. Liver glycogen depletion will occur within several hours in a fasting person. The net result of these metabolic pathways is to provide a constant supply of glucose to the blood for export to peripheral tissues to meet their energy requirements.

Protein metabolism in liver

Most serum proteins are synthesized in the liver, with two exceptions in the adult: gamma globulin and hemoglobin. In the infant the liver retains the ability to synthesize hemoglobin. As in carbohydrate synthesis, liver function must be extensively impaired before a decrease in protein synthesis can be unequivocally demonstrated. The normal concentrations of the major electrophoretic subgroups of proteins are quite variable and depend at least in part on the person's age.

Many liver enzymes exhibit half-lives of several weeks, though structural proteins are stable nearly indefinitely. Plasma proteins synthesized by the liver exhibit quite varied rates of synthesis and degradation (that is, turnover rates). Under normal conditions, the rate of synthesis of each protein equals its rate of degradation, since its concentration in plasma remains constant. Many proteins synthesized by the liver are excreted into *extravascular fluid* to carry out specific functions. These functions include nutrition, blood pressure control (oncotic pressure), and transport. Table 27-1 lists some liver proteins found in plasma and some of their properties.

One of the most important serum proteins produced in the liver is albumin. Present in concentrations of 40 to 50 g/L, albumin represents 50% to 60% by weight of all plasma protein. This molecule has an extraordinarily wide range of functions, including nutrition; maintenance of oncotic pressure; and serum transport of Ca^{++}, unconjugated bilirubin, free fatty acids, drugs, and steroids. Its multifactorial role in human physiology makes it an important analyte in the monitoring of liver disease.

The liver is also the site for the synthesis of several *acute phase reaction* proteins. When the body is stressed (as by an infectious disease), the serum levels of these proteins may become elevated. Some of these acute phase reaction proteins are used as markers for infectious disease, such as *C-reactive protein*. Others, such as *transthyretin (prealbumin),* are used as markers for the protein-nutritional status of an individual. When the body is protein malnourished, serum prealbumin levels are decreased, and measurement of prealbumin and albumin can be useful for the diagnosis and monitoring of malnutrition (see Chapter 37).

Metabolic pools of amino acids are present in the liver. From these pools amino acids are drawn for the synthesis of proteins. When a protein is degraded, the bulk of the constituent amino acids are returned to these intracellular pools. The released amino acids can also be used in gluconeogenesis, transamination, or deamination reactions or be reincorporated into new proteins. Important transamination reactions are catalyzed by the enzymes alanine aminotransferase (ALT, or formerly SGPT) and aspartate aminotransferase (AST, or formerly SGOT). In the healthy person who is in nitrogen equilibrium or positive nitrogen balance, the amino groups of excess amino acids in serum are converted to ammonia or urea for excretion.[2] Some amino acids are also excreted unchanged in the urine. Negative nitrogen balance (that is, insufficient dietary nitrogen) leads to a diminution of amino acid pools and thus decreased urea excretion.

Urea, creatinine, ammonia, and uric acid account for 70% to 75% of the serum nonprotein nitrogen; urea accounts for

Table 27-1   Major representative plasma proteins and their properties

Electrophoretic fraction	Protein	Approximate concentration (g/L)	Principal function
	Transthyrethin (prealbumin)	0.1-0.4	Binds retinol-binding protein, T_4
	Albumin	40-50	Binds Ca^{2+}, T_4, bilirubin
α_1	Antitrypsin	2-4	Inhibits some proteolytic enzymes
	Lipoprotein, high density (HDL)	3-8	Transport of cholesterol from peripheral tissue to liver
	Retinol binding	0.03-0.06	Transport of retinol
α_2	Thyroxine binding globulin	0.01-0.02	Transport of thyroxine
	Haptoglobins (three types)	1-3	Transport of free hemoglobin from destroyed red blood cells
	Lipoprotein, very low density (VLDL)	1.5-2.0	Transport of cholesterol and triglycerides
	Ceruloplasmin	0.2-0.6	Transport of copper, increases use of iron as ferroxidase
	Prothrombin (bovine)	0.1	Proenzyme of thrombin
	Angiotensinogen	—	Precursor of angiotensin I
	Erythropoietin	<0.05	Erythropoietic hormone
β_1	Lipoprotein, low density (LDL)	4-10	Transport of cholesterol and other lipids
	Plasminogen	0.3	Profibrinolysin, precursor of fibrinolysin
	Fibrinogen	3	Coagulation factor I
$\beta_1\beta_2$	Complement (C_4)	0.5-1.8	Lysis of foreign cells
	Transferrin	2-4	Transport of iron
β_2	Glycoproteins	0.3	Unknown
γ	Blood group globulins and immunoglobulins	7-15	Contain various antibodies, blood globulins, complement C_1, C_2, and so on

Modified from Orten JM, Neuhaus OW: *Human biochemistry,* ed 10, St. Louis, 1982, Mosby.

60% of the total. Most of the metabolism of nonprotein nitrogen occurs in the liver. Urea is produced in the liver because arginase, the enzyme that converts arginine to urea and ornithine, is present only in the liver. Although blood ammonia concentration is normally quite low, 500 μg/L, ammonia is an important intermediate in amino acid synthesis. Sources of ammonia include hepatic oxidation of glutamate to oxoglutarate, the transamination and oxidative deamination of amino acids and catecholamines, and bacterial breakdown of urea in the gut. Most blood ammonia is formed from the gut. The primary mechanisms for the metabolic disposal of ammonia is the synthesis of glutamate, glutamine, and carbamyl phosphate. Carbamyl phosphate may be used to synthesize orotic acid and ultimately pyrimidines for nucleic acids or to synthesize urea, which is the principal pathway for the excretion of excess nitrogen.

Lipid biosynthesis and transport in liver function

Lipids, for the sake of this discussion, include only free fatty acids, triglycerides, glycerophosphatides, sphingolipids, cholesterol, and cholesterol esters. General chemical structures for these lipids are shown in Chapter 53, and their metabolism is discussed in Chapter 33.

Lipids are synthesized in the liver in response to excess carbohydrate intake and to normal intake of dietary lipids. Excess carbohydrate is converted to acetyl coenzyme A (acetyl CoA), and a cytoplasmic enzyme system converts it

to the fatty acid palmitate, using reduced nicotinamide adenine diphosphonucleotide (NADPH) and adenosine triphosphate, which are also produced from glucose metabolism.

In the liver, fatty acids are broken down to acetyl CoA, which can then be oxidized to CO_2 by the citric acid cycle. However, a small portion of acetyl CoA is converted to ketone bodies, such as acetoacetate, beta-hydroxybutyrate, and acetone. In normal persons, these products are present in blood to the extent of only about 30 mg/L. In the presence of excess mobilization of fatty acids, as in diabetic ketoacidosis or alcohol intoxication, limiting amounts of NAD and NADP result in an increased hepatic synthesis of the ketone bodies.

The liver repackages dietary lipids and secretes them in the form of triglyceride-rich, very-low-density lipoproteins. These are eventually converted to low-density lipoprotein for delivery of cholesterol to peripheral cells. Cholesterol is also synthesized in the liver microsomes from acetyl CoA. Approximately 70% of the total cholesterol in plasma is esterified with fatty acids by the enzyme lecithin-cholesterol acyltransferase, which is also produced by the liver. Bile acids are produced from cholesterol by the cells lining the biliary canaliculi and ductules of the liver.[2] The bile acids are the final excretory metabolites of cholesterol. They also serve as aids in the digestion of dietary lipids (see Chapter 30). Approximately 80% of the available cholesterol is converted into the four major bile acids (Table

Table 27-2 Names of bile acids, their relative contribution to the total bile acid pool, and normal serum concentrations

Name	Relative content (%) in bile	Normal serum concentration (mmol)
Cholylglycine	38	0.2-0.9
Deoxycholylglycine	20	0.08-0.7
Lithocholylglycine	4	0.07-0.3
Chenodeoxycholylglycine	38	0.05-0.2

From Shaw LM: *Lab Management* 20:56-63, 1982.

27-2). Cholic acid and chenodeoxycholate are the primary bile acids and are present in a fivefold to tenfold excess over the secondary bile acids, deoxycholic acid and lithocholic acid, which are produced by metabolism of the primary hepatic bile acids by intestinal bacteria.

Bile acids are collected in the biliary canaliculi and ductules and stored in the gallbladder. They are then transported to the intestinal lumen, where they emulsify ingested lipids. This emulsification of the lipids permits the intestinal mucosa to digest the lipids and absorb the liberated triglycerides and cholesterol. More than 90% of the secreted bile acids are reabsorbed and returned to the liver through the portal circulation.[2]

Liver function as a storage depot

The liver is an important site for the storage of iron, glycogen, amino acids, and some lipids and vitamins. The adult liver contains about 700 mg of iron. Nutritional iron is absorbed primarily in the intestine. To be absorbed, ferric iron (Fe^{3+}) must be converted to ferrous iron (Fe^{2+}). Immediately after absorption, the Fe^{2+} is reconverted to Fe^{3+} and temporarily stored in the intestinal mucosa as the ferritin complex. The ferritin apoprotein is synthesized in the liver. The iron is then released once more as Fe^{2+} into the plasma and is rapidly oxidized into Fe^{3+} and complexed with transferrin, a hepatic synthesized α_1-globulin. In the healthy adult, transferrin is 25% to 30% saturated with Fe^{3+}. In the liver, transferrin releases iron, and a new ferritin-Fe^{3+} complex is formed. Ferritin is the primary storage form of iron; apoferritin binds iron as a colloidal hydrous ferric oxide. However, a small amount of iron is stored as hemosiderin, which is an insoluble cellular inclusion of Fe^{3+} complexed with ferritin. Hemosiderin granules serve as a storage form for iron when there are insufficient levels of apoferritin. The ratio of iron to protein is much greater in hemosiderin than in ferritin. Additional details of iron metabolism are found in Chapter 35.

Lipid is stored, primarily as triglyceride, in subcutaneous adipose tissue. Lipid is also stored in the liver, where it functions as an energy reservoir. Under normal circumstances the liver functions as a temporary storage site for lipids as they are synthesized in the liver or absorbed from the intestine after a meal.

Bile pigment formation

About 126 days after emergence from the reticuloendothelial tissue, the senescent erythrocytes are phagocytized and the hemoglobin is released. The heme portion of hemoglobin is converted to bilirubin, with the release of iron and the globin proteins. The liberated iron is bound by transferrin and returned to the iron stores of the liver or bone marrow; the globin is degraded to its constituent amino acids. The conversion of heme to bilirubin requires 2 to 3 hours (Fig. 27-2). Bilirubin, bound to albumin, is transported from the reticuloendothelial cells to the hepatocytes. In the liver, bilirubin is transported through the cellular microvilli of the sinusoids to the hepatocytes. Bilirubin is dissociated from albumin and taken up into the hepatocytes by specific proteins. Within the hepatocyte, bilirubin glucuronide is formed by reaction of bilirubin with uridine diphosphoglucuronate (UDP-glucuronate) in the presence of UDP-glucuronyltransferase. Approximately 8 to 10 mg/L of unconjugated bilirubin is present in normal adult serum; normal adult serum contains no conjugated bilirubin. Formation of bilirubin diglucuronide represents the usual (85% to 90%) conjugation reaction, but in disease states, monoglucuronides of bilirubin form as a result of the accumulation of unconjugated bilirubin in the face of a limited supply of glucuronate. In disease states, a small fraction of unconjugated bilirubin is also covalently conjugated to albumin. This fraction of bilirubin, termed *delta-bilirubin*, reacts like conjugated bilirubin in most chemical assays used to measure this fraction.

After formation, the bilirubin-diglucuronide is excreted by the hepatocyte into the biliary canaliculi. Any disease resulting in a decreased secretion of the conjugated bilirubin will result in an increased serum concentration of this analyte. As part of the bile, these water-soluble conjugates are secreted into the lumen of the small intestine. The bilirubin conjugates are hydrolyzed by a beta-glucuronidase, and the regenerated bilirubin is converted to *d*-urobilinogen

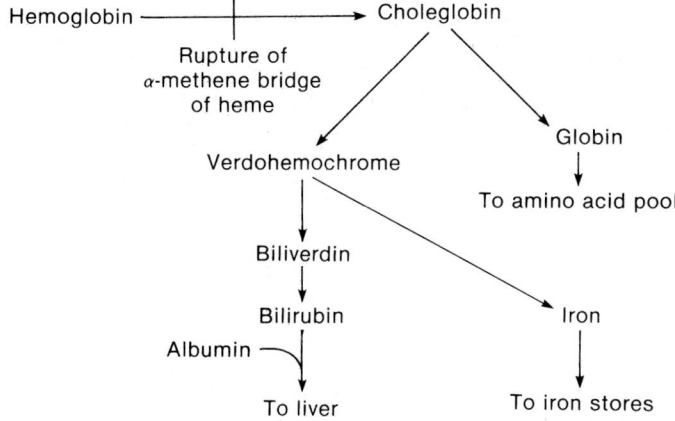

Fig. 27-2 Formation of bilirubin from hemoglobin occurs primarily in reticuloendothelial tissues.

and further reduced to *l*-urobilinogen and *l*-stercobilinogen by the anaerobic bacteria of the intestinal lumen. The urobilinogens are reabsorbed from the intestine and recirculated in the extrahepatic circulation, where they are ultimately excreted in the urine. Stercobilinogen is not reabsorbed from the intestine but is a normal constituent of the feces. These bilinogens oxidize spontaneously in air to the corresponding bilins and thereby contribute to the color of both urine and feces (Fig. 27-3). (See Chapter 35 for additional details on bilirubin metabolism.)

Metabolic end-product excretion and detoxification

Humans have two mechanisms for detoxification of foreign (xenobiotic) materials, such as drugs and poisons, and toxic metabolic products, such as ammonia and bilirubin. The first is to bind the compound reversibly to a protein so that the material is inactivated; thus bilirubin is bound to albumin and lead is bound to hemoglobin. The second mechanism is to modify the compound chemically so that it is readily excreted; thus ammonia is converted to urea and bilirubin is converted to bilirubin-glucuronide.

The inactivation and detoxification of exogenous compounds are usually accomplished by hydroxylation mediated by one of the cytochrome P-450 enzymes or by conjugation of the parent compound or its metabolite with sulfate or carbohydrate. These reactions are localized in the microsomes of the liver. The sulfated compounds are more water soluble than the parent compounds and are excreted directly in the urine. Carbohydrate conjugates are commonly excreted into the intestinal lumen as part of the bile.

LIVER-FUNCTION ALTERATIONS DURING DISEASE
Jaundice

Jaundice is a general condition that results from abnormal metabolism or retention of bilirubin. Jaundice causes a yellow discoloration of the skin, mucous membranes, and sclera. Jaundice can typically be seen at serum bilirubin levels of approximately 50 mg/L. The three principal types of jaundice are prehepatic, hepatic, and posthepatic.

Prehepatic jaundice is the result of acute or chronic hemolytic anemias. *Hepatic jaundice* includes disorders of bilirubin metabolism and transport defects, such as Crigler-Najjar disease, Dubin-Johnson syndrome, and Gilbert's disease, as well as neonatal physiological jaundice and diseases resulting in hepatocellular injury or destruction.

Each of the specific diseases of bilirubin metabolism represents a defect in one of the steps in the hepatic processing of serum bilirubin (Fig. 27-4). Thus *Gilbert's disease* is caused by a defect in the transport of bilirubin from plasma albumin into the hepatocyte. Although levels of unconjugated bilirubin are elevated in this familial disorder, levels of conjugated bilirubin are not. Impairment in the conjugation step by UDP-glucuronide caused by a defi-

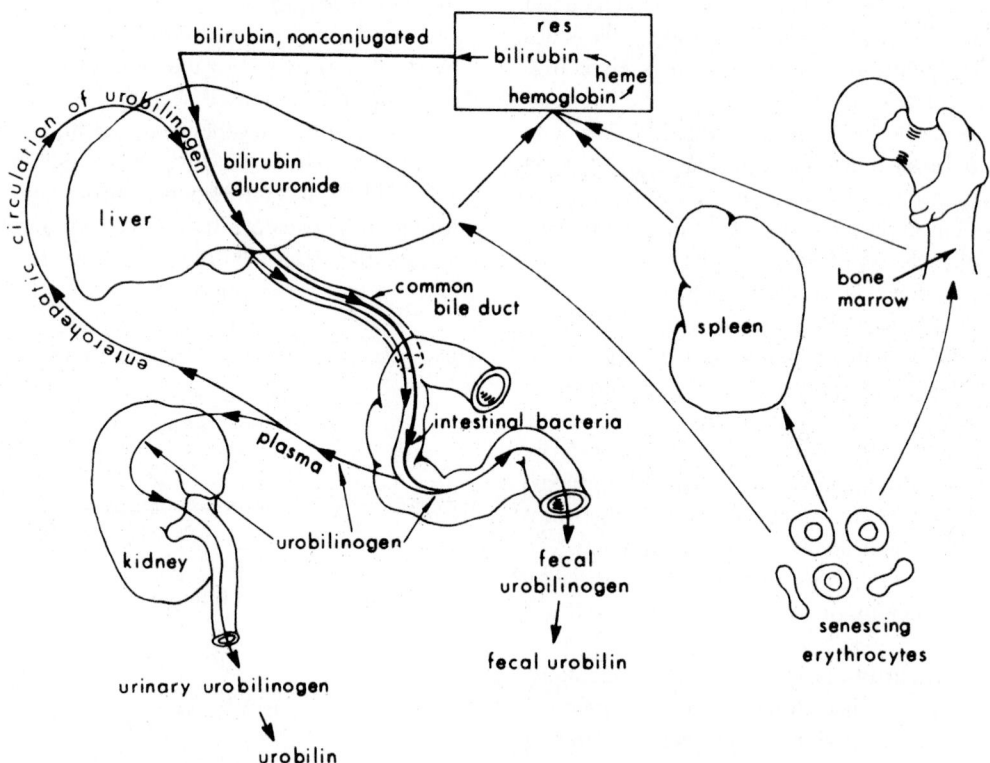

Fig. 27-3 Bilirubin metabolism. (From Bauer JD, editor: *Clinical laboratory methods,* ed 9, St. Louis, 1982, Mosby.)

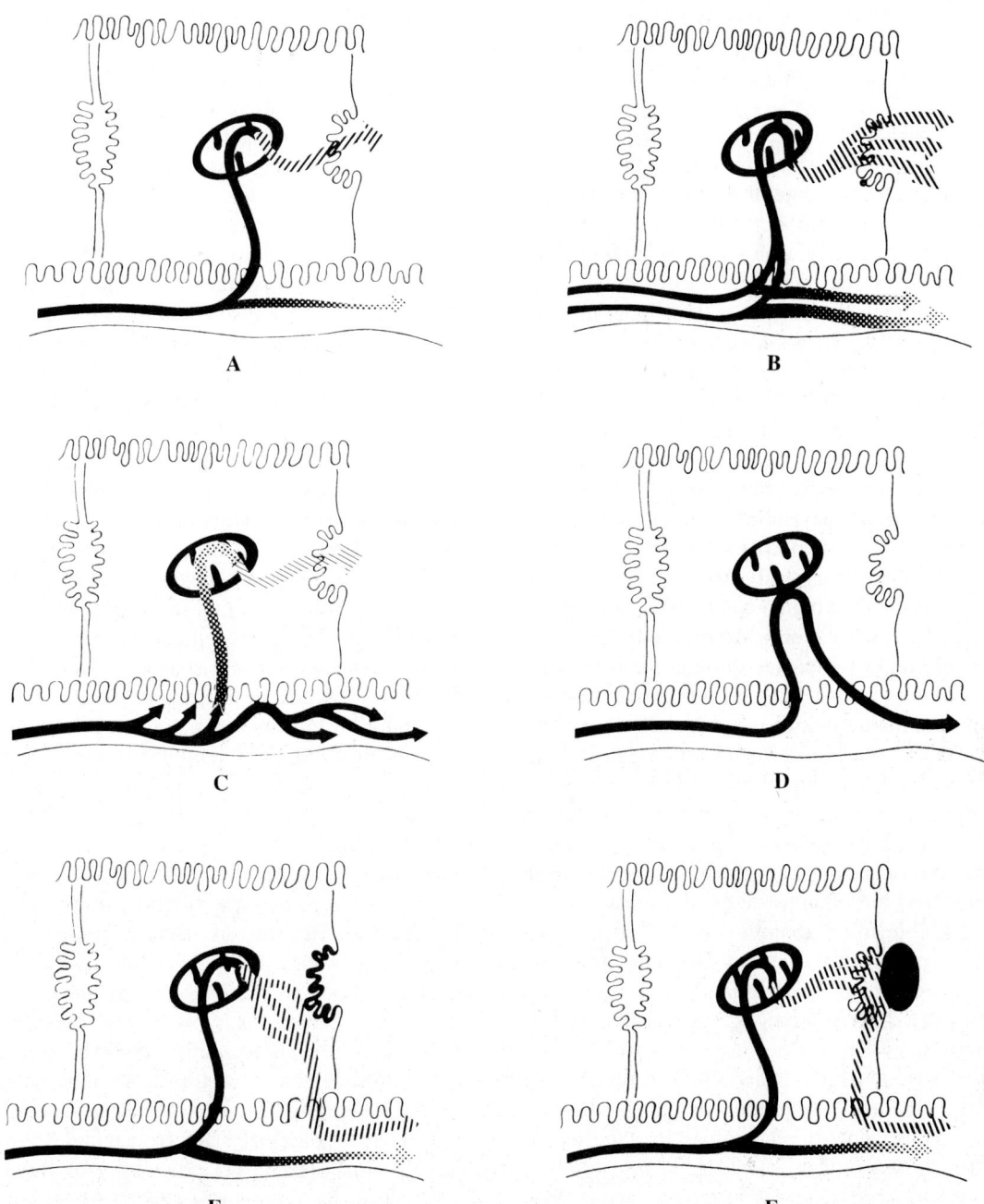

Fig. 27-4 Mechanisms of hyperbilirubinemia. **A,** Normal bilirubin metabolism with hepatocyte uptake of unconjugated bilirubin *(dark arrow)* and microsomal conjugation and excretion of conjugated bilirubin *(striped arrow)*. **B,** Hemolytic jaundice in which increased bilirubin production results in increased excretion of conjugated bilirubin and a rise in excess (exceeding liver capacity) unconjugated bilirubin in blood. **C,** Gilbert's disease in which decreased hepatic uptake results in a large increase in blood levels of unconjugated bilirubin. **D,** Physiological jaundice in which microsomal conjugating system is not functional, resulting in a large increase in unconjugated bilirubin. Congenital deficiency is the Crigler-Najjar syndrome. **E,** Dubin-Johnson syndrome in which there is a biochemical defect preventing secretion of conjugated bilirubin, resulting in a backflow into blood. **F,** Intrahepatic or extrahepatic obstruction in which a physical block prevents secretion of conjugated bilirubin. Hepatocellular disease results in a pattern similar to a combination of **C** and **D.** (From Leevy CM, editor: *Evaluation of liver function,* ed 2, Indianapolis, 1974, Lilly Research Laboratories.)

ciency in the enzyme UDP-glucuronyl transferase will also lead to a large increase in unconjugated bilirubin. When this enzyme deficiency is congenital, it is known as *Crigler-Najjar disease.*

However, deficiencies in glucuronyl transferase are most frequently encountered as *neonatal,* or *physiological, jaundice.*[3] This enzyme activity is one of the last liver functions to be activated in prenatal life, since unconjugated bilirubin formed in the fetus is cleared by the placenta into maternal blood. However, in premature births, infants are sometimes born without the enzyme activity present. This leads to a rapid buildup of unconjugated bilirubin, which can be life threatening. The unconjugated bilirubin, which is much more lipid soluble than water soluble, readily passes into the brain and nerve cells and is deposited in the nuclei of these cells, resulting in *kernicterus.* Kernicterus often results in cell damage and death. Neonatal jaundice will persist until the glucuronyl transferase is produced by the newborn's liver.[3] The newborn's blood must be monitored frequently so that dangerously high levels of unconjugated bilirubin (about 200 mg/L) can be detected. At this point the infant is treated either with ultraviolet radiation to destroy the bilirubin as it passes through the capillaries of the skin or with exchange transfusion.[3] Monitoring serum bilirubin in premature infants is particularly important. These infants are at greater risk for bilirubin-induced encephalopathy because (1) the blood-brain barrier may be incomplete, (2) these infants often have lower concentrations of albumin than normal, (3) there is an acidosis, whereby the increase in hydrogen ions can displace bilirubin from albumin, and (4) they are often treated with substances that may displace bilirubin from albumin such as free fatty acids in hyperalimentation fluids or drugs such as phenytoin (Dilantin) or phenobarbital. In hospitals where babies are at risk for hepatitis, measurements of conjugated bilirubin may also be needed (see below).

The last step in the hepatic processing of bilirubin is the postconjugation step of excretion of the bilirubin-glucuronide from the hepatic microsomes into the canaliculi. Impairment of this process, called the *Dubin-Johnson syndrome,* results in large increases in the conjugated bilirubin fraction of serum and a urine showing the presence of bilirubin.

The measurement of delta-bilirubin (δ-bili) has been advocated as a means of better assessing hyperbilirubinemia resulting from obstructive hepatic disease.[4] The δ-bili fraction has a much longer serum half-life than that of the other fractions. If elevated to significant concentrations, it may result in an apparent slowed decrease in the drop in serum bilirubin, giving a false impression of a lack of progress as the liver disease responds to treatment.

Hepatic jaundice also encompasses the disorders characterized by hepatocellular damage or necrosis, such as hepatitis and cirrhosis. *Posthepatic jaundice* is generally caused by biliary obstructive disease resulting from spasms or strictures of the biliary tract, ductal occlusion by stones, or compression by neoplastic disease. Since the hepatic functions of transport and conjugation of bilirubin are normal in these diseases, the major increase in serum bilirubin involves the conjugated fraction. Unable to be properly excreted by the liver in these disorders, the conjugated bilirubin fraction increases in serum, resulting in the appearance of bilirubin in the urine. If the hepatocellular disease is severe enough to cause jaundice, both the conjugated and the unconjugated bilirubin fractions are increased. The reason is the general disruption of bilirubin metabolism. The laboratory findings for bilirubin and its metabolites in these diseases are summarized in Table 27-3.

Hepatitis

Hepatitis, a general term meaning 'inflammation of the liver,' is used to describe diseases resulting in hepatocellular damage. Hepatitis is usually caused by infections or toxic agents. Viral hepatitis is the most common cause of acute hepatocellular disease. Four types of hepatitis virus have been recognized: type A virus; type B virus; type C virus; and the delta hepatitis virus. The last virus had been considered defective, requiring the presence of type B virus for infectivity. However, the delta virus is no longer believed to be biologically defective but may require the hepatitis B virus (HBV) for production of disease. Certainly, coinfection by both viruses results in a more aggressive

Table 27-3 Concentrations and changes in concentration of bilirubin and its metabolites in healthy persons and those with jaundice

| Condition | Serum | | Urine | | Feces pigment |
	Total bilirubin	Conjugated bilirubin	Bilirubin	Urobilinogen	
Healthy	2-10 mg/L	0-2 mg/L	Negative	0.5-3.4 mg/day	Brown
Prehepatic jaundice	Increased	Normal	Negative	Increased	Normal
Hepatic jaundice					
Hepatocellular disease	Increased	Increased	Positive	Decreased (normal)	Light brown
Gilbert's disease	Increased	Normal	Negative	Decreased (normal)	Normal
Crigler-Najjar syndrome	Increased	Decreased	Negative	Decreased	Light brown
Dubin-Johnson syndrome	Increased	Increased	Positive	Decreased (normal)	Light brown
Posthepatic obstructive jaundice	Increased	Increased	Positive	Decreased	Light brown

chronic liver disease than infection by HBV alone.[5] The clinical symptoms of the four types are similar, and the majority of hepatitis cases are anicteric because despite the hepatic necrosis the liver retains sufficient residual functional capacity to handle the bilirubin load from normal hemoglobin turnover. Other viruses known to cause hepatitis include cytomegalovirus, coxsackievirus B, and Epstein-Barr virus.

Serum levels of ALT and AST rise rapidly during the early course of hepatitis because of hepatic necrosis. In patients who develop jaundice, the rise in the transaminases precedes the increase in bilirubin, which persists for 2 to 8 weeks. AST is usually more elevated than ALT. Serum alkaline phosphatase and γ-glutamyltransferase (GGT) are elevated during the early cholestatic portion of the disease and remain elevated until the disease has resolved. Diagnosis of the type of viral hepatitis is accomplished by measurement of the specific hepatitis antigen during the prodromal phase of the illness. Specific antibodies to virus antigens are detectable for several weeks after the antigen is no longer detectable. Chronic hepatitis is generally the result of a persistence of hepatitis B infection. It is associated with elevation of serum bilirubin, minimally but persistently elevated serum transaminases (with ALT now greater than AST) caused by hepatic necrosis, and, occasionally, elevated alkaline phosphatase.

Drug-induced hepatic damage

The most common cause of drug-induced hepatic damage is chronic excessive ingestion of alcohol. Laboratory findings associated with this damage are an elevation of GGT, a mild elevation of the transaminases, an increase in the globulin with a decrease in the albumin fractions of the serum proteins, and a decrease in sulfobromophthalein (Bromsulphalein, BSP) or indocyanine green clearance. (See Chapter 34 for a detailed review of alcoholic liver disease.)

Other classes of drugs that induce hepatic damage include barbiturates, tricyclic antidepressants, antiepileptics, isoniazid, and acetaminophen. These drugs typically cause an increase in serum GGT. Acetaminophen is highly hepatotoxic. Overdoses require careful monitoring to prevent death from liver failure. Drug withdrawal permits liver regeneration. Chemotherapeutic drugs such as vincristine, vinblastine, actinomycin D, and 5-fluorouracil will typically cause an elevation of the serum transaminases and lactate dehydrogenase because of hepatic tissue damage and enzyme release.

Reye's syndrome

Reye's syndrome typically occurs in children between 2 and 13 years of age. The liver has fatty infiltration with necrosis and cholestasis, and encephalopathy occurs because of accumulation of ammonia. Laboratory findings include an elevated blood ammonia, elevated serum transaminases, and a prolonged prothrombin time.

Congenital deficiency syndromes with altered liver function

Porphyrias. The porphyrias are caused by congenital enzyme deficiencies in the pathways leading to the synthesis of the heme moiety of hemoglobin and other heme proteins, such as myoglobin and the cytochromes. Increased excretion of specific porphyrin metabolites, varying with the enzyme defect, is seen. The five types of porphyria are acute intermittent porphyria, acquired congenital hepatic porphyria, erythropoietic porphyria, and erythropoietic protoporphyria. Chapter 35 summarizes porphyrin metabolism and has a discussion of the enzyme defects.

Wilson's disease. Wilson's disease is an autosomal recessive disorder of copper metabolism. The accumulation of copper in the liver results in jaundice followed by liver cirrhosis. Wilson's disease is characterized by a low serum concentration of ceruloplasmin, glycosuria, phosphaturia, aminoaciduria, and an elevated urinary copper concentration with excretion greater than 50 μg/day.

Hemochromatosis. Hemochromatosis is another genetic disorder of metal metabolism. In this disease, iron accumulates in the liver, and the resulting cirrhosis is similar to alcoholic cirrhosis. An elevated serum iron, a low iron-binding capacity, and an elevated serum ferritin value in the presence of normal dietary iron intake are characteristic of this disorder.

Alpha$_1$-antitrypsin deficiency

Alpha$_1$-antitrypsin deficiency is an inborn error of protein metabolism that results in emphysema and liver cirrhosis. Numerous alpha$_1$-antitrypsin phenotypes have been identified and carry varying risks of disease.[6] The tissue damage seen in alpha$_1$-antitrypsin deficiencies may well be caused by hydrolytic damage to structural protein by trypsin-like enzymes that have not been neutralized by alpha$_1$-antitrypsin. Since alpha$_1$-antitrypsin represents approximately 80% of the alpha$_1$ fraction of serum proteins on electrophoresis, a severe deficiency is often diagnosed by the absence of this fraction in the electrophoretogram. Phenotyping of the various alpha$_1$-antitrypsin deficiencies is best done by isoelectric focusing.

Other genetic disorders that are associated with liver disease include the lipid-storage diseases and the glycogen-storage diseases. These are discussed in detail in Chapter 48.

Liver tumors and other hepatic disorders

Congenital hepatic fibrosis, hepatic cysts, and liver abscesses are generally best diagnosed by liver biopsy. However, nonspecific changes in liver enzymes and indocyanine green retention can accompany these disorders. Liver tumors frequently alter liver function as a result of tissue compression during tumor growth and infiltration. This results in an increase in serum alkaline phosphatase, 5'-nucleotidase, and especially GGT. BSP and indocyanine green

Table 27-4 Change of serum analyte with disease

	Alkaline phosphatase	GGT	5'-Nucleotidase	AST	ALT	Bile acids	Albumin	NH$_3$
Acute hepatitis (viral and so on)	↑	↑	↑	↑↑↑	↑↑	↑↑	N	N, ↑
Alcoholic (drug) hepatitis	N, ↑	↑↑↑	↑	↑	↑	↑	N	N, ↑
Chronic hepatocellular disease	N, ↑	N, ↑	N, ↑	↑	↑	↑	↓	N, ↑
Cirrhosis	N, ↑	N, ↑	N, ↑	N, ↑	N, ↑	↑	↓	N, ↑
Reye's syndrome	N			↑	↑			↑↑
Hepatomas	↑↑	↑↑↑↑	↑↑	↑	↑		N, ↓	N
Cholestatic disease	↑	↑↑	↑↑↑	↑	↑	↑	N	N

N, Normal; ↑, elevated; ↓, lowered.

clearances are frequently prolonged. The demonstration of an elevation of serum alpha-fetoprotein is diagnostic of hepatic tumor in the presence of an abnormal liver scan.

Liver transplantation

Liver transplantation is becoming increasingly common, and between 85% and 90% of patients survive their first transplant at least 1 year. It is important to monitor these patients for function as well as early signs of rejection.[11,12] Both cyclosporin A and FK-506 (Tacrolimmus) are used as immunosuppressive agents that aid in graft acceptance. Monitoring whole blood concentrations of these drugs is important for maintaining effective drug concentrations.

Measurement of both tissue necrosis factor-alpha[13] and plasma endotoxin have been reported to produce good early indication of graft rejection. Measurement of monoethylglycinexylidide after lidocaine administration has been reported to be useful in the assessment of donor liver function as well as recipient loss of graft hepatic function.[14] In patients receiving a liver transplant because of viral hepatitis, the measurement of delta hepatitis can be helpful in determining whether the transplanted liver is infected after transplantation.[11] Often evidence of the delta virus reinfection can occur months before evidence of the spread of HBV.

Maintenance of posttransplantation liver function can be assessed by measurement of the traditional liver-function enzymes such as ALT, lactate dehydrogenase (LD), GGT, and alkaline phosphatase in conjunction with other tests, such as prothrombin time. The interpretation of these is the same as that in other patients.

LIVER-FUNCTION TESTS

Liver-function tests are generally used to identify liver disease in the absence of jaundice or when the jaundice is the result of hemolytic disease and the existence of complicating liver disease is suspected. Liver function is tested by injection of a dye intravascularly and observation of the retention of the dye in the serum. It is essential that a dye that is excreted into the bile rather than filtered by the kidney be chosen. Thus indocyanine green is acceptable,

whereas phenolsulfonphthalein, which is excreted preferentially in the urine, is not. Indocyanine green retention depends on hepatic blood flow, biliary duct function, and liver cell function. Therefore these tests cannot distinguish between hepatocellular disease and obstructive liver disease. In the normal person the percentage of retention is less than 5% at 45 minutes. An increase in the retention is consistent with liver dysfunction resulting from hepatocellular disease, biliary obstructive disease, and space-filling lesions such as tumors in the liver. It should be emphasized that BSP testing is not done routinely any longer, in part because it is known to cause anaphylaxis in some patients.

A second group of liver function tests related changes in the liver's ability to metabolize drugs to changes in serum concentration of the parent drug or its metabolite, or in the rate of drug metabolite excreted into urine.

CHANGE OF ANALYTE IN DISEASE

Changes of serum analyte with disease are summarized in Table 27-4.

Enzymes

In this section, six serum enzymes are described and their value in the differential diagnosis of liver disease is examined. The enzymes discussed are alkaline phosphatase, GGT, AST, ALT, 5'-nucleotidase, and lactate dehydrogenase. Numerous other enzymes that are useful in the evaluation of liver function have been identified. However, these six enzymes are those generally used. Examples of the change in activity with time for several of these enzymes in hepatic disease are shown in Figs. 27-5 to 27-7.

Alkaline phosphatase (EC 3.1.3.1). Alkaline phosphatase is actually a group of enzymes that hydrolyze monophosphate esters at an alkaline pH. pH optima of these enzymes are generally about 10. The natural substrates for alkaline phosphatase are not known. The enzyme has been identified in most body tissues and is generally localized in the membranes of cells. Alkaline phosphatase activity is highest in the liver, bone, intestine, kidney, and placenta, and as many as 11 different isoforms of alkaline phosphatase have been identified in serum. Since alkaline phos-

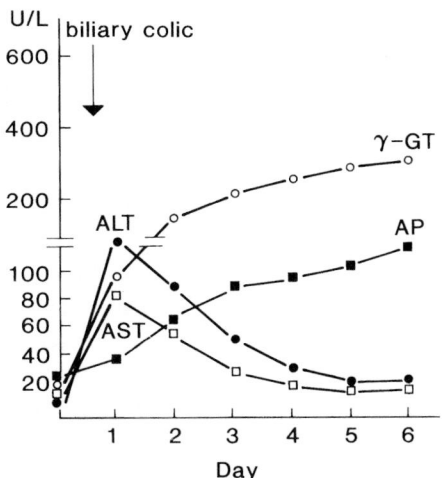

Fig. 27-5 Course of serum enzyme activities in obstructive jaundice. (From Schmidt E, Schmidt FW: *Brief guide to practical enzyme diagnosis,* Houston, 1977, Boehringer Mannheim Diagnostics.)

phatase normally contains significant amounts of sialic acid, most of these multiple enzyme forms are the result of different degrees of sialation. The enzyme produced by the placenta is known to have a protein composition different from the other enzyme compositions.

Measurement of serum alkaline phosphatase is useful in differentiating hepatobiliary disease from osteogenic bone disease. Alkaline phosphatase activity increases greatly (10 times) as a result of membrane-localized enzyme synthesis after extrahepatobiliary obstruction such as cholelithiasis or gallstones. Intrahepatic biliary obstruction is also accompanied by an increased serum alkaline phosphatase activity, but the degree of increase is smaller (two to three times).

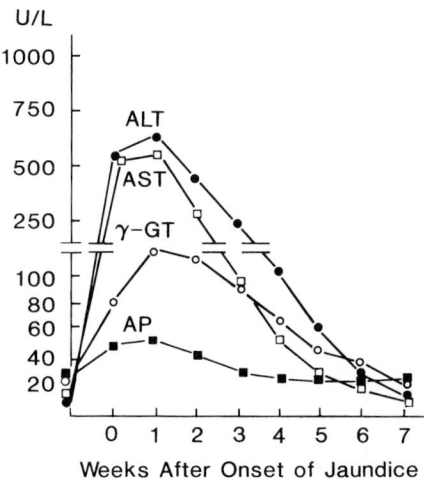

Fig. 27-6 Course of serum enzyme activities in acute viral hepatitis. (From Schmidt E, Schmidt FW: *Brief guide to practical enzyme diagnosis,* Houston, 1977, Boehringer Mannheim Diagnostics).

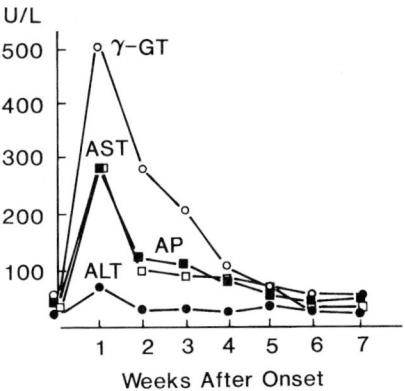

Fig. 27-7 Course of serum enzyme activities in acute alcoholic hepatitis. (From Schmidt E, Schmidt FW: *Brief guide to practical enzyme diagnosis,* Houston, 1977, Boehringer Mannheim Diagnostics.)

Liver disease resulting in parenchymal cell necrosis does not elevate serum alkaline phosphatase unless the liver disease is associated with damage to the canaliculi or biliary stasis.

Interpretation of serum alkaline phosphatase measurements is complicated by the fact that enzyme activity can increase in the absence of liver disease. The most common disorders causing elevation of alkaline phosphatase are bone diseases, such as Paget's disease, rickets, and osteomalacia. Serum alkaline phosphatase activity also rises during puberty because of rapid bone growth and during the third trimester of pregnancy because of alkaline phosphatase released from the placenta (see p. 521 for methods).

Gamma-glutamyltransferase (EC 2.3.2.2). GGT (or γ-GT) is a membrane-localized enzyme that plays a major role in glutathione metabolism and resorption of amino acids from the glomerular filtrate and from the intestinal lumen. Glutathione (γ-glutamylcysteinylglycine) in the presence of GGT and an amino acid or peptide transfers glutamate to the amino acid forming a peptide bond on the γ-carboxylic acid, thereby forming cysteinylglycine and the corresponding γ-glutamyl peptide.

Although the GGT activity is highest in renal tissue, serum GGT is generally elevated as a result of liver disease. Serum GGT is elevated earlier than other liver enzymes in diseases such as acute cholecystitis, acute pancreatitis, acute and subacute liver necrosis, and neoplasms of multiple sites at which liver metastases are present. Since GGT is a hepatic microsomal enzyme, chronic ingestion of alcohol or drugs such as barbiturates, tricyclic antidepressants, and anticonvulsants induces microsomal enzyme production. These drug-induced elevations precede any change in other liver enzymes, and if drug ingestion is stopped at this point, the liver changes are generally reversible. GGT permits differentiation of liver disease from other conditions in which serum alkaline phosphatase is elevated because serum GGT levels are usually normal in Paget's disease, rickets, and osteomalacia and in children and pregnant women without liver disease. Since the prostate contains significant GGT activity, serum activity is higher in healthy men than in women. Serum GGT is most useful in the diagnosis of cholestasis caused by chronic alcohol or drug ingestion, mechanical or viral cholestasis, liver metastases, bone disorders in which alkaline phosphatase is elevated but GGT is normal, and skeletal muscle disorders in which the transaminase AST is elevated but GGT is normal.

5′-Nucleotidase (EC 3.1.3.5). 5′-Nucleotidase (NTD) is a microsomal and cell membrane–localized enzyme that catalyzes the hydrolysis of nucleoside-5′-phosphate esters. The serum enzyme has an apparent pH optimum of 7.5:

$$\text{Nucleoside-5′-monophosphate} + H_2O \xrightarrow{\text{NTD}} \text{Nucleoside} + P_i$$

Like GTT, serum NTD is increased in hepatobiliary diseases such as gallstone obstruction of the bile duct, cholestasis, biliary cirrhosis, and obstructive disease caused by neoplastic growth. Serum NTD is not generally elevated in drug-induced liver damage.[7] Therefore it is useful to measure NTD in conjunction with GGT as one follows the course of chemotherapy for liver neoplasms. Since NTD is not elevated in bone disease, it, like GGT, is useful in differentiating hepatic causes of alkaline phosphatase increase from other causes, such as bone disease, pregnancy, and normal childhood growth.

Lactate dehydrogenase (EC 1.1.1.27). Lactate dehydrogenase is present in many tissues. LD catalyzes the interconversion of pyruvate and lactate:

$$NAD + H^+ + \text{Lactate} \xrightleftharpoons{\text{LD}} \text{Pyruvate} + NADH^+$$

LD activity is highest in the kidney and heart and lowest in the lung and serum. LD is localized in the cytoplasm of cells and thus is extruded into the serum when cells are damaged or necrotic (see p. 608 for methods).

When only a specific organ, such as the liver, is known to be involved, the measurement of total LD can be useful. Total LD is increased in viral or toxic hepatitis, extrahepatic biliary obstruction, acute necrosis of the liver, and cirrhosis of the liver. However, in conditions in which multiple organs are involved, the measurement of total LD is less useful than the measurement of LD isoenzymes. LD_5 and LD_4 account for the primary activity of liver LD, whereas LD_1 and LD_2 account for the predominant activities of heart and kidney LD. Since red blood cells also contain significant LD_1, analysis of hemolyzed serum specimens should be avoided. In these hepatic conditions, LD electrophoresis indicates that the increased total LD is caused by the release of LD_4 and LD_5 into the serum.

Aspartate aminotransferase (EC 2.6.1.1) and alanine aminotransferase (EC 2.6.1.2). The transaminases AST and ALT catalyze the conversion of aspartate and alanine to oxaloacetate and pyruvate respectively. (See pp. 518 and 523 in the methods section for discussion of the measurement of the transaminases.) The highest ALT levels are found in the liver, whereas AST is present in heart, skeletal muscle, and liver to nearly the same extent. Serum activity of both AST and ALT increases rapidly during the onset of viral jaundice and remains elevated for 1 to 2 weeks. In toxic hepatitis, ALT and AST are also elevated, but LD is elevated to an even greater extent as a result of hepatic cell necrosis. Patients with chronic active hepatitis also exhibit increased AST and ALT.

Acute liver necrosis is accompanied by significant increases in the activity of both ALT and AST. The increase in ALT activity is usually greater than the increase in AST activity. In cirrhotic liver disease, serum transaminase activities are generally not elevated above 300 U/L, regardless of the cause of the cirrhotic disease. The elevations of serum ALT and AST seen in Reye's syndrome are directly attributable to hepatic damage, and the increase in ALT is generally greater than the increase in AST. Neoplastic disease also elevates serum transaminase activity.

Measurement of ALT and AST serum levels is valuable in the diagnosis of liver disease. However, these laboratory tests are best used with other enzyme assays, such as LD and creatine kinase, and with other measures of liver and kidney function, such as blood urea, creatinine, ammonia, and bilirubin.[8] This is important when one establishes a diagnosis because ALT and AST are present in tissues other than the liver, and serum activity of these enzymes can reflect organic disease in tissues other than the liver. ALT and AST serum activities are elevated in myocardial infarction, renal infarction, progressive muscular dystrophy, and numerous diseases that only secondarily affect the liver, such as Gaucher's disease, Niemann-Pick disease, infectious mononucleosis, myelocytic leukemia, diabetic ketoacidosis, and hyperthyroidism.

Other hepatic analytes

Bilirubin (see Chapter 35). Serum bilirubin analysis is helpful in differentiating the cause of jaundice. *Prehepatic jaundice* results in a large increase in unconjugated bilirubin because of the increased release and metabolism of hemoglobin after hemolysis. No increase or only a slight increase in conjugated bilirubin is observed because the transport of bilirubin into the liver and the formation of the glucuronide conjugate become rate limiting. Additionally, because of the increased levels of conjugated bilirubin excreted by the liver, urinary urobilinogen and fecal urobilin concentrations are elevated, but urinary bilirubin (which is only the freely soluble, conjugated form) is absent. In contrast, *posthepatic obstructive jaundice* is characterized by large increases in serum-conjugated bilirubin. Delta bilirubin, bilirubin covalently bound to albumin, also increases in this disorder. The measurement of delta bilirubin as a diagnostic tool has not achieved widespread acceptance. The accumulation of bilirubin in the serum is the result of decreased biliary excretion after the conjugation of bilirubin in the liver rather than the result of an increased bilirubin load caused by hemolysis. Hepatic excretion of bilirubin metabolites is low, and urinary bilirubin can usually be demonstrated. *Hepatic jaundice* presents an intermediate pattern wherein both conjugated and unconjugated serum bilirubin are increased to the same degree and conjugated bilirubin is present in the urine. However, the fecal concentration of urobilin is generally decreased (see p. 523 for methods).

Cholesterol. Serum cholesterol comprises two forms, free cholesterol and esterified cholesterol. Since this esterification takes place in the liver, intrahepatic disease or biliary obstruction is characterized by an increase in the free cholesterol and occasionally a shift in the serum free fatty acid profile, though the total cholesterol usually remains unchanged. In chronic disease associated with parenchymal cell destruction, the total cholesterol may fall below the reference range.

Bile acids. Bile acid secretion and production is altered in disease.[2,8] In the healthy adult, serum contains 1 to 2 μg/mL of bile acids. In hepatobiliary disease, serum bile acid concentrations may rise as much as a thousandfold. Other diseases that can cause a significant rise in serum bile acid concentrations are hepatitis, cirrhosis, drug-induced liver disease, and hepatoma. Serum bile acid concentrations are normal in Gilbert's disease, hemochromatosis, and polycystic liver disease. Measurement of serum bile acids is useful in the diagnosis of minimal liver dysfunction when other biochemical parameters are still unchanged.

Triglycerides. Serum triglycerides should be measured in a fasting sample. Increases are relatively nonspecific[8]; liver dysfunction resulting from hepatitis, extrahepatic biliary obstruction, and cirrhosis is associated with an increase in serum triglycerides, but so are such disorders as acute pancreatitis, myocardial infarction, renal failure, gout, pernicious anemia, and diabetes mellitus. Free fatty acids exhibit a similar nonspecificity. They are decreased in chronic hepatitis, chronic renal failure, and cystic fibrosis. Serum free fatty acid concentrations are elevated in Reye's syndrome, hepatic encephalopathy, and chronic active hepatitis but also in myocardial infarction, acute renal failure, hyperthyroidism, and pheochromocytoma.

Serum proteins in evaluation of liver function. A healthy functioning liver is required for the synthesis of the serum proteins, except for the gamma globulins. The liver has the ability to increase protein output approximately twofold during diseases associated with protein loss. Therefore it is not surprising that total protein measurements are not altered until an extensive impairment of liver function has occurred.

Albumin (see p. 518, methods section) is decreased in chronic liver disease and is generally accompanied by an increase in the beta and gamma globulins as a result of production of IgG and IgM in chronic active hepatitis and of IgM and IgA in biliary or alcoholic cirrhosis respectively. It should be emphasized that these immunoglobulins are not produced by the liver but by the plasma cells of the reticu-loendothelial system. Immunoelectrophoresis may facilitate the identification of these subclasses of gamma globulin. However, a decrease in serum albumin is not specific for liver disease, since decreases are also seen in malabsorption, malnutrition, renal disease, alcoholism, and malignant diseases.

The alpha$_1$ fraction of the serum protein globulin is decreased in chronic liver disease, and when this fraction is absent or nearly so, it indicates that alpha$_1$-antitrypsin deficiency may be the cause of the liver disease. Serum alpha$_2$ globulin and beta globulin are increased in obstructive jaundice. The increase in alpha$_2$-globulin and beta globulin in obstructive jaundice is largely associated with interferences with normal lipoprotein metabolism. Thus one cannot phenotype a lipid disorder accurately in the presence of liver disease. The use of high-density lipoprotein cholesterol for assessment of the risk of coronary heart disease is obviated in patients with alcoholic liver disease, biliary obstruction, and acute liver necrosis.

Coagulation factors are produced by the liver and can decrease significantly in the presence of liver disease. Plasma fibrinogen is normally present in a concentration of 2 to 4 g/L. A decrease in plasma fibrinogen is usually an indication of severe liver disease and is associated with decreased concentrations of other clotting factors, most notably prothrombin. Since prothrombin synthesis occurs in the liver and requires the fat-soluble vitamin K, prothrombin time may be increased in biliary obstructive disease, liver cirrhosis or necrosis, hepatic failure, Reye's syndrome, liver abscess, vitamin K deficiency, and hepatitis. The response of the prothrombin time to exogenous vitamin K is useful in differentiating intrahepatic disease associated with a decrease in clotting factor from extrahepatic obstructive disease with decreased absorption of vitamin K.

Urea and ammonia in evaluation of liver function. Blood ammonia concentration is higher in infants than in adults because the development of the hepatic circulation is completed after birth. Hyperammonemia results infrequently from congenital defects of the urea cycle. The most common of these inborn errors of metabolism is ornithine transcarbamylase deficiency. A much more frequent cause of hyperammonemia in infants is hyperalimentation.[9] Reye's syndrome is frequently diagnosed by an elevated blood ammonia in the absence of any other demonstrable cause.

Adult patients exhibit elevated blood ammonia in the terminal stages of liver cirrhosis, hepatic failure, and acute and subacute liver necrosis. The onset of hepatic encephalopathy is presaged by an elevated blood ammonia. The measurement of cerebrospinal fluid (CSF) glutamine has been demonstrated to correlate well with the development of hepatic encephalopathy. Measurement of CSF glutamine can also be used to differentiate hepatic from septic encephalopathy.[11] Nonetheless, the measurement of CSF glutamine is not common. Urinary ammonia excretion is increased in acidosis and decreased in alkalosis, since ammonia salt formation is a significant mechanism for excretion of excess hydrogen ions. Damage to the renal distal tubules, as occurs in renal failure, glomerulonephritis, hypercorticoidism, and Addison's disease, results in decreased ammonia excretion but no changes in blood ammonia levels.

Since urea is synthesized in the liver, liver disease without renal impairment results in a low serum urea nitrogen, though the urea-to-creatinine ratio may remain normal.[10] An elevated serum urea nitrogen does not necessarily imply renal damage, since dehydration may result in a urea nitrogen as high as 600 mg/L, and infants receiving high-protein formula may exhibit a urea nitrogen level of 250 to 300 mg/L. Naturally, renal diseases such as acute glomerulonephritis, chronic nephritis, polycystic kidney, and renal necrosis result in an elevated urea nitrogen.

METHODS OF ANALYSIS

Alanine aminotransferase

STEVEN C. KAZMIERCZAK

Principles of analysis and current usage Alanine aminotransferase catalyzes the transfer of an amino group between the amino acids L-alanine and L-glutamate. The keto acids formed in this process are α-ketoglutarate and pyruvate as follows:

$$\text{L-Alanine} + \alpha\text{-Ketoglutarate} \overset{\text{ALT}}{\rightleftharpoons} \text{Pyruvate} + \text{L-Glutamate}$$

Early methods for ALT analysis utilized the ability of pyruvate formed in the above reaction to react with dinitrophenylhydrazine (DNPH) to produce the corresponding hydrazone (Table 27-5, method 1).[15] Alkalinization of the reaction mixture results in the formation of a blue color, which can be measured at 505 nm. α-Ketoglutarate also can react with DNPH to form the corresponding hydrazone. However, the amount of color produced is negligible and is usually ignored.[16] One drawback to this procedure is that pyruvate, which is a normal component of serum, also will react to produce hydrazones resulting in high initial absorbance readings. Although once widely used in clinical laboratories, this method is now considered obsolete.

The most common methods in use today for measurement of ALT are continuous monitoring methods. These methods couple the production of pyruvate in the reaction catalyzed by ALT to a second reaction whereby pyruvate is reduced by NADH in a reaction catalyzed by lactate dehydrogenase (LD) (Table 27-5, method 2).[17] The disappearance of

NADH because of its oxidation to NAD is monitored at 340 nm. With continuous monitoring methods, α-ketoglutarate L-alanine, NADH, and the indicator enzyme LD are present in excess quantity so that the rate-limiting step is the reaction catalyzed by ALT.

ALT requires a coenzyme cofactor for full catalytic activity. The cofactor pyridoxal-5'-phosphate (P-5'-P) is bound to the apoenzyme where it functions to accept the amino group from the alanine substrate. The P-5'-P (vitamin B_6) accepts the amino group from alanine to form enzyme-bound pyridoxamine-5'-phosphate and pyruvate. The pyridoxamine-5'-phosphate enzyme complex then transfers its amino group to α-ketoglutarate to form L-glutamate and regenerate P-5'-P as shown below:

1. L-Alanine + Pyridoxal-5'-phosphate–enzyme complex
   $\rightarrow$ Pyridoxamine-5-phosphate–
   enzyme complex + Pyruvate

2. α-Ketoglutarate + Pyridoxamine-5'-phosphate-enzyme complex $\rightarrow$ Pyridoxal-5'-phosphate–enzyme complex
   + L-Glutamate

Because the coenzyme may not be present in sufficient quantities in sera to produce maximal enzyme activity, addition of the P-5'-P coenzyme to reagent systems designed to measure ALT activity is sometimes performed.

Specimen Although serum or plasma may be used for measurement of ALT activity, serum is the preferred specimen. Plasma that has been anticoagulated with oxalate, heparin, or citrate may result in sample turbidity. Since erythrocytes contain three to five times more ALT than that present in normal blood, hemolyzed samples are unacceptable for analysis. The enzyme is stable for up to 24 hours at 20° to 25° C and up to 7 days if refrigerated at 2° to 8° C.[18]

Reference interval ALT, measured in adults at 37° C, using reagents employing P-5'-P typically yields activities of 10 to 50 U/L. Both newborns and infants have ALT activities in sera that are two to three times that found in adult sera. The greater activity in the serum of newborns and infants may be attributable to seepage of the enzyme across the more permeable hepatocyte membrane of newborns and infants.

Albumin

KEE CHEUNG
PETER E. HICKMAN

Principles of analysis and current usage Measurement of albumin concentrations in serum and other body fluids is a commonly performed laboratory test, useful for the evalua-

---

Table 27-5 Methods of alanine aminotransferase (ALT) analysis

Method	Type of analysis	Principle	Usage
1. Colorimetric	Quantitative	End-point absorbance measurement at 505 nm: Ala + α-KG $\rightarrow$ Gl + Pyr Pyr + DNPH $\rightarrow$ Pyr-DNP-hydrazone	Serum, historical
2. Enzymatic (ultraviolet monitoring)	Quantitative	UV monitoring of NADH disappearance at 340 nm: Ala + α-KG $\rightarrow$ Gl + Pyr Pyr + NADH + H$^+$ $\overset{\text{LD}}{\rightarrow}$ Lac + NAD$^+$	Serum, most frequently employed procedure. Some use P-5'-P cofactor

Ala, Alanine; *DNPH*, dinitrophenylhydrazine; *Gl*, glutamate; α-*KG*, α-ketoglutarate; *Pyr*, pyruvate; *P-5'-P*, pyridoxal-5'-phosphate.

tion of nutritional status, as an indicator of hepatic function, and in urine for monitoring renal impairment. Albumin possesses some unique characteristics when compared to other serum proteins and such characteristics have been used as a basis for its measurement. Two of these unique characteristics include the low content of the amino acid tryptophan and the finding that albumin exists as an anion at pH 7.4.[19]

One method of analysis for albumin utilizes the differences between the tryptophan content of this protein (0.2%) and the higher tryptophan content (2% to 3%) found in the globulin fractions.[20] One derives the albumin concentrations by subtracting the concentration of globulin present in the sample from the total protein concentration. An example of an albumin method based on the determination of tryptophan content is the one that employs glyoxylic acid (Table 27-6, method 1). In the presence of Ca^{++} in an acid medium, glyoxylic acid reacts with the tryptophan residues to produce a purple color.[21] One can compensate for the inter-

Table 27-6   Methods of albumin analysis

Method	Type of analysis	Principle	Usage	Comment
1. **Tryptophan content**	Quantitative	Glyoxylic acid and tryptophan in globulin → *purple chromogen* (A$_{max}$, 540 nm) Total protein = Globulin = Albumin	Serum, manual, and automated	Correlates well with electrophoresis but requires total protein measurement
2. **Dye binding**				
a. BCG (bromocresol green)	Quantitative	Dye-albumin complex causes shift of dye's spectra (A$_{max}$, 628 nm)	Serum, manual, or automated (most often used method)	Nonspecific for albumin if absorbance reading taken after 30 seconds
b. BCP (bromocresol purple)	Quantitative	Same as above (A$_{max}$, 603 nm)	Serum, manual or automated	Specific for albumin; low sensitivity; albumins from animal sources do not bind equivalently to human albumin
c. BPB (bromphenol blue)	Semiquantitative	Bromphenol blue in test strip changes color from yellow to blue in presence of albumin	Urine	Nonspecific; most sensitive with albumin; most commonly used test for urine protein
3. **Electrophoresis**	Quantitative	Albumin is separated from other proteins in electrical field	Serum, manual, and automated	Very labor intensive, but if albumin is eluted for measurement, very accurate
4. **Immunochemical**	Quantitative	Percent staining of albumin fraction multiplied by total protein value Protein migrates in electrical field through medium containing a specific antibody	Serum; manual	Candidate reference method; somewhat labor intensive
a. Nephelometry	Quantitative	Antigen-antibody complexes scatter light more than free antigen	Serum, CSF, urine automated	Reagent cost high
b. Turbidimetry	Quantitative	Antigen-antibody complexes decrease light transmission through sample	Serum, CSF, urine; manual or automated	Reagent cost high
c. Radioimmunoassay	Quantitative	Radiolabeled albumin competes with test albumin for limited amount of antibody	Serum, CSF, urine	Primarily used for urine
d. Enzyme immunoassay	Quantitative	Sandwich assay uses antibody bound to surface and peroxidase-labeled antibody	Serum, CSF, urine	New
e. Radial immunodiffusion	Quantitative	Protein diffuses through medium containing specific antibody	Serum, CSF, urine; manual	Reference method, very long incubation time
f. Electroimmunodiffusion				

A$_{max}$, Maximum absorbance; *CSF,* cerebrospinal fluid.

ference from albumin by standardizing the assay with serum. Although this method has been automated for use, methods for albumin based on determination of tryptophan content are rarely used because of the greater ease and specificity of dye-binding methods for albumin.

The most common methods in use for the determination of albumin concentrations in serum are dye-binding procedures (Table 27-6, method 2). These are based upon the ability of albumin to bind a wide variety of organic ions, including dye molecules. The dyes most commonly used for albumin determinations are bromocresol green ($3',3'',5',5''$-tetrabromo-*m*-cresolsulfonphthalein, BCG) or bromocresol purple ($5',5''$-dibromo-*o*-cresolsulfonphthalein, BCP). When these dyes become bound to albumin, they undergo a shift in their absorption maxima. This shift in the absorption maximum allows for the measurement of albumin-bound dye to be made in the presence of excess unbound dye present in the reaction mixture. Dye-binding methods have also been adopted for use with the dry film technology. Bromocresol green dye is incorporated into a reagent layer along with buffer and surfactants. Serum or plasma is applied onto the top layer of the slide where it is evenly distributed before diffusing into the reagent layer where it reacts with the BCG dye. The amount of albumin-bound dye is proportional to the concentration of albumin in the sample and is measured by reflectance spectrophotometry.

Methods that use BCG are fairly specific for albumin, with no interference from bilirubin and slight to moderate lipemia. Hemoglobin interferes with the binding of BCG to albumin and will decrease the albumin value by 1 g/L for each 100 g/L of hemoglobin present. Specificity of the BCG procedure is also improved by measurement of the absorbance of the BCG-albumin complex shortly after mixing of the specimen and BCG reagent.[22] Absorbance readings taken shortly after mixing eliminate the interference from other proteins such as ceruloplasmin and orosomucoid, which also bind BCG—the binding of which does not occur to any appreciable extent for up to 5 minutes after the start of the assay.

Although both BCG and BCP are commonly used in dye-binding methods, BCG does offer some advantages as compared to BCP. The molar absorptivity of the BCP-albumin complex is approximately half of that observed for the BCG-albumin complex. As a result, the sensitivity and precision of BCP methods are much less than that of methods using BCG. Another disadvantage of methods that employ BCP is the finding that albumin concentrations are underestimated in patients with renal insufficiency[23] or obstructive jaundice.[24] Finally, BCP methods are unsuitable for use with nonhuman specimens because BCP binds with much less affinity with nonhuman albumin. The most common method of monitoring for the presence of albumin in urine uses a dye displacement method (method 2C). This is the basis for urine dipsticks.

Although dye-binding methods are frequently used for determining albumin concentrations in serum or plasma, this technique finds little application in the measurement of albumin in other body fluids such as urine and cerebrospinal fluid because of the low concentrations of albumin normally seen in these specimens and the high concentrations of in-

terfering substances that may be present. Measurement of albumin concentrations in fluids other than serum or plasma is usually accomplished by alternative methods such as electrophoresis or immunochemical methods.

Separation of albumin from major proteins by electrophoretic techniques (Table 27-6, method 3) is one method that is used for its determination in both serum and other body fluids. After the separation of the major classes of proteins by electrophoresis, the different protein fractions are stained and the percentage of each fraction is determined by use of a densitometer (see Chapter 10 for additional information on protein electrophoresis). One calculates the concentration of albumin by multiplying the concentration of total protein present in the sample by the percentage of albumin present as determined by the densitometer. The various stains that may be used to dye the protein fractions have different affinities with which they interact with the protein fractions. Since albumin possesses the greatest affinity for these dyes, electrophoretic procedures will show an overestimation of the concentration of albumin because of its greater affinity for stains when compared to the other protein fractions.

A more common technique for quantitation of albumin in fluids such as cerebrospinal fluid and urine is an immunological method. Immunologic techniques used for quantitation of albumin include both immunonephelometric and immunoturbidimetric techniques, radioimmunoassay (RIA), enzyme-linked immunosorbent assays (ELISA), radial immunodiffusion (RID), and electroimmunodiffusion (EID) methods.

Immunonephelometric[25] and immunoturbidimetric[26] techniques (Table 27-6, methods 4a and 4b) are the most common immunologic methods used for quantitation of albumin in CSF and urine. These methods are based on the ability of an albumin–antialbumin antibody complex to either block (turbidimetry) or scatter (nephelometry) a beam of light directed on the sample. The amount of light that is blocked or scattered is related to the albumin concentration in the sample by comparison to standard solutions with known albumin concentrations.

Sensitive and specific RIA procedures (Table 27-6, method 4c) for determination of albumin in urine as an aid for monitoring the progress of diabetic nephropathy have been developed.[27] ELISA methods (Table 27-6, method 4d) are based upon the formation of a "sandwich" comprising an antibody coated onto a solid surface, albumin, and a second antibody conjugated to an enzyme.[28,29] The final addition of substrate to the system results in the development of a colored product that is proportional to the concentration of albumin in the sample.

Albumin quantitation by use of RID and EID is infrequently performed in clinical laboratories because of the technical nature of the procedures. In RID, albumin passively diffuses through an antibody-containing agar gel.[30] The concentration of albumin in the sample is determined by measurement of the distance that the albumin must diffuse before reaching equilibrium. Equilibrium in this system is defined as that area in the gel where the albumin-antibody complexes precipitate because of the presence of excess antibody. The albumin-antibody complex that precipitates is stained with a suitable dye. The diameter of the stained ring of albumin-antibody complexes is proportional to the albumin concentration in the sample.

Specimen Serum is the specimen of choice for albumin determinations. Use of heparinized plasma can lead to an overestimation of albumin concentrations with some dye-binding methods that use BCG.[31] Heparin can also interfere in dye-binding methods that use BCP; however this interference can be eliminated by the addition of hexadimethrine bromide to the reagent.[32]

Pronounced lipemia has also been found to interfere in assays that employ BCG as reagent; a fasting sample may be desirable. Hemoconcentration caused by venostasis can result in an increase in apparent concentration of albumin as well as other plasma proteins.

Proper storage of urine specimens collected for measurement of albumin is controversial. Recent studies suggest that storage of urine specimens at $-70°$ C should be adequate to prevent loss of albumin for at least 160 days.[33]

Albumin concentrations in serum are dependent on both sex and age as shown below.[34] Children and neonates reportedly have lower values than those seen in adults.[35] In addition, preterm infants have been reported to have lower values than full-term infants have.[36]

Posture will affect albumin concentrations; values are lower by approximately 5 g/L in recumbent patients when compared to the values obtained from ambulant patients.[37]

Albumin concentrations of urine in healthy individuals are generally less than 15 to 30 mg/L. Urine albumin values that consistently exceed these values should be interpreted as abnormal.[38]

Reference interval

AGE	ALBUMIN (g/L)
Infants	29-55
Children	38-55
21-44 years	33-61 (males)
20-44 years	28-57 (females)
45-54 years	29-61 (males)
45-54 years	25-54 (females)
55-93 years	32-55 (males)
55-81 years	32-53 (females)

Alkaline phosphatase

JULIE RAYMOND-HABECKER
JOHN A. LOTT

Principles of analysis Phosphatases are a family of enzymes that transfer a phosphate moiety from a donor compound to an acceptor compound. The natural in vivo substrate for ALP is unknown, however, many nonphysiological phosphate esters can serve as substrates. Phosphatases that exhibit optimal activity at an alkaline pH are collectively called "alkaline phosphatase" (ALP). Optimal activity of these enzymes require Mg^{++} and Zn^{++} ions and a pH of approximately 10.0. Ca^{++} and inorganic phosphate inhibit ALP activity.

Human ALP consists of at least five tissue-specific isoenzymes, with additional enzyme forms being found in association with certain benign and malignant disorders. The individual enzyme types exhibit different catalytic

and physical properties. Reaction rates are dependent on variables such as the type of substrate and buffer used, and the incubation temperature. Since ALP is denatured slowly at 37° C, a reaction temperature of 25° to 30° C is often recommended for clinical assays. Methods for measurement of ALP activity usually represent a compromise, with minimal bias toward any one individual ALP isoenzyme.

The choice of buffer used in methods of ALP measurement is critical. Buffers that have been proposed include diethanolamine (DEA) and 2-amino-2-methyl-propanol (AMP). Both DEA and AMP have certain drawbacks that must be considered. DEA preparations have been found to contain significant amounts of monoethanolamine, a potent inhibitor of ALP, whereas AMP may contain inhibitor compounds that inactivate ALP by binding Zn^{++} ions. Recently, the buffer N-methyl-D-glucamine has been proposed for use in ALP assays because of its being free of inhibiting compounds.[39]

Historical methods for total serum ALP measured the release of inorganic phosphate from substrates such as β-glycerophosphate (Table 27-7, method 1) and phenyl phosphate (Table 27-7, methods 2 and 3). These methods were relatively insensitive and laborious.

Modern methods for ALP analysis are based upon the principles established by Bessey and associates (Table 27-7, method 4). This method utilizes colorless pNPP (*para*-nitrophenyl phosphate) as substrate, which is hydrolyzed by ALP to form the yellow salt, pNP (*para*-nitrophenol). This assay can be performed as a kinetic assay, or it can employ background correction by the addition of acid to the reaction mixture after its completion. The acid converts the yellow sodium salt into colorless free nitrophenol, and a second absorbance measurement is made.

A rapid continuous spectrophotometric assay that offers the convenience of measurement at 340 nm has also been described (Table 27-7, method 5). This method utilizes α-naphthyl phosphate as substrate, yielding α-naphthol as the hydrolysis product.

A highly sensitive fluorometric assay for ALP using 4-methylumbelliferyl phosphate as substrate has also been proposed (Table 27-7, method 6). The substrate is hydrolyzed by ALP to yield 4-methylumbelliferone, a highly fluorescent compound.

Various reference methods for measurement of ALP activity have been proposed. These methods represent the culmination of experiments designed to carefully select optimum conditions of pH, temperature, buffer type, and reagent concentrations. The pNPP method of Bowers and McComb (Table 27-7, method 7), which uses AMP as buffer, is widely used today because of its simplicity and sensitivity. The controversy over the optimal conditions for measurement of ALP activity has yet to be settled, and a universally accepted reference method has yet to be established.

Specimen It is preferable that blood samples be drawn after a fast of 8 hours. Serum and heparinized plasma yield comparable results. Complexing anticoagulants, such as citrate, oxalate, and EDTA, which bind Mg^{++} and Zn^{++}, must be avoided during collection of blood for ALP analysis. Slight hemolysis is acceptable, but grossly hemolyzed samples

Table 27-7   Methods of alkaline phosphatase (ALP) analysis

Type of analysis	Method source	Principle	Usage	Comments
1. Two-point spectrophotometric	Shinowara et al.	Substrate: β-glycerophosphate Measure rate of release of inorganic phosphate; 1 hour incubation	All body fluids; manual	Requires long incubation time; high phosphate background in samples Considered obsolete
2. End-point spectrophotometric	King and Armstrong	Substrate: phenyl phosphate Measure rate of release of phenol with Folin-Ciocalteu reagent; 30 min incubation	All body fluids; manual	Samples require deproteinization Considered obsolete
3. End-point spectrophotometric	King and King	Substrate: phenyl phosphate Measure rate of release of phenol with 4-aminoantipyrine as chromogenic reagent; 15 min incubation	All body fluids; manual/automated	Faster rate than King and Armstrong method Requires no deproteinization
4. End-point or kinetic spectrophotometric	Bessey et al.	Substrate: p-nitrophenyl phosphate (pNPP) Measure rate of formation of yellow p-nitrophenoxide ion	All body fluids; manual/automated	Rapid; linear change in absorbance with time
5. End-point or kinetic spectrophotometric	Moss	Substrate: α-naphthol monophosphate Measure rate of formation of α-naphthol at 340 nm	All body fluids; manual/automated	Rapid; convenience of measuring at 340 nm
6. Fluorescent	Cornish et al.	Substrate: 4-methylumbelliferyl phosphate	All body fluids; automated	Highly sensitive
7. Kinetic or end-point spectrophotometric	Bowers and McComb	Substrate: pNPP Measure rate of release of p-nitrophenoxide in transphosphorylating buffer	All body fluids; manual or automated	Proposed reference method; more sensitive than Bessey et al method

*Sources:
Bessey O, Lowry OH, Brock MJ: *J Biol Chem* 164:321-329, 1946.
Bowers GN Jr, McComb RB: *Clin Chem* 21:1988-1995, 1975, and Bowers GN Jr, McComb RB: Alkaline phosphatase: total activity in human serum. In Faulkner WH, Meites S, editors: *Selected methods for the small clinical chemistry laboratory,* Washington, D.C., 1982, American Association for Clinical Chemistry.
Cornish CJ, Neale FC, Posen S: *Am J Clin Pathol* 53:68-76, 1970.
Kind PRN, King EJ: *J Clin Pathol* 7:322-326, 1954.
King EJ, Armstrong AR: *Can Med Assoc J* 31:376-381, 1934.
Moss DW: *Enzymologia* 31:193-202, 1966.
Shinowara G, Jones LM, Reinhart HL: *J Biol Chem* 142:921-933, 1942.

should not be used. Bilirubin does not interfere with kinetic pNPP methods.

Blood storage conditions can adversely affect ALP activity. Slight increases in ALP activity (1% to 2%) have been observed in samples kept at room temperature up to 4 hours after collection.[40] Significant increases may be seen after warming of previously refrigerated or frozen sera. A similar effect can be seen after reconstitution of lyophilized serum. This phenomenon has been attributed to the dissociation of complexes formed between ALP and lipoproteins at low temperatures or during lyophilization, leading to an apparent increase in enzyme activity.

Reference interval   The following reference ranges were developed using a kinetic pNPP method:

FEMALES (age in years)	ALP (up to U/L)	MALES (age in years)	ALP (up to U/L)
Newborns	250	Newborns	250
1 to 12	350	1 to 12	350
10 to 14	280	10 to 14	275
15 to 19	150	15 to 19	155
20 to 24	85	20 to 24	90
25 to 34	85	25 to 34	95
35 to 44	95	35 to 44	105
45 to 54	100	45 to 54	120
55 to 64	110	55 to 64	135
65 to 74	145	65 to 74	140
75+	165	75+	190

Table 27-8   Methods of aspartate aminotransferase (AST) analysis

Method	Type of analysis	Principle	Usage
1. Dinitrophenylhydrazone	Quantitative	L-Aspartate + α-Ketoglutarate $\xrightarrow{AST}$ L-Glutamate + Oxaloacetate Oxaloacetate + Dinitrophenylhydrazine → Oa-dinitrophenylhydrazone (absorbance at 505 nm)	Historical interest only
2. Enzymatic (ultraviolet monitoring)	Quantitative	L-Aspartate + α-Ketoglutarate $\xrightarrow{AST}$ L-Glutamate + Oxaloacetate Oxaloacetate + NADH $\xrightarrow{MD}$ Malate + NAD	Most frequently performed method
3. Enzymatic leuco dye (visible)	Quantitative	Aspartate + α-Ketoglutarate $\xrightarrow{AST}$ Oxaloacetate + Glutamate Oxaloacetate $\xrightarrow{Oxaloacetate\ decarboxylase}$ Pyruvate + CO_2 Pyruvate + Phosphate + O_2 $\xrightarrow{Pyruvate\ oxidase}$ Hydrogen peroxide + Acetyl phosphate Hydrogen peroxide + Leuco dye $\xrightarrow{Peroxidase}$ *Colored dye*	Thin-film procedure Infrequently used

MD, Malate dehydrogenase; *Oa*, Oxaloacetate.

Nondisease factors that can result in elevations of serum ALP levels include excercise, periods of rapid bone growth in prepubertal children, and pregnancy.

Aspartate aminotransferase
STEVEN C. KAZMIERCZAK

Principles of analysis   Aspartate aminotransferase catalyzes the interconversion of the amino acids L-aspartate and L-glutamate by the transfer of amino groups. The general reaction scheme catalyzed by AST is shown in reaction 1:

L-Aspartate + α-Ketoglutarate $\overset{AST}{\longleftrightarrow}$ Oxaloacetate
    + L-Glutamate   *Reaction 1*

Oxaloacetate + NADH $\overset{MD}{\longleftrightarrow}$ Malate + NAD + H^+
    Reaction 2

Although the equilibrium of the AST reaction at physiological pH favors the formation of aspartate, in vivo the reaction proceeds to the right to produce glutamate as a source of nitrogen for the urea cycle.

Early methods for AST analysis employed the coupling of oxalacetate with 2,4-dinitrophenylhydrazine (DNPH) to produce a blue colored hydrazone (Table 27-8, method 1).[42] The reaction is stopped by the addition of DNPH, which reacts with oxaloacetate to form an oxaloacetate-dinitrophenylhydrazone complex. Alkalinization of the reagent mixture converts the complex to a blue color, which is measured at 505 nm. Although this method was once widely employed, it has been replaced by enzymatic methods for AST and is of historical interest only.

Enzymatic determination of AST also makes use of oxaloacetate formation as a means for quantitating enzyme activity (Table 27-8, method 2).[43] In this procedure, the oxalate produced by the action of AST in reaction 1 is reduced to malate by the enzyme malate dehydrogenase (MD) in an indicator reaction (reaction 2). In the process, the oxidation of NADH to NAD^+ is monitored at 340 nm. Most laboratories today use the Karmen method for AST determinations. Its simplicity, specificity, ease of automation, and rapid analysis time make it the preferred method.

The inclusion of pyridoxal phosphate (P-5'-P) as a cofactor for AST is available by many manufacturers of AST reagent. The need to add this cofactor to AST reagent is still unsettled. Normal serum usually contains adequate amounts of P-5'-P (vitamin B_6), and so inclusion of the cofactor in the AST reagent is not usually essential. However, individuals who are vitamin B_6 deficient, such as chronic ethanol abusers, may show AST concentrations that are abnormally low. Addition of P-5'-P may produce increases in the measured AST activity of these individuals up to 50%.[44]

A colorimetric method for AST is also available. This method, employed in a dry film assay available for AST measurement (Table 27-8, method 3), uses two coupling reactions and a final indicator reaction. In this procedure, oxaloacetate formed in the deamination of L-aspartate is converted to pyruvate and carbon dioxide by oxaloacetate decarboxylase. The pyruvate is next oxidized by pyruvate oxidase to acetyl phosphate and hydrogen peroxide. The final indicator reaction step involves the oxidation of a leuco dye by peroxidase to produce a colored dye. Samples that contain increased concentrations of pyruvate will result in substrate depletion and must be diluted. The thin-film assays are also interfered with by the presence of increased protein concentrations, such as those found in patients with multiple myeloma.[45]

Specimen   Serum or plasma anticoagulated with heparin, oxalate, EDTA, or citrate are acceptable specimens[46] for use with enzymatic procedures utilizing MD. For the colorimetric thin-film procedure, only serum or heparinized plasma are acceptable specimens. Anticoagulants that use the ammonium salt (that is, ammonium heparin) should be avoided. Also, since red blood cells contain approximately 15 times as much AST activity as seen in normal sera, samples that are usually hemolyzed are unsuitable for analysis.

Reference intervals   Normal reference intervals for AST in serum and plasma are 5 to 34 U/L for adults when the assay is performed at 37° C. Enzyme activities in newborns and infants are approximately twice those found in adults. By 6 months of age, enzyme activities in this group approach those found in adults.[47]

Total bilirubin
STEVEN C. KAZMIERCZAK

Principles of analysis and current usage   As described above, bilirubin is present in three forms: unconjugated, conjugated, and covalently bound to albumin. These three forms have different solubilities in water and therefore different abilities to undergo a chemical reaction. Unconjugated bilirubin has extremely limited solubility in water, whereas the two other fractions are much more soluble. The solubility properties of the bilirubin fractions have affected both how we measure bilirubin and how we commonly describe the fractions.

Historically it was known that serum bilirubin reacted in a slow and a fast reaction and that the slow reaction could be greatly speeded up if an "accelerator" as added to the reaction mixture. The bilirubin fraction that reacted directly and rapidly in the absence of an accelerator was known as "direct" bilirubin, whereas the fraction that required the "accelerator" for rapid reaction was known as "indirect" bilirubin. Accelerators act by solubilizing the unconjugated bilirubin and increasing its availability for reaction.

We now know that the "direct" bilirubin is the readily soluble conjugated bilirubin and delta-bilirubin fractions and the "indirect" fraction is the unconjugated bilirubin. Since all bilirubin fractions react in the presence of an accelerator, this bilirubin is called *total bilirubin*. By measuring the total and direct-reaction bilirubin, one can calculate the amount of unconjugated (or indirect) bilirubin by subtraction.

$$\text{Total bilirubin} - \text{Conjugated bilirubin}$$
$$= \text{Unconjugated bilirubin}$$

Almost all methods commonly used to measure the bilirubin fractions are based on the reaction of bilirubin with some diazonium salt, as described in Fig. 27-8 for diazonium chloride. Historically the methods employed for this reaction differed in the pH of the reaction. The Jendrassik-Grof method (Table 27-9, method 2) was run at a near-neutral pH, but the reaction was measured after alkalinizing the reaction to pH 13 to produce a more intense chromophore, which absorbed at 600 nm. The Malloy-Evelyn procedure (Table 27-9, method 1) was carried out at a pH of approximately 1, and the red-purple color of the reaction product was measured at 560 nm. Variation of these two procedures depended on the diazonium salt used in the reaction and in the accelerator used in the total bilirubin reaction. Accelerators that have been used include sodium benzoate–caffeine, methanol, dimethyl sulfoxide, urea, and detergents.

Measurement of conjugated bilirubin in urine also employs the diazonium reaction. For example, the dipsticks sold by Miles Ames (Ames Co., Elkart, Ind.) are impregnated with a 2,4-dichloroanilinediazonium salt, whereas the Ames Ictotest uses *p*-nitrobenzenediazonium salt in the reaction. The Ictotest (sensitivity approximately 10 mg/L) is two to four times more sensitive than the dipstick method, though both tests are subject to false-positive results because of endogenous color.

Methods for measurement of total bilirubin by direct spectrophotometry are also available (Table 27-9, method 3). Bilirubinometers relate the absorbance of serum near 454 nm directly to bilirubin concentration. Reflectance meters can be used directly to measure levels of bilirubin in whole blood transcutaneously. In both cases, interference from oxyhemoglobin is minimized when one also takes measurements at a second wavelength (540 nm). Carotenoids strongly interfere in all direct methods, limiting their use to neonates who have not received foods containing these compounds. Bilirubin results obtained by the transcutaneous devices are, however, less accurate and consistent when compared to chemical methods. Differences in skin pigmentation between individuals make standardization of these instruments difficult.

The development of a high-performance liquid chromatography (HPLC) procedure (Table 27-9, method 4) that can quantitate the various fractions of bilirubin has led to a better understanding of the composition of bilirubin in normal blood. Measurement of bilirubin by HPLC shows that plasma from healthy individuals contains very little (that is, less than 5%) conjugated bilirubin. These findings indicate that most diazo methods for measurement of conjugated bilirubin greatly overestimate the actual concentration of this fraction. Measurement of bilirubin using chemical assays that give a low proportion (15% or less) of direct-reacting bilirubin in the serum of healthy individuals probably gives the most accurate results. The amount of direct-reacting bilirubin in a particular diazo method is dependent on the time and temperature of the reaction.

Determinations of total bilirubin using the enzyme bilirubin oxidase have also been performed (Table 27-9, method 5). Good agreement has been demonstrated between total and direct bilirubin measured by the enzyme-based method and the results of diazo-based methods. One major advantage of this assay is the high specificity of the enzyme for bilirubin. Techniques have also been developed for measuring both total and conjugated bilirubin using bilirubin oxidase.[48,49]

The measurement of bilirubin using dry-film technology is employed in the Johnson and Johnson Ektachem analyzers (Table 27-9, method 6). Bilirubin in the serum diffuses through the film into a layer that contains a hydrophobic cationic polymer that complexes with bilirubin, resulting in a shift in the bilirubin spectrum from 440 to 460 nm. The reaction is monitored by reflectance spectrophotometry at 455 nm. In one set of reaction conditions protein-complexed bilirubin, also called *delta bilirubin*, is unable to react in the Johnson and Johnson total bilirubin reaction. The Johnson and Johnson Ektachem method provides for measurement of direct bilirubin that is the sum of conjugated and delta bilirubin. The delta and direct bilirubin can be calculated by subtraction of the results.

Specimen Serum or plasma can be used in the diazo methods for measurement of total bilirubin. Serum is preferred for the Malloy-Evelyn procedure because the addition of alcohol can precipitate proteins from plasma. Hemolysis can falsely depress bilirubin results in most assays because of an increase in absorbance of the blank. Lipemic specimens may show falsely increased bilirubin concentrations because of the effects of turbidity. Bilirubin is readily destroyed by light and heat. Care should be taken to perform bilirubin analyses with no exposure to these factors.

Determinations of conjugated bilirubin are usually performed in serum because total bilirubin can be determined concomitantly. Both spinal fluid and urine are also acceptable sample types for bilirubin determinations.

Reference interval Total bilirubin levels in healthy adults are up to 15 mg/L (25.7 μmol/L), with a median of 7.0 mg/L (12 μmol/L). In both sexes the median concentration rises after puberty, falls during the third decade, and thereafter remains stable.

Conjugated bilirubin levels up to 2 mg/L are found in infants by 1 month of age, and conjugated bilirubin remains at this level thereafter.

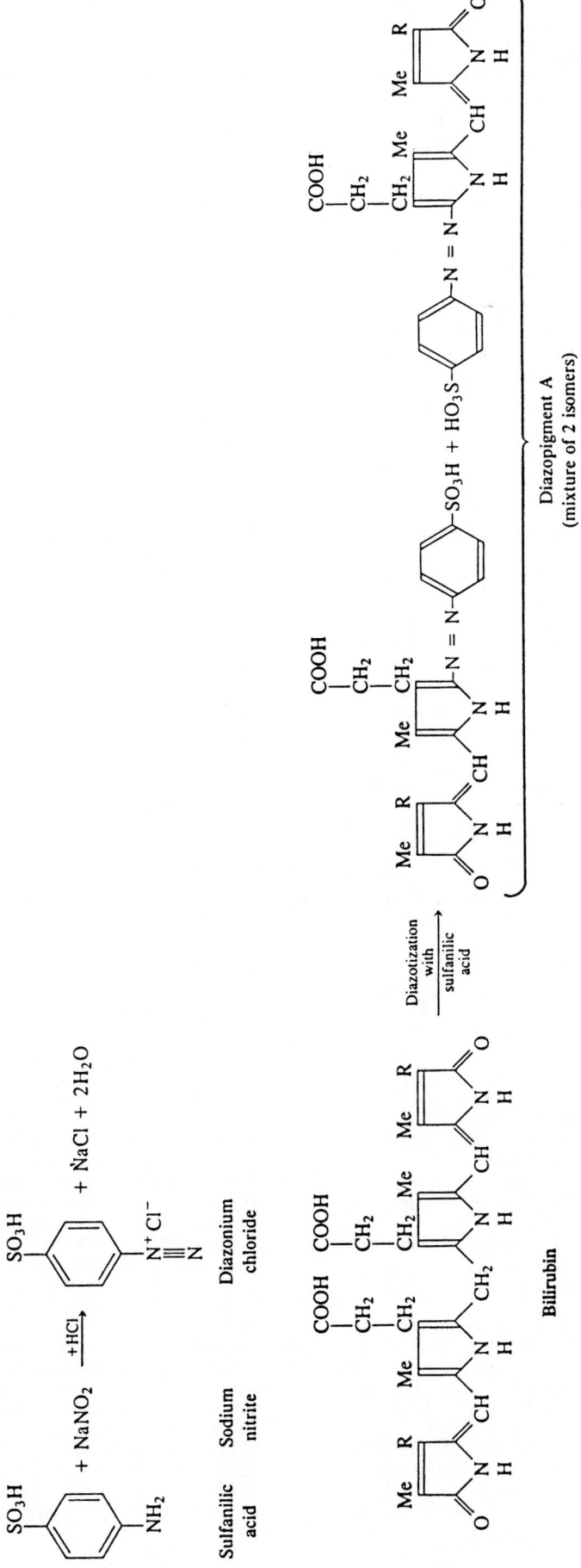

Fig. 27-8 Formation of diazotized sulfanilic acid and its reaction with esterified and nonesterified forms of bilirubin to form azobilirubin derivatives. *Me*, —CH₃ group; *R*, —CH=CH₂ group.

Table 27-9 Methods of bilirubin analysis

Method	Type of analysis	Principle	Usages	Comments
1. Malloy-Evelyn	Kinetic, end point, with or without blank	Reaction shown in Fig. 27-2 is performed at pH 1.2; azobilirubin measured at 560 nm.	Very frequently used, especially as automated procedure	Susceptible to significant hemoglobin interference
2. Jendrassik-Grof	Kinetic, end point, with or without blank	Reaction shown in Fig. 27-2 is performed near neutral pH, but chromophore is measured at alkaline pH (approximately 13) at 600 nm.	Most frequently used method	Has higher molar absorptvity and thus is more sensitive and precise at low bilirubin concentrations than Malloy-Evelyn method
3. Bilirubinometer	Direct spectrophotometric	Bilirubin concentration is directly determined by its absorbance at 454 nm; HbO_2 interference is corrected by subtraction of absorbance at a second wavelength (540 nm).	Not frequently used; primarily for neonatal analysis	Very simple to perform but very strong interference from carotenoids
4. High-performance liquid chromatography	Chromatographic separation	Methyl esters of conjugated and unconjugated bilirubin are detected at 430 nm.	Research use only	May become future reference method
5. Bilirubin oxidase	Kinetic, end point	Enzymatic oxidation of bilirubin to biliverdin and water; reaction is monitored at 405 to 460 nm.	Rarely used	May become future reference method; no hemoglobin interference
6. Spectral shift	End point	Binding of bilirubin by hydrophobic cationic polymer causes shift in spectrum of bilirubin. Magnitude of change, as measured by reflectance photometry, is related to bilirubin concentration.	Available on the Johnson and Johnson Ektachem only	No hemoglobin interference; can measure δ-bilirubin concentration

HbO_2, Oxyhemoglobin.

REFERENCES

1. Johnson TR: Development of the liver. In Johnson TR, Moore WM, Jefferies SE, editors: *Children are different: developmental physiology,* ed 2, Columbus, 1978, Ross Laboratories.
2. Demers LM: Serum bile acids in health and in hepatobiliary disease. In Demers LM, Shaw LM, editors: *Evaluation of liver function,* Baltimore, 1978, Urban & Schwarzenberg.
3. Stoner JW: Neonatal jaundice, *Am Fam Physician* 24:226-232, 1981.
4. Doumas BT, Wu FW: The measurement of bilirubin fractions in serum, *Crit Rev Clin Lab Sci* 28:415-445, 1991.
5. Craig JR: Hepatitis delta virus, editorial, *Am J Clin Pathol* 98:552-555, 1992.
6. Jeppson JO, Franzen B, Cox DW, et al: Typing of genetic variants of alpha-1-antitrypsin by electrofocusing, *Clin Chem* 28:219-225, 1982.
7. Ellis G, Goldberg DM, Spooner RJ, Ward AM: Serum enzyme tests in diseases of the liver and biliary tree, *Am J Clin Pathol* 70:248-258, 1978.
8. Friedman RB, Anderson RE, Entine SM, Hirschberg SB: Effects of diseases on clinical laboratory tests, *Clin Chem* 26:1D-476D, 1980.
9. Lloyd-Still JD: Disorders of the liver in childhood. In Demers LM, Shaw LM, editors: *Evaluation of liver function,* Baltimore, 1978, Urban & Schwarzenberg.
10. Nanji AA, Blank D: The serum urea nitrogen/creatinine ratio and liver disease, *Clin Chem* 28:1398-1399, 1982.
11. Ottobrelli A et al: Patterns of delta virus reinfection and disease in liver transplantation, *Gastroenterology* 101:1649-1655, 1991.
12. Todo S, Fung JJ, Tzakis A, et al: One hundred ten consecutive primary orthotopic liver transplants under FK-506 in adults, *Transplant Proc* 23:1397-1402, 1991.
13. Imagawa DK, Millis JM, Olthoff KM, et al: The role of tumor necrosis factor in allograft rejection. I. Evidence that elevated levels of tumor necrosis factor–alpha predict rejection following orthotopic liver transplantation, *Transplantation* 50:219-225, 1990.
14. Schroeder TJ, Gremse DA, Mansour ME, et al: Lidocaine metabolism as an index of liver function in hepatic transplant donors and recipients, *Transplant Proc* 21:2299-2301, 1989.
15. Reitman S, Frankel S: A colorimetric method for the determination of serum glutamic oxalacetic and glutamic pyruvic transaminases, *Am J Clin Pathol* 28:56-63, 1957.
16. Brétaudière JP, Burtis C, Pasching J, et al: Study of the alanine aminotransferase kinetic assay by response surface methodology, *Clin Chem* 26:1023, 1980 (Abstract).

17. Wróblewski F, LaDue JS: Serum glutamic-pyruvic transaminase in cardiac and hepatic disease, *Proc Soc Exp Biol Med* 91:569-571, 1956.
18. Tietz NW, editor: *Clinical guide to laboratory tests*, ed 2, Philadelphia, 1990, Saunders.
19. Peters T Jr: Serum albumin. In Putnam FW, editor: *The plasma proteins*, New York, 1975, Academic Press, vol 1.
20. Block RJ, Weiss KW, Carroll DB: In Block RJ, Weiss KW, editors: *Amino acid handbook*, Springfield, Ill., 1956, Charles C Thomas.
21. Goldenberg H, Drewes PA: Direct photometric determination of globulin in serum, *Clin Chem* 17:358-362, 1971.
22. Gustafsson JEC: Improved specificity of serum albumin determination and estimation of "acute phase reactants" by use of the bromocresol green reaction, *Clin Chem* 22:616-622, 1976.
23. Maguire GA, Price CP: Bromocresol purple method for serum albumin gives falsely low values in patients with renal insufficiency, *Clin Chim Acta* 155:83-88, 1986.
24. Bush V, Reed RG: Bromocresol purple dye-binding methods underestimate albumin that is carrying covalently bound bilirubin, *Clin Chem* 33:821-823, 1987.
25. Stamp RJ: Measurement of albumin in urine by end-point immunonephelometry, *Ann Clin Biochem* 25:442-443, 1988.
26. Barlow IM, Harrison SP, Sykes MO: Immunoturbidimetric microalbumin kit adapted to the Technicon RA-1000, *Clin Chem* 34:177-178, 1988.
27. Jury DR, Speed JF, Dunn RJ: Urinary albumin radioimmunoassay using a solid phase second antibody and solid phase iodination, *Clin Chim Acta* 148:63-67, 1979.
28. Puri A, Casburn-Budd R, Eisen V, Slater JDH: Simpler measurement of albumin in urine or plasma, *Clin Chem* 31:1241-1242, 1985.
29. Townsend JC: A competitive immunoenzymatic assay for albumin in urine, *Clin Chem* 32:1372-1374, 1986.
30. Watts GF, Bennett JE, Rowe DJ, et al. Assessment of immunological methods for determining low concentrations of albumin in urine, *Clin Chem* 32:1544-1548, 1986.
31. Hallbach J, Hoffmann GE, Guder WG: Overestimation of albumin in heparinized plasma, *Clin Chem* 37:566-568, 1991.
32. Duggan J, Duggan PF: Albumin by bromcresol green: a case of laboratory conservatism, *Clin Chem* 28:1407-1408, 1982.
33. MacNeil MLW, Mueller PW, Caudill SP, Steinberg KK: Considerations when measuring urinary albumin; precision, substances that may interfere, and conditions for sample storage, *Clin Chem* 37:2120-2123, 1991.
34. Denko CW, Gabriel P: Age and sex-related levels of albumin, ceruloplasmim, α_1-antitrypsin, α_1-acid glycoprotein, and transferrin, *Ann Clin Lab Sci* 11:63-68, 1981.
35. Meites S, editor: *Pediatric clinical chemistry*, Washington, D.C., 1977, American Association of Clinical Chemistry, p 20.
36. Zlotkin SH, Casselman CW: Percentile estimates of reference values for total protein and albumin in sera of premature infants (37 weeks of gestation), *Clin Chem* 33:411-413, 1987.
37. Jacobs DS, Kasten BL Jr, Demott WR, Wolfsen WL: *Laboratory test handbook with DRG index*, St. Louis, 1984, Mosby Lexi-comp, pp 32-33.
38. Tietz NW, editor: *Clinical guide to laboratory tests*, Philadelphia, 1983, Saunders.
39. Schmidt E, Henkel E, Klauke R, et al: Proposal for standard methods for the determination of enzyme catalytic concentrations in serum and plasma at 37° C, *J Clin Chem Clin Biochem* 28:805-806, 1990.
40. Bowers GN, McComb RB: Measurement of total alkaline phosphate activity in human serum, *Clin Chem* 21:1988-1995, 1975.
41. Proceedings of the 1992 international symposium on recent developments in alkaline phosphatase research, *Clin Chem* 38:2484-2551, 1992.
42. Reitman S, Frankel S: A colorimetric method for the determination of serum glutamic oxalacetic and glutamic pyruvic transaminase, *Am J Clin Pathol* 28:56-63, 1975.
43. Karmen S: A note on the spectrophotometric assay of glutamic oxalacetic transaminase in human blood serum, *J Clin Invest* 34:131-135, 1955.
44. Bruns D, Savory J, Titheradge A, et al: Evaluation of the IFCC-recommended procedure for serum aspartate aminotransferase as modified for use with the centrifugal analyzer, *Clin Chem* 27:156-159, 1981.
45. Tang M, Sullivan M, Gibson D, Truskolawski C: Kinetic error on Kodak Ektachem: a clue in diagnosis of myeloma, *Clin Chem* 40:166, 1994.
46. Demetriou JA, Drewes PA, Gin JN: Enzymes. In Henry RJ, Cannon DC, Winkelman JE, editors: *Clinical chemistry: principles and technics*, ed 2, Hagerstown, Md., 1974, Harper & Rowe.
47. Meites S, editor: *Pediatric clinical chemistry*, Washington, D.C., 1981, American Association for Clinical Chemistry.
48. Mullon CJ, Langer R: Determination of conjugated and total bilirubin in serum neonates, with use of bilirubin oxidase, *Clin Chem* 33:1822-1825, 1987.
49. Doumas BT, Perry B, Jendrzejczak B, Davis L: Measurement of direct bilirubin by use of bilirubin oxidase, *Clin Chem* 33:1349-1353, 1987.

BIBLIOGRAPHY

Bishop ML, Duben-Engelkirk JL, Fody EP, editors: *Clinical chemistry: principles, procedures, correlations*, ed 2, Philadelphia, 1992, Lippincott.
Gitnick G: *Hepatology*, New York, 1986, Medical Examination Publishing Co.
Halsted JA: *The laboratory in clinical chemistry: interpretation and application*, Philadelphia, 1976, Saunders.
Meites S, editor: *Pediatric clinical chemistry: reference (normal) values*, ed 3, Washington, D.C., 1989, American Association of Clinical Chemists.
Orton SM, Neuhaus OW: *Human biochemistry*, ed 10, St. Louis, 1982, Mosby.
Tilton RC, Balows A, Hohnadel DC, Reiss RF, editors: *Clinical laboratory medicine*, St. Louis, 1992, Mosby.

CHAPTER 28

Bone disease

Oussama Itani
Reginald C. Tsang

KEY TERMS

calcidiol 25-Hydroxyvitamin D (25-OHD) is cholecalciferol hydroxylated at the carbon-25 position in the liver.

calcitriol 1,25-Dihydroxyvitamin D (1,25-$(OH)_2$D), the active vitamin D metabolite, is cholecalciferol hydroxylated at both the carbon-1 and carbon-25 positions.

cholecalciferol The parent vitamin D compound.

cortical bone Dense compact bone that provides structural support.

diaphysis Shaft of a long bone.

epiphysis End of a long bone.

metaphysis Region in which diaphysis and epiphysis converge.

osteoblasts Cells that synthesize bone matrix.

osteoclasts Cells that resorb bone.

osteocytes Mature bone cells that have limited function and are encased in bone matrix, the composition of which they help to maintain.

osteoid Bone matrix.

osteomalacia Disorder in which bone contains normal amounts of osteoid but deficient amounts of mineral.

osteopenia The roentgenographic appearance of subnormally mineralized bone.

osteoporosis A generalized reduction in bone mass involving both mineral and osteoid.

rickets Osteomalacia in childhood.

trabecular bone Interlacing delicate spicules of bone that are predominantly involved in mineral homeostasis.

OBJECTIVES

- Describe the structure and function of normal bone.
- Describe effects of vitamin D metabolites, parathyroid hormone, magnesium, and phosphorus on calcium metabolism and regulation.
- Define osteopenia, osteoporosis, osteomalacia, rickets, osteitis fibrosa, and Paget's disease.
- State expected levels of calcidiol, parathyroid hormone, calcium, phosphorus, magnesium, calcitonin, alkaline phosphatase, and urinary hydroxyproline in the disease states listed above.

BONE STRUCTURE AND FUNCTION

Over 90% of the cells in bone are encased in calcified tissue and separated by great distances from a vascular supply. This gives the cells the appearance of inactivity. However, it is now clear that the skeletal system is a dynamic organ. The modern theory of skeletal system function proposes that bone has two interdependent roles: provision of support and maintenance of mineral homeostasis. Both functions are successfully achieved by continuous bone remodeling. Disturbances in the balance and nature of bone formation and resorption produce the common bone diseases.

Bone structure

Macroscopically, the major bones are classified as long bones or flat bones.[1] Long bones are confined to the limbs and consist of a shaft *(diaphysis)*, two ends *(epiphyses)*, and a region in which the two converge *(metaphysis)* (Fig. 28-1, *A*). Seen in cross section, the diaphysis is lined by dense, compact *(cortical)* bone, whereas the metaphysis contains interlacing bony spicules that resemble the structure of a sponge *(trabecular or cancellous bone)* (Fig. 28-1, *B*). Flat bones, typified by the bones of the skull, consist of two thin layers of cortical bone that enclose a layer of trabecular bone. Dense cortical bone provides strength needed for structural support, and the spicules of trabecular bone provide a large surface area for bone synthesis and resorption and provide a reservoir of minerals for the maintenance of mineral homeostasis.

Bone contains three major types of mature cells, *osteoblasts, osteocytes,* and *osteoclasts.*[2] *Osteoblasts,* found along surfaces of both cortical and trabecular bone, synthesize bone matrix. The plasma membrane of the osteoblast is very rich in alkaline phosphatase, the activity of which is an index of bone formation. Osteoblasts have receptors for parathyroid hormone (PTH), 1,25-dihydroxyvitamin D, $(1,25(OH)_2D)$ and estrogen but not for calcitonin. Stimulation by PTH, $1,25(OH)_2D$, growth hormone, and estrogen causes osteoblasts to produce insulin-like growth factor I (IGF-I), which has a significant role in local bone regulation and modeling. As osteoblasts become embedded in bone matrix, they differentiate into mature *osteocytes.* Osteocytes synthesize small amounts of matrix continuously to maintain bone integrity, and they are able to resorb bone (osteocytic osteolysis) in exceptional circumstances when normal mineral homeostasis is altered.

Osteoclasts contain enzymes that demineralize and digest bone matrix. The process of osteoclastic bone resorption has been understood only recently. Bone resorption occurs at a special part of the osteoclast cell membrane, "the ruffled border," which comprises a sealed lysosomal compartment. Because of their acidic pH, lysosomes dissolve bone crystals, and their proteolytic enzymes digest bone matrix.[1] Although bone resorption is primarily effected by the osteoclast, other cells influenced by bone resorbing hormones can direct the osteoclasts. Both osteoblasts and osteoclasts have receptors for bone resorbing hormones and appear to play a significant role in bone resorption. The moth-eaten

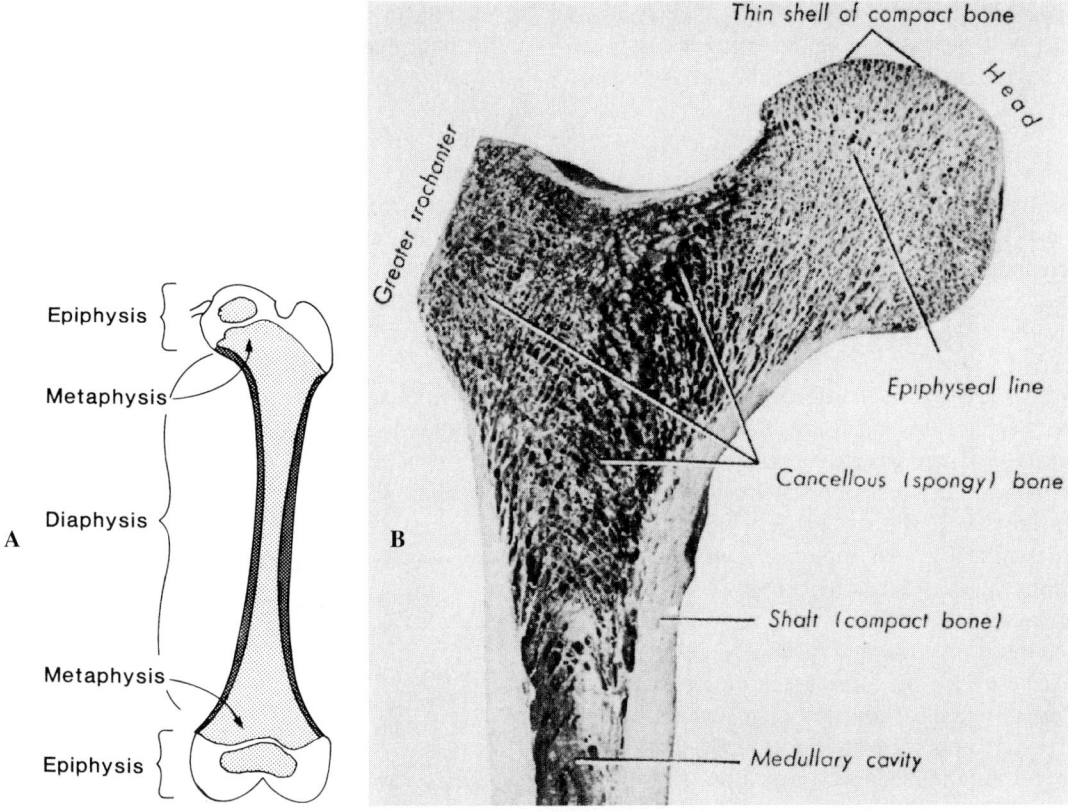

Fig. 28-1 **A,** Parts of a long bone. **B,** Long bone in cross section: notice predominance of trabecular, cancellous bone in diaphysis. (From Copenhaver WM, Kelly DE, Wood RL, editors: *Bailey's textbook of histology,* ed 17, Baltimore, 1978, Williams & Wilkins.)

appearance of bone that indicates bone resorption is evident in histological sections of areas in which osteoclasts are numerous.

Only a small portion of bone is cellular; calcified matrix predominates. This matrix is primarily composed of collagen fibers (mostly type I), a glycosaminoglycans-containing ground substance, and noncollagenous proteins. Type I collagen is the major collagen produced by osteoblasts and represents more than 90% by weight of the nonmineral component of bone. *Osteocalcin* is the major component of bone's noncollagen proteins (see below). Although most bone proteins are synthesized by osteoblasts, some proteins, such as alpha$_2$-HS-glycoprotein, are produced by the liver and absorbed by bone matrix. Spindle-shaped hydroxyapatite, $Ca_{10}(PO_4)_6(OH)_2$, crystals are present in the ground substance and aligned on and within collagen fibers. Glycosaminoglycans are highly anionic complexes that may play a major role in the calcification process and the fixation of hydroxyapatite crystals to collagen fibers. Approximately one fourth of the amino acids present in collagen are either proline or hydroxyproline, neither of which is present to any great extent in other tissues. When collagen is metabolized, hydroxyproline-containing oligopeptides are excreted in the urine, and the amount present correlates with the amount of bone turnover. The mineral elements of bone consist mostly of crystals of calcium and phosphate arranged either amorphously or as hydroxyapatite. A wide range of other elements may be present, including sodium, magnesium, copper, zinc, lead, and fluoride.

Bone mass

About 45% of the adult skeleton is built and enlarged during adolescence. The concept of peak bone mass has become crucial in understanding osteoporosis, especially postmenopausal osteoporosis. Peak bone mass is determined by several factors including genetic, nutritional, mechanical, and environmental.[13] The genetic effect on adult bone mass may be mediated largely through effects on bone formation premenopausally and postmenopausally, rather than through effects on resorption. There is a strong positive relationship between current and past calcium intake and the peak bone mass achieved.[14] Higher calcium intake during adolescence theoretically may optimize, within genetic limits, peak bone mass.[15] Physical activity, use of estrogenic oral contraceptives, and dietary calcium intake exert a positive effect on bone gain in young adult women.[16] Androgens and estrogen are important determinants of peak bone density in young women.[17] The optimal dietary calcium intake for bone growth is a debatable issue. Calcium retention requirements for growth are as follows: an average of 100 mg/day must be retained during childhood, 220 mg/day during adolescence, and probably 20 to 30 mg/day during early adulthood from 20 to 30 years of age.

Bone function

The large surface area and excellent blood supply of trabecular bone permit a quick response to perturbations in plasma mineral concentrations. In contrast, the abundant calcified matrix of cortical bone provides the strength to support body weight. Despite this segregation of structure and function, disturbances in both often coexist. Examples include vitamin D deficiency, which causes both hypocalcemia and easily fractured bone, and immobilization, which causes bone resorption, osteoporosis, and hypercalcemia. Under normal circumstances, such disturbances do not occur because, in *bone remodeling* that occurs throughout the body, bone formation and bone resorption are "coupled," resulting in equal amounts of bone formation and resorption.[4] Most bone diseases result from alterations in coupling that are either new or secondary to hormonal imbalance, which produce either excessive bone formation or excessive resorption.

Biochemical markers of bone turnover

The processes of bone formation and resorption are accompanied by production of a plethora of proteins. Measurement of several of these molecules in serum provides a valuable indicator of ongoing homeostatic bone processes (see box). These markers serve as noninvasive indicators of osteoblastic or osteoclastic activities. The major markers of osteoblastic activities and thus of bone formation are alkaline phosphatase and bone matrix proteins, in particular osteocalcin.

Osteocalcin is the major noncollagenous bone protein. It is a 49–amino acid protein that is synthesized by osteoblasts. Osteocalcin can serve as a marker of osteoblastic activity and bone formation. It contains gamma-carboxyglutamic acid, which is a vitamin K–dependent calcium binding amino acid. Most of synthesized osteocalcin is incorporated in bone where it constitutes 1% of the organic matrix of bone. Minute amounts of osteocalcin in the circulation are derived from new protein synthesis rather than from resorption of bone matrix. The synthesis of osteocalcin is stimulated by $1,25(OH)_2D$.

Procollagen, osteonectin, and *bone sialoprotein (BSP, or osteopontin)* are secreted by osteoblasts into the circulation.

Markers of Bone Turnover

Proteins
   Osteocalcin
   Procollagen
   Osteonectin
   Bone sialoprotein
Derived amino acids
   Collagen pyridinoline
   Hydroxyproline

However, the latter proteins are also produced by platelets, and it appears that assay of procollagen propeptides as an indicator of bone formation is less sensitive and specific than assay of either serum osteocalcin or bone isoenzyme of alkaline phosphatase.[34]

Urine collagen pyridinoline cross-linking amino acids probably are the best available specific biomarkers of bone resorption.[37,38] These compounds include hydroxylysylpyridinoline and lysylpyridinoline.[39]

Bone modeling

Inherent to bone physiology is the physiological "coupling" of the processes of bone formation and resorption, called *remodeling*.[1] Remodeling continues throughout life and requires a balance between bone formation and resorption. At any time approximately 10% of bone mass participates in bone remodeling. Growth during infancy and adolescence is associated with predominance of bone formation over bone resorption, resulting in increased bone mass and bone deposition. In young adults, the processes of bone resorption and formation are equal. With aging, bone resorption exceeds bone formation thereby predisposing the older individual to net bone loss and osteoporosis. In bone disease states, this balance is altered. For instance, in osteoporosis the volume of bone resorbed outweighs the volume of bone formed, resulting in a net loss of bone at each remodeling site.

Hormonal regulation of bone remodeling[3]

The dynamic balance between bone formation and resorption is controlled by both systemic and local regulators. Systematic regulators of bone homeostasis include primarily the calcitropic (PTH and vitamin D) hormones. Local regulation of bone homeostasis involves prostaglandins and growth factors, such as IGF-I and -II,[3] which act as autocrine or paracrine effectors of bone formation by increasing osteoblastic proliferation and bone matrix biosynthesis.

Parathyroid hormone and $1,25(OH)_2D$ play an important role in activating bone remodeling. PTH has a biphasic effect on bone homeostasis: on the one hand, intermittent administration of PTH stimulates bone formation, possibly through production of local growth factors IGF-I and IGF-II; on the other hand, continuous PTH administration has a catabolic effect on bone and favors bone resorption. Prostaglandins, particularly of the E series, are potent local bone resorbing agents. $1,25(OH)_2D$ and thyroid hormones also have a biphasic effect on bone homeostasis.[9] Thyrotoxicosis is a significant risk factor for osteoporosis. Growth hormone also has an anabolic effect on bone metabolism; it increases bone formation by increasing local concentrations of IGF-I.[6] Estradiol and progesterone stimulate osteoblastic activity to increase bone formation,[7] and estrogen increases production of both IGF-I and IGF-II. Several cytokines have osteoclast-activating effects and promote osteoclastic bone resorption.[1,3-6] These cytokines include interleukin-1, tumor necrosis factors alpha and beta, and differentiation-inducing factor. Osteoclasts carry receptors for calcitonin. Calcitonin directly inhibits bone resorption by binding to specific receptors on osteoclasts to inhibit osteoclast formation, motility, and activity.[1]

BIOCHEMISTRY AND PHYSIOLOGY
Mineral physiology

Calcium and mineral metabolism represents a delicate and complex biological process comprising many intricate and interrelated components. Normal homeostatic metabolism depends on the availability of mineral substrates and the interactions of tissues such as bone, kidney, and the gastrointestinal tract with the calcitropic hormones PTH, calcitonin (CT), and $1,25(OH)_2D$.

Calcium and phosphorus. Calcium is the fifth most abundant inorganic element in the human body. The human body contains about 1200 g of calcium in the adult and approximately 28 g in a full-term newborn. Almost all the body's calcium (99%) resides in bone. The remainder resides in body fluids and serves a crucial role in a multitude of physiologic processes including muscular contraction, neurotransmission, membrane transport, enzyme reactions, hormone secretion, and blood coagulation. In the circulation, calcium exists in three forms: 45% of total serum calcium is the biologically active ionized calcium, 45% is protein-bound mainly to albumin, and 10% is complexed to anions (phosphate, lactate, citrate).[22]

Bone contains 80% to 85% of total body phosphorus; approximately 9% is in muscle, and the remainder is in the viscera and extracellular fluid. The intracellular concentration of phosphorus (phosphates and organic phosphorus) is greater than the extracellular levels.

Metabolism. In the adult, dietary calcium is absorbed by the gut by specific calcium-binding proteins. This process is under the active control of vitamin D (see the text following for details). Most absorbed calcium is deposited in bone. The major route for excretion of body calcium is through the kidneys. Both processes, deposition and renal excretion, are under the control of PTH, as described below. Control of serum calcium homeostasis is under control of PTH and will also be discussed below.

By an active energy-dependent process, the placenta transfers calcium ions from mother to fetus against a concentration gradient. This results in relative fetal hypercalcemia and a calcium concentration higher in cord blood than in maternal blood. An intrinsic placental calcium-binding protein (CaBP, calbindin) is present only in the presence of specific receptors for $1,25(OH)_2D$, which have been demonstrated in the human placenta and human fetal gut. It is likely that calbindin may play a significant role in the active transport of calcium transplacentally to the fetus.

Magnesium. Magnesium (Mg) is the fourth most abundant cation and the second most abundant intracellular cation within the body. Most of the total body Mg content

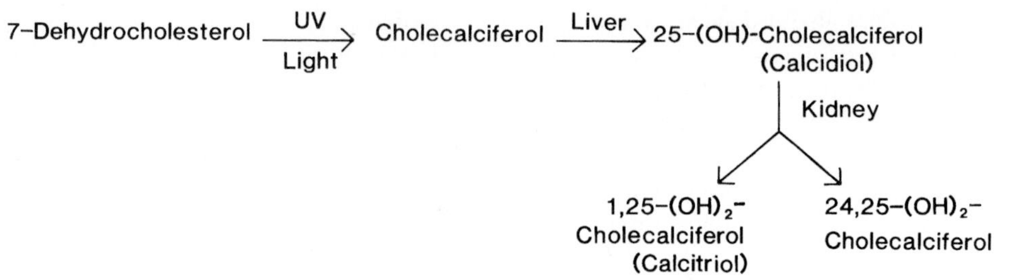

7–Dehydrocholesterol $\xrightarrow[\text{Light}]{\text{UV}}$ Cholecalciferol $\xrightarrow{\text{Liver}}$ 25–(OH)-Cholecalciferol
(Calcidiol)

Kidney

1,25–(OH)$_2$–
Cholecalciferol
(Calcitriol)

24,25–(OH)$_2$–
Cholecalciferol

Fig. 28-2 Conversion of 7-dehydrocholesterol to activated vitamin D by ultraviolet (UV) light and by liver and kidney.

(50% to 60%) is concentrated in bone tissue as an integral component of the hydroxyapatite lattice (30% to 40%) and as an exchangeable fraction (15% to 20%) adsorbed to apatite and in equilibrium with the extracellular fluid compartment. About 20% of total body Mg is concentrated in muscle and another 20% is in the intracellular compartment of blood cells and other body tissues. Changes in total body Mg content are largely reflected by changes in skeletal Mg and to a lesser extent in serum Mg concentrations. Only 1% of the body's magnesium is in blood. Magnesium serves as a cofactor for a multitude of enzymatic reactions involved in storage, transfer, and production of energy and the synthesis of nucleic acid. Further, Mg plays a significant role in calcium and bone homeostasis.

Metabolism. Magnesium is absorbed through the intestinal tract, with absorption rates ranging from 44% on an ordinary diet to 76% on a low-magnesium diet. There is an efficient conservation of magnesium in the kidney so that in magnesium deficiency extremely low magnesium-excretion rates occur. PTH appears to cause increases in serum magnesium concentrations, possibly by mobilizing magnesium from bone. In acute conditions an increase in the serum magnesium concentration results in suppression of the parathyroids, thus theoretically preventing further parathyroid hormone increase and completing a "feedback" loop for magnesium-parathyroid interrelationships.[22] This feedback mechanism is thus similar to that for calcium-parathyroid interrelationships (see p. 534).

Although acute lowering of serum magnesium appears to increase serum PTH concentrations, chronic magnesium deficiency results in *decreased* release of PTH. In addition to this impairment in parathyroid function, magnesium deficiency can decrease the response of target organs to PTH. Thus magnesium deficiency would lead to hypoparathyroidism and, secondarily, hypocalcemia. Hypocalcemia can also accompany magnesium deficiency because calcium release from bone is decreased. Under normal circumstances, magnesium and calcium undergo an exchange in bone related to their release into the circulation. Lowered magnesium content in bone would result in lowered interchange with calcium and lowered release of calcium from bone.[23]

Hormone physiology

Vitamin D. Attention has been focused on vitamin D, since its discovery in 1925 led to the elimination of the widespread problem of nutritional rickets. Initially considered a vitamin because rachitic patients were cured with oral supplementation of vitamin D, vitamin D is now considered to be a hormone.[5] The major source of vitamin D is not the diet, but its production in skin after exposure to sunlight.[6] Dietary vitamin D includes vitamin D$_2$ (derived from plant sterols) and D$_3$ (from animal or synthetic origin). Normally, in adults, at least 90% of vitamin D requirement is provided by endogenous photosynthesis in the skin, which may amount to 1.5 to 10 µg/day (100 to 400 IU/day). It is then transported in the bloodstream to the liver and kidneys for activation. It subsequently localizes at sites of activity in intestine and bone because of the presence of specific cellular receptors in these organs. Finally, as in other hormone systems, the plasma level of activated vitamin D is rigidly controlled by feedback regulation. Vitamin D is regarded as one of the three major hormones controlling calcium and phosphorus homeostasis and bone mineralization.[5,7]

Biochemistry and metabolism. Under the effect of small intestinal mucosal dehydrogenase, dietary cholesterol is converted into 7-dehydrocholesterol, which is then transported to the malpighian layer of the skin (Fig. 28-2). Ultraviolet radiation (of wavelengths 290 to 320 nm) penetrates the skin to break the C9-C10 bond of 7-dehydrocholesterol (provitamin D$_3$) to form pre–vitamin D$_3$. Pre–vitamin D$_3$ undergoes several reactions: it may be photoisomerized to lumisterol and tachysterol or converted by a temperature-dependent isomerization to cholecalciferol (vitamin D$_3$). Cholecalciferol is then released in the circulation where it is bound to vitamin D–binding protein and transported to the liver.

In the liver, cholecalciferol undergoes 25-hydroxylation to yield 25-hydroxyvitamin D, or 25(OH)D (calcidiol) (Figs. 28-2 and 28-3), which is released into the circulation once again before reaching the kidney. In the kidney mitochondrion, 25(OH)D undergoes 1-alpha-hydroxylation to produce 1,25-dihydroxyvitamin D (calcitriol), or 24-hydroxylation to form 24,25-dihydroxyvitamin D (24,25-(OH)$_2$D) (Fig. 28-2). Plasma calcitriol concentrations are

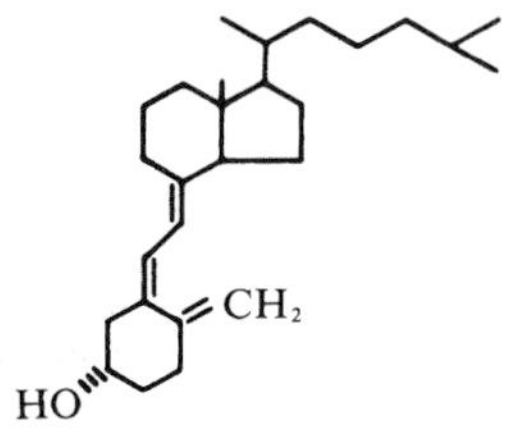

Vitamin D₃
(cholecalciferol)

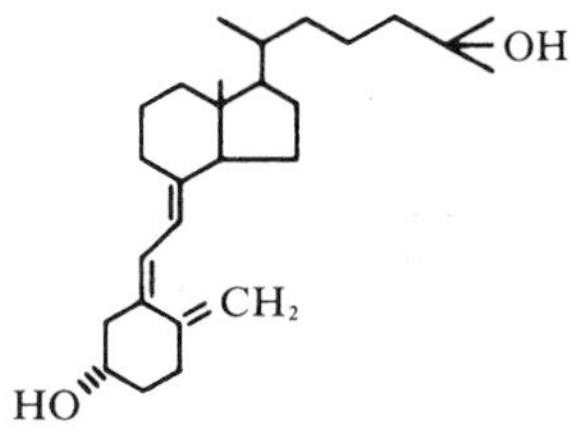

25-OH-Vitamin D₃

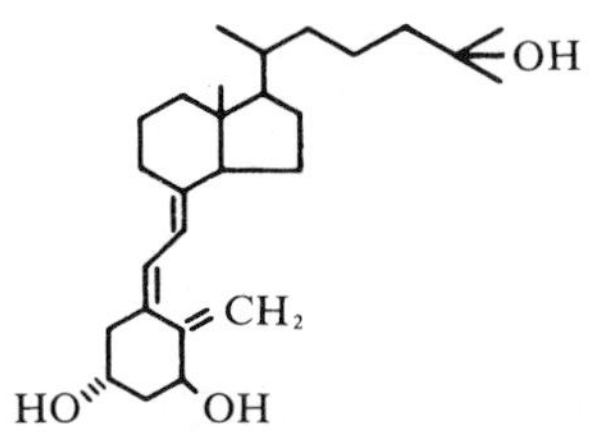

1α, 25-(OH)₂ Vitamin D₃

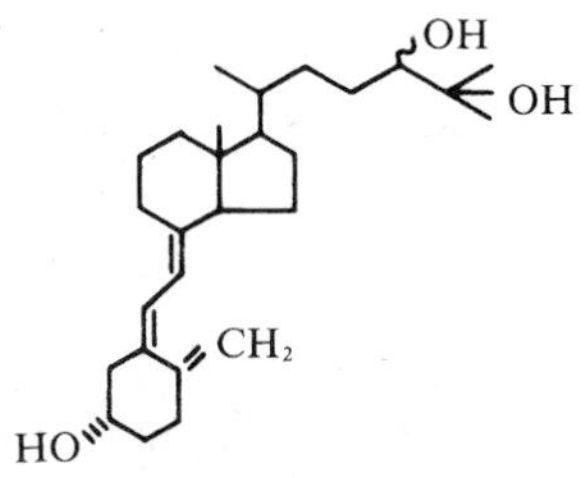

24,25-(OH)₂ Vitamin D₃

Fig. 28-3   Some common metabolites of cholecalciferol.

relatively low (approximately 30 pg/mL). Although normal plasma concentrations vary with age,[10] they are probably under strict feedback control.[11] The details of this control are discussed later. If plasma calcitriol concentrations are sufficient, calcidiol is hydroxylated in the kidney at the C-24 position to yield 24,25-dihydroxycholecalciferol (Fig. 28-2). This last metabolite is currently regarded by most investigators as a waste product of vitamin D metabolism. The role of 24,25(OH)₂D in mineral and vitamin D homeostasis is not very well known.

Although the human newborn has undetectable plasma vitamin D concentration, vitamin D metabolites are necessary for optimal human fetal and maternal bone mineralization. The fetus is totally dependent on maternal vitamin D.

Cholecalciferol and its metabolites pass through the circulation attached to vitamin D–binding protein.[12] Certain tissues contain an intracellular protein that serves as a specific receptor for calcitriol. This protein, located in the cytosol of the kidney, intestine, bone, and selected other tissues, functions like other established cellular steroid hormone receptors (see Chapter 40). It facilitates entry of calcitriol into cells and transports the calcitriol to the cell nucleus, where the hormone, in theory, directs protein synthesis to achieve its desired effect.

Mechanisms of action.[5,7,12] The three major target organs of calcitriol are intestine, bone, and kidney (see box). Calcitriol facilitates both calcium and phosphate absorption in the intestine and induces a specific calcium-binding protein in the intestines, calbindin D. Phosphate transport accompanies calcium transport, but it is also increased by an unknown, calcium-independent mechanism. Calcitriol works cooperatively with parathyroid hormone to increase bone resorption by increasing osteoclast activity.

Target Organs for Calcitriol

Intestine—increased calcium and phosphorus absorption
Bone—enhanced parathyroid hormone-induced bone resorption
Kidney—increased reabsorption of calcium and phosphorus

This may be considered paradoxical because vitamin D is believed to enhance bone mineralization. However, the net effect of the action of calcitriol at bone and intestine is to increase available blood calcium and phosphorus concentrations, which subsequently facilitate mineralization of newly formed bone matrix. Calcitriol increases the renal reabsorption of both calcium and phosphorus, but since 99% of filtered calcium is normally reabsorbed, the overall effect of alterations in plasma calcitriol concentrations on renal calcium reabsorption is small.

Calcitriol has a regulatory effect on PTH and CT gene transcription. In humans with secondary hyperparathyroidism, intravenous 1,25(OH)₂D administration leads to a sharp reduction in serum PTH concentration. Oral administration of calcitriol to children with hypophosphatemic rickets and secondary hyperparathyroidism also has an inhibitory effect on PTH secretion. Calcitriol upregulates its own receptor in the parathyroid glands; 1,25(OH)₂D administration increases the concentration of vitamin D receptor mRNA in the parathyroid gland.

Regulation of vitamin D metabolism. The regulation of vitamin D metabolism is easily understood once calcitriol function is known (see box on page 534). Although plasma calcidiol levels are poorly controlled,[10] there ap-

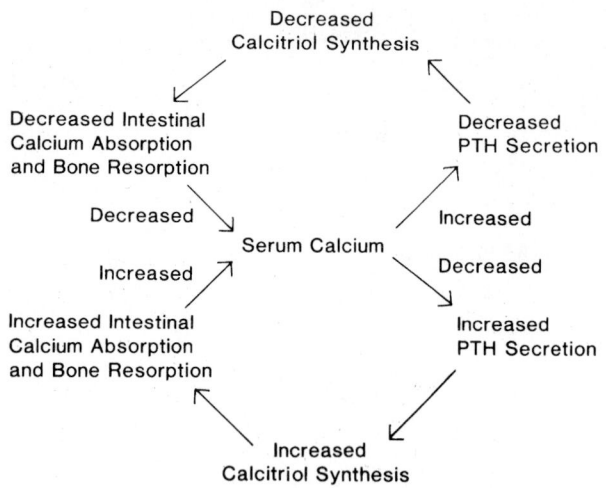

Fig. 28-4 Interrelationships of serum calcium concentrations and parathyroid hormone, *PTH,* and calcitriol.

pears to be relatively strict control of plasma calcitriol concentrations. The activity of renal 1-alpha-hydroxylase is stimulated by IGF-I, PTH, and hypophosphatemia and by periods of high calcium demand such as growth, pregnancy, or low calcium intake. Activity may be inhibited by $1,25(OH)_2D$ and other vitamin D metabolites.

PTH is the major stimulus for calcitriol formation. PTH administration is now used as a clinical tool to assess the ability of the kidney to produce calcitriol.[13] PTH may stimulate renal 1-alpha-hydroxylase, the enzyme that hydroxylates calcidiol at the C-1 position, indirectly by lowering intracellular phosphorus concentrations. Because phosphorus depletion increases calcitriol synthesis in normal or parathyroidectomized animals, decreased intracellular phosphorus levels may be the ultimate common stimulus for calcitriol synthesis.

Understanding the metabolic control of vitamin D allows one to comprehend control of serum calcium and phosphorus concentrations (Fig. 28-4). When the serum calcium concentration falls, PTH is secreted and acutely restores normal serum calcium concentrations by stimulating osteoclasts to resorb bone. Within hours, calcitriol production is increased, which causes enhanced intestinal calcium absorption, which subsequently restores the serum calcium concentration and indirectly the PTH concentration to normal. Elevations in serum calcium concentration produce the

opposite effect, that is, a reduction in both serum PTH concentrations and calcitriol synthesis.

Plasma calcitriol concentrations are altered by aging and pregnancy; they are elevated during adolescence and decline in old age.[14] Pregnancy and subsequent lactation are associated with elevated serum estrogen or prolactin concentrations; both hormones increase calcitriol synthesis.[15] It should be noted that the adolescent growth spurt, pregnancy, and lactation all increase requirements for calcium. Thus the elevated serum calcitriol concentrations represent an appropriate response to a physiological need.

Although the human newborn has undetectable plasma vitamin D concentration, vitamin D metabolites are necessary for optimal human fetal and maternal bone mineralization. The fetus is totally dependent on maternal vitamin D.

Parathyroid hormone

Biochemistry and metabolism. Parathyroid hormone is an 84-amino acid polypeptide (at 9500 daltons) synthesized in the parathyroid glands. The precursor protein for parathyroid hormone is *preproparathyroid hormone.* This precursor is sequentially converted in the gland, first to proparathyroid and then to parathyroid hormone, which is released into the circulation. Full biological activity resides in the amino-terminal 1-34 peptide; the middle and carboxy-terminal sequences (35 to 85 amino acids) are biologically inert though immunologically highly reactive. Thus fragments of parathyroid hormone bearing the N terminal generally are active, whereas those bearing the C terminal are inactive.

Mechanisms of action. Parathyroid hormone acts on two major target organs, bone and kidney, to produce three major effects: increase in serum calcium concentrations, decrease in serum phosphorus concentrations, and increase in the active hormonal form of vitamin D (calcitriol). In bone, parathyroid hormone predominantly mobilizes calcium and phosphorus to the extracellular fluid, thus raising serum calcium and phosphorus concentrations. PTH has a synergistic effect with $1,25(OH)_2D$ in stimulating bone resorption.

At the other target organ, the kidney, parathyroid hormone causes increased calcium retention, increased phosphorus excretion, stimulation of renal 1-alpha-hydroxylase activity (see above), and increased conversion of 25-hydroxycholecalciferol (calcidiol) to 1,25-dihydroxycholecalciferol (calcitriol). Calcitriol, in turn, as described earlier, predominantly causes increased intestinal calcium and phosphorus absorption. The effects of parathyroid hormone on the kidney are mediated through the formation of cyclic adenosine monophosphate (cAMP), and urinary levels of this substance rise when parathyroid hormone production is increased. The resultant effect of parathyroid hormone on the bone, kidney, and indirectly the intestine is to increase calcium concentrations in the blood. Although phosphorus concentrations may be elevated through parathyroid actions

---

Primary Stimuli for Calcitriol Synthesis
Decreased serum calcium concentration
Increased pathathyroid hormone secretion
Decreased intracellular phosphorus concentration

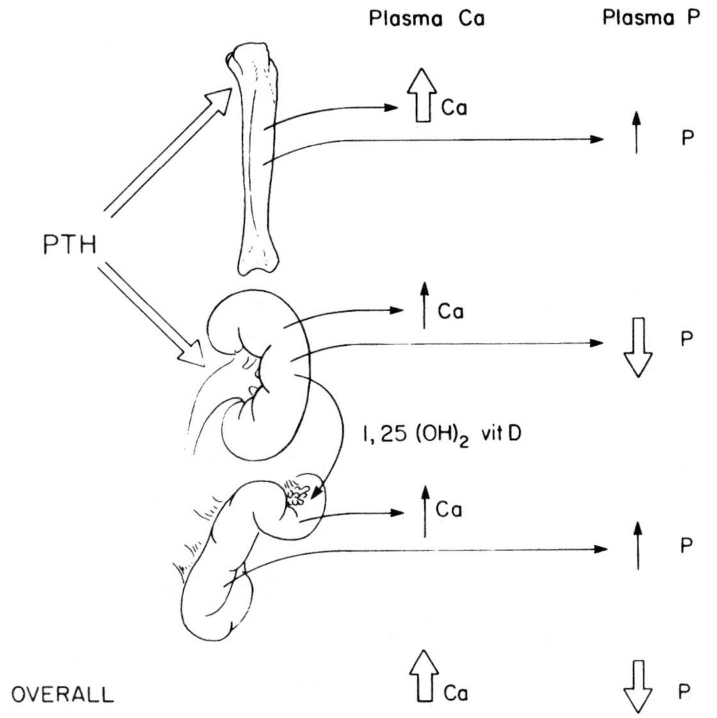

Plasma Ca   Plasma P

OVERALL

Fig. 28-5 Normal parathyroid hormone physiology. Parathyroid hormone action increases serum calcium concentrations predominantly through its bone and kidney effects but reduces plasma phosphorus concentrations, *P,* through increasing renal phosphorus excretion. (From Tsang RC, Noguchi A, Steichen JJ: *Pediatr Clin North Am* 26:223, 1979.)

on bone and indirectly the intestine, the effect on increased renal phosphorus excretion overwhelms the other effects and, overall, results in decreased serum phosphorus concentrations (Fig. 28-5).

Serum ionized calcium (iCa) concentration is the main determinant of PTH secretion: a drop in serum iCa concentration stimulates PTH secretion, whereas a rise in serum iCa concentration suppresses it. However, other ions and hormones influence PTH secretion by the parathyroid glands: for instance, a rise in serum 1,25(OH)$_2$D decreases PTH secretion. An acute drop in serum Mg concentration stimulates PTH secretion but to a much smaller extent (tenfold less on a molar basis) compared to the effect of acute hypocalcemia.[43] Chronic hypomagnesemia impairs PTH secretion and causes blunting of PTH action at target organs.[44-48] Magnesium ions are essential for adenylate cyclase–mediated secretion of secretory granules and subsequent release of PTH from the parathyroid chief cells. Therefore, magnesium deficiency may cause secondary hypocalcemia. Hypermagnesemia also suppresses PTH secretion.[49]

Perinatal PTH homeostasis. Theoretically, since PTH does not cross the placenta, the relative fetal hypercalcemia should suppress the fetal parathyroid glands. Paradoxically, fetal PTH secretion is not suppressed. A possible explanation for the nonsuppression of PTH secretion, despite relative fetal hypercalcemia, is that the negative-feedback

system regulating PTH secretion by calcium concentration operates with a higher "set point" in the fetus so that suppression of PTH secretion in the fetus requires higher serum calcium concentrations than those required after birth. Both PTH and PTHRP may have a significant role in placental transport of calcium, and PTHRP may significantly contribute to the PTH bioactivity in fetal serum.

Parathyroid hormone–related peptide

Biochemistry and metabolism. Parathyroid hormone–related peptide (PTHRP) and parathyroid hormone genes are members of the same gene family; the amino terminal of PTHRP has a sequence homology in 8 amino acids with the PTH amino terminal. PTHRP is also found to be equipotent to PTH when assessed by cytochemical bioassay and in situ biochemistry.[55] PTH synthesis is restricted to the parathyroid glands in normal subjects, but PTHRP messenger RNA is widely distributed in normal tissues, including the skin, thyroid, bone marrow, hypothalamus, pituitary, parathyroid, adrenal cortex, adrenal medulla, and stomach. Several studies suggest that PTHRP may have a significant physiological role. One of the major production sites of this peptide is lactating breast tissue, and PTHRP is present in large quantities in milk.

Mechanisms of action. In normal adults, plasma PTHRP concentrations range from less than 2 to 5 pmol/liter. Infusion of PTHRP causes an elevation in serum 1,25-

dihydroxy vitamin D concentration and an increase in bone formation parameters.[56-58] PTHRP may play a causal role in the cause of hypercalcemia of malignancies. It is possible that PTH and PTHRP act on the same bone receptor to cause increased bone resorption and formation and hypercalcemia and hypophosphatemia.[58] PTHRP, produced in the fetal parathyroid glands, may be responsible for stimulation of placental calcium transport.[60,61]

Calcitonin (CT)

Calcitonin,[16] discovered in 1962, is generally regarded as one of three hormones (along with vitamin D and parathyroid hormone) responsible for the control of calcium and phosphorus homeostasis. Despite great research efforts, a definitive role for calcitonin in calcium homeostasis has not yet been clarified. Neither calcitonin deficiency nor calcitonin excess is clearly associated with bone disease or alteration of serum calcium homeostasis.

Localization, biochemistry, and metabolism. Calcitonin is produced by the parafollicular C-cells of the thyroid gland, though the pituitary gland, gastrointestinal tract, and liver may also produce the hormone.[16] Calcitonin is secreted in a precursor form, with a molecular weight of 15,000 daltons, that is cleaved into the active 32–amino acid calcitonin polypeptide, which has a molecular weight of 3500 daltons.[16] Normal serum calcitonin concentrations are less than 100 pg/mL. Calcitonin is rapidly excreted, with a half-life of 10 minutes after intravenous administration.[17] Excretion is predominantly by the kidney, and serum calcitonin concentrations are increased in patients with renal failure.[18]

Biological effects. The best recognized physiologic effect of CT is to counteract the action of PTH at several organ sites in the human body. The biological effects of calcitonin may be divided into those related to calcium and phosphorus homeostasis and those related to gastrointestinal function. Intravenous calcitonin administration causes a prompt decline in the serum calcium and phosphorus concentrations. This occurs because of effects of calcitonin on both bone and kidney. Calcitonin alters cell function by increasing intracellular cAMP production.[19] Receptors specific for CT have been demonstrated on bone osteoclasts, and CT antagonizes PTH-mediated bone resorption by suppressing osteoclastic activity. Consequently, CT decreases the flux of calcium and phosphorus from bone into the circulation with urinary hydroxyproline excretion decreasing in parallel with the inhibition of bone resorption. Calcitonin also decreases the renal reabsorption of calcium, phosphorus, sodium, potassium, and magnesium.[19] CT also acts on vitamin D metabolism; it enhances $1,25(OH)_2D$ production by proximal renal tubules. These described effects on both bone and kidney have been produced with pharmacological calcitonin concentrations.

In the human fetus, the thyroid C-cells appear to be well developed by 14 weeks of gestation. However, the role of CT in fetal mineral and bone homeostasis is not very well understood. Calcitonin does not cross the placenta, and, as with PTH, fetal CT function may be autonomous from that of the mother and may play a role in fetal bone mineralization.

Regulation of calcitonin secretion. Calcitonin secretion is influenced by serum calcium concentrations; the gastrointestinal hormones gastrin, cholecystokinin, and glucagon; and sex steroids. Calcitonin release is affected primarily by the concentration of serum ionized calcium and is stimulated by hypercalcemia and inhibited by hypocalcemia.[21] Vitamin D has a direct inhibitory effect on CT gene expression and CT secretion; receptors for $1,25(OH)_2D$ have been demonstrated on parafollicular C-cells. Serum calcitonin concentrations may be higher in pregnant and lactating women than in controls. Men have higher circulating calcitonin concentrations than women.[21]

Calcitonin gene–related peptide (CGRP)

CGRP is another translation product of the calcitonin gene. CGRP is a 37–amino acid peptide that has little amino acid sequence homology with calcitonin. Receptors for this peptide are located primarily in neural tissues, and biosynthesis of CGRP is confined primarily to those neural tissues. It is likely that this peptide's prime role is in neurotransmission. It is not known up to now whether CGRP shares calcitropic activity with calcitonin.

BONE DISORDERS

Disorders of calcium, phosphorus, vitamin D, or parathyroid hormone homeostasis frequently produce *osteopenia,* a general term for the x-ray appearance of a subnormal amount of mineralized bone. Many illnesses are associated with osteopenia[24] (see box below). The bone histopathological condition of osteopenia can reveal decreased osteoid (bone matrix) formation, decreased osteoid mineralization, or increased bone resorption.[25] These histological categories correlate with the clinical diagnosis of *osteoporosis, osteomalacia,* or *osteitis fibrosa,* respectively. Osteopenia can result in the crush-fracture syndrome in adults and either fractures or growth failure in children. Trabecular bone is more frequently affected than cortical bone, and so fractures most often occur in vertebrae, the femoral neck, and the distal ends of the long bones, where trabecular bone is abundant. Whereas specific diagnoses of osteopenic bone are best made histologically, occasionally, characteristic laboratory abnormalities will permit differentiation among osteoporosis, osteomalacia, and osteitis fibrosa (Table 28-1).

Osteoporosis

Osteoporosis is characterized by a disturbed balance between bone resorption and bone formation, which results in a progressive decrease in bone mass and a decrease in the amount of normally mineralized bone; the mineral-collagen ratio is normal. The major sequelae are fragility

Table 28-1   Common serum abnormalities associated with metabolic bone disease

Disease	Ca	P	PTH	Alk PO$_4$	Calcidiol	Calcitriol
Osteoporosis	NL	NL	NL	NL	NL	LO
Osteomalacia	LO	LO	HI	HI	NL or LO	NL or LO
Osteitis fibrosa	HI or NL	LO or NL	HI	HI	NL	HI or NL

Alk PO$_4$, Alkaline phosphatase; *HI*, increased; *LO*, decreased; *NL*, normal; *PTH*, parathyroid hormone.

of bone and predisposition to fractures; particularly spine-vertebral crush fracture, hip-femoral neck fracture, and distal radius fracture, which may occur either spontaneously or in response to minor trauma. Primary osteoporosis is frequently diagnosed in older men and women (senile osteoporosis) and postmenopausal women. It occurs only rarely in childhood as an idiopathic illness and can also accompany certain systemic diseases (see box below). Environmental factors that predispose to bone loss and osteoporosis include cigarette smoking, chronic low dietary calcium intake, a sedentary life style, excessive caffeine intake, high-acid animal protein diet, and alcohol intake.[13]

Senile osteoporosis. Progressive bone loss normally occurs during aging. This process begins at 50 years of age in women and 65 to 70 years of age in men and results in a loss of 0.5% of total bone mass per year and approximately 20% in a lifetime.[28] Patients with senile osteoporosis experience accelerated losses of 1% to 2% per year, with symptoms of osteoporosis beginning when 30% of bone mass is lost. It has been suggested that osteoporosis is a natural part of the aging process manifested earlier in those persons who have accrued less skeletal mass during early adult life. The causes of senile osteoporosis are largely unknown. Hormonal alterations that occur during senescence undoubtedly potentiate bone loss (see box below). Decreased serum calcitriol concentrations found in elderly persons[29] probably result from a blunted synthetic response to parathyroid hormone.[30] In addition, serum parathyroid hormone concentrations increase[31] and serum calcitonin concentrations decrease[32] with aging. The net effect of these hormonal alterations is diminished intestinal calcium absorption and increased bone resorption.

There also appears to be a significant role for vitamin D deficiency in the cause of osteoporosis. Up to 60% of elderly people living in nursing homes develop vitamin D deficiency by the end of the winter season; also a significant number of elderly subjects with hip fractures (40% of males and 30% of females) are vitamin D deficient. Evidence supports a defective renal 1-α-hydroxylase activity with aging and secondary hyperparathyroidism as a cause of vitamin D deficiency in elderly people and secondary osteoporosis.

Postmenopausal osteoporosis. Postmenopausal osteoporosis, which occurs in females at a younger age than senile osteoporosis does, is caused by estrogen deficiency. Affected women have diminished intestinal calcium absorption and lower serum calcitriol concentrations than their normal age-matched peers.[29] Although serum PTH concentrations are normal when compared to controls with normal serum calcitriol concentrations, they are low when viewed in the context of calcitriol deficiency.[29] Estrogen supplementation increases intestinal calcium absorption and serum calcitriol and PTH concentrations.[33] These data have been interpreted to indicate that estrogen deficiency produces postmenopausal osteoporosis by causing bone resorption, which releases calcium into the extracellular space and

---

A Partial Differential Diagnosis of Osteopenia

Osteoporosis
    Aging (senile)
    Postmenopausal
    Juvenile
    Immobilization
    Cushing's syndrome
    Multiple myeloma
    Leukemia
    Turner's syndrome
    Alcoholism
    Chronic liver disease
Osteomalacia
    Vitamin D deficiency
    Chronic gastrointestinal disease
    Anticonvulsant medication induced
    Vitamin D dependency
    Vitamin D resistance (hypophosphatemia)
    Chronic acidosis
    Fanconi's syndrome
    Chronic renal failure
    Phosphorus and calcium deficiency
Osteitis fibrosa
    Primary hyperparathyroidism
    Chronic renal failure
Paget's disease

Calcium-Regulating Hormone Abnormalities Associated with Aging

Decreased serum calcitriol concentration and calcitriol secretory reserve
Increased serum parathyroid hormone concentration
Decreased serum calcitonin concentration

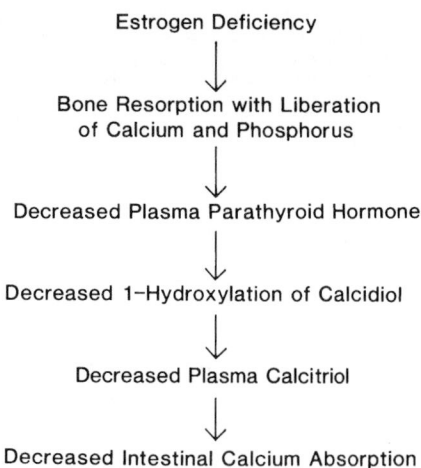

Estrogen Deficiency

↓

**Bone Resorption with Liberation
of Calcium and Phosphorus**

↓

Decreased Plasma Parathyroid Hormone

↓

Decreased 1–Hydroxylation of Calcidiol

↓

Decreased Plasma Calcitriol

↓

Decreased Intestinal Calcium Absorption

Fig. 28-6 Hypothesized pathogenesis of postmenopausal osteoporosis.

which in turn suppresses PTH secretion, calcitriol synthesis, and intestinal absorption of calcium (Fig. 28-6). It has been suggested that magnesium deficiency may play a role in postmenopausal osteoporosis.

Approximately 30% of postmenopausal white women sustain at least one osteoporotic fracture. However, the true incidence of these fractures is difficult to assess because a large number of vertebral fractures remain asymptomatic. Osteoporotic hip fractures occur in the third and fourth decades after menopause; they are twice as common in women as in men. By 90 years of age, about 33% of women and at least 17% of men sustain a hip fracture.

Idiopathic juvenile osteoporosis. Idiopathic juvenile osteoporosis is a rare form of bone demineralization that affects prepubertal children. Clinical features manifest as fractures of long bones and vertebrae, in addition to bone pain. It is characterized by spontaneous recovery after puberty. In severe cases, characteristic metaphyseal compression fractures of the lower extremities occur because of compaction of osteoporotic newly formed bone, a pathognomonic feature of this disease. The etiology of the disease is unknown to date. Some patients have transient calcitriol deficiency, which correlates with the clinical course of the disease. Treatment of these patients with calcitriol reduces bone fracture rate and increases bone mineralization within a year. Other patients may have a negative calcium balance, low 25(OH)D and high 1,25(OH)$_2$D, or possible calcitonin deficiency.

Corticosteroid-induced osteoporosis. There is a loss of bone substance and an increased incidence of pathological fractures in patients treated with corticosteroids for prolonged periods. The mechanism of steroid-induced bone resorption is not completely known. Corticosteroids do exert direct inhibitory effects on osteoblast function, decreasing bone formation. Serum osteocalcin concentration, an indicator of bone formation, is signifi-

cantly reduced in steroid-treated patients. Corticosteroid therapy reduces intestinal calcium and phosphorus absorption.

Hyperthyroidism. Both deficient and excessive circulating thyroid hormones can have deleterious sequelae on bone. The major role of thyroid hormone is to increase the number of bone remodeling units, thereby increasing bone-remodeling activity. Thyrotoxicosis causes increased bone resorption and a decrease in bone mineral density.

Osteomalacia

Osteomalacia is diagnosed when bone contains normal quantities of osteoid that fail to mineralize. When seen in the growing child, osteomalacia is termed *rickets*. The terms *rickets* and *osteomalacia* are used interchangeably in this chapter. The major causes of osteomalacia are listed in the box on p. 537 and their associated biochemical abnormalities are summarized in Table 28-2.

Clinically the earliest rachitic features in infancy may be hypocalcemic tetany or seizures, particularly in vitamin D–unsupplemented, exclusively human milk–fed infants and in infants with congenital rickets born to vitamin D–deficient osteomalacic mothers. Acute infection may precipitate hypocalcemic tetany, possibly by mobilizing bone phosphate into the circulation and therefore decreasing serum calcium concentration. In the first 6 months of life, abnormal bones will be seen on x-ray film. The wrist and the knee are most useful in demonstrating even the earliest signs of rickets. "Rachitic lungs" indicate rib-cage weakening, with secondary defective pulmonary ventilation. This feature occurs in the very young child, particularly among preterm infants. Beyond infancy, increased weight bearing aggravates rachitic changes particularly in vertebral, pelvic, and lower limb bones, resulting in spinal and pelvic deformities that cause a waddling gait and bowed legs, or "knock knees." Muscular weakness and hypotonia frequently involve proximal muscle groups in rickets and contribute to waddling gait, protuberance of the abdomen, and inefficient lung ventilation in rachitic children. The muscular weakness is believed to be caused by decreased calcium uptake by myocytes.

Vitamin D–deficient osteomalacia. Historically the most common cause of osteomalacia was *vitamin D deficiency* caused by a combination of insufficient sunlight exposure and inadequate dietary intake of vitamin D–containing foods.[34] Serum calcidiol concentrations, which reflect the adequacy of vitamin D in the body, are low in osteomalacia. Supplementation of foods with vitamin D has virtually eliminated the problem in industrialized countries, but it may still be seen in underdeveloped nations, particularly among dark-skinned people because skin pigment decreases the production of cholecalciferol, which normally occurs after ultraviolet-radiation exposure. It is also encountered in exclusively human milk-fed infants and in strict vegetarian adults, even in developed countries. These indi-

Table 28-2   Biochemical abnormalities associated with rickets

	Serum calcium	Serum phosphorus	Parathyroid hormone	Calcidiol	Calcitriol
Vitamin D deficiency	LO	LO	HI	LO	LO, NL, or HI
Vitamin D dependency					
I	LO	LO	HI	HI	LO
II	LO	LO	HI	HI	HI
Vitamin D resistance	NL	LO	NL	NL	NL or LO
Dietary phosphorus deficiency	NL	LO	NL	LO	HI

HI, Increased; *LO*, decreased; *NL*, normal.

viduals have limited exposure to sunshine and do not ingest vitamin D–fortified milk.

Alterations of vitamin D metabolism that can lead to rickets range from conditions of insufficient intake or production of cholecalciferol to disturbances in its activation by the liver and kidneys. Generally one can predict the biochemical response to a deficiency of calcitriol (see Fig. 28-4). The absorption of intestinal calcium will decrease and produce hypocalcemia. This will stimulate PTH release (secondary hyperparathyroidism), which will mobilize calcium from bone and increase phosphorus excretion by the kidney. Initially, serum calcium concentrations will be maintained at the expense of bone resorption, but as minerals are depleted, hypocalcemia occurs. Hypophosphatemia occurs because of increased urinary phosphorus losses. Thus the characteristic serum abnormalities associated with calcitriol deficiency are hypocalcemia, hypophosphatemia, and hyperparathyroidism (Table 28-2). In addition, hyperphosphaturia, aminoaciduria, rachitic bone disease, and elevated serum alkaline phosphatase concentration will be observed.

Osteomalacia also results from phosphorus deficiency. In this situation, low intracellular phosphorus concentrations should stimulate calcitriol synthesis, which will increase both intestinal and renal phosphate absorption. Serum calcium and PTH concentrations should be unaffected (Table 28-2).

Osteomalacia secondary to gastrointestinal disorders. Patients with gastrointestinal disease, particularly those with hepatobiliary disease, often develop osteomalacia. Vitamin D is fat soluble and requires bile acids for absorption (see Chapter 30). Patients with hepatobiliary disease have low serum calcidiol levels that appear to be caused in part by defective intestinal cholecalciferol or ergosterol absorption, impaired calcidiol production by the liver, and enhanced calcitriol metabolism. Osteopenia also may be seen after gastric surgery, though the pathogenesis is not understood.

Hepatic rickets. Hepatobiliary disease predisposes to rickets, presumably because of decreased 25-hydroxylase activity, vitamin D malabsorption, and decreased enterohepatic circulation of 25(OH)D. Malabsorption of vitamin D is probably a major factor in the pathogenesis of hepatic rickets. Biochemically, serum 25(OH)D and 1,25(OH)$_2$D

concentrations are low. Clinically, signs of rickets are superimposed on the primary hepatic disease. Infants with hepatitis and infants who require prolonged parenteral hyperalimentation may develop varying degrees of hepatic dysfunction and secondary rickets.

Osteomalacia secondary to anticonvulsant medication. Rickets may occur in up to 30% of children receiving anticonvulsant medications, such as phenytoin (Dilantin) and phenobarbital, that induce the hepatic microsomal mixed-oxidase enzyme system.[35] This enzyme system, when stimulated, converts calcidiol to polar inactive metabolites, which results in calcidiol deficiency. Other biochemical effects of the therapy can include hypocalcemia, hypophosphatemia, hypocalciuria, and elevated serum concentrations of alkaline phosphatase and PTH. In addition, anticonvulsants inhibit calcitriol-dependent intestinal calcium uptake.

Vitamin D–dependent osteomalacia (types I and II).
After foods were fortified with vitamin D, it became apparent that normal antirachitic doses of analogs of vitamin D failed to heal the rickets of a small subpopulation of rachitic patients. One group of such patients had the classical signs and symptoms of vitamin D deficiency, including early infantile hypocalcemia, hypophosphatemia, and tetany, but these patients required up to 100 times the normal intake of vitamin D to heal their rickets. This group of patients with *vitamin D–dependent rickets* has recently been classified into two subgroups with distinct pathophysiological bases.

Patients with vitamin D–dependent rickets type I have the classical biochemical abnormalities of vitamin D–deficient rickets, but their serum calcidiol concentrations are normal and they lack circulating calcitriol.[36] The presumed defect is an abnormal or absent renal 1-α-hydroxylase enzyme. Clinically, the disease presents before 2 years of age, most often in the first 6 months of life. A sporadic form of the disease has been described less often, and its onset is in late childhood and adolescence. The osteomalacia of these patients heals when physiological doses of calcitriol are administered.

Patients with vitamin D–dependent rickets type II have normal calcidiol and calcitriol levels and are resistant to physiological doses of calcitriol. The cause of the disease is an end-organ resistance to the effect of 1,25(OH)$_2$D because of a defective calcitriol-receptor effector system, and mechanistically should be called "calcitriol (1,25[OH]$_2$D)-resistant rickets." Clinically, the disease manifests as rickets and osteomalacia, most commonly before 2 years of life, rarely later in life. Biochemically, these patients have low serum calcium and phosphorus concentrations, normal serum 25(OH)D concentration, and elevated serum 1,25(OH)$_2$D and PTH concentrations. Both types of vitamin D–dependent rickets are inherited in an autosomal recessive pattern.

There are five classes of defective calcitriol receptors: (1) Defect in the hormone-binding domain. Calcitriol concentration is elevated but does not evoke a biochemical response. This is the most common defect. (2) Hormone-binding affinity is normal, accompanied by reduction in the number of receptors and hormone-binding sites (10% of normal). (3) Hormone-binding affinity is reduced twenty- to thirtyfold while the number of binding sites is normal. (4) Defective nuclear localization. In this form, calcitriol does not localize to the cell nucleus. (5) Decreased affinity of hormone-receptor complex to DNA. Intracellular defect categories 1, 2, and 5 do not respond to therapy with high vitamin D doses. In contrast, intracellular defects types 3 and 4 can be cured with high vitamin D doses. Prenatal diagnosis of this disease is now feasible and is indicated in high-risk families.

Vitamin D–resistant osteomalacia. Patients with *vitamin D–resistant rickets* lack most of the usual biochemical markers associated with rachitic patients. Serum phosphorus is severely decreased, whereas serum calcium concentrations may be normal or decreased. Serum PTH concentration is either normal or increased, and serum 1,25(OH)$_2$D concentration is either normal or low. This disorder is caused by a congenital defect in phosphate resorption in the proximal renal tubules, resulting in massive phosphaturia and hypophosphatemia. The defective gene responsible for this disease has been mapped to the short arm of the human X chromosome. Because low intracellular phosphorus concentrations are a major stimulus for calcitriol synthesis, serum calcitriol concentrations should be elevated in this disorder; however, when measured, serum calcitriol concentrations have been found to be low or low-normal.[36,39] This finding is suggestive of a potential second defect in this condition, that is, dysfunction of the renal 1-α-hydroxylase enzyme. Vitamin D–resistant rickets may be inherited in a sex-linked recessive or an autosomal dominant pattern. The most frequent type is the X-linked concomitant pattern and affects males. Traditionally, patients with vitamin D–resistant rickets have been treated with cholecalciferol and phosphate supplements.

Calcium-deficiency rickets. Also termed *calcipenic rickets,* this form of osteomalacia occurs when the diet is low in calcium or when the bioavailability of the calcium is reduced. Children who are following strict vegetarian or high cereal diets are at risk of developing rickets. Some of these children have clinical and biochemical features of vitamin D deficiency, attributed to vitamin D binding by dietary phytates in the intestinal lumen.

Clinically, affected children have rachitic features with "knock" knees, bow legs, or "wind-swept" deformities but no muscular weakness. Radiological features correspond to clinical findings of rachitic changes (see above). The bone histological pattern reveals features of osteomalacia and secondary hyperparathyroidism. Biochemical features of calcipenic rickets include hypocalcemia and hypocalciuria, normal serum 25(OH)D, elevated serum alkaline phosphatase, and elevated serum calcitriol and PTH concentrations.

Hyperalimentation-induced osteopenia. Long-term parenteral alimentation (TPN) has been associated with osteopenia and bone demineralization. The main feature seen in this metabolic bone disease is hypercalciuria. Several factors have been implicated in the cause of hypercalciuria including cyclic infusion of TPN solutions, sulfur-containing acidic amino acids, hypertonic dextrose infusions, which result in hyperinsulinemia and decreased tubular resorption of calcium, acidosis, and low phosphate in infused solutions. Hypercalciuria may be ameliorated by phosphate supplementation.

Aluminum-containing parenteral hyperalimentation solutions are responsible for causing a peculiar metabolic bone disease characterized by reduced bone formation. The degree of aluminum accumulation in bone correlates with decreased bone formation.

Other causes of osteomalacia. Chronic acidosis causes osteomalacia, hypercalciuria, and hyperphosphaturia because of neutralization of acids by bone with subsequent release of bone mineral. Patients with renal Fanconi's syndrome have diminished proximal tubule reabsorption of bicarbonate (resulting in chronic acidosis), phosphorus, glucose, and amino acids. Osteomalacia may be severe because of the chronic acidosis and severe hypophosphatemia. In addition, as part of the proximal tubulopathy, there may be subnormal activity of the renal 1-α-hydroxylase enzyme.[40]

Sufficient substrate must be supplied in the diet for proper bone mineralization. Delayed bone mineralization commonly occurs in very-low-birth-weight, premature infants who are fed normal infant formulas or breast milk,[41] both of which contain insufficient quantities of calcium and phosphorus for the rapid bone mineralization of premature infants.

Drug-induced osteomalacia. Prolonged administration of *heparin* has been associated with osteoporosis and decreased bone density. The incidence of heparin-induced osteopenia is unknown. It appears that an individual has to receive a dose of at least 15,000 units/day for 6 months before osteopenia occurs. The symptoms are nonspecific and basically manifest as back pain and vertebral fractures and are reversible after withdrawal of heparin. *Methotrexate* is a commonly used antineoplastic agent, particularly in child-

Pathological Forms of Renal Osteodystrophy

Predominant osteitis fibrosa
    Normal serum calcium level—calcitriol responsive
    Pretreatment hypercalcemia—exacerbated by calcitriol
Predominant osteomalacia
    Small amount of fibrosis present—calcitriol responsive
    Pure osteomalacia—hypercalcemia with calcitriol treatment
Mixed osteitis fibrosa and osteomalacia—calcitriol responsive
Mild—calcitriol responsive

hood leukemias. It has been shown to decrease osteoblastic activity in animals and to increase bone resorption in humans. Consequently, prolonged use of this agent may induce osteopenia.

Osteitis fibrosa

Osteitis fibrosa is the histopathological bone lesion produced by excessive parathyroid hormone secretion. It is primarily seen in two conditions, primary hyperparathyroidism and chronic renal failure. Bone disease is of lesser significance in primary hyperparathyroidism because surgical removal of the involved parathyroid glands cures the disease. The pathophysiological condition of secondary hyperparathyroidism associated with chronic renal failure is more complex and less amenable to treatment. Thus uremic patients frequently suffer from severe bone disease.

The complex bone abnormality associated with chronic renal failure is termed *renal osteodystrophy*. Two distinct histopathological forms of renal osteodystrophy, osteomalacia, and osteitis fibrosa (see box), frequently coexist in the same patient. Osteomalacia is probably caused by decreased synthesis of calcitriol secondary to renal parenchymal disease. Serum concentrations of calcitriol and 24,25-dihydroxyvitamin D are decreased in both children and adults with chronic renal failure, and calcidiol concentrations are normal.[42] Factors that contribute to secondary hyperparathyroidism of renal disease include (1) decreased phosphorus excretion and hyperphosphatemia, which directly decreases renal calcitriol synthesis (Figs. 28-7 and 28-8), (2) decreased renal hydroxylase activity because of renal damage, (3) a higher set point for PTH secretion in uremia possibly because of a decrease in the number of vitamin D receptors in parathyroid cells, (4) hypocalcemia, and (5) skeletal resistance to PTH.

Paget's disease

Paget's disease is a disorder of bone metabolism characterized by increased osteoclastic bone resorption followed by disordered bone formation. The incidence of this disease is difficult to determine because the majority of affected patients are asymptomatic. The incidence of Paget's disease varies with age and geographic location. It is more com-

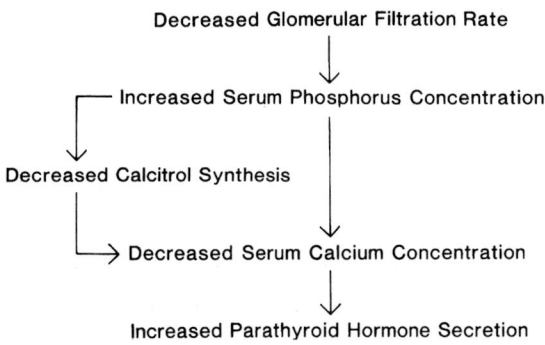

Fig. 28-7 Pathogenetic mechanism of secondary hyperparathyroidism in renal failure according to phosphate theory.

mon among elderly than among middle-aged people. In an autopsy series of persons over 40 years of age, 3% of this group is affected. Family history is positive in 14% of cases. Males are more prone to have the disease than females (3:2). The disease occurs more frequently among people of European ancestry. It is uncommon among Scandinavians, Asians, and black Africans. The cause of the disease is unknown.

The histological pattern of patients with Paget's disease proceeds through three stages. In the early phase of the illness, resorption predominates and the bone marrow is replaced with a highly vascular fibrous connective tissue. In the second phase of the disease, bone formation predominates. The pagetic bone is coarse-fibered, dense trabecular bone. In the final phase the rate of bone resorption declines, and continued bone formation produces hard, dense bone. The largest amount of bone resorption that initially occurs produces greatly elevated urinary hydroxyproline concentrations, and the subsequent rapid rate of bone formation results in dramatically elevated serum alkaline phosphatase concentrations. Serum calcium and phosphorus concentrations are normal. However, pathological fractures occur and are treated by immobilization of the patient. Hypercalcemia

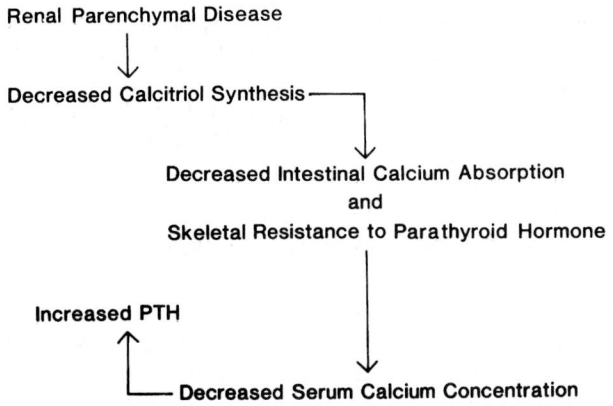

Fig. 28-8 Pathogenetic mechanism of secondary hyperparathyroidism in renal failure according to vitamin D theory.

frequently occurs because immobilization increases the rate of bone resorption. Paget's disease is treated successfully with calcitonin, which inhibits osteoclastic bone resorption.[45]

Heritable bone disease

Hypophosphatasia. Hypophosphatasia is a rare heritable bone disease characterized by generalized reduction in alkaline phosphatase activity in liver, bone, and kidney tissues. Placental and intestinal alkaline phosphatase isoenzyme activities remain normal. The disease occurs in all races but is especially common among Mennonites in Canada, where the incidence is up to 1 per 100,000 live births. Clinically, the disease affects bone and dentition and ranges from a severe, lethal in utero form to an asymptomatic adult disease. Four clinical forms of the disease are known: *perinatal (lethal) form,* commonly associated with stillbirth and polyhydramnios; *infantile form,* usually seen during the first 6 months of life; *childhood form;* and the *adult form,* usually appearing in middle age.

Osteogenesis imperfecta. The condition osteogenesis imperfecta is a heritable disorder of connective tissue involving abnormal synthesis of type I collagen fibers, the most abundant protein in bone matrix. The prime clinical manifestations of this disease are pronounced bone fragility, generalized osteopenia, and recurrent fractures in response to mild trauma. Hearing loss, which occurs in about 50% of patients less than 30 years of age, is most often conductive and rarely sensorineural. The pathogenesis of the disease involves defective mutations in the genes coding for pro–alpha 1 and pro–alpha 2 chains of type I collagen, resulting in bone fragility.

Osteopetrosis. Osteopetrosis encompasses a group of diseases characterized by failure of osteoclast-mediated bone resorption. The mechanism of osteoclast malfunction is poorly understood. The disease is classified into eight types according to clinical and genetic factors. The main two forms of osteopetrosis are a more common benign type, often asymptomatic and inherited as an autosomal dominant mode, and the rare malignant form, which typically presents in infancy and childhood and is inherited in an autosomal recessive mode. Rare forms of osteopetrosis may be associated with renal tubular acidosis, carbonic anhydrase deficiency, or neuronal storage disease.

CHANGE OF ANALYTE IN DISEASE
Vitamin D

Serum concentrations of vitamin D metabolites may be altered in a variety of disease states (see box). Decreased concentrations result from deficient intake, defective metabolic regulation, or increased excretion. Serum calcidiol concentrations are low in patients who have both an insufficient exposure to sunlight and a low intake of foods that contain vitamin D. Patients who receive anticonvulsant drugs convert calcidiol into biologically inactive polar metabolites.[35]

Diseases and Conditions Associated with Changes in Serum Concentrations of Vitamin D Metabolites
Calcidiol (25-hydroxycholecalciferol) deficiency
Nutritional osteomalacia
Anticonvulsant-induced osteomalacia
Liver disease
Nephrotic syndrome
Calcitriol (1,25-dihydroxycholecalciferol) deficiency
Vitamin D–dependent rickets type I
Postmenopausal and senile osteoporosis
Hypoparathyroidism
Pseudohypoparathyroidism
Vitamin D–resistant rickets
Nephrotic syndrome
Calcidiol (25-hydroxycholecalciferol) excess
Vitamin D intoxication
Excessive sunlight exposure
Calcitriol (1,25-hydroxycholecalciferol) excess
Childhood
Pregnancy and lactation
Sarcoidosis
Hyperparathyroidism

Production of calcidiol is impaired in patients with liver disease.[46] Inactive or absent renal 1α-hydroxylase activity and secondary low serum calcitriol concentrations are associated with vitamin D–dependent rickets type I,[36] postmenopausal and senile osteoporosis,[28-33] hypoparathyroidism,[47] pseudohypoparathyroidism,[48a] vitamin D–resistant rickets,[36-39] and chronic renal failure.[48b] Patients with nephrotic syndrome have low serum concentrations of both calcidiol and calcitriol because of urinary losses of both metabolites, as well as the serum protein (vitamin D–binding protein) to which they are attached.[49]

High serum calcidiol concentrations result from either increased exogenous intake or increased endogenous production secondary to an unusually large sunlight exposure. High serum calcitriol concentrations occur in physiological states of increased calcium requirements such as growth[50] and pregnancy and lactation.[51] High serum calcitriol concentrations are also seen in sarcoidosis, in which an extrarenal source of calcitriol production has been implicated, and in hyperparathyroidism, in which the serum concentrations of PTH, a major stimulus for calcitriol production, are elevated.

Parathyroid hormone

Hypoparathyroidism

Primary Idiopathic hypoparathyroidism. *Idiopathic hypoparathyroidism* describes the condition of a decreased production of PTH whose cause is not known. In pseudohypoparathyroidism, production of PTH is intact, but there is target organ resistance to PTH; in other words, PTH, though

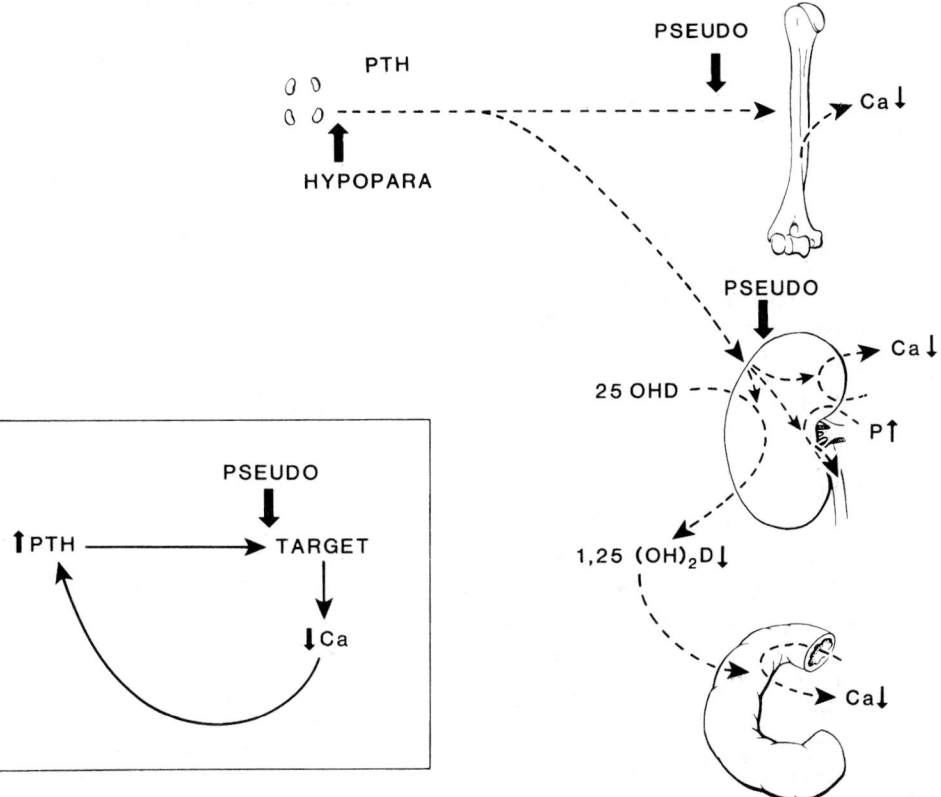

Fig. 28-9 In idiopathic hypoparathyroidism, decreased parathyroid hormone results in decreased serum calcium, increased serum phosphorus, and decreased production of 1,25-dihydroxy-vitamin D. In pseudohypoparathyroidism, although there is sufficient hormone, target organs are unresponsive and biochemical result is similar. *Inset,* In pseudohypoparathyroidism, resultant low serum calcium concentrations serve as a stimulus to parathyroid hormone production. Since parathyroid glands are intact, in contrast to idiopathic hypoparathyroidism, serum parathyroid hormone concentrations will be *elevated* in an attempt to overcome target organ resistance and rectify hypocalcemia.

present, does not exert its physiological actions because the target organs are not responsive. In current terminology, there may be a "receptor defect" for PTH. Another way of describing idiopathic hypoparathyroidism would be *hormone-deficient hypoparathyroidism,* and pseudohypoparathyroidism would be described as *hormone-sufficient, receptor-deficient hypoparathyroidism* (Fig. 28-9). Hypoparathyroidism classically manifests itself with hypocalcemia and hyperphosphatemia, usually in childhood.

Secondary hypoparathyroidism. Hypoparathyroidism may result from other disorders. Inadvertent surgical removal of the parathyroids may occur during thyroidectomy. Since magnesium is important for PTH secretion, magnesium deficiency may result in hypoparathyroidism. An interesting physiological hypoparathyroidism occurs in infants. In utero, calcium is transferred actively across the placenta, and serum calcium concentrations in the fetus are extremely high. These high serum calcium concentrations appear to inhibit fetal parathyroid function. Inhibited parathyroid function persists for a short interval after birth and

appears to be a cause of hypocalcemia in the first 3 days of life, especially in the premature infant.[48a]

The diagnosis of hypoparathyroidism is made from the clinical presentation of lowered serum calcium and elevated serum phosphorus concentrations. PTH concentrations will be low in hypoparathyroidism but elevated in pseudohypoparathyroidism. To further distinguish idiopathic hypoparathyroidism from pseudohypoparathyroidism, PTH infusion is administered. After the infusion, serum calcium and urinary phosphorus and cAMP concentrations are measured. Patients with pseudohypoparathyroidism may have varying "degrees of block" in response to PTH, at the bone site or at various "levels" in the kidney.[52] Patients with hypoparathyroidism are treated with supplements of calcium salts and calcitriol.

Hyperparathyroidism

Primary hyperparathyroidism. Primary hyperparathyroidism is often described as being related to hyperplasia or adenoma of the parathyroids. In contrast to hypoparathyroidism, which usually begins in childhood, hyperparathyroidism is usually discovered in adulthood. As expected from the physiological action of PTH, excess concentrations of the hormone result in increased serum calcium concentrations and decreased serum phosphorus concentrations. Demineralization occurs as a consequence of the bone lytic action of PTH and is associated with areas of extensive resorption (osteitis fibrosa, see p. 541). Many clinical problems are associated with the high serum calcium concentrations. The major organ systems adversely affected by hypercalcemia are the nervous system and the kidney.

Secondary hyperparathyroidism. Conditions that are associated with chronic hypocalcemia will result in chronic stimulation of the parathyroids and secondary hyperparathyroidism. The two major factors resulting in chronic hypocalcemia of nonparathyroid cause are vitamin D–metabolite deficiencies and high phosphorus loads. Any deficiency of vitamin D or its major metabolites will result in decreased intestinal absorption of calcium and hypocalcemia. The initial response to this hypocalcemia will be secondary hyperparathyroidism, which helps maintain serum calcium concentrations in the normal range. High phosphorus loads occur with infusion of phosphorus-containing fluids, ingestion of high phosphorus-containing milk (such as cow milk given to newborn infants), or retention of phosphorus by failing kidneys. High serum phosphorus concentrations result in a secondary decrease in serum calcium concentrations. With decreased serum calcium concentrations there is compensatory secondary hyperparathyroidism.[53]

The diagnosis of primary hyperparathyroidism is based on the findings of high serum calcium, low serum phosphorus, and high serum PTH concentrations. However, not all hyperparathyroid patients will have increased serum calcium concentrations or increased serum PTH concentrations. Ionized calcium measurements in blood may provide additional diagnostic help because the ionized calcium fraction is the physiologically active calcium.

In secondary hyperparathyroidism, serum calcium concentrations are low or normal because the parathyroid overactivity results from an initial decline in serum calcium. Serum phosphorus concentrations would be low except in situations of phosphorus overload, when they would be high. Serum PTH concentrations should be elevated in secondary hyperparathyroidism.

Calcium (see p. 549)

Hypercalcemia. Hypercalcemia resulting from primary hyperparathyroidism has been described earlier. Other causes of hypercalcemia are listed in the box.

Endocrine and tumor-related hypercalcemia. Hypercalcemia may occur with disorders of endocrine organs other than the parathyroids. Overproduction of thyroid hormone (thyrotoxicosis) and underproduction of corticosteroids (Addison's disease or abrupt withdrawal of steroid hormones) are associated with hypercalcemia. A wide variety of tumors appear to produce PTH-like substances with

---

Causes of Hypercalcemia
Primary hyperparathyroidism
Thyrotoxicosis
Addison's disease
Withdrawal of steroids
Tumors
Vitamin D and vitamin A intoxication
Sarcoidosis
Idiopathic hypercalcemia of infancy
Immobilization
Subcutaneous fat necrosis in infants
Thiazide diuretics
Milk-alkali syndrome
Benign familial hypercalcemia

---

osteoclast-stimulatory activity, which results in hypercalcemia. Hypercalcemia and hyperparathyroidism are sometimes associated with *pheochromocytoma* or multiple endocrine neoplasia type II syndrome. Pancreatic *VIPoma* tumors secrete vasoactive intestinal peptide (VIP), which causes severe diarrhea. About 50% of these cases have hypercalcemia possibly because of VIP-induced bone resorption. The mechanism of hypercalcemia in malignancy may, in part, be the result of the production of PTHRP (humoral hypercalcemia of malignancy), $1,25(OH)_2D$ in lymphoma, lymphotoxin in multiple myeloma, or other substances that cause bone resorption.

Vitamin A– and vitamin D–related disorders. Excessive intake of vitamin A or vitamin D may result in hypercalcemia. Hypercalcemia may be a feature of granulomatous diseases such as *tuberculosis* and *sarcoidosis,* which are associated with abnormal vitamin D metabolism and increased serum levels of $1,25(OH)_2D$. In sarcoidosis, elevated calcitriol concentrations appear to be the cause of the hypercalcemia. Vitamin A in high doses appears to have a direct effect on bone resorption. Therapy for vitamin D–resistant rickets or hypoparathyroidism with high doses of vitamin D is a common cause of hypercalcemia. Idiopathic hypercalcemia of infants is believed to be related to disordered vitamin D metabolism, possibly increased sensitivity to vitamin D.[54]

Iatrogenic causes. Immobilization of patients, especially male adolescents, results in rapid mobilization of calcium from bone and resultant hypercalcemia. Lactation causes a transient increase in bone resorption and secondary hypercalcemia, reversed by weaning. In infants born after traumatic deliveries, a curious condition of hypercalcemia can occur related to subcutaneous fat necrosis. Use of thiazide diuretics is classically associated with hypercalcemia. *Thiazides* act directly to increase calcium release from the skeleton and promote renal tubular reabsorption of calcium. Chronic *lithium* intake may cause hyperparathyroidism and mild hypercalcemia and hypermagnesemia. Excessive ingestion of milk and alkali in the treatment of peptic ulcer (the milk-alkali syndrome) also results in hypercalcemia.

Neonatal hypercalcemia (total serum calcium concentration >110 mg/L or serum ionized calcium concentration >58 mg/L) can be the result of prolonged *maternal hypocalcemia* resulting from a multitude of causes. Consequently a variable degree of congenital, transient hyperparathyroidism results. Neonatal hypercalcemia in the *phosphorus-deficiency syndrome* has been reported in preterm infants fed human milk.

Familial form. There is a benign form of familial hypercalcemia that is inherited as a dominant trait. Mild hypercalcemia (less than 130 mg/L) occurs and apparently is without adverse effects.

Hypocalcemia. The causes of hypocalcemia are currently classified in relation to the major hormone or biochemical involved: vitamin D, PTH, calcitonin, calcium, magnesium, and phosphate (see box at right).

Vitamin D deficiency, which has been covered earlier, occurs as a result of reduced synthesis or intake of the parent vitamin D, altered hepatic metabolism of vitamin D, and decreased renal synthesis of calcitriol, the final active metabolite of vitamin D.

Hypoparathyroidism (primary and secondary) and pseudohypoparathyroidism have been discussed previously. Calcitonin or mithramycin infusions will decrease calcium transport from bone to extracellular space and result in hypocalcemia. Intestinal malabsorption of calcium may lead to hypocalcemia. Acute pancreatitis is associated with fatty acid–calcium complex precipitates in the pancreas and hypocalcemia. Decreased blood ionized calcium occurs with infusion of agents complexing calcium (citrate and acid-citrated blood for transfusion, or EDTA), or alkalosis, which shifts the fraction of calcium that is ionized to that which is protein bound. Hypomagnesemia results in hypocalcemia mostly related to the adverse effect of hypomagnesemia on parathyroid function. Conditions whereby phosphorus concentrations in blood are elevated, as in renal failure (see earlier discussion), phosphate infusion, or infants receiving cow milk formulas with their high phosphate content, will result in decreased serum calcium concentrations because calcium is shifted from the extracellular space into bone and soft tissues and probably because there is a blunted bone response to the effects of PTH.[55]

Neonatal hypocalcemia is defined as a total serum calcium concentration of less than 70 mg/L for preterm infants or 80 mg/L for term infants (serum ionized calcium concentration less than 44 mg/L). Neonatal hypocalcemia is the direct result of the relatively high PTH set point (see p. 535) established in the fetus. After birth, this PTH set point is lowered, with a commensurate lowering of serum calcium. At birth, termination of the high transplacental calcium influx to the fetus can result in a transient hypocalcemia.

Prematurity is the major cause of neonatal hypocalcemia, which may develop in a large proportion (30% to 90%) of

---

Causes of Hypocalcemia

Vitamin D
  Decreased solar exposure and endogenous synthesis
  Decreased intestinal intake (malabsorption, dietary deficiency)
  Altered hepatic metabolism of vitamin D (hepatic disease, anticonvulsant therapy)
  Decreased renal synthesis of calcitriol (vitamin D dependency, renal failure)
Parathyroid
  Hypoparathyroidism (primary and secondary)
  Pseudohypoparathyroidism
Calcitonin
  Calcitonin or mithramycin infusion
Calcium
  Intestinal malabsorption
  Acute pancreatitis
  Infusion of agents complexing calcium
  Alkalosis decreasing ionized calcium
Magnesium
  Magnesium deficiency (see box, p. 547)
Phosphorus
  Renal failure
  Phosphate infusion
  Cow milk formulas

---

preterm infants. The incidence of hypocalcemia correlates inversely with gestational age and birth weight. Its cause is uncertain. About 30% of infants with *birth asphyxia* may develop hypocalcemia in the neonatal period.

Parathyroid gland adenoma is the most common cause of *maternal hyperparathyroidism* and hypercalcemia. Maternal hypercalcemia suppresses the fetal parathyroid glands, resulting in transient neonatal, or congenital, hypoparathyroidism. At least 50% of infants born to hyperparathyroid mothers present with hypocalcemic tetany.

Mothers with *insulin-dependent diabetes mellitus* have excessive urinary magnesium losses, especially if euglycemia is not maintained. Consequently, these mothers, and theoretically their fetuses, may be magnesium depleted. *Hypomagnesemia* impairs PTH secretion and may explain the transient neonatal hypoparathyroidism and hypocalcemia that may develop in about 50% of infants of diabetic mothers.

Hypocalcemia in infants born to mothers with gestational exposure to *anticonvulsant* therapy may be related to the effect of phenobarbital or phenytoin in enhancing accelerated hepatic metabolism of 25(OH)D (see p. 539). Hypocalcemia has also been described in a few infants born to hypercalcemic women with familial hypocalciuric hypercalcemia.

Changes in parathyroid hormone: vitamin D–axis analytes in hypercalcemia and hypocalcemia. Changes in the serum concentrations of phosphorus, the PTH–vitamin D axis, and vitamin D status help in evalua-

Table 28-3   Parathyroid hormone–vitamin D axis analytes in hypercalcemia

| Disorder | Serum phosphorus | Parathyroid hormone (PTH) | Parathyroid hormone–vitamin D axis | | Vitamin D status |
			Nephrogenous cyclic AMP	Calcitriol (1,25-dihydroxycholecalciferol)	Calcidiol (25-hydroxycholecalciferol)
Hyperparathyroidism	LO	HI	HI	HI	NL
Vitamin D disorders					
Vitamin D intoxication	NL	LO	LO	HI or NL	HI
High calcitriol in sarcoidosis	NL	LO	LO	HI	NL
Sensitivity to vitamin D: idiopathic hypercalcemia of infancy	NL	LO	LO	NL	NL
Non–parathyroid hormone, non–vitamin D disorders					
Malignancy	NL	LO	HI/LO	LO or HI	NL
Immobilization	NL	LO	LO	LO	NL
Thyrotoxicosis	NL	LO	NL	LO	NL

HI, Increased; *LO,* decreased; *NL,* normal.

tion of the causes of hypercalcemia and hypocalcemia. If the PTH–vitamin D axis is intact, two effects are seen: (1) cAMP production by the kidney is active; renal cAMP is best determined as "nephrogenous" cAMP, which takes into account the cAMP not produced in the kidney,[56] and (2) 1,25-dihydroxycholecalciferol (calcitriol) production is also active (Tables 28-3 and 28-4).

Of the *hypercalcemic* disorders listed in Table 28-3, serum phosphorus concentrations are decreased in hyperparathyroidism because of the phosphaturic effects of PTH; in the remaining hypercalcemic disorders, little effect on serum phosphorus is evident. In hyperparathyroidism, serum PTH concentrations and the PTH–vitamin D axis analytes are increased. In hypercalcemia from other causes, serum

PTH is suppressed. In turn the PTH–vitamin D axis may be suppressed, except in sarcoidosis, in which elevation of serum calcitriol concentrations appears to be a primary problem.

Vitamin D status is best assessed through measurement of serum 25-hydroxycholecalciferol (calcidiol) concentrations. Thus serum 25-hydroxycholecalciferol concentrations are elevated in vitamin D intoxication, with or without elevations in the serum 1,25-dihydroxycholecalciferol (calcitriol) concentrations.

In *hypocalcemia* (Table 28-4) related to parathyroid disorders, hypoparathyroidism or pseudohypoparathyroidism, serum phosphorus is elevated because of decreased urinary phosphorus excretion. The PTH–vitamin D axis is gen-

Table 28-4   Parathyroid hormone–vitamin D axis analytes in hypocalcemia

| Disorder | Serum phosphorus | Parathyroid hormone (PTH) | Parathyroid hormone–vitamin D axis | | Vitamin D status |
			Nephrogenous cyclic AMP	Calcitriol (1,25-dihydroxycholecalciferol)	Calcidiol (25-hydroxycholecalciferol)
Parathyroid disorders					
Hypoparathyroidism	HI	LO	LO	LO	NL
Pseudohypoparathyroidism	HI	HI	LO	LO	NL
Vitamin D disorders					
Vitamin D deficiency	LO	HI	HI	HI*; NL or LO	LO
Hepatic disease and anticonvulsant therapy	LO	HI	HI	NL or LO	LO
Renal					
Vitamin D–dependent rickets	LO	HI	HI	LO	NL
Osteodystrophy	HI	HI	—	LO	NL
Resistance to 1,25-dihydroxycholecalciferol	LO	HI	HI	HI	NL
Mineral disorders					
Calcium malabsorption	NL	NL or HI	—	—	—
Hypomagnesemia	NL	LO, NL, or HI	—	—	NL
High phosphate load	HI	NL or HI	—	—	NL

HI, Increased; *LO,* decreased; *NL,* normal.
*Especially in childhood.

Causes of Hypermagnesemia
Magnesium sulfate therapy Magnesium-containing antacids and purgatives Renal failure

Causes of Hypomagnesemia

Decreased intake of magnesium
   Steatorrhea
   Malabsorption syndromes
   Gut resections
   Specific intestinal malabsorption of magnesium
   Protein-calorie malnutrition
Increased loss of magnesium
   Renal tubular loss
   Dialysis with low magnesium dialysate
   Hyperaldosteronism
   Hyperparathyroidism
   Diabetes mellitus
   Alcoholism
   Diuretic therapy
   Aminoglycoside therapy

erally hypofunctioning, except in pseudohypoparathyroidism, in which serum PTH concentrations will be elevated because of target-organ resistance to the hormone.

In the vitamin D disorders, serum phosphorus concentrations are generally low because one of the major actions of vitamin D is to raise serum phosphorus concentrations. However, in renal osteodystrophy (renal failure) serum phosphorus concentrations are elevated because of decreased renal phosphorus excretion. The PTH-cAMP axis in this circumstance may be increased because of hyperparathyroidism secondary to hypocalcemia; however, serum 1,25-dihydroxycholecalciferol concentrations will remain decreased because of deficiency of vitamin D or blocks in vitamin D metabolism. In the condition of increased resistance to 1,25-dihydroxycholecalciferol, high serum concentrations of the metabolite are found, analogous to elevated PTH concentrations in pseudohypoparathyroidism. Serum 25-hydroxycholecalciferol measurements will be low in vitamin D deficiency or when there is a block in 25-hydroxylation of vitamin D but normal in vitamin D disorders caused by metabolic blocks beyond the liver step of hydroxylation.

In the mineral disorders causing hypocalcemia, little effect on the PTH–vitamin D axis has been reported. Secondary hyperparathyroidism can be a consequence of hypocalcemia. In hypomagnesemia, however, hypoparathyroidism can occur secondary to the magnesium deficiency.

Magnesium (see p. 550)

Hypermagnesemia. Excess of magnesium is usually a consequence of increased medicinal intake of magnesium. Magnesium ($MgSO_4$) is used in the treatment of hypertension induced by pregnancy (preeclampsia). The mother will become hypermagnesemic (up to 110 mg/L), as will her infant. Recent clinical studies demonstrated the apparent benefits of maternal magnesium supplementation in reducing the incidence of preterm labor and allowing greater fetal growth. Reduced magnesium excretion may occur in severe renal failure, and the use of medicines that contain magnesium (antacids, purgatives) in this situation may result in hypermagnesemia[57] (see box above).

Hypomagnesemia and magnesium deficiency. Severe magnesium deficiency in humans is uncommon, possibly because of the body's highly developed ability to conserve magnesium. Decreased uptake of magnesium caused by gastrointestinal disorders (steatorrhea, malabsorption

syndromes, gut resections) can cause magnesium deficiency. Specific intestinal malabsorption of magnesium also occurs and can cause hypomagnesemia in infancy. Protein-calorie malnutrition is often associated with magnesium depletion. Increased urinary magnesium losses may result from generalized renal disease or a specific renal defect in reabsorption of magnesium. Dialysis of patients may result in magnesium depletion if a low magnesium-content dialysate is used. High rates of production of aldosterone (hyperaldosteronism), hyperparathyroidism, and diabetes mellitus cause increased urinary magnesium losses. Alcoholism, intensive diuretic therapy, and treatment with the antibiotic gentamycin also result in increased urinary magnesium losses[58] (see box above).

Magnesium deficiency is often associated with hypocalcemia, and the signs and symptoms of magnesium deficiency normally are the signs of hypocalcemia. Although serum magnesium concentrations can be low, since magnesium is predominantly an intracellular mineral, serum measurements may not reflect intracellular concentrations. Red blood cell magnesium concentrations have been advocated as a measure of intracellular magnesium status.

Phosphate (see p. 551)

Hyperphosphatemia. Hyperphosphatemia is most often the result of decreased renal excretion of phosphate anions as encountered in acute or chronic renal failure, particularly when the glomerular filtration rate is reduced to less than 25% of normal. Hyperphosphatemia can also result from an increased body phosphate load, which can in turn result from phosphate-containing laxatives and enemas, blood transfusions, or hyperalimentation, or as the result of massive cell destruction after cell lysis by cytotoxic therapy (the tumor lysis syndrome), or tissue injuries (hyperthermia, hypoxia, or crush injuries), which result in rhabdomyolysis and hemolysis. Increased renal tubular reabsorption of

---

Diseases Associated with Abnormal Serum Calcitonin Concentrations

Excess
    Medullary thyroid carcinoma
    Bronchogenic carcinoma
    Zollinger-Ellison syndrome
    Renal failure
Deficiency
    Thyroid agenesis
    Thyroidectomy
    Osteoporosis

Sources of Alkaline Phosphatase

Osteoblasts
Bile canalicular cells
Placenta
Leukocytes
Proximal renal tubule cells
Active mammary gland

---

phosphate is responsible for the hyperphosphatemia seen in hypoparathyroidism, hyperthyroidism, hypogonadism, and growth hormone excess.

Hypophosphatemia. Moderate hypophosphatemia, which is defined as a serum phosphorus concentration between 10 and 25 mg/L in adults, is usually asymptomatic. In children, serum phosphorus concentrations below 40 mg/L are often considered abnormal. Hypophosphatemia may be caused by decreased intestinal absorption of phosphate or by increased urine losses of phosphate and an endogenous shift of inorganic phosphorus from extracellular to intracellular fluid compartments.

Calcitonin

Abnormal serum calcitonin concentrations are rarely found (see top box). Serum measurements are most useful in patients suspected of having medullary thyroid carcinoma, a malignancy of the thyroid C-cells. This cancer is frequently seen in different members within families and is often associated with a tendency for other malignancies (termed *multiple endocrine neoplasia syndrome type II*).[59] Serum calcitonin measurements are useful both in the screening of family members who are potentially at risk of developing the disease and in the follow-up examination of previously treated patients suspected of recurrent metastatic disease. Serum calcitonin elevations are produced by a wide variety of other neoplasias, the most frequent one being bronchogenic carcinoma.[60] Because gastrin is a potent stimulus for calcitonin secretion, serum calcitonin concentrations are el-

evated in Zollinger-Ellison syndrome, a pancreatic tumor of gastrin-secreting cells. Finally, calcitonin excretion is decreased in patients with renal failure, and that decrease results in secondary elevation of serum concentrations of calcitonin in these patients.

Because the thyroid gland is usually the sole source of calcitonin production, athyroid patients lack circulating calcitonin. Calcitonin levels are also decreased in some patients with osteoporosis. This may be caused by altered regulation of calcitonin synthesis or release.[61]

Alkaline phosphatase (ALP) (see p. 521)

In clinical practice, ALP determinations measure a group of enzymes that catalyze the hydrolysis of phosphate esters in an alkaline medium.[62] Alkaline phosphatase is produced by many tissues (see lower left box), but only the portion produced by bone and liver is usually detected in serum from healthy persons. The box below lists causes of abnormal serum bone alkaline phosphatase concentrations. Note that ALP lacks sensitivity and specificity for bone disease, particularly in patients with osteoporosis, when serum ALP is usually within reference ranges. Alkaline phosphatase is produced by osteoblasts and, as previously discussed, lowers bone pyrophosphate levels, which probably facilitates mineralization. Alkaline phosphatase synthesis is deficient in hypophosphatasia, a rare hereditary illness associated with undermineralized bones and pathological fractures, and achondroplasia, an inherited disorder of endochondral bone growth. Production is also decreased with generalized malnutrition or scurvy.

Far more common than decreased concentrations are diseases associated with elevated bone serum alkaline phosphatase concentrations. Such elevations signify increased osteoblastic activity, as seen in osteoblastic sarcoma, rickets, Paget's disease, and acromegaly. The elevated levels associated with hyperparathyroidism result from secondary bone mineralization rather than PTH-induced osteoclastic activity. One should exercise caution when considering the

---

Bone Diseases Associated with Abnormal Serum Alkaline Phosphatase Concentrations

Deficiency
    Hypophosphatasia
    Achondroplasia
    Severe malnutrition
    Scurvy
Excess
    Osteoblastic sarcoma
    Ostemalacia
    Paget's disease
    Hyperparathyroidism
    Growing children

Conditions Associated with Elevated Urinary Hydroxyproline Concentrations	
Paget's disease	Acromegaly
Osteomalacia	Rheumatoid arthritis
Neoplastic bone disease	Osteoporosis
Hyperthyroidism	Aseptic bone necrosis
Osteomyelitis	Chronic renal failure
Burns	

pathological significance of alkaline phosphatase increases in childhood because growth is an important physiological cause of such elevations.[63] Liver alkaline phosphatase elevations reflect biliary obstruction and do not occur to any great extent with pure hepatocellular disease (see p. 514).

Osteocalcin

Clinically, serum osteocalcin concentration is elevated in bone diseases characterized by increased osteoblastic activity including Paget's disease, osteomalacia, osteitis fibrosa, and renal osteodystrophy. Serum osteocalcin levels in these diseases correlate with other markers of bone formation, such as serum alkaline phosphatase and bone histomorphometry. Decreased serum concentrations of PTH, thyroid hormone, or growth hormone are associated with a decrease in the serum osteocalcin concentration, whereas the reverse is true; hyperparathyroidism, thyroxicosis, and acromegaly are associated with elevated serum osteocalcin concentrations. Puberty is associated with a rise in serum osteocalcin concentration, consistent with the increase in osteoblastic activity that accompanies the pubertal growth spurt and gonadal hormone surges. Circadian variation in serum osteocalcin concentration (peak levels at 4 A.M. and nadir at 5 P.M.) as well as in other serum markers of bone formation and resorption have been reported, but the etiology and physiological implications of these observations are unknown.[32]

Hydroxyproline (HP)

Collagen, which is present predominantly in bone and skin, is the sole source of the amino acid hydroxyproline, which, together with proline, makes up approximately one third of the total amino acid content of collagen. Collagen digestion, associated with either bone or skin breakdown, results in elevated urinary hydroxyproline (UHP) concentrations (see box above).[64] However, the determination of UHP concentration is not a specific test because sources of hydroxyproline include bone, diet, connective tissues, serum proteins, and degradation of propeptides from collagen biosynthesis. UHP correlates poorly with bone resorption as assessed by bone histomorphometric and calcium kinetic studies.[27]

METHODS OF ANALYSIS

Calcium

STEVEN C. KAZMIERCZAK

Principles of analysis Methods for calcium analysis in biological fluids can be divided into techniques of precipitation, chelation, or atomic absorption spectrophotometry. The historical methods for determination of total serum calcium (Ca) concentration were precipitation procedures. These include the method of Clark and Collip[65] (Table 28-5, method 1) and the calcium chloranilate and calcium naphthyl hydroxamate procedures (Table 28-5, method 2). Quantitation of the precipitated Ca in the Clark and Collip procedure was by titration, whereas the latter techniques were colorimetric assays.

Sensitive fluorescent methods[66] for analysis of calcium in serum or urine have the advantage of requiring small sample volumes. In one method, calcium is added to an alkaline solution containing calcein (Table 28-5, method 3). Calcium and calcein form a complex that at high pH fluoresces at 520 nm (excitation at 490 nm). The fluorescent complex is titrated with ethylene glycol-bis(β-aminoethyl ether)-N,N'-tetraacetic acid (EGTA). This complex binds the calcium from the complex with a resulting decrease in fluorescence. The volume of EGTA required to titrate the complex is directly proportional to the concentration of calcium. Magnesium and phosphate reportedly do not interfere with this method.

The use of specific calcium-binding compounds provide the basis of most routine methods in use today. The most widely used of these binding compounds is cresolphthalein complexone. The cresolphthalein complexone forms a red complex at a pH of 10 to 12 (Table 28-5, method 4). Interference by magnesium is eliminated by the addition of 8-hydroxyquinoline to the reaction mixture.[67] Potassium cyanide may also be added to the reaction mixture to stabilize the red complex and to eliminate interference from heavy metals. Dialysis of the sample with an acidic solution to release bound calcium and to reduce interference from serum protein was also used on some systems (Table 28-5, method 4b). Arsenazo III dye, an indicator that similarly changes color after complexing with calcium, is another frequently used Ca-complexing agent. Citrate has been reported to cause significant decreases in calcium concentrations in some systems that use this indicator.[68]

A highly sensitive and specific method for measurement of calcium is atomic absorption spectroscopy[69,70] (Table 28-5, method 5). This technique measures the amount of light that is absorbed by free calcium atoms at a characteristic wavelength (422.7 nm). Calcium is dissociated from protein and inorganic complexes by a variety of techniques. Acid is used to dissociate protein-bound calcium, and lanthanum or strontium ions are added to displace calcium from phosphate, oxalate, citrate, sulfate, and other calcium chelators. Interference from other elements such as magnesium is reduced by the use of the specific atomic absorption line of calcium at 422.7 nm. See pp. 95 for more detail on this technique.

The definitive method for calcium measurements is isotope-dilution mass spectroscopy (Table 28-5, method 6). This method, available in only a few institutions, is the ac-

Table 28-5   Methods of chloride measurement

Method	Principle	Usage	Comments
1. Precipitation by oxalate and redox titration	$Ca^{++} + Oxalate \rightarrow Ca\ oxalate\ (ppt)$ $Ca\ oxalate\ (ppt) + H_2SO_4 \rightarrow Oxalate + CaSO_4$ $2KMnO_4 + 5\ Oxalate + 3H_2SO_4 \xrightarrow{70°C} K_2SO_4 + 2MnSO_4 + 10CO_2 + 8H_2O$	Historical	Initial reference method
2. Precipitation by colored anions; spectrophotometric	$Ca^{++} + Chloranilate \rightarrow Ca\ chloranilate\ (ppt)$ $Ca\ chloranilate\ (ppt) + EDTA \xrightarrow{OH^-} Ca\ EDTA + Chloranilic\ acid\ (purple)$	Historical	Labor intensive, imprecise; many other dyes available
3. Titration of fluorescent Ca++ complex	$Ca^{++} + Calcein \rightarrow Ca\text{-}calcein\ (fluorescent)$ $EGTA + Ca\text{-}calcein \rightarrow Ca^+\text{-}EGTA + Calcein\ (decreased\ fluorescence)$	Stat. or small labs	Small sample size, dedicated instrument
4. Spectrophotometric measurement of Ca++ complexes			
a. Direct	$Ca^{++} + o\text{-}Cresolphthalein \xrightarrow{OH^-} Red\ complex\ (520\ nm)$	Most common	Early adapted to a variety of automated instruments; positive bias compared to atomic absorption
b. Indirect	$Ca^{++}\ complex + H^+ \xrightarrow{Dialysis} Ca^{++}\ in\ recipient\ stream$ $(Ca^{++}\ detected\ as\ in\ 4a)$	On Technicon AutoAnalyzer	
5. Atomic absorption	$Ca^{++} \xrightarrow{2e^-} Ca^0$ $Photon + Ca^0 \rightarrow Ca^*$	Reference method	Excellent accuracy and sensitivity
6. Isotope-dilution	Ca and known amount of Ca isotope; isolate Ca^{++} and record ratio of two isotopes on mass spectrometer	Definitive method	Available in reference centers only

Ca*, Calcium atom in excited state; *Ca⁰*, Calcium atom in ground state; *EGTA*, ethylene glycol-bis(β-aminoethyl ether) -N,N'-tetraacetic acid; *ppt*, precipitate.

curacy standard against which all methods must be compared.

Specimen Serum or heparinized plasma should be promptly separated to avoid the uptake of calcium by erythrocytes.[71] Anticoagulants that contain calcium or that would chelate or precipitate calcium, such as EDTA, oxalate, and fluoride, should not be used.[72] Centrifuged samples may be stored at room temperature for up to 8 hours, at 4° C for 1 day, or frozen for up to 1 year.[73] Venous stasis and erect posture can increase calcium by 4 to 6 mg/L.[74]

Calcium in urine can be kept from precipitating or can be redissolved by the addition of 10 mL of 6 M HCl to the collection container. Mix thoroughly.

Reference intervals

Population	Serum Ca mg/L (mmol/L)	Urine Ca mg/24 hr (mmol/24 hr)
Adults		
		Men, <275 (<6.87)
Atomic absorption	80-105 (2.0-2.6)	Women, <250 (<6.25)
		Hypercalcemic, >300 (>7.50)
Cresolphthalein complexone	80-105 (2.0-2.6)	Average diet, 100-250 (2.5-6.25)
Pediatric (by atomic absorption)		
Premature infants	60-100 (1.5-2.5)	
Full-term infants	73-120 (1.8-3.0)	
1 to 2 years	100-120 (2.5-3.0)	

Magnesium
STEVEN C. KAZMIERCZAK

Principles of analysis A variety of methods have been reported for measurement of magnesium[75] including precipitation techniques,[76] complexometric techniques using EDTA,[77] fluorometric assays,[78] and flame photometry.[75] These methods are rarely used today to measure magnesium concentrations. The majority of clinical laboratories utilize colorimetric methods, most frequently employing either calmagite or methylthymol blue as the chromophore. These and other colorimetric methods compare favorably with atomic absorption spectroscopy, which is the reference method for magnesium.[75]

The use of calmagite (1-[1-hydroxy-4-methyl-2-phenyl-azo]-2-naphthol-4-sulfonic acid) was introduced for the direct determination of magnesium without deproteinization[79] (Table 28-6, method 1). In this procedure, magnesium reacts with the blue-colored calmagite reagent forming a pink magnesium-calmagite complex. The color change of the reagent, from blue to a reddish violet, is monitored at 532 nm. Interference from calcium ion is prevented with the use of EGTA, and KCN (potassium cyanide) is used to inhibit the reaction of heavy metals with calmagite. Another colorimetric method for magnesium determinations utilizes the reaction between magnesium and methylthymol blue. The resulting complex is quantitated biochromatically at 510 and 600 nm (Table 28-6, method 2). The specificity of the assay is enhanced by the use of chelators to prevent calcium from interfering in the reaction.

The use of magon and xylidyl blue are other frequently used colorimetric methods for magnesium determina-

Table 28-6   Methods for magnesium analysis

Method	Principle	Usage	Comments
1. Calmagite	Mg^{++} + Calmagite $\rightarrow$ Reddish-violet complex (532 nm)	Most commonly used method	EGTA added to prevent Ca^{++} interference
2. Methylthymol Blue	Mg^{++} + Methylthymol Blue $\rightarrow$ *Complex* (510 and 600 nm)	Frequently used	Chelators added to prevent Ca^{++} interference
3. Chlorophosphonazo III (CPZ)	Mg^{++} + CPZ $\rightarrow$ Mg-CPZ complex $\xrightarrow{EDTA}$ Mg-EDTA + CPZ (550 nm)	Frequently used	Minimal interference from Ca^{++}
4. Ion-selective electrodes (ionized Mg only)	Ionophores selectively bind magnesium, resulting in a potentiometric signal	Infrequently used	Available on some whole blood analyzers

tions.[75,80] Magnesium forms a colored complex with magon under alkaline conditions. The intensity of the color, measured at 520 nm, is proportional to the magnesium concentration of the sample. The xylidyl blue magnesium method is based upon the formation of a red complex of magnesium and xylidyl blue. The absorbance of the resulting complex at 500 nm is directly proportional to the magnesium concentration.

The chelating agent chlorophosphonazo III (CPZ) is used to measure magnesium in serum and urine (Table 28-6, method 3).[81] The reaction is initiated by the introduction of sample to a dye reagent containing CPZ and EGTA. The CPZ selectively complexes the magnesium present in the sample while EGTA chelates the calcium. This first step results in an absorbance decrease at 550 nm and an absorbance increase at 675 nm. In the second phase of the assay, the reaction is backtitrated by the addition of EDTA, which removes magnesium from the dye complex with a resultant absorbance change. Less than 5% interference has been reported from samples containing up to 200 mg/L calcium.[81]

The majority of magnesium determinations performed in clinical laboratories measure the concentration of total magnesium that is present. However, the free, or ionized, magnesium is the physiologically active fraction. Significant progress has been made in the development of ionophores for ion-selective electrodes for measurement of either intracellular or extracellular magnesium (Table 28-6, method 4). For extracellular fluids, such as blood, which have calcium concentrations greater than those of magnesium, the ionophore cannot show significant interference from calcium. For intracellular determinations of magnesium, interference by calcium with the ionophore is generally ignored, since the ratio of magnesium to calcium within the cell is approximately 1000:1.[75]

Specimen   Either serum or plasma anticoagulated with heparin is an acceptable specimen. Blood anticoagulated with citrate, oxalate, or EDTA is unacceptable, since these compounds chelate magnesium. Because erythrocytes contain approximately three times the magnesium concentration found in normal serum, samples with more than faint hemolysis are unacceptable for magnesium analysis. Serum should be separated from red blood cells as soon as possible after blood collection.[82]

If urine is to be analyzed for magnesium concentrations, the sample should be acidified to pH 1.0 with concentrated HCl to prevent magnesium precipitation.

Reference interval   Changes in the concentration of magnesium in serum are determined by the dietary intake and urinary excretion of magnesium. The reference interval for magnesium in sera of adults is 1.5 to 1.9 mEq/L (18.0 to 23 mg/L).[83]

Phosphorus
STEVEN C. KAZMIERCZAK

Principles of analysis and current usage   Phosphorus is present in plasma in two main forms; an organic form associated mainly with lipids and an inorganic form. The inorganic forms can occur in serum as either monovalent or divalent anions. The ratio of the two forms is dependent on the blood pH. Equal concentrations of monovalent and divalent forms are present in acidosis, a ratio of 1:9 is seen in alkalosis, and a ratio of 1:4 occurs at pH 7.4. The pH dependence of the ratio of monovalent and divalent forms of phosphorus makes it difficult to calculate what the molecular weight of inorganic phosphate is in a particular specimen. Thus phosphorus is reported in units of milligrams or millimoles per volume of specimen but not in milliequivalents since this would change with variations in the ratio of monovalent to divalent forms.

The oldest and still the most common method in use for measuring phosphorus is the phosphomolybdate method. Phosphate ions react with ammonium molybdate to form molybdenum-phosphate complexes. These complexes can be quantitated directly by measurement of their absorbance at 340 nm, or by converting them with reducing agents to molybdenum blue, which absorbs at 660 nm (Table 28-7, method 1). Many variations of this method have been described including changing the type of reducing agent used, the temperature that the reaction takes place, the concentration of molybdate, and the acidity of the reaction (Table 28-7, methods 2 to 5). Reducing substances that have been used include hydroquinone, 1-amino-2-naphthol-4-sulfonic acid (ANS), stannous chloride, and ferrous ammonium sulfate.[84-86]

Certain compounds, such as oxalate, citrate, tartrate, sorbitol, mannitol, and silica, can interfere with the molybdate method by forming a complex with molybdate.[87] In addition, the acid conditions of the procedure may cause hydrolysis of organic phosphate compounds.

Another common method for measuring phosphorus involves monitoring the absorbance of the unreduced phosphorus-molybdate complex at 340 nm (Table 28-7,

Table 28-7 Methods of phosphate measurement

Method	Principle	Usage	Comments
1. Hydroquinone*	Reduction of phosphomolybdate to molybdenum blue	Historical	Irregular, rapid fading of color
2. ANS (1-amino-2-naphthol-4-sulfonic acid)	(Same as above)	Historical	Better than hydroquinone
3. ANS + 100° C, 5 min	(Same as above)	Historical	Intensified color
4. SnCl$_2$	(Same as above)	Early continuous flow	Replaced by improved methods because of reagent instability, poor linearity, and lack of precision
5. SnCl$_2$ + Hydrazine	(Same as above)	Continuous flow	Good accuracy, limited linearity, better reagent stability than method 4
6. No reduction	340 nm, monitoring	Discrete and continuous flow sensitivity	Good accuracy, precision, sensitivity
	Bichromatic	Some discrete analyzers	Bichromatic (340 and 380 nm); blanking problems with hemolysis and lipemia
7. Enzymatic	HPO_4^{2-} + Inosine $\xrightarrow{PNP}$ Hypoxanthine + Ribose-1-phosphate Hypoxanthine + $2H_2O$ + $2O_2$ $\xrightarrow{XOD}$ Uric acid + $2H_2O_2$ H_2O_2 + Chromogenic substrate $\xrightarrow{Peroxidase}$ *Reddish purple complex* ($A_{maximum}$, 555 nm)	Discrete analyzers	Not widely used

*Reaction: PO_4 + H_2SO_4 + $(NH_4)_6Mo_7O_{24}\cdot 4H_2O$ → $Mo-PO_4$ complex. $Mo-PO_4$ complex + Reducing agent → Heteropolymeric blue complex.
PNP, Purine nucleoside phosphorylase (EC 2.4.2.1); *XOD*, xanthine oxidase (EC 1.2.3.2); chromogenic substrate is *N*-ethyl-*N*-(3-methylphenyl)-*N*-acetyl-ethylenediamine.

method 6).[88] Lack of a reducing agent allows for faster reaction times and also improves reagent stability. In addition, the absorbance change that occurs is three to four times greater in this method than in those assays that use a reducing agent.

Various enzymatic approaches have been described to measure phosphorus (Table 28-7, method 7). One method utilizes purine nucleoside phosphorylase and xanthine oxidase to produce H_2O_2 from phosphate and inosine.[89] Another enzymatic procedure employs the phosphorylation of glycogen, using phosphorylase A, coupled with phosphoglucomutase and glucose-6-phosphate dehydrogenase to measure the change in NADH at 340 nm.[90] This procedure has the advantage of lack of bilirubin interference and use of a neutral pH, which minimizes hydrolysis of phosphate esters.[91]

Specimen Serum or heparinized plasma is suitable for analysis. Anticoagulants such as citrate, oxalate, and EDTA should not be used because they inhibit the formation of the phosphomolybdate complex. Serum or plasma should be separated promptly from red blood cells because erythrocytes contain phosphate concentrations several times greater than those found in the sera. A transient decrease in phosphorus is noted after the ingestion of food or administration of intravenous glucose. This decrease is attributable to the increase in blood pH after a meal, commonly referred to as the "alkaline tide," which enhances in vivo formation of calcium-phosphate complexes, which subsequently increase bone deposition. Another mechanism for the decrease in phosphorus after meals is the insulin-induced uptake of serum phosphate by muscle and liver cells, which allows formation of glucose-phosphate intermediates.

Reference interval Adult males and females, 25 to 48 mg of phosphorus/L (0.81 to 1.55 mmol of phosphorus/L).

SUGGESTED READINGS

Itani O, Tsang R: Calcium, phosphorus and magnesium in the newborn: pathophysiology and management. In Hay W, editor: *Neonatal nutrition and metabolism,* St. Louis, 1991, Mosby.

Itani O, Tsang RC: Calcium and mineral metabolism in the fetus. In Thorburn GD, Harding R, editors: *Textbook of fetal physiology,* Oxford, 1994, Oxford University Press.

Favus M, editor: *Primer on the metabolic bone diseases and disorders of mineral metabolism,* ed 2, New York, 1993, Raven Press.

Schrier R, editor: *Renal and electrolyte disorders,* ed 4, Boston, 1992, Little, Brown & Co.

Christakos S, Gabrielides C, Rhoten W: Vitamin D–dependent calcium binding proteins: chemistry, distribution, functional considerations, and molecular biology, *Endocr Rev* 10:3-26, 1989.

Mughal M, Tsang R: Calcium, phosphorus, and magnesium transport across the placenta. In Polin RA, Fox WW, editors: *Fetal and neonatal physiology,* vol 2, Philadelphia, 1992, Philadelphia, pp 1735-1744.

Broadus AE, Stewart AF: Parathyroid hormone–related protein: structure, processing and physiologic actions. In Bilezikian JP, editor: *The parathyroids,* New York, 1994, Raven Press.

REFERENCES
Bone structure and function

1. Shipman P, Walker A, Bichell D, editors: *The human skeleton,* Cambridge, Mass., 1985, Harvard University Press.

2. Ham AW, Cormack DH: *Histology,* ed 8, Philadelphia, 1979, Lippincott.

3. Potts JT, Deftos LJ: Parathyroid hormone, calcitonin, vitamin D,bone and bone mineral metabolism. In Bondy PK, Rosenberg LE, editors: *Duncan's diseases of metabolism,* Philadelphia, 1974, Saunders.

4. Baylink DJ, Lin CC: The regulation of endosteal bone volume, *J Periodontol* 50:43-49, 1979.

Biochemistry and physiology

5. DeLuca HF: The kidney as an endocrine organ for production of 1,25-dihydroxyvitamin D_3, a calcium-mobilizing hormone, *N Engl J Med* 289:359-365, 1973.

6. Hollick MF, Frommer JE, McNeill SC, et al: Photometabolism of 7-dehydrocholesterol to previtamin D_3 in skin, *Biochem Biophys Res Commun* 176:107-114, 1977.

7. Avioli LV: Hormonal aspects of vitamin D metabolism and its clinical implications, *Clin Endocrinol Metab* 8:547-577, 1979.

8. Haddad JG, Stamp TCB: Circulating 25-hydroxyvitamin D in man, *Am J Med* 57:57-62, 1974.

9. Avioli LV, Haddad JG: Vitamin D: current concepts, *Metabolism* 22:507-531, 1973.

10. Chesney RW, Rosen JF, Hamstra AJ, DeLuca HF: Serum 1,25-dihydroxyvitamin D levels in normal children and in vitamin D disorders, *Am J Dis Child* 134:135-139, 1980.

11. Chesney RW, Rosen JF, Hamstra AJ, et al: Absence of seasonal variation in serum concentrations of 1,25-dihydroxyvitamin D despite a rise in 25-hydroxyvitamin D in summer, *J Clin Endocrinol Metab* 53:139-142, 1981.

12. DeLuca HF: The vitamin D system in the regulation of calcium and phosphorus metabolism, *Nutr Rev* 37:161-193, 1979.

13. Eisman JA, Pounce RL, Ward JD, Moseby JM: Modulation of plasma 1,25-dihydroxyvitamin D in man by stimulation and suppression tests, *Lancet* 2:931-933, 1979.

14. Gallagher JC, Riggs LB, Eisman J, et al: Intestinal calcium absorption and serum vitamin D metabolites in normal subjects and osteoporotic patients: effect of age and dietary calcium, *J Clin Invest* 64:729-736, 1979.

15. Kumar R, Cohen WR, Silva P, Epstein FH: Elevated 1,25-dihydroxyvitamin D levels in normal human pregnancy and lactation, *J Clin Invest* 63:342-344, 1979.

16. Austin LA, Heath H III: Calcitonin physiology and pathophysiology, *N Engl J Med* 304:269-278, 1981.

17. Huwler R, Born W, Ohnhaus EE, Fischer JA: Plasma kinetics and urinary excretion of exogenous human and salmon calcitonin in man, *Am J Physiol* 236:15-19, 1979.

18. Ardaillou R: Kidney and calcitonin, *Nephron* 15:250-260, 1975.

19. Heersche JNM, Marcus R, Aurbach GD: Calcitonin and the formation of 3',5'-AMP in bone and kidney, *Endocrinology* 94:241-247, 1974.

20. Deftos LJ: Calcitonin. In Gray CH, James VHT, editors: *Hormones and blood,* New York, 1979, Academic Press.

21. Cooper CW: Recent advances with thyrocalcitonin, *Ann Clin Lab Sci* 6:119-129, 1976.

22. Alkawa JK: *Magnesium: its biologic significance,* CRC series on cations of biological significance, Boca Raton, Fla., 1981, CRC Press.

23. Tsang RC: Neonatal magnesium disturbances, *Am J Dis Child* 124:282, 1972.

Bone disorders

24. Chase L: Osteopenia, *Am J Med* 69:915-922, 1980.

25. Parfitt AM, Oliver I, Villanueva AR: Bone histology in metabolic bone disease: the diagnostic value of bone biopsy, *Orthop Clin North Am* 10:329-345, 1979.

26. Ivey JL, Baylink DJ: Postmenopausal osteoporosis: proposed roles of defective coupling and estrogen deficiency, *Metab Bone Dis Rel Res* 3:3-7, 1981.

27. Avioli LV: Postmenopausal osteoporosis: prevention versus cure, *Fed Proc* 40:2418-2422, 1981.

28. Wallach S: Management of osteoporosis, *Hosp Pract* 13:91-98, 1978.

29. Gallagher JC, Rigg BL, Eisman J, et al: Intestinal calcium absorption and serum vitamin D metabolites in normal subjects and osteoporotic patients: effect of age and dietary calcium, *J Clin Invest* 64:729-736, 1979.

30. Slovik DM, Adams JS, Neer RM, et al: Deficient production of 1,25-dihydroxyvitamin D in elderly osteoporotic subjects, *N Engl J Med* 305:372-374, 1981.

31. Gallagher JC, Riggs BL, Jerpbak CM, Arnaud CD: Effect of age on serum immunoreactive parathyroid hormone in normal and osteoporotic women, *J Lab Clin Med* 95:373-385, 1980.

32. Shamonki IM, Fumar AM, Tataryn IV, et al: Age-related changes of calcitonin secretion in females, *J Clin Endocrinol Metab* 50:437-439, 1980.

33. Gallaher JC, Riggs BL, DeLuca HF: Effect of estrogen on calcium absorption and serum vitamin D metabolites in postmenopausal osteoporosis, *J Clin Endocrinol Metab* 51:1359-1364, 1980.

34. Avioli LV: Hormonal aspects of vitamin D metabolism and its clinical implications, *Clin Endocrinol Metab* 8:547-577, 1979.

35. Winnacker JL, Yeager H, Saunders JA, et al: Rickets in children receiving anticonvulsant drugs, *Am J Dis Child* 31:286-290, 1977.

36. Scriver CR, Reade TM, DeLuca HF, Hamstra AJ: Serum 1,25-dihydroxyvitamin D levels in normal subjects and in patients with hereditary rickets and bone disease, *N Engl J Med* 299:976-979, 1978.

37. Brooks MH, Bell NH, Love L, et al: Vitamin D–dependent rickets type II: resistance of target organs to 1,25-dihydroxyvitamin D, *N Engl J Med* 298:996-999, 1978.

38. Scriver C: Rickets and the pathogenesis of impaired tubular transport of phosphate and other solutes, *Am J Med* 57:43-49, 1974.

39. Drezner MK, Lyles KW, Haussler MR, Harrelson JM: Evaluation of a role for 1,25-dihydroxyvitamin D_3 in the pathogenesis and treatment of X-linked hypophosphatemic rickets and osteomalacia, *J Clin Invest* 66:1020-1032, 1980.

40. Chesney RW, Rosen JF, Hamstra AJ, DeLuca HF: Serum 1,25-dihydroxyvitamin D levels in normal children and in vitamin D disorders, *Am J Dis Child* 134:135-139, 1980.

41. Steichen JJ, Tsang RC, Greer FR, et al: Elevated serum 1,25-dihydroxyvitamin D concentrations in rickets of very low-birth-weight infants, *J Pediatr* 99:293-298, 1981.

42. Chesney RW, Hamstra AJ, Mazess RB, et al: Circulating vitamin D metabolite concentrations in childhood renal diseases, *Kidney Int* 21:65-69, 1982.

43. Massry SG, Ritz E: The pathogenesis of secondary hyperparathyroidism of renal failure: is there a controversy? *Arch Intern Med* 138:853-856, 1978.

44. Singer FR, Schiller AL, Pyle EB, Krane SM: Paget's disease of bone. In Avioli LV, Krane SM, editors: *Metabolic bone disease,* vol 2, New York, 1978, Academic Press.

45. Singer FR: Huma calcitonin treatment of Paget's disease of bone, *Clin Orthop* 127:86-93, 1977.

Change of analyte in disease

46. Kooh SW, Jones G, Reilly BJ, Fraser D: Pathogenesis of rickets in chronic hepatobiliary disease in children, *J Pediatr* 94:870-874, 1979.

47. Drezner MK, Neelon FA, Jowsey J: Hypoparathyroidism: a possible cause of osteomalacia, *J Clin Endocrinol Metab* 45:114, 1977.

48a. Drezner MK, Neelon FA, Haussler, M: 1,25-Dihydroxycholecalciferol deficiency: the probable cause of hypocalcemia and metabolic bone disease in pseudohypoparathyroidism, *J Clin Endocrinol Metab* 42:621, 1976.

48b. Juttmann JR, Buurman CJ, De Kam E, et al: Serum concentrations of vitamin D in patients with chronic renal failure: consequences for the treatment with 1-α-hydroxy derivatives, *Clin Endocrinol* 14:225-236, 1981.

49. Goldstein DA, Haldimann B, Sherman D, et al: Vitamin D metabolites and calcium metabolism in patients with nephrotic syndrome and normal renal function, *J Clin Endocrinol Metab* 52:116-121, 1981.

50. Chesney RW, Rosen JF, Hamstra AJ, DeLuca HF: Serum 1,25-dihydroxyvitamin D levels in normal children and in vitamin D disorders, *Am J Dis Child* 34:135-139, 1980.

51. Kumar R, Cohen WR, Silva P, Epstein FH: Elevated 1,25-

dihydroxyvitamin D levels in normal pregnancy and lactation, *J Clin Invest* 63:342-344, 1979.

52. Tsang RC, Brown, DR: The parathyroids. In Kelley V, editor: *Practice of pediatrics,* vol 1, New York, 1979, Harper & Row.

53. Tsang RC, Venkataraman P: Pediatric parathyroid and vitamin D–related disorders. In Kaplan LA, editor: *Clinical pediatric and adolescent endocrinology,* Philadelphia, 1982, Saunders.

54. Taylor AB, Stern PH, Bell NH: Abnormal regulation of circulating 25-hydroxyvitamin D in the Williams syndrome, *N Engl J Med* 306:972-975, 1982.

55. Juan D: Hypocalcemia differential diagnosis and mechanisms, *Arch Intern Med* 139:1166-1171, 1979.

56. Broadus AE: Nephrogenous cyclic AMP, *Recent Prog Horm Res* 37:665, 1981.

57. Tsang RC: Neonatal magnesium disturbances, *Am J Dis Child* 124:282, 1972.

58. Aikawa JK: *Magnesium: its biologic significance,* CRC series on cations of biological significance, Boca Raton, Fla., 1981, CRC Press.

59. Grace K, Spiler IJ, Tashjian AH Jr: Natural history of familial medullary thyroid carcinoma: effect of a program for early diagnosis, *N Engl J Med* 229:980-985, 1978.

60. Silva OL, Brode LE, Doppman JL: Calcitonin as a marker for bronchogenic cancer, *Cancer* 44:680-684, 1979.

61. McTaggert H, Ivey JL, Sisom K, et al: Deficient calcitonin response to calcium stimulation in post-menopausal osteoporosis, *Lancet* 1:475-477, 1982.

62. Kaplan M: Alkaline phosphatase, *N Engl J Med* 286:200-201, 1972.

63. Root AW, Harrison HE: Recent advances in calcium metabolism, *J Pediatr* 88:1-18, 1976.

64. Niejadlik DC: Hydroxyproline, *Postgrad Med* 51:214-216, 1972.

65. Clark EP, Collip JB: A study of the Tisdall method for the determination of blood serum calcium with a suggested modification, *J Biol Chem Balt* 63:461-464, 1925.

66. Jackson JE, Breem M, Cheng C: Fluorometric titration of calcium, *J Lab Clin Med* 60:700-708, 1962.

67. Walmsley TA, Fowler RT: Optimum use of 8-hydroquinoline in plasma calcium determinations, *Clin Chem* 27:1782, 1981.

68. Beilby J, Randall A, Davis J: Variable citrate interference in arsenazo III dye assays of total calcium in serum, *Clin Chem* 36:824-825, 1990.

69. Kaplan LA, Pesce AJ: *Clinical chemistry: theory, analysis, and correlation,* St. Louis, 1984, Mosby, Chapt 3.

70. Cali JP, Bowers GN, Young DS, et al: A reference method for the determination of total calcium in serum. In Cooper GR, editor: *Selected methods of clinical chemistry,* vol 8, Washington, D.C., 1977, American Association for Clinical Chemistry.

71. Cadeau BJ, MacKay JS: *Serum calcium: review of methods,* ASCP Check Sample, vol 4, no 8, 1992, PTS 92-1 (PTS-59), American Society of Clinical Pathologists.

72. Lum G, Gambino SR: A comparison of serum versus heparinized plasma for routine chemistry tests, *Am J Clin Pathol* 61:108-113, 1974.

73. Winsten S: Collection and preservation of specimens, *Stand Methods Clin Chem* 5:1, 1965.

74. Caraway WT: Chemical and diagnostic specificity of laboratory tests, *Am J Clin Pathol* 37:445-464, 1962.

75. Elin RJ: Laboratory tests for the assessment of magnesium status in humans, *Magnes Trace Elem* 10:172-181, 1992.

76. Denis W: The determination of magnesium in blood, plasma and serum, *J Biol Chem* 52:411-415, 1922.

77. Schwartzenbach G, Bidermann W, Banserter F. Komplex-one VI: neue einfache Titriermethoden zur Bestimmung der Wasserhärte, *Helv Chim Acta* 29:811-818, 1946.

78. Brien M, Marshall RT: An automated fluorometric method for the determination of magnesium in serum and urine using o-o-dihydroxyazobenzene: studies on normal and uremic subjects, *J Lab Clin Med* 68:701-712, 1966.

79. Gindler EM, Heth DA: Colorimetric determination with bound "calmagite" of magnesium in human blood serum, *Clin Chem* 17:663, 1971 (abstract).

80. Baginski ES, Marie SS: Magnesium in biological fluids, *Selected Methods Clin Chem* 9:277-281, 1982.

81. Dixon DJ, Denton J, Kaufman RA: New magnesium method for the Cobas™ Chemistry Systems using chlorophosphonazo III, *Clin Chem* 36:1068, 1990.

82. Martin BJ, McGregor CW: Measurement of serum magnesium: effect of delay in separation from erythrocytes, *Clin Chem* 32:564, 1986.

83. Lowenstein FW, Stanton MF: Serum magnesium levels in the United States, 1971-1974, *J Am Coll Nutr* 5:399-414, 1987.

84. Bell RD, Doisey EA: Rapid colorimetric methods for the determination of phosphorus in urine and blood, *J Biol Chem* 44:55-67, 1920.

85. Fiske CH, Subbarow Y: The colorimetric determination of phosphorus, *J Biol Chem* 66:375-400, 1925.

86. Bartlett GR: Phosphorus assay in column chromatography, *J Biol Chem* 234:466-468, 1959.

87. Scott MG: *Inorganic phosphorus: review of methods,* ASCP Check Sample vol 8, no 5, 1992, PTS 92-5 (PTS-63), American Society of Clinical Patholgists.

88. Simonsen DG, Wertman M, Westover LM, Mehl JW: The determination of serum phosphate by the molybdivanadate method, *J Biol Chem* 166:747-755, 1946.

89. Adam A, Boulanger J, Azzouzi M, Ers P: Colorimetric versus enzymatic determination of serum phosphorus, *Clin Chem* 30:1724-1725, 1984 (letter).

90. Baginski ES, Epstein E, Zak B: Review of phosphate methodologies, *Ann Clin Lab Sci* 5:399-416, 1975.

91. Schultz DW, Passanneau JV, Lowry OH: An enzymatic method for the measurement of inorganic phosphate, *Anal Biochem* 19:300-314, 1967.

CHAPTER 29

The pancreas: function and chemical pathology

John A. Lott

OBJECTIVES

- Describe the anatomy of the pancreas.

- Describe the normal endocrine (islets) and exocrine (digestive) physiology of the pancreas; emphasize the functions of the endocrine organelles and the exocrine secretions of the organ.

- Describe the factors controlling normal exocrine pancreatic secretions and how food and alcohol stimulate the normal pancreatic functions.

- List the major disease groups of the endocrine and exocrine pancreas and how they affect laboratory measurements made on body fluids.

- Discuss exocrine pancreatic insufficiency, its causes, clinical findings, and specific changes that occur in clinical laboratory tests.

- Outline the presumed causes of acute pancreatitis, the clinical findings, the factors portending a bad outcome, and the effects on serum and urine tests.

- Discuss the sensitivity and specificity of the commonly performed pancreatic enzymes for the diagnosis of pancreatitis and the use of ROC (receiver-operating characteristic) curves in choosing optimal decision points.

- Discuss cystic fibrosis and the laboratory tests, especially those of pancreatic function, that aid in the diagnosis of this disease.

- Briefly discuss pancreatic adenocarcinoma, its prognosis, and tests that are used to follow disease progression.

- Outline the current knowledge of islet-cell tumors and the role of the laboratory in their diagnosis.

KEY TERMS

acinar From the Latin word *acinus,* meaning a 'berry' or 'grape.' In anatomy, the term refers to a small sacklike dilatation. (It is accented on the first syllable.)

adenocarcinoma A malignant growth that begins in the epithelial cells; for the pancreas, it is those that line the pancreatic ductules and duct. Nearly all pancreatic cancers are adenocarcinoma.

ampulla of Vater A flasklike dilatation at the point where the biliary and pancreatic ducts join. The ampulla joins the duodenal papilla (a nipple-shaped structure), and its orifice is encircled by a ring of smooth muscles called the "sphincter of Oddi." Note that the ampulla and the sphincter are two distinct structures.

cachexia A state of progressive weakness, loss of appetite, malnutrition, and weight loss that is observed in some chronic disorders, such as advanced cancer.

cholangiopancreatography Also known as *endoscopic retrograde cholangiopancreatography* (ERCP). It is an invasive diagnostic technique whereby the pancreatic duct is cannulated and an x-ray contrast medium is injected into the duct to visualize the biliary and pancreatic ducts.

cholecystitis Inflammation of the gallbladder.

cholecystokinin Cholecystokinin (CCK) is a gastrointestinal hormone that is released when the duodenum is distended by food or after alcohol ingestion. It is a powerful secretagogue for the pancreas, producing a high-volume secretion that is high in bicarbonate concentration but low in proteins and enzymes. CCK and secretin potentiate each other's actions.

enterokinase An enzyme produced by the mucosa of the small intestine that converts the inactive, digestive proenzymes from the pancreas into their active forms.

gastrin A hormone produced primarily by the mucosa of the small intestine that stimulates the secretion of HCl by the parietal cells in the stomach. Plasma gastrin is greatly increased in Zollinger-Ellison syndrome, usually a pancreatic neoplasm, but it is not normally present in the pancreas.

glucagon An islet-cell hormone that has multiple actions to raise plasma glucose.

gluconeogenesis A biochemical process whereby glucose is synthesized from amino acids, lactate, or glycerol.

glycogenolysis The biochemical breakdown of glycogen in liver and muscle to glucose.

hypoglycemia A low blood glucose concentration, generally <2.8 mmol/L (<500 mg/L), causing some individuals to become symptomatic.

insulin An islet-cell, anabolic hormone that controls glucose uptake, fat synthesis, and synthesis of proteins.

immunoreactive trypsin A form of the digestive enzyme found in blood. Because of the presence of potent antiproteases in blood, the enzyme must be measured in serum as a protein. It has little or no enzymatic activity in blood.

islets of Langerhans Clusters of cells in the pancreas that produce the endocrine secretions of the gland. They constitute about 1% of the pancreatic mass.

laparoscopy A technique used to view the pancreas or any other abdominal organ. A small incision is made in the abdomen to allow the insertion of the viewing instrument. It is probably the most objective and reliable method for diagnosing pancreatitis.

multiple endocrine neoplasias Also known as *MEN,* the type I MEN disorder often involves the pancreas and other endocrine organs such as the pituitary, adrenals, thyroid, and parathyroid glands. It is an inherited disorder and has many different clinical presentations.

pancreatic duct A conduit that passes through the pancreas, collects the pancreatic exocrine secretions of enzymes, water, and electrolytes, and carries them to the ampulla.

pancreatic polypeptide An islet-cell hormone (PP) that slows the absorption of food, stimulates gastric and intestinal secretions, and inhibits intestinal mobility.

peripancreatic fat necrosis A phenomenon occurring in acute, necrotizing pancreatitis whereby the lipolytic enzymes from the pancreas leak out of the gland and attack the fat surrounding the pancreas.

proteolytic Having the ability to break down proteins to peptides and amino acids.

secretin A gastrointestinal hormone that is released when the duodenum is distended by food or after alcohol ingestion. It is a powerful secretagogue for the pancreas producing a secretion high in protein and enzymes but low in volume.

somatostatin An islet-cell hormone that has largely inhibitory effects on insulin and glucagon secretion, gastric secretions, and exocrine pancreatic secretions.

trypsin A potent proteolytic enzyme produced in the pancreas but stored there in zymogen granules as the enzymatically inactive protrypsin form.

trypsinogen The enzymatically inactive or zymogen form of trypsin; also called *protrypsin.*

vagus nerve The tenth cranial nerve that carries motor, sensory, and autonomic nerve fibers to the neck, thorax, and abdomen including the pancreas. Vagal stimulation of the pancreas causes release of pancreatic fluid that is high in enzymes but low in volume and electrolytes.

vasoinhibitory polypeptide A hormone (VIP) from the intestinal mucosa that has a secretin-like effect on the pancreas.

Zollinger-Ellison syndrome It is the clinical picture of a patient with a gastrinoma in the pancreas, duodenum, or both. This frequently malignant tumor secretes gastrin and stimulates the parietal cells in the stomach to secrete HCl in uncontrolled amounts.

zymogen granules The storage form of the digestive enzymes in the pancreatic acinar cells. Some of the enzymes, especially the proteolytic and lipolytic forms, are present as their zymogens or inactive precursors.

ANATOMY

The pancreas is about the size and shape of the hand; the tail points to the spleen, and the head is nestled in the duodenal loop (Fig. 29-1). This soft, easily traumatized gland lies behind the peritoneum, which is behind the serous membrane lining the abdominal walls. The pancreas receives an ample blood supply from an artery branching from the aorta. Blood from the islets drains into the hepatic portal vein, like that from the gastrointestinal tract. The pancreatic exocrine functions are located in the acinar, centroacinar, and ductular cells. The exocrine acini (Fig. 29-2) are drained by ductules that combine into a single duct (pancreatic duct) that joins the common bile duct to form the *ampulla of Vater.* The latter opens through the duodenal papilla, the orifice of which is encircled by the *sphincter of Oddi,* so that pancreatic exocrine secretions can flow into the gastrointestinal tract.[1] Except when pancreatic fluid is secreted, the sphincter is tightly closed preventing stomach and duodenal contents from reaching the pancreas. Exocrine acinar cells and their associated structures account for more than 98% of the 60 to 140 g pancreatic mass.

About 1% (1 to 1.5 g) of the pancreas consists of unique cell clusters, the *islets of Langerhans,* that produce the endocrine secretions. A normal pancreas contains 1 to 2 million islets (Fig. 29-3).[2] Nerve fibers are present in pancreatic tissue that produce vasoactive intestinal peptide (VIP), substance P, somatostatin, enkephalin-related peptides, and bombesin-like peptides (see also p. 577).[3]

ENDOCRINE PHYSIOLOGY

Pancreatic endocrine secretion from the islets of Langerhans includes the hormones glucagon from the alpha-cells, insulin from the beta-cells, somatostatin from the delta-cells, and pancreatic polypeptide from the F-cells. Their action and control of these hormones are summarized in Table 29-1.[4] Gastrin was once believed to be present in the normal pancreas; current thinking is that, normally, gastrin comes only from glands in the intestinal mucosa.[5]

Alpha-cells, constituting 20% to 30% of the islet cells, produce *glucagon,* a hormone that acts to increase glucose concentrations in blood (see Chapter 32); it has a half-life in blood of 5 to 10 minutes. The release of glucagon is stimulated by the factors shown in Table 29-1.

Beta-cells produce *proinsulin,* which consists of A and B

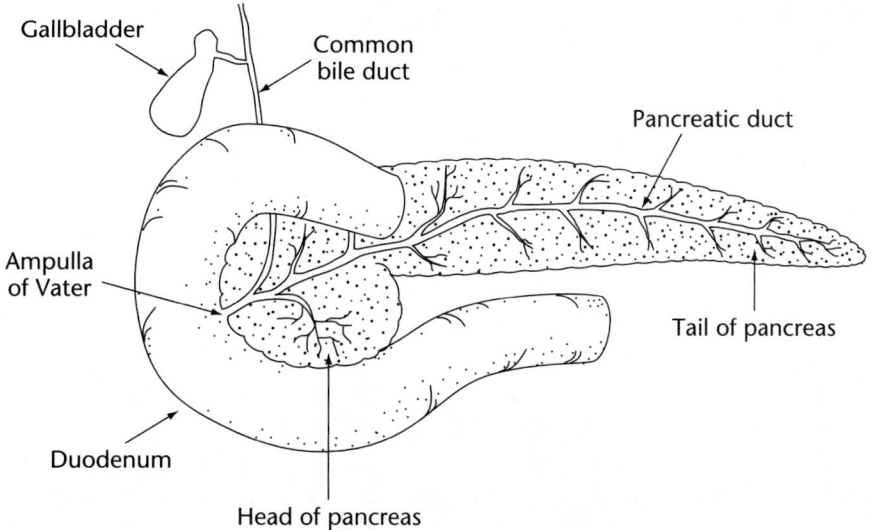

Fig. 29-1 Structure of pancreas including nearby organs. The pancreatic duct carries the exocrine secretions to the ampulla of Vater where it empties into the duodenum at the sphincter of Oddi. Notice that the sphincter is closed except during periods of secretion. The common bile duct joins the pancreatic duct before the latter reaches the duodenum.

chains and the C-peptide (see Chapter 32). *Insulin* is stored in secretory granules; these particles migrate to the cell wall and with appropriate stimuli, that is a high level of plasma glucose, are released by exocytosis. Proinsulin is normally converted to insulin, C-peptide, and other proteins before release. Insulin has a half-life in blood of about 10 to 25 minutes. C-peptide has no insulin-like action but can be measured in blood in patients receiving insulin to estimate residual beta-cell function.

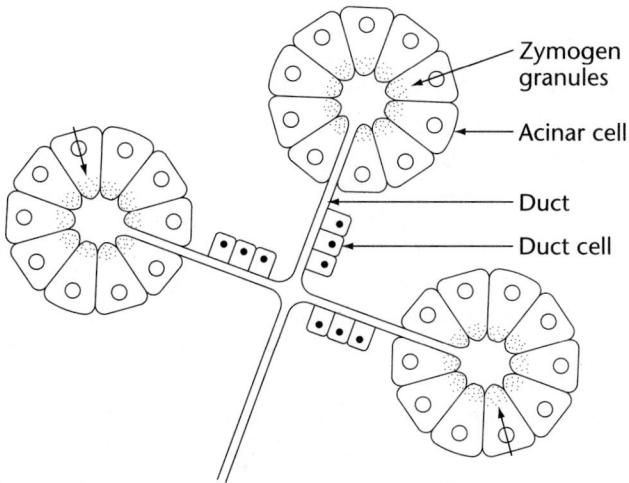

Fig. 29-2 Diagram of acinar cells and associated ductules. The exocrine acini terminate with a collection of acinar cells that contain zymogen granules; the latter contain the proenzymes and other digestive enzymes described in Fig. 29-4. Special cells line the ductules that secrete fluid and electrolytes, especially bicarbonate.

Delta-cells, constituting about 2% to 8% of the islets, produce somatostatin, a hormone that inhibits the action of insulin and of gastrin, inhibits the secretion of exocrine pancreatic enzymes, inhibits the release of growth hormone, and decreases the flow of bile. Somatostatin plays a role in glucose metabolism by inhibiting insulin secretion; an abnormal increase of somatostatin may lead to diabetes mellitus (DM) by inhibiting insulin secretion. The F-cells produce *pancreatic polypeptide,* a hormone that stimulates gastric and intestinal enzyme secretion and inhibits intestinal mobility.[2]

EXOCRINE PHYSIOLOGY
Normal pancreatic exocrine secretions

The pancreas produces at least 22 digestive enzymes, 15 of which are proteases, that act on three major sources of energy: proteins, digested by the enzymes trypsin, chymotrypsin, and elastase; lipids, digested by the enzymes lipase, phospholipase A_2, and carboxyl esterase; and complex carbohydrates digested by α-amylase.[6] Humans only produce α-amylase, an enzyme that breaks α-1,4-glycolytic linkages in starch and other complex polysaccharides. We cannot digest cellulose, a complex carbohydrate that requires β-amylase to break it down. The functional units of the exocrine pancreas consist of clusters of acini that store the digestive enzymes as *zymogen granules;* the free enzymes are not normally present in the acinar cell cytoplasm (see Fig. 29-2). The granules are released from the acinar cells by exocytosis into the collecting ductules and finally reach the pancreatic duct. Most of the enzymes are present as inactive zymogens or *proenzyme* forms; ribonuclease, deoxyribonuclease, carboxyl-

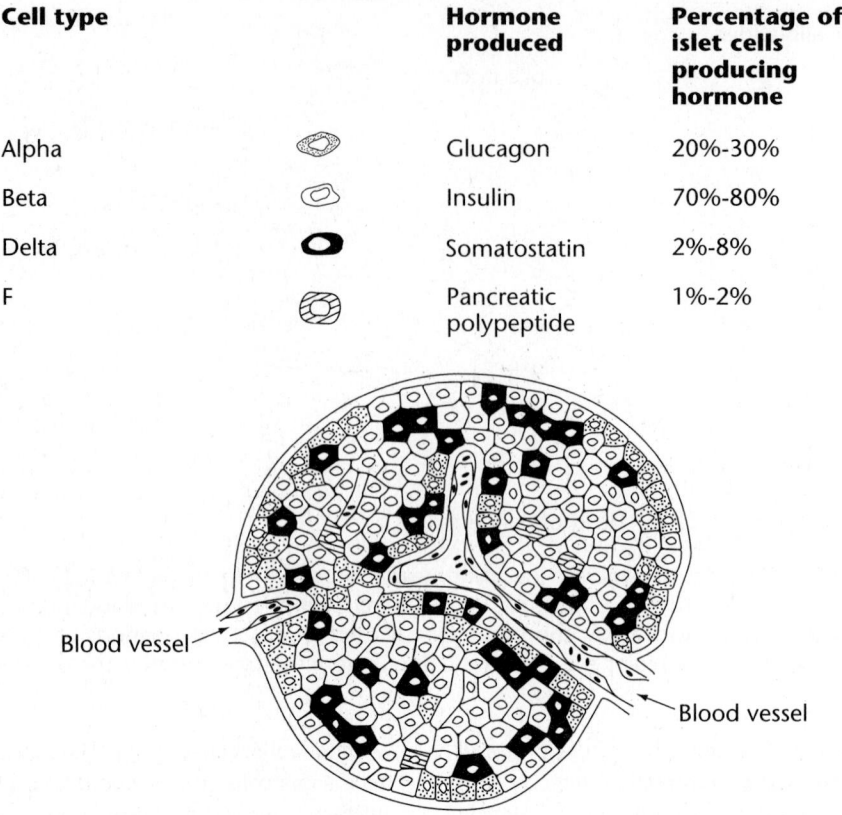

Cell type		Hormone produced	Percentage of islet cells producing hormone
Alpha		Glucagon	20%-30%
Beta		Insulin	70%-80%
Delta		Somatostatin	2%-8%
F		Pancreatic polypeptide	1%-2%

Blood vessel

Blood vessel

Fig. 29-3 Diagram of an islet of Langerhans. There are at least four types of cells secreting hormones into the blood. Most of the cells (beta-cells) produce insulin, and only a small fraction of the islets is composed of F-cells, which produce pancreatic polypeptide. (Adapted from Unger RH, Orci L: *N Engl J Med* 304:1518-1524, 1981.)

esterase, amylase, lipase, and colipase are exceptions to this.

The modification of exocrine digestive enzymes from zymogen granules in the acinar cells to their active forms after entry into the duodenal lumen is shown in Fig. 29-4. The potent proteolytic enzymes trypsin, chymotrypsin, carboxypeptidase A and B, and elastase constitute more than 75% of the mass of the digestive enzymes secreted. The proenzyme forms of the proteolytic enzymes contain a small amino acid chain that blocks their proteolytic site. This propitious arrangement of nature prevents the autodigestion of the zymogen granules, the acinar cells, and of course the pancreas itself; unfortunately the reverse is true in some diseases of the pancreas, such as pancreatitis. The pancreas also secretes protease inhibitors to neutralize any prematurely activated enzymes.

Upon entering the duodenum, *enterokinase* (also called *enteropeptidase*), a peptidase from the duodenal mucosa, cleaves off the small amino acid chains from the proenzymes; for example, it converts protrypsin to fully active trypsin. Free trypsin activates the other proenzymes in a cas-

cade or chain reaction–like fashion and, to a small degree, protrypsin itself (see Fig. 29-4).

Normal pancreatic fluid secretions

A normal adult weighing 75 kg produces about 2 to 3 liters of water-clear, colorless pancreatic juice per day containing the enzyme described above and 120 to 300 mmol/day of bicarbonate.[7] Amylase and lipase, for example, are present in pancreatic juice in huge activities of about 500,000 to 1 million U/L.[8,9] There is an approximately 10,000:1 gradient in the enzyme activities between pancreatic fluid and normal blood; hence the minimal intrusion of pancreatic juice into blood can produce considerable increases of serum amylase, lipase, trypsin, and other digestive enzymes. The principal cations in pancreatic fluid, totaling about 150 mmol/L, are Na^+, K^+, Ca^{++}, and Mg^{++}. The principal anions are bicarbonate at about 120 mmol/L, compared to a plasma concentration of about 25 mmol/L, and Cl^- at about 30 mmol/L, compared to a plasma concentration of about 100 mmol/L.

Water and electrolytes in pancreatic fluid are secreted by

Table 29-1   Normal pancreatic islet-cell hormones[1,4,5]

Cell of origin	Hormone*	Release stimulated by:	Release inhibited by:	Hormone causes:
Alpha	Glucagon (3500)	Low plasma glucose, sympathetic nervous system, epinephrine, any factors lowering plasma glucose	Somatostatin, glucose, secretin, insulin	Increased plasma glucose by stimulating hepatic glycogenolysis, gluconeogenesis; adipose tissue lipolysis; mobilizes amino acids
Beta	Proinsulin (11,500) Insulin (5734) C-peptide (31 amino acids)	Plasma glucose above 1000 mg/L, keto acids, arginine, leucine, sympathetic and parasympathetic nervous system stimulation, gastric inhibitory polypeptide, gastrin, secretin, CCK, glucagon, cortisol, growth hormone, thyroxine, progesterone, sex hormones, sulfonylureas	Alpha-adrenergic agonists, somatostatin, insulin, thiazide diuretics, phenytoin	Glucose uptake by liver, muscle, adipose tissue; inhibition of gluconeogenesis; glycogen formation; fat synthesis and storage; inhibition of mobilization and oxidation of fats; conversion of glucose to fatty acids or cholesterol; production of acetyl CoA; synthesis of proteins; inhibition of protein breakdown; increased RNA synthesis; entry of K, phosphate, Mg into muscle and liver cells
Delta	Somatostatin (1640)	Food intake, increased plasma glucose, arginine, leucine, CCK	Unknown	Inhibition of insulin and glucagon release, inhibition of gastric and exocrine pancreatic secretions
F	Pancreatic polypeptide (36 amino acids)	Food intake, especially protein; fasting; exercise; hypoglycemia	Hyperglycemia	Decreased rate of food absorption, stimulation of gastric and intestinal enzyme secretion, inhibition of intestinal mobility

CCK, Cholecystokinin.
*In parentheses molecular weight in daltons.

the ductal and centroacinar cells. The healthy pancreas can secrete bicarbonate into the pancreatic juice and hydrogen ions into blood. There is normally more than enough pancreatic bicarbonate to neutralize the acid coming from the stomach.

Control of exocrine pancreatic secretions

Exocrine secretions from the pancreas have both neural and hormonal controls; they are summarized in Table 29-2.[10-13] Three hormones in the mucosa of the upper gastrointestinal tract, cholecystokinin (CCK), secretin, and gastrin, affect pancreatic juice secretion.[14,15] Distension of the duodenum by food or by alcohol leads to the release of all three hormones. Fats and alcohol are particularly active stimulators of secretin production.[8] A negative-feedback loop exists; trypsin released as a consequence of CCK release has an inhibitory action on further CCK secretion.[16] VIP is structurally similar to secretin and glucagon; this probably explains the similar action of VIP on the pancreas. All pan-

creatic exocrine secretions and other gastrointestinal functions are inhibited by somatostatin.

PATHOLOGICAL CONDITIONS

Diseases of the pancreas can be broadly grouped into certain areas: endocrine disorders, such as diabetes mellitus and disorders of glucagon secretion; exocrine, such as pancreatic insufficiency and associated malabsorption; inflammatory, such as acute pancreatitis; destructive lesions, such as those resulting from cystic fibrosis and chronic pancreatitis; infectious disorders of many types including human immunodeficiency virus (HIV); atherosclerotic and atrophic diseases; and neoplastic, such as adenocarcinomas and islet cell tumors. The emphasis here is on those disorders in which chemical changes in body fluids or chemical responses to certain stimuli are abnormal. Laboratory tests are one of the tools used in defining pancreatic diseases. A carefully obtained history, physical examination, and imaging techniques such as endoscopic retrograde cholangiopancreatography (ERCP), ultrasonography, computerized tomography, magnetic resonance imaging, and roentgenography are of great importance when used in the diagnostic process.[17] Estimating the size of the pancreas by imaging methods is important. An inflamed, edematous gland is generally larger than normal, an important diagnostic finding. Even *laparotomy* or laparoscopy with visual observation and palpation are used; in fact, they are the standard for diagnosing disorders such as pancreatitis.

Endocrine pancreatic disorders

The major endocrine disorder is diabetes mellitus (DM), a disease with greater morbidity and mortality, by far, than all other pancreatic disorders combined.[3] Insulin is necessary for life, and a relative or absolute lack of insulin leads to DM. Diabetes and the laboratory tests used to diagnose and monitor this disease are discussed more fully in Chapter 32.

An abnormal serum amylase in the absence of pancreatitis is common in uncontrolled DM, especially in the presence of diabetic ketoacidosis. The release of amylase may be a consequence of the acidemia in these individuals. Kidney and pancreas allograft transplantation is currently being used with excellent success for patients with DM and end-stage renal disease.[18,19] (See Chapter 50.) Restoration of normal renal and endocrine pancreatic function occurs in most patients receiving kidney and pancreas transplants.

Exocrine pancreatic disorders

Reduction or loss of pancreatic exocrine (digestive) function leads to severe gastrointestinal disturbances such as di-

arrhea, constipation, and malabsorption. With advanced disease, a catabolic state leading to weight loss and *cachexia* appears. The exocrine pancreas has huge reserves; symptoms generally appear only after about 85% to 90% of the acinar tissue has been lost. Important causes of acinar cell loss are listed in the box on page 561.

Pancreatic function tests

Tests for volumes or analytes in pancreatic fluid.

Pancreatic function tests represent an attempt to measure the ability of the pancreas to produce enzymes, proteins, and bicarbonate and to secrete an adequate volume of fluid into the duodenum. Contemporary pancreatic function tests can be classified into four groups (Table 29-3). There are tests that measure fluid volume and bicarbonate output or residual enzymatic activity in pancreatic fluid. Tests on feces measure undigested fat, meat, or enzymes; tests on duodenal fluid, blood, or urine measure endogenous or exogenously administered agents; and tests on breath measure $^{13}CO_2$ or $^{14}CO_2$ produced by the action of pancreatic enzymes on labeled compounds, commonly fats or other esters.

After intubation with a double-lumen tube through the esophagus and stomach to a point in the duodenum below the ampulla the patient is then stimulation with intravenous CCK, secretin, or both. Duodenal fluid is collected to measure bicarbonate, fluid volume, and enzymes such as amylase, lipase, trypsin, or chymotrypsin. The bicarbonate production and fluid volume are reasonably sensitive tests for pancreatic function, but the fluid enzymes are less so. Patients with significant losses of pancreatic function may

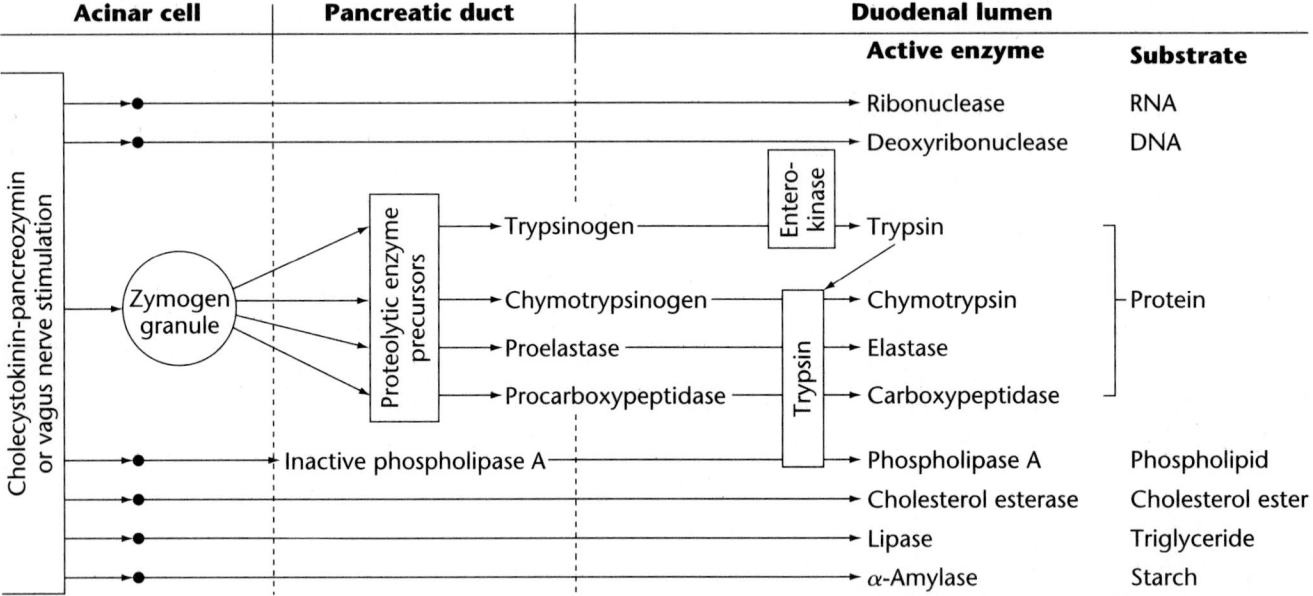

Fig. 29-4 The pancreatic enzymes and their conversion to active forms in the duodenum. The enzymes are stored in zymogen granules that reach the pancreatic duct by exocytosis. Upon reaching the duodenum, the proenzymes are converted to their active form by enterokinase and to a lesser extent by trypsin.

Table 29-2 Factors that control the normal exocrine pancreatic secretions[4,10-12,15]

Event or release of factor	Result
Vagal nerve stimulation of pancreas	Secretion of fluid high in protein and enzymes (such as trypsin), low in bicarbonate, low in volume; release of pancreatic polypeptide
Distension of duodenum by food; alcohol ingestion	CCK and gastrin secretion by duodenum
CCK or gastrin release	Release of zymogen granules from acinar cells; secretion of fluid high in protein and enzymes, low in bicarbonate, low in volume; release of pancreatic polypeptide
Secretin release	Secretion of fluid high in bicarbonate and volume but low in enzymes
Fatty acids or acid food ingestion	CCK release
Amino acids or Ca^{++} ingestion	CCK, gastrin release
Vasoinhibitory polypeptide (VIP) release	Secretin-like effect on gland
Somatostatin release	Inhibition of basal pancreatic secretions, increased fecal fat, decreased intestinal mobility
Trypsin in duodenum	Inhibition of CCK release
Thyroid hormone release	Maintenance of normal pancreatic function and response to stimuli

CCK, Cholecystokinin.

Causes of Acinar Cell Loss

Repeated bouts of pancreatitis, especially that caused by chronic alcoholism
Cystic fibrosis (CF)
Atherosclerosis and subsequent pancreatic atrophy
Any obstruction of the pancreatic ductules or duct as caused by a stone or stones or calcification of the gland, a benign or malignant tumor pressing on the pancreas, or other types of mechanical blockage

---

show a normal bicarbonate and volume because of the large reserve capacity. Enzyme tests on pancreatic fluid can be completely normal in patients with moderate loss of pancreatic acinar tissue; abnormalities appear when the pancreas is nearly exhausted of its enzyme synthetic ability. Thus the testing for pancreatic enzymes in tubal aspirates has limited value in patients with mild to moderate pancreatic insufficiency. In those with extensive exocrine pancreatic impairment as in patients with repeated bouts of pancreatitis or children with cystic fibrosis, tests on duodenal fluid have good sensitivity.

Tests on feces. An abnormal fecal fat test on a 72-hour collection remains as the standard for the diagnosis of pancreatic insufficiency. The patient *must* consume 80 to 100 g of fat per day for at least 1 week before the sample is collected. Undigested fat in feces is measured by qualitative or quantitative tests. Confounding the test are intestinal disorders that impair fat absorption, and fecal fat excretion generally becomes abnormal only after 85% to 90% of pancreatic acinar tissue loss.[20] Tests for trypsin and chymotrypsin in feces are unreliable.[21] (See Chapter 30 for additional information.)

Serum, urine, and breath tests. Because they lack sensitivity, serum amylase, lipase, and phospholipase A_2 are essentially useless for estimating pancreatic function. Im-

---

Table 29-3 Tests of pancreatic function

Test	Patient preparation	Specimen	Normal finding
Secretin/CCK stimulation test	Secretin or CCK (or both) given IV	Duodenal aspirate	Adequate fluid output containing bicarbonate, enzymes, proteins
Fecal fat excretion	80 to 100 g of fat/day and meat for at least 1 week	Feces, 72-hour collection	Less than 7 g of fat excretion per day; no obvious meat fibers observed microscopically on smear
Urinary amylase excretion	24-hour urine collection	Urine	Healthy amylase; greatly increased amylase in pancreas transplant recipients
Pancreatic enzymes in serum	None	Serum	Healthy IRT, trypsinogen
Fat or cholesterol labeled with ^{13}C or ^{14}C	^{13}C- or ^{14}C-labeled fats or cholesterol given by mouth in a controlled meal	Breath	Healthy $^{13}CO_2$ or $^{14}CO_2$ excretion
β-Carotene in serum	Controlled β-carotene in diet	Serum	Normal β-carotene

IRT, Immunoreactive trypsin; *IV,* Intraveneously.

munoreactive trypsin (IRT) consists of at least two unique proteins, an anionic and a cationic form, that differ in their isoelectric pH and electrophoretic mobility at pH 8.6. Cationic trypsin, anionic trypsin, or chymotrypsin measured in serum as proteins are better tests, and IRT on dried blood spots has been recommended as a screening test for cystic fibrosis in newborns.[22,23] The NBT-PABA test (Bentiromide) is used in a few centers for estimating pancreatic digestive function. The drug is *p*-aminobenzoic acid linked to a short chain of synthetic amino acids. In normal individuals, proteolytic enzymes in pancreatic fluid split the molecule, and PABA is absorbed by the small intestine and then excreted in urine where it is measured. Unfortunately the test has poor specificity and is affected not only by pancreatic enzyme secretion but also by intestinal absorption, liver function (conjugation), and renal excretion. PABA can be measured in serum thereby eliminating the renal component in patients with kidney diseases.

Fats labeled with ^{131}I, ^{13}C, or ^{14}C have been advocated as pancreatic function tests. If the pancreatic enzymes hydrolyze the fat or cholesterol esters, ^{131}I can be measured in urine with a gamma counter or, alternatively, $^{13}CO_2$ or $^{14}CO_2$ is measured in the breath with a mass spectrometer or beta counter respectively.[22] A similar strategy employs the fluorescein ester of lauric acid. Pancreatic lipase will split the ester, and the fluorescein is measured in urine or blood. Nearly all pancreatic function tests, whether they use endogenous (such as IRT) or exogenous (such as NBT-PABA) analytes, have limited sensitivity.

Inflammatory or necrotic pancreatic injury

Acute pancreatitis. Acute pancreatitis can be a life-threatening emergency; it must be distinguished from other disorders with a similar presentation. The box below lists several of the leading differential diagnoses of patients with abdominal pain and generally abnormal pancreatic enzymes.

Severe, knife-like pain associated with nausea and vomiting are common presenting features in acute pancreatitis. The disease varies from a mild, self-limiting, edematous form to full-blown necrotizing, hemorrhagic pancreatitis

---

Clinical Problems Associated with Abdominal Pain and Elevated Pancreatic Enzymes

Pancreatitis, perforated stomach ulcer, mesenteric artery infarction, biliary tract disorders, an inflamed gallbladder, gangrenous gallbladder, inflammation or obstruction anywhere along the gastrointestinal tract or abdominal cavity, an abscess anywhere in the abdomen, peritonitis, renal failure, volvulus, dissecting aortic aneurysm, diabetic ketoacidosis, connective tissue disorders with vasculitis, ectopic pregnancy, inflammation of the fallopian tubes[7,9]

---

that often has a fatal outcome. Any factors that obstruct the pancreatic afferent (incoming) or efferent (outgoing) blood supply, the pancreatic ducts, or the ampulla of Vater can precipitate pancreatitis. A proposed mechanism for the evolution of pancreatitis is shown in Table 29-4, though the precise factors leading to pancreatitis are unknown. Leading causes of pancreatitis are alcohol abuse, especially the chronic type, and biliary tract diseases. Alcohol has a double effect of stimulating pancreatic secretion and at the same time irritating the duodenal mucosa, possibly to the point of occluding the pancreatic duct or the duodenal sphincter. There may even be alcohol-caused protein plugs in the pancreatic ductules that lead to pancreatic obstruction.

Although autopsy studies indicate that a stone or obstructing tumor in the common bile duct can lead to the reflux of bile into the pancreas, which may lead to pancreatitis, these are infrequent causes of the disorder. Rather, gallstones tend to promote the development of cholecystitis that

Table 29-4 Proposed events in the development of acute pancreatitis

Event	Likely causes
Injury to acinar cell membranes	Reflux of bile or pancreatic juice into pancreas, alcoholic irritation of duodenum or precipitation of protein plugs in gland, infection or inflammation in gallbladder spreading to pancreas, viral and other microbiological infections of pancreas, ischemia, circulatory failure, trauma, surgery
Biochemical changes in gland	Activation of proenzymes such as protrypsin, proelastase, prophospholipase A_2 to their biochemically active forms; occlusion of pancreatic ductules or duct; conversion of kallikreinogen to kallikrein
Edema, swelling of pancreatic capsule	Inflammation of gland, disturbance of gland's afferent or efferent blood flow
Tetany and cardiac arrhythmias, respiratory distress	Peripancreatic fat necrosis, Ca^{++} sequestration by fatty acids, refractory hypocalcemia, unknown toxic substance(s) (phospholipase A_2?) acting on lung and other organs
Hemorrhagic necrosis of gland, shock, circulatory collapse, profound reduction of plasma volume	Autolysis and digestion of gland with bleeding into retroperitoneal space, release of hypotensive kinins, cytotoxic effect of lysolecithin (from bile)
Death	Acute circulatory and respiratory failure, refractory hypotension

spreads to and inflames the pancreas. Gallstone pancreatitis is especially common in elderly women. A history of alcohol abuse or biliary tract diseases is present in about 75% of patients with pancreatitis; other important causes are listed in the box below.

Prevalence of pancreatitis. Inflammatory diseases of the pancreas including acute pancreatitis, pancreatic pseudocyst, or pancreatic abscess are uncommon. In one series,[17] pancreatitis was suspected in 1800 patients because of abdominal pain or other suggestive symptoms, and serum amylase and lipase were ordered; of these, 188 patients had either or both tests reported as abnormal, and only 25 (1.4%) had confirmed inflammatory pancreatic disease. Nevertheless, the correct diagnosis of patients with pancreatitis may determine survival of the patient given the life-threatening state early on in some with the acute disease. The death rate from pancreatitis is about 1.5 per 100,000 population.

Patients with Frederickson-Levy type I hyperlipidemia (high triglycerides) are at increased risk for developing pancreatitis. The old notion that high triglycerides obscure an increased serum amylase is no longer true with modern methods for amylase, such as those using defined substrates in colorimetric assays (see p. 567).

Drugs associated with pancreatitis. The drugs listed in the box below are linked to pancreatitis, occasionally causing the disorder. A drug effect is generally confirmed if after withdrawal and readministration of the drug pancreatitis recurs. This has been shown several times with valproic acid.[24] There are many other drugs with a less-clear association with pancreatitis.[25]

Pathogenesis of pancreatitis. A likely important mechanism in the pathogenesis of acute pancreatitis is the activation of protrypsin in the gland. This can be caused by infections in the pancreas or in organs proximal to it, reflux of pancreatic fluid, pancreatic anoxia, and other factors. The release of active proteolytic enzymes in the gland results in a self-digestive, proteolytic attack on the gland's structure and blood vessels. Acinar cell injury and activation of the proteolytic enzymes may also occur as a consequence of viral infections, endotoxins, ischemia, and

trauma. Lysosomal enzymes such as cathepsin B may cause intracellular coalescence of zymogen granules leading to premature acinar cell activation of protrypsin and other proenzymes. Activation and release of vasoactive substances probably produce shock, circulatory collapse, and death in some patients. Conversion of prekallikrein to kallikrein in the pancreatic islets activates kinin and the clotting and complement systems; these act to promote inflammation, thrombosis, tissue damage, and bleeding.[8] If there is sufficient damage to the pancreatic blood vessels with bleeding into the peritoneal cavity, hemorrhagic pancreatitis can ensue. Lecithin from bile may be converted by phospholipase A_2 in the pancreas to the highly toxic substance lysolecithin, which promotes the destruction of acinar cell membranes.

The adult respiratory distress syndrome, a grave complication of pancreatitis, may be caused by autodigestive injury to the pulmonary capillaries by circulating lipolytic enzymes from the pancreas, such as phospholipase A_2.[6,7] Fatal, acute pancreatitis has been described as an internal "burn" because of the autopsy findings of extensive necrotic and inflammatory injury to the pancreas, peritoneum, and associated structures in patients who have died of pancreatitis. In most cases the pancreas is completely autolyzed. If the activated enzymes enter the peritoneal space and the systemic circulation, host antiprotease defenses such as α_1-antitrypsin and α_2-macroglobulin may be overwhelmed, and dysfunctions in distant organs such as the lung, kidneys, and parathyroids may occur.

It is possible to give only a very rough estimate of the severity of pancreatitis from the magnitude of the pancreatic enzymes in serum. In some patients, trivial inflammation and edema can lead to large increases in the serum activities of the pancreatic enzymes; in others with end-stage pancreatitis, the serum enzymes may be relatively low because of gland destruction. A host of disorders other than pancreatitis increase both amylase and lipase, though many of these afflicted patients may have undiagnosed secondary pancreatitis. The disorders that are often associated with secondary pancreatitis and with an increased serum amylase and lipase are listed in the box below and on p. 562.

In renal failure, amylase and lipase are typically both increased, not because of pancreatic disease, but because the kidneys fail to excrete amylase, the normal path, and fail

---

Causes of Acute Pancreatitis

Alcoholism, biliary tract diseases, surgery to the pancreas or nearby organs, atherosclerotic plaques in the pancreatic arteries, abdominal trauma, post-ERCP as a complication, metabolic disorders such as hypertriglyceridemia (especially with triglyceride concentrations above 10,000 mg/L), and infections.
Drugs associated with or possibly causing pancreatitis are: azathioprine, cimetidine, cytarabine, didanosine, estrogens, furosemide, 6-mercaptopurine, methyldopa, metronidazole, nitrofurantoin, pentamidine, sulfonamides, sulindac, tetracycline, and valproic acid[6,7,24]

Diseases Associated with Secondary Pancreatitis

All types of biliary tract disorders, any inflammatory process or abscess in the abdomen, renal failure, burns, shock, sepsis, diabetic ketoacidosis, status after surgery, volvulus, gastrointestinal perforation of any kind, pancreas and kidney transplantation

to metabolize lipase in the renal tubules, a normal catabolic process for lipase.

Harbingers of a poor outcome in patients with pancreatitis are hyperglycemia, because of decreased insulin secretion or insulin resistance, hypotension, abnormal pulmonary function tests, bloody or "prune-colored" peritoneal fluid that contains high activities of amylase, leukocytosis, a dropping hematocrit caused by internal bleeding, hypocalcemia, a Po_2 of less than 60 mm Hg, hypoalbuminemia, increased lactate dehydrogenase, azotemia, and an age over 55 years. When several of these factors are present, the prognosis is worse. A prolonged disease course and persistently increased pancreatic enzymes are suggestive of the presence of a pancreatic pseudocyst. Patients with chronic pancreatitis who show laboratory signs of biliary obstruction such as increased serum alkaline phosphatase, gamma-glutamyl transferase, and direct bilirubin probably have compression of the common bile duct as it passes through the fibrotic head of the pancreas.[9]

Sensitivity and specificity of tests in pancreatitis. The sensitivity, specificity, and diagnostic efficiency, that is, how well the tests agree with the diagnosis, is known for most of the commonly available laboratory tests. When pancreatitis is suspected, the commonly ordered studies are amylase and lipase. A somewhat arbitrary but useful ranking of tests from least to most efficient for diagnosing pancreatitis is as follows: urinary amylase, urinary amylase/creatinine ratio, serum phospholipase A_2, serum amylase, pancreatic elastase 1, lipase, pancreatic amylase, pancreatic lipase, lipase L2 isoenzyme, trypsinogen, and immunoreactive trypsin.[22,26]

Urine amylase is a poor test for pancreatitis because of the enormous range of values observed in healthy persons and its poor specificity. Serum phospholipase A_2, amylase, and lipase have good sensitivity but poor specificity, particularly the first of these. A single, moderately abnormal amylase or lipase is usually of no help in a patient with abdominal pain; only about 15% of such patients have pancreatitis.[17] Appropriate use of the pancreatic enzymes to diagnose pancreatitis includes repeat studies during the first 24 to 48 hours after admission. In a patient with signs and symptoms suggestive of acute pancreatitis with serum amylase or lipase values greater than four to five times the assay's upper reference limit and with amylase and lipase values that move in parallel over time, a diagnosis of acute pancreatitis is highly likely.[9,26] Whether amylase is higher than lipase depends on the methods used for the assays. For example, with the du Pont (Wilmington, Delaware) aca instrument, amylase tends to be higher than lipase in pancreatitis, but with the Johnson and Johnson (Rochester, New York) dry-slide technology, the reverse is usually the case.

The sensitivity and specificity of any tests including amylase and lipase in pancreatitis depend on an accurate diagnosis based on objective criteria, something that is not always possible. The sensitivity and specificity values are affected by how the patients were chosen, the time of blood collection since the onset of symptoms, and the methods used for the tests. Reported sensitivities and specificities for amylase are 70% to 100% and 33% to 89% respectively; for lipase they are 63% to 100% and 34% to 100%.[27] The general consensus is that amylase and lipase above the upper reference limit (URL) have good sensitivity but only fair specificity. Fig. 29-5 shows an ROC curve for total amylase, P3 isoenzyme of amylase, total lipase, and the L2 isoform for lipase.[26,28] From this figure, we can conclude that decision or cut-off points affect both the sensitivity and specificity, and P3 amylase or total amylase are inferior to total lipase or L2 lipase. For lipase, increasing the cut-off point between normal and abnormal improves the specificity of the test with little effect on the sensitivity. The URLs for amylase and lipase do not serve well as limits to separate the healthy from the sick.

For amylase and lipase in the diagnosis of acute pancreatitis, the number of false-positive and false-negative diagnoses is smallest when the decision point is set above the URL for amylase (such as 2 × URL) and above the URL for lipase (such as 3 × URL).[27] The predictive value of a moderately increased amylase or lipase (for pancreatitis) is low. The reasons are the low prevalence of pancreatitis in such patients and the poor specificity of these tests when they are only slightly above the upper reference limit.

Amylase has six isoenzymes, though not all are expressed in most individuals.[29] The major groupings of the amylase isoenzymes are salivary and pancreatic; they are readily separated by electrophoresis on cellulose acetate or agarose. The isoenzymes are of limited diagnostic utility. The pancreatic forms cannot be used to discriminate between various types of abdominal causes of an increased total amylase or between edematous and necrotizing pancreatitis. A possible exception is fallopian tube disorders in which salivary rather than the pancreatic isoamylases predominate. Unfortunately, even with serous ovarian carcinoma in which an increase in salivary amylase would be expected, no consistent increase is found, that is, the test has poor sensitivity.[30] Isoamylases assayed by electrophoresis are rarely performed because of the time-consuming nature of the test. Pancreatic amylase, obtained by inhibiting salivary amylase with a wheat protein or an antibody to salivary amylase appear to be better tests than the total serum amylase.

Miscellaneous causes of increased serum amylase. Diseases of the salivary gland, fallopian tubes, renal failure, some lung cancers, and macroamylasemia increase the serum amylase. Amylase has a broader tissue distribution than lipase has; organs containing amylase but not lipase include the salivary glands and fallopian tubes. The amylase activity in saliva is at least 10,000 times that in normal plasma. An increased serum amylase is common in mumps (sialoadenitis) and other inflammatory disorders of the salivary glands. The salivary form of amylase is generally increased in radiation injury of the salivary glands and in

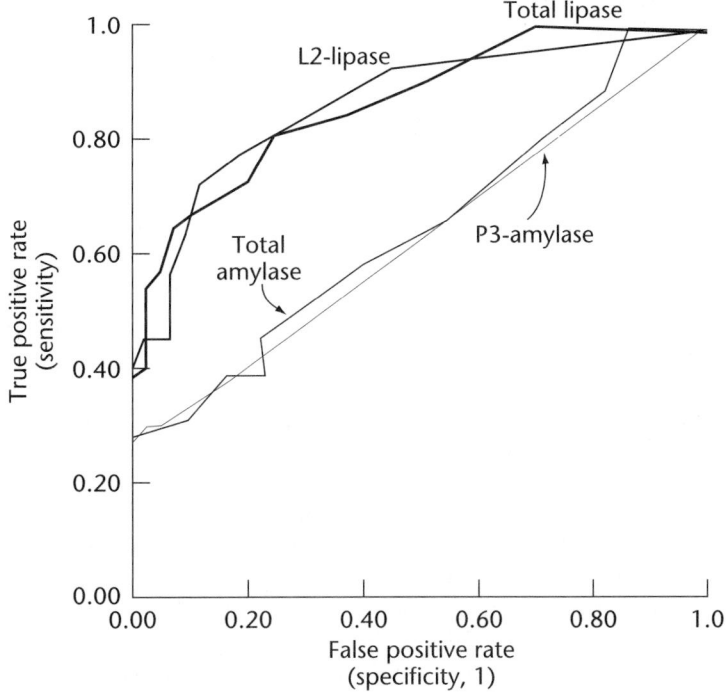

Fig. 29-5 Receiver-operating-characteristics (ROC) curves for amylase, P3-amylase, lipase, and L2-lipase in the diagnosis of pancreatitis. The lipase and L2-lipase tests are significantly better than amylase or P3-amylase. The ideal test should show a sensitivity of 1 and a false-positive rate of zero. The closer the curve gets to the top left corner of the figure, the better the test is. (Adapted from Zweig MH, Campbell G: *Clin Chem* 39:561-577, 1993.)

many ovarian disorders including ectopic pregnancy. After coronary artery bypass surgery, amylase is often increased because of entry of saliva into the lungs during intubation and surgery and absorption of amylase into the bloodstream; the patients usually do not have pancreatitis, and the amylase returns to normal in about 48 hours. In a few patients with lung cancer, an increased amylase may be observed because their tumors produce salivary amylase.[29]

A persistently abnormal amylase in an asymptomatic patient may be macroamylasemia, a laboratory curiosity, usually consisting of amylase bound to an immunoglobulin.[31] The normal clearance mechanisms for amylase are blocked, and the macroamylase accumulates in the blood. It is important to identify macroamylase when present to avoid unnecessary and costly diagnostic studies. After electrophoresis of amylase, macroamylase gives a smear; normally, distinct salivary and pancreatic amylase bands are seen. In the presence of macroamylasemia, the urinary amylase is usually low.

Chronic pancreatitis. Chronic pancreatitis is often a consequence of repeated bouts of acute pancreatitis and extensive destruction of the gland; usually much of the pancreas has been replaced with scar (fibrotic) tissue. Protein plugs in the small ductules may be present and lead to pancreatic fibrosis, calcification, loss of acinar cell function, and even destruction of the islets. DM and pancreatic in-

sufficiency may be present. These patients may be in acute distress but show no or trivial laboratory abnormalities because of the loss of much of the functional pancreatic tissue. Chronic alcohol abuse is the most common cause of chronic pancreatitis, yet most alcoholics do not develop chronic pancreatitis.[6] Nonalcoholic forms include tropical pancreatitis and familial hereditary pancreatitis. A calorie- and protein-deficient diet appears to predispose patients to tropical pancreatitis. Attacks may also be provoked by overeating. Considerable weight loss, a reduced serum albumin, abnormally low vitamins in blood, and other signs of undernutrition are characteristic of chronic pancreatitis.

Atherosclerotic lesions of the pancreatic artery are uncommon. When present, they lead to the gradual, chronic loss of pancreatic endocrine function and finally gland atrophy and total loss of pancreatic activity.

Destructive disorders

Cystic fibrosis. Exocrine pancreatic malfunction is a hallmark of cystic fibrosis (CF), an autosomal, recessively inherited disease of infants and children. CF is the result of a missing or nonfunctional cell-membrane protein that plays a role in the selective cellular uptake of ions. In CF, the pancreatic secretions as well as those of the lungs and other organs are viscous and of low volume. In the pancreas this leads to greatly reduced pancreatic flow and even pancreatic duct obstruction and atrophy. Malabsorption syndromes (see p. 580) and malnutrition can occur in the face of an adequate diet. The diagnosis of CF is based on finding genotypic defects using polymerase chain reaction (PCR) technology,[32] an abnormal sweat chloride test, abnormal pancreatic function tests, the characteristic pulmonary disease, and a history of a blood-related kin with the disease. The chromosome defects are multifaceted, and depending on the genetic error, CF can present in varying severity, from mild to lethal.

Infectious disorders. Infections are both a cause and a complication of pancreatitis. Causative agents are believed to include the mumps virus, echovirus, hepatitis A and B virus, Epstein-Barr virus, coxsackievirus B, HIV, *Ascaris* worms (producing ascariasis, a roundworm infection), and *Mycoplasma* bacteria. Acute pancreatitis has been observed in some HIV-infected children in whom pancreatitis is normally rare.[33] The onset of pancreatitis in a child with AIDS portends imminent death. Drugs given to AIDS patients such as pentamidine isethionate and didanosine also tend to provoke pancreatitis.[34,35]

Pancreatic neoplasms

Adenocarcinoma. Most pancreatic cancers are adenocarcinomas, arising from the ductal epithelial cells and carrying an ominous prognosis. Only about 1% of pancreatic cancers originate in the acinar cells. Pancreatic cancer is the fifth most lethal malignancy in the developed world after colorectal, breast, lung, and prostate cancer.[36] Predisposing factors are smoking; diabetes mellitus; a diet high in fat; and exposure to certain carcinogens such as coal tar, coke, benzidine, and β-naphthylamine. It may be possible to reduce the risk of pancreatic cancer by stopping cigarette smoking and reducing fat intake. Pancreatic cancer is extremely rare in vegetarians. Smokers have a two- to threefold greater incidence of pancreatic carcinoma. The earlier presumed association of coffee consumption and pancreatic cancer has not been confirmed.

Most pancreatic cancers are invasive and inoperable when clinically apparent. Death within 1 year of diagnosis is common, and the 5-year survival rate is a dismal 1%. Jaundice develops early on in 60% to 70% of patients with cancer in the head of the pancreas because of tumor-caused occlusion of the bile duct. In carcinoma of the body or tail of the pancreas, jaundice usually manifests late in the disease. Malabsorption of fats and proteins with weight loss is common. Rarely, a search for the cause of the jaundice may reveal surgically curable pancreatic cancer. The death rate in the United States is about 12 per 100,000 and is increasing.

Testing for the recurrence of pancreatic cancer is possible with the fetoacinar pancreatic protein; pancreatic cancer-associated antigen (CA-19-9), carcinoembryonic antigen, galactosyltransferase, CA-50, or DU PAN-2. There are no satisfactory screening tests for pancreatic cancer, and many acute but benign conditions will give abnormal results for the above tests.[21]

Islet-cell tumors. Ectopic production of hormones is very common in islet-cell tumors; about 20% of islet-cell tumors are biochemically silent and do not secrete. Islet-cell tumors have been found that secrete one or more of the following hormones: ACTH, β-chorionic gonadotropin, C-peptide, calcitonin, gastrin, glucagon, insulin, parathormone, prostaglandins, secretin, serotonin, somatostatin, and VIP.[5,7,37] In nearly all cases the patients have significant endocrine disturbances.

Gastrin-producing, or G-cell islet-cell, tumors are the most common; G-cell tumors, or gastrinomas, produce gastrin in the well-known Zollinger-Ellison syndrome (ZES), which includes uncontrolled stimulation of the stomach's parietal cells and excessive and continuous HCl secretion. The latter generally leads to severe stomach and duodenal ulceration usually to the point of bleeding and perforation.[5,7] Most gastrinomas are malignant and usually metastasize to the liver, abdominal aorta, and other nearby structures. About 10% of gastrinomas are exclusively in the duodenum; most are in the pancreas, and some are in both. A provocative test in patients with ZES with intravenous secretin produces dramatic increases in the plasma gastrin; this does not occur in normal persons (see p. 582). G-cell tumors probably originate from normal α-, β-, or δ-cells.

Beta-cell tumors are next in prevalence, and a few of these secrete insulin in uncontrolled amounts. Because there is no feedback mechanism that turns off the insulin secretion, plasma glucose concentrations may fall below 2.8 mmol/L (500 mg/L). Symptomatic hypoglycemia is common after a time of fasting. Most β-cell tumors are benign, though the profound hypoglycemia may be life threatening. Diagnosis of these tumors is made, in part, by demonstration of increased insulin concentrations in plasma after a period of fasting.

Glucagon-secreting α-cell tumors are rare; the patients usually present with mild DM, weight loss, anemia, and high concentrations of circulating glucagon. More than half of the neoplasms are malignant. Delta-cell tumors are very rare. Some secrete somatostatin, leading to the inhibitory action of this hormone on other cells of the pancreatic islets and on the cells in the gastrointestinal tract that secrete CCK and gastrin. About one half of the cases are malignant and show metastases to the liver.

D1 tumors, or vipomas, secrete VIP, a hormone not normally produced by the pancreas. The patients have profuse, watery diarrhea, hypokalemia, acidosis, a low plasma bicarbonate, and low HCl secretion in the stomach. A few are malignant. Somatostatinomas are rare. The tumors contain δ-cell–like granules and occur in the pancreas in about 60% of patients. Hypersomatostatinemia usually leads to mild DM, steatorrhea, malabsorption, low HCl in the stomach, and watery diarrhea reflecting the inhibitory effect of somatostatin on endocrine cells and on gastrointestinal function. The diagnosis is facilitated by demonstration of large concentrations of circulating somatostatin. Pancreatic carcinoid tumors produce serotonin and the typical carcinoid syndrome; they are rare.[2]

Multiple endocrine neoplasia. The endocrine pancreas is nearly always involved with the type I form of multiple endocrine neoplasias (MEN), a devastating disorder. Common features of this frequently malignant syndrome are listed in the box below.

The MEN I syndrome is inherited as an autosomal dominant trait; that is, the disease is expressed when the patient is heterozygous or homozygous for the abnormal gene. Diagnosis is difficult because the clinical presentation of type I (and type II MEN where the pancreas is usually not involved) is highly diverse,[2] but findings of abnormal concentrations of the endocrine secretions from the above organs is helpful. A standard meal in some type I MEN patients produces an exaggerated pancreatic polypeptide and gastrin response.[38] Also, there is interaction of the hormonal secretions as in the normal state: large concentrations of ACTH drive up the concentration of cortisol, which has an anti-insulin effect, and thus stimulate the pancreatic islets to secrete yet more insulin.

SUMMARY

The pancreas may be the body's "master gland" because of the profound metabolic and digestive disturbances that occur with the loss of endocrine or exocrine pancreatic functions. The major disorder involving loss of endocrine function is diabetes mellitus; it accounts for more morbidity and mortality than all the other pancreatic diseases combined. Important laboratory tests here are serum glucose, fructosamine, and hemoglobin A_{1c} to estimate short- and long-term glycemic control. Loss of exocrine function is common in cystic fibrosis and in some individuals after repeated attacks of pancreatitis commonly caused by chronic alcohol abuse. The pancreas has tremendous reserves, and loss of function leads to symptoms only after about 85% of the acinar cells are lost. There are many pancreatic function tests with the fecal fat test being the most important. Tests on serum, such as immunoreactive trypsin, are less sensitive and less specific though easier to perform.

Acute pancreatitis is a first-class medical emergency; alcoholism and biliary tract diseases are the major causes, though we have only some conjectural evidence on how pancreatitis begins. The changes of the familiar pancreatic enzymes amylase and lipase may be mild to profound; un-

fortunately, it is possible to obtain only a crude estimate of disease severity from laboratory studies. Chronic pancreatitis is usually the sequel of multiple bouts of the acute disease, and laboratory data may not be helpful in making a diagnosis. Pancreatic adenocarcinoma, the common form of the disease, is a disaster for nearly all patients because of the invasive nature of the cancer and its rapid and usually silent progression. There are no adequate screening tests for pancreatic cancer, and death within 6 months to 1 year is typical. Neoplasms of the islets of Langerhans present biochemical challenges for their diagnosis. Except for gastrinomas that produce the Zollinger-Ellison syndrome, most are not malignant but can be life threatening because of the usual uncontrolled release of their endocrine factors and untoward stimulation of their target organs. Tests for the hormones produced by the normal islet cells and other factors are needed to make the diagnosis.

METHODS OF ANALYSIS

Amylase
STEVEN C. KAZMIERCZAK

Principles of analysis and current usage Numerous techniques for measurement of amylase activity have been devised. Whatever method is employed for use, strict adherence to a pH optimum of 6.9 to 7.0 and the inclusion of calcium and chloride ion as enzyme cofactors is important. The various techniques used for amylase determinations are typically grouped into one of several categories.

Of historical interest only are the viscosimetric techniques, which determine amylase activity based on the ability of the enzyme to break down a suspension of starch molecules into smaller fragments. As the starch substrate is broken down into smaller fragments, the viscosity of the solution decreases. The change in viscosity measured before and after a timed incubation period is proportional to enzyme activity.

Iodometric, also called amyloclastic, techniques constitute another procedure that is mainly of historical interest only. These methods are based on the color produced after the reaction of iodine with starch.[39] A starch solution that has been allowed to react with amylase will produce a less intense color change after the addition of iodine. Thus the greater the amount of amylase present in the sample, the lighter is the color produced after the addition of iodine to the starch substrate.

Turbidimetry methods for amylase (Table 29-5, method 1) employ a starch substrate suspended in an aqueous medium to produce a turbid solution with an absorbance of approximately 1.000. Amylase degrades the substrate, resulting in a decrease in turbidity. Unfortunately, variations in substrate consistency make it difficult to standardize the assay. The action of amylase on the substrate may also be followed by use of nephelometry.[40]

A popular technique for amylase determinations employs saccharogenic procedures, which measure the monosaccharides or disaccharides liberated from the reaction of amylase with a defined polysaccharide substrate. In one approach (Table 29-5, method 2), amylase reacts with substrate to produce the disaccharide maltose. The maltose next re-

---

Common Features of Type I Multiple Endocrine Neoplasia Syndrome

Hyperpituitarism, medullary thyroid carcinoma and occasionally extraordinary concentrations of circulating calcitonin, hyperparathyroidism, adrenocortical hyperplasia, hyperinsulinism, peptic ulceration

Table 29-5 Methods of amylase measurement

Method	Principle	Usage	Comments
1. Turbidimetric or nephelometric	Enzymatic hydrolysis of starch solution by amylase causes decrease in both turbidity and amount of scattered light	Rare	Of historical interest
2. Saccharogenic	Reaction of amylase with polysaccharide substrate causes release of glucose. Glucose is quantitated and directly related to amylase activity	Frequent usage	Easily automated
3. Chromolytic	Dye or chromogen linked to substrate is released after reaction of amylase with substrate	Frequent usage	Easily automated
4. Fluorescence polarization	Fluorescein-labeled starch substrate is degraded by amylase into smaller and smaller fragments. Degraded fragments have more rapid spin rotation than parent molecule and cause polarized light to be emitted as depolarized fluorescence	Rare	Specialized instrumentation required

acts with the enzyme maltase to produce glucose, which in turn can be measured by a variety of enzymatic techniques. The amount of glucose that is produced is indicative of amylase activity. The endogenous glucose present in the patient's sample must be taken into consideration when using these methods.

The most frequently used methods for amylase determinations are collectively known as "chromolytic techniques" (Table 29-5, method 3). These methods are based on the ability of amylase to liberate a dye that has been linked to a defined polysaccharide substrate. In one procedure, the dye *p*-nitrophenol is linked to a maltoheptaoside substrate.[41] Cleavage of the yellow-colored *p*-nitrophenol from the glucoside substrate can be monitored at 405 nm. A somewhat similar approach is utilized with the dry-film procedures in which amylase activities are monitored after the hydrolysis of a red dye from a starch substrate. The released dye fragments diffuse into a reagent layer where they are measured photometrically. Dye that is not released from substrate remains hidden in another layer within the gel.

A final, although infrequently used technique for measurement of amylase activity makes use of fluorescence polarization (Table 29-5, method 4).[42] In this procedure, a high-molecular-weight fluorescein-labeled amylose molecule is used as substrate. Since the molecule is relatively large, its rotation in solution is relatively slow, and polarized light that interacts with the fluorescein label will be re-emitted as polarized fluorescent light. Amylase present in a sample will degrade the amylose molecule into smaller molecules. These smaller amylose molecules rotate more rapidly, causing the fluorescent light that is emitted from the fluorescein molecule to be depolarized. Thus the greater the amylase activity present in the sample, the greater the amount of emitted fluorescent light that is depolarized.

Specimen Either serum or heparinized plasma may be used as the sample.[43] However, one study found that when amylase activity is measured using the dry-film procedure, plasma samples anticoagulated with heparin yielded significantly higher results than serum samples.[44] Amylase requires calcium and chloride ions as cofactors. Thus chelating anticoagulants such as citrate, oxalate, and ethylenediaminetetraacetic acid are unacceptable for use. If urine is to be used as the specimen for amylase determinations, the sample should not be acidified.

Amylase is an extremely stable enzyme. In serum and urine specimens that are free of bacterial contamination, amylase is stable for up to 1 week at room temperature. The enzyme is stable for several months at 4° C.[45]

Reference interval Reference intervals differ between the various commercially available assays because of differences in the substrate used and the reagent preparations.[46] Reference ranges given for a commercially available colorimetric procedure is <88 U/L. Amylase activities in newborns are approximately one fifth of that found in adults, with adult levels usually being achieved by 3 to 4 years of age.[43] No sex-related differences in amylase activity have been noted.[43]

Lipase
STEVEN C. KAZMIERCZAK

Principles of analysis and current usage Lipases hydrolyze the long-chain fatty acids of triglycerides by acting on the glycerol–fatty acid ester bonds that exist *only* at an ester-water interface. The greater the surface area of the fatty acid emulsion, the more readily will be the reaction of the enzyme with its substrate.

The first practical assays for lipase measurements used titration of the fatty acids released by the action of lipase on an emulsion of olive oil and gum acacia. The titration was performed with 0.05 M NaOH, using a phenolphthalein indicator.[47] The original titration procedure took 24 hours to complete and was thus not intended as a "stat." procedure. A pH-meter end-point measurement has been developed,[48] as well as the development of a rate technique, which involves the determination of the rate of change in pH as fatty acids are released from an olive oil substrate.[49] Unfortunately, these titration techniques require special skills and equipment, making them unsuitable for most laboratories.

One of the most frequently used methods today employs turbidimetric or nephelometric monitoring of the decrease in turbidity of an olive oil emulsion as the result of the action of lipase on the substrate (Table 29-6, method 1).[50] A highly stable, reproducible substrate that demonstrates an appropriate initial absorbance is required. Approximately 3% to 5% of specimens analyzed by the emulsion-clearing technique will show an anomalous increase in absorbance because of the aggregation of sample components.[51] Rheumatoid factor has been shown to be one such factor that can aggregate sample components. To mitigate this phenomenon, one may pretreat samples with polyethylene glycol to precipitate immunoglobulins.

Table 29-6   Method of lipase measurement

Method	Principle	Usage	Comments
1. Turbidimetry or nephelometry	Action of lipase on substrate emulsion causes decrease in size of emulsion particles. Decrease in turbidity or light scatter is proportional to enzyme activity.	Frequently used	Stable, reproducible substrate required

2. Coupled enzymatic
   a. Glycerol production
   b. Colorimetric measurement of glycerol
	Lipase hydrolyzes triglyceride substrate resulting in production of free glycerol. Free glycerol is quantitated using various techniques.	Frequently used	Endogenous glycerol must be accounted for

Another procedure commonly used to measure lipase employs a coupled enzymatic approach. Lipase hydrolyzes fatty acids from a diglyceride or triglyceride substrate to form free glycerol. The glycerol that is produced can be quantitated and related to lipase activity within the sample (Table 29-6, method 2a).

One coupled-enzymatic assay utilizes a solubilized long-chain fatty acid 1,2-diglyceride obtained from egg lecithin.[53] Lipase cleaves the substrate to form 2-monoglyceride and fatty acid. The 2-monoglyceride is hydrolyzed to glycerol by a specific 2-monoglyceride lipase. In the final indicator reaction step, the chromogen substrate, which is 4-aminophenazone / N-ethyl-N-(2-hydroxy-3-sulfopropyl-m-toluidine), or TOOS, is oxidized to a violet dye, with an absorption maximum at 550 nm (Table 29-6, method 2b).[52]

These coupled-enzymatic assays, which are based upon the measurement of free glycerol, can be adversely affected if the patient's sample contains increased concentrations of free glycerol. Certain drugs and medications have been found to contain high concentrations of free glycerol.[53] However, if a suitable lag period is employed before the measurement of formed glycerol, endogenous glycerol should be consumed and thus not interfere with the assay.

Several immunochemical procedures have been developed. These include a semiquantitative latex-agglutination procedure in which antilipase antibodies are bound to latex particles, which are then mixed with the sample. If lipase is present, agglutinated clumps of particles appear on the reaction slide.[55] A noncompetitive immunoactivation procedure that is specific for pancreatic lipase has also been described.[56] This assay utilizes Fab-antibody fragments against pancreatic lipase, which are covalently bound to the enzyme horseradish peroxidase. In the presence of pancreatic lipase, the peroxidase catalyzes a color-producing reaction; the rate of which is proportional to lipase activity within the sample.

Almost all lipase assays available today employ the cofactor colipase. Colipase enhances the reaction of lipase by enabling the enzyme to interact more effectively with its substrate. Calcium chloride (8.5 mmol/L) and sodium glycocholate (35 mmol/L), a bile salt, are also added to most commercial kits to enhance the activity of lipase.[57]

When performing lipase measurements with current instrumentation that utilizes reusable reaction cuvettes, one must take special precautions to prevent contamination from lipase that may be present in many commercial reagents. The lipase is added as a "clearing factor" in many reagents to reduce interference from sample turbidity. Therefore, before performing the lipase analysis, a special cuvette wash with an alkaline solution is usually needed to remove traces of lipase from previous reagents.

Specimen Serum and plasma samples are suitable for use, since both give equivalent results.[58] Specimens should be stored at 4° C until analysis. Repeated freezing and thawing should be avoided. Lipase activity is normally absent in urine unless the integrity of the glomerular apparatus has been compromised.

Reference intervals Reference ranges for lipase activity in normal healthy individuals are method dependent. The upper references limit for the turbidimetric procedures is approximately 200 U/L, whereas the upper reference limit for the colorimetric assays is approximately 60 U/L. Lipase activity in serum remains relatively constant until about the sixth decade of life when values may increase by as much as 20% over the normal baseline level. No sex-related differences in lipase activity have been found.

ACKNOWLEDGMENTS
With acknowledgment to the previous author for the methods amylase and lipase, Michael D.D. McNeely.

REFERENCES
1. Ganong WF: Endocrine functions of the pancreas and the regulation of carbohydrate metabolism. In *Review of medical physiology,* ed 15, Norwalk, Conn., 1991, Appleton & Lange.
2. Cotran RS, Kumar V, Robbins SL: The endocrine pancreas. In *Robbins pathologic basis of disease,* Philadelphia, 1989, Saunders.
3. Go VLW: Pancreatic secretion. In Stein JH, editor: *Internal medicine,* Boston, 1990, Little, Brown & Co, pp 434-438 and 446-450.
4. Ackermann U: *Essentials of human physiology,* St. Louis, 1992, Mosby, pp 121-123.
5. Scarpelli DG: The pancreas. In Rubin E, Farber JL, editors: *Essential pathology,* Philadelphia, 1990, Lippincott, pp 445-455.
6. Steinberg W: Pancreatitis. In Wyngaarden JB, Smith LH Jr, Bennett JC, editors: *Cecil textbook of medicine,* ed 19, Philadelphia, 1992, Saunders, vol 1.
7. Greenberger NS, Toskes PP, Isselbacher KJ: Acute and chronic pancreatitis. In Wilson JD, Braunwald E, Isselbacher KJ, et al, editors: *Harrison's principles of internal medicine,* ed 12, New York, 1991, McGraw-Hill.
8. Cotran RS, Kumar V, Robbins SL: The exocrine pancreas. In *Robbins pathologic basis of disease,* Philadelphia, 1989, Saunders.
9. Lott JA, Patel ST, Sawhney K, et al: Assays of serum lipase: analytical and clinical considerations, *Clin Chem* 32:1290-1302, 1986.
10. Ganong WF: Regulation of gastrointestinal function. In *Review of medical physiology,* ed 15, Norwalk, Conn., 1991, Appleton & Lange.
11. Gullo L, Pezzilli R, Bellanova B, et al: Influence of the thyroid on exocrine pancreatic function, *Gastroenterology* 100:1392-1396, 1991.

12. Lembcke B, Creutzfeldt W, Schleser S, et al: Effect of the somatostatin analogue Sandostatin (SMS 201-995) on gastrointestinal, pancreatic and biliary function and hormone release in normal men, *Digestion* 36:108-124, 1987.

13. Sarles J. Current techniques for investigating exocrine pancreatic function in children, *Ann Pediatr Paris* 39:221-225, 1992.

14. Lu L, Louie D, Owyang C: A cholecystokinin releasing peptide mediates feedback regulation of pancreatic secretion, *Am J Physiol* 256:G430-G435, 1989.

15. Schmidt WE, Creutzfeldt W, Hocker M, et al: Cholecystokinin receptor antagonist loxiglumide: influence on bilio-pancreatic secretion and gastrointestinal hormones in man, *Digestion* 46(suppl 2):232-239, 1990.

16. Owyang C, Louie DS, Tatum D: Feedback regulation of pancreatic enzyme secretion: suppression of cholecystokinin release by trypsin, *J Clin Invest* 77:2042-2047, 1986.

17. Lott JA, Ellison EC, Applegate D: The importance of objective data in the diagnosis of pancreatitis, *Clin Chim Acta* 183:33-40, 1989.

18. Bolinder J, Wahrenberg H, Persson A, et al: Effect of pancreas transplantation on glucose counterregulation in insulin-dependent diabetic patients prone to severe hypoglycaemia, *J Intern Med* 230:527-533, 1991.

19. Landgraf R, Nusser J, Riepl RL, et al: Metabolic and hormonal studies of type 1 (insulin-dependent) diabetic patients after successful pancreas and kidney transplantation, *Diabetologia* 34(suppl 1):S61-S67, 1991.

20. Speicher CE: *The right test, a physician's guide to laboratory medicine,* ed 2, Philadelphia, 1993, Saunders, pp 122-126.

21. Lott JA: Enzyme tests in gastroenterology. In Moss DW, Rosalki SB, editors: *Principles and practice of diagnostic enzymology,* ed 2, London, 1995, Edward Arnold Publishers.

22. Lott JA: Pancreatic disorders, *Anal Chem* 63:176R-180R, 1991.

23. Waters DL, Dorney SFA, Gaskin KJ, et al: Pancreatic function in infants identified as having cystic fibrosis in a neonatal screening program, *N Engl J Med* 322:303-308, 1990.

24. Lott JA, Bond LW, Bobo RC, et al: Valproic acid–associated pancreatitis: report of three cases and a brief review, *Clin Chem* 36:395-397, 1990.

25. Young DS: *Effects of drugs on clinical laboratory tests,* ed 4, Washington, D.C., 1995, American Association for Clinical Chemistry Press, pp 3.34-3.36.

26. Lott JA, Lu CJ: Lipase isoforms and amylase isoenzymes: assays and application in the diagnosis of acute pancreatitis, *Clin Chem* 37:361-368, 1991.

27. Wong ECC, Butch AW, Rosenblum JL, et al. The clinical chemistry laboratory and acute pancreatitis, *Clin Chem* 39:234-243, 1993.

28. Zweig MH, Campbell G: Receiver-operating characteristic (ROC) plots: a fundamental evaluation tool in clinical medicine, *Clin Chem* 39:561-577, 1993.

29. Lott JA: Amylase. In Lott JA, Wolf PL, editors: *Clinical enzymology: a case-oriented approach,* St. Louis, 1986, Mosby.

30. Bruns DC, Mills SE, Savory J: Amylase in fallopian tube and serous ovarian neoplasms: immunohistochemical localization, *Arch Pathol Lab Med* 106:17-20, 1982.

31. Mifflin TE, Forsman RW, Bruns DE: Interaction of immobilized anti–salivary amylase antibody with human macroamylases: implications for use in a pancreatic amylase assay to distinguish macroamylasemia from acute pancreatitis, *Clin Chem* 35:1651-1654, 1989.

32. Beaudet A, Bowcock A, Buchwald M, et al: Linkage of cystic fibrosis to two tightly linked DNA markers: joint report from a collaborative study, *Am J Hum Genet* 39:681-693, 1986.

33. Miller TL, Winter HS, Luginbuhl LM, et al: Pancreatitis in pediatric human immunodeficiency virus infection, *J Pediatr* 120:223-227, 1992.

34. Shelton MJ, O'Donnell AM, Morse GD: Didanosine, *Ann Pharmacother* 26:660-670, 1992.

35. Bonacini M: Pancreatic involvement in human immunodeficiency virus infection, *J Clin Gastroenterol* 13:58-64, 1991.

36. DiMagno EP: Carcinoma of the pancreas. In Wyngaarden JB, Smith LH Jr, Bennett JC, editors: *Cecil textbook of medicine,* ed 19, Philadelphia, 1992, Saunders.

37. Grünfeld C: Pancreatic islet cell tumors. In Wyngaarden JB, Smith LH Jr, Bennett JC, editors: *Cecil textbook of medicine,* ed 19, Philadelphia, 1992, Saunders.

38. Skogseid B, Oberg K, Benson L, et al: A standardized meal stimulation test of the endocrine pancreas for early detection of pancreatic endocrine tumors in multiple endocrine neoplasia type 1 syndrome: five years' experience, *J Clin Endocrinol Metab* 64:1233-1240, 1987.

39. Caraway WT: A stable starch substrate for the determination of amylase in serum and other body fluids, *Am J Clin Pathol* 32:97-99, 1959.

40. Liu TZ, Wei JS: Rapid laser nephelometric determination of amylase activity in serum and urine, *J Formosan Med Assoc* 90:217-220, 1991.

41. Okabe H, Uji T, Netsu K, Noma A: Automated measurement of amylase with 4-nitrophenylmaltoheptaoside as a substrate and use of a selective amylase inhibitor, *Clin Chem* 30:1219-1222, 1984.

42. Hofman M, Shaffer M: Fluorescence depolarization assay for quantitative α-amylase in serum and urine, *Clin Chem* 31:1478-1480, 1985.

43. Gillard BK, Simbala JA, Goodglick L: Reference intervals for amylase isoenzymes in serum and plasma of infants and children, *Clin Chem* 29:1119-1123, 1983.

44. Doumas BT, Hause LL, Simuncak DM: Differences between values for plasma and serum in tests performed in the Ektachem 700 XR analyzer, and evaluation of "plasma separator tubes (PST)," *Clin Chem* 35:151-153, 1989.

45. Henry RJ: *Clinical chemistry: principles and techniques,* ed 4, New York, 1964, Harper & Row.

46. Chen CT, Dineen H, Newton JD: Specificity of different substrates used in three amylase assays, *Clin Chem* 34:1363-1364, 1988.

47. Cherry IS, Crandall IA Jr: The specificity of pancreatic lipase: its appearance in the blood after pancreatic injury, *Am J Physiol* 100:266-273, 1932.

48. Tietz NW, Fiereck EA: Measurement of lipase in serum. In Cooper GR, editor: *Standard methods of clinical chemistry,* vol 7, New York, 1972, Academic Press.

49. Cerolotti F, Bonini PA, Murone M, et al. Measurement of lipase activity by differential technique, *Clin Chem* 31:257-260, 1985.

50. Zinterhofer L, Wardlaw S, Jatlow P, Seligson D: Nephelometric determination of pancreatic enzymes. II. Lipase, *Clin Chim Acta* 44:173-178, 1973.

51. Kannisto J, Lalla M, Lukkari E: Characterization and elimination of a factor in serum that interferes with turbidimetry and nephelometry of lipase, *Clin Chem* 29:96-99, 1983.

52. Robbrecht JH, DeBuyzere ML, Delanghe JR: Wake UV colorimetric pancreatic lipase assay with 1,2-dilinoleoylglycerol as substrate evaluated, *Clin Chem* 35:1540-1541, 1989.

53. Fassati P, Ponti M, Paris P, et al: Kinetic colorimetric assay of lipase in serum, *Clin Chem* 38:211-215, 1992.

54. Bilodeau L, Grotte DA, Preese LM, et al: Glycerol interference in serum lipase assay falsely indicates pancreas injury, *Gastroenterology* 103:1066-1067, 1992.

55. Møller-Peterson J, Klaerke M, Dati F, et al. Immunochemical qualitative latex agglutination test for pancreatic lipase in serum evaluated for use in diagnosis of acute pancreatitis, *Clin Chem* 31:1207-1210, 1986.

56. van Ingen HE, Sanders GTB: Clinical evaluation of pancreatic lipase mass concentration assay, *Clin Chem* 38:211-215, 1992.

57. Tietz NW, Astles JR, Shuey DF: Lipase activity measured in serum by a continuous-monitoring pH-stat technique—an update, *Clin Chem* 35:1688-1693, 1989.

58. Doumas BT, Hause LL, Simuncak DM, et al: Differences between values for plasma and serum in tests performed in the Ektachem 700 XR analyzer, and evaluation of "plasma separator tubes (PST)," *Clin Chem* 35:151-153, 1989.

CHAPTER 30

Gastrointestinal function and digestive disease

Michael D.D. McNeely

OBJECTIVES

- Describe the anatomy of the normal digestive tract.
- Outline the digestive and absorptive functions of the normal digestive tract.
- List the major pathological conditions of the gastrointestinal tract and the causes of these conditions.
- Describe the gastrointestinal function tests and the expected test results in disease states.
- State expected results of the following laboratory tests in gastrointestinal disease states: gastrin, carotene, vitamin A, trypsin, fecal fat, fecal occult blood, CEA, 5-HIAA, and urinary oxalate.
- In general terms, define gastrointestinal hormones and describe their role in gastrointestinal function.
- State the site of origin, the action, and the clinical significance of the following hormones: gastrin, CCK-PZ, secretin, VIP, PP, GIP, motilin, enteroglucagon, and somatostatin.

KEY TERMS

achlorhydria Literally 'without hydrochloric acid'. Refers to lack of acid production by the stomach.

anticholinergic A drug that opposes the action of the cholinergic nervous system.

APUD cells Acronym for cytochemical properties of an endocrine cell that has an *a*mine content, an amine *p*recursor *u*ptake, and *d*ecarboxylation.

brain-gut axis Similar peptides that are found in the gut, nerves, and central nervous system.

chyme The semisolid end product of gastric action on food. Chyme consists of mucus, gastric secretions, and broken-down food.

gastrointestinal hormones Substances that are produced by gastrointestinal cells and then travel through the bloodstream to act at a separate site. These hormones include cholecystokinin, secretin, glucagon, gastric inhibitory polypeptide, vasoactive intestinal polypeptide, bombesin, somatostatin, motilin, bulbogastrone, entero-oxyntin, and pancreatic polypeptide.

gluten A protein found in wheat and wheat products.

intubation The procedure of introducing a tube-shaped instrument into the body, usually through an anatomical opening, such as the mouth.

pancreatic exocrine enzymes Enzymes required for digestion. Often released in a precursor form. These enzymes include trypsinogen, chymotrypsinogen, proelastase, procarboxypeptidase, ribonuclease, deoxyribonuclease, amylase, lipase, phospholipase A, and cholesterol esterase.

pancreatic hormones Endocrine hormones mainly concerned with carbohydrate intermediary metabolism and include glucagon, insulin, and gastrin.

pyrexia Fever. A body temperature above 37.5° C.

The gastrointestinal tract is a muscular tube lined with epithelial cells and extending 10 m from the mouth to the anus. Along its course its structure is modified to suit particular requirements for the digestion and absorption of food.

The old view of the gastrointestinal tract described it as an inert conduit, across which digested food molecules were allowed to pass into the bloodstream. Today physicians realize that the absorptive surface of the intestine is an extremely elaborate organ covered with minute microvilli that are invested with complex enzyme systems. This intricate microstructure creates an extremely efficient and highly selective absorptive mechanism.[1] In addition, the gastrointestinal tract is controlled by an elaborate hormonal and neural regulatory network.[2]

To complement this enhanced physiological knowledge, new diagnostic techniques, including imaging procedures, fiberoptic intubation, and chemical analyses, have introduced a new era of gastrointestinal diagnoses.

ANATOMY AND GENERAL FUNCTIONS

The gastrointestinal tract has five distinct regions: mouth, stomach, duodenum, jejunum-ileum, and large bowel (Fig. 30-1).

The mouth contains teeth, tongue, salivary glands, and an elaborate swallowing mechanism. It is responsible for tasting, grinding, and lubricating food. The swallowing mechanism propels the food down the esophagus, through the thoracic cavity, and into the stomach.

The stomach is a rough-surfaced, muscular bag coated with a protective mucus layer. The vigorous churning action of the stomach is responsible for the mixing and breakdown of food. Hydrochloric acid and the enzyme pepsin are also secreted and continue the digestive breakdown. These actions convert food into chyme.

The chyme enters the duodenum, into which bile and pancreatic enzymes are secreted. Further enzymatic degradation of the basic food materials takes place in the duodenum and continues as the food material enters the small intestine.

The small intestine is 4 m long. Its absorptive capacity is enhanced by its microvillous substructure. The small intestine consists of two parts—the jejunum proximally and the ileum distally. Here the fragmented food materials are finally broken down and absorbed into the bloodstream.

When the nutrients have been absorbed, the residual matter enters the large intestine, where a process of selective water and electrolyte balance occurs. The digestive process terminates with the formation of feces.

The entire absorptive surface of the gastrointestinal tract is drained by the portal venous blood vessels. These convey the newly absorbed materials directly to the liver so that they may be immediately converted into usable forms.

The intestinal tract, from the stomach to the small bowel, contains endocrine cells. The gastrointestinal hormones produced by these cells are a heterogeneous group of biologically active peptides that are involved in the regulation of gastrointestinal function. In addition, a significant number

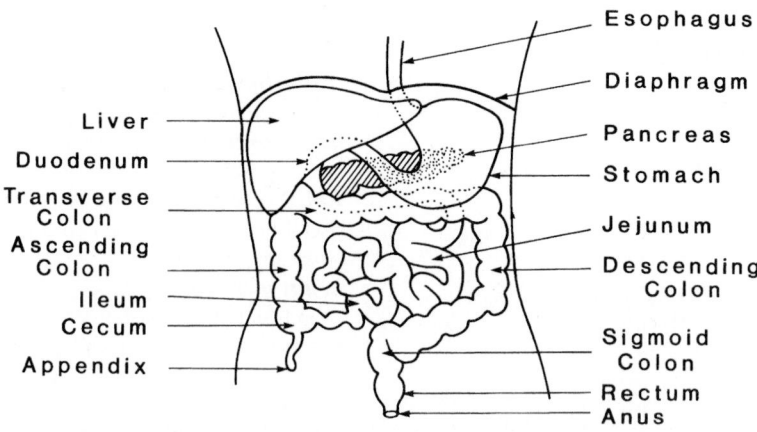

Fig. 30-1   Diagram of gastrointestinal tract.

of these peptides are present in the nerves of the gastrointestinal tract[2] and in the central nervous system,[3] thus establishing the "brain-gut axis" for these hormones. The knowledge that gut hormones are distributed not only in endocrine cells but also in peripheral and central nerves has established the fact that these peptides function not only as hormones but also as neurotransmitters.[4]

DIGESTION

Digestion is the chemical process of rendering food into a form that can be absorbed by the body. The digestive process begins in the mouth and is generally completed in the proximal portion of the small intestine. The digestive process for various foods is summarized in Table 30-1.

Digestive action of mouth

Food is tasted in the mouth by the combined action of the taste receptors on the dorsal surface of the tongue and on the palate, pharynx, and tonsils. Four fundamental tastes are recognized: sweet, salt, sour, and bitter. The taste of food also depends on its smell. The integration of these various neural inputs produces the sensation known as *taste*. The taste of a food substance is important to protect us from disagreeable foods, to encourage eating, and to initiate a complex psychoneurogenic reflex that acts on the rest of the gastrointestinal tract.

Part of this reflex stimulates the production of saliva from the three pairs of salivary glands: parotid, mandibular, and sublingual. These glands produce viscid, water-based, mucin-containing secretions that act as a lubricant. They also release salivary amylase to initiate the digestion of starch.

Food is masticated by the complex interaction of the teeth, tongue, and mouth. The resulting bolus of food is then propelled to the stomach.

Digestive action of stomach

The stomach is a thin-walled, muscular sac that one can roughly divide into three zones (Fig. 30-2). The very top part of the stomach is known as the *fundus*. The main portion of the stomach is known as the *body*. The outlet of the stomach is known as the *antrum* and is segregated from the duodenum by the pyloric region, which contains a strong, muscular sphincter.

The gastric mucosa is covered with numerous coarse

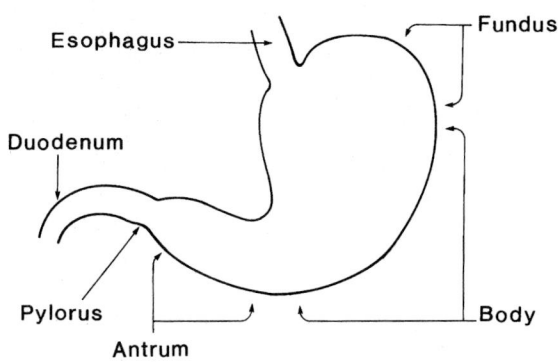

Fig. 30-2   Diagram of stomach.

folds known as *rugae*. The rugae assist in mixing food substances during the churning action of the stomach.

The gastric mucosa contains four types of cells. Mucous cells are found throughout the entire stomach and secrete mucus to protect the surface from attack by acid and enzymes. Also found in all parts of the stomach are the surface epithelial cells, which are also capable of secreting mucus but which proliferate rapidly and shed readily, producing a continually viable surface for the stomach. Parietal cells produce hydrochloric acid and intrinsic factor. Chief cells produce the enzyme pepsinogen. These last two cell types are found throughout the body of the stomach.

The antral cells secrete mainly mucus but also some pepsinogen. The hormone gastrin is synthesized and stored in the G cells of the antrum.

There are three phases of gastric activity. The first of these is the cephalic phase, which is initiated by the sight and smell of food. This sensation triggers a direct vagus nerve message from the brain to the stomach to initiate the digestive process.

Next is the gastric phase of digestion, in which a variety of mechanisms interplay to create the digestive milieu (Fig. 30-3):

1. The vagus nerve directly stimulates the parietal cells to release hydrochloric acid.
2. The antral cells are also stimulated by the vagus nerve to secrete gastrin. Gastrin in turn stimulates the parietal cells to produce more hydrochloric acid.
3. Local distension of the gastric antrum also stimulates the production of gastrin and thus the secretion of hydrochloric acid.

Table 30-1   Chemical processes for digestion of food

Food material	Digestive action	End product
Starch	Pancreatic amylase	Disaccharides (mainly maltose)
Disaccharides	Mucosal disaccharidases	Monosaccharides
Monosaccharides	None	
Protein	Gastric hydrochloric acid and pepsin	Partial degradation into large polypeptides
	Pancreatic trypsin, chymotrypsin, and carboxypeptidase	Polypeptides, depeptides, and amino acids
Long-chain triglycerides	Emulsification with bile, hydrolysis by lipase	Fatty acids and glycerol

4. Cholinergic (vagus) reflexes are further enhanced by distension of the fundus of the stomach.
5. The chief cells contain receptors that respond to the acid environment by secreting the enzyme precursor pepsinogen. Pepsinogen is rapidly converted into its active form (pepsin) at pH 3. Lipase and other enzymes are also liberated, but these enzymes are of little consequence in the digestive process.

The combined action of antral contractions, pyloric sphincter activity, and chemical secretions render the food into a much degraded, mucus-containing solution known as *chyme.*

Stomach activity subsides with time, and the fragmented material is then permitted to pass into the duodenum.

Digestive action of duodenum

The next step in digestion occurs in the duodenum. As chyme enters this portion of the intestine, several gastrointestinal hormones are released by both neural and local stimulation (Table 30-2). These hormones enter the portal blood system and act primarily on various regions of the gastrointestinal tract. See below and reference 3 for a review of the actions of these hormones.

As a result of intricate hormonal feedback activity, bile salts, bicarbonate, the enzymes amylase and lipase, and a variety of protein-degrading enzymes are secreted into the duodenum. The action of these agents on the primary food substances is now considered.

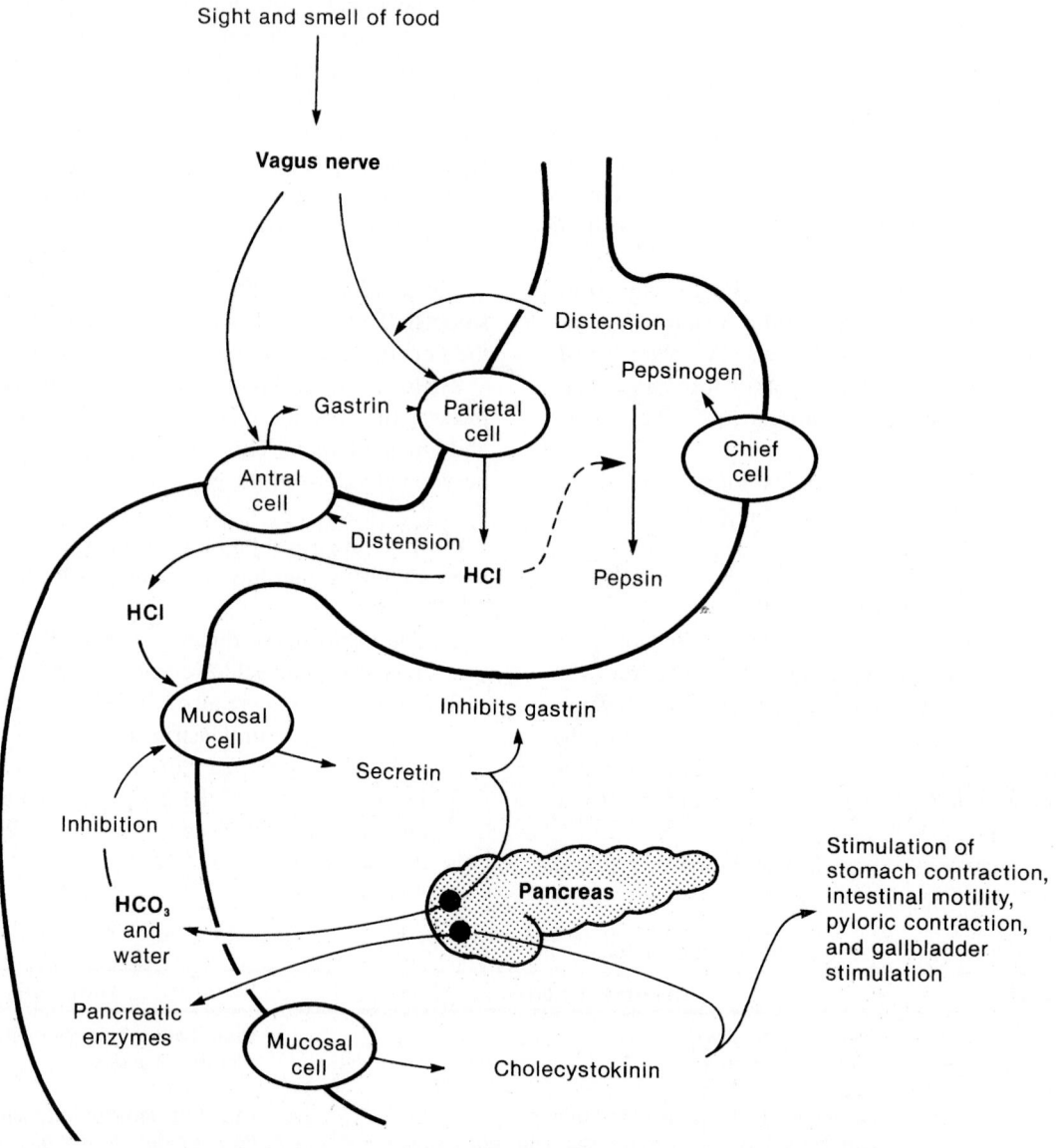

Fig. 30-3   Schema demonstrating various stimuli of stomach and duodenum.

Table 30-2   Intestinal hormones

Hormone	Number of amino acids	Source	Stimulating factor	Function
Cholecystokinin	33	Mucosa of upper small intestine	Amino acids, fatty acids, hydrochloric acid, and food in duodenum	Stimulates pancreatic enzyme secretion, gallbladder contraction, contraction of stomach and pylorus, intestinal motility
Gastrin	14-34	Stomach, gut lumen	Protein digestion products, food in duodenum	Stimulates stomach acid secretion, gastric mobility, gastral mucosal growth
Secretin	27	Throughout gut mucosa but concentrated in duodenum	Acid in duodenum	Stimulates pancreatic secretion of water and bicarbonate, gastric pepsin secretion; relaxes pyloric sphincter
Motilin	22	Upper small intestine	High-fat meal, duodenal acidification	Stimulates motility of small intestines and duodenum
Glucagon	29	Pancreatic and intestinal mucosa	Arginine, alanine, stress	Stimulates gluconeogenesis; raises blood glucose
Gastric inhibitory polypeptide (GIP)	43	Duodenal mucosa	Glucose and fat	Cholecystokinin-like activity
Vasoactive intestinal polypeptide (VIP)	28	Wide distribution throughout gut		Vasodilatation and hypotensive effects; inhibits histamine, pentagastrin acid release, and pepsin secretion; stimulates electrolyte and water secretion from pancreas; stimulates bile flow
Enteroglucagon (glucagon-like peptides)	29	Lower small intestine	Meal	Inhibits intestinal transit; enhances mucosal growth
Bombesin	14			Stimulates pancreatic secretion and gastrin release

Carbohydrate digestion[5]

Carbohydrates are present in the diet as monosaccharides, disaccharides, or complex polysaccharides. Only the polysaccharides require extensive digestion in the duodenum.

Starch is the most common complex polysaccharide. It has a branching structure based on 1,4-carbohydrate or 1,6-carbohydrate linkages. Amylase is capable of hydrolyzing starch into oligosaccharides and ultimately into disaccharides. The dominant disaccharide produced from starch is maltose. Thus, as the food leaves the duodenum, monosaccharides and disaccharides from the diet and disaccharides resulting from the action of amylase are passed to the jejunum and ileum, wherein absorption takes place.

Protein digestion[6]

Dietary protein is partially degraded in the stomach by hydrochloric acid and pepsin. In the duodenum, trypsin, chymotrypsin, and carboxypeptidase secreted by the pancreas act on the partially degraded protein to yield polypeptides, dipeptides, and amino acids. These tiny molecules then pass into the ileum and jejunum for assimilation.

Fat digestion[7]

Fat digestion is more complex than digestion of other basic food substances. Most dietary fats are long-chain triglycerides (palmitic, stearic, oleic, and linoleic acids). The stomach decreases the particle size of the fatty substances by its churning action. In the duodenum, fats are emulsified by the detergent action of bile. Emulsification allows the pancreatic enzyme, lipase, to attack the otherwise water-insoluble lipids. Lipase causes stepwise hydrolysis, which first forms a diglyceride, then a monoglyceride, and finally a fatty acid and glycerol (see Chapter 33).

The bile salts, which are so important for fat digestion, are synthesized in the liver from cholesterol and are conjugated to taurine or glycine. The main bile salts are conjugates of cholic and chenodeoxycholic acid.

ABSORPTION

Absorption is the process whereby digested food substances enter the body.[4] Having traversed the duodenum, these digested food substances enter the jejunum and ileum, wherein the final absorption process takes place.

The intestinal mucosa is thrown into many folds, which assist in propelling its contents distally. The surface of each fold is drawn up into fingerlike projections known as *villi* (Fig. 30-4). Each villus increases the absorptive surface many times. Electron microscopic studies have shown that each villus is covered by hairlike projections known as *microvilli*. There are 200 million microvilli per centimeter of epithelium. Thus the intestine is given a massive absorptive surface area measuring 500 m^2.

It was once believed that enzymes were secreted by the small intestine to produce a digestive juice known as *succus entericus*. We now know that the main enzymatic action occurs in intimate association with the epithelial surface. Rather than being a purely passive sieve through which food substances are permitted to pass, the intestinal mucosa contains a highly selective mechanism for the absorption of each nutrient.

Although there are regional differences in the ability of the intestine to absorb different food substances, these details are not considered here.

Carbohydrate absorption

The digestive process degrades carbohydrate into monosaccharides and disaccharides. The monosaccharides—glucose, galactose, and fructose—are absorbed by specific active-transport mechanisms; that is, they are conveyed from the intestinal lumen into the bloodstream against a concentration gradient. Energy is required for this to occur.

The disaccharides are split into monosaccharides by the enzymatic activity of disaccharidase enzymes located on the microvilli. For example, the milk sugar, lactose, is split by the enzyme lactase into its component sugars, glucose and galactose. These are then actively absorbed. The disaccharide sucrose is split by the enzyme sucrase into glucose and fructose. Maltose, which is the common product of starch hydrolysis, is split by a surface maltase into two molecules of glucose.

Protein absorption

The digested products of protein are small polypeptides, dipeptides, and amino acids. Dipeptides are absorbed more rapidly than amino acids because of special transport mechanisms. Proteins are not absorbed directly. A very large number of specific absorptive mechanisms designed for various types of amino acids are located in the mucosal surface.

Fat absorption (see also Chapter 33)

The successfully digested fat enters the intestine as a micelle. By diffusion the fatty acids and monoglycerides en-

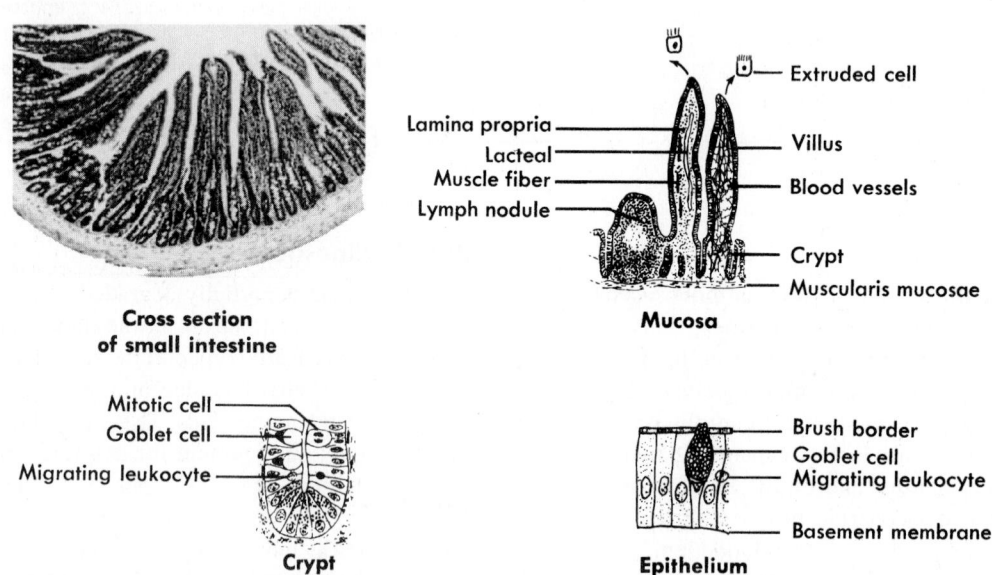

Fig. 30-4 Structures of functional components of small intestine. (From Arey LB: *Human histology: a textbook in outline form,* ed 4, Philadelphia, 1974, Saunders.)

ter the intestinal epithelial cells, where they then interact with a binding protein. Long-chain fatty acids of 16 to 18 carbons are reesterified to form triglycerides and then bound to apolipoproteins to form chylomicrons. These tiny lipid droplets are released into the lymphatic system and transported to the thoracic duct before entry into the bloodstream. Medium-chain fatty acids (8 to 10 carbons) are not reesterified and rapidly enter the portal bloodstream bound to albumin.

Vitamins D, E, A, and K[8,9]

Vitamins D, E, A, and K (see also Chapter 39) are not water soluble and must therefore be absorbed with lipids. Thus they depend on normal lipid absorption. Vitamin D absorption is modified by calcium intake and metabolism.

Water and sodium absorption

The control over water absorption is not fully understood, but it is believed that bulk flow with sodium absorption is the mode for water transport in the intestine. Sodium is absorbed by an active-transport mechanism that is linked to the absorption of amino acids, bicarbonate, and glucose.

Calcium

Calcium transport (see also Chapter 28) is under the influence of vitamin D and parathyroid hormone and is regulated by a calcium-binding protein in the mucosal cells.[10]

Iron absorption (see also Chapter 35)

Gastric acid is required to convert iron to the absorbable ferrous form.[11] Iron then enters the mucosal cells and is transported across these cells before being picked up by carrier proteins in the circulation.

Formation of stool

Having passed through the ileum and jejunum, the intestinal contents enter the large bowel. Very little absorption of nutrients occurs in this region. It is here that water is actively absorbed and returned to the circulation. In addition, the balance of electrolytes is regulated. Progressive dehydration of undigested food substances and the action of the bacteria that normally inhabit the colon lead to the formation of feces.

HORMONE PHYSIOLOGY
Gut hormone structure

The two main families of gut hormones are the gastrin and the secretin families. The *gastrin* family consists primarily of gastrin and cholecystokinin, but, in addition, motilin and enkephalin share several structural identities. The *secretin* group includes secretin, gastric inhibitory polypeptide (GIP), vasoactive intestinal polypeptide (VIP), glucagon, and bombesin.[12] Many of these hormones are present in multiple forms of varying molecular size.

Gut hormones are regarded as regulators of digestion and absorption. They are released in response to the presence of nutrients in the lumen of the gastrointestinal tract and stimulate the release of acid, bicarbonate, and enzymes for digestion of food. Once the nutrients enter the blood, the pancreatic metabolic hormones are released. This link has led to the term *enteroinsular axis*. Different steps of digestion, absorption, and storage can be both stimulated and inhibited by different gastroenteropancreatic peptides.

Each gastrointestinal function has several agonists and antagonists. Final control thus depends on a fine balance of numerous influences. In the case of gastric acid secretion, at least 21 different factors appear important in its normal control. Motilin, gastrin, VIP, and glucagon are the major hormones involved in the control of secretion, absorption, motility, and growth in the stomach and intestine. Secretin, cholecystokinin (CCK), VIP, and pancreatic polypeptide (PP) control exocrine pancreatic function, whereas insulin and GIP are involved in the enteroinsular axis. Insulin, glucagon, and somatostatin are primarily involved in the metabolism of carbohydrate, fats, and protein. Substance P, VIP, and the enkephalins have a major neurotransmitter involvement in the central, peripheral, and autonomic nervous systems.

Gastrin[13,14]

Gastrin exists in multiple molecular forms, containing from 14 to 34 amino acids. The cellular origin of gastrin is the G cell of the gut. These cells extend into the gut lumen, where they terminate in a tuft of microvilli.

Gastrin stimulates acid secretion, gastric motility, and the growth of fundic small bowel and mucosa.[15] Secretion of gastrin is mediated by luminal, nervous, and blood-borne stimuli. The principal luminal stimuli are the amino acid products of protein digestion.[16] Other luminal stimuli include calcium, alcohol, and intragastric pH. Excess acid provides a feedback mechanism for autoregulation of gastrin release. Secretin, GIP, VIP, glucagon, calcitonin, and somatostatin are known to inhibit the release of gastrin.

Cholecystokinin

The molecule is a basic peptide of 33 amino acid residues. Cholecystokinin (CCK) is found in the brain and in the K cells of the upper small intestinal mucosa.

The finding of CCK-like peptides in the central nervous system and in the gut indicates that these peptides may function as both neurotransmitters and hormones. The physiological role of CCK is the regulation of the motility of the gallbladder and intestine and the regulation of secretion by the pancreas. Physiological actions of CCK in the pancreas include the stimulation of the release of enzymes, the potentiation of the action of secretin, and stimulation of the growth of the pancreas. A mixture of polypeptides and amino acids is a strong stimulus for the release of CCK. Fatty acids with chains longer than nine carbons also stimulate CCK release.

Secretin

Secretin is a basic peptide of 27 amino acid residues with strong similarities in sequence to glucagon. Secretin is predominantly located in the S cells of the mucosa of the duodenum and jejunum.[17]

Secretin inhibits smooth muscle contraction, decreases gastric acid secretion, lowers the lower esophageal sphincter pressure, and stimulates pancreatic growth. In addition to these effects, it stimulates water and bicarbonate secretion from the pancreas and Brunner's glands and augments gallbladder contraction. It has a synergistic action with CCK in the stimulation of gallbladder contraction and pancreatic enzyme secretion.[18] The primary physiological role of secretin appears to be the modulation of pancreatic bicarbonate secretion.

A principal stimulus for duodenal secretin release is stomach acid, but in the adult jejunum there is seldom if ever likely to be sufficient acid to liberate secretin.[19] Fatty acids with 10 or more carbons in the chain weakly stimulate secretin release.

Vasoactive intestinal polypeptide

Vasoactive intestinal polypeptide (VIP) has 28 amino acids and has been shown to be present in both endocrine cells and nerves of the gut and central nervous system.[20] VIP has a wide range of gastrointestinal activities, including inhibition of gastric acid secretion, stimulation of insulin release, stimulation of pancreatic water and bicarbonate secretion, and stimulation of intestinal fluid and electrolyte secretion.

Pancreatic polypeptide

Pancreatic polypeptide (PP) contains 36 amino acids, but its entire biological activity is displayed by the last 6 amino acids. PP is found almost entirely in the pancreas, where it is distributed in the D_2 cells of the islets.

Pharmacological studies show that PP opposes the effects of cholecystokinin.[21] It therefore inhibits the pancreatic output of enzymes and gallbladder contraction. At somewhat higher doses it has a biphasic effect, initially stimulating and then later inhibiting pancreatic bicarbonate output. PP may play a role in the modulation of insulin and glucagon secretion by the islets. Fat and protein appear to be the main dietary constituents that are responsible for PP release after a meal.

Gastric inhibitory polypeptide

Gastric inhibitory peptide (GIP) contains 43 amino acids and is found in the K cells of the jejunal mucosa and to a lesser extent in the duodenum and ileum.

There is a relatively prolonged rise in GIP after a meal.[22] In the presence of oral ingestion of food, GIP causes an enhancement of glucose-induced insulin release. GIP is also a potent stimulant of small intestine fluid and electrolyte secretion.

Motilin

Motilin is a 22–amino acid peptide found in the enterochromaffin cells of the small intestine, predominantly in the upper portion.

Motilin is released into the plasma after a meal, particularly if the fat content is high. In humans duodenal acidification causes an increase in plasma motilin. The actions of motilin include stimulation of small intestine and gastric motility, increase in lower esophageal sphincter pressure, and stimulation of pepsin output. Motilin accelerates gastric emptying in humans, and it also may be responsible for emptying the small intestine between meals.

Glucagon-like immunoreactive peptides

Several molecular forms of this family of hormones, which includes pancreatic glucagon, have been identified. Each intestinal peptide probably has a separate physiological role, though only one cell type containing glucagon-like immunoreactivities is found in the intestine.[23]

Glucagon and the glucagon-like immunoactive peptides have several biological actions, which include relaxation of smooth muscle, inhibition of pancreatic enzyme secretion, inhibition of gastric acid secretion, stimulation of intestinal fluid and electrolyte secretion, and stimulation of cardiac output. Pancreatic glucagon is secreted primarily in response to hypoglycemia and is important in the mobilization of hepatic glycogen stores and carbohydrate homeostasis (see Chapters 27 and 32).

Somatostatin

Somatostatin is a peptide composed of 14 amino acids. Somatostatin is found throughout the brain, but the highest concentrations of somatostatin are found in the hypothalamus. In the gut the greatest amounts are found in the antrum of the stomach, in the mucosa of the upper small intestine, in the cells of the islets of Langerhans of the pancreas, and in a small number of fine nerve fibers.[24]

In the gastrointestinal tract, somatostatin inhibits gastric emptying, pepsin secretion, gallbladder contraction, and bile and pancreatic enzyme secretion.[25] Somatostatin is also one of the most potent inhibitors of endocrine secretions known.[26] It completely inhibits the release of growth hormone and also inhibits the release of thyroid-stimulating hormone, insulin, glucagon, pancreatic polypeptide, gastrin, secretin, motilin, enteroglucagon, and neurotensin.[27] In addition, somatostatin will prevent acid secretion during pentagastrin infusion and pancreatic bicarbonate secretion during secretin infusion.[25]

Peptides found in both gut and nervous system (brain-gut axis)

Several of these peptides have been discussed previously; the list includes gastrin, cholecystokinin, VIP, motilin, somatostatin, neurotensin, bombesin, substance P, and enkephalin. Other peptides in this group are neurotensin, substance P, and the endogenous opiate group, including the enkephalins and endorphins.

PATHOLOGICAL CONDITIONS
Malnutrition (see also Chapter 37)

Malnutrition is caused by an abnormal food intake. On a worldwide basis, malnutrition is one of the leading causes of death. In North America, overnutrition is the most common malnutrient state. Obesity contributes to the mortality of all diseases but is closely related to diabetes, hypertension, cardiovascular disease, and emotional disorders. Undernutrition may be caused by lack of food, bizarre diets, malabsorption, and hypermetabolic states. There is increasing awareness that many elderly persons in the United States are malnourished. Alcoholics, drug addicts, or mentally impaired persons may suffer from various forms of undernutrition. Chronically ill patients may suffer from anorexia, the loss of appetite. Occasionally, persons will adopt bizarre diets that lack the basic nutritional requirements. Disease of the gastrointestinal tract may prevent nutrients from being absorbed. Malignancy, pyrexia, and endocrine abnormalities may consume food energy at a faster rate than assimilation can occur.[28]

Stomach pathological conditions

Ulcers. The cause of ulcer disease[29] is multifactorial and relates to genetic and psychological makeup. For example, there is increased incidence of ulcer disease in persons with the blood group O. Some workers have claimed that an increased serum pepsinogen occurs in association with a high duodenal ulcer risk.[30] There has been a decrease in the incidence of ulcer disease in the last 20 years, and afflicted persons are now older. Duodenal and gastric ulcers are different disorders.

The pathogenesis of duodenal ulcer has been studied extensively.[31] Patients with duodenal ulcers, as a group, have an increased capacity to secrete acid and pepsin. They have an increased responsiveness to gastrin and tend to have higher-than-normal basal and maximal acid secretion, and therefore deliver an increased gastric load to the duodenum.

Other factors have been implicated in the pathogenesis of duodenal ulcers, including mucosal prostaglandins, the mucosal lining, and the presence of the bacteria *Helicobacter pylori*. *H. pylori* is now considered to be the direct cause of most cases of chronic active gastritis, and strong evidence has linked it to peptic ulcers, gastric cancer, and primary gastric lymphoma.[32] Certainly, eradication of *H. pylori* is associated with reduced symptoms of ulcers.[33]

The pathophysiology of gastric ulceration has not been definitely determined. Patients with gastric ulcer have elevations in both basal and postprandial serum gastrin concentrations. These patients have a lower basal and maximal acid output than normal, and it seems likely that the higher serum gastrin is the result of a decreased inhibition. What seems to be clear is that gastric ulcers are not associated with increased acidity.

An ulcer diagnosis is generally made on clinical grounds, with roentgenographic and endoscopic examinations being of prime importance. The patient's response to therapy is also very helpful. The patient is generally treated with antacids or anticholinergic agents, such as cimetidine. Surgery, which usually includes a vagotomy and antral drainage, is generally considered a second line of therapy and is used in cases of repeated ulceration.

After gastric surgery, several physiologically based complications can occur shortly after eating. Some persons with gastric surgery will absorb glucose at an abnormally fast rate. This triggers an extremely rapid release of insulin, which may overshoot and cause hypoglycemia.

Another problem is caused by the rapid entry of osmotically active food particles into the intestine. This causes a fluid and electrolyte shift into the intestine. Hypovolemia and transient hypokalemia cause a generalized nausea and dizziness. The activation of the kallikrein-kinin system has an important but not fully understood role in this dumping syndrome.

Pyloric obstruction. In pyloric obstruction, the outlet of the stomach is constricted by the contraction of an ulcer, malignancy, or congenital abnormality. Obstruction is characterized by vomiting (often projectile), abdominal distension, and loss of hydrochloric acid, leading to severe hypochloremic metabolic alkalosis.

Cancer. The incidence of stomach cancer[34] is declining in the United States, but it remains high in the Soviet Union and in Japan (54% of all cancers). It appears most often in the seventh and eighth decades of life, and the 5-year survival remains at 15%. Over half of all gastric cancers are found in the pylorus or antrum. Surgery in combination with radiotherapy or chemotherapy is used to treat the lesion. *Helicobacter pylori* infections of the stomach are associated with an approximately sixfold increase in the incidence of gastric cancer.[35]

Zollinger-Ellison syndrome. The Zollinger-Ellison syndrome is an extreme form of peptic ulcer disease caused by a gastrin-secreting tumor of the pancreas (gastrinoma).[36] The unrelenting gastrin release stimulates hypersecretion of hydrochloric acid by the stomach.[37] The typical clinical presentation (not seen in all patients) is recurrent peptic ulceration. Seventy-five percent of patients with this syndrome have ulcers in the duodenal bulb or immediate postbulbar area. The tumors are often very small and can be difficult to identify. Sixty percent of tumors metastasize, and multiple tumors are common. Some tumors (10%) arise in the duodenal wall. The excess secretion of hydrochloric acid accounts for most of the clinical manifestations of the syndrome. The large amount of gastric acid entering the duodenum interferes with the digestion of fat and leads to steatorrhea. The prolonged secretion of gastrin causes hypertrophy of the stomach, with parietal cell hyperplasia. The secretion of pancreatic bicarbonate is increased in compensation for the acid load delivered to the duodenum. Often the intestine becomes ulcerated. The proximal intestinal lining often displays abnormal villi, submucosal edema, and hemorrhage. Since gastrin also inhibits salt and water absorption by the intestine, diarrhea will occur in 50% of patients. The diarrhea is enhanced by the very large volumes of gastric contents that are presented to the intestine. The Zollinger-Ellison syndrome is associated with hyperparathyroidism in 20% of patients. Other endocrine abnormalities that appear less commonly include pituitary, adrenal, ovarian, and thyroid tumors. This cluster of endocrine adenomas and carcinomas is known as the *multiple endocrine neoplasia (MEN) syndrome I*. It may occur with autosomal dominant inheritance, as described originally by Werner, or it may occur sporadically (see also below).[38]

A fasting serum gastrin concentration four times the upper limit of normal in the absence of achlorhydria or renal failure is strongly suggestive of the Zollinger-Ellison syndrome. This criterion is not met in 40% of cases.

Provocative testing has been used. Serum gastrin is measured after administration of (1) intravenous secretin, 1 to 2 units/kg, (2) intravenous calcium gluconate, or (3) a standard meal. The secretin test, with a postinjection increase of gastrin of 110 pg/mL, is the most reliable.[39,40] A negative secretin response occurs in 5% of patients. Thus the sensitivity of the test is 95% and specificity virtually 100%.

In summary, for diagnosis of the Zollinger-Ellison syndrome, first, appropriate patients are screened with fasting serum gastrin measurements. Next the secretin test is administered to those patients with fasting serum gastrin values over 100 pg/mL.

Pernicious anemia. Pernicious anemia is a disease that consists of gastric achlorhydria, gastric atrophy, and failure to secrete intrinsic factor. The intrinsic-factor deficiency prohibits absorption of vitamin B_{12}. This leads to the sequelae of mucosal epithelial insufficiency, degeneration of the posterior columns of the spinal cord, and macrocytic anemia. It is covered in greater detail in Chapter 39.

Multiple endocrine neoplasia

Multiple endocrine neoplasia describes a group of syndromes, often familial, in which two or more endocrine glands undergo hyperplasia or tumor formation in the same individual, either at the same time or consecutively. The hyperfunctioning glands secrete their normal major hormones (orthoendocrine syndromes) and abnormal hormones (paraendocrine syndromes). There are two main types of multiple endocrine neoplasia syndromes.

Multiple endocrine neoplasia type I (MEN I, or MEA I), or Werner's syndrome. This syndrome manifests from the second decade to old age with an equal sex distribution. The areas involved in order of frequency are parathyroids (88%), pancreatic islets (81%), anterior pituitary (65%), adrenal cortex (38%), and thyroid follicular cells (19%).

Changes in the thyroid vary, and occasionally carcinoid tumors are present in the lungs, pancreas, or intestines. Peptic ulceration, especially duodenal, is a common feature in some families and may affect more than half the patients. These may form part of the Zollinger-Ellison syndrome as a result of an associated pancreatic gastrinoma or hyperparathyroidism. Many of these lesions are APUDomas, and the syndrome may result from a widespread dysplasia of the APUD cells.

Multiple endocrine neoplasia type II (MEN II, or MEA II), or Sipple's syndrome. The syndrome multiple endocrine neoplasia type II is usually inherited, affects sexes equally, and may manifest itself from the first decade onward, most commonly from 20 to 40 years. Three forms of the syndrome are recognized. The most common tumor is medullary carcinoma of the thyroid with a pheochromocytoma in one or both adrenal glands. Hyperparathyroidism resulting from hyperplasia or adenoma may be present and is probably caused by hypercalcemia. Another variant is a medullary carcinoma of thyroid and pheochromocytoma with multiple small subcutaneous and submucous neuromas of the eyelids, tongue, and buccal mucosa with a diffuse hypertrophy of the lips. These lesions are present from birth. In the last type, all features are present together with autonomic ganglioneuromatosis and various other congenital abnormalities.

Malabsorption syndromes

In malabsorption syndromes the gastrointestinal tract is impaired so that it cannot absorb a variety of nutrient materials. This inability is generally the result of a disorder that causes damage to the mucosal lining. Patients suspected of having a generalized malabsorption syndrome should be evaluated with serum iron, vitamin B_{12}, albumin, and calcium determinations. In addition, immunoglobulin determinations can be useful to rule out IgA deficiency, a condition that permits parasitic infestations to occur. The D-xylose absorption test can be used as a screening procedure for generalized malabsorption.

The other category of malabsorption syndrome should in fact be called *maldigestion*. In this group of disorders one of the important factors for the digestive process is in some way impaired. This is most commonly caused by some form of pancreatic insufficiency (see Chapter 29) or surgical procedure. The most common maldigestion syndrome leads to fat malabsorption and steatorrhea.

Steatorrhea. Steatorrhea is a clinical syndrome caused by the malabsorption of dietary fat. The undigested fat travels into the large bowel, and the stools contain an excess amount of lipid and are characteristically pale, bulky, and greasy with a repugnant odor. It is important to distinguish clinically the stools produced in steatorrhea from those produced in diarrhea. When steatorrhea is suspected, testing should be undertaken to estimate the actual amount of fat in the stool. When excess fat has been identified, the specific cause is sought. A deficiency of any factor important for lipid digestion and absorption can cause steatorrhea. Conditions producing steatorrhea include the Zollinger-Ellison syndrome, increased duodenal acid (postgastrectomy syndromes), abnormal bile output, pancreatic insufficiency, intestinal mucosal impairment, and disease of the large bowel that has caused an interruption of bile-salt enterohepatic circulation.

Celiac disease. Celiac disease is an extremely important cause of malabsorption. In this condition persons appear to have an abnormal immunological response to the presence of gluten in the diet. Up to 90% of celiac patients have circulating antibodies to gluten. The response to gluten is shedding of the microvillous mucosal surface of the intestine. This drastically reduces the absorptive surface area and causes malabsorption. Celiac disease may manifest in very subtle ways and may be definitely diagnosed only by the response to a gluten-free diet.[41]

Lactose intolerance and other carbohydrate malabsorption disorders. The most common carbohydrate malabsorption disorder is lactose intolerance.[42] All infants have the intestinal enzyme mechanism necessary to break the milk sugar disaccharide, lactose, into its components glucose and galactose, thereby allowing absorption to occur. In those population groups who characteristically feed on animal milk throughout life, these enzyme mechanisms persist into adulthood. However, in those groups who are historically not milk drinkers, the enzyme system regresses (African blacks and Orientals). If persons lacking the enzyme lactase ingest milk or milk products, they will fail to split the lactose in the proper fashion. This unabsorbed sugar will create an osmotic force that pulls fluid into the intestinal lumen. This causes cramping, bloating sensations, and diarrhea. Moreover, large-bowel bacteria can metabolize the sugar to produce gas. Although most people with lactose intolerance are aware of their problem and avoid milk products, there are persons with milder forms who experience discomfort in much more subtle ways. The diagnosis of lactose malabsorption is made by use of the lactose-tolerance procedures discussed later in this chapter. Malabsorption syndromes of other disaccharides have been reported but are extremely rare. The malabsorption of monosaccharides is seen only in extreme impairment of the mucosal surface.

Carcinoid syndrome[43]

A syndrome manifesting as vascular flushing, diarrhea, a carcinoid tumor of the bowel, occasional tricuspid insufficiency, and, rarely, pellagra is called the *carcinoid syndrome*. Carcinoid tumors, which are the most common of small bowel tumors, are located predominantly in the distal ileum. The remainder of the extra-appendicular gastrointes-tinal carcinoid tumors are found in the rectum and stomach. These tumors metastasize most commonly to the regional lymph nodes, liver, and skeleton. Primary carcinoid tumors of the appendix are common but rarely metastasize, whereas those that arise from other parts of the gastrointestinal tract do metastasize. The tumors produce serotonin and kinins in vast excess. It is these hormonal substances that are responsible for the characteristic clinical syndrome. One can detect the presence of the disorder by measuring serotonin or its metabolites.

Large intestine disease

Diarrhea. Diarrhea[44] is defined as the excessive production of feces, usually as a result of the overabundance of water in the stool. The causes of diarrhea are many. Diarrhea should be clinically distinguished from steatorrhea.

Severe diarrhea causes sodium and water depletion. Potassium is also lost. The acid-base disturbances caused by diarrhea are variable. However, the most common disorder is acidosis, which results from the increased fecal loss of bicarbonate. In chronic, mild diarrhea, hypokalemic alkalosis may be found.

There are three main reasons for diarrhea: solute malabsorption, secretion of fluid into the intestine, and motility disturbance.

Solute malabsorption is caused by the ingestion of poorly absorbed substances, "dumping," or intestinal malabsorption, such as lactose intolerance.

The secretion of fluid occurs in many conditions. Passive secretion will occur if the epithelial permeability is increased by obstruction or inflammation. The secretion of anions will occur through the activity of $3',5'$-cyclic adenosine monophosphate as stimulated by cholera toxin, endotoxin, prostaglandins, bile acids, and certain tumor products (such as vasoactive intestinal polypeptide). Another secretory mechanism is the replacement of absorptive epithelium by crypt epithelium (as occurs with viral gastroenteritis).

Motility disturbances are caused by cathartics and nervous tension. These will increase the motility and decrease the transit time and therefore the absorptive efficiency.

Cancer. Malignancies of the colon and rectum[44] account for over half the malignancies of the entire gastrointestinal system. The 5-year cure rate for these lesions runs between 25% and 50%. The cure rate is directly proportional to how early the lesion is detected and is therefore correlated with its proximity to the anus. Thus early detection through screening is the most effective approach to curing this often fatal disorder. Digital and sigmoidoscopic examination of the rectum is supplemented by screening for the presence of occult blood. Roentgenological studies are useful only in screening patients with a high risk of cancer. Colonoscopy is becoming the preferred method of examining high-risk patients.

Blind-loop syndromes. A variety of inflammatory and anatomical disorders of the gastrointestinal tract may cause regional outpouchings to occur in the large bowel.[45] These pockets can trap intestinal material and allow bacterial overgrowth. If this happens, the overabundant bacteria can cause excessive breakdown of bile conjugates. When these materials have been deconjugated, they cannot be reabsorbed by the body and are lost in the feces. This may be the cause of diarrhea. The bile acid breath test can be used in the diagnosis of this condition.

Common bowel disorders. Rarely a chemical diagnostic problem, the most common disorders of the bowel are associated with abnormal motility. Such symptoms as bloating, cramps, and excess flatus production are common clinical problems. Colonic inflammatory disease can also result in diarrhea. Colitis may be caused by replacement of normal colon flora by *Clostridium difficile*[46] and by increased nitric oxide synthesis.[47]

Hyperalimentation (see also Chapter 37)

In recent years, techniques for providing nutrition to persons who are otherwise unable to eat[48] have been highly refined. Such techniques employ tube feeding or intravenous alimentation. In the case of those who are undergoing tube feeding, it is important that the material not cause an osmotic load on the gastrointestinal tract and hence produce diarrhea.

The assessment of persons receiving such artificial nutrition is not highly refined. In general, the tests must first allow assessment of whether complications have occurred or whether undernutrition of one or more substances is present. Patients should be monitored carefully by clinical assessment. Biochemical monitoring of the urine is useful and includes measurement of the urine osmolality to evaluate hydration, sodium and potassium measurements to indicate electrolyte load, urea concentration to provide a rough guide to overall nitrogen balance, and ketones and glucose to indicate poor carbohydrate control and caloric loss. Blood analyses are also useful but should be interpreted with caution because the intravenous solution administered at the time of the blood collection can drastically influence the results by affecting lipemia or hyperosmotic forces.

GASTROINTESTINAL FUNCTION TESTS

There are many gastrointestinal function tests that have been designed for critical evaluation of various gastrointestinal physiological functions.

Tests of gastric acidity

Tests of gastric acidity are used to screen for the ability of the parietal cells to produce hydrochloric acid. The discovery of achlorhydria (anacidity) is strong evidence for the presence of pernicious anemia and rules out peptic ulcer disease, casting suspicion on gastric ulcer or gastric carcinoma. The presence of acid in the stomach is very strong evidence against pernicious anemia. Acid detection must be carried out to determine the significance of raised serum gastrin determinations.

The only suitable test for the presence of gastric acid is intubation and withdrawal of stomach juice. A pH measurement may then be made directly and should be less than 3. Anacidity is confirmed only by a pH over 6.

Gastric stimulation tests

Gastric analysis. The gastric analysis test involves draining stomach secretions for a baseline period to determine basal or unstimulated acid production. Next, a parietal cell stimulant is administered and gastric juice is collected to evaluate maximum secretory ability. Currently, pentagastrin, the active 5–amino acid portion of gastrin, is the recommended stimulant.[49-51]

Thus the protocol is (1) collect residual gastric fluid from a fasting patient by intermittent suction on a nasogastric tube positioned within the stomach by fluoroscopy, (2) collect basal secretions for four 15-minute periods, (3) administer pentagastrin intramuscularly in a dose of 5 μg/kg of body weight, and (4) collect further stomach secretions for six consecutive 15-minute time periods. All collections are then evaluated for appearance, blood, bile, pH, volume, millimoles of H^+ per liter, millimoles of H^+ per total volume, and millimoles of H^+ per hour for each collection.

The pH measurement is useful. Basal pH over 6 is almost certainly caused by anacidity; pH less than 3 indicates normal or excessive parietal cell function; intermediate values (pH 3 to 6) are not diagnostic and merely indicate a balance between hydrochloric acid and buffer. After stimulation, pH values should fall to less than 2. Failure to do so indicates inadequate parietal cell function, which may be found in pernicious anemia, gastric carcinoma, hypochromic anemia, rheumatoid arthritis, and myxedema. Next, one should compute the basal acid output (BAO) by averaging the millimole-per-hour output for the closest three basal collections. The maximum acid output (MAO) is also calculated as the mean of the two highest poststimulation values in millimoles per hour.

Healthy adult men have a BAO of 2.2 to 2.7 mmol/hour, with 5 mmol/hour being the absolute upper limit. The MAO for men under 30 years of age is 14 to 42 mmol/hour, and it is 3 to 33 mmol/hour for men over 30 years of age. The values for women are approximately 50% of those for men. Detailed tables of reference intervals have been published[52] and are reviewed in Table 30-3.

The Zollinger-Ellison syndrome is characterized by high BAO (Table 30-3). The MAO is generally only 40% to 60% higher than the BAO because the stomach is close to maximal stimulation. Indeed, a BAO/MAO greater than 60% is virtually pathognomonic for the Zollinger-Ellison syndrome. If the MAO is over 35 mmol/hour, an ulcer predisposition is likely. In persons over 45 years of age it is highly likely. An MAO less than 11 mmol/hour in a man under 30 years of age is suggestive of a very low peptic ulcer risk.[52]

Table 30-3 Pentagastrin stimulation test

	Basal acid output (BAO) (mmol/hour)	Maximal acid output (MAO) (mmol/hour)
Healthy adult men		
Under 30 years old	2.2-2.7	14-42
Over 30 years old	2.2-2.7	3-33
Healthy adult women	1-1.5	7-20
Zollinger-Ellison syndrome	10-100 (or more)	40%-60% above BAO
Ulcer predisposition		
Likely		>35
Highly likely		>45
Low risk		<11

Gastric analysis is used by some surgeons to indicate the nature of surgery to be used for ulcer treatment.

Hollander insulin test. The Hollander insulin test[53] is used to assess whether a surgical vagotomy has successfully denervated the stomach. In this procedure regular insulin (0.15 unit/kg of body weight) is administered intravenously to render the patient hypoglycemic (plasma glucose less than 300 mg/L). Vagus stimulation is a normal response to hypoglycemia. Those with an intact gastric vagus will release acid in response to hypoglycemia. A successful denervation will cause an MAO less than 0.05 mmol/hour, and the pH will remain over 3.5. The test is not often performed because clinical evaluation is generally sufficient.

Gastrin stimulation test. The principle of the gastrin stimulation test was described earlier.[39,40]

Blood for serum gastrin is collected from a fasting patient. Secretin (2 units/kg as an intravenous bolus) is then administered and serum gastrin collected at 2, 5, 10, 15, 30, and 60 minutes. An absolute increase of gastrin greater than 110 pg/mL is positive for the Zollinger-Ellison syndrome. Secretin administration has little or no effect on plasma gastrin levels when hypergastrinemia results from other causes.

Schilling test (see also p. 590)

The Schilling test of vitamin B_{12} absorption is an elegant evaluator of both gastric and intestinal function.[54] Radioactively tagged vitamin B_{12} is taken orally by the patient. If absorption is successful, the radioactive material will be excreted in the urine. The vitamin B_{12} is administered with and without intrinsic factor to determine whether that substance is absent. More specifically, the test is carried out in the following way.

The fasting patient is given an oral preparation containing radioactively labeled vitamin B_{12}. One hour later, an intramuscular injection of unlabeled vitamin B_{12} is given. This cold B_{12} saturates the body's binding sites for B_{12}, preventing the labeled oral dose from being stored. Urine is collected for 24 hours. The amount of radioactivity in the urine is determined as a percentage of the original dose.

After several days, the test may be repeated. This time, the radioactively labeled vitamin B_{12} is given with intrinsic factor. Again, a 24-hour urine collection is carried out and the amount of vitamin B_{12} excreted is determined. There are three possible results (Table 30-4).

If both stages of the test show greater than 15% excretion, vitamin B_{12} absorption is within the reference interval and any deficiency of serum vitamin B_{12} must be the result of a dietary problem.

If the absorption of vitamin B_{12} is low when it is given alone but within the reference interval when it is administered in association with intrinsic factor, one can presume a deficiency of intrinsic factor. Such a situation is found in classic pernicious anemia, gastrectomy, and the rare occurrence of nonfunctional intrinsic factor.

If vitamin B_{12} excretion in the urine is low after administration of both preparations, an absorptive defect of the terminal ileum is presumed to be present. This may be found in tropical sprue, nontropical sprue, regional enteritis, intestinal resection, neoplasm or granuloma, selective ileal vitamin B_{12} malabsorption (Imerslund syndrome; rare), fish tapeworm *(Diphyllobothrium latum)*, bacterial overgrowth, and chronic vitamin B_{12} deficiency.

A two-capsule test has been devised (Dicopac, Amersham Corp., Arlington Heights, Illinois). In this preparation, two forms of vitamin B_{12} are radioactively labeled using different isotopes of cobalt (^{57}Co, ^{58}Co). The advantage of the procedure is that one can give both the bound and unbound forms of vitamin B_{12} at essentially the same time. Absorption may then be determined by use of a single 24-hour urine collection. Special counting techniques to subtract the influence of one isotope from the other are required.

Table 30-4 Schilling test

Group	Absorption of intrinsic factor–bound vitamin B_{12}	Absorption of unbound vitamin B_{12}	Ratio of bound to unbound
Healthy	>15%	>15%	0.5-1.5
Gastric lesion group	>10%	<5%	>2
Pernicious anemia			
Gastrectomy			
Congenital absence of functional intrinsic factor			
Disorders of terminal ileum (see text)	<15%	<15%	0.5

Pancreatic challenge tests

The elucidation of malabsorptive disorders depends on the evaluation of pancreatic secretory ability. This is best performed using the pancreatic stimulation tests described in Chapter 29.

Fat absorption tests

The definitive test of fat absorption is the quantitative measurement of fat in timed collections of feces obtained while the patient is maintained on a diet containing a known amount of fat. Because the collection is extremely difficult for the patient, a variety of alternative approaches have been promoted. Unfortunately, none of these entirely replaces the diagnostic ability of the quantitative fecal fat measurement.

Fat screening. Fat screening[55] is carried out first by evaluation of the weight and appearance of the stool. A pale, frothy appearance is virtually diagnostic of excessive fat. More reliable than this is the application of a small amount of the fecal material onto a standard microscopic slide, followed by staining with a fat-specific stain. Trained observers are able to identify excessive fat in 80% of persons with fat malabsorption.

Quantitative fecal fat estimation. Quantitative fecal fat estimation[56] is performed after collection of feces for 3 consecutive days. In the 2 days preceding the collection and during the period of collection, patients must include approximately 100 g of medium-chain triglycerides in their diet.

The easiest way to ensure this intake is to supplement the patient's normal diet with four glasses of whole milk each day and 2 tablespoons of corn oil with each meal.

Feces can be collected in plastic bags. The plastic bags may then be closed with a tin tie and held in a preweighed, 5-gallon paint can. On arrival in the laboratory the can and contents are weighed and the weight of the collection is determined. The chemical analysis is then carried out on a thoroughly mixed aliquot of this 3-day collection.[57]

Serum fat estimations. Another rough screening test for fat absorption is the fat tolerance test.[58] A fasting blood sample is collected. The patient is then given a high-fat meal consisting of 6 ounces of corn oil. Serum is collected at 3 and 6 hours. Estimations of total fat in these samples are then made. The postfat specimens should exhibit a minimum of 50% increase in fat content over the fasting value. This test has poor diagnostic ability.

Isotope tests. Radioactively labeled, medium-chain triglyceride is administered to patients in whom fat malabsorption is suspected.[58] After a suitable time interval, blood is collected and its radioactivity determined. It is assumed that the radioactivity that finds its way into the bloodstream is a result of the successful digestion and absorption of the radioactive fat. Unfortunately, radioactive iodine tags are not suitable for this procedure because they must be linked to unsaturated fats and because the size of the iodine tag gravely distorts the triglyceride molecule, making it suscep-

tible to incidental breakdown. Thus the absorption of the radioactive iodine from these materials might not indicate successful fat absorption. A ^{14}C-labeled triglyceride has been tested and is measurable in the bloodstream or in the feces.[59]

D-Xylose absorption test[60]

D-Xylose is an aldopentose that is absorbed by the small intestine. It is postulated that D-xylose is absorbed passively; its successful absorption is therefore a reflection of the integrity of the surface area of the small intestine. Once D-xylose is absorbed into the bloodstream there is a small amount of metabolic alteration, but at least 50% is excreted in the urine within the next 24 hours. It has been shown that the amount of D-xylose excreted into the urine over a 5-hour period is closely correlated with the amount of D-xylose absorbed in the gastrointestinal tract.

Several options are available for the performance of this test. The patient is instructed to fast overnight but is encouraged to drink an ample amount of water during this time.

Two doses have been advocated. Most authors suggest that 25 g of D-xylose dissolved in approximately 300 to 500 mL of water is a suitable dose. Smaller subjects are given 1 g/kg of body weight to a maximum of 25 g. We have found that a 5 g dose is adequate.[61] This dose is less likely to cause abdominal cramps and is probably more sensitive because some persons with absorptive defects are capable of absorbing sufficient amounts of the larger dose.

After administration of the sugar, urine is collected for a 5-hour period. A quantitative assay for D-xylose is carried out on this sample. At least 25% of the administered dose will appear in the urine over a 5-hour period if renal function is within the reference interval.

For children who cannot be relied on to collect a urinary sample, blood collections at 1 and 2 hours may be substituted. Most persons demonstrate plasma levels greater than 300 mg/L in one of the samples. In children, values above 100 mg/L should be considered within the reference interval.

Low levels of urine or plasma xylose are suggestive of an absorptive defect in the jejunum. Low levels are also seen in ascites, vomiting, delayed gastric emptying, improper urine collection, and high-dose aspirin therapy and with neomycin, colchicine, indomethacin, atropine, and impaired renal function. Values within the reference interval are seen in persons who have absorptive defects occurring in a skip pattern. Such a disease distribution allows a sufficient amount of healthy mucosa to remain and absorb an amount of D-xylose within the usual interval.

Lactose tolerance test

Some persons do not have a fully developed mucosal lactase system. This deficiency prevents the usual hydrolysis of lactose, resulting in gastrointestinal bloating, cramps, and diarrhea. The lactose tolerance test is useful for the quick identification of such persons.

In this test, 50 g of lactose dissolved in water is administered orally to the patient, who is observed carefully for the onset of symptoms.

The standard protocol includes the collection of a baseline specimen and 5-, 10-, 30-, 60-, 90-, and 120-minute specimens of blood. The blood sample is analyzed for the concentration of glucose. Glucose levels will be increased in the bloodstream if lactose has been successfully cleaved and its components absorbed. The galactose moiety of the lactose is converted quickly into glucose by the liver. Healthy persons will demonstrate a glucose rise of greater than 200 mg/L over the baseline sample. Those with lactase deficiency will exhibit notable abdominal discomfort and will have less than a 100 mg/L increase in the serum glucose concentration.

It has been shown that the most reliable method of determining lactose absorption is the measurement of the amount of hydrogen appearing in exhaled breath after the oral administration of lactose.[62] Lactase-deficient persons will not absorb lactose, and it will find its way into the large bowel, where bacteria will metabolize it. Hydrogen is one of the by-products of this bacterial action. Hydrogen passes quickly into the bloodstream and is removed in the exhaled breath. Special-purpose gas chromatographs can detect the presence of postlactose hydrogen. A healthy person allows no lactose to enter the colon and therefore has less than 10 parts per million (ppm) of hydrogen in the exhaled breath. Persons with lactase deficiency demonstrate at least 50 ppm of hydrogen. Intermediate amounts of hydrogen in the breath can be caused by large doses of lactose and are of questionable significance.

The definitive diagnosis is made by tissue enzyme assays carried out on biopsy samples of the intestinal mucosa.

CHANGE OF ANALYTE IN DISEASE (Table 30-5)
Gastrin

The reference interval fasting serum gastrin concentration[40] is between 30 and 100 pg/mL. Increased serum gastrin may be caused primarily by hyperplasia of the G cells of the antrum, abnormal acid production, such as achlorhydria with compensatory hypergastrinemia or isolated retained antrum after gastrectomy, gastrinomas, and renal disease (see accompanying box).

Low gastrin concentrations are observed in persons with hypothyroidism and after the administration of oral acid, streptozocin, and phenformin.

Minimum elevations up to 500 pg/mL are not diagnostic of any specific disorder and are occasionally found in healthy persons. Such values are sometimes produced by the ingestion (or even by the thought or smell) of food, insulin administration, malignant carcinoma of the stomach, pheochromocytoma, hyperthyroidism, hyperparathyroidism, peptic ulceration, gastritis, cirrhosis of the liver, re-

---

Serum Gastrin Concentrations in Disease

Reference interval (30 to 100 pg/mL)
Low (<30 pg/mL)
  Hypothyroidism; administration of oral acid, streptozocin, phenformin
Minimum elevations (100 to 500 pg/mL)
  Normal persons (occasionally), ingestion of food, insulin administration, malignant carcinoma of the stomach, pheochromocytoma, hyperthyroidism, hyperparathyroidism, peptic ulceration, gastritis, cirrhosis of the liver, renal failure, rheumatoid arthritis, Zollinger-Ellison syndrome (unusual), pernicious anemia (unusual)
Significant increase (500 to 1000 pg/mL)
  Food ingestion, insulin administration, pheochromocytoma, hyperparathyroidism, renal failure, pernicious anemia, Zollinger-Ellison syndrome
Dramatic increase (>1000 pg/mL)
  Zollinger-Ellison syndrome, pernicious anemia, parietal cell antibody–positive chronic atrophic gastritis (rare)

---

nal failure, and rheumatoid arthritis. Some cases of Zollinger-Ellison syndrome and pernicious anemia may be found with serum gastrin values in this range, but this is unusual. Values between 500 and 1000 pg/mL are significant and, when accompanied by gastric acid hypersecretion, virtually diagnostic for gastrinoma. Patients with achlorhydria (decreased HCl output) may have serum gastrin in the gastrinoma range[34] but can be readily distinguished on the basis of acid secretory tests. Such results can also be associated with food ingestion, insulin administration, pheochromocytoma, hyperparathyroidism, renal failure, pernicious anemia, and Zollinger-Ellison syndrome. Serum gastrin concentrations are also raised in patients after massive small bowel resection as a result of either decreased gastrin clearance or removal of an intestinal factor that normally suppresses gastrin release.

Results over 1000 pg/mL are probably caused by either the Zollinger-Ellison syndrome, pernicious anemia, or, rarely, parietal cell antibody–positive chronic atrophic gastritis. Most cases of the Zollinger-Ellison syndrome have values greater than 2000 pg/mL.

If the Zollinger-Ellison syndrome is considered, a fasting serum gastrin should be obtained. Results under 100 pg/mL essentially rule out the Zollinger-Ellison syndrome. Results greater than this in persons with healthy renal function warrant stimulation testing as described on p. 583.

Other gastrointestinal hormones

Vasoactive intestinal polypeptide. Elevated levels of VIP are found in the plasma in some patients with watery diarrhea syndrome (Verner-Morrison syndrome). This syndrome was subsequently named "WDHA" after the initial letters of its main characteristics: *w*atery *d*iarrhea, *h*ypoka-

Table 30-5   Change of analyte and function tests in disease.

Disease	Fecal fat	Lactose intolerance	S-carotene S-vitamin A	S-vitamin B_{12} S-folate	Schilling test	D-Xylose absorption	Stool occult blood	Carcino-embryonic antigen	5-HIAA	Pancreatic enzyme testing	Stool examination
Steatorrhea	↑↑	N	↓	N,↓	AB	AB	Neg	N	N	AB	Foul smelling, greasy
Celiac disease	N,↑	N	N,↓	N	N, AB	N, AB	Neg	N	N	N	Variable
Lactose intolerance	N	AB	N	N	N	N	Neg	N	N	N	Loose in association with abdominal cramps
Carcinoid syndrome	N	N	N	N,↓	N, AB	N	Neg, pos	N,↑	↑↑	N	Loose in association with cutaneous flushing
Functional diarrhea	N	N	N	N	N	N	Neg	N	N	N	Loose
Bowel carcinoma	N	N	N	N,↓	N	N	Neg or pos	N,↑	N	N	Change in bowel habits
Inflammatory bowel	N	N	N	N,↓	N	N	Pos	N,↑	N	N	Loose, bloody

AB, Abnormal; *N*, normal (within the reference interval); *S*, serum; ↑, increase; ↓, decrease.

lemia, and *h*ypochlorhydria or *a*chlorhydria. The syndrome is rare; about one tenth as common as Zollinger-Ellison syndrome. It is sometimes part of the multiple endocrine neoplasia syndromes (see p. 580).

In patients with WDHA syndrome, a non–beta islet cell tumor (vipoma) of the pancreas is usually present (D_1 cells); about half of these tumors are malignant. Tumors can occur elsewhere (such as bronchial, probably oat cell carcinoma, or retroperitoneal neuroblastoma) and secrete VIP. In large doses, VIP causes vasodilatation with facial flushing, increases intestinal blood flow, induces watery diarrhea, and inhibits gastric secretion. The diarrhea, which is explosive and consists of up to 30 stools per day, causes a profound hypokalemia (1 to 3 mmol/L).

The diagnosis is made by elimination of the common causes of watery diarrhea and hypokalemia. Gastric secretion tests often show the presence of hypochlorhydria, and the diagnosis is confirmed by measurements of elevated blood levels of immunoreactive VIP.[63] The pseudo–Verner-Morrison syndrome refers to patients with watery diarrhea, hypokalemia, and achlorhydria who have serum VIP levels within the reference interval and no obvious tumor.

Secretin. Although serum secretin levels are elevated in patients with gastric hypersecretion, measurement of secretin is not usually required for a diagnosis.

Pancreatic polypeptide. Considerably elevated plasma pancreatic polypeptide levels have been documented in a high percentage of patients with vipomas, insulinomas, gastrinomas, and glucagonomas. Pure pancreatic polypeptide APUDomas (PPomas) are rare, though elevated plasma PP levels are found in one third of pancreatic APUDomas.

Glucagon-like immunoreactive peptides. A glucagon-secreting tumor of the pancreas is associated with diabetes, skin rash, and a high concentration of plasma glucagon. The diagnosis is easily confirmed by radioimmunoassay measurement of elevated plasma glucagon levels.

Somatostatin. Several somatostatin-producing tumors of the pancreas have been described and are known as *somatostatinomas*. These tumors produce an ill-defined clinical syndrome that includes diarrhea, gallbladder disease, and diabetes. Because somatostatin is a potent inhibitor of peptide hormone release, it is used as a therapeutic agent in the management of tumors. The administration of long-acting somatostatin analogs has resulted in inhibition of peptide secretion in many patients with gastrinomas, glucagonomas, and VIPomas, with amelioration of the clinical symptoms.

Malabsorption testing

Screening approach. Screening for persons with malabsorption syndromes in North American society is best done clinically. Elderly persons are at greatest risk for occult malabsorption. Laboratory screening for malabsorption is not very sensitive; however, measurement of serum albumin, calcium, vitamin B_{12}, and a peripheral smear looking for evidence of macrocytosis and iron-deficiency anemia constitute a reasonable general laboratory screen for malabsorption. If necessary, more specific tests for iron deficiency can be carried out. Measurements of the B vitamins are not generally available but would be particularly useful in elderly persons and in the indigent alcoholic population.

Persons believed to have specific malabsorption syndromes should be tested accordingly. Those with steatorrhea and suspected fat malabsorption should first have their feces examined visually. Next, one should carry out a rapid slide evaluation of a stool sample looking for meat fibers and excess fat. A carotene determination is easily performed and reflects gross abnormalities of fat absorption. A D-xylose absorption test will indicate whether significant generalized absorptive problems are present. Protein malabsorption is difficult to assess biochemically, and only when there is serious amino acid malabsorption will the serum albumin be depressed.

Carotene. Beta-carotene,[64] a naturally occurring pigment, is a common constituent of vegetables and fruit. Collectively, these pigments are called *carotenoids*. The carotenoid chemical structure consists of two 6-member carbon rings joined by a polyunsaturated 18-member carbon chain. Carotenoids are hydrophobic and insoluble in water. Consequently they must be absorbed into the body in association with fats. Therefore in clinical conditions in which fat malabsorption is impaired, the absorption of carotenoid pigments will be reduced, and the serum carotene will be lower than normal. The reference interval for serum carotene is 500 to 2500 $\mu g/L$.

Serum carotene is decreased in low carotene diets (low vegetable diets), abetalipoproteinemia, Tangier lipoprotein abnormality, liver failure, and 86% of patients with clinically significant fat malabsorption.

A serum carotene concentration within the reference interval is found in 14% of patients with fat malabsorption. The concentration of carotene is determined by the balance between the degree of malabsorption and the oral carotene intake.

Vitamin A. Vitamin A[63] is an alcohol derived from beta-carotene by hydrolytic cleavage at the midpoint of the C-18 polyene chain. Vitamin A is found only in animal tissue and animal products such as milk and egg yolk. Because it is chemically similar to carotene, it is also hydrophobic and must be absorbed into the body along with fat. Thus its presence in serum is also a reasonable estimate of the ability of the body to absorb fat. Serum vitamin A concentrations are less dependent on diet than serum carotene concentrations are. Reduced serum vitamin A concentrations are seen in association with fat malabsorption and liver disease.

Because the serum vitamin A determination is significantly more difficult to perform than the serum carotene and because its diagnostic ability is not significantly greater, it has never achieved popular acceptance as a screening test for fat malabsorption.

Trypsin. The measurement of trypsin in stool has been advocated as a screening test of pancreatic insufficiency.[65] Trypsin determination is much more reliable in infants and young children than in adults because there is less colonic degradation of pancreatic enzymes. The simplest test of tryptic activity is the application of a smear of fecal material to a thin film of gelatin. If trypsin is present, an enzymatic breakdown of the film will be seen. The test will be abnormal in all patients with significant pancreatic insufficiency, except in unusual cases of isolated defects of amylase and lipase. Some healthy infants, however, will fail to produce sufficient trypsin to degrade the gelatin layer. Although such tests have some validity in screening, a strong clinical suggestion of pancreatic insufficiency warrants specific testing, as outlined in Chapter 29.

Fecal fat determinations.[56] Persons taking a 100 g fat diet will excrete no more than 5 g of fecal fat per day. More than 10 g per day is certain evidence of fat malabsorption.

Failure to adhere to the diet may invalidate the results. Low fat intake will mask minimum fat malabsorption. Grossly excessive fat intake will raise the fecal content above 5 g.

Tests related to specific disorders

Occult blood in stool. Because the survival of persons with cancer of the bowel depends on early diagnosis, reliable methods for detecting carcinoma of the bowel are extremely important.[66] Several color reagents that react to trace amounts of hemoglobin in feces are available. Most rely on the ability of hemoglobin and its derivatives to act as peroxidases and catalyze the reaction between hydrogen peroxide and a chromogenic, organic compound. Benzidine has been used but is carcinogenic and therefore not currently recommended as a laboratory-prepared reagent.

Various commercial systems for stool occult blood measurement are available.[67] These have been evaluated by Morris et al.,[68] who recommend the Hemoccult test (Smith-Kline Beecham, Pittsburgh) as the most suitable. In any test of fecal blood loss, a reagent must be suitably sensitive so that it will detect the presence of all gastrointestinal malignancies and specific enough so that investigators are not burdened with large numbers of false-positive reactions.

The Hemoccult test is based on the guaiac-peroxide reaction and is not made positive by insignificant blood loss or meat ingestion. Moreover, it is suitable for patient use because it provides a convenient sample-handling envelope. Those laboratories wishing to use their own reagent system may employ the method of Woodman.[69] Whatever method is employed, the evaluation of occult blood in three separate stool aliquots is recommended for optimum diagnostic detection.

Carcinoembryonic antigen. Carcinoembryonic antigen (CEA) is a glycoprotein that is abundant in entodermally derived tissues (gastrointestinal mucosa, pancreas, lung).[70] In the gastrointestinal tract it is located in the glycocalyx of the cell. It is found in fetal tissues at 12 weeks of gestation, and peak levels are observed at 22 weeks. The value decreases near the end of the third trimester. It is not known how CEA enters the circulation. After removal of a CEA-producing tumor, the material disappears within 2 to 4 weeks, most likely because of hepatic breakdown.

Numerous glycoproteins have been found that have immunological cross-reactivity with CEA. They include fetal sulfoglycoprotein, normal colonic antigen, and normal glycoprotein. This latter antigen is also known as colonic antigen Be, colonic antigen X, colonic CEA II, and colonic cancer antigen III.

There are three possible clinical uses of CEA: for screening, for diagnosis, and for management of colonic carcinomas.[71]

CEA determination had been advocated as a method of screening for the presence of occult carcinomas of the gastrointestinal tract. Unfortunately, this is a very difficult proposition because CEA is increased in a variety of colonic disorders, some of which predispose to colonic carcinoma. For example, CEA is increased in 20% of patients with colorectal polyps. Thus it is not specific enough to be recommended as a screening procedure.

A variety of studies have been carried out to determine whether the CEA determination is useful to confirm the diagnosis of colonic cancer in individual patients. Unfortunately, the test is not sufficiently reliable to assist in the diagnosis of this potentially fatal disorder. For example, if a person has a 50% chance of colonic cancer, a positive CEA test result will increase the chance to 80%. Thus the CEA is not recommended as a preoperative indication of whether a malignancy is present. Indeed, the consensus statement of the U.S. Cancer Institute is as follows:

> We cannot recommend, based upon the available data, that CEA be used independently to establish a diagnosis of cancer. However, in a patient with symptoms, a value greater than five to ten times the upper limit of referenced normal should be strongly suggestive for the presence of cancer. . . . Further diagnostic efforts are indicated.[72]

The CEA test plays a well-established role in monitoring the course of disease in persons who have been treated for colonic cancer. For this purpose the CEA should be measured at the time of surgery to establish a baseline level. Six weeks must then be allowed to pass before the next measurement is taken. If the value is elevated, a rising titer over the next few weeks must be noted before residual cancer is considered. If the value is low at the 6-week measurement, one can presume that the original lesion has been removed in its entirety and further measurements at regular intervals should be carried out. Some authors believe that a rising CEA titer requires a second-look operation. However, although some patients will have a rising titer caused by surgically manageable local spread, others will exhibit inoperable metastases.

The CEA concentration approximates the tumor burden and correlates approximately with the clinical course of metastatic disease. Unfortunately, despite many excellent and supportive reports for the use of this test, it has not proved consistently reliable in individual cases.

The reference interval for CEA is 0 to 5 ng/mL. However, rising titers significant of disease may be seen within this range. A CEA value within this interval does not exclude an underlying neoplasm. Mild elevations of 5 to 10 ng/mL may be caused by malignancy or by heavy smoking, chronic liver disease, chronic chest disease, inflammatory bowel disease, or chronic renal failure. When the value reaches 10 to 15 ng/mL, malignancy is quite likely because less than 5% of the CEA-inducing, nonmalignant conditions produce results in this range. Values over 15 ng/mL are strongly suggestive of malignancy.

5-Hydroxyindoleacetic acid. The presence of cutaneous flushing and diarrhea is a sufficiently common syndrome to warrant the frequent request for tests that will identify the possibility of the carcinoid syndrome. The most commonly performed biochemical test for this purpose is the 5-hydroxyindoleacetic acid (5-HIAA) determination.[73] This test is performed because the most common biochemical product of this tumor is serotonin, which is formed by the conversion of tryptophan to 5-hydroxytryptamine (serotonin), which is ultimately converted to 5-HIAA.

The amount of 5-HIAA found in the urine is highly method dependent. Many screening procedures for this substance are very nonspecific and should therefore not be used to make diagnoses. An appropriate approach is the use of a screening procedure for all requests for 5-HIAA; those that exhibit an elevated value should be subjected to a somewhat more specific test.[73]

In healthy adults, up to 15 mg of 5-HIAA is excreted per 24 hours. In the carcinoid syndrome more than 25 mg is usually excreted. False-negative results are produced by many drugs, including *p*-chlorophenylalanine, corticotropin, ethanol, imipramine, isoniazid, monoamine oxidase inhibitors, methenamine, methyldopa, and phenothiazines. Reduction of an elevated value is also seen in renal disease and in phenylketonuria.

In the carcinoid syndrome, results are usually between 25 and 1000 mg/day. False-positive results have been reported in nontropical sprue, intestinal obstruction, pregnancy, sleep deprivation, oat cell carcinoma of the lung, and with ingestion of avocados, bananas, eggplants, pineapples, plums, and walnuts. Drugs that are known to cause an increase in 5-HIAA value are acetanilid, ephedrine, mephenesin, nicotine, phenacetin, phenobarbital, phentolamine, rauwolfia, reserpine, methocarbamol, and glycerol guaiacolate cough medicines.

^{14}C-bile acid breath test. The use of breath analysis in gastroenterology has been extensively reviewed by Newman.[74] The most common radioactive breath-testing procedure in current use is the ^{14}C bile acid breath test.[75] In this procedure, glycine-1-[^{14}C]cholate is administered orally. If the patient has an intestinal blind loop or other source of bacterial overgrowth, deconjugation of the tracer will occur, allowing ^{14}C to enter the bloodstream. Here it is metabolized to ^{14}CO$_2$. Breath CO$_2$ is trapped in an alkaline solution, and the subsequent detection of radioactivity is a sensitive indication of the presence of bacterial overgrowth.

Tests of celiac disease. The detection of circulating gluten antibodies has been suggested as a means of identifying persons with celiac disease.[76] The test is not sufficiently sensitive or specific to be recommended for routine testing.

IgA. A very good test to perform in persons with chronic undiagnosed diarrhea is the serum concentration of immunoglobulin A (IgA). Approximately 1 in 800 persons suffers from idiopathic deficiency of IgA. Such persons do not have a healthy immunodefense of their mucosal membrane system. They are therefore susceptible to infestations of parasites.[77] If a person is discovered to be suffering from a deficiency of IgA, an intestinal intubation with vigorous mucosal biopsy is warranted in search of such parasites as *Giardia lamblia*.

Urine oxalate. The metabolism of oxalate is very complex. A major component of its biochemistry is the enterohepatic circulation of glyoxalate materials secreted in the bile and subsequently reabsorbed by the bowel. In persons who have had gastrointestinal surgery, who have chronic inflammatory disease of the bowel, or who have chronic abnormalities of the gastrointestinal tract, it is possible to have excessive reabsorption of oxalate material, which has been split from the excretory products. Such persons secrete large amounts of oxalate in the urine and are prone to the formation of oxalate renal calculi. Thus the evaluation of urinary oxalate is recommended in anyone who has a chronic anatomical or physiological intestinal abnormality.[78]

Indican. Some intestinal bacteria (including *Escherichia coli* and the *Bacteroides* species) contain the enzyme tryptophanase, which can metabolize dietary tryptophan to indole. This product is then absorbed, converted to indican in the liver, and excreted in the urine.[79] Thus the estimation of indican in a 24-hour specimen of urine has been suggested as a means of diagnosing small bowel bacterial contamination. An increased urinary indican is not always found, however, because the predominant bacteria may not contain the appropriate enzyme. In addition, other small bowel diseases causing malabsorption may encourage indican excretion as a result of absorbed dietary tryptophan. Therefore estimations of urinary indican correlate only roughly with abnormalities in the gastrointestinal tract, and the test is not recommended for regular use in the diagnosis of gastrointestinal pathological conditions. The test is commonly requested by naturopathic physicians who ascribe their own particular interpretation to the results. It is of interest that this was the test that identified the first case of Hartnup's disease.

Serum folate.[80] Folate determinations are widely available and are often used in the assessment of malabsorption. The folate value obtained in red cells reflects a chronic situation, whereas the serum level reflects the day-to-day nutritional impact of folate. Increased serum folate is seen occasionally in pernicious anemia. Decreased serum folate is seen in a series of disorders in which the absorptive capacity of the small intestine is impaired, including Whipple's disease, myelofibrosis, hypothyroidism, celiac sprue, abetalipoproteinemia, vitamin B_6 deficiency, regional enteritis, ileitis, ulcerative colitis, acute and subacute necrosis of the liver, malignancy, and Down's syndrome.

Vitamin B_{12}. The validity of serum vitamin B_{12} determinations has been called to question[81] because many tests of vitamin B_{12} may detect the presence of nonphysiologically active analogs of vitamin B_{12}. Thus they may give false-normal vitamin B_{12} results in B_{12}-deficient persons. Most current methods recognize this potential problem.

Low vitamin B_{12} concentrations (less than 150 pg/mL) are found in pernicious anemia, gastric disease, thyroid disease, ileal disease, malabsorption, and vegetarian diets. Increased vitamin B_{12} is seen with vitamin B_{12} administration, liver tissue damage, leukemia, and lymphoma (see pp. 783 and 790).

METHODS OF ANALYSIS
Schilling test
REVISED BY STEVEN C. KAZMIERCZAK

Principles of analysis and current usage Deficiency of vitamin B_{12} may occur as the result of several mechanisms. The Schilling test is a procedure for determining the pathogenesis of a vitamin B_{12} deficiency. Normally, vitamin B_{12} that has been ingested is bound to intrinsic factor, secreted by parietal cells in the stomach. The vitamin B_{12}-intrinsic factor complex is then bound by specific protein receptors located in the terminal portion of the ileum. Vitamin B_{12} that has made its way into the portal blood is stored in the liver. Once the liver storage sites have been saturated, excess vitamin B_{12} is excreted unchanged into the urine.

The original test described by Schilling in 1953[82] to quantitate the absorption of vitamin B_{12} has undergone various modifications. The test may be performed in up to three different stages to determine the exact mechanism responsible for the vitamin B_{12} deficiency. Recent reviews outlining the physiologic basis and use of the Schilling test as a diagnostic test are available.[83]

In the classic, or first-stage, Schilling test the patient is given an intramuscular injection of nonlabeled vitamin B_{12}. This bolus or flushing dose of vitamin B_{12} saturates the body storage sites for the vitamin. The flushing dose may be given before or after the administration of labeled vitamin B_{12}. Ideally, the flushing dose should be administered 6 hours after the oral dose. This is because orally administered vitamin

B_{12} does not begin to cross the ileal wall for up to 6 hours after ingestion. If however the flushing dose is given more than 6 hours after administration of the oral dose, the tissue sites may not be saturated before the absorption of the labeled vitamin B_{12}. Generally, for the sake of convenience, the flushing dose is administered at the same time as the oral dose, or up to 1 hour later. Patients who are currently undergoing therapy with vitamin B_{12} may have the Schilling test performed, though treatment should be discontinued for 1 week before the performance of the test.

The patient is given a dose of vitamin B_{12} radiolabeled with ^{57}Co. If the patient's vitamin B_{12}–absorption mechanisms are functioning correctly, the labeled vitamin B_{12} will enter the patient's circulation and, because all the available storage sites for the vitamin are saturated, will be excreted into the urine. The amount of ^{57}Co labeled vitamin B_{12} excreted in urine collected for 24 to 72 hours after the ingestion of the vitamin B_{12} is proportional to the amount of vitamin absorbed.

Individuals who show normal absorption of vitamin B_{12} after this first-stage test may be assumed to have a healthy absorption mechanism for vitamin B_{12}. In those instances where the absorption of vitamin B_{12} is inadequate, a second-stage Schilling test may be performed.

The second-stage Schilling test is similar to the first-stage test except that radiolabeled vitamin B_{12} is administered with intrinsic factor. If the absorption of vitamin B_{12} is now judged to be adequate, the defect in absorption of vitamin B_{12} is presumed to be the result of deficiency or defect in intrinsic factor. However, if vitamin B_{12} is still not absorbed after the second-stage test, a third-stage test may be performed.

The third-stage Schilling test is performed to determine if there is a problem with ileal absorption attributable to bacterial overgrowth, blind-loop syndrome, or tapeworm (*Diphyllobothrium latum*) infestation.[84] The patient is given a full course treatment with antibiotic or antihelminthic therapy for several weeks before being tested. Once the treatment regimen has been completed, the first-stage Schilling test is repeated. If absorption of vitamin B_{12} is now judged to be within the healthy reference interval, the cause of the vitamin deficiency is presumed to be the result of bacterial overgrowth or tapeworm infestation.

Techniques that permit the simultaneous determination of the stage-one and stage-two Schilling test have been developed.[85] With this approach, B_{12} radiolabeled with ^{58}Co is administered with ^{57}Co-labeled vitamin B_{12} bound to intrinsic factor. This allows for the simultaneous determination of a stage-one and stage-two Schilling test. The gamma-ray scintillation counter must be optimized for each isotope to differentiate between ^{57}Co and ^{58}Co.[86]

Specimen A 24-, 48-, or 72-hour urine collection may be used, though urine collected for a 24-hour period is most frequently used. Incomplete urine collection is frequently cited as a reason for inaccurate test results.[86] Determination of urine creatinine can provide information as to the adequacy of a 24-hour urine collection.[87]

Reference intervals Suggested reference intervals for stage-one and stage-two Schilling tests are as follows:

1. *Stage-one test.* Excretion of vitamin B_{12} should be greater than 8% to 15%.
2. *Stage-two test.* Excretion of labeled vitamin B_{12} should be greater than 8% to 15%.

REFERENCES

1. Moog F: The lining of the small intestine, *Sci Am* 245:154-176, 1981.
2. Track NS: The gastrointestinal endocrine system, *Can Med Assoc J* 122:287-291, 1980.
3. Rayford PL, Miller TA, Thompson JC: Secretin, cholecystokinin and newer gastrointestinal hormones, *N Engl J Med* 294:1093-1101, 1157-1164, 1976.
4. Ingelfinger FJ: Gastrointestinal absorption, *Nutrition Today,* pp 2-10, March 1967.
5. Dawson AM: The absorption of disaccharides. In Card WI, Creamer B, editors: *Modern trends in gastroenterology,* vol 4, London, 1970, Butterworth.
6. McColl I, Sladen GEC, editors: *Intestinal absorption in man,* New York, 1975, Academic Press.
7. Wilson FA, Dietschy JM: Differential diagnostic approach to clinical problems of malabsorption, *Gastroenterology* 61:911-921, 1971.
8. Wiss O, Gloor U: Absorption, distribution, storage and metabolites of vitamin K and related quinones, *Vitam Horm* 24:576-586, 1966.
9. DeLuca HF, Suttie JW, editors: *The fat soluble vitamins,* Madison, Wisc., 1970, University of Wisconsin Press.
10. Holdsworth CD: *Calcium absorption in man.* In McColl I, Sladen GEG, editors: New York, 1975, Academic Press.
11. Martiner-Torres C, Layrisse M: Nutritional factors in iron-deficiency: food iron absorption, *Clin Hematol* 2:339-352, 1973.
12. Bloom SR, Polak JM: In Glass B, editor: *Progress in gastroenterology,* New York, 1977, Grune & Stratton.
13. McGuigan JE: Gastrointestinal hormones, *Annu Rev Med* 29:307, 1978.
14. Rehfeld JF: Gastrointestinal hormones. In Crane RK, editor: *International review of physiology: gastrointestinal physiology III,* vol 19, Baltimore, 1979, University Park Press.
15. Dockray GJ: Gastrin overview. In Bloom SR, editor: *Gut hormones,* Edinburgh, 1978, Churchill Livingstone.
16. Strunz UT, Walsh JH, Grossman MI: Stimulation of gastrin release in dogs by individual amino acids, *Proc Soc Exp Biol Med* 157:440-441, 1978.
17. Polak JM, Pearse AGE, Joffe SN, et al: Quantification of secretin release by acid using immunocytochemistry and radioimmunoassay, *Experientia* 31:462-464, 1975.
18. Rayford PL, Miller TA, Thompson JC: Secretin cholecystokinin, and newer gastrointestinal hormones, *N Engl J Med* 294:1093-1101, 1976.
19. Schaffalitzky de Muckadell OB, Fahrenkrug J, Watt-Boolsen S, et al: Pancreatic response and plasma secretin concentration during infusion of low dose secretin in man, *Scand J Gastroenterol* 13:305-311, 1978.
20. Bryant MG, Bloom SR, Polak JM, et al: Possible dual role for vasoactive intestinal peptide as gastrointestinal hormone and neurotransmitter substance, *Lancet* 1:991-993, 1976.
21. Lin TM, Evans DC, Chance RE, et al: Bovine pancreatic polypeptide: action on gastric and pancreatic secretion in dogs, *Am J Physiol* 232:E311-E315, 1977.
22. Anderson D, Elahi D, Brown JC, et al: Oral glucose augmentation of insulin secretin, *J Clin Invest* 62:152-161, 1978.
23. Grimelius L, Polar JM, Solcia E, et al: *Gut hormones,* Edinburgh, 1978, Churchill Livingstone.
24. Polak JM, Pearse AGE, Grimelius L, et al: Growth hormone release–inhibiting hormone in gastrointestinal and pancreatic D cells, *Lancet* 1:1220-1222, 1975.
25. Creutzfeldt W, Arnold R: Somatostatin and the stomach: exocrine and endocrine aspects, First International Somatostatin Symposium, Freiburg, Germany, 1977, *Metabolism* 27:1309-1315, 1978.
26. Raptis S, Gerich JE: Foreword, First International Somatostatin Symposium, Freiburg, Germany, 1977, *Metabolism* 27:1129-1130, 1978.
27. Vale W, Rivier C, Brown M: Regulatory peptides of the hypothalamus, *Annu Rev Physiol* 39:473-527, 1977.
28. Pearson WN: Assessment of nutritional status: biochemical methods. In Beaton GH, McHenry EW, editors: *Nutrition: a comprehensive treatise,* New York, 1966, Academic Press.
29. Mirsky IA: Physiologic, psychologic, and social determinants in the etiology of duodenal ulcer, *Am J Dig Dis* 3:285-314, 1958.
30. Grossman MI: Elevated serum pepsinogen I: a genetic marker for duodenal ulcer disease, *N Engl J Med* 300:89, 1979.
31. Grossman MI, Guth PH, Isenberg JI, et al: A new look at peptic ulcer, *Ann Intern Med* 84:57-67, 1976.
32. Genta RM: Counting angels and bacteria: the quest for a unifying theory of ulcerogenesis: an editorial, *Am J Clin Pathol* 98:549-551, 1992.
33. Forbes GM, Glaser ME, Cullen DJE, et al: Duodenal ulcer treated with *Helicobacter pylori* eradication: seven year follow-up, *Lancet* 343:258-260, 1994.
34. Shahon BB, Horowitz S: Cancer of the stomach: analysis of 1152 cases, *Surgery* 39:204-221, 1956.
35. The Eurogastric Study Group: An international association between *Helicobacter pylori* infection and gastric cancer, *Lancet* 341:1359-1362, 1993.
36. Deveney CW, Deveney KS, Way LW: The Zollinger-Ellison syndrome—23 years later, *Ann Surg* 188:384-393, 1978.
37. Walsh JH, Grossman MT: Gastrin, *N Engl J Med* 292:1324-1334, 1377-1384, 1975.
38. Johnson GJ, Somerskill WHK, Anderson VE: Clinical and genetic investigation of a large kindred with multiple endocrine adenomatosis, *N Engl J Med* 277:1379-1386, 1967.
39. Ippoliti AF: Zollinger-Ellison syndrome: provocative diagnostic tests, *Ann Intern Med* 87:787-788, 1977.
40. Deveney CW, Deveney KS, Jaffe BM, et al: Use of calcium and secretin in the diagnosis of gastrinoma, *Ann Intern Med* 87:680-686, 1979.
41. Trier JS: Celiac sprue (review article), *N Engl J Med* 325:1709-1719, 1992.
42. Gray GM: Congenital and adult intestinal lactose deficiency, *N Engl J Med* 294:1057-1058, 1976.
43. Kuehn PG, Coley GM, Christine B: Carcinoid syndrome: a study of 16 cases, *Hartford Hosp Bull* 28:305-307, 1973.
44. Jeejeebhoy KN: Symposium on diarrhea. I. Definition and mechanisms of diarrhea, *Can Med Assoc J* 116:737-738, 1977.
45. Gilbertson VA: The earlier diagnosis of adenocarcinoma of the large intestine, *Cancer* 27:143-149, 1971.
46. Kelly CP, Pothoulakis C, LaMont JT: *Clostridium difficile* colitis (review article), *N Engl J Med* 330:257-262, 1994.
47. Middleton SJ, Shorthouse M, Hunter JO: Increased nitric oxide synthesis in ulcerative colitis, *Lancet* 341:465-466, 1993.
48. Walravens PA: Keeping TPN on course with lab monitoring, *Diagn Med* 4:38-43, 1981.
49. Ward S, Gillespie IE, Passaro ER, et al: Comparison of Histalog and histamine as stimulants for maximal gastric secretions in human subjects and in dogs, *Gastroenterology* 44:620-626, 1963.
50. Abernethy RJ, Gillespie IE, Lowrie JH, et al: Pentagastrin as a stimulant of maximal gastric acid response in man: a multicentre pilot study, *Lancet* 1:291-295, 1967.
51. Kirsner JB, Ford H: The gastric secretory response to Histalog: one-hour basal and Histalog secretion in normal persons and in patients with duodenal ulcer and gastric ulcer, *J Lab Clin Med* 46:307-311, 1955.
52. Blackman AH, Lambert DL, Thayer WR, et al: Computed normal values for peak acid output based on age, sex and body weight, *Am J Dig Dis* 15:783-789, 1970.
53. McNeely MDD: Gastrointestinal function. In Sonnenwirth AC, Jarett L, editors: *Gradwohl's clinical laboratory methods and diagnosis,* ed 8, St. Louis, 1980, Mosby.

54. Herbert V: Detection of malabsorption of vitamin B_{12} to gastric or intestinal dysfunction, *Semin Nucl Med* 2:220-234, 1972.

55. Drummey GD, Benson JA, Jones CM: Microscopical examination of the stool for steatorrhea, *N Engl J Med* 264:85-87, 1961.

56. Massion CG, McNeely MD: Accurate micromethod for estimation of both medium- and long-chain fatty acids and triglycerides in fecal fat, *Clin Chem* 19:499-505, 1973.

57. Schwartz L, Woldow A, Dunsmore R: Determination of fat tolerance in patients with myocardial infarction: method utilizing serum turbidity changes following a fat meal, *JAMA* 149:364-366, 1952.

58. Silver S: *Radioactive isotopes in medicine and biology,* Philadelphia, 1962, Lea & Febiger.

59. Kaihara S, Wagner HN Jr: Measurement of intestinal fat absorption with carbon-14 labeled tracers, *J Lab Clin Med* 71:400-411, 1968.

60. Benson JA, Culver PJ, Ragland S, et al: The D-xylose absorption test in malabsorption syndromes, *N Engl J Med* 256:335-339, 1957.

61. Santini R, Sheehy TW, Martínez-de-Jesús J: The xylose tolerance test with a five-gram dose, *Gastroenterology* 40:772-774, 1961.

62. Newcomer AD, McGill DB, Thomas PJ, Hofmann AF: Prospective comparison of indirect methods for detecting lactase deficiency, *N Engl J Med* 293:1232-1235, 1975.

63. Parkinson CE, Gal I: Factors affecting the lab management of human serum and liver vitamin A analysis, *Clin Chim Acta* 40:83-90, 1972.

64. Onstad GR, Zieve L: Carotene absorption: a screening test for steatorrhea, *JAMA* 221:677-679, 1972.

65. Erlanger BF, Kokowsky N, Cohen W: The preparation and properties of two new chromogenic substrates of trypsin, *Arch Biochem Biophys* 95:271-278, 1961.

66. Winawer SJ, Sherlock P, Schottenfeld D, Miller DG: Screening for colon cancer, *Gastroenterology* 70:783-789, 1976.

67. Christensen F, Anker N, Mondrop M: Blood in feces: a comparison of the sensitivity and reproducibility of five chemical methods, *Clin Chim Acta* 57:23-27, 1974.

68. Morris DW, Lee CS, Hansell JR: Presentation at the annual meeting of the American Gastroenterological Society, San Francisco, 1974.

69. MaKarem A: Hemoglobins, myoglobins and haptoglobins. In Henry RJ, Cannon DC, Winkelman J, editors: *Clinical chemistry principles and technics,* New York, 1974, Harper & Row.

70. Gold P, Freedman SO: Specific carcinoembryonic antigens of the human digestive system, *J Exp Med* 122:467-481, 1965.

71. Meeker WR: The use and abuse of the CEA test in clinical practice, *Cancer* 41:854-862, 1978.

72. National Institutes of Health Consensus Conference: Carcinoembryonic antigen: its role as a marker in the management of cancer, *Br Med J* 282:373-375, 1981.

73. Tracy RP, Wold LE, Jones JD, Burritt ME: Colorimetric vs. liquid-chromatographic determination of urinary 5-hydroxyindole-3-acetic acid, *Clin Chem* 27:160-162, 1981.

74. Newman A: Breath-analysis tests in gastroenterology, *Gut* 15:1-15, 1974.

75. McNeely MDD: Breath test $^{14}CO_2$. In Pesce AJ, Kaplan LA, editors: *Clinical chemistry: a laboratory and managers' infobase,* Cincinnati, 1996, Pesce Kaplan Publishers.

76. Baker PG, Barry RE, Read AE: Detection of continuing gluten ingestion in treated coeliac patients, *Br Med J* 1:486-488, 1975.

77. Jones EA: Immunoglobulins and the gut, *Gut* 13:825-835, 1972.

78. Stauffer JQ, Humphreys MH, Weir GJ: Acquired hyperoxaluria with regional enteritis after ileal resection, *Ann Intern Med* 79:383-391, 1973.

79. Holdsworth CD: Intestinal and pancreatic function. In Brown SS, Mitchell FL, Young DS, editors: *Chemical diagnosis of disease,* New York, 1980, Elsevier/North Holland.

80. Rosenberg IH, Godwin HA: The digestion and absorption of dietary folate, *Gastroenterology* 60:445-463, 1970.

81. Kolhouse JF, Kondo H, Allen NC, et al: Cobalamin analogues are present in human plasma and can mask cobalamin deficiency because current radioisotope dilution assays are not specific for true cobalamin, *N Engl J Med* 299:785-792, 1978.

82. Schilling RF: Intrinsic factor studies. II. The effect of gastric juice on the urinary exretion of radioactivity after the administration of vitamin B_{12}, *J Lab Clin Med* 42:860-866, 1953.

83. Nickoloff E: Schilling test: physiologic basis for and use as a diagnostic test, *Crit Rev Clin Lab Sci* 26:263-276, 1988.

84. Streeter AM, Bathur FA, Arnold BJ, et al: Limitations of the Schilling test, *Lancet* 1:39-40, 1981.

85. Katz JH, DiMase J, Donaldson RM Jr: Simultaneous administration of gastric juice–bound and free radioactive cyanocobalamin, *J Lab Clin Med* 82:266, 1963.

86. Atrah HI, Davidson RJ: A survey and critical evaluation of a dual isotope (Dicopac) vitamin B_{12} absorption test, *Eur J Nucl Med* 15:57-60, 1989.

87. Heironimus JD, Borchert RD, Weiland FL: The value of urine creatinine analysis in the evaluation on Schilling tests, *Clin Nucl Med* 15:181-182, 1990.

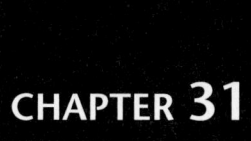

CHAPTER 31 — *Cardiac and muscle disease*

John F. Chapman
Robert H. Christenson
Lawrence M. Silverman

OBJECTIVES

■ Briefly describe myocardial energy metabolism and the important myocardial proteins involved in cell metabolism and function.

■ List proteins and enzymes (and their isoforms and isoenzymes) that are routinely measured in serum to assess myocardial disease, and state the time periods for the expected enzyme elevations following myocardial infarction.

KEY TERMS

actin One of the proteins involved in myocardial and arterial smooth muscle contraction.

atherosclerosis "Hardening of the arteries." A process that results in gradual deposition of lipid, fibrin, and calcium in the walls of arteries. The most common cause of death in Western countries.

atrium The chamber of the heart that collects blood from the veins and contracts to expel the blood into one of the two ventricles. There are two atria: the right collects blood from the systemic veins and fills the right ventricle; the left collects blood from the pulmonary veins and fills the left ventricle.

cardiac failure Failure of the heart to maintain blood circulation, with resultant accumulation of salt and water and inadequate perfusion of essential organs.

cardiomyopathy A heterogeneous group of disorders that have in common a toxic or genetic insult that affects contracting myocardial cells directly.

Embden-Meyerhof pathway The pathway of anaerobic glycolysis that will convert glucose or glycogen to lactate.

embolus A portion of a blood clot that breaks off from the main clot and travels through the circulation to settle in the lungs (pulmonary embolus) or in one of the systemic arteries (systemic embolus), depending on where the embolus originates.

glycoside A generic term for a group of drugs originally obtained from the foxglove plant. These drugs improve the contractility of the failing heart and slow the rate of ventricular contraction in atrial fibrillation. Digoxin is a member of this family of drugs.

infarction A process of tissue damage caused by a loss of blood supply. Thus myocardial infarction or heart attack occurs when one of the coronary arteries is occluded and the tissue distal to the occlusion dies.

ischemia A reduction of blood supply to tissue that is large enough to prevent the tissue from functioning normally.

Krebs citric acid cycle The pathway of intermediary metabolism that will accept metabolic products from the Embden-Meyerhof pathway and oxidize, decarboxylate, and reduce them, with the production of a relatively large amount of adenosine triphosphate.

myosin One of the contractile proteins involved in cardiac and arterial smooth muscle contraction.

technetium 99m (^{99m}Tc) An isotope injected intravenously to measure left ventricular output or to detect an acute myocardial infarction (*m* means *metastable*).

thallium 201 An isotope injected intravenously to delineate part of the ventricular muscle mass that is ischemic or a scar caused by an old infarction.

troponin Protein component of thin filaments that, together with tropomysin, regulates actin and myosin interactions.

ventricles The main pumping chambers of the heart that expel blood into the pulmonary artery and aorta. The left ventricle is more massive and powerful than the right ventricle because the pressure in the systemic circulation is higher than that in the pulmonary circulation; thus a stronger pump is required for the systemic side of the circulation.

ANATOMY AND FUNCTION
Muscle

Anatomy. There are three distinct groups of muscle: skeletal, cardiac, and smooth. The *skeletal muscle* consists of parallel bundles of unbranched, cylindrical muscle cells, or myotubes, fibers with multiple nuclei as a result of the fusion of many single cells during myogenesis. The fibers run the whole length of the muscle and microscopically show characteristic crossbanding. They have well-defined nerve end plates and are under voluntary control. Contractions are initiated by nerve impulses and are termed *neurogenic*.

In each muscle cell there is a bundle of cylindrical *myofibrils,* which are surrounded by an extensive network of tubular channels, the *sarcoplasmic reticulum. Nerve endings* are attached to the outer surface of the sarcolemma through the motor end plate of an axon. Within the sarcolemma-enclosed space the fibrils are bathed by the intracellular fluid of muscle, the *sarcoplasm.* Within the myofibrils the contractile material is organized into repeating units, termed *sarcomeres.* The organized contractile material within the fibrils is composed largely of the proteins *myosin* and *actin* in an alternating filamentous form in each sarcomere. The proteins found in the myofibrillar structure are listed in Table 31-1.

Cardiac muscle is found only in the heart. It is similar in structure to skeletal muscle except that the cells are branched and interconnected. There are no defined end plates in cardiac muscle, and in normal conditions it is not under voluntary control; that is, it does not require nerves to initiate and maintain its contraction and therefore it is termed *myogenic.*

Smooth muscle is composed of narrow, fusiform cells with a single nucleus. The smooth muscle cell does not have a structurally defined end plate and is not under voluntary control; therefore it is also termed *involuntary* muscle. Smooth muscle is found usually in walls of tubes or sacs such as blood vessels, the wall of the uterus, the urinary bladder, the intestines, and the bronchioles. It is characterized by slow contraction, and it can maintain tension or a given length without fatigue at low energy cost.

Table 31-1 Myofibrillar proteins and their localization in vertebrate skeletal muscle

Proteins	Localization	Amount of protein as percentage of total cellular protein
Contractile proteins		
Myosin	A band	60
Actin	I band	20
Regulatory proteins		
Tropomyosin	I band	3
Troponin	I band	4.5
M protein	M line (M band)	Less than 1
C protein	A band	Less than 1
Actinin	Z line, I band	1
Other minor proteins		
Connectin	A and I bands	Less than 1
Z protein	Z line	Less than 1
Desmin	Z line	Less than 1

Function and mechanism. The general function of the muscles is a mechanical response to stimulation that produces shortening and force development, both usually occurring together. The skeletal muscle function is modified by leverage as a result of its attachment to the skeleton. In cardiac muscle the force development is manifested by the development of pressure within the chambers of the heart during cardiac muscle shortening, which results in reduced chamber size.

Smooth muscle shortening is seen when smooth muscle sacs or cavities are emptied, as in the expulsion of urine from the bladder or of a child from the uterus. It is apparent that considerable force is developed during such smooth muscle activity.

The hydrolysis of adenosine triphosphate (ATP) supplies the immediate energy for muscle contraction. The amount of ATP hydrolyzed in contraction is not constant but depends on the duration of contraction and on the amount of work done by the muscle. The ATP-hydrolysis sites are on the cross-bridges formed between the interacting myosin and actin elements of the sarcomere, and the ATPase is highly active only when myosin and actin interact.

Relaxation of the muscle is a passive process. When there is no ATP hydrolysis by the myosin-actin complex, the sarcomere returns to its resting length. The interdigitated filaments slide back to a less overlapped position, thereby increasing the length of the muscle. The same basic principle applies to skeletal and cardiac muscle and even to smooth muscle contraction.

Acetylcholine as neuromuscular transmitter

Motor nerve endings differ, depending on the main fiber type. "Slow-twitch" fibers, which respond to nerve stimuli with prolonged contractions, are in general innervated by multiple nerve endings. "Fast-twitch" fibers are usually innervated by individual end plates. At both types of motor nerve terminals acetylcholine is synthesized and stored in vesicles. Acetylcholine, which serves as a neurotransmitter, is released from the nerve ending and is bound to receptors in the sarcolemma, depolarizing the muscle plasma membrane and initiating the biochemical events that result in muscle contraction. The events include the use of Ca^{++} ions as a second messenger, activating the ATPase in the troponin complex and triggering the interaction between myosin and actin.

Anatomy and function of the heart

The pumping action of the heart[1] is the prime factor in the maintenance of the body's circulation. The heart is a muscular organ composed of four chambers, the two atria and the two ventricles. The atria collect blood from the systemic circulation and pump it into the ventricles. The right ventricle pumps blood to the lungs for reoxygenation, and the left ventricle pumps blood to the rest of the body, including the heart itself. Cardiac output is determined primarily by the rate at which the heart pumps, by the systemic blood pressure, and by the contractile force developed in the wall of the left ventricle. Cardiac muscle, which is extremely active, requires large quantities of oxygen for metabolism. Delivery of the oxygen needed to fuel the heart requires a rich capillary bed. Normally, some 75% of the oxygen is extracted from the blood that passes through the heart, and changes in metabolic demand, particularly changes in heart rate, are met by alterations in coronary blood flow.

MUSCLE AND MYOCARDIAL BIOCHEMISTRY
Energy metabolism

Various substrates are used by muscle cells as fuels. Energy is liberated from these fuels by several pathways, including the Embden-Meyerhof glycolytic pathway, the pentose phosphate shunt, fatty acid oxidation, and the Krebs citric acid cycle (see Chapter 32). The energy produced by the breakdown of substrates is then transported through the electron-transport system of the mitochondria to produce adenosine triphosphate, the chemical form of stored energy that is used by muscle tissue to perform work. To perform their function, muscle cells must maintain a high [ATP]/[ADP] ratio, and all muscles require an effective storage method to maintain a reserve of ATP. This is achieved through the synthesis of creatine phosphate (CP), which acts as a backup storage source that can be used for rapid regeneration of ATP when levels fall as a result of increased demand.

This high-energy reservoir uses the enzymes creatine kinase (CK) and myokinase (MK) to maintain an equilibrium concentration of ATP, ADP, and CP. The immediate effect of increased ADP concentrations caused by the hydrolysis of ATP during contraction is a disturbance of the equilibrium of the creatine kinase–catalyzed reaction:

$$\begin{array}{c}
O \\
\parallel \\
HO\!-\!P\!-\!OH \\
\mid \\
NH \\
\mid \\
C = NH \\
\mid \\
N\!-\!CH_3 \\
\mid \\
CH_2 \\
\mid \\
COOH
\end{array}
\quad + \quad ADP \;\overset{CK}{\rightleftharpoons}\; ATP \; + \;
\begin{array}{c}
NH_2 \\
\mid \\
C\!=\!NH \\
\mid \\
N\!-\!CH_3 \\
\mid \\
CH_2 \\
\mid \\
COOH
\end{array}$$

Creatine   **Creatine**
phosphate

The equilibrium is reestablished by the phosphorylation of ADP to ATP by this reaction, thus preserving a high [ATP]/[ADP] ratio.

Another enzyme, *myokinase*, catalyzes the reaction:

$$2\;ADP \;\overset{MK}{\rightleftharpoons}\; ATP \; + \; AMP$$

This reaction also assures the re-establishment of the original high [ATP]/[ADP] ratio.

A third enzyme present in the muscle, *adenosine deaminase* (AD), prevents the accumulation of AMP produced by the myokinase reaction by deamination of the AMP:

$$AMP \;\overset{AD}{\rightleftharpoons}\; IMP \; + \; NH_3^+$$

Inosine monophosphate (IMP) then either returns to the nucleoside pool as inosine or is degraded further to uric acid. For a single contraction (twitch) or for short periods of muscle activity, the only measurable change in the high-energy phosphate pool is a small change in CP.

Myoglobin

The heart is critically dependent on oxygen, consuming between 6.5 and 10 mL/100 g of tissue per minute at rest. There is a dramatic increase in oxygen requirements with exercise. Normally, some 70% of the oxygen reaching the heart is extracted by *myoglobin*, a single-chain globular hemoprotein. All muscle cells contain myoglobin; the myocardium contains 1.4 mg of myoglobin per gram of tissue. Myoglobin's oxygen dissociation curve is different from that of hemoglobin and thus facilitates entry of oxygen into all muscle cells, provides local storage for oxygen, and is essential for maintaining cardiac function. Myoglobin, with a molecular weight of 17,000 daltons, is small enough to be freely filtered by the glomerulus and is excreted in the urine.

Energy demands of different muscle types

Skeletal. Human skeletal muscle contains both red and white fibers, which differ in their metabolic properties. Red, or slow, fibers are rich in myoglobin and mitochondria. In these fibers the main metabolic pathway is oxidative phosphorylation. White, or fast, fibers contain little myoglobin and mitochondria, and the main route for energy metabolism is glycolysis.

At maximal activity, skeletal muscle can increase its oxygen uptake twentyfold or more during the transition from rest to full activity to supply the oxygen needed for the oxidative process. However, at maximal activity the skeletal muscles still are relatively oxygen-poor (anoxic), and lactate, as the end product of anaerobic metabolism, increases in blood.

Acidosis occurs when either metabolic or other abnormal processes result in a lower than normal pH of the arterial blood. Lactic acidosis, which results from an excessive production of lactic acid, can occur in normal skeletal muscles after excessive exercise. The localized acidosis in skeletal muscle contributes to fatigue and can result in muscle cramps and pain, especially when it is accompanied by excessive sodium chloride loss.

Cardiac. The highly aerobic metabolism of the heart allows it to use as fuel many substrates normally present in plasma, and cardiac uptake of most of these substances is proportional to their arterial concentration once certain levels are exceeded. In general terms, the heart uses free fatty acids as its predominant fuel. It also consumes significant quantities of glucose and lactate, as well as lesser amounts of pyruvate, ketone bodies, and amino acids. Most of the energy for cardiac function is obtained from the breakdown of metabolites through the citric acid cycle and oxidative phosphorylation. These enzyme pathways are found principally in the mitochondria, which make up some 35% of the total volume of cardiac muscle.

Enzymes in myocardial cells

Several enzymes found in myocardial tissue[2] are clinically important because detection of their release into the bloodstream can be related to myocardial cell damage and death. Enzymes measured routinely in the clinical laboratory for the assessment of myocardial disease are discussed below.

Creatine kinase. The enzyme responsible for regeneration of ATP is creatine kinase.[2] It has a molecular weight of 85,000 daltons and exists in several isoenzymatic forms (see the following text and Chapter 55). CK is a dimer, composed of the two subunits M (muscle) and B (brain). The three isoenzymes formed from these subunits are found in the cytosol. These isoenzymes are given the abbreviations MM, MB, and BB. If one compares the activity of the enzyme in various tissues, skeletal muscle has by far the highest activity, possessing some 50,000 times the concentration of serum CK. The predominant skeletal isoenzyme is the MM isoenzyme, with only traces of MB and BB isoenzymes in most muscle fibers. The MB component, however, is increased in certain muscle disorders, particularly the Duchenne type of muscular dystrophy and polymyositis. The skeletal muscle CK activity measured in international units is around 2000 U/g, which compares with the cardiac muscle activity of 500 U/g. In normal serum, at least 95% of the CK present is of the MM type and is probably largely the result of leakage from skeletal muscle, particularly during physical activity. Because of this, serum CK activity in healthy, active persons shows an asymmetrical distribution skewed toward higher values. In addition, values are lower in women than in men and are lower in the morning than in the evening. Values tend to be lower in hospitalized patients, possibly because bed rest reduces the amount of enzymes released from muscle.

CK isoforms.[3-5] The CK-MM and CK-MB isoenzymes in serum can be fractionated into subtypes, or "isoforms," by high resolution techniques such as high-voltage electrophoresis or chromatofocusing. The isoforms of CK-MM and CK-MB are formed in blood by irreversible enzymatic cleavage of the COOH-terminal amino acid, a lysine residue, from the M subunit or subunits of the tissue isoenzymes. For CK-MM, this cleavage involves successive removal of the terminal lysine residues from *each* M subunit, giving rise to three isoforms called MM_3 (tissue form, or $M_{lysine}M_{lysine}$), MM_2 (or $M_{lysine}M$), and MM_1 (or MM). CK-MB, which has a single M subunit, consists of two isoforms in circulation, termed MB_2 (tissue form, or $M_{lysine}B$) and MB_1 (or MB). It is of note that the terminal amino acid sequence of the B subunit of CK is similar to that of the M subunit; however, cleavage of the terminal lysine of the B subunit of CK-MB is not fully accepted.

Lactate dehydrogenase. Lactate dehydrogenase $(LD)^2$ (see below and Chapter 55) is a ubiquitous tissue enzyme that catalyzes the reduction of pyruvate to lactate using nicotinamide adenine dinucleotide (NAD). LD has a molecular weight of about 140,000 daltons and is a tetramer composed of four subunits of molecular weight 35,000 daltons each. The subunits, which are of two forms, H (heart) and M (muscle), combine to form the five isoenzymes of LD. The principal isoenzyme in heart (HHHH) is maximally active in the presence of low concentrations of pyruvate but is inhibited by excess pyruvate. In contrast, the major muscle isoenzyme (MMMM) is maximally active in the presence of a higher pyruvate concentration and is less inhibited by excess pyruvate. The heart metabolizes fatty acids and carbohydrates at a fairly constant rate with complete oxidation of pyruvate through the Krebs citric acid cycle. The heart thus has a low tissue concentration of pyruvate and lactate and rapidly converts plasma lactate to pyruvate. In contrast, muscle, with rapid demands for increased energy during exercise, has to deal with rapid increases in tissue pyruvate and lactate caused by anaerobic metabolism (see Chapter 32).

LD is found in the cytosol of all human cells and thus would have little diagnostic specificity were it not for the fact that isoenzymes are present in different proportion in each tissue (Chapter 55). Heart and red blood cells contain mostly LD_1 and LD_2, whereas skeletal muscle and liver contain LD_5 and to a lesser degree LD_4. Normal serum contains mostly LD_2, with lesser amounts of LD_1 and the other isoenzymes. If the enzymes are released from cardiac tissue into serum, one frequently sees a change in the ratio of

LD_1 to LD_2. The half-life of LD is different for each isoenzyme; isoenzyme 1 (HHHH) has a half-life of about 100 hours, but isoenzyme 5 (MMMM) has a half-life of only 10 hours. The significance of this is evident in the discussion of the release of enzymes during myocardial infarction.

Aspartate aminotransferase. Aspartate aminotransferase (AST, formerly SGOT)[2] catalyzes the transfer of an amino group between aspartic acid and pyruvate to form oxaloacetate (alpha-ketoglutarate) and alanine. This ubiquitous enzyme is critical in intermediary metabolism and permits the amino acids aspartic acid and glutamic acid to be broken down in the Krebs cycle. The enzyme exists in two structurally different forms; one is found principally in the cytoplasm and the other in the mitochondria. It is the cytosol form that is found in serum. Its half-life in serum is probably about 20 hours. Liver has the highest enzyme activity, with some 85 U/g of tissue, whereas heart muscle possesses 75 U/g and skeletal muscle about 50 U/g.

Aldolase. Aldolase is an enzyme of the lyase group. Its effect is a reversible cleavage of its substrate into two compounds without hydrolysis. The following reaction is catalyzed by aldolase (ALD):

$$\text{Fructose-1,6-diphosphate} \underset{}{\overset{\text{ALD}}{\rightleftharpoons}} \text{Dihydroxyacetone phosphate} + \text{Glyceraldehyde-3-phosphate}$$

Aldolase is a significant enzyme in the glycolytic pathway and is found in every living cell. In tissues in which glycolysis supplies a large part of the energy need, high aldolase activity can be found. As an example, about 300 mg of skeletal muscle contains as much aldolase as is found in normal circulating blood volume. The fructose diphosphate aldolases are present in different isoenzyme forms. The three major forms are aldolase A, predominantly in muscle; aldolase B, in the liver; and aldolase C, in the brain. All three aldolases contain four polypeptide subunits, which differ in amino acid composition.

Contractile proteins[2,6-8] (Table 31-1)

Most currently used biochemical markers of myocardial injury are involved with cell metabolism, are soluble, and are located in the cell's cytosolic compartment. Because of these properties, a large proportion of these cytosolic markers is readily released into circulation after cell injury. In contrast, the nature and function of structural proteins dictate that they be insoluble; thus a relatively minor proportion is unbound in the cytosol and available for rapid release shortly after cell injury. This minor proportion available for release is referred to as the "cytosolic pool."

Despite the theoretical disadvantage of their insolubility, great interest has been generated in the following structural proteins: troponin I, troponin T, and the myosin light chains. The basis of this clinical interest stems from the identification and purification of cardiac forms of these proteins with high tissue specificity, allowing development of immuno-

assays for assessment of myocardial injury. They are discussed in further detail below.

Myosin, actin, and troponin. Myosin and actin proteins form the major part of the contractile apparatus of muscle cells. Together they compose 80% of the muscle cells' protein (see Table 31-1). The regulatory proteins troponin and tropomysin, in association with polymerized actin, form the thin filaments of the sarcomere. Troponin consists of a complex of three subunits: troponin C, troponin I, and troponin T.

Troponin T (TnT).[6] The 37-kilodalton protein troponin T has a cytosolic pool composing about 6% of its total intracellular concentration. Although found in both skeletal and heart tissue, TnT is being successfully used as a marker for ischemic heart disease because one subtype found in myocardial tissue has only 60% homology with the skeletal muscle form. Highly specific antibodies that discriminate between the cardiac and skeletal muscle subtypes have been developed.

Troponin I (TnI).[8] Like TnT, TnI is an integral part of the structural contractile apparatus in both skeletal and myocardial muscle. TnI's cytosolic pool is believed to be the same as that for TnT, about 6% of the cell's total TnI concentration. TnI, with a molecular weight of 21 kilodaltons, is slightly smaller than TnT. The cardiac subtype of TnI has several amino acid regions that differ substantially from the skeletal muscle form. These regions serve as the basis for cardiospecific immunoassays.

Myosin light chains (MLCs).[9] Myosin is a large filamentous molecule (540 kD) made up of six peptide chains, two of which are heavy (230 kD) and four of which are light (MLCs), each with molecular weights in the range of 26 kD. The MLCs are composed of two components, myosin light chain–1 and myosin light chain–2, that together constitute the thick filament of the contractile apparatus in skeletal and myocardial muscle. MLCs from cardiac and noncardiac sources can be differentiated by using antibodies specific for cardiac MLCs.[10] It is of note that the cytosolic pool for the MLCs is 0.5% of the cell's total amount, and only about 10% of the cytosolic pool for either TnT or TnI.

PATHOLOGICAL CONDITIONS
Myocardial disorders

Pathological processes affecting the heart are generally classified into one of the four general categories listed below:

1. Ischemic heart disease
2. Cardiomyopathy
3. Arrhythmias
4. Congenital and valvular heart disease

Ischemic heart disease. Ischemia[1] is a condition in which an organ has a blood supply that is inadequate to maintain its essential functions. There are many causes of myocardial ischemia, but the most common cause by far is coronary atherosclerosis. This condition can develop over many years, sometimes even beginning in childhood, as the arteries supplying blood to the heart gradually narrow because of deposition of cholesterol and other material in the arterial wall (see Chapter 33). Coronary vasospasm can also produce ischemia. In coronary vasospasm the arterial wall constricts in an abnormal and prolonged fashion because of supersensitivity to normal vasoconstrictor signals. Other less common causes of myocardial ischemia are inflammation of the coronary arteries, thrombosis (blood clots), severe anemia, and severe hypotension.

Effects of occlusion on myocardium. Cessation of blood flow produces a complex series of consequences. Not only is there serious hypoxia because tissue oxygen concentration drops drastically, but also there is the problem of removal of toxic cellular metabolites from ischemic tissue and the production of free radicals after reperfusion of the damaged tissues. Sudden occlusion of the coronary artery leaves myocardial cells with only a few seconds of aerobic metabolism as they rapidly consume the oxygen supplies remaining in the microvasculature. Once the oxygen supply has been exhausted, mitochondrial oxidative phosphorylation is unable to continue. Myocardial metabolism then switches to the use of glycogen or glucose in the anaerobic Embden-Meyerhof pathway, instead of the aerobic Krebs cycle. Since the Krebs cycle is unable to function, the end product of anaerobic glucose metabolism, pyruvate, is reduced to lactate, and lactate accumulation is one of the earliest and most dramatic signs of myocardial ischemia.

As ischemia progresses, creatine phosphate reserves are used up, adenosine triphosphate levels fall, and cardiac tissue becomes more acidic as lactate and other acidic intermediates of glycolysis accumulate. Up to 15 to 20 minutes after an ischemic incident, the tissue will recover if it is reperfused. However, after about 20 minutes of occlusion, over 60% of the cellular adenosine triphosphate has been used up and the amount of lactate in wet myocardial tissue is 12 times its normal aerobic level. In addition, all cellular glycogen has been used. Once all the glycogen and creatine phosphate reserves have been used, dramatic ultrastructural changes occur, indicating irreversible cell damage. Cell membrane damage is also evident. If, at this point, the obstruction is relieved and the myocardial tissue is reperfused, it is unable to tolerate the arrival of fresh blood and cell lysis and contracture develop.

The point when reversible ischemic injury becomes irreversible ischemic injury is the point when the cell is no longer able to maintain membrane integrity. Damage to the cell membrane results in the release of intracellular contents. Of these contents, it is release of enzymes and soluble proteins that is particularly significant in the evaluation and confirmation of irreversible ischemic injury. Enzyme release reflects irreversible damage to myocytes and indicates that the patient has had a myocardial infarction rather than simply an anginal or transient ischemic episode.

The significant molecules that are released after ischemic irreversible injury are soluble enzymes and proteins such as creatine kinase, aspartate aminotransferase, lactate dehydrogenase, aldolase, myokinase, alanine aminotransferase, myosin light chains, troponins, and myoglobin.

Most enzymes released early in the infarction are cytoplasmic. Mitochondrial enzymes, if soluble, are released also, but there is usually some delay before they appear in plasma. Once membrane damage has occurred, the rate of appearance of an enzyme in the circulation appears to depend on the rate and extent of reperfusion of the damaged myocardium and on the size of the enzyme molecule. The more flow, the better the reperfusion, and the smaller the molecule, the sooner the molecule will be seen in peripheral blood. CK, with a molecular weight of 85,000 daltons, is released before AST, with a molecular weight of 120,000 daltons, which in turn is released before LD, with a molecular weight of 140,000 daltons.

Cardiomyopathy.[11,12] Cardiomyopathy represents a diverse group of disorders, generally falling into two categories: (1) disease originating in heart tissue and (2) disease that is secondary to other nonmyocardial disorders. Cardiomyopathy is characterized by inadequate muscle contraction caused by direct damage to myocardial cells and typically results in hemodynamic overload and heart failure. Although there are some specific forms of cardiomyopathy, most clinical cases are idiopathic; that is, the cause is unclear. Cardiomyopathy manifests as an enlargement of all four chambers of the heart and cardiac failure. The biochemical findings in most cases of cardiomyopathy are nonspecific and reflect the major clinical presentation, that is, cardiac failure. At least two forms of this disease, *familial hypertrophic cardiomyopathy* and *viral myocarditis,* can now be diagnosed using molecular genetic techniques.[13,14]

Arrhythmias. Although the structure of the heart as a pump is relatively simple, the neuroregulatory system that controls the pattern of contractions of each of its four chambers and regulates cardiac function in relation to the needs of body organs is necessarily much more complex and therefore more at risk of damage.

The anatomical changes that result in cardiac arrhythmias are relatively nonspecific and are frequently related to the disease process affecting the heart muscle. An important cause of arrhythmias is myocardial infarction. Whatever the source of the damage, this damage frequently distorts the transmission of the cardiac nerve impulse, producing abnormal and self-sustaining irregular contractile activity. In functional terms the rhythm abnormalities are classified as bradycardias (resulting in heartbeat rates less than 60 beats/min) or as tachycardias (producing heartbeat rates faster than 100 beats/min). The arrhythmias can affect atrial or ventricle contractions and can be acute or chronic. Atrial fibrillation is a fairly common rhythm abnormality in which the atria beat in an irregular and abnormally rapid fashion.

Chronic arrhythmias are controlled by drugs, the serum levels of which should be routinely monitored.

Congenital and valvular heart disease. The many congenital heart abnormalities that have been described are not discussed in this text. In general terms, all components of the heart can be affected by maldevelopment. Most causes are unknown, but one important exception is rubella infection of the mother during the first trimester of pregnancy.

Of the acquired valvular diseases of the heart, one large group is caused by rheumatic carditis. In susceptible subjects affected by the hemolytic streptococcus, the body develops an immune reaction against all myocardial tissue, but particularly the valves, which become damaged and deformed.

Skeletal muscle disorders

The diseases of muscle are all characterized by motor dysfunction, such as muscular weakness. The abnormality is in some part of the motor unit. The *motor unit* consists of a single lower motor neuron, the anterior horn cell, its efferent root, the peripheral nerve fiber, and its terminal arborization. It also includes the motor end plate at the neuromuscular junction together with the 10 to 600 muscle fibers innervated by the neuron.

The three major categories of muscle disorders, according to the part of the motor unit affected, are (1) neurogenic muscular atrophies, (2) muscle fiber disorders, and (3) disturbances of the neuromuscular junction. Within each major class there are further distinctions based on the loci, or known origins of the defects. These categories are listed below.

The *muscular atrophies* are caused by a loss of efferent innervation as a result of a degeneration of either an anterior horn cell or an axon at the level of an anterior efferent root or peripheral nerve cell.

The *myopathies* are characterized by major defects at the level of the muscle fiber. Certain hereditary progressive myopathies are called, by convention, *muscular dystrophies.* *Nonhereditary myopathies* can result from inflammation or from an endocrine or metabolic abnormality.

Anterior root and peripheral nerve involvements. *Acute polyneuropathy,* or Guillain-Barré syndrome, is a parainfectious and postinfectious disease and presumed to be caused by immunological attack on peripheral nerves.

Metabolic neuropathies are seen with metabolic diseases such as diabetes mellitus or malnutrition.

Disorders of muscle fibers: muscular dystrophies. Muscular dystrophy is a general name for a group of chronic diseases of muscle. The general characteristics are progressive weakness and degeneration of skeletal muscle with no evidence of neural degeneration. They are inherited diseases with different inheritance patterns. The age of onset, the course of disease, and the effect on the different fiber types differ among the individual diseases.

Pseudohypertrophic muscular dystrophy, or Duchenne muscular dystrophy, is a sex-linked recessive disorder. It is the most commonly seen of the muscular dystrophies. It affects boys typically between 3 to 7 years of age with steady progression of proximal muscle weakness, and most patients are confined to wheelchairs by 10 to 12 years of age. Serum enzymes are greatly elevated in the disease even before symptoms develop; especially noted is the rise in creatine kinase. The creatine kinase values in heterozygous females and normal persons overlap; unfortunately only about 50% to 70% of heterozygous females are positively identifiable as gene carriers. Nevertheless, diagnosis of this disease by DNA analysis and genetic counseling has significantly changed the occurrence of the disease in the last 10 years, which is fortunate, given the severity of the disease and the lack of therapy.

FUNCTION TESTS

The most important tests for assessment of cardiac function are the electrocardiogram (ECG)[15] and myocardial imaging techniques.[1] The ECG involves noninvasive recording of the electrical impulses through the heart and is an effective but not perfect means of assessing cardiac rhythm abnormalities and diagnosing a myocardial infarction. Although relatively specific for myocardial infarction, the diagnostic sensitivity of the ECG is believed to range from 43% to 65%. Data from a recent study on the diagnostic reliability of the initial ECG in the emergency department setting found the sensitivity and specificity for acute myocardial infarction to be 79% and 83% respectively.[16] Myocardial imaging techniques (technetium-99m pyrophosphate and thallium 201) are used to assess cardiac output and wall-motion abnormalities and to detect nonfunctioning regions of the myocardium caused by infarction. The diagnostic sensitivity of the technetium-99m pyrophosphate scan may be as high as 84% in transmural infarctions; however, the sensitivity may be as low as 32% in patients with nontransmural infarctions. The thallium-201 scan is not typically used for initial diagnosis of infarction.[17]

DRUG THERAPY

Two groups of drugs[18,19] have a direct effect on cardiac tissue and are therefore monitored by the clinical chemistry laboratory. These are the cardiac glycosides and the antiarrhythmic drugs. Table 31-2 lists the most frequently monitored cardiac drugs.

Glycosides (see p. 607, methods)

The glycosides increase contractility in the heart and are particularly useful in treating heart failure. The problem with glycosides is that the therapeutic-to-toxic ratio is very low. At toxic dosage levels, the glycosides can upset the electrical activity of the heart and induce fatal arrhythmias. Since they have long half-lives in the body, they tend to have cumulative effects, necessitating careful monitoring

Table 31-2   Common drugs for treatment of cardiac disease

Name	Class	Mode of action	Comments
Digoxin	Cardiac glycoside	Increases contractility; slows A-V impulse conduction	Narrow therapeutic range; long half-life can produce cumulative toxic effects; can cause arrhythmias
Lidocaine	Antiarrhythmic	Suppresses ventricular abnormalities; attenuates depolarization, automaticity, and excitability	Relatively safe with no cardiac side effects; may cause cerebral toxicity
Quinidine	Antiarrhythmic	Depresses myocardial excitability, conduction velocity, and contractility	Coadministration with digoxin can produce toxicity; can cause arrhythmias

of blood levels to reduce the possibility of toxic side effects.

Lidocaine

Lidocaine is an anesthetic compound that is given intravenously as a bolus or infusion to suppress ventricular irregularities and to prevent the induction of life-threatening arrhythmias, such as ventricular tachycardia. Lidocaine is a particularly attractive drug because it has few side effects and because it has little or no effect on myocardial function and cardiac conduction. Toxicity may be manifested by major convulsive seizures with no prior warning. Accordingly, it becomes important to try to prevent lidocaine toxicity by monitoring serum drug levels. Toxicity is particularly common in older patients.

Quinidine and other drugs (see p. 610)

Quinidine is an antiarrhythmic drug whose major side effect is its capacity to induce severe arrhythmias in its own right. Indeed, many antiarrhythmic drugs have this potential, and for this reason, drug blood levels are usually monitored so that one may use antiarrhythmic drugs as safely as possible. Besides quinidine, other frequently monitored antiarrhythmic drugs are *procainamide* and *disopyramide*.

CHANGE OF ANALYTE IN DISEASE

The analytes that are most frequently used as diagnostic indicators of cardiac disease are the enzymes creatine kinase and lactate dehydrogenase. Two additional tests, myoglobin and aspartate aminotransferase, have been used infrequently in the past; however, neither is currently recommended for routine use in the diagnosis of acute myocardial infarction. Structural proteins, such as troponin T, troponin I, and myosin light chains, have become the subject of much interest as markers of myocardial injury.

These serum markers are used only for the diagnosis of acute myocardial infarction (AMI). Currently there are no biochemical markers unique for the other cardiac diseases.

Myoglobin

The value of myoglobin assays[20,21] in AMI is limited by myoglobin's early and rather brief appearance in serum after a myocardial infarction and by the presence of large amounts of myoglobin in skeletal muscle, which reduces the specificity of this analyte for myocardial damage.

Myoglobin is rapidly excreted in urine, and, as may be expected, reduced renal clearance results in elevations of serum myoglobin. Practical experience with myoglobin has not led to an increased ability to detect AMI. Because myoglobin is cleared so rapidly, false-negative values have been obtained when an AMI has indeed occurred.[22] Thus this analyte is infrequently used to confirm or rule out AMI. The presence of myoglobinuria can be used to confirm massive muscle cytolysis (trauma or drug induced) and to raise the possibility of myoglobin-induced acute renal failure.

Enzymes and isoenzymes in acute myocardial infarction (see pp. 603 and 608 for methods)

After the onset of symptoms in AMI there is usually a so-called time window during which the enzymes released from the damaged myocardial tissue are found to be elevated in serum. This temporal relationship is unique for each analyte and varies somewhat between persons, though a typical pattern has been determined (Fig. 31-1). Usually, 4 to 6 hours are required after the onset of chest pain before CK-MB becomes elevated in the serum of patients with AMI.[23] Detection times as short as 2 hours and as long as 15 hours have been reported.[24] This activity peaks at 12 to 24 hours and usually returns to baseline levels within 24 to 48 hours. In a typical course for CK and LD isoenzymes, CK-MB peaks first, with LD_1 exceeding LD_2 5 to 20 hours later. The average peak times for enzyme release after infarction in a study of 47 patients were 18 hours for CK-MB and total CK, 24 hours for AST, and 48 hours for LD.[25] This time course represents the classic temporal sequence of enzyme changes and is often helpful in distinguishing uncomplicated AMI from extension or reinfarction. Whereas this complete pattern is highly sensitive and specific for infarction, slightly different temporal patterns have been reported in up to 25% of patients with AMI.[26] These workers also report that CK-MB levels are higher and persist longer in patients with cardiogenic shock after AMI.

It follows from the above discussion that proper clinical interpretation of enzyme values in the diagnosis of AMI requires that samples be collected and analyzed at appropri-

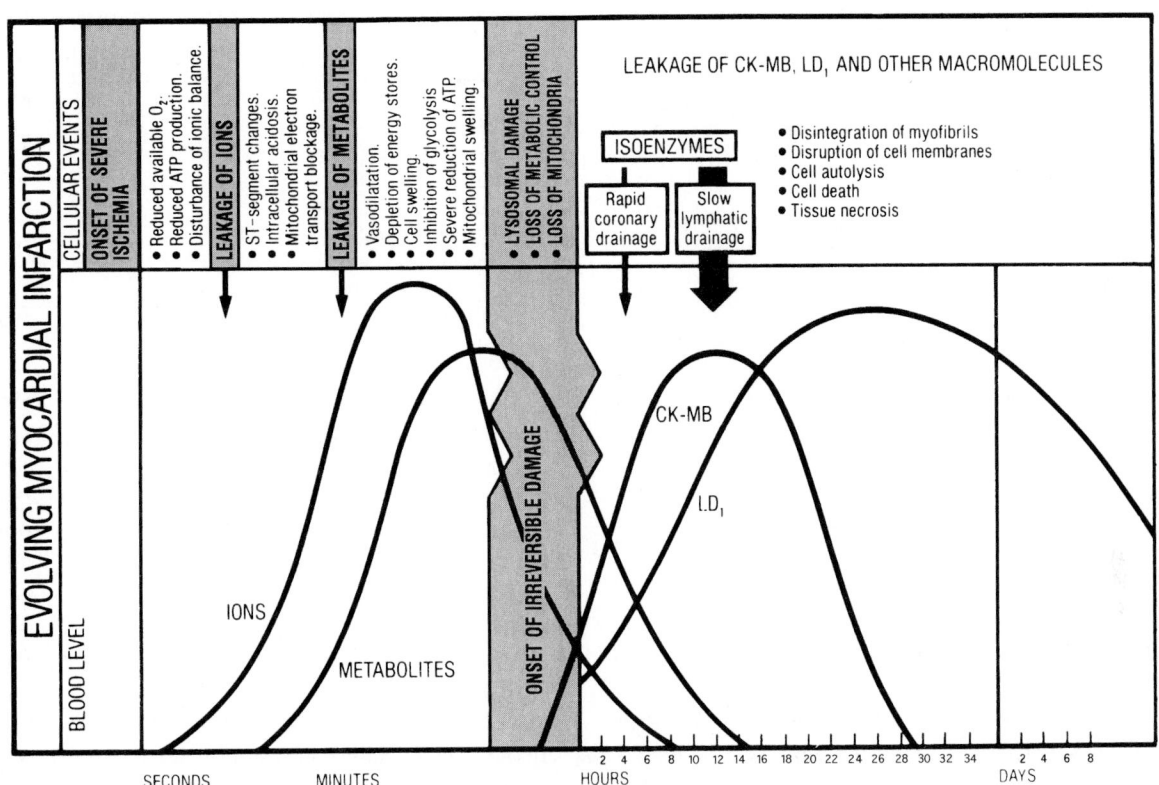

Fig. 31-1 Time course of biochemical events in a typical acute myocardial infarction (AMI). (Adapted from Usategui-Gomez M: *Lab World* 32:49-52, 1981.)

ate intervals. Since the temporal sequence of events is critical in the assessment of the biochemical changes after AMI, the diagnosis of an MI should normally not be made on the basis of a single isolated specimen. The recommended sampling sequence suggests that samples be drawn on admission and at 2-4 hours, 6-8 hours, and 12 hours after an AMI is suspected.[23,24,27] Results of total CK measurement should be available 24 hours a day, within several hours after receipt of a sample, whereas CK-MB measurements should be performed so that results are available every 3-4 hours, 7 days a week. The absolute minimum number of samples recommended for interpretation is two, obtained within 12 hours after the onset of symptoms. Normal results for CK-MB in samples obtained before 12 hours or after 24 hours should not be used to exclude the diagnosis of AMI. A sample collected in this fashion may reflect the period before or after CK-MB elevation occurs in some patients.[28] Keep in mind that normal values for total CK should not be used to rule out AMI or to exclude a request for CK-MB analysis.

Numerous cases in which elevated CK-MB levels are accompanied by normal total CK levels during the initial course of an AMI have been documented.[28] In most of these cases, however, there is a distinct rise and fall of the total CK values, though none ever exceeds the upper limit of normal. There is now some evidence that three subforms of

CK-MM, termed *isoforms*, may be elevated before CK-MB. Although the pattern is not totally specific for AMI, this approach may be useful in the future as an early indicator of this disease.[29]

CK isoforms.[3-5] Because the enzyme responsible for lysine cleavage is found in blood, only the unconverted MM and MB isoforms, MM_3 and MB_2, are found within cells; for this reason MM_3 and MB_2 are termed the *tissue isoforms*. As part of normal cell turnover, MM_3 and MB_2 are released into circulation where normally MM_3 constitutes only 30% of the CK-MM concentration in serum; MB_2 normally constitutes 50% of total serum CK-MB. After tissue injury, however, greater amounts of MM_3 and MB_2 isoforms are released from the intracellular compartment into circulation. Because the tissue/plasma ratios of CK-MM and CK-MB are very high and isoform conversion is not immediate, soon after cell death the plasma levels of unconverted MM_3 and MB_2 are present in great proportions relative to their respective seroconverted forms. For this reason, it is possible to formulate tissue to seroconverted isoform ratios, either MM_3/MM_1 or MB_2/MB_1, and to use increases in these isoform ratios to make early and sensitive diagnoses of myocardial injury. The MM_3/MM_1 ratio is easier to measure than the MB_2/MB_1 ratio because CK-MM constitutes the majority, about 75%, of the CK activity in the heart.

Elevated Serum CK-MB in Conditions Other Than Acute Myocardial Infarction

Severe angina
Chronic atrial fibrillation
Coronary insufficiency
Crush syndrome
Pericarditis
Defibrillation
Insertion of pacemaker
Coronary angiography
Open heart surgery
External cardiac massage or cardiopulmonary resuscitation
Carbon monoxide poisoning
Malignant hyperthermia
Muscular dystrophy, such as Duchenne's syndrome
Poliomyositis
Prostatic surgery or infarction
Dermatomyositis
Reye's syndrome
Malignancy

Causes of Increased LD_1/LD_2 Ratio ("Flip")

Acute myocardial infarction
Acute renal infarction
Hemolysis caused by
    Prosthetic heart valves
    Hemolytic anemias
    Megaloblastic anemias
    Sample processing
Malignancy

Isoenzymes in conditions other than myocardial infarction. Frequently the pattern of serum enzyme elevations in conditions other than myocardial infarction is different from that seen with myocardial infarction. In these conditions isoenzymes (see boxes) are often chronically elevated. These "false-positive" situations emphasize the importance of testing multiple samples obtained at appropriate intervals. The pattern of CK isoenzymes that is found in the developing fetus is duplicated in the adult in certain pathological states. This alteration is most commonly observed in skeletal muscle. In the adult, CK is predominantly present in the MM form. Fetal muscle, however, is predominantly BB until the sixteenth week of gestation,[30] at which time the expression of the gene coding for the M subunit is significantly increased. Diseases of skeletal muscle characterized by blood-perfusion regeneration are often associated with increased levels of the fetal isomeric forms of CK. Thus Duchenne muscular dystrophy, polymyositis, and some forms of rhabdomyolysis are examples of skeletal muscle diseases in which increased levels of CK-MB are frequently found in serum. These increases are in proportion to the degree of muscle fiber regeneration.[30] In these chronic diseases, the serum levels of total CK and CK-MB activities do not show the rise and fall characteristic of myocardial infarction but tend to remain constant over time. However, since skeletal muscle does contain CK-MB, the levels of CK-MB are frequently in the range associated with myocardial infarction. Since the absolute amount of CK in skeletal muscle is about 5 to 10 times that observed in cardiac tissue, the actual elevations of total CK observed in serum in skeletal muscle abnormalities are frequently dramatically higher than those observed in myocardial infarction though the proportion that is CK-MB is usually quite

low. Also, the LD isoenzyme pattern does not reflect myocardial injury or disease.

In addition to the pathological conditions discussed above, elevations of cardiac proteins, CK isoenzymes, LD isoenzymes, and AST are obviously present in any situation that increases leakage from myocardial cells. Examples include trauma such as surgery or flail chest and diseases involving the myocardium, such as myocarditis, congestive heart failure, and arrhythmias. Also, certain drugs may affect skeletal and cardiac muscle. Abuse of such drugs as alcohol and cocaine can result in elevation of the above analytes.

Sensitivity and specificity of CK and LD isoenzymes for myocardial infarctions. Clearly, the interpretation of serum enzymes in the diagnosis of AMI becomes obscured by the causes of false-positive and false-negative results. Galen and Gambino[31] have used the predictive value model to express mathematically the clinical usefulness of laboratory tests in various patient populations. Table 31-3 lists both positive and negative predictive values of CK-MB and LD ratio change ("flip") for high-prevalence and low-prevalence populations. The use of CK-MB in a coronary care population, with a 50% prevalence of disease assumed, clearly increases the predictive values of elevated enzyme levels. In comparison, in a low-prevalence population such as emergency room (5%) in which many conditions as outlined in the above left box may be seen, the usefulness of this same enzyme test to assess AMI is greatly diminished.

Table 31-3   Positive (PV+) and negative (PV−) predictive values for serum CK-MB and LD ratio change ("flip") with varying prevalence of acute myocardial infarction

	Test					
	CK-MB*		LD "flip"†		Both‡	
Prevalence	PV+	PV−	PV+	PV−	PV+	PV−
50%	96	100	100	91	100	96
5%	51	100	100	99.5	100	99.7

*Sensitivity = 100%; specificity = 95%.
†Sensitivity = 90%; specificity = 100%.
‡Sensitivity = 95%: specificity = 100%.

The MM isoforms are not cardiac specific and have a diagnostic sensitivity of only 70% within the first 6 hours after myocardial infarction. In contrast, the MB_2/MB_1 ratio is highly cardiospecific, though the MB isoforms are present in smaller concentrations than the MM isoforms are. Measurement of the isoforms has become feasible by use of a rapid high-voltage electrophoretic system (Helena REP and CardioREP, from Helena Laboratories, Beaumont, Texas). The MB_2/MB_1 ratio demonstrates excellent diagnostic sensitivity, at over 90%, within 4 to 6 hours after onset of symptoms in patients with MI. In addition, the MB_2/MB_1 ratio has also been proposed as a diagnostic tool for monitoring the success of cardiac reperfusion after thrombolytic therapy and for discriminating which patients should be admitted for further clinical workup of MI in the Emergency Department.

Diagnostic use of troponin T and I, and myosin light chains

Troponin T.[6-8] After myocardial infarction, TnT increases in serum after 4 hours, achieving an initial peak or plateau at 2 to 5 days. A second TnT peak is observed in many MI patients. This second peak occurs because TnT has both cytosolic and structurally bound TnT pools; the first peak is the result of the release of the cytosolic pool, and the second peak reflects the slower release of the structural component later during the myocardial necrosis process.

Use of TnT for early diagnosis of MI appears to offer no advantages over the use of CK-MB because the initial appearance in serum of CK-MB and TnT, and therefore the time frame in which the MI diagnosis can be made, appears to be very similar for the two proteins. On the other hand, TnT measurement offers advantages compared to CK-MB when there are both skeletal and myocardial muscle disease processes occurring. The reason is that TnT is truly cardiac specific and its appearance indicates cardiac muscle disorders whereas the interpretation of CK-MB in this case may be confounded since skeletal muscle contains a small proposition of CK-MB, up to about 3% of total. Because of TnT's long half-life in serum, TnT levels may provide important diagnostic information about an MI after serum CK-MB has achieved normal levels. In addition, TnT may offer substantial information about the recent history of myocardial dysfunction in ischemic patients. TnT has been used for prognostication of unstable angina patients. Prognostication in this context is the process of discriminating which of these patients are likely to go on to suffer a myocardial infarction.[32]

Troponin I. Although TnI has a low molecular weight compared to those of TnT (37 kilodaltons) and CK-MB (85 kilodaltons), its release characteristics and therefore its utilization as an early indicator of MI are quite similar to those of the other two proteins. TnI appears to be identical to TnT in essentially all possible clinical applications, and its mea-surement offers the same advantages over CK-MB as TnT does. Because they offer the same information, the choice between TnI or TnT will be based on the analytical performance, convenience, speed, and overall assay cost.

Myosin light chains.[10] MLC release after MI shows a pattern with two peaks; the first from the cytosolic pool occurring at 24 to 36 hours, the second from degradation of the contractile apparatus, occurring at 80 to 100 hours.

Cardiac-specific forms of the MLCs have been reported, and several assays were proposed in the early 1980s. The clinical information contributed by MLC measurement is the same as that provided by TnT and TnI for most applications. However, the MLC's smaller cytosolic pool and the nature of MLC release make it less advantageous than the use of the troponins. MLC measurement may prove useful for infarct sizing and prognostic applications because of the sustained release and slow clearance characteristics of this protein after myocardial cell necrosis.

Use of biochemical markers in triage of patients with chest pain

A wide variety of biochemical tests are currently available for the evaluation of patients in whom AMI is a diagnostic possibility. In such cases it is important that decisions regarding a patient's cardiac status be made rapidly and accurately. It has been suggested that CK-MB isoforms performed within 6 hours of the onset of chest pain may be useful in determining those patients that might benefit from thrombolytic therapy.[4] The utilization of the ECG in combination with appropriate biochemical markers over appropriate time periods (Fig. 31-2) may be useful in determining which patients require admission to the costly cardiac care unit, which may safely be monitored in intermediate care facilities, and which can safely be discharged.[5] To provide clinicians with the best support, these markers should be measured in accordance with the sampling and turn-around times discussed previously.

For patients who are first seen many hours after the onset of pain, measurement of LD isoenzymes, MLCs, or troponin T or I, may be helpful. An increase in LD_1 with concomitant reversal of the normal LD_1/LD_2 ratio, termed the *LD flip*, generally occurs at 12 to 24 hours after infarction and may persist for several days. Elevations in troponins or MLCs may likewise persist for many days after infarction and may demonstrate greater specificity for myocardial damage than LD.[33,34]

METHODS OF ANALYSIS
Creatine kinase
KORY M. WARD
JOHN A. LOTT

Principles of analysis and current usage Creatine kinase catalyzes the reversible phosphorylization of creatine using ATP as the donor of the phosphate group. The direction of the reaction is dependent on the pH; at neutral pH, forma-

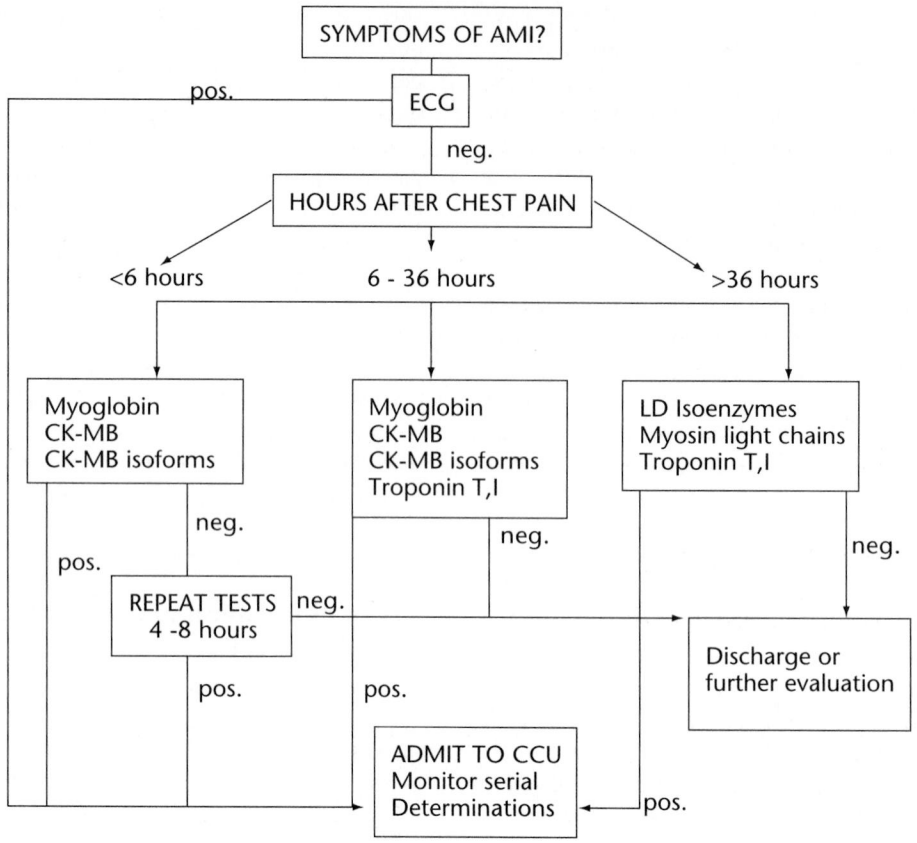

Fig. 31-2 Laboratory test algorithm for management of patients with suspected acute myocardial infarctions. (Adapted from Apple FS, Wu AH: Cardiac markers for diagnosis and monitoring therapy, *Clin Chem News* 19 (Suppl.), 1993.)

tion of ATP is favored, whereas formation of creatine phosphate is favored at pH 9.0.

$$\text{Creatine} + \text{ATP} \xrightleftharpoons[\substack{\text{pH } 6.8}]{\substack{\text{pH } 9.0 \\ \text{Mg}^{++}}} \text{Creatine phosphate} + \text{ADP}$$

Different enzyme reaction properties have been found for each of the CK isoenzyme fractions. Thus measurement of total CK activity in serum requires the use of reaction conditions that are a compromise.[35]

Methods for determination of total CK activity may be based on the measurement of products formed in either the forward or the reverse reactions. The "forward" reaction is that which results in the formation of creatine phosphate. Use of the forward reaction to measure CK activity has been carried out by measurement of the phosphate moiety of creatine phosphate formed in the reaction,[36] and determination of the ADP that is also produced in the forward reaction.[37] Various interferences along with the development of alter-

native methods have made these procedures essentially obsolete (see previous edition for details).

Almost all methods for measuring total CK activity utilize the reverse reaction of creatine phosphate to creatine (Table 31-4). This method is based on the principles proposed by Oliver[38] and modified by Rosalki[39] and others. The primary reaction catalyzed by CK results in the production of creatine and ATP. The ATP produced in the primary reaction is then employed in a coupled enzymatic glucose assay employing hexokinase (HK) and glucose-6-phosphate dehydrogenase (G6PD). The production of NADPH in the indicator reaction is monitored at 340 nm and is related to CK activity within the patient specimen.

$$\text{Creatine phosphate} + \text{ADP} \xrightarrow[\text{pH } 6.8]{\text{CK Mg}^{++}} \text{Creatine} + \text{ATP}$$

$$\text{Glucose} + \text{ATP} \xrightarrow{\text{HK}} \text{Glucose-6-phosphate} + \text{ADP}$$

$$\text{Glucose-6-phosphate} + \text{NADP}^+ \xleftarrow{\text{G6PD}}$$
$$\text{6-Phosphogluconate} + \text{NADPH} + \text{H}^+$$

Table 31-4 Methods of creatine kinase analysis

Method	Principle	Usage	Comments
Oliver and Rosalki	Creatine phosphate + ADP $\xrightarrow{\text{CK}}$ Creatine + ATP ATP is coupled to hexokinase and glucose-6-phosphate dehydrogenase reactions to produce NADPH	Most frequently used	Preferred method Readily automated

Table 31-5   Methods for creatine kinase (CK) isoenzyme analysis

Method	Principle	Usage	Comments
1. Electrophoresis	At pH 8.3, isoenzymes have different mobilities on 1% agarose; CK activity measured by enzymatic assay with densitometer	Previously most frequently used technique; still frequently used	Separates all three isoenzymes, aberrant bands also visualized, slow turnaround time, very small sample volume required
2. Ion-exchange chromatography	Separates isoenzymes through the utilization of minicolumns, CK isoenzymes eluted with NaCl	Rarely used	Subject to dilution effect and carryover of greatly increased CK-MM
3. Immunoinhibition	M subunits bound with polyclonal and monoclonal antibody; remaining B subunit activity is measured	Infrequently used for screening	CK-BB and macro-CK may interfere and result in false-positive results
4. Mass assay	IRMA, sandwich assay Polyclonal and monoclonal antibody bound to solid support binds CK-MB Second enzyme-labeled antibody forms antibody-CK-MB-antibody complex	Most frequently used for screening	Easily automated, specific for CK-MB; no interference by drugs, hemolysis

IRMA, Immunoradiometric assay.

Other procedures for determination of CK activity have been proposed, though rarely used. These alternative procedures include a fluorometric assay whereby creatine formed in the primary reaction is reacted with Ninhydrin (triketohydrindene hydrate) in the presence of KOH to form a fluorescent compound.[40] There has also been developed a bioluminescent assay in which ATP formed in the primary reaction is coupled to an indicator reaction employing the luciferin-luciferase reaction as follows:

1. Creatine phosphate + ADP $\xrightarrow{\text{CK}}$ Creatine + ATP

2. ATP + Luciferin + O_2 $\xrightarrow{\text{Luciferase}}$ AMP + Oxyluciferin + Phosphate + CO_2 + light

The intensity of light emitted in the indicator reaction is proportional to CK activity within the sample.[41] This method is extremely sensitive; however the need for specialized instrumentation and reagent costs limit its use.

Specimen Serum, plasma anticoagulated with heparin, cerebrospinal fluid (CSF), and amniotic fluid are acceptable specimens. Anticoagulants other than heparin are unacceptable because they inhibit CK activity.[42] Hemolysis should be avoided because of the interference by erythrocyte adenylate kinase, however, hemoglobin concentrations up to 320 mg/L have been found to not appreciably alter measured CK activities.[43] Icterus and lipemia can affect measured CK activities because of interference with instrument absorbance readings.

The cytoplasmic enzymes of CK exhibit varying degrees of stability during storage. CK-BB is the least stable isoenzyme fraction. The addition of a thiol-containing compound such as *N*-acetylcysteine or 2-mercaptoethanol can help stabilize CK-BB activity.[44] Loss of catalytic activity of CK isoenzymes may be caused by thermal inactivation, oxidation of reactive thiol groups, increasing pH from loss of CO_2, and irradiation with light.[45]

Specimens can be stored in the dark at 4° C for up to 2 weeks and at −20° C for up to 1 month with minimal loss of activity.[35]

Reference intervals Reference intervals for healthy individuals are dependent on the reaction conditions of the assay used for CK determinations. The various reference intervals and assay types for total CK activity have been recently reviewed.[46] CK activities in serum are affected by age, sex, and race.[47] Newborns usually exhibit increased CK activity resulting from skeletal muscle trauma during birth. Muscle mass can influence CK activities in serum; males generally show higher CK activities compared with females because of greater muscle mass. The 5th and 95th percentiles for the reference interval for total CK activity reported by 239 laboratories have been reported to be 130 U/L and 253 U/L respectively.[46]

Creatine kinase isoenzymes
MONIKA PAYNE
PETER HICKMAN

Principles of analysis and current usage Electrophoretic separation (Table 31-5, method 1) of the CK isoenzyme fractions has, until recently, been the most common technique for quantitation of CK isoenzymes. The M and B monomer subunits possess different charges, which allow for separation of the different isoenzyme fractions. Support media that have been used include agarose, cellulose acetate, and polyacrylamide. In agarose gel electrophoresis at pH 8.6, CK-BB migrates farthest from the point of application toward the anode, CK-MM remains slightly cathodic to the point of application, and CK-MB has an intermediate mobility between CK-BB and CK-MM. The mitochondrial CK isoenzyme migrates cathodally to the CK-MM fraction. Another CK variant that may be seen after electrophoresis is macro-CK type 1, a complex of an immunoglobulin, usually IgG, and CK-BB.

After the electrophoretic separation of the individual isoenzyme fractions, the support medium is incubated with CK substrate to allow formation of NADPH. The amount of NADPH formed can be measured directly, by its fluorescence, or by coupling the NADH with a diaphorase reaction to form a colored product. The amount of fluorescence or colored product formed is measured using a densitometer; the degree of fluorescence or color is proportional to the amount of CK present in each isoenzyme fraction.

One major advantage of using electrophoresis for the separation of CK isoenzymes is that atypical bands such as macro-CK and mitochondrial CK can be detected and may warrant further investigation. Unfortunately, however, CK isoenzyme analysis by electrophoresis has a fairly long turnaround time and therefore is unsuitable for the "stat." type of analysis. Also, skill is required in the interpretation of electrophoretic results, especially if atypically migrating bands are present.

Separation of CK isoenzymes on the basis of charge has been accomplished by ion-exchange chromatography (Table 31-5, method 2). One disadvantage of this procedure is that carryover of CK-MM into the CK-MB fraction can occur in specimens with greatly increased CK-MM activities, thus causing a falsely increased CK-MB result.[48] This technique is rarely used in clinical laboratories today.

Immunological methods have been developed for quantitation of CK-MB and are the techniques most frequently used today. Two types of immunological methods have been developed for CK-MB quantitation. One type of immunological procedure, termed *immunoinhibition* (Table 31-5, method 3), utilizes a specific antibody that inhibits the CK-M monomer subunit; the CK-B subunit is unaffected and thus retains its catalytic activity. CK-B activity is then measured. Since the CK-B fraction accounts for one half the activity exhibited by an uninhibited CK-MB enzyme, doubling the CK-B activity theoretically yields the CK-MB activity present in the sample. This method is based on the assumption that no CK-BB or macro-CK is contained in the sample. The presence of these isoenzymes will result in a falsely increased CK-MB result unless a blanking reaction is employed. Because of this interference from CK-BB and macro-CK, immunohibition methods are limited in their use and have been largely supplanted by use of immunological mass assays for CK-MB.

Mass assays (Table 31-5, method 4) are the most frequently used technique for determination of CK-MB. Antibody directed against CK-MB is covalently linked to a solid surface. CK-MB in the sample reacts with the bound antibody forming an antibody antigen complex. A second antibody, which is labeled, for example, by conjugation with an enzyme, such as alkaline phosphatase, is then added. This second antibody is directed against another antigenic site on the CK-MB molecule different from the first antibody. The enzyme-labeled antibody reacts with the antibody-bound CK-MB forming an antibody/antigen/labeled-antibody sandwich. After a wash step to remove any unbound labeled antibody, a substrate is added that reacts with the enzyme that

has been conjugated to the antibody to form a detectable product; the rate of product formation is proportional to CK-MB activity present in the specimen.

Mass assays for CK-MB have the advantage of minimal interference from specimens with CK-BB activity or greatly increased activities of CK-MM. In addition, hemolysis, drugs, or inhibitors of CK enzyme activity do not affect mass measurements of CK-MB. Because these assays have largely been automated and the analysis time is fairly short, mass measurements are well suited for the "stat." type of analyses.

Specimen Serum is usually the specimen of choice. The use of EDTA and citrated plasma, as well as specimens collected with oxalate or fluoride as preservative, should be avoided since these substances inhibit enzyme activity. Hemolyzed specimens may be unsuitable for some assays because of the presence of red blood cell adenylate kinase, which interferes with activity measurements of CK-MB. Most assays that measure CK activity now include inhibitors of adenylate kinase. However, grossly hemolyzed specimens may contain enough adenylate kinase to overcome the inhibitors that may be present.

Specimens may be stored for up to 5 days at 4° C, or frozen at −20° C for several weeks with minimal loss of activity. At room temperature, CK-MB can begin to dissociate into its monomer subunits within 2 hours.[49] Frequent freezing and thawing of specimens can also result in loss of enzyme activity.

Reference intervals The normal reference interval for CK-MB is dependent on the method of analysis used for its quantitation. For those methods, such as electrophoresis and immunohibition, that measure the activity of CK-MB, the percentage of total CK activity represented by CK-MB is usually reported along with total units of CK-MB.

Since skeletal muscle can contain varying amounts of CK-MB, a "normal" percentage of CK-MB is usually considered to range from 0 to 3%. Individuals with muscular dystrophy or other processes associated with regeneration of skeletal muscle may show greatly increased activities of CK-MB in the blood.[50] Patients with concomitant myocardial and skeletal muscle injury can have a percentage of CK-MB that falls into the normal reference interval because of the dilutional effect of CK-MM from skeletal muscle. Thus it is imperative that both the percentage of CK-MB and the total units of CK-MB activity that are present be used for evaluating patients with suspected myocardial infarctions.

Assays for CK-MB that measure the mass of enzyme present are less affected by concomitant skeletal muscle injury. However, significant increases of CK-MB mass concentrations have been noted in the blood of patients suffering severe muscle trauma.[51] Since total CK measurements are reported in units per liter (U/L), whereas mass concentration measurements are reported in micrograms per liter (μg/L), calculation of a new function, called a *relative index*, is used to relate CK-MB mass concentrations to total CK activities. The use of the relative index is necessary for the evaluation of patients with greatly increased total CK activities. Patients with greatly increased total CK activities may also have substantially increased CK-MB concentrations from the skeletal muscle injury. The relative index should not be used for assessment of patients with CK-MB values less than 10 μg/L or for those samples that have total CK activities within the normal reference interval. The relative index is calculated as follows:

$$\text{Relative index (RI)} = \frac{\text{CK-MB } (\mu g/L)}{\text{Total CK } (U/L)} \times 100$$

For a definitive diagnosis of myocardial infarction to be made, both the mass value of CK-MB and the relative index should be increased.

Digoxin and digitoxin
I-WEN CHEN
LINDA A. HEMINGER

Principles of analysis and current usage The cardiotonic glycosides, digoxin and digitoxin, occur naturally in a number of plants. The term *digitalis* is used to designate this whole group of compounds. These compounds are used for the treatment of heart failure, atrial flutter, atrial fibrillation, and supraventricular tachycardia through their ability to improve the strength of myocardial contractions and to slow the heart rate.

The decision to treat a patient with digoxin or digitoxin is primarily determined by the patient's ability to metabolize and excrete the drug. Elimination of digoxin is dependent upon renal function, especially the glomerular filtration rate. In subjects with normal renal function, digoxin has a half life of 1.5 to 2.0 days. The half-life is prolonged to 4 to

6 days in patients with renal insufficiency. Digitoxin differs from digoxin in that its primary site of metabolism is the liver. The only active metabolite of digitoxin is digoxin, which represents only a small fraction of the total metabolites. The portion of digitoxin that is not metabolized is excreted, through the billiary tract, into the intestines, reabsorbed by the enterohepatic circulation, and recycled to the liver until it is completely metabolized. Because digitoxin metabolism and excretion are largely independent of renal function, use of this drug is more appropriate in patients with renal insufficiency.

Digitalis compounds have a relatively narrow therapeutic range. In addition, sudden impairment of renal or liver function can result in toxicity if the dose is not adjusted. These two factors make frequent monitoring of digitalis concentrations necessary. The most frequent request is for determination of digoxin concentrations. Digitoxin analyses are performed much less frequently because of the less frequent use of the drug.

Chromatographic assays such as gas chromatography,[52] and bioassays based on inhibition of Na^+, K^+-ATPase in red blood cells[53] are labor intensive and time consuming and have been essentially discontinued. The most common methods in use today in the clinical laboratories are immunoassays. Until fairly recently, radioimmunoassay (RIA) (Table 31-6, method 1) was the most common method used for measuring digoxin concentrations in serum.[54] However, to eliminate the need for radionuclides, other immunoassay procedures have since replaced RIA. The most common immunoassay method used today is fluorescence polarization (FPIA)

Table 31-6   Methods of digoxin analysis

Method	Principle	Usage	Comment
1. Radioimmunoassay (RIA)	^{125}I-labeled and unlabeled digoxin in patient's sera compete for binding to antidigoxin antibody.	Plasma or serum	Most sensitive and precise; requires gamma counter
2. Fluorescence polarization (FPIA)	Fluorescein-labeled and unlabeled digoxin in patient's sera compete for binding to antidigoxin antibody. Degree of polarization of emitted fluorescence is inversely proportional to patient digoxin concentration.	Plasma or serum; most frequently used procedure	Older version required sample pretreatment; requires specialized instrumentation
3. Enzyme-multiplied immunoassay (EMIT)	Competitive binding for antibody between endogenous digoxin and enzyme-labeled digoxin. Binding of antibody to enzyme-labeled digoxin inhibits enzymatic activity.	Serum; commonly used	Older version required sample pretreatment; lacks sensitivity
4. Affinity column immunoassay	Free and digoxin-bound antibody-enzyme complexes separated by affinity chromatography. Amount of digoxin-bound antibody-enzyme complexes directly proportional to digoxin concentrations in patient's sera.	Plasma or serum	No sample pretreatment required; semiautomated

(Table 31-6, method 2). This method utilizes competitive binding of digoxin in patient's sera and fluorescein-labeled digoxin to antidigoxin antibody. See Chapter 4 for the principles of fluorescence polarization. A sample pretreatment step was necessary for the older version of this assay to minimize interferences from endogenous protein-bound fluorescent compounds in the sample. The addition of trichloroacetic acid to precipitate proteins followed by centrifugation results in a clear, protein-free supernatant suitable for analysis.

Other nonisotopic labels have been developed for use, including bioluminescent, time-delayed fluorescence and enzyme labels. In the homogeneous enzyme-multiplied immunoassay technique (EMIT) (Table 31-6, method 3) the enzyme glucose-6-phosphate dehydrogenase has been coupled to digoxin. Competition between patient's digoxin and labeled digoxin for antidigoxin antibody allows determination of the amount present in the patient's sera. This technique is more fully described in Chapter 13.

The CEDIA homogeneous enzyme immunoassay system utilizes two inactive subunits of the enzyme β-galactosidase produced by recombinant DNA technology.[55] One subunit is covalently attached to digoxin, which does not interfere with the spontaneous reassociation of the enzyme to form active enzyme. In the assay, digoxin present in patient's sera competes with enzyme-bound digoxin for binding to antidigoxin antibody. Binding of enzyme-bound digoxin to antidigoxin antibody results in the inability of the two enzyme halves to reassociate to form active enzyme. If, however, patient's sera contains digoxin, some antibody will combine with patient drug allowing for some of the enzyme-digoxin subunits to remain available for formation of active enzyme. The degree of enzyme activity is directly related to the concentration of digoxin present in the patient's sera.

An affinity column immunoassay technique (E.I. du Pont de Nemours, Wilmington, Delaware) separates free and digoxin-bound antibody-enzyme species by affinity chromatography[56] (Table 31-6, method 4). In this procedure, the $F(ab')_2$ fragment of the digoxin antibody is labeled with the enzyme β-galactosidase. An excess of the enzyme-antibody conjugate is present in the reagent so that all digoxin in the sample can bind to the antibody. After this initial incubation period, the sample is eluted through an affinity column located within the test pack. The affinity column contains ouabain, an analog of digoxin. Any antibody-enzyme conjugate not bound to digoxin from the patient's sera is retained within the column. The digoxin-enzyme-antibody complexes passes through the column into the test pack where the enzyme portion of the complex catalyzes the hydrolysis of the substrate *ortho*-nitrophenyl β-D-galactopyranoside (ONPG) to *ortho*-nitrophenol (ONP). The change in absorbance at 405 nm resulting from the formation of ONP is directly proportional to digoxin concentration in the patient's sample.[56]

Numerous interferences have been described for many digoxin assays. Certain drugs and metabolites can cross-react with the antibodies used in the immunoassays to measure digoxin. For example, accumulation of spironolactone and its metabolites, which occur in patients with renal or hepatic impairment, are a source of interference.[57] The presence of digoxin-like immunoreactive factors (DLIF) is another source of interference that makes interpretation of digoxin concentrations difficult. DLIF have been detected in samples from patients with certain normal and pathophysiological states, including renal or liver dysfunction, from pregnant women, and from neonates.[58]

Various techniques have been described to eliminate the interference caused by DLIF. These include attempts to develop more specific antibodies toward digoxin[59] and the use of centrifugal ultrafiltration to produce filtrates free of DLIF.[60] Use of ultracentrifugation has been found to help reduce DLIF interference in some specimens, but not all. Centrifugal ultrafiltration appears to be effective in removing DLIF from the serum of adult patients, however, similar reductions in interference from DLIF in pediatric patients have not been found.[58] Thus extreme caution should be taken when one is interpreting digoxin concentrations in ultrafiltrates produced by centrifugal ultrafiltration of serum from neonates and infants.

In an effort to identify samples containing DLIF more readily, attempts have been made to correlate various patient characteristics with concentrations of DLIF in the serum of neonates or infants. Conflicting reports have related concentrations of DLIF in serum to patient age[61,62] and to birth weight.[61,62] No correlation between sex and concentration of DLIF has been described.[61,62] A strong correlation has been described between DLIF concentrations and serum bilirubin concentrations in infants.[59,63]

Specimen Serum, or plasma collected using heparin or EDTA as anticoagulant, is acceptable for specimens. Samples may be stored at 2° to 8° C for up to 1 week. For longer periods of storage, samples should be kept frozen at −20° C.

Reference interval The usual therapeutic range for digoxin is 0.9 to 2.0 ng/mL. Concentrations above 2.0 ng/mL are generally considered toxic. However, patient response to the drug can vary widely. Thus individual patient results should be interpreted in conjunction with the clinical history and underlying disease state.

Lactate dehydrogenase
AMADEO J. PESCE

Principles of analysis and current usage Lactate dehydrogenase is an enzyme that has an almost ubiquitous distribution in tissues. The enzyme catalyzes the interconversion of pyruvate and L-lactate with NADH or NAD[+] respectively, acting as a cofactor. The direction of the reaction catalyzed by LD is pH dependent; the pyruvate to lactate reaction has a pH optimum near 7.0, whereas the reverse reaction proceeds most optimally at pH 8.7:

$$\text{Pyruvate} + \text{NADH} + \text{H}^+ \underset{\text{pH } 8.7}{\overset{\text{pH } 7.0}{\rightleftharpoons}} \text{L-Lactate} + \text{NAD}^+$$

Current methods for measurement of LD activity utilize the change in concentration of the NAD and NADH cofactors as the reaction proceeds. The rate of appearance or disappearance of the absorbance of NADH at 340 nm is proportional to LD activity (Table 31-7, methods 1 and 2).[64-67] The reaction can be followed in either the L-P or the P-L direction. However, it has been shown that when one is using the L-P reaction, the initial rate of the reaction is nonlinear and becomes linear only after about 20 seconds.[68]

Table 31-7 Methods for LD analysis

Method	Principle	Usage	Comments
1. Lactate to pyruvate (L-P)	L-Lactate + NAD $\xrightarrow{\text{pH 8.7}}$ Pyruvate + NADH Production of NADH monitored at 340 nm	Automated	Kinetic assay; suggested reference method
2. Pyruvate to lactate (P-L)	Pyruvate + NADH $\xrightarrow{\text{pH 7.0}}$ L-Lactate + NAD Disappearance of NADH monitored at 340 nm	Automated Most frequently used	Faster reaction rate than L-P
3. Tetrazolium	L-Lactate + NAD $\xrightarrow{\text{LD}}$ Pyruvate + NADH NADH reacts with tetrazolium dye forming reduced tetrazolium (colored)	Manual	Most commonly used for identification of LD isoenzyme fractions after electrophoretic separation

However, the P-L reaction is most frequently used because of certain considerations. In the P-L direction, only about 3% of the costly cofactor NADH is needed when compared to the L-P direction.[64] In addition, the P-L reaction proceeds at a faster rate than the reverse reaction does. Both the P-L and L-P reactions are commonly used because there is no generally accepted LD method. The reaction can be monitored by both kinetic and end-point absorbance measurements; however, kinetic monitoring is optimal and most frequently used.

In addition to monitoring changes in NADH concentrations, some older methods measured LD activities by using colorimetric assays of the reactants produced or consumed during the reaction. The only reaction of this type still in use today is the tetrazolium reaction, which is frequently used for the identification of LD isoenzyme fractions after electrophoretic separation (see Chapter 10). In this reaction, NADH reduces the tetrazolium dye to form a colored compound (Table 31-7, method 3). The intensity of the reduced tetrazolium dye is proportional to LD activity (see also below).

Specimen Analysis of LD should be performed using serum as the specimen, because plasma anticoagulated with some compounds, such as oxalate, can interfere with the assay. Erythrocytes contain high activities of LD. Thus any visible hemolysis can result in falsely increased LD activities. The different LD isoenzymes have varying degrees of stability. The stability is dependent on the temperature at which the sample is stored because no single method of storage will prevent some loss in LD activity. Consistency in the manner in which all samples are stored will yield the most accurate results. Specimens should not be frozen, since this storage technique results in loss of enzyme activity, especially the LD_4 and LD_5 isoenzyme fractions.

Reference range LD activity in serum is dependent on the method and temperature used for its analysis. Individuals up to 12 years of age generally show LD activities that are 10% to 15% higher than that in adults. Typical reference intervals for LD activity in adults measured using the P-L reaction at 37° C are approximately 90 to 320 U/L. LD may also be measured in CSF. LD activities in CSF are approximately 10% of that found in a corresponding serum sample drawn from the patient at the same time that CSF was obtained.

Lactate dehydrogenase isoenzymes
MONIKA PAYNE
PETER HICKMAN

Principles of analysis Lactate dehydrogenase is an enzyme present in virtually all tissues. Increases of the enzyme in serum may indicate injury to an organ or tissue. However, increases in total enzyme activity are nonspecific with respect to its origin. More specific information can be obtained by the measurement of the five isoenzyme fractions and the determination of each isoenzyme's contribution to the total LD activity. LD is a tetramer composed of subunits designated as H (LD_1; H_4), M (LD_5; M_4), or a combination of the H (heart) and M (muscle) subunits. The LD isoenzymes that contain both the H and M subunits include LD_2 (H_3M), LD_3 (H_2M_2), and LD_4 (HM_3).

The most common method in use for the separation and quantitation of the five LD isoenzyme fractions is electrophoresis. In some laboratories, specific determination of only the LD_1 isoenzyme fraction may be employed.

Electrophoretic separation of LD isoenzymes may be performed by use of agarose or cellulose acetate as support media (Table 31-8, method 1). The principle of electrophoretic fractionation of LD isoenzymes relies on the fact that the

Table 31-8 Methods for measurement of LD isoenzymes

Method	Principle	Usage	Comments
1. Electrophoresis	LD isoenzymes separated on agarose gel on basis of differing mobilities at pH 8.6. Amount of LD isoenzyme fractions determined densitometrically after fluorometric or colorimetric visualization	Most common	Separates all major isoenzyme fractions; allows determination of atypical LD fractions
2. Immunochemical	LD fractions containing M subunits, LD_2 through LD_5, are removed using double-antibody or solid-phase capture technique	Frequently used	Only LD_1 fraction is measured. Rapid and simple to perform

charges of the M and H subunits differ and also that each isoenzyme fraction contains a different proportion of the H and M subunits. Thus, when a sample containing LD is separated at a pH of approximately 8.6, LD_1, which exhibits the greatest negative charge, moves farthest toward the anode, whereas LD_5 migrates toward the cathode. The other LD isoenzymes migrate sequentially in positions between the LD_1 and LD_5 fractions.

Once separated by electrophoresis the relative concentration of each of the LD isoenzyme fractions may be determined by use of colorimetric or fluorometric techniques. Fluorometric determinations of LD isoenzymes can be performed with use of substrate containing lactate and NAD whereby LD catalyzes the following reaction:

$$\text{L-Lactate} + NAD^+ \overset{LD}{\rightleftharpoons} \text{Pyruvate} + NADH + H^+$$

The relative intensity of NADH is proportional to the LD activity of each isoenzyme fraction and can be determined at 340 nm. Visual determination of the individual LD isoenzyme fractions can be accomplished by coupling the formation of NADH in the reaction described above to the reduction of iodonitrotetrazolium chloride (INT) to a colored formazan compound as shown below:

$$NADH + INT \rightarrow NAD + \text{Formazan compound}$$

The intensity of the formazan compound that is formed is related to LD activity. The relative intensity of each of the LD isoenzyme fractions can be determined by scanning of the electrophoretic gel with a densitometer.

The relative percentage of total LD activity that is constituted solely by the LD_1 isoenzyme fraction can be determined with use of immunochemical methods (Table 31-8, method 2). These procedures use antibodies directed against the M subunit of LD to inhibit the LD_2 through LD_5 isoenzyme fractions selectively. In the first step of the procedure, anti-M antibody binds to the M subunit or subunits contained in LD_2 through LD_5. After this initial step, an antibody directed against the first antibody can be used to remove those isoenzymes containing an M subunit, leaving LD_1 in solution. The anti-M antibody can also be attached to a insoluble particle. This allows for the M-containing LD isoenzymes to be removed from solution by centrifugation. In both procedures, the LD_1 remaining in solution can be determined by means of the usual LD procedure. A comparison of LD activity present in the initial sample versus the activity remaining after removal of the M-containing LD isoenzymes allows the percentage of LD_1 as a function of total LD activity to be measured. These immunochemical procedures for LD_1 can be performed much more quickly compared to electrophoretic separation of LD isoenzymes.

Other methods to separate LD isoenzymes include anion-exchange procedures.[69,70] A sample is introduced into a column containing an ion-exchange resin such as diethylaminoethyl cellulose. At pH 8.0 LD_1 and LD_2 are bound to the resin with the greatest affinity. The LD isoenzymes are eluted from the column using salt solutions of increasing concentration; LD_5 is eluted first with LD_1 eluted at the highest

salt concentrations. This method is both tedious and time consuming and is rarely used today.

Specimen Serum is the preferred specimen. It should be separated from the red blood cells as quickly as possible to avoid the possibility of contamination of the specimen from LD present in the cells. Erythrocytes contain approximately 100 times the amount of LD present in normal serum, with the LD_1 and LD_2 isoenzyme fractions being most predominant. LD_4 and LD_5 are labile at lower temperatures. Therefore, samples should be kept at room temperature before analysis.

Reference intervals Reference intervals for the LD isoenzyme fractions are dependent on the support media used for their separation and the method used for visualization. Suggested reference intervals for LD isoenzyme fractionation using agarose gel electrophoresis and visualization using tetrazolium dye are given below.

ISOENZYME FRACTION	REFERENCE INTERVAL (relative %)
LD_1	17-31
LD_2	35-48
LD_3	15-29
LD_4	4-9
LD_5	3-10

Reference intervals for LD_1 measured using the immunochemical procedure are 0 to 102 U/L of LD_1 when total LD activity is less than 250 U/L. In patients with suspected acute myocardial infarction the following values may be observed:

LD VALUE	LD_1 VALUE
≤250 U/L	>102 U/L
>250 U/L	≥40% of total LD

Procainamide and *N*-acetylprocainamide

JOHN E. SHERWIN

Principles of analysis Measurement of procainamide and its pharmacologically active metabolite, *N*-acetylprocainamide (NAPA), is important for monitoring its therapeutic efficacy and for evaluating patient compliance with the medication regimen. The drug is prescribed for use in patients with cardiac arrhythmia.[71]

Quantitative measurement of procainamide and NAPA include a variety of techniques. Colorimetric[72] and fluorometric[73,74] methods were once used and are of historical interest only. These methods employed extraction of the drug followed by spectrophotometric measurement after diazotization or fluorescence measurements at 354 nm of both procainamide and NAPA.

Chromatographic procedures, including gas chromatography (GC)[75] and high-performance liquid chromatography,[76] have been used to measure these drugs. One advantage of these procedures is that procainamide and NAPA can be determined simultaneously. However, both of these procedures, especially GC, find limited use in laboratories today.

The most common methods in use for measurement of procainamide and NAPA are immunoassay procedures including fluorescence polarization immunoassay (FPIA) (Table 31-9, method 1) and enzyme-multiplied immunoassay (EMIT) techniques (Table 31-9, method 2). The tech-

Table 31-9 Methods of analysis for procainamide and NAPA

Method	Principle	Usage	Comments
1. Fluorescence polarization immunoassay (FPIA)	Competitive binding of patient drug and fluorescein-labeled drug to antibody	Most common	Procainamide and NAPA determined in separate assays
2. Enzyme-multiplied immunoassay technique (EMIT)	Competitive binding of patient drug and enzyme-labeled drug to antibody	Frequently used	Procainamide and NAPA determined in separate assays

niques utilized in both the FPIA and EMIT procedures have been previously described (Chapter 13). The precision of the FPIA procedure is generally better when compared to the assays using EMIT.

Specimen Both serum and plasma are acceptable specimens for both the EMIT and FPIA procedures. However, heparin is not recommended for use with FPIA. Samples should be refrigerated if analysis is delayed beyond 8 hours after collection. Procainamide and NAPA can be stored for up to 2 weeks at refrigerated temperatures. Specimens exhibiting severe hemolysis, lipemia, or icterus are unacceptable because of interference with photometric measurements.

Reference intervals The commonly accepted therapeutic range for procainamide is 4 to 10 μg/mL. The lower range for the combined serum concentration of procainamide and NAPA is around 5 μg/mL, whereas the upper limit for the total serum concentration is between 20 to 30 μg/mL.[77] Procainamide concentrations greater than 16 μg/mL are considered toxic.

ACKNOWLEDGMENTS

We would like to acknowledge the authors from the previous edition for the method creatine kinase isoenzymes: Lawrence M. Silverman, John F. Chapman, and Linda L. Woodard.

REFERENCES

1. Hurst JW et al, editors: *The heart, arteries, and veins,* ed 6, New York, 1986, McGraw-Hill.
2. Hearse DJ: *Enzymes in cardiology: diagnosis and research,* New York, 1979, Wiley & Sons.
3. Wu ABW: Creatine kinase isoforms in ischemic heart disease, *Clin Chem* 35:7-13, 1989.
4. Puleo PR, Guadagno PA, Roberts R, et al: Early diagnosis of acute myocardial infarction based on assay for subforms of creatine kinase-MB, *Circulation* 82:759-764, 1990.
5. Christenson RH, Ohman EM, Clemmenson P, et al: Characteristics of creatine kinase–MB and the MB isoforms in serum after reperfusion in acute myocardial infarction, *Clin Chem* 35:2179-2185, 1989.
6. Mair J, Dienstl F, Puschendorf B: Cardiac troponin T in the diagnosis of myocardial injury, *Crit Rev Clin Lab Sci* 29:31-57, 1992.
7. Apple FS: Acute myocardial infarction and coronary reperfusion, *Am J Clin Pathol* 97:217-226, 1992.
8. Bodor GS, Porter S, Landt Y, Ladenson JH: Development of monoclonal antibodies for an assay of cardiac troponin-I and preliminary results in suspected cases of myocardial infarction, *Clin Chem* 38:2203-2214, 1992.
9. Stryer L: *Biochemistry,* ed 3, New York, 1988, WH Freeman & Company, pp 924-926.
10. Nolan AC, Clark WA, Karoski T, Zak R: Patterns of cellular injury in myocardial ischemia determined by monoclonal antimyosin, *Proc Natl Acad Sci* 80:6046-6050, 1983.
11. Tears RD: Asymmetrical hypertrophy of the heart in young adults, *Br Heart J* 20:1-8, 1958.
12. Wigle ED: Hypercardiomyopathy, *Mod Concepts Cardiovasc Dis* 57:1-6, 1988.
13. Elstein E, Liew CC, Sole MJ: The genetic base of hypertrophic cardiomyopathy, *J Mol Cell Cardiol* 24:1471-1477, 1992.
14. Weiss LM, Liu XF, Chang KL, Billingham ME: Detection of enteroviral RNA in idiopathic dilated cardiomyopathy and other human cardiac tissues, *J Clin Invest* 90:156-159, 1992.
15. Chou TC: *Electrocardiography in clinical practice,* New York, 1979, Grune & Stratton.
16. Rouan GW, Lee TN, Cook EF, et al: Clinical characteristics and outcome of acute myocardial infarction in patients with initial normal or nonspecific electrocardiograms, *Am J Cardiol* 64:1087-1092, 1989.
17. Massie BM, Botvinick EH, Werner JA, et al: Myocardial scintigraphy with technetium-99m stannous pyrophosphate: an insensitive test for nontransmural myocardial infarction, *Am J Cardiol* 43:186-192, 1978.
18. Singh BN, Collett JT, Chew CYB: New perspectives in the pharmacologic therapy of cardiac arrhythmias, *Prog Cardiovasc Dis* 224:243-301, 1980.
19. Opie LH, editor: *Drugs for the heart,* ed 2, Orlando, 1987, Grune & Stratton.
20. Grenadier E, Keider S, Hahna L, et al: The rules of serum myoglobin, total CPK and CK-MB isoenzyme in the acute phase of myocardial infarction, *Am Heart J* 105:408-416, 1983.
21. Drexel H, Dworzak E, Kirchmair W, et al: Myoglobinuria in the early phase of acute myocardial infarction, *Am Heart J* 105:642-651, 1983.
22. Kagen L, Scheidt S, Butt A: Serum myoglobin in myocardial infarction: the "staccato phenomenon," *Am J Med* 62:86-92, 1977.
23. Guzy PM: Creatinine phosphokinase–MB (CPK-MB) and the diagnosis of myocardial infarction, *West J Med* 127:445-460, 1977.
24. Lott JA, Stang JM: Serum enzymes and isoenzymes in the diagnosis and differential diagnosis of myocardial ischemia and necrosis, *Clin Chem* 26:1241-1250, 1980.
25. Blomberg DJ, Kimber WD, Burker MD: Creatine kinase isoenzymes: predictive value in the early diagnosis of myocardial infarction, *Am J Med* 59:464-469, 1975.
26. Neufeld HN, Rabinowitz B, Clejan S, et al: Isoenzymes of creatine phosphokinase in acute myocardial infarction, *Angiology* 28:853-864, 1977.
27. Mair J, Morandell D, Genser N, et al: Equivalent early sensitivities of myoglobin, creatine kinase MB mass, creatine kinase isoform ratios, and troponin I and T for acute myocardial infarction, *Clin Chem* 41:1266-1272, 1995.
28. Irvin RG, Cobb FR, Roe CR: Acute myocardial infarction and creatine phosphokinase, *Arch Intern Med* 140:329-334, 1980.
29. Hashimoto H, Abendschein DR, Strauss AW, et al: Early detection of myocardial infarction in conscious dogs by analysis of plasma MM creatine kinase isoforms, *Circulation* 71:363-368, 1985.
30. Foxall CD: Changes in creatine kinase and its isoenzymes in human fetal muscle during development, *J Neurol Sci* 24:483-492, 1975.
31. Galen RS, Gambino SR: *Beyond normality,* New York, 1975, Wiley & Sons.
32. Hamm CW, Ravkilde J, Gerhardt W, et al: The prognostic value of serum troponin T in unstable angina, *N Engl J Med* 327:146-150, 1992.

33. Katus HA, Tsunehiro Y, Gold HK, et al: Diagnosis of acute myocardial infarction by detection of circulating cardiac myosin light chains, *Am J Cardiol* 54:964-970, 1984.

34. Mair J, Artner-Dworzak E, Lechleitner P, et al: Cardiac troponin T in diagnosis of acute myocardial infarction, *Clin Chem* 37:845-852, 1991.

35. Horder M, Elser RC, Gerhardt W, et al: IFCC methods for the measurement of catalytic concentrations of enzymes. Part 7. IFCC method for creatine kinase (ATP:creatine N-phosphotransferase, EC 2.7.3.2): IFCC recommendation, *Clin Chim Acta* 190:S4-S17, 1990.

36. Kuby SA, Noda L, Lardy HA: Adenosine triphosphate–creatine transphorylase, *J Biol Chem* 209:191-201, 1954.

37. Tanzer ML, Gilvarg C: Creatine and creatine kinase measurement, *J Biol Chem* 234:3201-3204, 1966.

38. Oliver IT: A spectrophotometric method for the determination of creatine phosphokinase and myokinase, *Biochem J* 61:116-122, 1955.

39. Rosalki SB: An improved procedure for serum creatine phosphokinase determination, *J Lab Clin Med* 69:696-705, 1967.

40. Sax SM, Moore JS: Fluorometric measurement of creatine kinase activity, *Clin Chem* 11:951-958, 1965.

41. Witteveen SAGJ, Sobel BE, DeLuca M: Kinetic properties of the isoenzymes of human creatine phosphokinase, *Proc Natl Acad Sci* 71:1384-1387, 1974.

42. Lott JA, Heinz JW: Creatine kinase in serum. In Faulkner WR, Meites S, editors: *Selected methods for the small clinical chemistry laboratory,* Washington, D.C., 1982, American Association for Clinical Chemistry.

43. Frank JJ, Bermes EW, Bickel MJ, Watkins BF: Effect of in vitro hemolysis on chemical values for serum, *Clin Chem* 24:1966-1970, 1978.

44. Abbott LB, Lott JA: Reactivation of serum creatine kinase isoenzyme BB in patients with malignancies, *Clin Chem* 30:1861-1863, 1984.

45. Morin LG: Creatine kinase: stability, inactivation, reactivation, *Clin Chem* 23:646-652, 1977.

46. Henderson AR, McQueen MJ, Patten RL, et al: Testing for creatine kinase and creatine kinase–2 in Ontario: reference ranges and assay types, *Clin Chem* 38:1365-1370, 1992.

47. Wong ET, Cobb C, Umehara MK, et al: Heterogeneity of serum creatine kinase activity among racial and gender groups of the population, *Am J Clin Pathol* 79:582-586, 1983.

48. Foreback CC: Biochemical diagnosis of myocardial infarction, *Henry Ford Hosp Med J* 39:159-164, 1991.

49. Lee TH, Goldman L: Serum enzyme assays in the diagnosis of acute myocardial infarction, *Ann Intern Med* 105:221-233, 1986.

50. Brownlow K, Elevitch FR: Serum creatine phosphokinase isoenzyme (CPK2) in myositis: a report of six cases, *JAMA* 230:1141-1144, 1974.

51. El Allaf M, Chapelle J-P, El Allaf D, et al: Differentiating muscle damage from myocardial injury by means of the serum creatine kinase (CK) isoenzyme MB mass measurement/total CK activity ratio, *Clin Chem* 32:291-295, 1986.

52. Watson E, Kalman SM: Assay of digoxin in plasma by gas chromatography, *J Chromatogr* 56:209, 1971.

53. Bertler A, Redfors A: An improved method of estimating digoxin in human plasma, *Clin Pharmacol Ther* 11:665, 1970.

54. Butler VP Jr, Chen JP: Digoxin specific antibody, *Proc Natl Acad Sci* 57:71, 1967.

55. Henderson DR, Friedman SB, Harris JD, et al. CEDIA™, a new homogenous immunoassay system, *Clin Chem* 32:1637-1641, 1986.

56. Leflar CC, Freytag JW, Powell LM, et al: An automated, affinity-column mediated, enzyme-linked immunometric assay for digoxin on the DuPont *aca* discrete clinical analyzer, *Clin Chem* 30:1809-1811, 1984.

57. Morris RG, Frewin DB, Taylor WB, et al: The effect of renal and hepatic impairment and of spironolactone on digoxin immunoassays, *Eur J Clin Pharmacol* 34:233-239, 1988.

58. Ray JE, Crisan D, Howrie DL: Digoxin-like immunoreactivity in serum from neonates and infants reduced by centrifugal ultrafiltration and fluorescence polarization immunoassay, *Clin Chem* 37:94-98, 1991.

59. Lacarelle B, Durand A, Labadie N, Cano JP: Comparison of digoxin-like immunoreactive substance cross-reactivity with two digoxin automated immunoassays, *Ther Drug Monit* 11:725-727, 1989 [Letter].

60. Christenson RH, Studenberg SD, Beck-Davis S, Sedor FA: Digoxin-like immunoreactivity from serum by centrifugal ultrafiltration before fluorescence polarization immunoassay of digoxin, *Clin Chem* 33:606-608, 1987.

61. Pudek MR, Seccombe DW, Jacobson BE, Whitfield MF: Seven different immunoassay kits compared with respect to interference by a digoxin-like immunoreactive substance in serum from premature and full-term infants, *Clin Chem* 29:1972-1974, 1983.

62. Phelps SJ, Kamper CA, Bottorff MB, Alpert BS: Effect of age and serum creatinine on endogenous digoxin-like substances in infants and children, *J Pediatr* 110:136-139, 1987.

63. Wolach B, Carmi D, Shilo L, et al: Endogenous digoxin-like factor in neonates: effect of age and relation to serum bilirubin levels, *Acta Paediatr Scand* 78:364-368, 1989.

64. Howell BF, McClure S, Schaffer R: Lactate-to-pyruvate or pyruvate-to-lactate assay for lactate dehydrogenase: re-examination, *Clin Chem* 25:269-272, 1979.

65. Keiding R, Horder M, Gerhardt W, et al: Recommended methods for determination of four enzymes in blood, *Scand J Clin Lab Invest* 33:291-306, 1974.

66. Demetriou JA, Drewes PA, Gin JB: Enzymes. In Henry RJ, Cannon DC, Winkelman JW, editors: *Clinical chemistry: principles and techniques,* New York, 1974, Harper & Row.

67. Freer DE, Statland BE, Johnson M, Felton H: Reference values for selected enzyme activities and protein concentrations in serum and plasma derived from cord-blood specimens, *Clin Chem* 25:565-569, 1979.

68. Buhl SN, Jackson KY: Optimal conditions and comparison of lactate dehydrogenase catalysis of the lactate-to-pyruvate and pyruvate-to-lactate reactions in human serum at 25°, 30°, and 37° C, *Clin Chem* 24:828-831, 1978.

69. Mercer DW: Simultaneous separation of serum creatine kinase and lactate dehydrogenase isoenzymes by ion-exchange column chromatography, *Clin Chem* 21:1102, 1975.

70. Mercer DS: Improved column method for separating lactate dehydrogenase isoenzymes 1 and 2, *Clin Chem* 24:480, 1980.

71. Lima JJ, Lewis RP: Procainamide therapeutic use and serum concentration monitoring. In Taylor WJ, Finn AL, editors: *Individualizing drug therapy: practical applications of drug monitoring,* vol 3, New York, 1981, Gross Townsend Frank, Inc.

72. Koch-Weser J, Klein SW: Procainamide dosage schedules, plasma concentrations, and clinical effects, *JAMA* 215:1454-1460, 1971.

73. Ambler PK, Masarei JRL: A new fluorometric method for procainamide, *Clin Chem Acta* 70:379-383, 1976.

74. Matusik E, Gibson TP: Fluorometric assay for N-acetylprocainamide, *Clin Chem* 21:1899-1902, 1975.

75. Karbson E, Molin L, Norlander B, Sjöqvist B: Acetylation of procainamide in man studied with a new gas chromatographic method, *Br J Clin Pharmacol* 1:457-467, 1974.

76. Baselt R: *Analytical procedures for therapeutic drug monitoring and emergency toxicology,* Davis, California, 1980, Biomedical Publications.

77. Atkinson AJ Jr, Strong JM: Effect of active drug metabolites on plasma level–response correlations, *J Pharmacokinet Biopharm* 5:95-109, 1977.

CHAPTER 32   *Diabetes mellitus*

Richard F. Dods

OBJECTIVES

- Describe normal glucose homeostasis.
- Differentiate between diabetes mellitus (types I and II), impaired glucose tolerance, and gestational diabetes.
- Describe common acute and chronic complications of diabetes mellitus.
- List steps in performing an oral glucose tolerance test.
- State expected levels of the following analytes in controlled diabetes mellitus I and II, ketoacidosis, and hyperosmolar coma: glucose, ketones, pH, bicarbonate, P_{CO_2}, insulin, C-peptide, sodium, potassium, glycohemoglobin, BUN, osmolality, and triglycerides.

KEY TERMS

acromegaly Growth hormone excess in adults and characterized by enlargement of features such as the head, hands, and feet.

adenosine 3',5'-cyclic monophosphate (cAMP) An organic molecule that is obligatory for the action of enzymes such as protein kinases.

aerobic glycolysis Glycolysis that is linked to the tricarboxylic acid cycle by the presence of oxygen. Aerobic glycolysis produces 36 moles of ATP per mole of glucose.

anaerobic glycolysis Glycolysis that occurs in the absence of oxygen. In this case glycolysis is not linked to the tricarboxylic acid cycle and only 2 moles of ATP are produced per mole of glucose.

angiogenesis A complication of diabetes mellitus. Abnormal proliferation of blood vessels in a tissue such as the eye lens.

angiopathy A complication of diabetes mellitus manifesting as damage to the basement membranes of blood vessels.

anorexia nervosa Loss of appetite because of psychological reasons and results in lowered blood insulin.

anoxia Lack of oxygen.

basement membrane A layer of noncellular material that underlies the epithelium.

diabetes insipidus A disorder caused by excessive secretion of arginine vasopressin. As in diabetes mellitus, a characteristic symptom of diabetes insipidus is polyuria.

diabetic ketoacidosis A complication of diabetes mellitus characterized by hyperglycemia, hyperosmolarity, low pH, ketonuria and ketonemia, and lethargy or coma.

disaccharide Two monosaccharides linked by a glycosidic bond.

gestational diabetes Glucose intolerance that occurs in some pregnancies.

glucagon A hormone produced by the alpha cells of the pancreas. Glucagon is primarily involved in energy release.

glucagonoma Excessive glucagon levels caused by a tumor.

gluconeogenesis Production of glucose from pyruvic acid.

glucose A six-carbon polyhydroxyl aldehyde; primary source of energy in living organisms. Its metabolism produces adenosine triphosphate.

glucosuria Excessive quantities of urinary glucose.

glucosylation Reaction in which glucose binds covalently to protein.

glycogen Highly branched, high-molecular-weight polysaccharide composed only of glucose units.

glycogenesis Formation of glycogen from glucose-6-phosphate.

glycolysis Metabolism of glucose-6-phosphate to pyruvic acid or lactic acid.

glycosylation Reaction in which monosaccharides such as glucose, mannose, galactose, xylose, ribose, and fructose covalently bind to proteins.

growth hormone Hormone produced by the anterior part of the pituitary. Also called somatotropin. Raises blood glucose.

hexose monophosphate shunt Metabolic pathway in which glucose-6-phosphate is metabolized to ribose and carbon dioxide.

histocompatibility antigen (human leukocyte antigen, HLA) Proteins responsible for rejection of tissue transplanted to an individual from another unrelated individual. Specific HLAs are present at a high frequency in persons who develop certain diseases.

hyperglycemia High blood glucose concentrations.

hyperglycemic, hyperosmolar nonketotic coma (HHNC) A complication of diabetes mellitus characterized by hyperglycemia, hyperosmolarity, low pH, normal ketoacid levels, and lethargy or coma.

islet cell antibodies (ICA) Antibodies frequently found in type I diabetics that are suggestive of an autoimmune cause.

islets of Langerhans Group of cells in the pancreas composed of alpha cells, which secrete glucagon; beta cells, which secrete insulin; and delta cells, which secrete somatostatin.

ketonemia Excess of ketones and derived ketoacids in the blood.

ketonuria Excess of ketones and derived ketoacids in the urine.

lactic acidosis Acidosis (low blood pH) caused by excess lactic acid.

lipolysis Hydrolysis of triglycerides to free fatty acids and glycerol.

monosaccharide A polyhydroxyl aldehyde or ketone, such as glucose, fructose, or mannose.

nephropathy A complication of diabetes mellitus referring to damage to the glomerulus and capillaries associated with the glomerulus.

neuropathy The most common complication of diabetes mellitus. It refers to reduced motor and sensory nerve conduction velocities caused by axonal degeneration and demyelination.

oxidative phosphorylation The process linking the tricarboxylic acid cycle with ATP formation.

polydipsia Excessive thirst. A symptom of diabetes mellitus.

polyphagia Constant hunger. A symptom of diabetes mellitus.

polysaccharide A carbohydrate composed of more than two monosaccharides linked by glycosidic bonds.

polyuria Excessive urinary output. A symptom of diabetes mellitus.

preproinsulin Precursor to proinsulin.

proinsulin Precursor to insulin.

protein kinases Enzymes that phosphorylate other proteins. Some protein kinases depend on adenosine monophosphate for activity.

receptor sites Sites on or in cells where hormones are bound. Hormone binding to the receptor site is the initial step for hormone action.

retinopathy A complication of diabetes mellitus. A disorder of the retina caused in diabetics by cataract formation or proliferation of small blood vessels (angiogenesis).

somatostatin A hormone produced in the delta cells of the pancreas. Inhibits insulin and glucagon secretion.

somatostatinoma A tumor that produces excess quantities of somatostatin, resulting in hyperglycemia.

thyroxine A hormone produced by the thyroid gland that increases blood glucose levels.

tricarboxylic acid cycle Metabolic pathway that converts glucose-6-phosphate via pyruvic acid to CO_2 and water. When coupled to oxidative phosphorylation, adenosine triphosphate is formed.

uronic acid pathway Converts glucose-6-phosphate to glucuronic acid.

Complications resulting from diabetes mellitus are the third leading cause of death attributable to disease in the United States according to statistics compiled by the National Commission on Diabetes.[1] A survey by the National Diabetes Data Group[2] estimates the prevalence of diabetes in the American population at 6.6%. Thus there are approximately 16.5 million diabetic Americans. Of this number only about 50% are diagnosed. Rates are equal by sex and greater for blacks than for whites. The cost of diabetes to the American economy exceeds $5 billion annually.

The implications of diabetes extend beyond its direct effects and long-term complications, since it has been established that diabetes is a risk factor for coronary heart disease[3] and cerebrovascular disease (stroke).[4] A diabetic has a twofold greater risk of suffering a myocardial infarction than a nondiabetic of the same age and sex.

Research has demonstrated that diabetes mellitus is not a single disease but an array of diseases that exhibit a common symptom, inability of the individual to handle glucose (glucose intolerance).

The primary symptoms of diabetes mellitus are abnormally high blood and urine glucose levels (hyperglycemia and glucosuria respectively), polyuria, excessive thirst (polydipsia), constant hunger (polyphagia), sudden weight loss, and, during acute episodes of diabetes mellitus, excessive blood and urinary ketones (ketonemia and ketonuria respectively). All these symptoms are the result of the inability to metabolize glucose and the consequences of high glucose levels.

GLUCOSE: PROPERTIES AND METABOLISM
Definition (see also p. 1052)

Carbohydrates are defined as polyhydroxyl aldehydes (aldoses) and ketones (ketoses). Simple carbohydrates such as glucose are also called monosaccharides. Two monosaccharides linked by a bond called a glycosidic bond form a disaccharide. More than two monosaccharides linked by glycosidic bonds form a polysaccharide. Dietary carbohydrates consist of monosaccharides such as glucose, fructose, and galactose; disaccharides such as sucrose, lactose, and maltose; and polysaccharides such as starch. Intestinal enzymes convert disaccharides and polysaccharides to monosaccharides (see p. 574).

Function

The principal biochemical function of glucose is to provide energy for life processes. *Adenosine triphosphate* (ATP) is the universal energy source for biological reactions. Glucose oxidation by the glycolytic and tricarboxylic acid pathways is the primary source of energy for the biosynthesis of ATP.

Glucose transport across cell membranes

The initial event in glucose metabolism is facilitated transport of glucose across the plasma membrane. Five glucose transporters, called GluT-1 through GluT-5, have been identified.[5] The glucose transporters are integral components of the cell membrane and are glycoproteins with molecular weights of approximately 55,000 daltons.

The glucose transporters vary with respect to tissue distribution and apparent Michaelis-Menten constant (K_m). GluT-1, GluT-3, and GluT-5 possess a low K_m of <1 to 2 mM, whereas GluT-4 has an intermediate K_m of 5 mM, and

GluT-2 has a high K_m of 17 mM. There is a considerable significance in the locations of the different forms of the glucose transporters. GluT-1 and GluT-3, predominantly located in glucose-sensitive, insulin-dependent cells, such as brain and erythrocytes, permit cell uptake of glucose at levels below the normal fasting range despite low levels of insulin and glucose. The highest K_m glucose transporter, GluT-2, is located in cells that are directly involved in blood glucose regulation and permit these cells to increase their glucose uptake, independent of insulin, in the presence of increased blood glucose levels. Thus small intestine, renal tubule and liver cells, and pancreatic beta cells possess GluT-2. High K_m transporters allow glucose uptake over a wide range of extracellular glucose levels. GluT-4, which has a K_m in the intermediate range, is found principally in the insulin-dependent muscle and adipose cells.

Principal glucose-6-phosphate metabolic pathways

Within the cell, glucose is rapidly converted to *glucose-6-phosphate* (G6P), a major intermediate in glucose metabolism. The enzyme catalyzing the phosphorylation of glucose by ATP is hexokinase (or glucokinase in the liver and beta cells of the pancreas). Glucokinase may play a key role in the regulation of glucose homeostasis by maintaining a gradient for glucose transport in hepatocytes.[6]

As shown in Fig. 32-1, glucose-6-phosphate serves as a starting point for five metabolic pathways. Glucose-6-phosphate is converted by glycolysis to pyruvate, a substance that is further metabolized by the tricarboxylic acid pathway to carbon dioxide and water. Glucose-6-phosphate is also oxidized by the hexose monophosphate shunt to ribose and carbon dioxide, converted by the uronic acid pathway to glucuronic acid, and incorporated into glycogen by glycogenesis.

Aerobic glycolysis

Glycolysis. Glucose-6-phosphate metabolism by the glycolytic pathway (also called the *Embden-Meyerhof cycle*) results in the formation of ATP (Fig. 32-2). Glycolysis converts the six-carbon glucose molecule to two molecules of a three-carbon compound called pyruvic acid. This process produces 2 moles of ATP per mole of glucose. An important aspect of glycolysis is the formation of pyruvic acid. In aerobic glycolysis, pyruvate is metabolized further by means of the tricarboxylic acid cycle.

Tricarboxylic acid cycle. Pyruvic acid enters the tricarboxylic acid cycle (citric acid cycle, Krebs cycle) where it is metabolized to carbon dioxide and water. Fig. 32-3 shows the intermediate steps in the tricarboxylic acid cycle and the steps that are used to reduce nicotinamide adenine dinucleotide (NAD) and flavin adenine dinucleotide (FAD) to their corresponding analogs, NADH and FADH$_2$. The tricarboxylic acid cycle does not directly produce ATP, but ATP is produced by the oxidation of NADH and FADH$_2$.

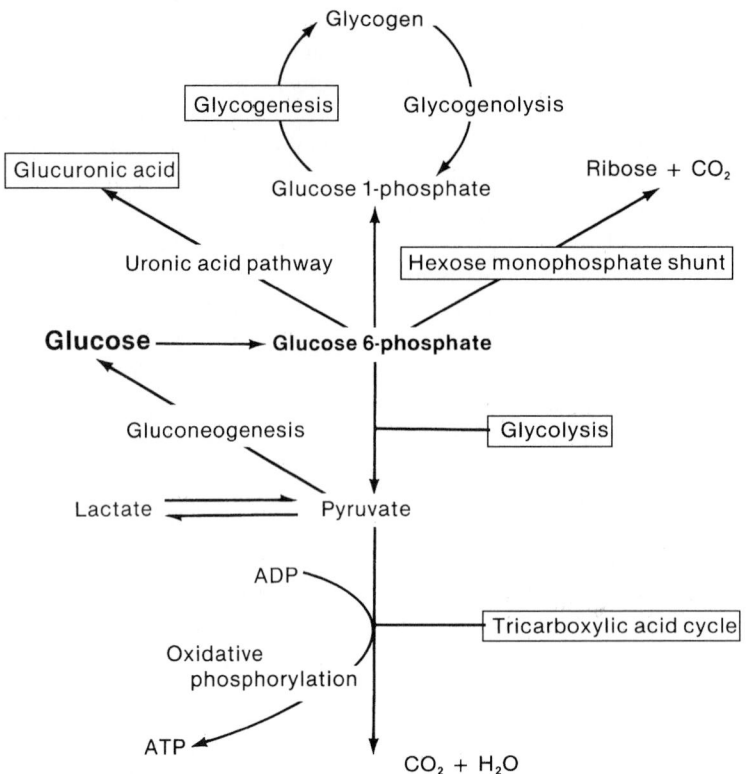

Fig. 32-1   The five principal pathways of glucose metabolism: glycolysis, tricarboxylic acid pathway, glycogenesis, hexose monophosphate shunt, and the uronic acid pathway.

Oxidative phosphorylation. Oxidative phosphorylation is a complex process that takes place in the mitochondria and that involves electron transfer from NADH and $FADH_2$ to a series of compounds, eventually ending up with the reduction of oxygen to yield a water molecule. Thus it is actually the reoxidation of NADH and $FADH_2$, compounds produced by the tricarboxylic acid cycle that produces ATP. In contrast to glycolysis, which produces 2 moles of ATP per mole of glucose, the tricarboxylic acid cycle linked with oxidative phosphorylation produces 36 moles of ATP per mole of glucose. The oxidative and ATP synthesis processes are tightly coupled because the availability of adenosine diphosphate (ADP) controls the rate of oxidation and oxygen availability regulates the rate of phosphorylation.

Anaerobic glycolysis

In fatigued muscle where there is a deficiency of oxygen, or *anoxia,* glucose converted by glycolysis to pyruvic acid cannot be further metabolized by the above pathways. Instead (Fig. 32-2) pyruvate is converted by the enzyme lactate dehydrogenase to lactate. This is called *anaerobic glycolysis.* In contrast to aerobic glycosis, only 2 moles of ATP per mole of glucose are produced by anaerobic glycolysis. Lactic acid produced by anoxic tissue is carried by the circulation to the liver, where it is reconverted to glucose in a process called *gluconeogenesis* (see the following text).

Alternate energy sources. As indicated in Fig. 32-3, amino acids and fatty acids also enter the tricarboxylic acid cycle to produce ATP and are therefore alternative sources of energy.

Glycogenesis, glycogenolysis, and gluconeogenesis

Glycogen. Excess glucose is stored in the cells as the polymer glycogen for later energy demands. Glycogen (Fig. 32-4) is a high-molecular-weight polysaccharide composed entirely of glucose units in 1,4-glycosidic bonds with 1,6-branches occurring approximately every 10 units. Glycogen is located in the cytoplasm of liver and muscle cells in granules that contain the enzymes involved in the synthesis (glycogenesis) and hydrolysis (glycogenolysis) of glycogen. Refer again to Fig. 32-1 to see how glucogenesis and glycogenolysis fit into the overall scheme of glucose metabolism. Fig. 32-5 presents a simplified representation of glycogenesis and glycogenolysis.

Glycogenesis. The first step in glycogenesis is conversion of glucose-6-phosphate to glucose-1-phosphate (Fig. 32-5). Reaction of glucose-1-phosphate with uridine-5′-triphosphate produces uridine diphosphate glucose, a substance that reacts with the preexisting glycogen molecule to form 1,4-glucosidic linkages. Synthesis of 1,4-glucosidic bonds is catalyzed by the enzyme *glycogen synthetase.* Gly-

Glyclosis

ATP balance

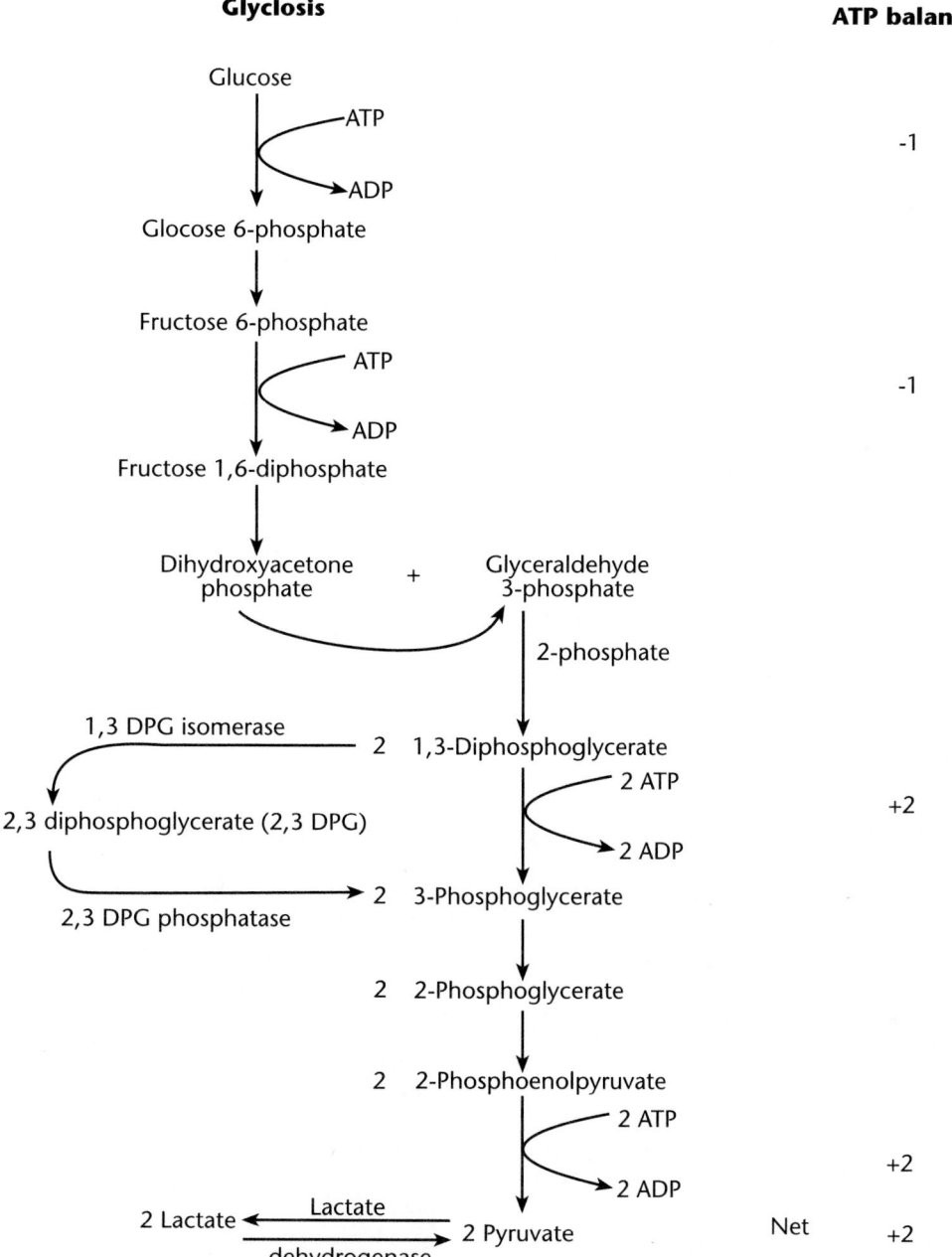

Fig. 32-2 Two stages of glycolysis. First stage proceeds from glucose to formation of 1,3-diphosphoglycerate and consumes 2 moles of ATP. Second stage proceeds from 1,3-diphosphoglycerate to pyruvate and produces 4 moles of ATP. Glycolysis therefore results in net gain of 2 moles of ATP per mole of glucose. The synthesis of 2,3-DPG by the Rapoport-Luebring cycle is important for the regulation of oxygen transport.

cogen synthetase exists in two forms: the phosphorylated, inactive enzyme form and the dephosphorylated, active enzyme form. Phosphorylation of the active enzyme is accomplished by any of several enzymes of the *protein kinase* class. Protein kinases are activated by low levels of adenosine 3′,5′-cyclic monophosphate (cAMP). Thus glycogen synthetase activity (and thereby glycogenesis) is regulated by intracellular cAMP levels. Glycogenesis is en-

hanced by low cAMP levels and inhibited by high cAMP levels; cAMP levels are in turn regulated by insulin, which causes decreased cAMP levels.

Branching of glycogen is accomplished by an enzyme called a *branching enzyme*. This branching enzyme hydrolyzes the 1,4-glycosidic bond of glycogen to form five to six glucose unit fragments, which are reattached to the glycogen molecule through 1,6-glycosidic bonds.

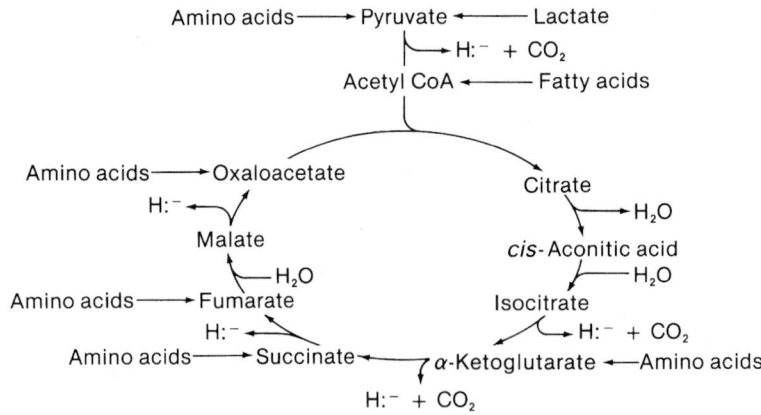

Fig. 32-3 Tricarboxylic acid cycle produces CO_2 and water from pyruvate, fatty acids, and amino acids, which enter the cycle at the points indicated. Hydride ions ($H:^-$) are produced and utilized in oxidative phosphorylation process to produce ATP from ADP and inorganic phosphate.

Glycogenolysis. Although glycogenolysis (Fig. 32-5) is the opposite of glycogenesis, it does not occur through a simple reversal of each step of glycogenesis but by a unique enzyme system. The *debranching enzyme* splits off trisaccharides from branches and reattaches them by 1,4-glycosidic bonds to the ends of the glycogen molecule. *Glycogen phosphorylase* hydrolyzes the 1,4-glycosidic bond producing glucose-1-phosphate:

Glycogen + P_i → Glycogen + Glucose-1-phosphate   *Eq. 32-1*
(*n* **residues**)   (*n* − 1 **residues**)

Like glycogen synthetase, glycogen phosphorylase exists in two forms. The active form, called phosphorylase a, is a tetramer. The inactive form, phosphorylase b, is the dimer. The active tetramer is formed in three steps; phosphorylation of the dimer by a protein kinase called *phosphorylase kinase* followed by binding of the phosphorylated dimer with another phosphorylated dimer. The third and final step in the activation process is the binding of one molecule of

pyridoxal phosphate to each subunit of the tetramer. Phosphorylase kinase is activated by cAMP. Note that high cellular cAMP levels favor glycogenolysis over glycogenesis. The activation of glycogen phosphorylase is under hormonal control (see below).

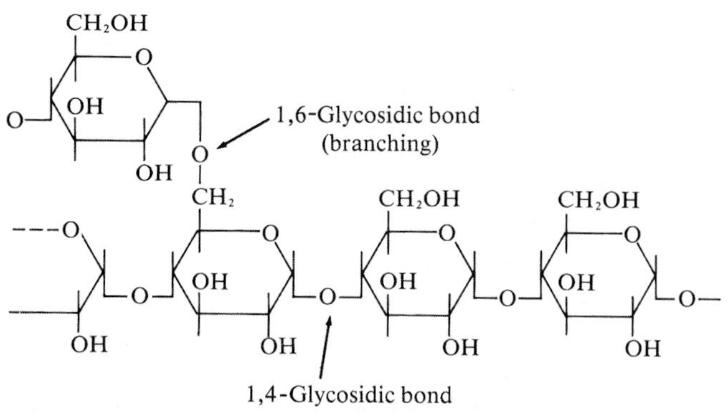

Gluconeogenesis. The steps in gluconeogenesis are shown also in Fig. 32-6. Gluconeogenesis produces glucose-6-phosphate from amino acids, fatty acids, glycerol, and lactate. Pyruvate is an important intermediary in gluconeogenesis (Fig. 32-6), since it can be formed directly from lactate oxidation (by lactate dehydrogenase) and from the amino acid alanine (via transamination by alanine transaminase). Glycerol, derived from hydrolysis of triglyceride

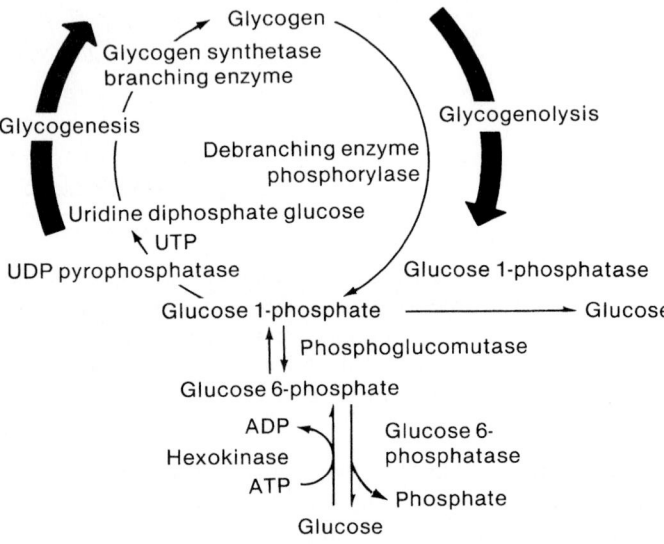

Fig. 32-5 Glycogen, storage molecule for glucose, is synthesized from glucose-1-phosphate by a process called *glycogenesis (left side)*. *Glycogenolysis* releases glucose units from glycogen. Debranching is first step in glycogenolysis *(right side)*.

Fig. 32-4 Glycogen is a 1- to 4-million dalton polysaccharide composed of glucose units in 1,4- and 1,6-glycosidic linkage. The 1,6-bonds produce branches at intervals of approximately 10 glucose units.

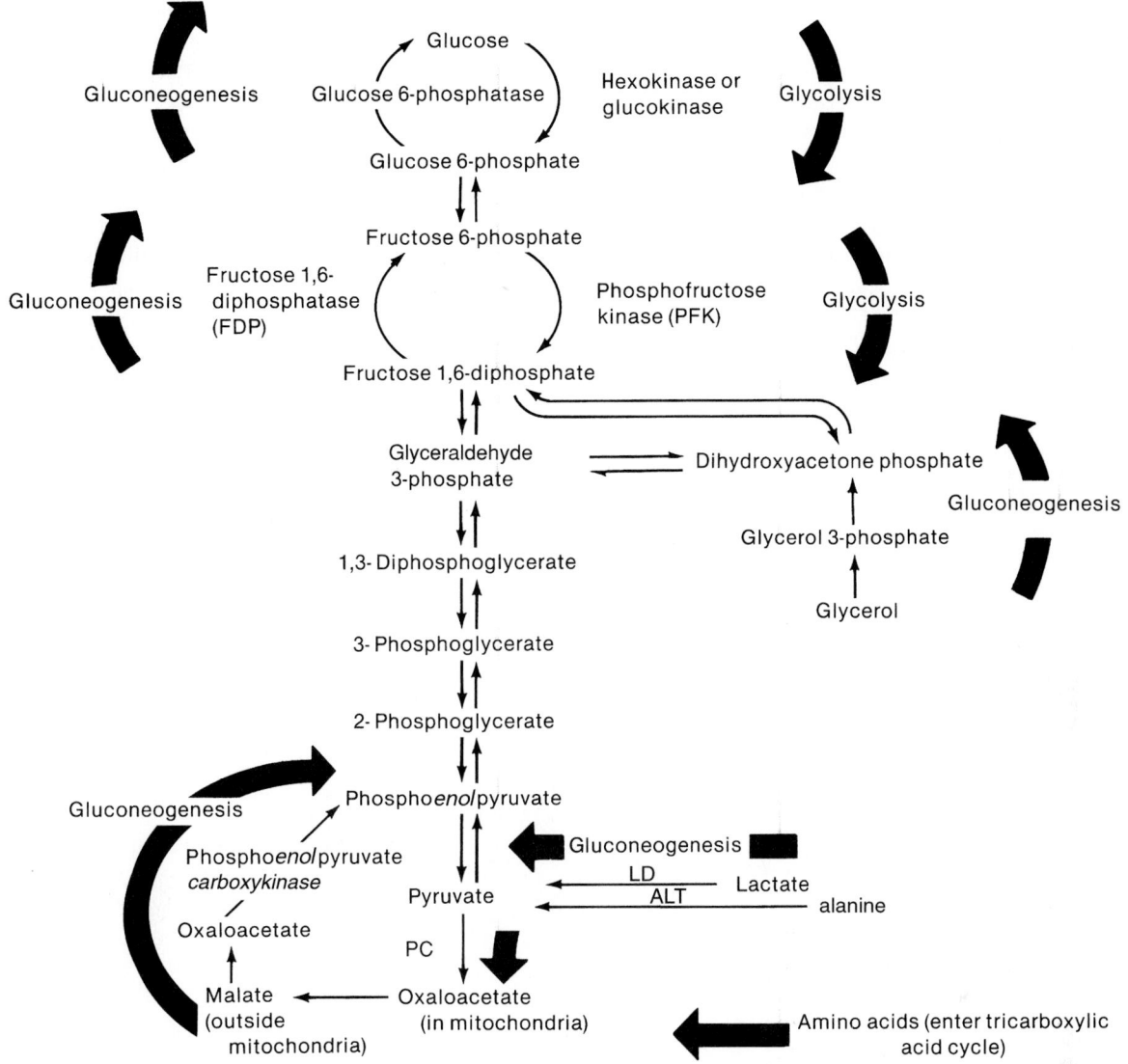

Fig. 32-6 Pathways involved in gluconeogenesis from amino acids, fatty acids, glycerol, and lactate. This pathway shares many of the enzymes of glycolytic and tricarboxylic acid pathways. Gluconeogenesis provides glucose whenever scarcity of glucose occurs and whenever lactate accumulates. *ALT,* Alanine transaminase; *LD,* lactate dehydrogenase; *PC,* pyruvate carboxylase.

(lipolysis), enters the gluconeogenic pathway after pyruvate as glycerol-3-phosphate. These three substances, lactate, alanine, and glycerol, are the primary precursors for glucose synthesis. Gluconeogenesis is not a simple reversal of glycolysis, though gluconeogenesis does share some of the enzymes of the glycolytic pathway. Glucose is formed only in the liver and kidney, which have the enzyme glucose-6-phosphatase, which hydrolyzes G6P to glucose. In fact, the liver is the major nondietary source of serum glucose of the body and is critical for maintaining blood glucose levels.

Hormone regulation of glucose metabolism[7]

The system for regulating blood glucose levels is designed to achieve two ends. The first is to store glucose in excess of the body's immediate needs in a compact reservoir (glycogen), and the second is to mobilize the stored glucose in order to maintain the blood glucose level. The regulation of blood glucose is essential to keep the brain, whose primary energy source is glucose, supplied with a constant amount of glucose. The role of insulin is to shift extracellular glucose to intracellular storage sites in the form of macromolecules (such as glycogen, fats, and proteins). Thus glucose is stored away in times of plenty for times of need.

In response to low blood glucose, as in periods of fasting, a series of hyperglycemic agents acts on intermediary metabolic pathways to form glucose from storage macromolecules. Thus proteins and glycogen are metabolized to form glucose-6-phosphate (gluconeogenesis), which in the liver is hydrolyzed to glucose and released into the blood to maintain blood glucose levels.

The most important hyperglycemic agents are glucagon, epinephrine, cortisol, thyroxine, growth hormone, and certain intestinal hormones. The behavior of each of these agents in regulating blood glucose is different; whereas insulin promotes anabolic metabolism (synthesis of macromolecules), these hormones in part induce catabolic metabolism to break down large molecules.

Insulin. Insulin is synthesized in the endocrine pancreas by the beta cells of the islets of Langerhans as a high-molecular-weight precursor called preproinsulin.[8] Preproinsulin (11,500 daltons) is shown in Fig. 32-7. Cleavage at the link marked by the arrow labeled *1* results in the for-

mation of proinsulin (9000 D). Proinsulin has only 5% of the activity of insulin. The proinsulin molecule consists of the A and B chains of insulin connected by disulfide bonds and by a connective peptide called *C-peptide*. During processing the C-peptide (3000 D) is removed from the molecule by cleavage at the links marked by arrows *2* and *3*. The resulting insulin molecule (6000 D) consists of chains A and B connected by two disulfide bonds. This entire process occurs within the beta cell. The initial synthesis of preproinsulin occurs at the Golgi apparatus. The molecule is packaged in a vesicle called a *beta granule*. Cleavage first to proinsulin and next to insulin occurs within the granule. Equal quantities of C-peptide and insulin are released into the circulation when the granule is dissolved at the plasma

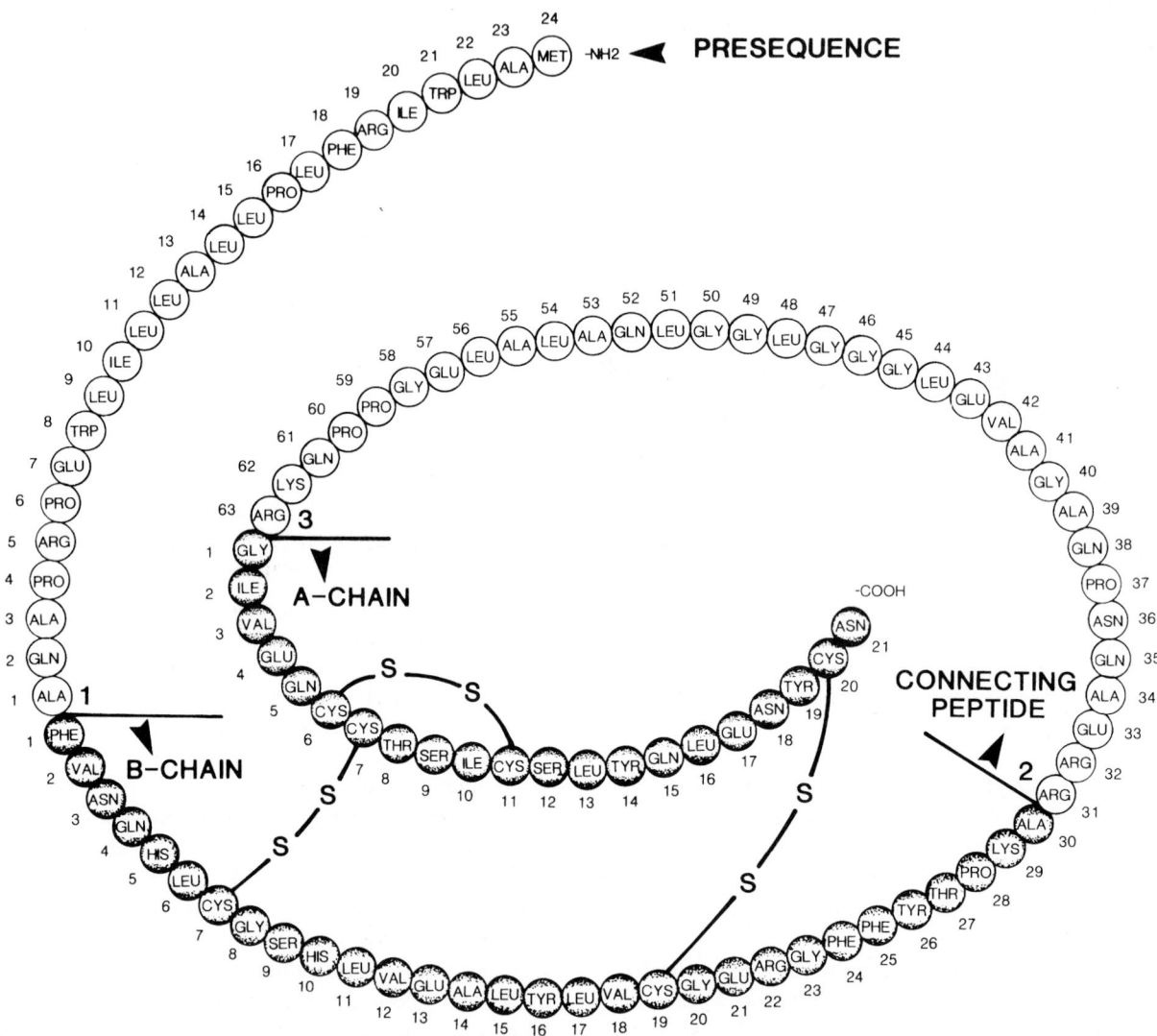

Fig. 32-7 Amino acid sequence of insulin. Amino acid sequence for this figure, a composite of sequences for bovine proinsulin and rat preproinsulin, probably does not differ too widely from amino acid sequence of human preproinsulin. The series of enzymatic cleavages of preproinsulin *(site 1)* to proinsulin and of proinsulin *(sites 2 and 3)* to insulin are described in text.

membrane of the beta cell after neural, dietary, or hormonal stimuli. Only small quantities of proinsulin are found in the circulation.

Glucagon and cortisol. Glucagon is a 3500-dalton polypeptide hormone that is synthesized in the alpha cells of the pancreas.[9] In diabetes mellitus, because of insulin deficiency, glucagon levels are elevated and are not suppressed by carbohydrate loading.[10]

Cortisol and the other adrenal corticosteroids increase the rate of gluconeogenesis from protein and amino acids, especially in the liver.

Epinephrine. Epinephrine raises glucose levels by inhibiting insulin secretion, stimulating glucagon secretion, stimulating glycogenolysis, and inhibiting gluconeogenesis.

Other hormones. *Growth hormone* and *thyroxine* also act to raise circulating levels of glucose. *Somatostatin* is a polypeptide hormone that is synthesized primarily in the delta cells of the pancreas. Somatostatin inhibits both insulin and glucagon release. *Gastric inhibitory polypeptide* stimulates insulin release. This hormone is located in the intestinal mucosa, and its release is stimulated by glucose and amino acids. Thus food ingestion results in increased levels of circulating insulin. Insulin-like growth factors are proteins with structured homology to proinsulin and somatomedin C. These factors may play a role in glucose control.

Opposite actions of insulin and glucagon. Insulin and glucagon have opposing effects. Insulin inhibits proteolysis, lipolysis, gluconeogenesis, and glycogenolysis and stimulates lipid synthesis and glycogenesis in the liver; increases protein synthesis in muscle; and accelerates triglyceride synthesis in fat cells (see the box). Insulin acts as the body's only hypoglycemic agent. In contrast, glucagon stimulates lipolysis, ketogenesis, gluconeogenesis, and glycogenolysis. A meal rich in carbohydrates induces insulin

secretion and suppresses glucagon release. Hypoglycemia stimulates the release of glucagon. Thus, in general, insulin and glucagon act oppositely to each other, with insulin promoting energy storage and glucagon promoting energy release. The net result of the hypoglycemic agent (insulin) and the hyperglycemic agents is glucose homeostasis.

Glucose metabolism in diabetes mellitus

Metabolic processes in the normal individual. The hormonal regulation of blood glucose levels and metabolic processes is abnormal in diabetics and results in the classic sign of diabetes mellitus: elevated blood glucose levels.

In the postabsorptive (fasting) state of normal individuals, the blood insulin/glucagon ratio is low, causing muscle and hepatic glycogen to be degraded as a source of glucose. Additional fasting results in the breakdown of protein to amino acids in skeletal muscle, and the lipolysis of triglycerides to fatty acids in adipose tissue. The amino acid alanine and glycerol are used to synthesize glucose by means of glucagon-stimulated gluconeogenesis. In addition, free fatty acids can be used as fuel by the heart, skeletal muscles, and liver.

Just minutes after ingestion of a meal, blood-insulin levels rapidly increase. Dietary glucose and amino acids, such as leucine, isoleucine, and lysine, are potent stimulants of the beta cells of the pancreas, causing them to secrete insulin. Most peripheral cells respond to the rise of blood glucose by rapidly increasing glucose transport into cells. Thus blood glucose levels increase by only 20% to 40% in nondiabetic individuals. However, approximately 80% of the glucose uptake is *not* insulin dependent, since the brain, red blood cells, liver, and intestines do not require insulin for increased glucose uptake in the presence of elevated blood glucose. Muscle is the most important insulin-dependent tissue. Increased blood insulin and glucose levels do inhibit lipolysis as well as approximately 60% of the normal hepatic release of glucose.

Metabolic processes in the diabetic.[7,11] In the diabetic, both the production and metabolism of glucose are increased. Thus, in the fasting state, hepatic glucose release is greatly elevated, causing the diagnostic, fasting hyperglycemia of diabetics.

In addition, both the release of insulin (type I diabetics) and the cellular response to insulin (insulin resistance in type II diabetics, see below) are decreased in diabetics, especially relative to a given blood glucose level. The decreased insulin control causes the diabetic to be in a semi-starvation state, with an increased dependence on triglycerides as a source of fuel and on protein as a source of glucose precursors. Thus, in the fasting state, the diabetic may have increased blood free fatty acids and ketones (see p. 625).

After a meal, the inhibition of hepatic glucose output is much smaller in the diabetic. Combined with both the diminished insulin output and insulin resistance, this results

---

Metabolic Action of Insulin

	Tissue		
	Liver	*Adipose*	*Muscle*
Inhibits:	Glyco-genolysis	Lipolysis	Protein break-down
	Gluconeo-genesis		Amino acid release
	Ketogenesis		
Stimulates:	Glycogen and fatty acid synthesis	Glycerol and fatty acid synthesis	Glucose uptake and metabolism
			Amino acid uptake
			Synthesis of protein
			Glycogenesis

in an abnormal and prolonged rise in blood glucose in diabetics after a meal (see Fig. 32-8).

In summary, the carbohydrate metabolism in a diabetic is strikingly similar to that of a nondiabetic in the fasting state. In both cases metabolism of fatty acids has replaced the metabolism of glucose-6-phosphate as the principal source of energy for the cell.

CLASSIFICATION OF DIABETES MELLITUS

In 1979 the National Diabetes Data Group of the National Institutes of Health (NIH) developed a classification scheme for diabetes mellitus and other types of glucose intolerance based on current knowledge of the biochemistry of this disease.[12] Table 32-1 summarizes the NIH classification system.

Type I diabetes

Type I diabetes, or insulin-dependent diabetes mellitus (IDDM), afflicts more than 2 million Americans. Its prevalence is 1 in 300 persons under 20 years of age, the time when this disease is usually diagnosed. This type of diabetes is caused by insufficient insulin secretion (insulinopenia). Insulin injections are necessary to maintain normal glucose metabolism. Individuals with type I diabetes are especially prone to ketoacidosis. *Ketoacidosis* refers to excessive formation of ketoacids and low blood pH (acidosis). This condition is discussed on p. 625. Other complications of type I diabetes include cataracts, diseases of nerves (neuropathy), kidney disease (nephropathy), and blood vessel diseases (angiopathy).

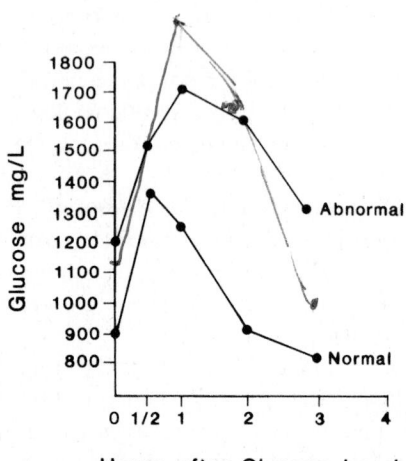

Fig. 32-8 Oral glucose tolerance test (OGTT, see p. 627). Diabetic's response to OGTT is compared to normal response. In diabetics, glucose curve is elevated and delayed. In normal response, peak is reached after 30 minutes and returns to baseline value after 2 hours. Type I diabetics produce a nearly flat insulin curve after glucose load. If there is a peak, it occurs late (greater than 1 hour). In type II diabetics, insulin response is often exaggerated, peak is late, and return to baseline value is later than 3 hours.

Type II diabetes

Type II diabetes, non–insulin-dependent diabetes mellitus (NIDDM), has no correlation with blood insulin levels. Type II diabetes afflicts nearly 10 million Americans. Onset is usually after 40 years of age. The type II individual is usually not dependent on insulin injection, is less prone to ketoacidosis, and is often obese.

Secondary diabetes

Diabetes mellitus caused by other conditions and diseases is called secondary diabetes. Secondary diabetes can be caused by pancreatic disease, acromegaly (growth hormone excess), Cushing's syndrome (elevated cortisol), pheochromocytoma (excessive catecholamines), glucagonoma (excessive glucagon because of a tumor), somatostatinoma (excessive somatostatin because of a tumor), primary aldosteronism, severe liver disease, and administration of certain drugs, hormones, and chemicals.

Impaired glucose tolerance

Impaired glucose tolerance (IGT) includes persons who have had an abnormal glucose tolerance test but no frank hyperglycemia. The oral glucose test is discussed later in this chapter. Estimates of IGT prevalence range from 4.6% to 11.2%.[2]

Gestational diabetes

Gestational diabetes refers to diabetes that occurs temporarily during pregnancy. One study[13] estimates that 39% of women with gestational diabetes manifest type II diabetes mellitus 20 years after delivery. Screening of pregnant women for gestational diabetes, to prevent perinatal complications associated with maternal hyperglycemia, has become a widespread, accepted practice.

PATHOGENESIS OF DIABETES MELLITUS [14]
Epidemiology

Epidemiologists have studied identical twins and offspring and siblings of diabetics.[14,15] These studies demonstrate clearly that diabetes mellitus develops from a complex interaction between environmental and genetic factors. If the development of diabetes were determined by hereditary factors alone, the disease should always afflict both identical twins. Three different studies show that when type I diabetes occurs in one twin its subsequent appearance in the other occurs only about 50% of the time. On the other hand, development of type II diabetes in one twin presages its appearance in the other nearly 100% of the time.

Studies of offspring of type II diabetic parents show that diabetes is transmitted to offspring at a frequency of only 6% to 10%. The prevalence of type II diabetes in the general American population is estimated at about 2%. However, a propensity to diabetes exists in the offspring since 25% to 40% of them have abnormal glucose tolerance test results. Similar results have been obtained using siblings of diabetics as subjects.

Table 32-1 NIH classification of diabetes and other categories of glucose intolerance

Class	Description

Type I diabetes mellitus (insulin-dependent diabetes mellitus [IDDM])	Deficiency of insulin (insulinopenia)
	 Dependence on injected insulin
	 Usually occurs below 40 years of age
	 Prone to ketoacidosis
	 Prone to diabetic complications:
	     Cataracts (6 times greater than in nondiabetics)
	     Neuropathy (all show some symptoms; 10% serious)
	     Nephropathy (40%-50% develop renal failure)
	     Angiopathy (high risk for heart attack and stroke)

Type II diabetes mellitus (non–insulin-dependent diabetes mellitus [NIDDM])	Variable levels of insulin Not dependent on exogenous insulin for control of hyperglycemia; often obese individuals Usually occurs after 40 years of age Not prone to ketoacidosis Not prone to diabetic complications
Secondary diabetes mellitus	Diabetes caused by various secondary conditions such as pancreatic disease, acromegaly, Cushing's syndrome, pheochromocytoma, glucagonoma, somatostatinoma, primary aldosteronism, severe liver disease, and certain drugs, chemicals, and hormones
Impaired glucose tolerance	Persons with plasma glucose levels intermediate between upper limit of normal and definitely diabetic levels (1100-1400 mg/L) and persons with an abnormal glucose tolerance test but no frank hyperglycemia
Gestational diabetes mellitus	Diabetes that occurs during pregnancy
Statistical risk classes; previous abnormality of glucose tolerance	Previous transient hyperglycemia that occurred either spontaneously or in response to specific stimuli but presently testing normally
Potential abnormality of glucose tolerance	Persons not presently exhibiting any indications of diabetes but at substantially increased risk to develop diabetes in the future; includes monozygotic twin of an NIDDM diabetic; person who has parent, sibling, or offspring who is NIDDM diabetic; obese individuals; members of certain racial or ethnic groups with a high prevalence of diabetes

The principal conclusions derived from these studies are as follows:

1. Offspring and siblings of diabetics are more likely to develop diabetes than those of nondiabetics.
2. The offspring of two diabetics is more likely to develop diabetes than an offspring having only one diabetic parent.
3. The lower-than-expected frequencies of diabetes in identical twins and offspring and siblings of diabetics are suggestive of the importance of environmental factors in the expression of the genetic component for diabetes.
4. A second event occurring early in life is postulated to trigger type I diabetes in genetically susceptible individuals. This event is likely to be a viral infection or a disturbance in the immune system. Type II diabetes occurs without such an event though its expression is modulated by factors such as obesity.
5. Diabetes is generally transmitted true to type. For example, diabetic siblings and offspring of type I diabetics are usually type I diabetics.
6. Inheritance plays a more important role in development of type II diabetes than type I diabetes.

Human leukocyte antigens and diabetes mellitus

Inherited susceptibility or resistance to type I diabetes mellitus is supported by studies that associate the production of specific human leukocyte antigens (HLAs) to the occurrence of the disease. HLAs are dimeric proteins produced by the major histocompatibility complex on chromosome 6. The *class II* HLA loci so far identified with susceptibility to type I diabetes are DP, DQ, and DR. HLAs DR3 or DR4, or both types, occur in 90% of type I diabetics. Resistance to type I diabetes is associated with DR2.[16] Recently it was determined that susceptibility to type I diabetes was greater when DR4 protein was produced in conjunction with a protein produced by the DQ locus, called DQw3.2.

The DQw3.2 allele has a gene frequency of 35.7% in type I diabetics as contrasted to 10.1% in nondiabetics. Individuals possessing the DQw3.1 allele are less likely to acquire type I diabetes than their DQw3.2 counterparts.[17] Susceptibility to type I diabetes is further increased when the DQ beta chain lacks aspartic acid at position 57 and has arginine present at position 52 of the DQ alpha chain.[18]

The autoimmune cause for type I diabetes mellitus has been suggested by observations of progressive lymphocyte infiltration of the islet cells of the pancreas with concomitant beta cell destruction and the appearance of antibodies to islet cell components before the manifestation of overt diabetes.

A role for T-cells in diabetes has been implicated by studies in which diabetes was induced in nondiabetic rat and mouse recipients by transfer of CD4 and CD8 T-cells from diabetic animals.[19]

Viruses

Viral infections have long been considered to be initiating factors in the autoimmune cause of type I diabetes. Epidemiological studies report a seasonal incidence for type I diabetes[15,20] and correlate the occurrence of viral infections such as mumps and measles with subsequent development of this type of diabetes.[21,22]

Further evidence for viral infection as a cause of type I diabetes comes from studies with coxsackievirus B4. Direct evidence that this virus causes diabetes in humans is derived from the isolation of coxsackievirus B4 from the pancreas of a child who had developed diabetic ketoacidosis shortly after the onset of a viral infection.[23] The child died of the disease, and autopsy showed extensive beta-cell destruction. Injection of the virus into mice produced diabetes. Since the coxsackievirus B4 reports, mumps virus, coxsackievirus B1, and rubella reovirus type 3 have been implicated in the transmission of type I diabetes.[24]

Receptor site defects

Insulin receptor proteins. Insulin binds reversibly to sites on cell membranes. Insulin-binding sites (called receptor sites) are found only on certain cell types (liver cells, monocytes, adipocytes, and muscle). The insulin receptor site is composed of two glycoprotein molecules.[25] One subunit is a tyrosine-specific protein kinase.[26] Insulin binding to the receptor site triggers a chain of events resulting in an increase of cell membrane permeability to glucose and amino acids, alteration of enzyme activities, and promotion of protein biosynthesis.

Insulin resistance. In type II diabetes, hyperglycemia is often associated with *hyper*insulinemia. This is in strong contrast to type I diabetes, in which hyperglycemia is always associated with insulin *deficiency*. In fact, whereas type I diabetics depend on insulin to maintain normal blood glucose, type II diabetics respond to relatively high doses of insulin with only small reductions in circulating glucose levels. Type II diabetics are said to be insulin resistant. Although cellular uptake of glucose does increase in response to a glucose load in type II diabetes, it is low relative to both the blood glucose and insulin levels. Insulin resistance in type II diabetes is directly related to a decreased number of insulin receptors.[27] Diabetes caused by decreased numbers of insulin-receptor sites is called *type A diabetes*. Type A diabetes occurs in obese persons. Obese individuals show a significant increase in the numbers of insulin-binding sites and a decrease in symptoms of diabetes when placed on a low-carbohydrate diet.[28] Type A diabetes in obese persons may derive directly from a high-carbohydrate diet rather than obesity per se.

Antibodies to receptor. The presence of circulating antibodies to the insulin receptor has also been reported.[25] Type II diabetes caused by such antibodies to insulin receptor sites is called *type B diabetes*. Type B diabetics usually have symptoms of autoimmune disorders such as antinuclear antibodies, arthralgia, and enlargement of the parotid gland. Type B diabetes has a lower incidence than type A.

Impaired glucose transport. Glucose transport is reduced in both type I and type II diabetics because of significantly reduced levels of the high K_m glucose transport protein, GluT-2.[29] The underlying defect appears to be an underexpression of the mRNA for GluT-2. The effect of this transport abnormality is a reduction in the insulin response to elevated glucose levels. This further aggravates the diabetic condition.

Summary

It is likely that type I diabetes mellitus is most commonly caused by destruction of islet cells resulting from an autoimmune response to viral infection, whereas most cases of type II diabetes are caused by receptor site defects that either reduce the numbers of insulin-binding sites or affect events after insulin binding. Other causes of diabetes described in this section are probably rare ($<10\%$).

COMPLICATIONS OF DIABETES MELLITUS[15,30]

The principal complications of diabetes mellitus are retinopathy, neuropathy, angiopathy, nephropathy, susceptibility to infection, hyperlipidemia, ketoacidosis, and hyperglycemic hyperosmolar nonketotic coma (HHNC). With the single exception of HHNC, these diabetic complications occur more frequently for type I diabetics than for type II diabetics.

Retinopathy

Opaque areas in the lens of the eye are called *cataracts*. Cataract formation is the principal retinopathy of diabetes. Retinopathy is also caused by proliferation of small blood vessels in the lens.

Neuropathy[31]

Neuropathy is the most common complication of diabetes mellitus. It is apparent in about 25% of diabetics and is recognized by a variety of symptoms that include pain, numbness, tingling or burning sensations in extremities, dizziness, and double vision. These symptoms are caused by decreased motor and sensory nerve conduction velocities caused by axonal degeneration and demyelination. Secondary manifestations of neuropathy include cardiac failure, excessive sweating, and male impotence.

Angiopathy

Angiopathy refers to damage to linings (basement membranes) of blood vessels. Angiopathy increases the risk of coronary heart disease and stroke and can lead to retinopathy and nephropathy.

Nephropathy

Nephropathy refers to damage to the glomerulus (filtering apparatus of the nephron) and capillaries associated with the glomerulus. Capillary damage is caused by angiopathy. The result is a reduction in the filtering capability of the kidneys. Proteinuria is often the first sign of diabetic nephropathy. Approximately 25% to 30% of individuals treated for end-stage renal failure are diabetics.

Infection

Diabetics are highly susceptible to infection, ulceration, and gangrene (especially in the extremities). Skin disorders are also more common in diabetics than in nondiabetics.

Hyperlipidemia and atherosclerosis

High triglyceride and cholesterol levels are often associated with type II diabetes.[32] Increased levels of very-low-density lipoprotein (VLDL) have been reported for type II diabetics.[33] High-density lipoprotein (HDL) has been reported to be significantly lower in diabetics than in nondiabetics.[34] These results are consistent with the higher incidence of coronary heart disease in diabetics and a poor survival rate for diabetics with myocardial infarction.[3]

Diabetic ketoacidosis (DKA)

Keto acid metabolism. As shown in Fig. 32-9, acetyl coenzyme A (acetyl CoA) is at the crossroads of glucose, protein, and lipid metabolism. It either enters the tricarboxylic acid cycle or is metabolized to 3-hydroxy-3-methylglutaryl coenzyme A (HMG CoA). HMG CoA can be metabolized to cholesterol, or it can be converted to acetoacetate. Acetoacetate has two possible fates, spontaneous decarboxylation to acetone (in the lungs) or enzymatic reduction to beta-hydroxybutyrate. Acetoacetate and beta-hydroxybutyrate are commonly called *ketoacids,* or *ketone bodies.* Ketoacids are normally a source of energy for the brain, kidneys, and cardiac muscle. A considerable quantity of acetoacetate and beta-hydroxybutyrate is excreted by the kidneys with concomitant loss of sodium and potassium. Kidney excretion of sodium and potassium results in the retention of hydrogen ions.

Ketoacids and insulin. In nondiabetics ketoacid formation is a minor pathway. In type I diabetics insulinopenia causes fat cells to mobilize fatty acids from triglycerides. Fatty acid degradation increases as it becomes the major source of energy for the cell. Increased fatty acid catabolism produces excessive quantities of acetyl CoA. Although

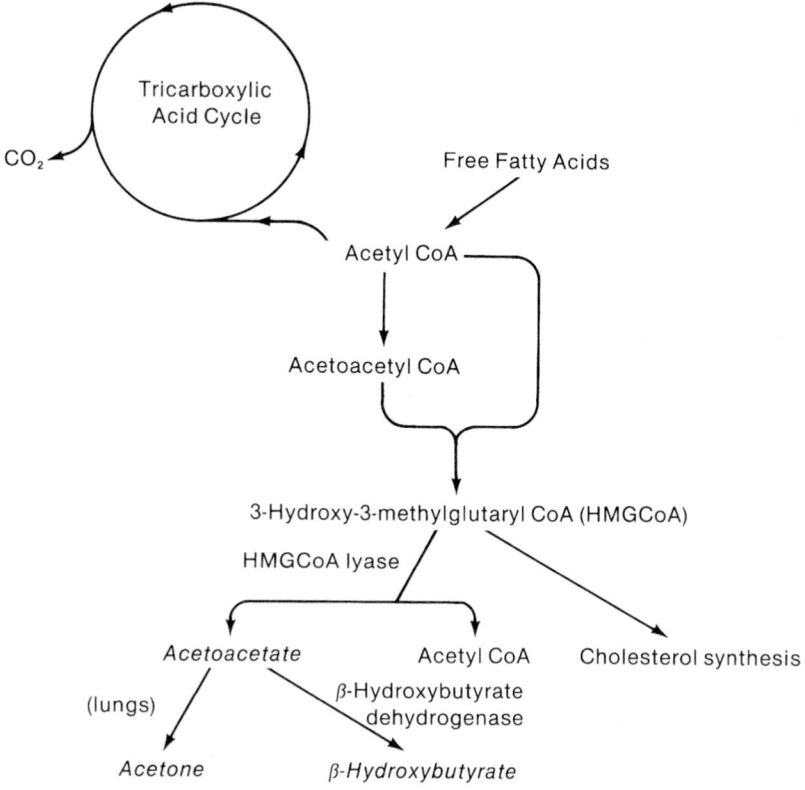

Fig. 32-9 Pathways involved in keto acid metabolism. Accumulation of keto acids, acetoacetate, and beta-hydroxybutyrate is a principal feature of diabetic ketoacidosis. Metabolic pathway leading from acetyl CoA to acetoacetate and beta-hydroxybutyrate is accelerated in diabetes because of free fatty acid mobilization.

a significant portion of the acetyl CoA is able to enter the tricarboxylic acid cycle to produce energy, an excess quantity of acetyl CoA is metabolized to produce abnormal levels of keto acids (ketosis). Increased production of keto acids consumes bicarbonate and thereby lowers blood pH (acidosis). This same metabolic pattern occurs in starvation except that hypoglycemia is present instead of hyperglycemia.

Diagnosis of ketoacidosis. Blood gases and blood glucose are useful in detecting diabetic ketoacidosis. Low pH, normal Pco_2, low bicarbonate, high anion gap, and high glucose are suggestive of uncompensated ketoacidosis. Low pH, low Pco_2, low bicarbonate, a high anion gap, and high glucose are suggestive of partially compensated diabetic ketoacidosis. The elevated anion gap is caused by the accumulation of keto acids (sodium salts).

Lactic acidosis. Lactic acidosis is caused by the accumulation of lactic acid resulting from tissue hypoxia (oxygen deficiency). Like the accumulation of keto acids, lactate accumulation causes increased blood hydrogen ions and therefore low pH. In the diabetic, lactic acidosis often occurs simultaneously with diabetic ketoacidosis, especially if the pH falls below 7.10, if renal insufficiency occurs, or if certain hypoglycemic agents such as phenformin (DBI) are administered.

Hyperglycemic, hyperosmolar nonketotic coma

Hyperglycemic, hyperosmolar nonketotic coma (HHNC) has been reported with increasing frequency over the past few years. It is characterized by a blood glucose level above 6000 mg/L, normal or slightly low blood pH, serum osmolality above 350 mOsm/kg, normal ketoacid levels, and lethargy or coma. Although diabetic ketoacidosis occurs primarily in type I diabetics, HHNC occurs primarily in type II diabetics. The absence of keto acids in HHNC is probably caused by the differential sensitivity of lipid and glucose metabolism to insulin. Lipolysis is inhibited by one tenth the insulin level that is required to enhance glucose metabolism.[35] In type I diabetics, insulinopenia enhances lipolysis with resulting accumulation of ketoacids and glucose utilization is blocked, resulting in hyperglycemia. In type II diabetics, although insulin resistance occurs, there is sufficient insulin activity to limit lipolysis and thus keto acid production but insufficient insulin activity to avoid hyperglycemia. HHNC is often brought on by stressful events and major illness.

Hypoglycemia

Hypoglycemia causes numerous neurogenic problems, ranging from the mild to severe coma, seizures, and death. The level of blood glucose when symptoms become obvious varies but will tend to be <500 mg/L for adults and <400 mg/L for newborns. This potentially life-threatening disorder is most often the result of treatment of hyperglycemia with insulin, usually because of mismanagement. However, aggressive use of insulin treatment to maintain normoglycemia can greatly increase this risk of hypoglycemia.[36]

There are several other causes of hypoglycemia[37] that are listed in the following box. Many of these are detected in emergency room cases as coma, treatable simply with intravenous glucose. Differential diagnosis may require measurement of blood glucose, insulin, and C-peptide. C-peptide is important in diagnosing surreptitious or overzealous insulin treatment because commercial insulin preparations contain no C-peptide.[38] In these cases, although blood insulin levels are elevated, C-peptide levels are low. Production of autoantibodies against insulin can also result in a similar pattern, though these cases are often associated with postprandial hyperglycemia.

The risk for hypoglycemia is increased for hospitalized patients. This risk is often unrelated to diabetes but is associated with advanced liver disease, renal insufficiency, and malnutrition. Such severely ill patients will have increased mortality.

Other complications of diabetes

The acutely ill diabetic, with ketoacidosis or hyperosmolar coma, is at risk for immediately life-threatening complications. The hypovolemia associated with these acute illnesses can result in shock and renal failure. Cerebral edema may arise in patients with ketoacidosis and hyperosmolar coma as a result of insulin and fluid administration. Loss of salts usually occurs in DKA and HHNC. Although patients' serum electrolytes may be elevated, normal, or low, they usually have a deficit of body potassium.

Effect of diabetes on the fetus. The fetus of a pregnant diabetic is at increased risks for adverse complications directly resulting from hyperglycemia. These include spontaneous abortion,[39] birth defects, and macrosomia.[40] The risk for these complications is directly related to the degree of maternal hyperglycemia and can be reduced if greater

---

Causes of Fasting Hypoglycemia

Depressed blood insulin/decreased glucose production
  Liver disease
  Alcoholism
  Renal insufficiency
  Galactosemia and glycogen storage disease
Malignancy (increases consumption of glucose or production of insulin-like growth factor)
Infection
Late pregnancy
Malnutrition
Overtreatment with insulin
  Insulinoma
  Factitious (exogenous) treatment with insulin
  Treatment with sulfonylurea drugs
  Anti-insulin antibodies

glycemic control is enforced, especially during the early weeks of pregnancy.[39,40]

PATHOGENESIS OF DIABETIC COMPLICATIONS
Protein glycosylation

Nonenzymatic protein glycosylation commonly occurs in red blood cells, glomeruli, and nerve cells as well as in other tissues. The extent of the glucosylation is proportional to extracellular glucose concentrations. Such glycosylation occurs by the mechanism shown for the glucosylation of hemoglobin (see p. 630). The carbonyl functional groups of glucose and other sugars react with free amino groups of proteins to form intermediates called *Schiff bases,* or *aldimines.* The amino group that reacts is either an N-terminal amino group or a lysine epsilon–amino group. The aldimine subsequently rearranges to form a ketamine. This rearrangement is called the Amadori rearrangement. The aldimine is labile; it can readily hydrolyze to re-form a free amino group and a carbonyl group. The ketamine is relatively stable, and its formation is not reversible.

Excessive glycosylation is known to produce significant alterations in a protein's physical and biochemical properties. For example, glycosylation of alpha-crystallin, a protein occurring in the lens of the eye, greatly reduces its solubility. Hyperglycemia in rats has been shown to increase alpha-crystallin glycosylation simultaneously with cataract formation.[41] Glycosylation of the basement membrane of blood vessels is known to cause basement membrane thickening similar to that found in most if not all diabetics.[42] Functional alterations of immunoglobulin G (IgG) by nonenzymatic glycosylation have been reported[43] to be associated with increased susceptibility to infection.

Based on these and other findings, a hypothesis has been proposed stating that many of the complications of diabetes are caused by glycosylation of specific proteins such as alpha-crystallin, IgG, and basement membrane protein, which impairs their function and results in disease such as diabetic nephropathy.[41-43]

Sorbitol accumulation

The intracellular accumulation of sorbitol is the basis for another hypothesis designed to explain diabetic complications.[44] Aldose reductase reduces glucose to sorbitol, which in turn is oxidized to fructose by sorbitol dehydrogenase. Sorbitol does not easily cross cell membranes. The removal of sorbitol from the cell depends on its conversion to fructose, which does pass freely through the cell membrane. However, when glucose levels are high, the quantities of sorbitol produced outstrip the cell's ability to convert sorbitol to fructose, resulting in the intracellular accumulation of sorbitol. Intracellular accumulation of ketones, glucose, and sorbitol causes osmotic swelling and injury to cell structures. Only cells that do not depend on insulin for glucose transport across the plasma membrane are affected. These cells include nerve, ocular lens, and glomerulus cells. This osmotic effect is the cause of life-threatening cerebral edema that can occur during treatment for DKA and HHNC. The decreased blood osmolality after treatment can increase the shift of extracellular water into brain cells. Supporting this hypothesis are reports of elevations in sorbitol and fructose levels in the nerve and ocular lens cells of diabetics. The strongest support for this hypothesis is derived from studies utilizing aldose reductase inhibitors. The aldose reductase inhibitors sorbinol and tolrestat are reported to improve nerve conduction in diabetic rats[45] and diabetic humans.

FUNCTION TESTS
Postprandial plasma glucose

Diabetes is more readily detected when the carbohydrate metabolic capacity is tested. One can do this by stressing the system with a defined glucose load. Measurement of the rate that the glucose load is cleared from the blood, as compared to the rate of glucose clearance in healthy persons, detects impairment in glucose metabolism. A meal high in carbohydrates is often used as the carbohydrate load, though a 75 g glucose drink is usually preferred over a meal. It is called the *postprandial test.*

Blood is drawn at 2 hours after ingestion of the meal or glucose drink. Glucose levels above 1400 mg/L are abnormal; levels of 1200 to 1400 mg/L are ambiguous; and levels below 1200 mg/L are normal. The postprandial glucose test, though widely used for detection of diabetes, is highly inaccurate because of several variables that are difficult to control or adjust for. These variables include age, weight, previous diet, activity, illness, medications, time of day that the test is conducted, and actual size of the glucose dose. When a meal is used as the load, the effective glucose load depends on the digestion of disaccharides and polysaccharides and their subsequent absorption from the intestinal tract.

O'Sullivan test

The O'Sullivan test is frequently used to detect gestational diabetes. A 50 g load of glucose is given to a fasting patient. Blood is drawn at 1 hour. Gestational diabetes is suggested by plasma glucose levels above 1500 mg/L (above 1300 mg/L for whole blood).

Oral glucose tolerance test

The oral glucose tolerance test (OGTT) evaluates glucose clearance from the circulation after glucose loading under defined and controlled conditions. The test has been standardized by the Committee on Statistics of the American Diabetes Association.[46]

Standard conditions call for a minimum carbohydrate intake of 150 g/day for 3 days before the test. Daily carbohydrate intake less than this lowers carbohydrate intolerance. There should be an 8- to 16-hour fast before testing. The patient must be ambulatory, since inactivity decreases

Table 32-2 Comparison of four criteria for evaluation of oral glucose tolerance test

| Time of blood drawing (hours) | Plasma glucose levels (mg/L) | | | |
	Wilkerson Point system	Fajans-Conn system	WHO	UGDP
Fasting	>1290 (1)*	—	>1390	Sum
1	>1940 (½)*	>1840	—	Sum
1½	—	>1640	—	—
2	>1390 (½)*	>1390	1400-2000 (IGT) >2000 (diabetes)	Sum
3	>1290 (½)*		—	Sum

UGDP, University Group Diabetes Program; *WHO,* World Health Organization.
*Points given in Wilkerson Point system.

glucose tolerance. However, exercise and emotional stress should be avoided.

Illness reduces glucose tolerance. Abnormalities of such hormones as thyroxine, growth hormone, cortisol, and catecholamines interfere. Drugs and medications such as oral contraceptives, salicylates, nicotinic acid (found in cigarettes, cigars, pipe tobacco, chewing tobacco), diuretics (including caffeine), and hypoglycemic agents (insulin, sulfonylureas) interfere. Testing time affects the test. The best time to conduct the test is between 7 AM and noon. Evaluation criteria should also be adjusted for age. If adjustments for age are not made, about 80% of persons over 60 years of age will be judged diabetic.[47]

The glucose load should consist of glucose only. Some commercial preparations labeled "100 grams glucose equivalent" contain disaccharides and polysaccharides. The rate that these saccharides are hydrolyzed and absorbed from the intestinal tract varies from person to person. Such a preparation is obviously not desirable for individuals with pancreatic or malabsorptive disorders. The size of the load is 40 g of glucose per square meter of body area. For most subjects 75 g of total glucose is sufficient. The drink can be flavored if caffeine or theophylline is not used.

Blood samples are drawn at fasting and 1, 2, and 3 hours after ingestion of glucose. Additional samples at ½, 1½, and 2½ hours after glucose ingestion are helpful and sometimes necessary for evaluation of the test.

The OGTT is commonly evaluated by several alternative scoring systems. All use criteria based on the glucose oxidase method for plasma glucose quantification. Plasma glucose values are converted to whole blood values by use of the following equation:

Glucose (whole blood, in mg/L) =
$\qquad$ Glucose (plasma, in mg/L) × 1.15 + 6 mg/L

The criteria for the Wilkerson Point system, the Fajans-Conn system, the University Group Diabetes Program (UGDP), and the World Health Organization (WHO) appear in Table 32-2.[48]

The *Wilkerson Point system* uses points as indicated by numbers in parentheses in Table 32-2. Two points or greater is a value suggestive of diabetes mellitus. A uniform dose

of 100 g of glucose is used. The *Fajans-Conn system* allows one to judge an individual diabetic if two or more criteria (Table 32-2) are exceeded. A dose of glucose based on 40 g of glucose per square meter of body surface area is employed. The WHO system suggests impaired glucose tolerance or diabetes when both fasting and 2-hour plasma glucose levels exceed 1390 mg/L (Table 32-2). When the 2-hour value is 1400 to 2000 mg/L, IGT is suggested. When the 2-hour value exceeds 2000 mg/L, diabetes mellitus is suggested. UGDP evaluates the oral glucose tolerance test by summing the fasting, 1-, 2-, and 3-hour plasma glucose values (Table 32-2). A sum exceeding 5990 mg/L is suggestive of diabetes mellitus. A glucose load of 30 g per square meter of body surface area is employed.

The National Diabetes Data Group[12] suggests administering the OGTT only to adults with fasting plasma glucose values less than 1400 mg/L. Virtually all persons with a fasting plasma glucose value greater than 1400 mg/L on more than one occasion will exhibit an abnormal OGTT. For nonpregnant adults, a glucose load of 75 g is recommended. In pregnancy, the dose is increased to 100 g. For children the dose is 1.75 g/kg of ideal body weight up to a maximum of 75 g. Blood samples are drawn while the patient is fasting and at 30-minute intervals after ingestion of the glucose dose for 2 hours, except in pregnancy, where a 3-hour sample is also drawn. IGT is indicated in nonpregnant adults by a 2-hour plasma glucose level between 1400 and 2000 mg/L and at least one other value greater than 2000 mg/L. Diabetes mellitus is indicated in nonpregnant adults by a 2-hour plasma glucose level and at least one other value of greater than 2000 mg/L. IGT is indicated in children by a 2-hour plasma glucose level between 1400 and 2000 mg/L. Diabetes mellitus is indicated in children by a fasting plasma glucose level of greater than 1400 mg/L, a 2-hour level greater than 2000 mg/L, and at least one other value greater than 2000 mg/L. Gestational diabetes is indicated when two or more of the following criteria are exceeded: 1-hour value greater than 1900 mg/L, 2-hour value greater than 1650 mg/L, and 3-hour value greater than 1400 mg/L.

The shape of the glucose tolerance curve is useful in evaluating OGTT (see Fig. 32-8). Healthy subjects peak at ½ hour and return to fasting levels at 2 hours. Diabetics peak late (approximately 1 hour) or even show a plateau at 2 to 3 hours and return to baseline value after 3 hours.

Insulin determinations performed along with glucose determinations are useful in evaluating the OGTT. Plasma insulin levels after a glucose load differentiate type I from type II diabetes. In nondiabetics, insulin levels peak 1 hour after a glucose load and return to fasting levels at 2 to 3 hours. Type I diabetics respond to a glucose load with little or no insulin increases above fasting levels. Type II diabetics respond to the challenge with an abnormally late and often excessive increase in insulin levels. Type I diabetics often have low fasting insulin levels. Type II diabetics have variable fasting insulin levels.

The OGTT has been criticized.[49,50] Since many of the variables affecting test results are difficult to control, the reproducibility of the test is poor. Different evaluation schemes for the same OGTT often produce different interpretations. In general, the test tends to greatly overdiagnose diabetes. One group of investigators suggests a more conservative evaluation scheme in which glucose levels must exceed 2590 mg/L at 1 hour and 2190 mg/L at 2 hours for the OGTT to be considered abnormal.[51] Others have suggested adding 95 mg/L to the 1-hour glucose value and 53 mg/L to the 2-hour value for each decade after 40 years of age. Nevertheless, it has been estimated that only 1% to 5% of individuals with one abnormal OGTT will become diabetics per year.[50] The OGTT is best used to assess individuals who have borderline fasting glucose levels or who are at risk for the development of diabetes and to distinguish type I from type II diabetes.

Intravenous glucose tolerance test

The intravenous glucose tolerance test is often used for persons with malabsorptive disorders or previous gastric or intestinal surgery. Glucose is administered intravenously over 30 minutes, using a 20% solution. A glucose load of 0.5 g/kg of body weight is used. Nondiabetics respond with a plasma glucose level of 2000 to 2500 mg/L. Discontinuation of the glucose loading leads to a decrease in plasma glucose levels with fasting levels reached at about 90 minutes. Diabetics demonstrate plasma glucose levels above 2500 mg/L during administration of the load. On discontinuation of the loading, plasma glucose levels of diabetics also return to fasting levels at about 90 minutes. An alternative procedure called the Soskin method uses 50% glucose delivered intravenously within 3 to 5 minutes. The glucose load used is 0.3 g/kg of body weight. Nondiabetics reestablish fasting levels less than 60 minutes after discontinuing the glucose infusion. In diabetics fasting levels are reestablished significantly later than 60 minutes.

CHANGE OF ANALYTE IN DISEASE

The following is a summary of analyte changes in diabetes mellitus. For each analyte, levels in controlled diabetes, diabetic ketoacidosis, and HHNC are compared.

Conditions and Diseases that Often Cause Both Hyperglycemia and Glucosuria or Glycosuria in Absence of Hyperglycemia

Hyperglycemia and glucosuria

Septicemia	Hypercortisolism
Pancreatic cancer	Glucagonoma
Acute pancreatitis	Somatostatinoma
Pheochromocytoma	Primary aldosteronism
Hyperthyroidism	Acute myocardial infarction
Acromegaly	Cerebral hemorrhage

Glucosuria and normal plasma glucose

Pregnancy (renal threshold is reduced)
Vitamin D–resistant rickets
Osteomalacia (proximal tubular malfunction)
Hepatolenticular degeneration

Fasting plasma glucose (see methods, p. 634)

Fasting plasma glucose and urinary glucose are the most commonly used markers for diabetes mellitus. In general, repeated fasting plasma glucose levels exceeding 1400 mg/L are strongly suggestive of diabetes, provided that drugs such as glucocorticoids are not being administered and diseases and conditions such as those listed in the box are not present. Repeated plasma glucose levels of 1150 to 1400 mg/L may indicate the presence of diabetes.

Fasting plasma glucose is directly proportional to the severity of diabetes mellitus. Levels above 1800 mg/L may produce glucosuria. Ketoacidosis can occur at almost any level above 1400 mg/L but is more common at levels above 1800 mg/L. HHNC is associated with glucose levels above 6000 mg/L.

Diabetics who are under control exhibit wide variations in their plasma glucose concentrations. Plasma glucose levels in controlled diabetics range during a typical 24-hour period from as low as 250 mg/L to as high as 3250 mg/L. These variations are considerably wider than those of nondiabetics.[52] Wide swings in plasma glucose contribute to the development of diabetic complications. Management of insulin therapy remains a significant challenge for the physician. Excessive quantities of insulin cause insulin-induced hypoglycemia, which often leads to coma. On the other hand, inadequate control of glucose levels causes diabetic complications such as those described earlier. Generally, fasting plasma glucose in diabetics is maintained at normal or slightly above normal concentrations.

Urinary glucose

Urinary glucose is a poor marker for diabetes mellitus. The normal renal threshold for glucose is 1800 mg/L. Blood glucose levels must exceed this value before excessive glucose is apparent in the urine. Further complicating this picture is the fact that the renal threshold in diabetics is often increased to above 3000 mg/L. Some diseases and conditions that produce both hyperglycemia and glucosuria are listed in the preceding box. This box also lists conditions that cause glucosuria in the absence of hyperglycemia.

Self- and bedside monitoring of blood glucose

The goal of therapy for diabetics is to maintain normal levels of glucose so as to minimize the acute and long-term complications of the disease. Aggressive therapy to achieve this goal has the primary side effect of an increased risk for hypoglycemia (see above). However, close monitoring of blood glucose levels has been aided by the development of increasingly accurate and reliable bedside glucose monitors (see Chapter 17). In a consensus statement on blood glucose monitoring, many insulin-treated populations have been recommended for self-monitoring programs.[53] These include pregnant women; patients with unstable diabetes; patients with histories of severe ketosis or hypoglycemia, especially those who do not demonstrate warning symptoms of hypoglycemia; patients receiving intensive insulin therapy; and patients with abnormal renal thresholds for glucose.

The consensus panel also had important recommendations on the blood-glucose monitoring devices, which are widely employed in hospitals for bedside monitoring and control of blood glucose levels. The correct use of such devices (see the methods, p. 319) should minimize the wide variations of blood glucose experienced by diabetics and, as a result, the hypoglycemic events and even the long-term complications of diabetes.

Glucosylated hemoglobin and plasma albumin

A minor hemoglobin derivative called Hb A_{1c} is produced by glucosylation. Since this reaction is nonenzymatic and since the red cell is completely permeable to glucose, the quantity of Hb A_{1c} formed is directly proportional to the average plasma glucose concentration that the red blood cell is exposed to during its 120-day life span, that is, the 4 to 6 weeks before sampling. Thus, in long-term hyperglycemia, Hb A_{1c} constitutes a higher percentage of total hemoglobin than in normoglycemia. Transient elevations in plasma glucose only mildly affect Hb A_{1c} levels.

Hb A_1 actually consists of four principal components, called Hb A_{1a_1}, Hb A_{1a_2}, Hb A_{1b}, and Hb A_{1c}.[54] As seen in Table 32-3, each consists of two components, a labile component, which is actually the aldimine, and a stable component, which is actually the ketamine. For normoglycemic persons, Hb A_{1a_1}, Hb A_{1a_2}, and Hb A_{1b} constitute 0.4% to 0.8% of the total hemoglobin. Hb A_{1c} constitutes 4% to 5% of total hemoglobin. Total Hb A_1 is normally 5.0% to 7.0% (see the methods, p. 635, Table 32-8). As shown in Table 32-3, diabetics have total Hb A_1 and Hb A_{1c} percentages that are significantly elevated. The elevations are directly

Table 32-3 Components of glycosylated hemoglobin in diabetics and nondiabetics

Glycosylated hemoglobin fraction	Percent of total hemoglobin	
	Nondiabetics	Diabetics
A_{1a_1} (labile + stable)	0.19 ±0.02	0.20 ±0.03
A_{1a_2} (labile + stable)	0.19 ±0.4	0.22 ±0.04
A_{1b} (labile + stable)	0.48 ±0.15	0.67 ±0.3
A_{1c} (by high-performance liquid chromatography)		
Labile + Stable	3.3 ±0.3	7.5 ±2.0
Labile	3.2	6.9
Stable	96.8	93.1

proportional to the long-term degree of hyperglycemia.[55] Glycosylated hemoglobins are most useful for monitoring of diabetes; they are not sufficiently sensitive to effectively detect borderline cases of diabetes mellitus.[56]

As stated above, serum albumin is also glucosylated to a degree proportional to plasma glucose levels. The relatively short half-life for albumin of 15 days makes it a good monitor of short-term blood plasma glucose levels.[57]

Insulin (see methods, p. 637)

Fasting plasma insulin levels in type I diabetics are usually low. Those of type II diabetics are low only when fasting plasma glucose levels exceed 2500 mg/L. Otherwise, they are normal.[58] A glucose challenge separates type I diabetics from type II diabetics. Glucose loading elicits no significant insulin response for type I diabetics and a delayed, often exaggerated response in type II diabetics.

Keto acids (see methods, p. 632)

Significant elevations of acetoacetate and beta-hydroxybutyrate cause diabetic ketoacidosis. It is important to measure both blood and urinary keto acid levels, since plasma keto acid levels can be normal even though urinary keto acid concentrations are high. This effect is caused by increased urinary keto acid excretion resulting from renal compensation to low pH. Both ketonemia and ketonuria are absent in HHNC. Controlled diabetics should have both normal plasma and normal urinary keto acid levels.

The nitroprusside test (commonly known as Acetest) is useful for the detection of acetoacetic acid (AcAc) in the blood or urine (see p. 632). Nitroprusside does not react with beta-hydroxybutyrate (β-HBA) and reacts only weakly (20%) with acetone. In the early stages of diabetic ketoacidosis, acetoacetate levels are often normal (AcAc:β-HBA, 1:3) or only mildly elevated. In later stages of ketoacidosis beta-hydroxybutyrate levels are highly elevated (AcAc:β-HBA, 1:30). Under these conditions the nitroprusside test can significantly produce an underestimate of the severity of the ketoacidosis. As the ketoacidosis becomes controlled, the beta-hydroxybutyrate is metabolized to acetoacetic acid, and the nitroprusside test can become strongly positive.

Urinary protein

One of the earliest signs of impending glomerular nephropathy is the increased excretion of albumin in the urine, also termed *microalbuminuria*. It has been suggested that diabetics be routinely monitored for microalbuminuria (see p. 492), and so this complication of diabetes can be treated early and prevented.

Lactic acid (see p. 481)

Plasma lactic acid levels are frequently elevated (lactic acidosis) during diabetic ketoacidosis.

Hydrogen ion (pH)

High plasma hydrogen-ion concentrations (low pH) occur in diabetic ketoacidosis, ketoacidosis with lactic acidosis, and HHNC. pH levels below 7.00 are associated with a poor prognosis.

Electrolytes

Uncontrolled diabetics can exhibit normal, low, or high plasma sodium levels. Plasma sodium levels in diabetics are influenced by three factors, described next.

Hyperglycemia causes an increase in the osmotic pressure of plasma. As a result water flows from cells to plasma. Plasma substituents are thereby diluted. Thus hyponatremia (low plasma sodium) is common in diabetes. In diabetic ketoacidosis excessive quantities of sodium are excreted in the urine, further lowering plasma sodium levels. However, complicating matters is the preferential excretion of water relative to sodium. This effect often compensates for sodium loss from high plasma glucose levels and ketosis, thus resulting in normal or even elevated plasma sodium levels.

The same factors described above affect plasma potassium levels. However, for potassium, two additional factors are operative. First, insulin causes the transport of intracellular potassium to the plasma. Thus hypokalemia (low plasma potassium) occurs in insulin deficiency (type I diabetes). Second, in acidosis, potassium moves out of cells. Thus, in diabetic ketoacidosis, significant quantities of potassium ion are shifted from cells to plasma. This produces hyperkalemia (high plasma potassium). Type II diabetics normally exhibit hypokalemia or normokalemia. However, because of urinary losses of potassium, diabetics in DKA always require potassium replacement and monitoring during therapy.

Plasma bicarbonate levels are normal in controlled diabetes. Ketoacidosis causes low plasma bicarbonate levels. The body responds to ketoacidosis by kidney retention of bicarbonate and rapid, deep respiration called *Kussmaul breathing*, which removes CO_2. Both of these compensatory mechanisms raise pH. Kussmaul breathing lowers the Pco_2. Both plasma bicarbonate and Pco_2 are low in diabetic ketoacidosis.

Osmolality

Serum osmolality is increased in both ketoacidosis and HHNC because of the water loss that accompanies glucose excretion. Serum osmolality in HHNC is usually above 350 mOsm/kg, a hallmark of the condition.

Body fluid volume

Renal loss of water in diabetic ketoacidosis produces severe volume depletion, often as much as 6 to 8 L. Patients with HHNC can have fluid deficits greater than 9 L. Low fluid volume (hypovolemia) often coexists with hyponatremia. Insulin therapy restores both fluid volume and plasma sodium to normal.

Anion gap

In ketoacidosis the anion gap is always increased because of the excessive formation of keto acids. Lactic acidosis further increases the gap because of the high lactate levels.

Blood urea nitrogen (BUN)

BUN levels are increased in both diabetic ketoacidosis and HHNC because of increased protein catabolism and prerenal azotemia secondary to loss of extracellular fluids. Prerenal azotemia refers to increased BUN caused by decreased renal flow. In diabetic ketoacidosis, prerenal azotemia is caused by hypovolemia.

Lipids

Elevated plasma triglyceride, cholesterol, and VLDL are commonly found in diabetics. On the other hand, HDL is usually low.

METHODS OF ANALYSIS

Total ketones, acetoacetic acid, and beta-hydroxybutyric acid
STEVEN C. KAZMIERCZAK

Acetoacetate, acetone, and beta-hydroxybutyric acid are metabolites of fat catabolism that are produced in excess amounts in individuals with insulin-dependent (type I) diabetes and in individuals who metabolize fat stores.[69] Serum ketone bodies include pyruvate, acetoacetate, and acetone and the reduced forms, lactic acid and beta-hydroxybutyric acid. The severity and type of illness can cause substantial variations in the proportion of ketones that are present. This finding and the fact that no current chemical or enzymatic procedure can measure all ketone bodies at one time limit the diagnostic utility of ketones.

Measurement of acetoacetic acid is important for the evaluation of ketosis. Determinations of this compound are performed most frequently for the diagnosis and management of patients with diabetes. Concentrations of acetoacetate are increased in diabetes, starvation, and any stress situation that results in the production of a hyperglycemic state.

Total ketones

STEVEN C. KAZMIERCZAK

Principles of analysis and current usage Several quantitative methods for ketones that are only of historical interest can be found in the second edition of this book. A significant drawback to these procedures is that they measure only acetone, which represents a very small proportion of the total ketone bodies normally present.

The colorimetric reaction that occurs between ketones and nitroprusside (sodium nitroferricyanide) is the most widely used method for the rapid semiquantitative measurement of ketones employed today (Table 32-4, method 1).[59,74] For the semiquantitative assessment of acetoacetic acid and acetone in serum or urine, the color change produced with the reagents embedded in the dipstick is compared with a color chart. Although both acetone as well as acetoacetic acid produce a color change in this reaction, the method is more sensitive to acetoacetic acid (50 to 100 mg/L) than to acetone (200 to 250 mg/L). This assay is commercially available in the form of a dipstick, usually paper impregnated with nitroprusside, glycine, and sodium phosphate (Ames Inc., Division of Miles Laboratories, Elkhart, Indiana). If used for ketones in urine, urine samples with a specific gravity of 1.010 to 1.020 yield the most accurate results. Highly colored urine or hemolyzed serum can cause false-positive results with this method. The dry chemical reagent must be protected from air to prevent deterioration. Methods for stabilizing the nitroprusside color complex include the addition of various buffers, metal salts, and organic stabilizers.

Enzymatic procedures that can measure either acetoacetic acid or beta-hydroxybutyric acid have also been developed (Table 32-4, method 2).[115] The general reaction that is used for the enzymatic determination of these ketones is the following:

$$\text{NADH} + \text{H}^+ + \text{Acetoacetic acid} \xrightleftharpoons[]{\substack{\beta\text{-Hydroxybutyrate} \\ \text{dehydrogenase}}} \beta\text{-Hydroxybutyrate} + \text{NAD}^+$$

When the above reaction is performed at a pH of 8.5 to 9.5, the reaction proceeds to the left. The concentration of β-hydroxybutyric acid can be quantitated by measurement of the increase in absorbance at 340 nm caused by the production of NADH. If the reaction is performed at a pH of 7.0, the reaction proceeds to the right and the amount of acetoacetic acid that is present can be determined by the decrease in absorbance at 340 nm caused by the disappearance of NADH. An advantage of the enzymatic procedures is that they are more specific for ketones as compared to the colorimetric procedures.

Both gas chromatography (GC; Table 32-4, method 3)[115] and HPLC as well[116] have been developed for quantitation of acetone and acetoacetic acid. Acetone can be quantified with use of a flame ionization detector. Acetoacetic acid is estimated by measurement of acetone before and after heating of the sample; heating converts the acetoacetic acid to acetone. Although GC and HPLC are not suitable for "stat." or even routine ketone determinations in most laboratories, the determination of acetone may be beneficial in identifying patients with isopropanol ingestion.[117]

Specimen Urine that has been centrifuged to remove particulates, serum, or plasma may be used for the semiquantitative colorimetric nitroprusside test. For enzymatic ketone assays, serum or plasma may be used.

Loss of ketones attributable to microbial action can cause false-negative test results. Because acetone is a volatile substance, both blood and urine specimens must be kept in a closed container to prevent loss from evaporation. Refrigeration of the specimen can stabilize the sample.

Reference intervals Reference ranges that have been established for acetoacetate in serum are 5 to 30 mg/L (0.09 to 0.52 mmol/L).[118] No age-related differences in ketone bodies have been reported.[119] For the other ketones, reference ranges are less than 10 mg/L (0.1 mmol/L), whereas reference ranges for beta-hydroxybutyrate have been reported to be less than 0.7 mmol/L.[77]

Table 32-4 Methods for ketone analysis

Method	Analyte	Type of analysis	Principle	Usage	Comments
1. Colorimetric	Acetoacetate, acetone	Semi-quantitative	$\text{Na}_2\text{Fe(CN)}_5\text{NO}$ + Acetone/acetoacetate $\rightarrow$ *purple color*	Most common; frequently used as a stat. procedure	Sensitivity for acetoacetate 5 times greater than that for acetone
2. Enzymatic	AcAc, β-HB	Quantitative	$\text{NADH} + \text{H}^+ + \text{AcAc} \xrightleftharpoons[\substack{\text{pH 8.5–9.5}}]{\substack{\text{pH 7.0} \\ \beta\text{-Hydroxybutyrate} \\ \text{dehydrogenase}}} \beta\text{-HB} + \text{NAD}^+$	Rare; not useful as a stat. procedure	Excellent precision; ease of automation; rapid, precise, small sample volume
3. Gas chromatography	Acetone (AcAc, β-HB by calculation)	Quantitative	Acetone is detected by flame ionization detector; AcAc is converted to acetone by heating.	Rare; not useful as stat. test	Acetoacetate quantitated by subtraction of nonheated acetone from heated acetone
4. Capillary electrophoresis	β-HB	Quantitative	Electrophoretic separation of β-HB	Rare	Specialized equipment

AcAc, Acetoacetate; β-HB, beta-hydroxybutyric acid.

Acetoacetic acid
STEVEN C. KAZMIERCZAK

Principles of analysis and current usage   Acetoacetic acid can be measured using a variety of techniques; however, the most common methods in use today are colorimetric assays and enzymatic procedures.

The most frequently performed procedure for acetoacetate is the colorimetric procedure, described above, based on the reaction of acetoacetate with sodium nitroprusside (Table 32-4, method 1).[149] In addition to the dipstick nitroprusside technology, a tablet formulation is also available (Ames Co., Division of Miles Laboratories, Elkhart, Indiana). The serum or urine is placed directly onto the tablet, and any observed color change is recorded. This procedure is more sensitive than the dipstick procedure. Although the dipstick and tablet procedures for the determination of acetoacetic acid are at best semiquantitative, they have the advantages of being rapid and convenient to perform and are readily available 24 hours a day. The nitroprusside reaction is not specific for acetoacetate (see above).

In addition, drugs containing free sulfhydryl groups, such as captopril, *N*-acetylcysteine, and penicillamine, also react with nitroprusside to produce a purplish red color.[60-62] A variety of techniques may be used to recognize false-positive reactions for ketones caused by free sulfhydryl compounds. These include the addition of glacial acetic acid to the reaction pad and the observation that false-positive ketone reactions, caused by free sulfhydryl compounds, result in an instantaneous color development after the addition of sample to the reagent pad, whereas acetoacetic acid results in the development of color that increases in intensity for at least 60 seconds.[63,64] Thus, correct timing is extremely important for correct interpretation of the nitroprusside reaction. The purple color produced in the nitroprusside reaction can also be measured spectrophotometrically at 550 nm for the quantitative assessment of acetoacetate concentrations.[65]

Although precise quantitative measurements of acetoacetate are generally not required clinically, procedures that enable quantitative determinations of acetoacetate to be performed have been developed. The most common method in use for quantitation of acetoacetate concentrations is the enzymatic procedure that utilizes beta-hydroxybutyrate dehydrogenase (Table 32-4, method 2).[66] This assay is based on the reduction of acetoacetate to beta-hydroxybutyrate by the enzyme beta-hydroxybutyrate dehydrogenase with concomitant oxidation of NADH to NAD. The decrease in NADH is measured spectrophotometrically at 340 nm and is related to acetoacetate concentrations present in the sample. Both end-point analysis[66] and kinetic analysis methods have been developed.[67]

Specimen   Serum, plasma, and urine are acceptable specimens. Serum or plasma concentrations of acetoacetate should be measured within 1 hour after phlebotomy, or samples should be kept on ice if analysis is delayed.[68] When kept in an ice bath, samples are stable for up to 6 hours.

Reference interval   Concentrations of acetoacetic acid in the serum of healthy individuals are less than 0.1 mmol/L when measured by use of an enzymatic procedure.

Beta-hydroxybutyric acid
STEVEN C. KAZMIERCZAK

Principles of analysis and current usage   Measurement of beta-hydroxybutyrate is infrequently performed in clinical laboratories; measurement of acetoacetate and acetone is the most common means for rapidly assessing ketoacidosis. However, measurement of beta-hydroxybutyrate can be useful for monitoring purposes in patients with ketoacidosis. In patients with severe acidosis, increased NADH production favors the formation of beta-hydroxybutyrate from acetoacetate, raising the ratio of beta-hydroxybutyrate to acetoacetate (β-HB/AcAc). As the patient is treated for the underlying cause of the ketoacidosis, the β-HB/AcAc ratio will decrease as beta-hydroxybutyrate is oxidized to acetoacetate. This oxidation of beta-hydroxybutyrate to acetoacetate can result in an increase in acetoacetate, even as the patient's condition improves.

Methods developed to measure beta-hydroxybutyrate include colorimetric methods based upon the oxidation of beta-hydroxybutyrate to acetone by acid, with subsequent measurement of the acetone formed.[70] GC measurement of beta-hydroxybutyrate is based upon the initial measurement of endogenous acetone in one aliquot followed by a second measurement performed on another aliquot after the oxidation of beta-hydroxybutyrate to acetone. The beta-hydroxybutyrate concentration in the specimen is obtained by subtraction of endogenous acetone measured in step 1 from that measured in step 2. The colorimetric procedure is of historical interest; poor recovery, nonspecificity, and length of the procedure limit its use.[71] The GC procedure is more accurate; however, the use of specialized instrumentation also limits its use.

An enzymatic method for determination of beta-hydroxybutyrate that is rapid, precise, and easily automated has been developed (Table 32-4, method 2). In this procedure, described above, hydrazine is added to remove the acetoacetate that is produced, which allows the oxidation of all available beta-hydroxybutyrate. This enzymatic procedure has been automated.

A newly developed isotachyphoretic technique uses an electric field to separate beta-hydroxybutyrate from other anionic compounds within a capillary tube (Table 32-4, method 4).[75] This method is sensitive and rapid to perform; however, specialized equipment is required, and poor results can occur if optimal pH conditions are not strictly adhered to.

Specimen   Both serum and plasma are acceptable specimens. Anticoagulants including oxalate, fluoride, EDTA, citrate, and heparin do not interfere with these assays. Collected specimens should be separated from red blood cells within 24 hours. Separated serum or plasma is stable for up to 1 week if stored at 4° C.[76]

Reference interval   The normal reference interval of beta-hydroxybutyrate in the serum of healthy adults appears to be dependent on the method used for its analysis. The range of values found in healthy adults using an enzymatic procedure for beta-hydroxybutyrate determinations was 0.02 to 0.27 mmol/L.[77]

Glucose

STEVEN C. KAZMIERCZAK

Principles of analysis A wide variety of methods for measurement of glucose have been developed. Early methods utilized some nonspecific properties of glucose as a means for its determination. These include the ability of the aldehyde group of glucose to reduce copper salts or ferricyanide and the ability of the aldehyde group of glucose to condense with an aromatic amine, such as *o*-toluidine, to form a colored glycosamine.

The copper reduction method is based on the ability of glucose to reduce cupric ions (Cu^{++}) to cuprous ions (Cu^+). In the presence of heat the reduced cuprous ions form cuprous oxide (CuO_2), which can be detected by a variety of techniques. The most popular copper reduction methods entail the reaction of cuprous oxide with phosphomolybdate (Folin-Wu) or arsenomolybdate (Somogyi-Nelson) to form colored molybdenum compounds. Chemical interferences by other sugars and metabolic compounds make these procedures nonspecific for glucose. As a result they are no longer in use.

A modification of the copper reduction method by Benedict[78] (Table 32-5, method 1) is currently widely used as a semiquantitative method to measure glucose in urine. The procedure is sensitive to all reducing compounds present in urine and is therefore not specific for glucose only. After the reaction of cupric ions with glucose in the presence of heat, this procedure yields red Cu_2O and yellow CuOH. The greater the glucose concentration, the more intense the color produced. Although this method is nonspecific for glucose, it can be used with a glucose-specific assay to screen for genetic diseases of carbohydrate metabolism in newborns and infants (see p. 960). A positive Benedict reaction in conjunction with a negative test for glucose using a glucose-specific assay is suggestive of such diseases (see Chapter 47 for further discussion on inherited disorders of carbohydrate metabolism).

The ferricyanide methods are based on the ability of glucose to reduce ferricyanide in alkaline solution to ferrocyanide and is subject to significant positive interference from compounds such as creatinine and uric acid. The *o*-toluidine procedure for measurement of glucose has been replaced by other methods because of the health hazard posed from *o*-toluidine, which is now classified as a carcinogen. This procedure also has problems with interference from urea and other hexose sugars such as mannose and galactose. Both the ferricyanide and *o*-toluidine methods are not in current use.

The most common procedure in current use for glucose measurement uses enzymes such as glucose oxidase or hexokinase, which allow for highly sensitive, accurate, and precise measurement of glucose concentrations. These enzymes have been used in the development of a wide variety of applications.

GLUCOSE OXIDASE. The enzyme glucose oxidase has been used in both polarographic and colorimetric assays. Most reagent preparations also include the enzyme mutarotase to

---

Table 32-5   Methods for glucose analysis

Method	Principle of analysis	Usage	Comments
1. Benedict's (copper reduction)	Based on ability of glucose to reduce cupric ion (Cu^{++}) to cuprous ion (Cu^+): Cu^{++} + Glucose $\rightarrow$ Cu_2O *(red)* + CuOH *(yellow)*	Frequently used as semiquantitative test for total reducing sugars in urine	Used with more specific glucose procedure to differentiate glucosuria from other sugars in urine
2. Glucose oxidase (oxygen consumption)	Glucose + O_2 $\rightarrow$ Gluconic acid + H_2O_2 H_2O_2 is consumed in side reactions. Consumption of O_2 is measured polarographically.	Frequently used	Accurate and precise Automated
3. Glucose oxidase coupled with enzymatic reaction ("Trinder")	Glucose + O_2 $\rightarrow$ Gluconic acid + H_2O_2 H_2O_2 + Reduced dye $\rightarrow$ Oxidized dye *(colored)* + H_2O	Frequently used Serum, urine Automated	Indicator reaction subject to interference; otherwise good accuracy and precision
4. Hexokinase coupled with enzymatic reaction	Glucose + ATP $\rightarrow$ Glucose-6-phosphate + ADP Glucose-6-phosphate + $NADP^+$ $\rightarrow$ 6-Phosphogluconate + NADPH + H^+ Increase in absorbance at 340 nm is directly related to glucose concentration.	Most common method in use	Very good accuracy and precision
5. Glucose dehydrogenase	Glucose + NAD^+ $\rightarrow$ D-Gluconolactone + NADH + H^+ Increase in absorbance at 340 nm is directly related to glucose concentrations.	Rarely used	Can be automated Good accuracy and precision

convert alpha-D-glucose to beta-D-glucose. This is necessary because glucose oxidase is specific for beta-D-glucose only.

Polarographic determination of glucose with an O_2 electrode and glucose oxidase allows for a rapid means of measuring glucose (Table 32-5, method 2). In this procedure glucose reacts with O_2 in a reaction catalyzed by glucose oxidase, producing gluconic acid and hydrogen peroxide. The hydrogen peroxide is eliminated by its reaction with catalase in a side reaction. The amount of O_2 consumed is measured by an oxygen electrode and directly related to glucose concentration in the sample.

The glucose oxidase reaction has also been coupled with a second enzyme-catalyzed reaction (Table 32-5, method 3). The initial reaction catalyzed by glucose oxidase produces gluconic acid and hydrogen peroxide. The hydrogen peroxide produced in the initial step can be reacted with a variety of dyes in a reaction catalyzed by horseradish peroxidase to produce an oxidized dye that is colored. The coupled glucose oxidase procedure is subject to interference from many compounds in serum and urine, including bilirubin, ascorbic acid, and uric acid. These substances can be oxidized by the hydrogen peroxide produced in the step catalyzed by glucose oxidase resulting in a negative bias.

The negative interference by bilirubin can be a severe problem in an acute care facility, where a large percentage of samples may be icteric.

Glucose measurements in cerebrospinal fluid (CSF) can have significant interference from ascorbate with this method because CSF normally contains higher concentrations of ascorbate and lower concentrations of glucose than serum does.[79,80] Use of an alternative method for CSF specimens is recommended.[81]

The glucose oxidase reaction has been automated on a variety of instruments and has also been adapted for use in a urine dipstick. When used in a dipstick format, this procedure is highly specific for glucose. However, strong oxidizing substances, such as hypochlorite and chlorine, can produce a positive reaction, whereas compounds, such as ascorbic acid, that interfere with the peroxidase step can give falsely low glucose values.

HEXOKINASE. Another frequently used enzymatic procedure for glucose determinations is the coupled hexokinase–glucose-6-phosphate dehydrogenase reaction (Table 32-5, method 4). In this method, hexokinase phosphorylates glucose in the presence of ATP to produce glucose-6-phosphate. The glucose-6-phosphate reduces NAD^+ or NADP in a reaction catalyzed by glucose-6-phosphate dehydrogenase to produce NADH or NADPH respectively. The increase in absorbance measured at 340 nm is directly related to glucose concentrations within the specimen. This coupled enzyme reaction is virtually specific for glucose and is not subject to interference from uric acid or ascorbate.[82] Comparison of the hexokinase enzymatic procedure versus the glucose oxidase enzymatic method has demonstrated the former to be the best method overall, especially useful in acute care facilities.[83]

Another enzymatic procedure for glucose utilizes the enzyme *glucose dehydrogenase,* obtained from *Bacillus megaterium* or *B. cereus.*[84] The assay requires only a single reaction step, since the enzyme is NAD^+ dependent (Table 32-5, method 5). Glucose dehydrogenase catalyzes the reduction of NAD^+, producing gluconolactone and NADH, which can be monitored at 340 nm. The only reported interfering compounds, D-xylose and mannose, are rarely encountered to any significant degree.[85] When compared with the glucose oxidase and hexokinase enzymatic procedures, the glucose dehydrogenase method has been shown to have better sensitivity and within-run precision.[86]

Specimen Serum or plasma, cerebrospinal fluid, and urine are all acceptable specimens. Glucose in whole blood stored at room temperature is metabolized at a rate of approximately 5% per hour. Thus samples should be centrifuged as soon as possible to remove the specimen from cells. Once separated, glucose in serum or plasma is stable for up to 3 days when refrigerated at 2° to 8° C. Specimens that cannot be rapidly separated should be collected into tubes containing fluoride or iodoacetate. These compounds inhibit glycolysis and thus preserve glucose in whole blood.

Reference intervals Glucose concentrations in children less than 5 years of age are approximately 10% to 15% below those levels found in adults. Newborns show glucose concentrations ranging from 200 to 800 mg/L (1.11 to 4.44 mmol/L), though blood glucose concentrations in premature infants are even lower.[87] Glucose concentrations in healthy adults range from 700 to 1050 mg/L (3.9 to 5.8 mmol/L). Cerebrospinal fluid glucose concentrations are approximately 40% to 80% of those values found in serum or plasma. Concentrations of glucose in serum are approximately 15% higher than glucose concentrations in whole blood. It must be noted that whole blood concentrations vary with the hematocrit. Whole blood glucose most closely approximates plasma glucose when the hematocrit is low. The 15% difference between whole blood glucose and plasma glucose described above is for hematocrit value of approximately 45%.

Urine does not normally contain any detectable glucose. However, newborns and those individuals with inborn errors of carbohydrate metabolism may excrete sufficient galactose to give a positive glucose result when glucose is measured using the nonspecific copper-reduction methods.[88]

Glycated hemoglobin
ANDREA ROSE

Principles of analysis and current usage Although the terms "glycated" and "glycosylated" are used interchangeably, glycated is the preferred term to describe the reaction product between a sugar and a protein.[89] In all individuals, glycation of normal adult hemoglobin (A_0) occurs under physiological conditions resulting in the nonenzymatic formation of several minor hemoglobin components. Initially the carbonyl group on sugars undergoes a rapid, reversible reaction with an amino group on sugars to form a Schiff base. This is followed by an Amadori rearrangement to form a stable product[90] (Fig. 32-10).

Assessment of glycemic control can be performed by measurement of combined hemoglobin A_1, which is composed of hemoglobin A_{1a} (products of fructose-1,6-diphosphate and glucose-6-phosphate with the N-terminal group of beta

Table 32-6 Methods of glycated hemoglobin (GHb) analysis

Method	Basis of Hb separation	Basis of analysis	Type of glycated Hb measured
1. Minicolumn (microcolumn)	Ion-exchange chromatography	Spectral absorbance of separated Hb components	A_1* or A_{1c}
2. Electrophoresis	Charge differences	Spectral absorbance of separated Hb components	A_1* or A_{1c}; S_1, C_1, S_1, C_{1c} can also be measured
3. HPLC	Ion-exchange chromatography	Spectral absorbance of separated Hb components	A_{1c}*
4. Immunoassay	Antibody affinity	EIA, TINIA, LIAI	A_{1c}†; labile GHb will not bind
5. Minicolumn	Affinity chromatography	Spectral absorbance of separated Hb components	A_{1c} + non-A_1 GHb; labile GHb will not bind
6. Colorimetric	Acid hydrolysis	Formation of colored product from 5-HMF and TBA	A_{1c} glycated A_0

EIA, Enzyme immunoassay; *5-HMF*, 5-hydroxymethyl furfural; *HPLC*, high-performance lipid chromatography; *LIAI*, latex immunoagglutination inhibition; *TBA*, thiobarbituric acid; *TINIA*, turbidimetric inhibition immunoassay.
*Methods 1, 2, and 3 now routinely include an agent in the hemolysis reagent to remove the labile GHb.
†Recognition of Hb variants, such as S_{1c}, is antibody specific.

chains), A_{1b}, and A_{1c}, or quantitation of A_{1c}, which is the most abundant hemoglobin A_1 component. Hemoglobin A_{1c} is the reaction product of glucose and the N-terminal group of beta chains. The designations assigned to hemoglobins A_{1a}, A_{1b}, and A_{1c} are derived from the order in which these minor hemoglobin components elute after cation-exchange chromatography of a hemolysate of whole blood.

In addition to measurement of combined hemoglobin A_1 or A_{1c}, measurement of total glycated hemoglobin may be used for evaluating glycemic control. Total glycated hemoglobin includes hemoglobin A_1 and hemoglobins with glucose linked to the N-terminal amino group of the α chain as well as the ϵ-amino group of several lysine residues in both the α and β chains.[91] In contrast to the components of hemoglobin A_1, glycation at these sites cannot be determined by ordinary chromatographic or electrophoretic means. However, these glycated hemoglobins can be readily isolated by use of boronate-affinity chromatography.

Methods used for the quantitation of the combined hemoglobin A_1 fractions include cation-exchange chromatography (Table 32-6, method 1)[92] and electrophoresis (Table 32-6, method 2).[93]

Cation-exchange chromatography for separation of combined hemoglobin A_1 is based upon the finding that glycated hemoglobin A_1 species are less positively charged at neutral pH than hemoglobin A_0. As a result of this charge difference, glycated hemoglobin A_1 will bind less readily to negatively charged resin contained within a chromatography column. When a hemolysate is applied to a column filled with resin, the less positively charged A_{1a}, A_{1b}, and A_{1c} fractions will elute together from the column before the main hemoglobin A_0 fraction. The amount of hemoglobin in each fraction is determined spectrophotometrically at 415 nm. This method, like most, reports the result as the percentage of glycated hemoglobin (%HbA$_1$; HbA$_1$/[HbA$_1$ + Hb$_0$] × 100).

Although chromatographic methods are cumbersome and time consuming, the availability of inexpensive disposable columns simplifies the performance of this method. The reproducibility of this technique is affected by the ability to maintain a uniform temperature (±1 Celsius degree) during analysis.[94] Other factors that can affect test results include pH and ionic strength of the buffers that are used and the column size.[95] The presence of abnormal hemoglobin variants such as hemoglobins S, C, D, and G, as well as increased concentrations of hemoglobin F (>0.5%), can also interfere with analysis. In addition, falsely increased hemoglobin A_1 concentrations can be obtained in patients with uremia[96] and in patients with alcoholism.[97]

The electrophoretic separation of combined hemoglobin A_1 is based on the ability of the free N-terminus of nonglycated hemoglobin to interact with negatively charged groups present in the support medium. Once separated by electrophoresis, the hemoglobin bands can be stained and quantitated by use of a densitometer. The presence of hemoglobin variants can interfere with test results. In addition, carbamylated and acetylated hemoglobins are measured as the hemoglobin A_{1c} fraction.[98]

Methods that may be used for measurement of hemoglobin A_{1c} include variations of the ion-exchange chromatography and electrophoresis procedures and immunochemical methods.[99]

Electrophoretic methods developed for the separation of hemoglobin A_{1c} include isoelectric focusing on polyacrylamide gel and electrophoresis on agar gel at pH 6.5. Isoelectric focusing provides a distinct separation of hemoglobin A_{1c} from hemoglobin A_0, but the method requires a skilled technician and a high-quality densitometer for quantitation. Electrophoretic separation on agar gel yields a much broader separation of hemoglobin A_{1c} from the other hemoglobin species, and quantitation is much easier.[93]

The application of high-performance liquid chromatography (HPLC) (Table 32-6, method 3) for the separation of glycated hemoglobin also uses cation-exchange resin as the stationary phase. The various hemoglobin fractions are separated as buffers of increasing ionic strength pass through the column. The concentrations of the separated hemoglobin fractions are measured spectrophotometrically at 415 nm as they leave the column. HPLC methods recognize the hemoglobin variants such as hemoglobins S, C, D, and G. As a

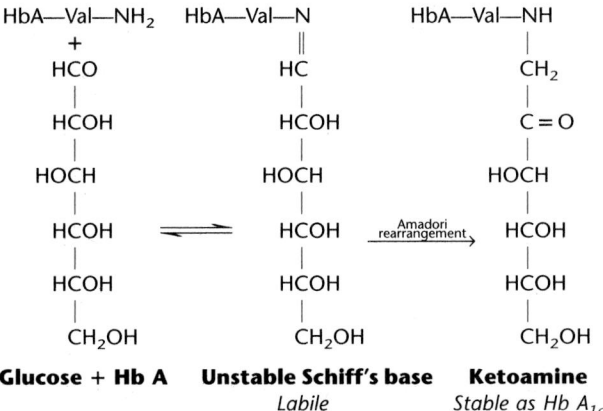

Fig. 32-10 Formation of Schiff base to produce a stable product.

Glucose + Hb A   Unstable Schiff's base   Ketoamine
                  Labile   *Stable as Hb A$_{1c}$*

result, mathematic corrections must be performed before interpretation to account for these hemoglobin variants.[98]

Immunologic methods (Table 32-6, method 4) for measurement of hemoglobin A_{1c} include radioimmunoassay,[99] enzyme immunoassay,[100] and latex immunoagglutination procedures.[101] Both monoclonal and polyclonal antibodies that recognize the sugary moiety and any number of amino acids at the N-terminus of the beta chain have been developed.[100]

Measurement of total glycated hemoglobin can be achieved by use of affinity chromatography with phenylboronic acid linked to an inert resin. Boronic acid forms a weak covalent linkage with hydroxyl groups of sugars. Nonglycated hemoglobins fail to bind to the resin and are eluted first. The bound glycated hemoglobin is then eluted by the application of a buffer containing a competing sugar, such as sorbital, which competes with the bound glycated hemoglobin for the boronic acid–binding sites. Glycated hemoglobins that bind to the resin include not only hemoglobin A_{1c} but other forms of glycated hemoglobin A_0. The method is simple to perform and is specific for glycated hemoglobin.

Colorimetric methods (Table 32-6, method 6) for hemoglobin A_{1c} are based upon the finding that when hemoglobin A_{1c} is subjected to mild acid hydrolysis, 5-hydroxymethylfurfural (5-HMF) is released and can combine with thiobarbituric acid to form a colored product.[102] This method is specific for ketamine-linked sugars; thus hemoglobin F and hemoglobin variants do not interfere. Drawbacks of the procedure include falsely increased values because of the formation of 5-HMF as a result of the condensation of glucose (in high concentrations) with hemoglobin.[103]

Specimen Specimens anticoagulated with EDTA are preferred. Most methods require hemolysate prepared using a cell-lysing agent. Whole blood specimens may be stored up to 5 days at 2° to 6° C.

Reference intervals Reference ranges for glycated hemoglobin are dependent on the hemoglobin species that is measured and the type of procedure that is used. Table 32-8 gives

Table 32-7 Reference ranges for different glycated hemoglobin methods

Method	Reference range (%)	Hemoglobin species measured
Affinity chromatography	4.0-7.7	Total glycated hemoglobin
Electrophoresis	4.7-7.6	Hemoglobin A_1
Immunologic	4.1-5.3	Hemoglobin A_{1c}
Ion exchange	4.2-5.9	Hemoglobin A_{1c}

representative reference ranges for several different types of methods.

Insulin and C-peptide
STEVEN C. KAZMIERCZAK

Principles of analysis and current usage. Competitive-binding immunoassay employing ^{125}I labeling (radioimmunoassay, RIA) is still the most widely used technique for measurement of insulin (Table 32-8, method 1). The determination of insulin in insulin-treated diabetics presents special problems because of interferences by exogenous insulin and circulating antibodies to insulin.[104] Nonprotein bound, or free, insulin is considered to be the biologically active form of the molecule. Thus, for assay of total insulin the bound insulin must be dissociated from antibodies before analysis. The dissociation of insulin from endogenous insulin antibodies can be performed by use of acid precipitation. Separation of the bound and free labeled insulin can be accomplished by a variety of techniques including precipitation using a second antibody, dextran-coated charcoal, and polyethylene glycol.[105]

Nonisotopic, competitive-binding immunoassays for insulin have also been developed, some of which are available commercially. These competitive immunoassays employ enzyme labels with fluorometric or luminometric measurements of enzyme activity, as well as fluorescence labels for use in fluorescence immunoassays.[106-108] The reagents used in the nonisotopic immunoassays are typically stable for longer periods of time when compared to RIA techniques.[109]

A two-site, solid-phase immunoenzymometric assay by TOSOH Medics Corp., Foster City, California (Table 32-8, method 2), employs mouse monoclonal antibody that has been immobilized on a magnetic solid-phase bead. The second, enzyme-labeled mouse monoclonal antibody creates an antibody/insulin/labeled-antibody sandwich. The rate of fluorescence produced by the hydrolysis of the substrate is directly proportional to the insulin concentration within the sample.

The Microparticle Enzyme Immunoassay (MEIA) technology by Abbott Laboratories (Table 32-8, method 3) employs anti-insulin monoclonal antibodies coated on microparticles. An aliquot of the reaction mixture containing insulin bound to the anti-insulin coated microparticles is transferred to a glass-fiber matrix. The matrix is washed to remove unbound materials, and the second anti-insulin antibody conjugated with alkaline phosphatase is dispensed onto the glass-fiber matrix where it binds to the antibody-antigen complex. After a wash step, the substrate, 4-methyl-

Table 32-8   Methods for measurement of insulin

Method	Principle	Usage	Comments
1. Radioimmunoassay (RIA)	Radioactive iodine (^{125}I)-labeled competes with insulin in specimen for limited number of binding sites on anti-insulin antibodies.	Most frequently used procedure	Interference from endogenous anti-insulin antibodies possible
2. Immunoenzymometric assay (IEMA)	Insulin bound to antibody immobilized to magnetic solid phase support. Addition of second antibody labeled with ALP added to form sandwich. Fluorogenic substrate added after wash step to remove unbound labeled antibody.	Frequently used	Interference from endogenous anti-insulin antibodies and human antimouse antibodies possible
3. Microparticle enzyme immunoassay (MEIA)	Similar to method 2 except insulin is bound to anti-insulin coated microparticles transferred to glass-fiber matrix where anti-insulin:ALP conjugate is added to form "sandwich" complex. 4-Methylumbelliferyl phosphate is added as substrate for ALP.	Frequently used	Same as for method 2

ALP, Alkaline phosphatase.

umbelliferyl phosphate, is added to the matrix, and the fluorescence produced is directly related to insulin concentrations within the specimen.

The determination of the connecting peptide (C-peptide) of proinsulin provides an assessment of endogenous insulin secretory reserves in patients with diabetes mellitus. Insulin and C-peptide are secreted by the pancreas in equimolar quantities into the portal blood, which passes through the liver. While the liver extracts a considerable and variable amount of insulin from blood,[110] almost all the C-peptide emerges from the liver to enter the systemic circulation. As a result, C-peptide in the peripheral blood is a more reliable indicator of insulin secretion than insulin itself. In addition, assays for C-peptide do not measure exogenous insulin and are not subject to significant interference from insulin antibodies seen in patients receiving insulin therapy.[111] The most common immunoassay technique in use for determination of C-peptide is RIA.

Questions still remain regarding the standardization of C-peptide assays.[110] In addition, even minor cross-reactivity of C-peptide antisera with human proinsulin can significantly interfere in C-peptide immunoassays if proinsulin secretion still persists in a diabetic patient who has circulating insulin antibodies induced by insulin therapy.[104,110]

Specimen   Serum is an acceptable specimen for all assays. Plasma (EDTA and heparin) can be used with some immunoassay procedures. The presence of an insulin-degrading enzyme in erythrocytes may result in falsely decreased insulin values in hemolyzed specimens.[112] Falsely increased results caused by heterophil antibodies or rheumatoid factors have been observed in immunoassays that use a sandwich technique.[113] Serum for insulin determinations should be separated from red blood cells within 5 hours af-

ter collection.[114] Once separated, insulin is stable for up to 12 hours at room temperature, for 1 week at 4° C, and for 1 month at −10° C.

Reference intervals   Reference ranges for insulin in serum are dependent on factors such as the type of assay used for its measurement and the clinical state of the patient in relationship to the blood glucose concentration. Insulin concentrations in fasting patients are typically less than 25 μU/mL (1042 pg/mL, 0.17 pmol/mL).

ACKNOWLEDGMENTS

The editors would like to acknowledge the previous contributors to methods: Nancy Gau, acetoacetic acid and beta-hydroxybutyric acid; Mary Ellen King, glycated hemoglobin; and Michael D.D. McNeely, insulin and C-peptide.

REFERENCES

1. National Commission on Diabetes: The long range plan to combat diabetes, U.S. Department of Health Education and Welfare, no 76-1018, Bethesda, Md., 1976, National Institutes of Health.
2. Harris MR, Hadden WC, Knowler WC, et al: Prevalence of diabetes and impaired glucose tolerance and plasma levels in the U.S. population aged 20-74 yr, *Diabetes* 36:523, 1987.
3. Smith JW, Marcus FI, Serokman R, et al: Prognosis of patients with diabetes mellitus after myocardial infarction, *Am J Cardiol* 54:719, 1984.
4. Oppenheimer SM, Hoffbrand BI, Oswald GA, et al: Diabetes mellitus and early mortality from stroke, *Br Med J* 291:1014, 1985.
5. Mueckler M, Caruso C, Baldwin SA, et al: Sequence and structure of a human glucose transporter, *Science* 229:941, 1985.
6. Froguel P, Zouali H, Vionnet N, et al: Familial hyperglycemia due to mutations in glucokinase, *N Engl J Med* 328:697-702, 1993.
7. Cryer PE, Gerich JE: Glucose counterregulation, hypoglycemia,

and intensive insulin therapy in diabetes mellitus, *N Engl J Med* 131:232-241, 1985.

8. Chan SJ, Keim P, Steiner DF: Cell-free synthesis of rat preproinsulin: characterization and partial amino acid sequence determination, *Proc Natl Acad Sci USA* 73:1964, 1976.

9. Unger RH, Orci L: Glucagon and the A cell, *N Engl J Med* 304:1518-1524, 1575-1580, 1981.

10. Hartmann H, Probst I, Jungermann K, et al: Inhibition of glycogenolysis and glycogen phosphorylase by insulin and proinsulin in rat hepatocyte cultures, *Diabetes* 36:551, 1987.

11. Dinneen S, Gerich J, Rizza R: Carbohydrate metabolism in non-insulin-dependent diabetes mellitus, *N Engl J Med* 327:707-713, 1992.

12. National Diabetes Data Group: Classification and diagnosis of diabetes mellitus and other categories of glucose intolerance, *Diabetes* 28:1039-1057, 1979.

13. O'Sullivan JB, Worshop Y: Subsequent morbidity among gestational diabetes women. In Sutherland HW, Stowers M, editors: *Carbohydrate metabolism in pregnancy and the newborn*, Edinburgh, 1984, Churchill Livingstone.

14. Atkinson MA, Maclaren NK: The pathogenesis of insulin-dependent diabetes mellitus, *N Engl J Med* 331:1428-1436, 1994.

15. Krolewski AS, Warram JH, Rand LI, Kahn CR: Epidemiologic approach to the etiology of type I diabetes mellitus and its complications, *N Engl J Med* 317:1390-1398, 1987.

16. Tiwari JL, Terasaki PI: *HLA and disease*, New York, 1985, Springer-Verlag.

17. Baisch JM, Weeks T, Giles R, et al: Analysis of HLA-DQ genotypes and susceptibility in insulin-dependent diabetes mellitus, *N Engl J Med* 322:1836, 1990.

18. Khalil I, d'Auriol L, Gobet M, et al: A combination of HLA DQ beta Asp 57-negative and HLA DQ alpha Arg 52 confers susceptibility to insulin-dependent diabetes mellitus, *J Clin Invest* 85:1315, 1990.

19. Wicker LS, Miller J, Mullen Y: Transfer of autoimmune diabetes mellitus with splenocytes from nonobese diabetic (NOD) mice, *Diabetes* 35:855, 1986.

20. Gamble DR, Taylor KW: Seasonal incidence of diabetes mellitus, *Br Med J* 3:631, 1969.

21. Hinden E: Mumps followed by diabetes, *Lancet* 1:1381, 1962.

22. Johnson GM, Tudor RB: Diabetes mellitus and congenital rubella infection, *Am J Dis Child* 120:453, 1970.

23. Yoon JW, Onodera T, Jenson AB, et al: Virus induced diabetes mellitus. XI. Replication of Coxsackie B3 in human pancreatic beta cell cultures, *Diabetes* 27:778, 1978.

24. Craighead JE: Does insulin dependent diabetes mellitus have a viral etiology? *Hum Pathol* 10:267, 1979.

25. Kasuga M, van Obberghen E, Yamada KM, Harrison LC: Autoantibodies against the insulin receptor recognize the insulin binding subunits of an oligomeric receptor, *Diabetes* 30:354, 1981.

26. Roth RA, Cassell DJ: Insulin receptor: evidence that it is a protein kinase, *Science* 219:299, 1983.

27. Moller DE, Flier JS: Insulin resistance—mechanisms, syndromes, and implications, *N Engl J Med* 325:938-948, 1991.

28. Bar RS, Gorden P, Roth J, et al: Fluctuations in the affinity and concentration of insulin receptors on circulating monocytes of obese patients, *J Clin Invest* 58:1123, 1976.

29. Unger RH: Diabetes hyperglycemia: link to impaired glucose transport in pancreatic beta cells, *Science* 251:1200, 1991.

30. Nathan DM: Long-term complications of diabetes mellitus, *N Engl J Med* 328:1676-1685, 1993.

31. Understanding diabetic neuropathy, editorial, *Lancet* 338: 1496-1497, Dec 14, 1991.

32. Bradley RF: Cardiovascular disease. In Marble A, White P, Bradley RF, Krall LP, editors: *Joslin's diabetes mellitus*, ed 11, Philadelphia, 1971, Lea & Febiger.

33. Goldberg RB: Lipid disorders in diabetes, *Diabetes Care* 4:561, 1981.

34. Lopes-Virella MFL, Stone PG, Colwell JA: Serum high density lipoprotein in diabetic patients, *Diabetologia* 13:285, 1977.

35. Zierler KL, Rabinowitz D: Effect of very small concentrations of insulin on forearm metabolism: persistence of its action on potassium and free fatty acids without its effect on glucose, *J Clin Invest* 43:950, 1964.

36. The OCCT Research Group: Epidemiology of severe hypoglycemia in the diabetes control and complications trial, *Am J Med* 90:450-459, 1991.

37. Polonsky KS: A practical approach to fasting hypoglycemia [editorial], *N Engl J Med* 326:1020-1021, 1992.

38. Fischer KF, Lees JH, Newman JH: Hypoglycemia in hospitalized patients, *N Engl J Med* 315:1245-1250, 1986.

39. Miodovnik M, Mimouni F, Tsang RC, et al: Glycemic control and spontaneous abortion in insulin-dependent diabetic women, *Obstet Gynecol* 68:366-369, 1986.

40. Schwartz R: Hyperinsulinemia and macrosomia, editorial, *N Engl J Med* 323:340-342, 1990.

41. Cerami A, Stevens VJ, Monnier VM: Role of nonenzymatic glycosylation in the development of the sequelae of diabetes mellitus, *Metabolism* 28:431, 1979.

42. Makita Z, Radoff S, Rayfield E, et al: Advanced glycosylation end products in patients with diabetic nephropathy, *N Engl J Med* 325:836-841, 1991.

43. Kaneshige H: Nonenzymatic glycosylation of serum IgG and its effect on antibody activity in patients with diabetes mellitus, *Diabetes* 36:822, 1987.

44. Gabbay KH: The sorbitol pathway and the complication of diabetes, *N Engl J Med* 288:831, 1973.

45. Notvest RR, Inserra JJ: Tolrestat, an aldose reductase inhibitor, prevents nerve dysfunction in conscious diabetic rats, *Diabetes* 36:500, 1987.

46. Report on the Committee on Statistics of the American Diabetes Association: Standardization of the oral glucose tolerance test, *Diabetes* 18:299, 1969.

46a. Judzewitsch RG, Jaspen JB, Polonsky KS, et al: Aldose reductase inhibition improves nerve conduction velocity in diabetic patients, *N Engl J Med* 308:119-125, 1983.

47. Davidson MB: The effect of aging on carbohydrate metabolism: a review of the English literature and a practical approach to the diagnosis of diabetes mellitus in the elderly, *Metabolism* 28:688, 1979.

48. Harris MI, Hadden WC, Knowler WC, et al: International criteria for the diagnosis of diabetes and impaired glucose tolerance, *Diabetes Care* 8:562, 1985.

49. Sherwin RS: Limitations of the oral glucose tolerance test in diagnosis of early diabetes, *Primary Care* 4:255, 1977.

50. Nelson RL: Subspecialty clinics: endocrinology: oral glucose tolerance test: indications and limitations, *Mayo Clin Proc* 63:263-269, 1988.

51. Unger RH: The standard two hour oral glucose tolerance test in the diagnosis of diabetes mellitus in subjects without fasting hyperglycemia, *Ann Intern Med* 47:1138, 1957.

52. Mauer AC: The therapy of diabetes, *Am Scientist* 67:422, 1979.

53. Consensus Development Panel: Consensus statement on self-monitoring of blood glucose, *Diabetes Care* 10:95-99, 1987.

54. Gonen B, Rochman H, Rubenstein AH: Metabolic control in diabetic patients: assessment by hemoglobin A1 values, *Metabolism* 28:448, 1979.

55. Larsen ML, Hørder MN, Mogensen EF: Effect of long-term monitoring of glycosylated hemoglobin levels in insulin diabetes mellitus, *N Engl J Med* 323:1021-1025, 1990.

56. Dods RF, Bolmey C: Glycosylated hemoglobin assay and oral glucose tolerance test compared for detection of diabetes mellitus, *Clin Chem* 25:764, 1979.

57. Guthrow CE, Morris MA, Day JF, et al: Enhanced nonenzymatic glucosylation of serum albumin in diabetes mellitus, *Proc Natl Acad Sci USA* 76:4528, 1979.

58. Ward WK, Beard JC, Halter JB, et al: Pathophysiology of insulin secretion in non-insulin-dependent diabetes mellitus, *Diabetes Care* 7:491, 1984.

59. Friedemann TE, Sheft BB, Miller VC: An assessment of the value of nitroprusside reaction for the determination of ketone bodies in urine, *Q Bull Northwestern Univ Med School* 20:301-310, 1946.

60. Csako G, Benson CC, Elin RJ: False-positive ketone reactions in CAP surveys, *Clin Chem* 39:915-917, 1993.

61. Poon R, Hinberg I: One-step elimination of interference of free-sulfhydryl-containing drugs with Chemstrip ketone readings, *Clin Chem* 36:1527-1528, 1990.

62. Poon R, Hinberg I, Peterson RG: N-Acetylcysteine causes false-positive ketone results with urinary dipsticks, *Clin Chem* 36:818-819, 1990.

63. Csako G: False-positive results for ketone with the drug mesna and other free sulfhydryl compounds, *Clin Chem* 33:289-292, 1987.

64. Csako G: Causes, consequences, and recognition of false-positive reactions for ketones, *Clin Chem* 36:1388-1389, 1990.

65. Schulke RE, Johnson RE: A colorimetric method for estimating acetoacetate, *Am J Clin Pathol* 43:539-543, 1965.

66. Williamson DH, Mellanby J, Krebs HA: Enzymatic determination of D(−)-β-hydroxybutyric acid and acetoacetic acid in blood, *Biochem J* 82:90-96, 1962.

67. Price CP, Lloyd B, Alberti KGMM: A kinetic spectrophotometric assay for rapid determination of acetoacetate in blood, *Clin Chem* 23:1893-1897, 1977.

68. Yamanishi H, Iyama S, Yamaguchi Y, Amino N: Stability of acetoacetate after venesection, *Clin Chem* 39:920, 1993.

69. Kundu SK, Judilla AM: Novel solid-phase assay of ketone bodies in urine, *Clin Chem* 37:1565-1569, 1991.

70. Greenberg LA, Lester D: A micromethod for the determination of acetone and ketone bodies, *J Biol Chem* 154:177-190, 1944.

71. Seigel L, Robin NI, McDonald LJ: New approach to determination of total ketone bodies in serum, *Clin Chem* 23:46-49, 1977.

72. Williamson DH, Mellanby J, Krebs HA: Enzymic determination of D(−)-beta-hydroxybutyrate acid and acetoacetic acid in blood, *Biochem J* 82:90-96, 1962.

73. Hansen JL, Frier EF: Direct assays of lactate, pyruvate, beta-hydroxybutyrate and acetoacetate with a centrifugal analyzer, *Clin Chem* 24:475-479, 1978.

74. Li PL, Lee JT, MacGilliray MH, et al: Direct fixed-time kinetic assays for beta-hydroxybutyrate and acetoacetate with a centrifugal analyzer or a computer-backed spectrophotometer, *Clin Chem* 26:1713-1717, 1980.

75. Dolnik V, Bocek P: Determination of pyruvate, lactate, acetoacetate and β-hydroxybutyrate in serum by capillary isotachophoresis, *J Chromatogr* 225:455-458, 1991.

76. Eckfeldt JH, Leindecker-Foster C, Kershaw MJ: Calibration of 3-hydroxybutyrate assays, *Clin Chem* 30:1116, 1984.

77. Koch DD, Feldbruegge DH: Optimized kinetic method for automated determination of β-hydroxybutyrate, *Clin Chem* 33:1761-1766, 1987.

78. Benedict SR: Analysis of whole blood: determination of sugar and of saccharoids (nonfermentable copper-reducing substances), *J Biol Chem* 92:141-159, 1931.

79. Macquire GA, Price CP: Evidence of interference by ascorbate in the measurement of cerebrospinal fluid glucose by a kinetic glucose oxidase/peroxidase procedure, *Clin Chem* 29:1810-1812, 1983.

80. Spector RN: Vitamin homeostasis in the central nervous system, *N Engl J Med* 296:1393-1398, 1977.

81. Price CP, Spencer K: A rapid kinetic assay for glucose using glucose dehydrogenase, *Ann Clin Biochem* 16:100-105, 1979.

82. Israngkun PP, Speicher CE: Glucose: review of methods, *Am Soc Clin Pathol* 7(3), 1991.

83. Giampietro O, Pilo A, Buzzigoli G, et al: Four methods for glucose assay compared for various glucose concentrations and under different clinical conditions, *Clin Chem* 28:2405-2407, 1982.

84. Banauch D, Brümmer W, Ebeling W, et al: Eine Glucose-Dehydrogenase für die Glucose-Bestimmung in Körperflüssigkeiten, *Z Klin Chem Klin Biochem* 13:101-107, 1975.

85. Pauly HEW, Pfleiderer G: D-Glucose dehydrogenase from *Bacillus megaterium* M 1286: purification, properties and structure, *Hoppe-Seylers Z Physiol Chem* 356:1613-1623, 1975.

86. Burrin JM, Price CP: Performance of three enzymic methods for filter paper glucose determination, *Ann Clin Biochem* 21:411-416, 1984.

87. Meites S, editor-in-chief: Pediatric clinical chemistry, reference values, Washington, D.C., 1989, American Association for Clinical Chemistry.

88. Breusch FL, Tulus R: Die Spezifität der Mikromethoden zur Citronensäurebestimmung als Pentabromaceton, *Biochim Biophys Acta* 1:77, 1947.

89. Roth M: "Glycated hemoglobin," not "glycosylated" or "glucosylated" [Letter], *Clin Chem* 29:1991, 1983.

90. Hodge JE: The Amadori rearrangement, *Adv Carbohydr Chem* 10:169, 1955.

91. Shapiro R, McManus MJ, Zalut C, et al: Sites of non-enzymatic glycosylation of human hemoglobin A, *J Biol Chem* 255:3120, 1980.

92. Abraham EC, Huff TA, Cope ND, et al: Determination of the glycosylated hemoglobins (HbA₁) with a new microcolumn procedure, *Diabetes* 27:931-937, 1978.

93. Menard L, Dempsey ME, Blankstein LA, et al: Quantitative determination of glycosylated hemoglobin A₁ by agar gel electrophoresis, *Clin Chem* 26:1598-1602, 1980.

94. Rosenthal MA: The effect of temperature on the fast hemoglobin test system, *Hemoglobin* 3:215, 1979.

95. Goldstein DE, Little RR, Wiedmeyer H, et al: Glycated hemoglobin: methodologies and clinical applications, *Clin Chem* 32:B64-B70, 1986.

96. Fluckiger R, Harmon W, Meier W, et al: Hemoglobin carbamylation in uremia, *N Engl J Med* 304:823, 1981.

97. Hoberman HD, Chiodo SM: Elevation of the hemoglobin A₁ fraction in alcoholism, *Alcoholism: Clin Exp Res* 6:260, 1982.

98. Weykamp CW, Penders TJ, Muskiet FAJ, et al: Influences of hemoglobin variants and derivatives on glycohemoglobin determinations as investigated by 102 laboratories using 16 methods, *Clin Chem* 39:1717-1723, 1993.

99. Javid J, Pettis PK, Koenig RJ, et al: Immunologic characterization and quantification of haemoglobin A₁c, *Br J Haematol* 38:329, 1978.

100. John WG, Gray MR, Bates DK, et al: Enzyme immunoassay: a new technique for estimating hemoglobin A₁c, *Clin Chem* 39:663-666, 1993.

101. Pope RM, Aps JM, Page MD, et al: Immunologic characterization and quantification of haemoglobin A₁c, *Diabetic Med* 10:260-263, 1993.

102. Fluckiger R, Winterhalter KH: Glycosylated hemoglobins. In Labie D, Poyart C, Rosa J, editors: *Molecular interactions of hemoglobin*, vol 70, Paris, 1977, Institut de la Santé et de la Recherche Médicale, pp 319-326.

103. Kennedy AL, Mehl TD, Merimee TJ: Non-enzymatically glycolated serum proteins: spurious elevation due to free glucose in serum, *Diabetes* 29:413, 1980.

104. Myrick JE, Gunter EW, Maggio VL, et al: An improved radioimmunoassay of C-peptide and its application in a multi-year study, *Clin Chem* 35:37-42, 1989.

105. Arnqvist H, Ollson PO, von Schneck H: Free and total insulin as determined after precipitation with polyethylene glycol: analytical characteristics and effects of sample handling and storage, *Clin Chem* 33:93-96, 1987.

106. Tsuji A, Maeda M, Arakawa H, et al: Enzyme immunoassay of hormones and drugs by using fluorescence and chemiluminescence reaction. In Dal SB, editor: *Enzyme labeled immunoassay of hormones and drugs*, Berlin, New York, 1978, Walter de Gruyter & Co.

107. Yamaguchi Y, Hayashi C, Miyai K: Fluorescence polarization immunoassay for insulin preparations, *Anal Lett* 15:731-737, 1982.

108. Toivonen E, Hemmilä I, Marniemi J, et al: Two-side time-resolved immunofluorometric assay of human insulin, *Clin Chem* 32:637-640, 1986.

109. Andersen L, Dinesen B, Jørgensen PN, et al: Enzyme immunoassay for intact human insulin in serum or plasma, *Clin Chem* 39:578-582, 1993.

110. Koskinen P: Nontransferability of C-peptide measurements

with various commercial radioimmunoassay reagents, *Clin Chem* 34:1575-1578, 1988.

111. Malmquist J, Birgerstam G: Assays of pancreatic B cell secretory products: utility in investigative and clinical diabetology, *Scand J Clin Lab Invest* 46:705-713, 1986.

112. Duckworth WC, Hamel FG, Bennett R, et al: Human red blood cell insulin degrading enzyme and rat skeletal muscle insulin protease share antigenic sites and generate identical products from insulin, *J Biol Chem* 265:2984-2987, 1990.

113. Boscato LM, Stuart C: Heterophilic antibodies: a problem for all immunoassays, *Clin Chem* 34:27-33, 1988.

114. Walters E, Henley R, Barnes I: Stability of insulin in normal whole blood, *Clin Chem* 32:224, 1986.

115. Kimura M, Kobayashi K, Matsuoka A, et al: Head-space gas chromatographic determination of 3-hydroxybutyrate in plasma after enzymic reactions, and the relationship among the three ketone bodies, *Clin Chem* 31:596-598, 1985.

116. Brega A, Villa P, Quadrini G, et al: High-performance liquid chromatographic determination of acetone in blood and urine in the clinical diagnostic laboratory, *J Chromatogr* 553:249-254, 1991.

117. Jerrard D, Verdile V, Yealy D, et al: Serum determinations in toxic isopropanol ingestion, *Am J Emerg Med* 10:200-202, 1992.

118. Drews PA: Carbohydrate derivatives and metabolites. In Henry RJ, Cannon D, Winkleman JW, editors: *Clinical chemistry: principles and techniques,* ed 2, Hagerstown, Md., 1974, Harper & Row.

119. Peden VH: Determination of individual serum "ketone bodies," with normal values in infants and children, *J Lab Clin Med* 63:332-343, 1964.

CHAPTER 33

Coronary artery disease and disorders of lipid metabolism

Herbert K. Naito

OBJECTIVES

- Describe digestion, absorption, and metabolism of cholesterol and triglycerides, including the role of the liver and adipose tissue.

- List the lipoproteins and their apolipoprotein content; state the primary function of each lipoprotein.

- Describe the synthesis and catabolism of HDL, LDL, VLDL, and chylomicrons.

- Discuss each of the six types of lipoproteinemias with respect to lipid and lipoprotein levels, appearance of the specimen, and genetic etiology.

- Discuss the initiation and development of atherosclerosis.

- Discuss the risk factors for coronary atherosclerosis.

- State the clinical significance of hyperlipidemia.

KEY TERMS

amphipathic From amphi- 'on both sides' and pathic 'of feeling' and pertaining to a molecule having two sides with characteristically different properties, or a detergent, which has both a polar (hydrophilic) end and a nonpolar (hydrophobic) end but is long enough so that each end demonstrates its own solubility characteristics.

apolipoprotein The protein component of lipoprotein complexes.

chylomicron Large lipid-protein complexes that are made by the gut and serve an important function in the transport of fats (mainly dietary triglycerides).

HDL High-density lipoprotein. This lipid-protein complex is also called *alpha-lipoprotein* and is the most dense of the lipoproteins.

IDL Intermediate-density lipoprotein. This lipid-protein complex has a density between VLDL and LDL, has a relatively very short half-life, and is in the blood in very low concentrations in a healthy person. In a dysbetalipoproteinemic person the IDL concentration in the blood is found to be elevated.

LDL Low-density lipoprotein. This lipid-protein complex is also called *beta-lipoprotein* and is the end product of VLDL catabolism. It is the major carrier of serum cholesterol.

lipoproteins Lipid (apoprotein)-protein complexes consisting of discrete families of macromolecules with known physical, chemical, and physiological properties.

VLDL Very-low-density lipoprotein, also called *pre-beta-lipoprotein.* It is a relatively large lipid-protein complex that transports mainly endogenously synthesized triglycerides.

Part I: Lipids
NORMAL PHYSIOLOGY OF LIPIDS
Lipid composition of foods

The fat found in food is composed mainly of triglycerides, about 98% to 99%, of which 92% to 95% is fatty acid and the remainder is glycerol. The remaining 1% to 2% of the lipids includes cholesterol, phospholipids, diglycerides, monoglycerides, fat-soluble vitamins, steroids, terpenes, and other fats. Most fats are mixtures of triglycerides containing four or five major fatty acids and many more minor or trace constituents. The individual glyceride molecules in most food fats contain both saturated and unsaturated fatty acids. Several polyunsaturated acids (linoleic, linolenic, and arachidonic acids) cannot be synthesized in the animal body and must be provided in the diet. These have been termed *essential fatty acids* (EFAs) (see Chapter 37).

The small amount of nonhydrolyzable matter in food fats consists of sterols, fatty alcohols, hydrocarbons, pigments, glycerol esters, and various other compounds. Cholesterol occurs in all animal fats. Most sterols are cholesterol, but depending on the diet, other sterols, such as phytosterols, can make up an appreciable percentage of the total sterols, particularly in people on vegetarian diets. The phytosterols are important because they compete with cholesterol for uptake by the mucosal cell. Thus the more phytosterols consumed, the less dietary cholesterol is absorbed by the mucosal cells of the gut.

Fat digestion, absorption, and metabolism of lipids

Fat absorption occurs in three phases: the *intraluminal,* or digestive, phase, during which the dietary fats are modified both physically and chemically before absorption; the *cellular,* or absorptive, phase, in which the digested material enters the intestinal mucosal cells where it is reassembled into its preabsorptive form; and the *transport* phase, during which the absorbed lipids are carried from the mucosal cell to other tissues through the lymphatics and blood.[1-4]

Intraluminal phase. Most digestion of food fat is carried on in the intestine through the action of intestinal and pancreatic enzymes (lipases) and bile acids (see Chapters 29 and 30 respectively). Because of their surface-active properties, the bile salts emulsify the dietary triglyceride into very small particles with a diameter of approximately 1 μm. The emulsification process thus forms particles that can be readily acted on by digestive enzymes.

In the intestinal lumen the action of pancreatic lipase on ingested fat results in the progressive digestion of triglycerides to 1,2-diglycerides and then to 2-monoglycerides and fatty acids. Only a small percentage of the fat is completely hydrolyzed to free fatty acids (FFAs) and glycerol. Cholesterol esters are hydrolyzed to free cholesterol and free fatty acid; the reaction is catalyzed by the enzyme cholesterol esterase.

Absorptive phase. After monoglycerides and fatty acids enter the endoplasmic reticulum of the mucosal cell, presumably by diffusion, the monoglycerides and fatty acids are reesterified into triglycerides by either of two pathways. The monoglyceride pathway is peculiar to the intestinal mucosa and involves the direct acylation of the absorbed monoglyceride from the lumen with activated FFA. The alpha-glycerophosphate pathway present in most tissues involves the formation of a coenzyme A (acyl CoA) derivative of the fatty acid. This reaction, which requires adenosine triphosphate (ATP), is catalyzed by the enzyme fatty acid:CoA ligase (AMP). This enzyme has a pronounced specificity for longer-chain fatty acids. Thus long-chain fatty acids appear in thoracic duct lymph transported as triglycerides in the chylomicrons, whereas short- and medium-chain fatty acids are transported bound to albumin in the portal circulation.

The percentage of cholesterol that is absorbed from the diet is self-regulating. Increased levels of triglyceride in the diet and an expanded bile acid pool tend to promote cholesterol absorption. When the continuous intake of cholesterol is less than about 300 mg/day, more is absorbed (about 40% to 60%). If the intake is increased to 2 to 3 g/day, as little as 10% may be absorbed. In a typical American diet, about 600 mg of steroids are consumed per day, and the coefficient of absorption of dietary cholesterol is generally 25% to 40%. It should be stressed that there is a large individual variation in cholesterol absorption. This could account partially for the difference in individual responsiveness or lack of responsiveness to diet-induced hypercholesterolemia.

Transport phase. Once triglycerides have been resynthesized within the intestinal mucosal cell, they are assembled in the mucosal cell endoplasmic reticulum and the Golgi apparatus into water-soluble macromolecules—*chylomicrons.* The intestinal lipoproteins leave the mucosal cells presumably by reverse pinocytosis. They first appear in the lymphatic vessels of the abdominal region and later in the systemic circulation. The intestinal release of chylomicrons persists for several hours after the ingestion of a fat meal. Because the chylomicrons are large enough to scatter light (up to 0.5 μm in diameter), the plasma becomes lactescent (turbid) so as to produce what is commonly called an *alimentary lipemic response*. These larger lipid-protein complexes are mixtures of triglycerides (82%), some proteins (2%, as apoproteins), small amounts of cholesterol (9%, mainly as ester), and phospholipids (7%). Although the amount of protein is small, there is a good deal of evidence that its presence is necessary for the release of the chylomicrons. For example, in abetalipoproteinemia (a genetically determined disease in which apoprotein B cannot be made in the body), triglyceride is not released from the intestinal cells.

The bloodstream transports chylomicrons to all tissues in the body, including adipose tissue, which is their principal site of uptake. The large chylomicrons, heavily laden with triglyceride (Fig. 33-1), are removed rather rapidly (within minutes). Chylomicrons are normally present in only trace amounts in blood samples taken from individuals after an overnight fast.

Under normal conditions, chylomicron catabolism proceeds in two known phases. In the first, triglycerides are hydrolyzed at extrahepatic tissue sites under the influence of *triglyceride* (or *lipoprotein*) *lipase*. The process results in a relatively triglyceride-poor, cholesterol-rich *remnant* particle. In the second catabolic phase, the remnant particle is removed by the liver.

The hydrolysis by lipoprotein lipase of triglyceride-rich, plasma proteins takes place at the luminal surface (bloodstream side) of the capillary endothelium. The enzyme is bound to the capillary endothelial cells in muscle and adipose tissue and can be released by intravenous administration of heparin (*postheparin lipolytic activity*, PHLA).

As a result of the first phase of chylomicron metabolism, unesterified fatty acids are released into the bloodstream, and the diglycerides and monoglycerides are taken up in vacuoles and transported across the capillary wall for hydrolysis.

Within tissue cells, the fatty acids derived from triglycerides (in chylomicrons or very-low-density lipoproteins, VLDL) can be stored or utilized for energy when needed, especially by the heart. FFAs are also used for cellular phospholipid synthesis, including the synthesis of prostaglandins, the ubiquitous local hormones.

Remaining chylomicron remnant particles are cleared by the liver. Further catabolism of the VLDL remnant occurs at an extracellular site and results in the formation

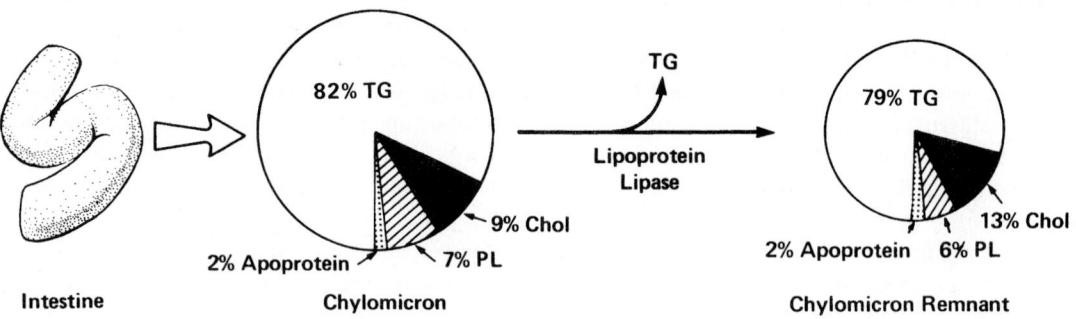

CATABOLIC PATHWAY FOR CHYLOMICRON AND VLDL

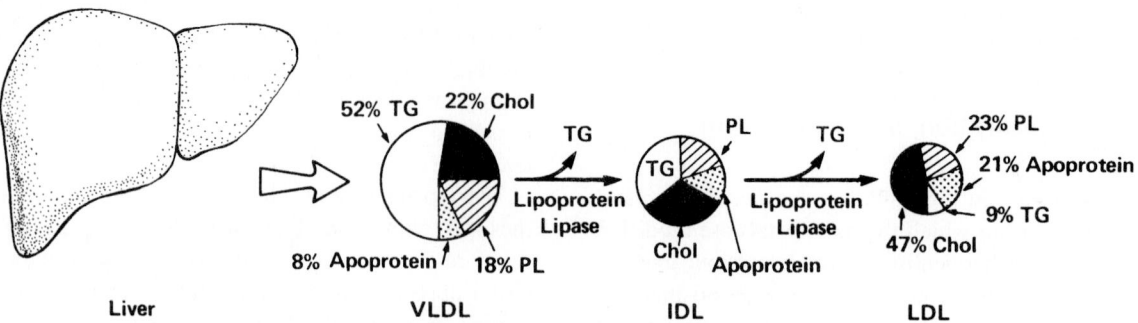

Fig. 33-1 Origin and catabolic pathway of chylomicron and very-low-density lipoprotein *(VLDL)*. End product of chylomicron is chylomicron remnant; end product of VLDL is LDL. *Chol,* Cholesterol; *PL,* phosphatidyllecithin; *TG,* triglyceride.

of low-density lipoprotein (LDL), a cholesterol-rich particle.

Role of liver in metabolism of lipids

In addition to the intestines and other organs, the liver can synthesize lipoprotein particles from recently absorbed dietary constituents. In fact, the liver is the major organ that synthesizes cholesterol; that is, about 70% of the daily cholesterol production comes from the liver. Newly synthesized hepatic triglycerides are coupled with phospholipid, cholesterol, and proteins to form VLDL. These macromolecules are then released into the circulation and transported to adipose tissue.

Hepatic triglyceride synthesis is accelerated when the diet is rich in excess calories. This results in VLDL overproduction, which may explain the hypertriglyceridemia observed when diets are particularly rich in simple sugars.

During fasting, the metabolic pathways in the liver are reversed. Blood glucose concentration falls, and insulin levels are diminished. Hepatic VLDL triglyceride synthesis is diminished during normal fasting. FFAs derived from adipose tissue are taken up by the liver, and their oxidation to ketone bodies provides energy for gluconeogenesis. FFAs of adipose tissue origin can be esterified to triglycerides, incorporated into hepatic VLDL, and then released into the bloodstream. During periods of stress and in certain metabolic conditions, such as uncontrolled diabetes, FFAs are the principal precursors of hepatic VLDL.

CHOLESTEROL METABOLISM
Biological functions

Cholesterol is a member of a large class of biological compounds called *steroids* that have a similar four-ring structure, a cyclopentanoperhydrophenanthrene ring (Fig. 33-2).

Because of the well-established positive association between plasma cholesterol concentration and coronary heart disease (CHD), we are apt to think of cholesterol as a harm-

ful substance. Contrary to that belief, cholesterol is essential for normal functioning of the organism because it is:

1. An essential structural component of membranes of all animal cells and subcellular particles
2. An obligatory precursor of bile acids
3. A precursor of all steroid hormones, including sex and adrenal hormones.

Physiology of cholesterol metabolism

Tissue cholesterol is in constant exchange with plasma cholesterol; the turnover rate and the amount of tissue cholesterol that is exchangeable with the plasma cholesterol will vary from one tissue to another.

Because of loss and replacement, about 2% of the body's cholesterol is renewed each day. The main channel for outflow from the pool is the gastrointestinal tract; the absolute rate of turnover (in grams per day) as estimated by measurement of the daily fecal output is 1 to 2 g/day for cholesterol, with excretion of bile acids accounting for about half the total turnover. Fig. 33-3 illustrates that the concentration of a given cholesterol pool is under the influence of cholesterol input, output, and turnover rates. It should be stressed that because of the continuous cycling of cholesterol into and out of the bloodstream, the plasma cholesterol concentration is not a simple additive function of dietary cholesterol intake and endogenous cholesterol synthesis. Rather, it reflects the rates of synthesis of the cholesterol-carrying lipoproteins and the efficiency of the receptor mechanisms that determine their catabolism. A detailed discussion of the dynamics of lipoprotein concentra-

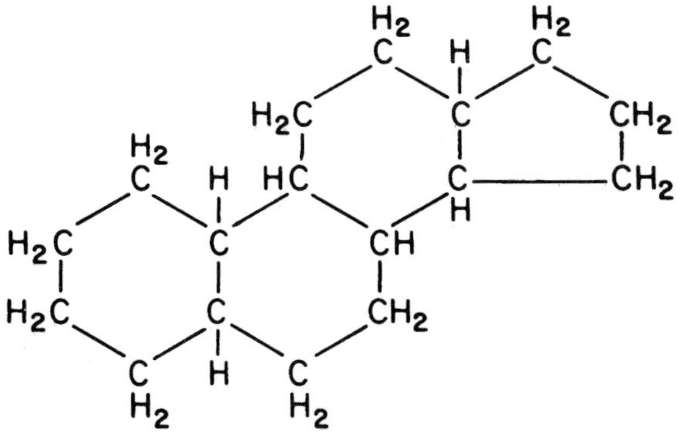

Cyclopentanoperhydrophenanthrene

Fig. 33-2 Chemical structure of cyclopentanoperhydrophenanthrene ring. This common four-ring structure is basic structure of all steroids.

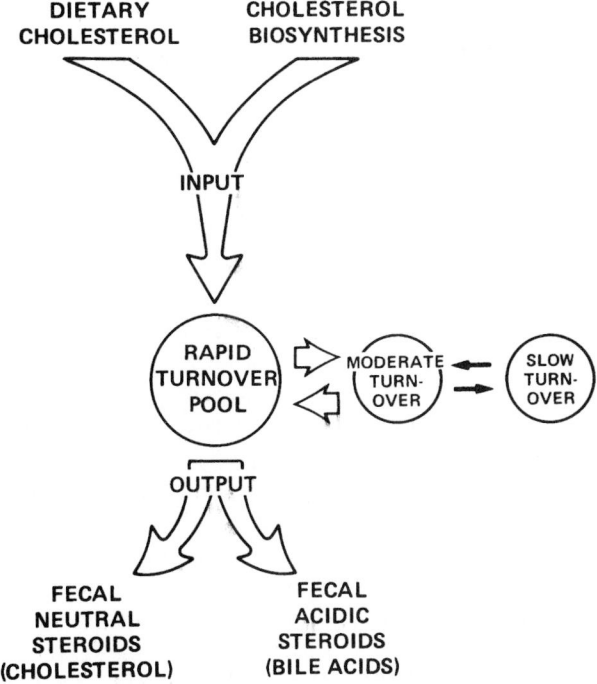

Fig. 33-3 Scheme of dynamics of cholesterol metabolism.

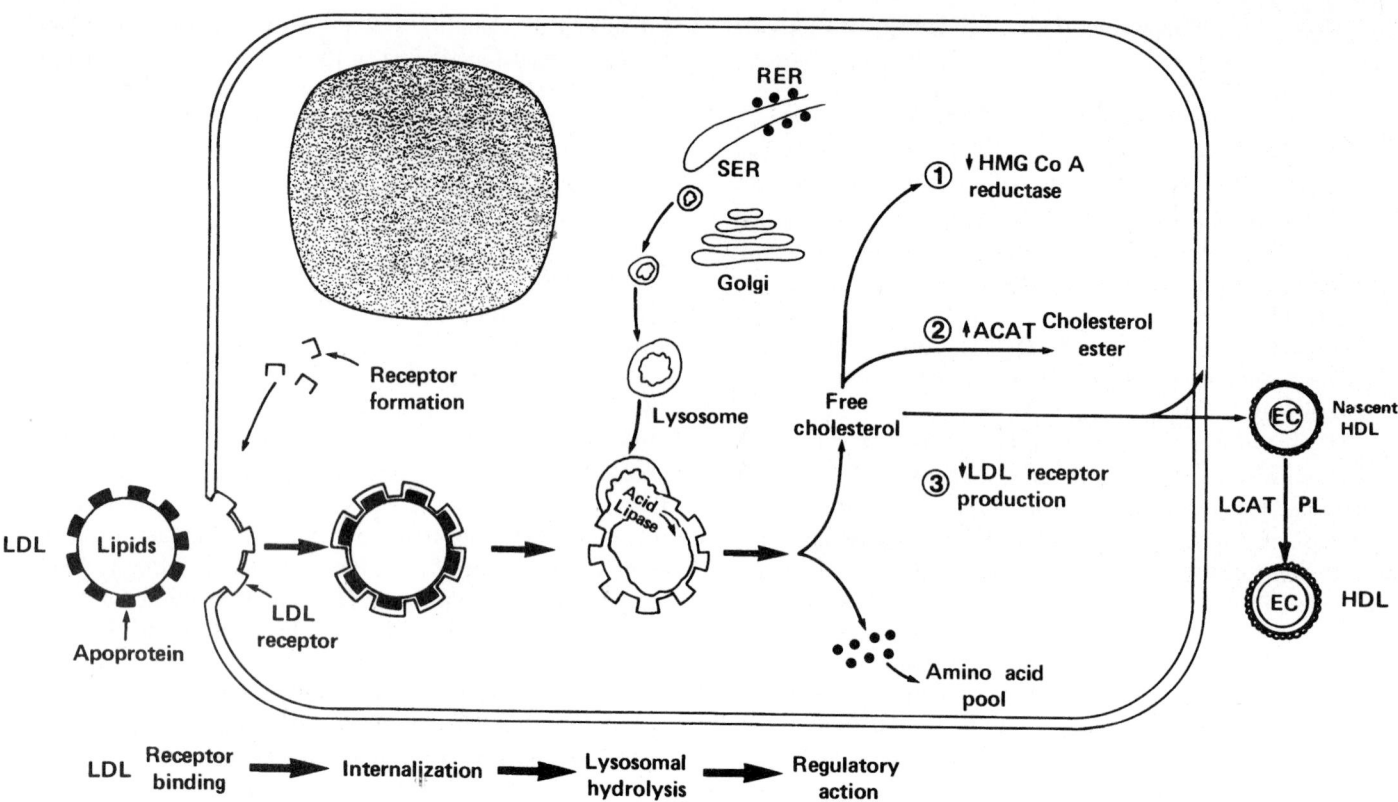

Fig. 33-4   Scheme of LDL uptake and catabolism by a cell. Mechanism not only clears LDL from circulation but also aids in regulation of cholesterol synthesis and storage. High-density lipoprotein, *HDL,* plays an integral role in removing cellular cholesterol, esterifying free cholesterol in blood and transporting cholesterol to liver for catabolism. *ACAT,* Acyl-CoA:cholesterol acyltransferase; *EC,* cholesteryl ester; *HMG-CoA reductase,* β-hydroxy-β-methylglutaryl-coenzyme A reductase; *LCAT,* lecithin:cholesterol acyltransferase; *PL,* phospholipid; *RER,* rough endoplasmic reticulum; *SER,* smooth endoplasmic reticulum.

tion can be found in the section on lipoprotein metabolism.

Cholesterol is present in all plasma lipoproteins, but about 60% of the total cholesterol in plasma from a fasting human subject is carried in the LDL.[5] About two thirds of the plasma total cholesterol is esterified with long-chain fatty acids, with linoleic acid being the predominant fatty acid in humans. The cholesteryl esters in the plasma are in a state of constant turnover because of their continual hydrolysis and resynthesis. Hydrolysis of cholesteryl esters takes place in the liver, but synthesis occurs mainly in the plasma by transfer of a fatty acid residue from lecithin to free cholesterol (Fig. 33-4). This reaction is catalyzed by a plasma enzyme known as *lecithin:cholesterol acyltransferase,* or LCAT. The preferred lipoprotein substrate for human LCAT is high-density lipoprotein (HDL), and it seems likely that the bulk of the esterified cholesterol in the plasma is formed on HDL.[6] The cholesteryl ester then is transferred from HDL to LDL and VLDL, partly in exchange for triglyceride.

It is believed that one of the functions of HDL is to transport cholesterol, in esterified form, from the tissues to the liver.[6] One might then envisage the following sequence of events. Free cholesterol from peripheral tissues is transferred to HDL; it is then esterified by LCAT, enabling HDL to take up more free cholesterol. The esterified cholesterol formed on HDL is transferred to LDL and VLDL, where it is incorporated into the nonpolar core of the lipoprotein molecules. LDL, carrying its load of cholesteryl ester to peripheral tissues, reaches the liver, where the cholesteryl esters are hydrolyzed, entering the pool of free cholesterol in the hepatocyte. The free cholesterol can leave the hepatic pool by secretion into the bile, directly or after conversion into bile acids, or by reincorporation into plasma lipoprotein (VLDL). Hepatic excretion of cholesterol via the biliary pool is one of the major mechanisms for removing cholesterol from the circulation.

Synthesis

Almost all animal tissues synthesize cholesterol from acetyl CoA. In adults the liver and intestinal wall probably supply over 90% of the plasma cholesterol of endogenous origin. Hepatic cholesterologenesis, unlike intestinal cholesterol synthesis, is inhibited by dietary cholesterol. Cholesterol production rate (absorbed cholesterol plus endogenously synthesized cholesterol) amounts to about 1 g/day. In most tissues the rate of synthesis of cholesterol is determined by the capacity of β-hydroxy-β-methylglutaryl CoA (HMG-CoA) reductase, which catalyzes a rate-limiting step in the biosynthetic sequence from acetyl CoA to cholesterol. Although this appears to be the main rate-limiting reaction, there appears to be other sites of suppression in the biosynthetic cholesterol pathway. Hepatic HMG-CoA reductase is subject to induction and repression by several hormones, dietary factors, and drugs. Feedback control of hepatic cholesterologenesis is also mediated by cholesterol itself and directly or indirectly by bile acids. A brief scheme of the control of hepatic cholesterologenesis is shown in Fig. 33-5.

Catabolism

In humans, increased absorption of cholesterol is followed by increased excretion of cholesterol from the exchangeable pool. Increased conversion of cholesterol into bile acids can be brought about by interruption of the enterohepatic circulation of bile salts. Bile salts returning to the liver

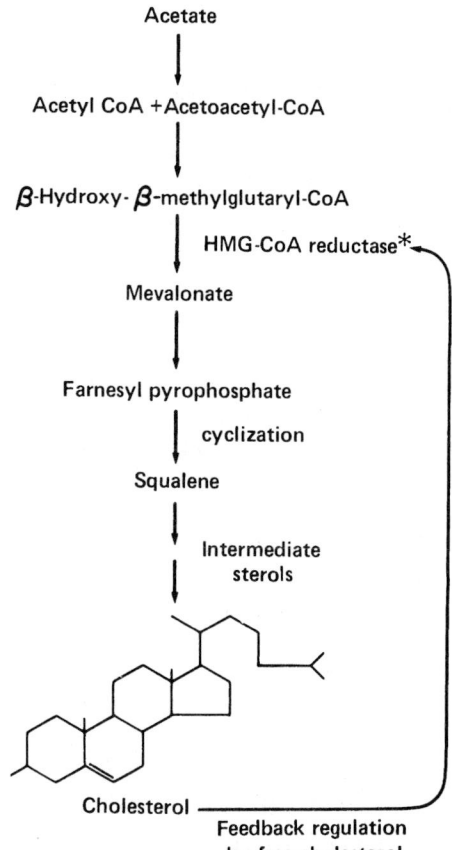

Fig. 33-5 Metabolic pathway of cholesterol synthesis, emphasizing negative feedback end-product inhibition step at β-hydroxy-β-methylglutaryl CoA step with the important enzyme HMG-CoA reductase.

from the intestine repress the formation of an enzyme catalyzing the rate-limiting step in the conversion of cholesterol into bile acids. When bile salts are prevented from returning to the liver, the activity of this enzyme increases and degradation of cholesterol to bile acids is stimulated. This effect may be exploited therapeutically in the treatment of hypercholesterolemia by the use of unabsorbable resins, which bind bile acids in the lumen of the intestine and prevent their return to the liver.

The mechanisms just stated for excretion of cholesterol by means of bile acids or cholesterol in the bile depend on the receptor-mediated activity in the hepatocytes. The hepatocytes have receptor sites that are specific for apoproteins (Apo) B and E. The major function of the liver in lipoprotein clearance is to remove lipoproteins containing Apo E (such as chylomicron remnants and VLDL remnants) and Apo B (such as LDL remnants) from plasma. However, the Apo E–containing lipoproteins are cleared with much greater efficiency than the Apo B–containing lipoproteins. For this reason chylomicron remnants and VLDL remnants (intermediate-density lipoprotein, IDL) are not normally measurable in healthy individuals (see Fig. 33-1).

The uptake of LDL by the peripheral tissues is also receptor-site dependent (see Fig. 33-4). The binding of LDL to the receptor site followed by internalization and hydrolysis of the LDL serves to deliver free cholesterol to the cell. The intracellular free cholesterol then functions (1) as a regulator for the rate of receptor synthesis, (2) as a regulator for cholesterol synthesis by the end-product negative-feedback mechanism, or (3) as a regulator for ACAT (acyl-CoA : cholesterol acyltransferase) activity, which determines how much cholesterol is stored in the cell as cholesteryl oleate, a cholesterol ester. It is believed that one of the factors that causes the efflux of cholesterol from the cell into the blood is the availability of HDL.[6] By this process, the cholesteryl oleate in the cell is hydrolyzed to free cholesterol and fatty acid. The liver and to some extent the gastrointestinal tract and other organs, such as the adrenal glands and gonadal tissues, take up the HDL and catabolize the HDL to its protein and lipid constituents (including cholesterol).

Normal expected cholesterol values

Unlike many of the blood analytes that we measure in the laboratory, lipids and lipoproteins require a different approach when normal expected values are being defined.[7] A problem arises in defining what levels of plasma lipids separate persons with elevated blood fats and who have or will develop CHD from the rest of the "normal" population. Before one can address the question of what is adequate dietary or drug therapy for the control of serum lipid and lipoprotein concentrations, one needs first to consider the degree to which blood lipids should be lowered. In other words, at what level should the clinician consider a sample "hyperlipidemic"? Many clinical laboratories and practicing physicians used reference intervals derived from the central 95% of values when classifying a sample as normal or abnormal. Unfortunately, because of the way we have defined "normal" in the past, many lipid and lipoprotein test results do not correlate very well with health-risk conditions on an individual basis. Thus a cholesterol value in the normal range for a given population may not represent a healthy cholesterol level. For example, a cholesterol value of 2500 to 2800 mg/L may be within the 95th percentile of the distribution of an apparently healthy male population between 51 and 59 years of age in the United States, but about 40% to 50% of these persons eventually will develop CHD.

Critical values for serum lipids and lipoproteins that are highly predictive of disease or disease risk, irrespective of the "normal" distribution, have been established (see the discussion of the National Cholesterol Education Program, p. 669).

Because of the positive correlation between blood cholesterol concentration and the increased risk for CHD, many investigators believed that the average cholesterol concentration for the entire population should be as low as possible. According to clinical data,[13] the individuals with plasma cholesterol values below 1800 mg/L had minimum CHD mortality (about 3.3/1000). However, the relative risk increased by 25% for those with values between 1800 and 2000 mg/L. Between 2000 and 2390 mg/L the relative risk increased about 80%; for values above 2400 mg/L, the relative risk increased almost two and one-half times, or 230%. For individuals with plasma cholesterol concentrations near 2600 mg/L, the relative risk increased by 400%. In simplistic terms, concentrations below 2000 mg/L can be considered to be more ideal than concentrations above 2000 mg/L for the adult population. Using such a definition, this means that about 58% of the adult population has undesirably elevated cholesterol concentrations. The plasma concentration in young American men is essentially within the ideal range. If it did not increase with age, the risk of CHD in the United States population would perhaps be much lower than it is now. Recent reports suggest that the mean cholesterol value of the United States population declined from 2200 to less than 2150 mg/L, and the CHD morbidity and mortality have decreased. Again, it should be remembered that the relationship of blood cholesterol concentration to CHD shows no threshold for the disease.

It is well known that as we age we become more susceptible to the atherosclerotic process. It has been calculated that, for an individual with a cholesterol level of 2000 mg/L and no other risk factors, a critical degree of atherosclerosis (greater than 60% stenosis) is reached in many people by the time they reach the age of 70 years. If the same individual had a cholesterol value of 2500 or 3000 mg/L, this degree of coronary artery disease (CAD) would probably be attained by 60 or 50 years of age respectively. This timetable is accelerated when one considers the inter-

action of risk factors for CHD. With the addition of a CHD risk factor, such as smoking, the critical age is reached by 60 years of age, and by further addition of another CHD risk factor, hypertension, this age drops to 50 years. A plasma cholesterol concentration of 2500 mg/L would move the critical age back to 50 years with one risk factor and to 40 years with two risk factors. It should be emphasized that a person's serum or plasma total cholesterol concentration is under the influence of many other factors, some of which are controllable and some uncontrollable.[11]

Genetics. Genetics probably has the most important influence on a person's cholesterol concentration. It is estimated that about half of the variability in blood cholesterol concentrations has a genetic basis.

Age. Serum cholesterol concentration starts out around 650 mg/L at birth and steadily increases with age (about 15 mg/L per year).

Sex. Cholesterol concentration in the blood of males is generally always higher than that in premenopausal females. After menopause, however, the cholesterol concentration is higher in females than in males. Serum cholesterol levels in males seem to plateau by 50 to 60 years of age.

Diet. Saturated fat in the diet increases serum cholesterol levels, whereas polyunsaturated fat decreases cholesterol concentration; monounsaturated fats have some lowering effect. Dietary cholesterol elevates serum cholesterol levels. Plant sterols and certain types of fiber decrease serum cholesterol concentration. Fish oils seem to lower triglycerides more than cholesterol.

Obesity. Although obesity is commonly regarded as an important contributor to the development of hypertriglyceridemia, it is well established that as the percentage of individuals with obesity increases with age so does the blood cholesterol concentrations.

Physical activity. Physical activity tends to lower serum total cholesterol. Much of this effect depends on the type, intensity, duration, and frequency of physical activity. Exercise also lowers LDL cholesterol and increases HDL cholesterol concentration.

Hormones. Growth hormone, thyroxine, and glucagon decrease serum cholesterol levels, whereas anabolic steroids and progestins increase cholesterol levels. The loss of estrogen in the postmenopausal women is associated with elevated blood cholesterol concentrations in older women.

Primary disease states. Diabetes mellitus, thyroid dysfunction, obstructive liver disease, acute porphyria, dysgammaglobulinemias, and nephrotic syndrome all have an effect on blood cholesterol concentrations.

TRIGLYCERIDE METABOLISM
Biological functions

Triglycerides are the major form of fat found in nature, and their primary function is to provide energy for the cell. One gram of fatty acids liberates about 9 kcal. The human body stores large amounts of fatty acids in ester linkages with glycerol in the adipose tissue. This form of storage of reserve energy is highly efficient because of the magnitude of the energy that is released when fatty acids undergo catabolism.

Physiology

Triglycerides are by far the most abundant subclass of neutral glycerides in nature. Mammalian tissues also contain some diglycerides and monoglycerides, but these occur in trace levels when compared to triglycerides. Most triglyceride molecules in mammalian tissues are mixed glycerides.

Because of their water insolubility, triglycerides are transported in the plasma in combination with other more polar lipids (phospholipids) and proteins, as well as with cholesterol and cholesteryl esters, in the complex lipoprotein macromolecules. It appears that the essentially nonpolar triglyceride (and cholesteryl ester) is largely in the center of the lipoprotein, with the more polar protein and phospholipid components at the surface, with their polar groups being directed outward to stabilize the whole structure in the aqueous plasma environment.

Synthesis

The concentration of triglyceride in the plasma at any given time is a balance between the rate of entry into the plasma and the rate of removal. A change in concentration may therefore be the result of a change in either or both of these factors. Moreover, a primary change in one may result in a secondary change in the other. Thus, perhaps the main problem to be considered in any situation where the plasma triglyceride concentration is abnormally high is whether this is attributable to a rise in the rate of entry or to a fall in the rate of removal of plasma triglycerides.

Plasma triglycerides are derived from two sources, intestinal and liver. Intestinal triglycerides are synthesized from dietary fat. The source of the fatty acids present in the triglyceride entering the blood from the liver depends greatly on the individual's nutritional state. Thus in the fasting state, fatty acids derived from adipose cell triglycerides are taken up by the liver and a portion is reexcreted as VLDL. Following a meal, dietary carbohydrates are taken up by the liver and converted to triglycerides, which are secreted as lipoproteins. It is important to realize that, except during the absorption of dietary fat, the liver is the main contributor of triglyceride to the plasma.

The size, triglyceride content, and particle density of the lipoprotein complexes formed by the intestines and liver varies according to the amount of triglyceride that is being released. Thus high rates of release result in large complexes with a higher triglyceride load and a correspondingly lower density. In fact, the lipoprotein complexes released from the liver under such conditions may reach a size not much below that of the intestinal chylomicrons, even though they normally have a somewhat lower triglyceride content and therefore a higher density.

Catabolism

The action of clearing-factor lipase at the endothelial cell surface not only facilitates the removal of triglyceride fatty acid from the blood but also determines where it is utilized, and this has important consequences. For example, in a state of caloric excess, the proportion of the triglyceride fatty acid in the bloodstream that is in excess of the immediate caloric needs is taken up by adipose tissue. Most fatty acids are reconverted to intracellular triglyceride and stored. In contrast, in a state of calorie deficit (as during fasting) the tissues derive their energy primarily from the oxidation of unesterified fatty acids, which are mobilized from adipose tissue and carried to the body tissues in the blood. There is still triglyceride in the blood in VLDL under these conditions, but instead of being taken up by adipose tissue for storage, it is now directed away from this tissue and toward muscle to supplement the supply of energy from the mobilized fatty acids. This switch in triglyceride fatty acid uptake is achieved through changes in the activity of intracellular lipase in the tissues concerned. Thus fasting results in a fall in the activity of the enzyme in adipose tissue and an increase in its activity in muscle.

The intracellular adipose triglyceride enzyme is distinct from the plasma enzyme and is called *hormone-sensitive lipase* because it is converted from an inactive to an active form by epinephrine, norepinephrine, adrenocorticotropin, thyroid-stimulating hormone, and glucagon. Moreover, its activity is promoted by growth hormone. On the other hand, insulin inhibits the activity of this lipase. Unlike the lipoprotein lipase of adipose tissue, hormone-sensitive lipase of other tissue exhibits increased activity during fasting, possibly because of falling insulin levels. It is believed that hormone-sensitive lipase plays an important role in fat mobilization from adipose tissue.

Normal expected triglyceride values

Rather than base triglyceride reference intervals on traditional 95th percentile ranges, an NIH consensus conference recommended that the most useful triglyceride value to remember is 10,000 mg/L or greater, which represents an increased risk for acute pancreatitis.[8] The adult upper limit of normal was defined as 2000 mg/L for both sexes, regardless of age. The difficulty in the interpretation of the triglyceride values is the "gray zone"; that is, does one treat for the mild hypertriglyceridemia if the values are between 2000 and 4000 mg/L? Clinically, it makes sense to treat for the mild hypertriglyceridemia only if the patient's HDL cholesterol concentration is depressed. The lack of convincing evidence that triglyceride is a primary risk factor for CHD does not warrant aggressive intervention with treatment for the mild hypertriglyceridemic patient. However, in many instances, the lowering of the triglycerides will nor-

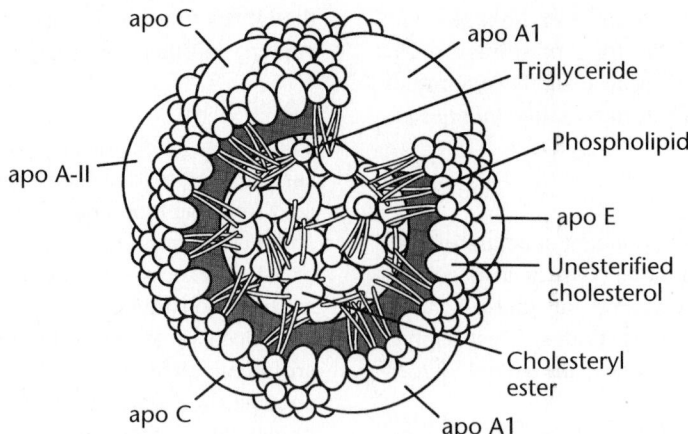

Fig. 33-6   Scheme of a lipoprotein complex showing polar outer surface and a core filled with neutral lipids. *HDL,* High-density lipoprotein. (Modified from Grundy SM: *Slide atlas of lipid disorders: cholesterol, atherosclerosis, and coronary heart disease,* New York, 1990, Gower Medical Publishing.)

malize the below-normal HDL cholesterol levels because of the existence of the reverse relationship between triglyceride and HDL cholesterol concentrations. On the other hand, if the HDL cholesterol concentrations are normal or above the normal limits (that is, 600 mg/L), there is no indication for treatment intervention for the patient with mild hypertriglyceridemia.

Part II. Lipoproteins

As discussed earlier, lipids are insoluble in aqueous media, including that of plasma.[3,4] It is only when the hydrophobic lipids are bound to protein-containing "lipoproteins" that they become soluble in the bloodstream. Because lipoproteins are generally viewed as a class of macromolecules associated with lipid transport, recommendations were made in about 1967 to transfer the diagnostic emphasis from hyperlipidemia to hyperlipoproteinemia.[1,2,5,9]

A lipoprotein can be visualized most simply as a globular structure with an outer solubilizing coat of protein and phospholipid and an inner hydrophobic, neutral core of triglyceride and cholesterol (Fig. 33-6). The protein and phospholipid impart solubility to the otherwise insoluble lipids. The binding of the inner lipid to the phospholipid and protein coat is noncovalent, occurring primarily through hydrogen bonding and van der Waals forces. The protein, free of lipid, is called *apolipoprotein.* Note that the lipids, which are weakly bound to the protein and phospholipid, are bound loosely enough to allow the ready exchange of lipid between the serum lipoproteins themselves, as well as between serum and tissue lipoproteins, yet strongly enough to allow the lipid and protein moieties to be separated in the analytical systems that are used to isolate and classify the lipoproteins.

CLASSIFICATION OF LIPOPROTEINS

The four most frequently used systems to isolate, separate, and characterize lipoproteins are based on analytical ultracentrifugation, preparative ultracentrifugation, electrophoresis, and precipitation techniques.[10] The most frequently used systems are those based on ultracentrifugation and electrophoresis (Fig. 33-7). With a paper or agarose support medium, electrophoretic patterns show that chylomicrons remain at the origin while pre-beta-lipoproteins and beta-lipoproteins migrate in the $beta_1$- and $beta_2$-globulin areas respectively and alpha-lipoproteins migrate in the $alpha_1$-globulin area.

Using the ultracentrifuge and taking advantage of the fact that lipoproteins are lighter than the other serum proteins, one can separate the lipoproteins into chylomicrons (the lightest lipoproteins, of a density less than plasma), VLDL at a density below 1.006 g/mL (after chylomicron removal), LDL of density 1.006 to 1.063 g/mL, and HDL of density 1.019 to 1.210 g/mL.[1-4,9] These lipoprotein classes correlate with electrophoretic patterns; for example, pre-beta-lipoprotein is generally synonymous with VLDL, beta-lipoprotein with LDL, and alpha-lipoprotein with HDL. Table 33-1 and Fig. 33-7 summarize the physical, chemical, and physiological characteristics of the major plasma lipoproteins.

Chylomicrons

Chylomicrons contain mainly triglyceride combined with cholesterol, small amounts of phospholipid, and specific apoproteins (Apo B-48, A-I, A-II, C-I, C-II, C-III, with small amounts of Apo B and E-II, E-III, E-IV) (see Table 33-3). Most models for chylomicron structure have been made under the assumption that the neutral lipids (triglycerides and cholesteryl ester) are partially surrounded by an outer shell

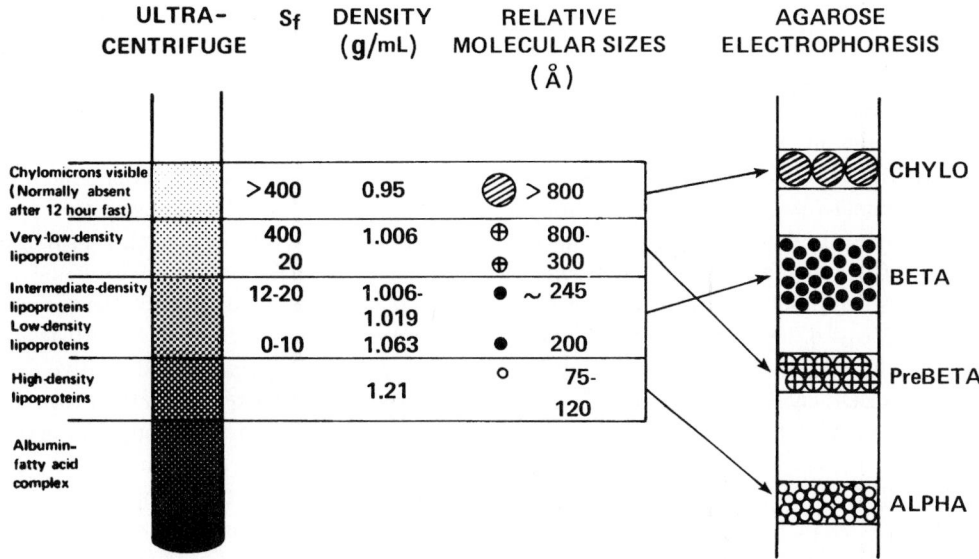

Fig. 33-7   Overview of major types of lipoproteins, showing some basic chemical and physical properties. *alpha,* Alpha-lipoprotein; *beta,* beta-lipoprotein; *chylo,* chylomicrons; *pre-beta,* a very-low-density lipoprotein; S_f, Svedberg flotation rate.

of phospholipid, free cholesterol, and protein. Under fasting conditions (more than 10 to 12 hours after a meal), no chylomicrons are generally found in the blood of healthy persons. The presence of chylomicrons makes the serum appear turbid or milky.

Very-low-density lipoprotein

An average preparation of VLDL contains 52% triglyceride, 18% phospholipid, 22% cholesterol, and about 8% protein. Cholesterol and cholesteryl esters occur in a ratio of about 1:1 by weight. Sphingomyelin and phosphatidylcholine are the major phospholipids. The larger the size of a VLDL particle, the greater the proportion of triglycerides and Apo C and the smaller the proportion of phospholipid, Apo B, and other apoproteins. Apo B appears to be present

in a constant absolute quantity in all VLDL fractions. Apo B-100 accounts for approximately 30% to 35%, with Apo C-I, C-II, and C-III making up over 50% of the apoprotein content in VLDL. Apo E-II, E-III, and E-IV and varying quantities of other apoproteins (A-I, A-II, B-48) may also be present. The relative quantity of each protein varies with the individual and with the degree of hyperlipidemia.

Low-density lipoprotein

LDL contains, by weight, 80% lipid and 20% protein. Consistent with this increased protein content, LDL is smaller (21 to 25 nm) and is of higher hydrated density (1.006 to 1.063 g/mL) than VLDL and chylomicrons are. About 50% of LDL lipid is cholesterol. LDL constitutes 40% to 50% of the plasma lipoprotein mass in humans. Its average con-

Table 33-1   Physical and chemical description of plasma lipoproteins in humans

Feature	Chylomicrons	VLDL	IDL	LDL	HDL
Density (g/mL)	<1.006	<1.006	1.006-1.019	1.019-1.063	1.063-1.21
Electrophoretic mobility	Origin	Pre-beta	Beta	Beta	Alpha
Flotation rate (S_t)	>400	20-400	12-20	0-10	—
Diameter (nm)	80-500	40-80	24.5	20	7.5-12
Lipids (% by weight)	98	92	85	79	50
Cholesterol	9	22	35	47	19
Triglyceride	82	52	20	9	3
Phospholipid	7	18	20	23	28
Apoproteins (% of weight)	2	8	15	21	50
Major	A-I, A-II	B-100	B-100	B-100	A-I, A-II
	B-48	C-I, C-II, C-III	C-I, C-II, C-III		C-I, C-II, C-III
	C-I, C-II, C-III	E	E		
Minor	B-100	A-I, A-II	B-48	C-I, C-II, C-III	B-100
	D	B-48		E-II, E-III, E-IV	D
	E-II, E-III, E-IV				E-II, E-III, E-IV

centration in normal adult American males is about 4000 mg/L, and in females it is 3400 mg/L. LDL is the major carrier of cholesterol and is considered an atherogenic lipoprotein. Apo B-100 is the major apoprotein of normal LDL, and LDL Apo B represents 90% to 95% of the total plasma Apo B-100. Experimental evidence suggests that the LDL Apo B in healthy humans is derived almost entirely from VLDL Apo B in plasma. LDL is frequently separated into two classes, LDL_1 (or intermediate-density lipoprotein, IDL) and LDL_2, on the basis of flotation density. The lower-density fraction, IDL (1.006 to 1.109 g/mL), is more lipid rich than LDL_2 (1.019 to 1.063 g/mL) and probably represents an intermediate in VLDL catabolism (see Fig. 33-1). Thus a comparison of IDL with LDL_2 demonstrates the gradual disappearance of triglyceride and of apoproteins more characteristic of VLDL (Apo C and Apo E) and an enrichment with Apo B-100 and cholesterol ester.

High-density lipoprotein

The HDL macromolecular complex (see Fig. 33-6) contains approximately 50% protein and 50% lipid. HDL is the smallest of the lipoproteins (9 to 12 nm) and floats at the highest density (1.063 to 1.21 g/mL) of any of the lipoprotein molecules. The quantitatively most important HDL lipid is phospholipid, though HDL cholesterol is of particular interest. The major phospholipid species is phosphatidylcholine (also known as lecithin), which accounts for 70% to 80% of the total phospholipid. It has an important functional role as a reactant in plasma cholesterol esterification, which is catalyzed by the enzyme lecithin:cholesterol acyltransferase (LCAT).

HDL may be further subfractionated by differential ultracentrifugation into HDL_2 (with a density of 1.063 to 1.110 g/mL) and HDL_3 (1.110 to 1.21 g/mL); the former is present in premenopausal women at about three times its concentration in men. Persons with lower HDL_2 levels are apparently more susceptible to premature CHD.

Other lipoproteins

Floating beta-lipoprotein, or beta-migrating VLDL. The lipoprotein fraction called *floating beta-lipoprotein* is found in persons with type III hyperlipoproteinemia, or "broad-beta disease" (derived from the broad smear from beta- to pre-beta-lipoprotein regions frequently present on whole plasma lipoprotein electrophoresis in these subjects); it is also called dybetalipoproteinemia.[11] This fraction has a density of 1.006 g/mL, which is a VLDL characteristic, but has a beta-lipoprotein migration pattern. The abnormal lipid composition of VLDL in type III hyperlipoproteinemic persons is attributable to a proportionately larger amount of cholesterol in that fraction. This is considered to be a very atherogenic lipoprotein; most individuals with this lipoprotein disorder usually die of CHD by 20 to 30 years of age.[11]

This is a very rare genetic disorder, affecting approximately 1:10,000 individuals, or less than 0.1% of the population. A hallmark clinical presentation of this disease is palmar xanthoma (also called xanthoma striatum palmare). Occasionally, tuberous or tuberoeruptive xanthomas occur on the arms and, less frequently, on the buttocks. In addition to premature CHD, dysbetalipoproteinemia causes cerebral and peripheral vascular disease. This biochemical abnormality is reflected by an increase in IDL and chylomicron remnants, a VLDL cholesterol–to–VLDL triglycerides ratio greater than 0.35, and an isoelectric focusing pattern demonstrating the presence of the E-II/E-II apolipoprotein isoform, which is presently the definitive diagnostic test.

Lp(a), or sinking pre-beta-lipoprotein. Similarities in lipid composition, concentration, and density (1.05 to 1.10 g/mL) between Lp(a) and LDL prevented clear discrimination of these two lipoproteins until immunological tests demonstrated the uniqueness of their protein moieties. Sixty-five percent of Lp(a) protein is Apo B-100, but another 15% is albumin, and the remainder is an apoprotein unique to Lp(a), called *Apo Lp(a)*. Despite its high frequency in the population, the functional significance of this lipoprotein is uncertain.

There is increasing evidence that high Lp(a) levels (that is, greater than 300 mg/L) are associated with an elevated risk for CHD.[12] It appears that a person can have a normal LDL cholesterol but an elevated Lp(a) concentration and be at increased risk for CHD. Familial hypercholesterolemic persons with elevated levels of Lp(a) are at very high risk for premature CHD. Although about a third of the American public have normal or low Lp(a) levels (less than 100 mg/L), about 50% of the population have elevated levels. The elevation of Lp(a) occurs early in childhood and persists throughout adulthood. Lp(a) levels are not affected by any dietary intervention techniques and are not responsive to most lipid-lowering drugs, except for nicotinic acid.

Lipoprotein X. Although lipoprotein X has a flotation density similar to that of LDL, the lipid and protein compositions are quite different, and this abnormal lipoprotein migrates electrophoretically differently from LDL. Lipoprotein X is characterized by an unusually high proportion of plasma phospholipid and unesterified cholesterol and by a low protein content consisting of Apo B, Apo C, and albumin. It is found most characteristically in plasma of patients with biliary obstruction.

Lp-X is not found in healthy persons but is often found in patients with a familial deficiency of the enzyme LCAT and in patients with obstructive liver disease. Lp-X has been used in Europe for differentiating cholestasis from hepatic parenchymal disease. It is not a useful marker for differentiating extrahepatic from intrahepatic cholestasis.

LIPOPROTEIN METABOLISM
Chylomicrons

As discussed previously, chylomicrons are made exclusively in the intestine and traverse the lymphatic system to the thoracic duct where they then enter the systemic circulation. The major function of the chylomicron is the transport of dietary or exogenous triglycerides.

It is postulated that the newly synthesized and secreted chylomicrons (80 to 500 nm) from the intestinal mucosal cells ultimately pick up Apo C-II from HDL. Apo C-II then catalyzes lipoprotein triglyceride hydrolysis by lipoprotein lipase. The hydrolysis results in the liberation of FFAs and monoglycerides.

As shown in Fig. 33-1 endothelial cell lipoprotein lipase–catalyzed hydrolysis results in progressive triglyceride depletion of the chylomicron molecule resulting in the chylomicron remnant particle. This transformation involves maintenance of lipoprotein structure by simultaneous removal of phospholipid, unesterified cholesterol, and Apo C peptides from the lipoprotein surface to plasma HDL. A reciprocal transfer of cholesteryl ester from HDL may occur; Apo D may aid in this transfer process. The circulating chylomicron remnant particle is then released from the capillary wall and cleared from circulation through the liver, where it is metabolized. This particle, now smaller (30 to 80 nm), retains its cholesteryl ester and Apo B and Apo E, which play an important role in the uptake of these particles by a high-affinity hepatic receptor uptake mechanism (see Fig. 33-4). When binding occurs, the remnants are immediately internalized by receptor-mediated endocytosis and degraded in hepatic lysosomes.

Very-low-density lipoprotein

After the postprandial rise in chylomicron triglyceride, a secondary rise in triglyceride concentration occurs 4 to 6 hours after a meal. This represents predominantly hepatic VLDL triglyceride synthesized from glucose and chylomicron triglyceride not hydrolyzed in the peripheral tissue. The relative contributions of glucose and dietary fat vary with diet composition. Consumption of a high-carbohydrate diet may lead to a phenomenon known as *carbohydrate-induced hypertriglyceridemia*. With high dietary carbohydrate, glucose influx into the hepatocyte is in excess both of energy demands and of glycogen-storage capacity. This results in the shunting of acetyl CoA into fatty acid synthesis and dihydroxyacetone phosphate into activated glycerol. This phenomenon may not persist in healthy persons, but others may be unusually susceptible to carbohydrate induction of VLDL synthesis. This is the basis for reduction of dietary carbohydrate (simple sugars and alcohol) in the treatment of hypertriglyceridemia, but this approach is not successful if the hypertriglyceridemia has other causes, such as overproduction or a clearance defect. Normally, VLDLs represent about 10% to 15% of the total circulating lipoproteins in a normal healthy individual.

VLDL triglycerides are believed to have a fate similar to that of the lipids from chylomicrons (see section on chylomicron catabolism, p. 652 and just above). During the catabolism of VLDL, more than 90% of Apo C is transferred to HDL, whereas essentially all the Apo B remains with the original lipoprotein particle. According to this postulated catabolic pathway, breakdown of VLDL leads to the formation of the cholesterol-rich particle LDL. HDL plays an important role by serving as an acceptor macromolecule for Apo C and unesterified cholesterol and phospholipids, the excess surface materials from a saturated VLDL. Apo C may recycle from HDL to newly synthesized chylomicrons or VLDL. The half-life of VLDL is 1 to 3 hours.

Intermediate-density lipoprotein

IDL is a transient particle (22 to 28 nm) usually present in very low concentrations in plasma from fasting persons. IDL, as discussed previously, is a lipoprotein derived from VLDL catabolism. The HDL particles interact with the plasma enzyme LCAT, which esterifies the excess HDL free cholesterol with fatty acids derived from the carbon-2 position of lecithin, the major phospholipid of plasma. The newly synthesized cholesteryl ester is transferred back to the IDL particles from HDL, apparently through the action of a plasma cholesteryl ester exchange protein (possibly Apo D). The net result of the coupled lipolysis and exchange reactions is the replacement of most of the original triglyceride core of VLDL with cholesteryl ester.

After lipolysis, the IDL particles are released from the capillary wall into the circulation. They then undergo a further conversion in which most of the remaining triglycerides are removed and all the apoproteins except Apo B are lost. The resultant particle, which contains almost pure cholesteryl ester in the core and Apo B at the surface, is LDL.

Low-density lipoprotein

As discussed previously, LDL formation occurs primarily from the catabolism of VLDL. In normal healthy persons, LDL cholesterol constitutes about two thirds of the total plasma cholesterol; LDL cholesterol concentration in women is slightly less than that in men (except after menopause). LDL delivers cholesterol to extrahepatic tissues (and to the liver), where it is utilized, deposited, or excreted.

Delivery of the LDL particles to peripheral tissue is accomplished when the LDL binds to high-affinity receptors located in regions of the plasma membrane called *coated pits*. These pits invaginate into the cell and pinch off to form endocytic vesicles that carry the LDL to the lysosomes (Fig. 33-4). Fusion of the vesicle membrane with the lysosomal membrane exposes the LDL to a host of hydrolytic enzymes, which degrade the Apo B to amino acids. The cholesteryl esters are hydrolyzed by an acid lipase, and liberated free cholesterol leaves the lysosomes for use in cellular reactions. As a result of this uptake mechanism, extrahepatic cells have low rates of cholesterol synthesis, relying instead on LDL-derived cholesterol. The free cholesterol thus released is used for membrane synthesis and serves to regulate, that is, depress cellular cholesterol synthesis by

HMG-CoA reductase. LDL internalization also regulates synthesis of the LDL receptor itself.

Excess cholesterol activates the enzyme acyl-CoA:-cholesterol acyltransferase (ACAT), leading to intracellular cholesteryl ester storage. Thus the net result of LDL binding and internalization is the reciprocal inhibition and activation of enzymes synthesizing and storing cellular cholesterol and a reduction in the number of receptors available to bind LDL.

The significance of this process for regulation of plasma cholesterol levels in humans is illustrated by patients with the homozygous form of familial hypercholesterolemia. These patients are deficient in LDL receptors and have excessive LDL production and defective LDL catabolism because of an inability of tissues to bind, internalize, degrade, and thus regulate cholesterol synthesis. Except for the receptor-deficient state of familial hypercholesterolemia, however, the role of the LDL receptor in the final control of plasma cholesterol levels is uncertain and is probably only complementary to other regulatory processes. It has been recognized that the specificity of the LDL receptor extends to lipoproteins containing Apo E and Apo B as well. It appears that although extrahepatic receptors take up LDL readily, hepatic receptors take up chylomicron remnants with greater efficiency (about 20 times greater) and LDL with much less efficiency. This difference is probably attributable to the Apo E content of chylomicron remnants and IDL, which has a higher receptor affinity than that of Apo B.

In addition to its normal degradation mechanism, the high-affinity LDL receptor pathway, plasma LDL can be degraded by less efficient mechanisms that require high plasma levels to achieve significant rates of removal. One of these mechanisms occurs in scavenger cells (macrophages) of the reticuloendothelial system. When the plasma level of LDL rises, these scavenger cells degrade increasing amounts of LDL. When overloaded with cholesteryl esters, they are converted into foam cells, which are classic components of atherosclerotic plaques. In humans, estimates of the proportion of plasma LDL degraded by the LDL receptor system range from 33% to 66%. The remainder is degraded by the scavenger cell system and perhaps by other mechanisms not yet elucidated.

High-density lipoprotein

Nascent HDL molecules are synthesized in intestinal mucosal cells and in hepatocytes by a process analogous to that of VLDL and chylomicron synthesis. This involves microsomal lipid and protein synthesis followed by secretion. During the synthetic process, phospholipid and free cholesterol are combined with specific apoproteins to form disklike structures that undergo extensive compositional and structural modifications after secretion. The most important of these modifications is the esterification of free cholesterol to form cholesteryl ester by an enzymatic reaction catalyzed by LCAT. In humans this is the major source of plasma ester cholesteryl. Persons with LCAT deficiency have an accumulation of these cholesteryl ester–deficient particles in plasma. This finding possibly indicates that the cholesteryl ester formed in the LCAT reaction allows the expansion of the disklike structures to form spheres characteristic of normal plasma HDL. Cholesteryl ester thus formed may be transferred to VLDL during catabolism.

The apoprotein profile of nascent HDL is modified concomitantly with changes in lipid content. Apo E is a major component of newly secreted (nascent) HDL, unlike the plasma HDL, which is characterized by a predominance of Apo A with minor contributions by Apo C and Apo E. The functional significance of this modification is not completely understood, but Apo A-I is an activator of LCAT, and its acquisition must facilitate all LCAT reactions. In addition, HDL participates in the regulation of triglyceride catabolism and cholesteryl ester formation by providing the respective cofactors, Apo C-II for activation and Apo C-III for inhibition of lipoprotein lipase activity. Also normal HDL may balance LDL transport by mediating cholesterol removal from peripheral sites to degradative and excretory sites. This role of HDL in reverse cholesterol transport may be the basis for the protection afforded by HDL against cardiovascular disease.

The plasma half-life of HDL in normal subjects ranges from 3.3 to 5.8 days. The Apo A-I catabolism and Apo A-II catabolism within HDL are similar. HDL catabolism is enhanced in nephrotic patients but decreased in hypertriglyceridemic subjects, especially those with hyperchylomicronemia. It is also increased in subjects on high-carbohydrate diets and is greatly enhanced in patients with familial HDL deficiency (Tangier disease). It appears that changes in HDL catabolism may play a major role in regulating HDL levels in plasma.

HYPERLIPIDEMIA

By definition, hyperlipidemia is an elevated concentration of lipids in the blood. The major plasma lipids of interest are total cholesterol (free cholesterol + cholesteryl ester) and the triglycerides. When one or more of these major classes of plasma lipids is elevated, a condition referred to as *hyperlipidemia* exists.

Cholesterol and triglyceride concentrations can be used to detect hyperlipoproteinemia. Over 90% of persons with hyperlipidemia, as defined previously, have hyperlipoproteinemia. The major exceptions are individuals with excessive amounts of LDL whose plasma cholesterol is kept within normal limits by a concomitant decrease in HDL.

The NIH suggests that treatment in the United States should be initiated when an adult has a serum cholesterol level above 2000 mg/L.[13,14] The upper limit of serum triglyceride levels is somewhat less clear. Patient triglyceride concentration above 4000 mg/L can be considered high, and levels in excess of 10,000 mg/L can be considered undesirable because of the increased risk for acute pancreatitis.[8,14] Dietary therapy should be initiated when the above limits are exceeded in order to prevent or minimize the development of CHD, since atherosclerosis seldom occurs with a total cholesterol concentration of less than 1500 mg/L over the life-span of a person, unless other risk factors such as genetics, high blood pressure, smoking, and obesity are present.

HYPERLIPOPROTEINEMIA

Hyperlipoproteinemia is an elevation of serum lipoprotein concentrations. The classification of hyperlipoproteinemia begins with the determination of the type of abnormal lipoprotein profile.[1-3,9-16] However, other differentiation and analyses are always necessary, for example:

1. Separation of hyperlipoproteinemia into primary and secondary forms (Table 33-2). The secondary form is caused by another known disease that can result in secondary hyperlipoproteinemia manifesting itself in any of the five major types of lipoprotein profiles.
2. Differentiation of primary hyperlipoproteinemia into heritable and nonheritable forms.
3. Determination of the relative concentration of the lipoprotein fractions, that is, VLDL cholesterol, LDL cholesterol, and HDL cholesterol.

There are numerous types of hyperlipoproteinemias, but the majority of the patients with heritable hyperlipidemia have one of six common abnormal lipoprotein patterns. These patterns are summarized in Fig. 33-8, where one can observe that three of the four lipoprotein families serve as determinants. These three families are (1) chylomicrons, (2) VLDL, and (3) LDL (including IDL). The original Fredrickson phenotyping system[1,2] disregarded the importance of HDL and other lipoproteins discussed in this chapter. Because of the fairly recent worldwide epidemiological finding that there is a statistically significant inverse relationship between HDL cholesterol concentration and risk for CHD, laboratories now do LDL-cholesterol and HDL-cholesterol determinations as part of the overall lipid-lipoprotein profile.

CLASSIFICATION OF HYPERLIPOPROTEINEMIAS

Although the classification of hyperlipoproteinemia is based on identification of elevated concentration of blood lipids and abnormal lipoprotein patterns (Fig. 33-8), it must be emphasized again that each form of dyslipoproteinemia is not a homogeneous entity from a genetic, clinical, or pathological point of view.

The hyperlipoproteinemias are now described in somewhat greater detail, with emphasis on distinctive clinical, diagnostic, genetic, biochemical-pathophysiological, and therapeutic aspects.[1-4,9-16]

Table 33-2   Causes of secondary hyperlipoproteinemia

Pattern	Causes
Hyperchylomicronemia	Insulinopenic diabetes mellitus Dysglobulinemia Lupus erythematosus Pancreatitis
Hyperbetalipoproteinemia	Nephrotic syndrome Hypothyroidism Obstructive liver disease Porphyria Multiple myeloma Portal cirrhosis Viral hepatitis, acute phase Myxedema Stress Anorexia nervosa Idiopathic hypercalcemia
Dysbetalipoproteinemia	Hypothyroidism Dysgammaglobulinemia Myxedema Primary biliary cirrhosis Diabetic acidosis
Hyperprebetalipoproteinemia	Diabetes mellitus Nephrotic syndrome Pregnancy Hormone use (oral contraceptives) Glycogen-storage disease Alcoholism Gaucher's disease Niemann-Pick disease Pancreatitis Hypothyroidism Dysglobulinemia
Mixed type of lipoproteinemia	Insulinopenic diabetes mellitus Nephrotic syndrome Alcoholism Myeloma Idiopathic hypercalcemia Pancreatitis Macroglobulinemia Diabetes mellitus (insulin independent)

Hyperchylomicronemia

This lipoprotein disorder is characterized by highly elevated plasma triglyceride concentration, generally greater than 10,000 mg/L, as the result of chylomicronemia. The occasional elevation in cholesterol is secondary to the pronounced elevation in chylomicron levels, since these particles also contain cholesterol. LDL and HDL are often low, whereas VLDL may be slightly elevated. Chylomicron removal is reduced, and subjects have deficiencies in lipase activities, such as postheparin lipolytic activity (PHLA) (specifically extrahepatic, protamine-inactivated lipoprotein lipase). Primary hyperchylomicronemia usually manifests itself early in childhood. Although this disorder is usually primary and familial, the lipoprotein pattern may be produced by several other disease or metabolic states. Thus sec-

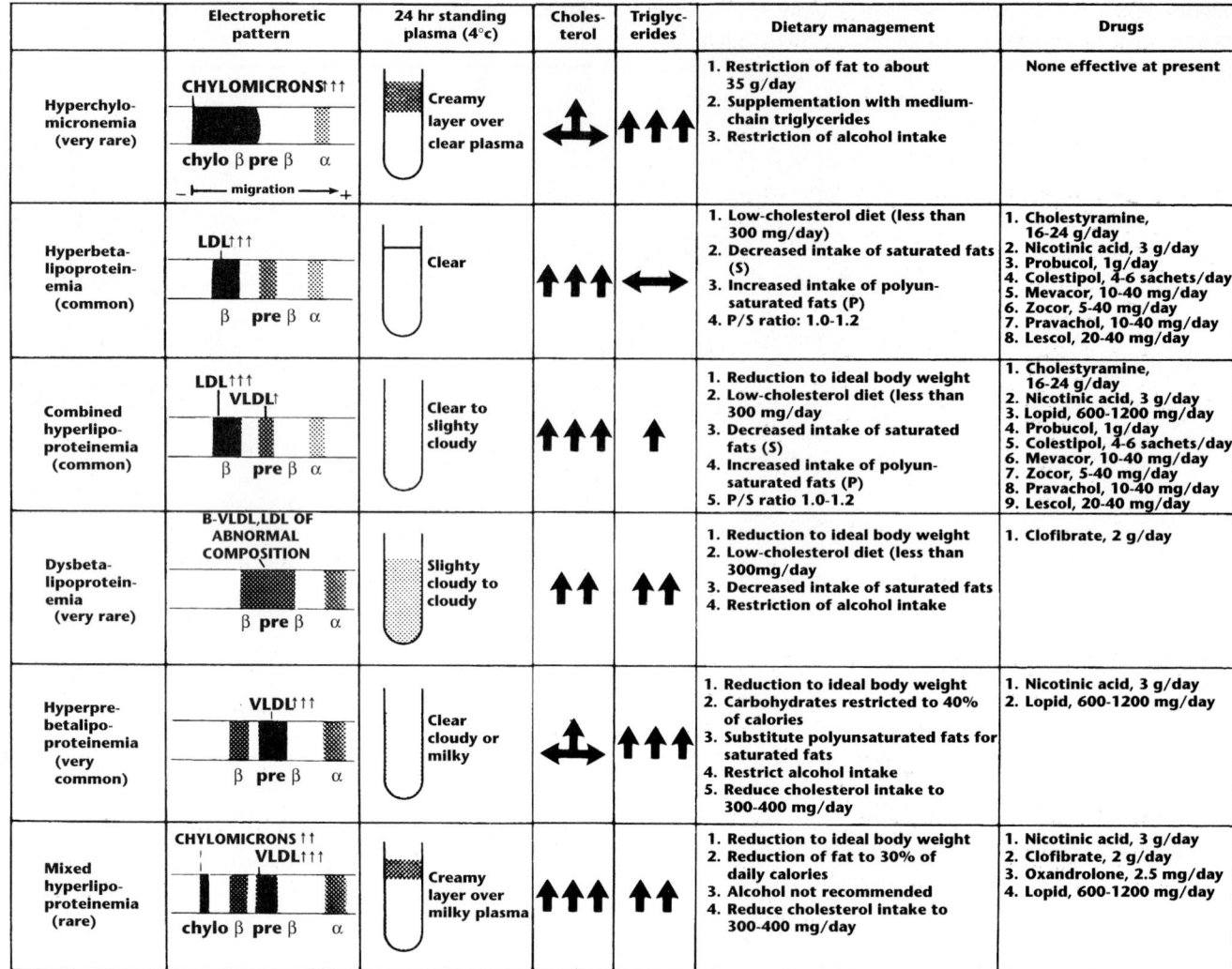

Fig. 33-8   Summary of six types of hyperlipoproteinemias. Abbreviations as in Fig. 33-7.

ondary forms of this dyslipoproteinemia should be ruled out (see Table 33-2).

Once the obvious secondary causes have been ruled out, the primary disorder can be confirmed by (1) presence of eruptive xanthomas, hepatosplenomegaly, lipemia retinalis, abdominal pain, and pancreatitis early in life, (2) intake of drugs that can cause secondary hypertriglyceridemia, (3) presence of reduced plasma levels of triglyceride lipases, (4) reduction in triglyceride levels and disappearance of chylomicronemia on a fat-free diet, and (5) confirmation by family screening of inheritance as an autosomal recessive trait.

Current lipid-lowering drugs are not effective in lowering serum triglycerides, therefore only a low-fat diet is effective in treating this disorder. Because chylomicrons are produced as a response to the ingestion of fat in the diet, the therapeutic approach is to reduce the amount of dietary fat to 10% of total calories. This intervention technique can result in a decrease in serum triglycerides within 24 hours.

The primary goal is to decrease serum triglycerides to less than 10,000 mg/L to reduce the patient's risk for acute pancreatitis. The secondary goal is to further reduce triglyceride levels to normalize the HDL-cholesterol levels. The NECP recommendation[8,14] for healthy triglyceride levels is less than 2000 mg/L (Table 33-3).

Hyperbetalipoproteinemia

The lipoprotein disorder hyperbetalipoproteinemia is characterized by elevated concentration of plasma cholesterol with mostly normal triglyceride levels and clear plasma. Primary hypercholesterolemia can be caused by (1) overproduction of VLDL, (2) increased rate of conversion of VLDL to LDL, (3) LDL enriched with cholesteryl esters, (4) defective LDL structure, and (5) decreased LDL receptor number or activity on each cell. It is estimated that about 50% of the variability in blood cholesterol concentrations in the general population has a genetic basis. The lipoprotein pattern is characterized by an elevation of the LDL with nor-

Table 33-3   National Cholesterol Education Program recommendations for triglyceride classification of risk

Triglyceride (mg/L)	Risk
Less than 2000	Normal
2000-4000	Borderline-high
4000-10,000	High
Greater than 10,000	Very high

From National Heart, Lung, and Blood Institute Consensus Conference on Treatment of Hypertriglyceridemia, *JAMA* 251:1196-1200, 1984, and from Second Expert Panel: Detection, Evaluation, and Treatment of High Blood Cholesterol in Adults (Adult Treatment Panel II), *Circulation* 89:1329-1445, 1994.

mal VLDL. This lipoprotein disorder is recognized as familial hypercholesterolemia, which exhibits the following features: (1) a deficient number of functional LDL receptors in the fibroblast cultures (the pathognomonic feature), (2) an expression of type II pattern in infancy, (3) xanthomatosis in severely affected members, and (4) premature CHD seen by the third and fourth decade.

Secondary hyperbetalipoproteinemic disorders, such as hypothyroidism, acute intermittent porphyria syndrome, dysgammaglobulinemia, obstructive liver disease, and highly saturated fat and cholesterol diets should be ruled out.

Once secondary hyperlipoproteinemia has been ruled out, the primary disorder can be confirmed by (1) family screening, including children; (2) persistent hypercholesterolemia even after 8 weeks of a low cholesterol (less than 300 mg/day), high polyunsaturated fat diet (polyunsaturated fat–to–saturated fat [P/S] ratio of 1:1.2); (3) presence of tendinous xanthomas, xanthelasma, and corneal arcus; and (4) determination of LDL receptor defect or deficiency or other genetically determined molecular defects.

Special treatment is often required for the highly elevated cholesterol levels of familial hypercholesterolemic (FH) individuals (5000 to 15,000 mg/L). In addition to the customary diet and drug approach (see below), most FH patients require plasmapheresis every 3 to 4 weeks for removal of LDL. In extreme cases, liver transplants are required. For non-FH hypercholesterolemics, a rigorous low-fat diet is the first treatment step. If the diet cannot sufficiently reduce serum cholesterol, lipid-lowering drugs are employed.

The goal of diet therapy is to reduce serum LDL cholesterol while maintaining a nutritionally adequate diet. The recommended dietary approach can be found in the NECP adult treatment panel (ATP) reports.[13,14] The ATP recommendations are for the intervention to occur in two steps, the step I and step II diets. These diets progressively reduce the intake of total and saturated fat and cholesterol and promote weight loss in patients who are overweight. These step diets reduce other risks for CHD by reducing blood pressure, raising HDL-cholesterol levels, and lowering the risks for diabetes. LDL- and HDL-cholesterol levels should be monitored after 4 to 6 weeks and then 3 months after

beginning step I diet therapy. If the cholesterol goals are not achieved, the patient may progress to the step II diet. If the step II intervention still does not achieve the cholesterol goals, drug therapy should be considered. The cholesterol-lowering agents include bile acid sequestrants (cholestyramine or cholestipol), HMG-CoA reductase inhibitors (such as lovastatin [Mevacor], pravastatin [Pravacol], simvastatin [Zocor], fluvastatin [Lescol], nicotinic acid, and probucol. The effect of lipid-lowering drug therapy should be monitored at 4 to 6 weeks and then again at 3 months.

Combined hyperlipoproteinemia

Another form of familial hyperlipidemia is familial combined hyperlipidemia. The important features include (1) no abnormality in the number of functional LDL receptors in the fibroblast culture, (2) absence of the hyperbetalipoproteinemic pattern in children, (3) early expression of hypertriglyceridemia, (4) multiple lipoprotein patterns in affected relatives in successive generations, and (5) hypercholesterolemia in the common hyperbetalipoproteinemic pattern.

This is the more common of the primary hyperlipoproteinemias. The characteristic feature of this disorder is a scatter of lipoprotein phenotypes within a family. Most commonly, patients will have an elevation in both LDL and VLDL; however, within a family, hyperbetalipoproteinemia and hyperprebetalipoproteinemia will also be found, affecting different persons. In contrast to familial hyperbetalipoproteinemia, subjects with familial combined hyperlipoproteinemia generally do not manifest their disease until adulthood. Clinically, these patients have an increased incidence of coronary artery disease (CAD). They also are frequently diabetic, have a tendency for hyperuricemia, and show a low incidence of tendinitis and tuberous xanthomas. These features are suggestive of a closer clinical relation to familial hyperprebetalipoproteinemia than to familial hyperbetalipoproteinemia. The mode of inheritance of familial combined hyperlipoproteinemia is still in doubt; however, it is clearly a familial disorder that is seen most commonly with this lipoprotein pattern.

Remember that subjects with hyperbetalipoproteinemia or hyperprebetalipoproteinemia may also belong within a family group that has familial combined hyperlipoproteinemia.

This lipoprotein disorder is characterized by elevated total cholesterol, LDL, triglycerides, and VLDL with the absence of floating beta-lipoprotein. Any secondary hypercholesterolemia and hypertriglyceridemia should be ruled out before confirmation of the primary lipoprotein disorder. Family screening is mandatory for recognition of this lipid abnormality. Accurate diagnosis of the lipoprotein profile also requires an appreciation of the factors that determine triglyceride levels. Studies in free-living populations in the United States have documented increases in triglyceride levels with age and have indicated that as many as one fourth of middle-aged men had triglyceride levels that exceeded previously published cutoff values. Thus, although statistically valid, the critical limits for triglyceride concentrations may not represent physiological limits. Therefore one might expect a greater prevalence of combined hyperlipoproteinemia in older age groups.

The possible effects of dietary carbohydrates should not be overlooked when one is assessing this lipoprotein disorder. It has been shown that fasting hypertriglyceridemia in patients with this metabolic lipoprotein profile could be attributable to an acute increase in dietary carbohydrates. It appears that triglyceride values greater than 4000 mg/L are rare in patients with this lipoprotein pattern. The few reported cases in the medical literature occurred in postmenopausal women.

Lipoprotein electrophoresis is rarely necessary for the diagnosis of this pattern. If the hyperbetalipoprotein profile is present, the elevated cholesterol and the normal triglyceride levels leave little for the lipoprotein electrophoretic pattern to clarify. If the familial combined hyperlipidemic pattern is present, the decisive diagnostic procedure is differentiation of this pattern from either the broad-beta pattern or hyperprebetalipoproteinemic pattern. This task is not easily done with lipoprotein electrophoresis. Also note that the total plasma cholesterol may be normal despite an elevated LDL cholesterol value. This relationship also occurs in familial hypercholesterolemia.

The broad-beta pattern described below is no longer considered unique and has been noted in cases homozygous for familial hypercholesterolemia. The presence of a discrete band attributable to high concentrations of Lp(a), or "sinking" pre-beta-lipoprotein, can cause diagnostic confusion with the familial combined hyperlipidemic profile. When the triglyceride value is normal, the appearance of the broad-beta pattern of electrophoresis is suggestive of the presence of Lp(a). Thus the electrophoretic pattern is insensitive and is not a highly specific tool for differentiating patterns.

Treatment for combined hyperlipoproteinemia should be focused on decreasing both the LDL cholesterol and the triglyceride concentrations. The strategy for lowering LDL cholesterol is discussed in the section on hyperbetalipoproteinemia (p. 657). The lowering of triglycerides and VLDL cholesterol is somewhat different. From a dietary standpoint, the focus is on carbohydrate and calories (if the patient is overweight), requiring alcoholic restriction, and increased physical activity and achieving an ideal body weight. Drug therapy is generally indicated in patients with very high triglyceride concentrations (see Table 33-3).[8,14] Both clofibrate and gemfibrizol are effective in lowering triglycerides (thus VLDL or VLDL cholesterol). The drug of choice for combined hyperlipoproteinemia is nicotinic acid, since it is very effective in lowering both cholesterol (LDL cholesterol) and triglycerides (VLDL cholesterol) while increasing HDL cholesterol.

Dysbetalipoproteinemia

Dysbetalipoproteinemia (also called broad-beta hyperlipoproteinemia) is characterized by an elevation of both plasma cholesterol and triglyceride concentrations and an abnormal LDL (more specifically IDL), which floats in the fraction with a density less than 1.006 g/mL. This abnormal LDL often merges with the pre-beta band on electrophoresis to produce a *broad-beta* band (see Fig. 33-8). For accurate diagnosis of dysbetalipoproteinemia an ultracentrifugal study with measurement of cholesterol and triglyceride in the fractions with a density below 1.006 g/mL is required to document the presence of the floating beta-lipoprotein.

Measurements of the lipid composition of lipoproteins of a density less than 1.006 appear to offer a more reliable means of identifying this dyslipoproteinemia than is afforded by the detection of the presence of floating beta-lipoproteins by electrophoresis alone. The ratio used clinically is that of the cholesterol content of the VLDL divided by the plasma triglyceride concentration. This ratio appears to be most useful for documenting this hyperlipoproteinemia when the triglyceride level is at least 1500 mg/L, but it may be subject to error when triglyceride exceeds 10,000 mg/L. It has been suggested that if the VLDL cholesterol–to–triglyceride ratio is 0.30 or more, the subject may have dysbetalipoproteinemia. However, when the ratio is between 0.25 and 0.29, a diagnosis of possible broad-beta hyperlipoproteinemia should be considered. Confirmation of this disorder is made by finding an apoE isoform pattern of E_2-E_2.

The clinical characteristics of subjects with this lipoprotein disorder vary widely as a function of age, sex, degree of adiposity, and presence of associated disorders such as hypothyroidism and alcoholism.

The most characteristic xanthoma in subjects with broad-betalipoproteinemia is called *xanthoma striatum palmare* (in the literature both "xanthoma striatum palmaris" and "xanthoma striata palmaris" are improper Latin). In their most subtle form these lesions produce an orange or yellowish discoloration of the palmar creases (xanthochromia striata palmaris), a phenomenon most easily detected in subjects of fair complexion. When more advanced, these lesions may produce planar elevations and even the virtual obliteration of the palmar and digital creases. Raised lesions can occasionally affect the remaining palmar surfaces and in the severe form produce tuberous, incapacitating xanthomas.

Various forms of CHD have been reported in association with broad-beta hyperlipoproteinemia. Hyperlipoproteinemia is readily treated by diet and drugs. The form of cardiovascular disease associated with this form of dyslipoproteinemia differs significantly from that associated with familial hyperbetalipoproteinemia in that peripheral and even cerebrovascular disease appears to be as common as CHD.

Secondary broad-beta hyperlipoproteinemia has been associated with hypothyroidism, gout, and diabetes mellitus and is found in patients with acute renal failure receiving maintenance hemodialysis.

Hyperprebetalipoproteinemia

The pre-beta form of hyperlipoproteinemia has also been called *endogenous hyperlipemia,* or *carbohydrate-induced hyperlipemia.* The latter term is no longer accepted by most workers, since carbohydrate induction of hypertriglyceridemia is also observed in normolipemic individuals. Endogenous hyperlipemia excludes the rare hyperchylomicronemia but includes the uncommon mixed endogenous and exogenous hyperlipemia (see below).

By definition, hyperprebetalipoproteinemia is an elevation of VLDL (and triglyceride) levels above an arbitrary cutoff point in the absence of either chylomicrons or the abnormal VLDL of dysbetalipoproteinemia. LDL levels are normal, and LDL cholesterol measurement is normal.

A tentative diagnosis of this lipoprotein disorder may be made if the triglyceride concentration is increased, the total cholesterol is normal or moderately elevated, and the standing plasma (at 4° C for 10 to 12 hours) reveals no chylomicrons. The biochemical diagnosis is confirmed if electrophoresis reveals a distinct pre-beta-lipoprotein band and the LDL cholesterol is within normal limits. Keep in mind that the presence of a pre-beta band with normal plasma triglyceride levels occurs with "sinking" pre-beta-lipoprotein, a triglyceride-poor, apparently normal lipoprotein variant observed in up to 35% of healthy subjects.

Once the biochemical pattern of hyperprebetalipoproteinemia has been confirmed (that is, based on more than one sample under standard conditions), it should be classified according to cause as a primary—either familial or sporadic—or secondary disorder (see Table 33-2).

The diagnosis of the primary disorder depends on the following criteria: (1) a hyperprebetalipoproteinemic electrophoretic pattern, (2) an increase in VLDL cholesterol, (3) one or more first-degree relatives with this disorder, and (4) no close relative with other primary lipoprotein disorders. Other common features are a normal cholesterol level if the triglyceride level is less than 4000 mg/L, a triglyceride level usually below 15,000 mg/L, and a family history of diabetes.

Since a large proportion of our society imbibes alcohol, a brief comment will be made. Although not regarded as a major cause of hyperlipidemia, ethanol is known to cause acute but transient hypertriglyceridemia with an elevation in primarily VLDL, causing mainly prebetahyperlipoproteinemia (sometimes mixed hyperlipoproteinemia).

In the hypertriglyceridemia produced by ethanol intake, the following features stand out:

1. The hypertriglyceridemia is usually moderate in extent and limited in duration. The level of triglyceridemia rarely exceeds 10,000 mg/L, and the lipemia peaks in 12 to 14 hours and disappears after 25 to 40 hours. This apparently transient effect appears to hold true, especially for normolipemic individuals.
2. This hypertriglyceridemia is, for the most part, the result of increased VLDL and possibly chylomicrons.
3. The fatty liver associated with alcohol intake plays a vital role in the form and extent of the induced hyperlipoproteinemia, and the resultant changes may be related to the stage of the hepatic damage.
4. The triglyceride concentration in alcoholic hyperlipidemia is intimately related to the quality and quantity of dietary fatty acid intake. It is well known that simultaneous ingestion of ethanol with fat (as in complex meals or singly as corn oil) produces a prolonged and augmented rise in serum triglyceride concentration.

Although it is obvious that hyperlipemia can be produced by an excessive production and release of lipids (hence lipoproteins) into circulation, by defective removal or clearance of lipids from the blood, or by a combination of these physiological processes, the precise mechanism of ethanol-induced hyperlipemia is still unknown.

The treatment protocol is described in the section on combined hyperlipoproteinemia (p. 658).

Mixed hyperlipoproteinemia

Another form of hyperchylomicronemia is a mixed hyperlipoproteinemia. It is distinguished by the presence of both elevated VLDL and chylomicrons in the plasma of fasting subjects on a regular diet. This disorder can occur as a primary genetic defect and thus represents a second form of familial hyperchylomicronemia. Triglyceride levels similar to those seen in hyperchylomicronemia may be observed. As in that disorder, the occurrence of abdominal syndromes, including pancreatitis, and the physical findings of eruptive xanthomas, lipemia retinalis, and hepatosplenomegaly are related to the level of plasma triglyceride. Although the pathophysiological characteristics of these manifestations of this form of hyperlipoproteinemia probably do not differ from those observed in hyperchylomicronemia, a variety of other differences exist in clinical, genetic, metabolic, and biochemical observations.

In sharp contrast to hyperchylomicronemia, most instances of this order occur in adulthood. Full appearance of the abnormality may not occur until the fifth or sixth decade of life, with the females presenting later than the males. Several children with familial hyperlipoproteinemia have been described.

Extremely high triglycerides and hyperchylomicronemia are usually not attributable to primary metabolic disorders but are found in the setting of several disorders that can lead to secondary metabolic disorder. These disorders are particularly prone to produce this form of dyslipoproteinemias if they occur in a patient with primary hyperprebetalipoproteinemias. For example, pancreatitis may be associated with pronounced hyperchylomicronemia, but later only mild hypertriglyceridemia is found when the patient is re-evaluated under stable conditions. It is also well known that hyperprebetalipoproteinemia can present as this disorder in poorly controlled, insulin-dependent diabetics and in alcoholics.

Although this form of hyperlipoproteinemia is associated with elevated triglycerides (that is, VLDL and chylomicrons), plasma cholesterol concentrations may be slightly to moderately increased. LDL and HDL cholesterols are usually normal to low. The plasma is usually opaque, and a floating cream layer above the turbid plasma may be observed.

When total triglyceride is over 10,000 mg/L, visual appreciation of a discrete floating "creamy" supernate over turbid plasma becomes difficult. The use of ultracentrifugation (to remove the chylomicrons) or refrigeration test (separation of chylomicrons after standing overnight at 4° C) will help differentiate this form of hyperlipoproteinemia. The ultracentrifuge may be used to separate the chylomicrons from the VLDL for individual quantification if needed. A qualitative assessment of the electrophoresis strip is sometimes sufficient to document elevated VLDL and chylomicrons. Since in practice some overlap of VLDL levels may occur between these two lipoprotein patterns, a postheparin lipoprotein lipase measurement should be made as a final characterization. This enzyme should be present in this lipoprotein disorder. In the absence of a specific assay for the enzyme, a reasonably reliable clue to its presence may be sought by observation of the change in the lipoprotein electrophoresis pattern obtained with a plasma sample drawn 10 minutes after heparin injection (10 U/kg of body weight). The plasma cholesterol-to-triglyceride ratio in this form of dyslipoproteinemia (0.23 ±0.02) is usually lower than in hyperprebetalipoproteinemia (0.86 ±0.03) because the chylomicrons incorporate less cholesterol than the VLDL does. Major qualitative difficulties can arise in distinguishing this lipoprotein disorder from hyperprebetalipoproteinemia (endogenous hypertriglyceridemia) because this pattern is often transient, with many subjects losing their chylomicron band with moderate reductions in triglyceride.

This form of hyperlipoproteinemia is often secondary to a wide variety of diseases, drugs, and dietary habits (see Table 33-2). Since there are many ways of acquiring this form of hyperlipoproteinemia, a careful distinction between primary and secondary causes must be made. A routine history of ethanol intake and estrogen or steroid administration, a urinalysis, and the measurement of a fasting or 2-hour postprandial blood glucose, and liver, thyroid, and renal function tests are all useful in this distinction. Superimposition of poorly controlled diabetes mellitus, alcoholic excess, or estrogens or estrogen-containing oral contraceptives in an individual with preexisting hyperprebetalipoproteinemia will often produce the mixed pattern. In familial cases, particularly with plasma triglycerides above 15,000 mg/L, lipemia retinalis, hepatosplenomegaly, and eruptive xanthomas may be present.

The biochemical defect in this form of hyperlipoproteinemia is still not clear. The presence of high levels of chylomicrons in the fasting plasma of a subject whose diet contains a usual or low content of fat clearly indicates that clearance mechanisms are inadequate. A primary defect in removal of plasma triglyceride could also explain the elevated VLDL. That this defect is not simply a variant of hyperchylomicronemia is established by detecting and often quantitating heparin-releasable plasma PHLA from these subjects. Thus a different type of problem must lead to this failure in lipoprotein uptake. One possibility is that the synthesis of endogenous triglyceride and the resulting secretion of VLDL from the liver may proceed at an abnormally high rate, sufficient to saturate pathways of removal that are shared by chylomicrons, thus leading to an elevation of both lipoproteins. Studies utilizing lipoproteins labeled with radioisotopes have indicated that many patients with endogenous hypertriglyceridemia have elevated synthesis of VLDL triglyceride.

Familial hyperchylomicronemia may be divided into hyperchylomicronemia and a mixed form of hyperlipoproteinemia. Both disorders are manifested by very elevated triglyceride levels and frequently present with eruptive xanthomas, lipemia retinalis, hepatosplenomegaly, and abdominal pain. Hyperchylomicronemia is caused by a pronounced deficiency of lipoprotein lipase. The triglyceride elevation appears with ingestion of dietary fat and is thus manifested in very young children. The mixed form may be detected in rare instances in childhood, but the usual presentation is in the adult. It also differs from hyperchylomicronemia in that lipoprotein lipase is measurable and glucose intolerance and hyperuricemia are commonly associated findings. The only effective treatment for hyperchylomicronemia is a low-fat diet. The mixed form of hyperlipoproteinemia is most effectively treated by diet-induced weight loss and will frequently respond to one of the following drugs: nicotinic acid, norethindrone, oxandrolone, benzafibrate, gemfibrizol, or clofibrate.

TRANSFORMATION OF HYPERLIPIDEMIA TO HYPERLIPOPROTEINEMIA
Limitation of classification of types of hyperlipoproteinemia

The limitations and potentials of the lipoprotein-typing system of Frederickson, Levy, and Lees are well recognized.[1,2] However, it should be stressed that plasma lipoprotein patterns are not a substitute for an etiological classification of the hyperlipoproteinemias. The approach of Fredrickson, Lees, and Levy is to be regarded as provisional, pending a more fundamental understanding of the causes of the hyperlipidemias.

Using quantitative measurements of cholesterol and triglyceride alone, one can divide patients into three major groups: those with hypercholesterolemia alone, those with hypertriglyceridemia alone, and those with a combination of the two. Subjects with pure hypercholesterolemia usually have the hyperbetalipoproteinemic pattern and those with pure hypertriglyceridemia without chylomicrons, the hyperprebetalipoproteinemic pattern. Subjects with relatively high cholesterol and triglyceride levels may have dysbetalipoproteinemic or hyperprebetalipoproteinemic patterns or profiles. Although lipoprotein-typing is no longer considered necessary or important today, there may be four areas where the typing system retains general validity for clinical research purposes:

1. Lipoprotein patterns are useful in sharpening the focus on the diverse metabolic abnormalities that underlie hyperlipidemia.
2. The types of hyperlipoproteinemias so identified are not disease states but are the result of disorders that similarly affect the concentrations of particular lipoproteins.
3. Each lipoprotein type is often associated with certain distinctive clinical features.
4. Each lipoprotein type, irrespective of cause, is generally more successfully handled by a specific diet and therapeutic approach.

The typing system has four major limitations:

1. For distinction of dysbetalipoproteinemia, the diagnosis requires substantiation by determination of the ratio of cholesterol in VLDL divided by the plasma triglyceride as well as electrophoretic confirmation of beta-migrating VLDL. In addition, in subjects with mixed elevations of cholesterol and triglyceride, quantitation of LDL (LDL cholesterol) is important for accurate distinction.
2. The second major area where the typing system has limitations is genetics. No specific type of hyperlipoproteinemia should be considered genotypic; lipid and lipoprotein determinations cannot provide the diagnosis of a specific genetic disorder in a single patient; and there is increasing evidence of strong heterogeneity in lipoprotein patterns in first-degree relatives from families with monogenic familial hyperlipidemia.
3. The third area that the typing system did not cover was the evaluation of alpha-lipoprotein in the classification. It is now known that a low concentration of HDL cholesterol is an independent risk factor for coronary heart disease, and genetic abnormalities such as hypoalphalipoproteinemia, though rare, does exist.
4. Finally, the present electrophoretic systems are limited in their ability to resolve other unusual lipoprotein fractions, such as lipoprotein variants, beta-migrating VLDL, and IDL.

From lipids to lipoproteins: laboratory considerations

In the transformation of hyperlipidemia to hyperlipoproteinemia, lipid analyses and the overnight refrigeration test can be used to determine the lipoprotein profile with a fair degree of accuracy. If the plasma is clear, the triglyceride level is most likely to be either normal or near normal (less than 2000 mg/L). When triglyceride increases to about 3000 mg/L or higher, the plasma is usually hazy to turbid in appearance and is not translucent enough to allow for clear reading of newsprint through the tube. When plasma triglyceride is over 10,000 mg/L, the plasma is usually opaque and milky (lipemic, lactescent). If chylomicrons are present, after an overnight incubation at 4° C a thick homogeneous "cream" layer may be observed floating at the plasma surface. As summarized in Fig. 33-8, a uniformly opaque plasma sample usually denotes a hyperprebetalipoproteinemia. An opaque plasma sample with a cream layer on top is usually consistent with the mixed form of hyperlipoproteinemia. A thick chylomicron cream layer with generally clear plasma infranate is usually consistent with a hyperchylomicronemic profile.

In patients with hypercholesterolemia without hypertriglyceridemia, most often with raised LDL levels, the plasma is clear but may have an orange-yellow tint, since carotene is carried with LDL. After visual observation, which is "simple and free," the diagnosis of the lipid abnormality can be made in as many as 90% of subjects by quantitation of plasma cholesterol and triglyceride alone.

The NECP ATP recommended protocol for the laboratory analyses needed to effectively assess CHD risk and detect common lipoprotein abnormalities includes measurement of total cholesterol, triglycerides, and LDL and HDL cholesterol.[13,14] These measurements can be performed by most clinical laboratories (see below). More demanding analytical techniques, such as analytical ultracentrifugation or apolipoprotein and lipoprotein subfraction measurements, may be needed to differentiate atypical lipoprotein abnormalities; these are usually available in specialized research laboratories. Most commonly, LDL cholesterol levels are conventionally measured by use of the preparative ultracentrifuge but can cheaply and conveniently be estimated by the Friedewald formula:

$$\text{LDL cholesterol} = \text{Total cholesterol} - \left(\frac{\text{Triglyceride}}{5} + \text{HDL cholesterol}\right)$$

This estimation requires measurement of HDL cholesterol by various precipitation techniques and is accurate in patients whose triglycerides are less than 4000 mg/L; triglyceride concentrations over 4000 mg/L lead to an inconsistency in the VLDL triglyceride; that is, the VLDL cholesterol-to-triglyceride ratio does not permit division by a fixed number, and the formula cannot be used with great accuracy. In addition, hypertriglyceridemia is a major cause of inaccurate measurements of HDL-cholesterol. The reason is that the triglyceride-rich, Apo B–containing lipoproteins are incompletely precipitated, resulting in falsely elevated HDL cholesterol values. New HDL cholesterol methods (see p. 674) are more robust and can tolerate triglyceride concentrations that exceed 15,000 mg/L[17] or even 43,000 mg/L (Naito, unpublished results) before this interference occurs.

Use of electrophoresis alone, without prior quantitation of cholesterol and triglyceride, is not a logical step for the following reasons:

1. Except under very controlled conditions, electrophoretic patterns are difficult to quantitate consistently so that they can provide relative or absolute concentrations for the lipoprotein classes. Most of these difficulties relate to differing intensities of dye, application problems, and other variables that are difficult to control routinely in electrophoresis.

2. A ubiquitous lipoprotein, Lp(a), often appears as a pre-beta band on electrophoresis but is not associated with any triglyceride elevation (see p. 652).

Secondary hyperlipoproteinemia

In general, lipoprotein quantification and typing alone will not distinguish the primary from the secondary forms (see Table 33-2). Even the diagnosis of a concurrent disorder that is likely to cause secondary hyperlipoproteinemia does not necessarily establish it as the cause of a patient's hyperlipoproteinemia. Reversal of the lipid abnormality accompanying treatment of the suspected causative disorder, however, is compelling evidence of the secondary nature of the hyperlipoproteinemia. Failure of such reversal to occur implies that the hyperlipoproteinemia may be primary and indicates the need for family screening.

Some disorders that are associated with hyperlipoproteinemia will be obvious from the patient's history and physical examination. Others will require blood or urine tests for diagnosis. If such a screening reveals no abnormalities, it is reasonable to assume that the patient has a primary hyperlipoproteinemia. Whether the hyperlipoproteinemia is established as being familial in origin will depend on the results of family screening.

Other forms of dyslipoproteinemias

In the familial lipoprotein disorders discussed in this chapter, one or more of the four lipoprotein fractions (chylomicron, VLDL, beta-migrating VLDL, and LDL) are present in elevated concentrations.

However, there are other lipoprotein abnormalities in addition to the hyperlipoproteinemias reviewed so far. There are three genetically determined disorders in which one or more of the lipoprotein families are absent from plasma or occur in concentrations that are extremely low.[1] The first of these to be discovered was *abetalipoproteinemia,* in which chylomicrons, VLDL, and LDL are missing. The probable inherited defect is one involving synthesis of the major protein moiety of LDL, Apo B. Another disease is *hypobetalipoproteinemia* (familial LDL deficiency), in which no lipoproteins are missing but LDL concentrations are far below normal. In the third disorder, *familial hypoalphalipoproteinemia,* HDL circulates but contains an abnormal proportion of the two major HDL apolipoproteins. A defect in the synthesis of Apo A-I is the probable locus affected by this rare mutation. With this abnormal high-density lipoprotein, patients with *Tangier disease* have low plasma HDL concentration, store cholesteryl esters in most parts of the body, and often have neuropathic changes for reasons that are not understood. Their large orange tonsils form an unforgettable part of the syndrome. All these diseases are usually detected initially because of a common manifestation, hypocholesterolemia.

Last, although not classified as a dyslipoproteinemia, *hyperalphalipoproteinemia* is a condition in which the HDL is elevated in the blood beyond two standard deviations for a given age and sex. This condition is under genetic influence, and these persons appear to have a longer life-span than those with "normal" concentrations of HDL. There are no other clinical symptoms associated with this lipoprotein feature. A more detailed discussion of each of these lipoprotein abnormalities is provided below.

Abetalipoproteinemia. The rare disorder abetalipoproteinemia has five basic features: undetectable plasma LDL concentration, malabsorption of fat, acanthocytosis, retinitis pigmentosa, and ataxic neuropathic disease. These are not specific for this lipoprotein condition. Acanthocytosis may occur in other diseases in which lipoproteins are not deficient. In abetalipoproteinemia LDL is absent, not merely deficient. The plasma cholesterol concentration does not exceed 800 mg/L and is likely to be no higher than 300 mg/L. This is accompanied by concentrations of triglycerides lower than those seen in any other disease, usually less than 200 mg/L. The total phospholipid concentration is also low, that is, less than 1000 mg/L. Both the phospholipid partition and the fatty acid composition of the plasma lipids are abnormal and are frequently reflected in similar abnormalities in erythrocytes and adipose tissue. The gastrointestinal problems of patients with abetalipoproteinemia are stereotypical. Fat malabsorption is present from birth, and the neonatal period is characterized by poor appetite, vomiting, loose voluminous stools, and little weight gain. The neuromuscular manifestations of abetalipoproteinemia are devastating. The cause of the neuromuscular abnormalities in abetalipoproteinemia is obscure. Attention has focused on the abnormal amount of ceroid pigment (lipofuscin) in the cerebellum and other tissues in this disorder.

In abetalipoproteinemia there is a functional disturbance in fat transport. Chylomicrons never enter the plasma, and net transport of endogenous glycerides in VLDL appears to be either absent or sustained at some unchanging minimum level. Heavy feeding of carbohydrate for days, which promotes a brisk rise in the level of plasma glycerides and VLDL in patients with Tangier disease and in nearly all other subjects, fails to do so in patients with abetalipoproteinemia. The defect in abetalipoproteinemia is not known. The most likely one is a failure to synthesize Apo B. The intracellular assembly point of Apo B–containing lipoprotein is another possible site of dysfunction, or the defect may possibly lie in the secretion process. Whichever of these may be primary, none of these defects allow one to explain the many secondary manifestations of the disease.

Diagnosis of abetalipoproteinemia can be made in a patient with one of the abnormalities listed at the beginning of this section. The possibility of dysglobulinemia producing antibodies to LDL should also be kept in mind. The single most important laboratory test for screening is the plasma cholesterol determination. The finding of a subnormal value, particularly any concentration below 1000 mg/L, should be followed by a triglyceride determination and lipoprotein electrophoresis. The definitive diagnosis depends on immunochemical demonstration of the absence of LDL Apo B in the plasma. In all patients in whom the diagnosis is made, it is also important to check, in all obligate heterozygotes, the concentration of LDL by immunochemical or ultracentrifugal analysis. In familial hypobetalipoproteinemia, the heterozygote has lower than normal concentrations of LDL and Apo B.

Hypobetalipoproteinemia. Apparently unrelated to abetalipoproteinemia is another genetic disorder, hypobetalipoproteinemia, in which plasma LDL concentrations are about one tenth of normal. This lipoprotein abnormality is inherited as an autosomal dominant trait. The plasma total cholesterol concentrations can be as low as those seen in abetalipoproteinemia. The percentage of cholesterol esterified is normal. The triglyceride levels may be well within the normal range, but sometimes these are in the lower limits of accurate measurement. The phospholipid concentrations may vary from 100 to 1800 mg/L and are usually in the low-normal borderline region in most patients. Vitamin A and E concentrations are normal or low but, if low, are not decreased to the level seen in abetalipoproteinemia. A faint beta-lipoprotein band is visible on electrophoresis. HDL concentrations as measured by precipitation, preparative ultracentrifuge, or analytic ultracentrifuge are normal; VLDL is usually modestly reduced but is present.

LDL is present in serum as measured by immunoprecipitin tests. These measurements have suggested concentrations of LDL that are one eighth to one sixteenth of normal.

Hypoalphalipoproteinemia or an alphalipoproteinemia. Tangier disease (familial HDL deficiency) is characterized by severe deficiency or absence of normal HDL in plasma and by the accumulation of cholesteryl esters in many tissues throughout the body, including liver,

spleen, lymph nodes, thymus, intestinal mucosa, skin, and cornea. A combination of two features is pathognomonic: a low plasma cholesterol concentration in combination with normal or elevated triglyceride levels and hyperplastic orange-yellow tonsils and adenoid tissue. Some persons may exhibit peripheral neuropathy. The small amounts of HDL in Tangier plasma differ qualitatively and quantitatively from normal HDL, particularly with respect to apolipoprotein content (Apo A-I). The disorder appears to be attributable to an autosomal recessive gene affecting HDL synthesis or catabolism. Heterozygotes in families with known homozygotes can usually be identified by low HDL concentrations (50% below normal); they do not develop neuropathy and cholesteryl ester accumulation. Among the lipoprotein-deficiency states and indeed among all known diseases, the combination of very low cholesterol and elevated triglyceride concentrations gives Tangier disease a unique signature. Some patients may have normal triglyceride levels in the postabsorptive state, however, and may superficially resemble those with LDL deficiency. The plasma total cholesterol level ranges from about 400 to 1250 mg/L, within the range also observed in abetalipoproteinemia and hypobetalipoproteinemia. Individual variation in the plasma triglyceride levels is considerable and is highly contingent on diet. Substitution of carbohydrate for fat often paradoxically lowers the plasma triglyceride concentration in this disorder. The plasma lipoprotein pattern is distinctive: the alpha-lipoprotein band is absent, irrespective of the support medium used. Immunoelectrophoresis may occasionally generate a faint precipitin line of alpha-globulin mobility against anti-HDL antiserum. Most useful for detecting the small amounts of the A apoproteins is immunoanalysis of plasma with specific antiserums to the A-I and A-II apolipoproteins. The reactivity with anti–Apo-A-lI is generally stronger than with anti–Apo-A-I. Estimation of the cholesterol content of the plasma lipoproteins after sequential preparative ultracentrifugation or after ultracentrifugation and selective heparin-manganese precipitation confirms the paucity of HDL.

In addition to HDL absence or deficiency, the following diseases must be excluded:

1. Familial deficiency of LCAT. Here HDL is very low, but the plasma cholesterol level is normal or high, and most of the cholesterol is unesterified.

2. Obstructive liver disease, in which the plasma HDL and Apo A may be reduced to levels as low as those seen in Tangier disease. In this disorder the cholesterol level is not low but high, and most of the cholesterol is not esterified. Appropriate tests of liver function should permit the correct diagnosis.

3. Severe malnutrition or hepatic parenchymal disease in which high-density lipoproteins are decreased. The decrease in cholesterol will also be associated with low triglyceride and LDL levels.

4. Acquired HDL deficiency attributable to dysglobu-

linemia, including possible development of antibodies to HDL.

5. Other storage diseases associated with foam cells and hepatosplenomegaly. In these conditions HDL levels are higher than those seen in Tangier disease, and typical tonsillar abnormalities are absent.

CLINICAL IMPLICATIONS OF HYPERLIPIDEMIA

Why should there be any concern for hyperlipidemia or hyperlipoproteinemia? Hyperlipidemia is usually a symptomless biochemical state that, if present for a sufficiently long time, may be associated with the development of atherosclerosis and its complications; including myocardial infarctions and vascular diseases. Occasionally hyperlipidemia may be associated with specific overt symptoms or signs directly attributable to the presence of hyperlipidemia. Examples are abdominal pain, pancreatitis, and the cutaneous manifestations of hyperlipidemia, such as xanthomas, corneal arcus, and xanthelasmas.

Coronary artery disease

CAD is almost always the result of atherosclerosis—hardening of the arteries. Coronary atherosclerosis primarily results from the accumulation of fatty deposits in the walls of coronary arteries, which leads to the formation of fibrous tissue in the vessel wall. CAD is the most common type of heart disease and the leading cause of death in the United States and many other countries. In the United States, an estimated 50% of the adult deaths each year are attributable to CAD.[7]

CAD affects middle-aged males; nearly 45% of all heart attacks occur in individuals younger than 65 years of age. Coronary heart disease (CHD) develops in men 60 years of age or younger at approximately twice the rate as that of women, whereas postmenopausal women have a higher incidence of CHD than premenopausal women of the same age.[18] For both men and women, the incidence of coronary vascular disease (CVD) and the rates of death from atherosclerosis increase with advancing age. About 75% of coronary-related mortalities are the result of atherosclerosis. Each year about 1.25 million Americans are afflicted with myocardial infarction (MI), and about 300,000 bypass operations are performed.[19] It is estimated that the annual cost of CHD to the American public is approximately $42 billion to $88 billion.[20]

Risk factors associated with coronary artery disease. Although the basic cause of CAD is unknown, scientists have identified several factors associated with a distinct increase in the likelihood that a person will develop a heart attack later in life.[20,21] These factors, which correlate with the presence of CHD, are spoken of as *risk factors*. The box lists the primary and secondary risk factors associated with coronary heart disease. Some risk factors are unavoidable, such as racial and genetic susceptibility, increased prevalence in males, and increased likelihood of having a heart attack as aging occurs. Many known risk fac-

---

Primary and Secondary Risk Factors Associated with Coronary Heart Disease (CHD)

Primary
Genetic predisposition for CHD
Hypertension
Cigarette smoking
Elevated total cholesterol (LDL cholesterol)
Decreased HDL cholesterol
Age
Male sex

Secondary
Lack of exercise
Obesity
Stress
Diabetes mellitus
Gout and hyperuricemia
Renal failure patients receiving hemodialysis
Postmenopausal state
Hypothyroidism
Certain thrombogenic disorders

---

tors are, however, susceptible to modification. Particularly important among these are high blood pressure, cigarette smoking, and elevated serum cholesterol. Approximately 50% of those who have heart attacks are persons who have one or more of these three risk factors. According to the Framingham data, there is a clear gradient of CHD incidence rates in relation to serum HDL-cholesterol concentrations. Persons with levels below 350 mg/L have eight times the CHD rate of persons with HDL-cholesterol levels of 650 mg/L or greater.

Important additional risk factors include lipoprotein (a) (Lp[a]), oxidized LDL, small lipoprotein particle size (or dense LDL), fibrinogen, homocyst(e)ine, specific apolipoprotein (Apo) A-I, B, E isoforms, and triglyceride-rich remnant lipoproteins.[22-28] No degree of risk has yet been assigned to these factors. Other possible factors whose relative importance is still being established include hypertriglyceridemia, level of physical activity, and personality types.

ATHEROSCLEROTIC PLAQUE FORMATION

The healthy blood vessel (artery) architecture consists of an *intima,* lined by endothelium on the inner, luminal side of the vessel, which is bound by the internal elastic lamina to the *media* (Fig. 33-9). The outermost layer is the adventitia, which is bound by the external elastic lamina and exterior to the vessel itself. The intima is the site at which the atherosclerotic lesions form. The endothelium serves as a barrier to blood-borne materials and as a site where at least two mitogens are synthesized and secreted (see p. 665). The tunica media is the muscular wall of the artery that consists of smooth muscle cells held together by a discontinu-

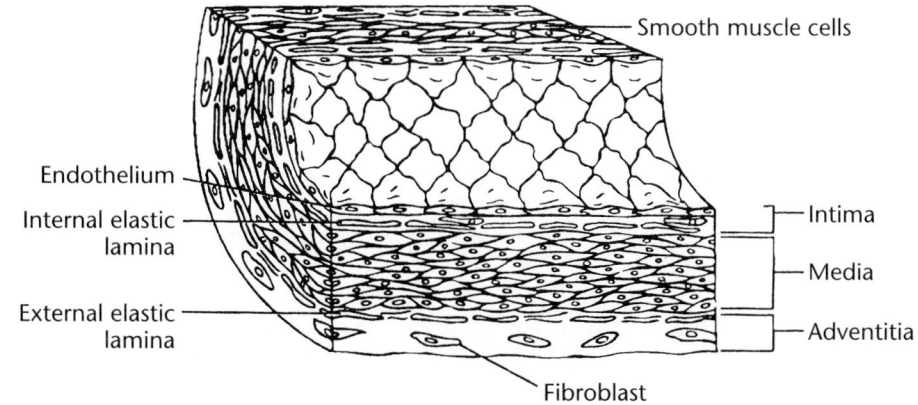

Fig. 33-9   Diagram of a healthy blood vessel (artery) with normal integrity of the intima, media, and adventitia. (Modified from Grundy SM: *Slide atlas of lipid disorders: cholesterol, atherosclerosis, and coronary heart disease,* New York, 1990, Gower Medical Publishing.)

ous basement membrane and by interspersed collagen fibrils and proteoglycan.[21,29,30] The smooth muscle cells that proliferate in the arterial intima to form the advanced lesions of atherosclerosis originate in the media. This smooth muscle cell proliferation represents the *sine qua non* of the lesions of advanced atherosclerosis. The smooth muscle cells, like the endothelium and fibroblasts, contain receptors for LDL and PDGF (see below). One characteristic feature of the smooth muscle cells found in the lesions of atherosclerosis is the accumulation of lipids that results in the formation of highly vacuolated cells, or *foam cells.*

There are three progressive stages of atherosclerotic plaque formation: (1) the *fatty streaks,* which gradually develop into raised lesions, which are called *fatty plaques;* (2) the *fibrous plaque,* which has a proliferation of smooth muscle cells and a collagen-rich fibrous cap that covers a lipid core that is lined by foam cells and surrounds an amorphous extracellular accumulation of cholesteryl esters; and (3) the *complicated lesion,* which can manifest calcification, hemorrhage, ulceration (rupture), and thrombosis (Fig. 33-10). It is the complicated lesion that frequently underlies the acute clinical event of arterial occlusion that leads to myocardial injury (MI).

The formation and accumulation of foam cells in the intima is the hallmark of the early atherosclerotic lesion. Currently it is believed that most of the foam cells are derived from blood-borne macrophages, though some may come from smooth muscle cells. A pivotal step in the development of foam cells is the accelerated uptake of modified LDL (see below), followed by proliferation of smooth-muscle cells (with and without lipid deposits in their cytoplasm) (Fig. 33-11). The smooth muscle cell proliferation is accompanied by increased synthesis of cellular elastin, collagen, and proteoglycans, which these cells deposit extracellularly in the developing plaque.

The development of the atherosclerotic lesion is promoted by the secretion of two key blood cells, macropha-

ges and platelets. The macrophages can secrete chemotactic agents (such as interleukin-1, superoxide anion, leukotriene B_4) and growth factors (such as platelet-derived growth factor [PDGF], interleukin-1, fibroblast growth factor, epidermal growth factor, transforming growth factor–β). These two macrophage-derived groups of factors are probably responsible for the promotion of connective tissue proliferation in the blood vessel during the disease process.[21]

The platelets play a smaller role in some atherosclerotic lesions but play a major role in the formation of thrombi. It is usually a mural or occlusive thrombus that leads to an MI. Platelets can also produce the same growth factors as activated macrophages. Thus, at sites of injury in which collagen exposure occur, numerous vasoactive, stimulatory, and proliferative responses can take place and probably play a role in the initiation of the atherosclerotic lesions.

The initial biochemical step in cell proliferation is the infiltration of lipoproteins (VLDL remnants, LDL, and IDL) into the subendothelial space. Here some lipoproteins are trapped in the intimal ground substance, modified, and ingested by macrophages to form foam cells. The uptake of LDL by the macrophages can be enhanced if the LDL is modified by oxidation or degradation of Apo B by reactive oxygen species (such as free radicals), or by derivitization of the Apo B by glycosylation or by reaction with malonaldehyde[31] (Fig. 33-12).

The fat-laden macrophages, together with varying numbers of lipid-filled smooth muscle cells, develop into the fatty streaks. Most of the lipid in the foam cells is free cholesterol and cholesteryl ester.

The fatty streaks are observed early in childhood, and their transformation into the complicated lesions usually takes four to five decades before the clinical manifestation of the disease, including angina pectoris, MI, or sudden cardiac death, are apparent.[29] In males, the first MI event usually occurs around 55 years of age, whereas in females there is a 10-year delay, occurring around 65 years of age. This

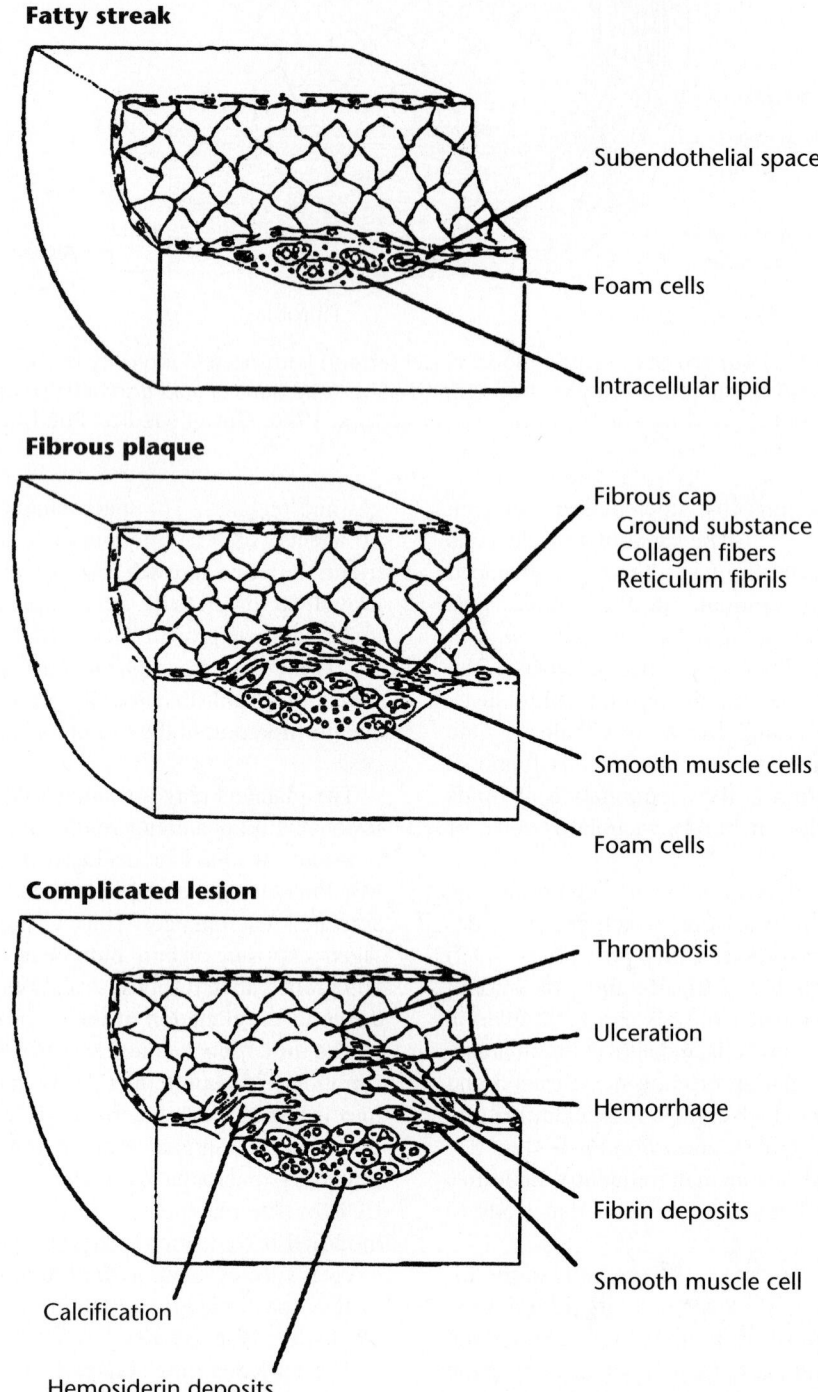

Fatty streak

Subendothelial space

Foam cells

Intracellular lipid

Fibrous plaque

Fibrous cap
  Ground substance
  Collagen fibers
  Reticulum fibrils

Smooth muscle cells

Foam cells

Complicated lesion

Thrombosis

Ulceration

Hemorrhage

Fibrin deposits

Smooth muscle cell

Calcification

Hemosiderin deposits

Fig. 33-10   The three stages of atherogenesis: formation of the fatty streak, fibrous plaque, and complicated lesion. Notice the development and accumulation of foam cells in the *fatty streak,* accumulation of smooth muscle cells in the *fibrous plaque,* and formation of calcification, ulceration, thrombosis, and hemorrhage in the advanced or *complicated lesion.* (Modified from Grundy SM: *Slide atlas of lipid disorders: cholesterol, atherosclerosis, and coronary heart disease,* New York, 1990, Gower Medical Publishing.)

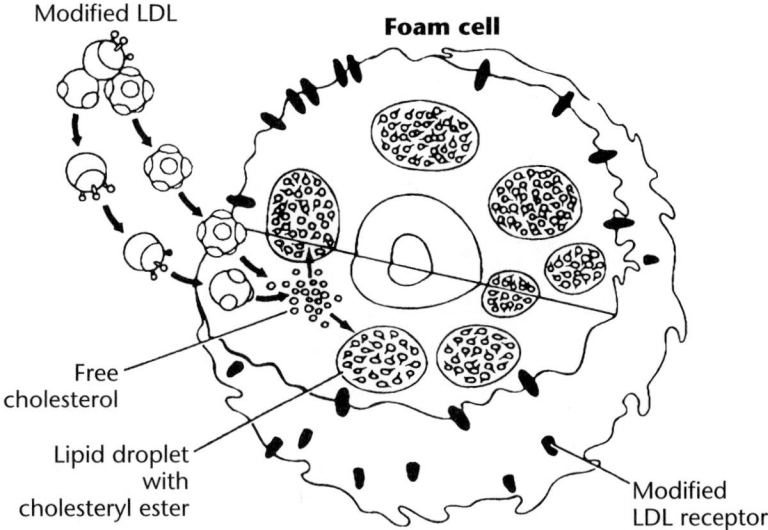

Fig. 33-11   Formation of the foam cell: *macrophage* uptake (ingestion) of *modified LDL* by the modified LDL receptor pathway, which results in the development of large *fat-laden droplets*. This process of foam cell formation is the hallmark of the fatty streak development in atherogenesis. (Modified from Grundy SM: *Slide atlas of lipid disorders: cholesterol, atherosclerosis, and coronary heart disease,* New York, 1990, Gower Medical Publishing.)

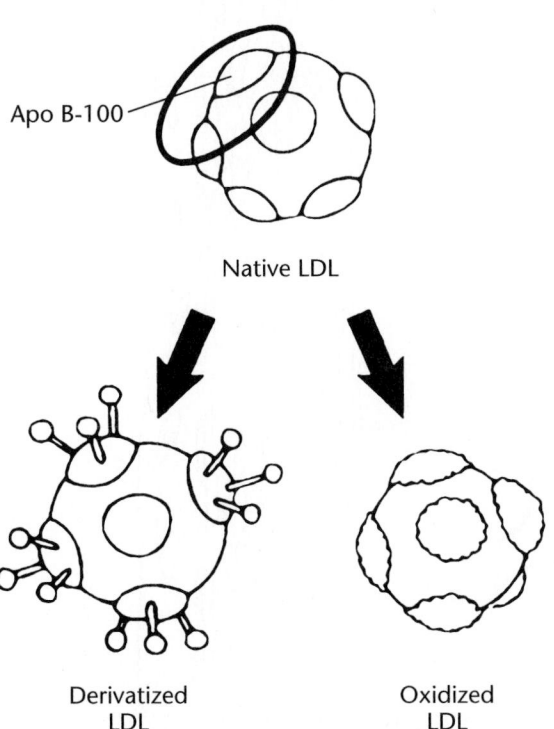

Fig. 33-12   Modification of LDL. Entrapped *native LDL* (in the subendothelial space) can undergo two types of modification—*derivatization* (malonaldehyde attachment to or glycosylation of Apo B-100) or *oxidation* (degradation of Apo B-100 by superoxides). (Modified from Grundy SM: *Slide atlas of lipid disorders: cholesterol, atherosclerosis, and coronary heart disease,* New York, 1990, Gower Medical Publishing.)

atherosclerotic process can be accelerated by having (1) additional CHD risk factors (see above), (2) endothelial injury, which removes the natural barrier to the entrance of lipoproteins into the arterial wall or causes thrombosis, and (3) a genetic predisposition for primary hypercholesterolemia.

Etiology of atherosclerotic lesions

Current thoughts on the pathogenesis of atherosclerotic lesions include the response-to-injury and monoclonal hypotheses. The first theory centers on the premise that an initial injury occurs to the endothelial cell lining of the arterial wall. The endothelial injury, caused by mechanical, chemical, immunologic, toxic, or infectious factors, results in an increased uptake of LDL-cholesterol. This, in turn, changes the surface characteristics of the endothelial cells and the circulating leukocytes (monocytes and platelets), leading to enhanced adhesion of monocytes to the endothelium.[21] The monocytes are then transformed to macrophages, which now have the ability to take up additional lipids. According to Steinberg et al.,[31] oxidized LDL may play a central role in atherogenesis in at least four ways (Fig. 33-13): (1) it acts as a chemoattractant for the blood-borne monocytes to enter the subendothelial space; (2) it causes the transformation of the monocytes to macrophages; (3) it causes the trapping of macrophages in the endothelial spaces by inhibiting their motility; and (4) it is toxic to the endothelial cells. The lipid-laden macrophage forms the foam cells that contribute to the development of the fatty streaks. Also, these activated macrophages can form at least

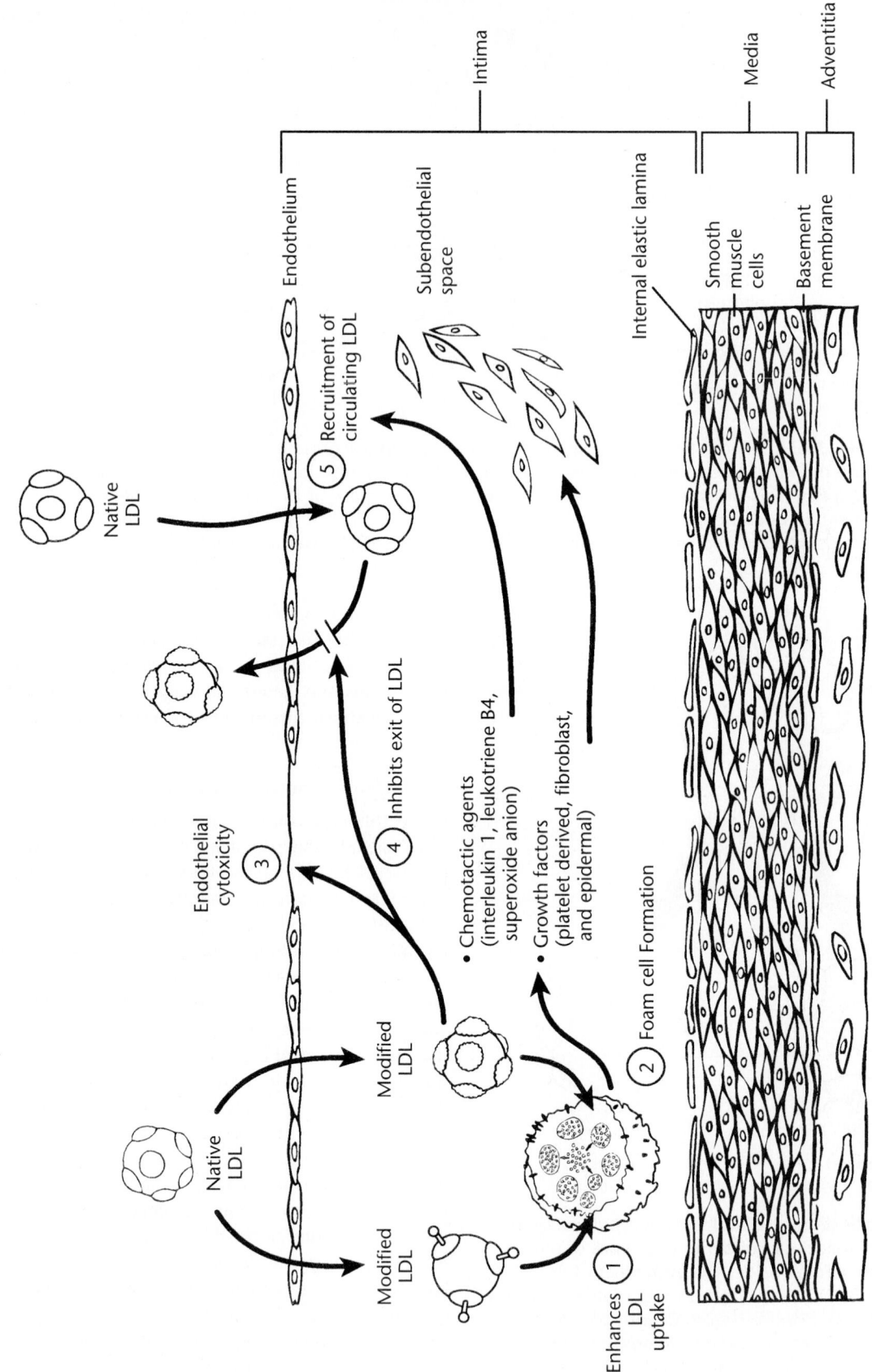

Fig. **33-13** Hypothesis of the multiple roles of *oxidized LDL* in atherogenesis. (From Steinberg D, Parthasarathy S, Carew TE, et al: *N Engl J Med* 320:915-923, 1989.)

four different growth factors, which could be responsible for the migration of smooth muscle cells and fibroblasts into the intima and for their subsequent proliferation. The platelets, in this hypothesis, are involved in atherogenesis by aggregating and forming mural thrombi at particular anatomical sites where the blood flow properties produce shearing effects and cause some sort of injury to the endothelium. This mechanism causes the platelets to release growth factors (similar to those released by activated macrophages) that could lead to the proliferative smooth muscle atherosclerotic lesions.

It should also be mentioned that other hemostatic factors have been investigated and have shown to have a reasonable association with ischemic heart disease (IHD).[32] These factors include fibrinogen, factor VII, factor VIII, antithrombin III, plasminogen activator inhibitor 1, Lp(a), and antiphospholipid antibodies. Of these various thrombogenic factors, the most convincing independent risk factor for CVD has been plasma fibrinogen. The Northwick Park Heart Study[32] indicated that the incidence of IHD was more strongly related to fibrinogen levels than to total cholesterol concentrations. The Leigh study[32] also concluded that the association between fibrinogen concentration and IHD was higher than that of total cholesterol, blood pressure, and smoking. Possible mechanisms for the role of fibrinogen as a thrombogenic risk factor include its role as a precursor of fibrin and subsequent thrombosis and its effect on increases in blood viscosity, which affects the blood flow hemodynamic characteristics that can lead to thrombosis.

The second hypothesis associated with the atherogenesis is the monoclonal hypothesis. This premise is based on a single smooth muscle cell that serves as a source of all the cells within the lesion. This benign neoplasm of the arterial wall is derived from a cell that has been transformed by viruses, chemicals, toxins, or some other mutagens.

THE NATIONAL CHOLESTEROL EDUCATION PROGRAM

In the late 1980s, health care workers realized that a unified effort was needed to standardize the approach for the detection and classification of individuals at high risk for CHD and to standardize treatment and monitoring of such individuals. This effort also required a major educational drive to inform both physicians and their patients of CHD risk factors. To fulfill this scientific and educational goal, the federal government and a broad range of professional health care groups worked together to formulate guidelines and recommendations with the intent of reducing CHD in America. This national campaign was called the National Cholesterol Education Program (NCEP).

As a result of this effort, the NIH in 1985[33] and in 1988 (the NIH Adult Treatment Panel [ATP] of the NCEP) recommended new medical decision levels for cholesterol and LDL cholesterol that should have a larger effect on reducing the CHD morbidity and mortality in the United States, where CHD is still a major disease. To simplify the classification system and to make it more convenient to remember the cutoff levels, the panel eliminated the age and sex stratification once recommended.[33] These new cutoff levels, shown in Table 33-4, apply to all adults 20 years or older.[13,14]

The goal of the NCEP program was to establish criteria that defined the high-risk person for medical intervention and to provide clear guidelines on how to detect, set goals for, treat, and monitor these patients over time. Some of the key features of this landmark report[13] on cholesterol are as follows:

- All adults 20 years of age or older should be screened for *hypercholesterolemia* by having their *total blood cholesterol* measured.
- After an elevation in total cholesterol is confirmed by repeated measurements, the *LDL and HDL cholesterol* should be determined.
- New, more aggressive upper limits of healthy for total and LDL cholesterol are defined for a *primary preventive medicine* strategy (Table 33-4).
- The *LDL cholesterol* and not the total cholesterol will serve as the key index for *classifying* a person's *CHD risk.*
- Along with lipid and lipoprotein testing, all adults should also be evaluated for the presence of *other CHD risk factors* (cigarette smoking, diabetes mellitus, severe obesity, or a history of CHD in the patient or of premature CHD in family members, or definite cerebrovascular or occlusive peripheral vascular disease). The patient is considered to have a *high-risk status* if he or she has either (1) definite CHD (that is, definite prior myocardial infarction or myocardial ischemia) or (2) the presence of two or more other CHD risk factors or (3) a lipid or lipoprotein abnormality with the presence of one other CHD risk factor.
- The selection of therapeutic intervention modalities (that is, diet with cholesterol-lowering agents), treatment goals, and methods of monitoring have been clearly outlined.

Table 33-4 Classifications of risk in adults based on total cholesterol and low-density lipoprotein cholesterol

Total cholesterol (mg/L)*	Classification of risk	LDL cholesterol (mg/L)
<2000	Desirable	<1300
2000-2390	Borderline high	1300-1590
≥2400	High	≥1600

From Report of the National Cholesterol Education Program Expert Panel on Detection, Evaluation, and Treatment of High Blood Cholesterol in Adults, *Arch Intern Med* 148:36-39, 1988, and from the Second Expert Panel: Detection, Evaluation, and Treatment of High Blood Cholesterol in Adults (Adult Treatment Panel II), *Circulation* 89:1329-1445, 1994.
*Milligrams of cholesterol per liter of blood; to convert mg/L of cholesterol to mmol/L, divide by 387 or multiply by 0.002586.

A subsequent report[14] with modifications to the recommended guidelines was published. Briefly the following was added:

- Increased emphasis on the CHD risk status as a guide to the type and intensity of a cholesterol-lowering therapy. Particular emphasis has been given to the patient with existing CHD or other atherosclerotic diseases, which is now being placed at the highest risk and the establishment of lower LDL target values.
- *Age* (45 years or older for males and 55 years or older in women) has been added to the list of major CHD risk factors (Table 33-5).
- Delayed use of pharmacological agents for lipid and lipoprotein therapy in most young adult men and premenopausal women with elevated LDL cholesterol levels.
- Enhanced recognition that high-risk postmenopausal women and high-risk elderly patients who are otherwise in good health are candidates for cholesterol-lowering therapy.
- More attention to *HDL cholesterol* as a CHD risk factor, which includes the addition of HDL cholesterol measurements to the initial cholesterol testing. A high HDL cholesterol (greater than 600 mg/L) level has been designated as a negative CHD risk factor, whereas a low HDL cholesterol (less than 350 mg/L) has been designated as a positive CHD risk factor (Table 33-6). In addition, when one is selecting a drug for lowering LDL cholesterol, consideration should be given to the effect of the drug on the patient's HDL cholesterol.
- Increased emphasis on *physical activity* and *weight loss* as components of the dietary therapy of high blood cholesterol.

It should be reiterated that the NCEP ATP strategy is based on *LDL-cholesterol* and *HDL-cholesterol* being the criteria used for the initial classification of the patient's CHD risk, which also depends on other risk factors (Table 33-5) that can influence the final category of risk.

This NIH Expert Panel on Blood Cholesterol Levels in

Table 33-5 Risk factors associated with the development of coronary heart disease

Positive risk factors

Age (years)
    Male ≥45
    Female ≥55 or premature menopause without estrogen
      replacement therapy
Family history of premature coronary heart disease
Current cigarette smoking
Hypertension
Diabetes mellitus
Low HDL cholesterol, <350 mg/L (0.9 mmol/L)

Negative risk factors

High HDL cholesterol, ≥600 mg/L (1.6 mmol/L)

Table 33-6 Cutoff values for risk of coronary heart disease based on HDL cholesterol levels

Classification	HDL cholesterol cutoff value
Positive coronary heart disease risk	<350 mg/L
Negative coronary heart disease risk	>600 mg/L

From Second Expert Panel: Detection, Evaluation, and Treatment of High Blood Cholesterol in Adults (Adult Treatment Panel II), *Circulation* 89:1329-1445, 1994.

Children and Adolescents[19] recommended the following (see Table 33-7):

- Selective screening of *high-risk children* and *adolescents* who have a *family history of premature cardiovascular disease* or at least one parent with *high blood cholesterol* (above 2400 mg/L). Screening was also advocated if the *parents* or *grandparents*, at 55 years of age or less, underwent diagnostic coronary arteriography and were found to have coronary atherosclerosis. This includes parents or grandparents who have undergone balloon angioplasty or coronary artery bypass surgery. This also includes parents or grandparents who suffered a documented MI, angina pectoris, peripheral vascular disease, cerebrovascular disease, or sudden cardiac death.
- *Universal screening* of children and adolescents for high blood cholesterol was not advocated.
- The goals for *treatment* for patients with borderline LDL cholesterol to lower the level to less than 1100 mg/L and for the patient with high LDL cholesterol to lower the level to less than 1300 mg/L as a minimal goal. Drug therapy should not be used in children who are less than 10 years of age and for those who have not been prescribed an adequate cholesterol-lowering diet for at least 6 months to 1 year.

The positive and negative CHD risk factors are used as a guide to the type and intensity of cholesterol-lowering therapy that should be used by the physician (Table 33-5). For example, a male subject who is over 45 years or a female over 55 years is at higher risk for CHD and should be treated more aggressively. Therefore the goals for lowering

Table 33-7 Recent recommendations from the NCEP for children and adolescents

Total cholesterol (mg/L)	Classification of risk	LDL cholesterol (mg/L)
<1700	Acceptable	<1100
1700-1990	Borderline high	1100-1290
≥2000	High	≥1300

NCEP, National Cholesterol Education Program.
From the Expert Panel: Report of the National Cholesterol Education Program Expert Panel on Blood Cholesterol Levels in Children and Adolescents, U.S. Department of Health and Human Services, NIH publ no 91-2732, Sept 1991, pp 1-119. Also from Scanu AM: *Clin Chem* 41:170-173, 1995.

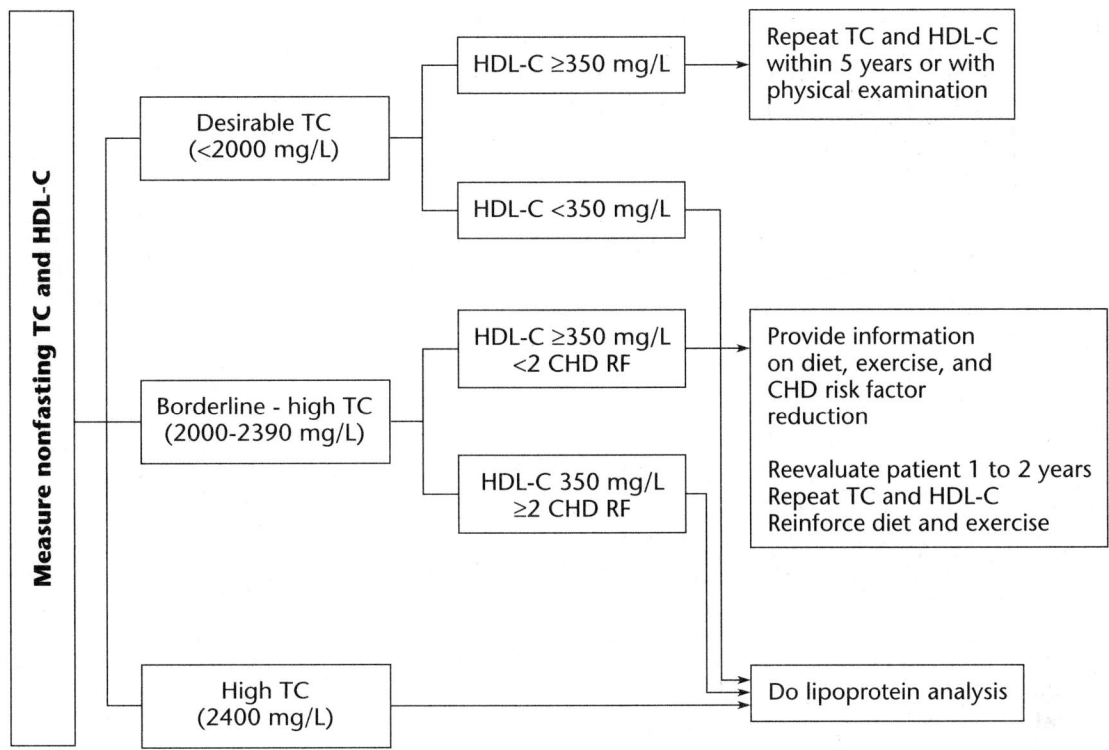

Fig. 33-14   Algorithm of coronary heart disease risk assessment, treatment, and monitoring using the NCEP Adult Treatment Panel II guidelines[14] for primary prevention in adults with and without evidence of CHD. Initial classification based on both the *TC* (total cholesterol) and *HDL-C* (high-density lipoprotein cholesterol) concentrations. *PE,* Physical examination; *RF,* risk factor.

serum levels of low-density lipoprotein (LDL) cholesterol and total cholesterol are more intensive.

It should be stressed that a person with two or more of the positive risk factors listed in Table 33-5 in addition to LDL cholesterol value would be classified as a high-risk individual for CHD. Keep in mind that a high amount of HDL cholesterol (greater than 600 mg/L) represents a negative risk factor.

Treatment strategies still focus on lowering the high blood level of LDL cholesterol in order to provide primary prevention of CHD. The algorithm of testing and treatment modality for primary prevention in adults *without* evidence of CHD is shown in Figs. 33-14 and 33-15. For example, for a person with a desirable total cholesterol (≤2000 mg/L) the HDL cholesterol value determines the follow-up strategy. If the HDL cholesterol is ≤350 mg/L, LDL analysis should be done. In most cases, the above example would not be of great clinical concern unless the HDL cholesterol was considerably depressed (that is, <100 mg/L), which could likely cause the LDL cholesterol concentration to be abnormal. Those with HDL cholesterol ≤350 mg/L should be given general educational materials about dietary modification, physical exercise, and other CHD risk-reduction activities and told to monitor their total and HDL cholesterol levels in 5 years. For individuals in the borderline

high-risk group (total cholesterol 2000 to 2390 mg/L), the concentration of HDL cholesterol and the presence or absence of multiple other CHD risk factors (see Table 33-7) determine the follow-up strategy. For example, those persons with HDL cholesterol concentrations ≤350 mg/L with less than two other risk factors should be given general educational materials as discussed above and told to have their total and HDL cholesterol levels monitored in 1 to 2 years. On the other hand, individuals with a total cholesterol of 2000 to 2390 mg/L and an HDL cholesterol of ≤350 mg/L or two or more other CHD risk factors should have additional lipoprotein analyses done. Since individuals with total cholesterol of 2400 mg/L or greater are considered at high risk, lipoprotein analyses should be done before any clinical decisions are made, Again, it should be emphasized that it is the LDL cholesterol and not the total cholesterol that more strongly affects a person's CHD risk. Persons with LDL cholesterol less than 1300 mg/L do not need further evaluation or active medical intervention; they should be given general information as described above and be reevaluated within 5 years. Persons with borderline high–risk LDL cholesterol concentrations (1300 to 1590 mg/L) who have fewer than two other CHD risk factors should be given general instructions and be reevaluated in 1 year. Patients with high-risk LDL cholesterol (>1600 mg/L) and those

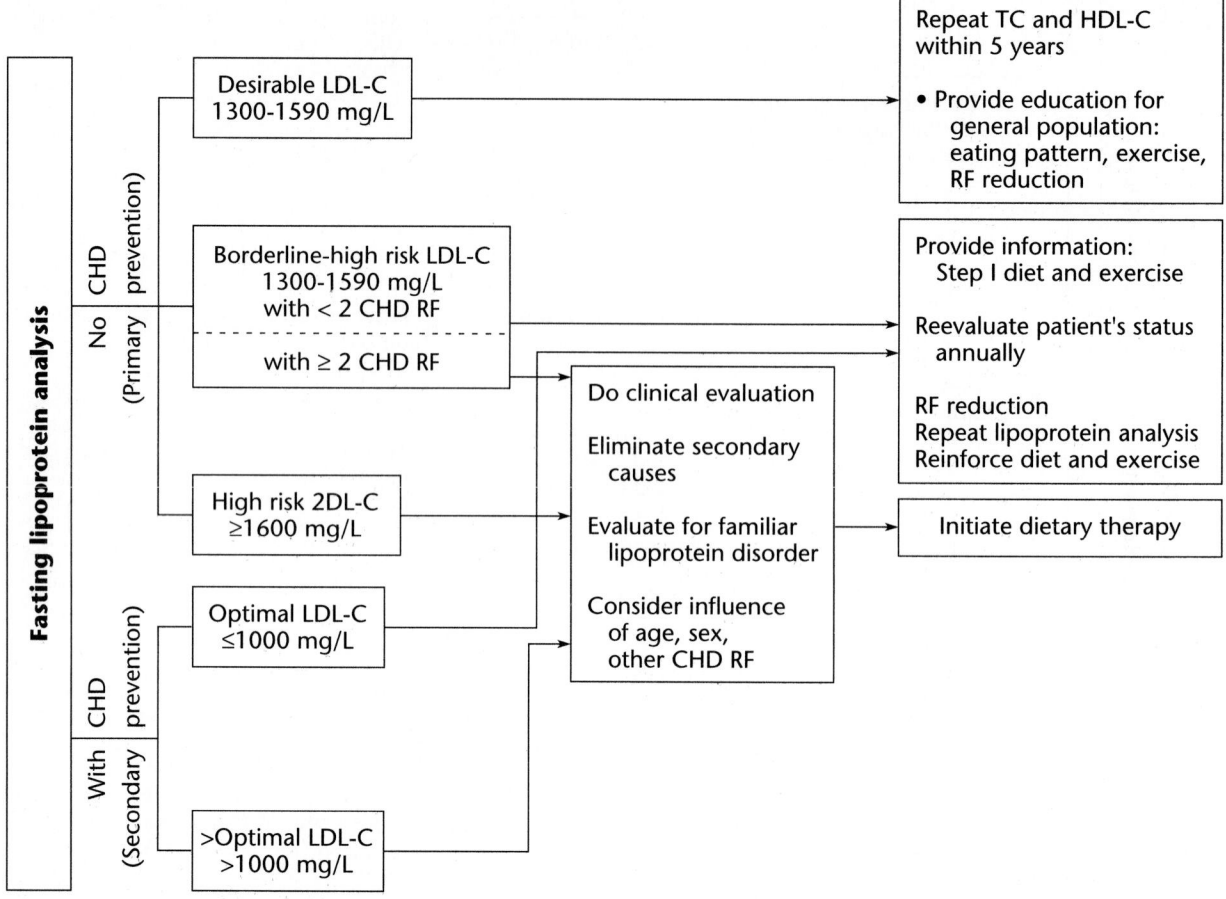

Fig. 33-15   Algorithm of CHD risk assessment, treatment, and monitoring for primary and secondary prevention of CHD in adults with and without evidence of CHD.[14] Subsequent classification of risk is based on low-density lipoprotein cholesterol (LDL-C) concentration. *RF,* Risk factor.

with borderline high risk who have two or more other risk factors should be evaluated clinically and begin active cholesterol-lowering intervention therapy.

For secondary prevention of disease in adults with evidence of CHD or other clinical atherosclerotic disease, lipoprotein analyses are required, and again the LDL cholesterol concentration is the key index for classification of CHD risk and therapy. For secondary prevention the optimum LDL cholesterol is <1000 mg/L, a far more aggressive goal than that of the primary prevention group. Persons in this category with LDL cholesterol levels >1000 mg/L should have appropriate clinical work-up and cholesterol-lowering therapy started.

To achieve the LDL cholesterol targets described in Tables 33-4, 33-6, and 33-7 it cannot be emphasized enough that therapy should always start with dietary intervention. Weight reduction (if appropriate) and physical activity should be part of the intervention process. If the elevated LDL cholesterol persists after an appropriate trial of dietary therapy, drug intervention may be considered. The NCEP report is very specific as to when drug therapy should be

used (Table 33-8). In addition, the report recommended delaying of the use of drug therapy in most young adult men (less than 35 years of age) and premenopausal women who have LDL cholesterol concentrations below 2200 mg/L and who are not otherwise at risk.

A common mistake when classifying a patient's CHD risk is not differentiating secondary from primary dyslipidemias. Some of the more frequently occurring secondary dyslipidemias are listed in Table 33-2. It is imperative that the primary condition leading to secondary hyperlipidemia be treated first.

METHODS OF ANALYSIS
Cholesterol
HERBERT K. NAITO

Principles of analysis and current usage   Several reviews that describe the utility and limitations of various cholesterol methods are available.[35,36] In routine laboratory practice today, however, determination of cholesterol by enzymatic assays are virtually the only methods that are employed.

The oldest method for cholesterol analysis still in use is

Table 33-8 Treatment decisions based on LDL cholesterol concentrations

CHD and risk factor status	LDL cholesterol decision level mg/L (mmol/L)	Treatment modality
Without CHD and <2 risk factors	≥1600 (4.1)	Dietary
	≥1900 (4.9)	Drug
Without CHD and ≥2 risk factors	≥1300 (3.4)	Dietary
	≥1600 (4.1)	Drug
With CHD	>1000 (2.6)	Dietary
	>1300 (3.4)	Drug

Modified from Second Expert Panel: Detection, Evaluation, and Treatment of High Blood Cholesterol in Adults (Adult Treatment Panel II), *Circulation* 89:1329-1445, 1994.

that of Liebermann-Burchard (L-B)[36] (Table 33-9, method 1). An intense blue-green color is produced as the result of the reaction of acetic anhydride and sulfuric acid with a solution of cholesterol in chloroform. This reaction became the basis for many subsequent methods for measuring cholesterol. The chemical reaction responsible for the color change in the colorimetric cholesterol methods is a stepwise oxidation of cholesterol. Modifications to the L-B procedure enable measurement of either free cholesterol, cholesteryl ester, or both. Measurement of these different fractions can be performed by saponification (hydrolysis of an ester bond) with use of a saponin compound, such as digitonin. Digitonin reacts with nonesterified cholesterol and forms a precipitate. Measurement of the cholesterol remaining in the supernatant provides an estimate of esterified cholesterol. One calculates free cholesterol by subtracting the esterified cholesterol value from the total cholesterol, which is measured directly, without the use of digitonin.

The L-B method suffers from several drawbacks that can adversely affect results. For example, the color intensity produced by esterified cholesterol is much greater than that produced by nonesterified, or free, cholesterol. Thus a saponification step is necessary to ensure that total cholesterol concentrations are not overestimated because of the positive bias caused by the presence of cholesterol esters. Artifactual increases in measured cholesterol can also occur in the presence of increased bilirubin concentrations,[37] increased vitamin A (retinol), and unreacted digitonin. In addition, the accuracy of the L-B method is strongly dependent on strict adherence to uniform reaction times and temperature, and the wavelength used to measure the final color change. Slight variations in these parameters can produce erroneous results.

The reference method for cholesterol, utilized by the Centers for Disease Control and Prevention, is based upon a modification of the procedure of Abell et al.,[38] (Table 33-9, method 2) which, in turn, is a modification of the L-B reaction. This reference method involves the initial hydrolysis of cholesterol esters. The free cholesterol is then extracted into petroleum ether, and the color development is performed with use of an acetic acid–acetic anhydride–sulfuric acid reagent.

The most common methods in use for determination of cholesterol in serum, plasma, or whole blood are enzymatic procedures (Table 33-9, method 3). The first step in the en-

zymatic sequence makes use of the enzyme *cholesterol esterase* to hydrolyze cholesteryl esters to free cholesterol. The free cholesterol that is produced, along with the free cholesterol that was initially present in the sample, is then oxidized to cholest-4-en-3-one and H_2O_2 in a reaction catalyzed by *cholesterol oxidase*. The final step or steps of these assays makes use of the ability of H_2O_2 to oxidize various compounds to produce a colored product, with the magnitude of color produced being proportional to cholesterol concentrations in the sample. Various hydrogen peroxide–indicator reactions that have been employed, including Trinder's reaction, which is based on the formation of a quinoneimine dye (absorbance maximum, 500 nm; Table 33-9, method 3A). One drawback to this indicator reaction is the interference exerted by bilirubin.[39] In addition, turbid samples can interfere with absorbance readings, and use of Tygon tubing should be avoided because of adsorption of the quinoneimine dye by the tubing. Ultraviolet spectrophotometric indicator reactions, based upon the formation of NADPH, have also been developed (Table 33-9, method 3B). Other techniques that have been employed for monitoring the formation of H_2O_2 produced by cholesterol oxidase include the oxidation of homovanillic acid by H_2O_2 to form a fluorescent compound monitored at 470 nm[40] and the use of polarographic techniques for directly monitoring the production of H_2O_2.[41]

The Laboratory Standardization Panel (LSP) recommended the following guidelines for reliable cholesterol measurements[13]:

- *Intralaboratory goals* for *precision* should be ±3% CV (coefficient of variation) or less and *analytical bias* (accuracy) should be 3% or less from the reference-method target values.

- The *accuracy* of each analytical system should be verified by the use of certified *reference materials* from the National Institute of Standards and Technology (NIST, Gaithersburg, Md.), the Centers for Disease Control and Prevention (CDC, Atlanta, Ga.), or the College of American Pathologists (CAP, Chicago, Ill.) or other reference materials that are traceable to the National Committee for Clinical Laboratory Standards' National Reference System for Cholesterol (NCCLS, Villanova, Penna.; NRS/ Chol).

- All laboratories should participate in a proficiency testing (PT) program that provides target values for cholesterol that are traceable to the NCCLS NRS/Chol. The PT programs should use a *total error* goal of 9.5% or less (for single measurements) to evaluate survey participants' proficiency (precision and accuracy) for cholesterol measurements.

- Medical decisions should be based on at least two separate analyses, on at least two separate occasions, for total and LDL cholesterol measurements. The total cholesterol values should be within 300 mg/L before they are averaged to assess an individual's usual cholesterol level.

- Patient preparation and blood collection procedures must be standardized to minimize preanalytical factors that may lead to inaccurate cholesterol values.

Specimen Serum, plasma, or whole blood are suitable specimens for cholesterol determinations. If plasma or whole blood is used, the preferred anticoagulants are EDTA (1 mg/ mL) or heparin. Anticoagulants such as fluoride, citrate, and

Table 33-9   Methods for cholesterol analysis

Method	Method classification	Principle	Usage	Comments
1. Liebermann-Burchard (L-B)	Colorimetric	Cholesterol is extracted and reacted with strong acid (sulfuric acid) and acetic anhydride to form colored product with absorbance maximum of 410 nm.	Rarely used	Esterified cholesterol produces greater color change than nonesterified form does
2. Abell et al.[38]	Colorimetric	Cholesterol esters are chemically hydrolyzed (saponification), and total cholesterol is measured by Liebermann-Burchard reaction	Considered current reference method Rarely used	Laborious
3. Enzymatic end-point	Colorimetric	1. Cholesteryl esters $\xrightarrow{\text{Cholesterol esterase}}$ Cholesterol + Fatty acids 2. Cholesterol + O_2 $\xrightarrow{\text{Cholesterol oxidase}}$ Cholest-4-en-3-one + H_2O_2 H_2O_2 produced in reaction 2 utilized in reactions A or B: A. $2H_2O_2$ + Phenol + 4-Aminophenazone $\xrightarrow{\text{Peroxidase}}$ Quinoneimine dye + $4H_2O$ B. H_2O_2 + Ethanol $\xrightarrow{\text{Catalase}}$ Acetaldehyde + H_2O Acetaldehyde + NADP $\xrightarrow{\text{Aldehyde dehydrogenase}}$ Acetate + NADPH + H^+	Most common method	Accurate and easily automated Possible future reference method

oxalate may cause dilutional errors as a result of their osmotic effect of drawing water from erythrocytes into the plasma. Plasma cholesterol values have been reported to be 3% to 5% lower than serum cholesterol values.[34] It should be remembered that the NCEP cholesterol coronary heart disease risk values (see Table 33-4) are based on serum specimens. If plasma is used for analysis, the values should be multiplied by 1.03 to provide serum equivalency values.[34]

Samples for cholesterol determination need not be collected from fasting individuals. However, if triglyceride or HDL-cholesterol concentrations are to be measured using the same sample, blood should be collected only if the patient has been fasting for a minimum of 12 hours. Once collected, serum or plasma should be separated from red blood cells as soon as possible. Exchange of cholesterol between red blood cell membranes and serum or plasma can alter cholesterol concentrations. If analysis is to be delayed for several days, samples can be stored at 4° C. For longer periods of storage, freezing the samples at −60° C allows reproducible results to be obtained for up to 1 year.[42] Samples frozen at −20° C can be maintained for several months. Samples that have been stored at refrigerated or frozen temperatures should be adequately mixed before analysis; this reverses the layering of the various lipid fractions according to their densities within the specimen that can occur with storage over time.

Reference intervals   The reference intervals for total cholesterol concentrations have been based upon the relative risk of developing CHD (see Tables 33-4 and 33-7). Positive and negative risk factors that have been associated with the development of CHD and are therefore part of the classification-of-risk scheme are given in Table 33-5. Diagnostic and treatment decisions (see Figs. 33-14 and 33-15) are also based upon the concentration of HDL (see Table 33-6) and LDL (see Tables 33-4 and 33-7).

High-density lipoprotein (HDL) cholesterol
HERBERT K. NAITO

Principles of analysis and current usage   Serum high-density lipoprotein (HDL) concentrations are considered one of the primary risk factors for coronary heart disease.[43] Recent guidelines indicate that this analyte should be included along with measurement of total cholesterol as part of the initial screening process for risk of coronary heart disease. Measurement of HDL should be performed as part of the routine assessment after pharmacologic intervention of hypercholesterolemia. Intralaboratory analytic goals for precision are a percent coefficient of variation (%CV) of ≤4%, and goals for accuracy are an allowable bias of 10% from target values.

Although a variety of techniques have been employed for the measurement of HDL concentrations, one can perform most HDL determinations in the routine clinical laboratory using simple precipitation methods. Although these precipitation techniques are quick and easy to perform, they can yield highly disparate results when performed in different laboratories. Interlaboratory differences for HDL determination of HDL are high, with coefficients of variation ranging from 7% to 25%.

The reference method for HDL determinations employs ultracentrifugation (Table 33-10, method 1). With this technique, the sample to be analyzed is adjusted to a density of 1.063 g/mL by overlayering of the specimen with a solution of potassium bromide. The specimen is then centrifuged at 105,000 *g* for 24 hours at 16° C. Since the density of HDL is greater than 1.063 whereas that of both low-density (LDL) and very-low-density (VLDL) lipoproteins is less than 1.063, the LDL and VLDL fractions will partition into the supernatant fraction while HDL and a trace amount of other lipoproteins with densities greater than 1.063 will partition into the infranatant solution. The presence of these trace amounts of lipoproteins with densities greater than 1.063

Table 33-10 Methods for HDL cholesterol analysis

Method	Principle	Usage	Comments
1. Ultracentrifugation	Specimen adjusted to density of 1.063 g/mL with potassium bromide; centrifuged at high speeds for 24 hours; lipoproteins separated by density, with HDL fraction in 1.063 to 1.21 g/mL range	Research use	Reference method; laborious and time consuming
2. Precipitation	Precipitating agent used to precipitate larger, Apo B–containing lipoproteins; cholesterol remaining in supernatant is quantitated as HDL cholesterol	Most frequently used technique	Current method of choice
a. Heparin–manganese chloride		Infrequently used	Not compatible with all cholesterol procedures
b. Dextran sulfate		Commonly used	Use of lower molecular weight dextran can produce biased results; higher molecular weight dextrans produce excellent results. Compatible with enzymatic procedures
c. Phosphotungstate		Most commonly used	Underestimates HDL; sensitive to temperature fluctuations
d. Polyethylene glycol		Used frequently	Poorest accuracy and precision; not recommended

found in the infranatant is usually ignored. The supernatant fraction containing the LDL and VLDL fractions is removed by aspiration, and the HDL cholesterol in the infranatant solution is measured. An alternative approach is employed by the Lipid Standardization Laboratory at the Centers for Disease Control and Prevention in Atlanta, Georgia. This procedure entails the removal of the VLDL by ultracentrifugation and then the LDL fraction is precipitated by use of heparin–manganese chloride solution (see below). The HDL concentration is determined by measurement of the cholesterol content remaining in the solution.

The most common methods in use for HDL cholesterol determinations involve the selective precipitation of Apo B–containing lipoproteins with polyanion solutions (Table 33-10, method 2 and Fig. 33-16). The polyanion solutions most frequently used for this purpose include sodium phosphotungstate and dextran sulfate–magnesium chloride. These agents bind to and precipitate all the major lipoprotein fractions, except for HDL. The use of heparin–manganese chloride as the precipitating agent is infrequently employed, though it is considered to be the precipitating agent of choice. The routine use of heparin–manganese chloride is limited by two major factors. First, the presence of high concentrations of manganese in the sample renders the specimen unsuitable for cholesterol analysis by use of the commonly employed enzymatic cholesterol methods. Another drawback to the use of this agent is that there can be a large degree of heterogeneity of commercial heparin preparation, especially with respect to the variation in molecular weight. This, in turn, can lead to increased lot-to-lot variability in the HDL analysis.

Dextran sulfate procedures tend to underestimate the true HDL concentration. The use of higher molecular weight dextran sulfates (50,000 daltons) can yield HDL values that are consistent with those obtained using heparin–manganese chloride methods. In addition, dextran sulfate–magnesium chloride methods that are compatible with enzymatic cholesterol determinations have been developed.[44]

Sodium phosphotungstate can also produce an underestimation of HDL concentrations. Another disadvantage associated with use of this particular agent is that temperature fluctuations and differences in reagent concentrations can be major sources of error. However, modifications to this precipitation method have resulted in better precision and accuracy for HDL determinations.[5]

A problem that is common to all precipitation methods occurs with samples containing increased triglyceride concentrations (>4000 mg/L). The presence of hypertriglyceridemia can cause incomplete precipitation of the non-HDL lipoproteins, resulting in substantial quantities of LDL and VLDL remaining in solution with the HDL cholesterol. Measurement of cholesterol in these samples with incomplete precipitation will result in falsely increased HDL values. Samples with increased triglyceride concentrations can be utilized for HDL determinations if certain steps are taken to ensure that complete precipitation of all non-HDL lipoprotein fractions occurs. In routine practice, the precipitation of all LDL and VLDL in samples with hypertriglyceridemia can be accomplished by dilution of the samples with 0.9% saline and reprecipitation or use of twice the usual amount of precipitating agent in an undiluted sample.

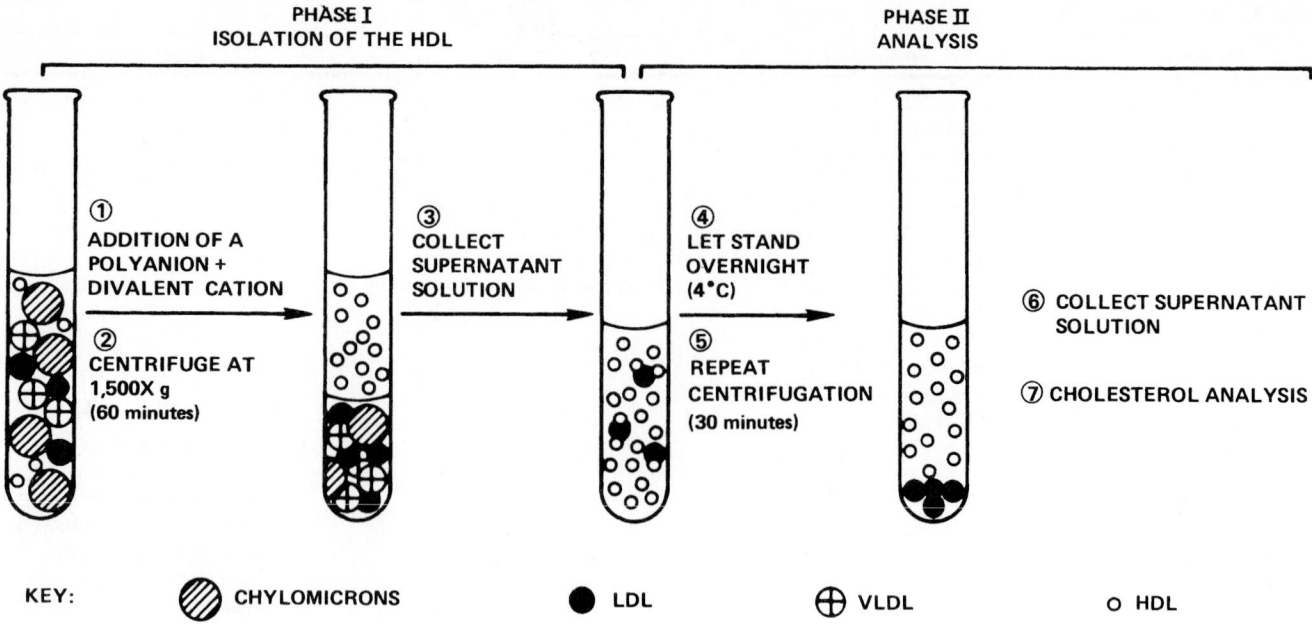

Fig. 33-16   Scheme of polyanion precipitation method (heparin-MnCl$_2$) for determination of HDL cholesterol.

Recently a precipitation technique for HDL determinations based on the use of dextran sulfate covalently linked to iron has been introduced. The principle of this method is similar to that of the traditional precipitating assays except that after the dextran sulfate–iron complex attaches to the LDL and VLDL lipoprotein fractions the bottom of the tube is placed near a magnetic source that "pulls" the LDL and VLDL fractions out of solution. Thus, this technique eliminates the need for centrifugation. In addition, this method is more robust and does not appear to be so readily affected by incomplete precipitation of the Apo B–containing lipoproteins caused by the presence of hypertriglyceridemia as compared to other precipitation methods.[17]

Other methods for HDL cholesterol determinations include ion-exchange chromatography and agarose gel electrophoresis (see following text). Neither of these methods is utilized in routine clinical laboratories for HDL determinations.

Specimen   Serum or plasma are acceptable for analysis of HDL concentrations. If plasma is used, the anticoagulant of choice is EDTA. Although fasting does not appear to influence HDL concentrations in blood, hypertriglyceridemia, which can occur with a nonfasting specimen, can interfere with some of the methods used for HDL determinations. Thus, use of a fasting specimen is preferred. Once collected, the sample should be removed from the clot within 2 hours and stored at 4° C until analysis.

Reference interval   The reference intervals for HDL cholesterol established for white males and females are given in Table 33-11. In addition, Table 33-6 gives the NCEP HDL cutoff values that may be used for the classification of individuals with respect to risk of developing coronary heart disease. Diagnostic and treatment strategies are summarized in Figs. 33-14 and 33-15.

Table 33-11   Fifth and 95th percentiles for plasma HDL cholesterol concentrations in white males and females in mg/L (mmol/L)

Age (years)	Percentiles			
	Males		Females	
	5	95	5	95
5-9	380 (0.98)	740 (1.91)	360 (0.93)	730 (1.89)
10-14	370 (0.96)	740 (1.91)	370 (0.96)	700 (1.81)
15-19	300 (0.78)	630 (1.63)	350 (0.91)	740 (1.91)
20-24	300 (0.78)	630 (1.63)	330 (0.85)	790 (2.04)
25-29	310 (0.80)	630 (1.63)	370 (0.96)	830 (2.15)
30-34	280 (0.72)	630 (1.63)	360 (0.93)	770 (1.99)
35-39	290 (0.75)	620 (1.60)	340 (0.88)	820 (2.12)
40-44	270 (0.70)	670 (1.73)	340 (0.88)	880 (2.28)
45-49	300 (0.78)	640 (1.66)	340 (0.88)	870 (2.25)
50-54	280 (0.72)	630 (1.63)	370 (0.96)	920 (2.38)
55-59	280 (0.72)	710 (1.80)	370 (0.96)	910 (2.35)
60-64	300 (0.78)	740 (1.91)	380 (0.98)	920 (2.38)
65-69	300 (0.78)	780 (2.02)	350 (0.91)	980 (2.53)
70+	310 (0.80)	750 (1.94)	330 (0.85)	920 (2.38)

Lipoprotein electrophoresis

HERBERT K. NAITO

Principles of analysis and current usage   The electrophoretic separation of the major lipoprotein fractions for the evaluation of an individual's lipoprotein profile is utilized infrequently in the clinical laboratory today because most dyslipoproteinemias can be classified by simple and inexpensive determinations of total cholesterol and triglyceride concentrations and a visual examination of the serum or plasma sample. This visual examination for the presence of floating

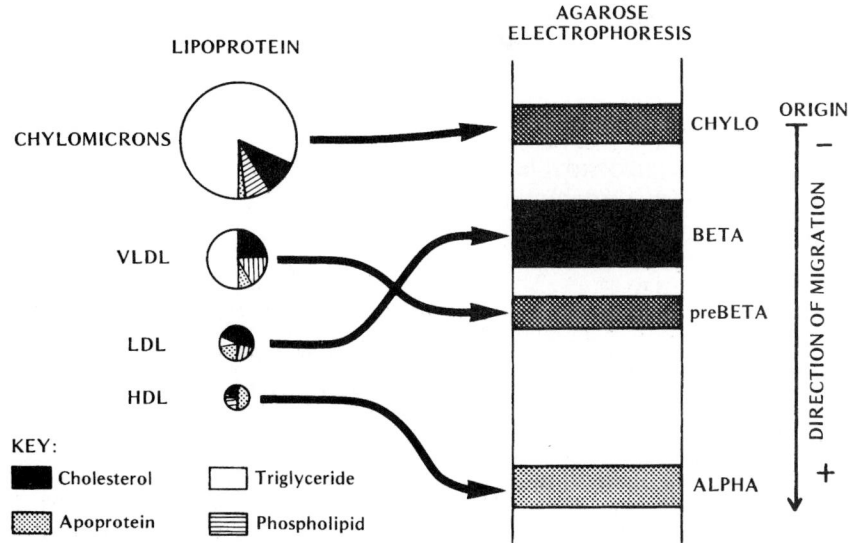

Fig. 33-17   Scheme of lipoprotein electrophoretic pattern on agarose support medium. *HDL,* High-density lipoprotein; *LDL,* low-density lipoprotein; *VLDL,* very-low-density lipoprotein.

chylomicrons or sample turbidity is performed after the sample has been allowed to sit undisturbed at 4° to 8° C for a period of time (usually overnight). These simple tests, coupled with the determination of HDL and LDL, have largely supplanted lipoprotein electrophoresis in the clinical laboratory. However, in certain situations lipoprotein electrophoresis can be of great utility in helping to identify individuals with the rare Fredrickson's type III hyperlipoproteinemia (also called dysbetalipoproteinemia) (see Fig. 33-8 and p. 658). This dysbetalipoproteinemia is characterized electrophoretically by a characteristic broad smear between the beta and prebeta bands. This finding can be of great diagnostic utility for identifying this dysbetalipoproteinemia.

The separation of lipoproteins by electrophoresis is similar in theory and technique to the electrophoretic separation of proteins (see Chapter 10) and thus is not discussed in detail here. Reviews of electrophoretic theory and technique can be found elsewhere.[10]

The support medium that is employed in the electrophoretic separation of lipoproteins is one of the most critical factors affecting this technique. Support media that have been used include paper, starch, agarose, polyacrylamide, agar, and cellulose acetate.

The use of paper as a support medium for lipoprotein electrophoresis has since been mostly replaced by agarose. However, the use of paper as a support medium is considered the classical method for lipoprotein electrophoresis, and the Fredrickson classification of hyperlipoproteinemia is based on the paper electrophoretic system.[1,2]

Starch gel has never been used to any great extent for lipoprotein electrophoresis. One may prepare these gels by using partially hydrolyzed potato starch, and such gels will separate lipoproteins on the basis of both electrical charge and molecular size.[10] When separated using starch gel electrophoresis, serum lipoproteins migrate in order of increasing mobility as alpha-lipoproteins, beta-lipoproteins, very-

low-density lipoproteins, and chylomicrons. In fact, the molecular size of the chylomicron fraction precludes its entering the starch gel. Today the use of starch gel electrophoresis is limited mainly to the preparation of lipoprotein fractions for additional investigations.

Agarose is the most widely used support medium for electrophoretic separation of lipoproteins (Fig. 33-17). Agarose gel enables much better separation of the pre–beta-lipoprotein and beta-lipoprotein fractions when compared to the other available support media. Separation of the lipoprotein fractions with agarose can be accomplished within 1 hour, whereas paper or starch gel electrophoresis may take up to several days. Also, the clear matrix of the agarose gel allows for quantitation of the lipoprotein fractions with use of a scanning densitometer. Finally, lipoprotein fractionation with an agarose medium most closely approximates those results obtained when lipoproteins are separated by ultracentrifugation, the reference method for lipoprotein analysis.

Polyacrylamide, like starch gel, separates lipoprotein fractions on the basis of both electrical charge and molecular size. The molecular sieving action of the polyacrylamide gel (and starch gel) causes the prebeta band to migrate more slowly than the beta-lipoprotein band (Fig. 33-18). The molecular sieving effect also results in lipoprotein fractions being separated with a higher degree of resolution on polyacrylamide gel when compared to other support media. In fact, the resolving power of polyacrylamide gel is so good that some specimens may show an excess of bands, making interpretation difficult. The use of polyacrylamide is best suited for samples that produce questionable or complicated lipoprotein patterns with other support media, such as agarose. Also, the time-consuming process of making polyacrylamide gels further limits the use of this technique in the routine clinical laboratory.

Other support media that have been used include cellulose acetate and agar gel. Although cellulose acetate is still

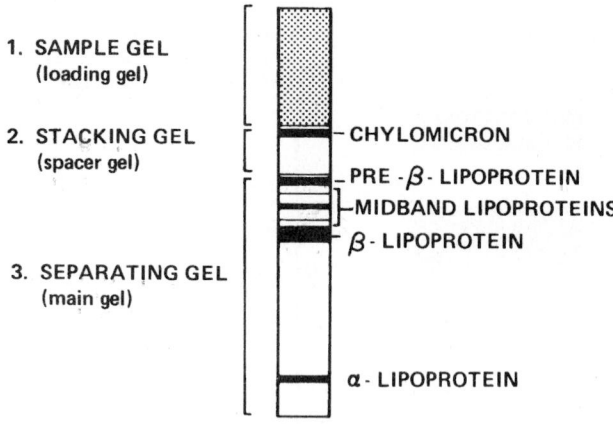

1. **SAMPLE GEL**
   (loading gel)

2. **STACKING GEL**
   (spacer gel)

   — CHYLOMICRON

   — PRE -*β* - LIPOPROTEIN

   —MIDBAND LIPOPROTEINS

   — *β* - LIPOPROTEIN

3. **SEPARATING GEL**
   (main gel)

   α - LIPOPROTEIN

Fig. 33-18 Scheme of a lipoprotein electrophoretic pattern on a polyacrylamide-gel support medium.

utilized for serum protein electrophoresis, it has disadvantages that include a tendency for this medium to yield a falsely increased beta-lipoprotein fraction, when compared to other established electrophoretic methods, and the need for clearing the gel before interpretation because of high background staining.

Agar gel is not generally used for routine electrophoretic separation of lipoproteins. However, the use of this medium does have utility in the identification of an abnormal serum lipoprotein termed *lipoprotein-X* (Lp-X). This lipoprotein variant is characterized by a high content of cholesterol and phospholipid and a low content of protein. The presence of Lp-X is associated with cholestatic liver disease. Although Lp-X migrates in the same position as beta-lipoprotein on other support media, in agar gel this species migrates cathodally to the beta-lipoproteins.[4] Thus the presence of Lp-X can be readily confirmed by electrophoresis using agar gel as the supporting medium.

Visualization of separated lipoproteins can be accomplished with use of any lipid-specific stains. Oil red O and fat red 7B are the most commonly used stains.

Specimen Either serum or plasma can be used for lipoprotein determinations by electrophoresis. If plasma is used, the preferred anticoagulant is EDTA. In addition to its use as an anticoagulant, EDTA also helps preserve specimen integrity by inhibiting metal-induced auto-oxidation of unsaturated fatty acids and cholesterol. Samples should be obtained from individuals who have fasted for at least 12 hours. Since lipoprotein metabolism is affected by a variety of pathophysical conditions, care must be taken to ensure that the sample obtained is representative of an individual's normal daily life-style and well-being. Thus, samples should not be collected from individuals who have recently experienced substantial changes in caloric intake, alcohol consumption, weight gain or loss, and changes in medication. In addition, factors such as acute illness or injury (such as myocardial infarction) or recent surgery can dramatically alter lipoprotein metabolism. Collection of samples for lipoprotein analysis should be deferred in individuals with these conditions.

Table 33-12 Percentage of distribution of lipoprotein fractions in children and adults

Age (years)	Sex	Lipoproteins (%), $X \pm SD$		
		Beta	Prebeta	Alpha
Children (4-14)	M, F	55 ± 5	12 ± 3	33 ± 3
Adults (18-65)	M	65 ± 8	12 ± 4	23 ± 4
Adults (18-65)	F	60 ± 6	8 ± 4	32 ± 5

Reference intervals The percent distribution of lipoproteins in serum of children and adults is give in Table 33-12.

Triglycerides
HERBERT K. NAITO

Principles of analysis and current usage The determination of triglyceride concentrations in serum or plasma is useful for the evaluation and differential diagnosis of primary or secondary hyperlipidemias and the assessment of risk factors for acute pancreatitis. In addition, accurate determination of triglycerides is important because of its role in estimating the concentration of LDL cholesterol by use of the Friedewald equation:

$$LDL \; Cholesterol = Total \; Cholesterol - \\ (VLDL \; cholesterol + HDL \; cholesterol)$$

where VLDL cholesterol equals triglycerides divided by 5. The recommended precision goal for triglyceride measurements is a %CV of ≤5%, and an accuracy goal of a bias from target values of no more than 5%. Similar goals for LDL cholesterol measurements are 4% CV and 4% bias.

The earliest methods for triglyceride determinations were indirect procedures based upon substraction of cholesterol and phospholipids from the concentration of total lipids present in the sample,[45] with the remaining lipid content being attributed to triglyceride. Current methods for triglyceride determinations use enzymatic procedures to measure the concentration of glyceride glycerol. The amount of glyceride glycerol is proportional to triglyceride concentrations in the sample. Glyceride glycerol concentrations can also be determined by chemical means; however, this method is rarely performed in clinical laboratories today (see Methods in *Clinical Chemistry*[36]).

Enzymatic methods for triglyceride quantitation first require the hydrolysis of fatty acids from glycerol, usually accomplished with the use of lipase. The use of enzymes for this step have made it possible to develop rapid and automated methods for triglyceride determinations. In addition to lipase, a protease enzyme is also usually employed in the hydrolysis step. The role of the protease enzyme in the hydrolysis of fatty acids from glycerol is not yet known; however, its inclusion in the reagent system helps ensure the complete hydrolysis of triglycerides. Alpha-chymotrypsin is one protease commonly employed for this purpose.[46] After the production of free glycerol by the enzymatic hydrolysis of triglycerides, a variety of techniques may be employed for the determination of glycerol that is liberated.

One common method employs lipase, glycerol kinase, pyruvate kinase (PK), and lactate dehydrogenase (LD)

Table 33-13   Method for triglyceride analysis

Method	Type of analysis	Principle	Usage	Comments
1. Pyruvate kinase	Enzymatic ultraviolet	1. Triglyceride $\xrightarrow[\text{Protease}]{\text{Lipase}}$ Glycerol + Fatty acids 2. Glycerol + ATP $\xrightarrow[\text{kinase}]{\text{Glycerol}}$ Glycerol-3-phosphate + ADP 3. ADP + Phospho*enol*pyruvate $\xrightarrow{\text{Pyruvate}}$ ATP + Pyruvate 4. Pyruvate + NADH $\xrightarrow[\text{dehydrogenase}]{\text{Lactate}}$ Lactate + NAD Decrease in absorbance at 340 nm because of disappearance of NADH proportional to triglyceride concentration	Serum, plasma	Good sensitivity, specificity, and precision; requires serum blank; frequently used
2. Glycerol phosphate oxidase (GPO)	Enzymatic colorimetric	Utilizes reactions 1 and 2 as described above, then: 3. Glycerol-3-phosphate + O_2 $\xrightarrow{\text{GPO}}$ Dihydroxyacetone phosphate + H_2O_2 4. H_2O_2 + 4-Chlorophenol + 4-Aminophenazone + K hexacyanoferrate (II) $\xrightarrow{\text{Peroxidase}}$ 4-*p*-Benzoquinone monoiminophenazone + K hexacyanoferrate (III) + HCl + H_2O Formation of quinone monoimine dye proportional to triglyceride concentrations	Serum, plasma	Good sensitivity, specificity, and precision; requires serum blank; frequently used
3. Glycerol-3-phosphate dehydrogenase (GPD)	Enzymatic colorimetric	Utilizes reactions 1 and 2 as described above, then: 3. Glycerol-3-phosphate + NAD^+ $\xrightarrow{\text{GPD}}$ Dihydroxyacetone phosphate 4. NADH + 2-*p*-Iodophenyl-3-*p*-nitrophenyl-tetrazolium (oxidized) diaphorase $\rightarrow$ 2-*p*-Iodophenyl-3-*p*-nitrophenyl-tetrazolium (reduced) + NAD^+ Production of formazan dye proportional to triglyceride concentration	Serum, plasma	Good sensitivity, specificity, and precision; requires serum blank; frequently used

(Table 33-13, method 1). In this assay, glycerol is liberated from triglycerides by the action of lipase, and then the free glycerol reacts with ATP in the presence of glycerol kinase to produce glycerol-3-phosphate and ADP. The ADP formed in this first reaction is rephosphorylated by phospho*enol*pyruvate, in a reaction catalyzed by PK, to produce ATP and pyruvate. In the final reaction of the sequence, pyruvate is enzymatically reduced in the presence of NADH by the LD, yielding lactate and NAD. The decrease in absorbance resulting from consumption of NADH is monitored at 340 nm and is proportional to triglyceride concentrations in the sample.

Another commonly used enzymatic method (Table 33-13, method 2) employs the enzyme L-alpha-glycerol phosphate oxidase (GPO), which reacts with the glycerol-3-phosphate formed by the sequential reaction of lipase and glycerol kinase described above. In the presence of GPO and O_2, glycerol-3-phosphate is oxidized to produce dihydroxyacetone phosphate and hydrogen peroxide. The hydrogen peroxide reacts with a chromogen in a reaction catalyzed by horseradish peroxidase, causing oxidation of the chromogen and a color change, which can be monitored.[47]

Another procedure for triglyceride determinations utilizes the glycerol-3-phosphate produced in the reaction catalyzed by glycerol kinase to yield a highly colored formazan (Table 33-13, method 3). Glycerol-3-phosphate is first oxidized by NAD in a reaction catalyzed by glycerol-3-phosphate dehydrogenase to form NADH. The NADH that is formed then reacts with 2-*p*-iodophenyl-3-nitrophenyl-5-phenyltetrazolium, in a reaction catalyzed by diaphorase, to produce a formazan dye.

Triglyceride methods based on absorbance measurements of NADH at 340 nm should utilize a serum blank as part of the assay procedure. The serum blank corrects for the presence of serum components that can absorb or scatter light at 340 nm. The colorimetric methods that are based on the reduction of tetrazolium salts by NADH and diaphorase and measurement of the resulting formazan dye in the visible spectrum do not require a sample blank measurement. However, these methods suffer from the spontaneous formation of the formazan dye, which results in an increase in the reagent blank reading.

Another factor that can adversely affect the accuracy of triglyceride measurements is the use of a blanking step to correct for the free glycerol present in serum. Blanking steps are typically carried out by performance of a two-part analysis. In the first part of the analysis, all the steps necessary to measure glycerol concentrations are performed, except that hydrolysis of triglyceride is not done; this step measures the free glycerol. In the second part of the analysis, the complete reaction is performed to measure total glycerol concentrations. The actual triglyceride concentration is based on and calculated from the corrected glycerol level, that is, total glycerol minus the free glycerol. The free glycerol present in serum is produced as a result of lipolysis of stored triglycerides and usually occurs in concentrations ranging from 80 to 200 mg/L.[48,49] However, situations such as stress or certain disease states can result in a substantial increase in the rate of adipose tissue lipolysis with a resultant increase in the amount of free glycerol present in the sera. In addition, glycerol or glycerol-like products may be present in certain intravenous infusates given to patients, with resultant increases in the free glycerol content of serum.[48,50] Thus, although various formulas have been developed as a means of correcting for the free glycerol content of serum, their use is mainly restricted to nonstressed, healthy individuals. It must be noted, however, that even in this population free glycerol concentrations greater than 750 mg/L are not uncommon.[48]

Specimen Serum or plasma may be used for determination of triglyceride concentrations. It must be noted, however, that plasma values are about 2% to 4% lower than serum because of the dilutional effect caused by the anticoagulant-induced efflux of water from erythrocytes. Anticoagulants such as fluoride, citrate, and oxalate can cause large shifts of water from erythrocytes to plasma and should be avoided.[51] Blood should be collected for triglyceride determinations only if the patient has been fasting for a minimum 10- to 12-hour period. Triglyceride concentrations increase within 2 hours after eating and reach a maximum after 4 to 6 hours. Thus, in the nonfasting patient who has had blood drawn for triglyceride analysis, an increased triglyceride concentration is impossible to interpret properly. In addition, the increased concentration of chylomicrons in nonfasting specimens can interfere with absorbance measurements in some colorimetric triglyceride determinations.

Reference interval The NCEP recommendations have eliminated the use of reference interval for triglycerides. Instead, the expert panel[13,14] has recommended a few cutoff values, like total cholesterol, to simplify the remembering of important medical decision numbers (see Table 33-3).

REFERENCES

1. Fredrickson DS, Lees RS: Familial hyperlipoproteinemia. In Stanbury JB, Wyngaarden JB, Fredrickson DS, editors: *The metabolic basis of inherited disease,* ed 3, New York, 1982, McGraw-Hill.
2. Fredrickson DS, Levy RJ, Lees RS: Fat transport in lipoproteins: an integrated approach to mechanisms and disorders, *N Engl J Med* 276:32-44, 94-103, 148-156, 215-224, 273-281, 1967.
3. Gotto AM Jr, editor: *Plasma lipoproteins,* New York, 1987, Elsevier Science Publishers.
4. Scanu AM, Spector AA, editors: *Biochemistry and biology of plasma lipoproteins,* New York, 1986, Marcel Dekker.
5. Levy RJ, Rifkind BM, Dennis BH, Ernst N, editors: *Nutrition, lipids, and coronary heart disease,* New York, 1979, Raven Press.
6. Miller ME, Lewis B, editors: *Lipoproteins, atherosclerosis and coronary heart disease,* New York, 1981, American Elsevier Publishing.
7. Naito HK, editor: *Nutrition and heart disease,* New York, 1982, Spectrum Publications, Inc.
8. National Heart, Lung, and Blood Institute Consensus Conference on Treatment of Hypertriglyceridemia, *JAMA* 251:1196-1200, 1984.
9. Lewis LA, Opplt JJ, editors: *Handbook of electrophoresis,* vol 1: *Lipoproteinemia: basic principles and concepts;* vol 2: *Lipoproteins in disease,* Boca Raton, Fla., 1980, CRC Press.
10. Lewis LA, editor: *Handbook of electrophoresis,* vol 3: *Lipoprotein methodology and human studies,* Boca Raton, Fla., 1983, CRC Press.
11. Havel RJ: Familial dysbeta-lipoproteinemia, *Med Clin North Am* 66(2):441-454, 1982.
12. Scanu AM: Structural and functional polymorphism of lipoprotein(a): biological and clinical implications, *Clin Chem* 41:170-172, 1995.
13. The Expert Panel: Report of the National Cholesterol Education Program expert panel on detection, evaluation, and treatment of high blood cholesterol in adults, *Arch Intern Med* 148:36-39, 1988.
14. Second Expert Panel: Detection, Evaluation, and Treatment of High Blood Cholesterol in Adults (Adult Treatment Panel II), *Circulation* 89:1329-1445, 1994.
15. Havel RJ: Approach to the patient with hyperlipidemia, *Med Clin North Am* 66(2):319-333, 1982.
16. Rifkind BM, Levy RI, editors: *Hyperlipidemia: diagnosis and therapy,* New York, 1977, Grune & Stratton.
17. Naito HK, Kwak YS: Evaluation of a new high-density lipoprotein cholesterol (HDL-C) technology: selective separation of lipoproteins by magnetic precipitation, *Clin Chem* 41:S135, 1995.
18. Kris-Etherton PM, editor-in-chief: Risk factors for coronary heart disease. In *Cardiovascular disease: nutrition for prevention and treatment,* Chicago, Ill., 1990, American Dietetic Association.
19. The Expert Panel: Report of the National Cholesterol Education Program Expert Panel on Blood Cholesterol Levels in Children and Adolescents, U.S. Department of Health and Human Services, NIH publ no 91-2732, Bethesda, Md., Sept 1991, pp 1-119.
20. Gotto AM Jr, Farmer JA: Risk factors for coronary artery disease. In Braunwald E, editor: Heart disease: a textbook of cardiovascular medicine, ed 3, Philadelphia, 1988, Saunders.
21. Ross R: The pathogenesis of atherosclerosis. In Braunwald E, editor: *Heart disease: a textbook of cardiovascular medicine,* ed 3, Philadelphia, 1988, Saunders.
22. Naito HK: 18th Annual Symposium, National Academy of Clinical Biochemistry. Atherogenesis: current topics on etiology and risk factors, *Clin Chem* 41:132-133, 1995.
23. Grundy SM: Role of low-density lipoproteins in atherogenesis and development of coronary heart disease, *Clin Chem* 41:139-146, 1995.
24. Roheim PS, Asztalos BF: Clinical significance of lipoprotein size and risk for coronary atherosclerosis, *Clin Chem* 41:147-152, 1995.
25. Malinow MR: Plasma homocyst(e)ine and arterial occlusive diseases: a mini-review, *Clin Chem* 41:173-176, 1995.
26. Srinivasan SR, Berenson GS: Serum apolipoproteins A-I and B as markers of coronary artery disease risk in early life: the Bogalusa Heart Study, *Clin Chem* 41:159-164, 1995.
27. Wilson WF: Relation of high-density lipoprotein subfractions and apolipoprotein E isoforms to coronary disease, *Clin Chem* 41:165-169, 1995.
28. Zilversmit DB: Atherogenic nature of triglycerides, postprandial lipidemia, and triglyceride-rich remnant, *Clin Chem* 41:153-158, 1995.
29. Strong JP: Natural history and risk factors for early human atherogenesis, *Clin Chem* 41:143-138, 1995.
30. Wissler RW: Theories and new horizons in the pathogenesis of atherosclerosis and the mechanisms of clinical effects, *Arch Pathol Lab Med* 116:1281-1291, 1992.
31. Steinberg D, Parthasarathy S, Carew TE, et al: Beyond cholesterol: modifications of low-density lipoproteins that increase its atherogenicity, *N Engl J Med* 320:915-923, 1989.
32. Meade TW, Miller GJ, Rosenberg RD: Characteristics associated with the risk of arterial thrombosis and the prethrombotic state. In Fuster V, Verstraete M, editors: *Thrombosis in cardiovascular disorders,* Philadelphia, 1992, Saunders.

33. NIH Consensus Development Conference: Lowering blood cholesterol to prevent heart disease, *JAMA* 253:2080-2086, 1985.

34. Current status of blood cholesterol measurement in clinical laboratories in the United States: a report from the Laboratory Standardization Panel of the National Cholesterol Education Program, *Clin Chem* 34:193-201, 1988.

35. Naito HK: *Cholesterol: review of methods, Check Sample PTS 85-I,* Chicago, 1985, American Society of Clinical Pathology, pp. 1-17.

36. Naito HK: Cholesterol. In the CD-ROM by Kaplan LA, Pesce AJ, editors: *Clinical chemistry: a scientific and management infobase,* Cincinnati, Ohio, 1996, Pesce Kaplan Publishers.

37. Kim E, Goldberg M: Serum cholesterol assay using a stable Liebermann-Burchard reagent, *Clin Chem* 15:1171-1179, 1969.

38. Abell LL, Levy BB, Brodie BB, Kendall FE: Simplified methods for the estimation of the total cholesterol in serum and demonstration of its specificity, *J Biol Chem* 195:357-366, 1952.

39. Pesce MA, Bodourian SH: Interference with the enzymic measurement of cholesterol in serum by use of five reagent kits, *Clin Chem* 23:757-760, 1977.

40. Huang HS, Kuan JC, Guilbault GG: Fluorometric enzymatic determination of total cholesterol in serum, *Clin Chem* 21:1605-1608, 1975.

41. Noma A, Nakayama K: Polarographic method for rapid microdetermination of cholesterol with cholesterol esterase and cholesterol oxidase, *Clin Chem* 22:336-340, 1976.

42. Cooper GR: High density lipoprotein reference materials. In Lipel K, editor: *Report of the high density lipoprotein methodology workshop,* DHEW publ no NIH 79-1661, Washington, D.C., 1979, U.S. Government Printing Office, p 178.

43. Kannel WB: Low high-density lipoprotein cholesterol and what to do about it, *Am J Cardiol* 70:810-814, 1992.

44. Kerscher L, Schiefer S, Draeger B, et al: Precipitation methods for the determination of LDL-cholesterol, *Clin Biochem* 18:118-125, 1985.

45. Van Handel E, Zilversmit BD: Micromethod for the direct determination of triglycerides, *J Lab Clin Med* 50:152-157, 1957.

46. Bucolo G, David H: Quantitative determination of serum triglycerides by the use of enzymes, *Clin Chem* 19:476-482, 1973.

47. Nägele U, Hägele EO, Sauer G, et al: Reagent for the enzymatic determinations of serum total triglycerides with improved lipolytic efficiency, *J Clin Chem Clin Biochem* 22:165-174, 1984.

48. Naito HK, David JA: Laboratory considerations: determination of cholesterol, triglyceride, phospholipid, and other lipids in blood and tissues. In Story JA, editor: *Lipid research methodology,* New York, 1984, Alan R Liss.

49. Stinshoff K, Weisshaar D, Staehler F, et al: Relation between concentrations of free glycerol and triglycerides in human sera, *Clin Chem* 23:1029-1032, 1977.

50. Lindblad BS, Settergren G, Feychting H, Persson B: Total parenteral nutrition in infants: blood levels of glucose lactate, pyruvate, free fatty acids, glycerol, D-beta-hydroxybutyrate, triglycerides, free amino acids, and insulin, *Acta Paediatr Scand* 66:409-419, 1977.

51. Alper C: Specimen collection and preservation. In Henry RJ, Cannon DC, Winkelman JW, editors: *Clinical chemistry: principles and techniques,* Hagerstown, Md., 1974, Harper & Row.

CHAPTER 34 *Alcoholism*

Charles L. Mendenhall
Robert E. Weesner

OBJECTIVES

- Describe the metabolism of ethanol and the alterations of lipid, protein, and carbohydrate biochemistry that result from excess alcohol consumption.
- List and describe nutritional alterations associated with alcoholism and alcoholic liver disease.
- Describe the systemic diseases associated with alcoholism.
- State expected changes in serum levels of the following laboratory analytes in alcoholic liver disease: aspartate aminotransferase, alanine aminotransferase, lactate dehydrogenase, gamma-glutamyltransferase, alkaline phosphatase, 5′-nucleotidase, bilirubin, albumin, globulins, cholesterol, triglycerides, bile acids, and glucose.

KEY TERMS

alcoholic cirrhosis Cirrhosis resulting from chronic excess alcohol consumption. The cirrhotic process in the liver is a pathological process in which progressive injury produces fibrotic bands or scar tissue that entraps liver cells and results in loss of normal microscopic lobular architecture (nodular regeneration).

alcoholic hepatitis Acute toxic liver injury associated with excess ethanol consumption. This is characterized by necrosis, polymorphonuclear inflammation, and in many instances Mallory bodies.

alcoholic ketoacidosis The fall in blood pH (acidosis) sometimes seen in alcoholics and associated with a rise in serum ketone bodies (acetone, beta-hydroxybutyric acid, and acetoacetic acid).

alcohol withdrawal syndrome The clinical symptoms associated with cessation of alcohol consumption. These may include tremor, hallucinations, autonomic nervous system dysfunction, and seizures.

fatty liver Excessive accumulation of fat in the liver parenchymal cells, primarily neutral lipids, triglycerides, and cholesterol. Fatty liver predictably develops after exposure to a variety of hepatotoxins, of which ethanol (ethyl alcohol) is the most common.

fetal alcohol syndrome A group of fetal abnormalities resulting from maternal alcohol consumption during gestation.

hemochromatosis A disorder of iron metabolism characterized by excess iron deposits in tissues, such as those composing the liver, pancreas, and heart, leading to organ injury. The organ injury may manifest itself as cirrhosis, diabetes mellitus, or heart failure.

hepatic fibrosis The deposition of collagen and fibrous tissue in the liver before the development of nodular regeneration and cirrhosis.

kwashiorkor A nutritional disease resulting from protein deprivation. It is characterized by depleted visceral proteins and immunological dysfunction. Total calorie consumption may be deficient, adequate, or even excessive.

Mallory bodies (alcoholic hyalin) An eosinophilic cytoplasmic inclusion that accumulates in the liver cells. It is typically but not always associated with acute alcoholic liver injury (alcoholic hepatitis).

marasmus A nutritional disease resulting from calorie deprivation. It is characterized by weight loss and wasting of muscle mass and fat stores.

Wernicke-Korsakoff syndrome A disease of the central nervous system occurring in alcoholics and attributed to thiamin deficiency. Wernicke's encephalopathy consists of ocular disturbances, ataxia, and impaired mental functions. If untreated, it may become Korsakoff's syndrome, which includes memory impairment, confabulations, and deranged perception of time.

Alcoholism represents one of the most serious worldwide socioeconomic and health problems. In the United States, alcohol-related liver disease is the sixth leading cause of death.[1] An alcoholic is a person who consumes an amount of ethanol (ethyl alcohol) capable of producing pathological changes.[2] The amount of ethanol capable of producing disease depends on a variety of factors, including genetic predisposition,[3] malnutrition,[4] and concomitant viral infection of the liver (viral hepatitis).[5] For a susceptible person this may be as low as 35 g/day,[6] which is equivalent to the daily consumption of three cocktails made with 100-proof whiskey. However, for most persons the amount of alcohol necessary to produce disease is in excess of 80 g/day for at least 10 to 15 years. When this amount is converted to the quantity of alcoholic beverages consumed, it represents eight 12-ounce 6% (alcohol by volume) beers, a liter of 12% (alcohol by volume) wine, or a half pint of 80-proof (approximately 40% alcohol by volume) whiskey per day. It should be pointed out that susceptible persons may develop disease with much smaller amounts of ethanol. When the ethanol level is below 7 g/day, however, a pathological condition does not develop even in susceptible persons.[6]

See Chapter 52 for a discussion of the general problem of addiction.

DIAGNOSIS OF ALCOHOLISM
Alcoholic intoxication

An elevated blood alcohol level demonstrates recent alcohol ingestion and intoxication. Although blood alcohol levels correlate with current signs of physical and mental impairment from ethanol intoxication, a blood alcohol level cannot be used to diagnose alcoholism. The general signs of ethanol intoxication are listed in the following box.

Signs of Ethanol Intoxication

History of alcohol consumption
Odor of alcohol on breath
Nystagmus (rapid horizontal eye movement)
Slurred speech
Diminished pain response
Poor motor coordination
Depressed level of consciousness

The well-established relationship between blood alcohol levels and the physical signs of intoxication in a sporadic drinker is summarized in Table 34-1. The decreased motor function associated with elevated levels of blood alcohol can lead to trauma of the intoxicated person (see p. 690). At blood alcohol levels between 400 and 600 mg/L, there is already significant impairment of driving skills, including motor, cognitive, and information-processing skills.[7] Drivers with blood alcohol levels between 500 and 900 mg/L are nine times as likely to be involved in a vehicular crash than individuals with undetectable blood alcohol.[8]

For chronic users of ethanol, the same signs and symptoms may be seen at higher blood alcohol levels, even at levels of alcohol as much as 1000 mg/L and higher. A current history of alcohol intoxication may lead a physician to suspect chronic alcoholism.

Alcoholism

Characteristically alcoholics may attempt to conceal their excessive drinking, and so the history of consumption may be unreliable. Verification from the spouse is frequently necessary to determine an accurate drinking history. However, signs and symptoms of current intoxication, such as those listed above, and the symptoms of drug withdrawal (for an alcoholic, *delerium tremens*), may raise the suspicion of chronic alcohol abuse.

Several laboratory tests have been proposed for use as diagnostic tools to confirm the excess consumption of ethanol.[9,10] As few as two drinks per day have resulted in significant increases in mean red blood cell volume (MCV)[9]; however, the changes are small, and it may be necessary to use baseline predrinking values to recognize the effect of ethanol.

Serum gamma-glutamyltransferase (GGT) has been shown to be readily inducible by a variety of compounds, including ethanol. In the absence of other abnormal laboratory tests for liver disease, elevated levels of GGT may be useful for recognition of the heavy drinker in the predisease state.

Table 34-1   Blood alcohol levels and symptoms

Blood alcohol level (mg/L)	Physical signs	Degree of intoxication
<500	Relaxed state	Generally, none
1000		*Legally intoxicated* in most states
2000-2500	Decreased alertness	
	Gross intoxication	
	Increasingly lethargic	
	Effort may be needed to have emotional and motor control	
3000-3500	Stupor to coma	
>5000	Death may ensue	

BIOCHEMICAL AND METABOLIC ALTERATIONS
Ethanol metabolism

In humans, ethanol is primarily an exogenous compound consumed in alcoholic beverages and readily absorbed from the entire gastrointestinal tract. Blood ethanol is cleared by the liver at a constant rate, decreasing at 150 to 200 mg/L per hour in a normal individual and at 300 to 400 mg/L in a chronic alcoholic. This translates to a clearance rate of approximately 3 ounces of ethanol per hour in an average adult.

Most of the absorbed ethanol is then degraded by oxidative processes, primarily in the liver, first to acetaldehyde and then to acetate. At least three enzyme systems are capable of ethanol oxidation: (1) alcohol dehydrogenase, (2) microsomal ethanol oxidizing system (MEOS), and (3) catalase. Only 2% to 10% is excreted unoxidized in the urine and lungs.

Alcohol dehydrogenase (ADH) appears to be the principal pathway for ethanol oxidation. This is especially true for acute intoxication:

$$\text{Ethanol} \xrightarrow[\substack{\text{NAD}^+ \qquad \text{NADH} + \text{H}^+}]{\text{Alcohol dehydrogenase}} \text{Acetaldehyde}$$

The initial step catalyzed by alcohol dehydrogenase appears to be rate limiting for the clearance of ethanol from the blood, but it is not specific for ethanol. Methanol, retinol (vitamin A), and several other alcohols are also oxidized by this enzyme. This fact is important clinically in the treatment of acute methanol poisoning.[11] In this instance, ethanol is given clinically to compete with methanol for binding sites on the ADH enzyme; thus oxidation of methanol to the toxic formaldehyde is delayed.

MEOS appears to be a secondary enzyme system for ethanol clearance:

$$\text{Ethanol} \xrightarrow[\substack{\text{NADP} + \text{H}^+ \qquad \text{NADP} + \text{H}_2\text{O}}]{\substack{\text{Oxygen} \\ \text{MEOS}}} \text{Acetaldehyde}$$

This microsomal enzyme is found in the smooth endoplasmic reticulum (SER) of the hepatocytes. In the chronic alcoholic, there is an increase in MEOS activity.[12] The induction of MEOS activity is associated with increased activity of various other constituents of the SER involved with drug metabolism, such as other enzymes (5′-nucleotidase and GGT), cytochrome P-450 reductase, and cytochrome P-450. These changes have clinical significance because they render the alcoholic more resistant to the effects of many common sedatives and barbiturates, resulting in the necessity for a larger-than-normal dose when sedation is required. If, however, ethanol and barbiturates are consumed simultaneously, competitive enzyme inhibition results in reduced clearance[13] and abnormally high blood levels of barbiturates. Indeed, death has resulted from this interaction.

The role of catalase in the biological oxidation of ethanol is controversial.[14] In vitro in the presence of a peroxide (H_2O_2)-generating system, catalase has been shown to be capable of oxidizing ethanol by the following reaction:

$$\text{Ethanol} + \text{H}_2\text{O}_2 \xrightarrow{\text{Catalase}} 2\text{H}_2\text{O} + \text{Acetaldehyde}$$

It appears that the slow rate at which peroxide can be generated from NADPH oxidase or xanthine oxidase prevents catalase from contributing to more than 2% of the in vivo ethanol oxidation.

Altered lipid, protein, and carbohydrate biochemistry

Lipids. Lipids accumulate in most tissues in which ethanol is metabolized, and such accumulation results in fatty liver, fatty myocardium, fatty renal tubules, and so on.[20a] The mechanism appears to be multifactorial, resulting from both increased lipid accumulation and decreased lipid oxidation.[15] Although the secretion of serum lipoproteins is low relative to the lipid load accumulating in the liver, the total amount secreted is increased above normal, and alcoholic hyperlipemia may result.[16] This is a type IV hyperlipemia with increases in both serum triglycerides and cholesterol esters, resulting in an increase in serum of hepatic very low-density lipoproteins and chylomicron-like particles.

Enzyme activities related to ethanol oxidation and drug metabolism are frequently altered. These changes may be produced either directly by enzyme induction or suppression or indirectly by the shift in reducing equivalents, that is, by increasing the ratio, NADH/NAD^+.

Protein. Once synthesized, the cellular release of proteins may be altered. As a consequence of the altered release of protein from the liver cell, one of the earliest liver changes seen in the alcoholic is the accumulation of protein,[17] which occurs concurrently with fat accumulation and contributes to the development of the enlarged liver (hepatomegaly) that is seen in more than 90% of alcoholics with liver disease.[18]

Carbohydrate. Gluconeogenesis is similarly impaired by ethanol by a variety of mechanisms. Gluconeogenesis is the process whereby glucose is formed from noncarbohydrate sources, that is, glycerol, pyruvate, and several amino acids. Because ethanol promotes glycerol-lipid formation and impairs amino acid transport, the availability of these compounds for gluconeogenesis is decreased. Glutamic acid dehydrogenase activity is also diminished by elevated NADH levels, decreasing the availability of alpha-ketoglutarate, which is necessary for the transamination of amino acids before their conversion into glucose. This further impairs gluconeogenesis.

The increase in NADH with a concomitant decrease in NAD^+ associated with ADH activity may also produce sequential changes of carbohydrate metabolism with clinical consequences. The increased availability of NADH results in increased lactate production, which decreases its availability for gluconeogenesis and can result in hyperlacticacidemia.[19] The hyperlacticacidemia reduces the capacity of the kidney to excrete uric acid, leading to a secondary hyperuricemia.[20] In susceptible persons this may aggravate or precipitate attacks of gout.[21]

Typically the storage of glycogen in the liver is also diminished in alcoholics. This results from both poor dietary intake and the liver diseases so frequently associated with chronic alcoholism (fatty liver, alcoholic hepatitis, and alcoholic cirrhosis). The clinical implications of these changes in liver glycogen and impaired gluconeogenesis are discussed later along with insulin and other hormonal involvement in the development of alcoholic hypoglycemia.

In the absence of liver disease, malnutrition, or other predisposing conditions, ethanol itself produces only a slight increase or no change in blood glucose. If it is present, the peak rise in glucose occurs 30 to 45 minutes after ingestion and represents usually no more than a 7% to 10% increase.

NUTRITIONAL ALTERATIONS ASSOCIATED WITH ALCOHOLISM AND ALCOHOLIC LIVER DISEASE
Protein-calorie malnutrition

Alcoholic beverages are high in calories. Each gram of ethanol yields 7 kcal, and ethanol may account for up to 10% of the total energy intake of moderate consumers of ethanol and up to 50% for alcoholics. However, alcoholic beverages are low in nutritive value.[22] In fact, chronic alcoholism has long been associated with both malnutrition and liver disease. Malnutrition in the form of protein-calorie deficiency results from a variety of causes: (1) poor dietary intake; (2) malabsorption of consumed nutrients as a result of alcohol-induced gastritis, pancreatitis, or diarrhea; and (3) altered biochemical and physiological processes.

Protein-calorie malnutrition (PCM) has been classified as marasmus or a kwashiorkor-like disease, depending on whether a caloric deficit (marasmus) or a protein deficit (kwashiorkor-like disease) predominates[23] (see Chapter 37). In a study of 284 alcoholics with alcoholic hepatitis, all patients had some degree of protein-calorie malnutrition, and 80% had features of both marasmus and kwashiorkor-like

disease.[4] Serum prealbumin measurements can be used to help diagnose and monitor PCM.[23]

Liver injury can develop in the absence of malnutrition. However, the more severe forms are invariably associated with severe malnutrition. Recognition of nutritional deficits appears to be important for the alcoholic with liver disease because correction of these abnormalities by appropriate nutritional therapy may increase survival and accelerate improvement of the liver injury.

Vitamin abnormalities

Excessive alcohol use commonly leads to vitamin deficiency.[24] Vitamin deficiency results because of the poor general nutrition associated with alcohol abuse and because of hepatic damage. Not only is the liver a major storage depot for vitamins but it also converts vitamins into metabolically useful forms (see Chapter 39). Therefore injury to the liver alters vitamin metabolism. Vitamins can be released from necrotic liver cells that are lost from the body and not adequately replaced.[25] In addition, fat-soluble vitamins (vitamins A, D, K, and E) may not be adequately absorbed by the intestine of alcoholics.[24]

Alcohol can increase the body's need for folic acid, vitamin B_{12}, and vitamin B_6 because of increased nucleic acid synthesis and liver regeneration.[26] Because of the many interactions between the liver, alcohol, and vitamins, vitamin and protein replacement plays a major role in the treatment of the alcoholic patient. Table 34-2 gives the incidence of low serum values of vitamins in persons with alcoholic cirrhosis. (See Chapter 39 for a discussion of the biochemistry and physiology of vitamins.)

Vitamin A. Vitamin A is absorbed as retinol, which must be oxidized to retinal with the help of alcohol dehydrogenase to be functional. Alcohol competitively inhibits the conversion of retinol to retinal in the liver.[27]

Vitamin B_1 (thiamin). Thiamin deficiency is encountered frequently in alcoholics.[24] The requirement for thiamin is greatest when carbohydrate is the major source of energy, which is sometimes found in the alcoholic. Thiamin deficiency can produce a neuropsychiatric disorder

Table 34-2 Vitamins in the alcoholic

Vitamin	Classification of vitamin	Effect of alcohol on intestinal absorption	Incidence (%) of low serum values in alcoholic cirrhosis
A	Fat soluble	Decrease	12
B_1 (thiamin)	Water soluble	Decrease	58
B_2 (riboflavin)	Water soluble	None	6
Nicotinic acid	Water soluble	Not evaluated	33
B_6 (pyridoxine)	Water soluble	None	60
Folic acid	Water soluble	None	78
B_{12} (cyanocobalamin)	Water soluble	Decrease	25
C (ascorbic acid)	Water soluble	Not evaluated	25
D	Fat soluble	Not evaluated	?
E	Fat soluble	Not evaluated	15
K	Fat soluble	Not evaluated	?

called *Wernicke-Korsakoff syndrome* in a small number of alcoholics; this syndrome can be genetically determined.[28] There is also increasing evidence that thiamin deficiency may contribute to other forms of brain injury in alcoholics.[27]

Vitamin B$_2$ (riboflavin). Vitamin B$_2$ is rarely a problem in the alcoholic.[24]

Nicotinic acid. A severe deficiency of nicotinic acid leading to pellagra can be found in the alcoholic population.[29]

Vitamin B$_6$ (pyridoxine). In alcoholic hepatitis the serum aspartate aminotransferase (AST) is greater than the serum alanine aminotransferase (ALT) in 90% of the patients.[30]

Folic acid. Folic acid deficiency is the most common vitamin deficiency among alcoholics.[24] Folate deficiency contributes to the megaloblastic anemia observed in alcoholics.[31] Alcohol does not inhibit intestinal absorption of food-associated folate.[32] Poor dietary intake, increased requirements, and increased excretion are believed to be the major causes of folate deficiency in the alcoholic.[27] In addition, alcohol may directly block folate metabolism.[33]

Vitamin B$_{12}$ (cyanocobalamin). Although alcohol in some way inhibits vitamin B$_{12}$ absorption at the ileum,[27] vitamin B$_{12}$ deficiency is rarely a problem.[24] Because vitamin B$_{12}$ is stored in the liver, acute liver cell necrosis of alcoholic hepatitis may actually produce a noticeable increase in serum B$_{12}$ levels that parallels the severity of the liver injury.

Vitamin C (ascorbic acid). Vitamin C deficiency is not common in alcoholics; low levels in alcoholics have been attributed to poor dietary intake.[34]

Vitamin D. Vitamin D deficiency is not a major problem among alcoholics.[29]

Vitamin E. Chronic alcoholics are susceptible to vitamin E deficiency because of low dietary intake and general malnutrition. Pure vitamin E deficiency is known to produce a testicular lesion, but whether this plays a role in alcoholic hypogonadism remains unclear.[27]

Vitamin K. Because the stores of vitamin K are small, biliary obstruction or severe parenchymal liver disease can produce bleeding abnormalities.[29] Alcoholics often have prolonged prothrombin time.[18] When these patients are given vitamin K parenterally, some show corrected prothrombin time, indicating vitamin K deficiency. Those who do not improve with vitamin K have liver disease too severe to use the vitamin.[29]

Mineral abnormalities (see Chapters 35 and 37)

Iron. The mechanism responsible for the mild to moderate iron accumulation in the liver of some patients with alcoholic liver disease is not clearly understood. First, some alcoholic beverages, especially red wines, contain iron. Making beer in iron kettles has led to hemochromatosis among the South African Bantu.[35] Finally, the effect of al-

cohol on folate could influence iron absorption. Folate deficiency is associated with ineffective red blood cell formation (erythropoiesis) and iron overloading.[36] Alcoholics with significant iron overload may, in fact, carry the gene for primary idiopathic hemochromatosis.[37] Some alcoholics have low iron levels because of poor dietary intake or chronic blood loss from the intestinal tract (gastritis), peptic ulcer, esophageal and gastric varices, and poor clotting.[29]

Zinc. Zinc, an essential micronutrient element, is important for RNA and DNA synthesis and for a variety of zinc-dependent enzymes, including alcohol dehydrogenase.[27] Vitamin A metabolism can also be altered in zinc deficiency.[38] Alcoholics can have low zinc levels from both reduced oral intake and increased urine loss and may suffer many symptoms seen in zinc-deficient states.[35] Further studies are needed to define the role of zinc in alcohol-related hypogonadism and other related problems.[27]

Lead. The lead content of some wines is high.[27] In addition, when old radiators or lead pipes are incorporated into homemade stills for the production of "moonshine" whiskey, lead poisoning can result.[35] Therefore an effort must be made to detect any signs or symptoms of lead poisoning (see Chapter 38) in alcoholics because of the increased risk.

Magnesium. Chronic alcoholics commonly have magnesium deficiency. This is a result of poor dietary intake, the increased urine loss that is a direct effect of alcohol, starvation ketosis, and vomiting. Magnesium is often low during the alcohol withdrawal syndrome and may contribute to the signs and symptoms of this disorder.[39]

Calcium (see Chapter 28). Patients with alcoholic liver disease may have low levels of calcium. Alcohol has been found to increase calcium excretion.[40] Patients with cirrhosis have lower calcium absorption, which may be a result of decreased liver hydroxylation of vitamin D (see p. 532).[41] If the alcoholic has fat malabsorption, the calcium in the intestinal lumen may form insoluble soaps with the fats, thus preventing intestinal absorption.

Phosphorus. Hypophosphatemia occurs in about 50% of hospitalized alcoholics.[42] Serum phosphorus is depressed acutely by as much as 10 to 15 mg/L after ingestion of carbohydrates. Alcoholics reach their lowest phosphorus levels on the second to fourth day of hospitalization.[27] The low phosphorus levels in alcoholics may be a result of alcohol itself, poor food intake, diarrhea, vomiting, magnesium deficiency, or use of aluminum-containing antacids.

PATHOLOGY: SYSTEMIC DISEASES OF THE ALCOHOLIC
Mechanisms of organ damage

Ethanol is a direct systemic toxin that produces injury to all tissues, depending on the dose and duration of exposure. The degree of injury varies among organ systems. The liver, the organ that is predominantly responsible for ethanol metabolism, develops the highest incidence and severity of injury.

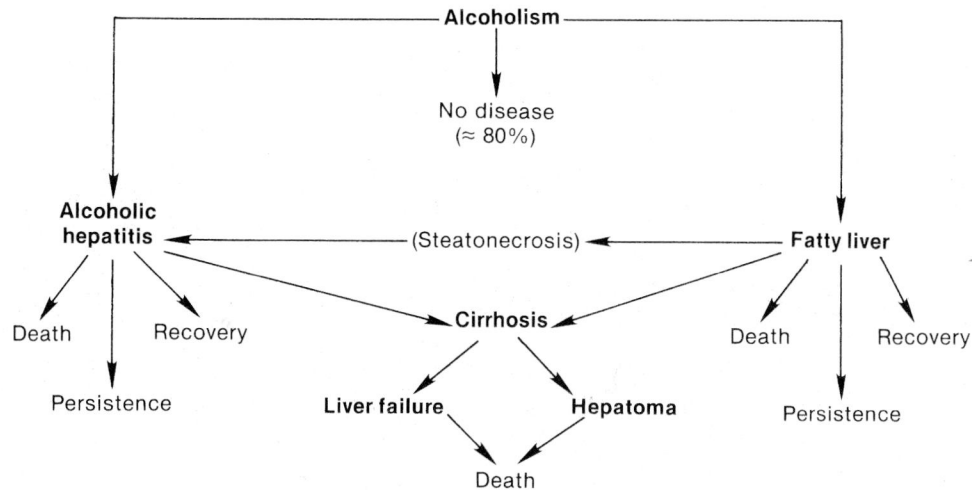

Fig. 34-1 Alcoholic liver disease.

The product of all three ethanol oxidation pathways described above is acetaldehyde. It appears that various organ disorders and biochemical alterations are induced by either ethanol or acetaldehyde but not necessarily by both. For example, fetal alcohol syndrome appears to be an ethanol effect independent of acetaldehyde,[43] whereas liver fibrosis and collagen formation may be more closely associated with acetaldehyde than with ethanol. Acetaldehyde readily forms adducts with components of cellular membranes. These adducts may directly cause cellular damage or may create new antigenic stimulants. Organ damage, especially of the liver, may be immunological in nature.[44]

Liver

Three types of pathological liver conditions develop, forming a continuum of disease from very mild reversible changes to life-threatening irreversible disease.[21a] The interrelationships among these changes are depicted in Fig. 34-1.

Fatty liver. The mildest form of liver damage is characterized by fatty infiltration (alcoholic fatty liver) and by some minimum degree of inflammation and necrosis. In more severe cases of fatty liver, fibrosis may be present, especially around central venous channels. Clinically this is manifested by liver enlargement (hepatomegaly), tenderness over the liver, and anorexia. Laboratory changes are minimum with slight elevation of AST, bilirubin, and alkaline phosphatase levels. When available, the serum bile acids and dye-clearance tests (indocyanine green) appear to be the most reliable parameters to detect early disease. Alcoholic fatty liver is usually considered a benign, reversible disease. However, sudden deaths have been observed in a small percentage of alcoholics, presumably from fat emboli.

Alcoholic hepatitis. The more severe toxic form of hepatic injury, alcoholic hepatitis, is also characterized by fatty liver and hepatomegaly. In addition, inflammation and

necrosis are more extensive, and fibrosis is a prominent feature. The mortality from acute alcoholic hepatitis is approximately 60% during the 6 weeks after hospital admission.

Alcoholic hepatitis is frequently a crucial stage toward the progression of cirrhotic disease. In the large Veterans Administration Cooperative Study[18] of patients with clinical alcoholic hepatitis, the disease had progressed to cirrhosis in 54.7% of 97 patients in whom histological specimens were available. In a high percentage of patients (76.2%) an irregularly outlined homogeneous meshwork of eosin-staining material could be seen in the cytoplasm of the liver cells (Mallory bodies or alcoholic hyalin). Its presence is not diagnostic for alcoholic hepatitis because it has been seen in a variety of other liver conditions. However, in an alcoholic with liver disease its presence most likely represents alcoholic hepatitis. It has been suggested that alcoholic hyalin results from degenerating microfilaments, which then act as immunological irritants and stimulate fibrosis.[45]

The clinical and laboratory manifestations of alcoholic hepatitis are shown in Table 34-3. None of the symptoms or changes are pathognomonic for this condition.

As the disease progresses, all standard laboratory tests for liver injury become abnormal to varying degrees. Of special note are the serum enzyme changes. Although AST is elevated in more than 75% of even the mild cases, the magnitude of the elevation rarely exceeds 10 times the upper limits of normal. The mean value observed was 84 ±6 mU/mL. Similarly ALT was only mildly elevated; the ALT value was usually less than 100 mU/mL and almost invariably less than the AST. ALT values of 200 mU/mL or ALT values that are greater than the AST indicate a chronic, persistent hepatitis or chronic, aggressive hepatitis rather than uncomplicated alcoholic hepatitis. In these instances only a liver biopsy can differentiate the cause of liver disease.

Although the histological presentation of hepatitis is the

Table 34-3   Initial clinical features and complications of alcoholic hepatitis*

Feature or complication	Severity of disease		
	Mild	Moderate	Severe
Anorexia†	46.2	63.0	65.7
Weight loss†‡	36.8	27.1	16.2
Fever	18.0	26.2	19.2
Hepatomegaly	85.9	97.1	88.9
Splenomegaly†	24.5	38.6	46.2
Infection	5.2	16.8	8.1
Pancreatitis	13.6	10.3	10.1
Gastrointestinal bleeding	10.4	7.5	14.1
Ascites			
Mild	18.7	19.4	17.2
Moderate	11.0	38.0	45.5
Severe	1.3	20.4	29.3
Combined†	31.0	77.8	92.0
Encephalopathy			
Grade 1	17.3	29.6	25.3
Grade 2	4.5	24.1	41.4
Grades 3 and 4	0.7	3.7	0
Combined†	2.5	57.4	66.7
Probability of surviving 1 yr§	0.91 ±0.027	0.75 ±0.045	0.46 ±0.055

From Mendenhall CL, Anderson S, Weesner RE, et al: *Am J Med* 76:221-222, 1984.
*The diagnoses of the various complicating features and conditions were not defined in the protocol but were determined by the clinical judgment of the participating investigator. Because *n* varied among severity groups (mild, 156; moderate, 108; severe, 99), values are expressed as a percentage of total. Data analysis consisted of an overall chi-squared test, which, when significant at the 0.05 level, was followed by Bartholomew's test for order. The hypothesized order was $p_{mild} < p_{moderate} < p_{severe}$ except for weight loss where the presence of ascites reversed the hypothesized order.
†$p < 0.005$ (Bartholomew's test).
‡The decreasing incidence of weight loss with increasing severity represented an increasing incidence of ascites.
§$p < 0.006$. All pairwise comparisons (mild, moderate, severe) determined by normal distribution test statistics.

best prognostic indicator of survival, the serum bilirubin level and prothrombin time are the laboratory tests that allow the most reliable prediction of the severity and survival prognosis of liver disease. These tests, however, are not sensitive enough to diagnose minimum disease. In very mild cases results may be normal or near normal. However, as the disease progresses, the usefulness of the tests increases. Patients are at high risk when the bilirubin level becomes greater than 200 mg/L and the prothrombin time becomes prolonged more than 4 seconds. In this group mortality exceeds 75%.

The bilirubin and prothrombin time results are used to classify the severity of disease as mild, moderate, or severe.[18] Mild disease is present when the bilirubin is less than 50 mg/L with a normal or only slightly increased prothrombin time. Moderate disease is present when the bilirubin is equal to or greater than 50 mg/L and the prothrombin time is normal to moderately elevated (less than 4 seconds prolonged). Severe disease is present when the bilirubin exceeds 50 mg/L and the prothrombin time is more than 4 seconds prolonged. As severity increases, the incidence of ascites and encephalopathy also increases, whereas 1-year survival decreases progressively from 91% to 46% (see Table 34-3).

Cirrhosis. The end stage of chronic alcoholic liver disease is the development of cirrhosis with extensive liver fibrosis, nodular regeneration, distortion of the liver archi-

tecture, and ultimately all the clinical complications of chronic liver disease, liver failure, and death. In some instances cirrhosis may be hard to diagnose clinically, especially when active alcoholic hepatitis with acute necrosis and inflammation are also present. Only the liver biopsy specimen provided an accurate diagnosis of cirrhosis.

Pancreas

The association between alcohol and pancreatitis is at least as strong as the relationship between alcohol and liver disease is. At postmortem examination 18% to 47% of alcoholics dying of causes other than pancreatitis have some histological evidence of pancreatitis.[46] Alcohol is responsible for at least 30%, in some studies 60% to 90%, of the cases of pancreatitis in the United States.[47] Although there is a wide range of individual variation, the average duration of alcohol consumption before the initial diagnosis of pancreatitis is made is 18 years in men and 11 years in women. This difference indicates that women have an increased susceptibility. With each approximately 50 g increase in daily alcohol consumption, the risk of developing pancreatitis doubles.[46]

Alcohol stimulates the secretion of at least some acid from the stomach. When acid comes into contact with duodenal mucosa, it stimulates the flow of pancreatic juice.[48] The pancreatic juice induced by alcohol early in the disease process has a high concentration of protein, which precipitates and forms protein plugs. These plugs form within the pancreatic ductules and subsequently obstruct the ductules. This obstruction leads to ductular dilatation, ductular proliferation, dilatation of acinar tissue, and ductal sclerosis. In time the protein plugs may calcify, giving the x-ray picture of chronic calcific pancreatitis. As scarring of the pancreas continues, the protein or enzyme concentration in the pancreatic juice decreases until not enough enzymes are present for food digestion, and malabsorption occurs.[48,49] For reasons that are not clear, acute painful attacks of pancreatitis characterized by elevations in amylase and lipase may be superimposed on this chronic process.

Because a long interval of steady alcohol consumption is required before the first clinical attack of pancreatitis, most patients develop the first attack of pancreatitis between 30 and 40 years of age.[48] Once pancreatitis has been established, a fairly high percentage of patients who continue to drink have chronic pain.[50] After 80% to 90% of the pancreas has been destroyed, pancreatic insufficiency develops, requiring oral enzyme replacement.[51] In addition to the enzyme-secreting cells being destroyed, insulin- and glucagon-producing cells may also be destroyed. When this occurs, the alcoholic develops diabetes mellitus and the need for insulin. Because the glucagon level is also decreased and is too low to stimulate glucose synthesis adequately, these patients are brittle diabetics and are prone to hypoglycemic attacks.[48] This makes treatment of these patients difficult, especially if alcohol consumption continues.[52]

Fetal alcohol syndrome

Alcohol readily crosses the placenta and is distributed throughout fetal tissue. However, it is well established that ethanol is a fetal toxin and teratogen. Thus, ethanol consumption during pregnancy is associated with a wide variety of adverse effects, including spontaneous abortion, premature delivery, low infant birth weight, stillbirth, and poor outcome of the newborn. The last effect includes poor mental and motor development and the *fetal alcohol syndrome.*

The fetal alcohol syndrome is characterized by a pattern of birth defects that include prenatal and postnatal growth retardation, facial abnormalities, renal and CNS dysfunction, and mental retardation. It has been estimated that the fetal alcohol syndrome is now the leading cause of mental retardation in the Western world.[53]

Less common systemic involvement

Heart. Among alcoholics the incidence of clinically significant heart disease appears to be much less than that of liver or pancreatic disease. It is estimated that 20% to 30% of alcoholics develop liver disease. In two large studies of alcoholics totaling 278 cases at autopsy, 11% to 15% had alcoholic cardiomyopathy.[54] The true incidence of cardiomyopathy is unknown. When it occurs, ethanol produces an acute depressant effect on myocardial function[55] with a progressive cardiac dilatation and a low output type of cardiac failure. When death occurs, it is most often a result of gross cardiomegaly and chronic intractable cardiac failure complicated by embolic phenomena.

Central and peripheral nervous system. The most common manifestations of altered brain function in the alcoholic are the symptoms of inebriation, followed in frequency by the withdrawal syndromes of tremor, confusion, hallucinations, delirium tremens, and convulsions. These are usually reversible functional changes. Much less common but frequently irreversible are the metabolic disorders associated with protracted steady drinking and, in most instances, nutritional deficiencies. These include Wernicke-Korsakoff syndrome, peripheral neuropathy, amblyopia (loss of vision), cerebellar degeneration, cerebral degeneration, central pontine myelinolysis, and progressive dementia with demyelination of the corpus callosum (Marchiafava-Bignami disease). Both clinical and animal studies on mnemonic brain function indicate an ethanol-induced impairment.[56] (Refer to a neurology text for details on each of these syndromes.)

Cancer. Primary liver cancer, a rare tumor, is seen in 5% to 10% of alcoholics with alcoholic cirrhosis.[57] This is believed to be caused by the cirrhotic process. In addition to the hepatomas associated with alcoholic cirrhosis, prospective and retrospective epidemiological studies indicate that chronic alcohol consumption by itself is a cancer hazard.[58] Numerous clinical studies of alcoholics have arrived at this conclusion. Heavy drinkers have an increased incidence of cancer of the mouth, pharynx, larynx, and esophagus.[58] Alcohol consumption may also be related to incidence of cancer of the pancreas, the cardia of the stomach, and the colon.[59] Such epidemiological evidence is most abundant in the case of cancers of the mouth and pharynx, and so a heavy drinker and heavy smoker has a 15 times greater risk of developing oral malignancy than a nondrinker and nonsmoker has. It appears that the cancer risk from ethanol is both time and dose related.[59]

Endocrine effects. The endocrine effects of alcohol vary depending on whether the alcohol intake is acute or chronic.[60] Moderate alcohol consumption has little effect on cortisol from the adrenal gland.[61] Alcohol blood levels in excess of 1 g/L, however, may produce an elevated plasma cortisol level. Occasionally chronic alcoholics will show clinical features of Cushing's syndrome and high cortisol levels.[62] Abstention causes the cortisol level to return to normal in 2 to 3 weeks.[60]

Some alcoholics have evidence of pituitary insufficiency. Low blood glucose normally produces a rise in cortisol. This response is decreased or absent in 25% of chronic alcoholics because the pituitary gland does not secrete enough adrenocorticotropic hormone to stimulate the adrenal gland.[60] Low levels of growth hormone and prolactin after low blood glucose stimulation are further evidence for pituitary insufficiency.[63] The low testosterone levels seen in alcoholics are now believed to be related to pituitary insufficiency.[60]

Hematopoietic effects. The effects of alcohol on the blood and bone marrow are the result of both a direct toxic effect and associated nutritional deficiencies[60] (see Chapters 37 and 39). Not only do alcoholics have low folate levels, but also vitamin B_{12} absorption is inhibited by alcohol. Each of these factors alone or in combination can lead to abnormally large red blood cells and megaloblastic anemia.[29,31]

Iron metabolism is affected by alcohol in several ways. Alcohol can produce chronic blood loss (ulcers, gastritis, variceal bleeding) leading to iron-deficiency anemia.[29] An increase in serum and tissue iron can also be seen with excess alcohol consumption and causes abnormal iron use within the bone marrow. Finally, alcohol excess can cause acute hemolytic anemia.

Inhibition of the bone marrow by alcohol can result in a low number of circulating white blood cells[64] and platelets.[65] Alcohol also can impair the function of white blood cells,[66] and alcoholic cirrhosis impairs platelet function,[67] which may lead to increased susceptibility to infection and bleeding. Vitamin K deficiency, seen in alcoholics, causes a prolonged prothrombin time because of the lack of vitamin K–dependent clotting factors normally produced in the liver. When liver disease is severe, inadequate clotting factors are produced even when vitamin K is present.

Immune system. Ethanol is known to affect the immune system. Increased circulating B-cell antibodies have been identified in most patients with alcoholic liver disease[18] (see discussion below). Specific antibodies against alcoholic hyalin have been identified in patients with alcoholic hepatitis,[68] which may explain the frequent elevation in IgA.[69] The primary changes have been observed in the cell-mediated immune system. Total numbers of T-cells are decreased[70]; their ability to synthesize DNA is impaired (lymphocyte transformation)[71]; their response to antigens and mitogens is suppressed[71]; and their cytotoxic properties are increased.[72] These are manifested clinically by a low lymphocyte count, anergy to skin tests,[4] altered response to vaccinations,[18,73] and increased susceptibility to infections.

These immunological alterations may be partly responsible for some of the liver cell injury and progression of the disease seen in patients with alcoholic hepatitis.[18,72]

PATHOLOGY: TRAUMA AND ALCOHOL ABUSE

Various studies have demonstrated that approximately 35% to 55% of trauma patients seen in emergency rooms have elevated blood alcohol levels.[74] Many of these patients also show evidence of drugs of abuse. Vehicular trauma is the most frequent cause of trauma. Half of all vehicular accidents, accounting for 25,000 deaths and over a half a million injuries a year, are associated with a car driver that has a positive blood alcohol.[75] Overall, males are twice as likely

as females to be the victim of a drunk-driving death. In the 18 to 45 year age group, however, the male to female ratio is 3 to 1.[76] These numbers certainly describe a pathological state that is endemic in American society.

The large number of trauma patients that are seen in the country's emergency rooms presents a challenge to laboratories. A patient presenting with trauma and altered mental status requires laboratory studies to determine the immediate cause of the altered mental status. Trauma, metabolic causes, infectious agents, and abuse of drugs must be ruled out as possible causes of the altered mental state. The screening test panel for abused drugs must include the measurement of blood alcohol. Treatment of the patient greatly depends on the outcome of these laboratory studies, which must be performed within a reasonably short time.

CHANGE OF ANALYTE IN DISEASE (Table 34-4)
Enzymes

Increases in serum enzyme levels in liver disease may result from leakage of enzymes into the serum because of damaged cell membranes (AST, ALT, and lactate dehydrogenase) or from increased enzyme production (alkaline phosphatase and GGT).

Aspartate aminotransferase and alanine aminotransferase. Serum AST and ALT are two serum enzymes that are found in the liver and readily leak from the cells during necrosis and cell injury. Although alcoholic liver injury is characterized by liver cell necrosis and inflammation, the increase in these enzymes is minimum to moderate, with the rise in AST almost always exceeding that observed in ALT. Abnormalities in AST are common and occur early, but the magnitude of the change may not parallel the clinical severity of the liver injury.[18] Explanations for this minimum response to injury are inadequate. Because pyridoxal phosphate is required for transamination reactions, deficiency in pyridoxine may in some alcoholics contribute to the diminished response (see p. 518, methods).

Alkaline phosphatase. In alcoholic liver disease the increase in alkaline phosphatase activity tends to parallel the changes seen in bilirubin.

5′-Nucleotidase. 5′-Nucleotidase is not so sensitive to liver injury as alkaline phosphatase. It is measured along with alkaline phosphatase to determine whether a rise in the latter enzyme is the result of hepatobiliary disease or bone disease.

Gamma-glutamyltransferase. Increases in serum levels of GGT have been reported in alcoholics with minimum or no liver disease. This has been attributed to microsomal enzyme induction rather than liver injury (see p. 515).

Bilirubin

Although alcohol does not directly alter bilirubin metabolism, the liver injury produced by alcohol does. Jaundice, the clinical sign of elevated bilirubin, is seen in about 60% of patients with alcoholic hepatitis.[18] Bilirubin elevation,

Table 34-4 Prevalence of laboratory changes in alcoholic hepatitis

Laboratory test	Direction of analyte change	Incidence of abnormal results, % (ULN × X̄ of group)*		
		Group I	Group II	Group III
Hemoglobin	Decrease	74 (0.70)	85 (0.66)	93 (0.60)
Hematocrit	Decrease	76 (0.80)	83 (0.76)	95 (0.70)
MCV	Increase	73 (1.1)	83 (1.1)	90 (1.1)
	Decrease	2	8	0
WBC	Increase	13	7 (1.1)	54 (1.24)
	Decrease	11 (0.8)	9	8
AST (SGOT)	Increase	79 (2.1)	98 (3.1)	91 (2.5)
ALT (SGPT)	Increase	62 (1.9)	73 (1.9)	56 (1.9)
Total bilirubin	Increase	53 (1.6)	100 (13.5)	100 (18.7)
Alkaline phosphatase	Increase	67 (1.4)	100 (2.3)	88 (1.9)
Prothrombin time	Increase	65	90	100
BUN	Increase	3	17 (0.7)	36 (1.4)
	Decrease	3 (0.5)	0	0
Creatinine	Increase	2 (0.60)	17 (0.76)	29 (1.35)
	Decrease			
Albumin	Decrease	36 (0.74)	90 (0.54)	96 (0.48)
Cholylglycine	Increase	85 (8.2)	100 (25.2)	100 (15.1)
Immunoglobulins				
IgG	Increase	49 (1.1)	72 (1.3)	83 (1.6)
IgA	Increase	84 (1.7)	98 (2.6)	93 (2.8)
IgM	Decrease	17 (0.66)	26 (0.73)	43 (0.95)

From Leevy CM, Cardi L, Frank O, et al: *Am J Clin Nutr* 17:259-271, 1965.
*Data are expressed as the change in analyte, and the incidence of abnormal occurrence is expressed as the percentage of total and the magnitude of the change (times upper limit of normal [ULN] for mean); n = 89 in group I, 58 in group II, and 37 in group III.

along with a prolonged prothrombin time unresponsive to vitamin K, and depressed serum albumin correlate well with the severity of alcoholic hepatitis. In some cases of alcoholic hepatitis the bilirubin will rise along with the alkaline phosphatase level so that common bile duct obstruction is suspected.[22] Because the patient with alcoholic hepatitis does not tolerate surgery well, a diagnostic procedure such as endoscopic or percutaneous cholangiography should be done to confirm the diagnosis of extrahepatic obstruction before surgery.

Proteins

Prealbumin and albumin. Many tests used to evaluate liver disease measure alterations in biochemical functions of the liver. Because serum albumin and prealbumin are synthesized and secreted by the liver, their serum concentrations have been used as tests of liver function. Serum levels of prealbumin are depressed in PCM and in all forms of liver disease, including those associated with alcoholism. It is not uncommon to find values below 160 mg/L in severe PCM.[77] Prealbumin is considered to be a more sensitive and specific test for PCM than serum albumin.

Depressed serum albumin levels in alcoholics may indicate either PCM or liver disease. Of 111 patients with severe alcoholic hepatitis in the Veterans Administration Cooperative Study,[18] 18% had values below 20 g/L, whereas only 1% had values within the normal range. However, many patients with alcoholic liver disease have ascites with expanded extravascular pools. The low serum albumin in these persons may represent a shift of albumin from the intravascular to the expanded extravascular space.

Globulins. Serum gamma globulin levels change during liver disease in response to antigenic stimulation, reflecting the immune changes associated with alcoholic liver disease. Of the three types of gamma globulins (IgG, IgA, and IgM), IgA is most frequently increased in alcoholic liver disease, being elevated in 90% of cases, with a mean increase of 118%.[18] IgM increases the least and is elevated in 25% of cases. IgG is intermediate at 64% with a mean increase of 25%.

Lipids

Triglycerides and cholesterol. Increases in serum triglyceride and cholesterol are frequently observed and are discussed on p. 654.

Bile acids. Because the liver is responsible for almost all phases of bile acid metabolism, bile acids are very sensitive indicators of even minimum liver injury. In alcoholic liver disease, serum bile acids, especially cholic acid conjugates, have been correlated with biopsy findings.[78] Fatty liver alone was not associated with elevated levels, whereas alcoholic hepatitis and cirrhosis were accompanied by significant increases in serum levels. In the Veterans Administration Cooperative Study[18] on alcoholic hepatitis, cholylglycine was abnormal more often than any other parameter of liver injury.

Carbohydrates

Hyperglycemia. Hepatocellular damage, regardless of its cause, is an important cause of glucose intolerance and may play a major role in the hyperglycemia found in some alcoholics.[79] However, alcohol is rarely responsible for producing gross glucose intolerance or frank diabetes.[52] Alcohol-induced elevation in cortisol, especially when sufficient to produce pseudo–Cushing's syndrome, is another contributing factor in alcoholic hyperglycemia.[80]

Hypoglycemia. Although hypoglycemia may occur in severe liver disease with fulminant hepatic failure, it may also occur in association with alcohol use and a relatively normal liver.[60] Hypoglycemia may be the cause of sudden death among alcoholics, with an 11% mortality in adults and a 25% mortality in children.[81] This form of hypoglycemia (alcohol-induced fasting hypoglycemia) occurs in chronically malnourished alcoholics or when moderate to large amounts of alcohol are consumed after a 6- to 36-hour fast.[52] The patients are stuporous or comatose, smell of alcohol, and are often hypothermic. The diagnosis is made on the clinical findings of hypoglycemia and elevated blood alcohol; lactic acidosis is not uncommon.[60] Plasma insulin levels are low and glucagon levels high.[82] Although growth hormone and cortisol levels are elevated, the elevation is still less than that expected for the severity of the hypoglycemia.[82] The mechanism for the hypoglycemia is probably multifactorial, with alcohol inhibition of gluconeogenesis playing a major role.[83] Other contributing factors include a relatively mild adrenocortical insufficiency and a defect in growth hormone secretion.[60]

Another form of hypoglycemia occurs when alcohol is consumed with carbohydrates (alcohol-induced reactive hypoglycemia).[52] Alcohol has the capacity to potentiate the insulin-stimulating properties of glucose.[84] Therefore alcohol consumed at a meal may potentiate insulin secretion and lead to nocturnal hypoglycemia. Thus large amounts of sweetened coffee used to sober up an alcoholic could cause a rapid and severe reactive hypoglycemia that could contribute to an accident during the drive home.

Alcoholic ketoacidosis. Ketoacidosis is an uncommon condition occurring in nondiabetic alcoholics.[60] Patients often have abdominal pain, vomiting, and a history of no recent food intake. The patients are acidotic but conscious, with high levels of serum ketones, salt and water depletion, and normal glucose levels.[85] The mechanism for alcoholic ketosis is uncertain.[60] Serum insulin concentrations are low with high cortisol levels and mild elevations of growth hormone.

TEST OF LIVER FUNCTION
Indocyanine green dye excretion

Indocyanine green is free of side effects and is rapidly excreted into the bile without being conjugated by the liver. This dye has the advantage of being monitored accurately and continuously with a dichromatic ear densitometer; thus one can eliminate venous blood sampling.[86] Disappearance of the dye is believed to be related to hepatic blood flow. Although the test is not used routinely, it is probably the current dye excretion test of choice.

METHODS OF ANALYSIS
Alcohol
K. MICHAEL PARKER

Principles of analysis and current usage Alcohol is a primary depressant of the central nervous system. If alcohol is taken in sufficient quantity, death can result from irreversible depression of respiration. Because of the serious consequences of ethanol intoxication, rapid analysis is required for initiation of appropriate therapy. Also, because of medicolegal ramifications of ethanol intoxication, analysis must be accurate.[87] In addition to ethanol, other alcohols, notably *methanol, isopropanol,* and *ethylene glycol,* may also be present. Techniques to quantitate these other alcohols have also been developed.

The measurement of ethanol by the clinical laboratory may be performed by chemical means, enzymatic assays, and chromatographic assays. In addition to these direct techniques for measurement of ethanol, indirect semiquantitative estimates of ethanol may be performed by use of freezing-point depression osmometry.

Early chemical methods for determination of ethanol were often based on the oxidation of ethanol by potassium dichromate, or other oxidizing agents, in a strongly acid medium (Table 34-5, method 1). Reduction of the dichromate results in a color change that can be measured to monitor the reaction. Most of the chemical methods are considered obsolete because of their poor specificity, tediousness, and lack of adaptation to automation.[87] It is important to remember that the chemical assays are not specific for ethanol but detect volatile reducing agents.

A variation of the chemical method was that of Widmark.[89] His method was based on the simultaneous distillation and quantitative oxidation of ethanol by dichromate. A microdiffusion method based on essentially the same principle has more recently been developed for commercial use.[90] In this procedure, chromic acid reagent, contained within a sheet of glass fiber paper, is reduced to blue-colored chromic oxide by ethanol. By heating of the sample at 80° to 120° C, the ethanol is released into the glass fiber sheet that is placed directly above the sample.

Enzymatic methods have become the most common means for measurement of ethanol. Alcohol dehydrogenase (ADH), the enzyme employed in these assays, is specific for ethanol and does not react with methanol or acetone. The enzyme does, however, show slight cross reactivity with propanol (6% for 2-propanol and 1% for 1-propanol). Although the high specificity of ADH for ethanol ensures no interference from methanol and little interference from isopropanol, enzymatic assays can be the source of misleading results in cases where intoxication results from the ingestion of isopropanol. Comparison of results from enzymatic assays with those from less specific assays (chemical or osmometric) can help in identifying the presence of these or other alcohols.

Table 34-5   Methods for alcohol analysis

Method	Type of analysis	Principle	Usage	Comments
1. Distillation-oxidation	Colorimetric	Alcohol diffuses into gas phase and reacts with oxidizing agent, changing its color: $2K_2Cr_2O_7 + 10H_2SO_4 + 3C_2H_5OH \rightarrow$ (yellow-orange) $2Cr_2(SO_4)_4 + 2K_2SO_4 + 3CH_3COOH +$ (blue-green) $11H_2O + 4H^+$	Rarely used	Nonspecific; gives reaction with all volatiles; all body fluids; tissue
2. Enzymatic	a. Spectro-photometric	$NAD^+ + Alcohol \xrightarrow{\text{Alcohol dehydrogenase}}$ $NADH + H^+ + Acetaldehyde$	Stat. or routine; serum; frequently used	Specific for ethanol; other alcohols not readily measured
	b. Fluorometric	Above reaction (2a) plus $NADH \rightarrow$ $NAD^+ +$ Reduced monotetrazolium dye (fluorescein fluorescence decreased)	Stat. or routine; serum; frequently used	Specific for ethanol; other alcohols not readily measured
3. Gas chromatography	Flame ionization	Alcohol separates on chromatographic column	Stat. or routine; all body fluids; frequently used	Specific for all alcohols
4. Osmometry	Freezing point depression	Alcohol in high concentration increases serum osmolality; difference between calculated and measured value is proportional to alcohol levels	Stat.; serum	Nonspecific; other volatile substances detected

The enzymatic ethanol assay (Table 34-5, method 2a) is based on the oxidation of alcohol to acetaldehyde with concomitant reduction of NAD^+ to NADH. The NADH that is produced may be measured directly at 340 nm, or may be coupled to an alternative, that is, indicator, reaction. One such variation (Abbott) that has been developed, termed *radiative energy attenuation*, measures the degree of inhibition of the fluorescence of fluorescein dye resulting from the production of a colored product (Table 34-5, method 2b).[91] In this assay, the initial reaction of ADH with ethanol is coupled with a second reaction between NADH and the tetrazolium salt, iodonitrotetrazolium (INT). This additional reaction, catalyzed by diaphorase, results in the reoxidation of NADH to NAD along with the generation of a colored formazon-INT. This product has an absorbance peak at 492 nm, which overlaps the excitation and emission spectral profile of fluorescein included in the reaction mixture. The decrease in fluorescence intensity is inversely related to ethanol concentrations present in the sample.

There is good agreement between enzymatic methods and chromatographic methods.[92] However, some enzymatic methods can give falsely increased ethanol concentrations with samples from patients with increased levels of serum lactic acid and lactate dehydrogenase.[93] Although the enzymatic methods are not absolutely specific for ethanol, these methods usually meet the requirements for accuracy, precision, and reliability.

Gas chromatography (GC; Table 34-5, method 3) is considered to be the reference method.[88] Chromatography is not as popular as enzymatic methods because of the need for specific expertise for performing the analysis and the concern that the purchase and maintenance of sophisticated instrumentation dedicated only to a single class of analytes is not cost effective. However, gas chromatography offers the distinct advantage for simultaneous detection of other alcohols and volatiles, such as methanol and isopropanol.

An important consideration when using GC is the type of injection method, direct or head-space analysis, which is to be used. The direct injection of blood or serum usually requires that the sample be diluted with an aqueous solution containing the internal standard, as one injects small volumes (0.5 µL), and thoroughly washes the syringe after each injection. Using these precautions substantially increases the life of the chromatographic column. Head-space procedures inject into the GC system an air sample removed from a confined space above blood in a closed container. Head-space analysis prevents contamination of the column and injector. Increased sensitivity of head-space analysis can be gained by the addition of a salt, such as sodium chloride, to the specimen. The addition of salt results in an increase in the concentration of the volatile substance in the vapor phase.

The presence of alcohol in serum leads to an increase in the osmolality of the serum when the osmolality is measured by use of the freezing point depression technique (Table 34-5, method 4). Osmometers that use the property of vapor pressure depression to measure osmolality cannot be used for the purpose of estimating alcohol concentrations because alcohols are volatile and contribute significantly to the vapor pressure above a solution. This phenomenon will result in a falsely low measurement for serum osmolality.

In the presence of alcohol, there will be an increased gap between the measured (by freezing point depression) and the calculated osmolality values (see Chapter 14 for a discussion of calculated osmolality). This osmolal gap correlates reasonably well with blood alcohol concentrations. However, an overestimation of alcohol concentrations of up to 30% has been reported.[94] This discrepancy has been attributed to the nonideal osmotic behavior of ethanol, which can alter the degree of dissociation of solutes within the specimen. Regardless of these shortcomings, osmolal gap evaluations can be helpful in the diagnosis of acutely intoxicated patients in emergency situations. In addition, the osmolal gap is nonselective with respect to the type of alcohol detected. Thus the osmolal gap can help reveal the presence of alcohols other than ethanol if the results of enzymatic ethanol measurements are available.

Specimen Serum, plasma, or urine may be used if ethanol is to be measured by use of an enzymatic procedure. Anticoagulants do not interfere with the enzymatic or gas chromatographic ethanol methods. When gas chromatography is used, any tissue or body fluid may be used as specimen. Regardless of what specimen is used, the samples must be well stoppered and preferably refrigerated to prevent loss of ethanol or other alcohols present. Specimens of whole blood that have been sealed did not show any loss of ethanol when stored at 0° to 3° C or at room temperature (22° to 29° C) for up to 14 days.[95]

Reference interval Ethanol as well as other volatiles methanol and n-propanol are normally not present in blood or tissues. A blood ethanol concentration of 3000 µg/mL (65.1 mmol/L) or greater may be associated with coma, whereas values greater than 4000 µg/mL (86.8 mmol/L) have been reported to be fatal. However, because alcohol metabolism can vary substantially between individuals, symptoms associated with ethanol consumption can present differently between persons.

REFERENCES

1. US Bureau of the Census: Statistical abstract of the United States, 1975, Washington, D.C., 1975, US Government Printing Office.
2. Criteria Committee, National Council on Alcoholism: Criteria for the diagnosis of alcoholism, *Ann Intern Med* 77:249-258, 1972.
3. Bailey RJ, Krasner N, Feddleston ALW, et al: Histocompatibility antigens, autoantibodies, and immunoglobulins in alcoholic liver disease, *Br Med J* 2:727-729, 1976.
4. Mendenhall CL, Anderson S, Weesner RE, et al: Protein-calorie malnutrition associated with alcoholic hepatitis, *Am J Med* 76:221-222, 1984.
5. Hall P, editor: *Alcoholic liver disease: pathobiology, epidemiology, and clinical aspects,* New York, 1985, Wiley & Sons.
6. Rydberg U, Skerfuing S: Toxicity of ethanol: a tentative risk evaluation. In Gross EM, editor: *Alcohol intoxication and withdrawal,* New York, 1977, Plenum Publishing Corp.
7. AMA Council on Scientific Affairs: Alcohol and the driver, *JAMA* 255: 522-527, 1986.
8. Zador PL: *Alcohol-related relative risk of fatal driver injuries in relation to driver age and sex,* Arlington, Va., 1989, Insurance Institute for Highway Safety.
9. Kristensson H, Trell E, Eriksson S, et al: Serum-γ-glutamyl-transferase in alcoholism, *Lancet* 1:609, 1977.
10. Lieber CS: Pathogenesis and early diagnosis of alcoholic liver injury, *N Engl J Med* 298:888-893, 1978.
11. Mendenhall CL, Weesner RE: Alcohols and glycols. In Hanenson IB, editor: *Quick reference to clinical toxicology,* Philadelphia, 1980, JB Lippincott Co.
12. Lieber CS, DeCarli LM: Effect of drug administration on the activity of the hepatic microsomal ethanol oxidizing system, *Life Sci* 9:267-276, 1970.
13. Lieber CS, DeCarli LM: The role of the hepatic microsomal ethanol oxidizing system (MEOS) for ethanol metabolism in vivo, *J Pharmacol Exp Ther* 181:279-287, 1972.
14. Freytmans E, Leighton F: Effects of pyrazole and 3-amino-1,2,4-triazole on methanol and ethanol metabolism by the rat, *Biochem Pharmacol* 22:349-360, 1973.
15. Suter PM, Schutz Y, Jequier E. The effect of ethanol on fat storage in healthy subjects, *N Engl J Med* 326:983-987, 1992.
16. Losowsky MS, Jones DP, Davidson CS, et al: Studies of alcoholic hyperlipemia and its mechanism, *Am J Med* 35:794-803, 1963.
17. Baraona E, Leo M, Borowsky SA, et al: Alcoholic hepatomegaly: accumulation of protein in the liver, *Science* 190:794-795, 1975.
18. Mendenhall CL, and the Cooperative Study Group on Alcoholic Hepatitis: Pathogenesis, diagnosis, and treatment of alcoholic hepatitis, *Clin Gastroenterol* 10:417-441, 1981.
19. Lieber CS, Jones DP, Losowsky MS, et al: Interrelation of uric acid and ethanol metabolism in man, *J Clin Invest* 41:1863-1970, 1962.
20. Olin JS, Devenyi P, Weldon KL: Uric acid in alcoholics, *Q J Study Alcohol* 34:1202-1207, 1973.
21. Newcombe DS: Ethanol metabolism and uric acid, *Metabolism* 21:1193-1203, 1972.
22. Pirola RC, Lieber CS: The energy cost of the metabolism in drugs, including ethanol, *Pharmacology* 7:185-196, 1972.
23. Blackburn GL, Bristrian BR, Maini BS, et al: Nutritional and metabolic assessment of the hospitalized patient, *J Parenter Ent Nutr* 1:11-22, 1977.
24. Leevy CM, Thompson A, Baker H: Vitamins and liver injury, *Am J Clin Nutr* 23:493-498, 1970.
25. Frank O, Baker H, Leevy CM: Vitamin binding capacity of experimentally injured liver, *Nature* 203:302-303, 1964.
26. Leevy, CM, ten Hove W, Frank O, et al: Folic acid deficiencies and hepatic DNA synthesis, *Proc Soc Exp Biol Med* 117:746-748, 1964.
27. Thomson AD, Majumdor SK: The influence of ethanol on intestinal absorption and utilization of nutrients, *Clin Gastroenterol* 10:263-293, 1981.
28. Leevy CML: *Liver regeneration in man,* Springfield, Ill., 1973, Charles C. Thomas.
28a. Blass JP, Gibson GE: Abnormality of a thiamine-requiring enzyme in patients with Wernicke-Korsakoff syndrome, *N Engl J Med* 297:1367-1370, 1977.
29. McIntyre N, Morgan MY: Nutritional aspects of liver disease. In Wright R, Alberti KGMM, Karran S, et al, editors: *Liver and biliary disease,* Philadelphia, 1979, Saunders.
30. Cohen JA, Kaplan MM: The SGOT/SGPT ratio: an indicator of alcoholic liver disease, *Dig Dis Sci* 24:835-838, 1979.
31. Herbert V, Zalusky R, Davidson CS: Correlation of folate deficiency with alcoholism and associated macrocytosis, anemia, and liver disease, *Ann Intern Med* 58:977-988, 1963.
32. Baker H, Frank O, Zetterman R, et al: Inability of chronic alcoholics with liver disease to use food as a source of folates, thiamin and vitamin B_6, *Am J Clin Nutr* 28:1377-1380, 1975.
33. Sullivan LW, Herbert V: Suppression of hematopoiesis by ethanol, *J Clin Invest* 43:2048-2062, 1964.
34. Beattie AD, Sherlock S: Ascorbic acid deficiency in liver disease, *Gut* 17:571-575, 1976.
35. Flink EB: Mineral metabolism in alcoholism. In Kissin F, Begleiter H, editors: *The biology of alcoholism,* vol 1, *Biochemistry,* New York, 1971, Plenum Publishing.
36. Celada A, Rudolph H, Donath A: Effect of experimental chronic alcohol ingestion and folic acid deficiencies on iron absorption, *Blood* 54:906-915, 1979.
37. Powell LW: The role of alcoholism in hepatic iron storage disease, *Ann NY Acad Sci* 252:124-134, 1979.
38. Smith JC, McDaniel EG, Fan FF, et al: Zinc: a trace element essential in vitamin A metabolism, *Science* 181:954-955, 1973.
39. Wolfe SM, Victor M: The relationship of hypomagnesemia to alcohol withdrawal seizures and delirium tremens, *Ann NY Acad Sci* 162:973-984, 1969.
40. Kalbfleisch JM, Lindeman RD, Ginn HE, et al: Effects of ethanol administration on urinary excretion of magnesium and other electrolytes in alcoholic and normal subjects, *J Clin Invest* 42:1471-1475, 1963.
41. Jung RT, Davie M, Chalmers JO, et al: Abnormal vitamin D metabolism in cirrhosis, *Gut* 19:290-293, 1978.
42. Knochel JP: The pathophysiology and clinical characteristics of severe hypophosphatemia, *Arch Intern Med* 137:203-220, 1977.
43. Mathinos PR: *Determination of the proximal teratogen of the fetal alcohol syndrome in CD/Mice,* doctoral dissertation, Cincinnati, 1982, University of Cincinnati.
44. Thomson AD, Bird GL, Saunders JB: Alcoholic liver disease, *Gut,* suppl: S97-103, Sept 1991.
45. Popper H: The problem of hepatitis, *Am J Gastroenterol* 55:335-346, 1971.
46. Durbec JP, Sarles H: Multicenter survey of the etiology of pan-

creatic diseases: the relationship between the relative risk of developing chronic pancreatitis and alcohol, protein, and lipid consumption, *Digestion* 18:337-350, 1970.

47. Camerson JL, Zuidema GD, Margolis S: A pathogenesis for alcoholic pancreatitis, *Surgery* 77:754-763, 1975.

48. Banks PA, editor: *Pancreatitis,* ed 1, New York, 1979, Plenum Publishing.

49. Sarles H: Chronic calcifying pancreatitis—chronic alcoholic pancreatitis, *Gastroenterology* 66:604-616, 1974.

50. Amman RW, Largiades F, Akovbiantz A: Pain relief by surgery in chronic pancreatitis? Relationship between pain relief, pancreatic dysfunction, and alcohol withdrawal, *Scand J Gastroenterol* 14:209-215, 1979.

51. DiMagno EP, Go VLW, Summerskill WHJ: Relationship between pancreatic enzyme outputs and malabsorption in severe pancreatic insufficiency, *N Engl J Med* 288:813-815, 1973.

52. Marks V: Alcohol and carbohydrate metabolism, *Clin Endocrinol Metab* 7:333-349, 1978.

53. Abel EL, Sokol RJ: Incidence of fetal alcohol syndrome and economic impact of FAS-related abnormalities, *Drug and Alcohol Dependence* 19:51-70, 1987.

54. Schnek EA, Cohen J: The heart in chronic alcoholism: clinical and pathologic findings, *Pathol Microbiol* 35:96-104, 1970.

55. Fisher VJ, Kavaler F: The action of ethanol upon the contractility of normal ventricular myocardium. In Rothschild MA, Oratz M, Schreiber SS, editors: *Alcohol and abnormal protein biosynthesis,* Elmsford, N.Y., 1975, Pergamon Press.

56. Tamarin JS, Weiner S, Poppen R, et al: Alcohol and memory, *Am J Psychol* 127:1659-1667, 1971.

57. Sherlock S: Alcohol and the liver: treatment, early recognition. In Sherlock S, editor: *Diseases of the liver and biliary system,* ed 6, London, 1981, Blackwell Scientific Publications.

58. Keller AZ, Terris M: The association of alcohol and tobacco with cancer of the mouth and pharynx, *Am J Public Health* 55:1578-1585, 1965.

59. Williams RR, Horm JW: Association of cancer sites with tobacco and alcohol consumption and socioeconomic status of patients: interview study from the Third National Cancer Survey, *J Natl Cancer Inst* 58:525-547, 1977.

60. Johnston DG, Alberti KGMM: The liver and the endocrine system. In Wright R, Alberti KGMM, Karran S, et al, editors: *Liver and biliary disease,* Philadelphia, 1979, Saunders.

61. Jenkins JS, Connolly J: Adrenocortical response to ethanol in man, *Br Med J* 2:804-805, 1968.

62. Merry J, Marks V: Hypothalamic-pituitary-adrenal function in chronic alcoholics. In Cross MM, editor: *Alcohol intoxication and withdrawal: experimental studies,* Advances in Experimental Medicine and Biology, New York, 1973, Plenum Publishing.

63. Chalmers RJ, Bennie EH, Johnson RH, et al: Growth hormone, prolactin and corticosteroid responses to insulin hypoglycaemia in alcoholics, *Br Med J* 2:745-748, 1978.

64. Liu YK: Leukopenia in alcoholics, *Am J Med* 54:605-610, 1973.

65. Cowan DH, Hines JD: Thrombocytopaenia of severe alcoholism, *Ann Intern Med* 74:37-43, 1971.

66. McFarland W, Leibre EP: Abnormal leukocyte response in alcoholism, *Ann Intern Med* 59:865-877, 1963.

67. Thomas DP, Ream VJ, Stuart RK: Platelet aggregation in patients with Laënnec's cirrhosis of the liver, *N Engl J Med* 276:1344-1348, 1967.

68. Chen T, Kanagasundaram N, Kakumu S, et al: Serum autoantibodies to alcoholic hyalin in alcoholic hepatitis [abstract], *Gastroenterology* A13:813, 1975.

69. Zinneman HH: Autoimmune phenomena in alcoholic cirrhosis, *Am J Dig Dis* 20:337-345, 1970.

70. Bernstein IM, Webster KH, Williams RC Jr, et al: Reduction in circulating T lymphocytes in alcoholic liver disease, *Lancet* 2:488-490, 1974.

71. Hsu CCS, Leevy CM: Inhibition of PHA-stimulated lymphocyte transformation by plasma from patients with advanced alcoholic cirrhosis, *Clin Exp Immunol* 8:749-760, 1971.

72. Kakumu S, Leevy CM: Lymphocyte cytotoxicity in alcoholic hepatitis, *Gastroenterology* 72:524-526, 1977.

73. Smith WI Jr, Van Thiel DH, Whiteside T, et al: Altered immunity in male patients with alcoholic liver disease: evidence for defective immune regulation, *Alcohol Clin Exp Res* 4:199-206, 1980.

74. Sloan EP et al: Toxicology screening in urban trauma patients: drug prevalence and its relationship to trauma severity and management, *J Trauma* 29:1647-1652, 1989.

75. Fell JC, Nash CE: The nature of the alcohol problem in the US fatal crashes, *Health Educ Q* 16:335-343, 1989.

76. National Highway Traffic Safety Administration: *Fatal traffic crashes in 1987,* Washington, D.C., 1988, NHTSA.

77. Kaplan LA, editor: *Standards of laboratory practice: assessment of nutrition of hospitalized patients,* Cincinnati, 1994, National Academy of Clinical Biochemistry.

78. Milstein HJ, Bloomer JR, Klatskin G: Serum bile acids in alcoholic liver disease, *Am J Dig Dis* 21:281-295, 1976.

79. Lundquist GAR: Glucose tolerance in alcoholism, *Br J Addict* 61:51-55, 1965.

80. Rees LH, Besser GM, Joffcoate WJ, et al: Alcohol-induced pseudo–Cushing's syndrome, *Lancet* 1:726-728, 1977.

81. Madison LL, Lochner A, Wulff J: Ethanol induced hypoglycemia. II. Mechanism of suppression of hepatic gluconeogenesis, *Diabetes* 16:252-258, 1967.

82. Joffe BI, Seftel HC, Van As M: Hormonal responses in ethanol-induced hypoglycaemia, *J Stud Alcohol* 36:550-554, 1975.

83. Arky RA, Freinkel N: Alcohol hypoglycemia. V. Alcohol infusion to test gluconeogenesis in starvation, with specific reference to obesity, *N Engl J Med* 274:426-433, 1966.

84. O'Keefe SJ, Marks V: Lunchtime gin and tonic, a cause of reactive hypoglycaemia, *Lancet* 1:1286-1288, 1977.

85. Cooperman MT, Davidoff F, Spark R, et al: Clinical studies of alcoholic ketoacidosis, *Diabetes* 23:433-439, 1974.

86. Leevy CM, Smith F, Longueville J, et al: Indocyanine green clearance as a test for hepatic function: evaluation by dichromatic ear densitometry, *JAMA* 200:236-240, 1967.

87. Caplan YH: Blood, urine, and other fluid and tissue specimens for alcohol analysis. In Garriott JC, editor: *Medicolegal aspects of alcohol determination in biological specimens,* Littleton, Mass., 1988, PSG (Mosby, St. Louis), pp 74-75.

88. Tagliaro F, Lubli G, Ghielmi S, et al: Chromatographic methods for blood and alcohol determination, *J Chromatogr* 580:161-190, 1992.

89. Widmark EMP: Modification of the Niclocex method for estimating ethyl alcohol, *Skand Arch Physiol* 35:125-130, 1916.

90. Bachand SS, Gaor MJ, Martel PA, O'Donnell CM: Alcohol detection by microdiffusion [Letter], *Clin Chem* 35:1269, 1989.

91. Yost DA, Boehnlein L, Shaffer M: A novel assay to determine ethanol in whole blood on the Abbott TDX, *Clin Chem* 30:1029A, 1984.

92. Jortani SA, Poklis A: Emit® ETS® plus ethyl alcohol assay for the determination of ethanol in human serum and urine, *J Anal Toxicol* 16:368-371, 1992.

93. Badcock NR, O'Reilly DA: False-positive EMIT®-st™ ethanol screen with post-mortem infant plasma, *Clin Chem* 38:434, 1992.

94. Bhagat CI, Beilby JP, Garcia-Webb P, Dusci LJ: Errors in estimating ethanol concentration in plasma by using the "osmolal gap," *Clin Chem* 31:647-648, 1985.

95. Winek CL, Paul LJ: Effect of short-term storage conditions on alcohol concentrations in blood from living human subjects, *Clin Chem* 29:1959-1960, 1983.

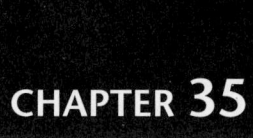

CHAPTER 35

Iron, porphyrin, and bilirubin metabolism

William E. Schreiber

OBJECTIVES

- List the physiological functions of iron and describe its absorption from the gut and its transport in the body.

- Describe the pathological conditions leading to iron deficiency and overload and describe changes in the following analytes in iron-deficiency anemia, anemia of chronic disease, thalassemia, hemochromatosis, and lead poisoning: ferritin, serum iron, iron-binding capacity, and free erythrocyte protoporphyrin.

- Define porphyria and distinguish between primary and secondary porphyrias.

- List porphyrin analytes that will be elevated in each of the primary and secondary porphyrias.

- Outline the formation and catabolism of bilirubin.

KEY TERMS

ampulla of Vater The junction of the common bile duct and pancreatic duct proximal to their opening into the duodenum.

anemia A reduction in the quantity of hemoglobin or number of red cells in blood.

bile The yellow-green fluid secreted by the liver and poured into the duodenum through the bile ducts.

bile canaliculi The fine tubular canals running between liver cells into which bile is discharged.

chelate A chemical compound in which a metallic ion is firmly bound to a chelating molecule.

cholestasis The stoppage of the flow of bile.

cirrhosis A liver disease characterized by the loss of the normal microscopic architecture, with fibrosis and nodular regeneration.

erythropoiesis The production of erythrocytes.

hemolytic anemia Anemia caused by shortened survival of mature red blood cells.

hypochromic Referring to erythrocytes that are paler than normal because of a decrease in hemoglobin content.

mean corpuscular hemoglobin (MCH) The average amount of hemoglobin per red blood cell.

mean corpuscular hemoglobin concentration (MCHC) The average concentration of hemoglobin per red blood cell.

mean corpuscular volume (MCV) The average red blood cell volume.

megaloblastic anemia Anemia characterized by large red cell precursors in the bone marrow.

microcytic Referring to erythrocytes that are smaller than reference interval.

parenchyma The functional tissue of an organ (excluding the fibrous framework).

pernicious anemia A megaloblastic anemia caused by failure to absorb vitamin B_{12}.

phagocyte Any cell that ingests microorganisms, other cells, or foreign particles.

photoisomers Isomers produced on exposure to light.

photosensitivity Abnormal reactivity of the skin to sunlight.

porphyrinuria The presence of excess porphyrin in urine.

reticuloendothelial system A functional system composed of highly phagocytic cells with both endothelial and reticular attributes, located in blood vessels, lymph nodes, liver, spleen, bone marrow, and other tissues.

sideroblastic anemia A heterogenous group of anemias in which iron stores of the reticuloendothelial tissues are increased and bone marrow normoblasts contain iron deposits within mitochondria (ringed sideroblasts).

tachycardia Rapid heart rate.

thalassemia A heterogeneous group of hereditary hemolytic anemias that have a decreased rate of synthesis of one or more hemoglobin polypeptide chains.

Part I: Iron metabolism
FUNCTION

Iron is one of the most abundant elements on earth, yet only trace amounts are present in living cells. Most of the iron in humans is located within the porphyrin ring of heme, which is incorporated into proteins such as hemoglobin, myoglobin, catalase, peroxidases, and cytochromes. There are also iron-sulfur proteins, such as NADH dehydrogenase and succinate dehydrogenase, in which iron is present in clusters with inorganic sulfur. In all these systems, it is the ability of iron to interact reversibly with oxygen and to function in electron-transfer reactions that makes it biologically indispensable.

An average adult male has about 4 g of body iron. About 65% to 70% of the total is found in hemoglobin, and about 10% is located in myoglobin and other iron-containing enzymes and proteins. The remaining 20% to 25% consists of a storage pool of iron. By comparison, the average adult woman has only 2 to 3 g of iron in her body. This difference is attributable in part to the much smaller iron reserves in women. There is also less hemoglobin iron because women have a lower hemoglobin concentration in blood and a smaller vascular volume than men have. Iron distribution is summarized in Table 35-1.

METABOLISM

Daily requirements for iron vary depending on the person's age, sex, and physiological status. Although iron is not excreted in the conventional sense, there is a daily loss of about 1 mg through the normal shedding of skin epithelial cells and cells lining the gastrointestinal and urinary tracts. Small numbers of erythrocytes are lost in urine and feces as well. An iron intake of 1 mg per day is therefore sufficient for men and postmenopausal women. However, since the blood lost in each menstrual cycle drains 20 to 40 mg of iron, women in their reproductive years need 2 mg of iron per day. The diversion of iron to the growing fetus during pregnancy, blood loss during delivery, and subsequent breast feeding of the infant consume 900 mg of iron on average. This increases daily iron demands to 3 or 4 mg in pregnant and lactating women.

Absorption

A healthy North American diet contains between 10 and 30 mg of iron per day. Only 5% to 10% of this amount is absorbed, mainly in the duodenum and upper small intestine. Most dietary iron is in the ferric (Fe^{3+}) state. Fe^{3+} is soluble at the acidic pH of the stomach but becomes insoluble at the more alkaline pH of the duodenum. Gastric acid, which converts Fe^{3+} to the more absorbable Fe^{2+} form, and dietary components that form soluble iron chelates (such as ascorbic acid, sugars, and amino acids) increase the absorption of iron. Substances that form insoluble complexes with iron, such as phosphates (in eggs, cheese, and milk), oxalates and phytates (in vegetables), and tannates (in tea), decrease iron absorption. Heme iron, which comes mainly from meat and fish, is processed differently. After it is re-

Table 35-1 Iron distribution and function in a normal adult male

Compound	Function	Iron (mg)
Hemoglobin	O$_2$ transport, blood	2500
Myoglobin	O$_2$ storage, muscle	
Enzymes		
Catalase	H$_2$O$_2$ decomposition	
Peroxidases	Oxidation	300
Cytochromes	Electron transfer	
Iron-sulfur*	Electron transfer	
Transferrin*	Iron transport	4
Ferritin* and hemosiderin*	Iron storage	1000

*Nonheme iron compounds

leased from the surrounding polypeptide chain, heme is absorbed intact by the mucosal cell, where the porphyrin ring is split and iron is liberated. This process is more efficient than the absorption of nonheme iron and is not affected by dietary factors.

Since iron loss is a continuous and largely unregulated process, iron balance is controlled by changes in absorption. The intestinal cells take in considerably more iron than the 5% to 10% that eventually will enter the circulation. Once inside the intestinal cell, iron is transferred directly into plasma or is incorporated into ferritin for storage. Stored iron can subsequently be mobilized as necessary, but most of this iron is lost when the mucosal cells are shed. New cells take their place, and the cycle of iron buildup starts again.

The mechanisms that control iron transfer from the intestinal mucosa to the plasma are not well understood (Fig. 35-1). Their overall effect is to prevent the absorption of excess iron while maintaining an adequate supply for current needs. The major factors affecting iron absorption are

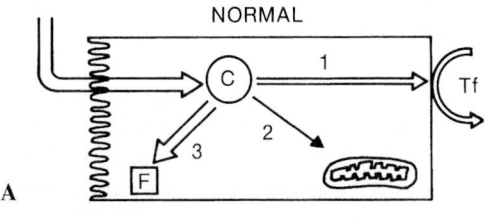

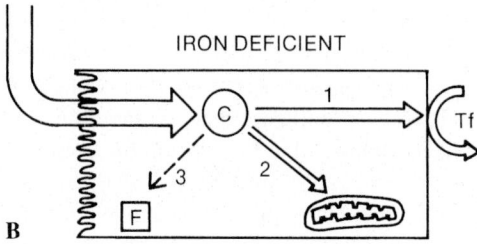

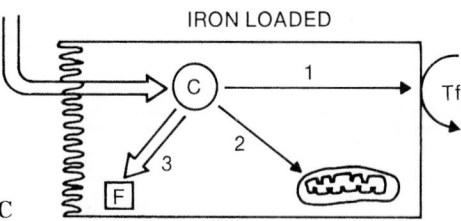

Fig. 35-1 Iron uptake and disposition within the small intestinal epithelial cell. **A,** Normal iron status. **B,** Iron deficiency: increased uptake and transfer of iron to plasma *(1)* and mitochondria *(2)*, with decreased transfer to ferritin *(3)*. **C,** Iron loaded: normal uptake with decreased transfer to plasma *(1)* and increased transfer to ferritin *(3)*. *C,* Intracellular iron carrier; *F,* ferritin; *Tf,* transferrin. (From Jacobs A: *Clin Haematol* 2:323, 1973.)

body iron stores and the rate of red blood cell production. When necessary, the efficiency of absorption can increase by threefold or more. Thus iron deficiency, pregnancy, and the accelerated erythropoiesis that occurs in anemia all stimulate increased iron absorption. On the other hand, absorption is reduced after the consumption of unusually large amounts of iron (such as, dietary supplementation or iron poisoning).

Red blood cell turnover

Absorbed iron represents only a fraction of the iron required for heme synthesis. Most of the needed iron, 20 to 25 mg/day, comes from the destruction of old erythrocytes by tissue macrophages, primarily in the spleen. Within these cells, heme oxygenase breaks open the porphyrin ring to release iron. Macrophages transfer most of the iron to plasma transferrin, which then carries it to the bone marrow for hemoglobin synthesis. In this manner, the reticuloendothelial system continuously recycles used iron from old red cells into new ones.

Macrophages also maintain a storage pool of iron. When red cell destruction exceeds the rate of production, iron accumulates within macrophages and the storage pool expands. When the balance shifts toward red cell production, macrophages release additional iron from their stores. Infection, inflammation, and malignancy interfere with the release of iron from macrophages and may cause a drop in red cell production despite the presence of adequate iron reserves.

Transport and cell uptake

Transferrin, a single-chain glycoprotein with a molecular weight of 79,500 daltons, is the transport protein for iron in blood. Each transferrin molecule has two binding sites for Fe^{3+}, and these sites are normally 20% to 50% saturated. The need for a specific carrier protein derives from the toxicity and insolubility of free iron; virtually all the 3 to 4 mg of plasma iron is protein bound. Iron transport is a dynamic process, and the half-life of an iron atom in plasma is between 60 and 120 minutes under normal circumstances.

Transferrin delivers iron to cells with specific surface receptors for this protein. After binding to the receptor, the transferrin receptor–transferrin complex is taken into the cell by endocytosis and formed into a vesicle. At the acidic pH of the vesicle, iron is released from transferrin. The receptor-apotransferrin complex is then returned to the cell surface, where both apotransferrin and the receptor become available for additional rounds of iron transport and uptake. Inside the cell, iron is utilized for heme synthesis within the mitochondria or is stored as ferritin.

Storage

Iron is stored in tissues in either of two forms, ferritin or hemosiderin. Ferritin consists of a multisubunit protein shell, known as *apoferritin*, surrounding a core of up to

4500 iron atoms. The iron in ferritin is deposited within its core as a ferric hydroxyphosphate complex. Ferritin is present in most cells and is a readily mobilized form of storage iron. It serves to package and isolate iron atoms from the intracellular environment, thus preventing any toxic action on cell constituents. *Hemosiderin* is an insoluble complex derived from ferritin that has lost some of its surface protein and become aggregated. It is present in granules 1 to 2 μm in diameter and is visible by light microscopy after being stained with Prussian blue. Hemosiderin has a higher iron concentration than ferritin has, but it releases iron more slowly.

About one third of the body's iron reserves is stored in the liver, one third in the bone marrow, and the remainder in the spleen and other tissues.

PATHOLOGICAL CONDITIONS
Iron deficiency

When iron intake falls below the amount required for red blood cell production, iron reserves become depleted and, in time, anemia develops. Iron deficiency is a common nutritional disorder in humans and is the most frequent cause of anemia. It is estimated that about 3% of adult men, 20% of women in their reproductive years, and 50% of pregnant women are deficient in iron.

The high prevalence of iron deficiency among women is the result of the blood loss that occurs during each menstrual cycle. Bleeding from the gastrointestinal tract is the usual cause of iron deficiency in men. The increased demand for iron in infants and young children, adolescents, and pregnant women may also lead to iron deficiency, especially if these individuals have diets that are low in iron. Impaired absorption of iron after a gastrectomy and in patients with chronic diarrhea or malabsorption also causes depletion of iron reserves.

Iron deficiency develops in stages, the first of which is depletion of storage iron in response to a prolonged negative iron balance. Once iron reserves have been exhausted, biochemical tests of iron metabolism become abnormal. Next, a drop in the hemoglobin concentration of blood is

seen, and in time the red blood cells become smaller and paler than normal. In fully developed iron-deficiency anemia, a complete blood count reveals a decrease in hemoglobin and in all the red blood cell indices: mean corpuscular volume (MCV), mean corpuscular hemoglobin (MCH), and mean corpuscular hemoglobin concentration (MCHC). Examination of a peripheral blood smear shows erythrocytes that are hypochromic and microcytic with an abnormal variation in size and shape. No stainable iron is visible in the bone marrow.

Laboratory tests of iron status can distinguish iron deficiency from other causes of hypochromic, microcytic anemia (Table 35-2). The concentration of serum iron decreases, while the total iron-binding capacity (TIBC), which measures the capacity of transferrin for iron, increases. The transferrin saturation, calculated as iron concentration divided by TIBC, is well below its healthy value. A decrease in serum ferritin, which is a reflection of body iron stores, is the single most reliable indicator of iron deficiency. Free erythrocyte protoporphyrin is increased, but this increase is not specific for iron deficiency, and measurement of this analyte is best used as a screening test.

Iron overload

Hemochromatosis. Hemochromatosis is a hereditary disorder characterized by a progressive increase in iron stores, leading to organ impairment and damage. Inheritance is autosomal recessive. Among populations of northern European descent, about 10% of people carry the gene and 0.3% are homozygotes. For reasons that are not clearly understood, only a fraction of homozygotes develop the full-blown disease. Men are affected five to 10 times more frequently than women are because of the protective effect of menstrual blood loss and pregnancy. Symptoms of the disease are not usually apparent before 40 years of age.

Patients with hemochromatosis absorb 4 mg of iron or more per day, even on a usual diet. The mechanism of enhanced iron absorption remains unknown. Under usual conditions, excess iron is processed by cells of the reticuloendothelial system. However, in individuals with hemochro-

Table 35-2   Laboratory measurements of iron status

Disease	Serum iron (μg/L)	TIBC (μg/L)	Transferrin saturation (%)	Serum ferritin (μg/L)	Free erythrocyte protoporphyrin (μg/L)	Tissue iron stores
Healthy	650-1750 (men) 500-1700 (women)	2500-4500	20-50 (men) 15-50 (women)	20-250 (men) 10-120 (women)	170-770	N
Storage iron depletion, no anemia	N	N	N	↓	N	↓
Iron-deficiency anemia	↓	↑	↓	↓	↑	↓
Anemia of chronic disease	↓	↓	↓	N or ↑	↑	N or ↑
Thalassemia trait	N	N	N	N	N	N
Sideroblastic anemia	↑	N	↑	↑	N or ↑	↑
Hemochromatosis	↑	↓	↑	↑	N	↑

N, Normal (within the reference interval); ↓, decreased; ↑, increased.

matosis, iron is deposited directly into parenchymal cells of the liver, pancreas, heart, and other organs. After accumulating for years, the excessive amounts of intracellular iron lead to tissue injury and ultimately organ failure. At this stage, the amount of storage iron may exceed 20 g.

Several systems are affected by hemochromatosis. The liver is nearly always enlarged and in time may become cirrhotic, predisposing patients to an unusually high risk of hepatocellular carcinoma. About two thirds of the patients develop diabetes mellitus; both a genetic predisposition and direct injury to the pancreas from iron overload appear to play a role in the development of diabetes. Most patients show an increase in skin pigmentation as a result of increased melanin production and iron deposition within the skin. Cardiac damage is expressed as congestive heart failure or arrhythmias. Testicular atrophy in men is caused by a drop in the production of gonadotropins by the pituitary gland, another site of iron deposition. Arthritis also occurs in up to half of the patients.

In hemochromatosis, the serum iron concentration increases and the total iron-binding capacity (TIBC) decreases, the opposite of the changes seen in iron deficiency. The transferrin saturation is much higher than the reference interval and is a particularly sensitive index of iron overload. Serum ferritin concentration is increased early in the course of disease, before signs and symptoms become apparent. The definitive test for hemochromatosis is the measurement and histochemical evaluation of hepatic iron in a liver biopsy specimen.

The gene for hemochromatosis has not yet been identified, but it is located on the short arm of chromosome 6 near the human leukocyte antigen (HLA) locus. In families with a known patient, it is often possible to identify other homozygotes and heterozygotes by testing family members for their HLA haplotypes and performing linkage analysis. Once the hemochromatosis gene is isolated and mutations causing the disease are defined, more specific and reliable tests based on DNA analysis will become available.

Acquired hemochromatosis. Iron overload can also be an acquired disorder. At first, excess iron is deposited in reticuloendothelial cells of the liver, spleen, and bone marrow, rather than directly in parenchymal cells. Tissues remain anatomically and functionally healthy. As the iron load increases, its distribution pattern changes, and iron is deposited in the parenchymal cells of the liver, pancreas, heart, and other organs. The clinical picture then resembles the hereditary form of hemochromatosis.

Acquired hemochromatosis may be a complication of anemias in which there is ineffective erythropoiesis, such as β-thalassemia major (see p. 727). Not only is iron absorption increased in this disorder, but patients are treated with multiple blood transfusions, further increasing their iron load. Alcoholics with chronic liver disease may also develop an increase in tissue iron stores, but those with mas-

sive iron overload probably have the genetic form of hemochromatosis. Use of medicinal iron supplements is rarely if ever, by itself, a cause of hemochromatosis.

CHANGE OF ANALYTE IN DISEASE

There are three iron compartments, accounting for 90% of the total body iron, that the clinical laboratory can measure. The largest of these pools is the iron contained in hemoglobin, which is measured as part of a complete blood count. Next largest is the tissue storage compartment, and the serum ferritin concentration is proportional to the size of this pool. Finally, circulating iron is evaluated by measurement of the serum concentrations of iron and its transport protein, transferrin. This combination of hematological and biochemical studies enables one to identify disorders of iron metabolism (see Table 35-2).

Hematological studies

A complete blood count gives the number of erythrocytes per liter, hemoglobin concentration, hematocrit, and red blood cell indices. When the hemoglobin concentration falls below about 130 g/L in men, below 120 g/L in women, and below 110 g/L in pregnant women, anemia is present. Iron deficiency causes a hypochromic, microcytic anemia, and so cell size (MCV), hemoglobin content (MCH), and the concentration of hemoglobin per cell (MCHC) are all reduced. The peripheral blood smear shows a wide variation in the size, shape, and hemoglobin content of erythrocytes, with a large proportion of cells that are smaller and paler than normal. This clear-cut picture will not be present at the early stages of iron depletion, when both hemoglobin concentration and red cell indices remain normal. Hypochromic, microcytic anemia is characteristic of the thalassemia trait, sideroblastic anemia, and anemia of chronic disease as well as iron deficiency. Red blood cell parameters thus define the presence or absence of anemia and its morphologic character, but other tests are required to identify the cause of anemia. Erythrocyte studies do not contribute to the diagnosis of hemochromatosis.

Serum iron (see p. 712, methods)

The circulating iron pool turns over 10 to 20 times per day; thus a typical iron atom spends no longer than 2 hours in plasma. Changes in serum iron concentration of 20% or greater may occur suddenly, even in healthy people, because of momentary imbalances in iron inflow and outflow. There is a diurnal variation, with a fall in iron concentration in the evening; significant day-to-day variations occur as well. All these factors limit the diagnostic usefulness of serum iron measurements.

The reference interval for men is 650 to 1750 μg/L and for women 500 to 1700 μg/L. Causes for abnormal levels of serum iron are listed in the left box on p. 701.

Serum iron values should always be interpreted in combination with TIBC and transferrin saturation.

Changes in Serum Iron

Decreased by:
  Iron deficiency
  Chronic disease
  Malignancy
  Inflammation
  Recent blood loss
  Menstruation
Increased by:
  Ineffective erythropoiesis
    Megaloblastic anemia
    Thalassemia major
    Sideroblastic anemia
  Hemolytic anemia
  Aplastic anemia
  Viral hepatitis
  Hemochromatosis
  Acute iron poisoning

Changes in Total Iron-Binding Capacity (TIBC)

Decreased by:
  Malignancy
  Inflammation
  Nephrotic syndrome
  Malnutrition
  Megaloblastic and hemolytic anemia
  Hemochromatosis
Increased by:
  Iron deficiency
  Hepatitis
  Pregnancy
  Use of oral contraceptives

Total iron-binding capacity (TIBC) and transferrin saturation (see p. 712, methods)

TIBC measures the maximum amount of iron that serum proteins can bind and is therefore an indirect way of assessing transferrin levels. Transferrin can also be measured directly by immunoassay and converted to TIBC by application of a conversion formula. The serum iron concentration divided by TIBC gives the transferrin saturation. The reference interval for TIBC is 2500 to 4500 μg/L, and transferrin saturation is 20% to 50% in men and 15% to 50% in women.

Causes of abnormal values for TIBC are listed in the box at the upper right.

The low serum iron and high TIBC in iron deficiency produce a low transferrin saturation; low values may also be seen in pregnancy and chronic disease. High transferrin saturation is characteristic of iron overload and is a sensitive test for hemochromatosis. Thalassemia major, sideroblastic anemia, and acute iron poisoning also cause the transferrin saturation to increase.

Serum ferritin

A small amount of ferritin circulates in plasma, mostly as iron-free apoferritin. Circulating ferritin is in equilibrium with tissue iron stores and, under most circumstances, accurately reflects the amount of storage iron present. The reference interval is dependent on the immunoassay used to measure ferritin but is approximately 20 to 250 μg/L in men and 10 to 120 μg/L in women.

A low serum ferritin concentration is diagnostic of iron deficiency. Ferritin levels drop early in the development of iron deficiency, before serum iron and transferrin saturation become abnormally low. The availability of this reliable blood test for iron deficiency has eliminated the need for bone marrow evaluation in nearly all cases. An increase in serum ferritin is seen in iron overload before the development of signs and symptoms of hemochromatosis. However, the release of ferritin from damaged tissues in hepatitis, acute inflammatory conditions, and a variety of tumors also dramatically increases the serum ferritin level. In these situations, normal ferritin values can mask the presence of iron deficiency, and examination of the bone marrow for stainable iron may be required to confirm the diagnosis.

Free erythrocyte protoporphyrin

In the course of heme synthesis, small numbers of protoporphyrin molecules escape from the pathway and do not complex with Fe^{2+}. Most of these molecules bind Zn^{2+} instead to produce zinc protoporphyrin, which then attaches to a heme site of hemoglobin and circulates in the mature erythrocyte. Assays of red cell porphyrins have traditionally involved an acid extraction step, which removes zinc and leaves behind the metal-free protoporphyrin. Thus the term *free erythrocyte protoporphyrin* (FEP) is actually a misnomer. Measurement of FEP indicates the amount of nonheme protoporphyrin in red cells, which is a clinically useful parameter. The reference interval is 170 to 770 μg/L of cells. Similar information is obtained by hematofluorometry, in which a single instrument measures both zinc protoporphyrin (ZPP) and heme concentrations and expresses the result as a ratio of the two values in μmol ZPP/mol heme.

A decrease in the iron available to developing red cells increases the formation of zinc protoporphyrin. Both iron deficiency (absolute lack of iron) and chronic disease (impaired utilization of iron) will increase FEP. Lead interferes with the final step in heme synthesis, and chronic lead poisoning may produce large increases in FEP. Protoporphyria, a hereditary deficiency of ferrochelatase, is associated with very high FEP values.

The FEP assay is most commonly used as a screening test for iron deficiency. FEP measurements have also been used to screen for lead poisoning, but it is no longer considered sensitive enough and is being replaced by direct measurement of blood lead. When performed with a hematofluorometer, the test is rapid, technically simple, reproducible, and requires only a drop of blood, making it especially useful in children. An increased FEP or ZPP/heme ratio should be followed by more specific tests of iron status.

Part II: Heme synthesis and the porphyrias
STRUCTURE AND FUNCTION

All porphyrins contain a nucleus of four pyrrole units joined by methenyl (=CH—) bridges into a macrocyclic ring structure (Fig. 35-2). The extended network of alternating single and double bonds causes porphyrins to absorb visible light; it is this group that imparts a red color to hemoglobin. Porphyrins also fluoresce a reddish-pink color under a long-wavelength ultraviolet light, a property that is very useful when one is detecting and measuring porphyrins in body fluids. Another unique property is the arrangement of four nitrogen atoms at the center of the ring, enabling porphyrin molecules to chelate metal atoms. In biological systems, iron is the most important metal that complexes with porphyrins.

Differences in porphyrin structure depend on the type and position of side chains located at the corners of the pyrrole rings. In humans, there are three major porphyrins: uroporphyrin (URO), coproporphyrin (COPRO), and protoporphyrin (PROTO) (Figs. 35-3 and 35-4). URO has four propionate and four acetate side chains, whereas COPRO has four propionate and four methyl side chains. These groups may be arranged in four different structural configurations, of which the type III isomer is normally produced. PROTO has two propionate, two vinyl, and four methyl groups that can be arranged in any of 15 different configurations. Only the type IX isomer is produced by the body.

Free porphyrins are by-products of the heme synthetic pathway and have no biological function of their own. Heme, the iron chelate of protoporphyrin, is the prosthetic group for many proteins and enzymes involved in oxygen metabolism and electron-transfer reactions (see Table

35-1). Trace amounts of zinc protoporphyrin also occur naturally, but no physiological role has been assigned to this compound.

BIOCHEMISTRY

Heme synthesis takes place in all cells but occurs to the greatest extent in the bone marrow (red cell precursors) and liver. It is helpful to consider the pathway in two halves: (1) formation of the ring structure by repeated condensations of precursors (Fig. 35-3), and (2) modification of the side chains and insertion of iron (Fig. 35-4). This arbitrary division simplifies an otherwise long and complex series of reactions.

Synthetic pathway

The synthetic pathway begins with the condensation of succinyl CoA and glycine, activated by pyridoxal phosphate, to form delta-aminolevulinic acid (ALA). This reaction, catalyzed by ALA synthase, is the rate-limiting step in heme synthesis. Two ALAs then condense to form porphobilinogen (PBG), a pyrrole with propionate and acetate side chains at its corners. Next, four PBG molecules condense in head-to-tail fashion to form a linear tetrapyrrole, hydroxymethylbilane, that cyclizes to form uroporphyrinogen. This is a critical step in which one of the pyrroles must change its orientation of propionate and acetate side chains to produce the type III isomer of uroporphyrinogen. Porphobilinogen deaminase catalyzes the condensation reaction, but uroporphyrinogen III cosynthase performs the isomerization of one pyrrole unit.

At this point the basic ring structure is in place. Modification of the side chains begins with the decarboxylation of the four acetate groups to form coproporphyrinogen III. Two propionate groups are then decarboxylated and dehydrogenated to vinyl groups, producing protoporphyrinogen IX. The bridging carbon atoms are oxidized from methylene (—CH$_2$—) to methenyl (=CH—) to yield protoporphyrin IX. In the final step, Fe^{2+} is inserted into the protoporphyrin ring to produce heme.

Within the liver, heme synthesis is controlled primarily by changes in the activity of ALA synthase, the first and rate-limiting enzyme. Small amounts of free heme are present within liver cells. An increase in this cellular pool inhibits the activity of ALA synthase, whereas a decrease stimulates the enzyme. Regulation of heme synthesis in red cell precursors appears to involve other enzymes within the pathway as well as the rate of cellular iron uptake.

Points of interest

Several aspects of porphyrin synthesis deserve a closer look. Two enzymes, ALA dehydratase and ferrochelatase, are inhibited by lead, resulting in the buildup of their respective substrates (ALA and protoporphyrin IX) in lead poisoning. Another interesting enzyme is uroporphyrinogen III cosynthase, which produces the type III isomer of uroporphyrino-

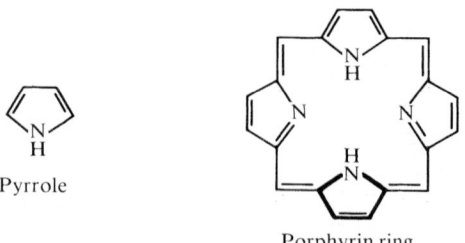

Fig. 35-2 Structures of pyrrole and the porphyrin ring. Structure in boldface is basic pyrrole ring.

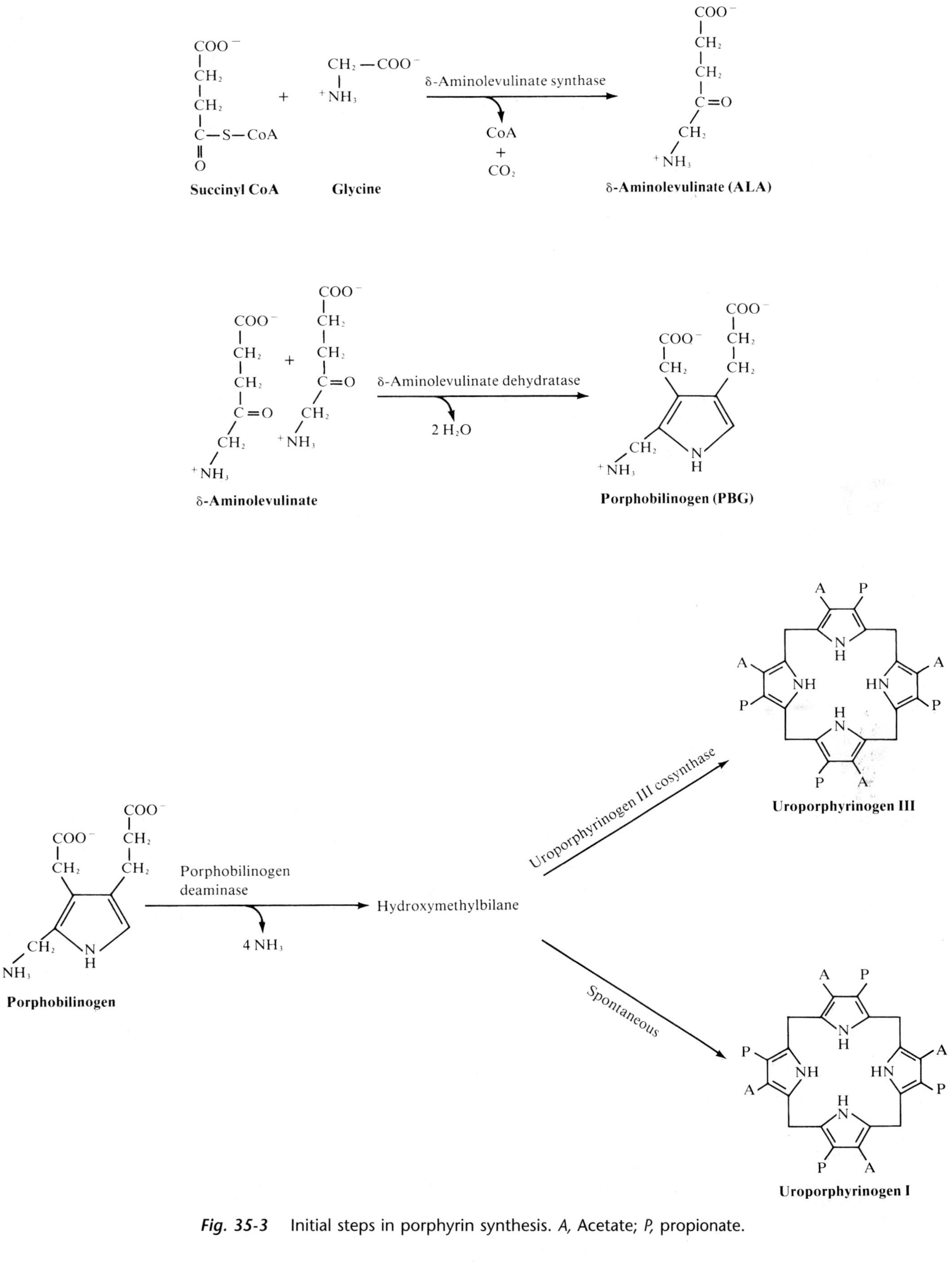

Fig. 35-3 Initial steps in porphyrin synthesis. *A,* Acetate; *P,* propionate.

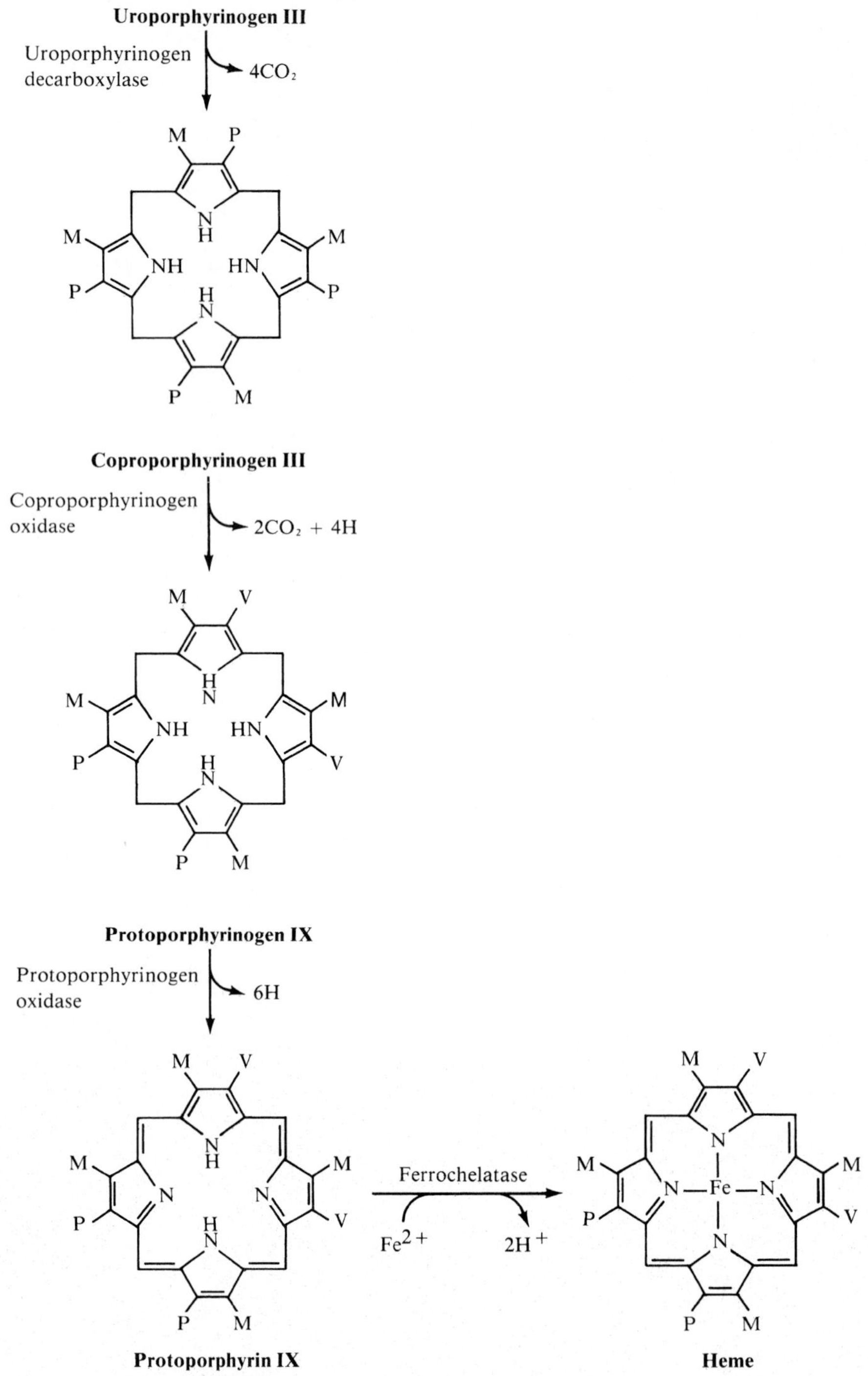

Fig. 35-4 Latter half of the heme biosynthetic pathway. *M,* Methyl; *P,* propionate; *V,* vinyl.

gen during the ring cyclization step. Without this enzyme only the type I isomer, which is not a precursor of heme, is formed.

Note also that during the latter half of the pathway porphyrinogen intermediates are formed. Porphyrinogens differ from porphyrins in that the bridging carbon atoms are fully reduced, and all four nitrogen atoms are protonated.

There is no network of alternating single and double bonds, and so these compounds are colorless and nonfluorescent. Porphyrinogens that are not used in the regular pathway, spontaneously and irreversibly oxidize to the corresponding porphyrins. That is the reason URO, COPRO, and PROTO, and not the porphyrinogens, are the major excretion forms.

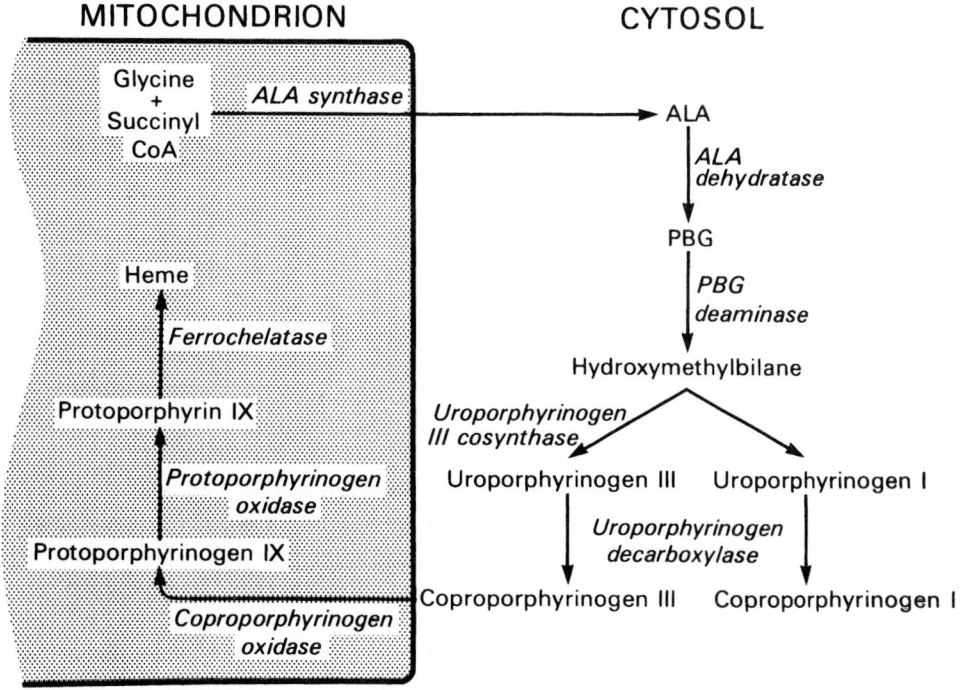

MITOCHONDRION   **CYTOSOL**

Fig. 35-5   Distribution of the porphyrin pathway between mitochondria and cytosol.

Finally, the porphyrin pathway begins and ends in mitochondria, but four of the intervening steps take place in the cytosol. The intracellular distribution of enzymes is shown in Fig. 35-5. Since erythrocytes lose their mitochondria as they mature, only half of these enzymes can be assayed in circulating red blood cells.

PATHOLOGICAL CONDITIONS

What would happen if the enzymes involved in heme synthesis did not function properly? The answer to that question can be found in the study of the porphyrias, a group of genetically determined disorders of heme synthesis. Five of the porphyrias are inherited as an autosomal dominant trait. Since the patient has only one gene producing a functional enzyme, there is about 50% of normal enzyme activity. This partial defect does not cause a deficiency of heme in red blood cells, and so patients do not develop anemia. However, porphyrins and their precursors build up behind the deficient enzyme and accumulate in body tissues and fluids. The photosensitizing properties of porphyrins are responsible for the cutaneous signs and symptoms seen in patients with these disorders.

The excretion of excess porphyrins and their precursors is the basis for diagnosing the porphyrias. The route of excretion is a function of solubility. URO, with eight carboxyl groups, is the most water soluble and is excreted almost entirely in urine. PROTO, with only two carboxyl groups, is excreted exclusively in feces. COPRO, which has four carboxyl groups, is excreted by either route. The porphyrin precursors ALA and PBG are both water soluble and are eliminated in urine.

Traditionally the porphyrias have been classified as erythropoietic or hepatic, based on the site of overproduction of the porphyrins and their precursors. A more useful approach is the classification of the porphyrias by signs and symptoms (neurological versus cutaneous), since this allows one to think in terms of clinical presentation.

Neurological porphyrias

There are three porphyrias characterized by acute attacks of abdominal pain, neuromuscular signs and symptoms, and psychiatric disturbances. The acute attacks, which may last from days to weeks, are accompanied by an increase in the excretion of ALA and PBG in urine. Despite the association of increased levels of porphyrin precursors with the attacks, their biochemical basis remains a mystery. Neither ALA nor PBG has been clearly shown to cause neurotoxicity. ALA is a structural analog of gamma-aminobutyric acid and, at high concentrations, could mimic or interfere with the actions of this neurotransmitter. Another theory maintains that heme deficiency within nerve cells is responsible for the attacks. Each enzyme defect is inherited as an autosomal dominant trait.

The signs and symptoms of the neurological porphyrias usually begin during adolescence or early adulthood and affect women more often than men. Abdominal pain is the most constant finding and is frequently accompanied by constipation, nausea, and vomiting. Abnormalities of the autonomic nervous system include tachycardia, hypertension, sweating, and urinary retention. Peripheral neuropathy may be expressed as pain in the extremities, areas of reduced or altered sensation, muscle weakness, and paralysis. Visual disturbances, seizures, and coma can also occur, and inappropriate secretion of antidiuretic hormone may contribute to a low serum sodium concentration. Some patients have a history of nervousness, mood disorders, or delusional thinking, suggestive of a primary psychiatric illness.

Acute attacks can be precipitated by many drugs, notably the barbiturates and sulfonamides. Fasting or dieting can precipitate an attack, and patients need to maintain an adequate intake of calories. Alcohol consumption and steroid hormones (such as oral contraceptives) are also associated with attacks. Between attacks, the signs and symptoms of porphyria are usually absent. Most gene carriers for one of these porphyrias never have an attack, and their disease remains clinically latent.

The unique features of each neurological porphyria are reviewed below and in Table 35-3.

Acute intermittent porphyria. Acute intermittent porphyria is the most common of the neurological porphyrias with an estimated prevalence of 1 to 10 per 100,000 population. Patients with this disease have a 50% deficiency of porphobilinogen deaminase, the enzyme that joins four PBG molecules to form uroporphyrinogen. The defect causes ALA and PBG to accumulate behind the enzyme block, and the partial interruption of the pathway induces the activity of ALA synthase. Thus ALA and PBG are excreted in the largest amounts in this porphyria. Since the defect does not involve the porphyrinogen portion of the pathway, porphyrins are not produced in excess, and photosensitivity does not occur.

The major diagnostic laboratory finding is an increase in urine ALA and PBG concentrations during acute attacks. However, between attacks their values may revert to normal. When PBG is present at high concentrations in urine, it spontaneously condenses and cyclizes to form uroporphyrinogen, which then oxidizes to URO. Large increases in URO may be present in any of the neurological porphyrias, particularly acute intermittent porphyria. By contrast, fecal porphyrins are normal. Porphobilinogen deaminase can be assayed in erythrocytes and is usually decreased to about 50% of normal, whether the patient is acutely ill or has the unexpressed latent form.

Variegate porphyria. Patients with variegate porphyria suffer from both acute neurological attacks and sensitivity of the skin to sunlight and mechanical trauma. The enzymatic defect is a partial deficiency of protoporphyrinogen oxidase. PROTO and COPRO accumulate in the body, giving rise to photosensitivity and cutaneous lesions. The disease is most common among South African whites and has been traced to a couple who emigrated from Holland in 1688. In an interesting but unproved historical footnote, several authors have speculated that King George III of England suffered from variegate porphyria.

The finding of increased ALA and PBG in urine during acute attacks establishes the presence of a neurological porphyria. Variegate porphyria is distinguished from the other two neurological porphyrias by the increased excretion of PROTO and COPRO in feces.

Coproporphyria. A partial deficiency of coproporphyrinogen oxidase in this disease causes COPRO to accumulate. In addition to the acute attacks, photosensitivity and skin lesions may occur, though less often than in variegate porphyria. Urinary levels of ALA and PBG are increased during acute attacks. The key diagnostic finding is an increase in the fecal excretion of COPRO.

ALA dehydratase deficiency. Several patients with a nearly complete deficiency of ALA dehydratase have been described. Homozygotes have neurologic symptoms but no photosensitivity; heterozygotes are asymptomatic. Increased excretion of ALA and COPRO in urine are the laboratory findings.

Table 35-3   Biochemical and clinical features of the porphyrias

Feature	Acute intermittent porphyria	Variegate porphyria	Coproporphyria	Porphyria cutanea tarda	Protoporphyria	Congenital erythropoietic porphyria
Enzyme defect	Porphobilinogen deaminase	Protoporphyrinogen oxidase	Coproporphyrinogen oxidase	Uroporphyrinogen decarboxylase	Ferrochelatase	Uroporphyrinogen III cosynthase
Inheritance	Autosomal dominant	Autosomal dominant	Autosomal dominant	Autosomal dominant	Autosomal dominant	Autosomal recessive
Abdominal pain and neurological symptoms	Yes	Yes	Yes	No	No	No
Photosensitivity and cutaneous lesions	No	Yes	Yes	Yes	Yes	Yes
Metabolic expression	Liver	Liver	Liver	Liver	Erythroid cells and liver	Erythroid cells

Cutaneous porphyrias

The three cutaneous porphyrias have in common an excess of porphyrins in body tissues, including skin. Porphyrin molecules absorb light at about 400 nm, which raises electrons to a higher energy state. As electrons return to their ground state, some of the energy they release may be transferred to molecular oxygen, generating excited oxygen species that can attack cellular constituents. These reactions at the molecular and cellular level ultimately translate into photosensitivity and skin lesions.

In cutaneous porphyrias, ALA and PBG are not excreted in excess as is the case for the neurological porphyrias, and no neurological signs or symptoms are present. One must remember that the two neurological porphyrias in which porphyrins accumulate (variegate and coproporphyria) may also have skin manifestations. Each of the cutaneous porphyrias is briefly discussed below and reviewed in Table 35-3.

Porphyria cutanea tarda. Porphyria cutanea tarda is a disorder of skin that does not usually appear until adulthood. It is the most common type of porphyria and is caused by a partial deficiency of uroporphyrinogen decarboxylase. Some cases of the disease are clearly familial and are inherited as an autosomal dominant trait, but most cases are sporadic and probably represent an acquired deficiency of the hepatic enzyme. Signs and symptoms of this disorder include fragile skin, blister formation, thickening and scarring of sun-exposed skin, and areas of hyperpigmentation. The disease remains dormant until some form of liver dysfunction develops, such as an overload of hepatic iron or alcoholic liver disease. Estrogen therapy may also activate the disease. The rare, homozygous form of this disease, called hepatoerythropoietic porphyria, produces severe photosensitivity.

The deficiency of uroporphyrinogen decarboxylase causes URO as well as 7-, 6-, and 5-carboxyl porphyrins to accumulate, and their concentrations in urine are greatly increased. Fecal porphyrins are only mildly elevated, but the presence of isocoproporphyrin, which is an isomer of COPRO, is distinctive for this porphyria. Red blood cell porphyrins are within the reference interval.

Protoporphyria. In protoporphyria there is a partial deficiency of ferrochelatase, the last enzyme in the synthetic pathway for heme. The resulting accumulation of PROTO causes photosensitivity beginning in childhood or adolescence. When exposed to sunlight, patients develop burning, itching, swelling, and redness of the skin. Sun-exposed areas such as the backs of the hands and face are affected, but skin changes are mild and scarring uncommon. A minority of patients develop liver disease or protoporphyrin-containing gallstones, since the liver is involved in excreting the unusually large amounts of PROTO.

The concentration of free erythrocyte protoporphyrin is greatly elevated. Fecal PROTO is usually increased as well, though the size of the increase is variable. Urine porphyrins and their precursors are normal.

Congenital erythropoietic porphyria. Congenital erythropoietic porphyria is a rare autosomal recessive disorder caused by deficiency of uroporphyrinogen III cosynthase. The enzyme defect is not complete, and enough uroporphyrinogen III is synthesized to meet metabolic needs. However, large amounts of the type I isomer series are also produced and are eventually oxidized to form URO I and COPRO I. The disease usually presents in early childhood with extreme photosensitivity. Light-exposed areas of the skin become scarred and, as patients grow older, extensive scarring and mutilation of the fingers, nose, and ears may occur. A unique finding of the disease is *erythrodontia,* the reddish-brown staining of teeth caused by porphyrin deposition. Patients also develop hemolytic anemia and enlargement of the spleen. Of all the porphyrias, this one has the worst prognosis.

Patients excrete urine that is pink or red because of the massive amounts of URO and COPRO present. Red blood cells contain large amounts of URO and COPRO and fluoresce when examined microscopically under ultraviolet light. Fecal porphyrins are also increased.

Secondary disorders of porphyrin metabolism

Alterations in porphyrin metabolism and excretion can occur in situations other than the porphyrias. Several common disorders are described below.

Lead poisoning. Lead poisoning may occur in young children who eat chips of paint containing lead or in adults who are exposed to lead compounds in an industrial setting or who drink "moonshine" whisky distilled in lead-containing equipment. The signs and symptoms include abdominal pain and neurological abnormalities that may mimic an acute attack of porphyria. Lead inhibits two enzymes in the porphyrin pathway: ALA dehydratase and ferrochelatase. Consequently, there is an increase in urine ALA (but *not* PBG) and in the erythrocyte concentration of zinc protoporphyrin; urine COPRO is also increased. Although these findings are typical of lead poisoning, the diagnosis is based on the demonstration of increased concentrations of lead in whole blood.

Iron deficiency. Patients with iron deficiency have an imbalance between protoporphyrin, which is produced in normal amounts, and iron, which is not readily available for heme synthesis. As a result, zinc protoporphyrin accumulates in red blood cells to above normal levels. Because it is such a widespread condition, iron deficiency is the most common cause of increased red blood cell porphyrins. Conditions that decrease the availability of iron, such as acute or chronic inflammation, also increase red cell porphyrins. Measurement of zinc protoporphyrin is a useful screening test for iron deficiency, but the diagnosis is confirmed by studies of serum iron, total iron-binding capacity, and ferritin.

Coproporphyrinuria. An isolated increase in urinary COPRO is the most common abnormal finding when urine is screened for porphyrins. Although this finding may indicate a porphyria, it is much more often caused by problems unrelated to heme synthesis, such as liver disease, acute illness, or exposure to toxic compounds. A small (less than twofold) isolated increase in urinary COPRO is usually a nonspecific finding of limited diagnostic value.

CHANGE OF ANALYTE IN DISEASE

The laboratory work-up of a suspected porphyria depends on the clinical presentation. For the neurological porphyrias, analysis of urine and feces samples is usually sufficient to make a diagnosis. Cutaneous porphyrias are diagnosed by analysis of urine, red blood cell, and fecal porphyrins. As a rule, screening tests are used to identify increases in PBG and in urine and fecal porphyrins. Positive screening tests should be confirmed by quantitative measurements on a 24-hour urine sample or random feces sample, as well as by the identification of which porphyrins are elevated. Negative screening tests require no further analysis.

The interpretation of results is complicated by several factors. In the traditional screening tests, porphyrins are extracted into an acidified organic solvent, and a positive result is indicated by a reddish pink fluorescence of the extract under long-wavelength ultraviolet light. The screening test for PBG is based on its reaction with *p*-dimethylaminobenzaldehyde to form a reddish purple compound. Both techniques require subjective judgement as to whether the expected color is present and may give false-positive and false-negative results because of interfering substances in urine and feces. Newer screening tests based on spectrophotometry and spectrofluorometry have eliminated these interferences and provide a numerical value for the amount of PBG or porphyrin that is present in the sample.

Another issue is the variable excretion of porphyrins and their precursors in health and disease. Urine, fecal, and red blood cell porphyrins are typically increased by five- to tenfold in patients with porphyria. The same is true for ALA and PBG in the acute phase of a neurologic porphyria. However, some analytes, notably ALA and PBG, are affected by current disease activity, and the range of values seen in any of the porphyrias can vary greatly. Isolated increases of porphyrins in urine (<twofold), feces (<threefold) and red blood cells (<fivefold) may also occur in people who do not have a porphyria. For these reasons, diagnosis must be based on a combination of clinical presentation, reliable analytical techniques, and careful interpretation of test results.

The key laboratory findings in the porphyrias are summarized in Table 35-4.

Porphobilinogen (PBG)

Urine PBG is elevated in acute intermittent porphyria, variegate porphyria, and coproporphyria. The screening test for PBG is positive during acute attacks but may be negative between attacks. A positive screening test is confirmed by a quantitative PBG analysis, performed on a 24-hour urine collection. The reference interval is ≤ 2 mg/day.

Delta-aminolevulinic acid (ALA)

Urine ALA values parallel the increase in PBG seen in the three neurological porphyrias. It is also elevated in lead poisoning and hereditary tyrosinemia and is therefore a less specific indicator of porphyria than PBG. Measurements are made on 24-hour urine collections, and the reference interval is 1.5 to 7.5 mg/day.

Urine porphyrins

Screening tests for urine porphyrins are usually positive in all the porphyrias except protoporphyria and the latent phase of acute intermittent porphyria. Positive urine screens are followed by identification of the porphyrin (URO or COPRO, or both) that is elevated. A slight to moderate el-

Table 35-4 Laboratory diagnosis of the porphyrias

Porphyria	Urine ALA and PBG*	Urine porphyrins	Fecal porphyrins	Red blood cell porphyrins
Neurological				
Acute intermittent porphyria	↑	URO ↑*	N	N
Variegate porphyria	↑	COPRO ↑	PROTO ↑ COPRO ↑	N
Coproporphyria	↑	COPRO ↑	COPRO ↑	N
Cutaneous				
Porphyria cutanea tarda	N	URO ↑ 7-carboxyl ↑	Isocoproporphyrin ↑	N
Protoporphyria	N	N	PROTO ↑	PROTO ↑
Congenital erythropoietic porphyria	N	URO ↑ COPRO ↑	COPRO ↑	URO ↑ COPRO ↑

N, Normal (within the reference interval); ↑, increased.
*May be increased only during acute attack.

evation of urinary COPRO concentration is seen in liver disease, lead poisoning, alcohol ingestion, and acute illness. Larger increases, especially in URO concentrations, require quantitative analysis of a 24-hour urine collection. Reference intervals are ≤ 50 μg/day for URO and ≤ 230 μg/day for COPRO.

Patients with congenital erythropoietic porphyria excrete huge amounts of URO and COPRO. In porphyria cutanea tarda, excretion of URO and a distinctive 7-carboxyl porphyrin, with smaller amounts of 6- and 5-carboxyl porphyrins and COPRO, is seen and depends on the current activity of the disease. Variegate porphyria and coproporphyria are characterized by an excess of COPRO in urine. Patients with acute intermittent porphyria sometimes excrete high levels of URO because of the nonenzymatic condensation of PBG molecules in urine. URO may be increased in the other two neurological porphyrias for the same reason.

Fecal porphyrins

Fecal porphyrins consist of COPRO, PROTO, and several other dicarboxylic porphyrins (meso-, deutero-, and pemptoporphyrin). The amount of porphyrins excreted by this route is a function of diet and the anaerobic flora of the colon. Consequently, increases in fecal porphyrin excretion up to threefold the upper reference limit may be seen in healthy individuals. The reference intervals are ≤ 30 μg/g dry weight for COPRO and ≤ 60 μg/g dry weight for PROTO.

Fecal porphyrins are usually increased in all the porphyrias except acute intermittent porphyria. A positive screening test for fecal porphyrins should be followed by an analysis to determine which porphyrins are elevated. The most important application of this test is to distinguish variegate porphyria (PROTO and COPRO both elevated) from coproporphyria (only COPRO elevated). An increase in PROTO is also seen in protoporphyria, whereas patients with congenital erythropoietic porphyria excrete large amounts of COPRO. Fecal porphyrins may be within the reference interval or only slightly increased in porphyria cutanea tarda, but fractionation reveals a range of porphyrins, including URO, 7-carboxyl porphyrin, and isocoproporphyrin, not normally seen in feces.

Red blood cell porphyrins

The concentration of red blood cell porphyrins, measured as free erythrocyte protoporphyrin (FEP), is greatly increased in congenital erythropoietic porphyria (URO and COPRO) and protoporphyria (PROTO) but is normal in other porphyrias. Fractionation of red blood cell porphyrins is not necessary, because these two disorders can be differentiated by urine porphyrin assays and clinical presentation. As previously mentioned, FEP is also increased in iron deficiency and lead poisoning. The reference interval for FEP is 170 to 770 μg/L of erythrocytes.

Enzyme assays

Only one heme pathway enzyme, porphobilinogen (PBG) deaminase, is routinely measured by clinical laboratories. Its activity is decreased to about 50% of normal in the red blood cells of most individuals with acute intermittent porphyria, whether the disease is latent or in an acute phase. The usefulness of this assay is diminished by two factors. First, there is an overlap of values between patients and healthy individuals at the lower end of the reference interval. Second, a small subset of patients with the disease have normal PBG deaminase activity in erythrocytes, caused by mutations in the gene that do not affect expression of the enzyme in red cells. Despite its shortcomings, PBG deaminase is frequently the only test that can identify asymptomatic individuals who carry the gene for acute intermittent porphyria.

Molecular genetics

Most of the genes that encode enzymes of the heme synthetic pathway have now been identified and are at least partially sequenced. This work has led to the discovery of mutations that cause acute intermittent porphyria, coproporphyria, porphyria cutanea tarda, protoporphyria, and congenital erythropoietic porphyria. Once the molecular basis for the porphyrias is more completely defined, accurate testing for these disorders with DNA-based assays will become possible.

Part III: Bilirubin
FORMATION AND STRUCTURE

Heme is degraded in cells of the reticuloendothelial system (Fig. 35-6). Heme oxygenase, in the presence of molecular oxygen and NADPH, opens the protoporphyrin ring to release iron, carbon monoxide, and a linear tetrapyrrole, biliverdin. Iron is recycled for future heme synthesis, and carbon monoxide is excreted by the lungs. Biliverdin is metabolized one step further; the double bond at the center of the molecule is reduced to form bilirubin.* This yellow-orange pigment is the major waste product of heme metabolism.

The structure of bilirubin appears in Fig. 27-8, p. 525. The molecule consists of two nearly identical halves joined by a —CH_2— group at its center. Because the central carbon atom is fully saturated, there is free rotation about its bonds. This enables the polar groups to form internal hydrogen bonds, leaving a hydrophobic exterior to the molecule. The double bonds between carbon 4 and carbon 5 in

---

*Bilirubin is more properly referred to as *bilirubin IXα*, since it is derived from the type IX isomer of protoporphyrin and ring cleavage takes place at the α-methene bridge. For convenience, the term IXα is omitted in this section.

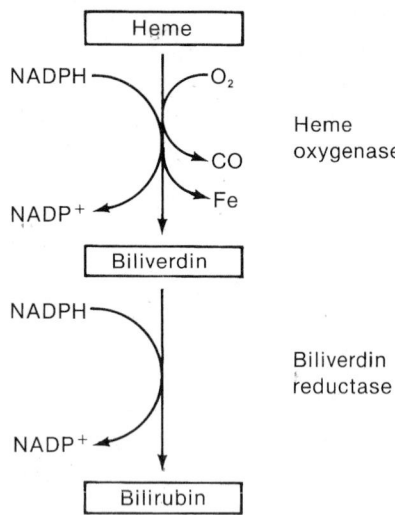

Fig. 35-6 Formation of bilirubin from heme.

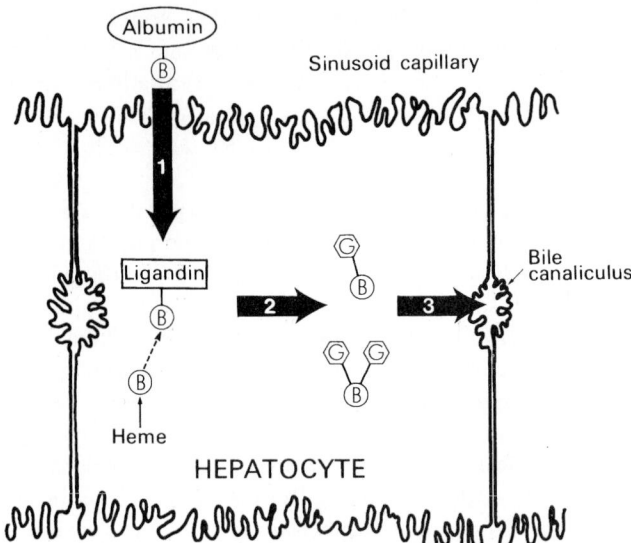

Fig. 35-7 Hepatic metabolism of bilirubin. The indicated steps are *(1)* uptake, *(2)* conjugation, and *(3)* excretion. A small amount of bilirubin is produced by breakdown of heme-containing proteins within hepatocytes. *B*, Bilirubin; *G*, glucuronic acid.

one half of the molecule and carbon 15 and carbon 16 in the other half are normally in the *trans,* or "Z," configuration. On exposure to light, either of these double bonds may flip to the *cis,* or "E," configuration, thereby forming E-Z, Z-E, or E-E isomers. The E configuration interferes with internal hydrogen bonding and makes the molecule more polar.

The chemical structure of bilirubin explains its extremely low solubility in aqueous solutions. It also provides a rationale for treating jaundiced infants with phototherapy, since the photoisomers of bilirubin are more polar and can be excreted directly into bile without conjugation.

METABOLISM
Production

The breakdown of heme-containing proteins generates about 250 to 300 mg of bilirubin per day. Approximately 80% to 85% of bilirubin is derived from the hemoglobin in aged erythrocytes. Most erythrocytes are destroyed within reticuloendothelial cells, mainly in the spleen. A small percentage of erythrocytes is destroyed within the circulatory system as well. The remaining 15% to 20% of bilirubin comes from the destruction of red blood cell precursors in the bone marrow and from the turnover of hemoproteins in other tissues.

Transport

Once bilirubin is released into plasma, it binds very tightly to albumin. Each albumin molecule has one high-affinity binding site for bilirubin and one or two sites of weaker affinity. Transport of bilirubin in the bound state prevents it from crossing cell membranes and entering tissues, where it would exert toxic effects. Certain anionic drugs, such as sulfonamide antibiotics, barbiturates, and salicylates, as well as free fatty acids, compete for the bilirubin-binding sites on albumin. This is not usually a problem in adults,

but infants have a lower binding capacity for bilirubin. In the presence of competing substances, bilirubin may be displaced from albumin, cross the blood-brain barrier, and enter brain cells to cause *kernicterus.*

In addition to the usual reversible binding, bilirubin may also become covalently bound to albumin in patients with impaired hepatic excretion of bilirubin. The covalently bound form, *delta-bilirubin,* continues to circulate with its albumin carrier until the albumin itself is removed from the circulation. The mechanism of attachment and physiologic purpose of delta-bilirubin, if any, are not known.

Hepatic uptake, conjugation, and excretion

During passage through the microcirculation of the liver, albumin releases bilirubin to hepatocytes (Fig. 35-7). After bilirubin diffuses across the cell membrane, it binds mainly to *ligandin,* a cytosolic protein that binds organic anions. Ligandin does not appear to be involved in the cellular uptake of bilirubin. Its function is probably to prevent the diffusion of bilirubin out of the hepatocyte or into other cellular compartments.

In the endoplasmic reticulum, glucuronic acid residues are added to the propionate side chains of bilirubin. The reaction is catalyzed by bilirubin UDP-glucuronyl transferase, and UDP-glucuronic acid is the carbohydrate donor. The addition of the sugar residues increases the water solubility of bilirubin so that it can be excreted into the biliary system. About 85% to 90% of bilirubin appears in bile as the diglucuronide and about 10% to 15% appears as the monoglucuronide. Small amounts of other bilirubin-sugar conjugates (glucosides, xylosides), as well as free bilirubin (water-soluble photoisomers), are also found in bile. Excretion into bile is the rate-limiting step in the hepatic metabolism of bilirubin. It is an energy-dependent process in which bilirubin is transported against a concentration gradient.

Intestinal transit

After excretion into bile, conjugated bilirubin passes through the hepatic and common bile ducts and into the intestinal lumen. In the distal small intestine and colon, anaerobic bacteria hydrolyze the glucuronic acid residues and reduce bilirubin to a variety of compounds known collectively as *urobilinogens*. Unlike the more polar bilirubin glucuronide, urobilinogens may be reabsorbed by the intestine and returned by means of the portal circulation to the liver. More than 90% of recirculated urobilinogens are taken up by liver cells and reexcreted into bile; the remainder are filtered by the kidneys and excreted in urine. Urobilinogens are colorless, but in the presence of air they oxidize spontaneously to the corresponding urobilins. These colored compounds contribute to the normal color of feces and urine.

PATHOLOGICAL CONDITIONS: HYPERBILIRUBINEMIA

Diseases or conditions that interfere with bilirubin metabolism may cause a rise in its serum concentration. Jaundice, a yellowish discoloration of the sclera and skin, appears when the serum bilirubin concentration reaches about 25 mg/L. By itself, hyperbilirubinemia is usually not a threat to health, since adequate mechanisms exist for binding and detoxifying bilirubin. However, hyperbilirubinemia does indicate an abnormality in the production or subsequent metabolism of bilirubin.

There are five mechanisms that can lead to hyperbilirubinemia and jaundice:
1. Overproduction
2. Impaired uptake by liver cells
3. Defects in the conjugation reaction
4. Reduced excretion into bile
5. Obstruction to the flow of bile

The first three mechanisms cause an increase in unconjugated serum bilirubin, whereas the latter two mechanisms produce an elevation of both unconjugated and conjugated bilirubin in serum. For a pictorial description of the mechanisms of hyperbilirubinemia, see p. 511.

Overproduction

Increased production of bilirubin is usually the result of accelerated red blood cell breakdown. When the rate of hemolysis exceeds the liver's capacity to clear bilirubin from blood, the patient develops hyperbilirubinemia. Serum bilirubin does not usually exceed 50 mg/L in hemolytic states, and the bilirubin is almost entirely unconjugated. In chronic hemolytic anemias such as sickle cell disease or hereditary spherocytosis, prolonged overproduction of bilirubin may lead to the formation of bilirubin-containing gallstones. Ineffective erythropoiesis, which occurs in thalassemia major, pernicious anemia, and other disorders, causes a similar increase in bilirubin production.

Impaired uptake

The hepatic phase of bilirubin metabolism begins with its uptake by liver cells. Several drugs interfere with this process, possibly by competing with bilirubin for binding to ligandin. *Gilbert's syndrome* is a hereditary disorder characterized by a small increase in serum unconjugated bilirubin. Some cases appear to involve a defect in hepatic uptake, but more commonly there is a partial deficiency of the conjugating enzyme glucuronyltransferase. The degree of hyperbilirubinemia in patients with Gilbert's syndrome is variable; it is exacerbated by prolonged fasting. There are no other signs, symptoms, or laboratory abnormalities, and the prognosis is excellent.

Defective conjugation

Defects in the conjugation reaction may be hereditary, acquired, or developmental. Hereditary deficiency of the conjugating enzyme is known as the *Crigler-Najjar syndrome*. In the rare type I disorder, there is a complete absence of glucuronyltransferase activity. Serum bilirubin levels are exceedingly high from birth, since failure to conjugate bilirubin prevents it from being excreted into bile. Most affected infants die from kernicterus before reaching 1 year of age. Patients with type II disease have a partial deficiency of glucuronyltransferase. The serum concentration of bilirubin is lower, and neurologic complications are unusual. Inheritance is autosomal recessive for the type I disorder and autosomal dominant for type II.

Neonatal jaundice refers to the mild hyperbilirubinemia seen in newborns at 2 to 5 days of life. It is caused in part by immaturity of the glucuronyltransferase system. Other factors include an increase in red blood cell destruction and possibly a deficiency of ligandin. As the hepatocytes mature, jaundice resolves spontaneously, usually within 7 to 10 days of birth. Glucuronyltransferase is inhibited by certain drugs, and its activity is decreased in hepatocellular diseases such as hepatitis.

Reduced excretion

Excretion of bilirubin into bile is the rate-limiting step in its metabolism and the one most sensitive to injury. Therefore, damage to liver cells is associated with an increase in conjugated bilirubin. Hepatocellular damage also affects uptake and conjugation, which contributes to a rise in unconjugated bilirubin as well. Hepatitis and cirrhosis are the most common disorders that produce liver cell injury and jaundice. Some drugs may exert a direct toxic effect on liver cells. Oral contraceptives and other synthetic sex steroids cause a drug-induced *cholestasis* in some people.

The *Dubin-Johnson* and *Rotor* syndromes are two hereditary disorders of bilirubin excretion. Both are characterized by increased levels of conjugated bilirubin, whereas other routine liver function tests remain normal. The Dubin-Johnson syndrome is distinguished by the dark pigment that accumulates in hepatocytes. Inheritance of these rare disorders is autosomal recessive, and the prognosis is excellent.

Obstruction

Mechanical obstruction to the flow of bile is most often produced by gallstones in the common bile duct or by tumors. Cancer of the head of the pancreas compresses the major bile ducts, whereas cancers of the bile duct or ampulla of Vater directly occlude the final portion of the biliary tree. Postoperative strictures of the common bile duct narrow this passageway and impair bile flow. Serum bilirubin increases in proportion to the extent of obstruction and is largely conjugated.

CHANGE OF ANALYTE IN DISEASE

An increase in serum bilirubin accompanies a wide variety of pathological states. The majority of diseases or conditions causing jaundice originate in the liver and biliary tree; a smaller percentage are the result of hematological disorders. The clinical laboratory can measure both conjugated and unconjugated fractions of bilirubin, an important first step in the diagnosis of the cause of jaundice. Other first-line laboratory investigations include measurement of aspartate and alanine aminotransferase activities, alkaline phosphatase activity (see pp. 518, 521-523), prothrombin time, and a complete blood count with peripheral smear evaluation. This group of tests can usually identify the pathophysiological basis of jaundice. More specialized tests, such as serological tests for hepatitis or radiological studies of the biliary tree, are then performed to make a specific diagnosis.

Bilirubin (see p. 523, methods)

Serum bilirubin is most commonly measured by its reaction with diazotized sulfanilic acid to form two azodipyrroles. Conjugated bilirubin reacts in aqueous solution to give the amount of "direct" bilirubin. Total bilirubin is rapidly measured after the addition of an "accelerator," such as methanol or caffeine, that disrupts internal hydrogen bonding and allows the unconjugated fraction to react as well. One can obtain the unconjugated, or "indirect," bilirubin by subtracting the direct from the total bilirubin. Reference intervals are 2 to 10 mg/L for total bilirubin and 0 to 2 mg/L for direct bilirubin.

A portion of the conjugated bilirubin in blood is filtered by the kidneys and excreted in urine. One can easily test for urine bilirubin with commercial dipsticks (see p. 1123 in Chapter 57), and it is usually undetectable. The presence of bilirubin in urine indicates an elevation in the conjugated fraction of serum bilirubin.

Delta-bilirubin

Delta-bilirubin is measured in conventional assays as part of the direct bilirubin fraction. Because it is covalently bound to albumin, delta-bilirubin continues to circulate in blood for a week or more after urine bilirubin has disappeared. Clinical studies show that during recovery from hepatocellular jaundice, the percentage of delta-bilirubin may increase to 80% to 90% of total bilirubin. This level is suggestive of a role for delta-bilirubin in monitoring the recovery phase of hepatic disease. Up to now, measurement of delta-bilirubin has not become a routine clinical test.

Urobilinogen

The usual excretion of urobilinogen in urine is 1 to 4 mg/day. Overproduction of bilirubin, as occurs in hemolytic anemia, increases the amount of urobilinogen formed in the intestine and therefore the amount that is reabsorbed and excreted into urine. Hepatocellular disease may also increase urinary urobilinogen by interfering with its uptake and excretion into bile. Processes that reduce the flow of bilirubin into the intestine, such as common bile duct obstruction, limit the formation of urobilinogen and reduce the amount excreted in urine.

Urobilinogen can be detected with commercial dipsticks (see p. 1123), and an increase provides evidence of a hemolytic cause of jaundice. However, urobilinogen is of little use in the diagnosis of liver disease.

METHODS OF ANALYSIS

GERARDO PERROTTA

Iron and total iron binding capacity

Principles of analysis and current usage Many methods are available for determination of serum iron concentrations. The most common methods in use are colorimetric procedures that are based on the formation of a colored complex after the interaction of iron with an iron-complexing chromogenic agent. Iron must be unbound and in the ferrous (Fe^{2+}) state before it will react with a chromogen. Thus, all colorimetric procedures must first dissociate the ferric (Fe^{3+}) iron that is bound to transferrin by use of an acidic releasing substance. The released ferric iron is then reduced to the ferrous state by use of a strong reducing agent. Reducing agents that are used include hydrazine, ascorbic acid, thioglycolic acid, and hydroxylamine.[1,2] Chromogenic ligands include bathophenanthroline sulfonate, ferrozine, ferene, and pyridylazo dye. The three steps employed by spectrophotometric methods can be summarized as follows (Table 35-5, method 1):

$$\text{Transferrin (Fe}^{3+})_2 \xrightarrow{\text{Acid}} 2Fe^{3+} + \text{Transferrin}$$

$$Fe^{3+} + \text{Reducing agent} \rightarrow Fe^{2+}$$

$$Fe^{2+} + \text{Ligand} \rightarrow \text{Chromogen}$$

The absorbance of the chromogen at its characteristic wavelength is then measured. The chromogens that are used

Table 35-5 Methods of iron analysis

Type of analysis	Principle	Usage	Comments
1. Colorimetric	Transferrin (Fe^{3+})$_2$ $\xrightarrow[\text{Reducing agent}]{\text{Buffer}}$ $2Fe^{2+}$ + Transferrin Fe^{2+} + Chromogen colored complex	Serum	Good coefficient of variation; no prior protein removal is necessary; manual assay Good for stat. tests; automated
2. Coulometry	Voltage at each of two electrodes held constant. Reaction at each electrode is: E1: $Fe^{2+} - e \rightarrow Fe^{3+}$ E2: $Fe^{3+} + e \rightarrow Fe^{2+}$ Loss of electron at E1 and gain of electron at E2 constitutes current flow, which is proportional to iron concentration	Serum	Correlates well with chromogenic method. Has very good accuracy and precision. Excellent for microsamples and stat. tests; can be automated
3. Atomic absorption	Iron is concentrated by chelation with bathophenanthroline and is extracted into methylisobutyl ketone (MIBK). Extract is analyzed by atomic absorption at 248.3 nm.	Serum	Not practical for routine use

most frequently are ferene and ferrozine, which have absorption peaks at 600 and 560 nm respectively.

Measurement of iron based on the principles of coulometry (Table 35-5, method 2) has also been used. Coulometric determination of iron is based upon the finding that an electrochemical potential develops at the interface of a salt solution (that is, serum) and an electrode. An electrode is maintained at a constant potential selected with respect to the electropositivity of the metal being measured. The electropositivity of a metal is an inherent chemical property and is a measure of the tendency of a metal atom to lose one or more electrons.[3] The amount of current that is required to maintain the electrical potential of the electrode at a constant value depends on the electropositivity of the metal being measured as well as the concentration of the metal. Because the electropositivity of iron is known and is a constant, the current required to maintain a constant electrical potential is proportional to the iron concentration. One commercially available instrument (ESA, Inc., Bedford, Mass.) makes use of the above principle to measure iron in serum. Other methods that are infrequently used to measure iron include radiometry and atomic absorption spectrophotometry. Although atomic absorption (Table 35-5, method 3) is rarely used for measurement of iron in serum, this method is used to measure the iron content present in liver biopsy specimens obtained in the evaluation of hemochromatosis.

In order to interpret the result of total serum iron measurement, an assessment of the total iron-binding capacity (TIBC) is also needed. The TIBC is the amount of iron that serum transferrin (TR) can bind when its iron-binding sites are completely saturated. One can estimate the TIBC by either a subtractive or an additive process. In the subtractive method, excess iron is added to serum to saturate TR. The excess iron is precipitated from the sample and the total iron remaining is measured. In the additive method, a known amount of iron is added to serum to saturate serum TR. The regular iron procedure is then used to measure the *unbound* iron. The concentration of the iron standard minus the unbound iron is the unbound iron-binding capacity

(UIBC), which can be used to calculate the TIBC as follows: TIBC = UIBC + total serum iron.

Because iron is a ubiquitous element, contamination of reagents, plastics, and glassware used in the measurement of iron must be avoided. Contamination can also occur as a result of hemolysis because of the high iron content of erythrocytes. The presence of other potentially interfering metal ions such as copper must be avoided. A chelating agent is often employed in spectrophotometric methods to prevent copper from reacting with the chromogenic ligand. Thiourea and thioglycolic acid are chelating agents frequently used. Interference from copper with coulometric determinations of serum iron is accomplished by careful selection of the potentials of each electrode so that the electrochemical reactions of copper are identical at each electrode: Because the reactions of copper are identical at each electrode, there is no net movement of electrons associated with the reactions of copper thus eliminating the effect of this metal on iron measurements.

Certain pharmacologic agents and physiologic conditions can adversely affect some methods. For example, iron-dextran is frequently used to treat iron deficiency in patients receiving chronic hemodialysis. After parenteral administration of this compound, the concentrations of iron in serum can remain substantially increased for several weeks. Most colorimetric methods detect only very small quantities of dextran-bound iron in serum because iron-dextran is quite stable in acid media, unlike transferrin-bound iron, which readily dissociates in an acid medium.[4] In addition, coulometric procedures detect only part of the dextran-bound iron.[5] Accurate measurement of iron in patients who have received iron-dextran therapy can be performed by use of atomic absorption spectroscopy,[6] which quantitatively measures total circulating iron bound to transferrin and dextran. Dry chemistry slide methods exclude iron-dextran from the reaction layer and therefore measure only transferrin-bound iron.[10]

Turbidity attributable to hypertriglyceridemia in specimens used for iron analysis can cause a positive bias in test

Table 35-6 Reference intervals for serum iron

Age	Iron, μmoL/L (μg/L)
Newborn	17.9-44.8 (1000-2500)
Infant	7.2-17.9 (400-1000)
Child	9.0-21.5 (500-1200)
Adult male	11.6-31.3 (650-1750)
Adult female	9.0-30.4 (500-1700)

results if a blanking method is not used.[7] The presence of monoclonal immunoglobulins in serum has also been found to cause artifactual increases in colorimetric methods for iron.[8,9]

Specimen Serum or heparinized plasma are acceptable specimens. Serum iron concentrations show a diurnal variation with peak values seen in the early morning. Because of this diurnal variation, serum iron may vary by up to 30% during the course of a day.

Reference interval Reference intervals for iron are dependent on both age and sex (Table 35-6).[3] As previously mentioned, a diurnal variation in serum iron levels, which is attributed to the circadian variation in the uptake and release of iron by peripheral tissues, is also observed.[11] Morning is the preferred time for collection of specimens for determination of iron concentrations.

Porphobilinogen
STEVEN C. KAZMIERCZAK

Principles of analysis and current usage One of the most frequently used methods for the detection of porphobilinogen in urine is the method devised by Watson and Schwartz.[12] This qualitative test is based upon the reaction between porphobilinogen and Ehrlich's aldehyde reagent (*p*-dimethylaminobenzaldehyde in strong acid). This reaction results in the formation of a red compound. Once formed, the color slowly fades as the initial condensation product reacts with a second molecule of porphobilinogen to form colorless dipyrrylphenyl methane.

The test is not totally specific for porphobilinogen; urobilinogen, indole, and indican in urine will also result in a color change. Specificity of the assay is increased by a chloroform extraction of the interfering colored adducts after the addition of sodium acetate to the reaction mixture to increase pH, which makes these interferents preferentially soluble in chloroform. Thus, if a color change is observed after the addition of Ehrlich's reagent and sodium acetate, a chloroform extraction is carried out. The color remaining in the supernatant aqueous phase is assumed to be caused by the presence of porphobilinogen.

Modifications to the Watson-Schwartz test have been described including direct application of the Ehrlich's aldehyde reagent to a pad[13] and dual-wavelength spectrometry.[14]

The Hoesch test is a simplified version of the Watson-Schwartz test in which Ehrlich's aldehyde reagent is used without sodium acetate and chloroform extraction.[15] Although this test is easier to perform, it is less specific for porphobilinogen. Indoles, indole-3-acetic acid, alpha-methyldopa, phenazopyridine hydrochloride, and patients with end-stage alcoholic malnutrition can cause false-positive test results.[16] A limit of all these tests is the poor sensitivity.[17] The sensitivity of the assay can be improved by the use of ion-exchange chromatography.[17]

Specimen Intermittent acute porphyria occurs episodically and, as a result, urine should be collected during or immediately after an attack. Urine collected at other times may not show porphobilinogen to be present. A freshly voided urine specimen is preferred, which should be cooled to room temperature before testing. Cooling the specimen helps prevent the occurrence of a "warm aldehyde" reaction. Porphobilinogen degrades in urine fairly rapidly. Both random and timed urine samples should be protected from light; 24-hour samples should be collected in a container containing 5 g of Na_2CO_3.[18] Thus, analysis for porphobilinogen should be performed within several hours after collection or stored frozen.[9]

Reference interval Healthy individuals typically excrete less than 4 mg of porphobilinogen per day. At these concentrations, the qualitative screening test should be negative.

ACKNOWLEDGMENTS
The editors wish to acknowledge the previous version of the *Porphobilinogen* section written by Michael D.D. McNeely.

REFERENCES
1. Perrota G: Iron and iron binding capacity. In Kaplan LA, Pesce AJ, editors: *Methods in clinical chemistry*, St. Louis, 1987, Mosby.
2. Zak B, Baginski ES, Epstein E: Modern iron ligands useful for the measurement of serum iron, *Ann Clin Lab Sci* 10:276-289, 1980.
3. Kohll DE, Schreiber WE: *Serum iron: review of methods.* ASCP Check Sample Core Analyte no. PTS 93-5 (PTS-71), pp 1-8, Chicago, 1993, American Society of Clinical Pathologists.
4. Huisman W: Interference of Imferon in colorimetric assays for iron, *Clin Chem* 26:635-637, 1980.
5. Jacobs JC, Alexander NM: Colorimetry and constant-potential coulometry determinations of transferrin-bround iron, total iron binding capacity, and total iron in serum containing iron-dextran, with use of sodium dithionite and alumina columns, *Clin Chem* 36:1803-1807, 1990.
6. McIntosh ME, Lynn JK, Meyerriecks N, et al: Serum iron determination in patients receiving therapy with iron dextran ("Imferon"), *Clin Chem* 22:524-527, 1976.
7. Labbe D, Phung HT, Vassault A, et al: Direct methods vs blanking methods for iron determination: effect of serum turbidity, *Clin Chem* 38:782-783, 1992.
8. Dorizzi R, Battaglia P, Lora A: Iron measurement in patients with monoclonal immunoglobulin: a further caution, *Clin Chem* 37:589-590, 1991.
9. Bakker AJ: Influence of monoclonal immunoglobulins in direct determinations of iron in serum, *Clin Chem* 37:690-694, 1991.
10. Vercammen M, Goedhuys W, Boeyckens A, et al: Iron and total iron-binding capacity in serum of patients receiving iron-dextran: Kodak Ektachem methodologies, spectrophotometry, and atomic-absorption spectrometry compared, *Clin Chem* 36:1812-1815, 1990.
11. Bothwell TH, Charlton RW, Motulsky AG: Hemochromatosis. In Scriver CR, Beaudet AL, Sly WS, Walli D, editors: *The metabolic basis of inherited disease*, ed 6, New York, 1989, McGraw-Hill.
12. Watson CJ, Schwartz S: Simple test for urinary porphobilinogen, *Proc Soc Exp Biol Med* 47:393-394, 1941.
13. With TK: Screening for acute porphyria, *Lancet* 2:1187-1188, 1970.
14. Moore DJ, Labbe RF: A quantitative assay for urinary porphobilinogen, *Clin Chem* 10:1105-1111, 1964.

15. Hoesch K: Über die Pantothensäurebehandlung der Porphyrie, *Dtsch Med Wochenschr* 72:252-254, 1947.
16. Pierach CA, Cardinal R, Bossenmaier I, Watson CJ: Comparison of the Hoesch and the Watson-Schwartz tests for urinary porphobilinogen, *Clin Chem* 23:1666-1668, 1977.
17. Schreiber WE, Jamani A, Pudek MR: Screening tests for porphobilinogen are insensitive: the problem and its solution, *Am J Clin Pathol* 92:644-649, 1989.
18. Schreiber WE: ASCP Check Sample cc-252, Chicago, 1994, American Society of Clinical Pathologists.
19. Watson CJ, Bossenmaier I, Cardinal R: Acute intermittent porphyria, *JAMA* 175:1087-1091, 1961.

BIBLIOGRAPHY

Iron metabolism

Bothwell TH, Charlton RW, Motulsky AG: Hemochromatosis. In Scriver CR et al, editors: *The metabolic basis of inherited disease,* ed 6, New York, 1989, McGraw-Hill.
Bridges KR, Bunn HF: Anemias with disturbed iron metabolism. In Wilson JD et al, editors: *Harrison's principles of internal medicine,* ed 12, New York, 1991, McGraw-Hill.
Cavill I, Jacobs A, Worwood M: Diagnostic methods for iron status, *Ann Clin Biochem* 23:168-171, 1986.
Crosby WH: Hemochromatosis: current concepts and management, *Hosp Pract* 22:173-192, 1987.
Fairbanks VF, Beutler E: Iron metabolism. In Williams WJ et al, editors: *Hematology,* ed 4, New York, 1990, McGraw-Hill.
Fairbanks VF, Beutler E: Iron deficiency. In Williams WJ et al, editors: *Hematology,* ed 4, New York, 1990, McGraw-Hill.
Jacobs A, Worwood M, editors: *Iron in biochemistry and medicine,* II, London, 1980, Academic Press.
Kushner JP: Hypochromic anemias. In Wyngaarden JB et al, editors: *Cecil textbook of medicine,* ed 19, Philadelphia, 1992, Saunders.
Powell LW, Isselbacher KJ: Hemochromatosis. In Wilson JD et al, editors: *Harrison's principles of internal medicine,* ed 12, New York, 1991, McGraw-Hill.

Heme synthesis and the porphyrias

Anderson KE: The porphyrias. In Wyngaarden JB et al, editors: *Cecil textbook of medicine,* ed 19, Philadelphia, 1992, Saunders.
Deacon AC: Performance of screening tests for porphyria, *Ann Clin Biochem* 25:392-397, 1988.
Kappas A, Sassa S, Galbraith RA, Nordmann Y: The porphyrias. In Scriver CR et al, editors: *The metabolic basis of inherited disease,* ed 6, New York, 1989, McGraw-Hill.

Kauppinen R, Mustajoki P: Prognosis of acute porphyria: occurrence of acute attacks, precipitating factors, and associated diseases, *Medicine* 71:1-13, 1992.
Meyer UA: Porphyrias. In Wilson JD et al, editors: *Harrison's principles of internal medicine,* ed 12, New York, 1991, McGraw-Hill.
Moore MR, McColl KEL, Rimington C, Goldberg A: *Disorders of porphyrin metabolism,* New York, 1987, Plenum Publishing.
Nordmann Y, de Verneuil H, Deybach J-C, et al: Molecular genetics of porphyrias, *Ann Med* 22:387-391, 1990.
Pudek MR, Schreiber WE, Jamani A: Quantitative fluorometric screening test for fecal porphyrins, *Clin Chem* 37:826-831, 1991.
Schreiber WE, Jamani A, Pudek MR: Screening tests for porphobilinogen are insensitive: the problem and its solution, *Am J Clin Pathol* 92:644-649, 1989.
Westerlund J, Pudek M, Schreiber WE: A rapid and accurate spectrofluorometric method for quantification and screening of urinary porphyrins, *Clin Chem* 34:345-351, 1988.

Bilirubin

Chowdhury JR, Wolkoff AW, Arias IM: Hereditary jaundice and disorders of bilirubin metabolism. In Scriver CR et al, editors: *The metabolic basis of inherited disease,* ed 6, New York, 1989, McGraw-Hill.
Isselbacher KJ: Bilirubin metabolism and hyperbilirubinemia. In Wilson JD et al, editors: *Harrison's principles of internal medicine,* ed 12, New York, 1991, McGraw-Hill.
Isselbacher KJ: Jaundice and hepatomegaly. In Wilson JD et al, editors: *Harrison's principles of internal medicine,* ed 12, New York, 1991, McGraw-Hill.
Ostrow JD, editor: Bile pigments and jaundice: molecular, metabolic, and medical aspects, New York, 1986, Marcel Dekker.
Sherlock S, Dooley J: Diseases of the liver and biliary system, ed 9, Oxford, 1993, Blackwell Scientific.
Weiss JS, Gautam A, Lauff JJ, et al: The clinical importance of a protein-bound fraction of serum bilirubin in patients with hyperbilirubinemia, *N Engl J Med* 309:147-150, 1983.
Wu T-W: Delta bilirubin—the state of the art and future prospects. In Goldberg DM, Walker WHC, editors: *Clinical biochemistry reviews,* vol 1, New York, 1987, Pergamon Press.
Zimmerman HJ, Deschner KW: Differential diagnosis of jaundice, *Hosp Pract* 22:99-122, 1987.

CHAPTER 36

Hemoglobin

Harold R. Schumacher
Patricia A. Miller-Canfield

All globin genes are believed to have arisen from a common globin-like heme protein. The earliest duplication of this progenitor gene led to the divergence of myoglobin and the globins that compose hemoglobin. From this ancestral globin gene diverged the α-globin genes, which include the zeta gene. The ancient β-globin gene evolved to form hemoglobin gene families. In estimated order of appearance, they are the γ-globin, the ϵ-globin, and the δ-globin genes. Modern globin proteins are the result of an evolutionary process that began over 700 million years ago (Fig. 36-1). Mutations continue to occur, often resulting in disease states called *hemoglobinopathies.*

STRUCTURE AND FUNCTION OF HEMOGLOBIN
Structure

Hemoglobin (Hb) is a red-pigmented, oxygen-carrying protein found in red blood cells. It is a globular tetramer (molecular weight 68,000 daltons) consisting of two pairs of unlike polypeptide chains (Fig. 36-2). Each chain carries an iron-containing porphyrin derivative called *heme,* a ferroprotoporphyrin IX in which one iron atom is bound in the center of the porphyrin ring. The polypeptide chains (without heme) are collectively called the *globin* moiety of hemoglobin. Each polypeptide chain is designated by a Greek letter: α (alpha), β (beta), γ (gamma), δ (delta), ϵ (epsilon), and ζ (zeta). Normal mammalian hemoglobin contains two pairs of chains: two α- and two non-α (β, γ, or δ) chains. The α chains bind with β chains to produce normal adult Hb (HbA = $\alpha_2\beta_2$), they bind with the γ chain to produce fetal Hb (HbF = $\alpha_2\gamma_2$), and they bind with the δ-chain to produce HbA$_2$ (HbA$_2$ = $\alpha_2\delta_2$). The latter accounts for only 2.5% of normal adult Hb. The two early embryonic Hbs, termed Hbs Gower 1 and Gower 2, consist of alpha-like ζ-chains and beta-like ϵ-chains.

The primary, secondary, tertiary, and quaternary structures of all the hemoglobins have been determined. The β-,

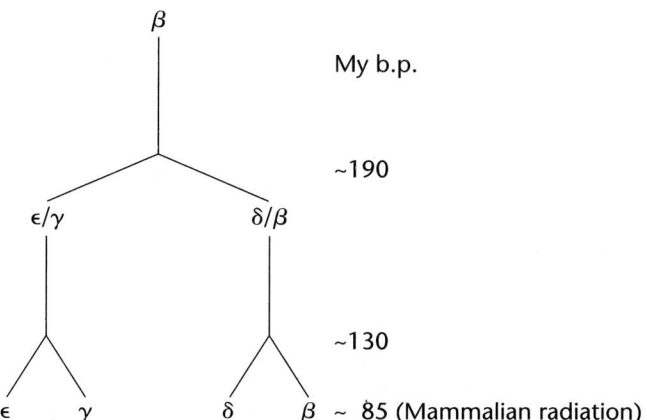

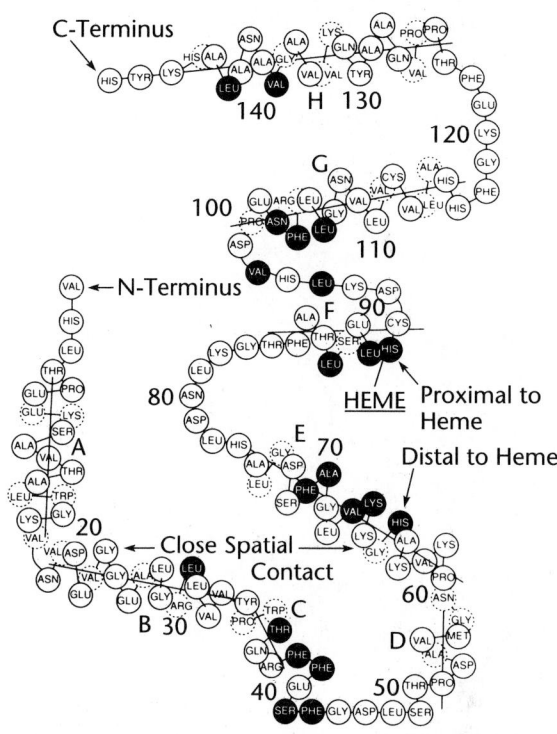

Fig. 36-1 The evolutionary history of the globin gene. *M.y.b.p.* = million years before present. (From Steinberg MH, Adams JG III: Hemoglobin A₂: origin, evolution and aftermath, *Blood* 78:2165, 1991.)

Fig. 36-3 The β-globin chain showing helical and nonhelical segments. The helical segments are labeled *A* through *H*, whereas nonhelical segments are designated *NA* for those residues between the N terminus and the A helix, *CD* for residues between the C and D helices, etc. (From Huisman THJ, Schroeder WA: *New aspects of the structure, function and synthesis of hemoglobin*, Boca Raton, Fla., 1971, CRC Press.)

γ-, δ-, and ε-chains have similar amino acid sequences, as the α- and ζ-chains have. The α-chain contains 141 amino acid residues, and the β-, δ-, and ε-chains each contain 146.

In all hemoglobin and myoglobin chains, approximately 75% of the amino acids are arranged in an α-helix with 3 to 6 amino acids per turn (Fig. 36-3). The tertiary structure of hemoglobin is depicted in Fig. 36-4. The folding pattern places polar amino acid residues on the outside of the molecule and provides a pocket with a deep hydrophobic niche for the heme ring between the E and F helices in each protein subunit. Many noncovalent bonds are formed between the heme moiety and the surrounding amino acids. An iron atom, in the ferrous (Fe^{2+}) state, in the center of the ferroprotoporphyrin IX ring forms an important bond with the F8, or proximal, histidine and via the bound oxygen with the E7, or distal, histidine. This heme iron is critical since oxygenation and deoxygenation occur at this site.

The complete hemoglobin tetramer composed of two α-globin and two non–α-globin chains fits together to form a quaternary structure (Fig. 36-5). The central cavity is filled with water and allows the entrance of small molecules such as 2,3-diphosphoglycerate (2,3-DPG) and salts. The motion of individual globin chains, including the movement of globin chains relative to one another during oxygenation and deoxygenation, gives hemoglobin its unique ability to serve as a carrier of oxygen. The substitution of a single amino acid can change the secondary, tertiary, and quaternary structures of hemoglobin, causing severe and even fatal pathophysiological changes.

Ontogeny

The hemoglobin composition of a red blood cell (RBC) varies widely depending on when, during gestation or postnatal development, the RBC is produced. The first globin chains formed in embryonic red cells are ε-chains, which resemble β-chains in their primary structure.[1] Almost immediately, the synthesis of ζ-, α-, and γ-chains begins. The sequential activation and inactivation, or switching, among genes within the α- and non–α-globin gene clusters results in the formation of four commonly encountered embryonic

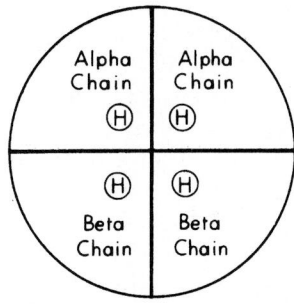

Fig. 36-2 Diagram of structure of HbA molecule. Four heme groups are attached to one globin molecule, which consists of four polypeptide chains, two of which have an identical amino acid sequence of one type (α-chain) and the other two an identical amino acid sequence of another type (β-chain). Each polypeptide chain is conjugated to one heme moiety. *H*, Heme. (From Bauer JD: *Clinical laboratory methods*, ed 9, St. Louis, 1982, Mosby.)

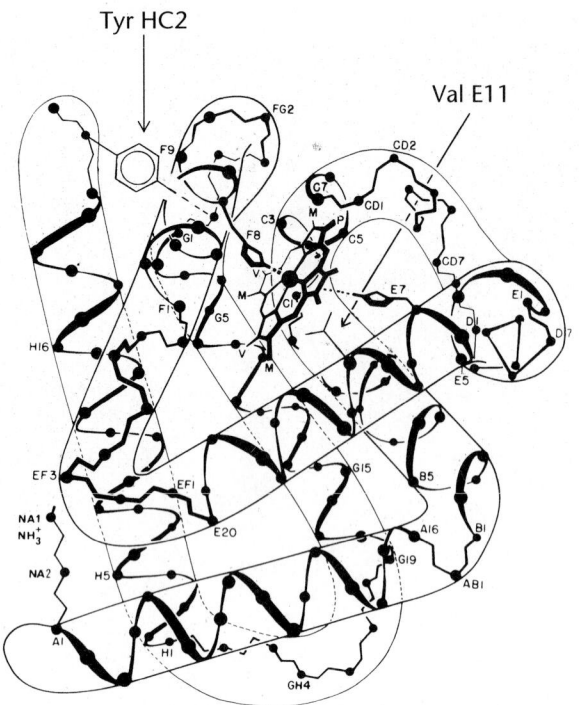

Tyr HC2

Val E11

Fig. 36-4 Secondary and tertiary structure of the hemoglobins showing α carbons and coordination of hemes. The diagram shows the proximal histidine F8 linked to the heme iron, the distal residues His E7 and Val E11, and also Tyr HC$_2$, which are important in the mechanism of the mammalian hemoglobins. The exact numbers of residues in the different segments are the same in all mammals but vary in other vertebrates. The letters *M*, *V*, and *P* refer to the methyl, vinyl, and propionate side chains of the heme. (From Perutz MF: Molecular, anatomy, physiology and pathology of hemoglobin. In *The molecular basis of blood disease*, Philadelphia, 1987, Saunders.)

hemoglobins. These are Gower 1, $\zeta_2\epsilon_2$, Gower 2, $\alpha_2\epsilon_2$, Portland, $\zeta_2\gamma_2$, and fetal hemoglobin, $\alpha_2\gamma_2$. Gower 1 and Gower 2 hemoglobins constitute 42% and 24% of the total hemoglobin, respectively, at five weeks of gestation. The rest is fetal hemoglobin. Hemoglobin switching during embryonic, fetal, and adult development is shown in Fig. 36-6.

NORMAL HEMOGLOBIN BIOCHEMISTRY
Assembly of hemoglobin

The α-like globin genes of man are located on the short arm of chromosome 16, between band P 13.2 and the terminus, whereas the β-like genes are located on the terminal portion of the short arm of chromosome 11 (P15).[2] The α and β polypeptide chains of an adult hemoglobin are synthesized in equal amounts, though there may be an excess of α-chains in the cytoplasm of young red cells. The assembly process starts with the release of α- and β-chains from the ribosomes into the cytoplasm. They immediately incorporate heme (see Chapter 35, for discussion on the syn-

thesis of heme) and form monomer combinations and dimer aggregates followed by the synthesis of tetramers. In the hemoglobinopathies, the concentrations of the two like chains, such as βA and βS; βA and βC; and βA and βE, may differ even though their rates of synthesis are the same. There is evidence that the relative rates of assembly in relation to synthesis of hemoglobins A and S may differ because of differences in affinities of βA and βS for α-chains. The α-chains, if in short supply, prefer to combine with normal β-chains rather than with the variant chains,[3] and excess variant chains are then removed by proteolysis.

The synthesis of hemoglobin is normally stimulated by tissue *hypoxia* (low Po$_2$ in tissues). Hypoxia causes the kidneys to produce increased amounts of erythropoietin (see p. 490), which in turn stimulates the production of hemoglobin and RBCs.

Functional and structural interrelationships

Hemoglobin and oxygen: the oxygen-dissociation curve. The four subunits of hemoglobin each contain a heme moiety deep in the pocket of the globin chains, leaving one edge of the heme exposed to receive the oxygen. Each of the four heme iron atoms can reversibly bind one oxygen molecule. Since the iron remains in the ferrous form, the reaction is an oxygenation, not an oxidation.

To fulfill its function as a respiratory pigment, hemoglobin must specifically bind oxygen molecules with high affinity, transport them, and unload them at the oxygen tension of tissues. Approximately 1.34 mL of oxygen is bound by each gram of hemoglobin. The tetrameric structure of hemoglobin is responsible for its unique oxygen-binding capacity and renders it physiologically superior to single hemoglobin subunits or to myoglobin. The heme iron has six valence bonds, four of which are occupied by the four pyrrole rings of heme. The fifth iron valency bond attaches heme to globin, leaving the sixth iron valency bond available for a reversible combination with oxygen or other ligands.

The affinity of hemoglobin for oxygen depends on the partial pressure of oxygen (Po$_2$). A plot of the oxygen content (percentage of hemoglobin saturated with oxygen) against Po$_2$ in myoglobin subunits results in a hyperbolic oxygen-dissociation curve, but a similar plot using hemoglobin gives a sigmoid curve (Fig. 36-7). The hyperbolic curve indicates appreciable release of oxygen at very low partial pressures only, whereas the sigmoid curve indicates a much earlier release of oxygen even at relatively high oxygen tensions, allowing adequate oxygenation of tissues. The curve has a sigmoid shape because oxygenation of one heme group increases oxygen affinity of the others, a phenomenon called *heme-heme interaction* (or *subunit cooperativity*), which is responsible for the physiologically efficient uptake and release of oxygen. There is a progressive change in oxygen affinity as each heme molecule becomes oxygenated; the affinity for oxygen is low at first but in-

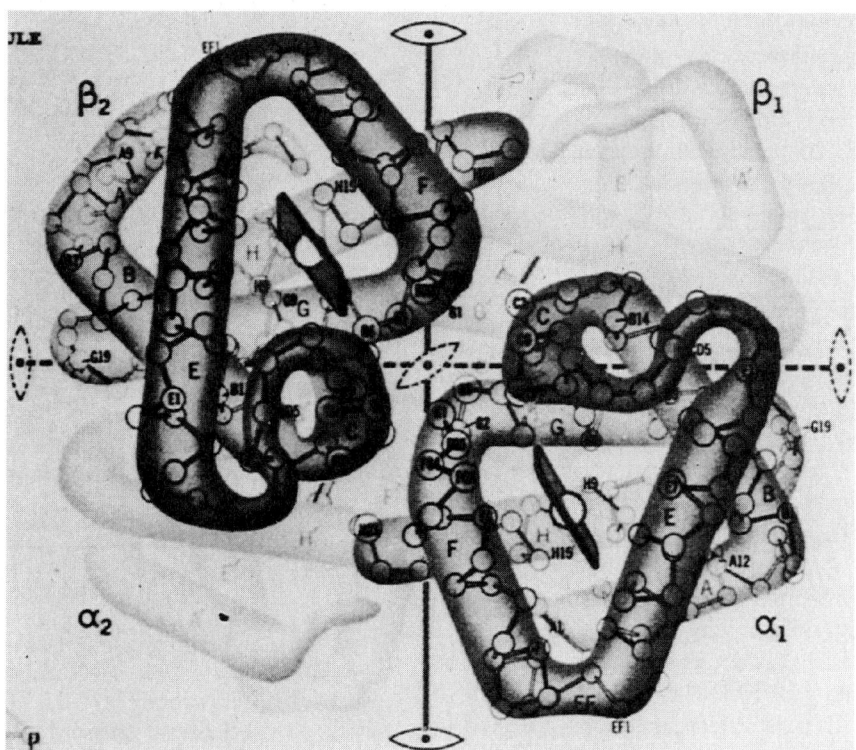

Fig. 36-5   Quaternary structure of hemoglobin. The α_1 and β_2 chains are in foreground, and $\alpha_1\beta_2$ contact is at center. (From Dickerson RE, Geis I: *The structure and action of proteins,* Menlo Park, Calif., 1969, Benjamin/Cummings.)

Hemoglobins (embryonic)	Hemoglobins (% at birth)	Hemoglobins (% in adults)
Gower 1 $\zeta_2\varepsilon_2$	HbF $\alpha_2\gamma_2$ (75)	HbA $\alpha_2\beta_2$ (97)
Portland 1 $\zeta_2\gamma_2$	HbA $\alpha_2\beta_2$ (25)	HbA$_2$ α_2s_2 (2.5)
Gower 2 $\alpha_2\varepsilon_2$		HbF $\alpha_2\gamma_2$ (<1)

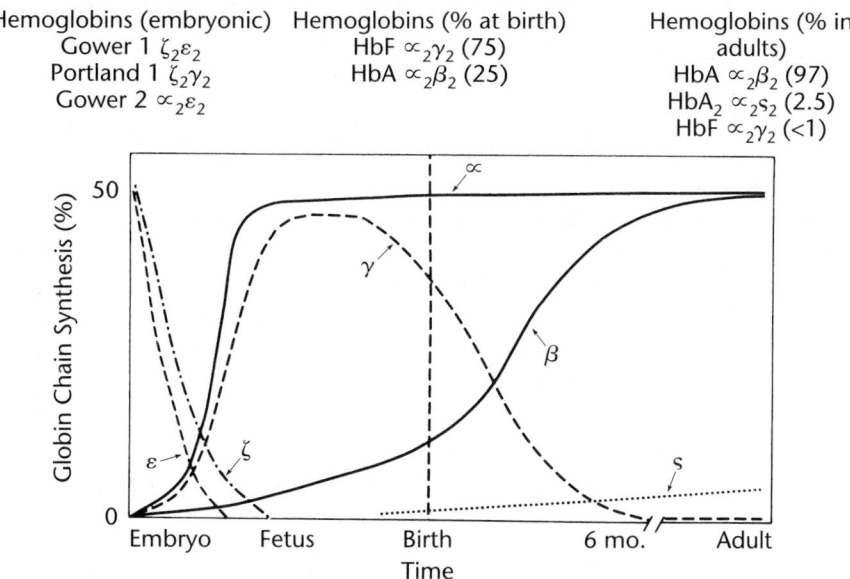

Fig. 36-6   Hemoglobin switching during embryonic, fetal, and adult development. The ζ and ϵ genes are transcribed during embryonic development and soon replaced by the fetal γ-globin and adult α-globin gene. At birth, fetal hemoglobin forms about 75% and hemoglobin A 25% of the total. Transcription of the γ gene begins to fall before birth, and by 6 months of age this gene is expressed only at very low levels. Expressions of the δ-globin gene begin near birth. In adults, hemoglobin A makes up about 97%, hemoglobin A$_2$ about 2.5%, and fetal hemoglobin less than 1% of the total. (From Steinberg MH: Hemoglobinopathies and thalassemias. In Stein JH, editor: *Internal medicine,* ed 3, Boston, 1990, Little Brown & Co.)

creases as each heme molecule takes up oxygen. In myoglobin, the hyperbolic dissociation curve indicates that each molecule is oxygenated independently. In the lung, at a Po_2 of about 95 mm Hg, arterial blood becomes 97% saturated with oxygen and carries 20 volumes of oxygen per 1000 mL of blood. In the capillary bed, venous blood at a Po_2 tension of about 40 mm Hg is still about 75% saturated with oxygen but is nevertheless able to give up 46 volumes of oxygen per 1000 mL of blood. The 75% of hemoglobin returned to the lung in an oxygenated form establishes a large reservoir for improved oxygen delivery to tissues.

The position of the oxygen-dissociation curve is determined by several factors affecting the affinity of hemoglobin for oxygen. The oxygen-dissociation curve is conventionally indexed by the P_{50} value, the Po_2 at which the hemoglobin is 50% saturated with O_2; this normally occurs at a Po_2 of 27 mm Hg. The higher the P_{50}, the lower is the affinity of hemoglobin for oxygen. A decreased P_{50} indicates a shift to the left of the oxygen-dissociation curve, an increased oxygen affinity of hemoglobin, and an impaired oxygen release to tissues. P_{50} is decreased in the presence of (1) a high concentration of HbF, the γ-chain of which binds 2,3-DPG poorly; (2) a modified hemoglobin, such as methemoglobin and carboxyhemoglobin; (3) certain hemoglobin variants, such as Hb Rainier; and (4) 2,3-DPG–depleted blood found after massive transfusions (Fig. 36-7). Obviously, 2,3-DPG binding to hemoglobin decreases the affinity of hemoglobin for oxygen (see below). A *shift to the right* indicates a decreased oxygen affinity, which eases the delivery of oxygen to tissues. It is seen in various types of hypoxia, such as that occurring at high altitude, with severe anemia and heart and lung disease.[2]

Oxygen affinity and transport

Oxygen affinity and transport depend not only on Po_2 (see above) but also on temperature, pH (Bohr effect), and 2,3-DPG concentration.

Bohr effect. The Bohr effect expresses the fact that the oxygen affinity of hemoglobin varies with the pH. Protons lower the affinity of hemoglobin for oxygen mass and, conversely, oxygen lowers the affinity of hemoglobin for protons.

$$HB(O_2)_4 + 2H^+ \rightleftharpoons 2HbH^+ + 4O_2 \qquad \textit{Eq. 36-1}$$

At physiological pH in the tissues, about two protons are taken up for every four molecules of oxygen released; whereas in the lungs two protons are liberated again when four molecules of oxygen are bound to hemoglobin. This reciprocal action is known as the *Bohr effect* and is essential to the mechanism of oxygen transport and the buffering of carbon dioxide (see Chapter 25).

In the physiological pH range, the affinity of hemoglobin for oxygen decreases in the tissues as the acidity increases and the dissociation curve shifts to the right (see Fig. 36-7). The Bohr effect aids in the transport of oxygen and buffering of carbon dioxide in the acid milieu of the

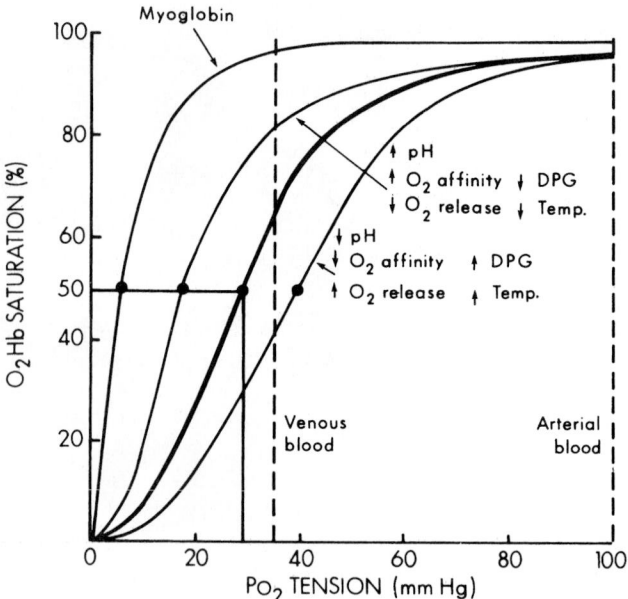

Fig. 36-7 Oxygen-dissociation curves of normal human hemoglobin. *Heavy middle line,* dissociation curve of normal adult blood (temperature 37° C, pH 7.4, Pco_2 35 mm Hg). *Dots,* P_{50} values, partial pressure of oxygen (27 mm Hg) at which hemoglobin solution is 50% oxyhemoglobin and 50% deoxyhemoglobin. If temperature increases, pH decreases, or carbon dioxide tension (Pco_2) increases, the curve shifts to the right. This shift increases release of oxygen from hemoglobin at given oxygen tension by decreasing its oxygen affinity. If temperature decreases, pH rises, or carbon dioxide tension decreases, oxygen-dissociation curve moves to the left. This shift increases oxygen-binding capacity of hemoglobin at given oxygen tension: thus there is a decrease in oxygen release. (From Bauer JD: *Clinical laboratory methods,* ed 9, St. Louis, 1982, Mosby.)

tissues in which carbon dioxide and acid metabolites accumulate and in the more alkaline milieu of the lungs where carbon dioxide is released and oxygen is picked up. The Bohr effect is enhanced by both 2,3-DPG and chloride.

2,3-Diphosphoglycerate

Other molecules influence the structure and function of hemoglobin. Of the factors that affect oxygen release from hemoglobin (temperature, pH, Po_2, Pco_2, and 2,3-DPG), 2,3-DPG is the most important. It is the most abundant glycolytic intermediate in red blood cells and is present at a concentration equimolar with that of deoxyhemoglobin. In oxyhemoglobin the helices of the β-chains are not open enough to permit firm stereospecific binding of 2,3-DPG within the central cavity of the hemoglobin tetramer to the N-terminal valine, the H21 histidine (position 143) and the EF6 lysine (position 82) of the β-chain. Thus, 2,3-DPG binding stabilizes the deoxygenated form at the expense of the oxyhemoglobin form. This, along with other conformational changes in the oxygenated molecule, favors binding

2,3-DPG to the deoxygenated rather than the oxygenated form, reducing the affinity of hemoglobin for oxygen and shifting the oxygen dissociation curve to the right.

$$HBO_2 + DPG \rightleftharpoons Hb \cdot DPG + O_2 \qquad \textit{Eq. 36-2}$$

During anaerobic metabolism, peripheral cells increase production of 2,3-DPG, facilitating oxygen release.

When the pH drops, as in acidosis, the oxygen-dissociation curve moves to the right, but the resulting inhibition of 2,3-DPG corrects the shift by an equal change to the left. An elevated red blood cell pH shifts the dissociation curve to the left, but the rising 2,3-DPG concentration shifts it to the right, returning it to base position (Fig. 36-7). The common denominator of the 2,3-DPG–Bohr effect is the rate of glycolysis, which is stimulated by alkalosis and suppressed by acidosis because the former stimulates phosphofructokinase activity and the latter suppresses it. 2,3-DPG is formed from 1,3-DPG, an intermediary of the Embden-Meyerhoff pathway (Rappaport-Leubering cycle, see Fig. 32-2).

Other chemical derivatives of hemoglobin

Besides oxyhemoglobin and deoxyhemoglobin (see above and in Chapter 25), other chemically modified forms of hemoglobin exist.

Hemoglobin A_1. Hemoglobin A_1 is formed by the postsynthetic, nonenzymatic reaction of various sugars with amino groups of the globin chains. HbA_1 actually consists of four principal components, called HbA_{1a1}, HbA_{1a2}, HbA_{1b}, and HbA_{1c}. Hemoglobin A_{1c}, the major sugar derivative, is produced by the reaction of glucose with the terminal amino group (valine) of the β-chain. The glycosylated hemoglobins are useful for the monitoring of diabetes; other hemoglobins are the adducts of glucose-6-phosphate or fructose-1,6-diphosphate and the β-chain. See Chapter 32 for further discussion of glycosylated hemoglobins.

Carboxyhemoglobin. Carbon monoxide (CO) is a ligand that, like oxygen, binds reversibly to the ferrous ion of hemoglobin. However, it forms a toxic compound, carboxyhemoglobin (CO-Hb). It also binds to other heme-containing proteins, such as myoglobin, cytochrome P-450, and cytochrome oxidase.[4] CO combines with hemoglobin more slowly than oxygen, but, since the union is much firmer, the release of CO is 10,000 times slower than the release of oxygen from oxyhemoglobin. Also, the affinity of hemoglobin for CO is 218 times greater than that for oxygen. Because both CO and O_2 compete for the same binding sites on heme, the presence of CO reduces the concentration of oxyhemoglobin. At a CO concentration of 0.1% in the inhaled air, more than 50% of the hemoglobin is unavailable for O_2 transport. In the presence of CO, the oxyhemoglobin dissociates more slowly because the iron atoms not bound to CO have a higher affinity for O_2, causing the oxygen-dissociation curve to shift to the left. CO-Hb can be identified in blood by spectroscopic, spectrophotometric, chemical, or gas chromatographic techniques.[5] The presence of CO-Hb in blood does not cause substantial error in pulse oximetry,[6] a determination that has great clinical importance.

Methemoglobin. Methemoglobin (Met-Hb) is a form of hemoglobin (with oxy- or deoxy- forms) in which the ferrous ion (Fe^{++}) of hemoglobin has been oxidized to the ferric state (Fe^{+++}) to form ferrihemoglobin. Met-Hb cannot bind oxygen reversibly and is unable to act as an effective oxygen transporter. If Met-Hb is present in high enough concentrations (over 30% of total hemoglobin), *hypoxia* and *cyanosis* (methemoglobinemia) will result. Normally, a small amount of methemoglobin forms continuously in red blood cells; however, this does not exceed 1% of the total hemoglobin because the methemoglobin is reduced back to Hb (see p. 728).

After prolonged exposure to the air, the oxyhemoglobin in normal blood is auto-oxidized and the blood turns brown as methemoglobin is formed. This process is also responsible for the brown color of blood in acid urine.

Hemichromes. Hemichromes are greenish ferric compounds with characteristic absorption spectral profiles. During the oxidation of hemoglobin to Met-Hb superoxide anions are formed, and hydrogen peroxide is produced. As a result, more Met-Hb is formed, and oxidative changes occur in the globin protein. These changes, in the heme group and in the protein, alter the stereochemical binding of the heme to the protein, and the heme iron may form ligands with various side chains in the proteins *(hemichromes)* rather than with the proximal histidine or with oxygen. The heme group can be physically displaced from the protein and precipitate as free ferriheme (or hematin) onto the interior of the red blood cell membrane. Polypeptide chains also precipitate when they are denatured. These hemoglobin breakdown products form inclusions on the interior of the red blood cell membrane, called Heinz bodies, which are responsible for the lysis of the affected red cells.[7] The steps leading to cell lysis are as follows:

Oxyhemoglobin
↓
Methemoglobin
↓
Hemichrome 1, reversible
↓
Hemichrome 2, irreversible
↓
Heinz bodies
↓
Lysis

Hematologists use supravital stains to identify Heinz bodies, which are found in a group of anemias known as Heinz body anemias.

Sulfhemoglobin. Sulfhemoglobin (S-Hb) is a stable compound resulting from the linkage of sulfur to hemoglobin. The toxic effects of certain drugs on hemoglobin lead not only to the formation of methemoglobin, but also to concomitant S-Hb production.[8] Sulfhemoglobinemia appears in some persons after exposure to sulfonamides, phenacetin, acetanilid, and trinitrotoluene. It is not clear why Met-Hb is found in the blood of some individuals whereas S-Hb is seen in the blood of others after exposure to these drugs. The structure of S-Hb is unknown, but sulfur is probably linked to heme. The S-Hb complex is stable and irreversible (thus differing from Met-Hb) and does not disappear from the circulation until affected red blood cells complete their life cycle. Sulfhemoglobin produces anoxia and cyanosis, which clinically are indistinguishable from the anoxia and cyanosis of Met-Hb. Sulfhemoglobin shows a characteristic absorption of light at 620 nm that does not shift when cyanide is added. Rarely, sulfhemoglobin causes Heinz body formation.

NORMAL HUMAN HEMOGLOBINS (Table 36-1)
Hemoglobin A ($\alpha_2\beta_2$)

Hemoglobin A makes up the major portion (95% to 98%) of the adult hemolysate. Small amounts of HbA are produced in the last 6 weeks of fetal life (see Chapter 40), along with the predominant fetal hemoglobin. During the 6 to 12 months post partum, the shift to the adult form of hemoglobin is completed (see below).

Hemoglobin A₂ ($\alpha_2\delta_2$)

Hemoglobin A_2 is a minor component of hemoglobin that makes its first appearance before the completion of intrauterine development (0.2% of cord blood hemolysate) and remains at low concentration (2.5%) throughout adult life. Its exact function is unknown but is probably similar to that of HbA.

Fetal hemoglobin ($\alpha_2\gamma_2$)

Hemoglobin F is the major hemoglobin of fetal life, preceded by the embryonic hemoglobins Gower 1, Gower 2, and Portland. HbF is a mixture of two molecular species in which the γ-chains have either glycine (Gγ) or alanine (Aγ) at position 136. At birth, the HbF GγAγ ratio is about 3:1, whereas in the normal adult the Gγ/Aγ ratio of the small

amount of HbF (less than 1%) is 2:3. In the first months of fetal life, small amounts of HbF are produced along with the Gower hemoglobins, which are replaced by HbF at the end of the second month. From this time to just before birth, the percentage of fetal hemoglobin is about 90%. At birth, the red blood cells contain about 70% to 90% HbF, though higher concentrations have been reported. After birth, HbF decreases rapidly to about 50% to 70% at the end of the first month, 25% to 60% at the end of the second month, and 10% to 30% at the end of the third month. Between 6 months and 12 months, the HbF concentration falls from 8% to 2%; in the second year it falls to 1.8%; and in the third year it falls to 1%. It finally levels off to the adult level of less than 0.4%, a level not detectable by routine laboratory methods.

The functions and molecular characteristics of HbF are as follows:

1. Electrophoretically it is slower than HbA.
2. It resists alkali denaturation, a feature that is the basis of the Singer test for HbF.[28]
3. It is twice as resistant to acid elution as HbA, a characteristic that forms the basis of the Kleihauer elution technique.[29]
4. HbF is oxidized to Met-Hb twice as quickly as HbA, predisposing the newborn to cyanosis.
5. It has a higher oxygen affinity than HbA has, since it binds 2,3-DPG to a lesser degree than adult hemoglobin because of its γ-chain. This characteristic allows oxygen transport across the placental villi, despite their low oxygen concentration (80%).[30]

The molecular properties of HbF allow HbF to function as the primary oxygen carrier for the fetus. The other embryonic hemoglobins have similar properties and are able to combine with oxygen at the low oxygen tension and low pH of interstitial fluid, facilitating fetal growth and development. Embryonic hemoglobins are detectable in red cells by a modification of the Kleihauer method for HbF.

PATHOLOGIC CONDITIONS
Hemoglobinopathies

The inherited disorders of hemoglobin, the *hemoglobinopathies,* are genetic disorders involving the structure and synthesis of one or more of the globin polypeptide chains. Hemoglobinopathies may be divided into several overlapping groups[9]: (1) the structural hemoglobin variants that involve substitution, addition, or deletion of one or more amino acids of the globin chain; (2) the *thalassemias,* a group of disorders in which there is a quantitative defect in globin chain production; (3) combinations of types 1 and 2 that result in complex hemoglobinopathies; and (4) hereditary persistence of fetal hemoglobin, an asymptomatic disorder.

Structural hemoglobin variants

Nomenclature. Hemoglobins A, F, and S were the first hemoglobins to be discovered and were assigned letters. As

Table 36-1   Normal human hemoglobins

Designation	Tetrameric structure	Hemolysate (%) Adult	Hemolysate (%) Newborn
Adult			
HbA	$\alpha_2\beta_2$	95-98	20-30
HbA₂	$\alpha_2\delta_2$	2-3	0.2
Fetal			
HbF	$\alpha_2\gamma_2$	<1	80
Embryonic			
Gower 1	$\zeta_2\epsilon_2$	0	0
Gower 2	$\alpha_2\epsilon_2$	0	0
Hb Portland	$\zeta_2\gamma_2$	0	0

additional variants were discovered, they were assigned successive letters of the alphabet beginning with HbC. Subsequently, hemoglobins were discovered so rapidly that the letters of the alphabet were depleted. Therefore, hemoglobins with similar electrophoretic mobility, but with different structures were distinguished by adding (properly as a subscript) the place of discovery of the new hemoglobin, such as HbC$_{Georgetown}$, HbD$_{Punjab}$. Finally, some hemoglobins are called by the names of the families in which they were first discovered, such as Hb$_{Lepore}$. When the exact amino acid substitution of the new variant and the spatial structure of hemoglobin were determined, the expression became more complex. For instance, HbS evolved into the scientific designation: HbS B6 (A3) Glu → Val. This designation reveals that the substitution is located at the sixth position of the amino acid sequence, in the A3 position of the β-chain. It also shows that the glutamine (Glu) has been replaced by a valine (Val). There are approximately 500 variant hemoglobins identified at present. Some of the more important ones demonstrating clinical disorders are shown in Table 36-2.

Excellent tables on nomenclature, molecular structure, clinical manifestations, and electrophoretic mobility of hemoglobin variants are found in reference 10.

Classification

Hemoglobin variants are classified according to (1) molecular mechanism; (2) clinical and functional manifestations; and (3) electrophoretic behavior.

Molecular mechanisms responsible for structural hemoglobin variants.
Five basic molecular mechanisms are responsible for the structural changes found in most hemoglobin variants: (1) amino acid substitution, (2) deletions and insertions, (3) unequal crossing over (fusion genes), (4) chain elongation, and (5) frame shift variance.[11]

Clinical consequences of structural alterations of hemoglobin molecules.
Structural alterations of the hemoglobin molecule are responsible for a wide range of clinical manifestations. Most mutations are asymptomatic because they do not interfere with hemoglobin function. Others produce disease because they affect the stability, shape, or function of the hemoglobin molecule. A person homozygous for an abnormal hemoglobin may have striking clinical manifestations such as sickle cell anemia, whereas a person heterozygous for abnormal hemoglobin (HbA-HbS) is usually asymptomatic. Some hemoglobins (HbC, HbD, HbE) even in the homozygous state produce only mild symptoms, whereas others are responsible for almost spe-

Table 36-2 Clinical manifestations associated with some abnormal hemoglobins

Disorder	Abnormal Hb	Structural change	Comments
Hemolytic anemia	H	alpha$_2$beta$_2$ → beta$_4$	Unstable hemoglobin occurring in some forms of alpha-thalassemia; precipitation of hemoglobin and hemolysis are accelerated by certain drugs
	S	beta 6 glu → val	Forms molecular aggregates when deoxygenated, producing sickle cell anemia in homozygotes
	C	beta 6 glu → lys	Low solubility lessens plasticity of red cells, causing hemolytic anemia in homozygotes
	D$_{Punjab}$	beta 121 glu → gln	Mechanism unknown
	E	beta 26 glu → lys	
	Zurich	beta 63 his → arg	Unstable hemoglobin precipitated by certain drugs, producing hemolytic anemia in heterozygotes
	Köln	beta 98 val → met	
	Sydney	beta 67 val → ala	
	Santa Ana	beta 88 leu → pro	
	Philly	beta 35 tyr → phe	Unstable hemoglobin causes congenital nonspherocytic
	Gun Hill	beta deletion of 5 residues between 90 and 96	hemolytic anemia in heterozygotes; precipitated hemoglobin tends to form inclusion bodies with red cells, under certain conditions
Cyanosis caused by methemoglobinemia	M$_{Boston}$	alpha 58 his → tyr	Methemoglobin causes cyanosis in heterozygotes; some also have evidence of hemolytic anemia
	M$_{Iwate}$	alpha 87 his → tyr	
	M$_{Hyde Park}$	beta 92 his → tyr	
Cyanosis caused by increased deoxyhemoglobin	Kansas	beta 102 asn → thr	Decreased oxygen affinity of hemoglobin causes cyanosis in heterozygotes
Polycythemia	J$_{Capetown}$	alpha 92 arg → gln	
	Chesapeake	alpha 92 arg → leu	Increased oxygen affinity of hemoglobin hinders release of oxygen to tissues, causing compensatory polycythemia in heterozygotes
	Rainier	beta 145 try → cys	
Hydrops fetalis	Bart's	alpha$_2$gamma$_2$ → gamma$_4$	Unstable hemoglobin with high oxygen affinity occurring in high concentration in stillborn fetuses with homozygous alpha-thalassemia

From Schmidt RM, Brosious EM: *Basic laboratory methods of hemoglobinopathy detection,* Atlanta, 1978, Centers for Disease Control.

cific pathophysiological changes, such as cyanosis and erythrocytosis.

The clinical disorders can be grouped as follows[12] (Table 36-2):

Hemolytic anemias. Intraerythrocytic crystals of HbS and HbC may be formed and cause deformity of the red blood cells. Such deformities are easily recognized by light microscopy, such as the sickle-shaped cells of sickle cell anemia. Unstable hemoglobins and enzyme abnormalities of the hexose-monophosphate shunt are also responsible for intraerythrocytic Heinz body inclusions. The affected cells are prematurely destroyed in the spleen, resulting in a greatly shortened red cell life-span.

Cyanosis. Amino acid substitution near the heme pocket produces *M-hemoglobins,* which result in methemoglobinemia and cyanosis. Cyanosis may also occur because of hemoglobin mutants that result in increased deoxyhemoglobin, that is, Hb Kansas, Hb Beth Israel. Both types of hemoglobin show decreased oxygen affinity.

Erythrocytosis. Amino acid substitution causes high oxygen affinity and tissue hypoxia. Because of the hypoxia, erythropoietin synthesis is stimulated, resulting in an increased production of red blood cells *(erythrocytosis).* Examples are Hb Rainier, Hb Chesapeake, and Hb Ypsilanti.

Hypochromic anemias. The mutation reduces the hemoglobin output. Examples are Hb Lepore and Hb Constant Spring.

Electrophoretic behavior of hemoglobins. Hemoglobin electrophoresis is the most important laboratory test used to diagnose and classify a hemoglobin abnormality (see p. 732). However, no single test can accurately distinguish an abnormal hemoglobin from a thalassemic disorder.

Sickle cell disorders: sickle hemoglobin

Sickling disorders are caused by the homozygous form of the sickle cell gene (sickle cell anemia), the heterozygous form of the sickle cell gene (sickle cell trait), and the combination of either with other structural hemoglobin variants or thalassemias.

Sickle hemoglobin (HbS) results when valine is substituted for the normally occurring glutamine residue and intracellular crystals of deoxygenated HbS form, causing the RBC to sickle.

HbS is not the only hemoglobin that causes RBC to sickle, since red blood cells containing HbC Georgetown, HbI, and Hb Bart's also sickle. Nevertheless, in America and Africa, HbS is the most common hemoglobin variant, with an incidence of the heterozygous form of approximately 8% in American blacks and 30% in African blacks. HbS can also be found in nonblack inhabitants in the areas bordering Africa. In Africa the high frequency of the sickle cell gene has persisted because heterozygotes for HbS are somewhat protected from malaria since *Plasmodium* organisms fail to grow in HbS-containing red blood cells.[13]

Molecular mechanism of sickling

The substitution of valine for the normal glutamic acid at position 6 in the β-chain results in a hemoglobin whose deoxy form (deoxy-Hbs) polymerizes within the red blood cells and forms long fibers readily visible on electron microscopy of red cells from patients homozygous for the β^S mutation. Oxyhemoglobin S does *not* form such fibers.

Several facts about the polymerization are relevant to the pathogenesis of the sickle configuration—and to possible therapeutic intervention. The polymerization occurs in two phases. The first of these, the slow-nucleation (or "delay") phase, reflects the initial association of a few molecules of deoxy-HbS. This phase varies in duration from milliseconds to a few minutes, depending on several factors, including temperature and the presence of hemoglobins other than HbS.

The duration also depends, exponentially, on the concentration of HbS. Thus, a prolonged delay time, resulting from a decreased concentration of HbS within the red blood cell, might permit the deoxygenated cell to traverse the microcirculation without sickling. Factors that favor increasing polymerization of HbS within red cells and thus the severity of the disease have their effect by increasing the relative abundance of deoxy-HbS. Such factors include a decrease in Po_2, increased organic phosphates, increased hydrogen-ion concentrations, and increased temperature.[14] The varying clinical severity of the different sickle syndromes is depicted in Table 36-3.

Pathophysiology of sickle cell disease

HbS is inherited as an autosomal codominant trait. The sickle-shaped cells temporarily or permanently block microcirculation, and the resulting stasis leads to hypoxia and ischemic infarcts of various organs including liver, kidneys, spleen, lungs, heart, bones, and nervous system. Such infarcts lead to increased morbidity and, if located in a vital area, cause death.[15] The vascular endothelial lining, damaged by lack of oxygen, attracts platelets, which initiate the process of disseminated intravascular coagulation.[16]

Sickled cells have a greatly shortened life-span. The ensuing hemolytic anemia is augmented by the inability of the

Table 36-3 Varying clinical severity of the different sickle syndromes

Genotype	% of hemoglobin S	% of non-S hemoglobin	Clinical severity
SA	30-40	60-70 (A)	0
SF*	70	30 (F)	0
SS	80-90	5-15 (F)	++/++++
S-thalassemia	80	20 (A + F)	+/+++
SC	50	50 (C)	+/+++
SO.SD	30-40	60-70 (O.D)	++/++++

From Bunn HF: Sickle cell anemia and other hemoglobinopathies. In Beck WS, editor: *Hematology,* Cambridge, Mass., 1981, MIT Press.
*Double heterozygous state for hemoglobin S and hereditary persistence of fetal hemoglobin.

bone marrow to respond adequately to the anemia because of ineffective erythropoiesis. The increased red blood cell destruction is responsible for hyperbilirubinemia, reticulocytosis, bone marrow erythroid hyperplasia, gallbladder pigment stones, and osteoporosis as a result of the expanding bone marrow.

Sickle cells exhibit oxygen-transport abnormalities.[16] In sickled cells the oxygen-dissociation curve is shifted to the right. The resulting decreased oxygen affinity favors the release of oxygen at higher oxygen tensions but also supports the formation of deoxyhemoglobin and sickling.[9] The shift to the right of the oxygen equilibrium is caused by an elevated 2,3-DPG concentration and by an HbS polymerization–mediated defect.

Sickle cell trait (HbAS)

Persons with sickle cell trait are usually asymptomatic and have a normal hemogram (red blood cell profile, including red blood cell count, mean corpuscular volume [MCV], and mean corpuscular hemoglobin [MCH]) and red blood cell survival. The demonstration of HbS is usually of no clinical significance, since a normal HbA gene has been inherited along with the HbS gene, but should indicate the need for genetic counseling. There are rare reports of sickling complications in HbAS patients. They include (1) spontaneous hematuria in about 3% of patients and more frequently hyposthenuria because of the impairment of the concentrating power of the kidneys, both signs pointing to sickling within the blood vessels of the medulla; (2) rupture of the infarcted spleen; (3) sickling crisis at elevated altitudes; and (4) rarely, proliferative retinopathy. Recently, a large study on military personnel with the sickle cell trait undergoing basic training showed a significant increase in sudden death.[17] The exact cause of this in individuals with the sickle cell trait is not known.

Sickle cell anemia (HbSS)

Sickle cell anemia is a chronic, moderate to severe, hemolytic anemia in a person homozygous for HbS having inherited the HbS gene from both parents. The finding of HbSS is useful in order to differentiate sickle cell anemia from sickle cell–β-thalassemia or HbS hereditary persistence of HbF. The disease is not evident at birth and does not manifest itself until the γ-chains of the newborn are replaced by βS-chains after 3 to 6 months of life.

The clinical severity of HbSS disease varies from patient to patient. Such variation has been further clarified by the investigation of haplotypes. These genetic variations (Benin, Bantu, Senegal) are of hematologic, genetic, and anthropologic interest, since they offer new insights in the sickling disorders.[18] Clinical manifestations may be divided into acute and chronic episodes. Acute problems result from vaso-occlusive crises involving several areas, as well as acute hematologic crises (see box below).

Splenic crisis may result from sudden trapping of blood in the spleen. Chronic manifestations of sickle cell disease usually appear after midchildhood. These include disturbances in growth and development, bone and joint disease, and organ damage involving cardiovascular, pulmonary, hepatobiliary, genitourinary, ocular, and dermatologic systems. Renal failure may occur in many patients with sickle cell anemia, probably as the result of glomerular capillary disease.

Hemoglobin values hover around 70 to 80 g/L accompanied by a greatly elevated reticulocytosis (10%). The hemoglobin electrophoretogram shows absence of HbA (no βA-chains), 80% to 95% HbS, 2% to 4% HbA$_2$, and 2% to 20% HbF. Three outstanding biochemical findings include hyperuricemia in patients with altered tubular function; reduced zinc levels in plasma, red cells, and hair; high lactate dehydrogenase levels in patients in crisis. Treatment of HbSS is designed to (1) inhibit HbS polymerization, (2) decrease intracellular levels of total Hb, and (3) increase the concentration of HbF. Hydroxyurea has been the most effective drug to affect increased HbF production and decreased sickling.

Sickle cell–HbC disease

Sickle cell–HbC disease has a relatively high incidence (1:833 births among blacks in the United States) because HbS and HbC are common hemoglobin variants. The patient inherits one abnormal gene from each parent, and the resulting disease is a mild to moderate hemolytic anemia associated with the same vaso-occlusive complications seen in sickle cell disease. However, these complications usually occur with a lower frequency. Since genes in this disease are allelic β-chain mutations, no normal β-chains are formed and HbA is absent.

Peripheral blood smear reveals many *target cells,* rare sickle cells and red cells with straight or curved crystals. The hemoglobin values range from 100 to 130 g/L, with

---

Acute Clinical Manifestations of HbSS

Hematological
Accelerated hemolytic anemia
Megaloblastic anemia
Aplastic crisis

Vaso-occlusive
Bone and joints
Abdomen, spleen
Lungs
Central nervous system
Back

only HbC and HbS bands seen on electrophoresis. The reticulocyte count varies from 3% to 10%.

HbC trait and disease

HbC trait (HbAC) affects about 3% of American blacks. It is asymptomatic, and the peripheral blood smear is normal, except for a few target cells. Electrophoresis patterns show about 30% to 40% HbC, 50% to 60% HbA, 3% to 4% HbA_2, and 7% HbF.

Hemoglobin C disease (HbCC)

The homozygous form is rare, occurring in 1 out of 10,000 American blacks, and is asymptomatic.

Hemoglobin E trait and disease

The variant HbE, or B26 Glu $\rightarrow$ Lys, is the second most common hemoglobin abnormality worldwide. Because of the large influx of refugees from Southeast Asia, an increasing number of patients with HbE are encountered in the United States. HbE trait, though clinically silent, exhibits moderately severe *microcytosis* and no anemia. The amount of HbE in HbE trait is 30% to 35%. This is lower than expected for a heterozygous condition; for example, 45% HbS is observed in patients with sickle cell trait. This discrepancy is attributable to the thalassemia-like defect of the HbE gene.

Patients with HbE disease exhibit mild microcytic, normochromic anemia with many target cells, conferring a thalassemic phenotype.

Since many Southeast Asians have α and β thalassemic gene abnormalities, combinations of HbE with these genes become much more clinically significant. For example, patients with HbE-β^0 thalassemia have significant anemia and require transfusions; a clinical situation similar to that seen with thalassemia intermedia.[19]

Unstable hemoglobin disorder

The unstable hemoglobins are structural variants of HbA, in which the mutant hemoglobin is less stable than normal hemoglobin. Approximately 150 variants of HbA have been shown to be unstable in in vitro tests. However, only 70 have been shown to have significant clinical manifestation, usually hemolysis.[20] The molecular distortion responsible for unstable hemoglobin produces a series of pathophysiologic effects that one can evaluate by laboratory methods, though they are not equally expressed by all unstable hemoglobins. They are (1) hemolytic anemia, (2) increased methemoglobin and sulfhemoglobin production, (3) hemichrome formation, (4) inclusion (Heinz) body formation, (5) altered oxygen dissociation, (6) drug sensitivity, (7) altered electrophoretic mobility (rare), (8) altered response to hemoglobin stability tests, and (9) passage of dark urine. The deeply pigmented urine is caused by mesobilifuscin, a dipyrrole derived from the catabolism of Heinz bodies or free heme.[21]

THALASSEMIAS

Definitions

Thalassemias are inherited hemoglobinopathies resulting from a decreased rate of production of one or more globin chains of hemoglobin.[9,22] They are quantitative hemoglobinopathies that differ from the qualitative hemoglobinopathies by the fact that the structure of the affected globin chain (or chains) is normal, but its synthesis is reduced or absent. The decreased hemoglobin synthesis results in decreased red blood cell hemoglobin, hypochromia, microcytosis, and a variable degree of hemolysis.

Defective synthesis of one set of globin chains results in excess production of the unaffected pair[9] (imbalanced globin-chain synthesis), which precipitates in the red blood cells in the form of inclusion bodies, which causes the hemolysis.

Classification

The older classification of thalassemias as *thalassemia major, intermedia, minor,* and *minima* describes the clinical severity of the disorder and disregards the genetic makeup. The preferred genetic classification is based on the particular deficient polypeptide chain. In α-thalassemia, the synthesis of α-chains is diminished, in β-thalassemia the synthesis of β-chains is diminished. The major forms of thalassemia are depicted in Table 36-4.

Thalassemias involving γ, ϵ, or ζ genes may lead to fetal or embryonic death.[22] A thalassemia-like condition that is asymptomatic is the hereditary persistence of fetal hemoglobin (HPFH). The inheritance of thalassemia is autosomal and is similar to that of HbS. From the clinical viewpoint, it is recessive because the heterozygous form is asymptomatic. Similar to the HbS(β^S) gene, the thalassemia gene may express itself in homozygous, heterozygous, and doubly heterozygous states.

The clinical range varies from normal to a severe, life-threatening condition and can include growth retardation, hepatomegaly, bone overgrowth, bone pain, and jaundice.

Alpha-thalassemias

The alpha (α)-thalassemias are a group of genetic disorders that result in defective α-chain synthesis. The α-thalassemias are more difficult to diagnose since characteristic elevations in HbA_2 or HbF seen in the β-thalassemias are not observed. Diminished α-chain synthesis depresses the production of HbA, HbF, and HbA_2 because they contain α-chains, and it leads to excess β- and γ-chains, which polymerize to the tetrameric forms γ_4 (Hb Bart's) and β_4 (HbH). The presence of these hemoglobins is the hallmark of α-thalassemia. Four classical α-thalassemias include α-thalassemia-2 trait (silent carrier) in which one of the four α-globin gene loci fails to function; α-thalassemia-1 trait (mild hypochromic anemia) with two dysfunctional loci; HbH (moderate severe hemolytic anemia) with three loci affected; and Hb Bart's (hydrops fetalis incompatible with

Table 36-4   Laboratory findings in α-thalassemias

Genotype	Anemia (hypochromic)		Hb types	α-Chain deletion
α-Thalassemia 1 trait	±	Birth:	Hb Bart's 5%-10%	2
			HbCS 1%-2%	
		Adult:	HbA,A$_2$,F	
α-Thalassemia 1/α-thalassemia 1 (hydrops)	+++	Birth:	Hb Bart's 80%	4
			Traces of HbH and Portland	
		Adult:	Not compatible with life	
α-Thalassemia 2/trait	±	Birth:	Hb Bart's 1%-2%	1
			HbCS 1%-2%	
		Adult:	HbA,A$_2$,F	
α-Thalassemia 1/α-thalassemia 2 (HbH disease)	± (Inclusions)	Birth:	Hb Bart's 1%-15%	3
			HbH 4%-30%	
		Adult:	HbA,A$_2$,F	
			HBH 8%-10%	
α-Thalassemia 1/HbCS (Hb H/CS)	++ (Inclusions)	Birth:	Hb Bart's	2 plus α-chain termination mutation
			HbH, HbCS	
		Adult:	HbH	
			HbA,A$_2$,F,CS	
α-Thalassemia 2/HbCS	+	Birth:	Hb Bart's	1 plus α-chain termination mutation
		Adult:	HbA, CS	
HbCS/HbCS	+	Birth:	Hb Bart's	α-chain termination mutation
		Adult:	HbA,A$_2$,F,CS	

life) in which all four loci are affected. α-thalassemia may also result from the production of Hb Constant Spring (HbCS). This hemoglobin is the result of a mutation in the terminal codon of the 3′ portion of DNA that normally stops α-chain production. Therefore, HbCS contains 172 amino acids in the α-chain rather than 141. Production of this elongated α-chain causes an inadequacy of α-chains relative to non–α-chains with a resultant thalassemic condition (Table 36-4).

Beta-thalassemias

The beta (β)-thalassemias are a group of genetic disorders that result in diminished (β$^+$ and β^{++} thalassemias) or absent (β^0-thalassemia) β-chain synthesis. They are inherited in a multitude of genetic combinations responsible for a heterogeneous group of clinical syndromes. Like α-thalassemia, β-thalassemia is transmitted as a mendelian autosomal recessive characteristic. The output of β-chains is reduced or absent because of a defect in transcription of the β-thalassemia genes. Currently point mutations that result in the various β-thalassemias number approximately 90. β-thalassemia major, also known as Cooley's anemia, or homozygous β-thalassemia, is a clinically severe disorder caused by the inheritance of two β-thalassemia alleles, one on each copy of chromosome 11. The hypochromic anemia of thalassemia major is so severe that lifetime blood transfusions are usually required.

β-thalassemias are widely distributed throughout the world but occur most frequently in the Mediterranean population; they also occur in Southeast Asia, the Middle East, India, and Pakistan. In Greeks and in American blacks the β$^+$-thalassemia is most common, whereas in Italy the β^0 is predominant.

Heterozygous β-thalassemia, whether β$^+$ or β^0, is an asymptomatic disorder that may or may not be associated with a mild degree of anemia.[23] It is the most commonly found thalassemia in North America.[22] Characteristically there is a slight to moderate erythrocytosis of poorly hemoglobinized red blood cells. The MCH and the MCV are always strikingly decreased. The mean corpuscular hemoglobin content is variable.

The heterozygous carrier states have also been called thalassemia minor and thalassemia minima. The designation thalassemia intermedia describes clinical manifestations of a form of β-thalassemia more severe than the traits and milder than the homozygous form.

Homozygous β^0-thalassemia leads to complete suppression of β-chain synthesis and to complete absence of HbA. It is the cause of a severe lethal transfusion-dependent hemolytic anemia accompanied by characteristic clinical and hematological findings. Homozygous β$^+$ thalassemia is a heterogeneous disorder that, on the basis of the amount of HbA synthesized, is best divided into three main types. Type 1, in which 5% to 15% HbA is synthesized, is the Mediterranean and Oriental form characterized by a severe transfusion-dependent anemia. Type 2, of African background, has 20% to 30% HbA and is responsible for a milder disease. Type 3 leads to a mild form of thalassemia intermedia.[9]

Pregnancy may lead to severe anemia in patients with thalassemia trait.[23] The hemoglobin electrophoretogram shows a slightly elevated HbF (1% to 7%) in 50% of cases and a diagnostic elevation of A$_2$ (3.5% to 7.5%).[22] Distribution of HbF within the red blood cells demonstrated by acid elution technique reveals a heterogeneous pattern.

Hereditary persistence of fetal hemoglobin (HPFH)

HPFH consists of a group of rare conditions characterized by continued synthesis of high levels of HbF in adult life. No deleterious effects on patients are observed, and such an absence supports the concept that prevention or reversal of the switch from the fetal hemoglobin to the adult hemoglobin would benefit patients with sickle cell anemia and β-thalassemia. It is considered to be a form of δβ-thalassemia[24] because the persistence of the γ-chain synthesis compensates for the deficient δ- and β-chain production.

Two major types of HPFH exist: (1) pancellular and (2) heterocellular. The pancellular type has very high levels of fetal hemoglobin synthesis and uniform distribution of HbF among all red blood cells. It can be further divided by mutation type into deletional and nondeletional forms. HPHF shows ethnic differences in that blacks with heterozygous pancellular deletional disease have HbF ranges between 15% and 35% and contains γ^{Gly} and γ^{Ala} chains in a ratio of 2:3. On the other hand, Greeks with pancellular nondeletional HPFH demonstrate lower HbF levels (10% to 20%) and contain 90% γ^{Ala}.[24]

A few black patients may have homozygous HPFH. All the Hb within the red cells is HbF. These patients demonstrate mild microcytic hypochromic erythrocytes but no anemia.

HPFH–β-thalassemia is similar to the β-thalassemia trait except for a greater proportion and regular distribution of HbF in the red blood cells.[25] Some patients with HPFH–δβ-thalassemia may have a more severe clinical condition similar to thalassemia intermedia.

Heterocellular HPFH seems to result from mutations outside the globin gene cluster and results in a variable increase in the number of F cells. HbF levels are usually lower than those in the pancellular forms.

Methemoglobinemia

Methemoglobinemia is classified into acquired and hereditary forms.

Acquired methemoglobinemia. Normal individuals develop methemoglobinemia after exposure to agents that increase methemoglobin production beyond the capacity of the methemoglobin-reducing pathways. Most agents capable of producing methemoglobinemia are aromatic compounds containing amino, hydroxy, or nitro functional groups. Some of the agents responsible for methemoglobinemia include nitrites, nitrates, sulfonamides, aniline dyes (laundry markings), acetanilid, phenacetin, and Pyridium (phenazopyridine HCl). The nitrites and nitrates account for the majority of the occurrences. The blood may be chocolate-brown in color. Symptoms vary in intensity, depending on the level of methemoglobin.

Hereditary methemoglobinemia. Hereditary methemoglobinemia can be subdivided into two forms: one resulting from mutations leading to NADH methemoglobin reductase deficiency and the other resulting in M hemoglobin accumulation because of an amino acid substitution in the globin chain that stabilizes methemoglobin, rendering it poorly susceptible to subsequent reduction.

Four metabolic pathways for the reduction of the methemoglobin to hemoglobin are available[26]: (1) The NADH methemoglobin reductase pathway, (2) the reverse (NADPH) methemoglobin reductase pathway, (3) the reduction by ascorbic acid, and (4) the reduction by reduced glutathione. Methemoglobinemia caused by an inherited deficiency of NADH methemoglobin reductase is transmitted as an autosomal recessive trait. M hemoglobins show a recessive inheritance pattern and, unlike many hemoglobinopathies, do not produce hemolytic anemias. The mutation causes the formation of an abnormally stable methemoglobin. This stability is attributable to amino acid substitution in or near the heme pocket resulting in direct hemeglobin bonding. Tyrosine is substituted for histidine at or across from the heme-binding site in many of the M hemoglobins. HbM_{Iwate} and M_{Boston} have this substitution in the α-chain, whereas HbS $M_{Hyde\ Park}$ and $M_{Saskatoon}$ have it in the β-chain. Methemoglobin rarely exceeds 25% to 30% in these individuals. If α-chains are involved, the cyanosis may be present at birth, whereas β-chain substitutions are responsible for cyanosis in later months because of the later appearance of these chains.[27]

Clinically, patients with hereditary methemoglobinemia have erythrocytosis and slate gray cyanosis from birth, which is not associated with cardiopulmonary disease. Methemoglobin concentrations of 10% to 20% of the total hemoglobin produce cyanosis but no other ill effects. Methemoglobin concentrations of 30% may be responsible for headache and dyspnea, and concentrations of 70% and over may be fatal. A low incidence of mental retardation and early death can be observed in cases of methemoglobinemia caused by NADH methemoglobin reductase deficiency, a disease that lends itself to prenatal diagnosis.[27]

CHANGE OF ANALYTE IN DISEASE
Interpretation of hemoglobin values

The mean and reference intervals for hemoglobin in healthy adults are 151 (136 to 163) g/L for men and 135 (120 to 150) g/L for women. The values of hemoglobin vary greatly for newborns, infants, children up to puberty, and adults (Table 36-5).

Hemoglobin concentrations are influenced by physiological variations and pathological processes. The physiological variations include age, sex, physical exercise, posture, dehydration, and altitude. The influence exerted by age is readily apparent in Table 36-5. During puberty the male hemoglobin level increases over the female value secondary to the influence of testosterone. Strong exercise raises the hemoglobin level probably through fluid loss, and a transient increase is also experienced after one changes from

Table 36-5 Reference intervals for hemoglobin in grams per liter in "apparently healthy" subjects, white and black

Subjects	Mean (reference interval)
Adult men	151 (139-163)
Adult women	135 (120-150)
Boys	
Birth	200 (185-215)
1 mo	170 (155-185)
3 mo	150 (135-165)
6 mo	140 (130-160)
9 mo	130 (120-140)
1 yr	121 (100-140)
2 yr	123 (105-142)
4 yr	126 (112-143)
8 yr	134 (120-148)
14 yr	140 (125-150)
Girls	
Birth	195 (180-210)
1 mo	170 (158-189)
3 mo	148 (133-164)
6 mo	138 (128-148)
9 mo	128 (117-139)
1 yr	122 (100-140)
2 yr	122 (105-142)
4 yr	127 (113-142)
8 yr	130 (115-145)
14 yr	132 (116-148)

From Miale JB: *Laboratory medicine: hematology*, ed 6, St. Louis, 1982, Mosby.

the recumbent to the standing position. Dehydration is responsible for a rise in hemoglobin concentration of such magnitude as to mask a significant anemia. High altitude is responsible for increased hemoglobin levels because of the erythropoietin-stimulating effect of hypoxia.

There are three main causes of anemia: an impaired production, increased destruction, and excessive blood loss. Impaired production occurs with aplastic anemias; increased destruction occurs with the hemolytic anemia; and excessive blood loss usually occurs in iron-deficiency anemia. The reticulocyte count is usually depressed in chronic iron deficiency, reflecting the effect of iron lack on erythropoiesis.

Increased hemoglobin values are encountered in polycythemia vera, erythrocytosis, dehydration, newborn chronic heart and lung disease, high altitude, renal cysts, and numerous erythropoietin-producing tumors.

HbF

In normal adults, the concentration of F cells is fairly constant at 0.2% to 0.7%, but there are both genetic and acquired hematological conditions in which the concentration is increased. The genetic disorders include thalassemias (β and $\delta\beta$), hereditary persistence of HbF, sickle cell anemia, and unstable β-chain variants. The acquired conditions include pregnancy at about midterm, recovery from bone marrow depression,[28] leukemias (highest values in Philadelphia

chromosome–negative juvenile chronic myelocytic leukemia), thyrotoxicosis, and hepatoma.[29,30]

HbA$_{1c}$

HbA$_{1c}$ levels depend on the time-integrated blood levels of glucose. See Chapter 32 for a more detailed discussion. HbA$_{1c}$ levels are decreased in hemolytic anemia because the red blood cell life-span is shortened by lysis[31] and in hemoglobinopathies in which there is decreased HbA (though the percentage of HbA$_{1c}$ in relation to total HbA may be normal).

Carboxyhemoglobin (CO-Hb)

Some carboxyhemoglobin produced endogenously as 1 mole of CO is generated by the degradation of 1 mole of heme to bilirubin (see Chapter 35). Although this endogenous production of carboxyhemoglobin can present a hazard when exhaled air is concentrated in poorly ventilated, small spaces, the exogenous generation of CO from combustion of organic material in confined spaces causes intoxication. Exogenous CO is derived from the exhaust of automobiles and from industrial pollutants such as coal gas, charcoal burning, and tobacco smoke. In the absence of exogenous CO, the endogenous CO-Hb concentration is 0.2% to 0.8%. Co-Hb levels can be elevated in hemolytic anemias,[32] and in smokers the Co-Hb may vary from 4% to 20%. In smokers who have a greater exposure to CO, the average level may be 10%.

Because of the firm binding of CO to hemoglobin, long exposure to even low CO concentrations can lead to toxic accumulations to which the most oxygen-dependent organs, such as brain and heart, are most susceptible. Mild symptoms such as slight headache and slight dyspnea on exertion can occur at levels of 10% to 15% saturation. At levels of 20% to 30%, the headaches will be more severe and will be accompanied by impaired vision and judgment. Levels of more than 50% cause increasingly severe symptoms, coma, and convulsions, and levels of 60% and over are usually fatal, though death has occurred at levels as low as 20%. The half-life of elimination of CO is about 4 hours for a person breathing atmospheric air, but in smokers the level may remain high.[33] Chronic exposure to CO may be responsible for a relative polycythemia.[34] Carboxyhemoglobin produces a cherry-red color of the blood and skin. Sometimes the blood may have a violet tinge because of the simultaneous presence of moderate quantities of reduced hemoglobin. Exposure to toxic levels of CO is treated with oxygen, often at elevated pressures (hyperbaric treatment), in order to displace CO from hemoglobin. Both exposure and therapy are closely followed by blood-gas analysis for CO-Hb.

Oxygen saturation

Clinically, oxygen saturation is used as an indicator of tissue hypoxia or hyperoxia. Tissue hypoxia is produced by decreased oxygen content of inspired air, as in high altitude, or by decreased alveolar capillary oxygen exchange in the lungs, as in pulmonary fibrosis, emphysema, and chronic heart disease with a left-to-right shunt. Tissue hypoxia is also produced (1) by a defect in the erythrocytic oxygen transport as in severe anemia, (2) when hemoglobin ligands are present that prevent oxygen binding, such as carboxyhemoglobin, sulfhemoglobin, and methemoglobin, (3) in hemoglobinopathies, (4) in inappropriate concentrations of erythrocytic 2,3-DPG, and (5) in intraerythrocytic enzyme deficiencies. Therapeutic hyperoxia must be carefully monitored because of danger of oxygen toxicity. In newborns it can be responsible for retrolental fibroplasia and in adults for hyaline membrane disease of the lungs (adult respiratory distress syndrome).

2,3-Diphosphoglycerate

DPG and hemoglobin interaction in hypoxia are related to the increased intraerythrocytic levels of deoxyhemoglobin, which bind large amounts of DPG. This binding results in a feedback mechanism that stimulates glycolysis and DPG synthesis. Increased deoxyhemoglobin concentrations raise the pH, which in turn also stimulates the synthesis of DPG. Carrell and Lehman (1979) emphasize that there is a reciprocal relationship between hemoglobin and DPG concentrations. Pyruvate kinase deficiency leads to a buildup of DPG, decreased oxygen affinity, and a low hemoglobin concentration. Hexokinase deficiency leads to a decrease in DPG and to a compensatory erythropoietic response with increased hemoglobin values. Many hemoglobin mutations result in an increased oxygen affinity by the abnormal hemoglobin, and some increase this affinity further by impairing DPG binding, such as $HbS_{Shepherds\ Bush}$, HbS_{Ohio}, $HbS_{Little\ Rock}$.

Other hemoglobins

The HbF concentration can vary from 10% to 90%, and the HbF distribution in the red blood cells as determined by the Kleihauer technique can be heterogeneous. Possible abnormal cellular distribution patterns are as follows:

- *Separate cell patterns.* Red blood cells containing HbA or HbF are observed in cases of fetal-maternal hemorrhage if the mother's blood is examined or in cases of maternal-fetal hemorrhage if the infant's blood is examined.
- *Even distribution.* HbA and HbF are equally distributed in all the red blood cells. This distribution is observed in hereditary persistence of HbF (HPF).
- *Uneven distribution.* Red blood cells have varying amounts of HbA and HbF. This pattern is seen in thalassemia, sickle cell disease, Fanconi's anemia, and hereditary spherocytosis.

The HbA_2 concentration may vary from 1.4% to 20%, including low, normal, elevated, and very high values. The concentration of HbA_2 is increased in β-thalassemia, β-chain unstable hemoglobinemias, sickle cell trait, megaloblastic anemias, and hyperthyroidism. Normal or decreased values are seen in α-thalassemias, δβ-thalassemias (Lepore heterozygotes), δ-thalassemia, and hereditary persistence of fetal hemoglobin. In hemoglobin Lepore homozygotes, HbA_2 is absent because there is no δ-chain synthesis. HbA_2 is decreased in acquired disorders such as iron deficiency, sideroblastic anemias, and lead poisoning.

In homozygous β-thalassemia, the A_2 value, even if it is low or normal in the patient, will be high in both parents. If the HbA_2 level in the patient is expressed as a percentage of the total hemoglobin, it spans the previously mentioned range from low to high, but if it is expressed in relation to the HbA value only, the ratio is decreased in all cases of β-thalassemia, that is, the A/A_2 ratio is about 10:1 as compared to the normal A/A_2 ratio of about 40:1. If the HbA_2 level is greatly increased, HbF is normal or only slightly elevated and vice versa. In $β^0$-thalassemia, there is a total absence of HbA, and so the patient's hemoglobin consists only of HbF and HbA_2, whereas in $β^+$-thalassemia diminished amounts of HbA are found (5% to 20%). In both these β-thalassemias, free α-chains may be seen close to the application point of the electrophoretogram at alkaline pH. The severe reduction in β-globin chains leads to a β/α ratio of less than 0.25:0.3. Some of the more common hemoglobinopathies evaluated by cellulose acetate, pH 8.6, and citrate agar, pH 6.0 to 6.2, electrophoresis are depicted on p. 733.

Other related biochemical findings

Because of the hemolytic components of the anemia in most hemoglobinopathies, serum unconjugated bilirubin levels are elevated, and haptoglobin is decreased or absent. Serum aspartate aminotransferase, lactate dehydrogenase, and erythropoietin concentrations are also raised. The erythropoietin elevation is responsible for the 20% to 30% increase in erythropoietic marrow and is a result of the anemia and high oxygen affinity of HbF, which further increases the tissue anoxia. The liver involvement (transfusion hemosiderosis) can lead to a bleeding tendency. Gross examination of the urine may show the brown color of dipyrroles caused by excessive hemolysis.

Use of hemogram results to differentiate iron deficiency from thalassemias

Various formulas exist to differentiate iron deficiency from milder forms of thalassemia. One such formula is the discriminant function (DF):

$$DF = MCV - RBC - (5 \times Hb) - 3.4 \qquad \textit{Eq. 36-3}$$

where MCV is in fL, RBC is in millions/mm^3, and Hb is in g% (g/dL). The 3.4 is an instrument constant and varies with the instrument. A positive DF result is suggestive of iron deficiency, whereas a negative DF result is suggestive of a

Table 36-6   Methods of haptoglobin measurement

Method	Principle	Usage	Comments
1. Nephelometry	Reaction of haptoglobin with antihaptoglobin antibody results in formation of antigen-antibody complexes which scatter light	Most common method in use	Precise, automated; requires specialized instrumentation
2. Radial immunodiffusion (RID)	Diffusion of serum containing haptoglobin into gel containing antihaptoglobin antibody results in formation of precipitin ring. Diameter or area of ring is directly related to haptoglobin concentration	Frequently used	Not automated; less precise than nephelometry

thalassemia. EXAMPLE: A patient with MCV of 65 fL, Hb of 13 g/dL, and RBC of 6 million/mm^3: DF = 65 − 6 − (5 × 13) − 3.4 = −9.4. The example indicates a diagnosis of thalassemia minor. A simpler formula is the ratio $\dfrac{\text{MCV}}{\text{RBC}}$. Values of this ratio greater than 13 are associated with iron-deficiency anemia; values less than 13 are associated with thalassemias. In the above example the ratio would be 10.8.

METHODS OF ANALYSIS
Haptoglobin
STEVEN C. KAZMIERCZAK

Principles of analysis and current usage   Haptoglobin is an acute-phase glycoprotein that becomes increased in blood after acute disease or shock. The protein binds free hemoglobin thereby facilitating removal of hemoglobin by the reticuloendothelial system. Thus haptoglobin becomes decreased in intravascular hemolysis as a result of binding with hemoglobin and its subsequent removal. Decreased haptoglobin concentrations are generally indicative of erythrocyte destruction. However, individuals with simultaneous inflammation and hemolysis may show low, normal, or even increased haptoglobin concentrations.

The methods of choice for measuring haptoglobin concentrations are immunological. These include immunonephelometry (Table 36-6, method 1) and radial immunodiffusion (RID) (Table 36-6, method 2). Immunonephelometric techniques for haptoglobin are based on the amount of light scatter that occurs when serum containing haptoglobin is mixed with reagent containing antihaptoglobin antibody; the amount of light scatter is directly proportional to haptoglobin concentrations within the sample.[35] A nephelometric method based on the rate of formation of the antibody-antigen complex has also been described.[36] The immunonephelometric methods have the advantages of small sample-size requirements, fast turnaround time, and good precision. Drawbacks to the technique include high reagent costs and the need for specialized instrumentation. See Chapter 12 for further discussions of these two techniques.

The RID method for serum haptoglobin is based on measurement of a precipitin ring that is formed as serum containing haptoglobin diffuses into a thin, two-dimensional gel containing antihaptoglobin antibody. The concentration of haptoglobin in the sample is proportional to the diameter of the precipitin ring that is formed (see also Chapter 11). Measurement of the precipitin rings may be performed by one of two methods. In the first technique, the RID plate is incubated until enlargement of the precipitin ring ceases and equilibrium is reached.[37] The concentration of haptoglobin is obtained by comparison of the ring diameter to a standard curve obtained with reference sera. Unfortunately, this method takes approximately 48 hours for full development of the precipitin rings to occur.

In an effort to obtain results more quickly, before full development of the rings occurs, a nonequilibrium technique may be utilized. In this technique the precipitin rings are measured before they reach their full size and results can usually be obtained within 18 hours. However, the precision of the nonequilibrium technique is much worse than the equilibrium method.

The RID technique has the advantage of small sample-size requirements, ease of use, minimal equipment costs, and acceptable precision. The main disadvantage is the relatively long incubation time required for development of the precipitin rings.

Specimen   Serum free of hemolysis is the required specimen. Serum may be stored for several days at 2° to 8° C. If longer storage is required, specimens should be frozen at −20° C. Repeated freeze-thaw cycles should be avoided to minimize the risk of haptoglobin denaturation.

Reference interval   The normal reference interval for haptoglobin in adults is 600 to 2700 mg/L (7.0 to 31.8 μmol/L). Haptoglobin concentrations in newborns is low to undetectable; however, adult concentrations are usually attained by 4 months of age. No sex-related differences for haptoglobin have been detected.[39]

Hemoglobin F
STEVEN C. KAZMIERCZAK

Principles of analysis   Quantitation of HbF can be accomplished by a variety of methods. Perhaps the simplest procedure is the alkali denaturation test (Table 36-7, method 1). This method is based on the relative resistance of HbF to denaturation by an alkali.[40,41] Sodium hydroxide is typically added to the test solution to convert oxyhemoglobin to hematin. After the addition of alkali, the blood of adults, which contains low concentrations of HbF, quickly changes from a pinkish color (from the oxy-HbA) to a brownish yellow (from the alkaline hematin). The denatured HbA can be precipi-

Table 36-7   Methods of hemoglobin F analysis

Method	Principle	Usage	Comments
1. Alkali denaturation	Hemoglobins other than HbF are denatured by addition of alkali (NaOH). Denatured hemoglobins may be precipitated with ammonium sulfate.	Commonly used	Not accurate at low HbF concentrations
2. Electrophoresis	Hemoglobins are separated electrophoretically and quantitated by densitometric scanning.	Frequently used	Method shows poor correlation with alkali denaturation method
3. Immunological (RIA, RID, ELISA, IFMA)	HbF reacts with a specific antibody directed against γ subunit chains. Method of detection is dependent on specific method used.	Commonly used	Accurate and reproducible
4. HPLC	Hemoglobins separated according to net ionic charge and charge distribution at a particular pH.	Infrequently used	Commercially available dedicated systems may allow for more common usage of this method

tated with ammonium sulfate and removed by filtration. The measurement of the unprecipitated, alkali-resistant hemoglobin provides for an estimate of the amount of HbF present. Various modifications to this procedure have been described to help improve the accuracy of this procedure.[42]

A common method in use for HbF measurement is electrophoretic separation of this hemoglobin from the other hemoglobin fractions (Table 36-7, method 2) (see the following discussion of hemoglobin electrophoresis). One can measure the separated HbF fraction by scanning the electrophoretic gel with a densitometer.[40] Unfortunately, measurement of HbF by this method is only semiquantitative at best and suffers from lack of sensitivity.

Immunologic techniques (Table 36-7, method 3) such as radioimmunoassay (RIA),[43] radial immunodiffusion (RID),[44] enzyme-linked immunosorbent assay (ELISA),[45] and time-resolved immunofluorometric assay (IFMA)[46] have been described. The use of polyclonal, or more recently, monoclonal antibodies directed against the γ-chain subunits of HbF allow this hemoglobin fraction to be quantitated. The immunological methods are generally very accurate with a relatively large analytical range. In addition, the ELISA and IFMA procedures can be performed fairly rapidly.

Chromatographic procedures such as high-performance liquid chromatography (HPLC) with use of cation-exchange columns have been developed (Table 36-7, method 4). These procedures enable the separation of HbF from normal and variant hemoglobins.[47] The HPLC methods have been devised and are rapid, technically easy, and give good precision and reproducibility.[48]

Specimen   Whole blood anticoagulated with the disodium salt of ethylenediaminetetraacetic acid (EDTA), heparin, or ammonia oxalate are acceptable specimens. Whole blood may be stored for 1 week at 4° C with no appreciable loss of HbF. Storage for 1 year at 4° C results in a decrease in HbF of approximately 10%.[49]

Reference interval   In newborns HbF accounts for 60% to 95% of the total hemoglobin present. The proportion of HbF decreases to less than 10% by 28 weeks post partum. Healthy adults contain low concentrations of HbF, ranging from 0.6%

to 1.0%. The largest reference interval of 0 to 2.8% has been obtained with use of RIA.[50]

Hemoglobin separation and quantitation
GERARDO PERROTTA

Principles of analysis   Erythrocytes contain different species of hemoglobin, the identification of which can help in the diagnosis of individuals with hemoglobinopathies. Usually a combination of methods, including both qualitative and quantitative procedures, is necessary for positive identification of the presence of abnormal hemoglobins.

Electrophoretic separation of hemoglobins utilizes the difference in charge of most hemoglobin species. The various electrophoretic procedures may differ in pH, the type of buffer used, the support medium, or the strength of the electric field. The most common electrophoretic method used for hemoglobin fractionation employs a cellulose acetate support medium with an alkaline buffer at pH 8.4 (Table 36-8, method 1). This technique readily resolves most of the major hemoglobin fractions, such as hemoglobins A_1, A_2, F, and S. However, this technique cannot resolve HbS from HbD and HbG, since those three fractions have the same mobility with this procedure. Likewise, hemoglobins C, E, and O have the same mobility as HbA_2 (Fig. 36-8).

Many laboratories also employ electrophoretic separation of hemoglobins at an acid pH (6.0) with an agar gel support medium (Table 36-8, method 2). When this technique is used with the cellulose acetate-alkaline buffer procedure, confirmation of the presence of hemoglobins D, G, C, and E can be accomplished (Fig. 36-9).

Once the electrophoretic separation of hemoglobin has been performed, the position and relative intensity of the hemoglobin fraction must be determined. This can be accomplished by fixation (denaturation) of the hemoglobin fractions followed by visualization of the hemoglobin protein with a specific stain. Typically, stains such as Paragon Blue, Ponceau S, or Amido Black 10 are used to visualize the separated fractions. The relative staining intensity of each fraction is quantitated with use of a densitometer.

In addition to electrophoretic determination of hemoglobins, several nonelectrophoretic methods are used to quan-

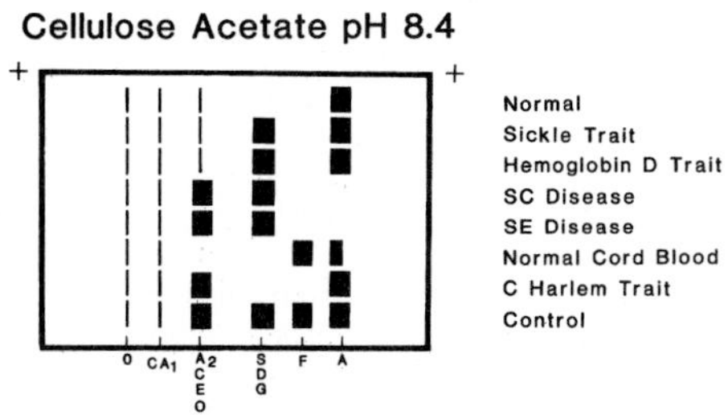

Cellulose Acetate pH 8.4

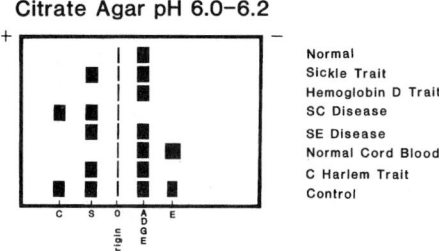

Fig. 36-8   Representation of hemoglobin electrophoresis on cellulose acetate strips, pH 8.4. CA_1, Carbonic anhydrase; others are hemoglobin variants discussed in text. (From CDC77-8266; Atlanta, 1976, DHEW.)

Citrate Agar pH 6.0–6.2

Fig. 36-9   Representation of hemoglobin electrophoresis on citrate agar, pH 6. On some plates the origin may not be as visible or as separated from HbS as shown here. (From CDC77-8266; Atlanta, 1976, DHEW.)

Table 36-8   Methods of hemoglobin analysis

Method	Principle	Usage	Comments
1. Electrophoresis (alkaline)	Electrophoretic separation of hemoglobin fractions on cellulose acetate support at pH 8.4 A_2 S F A_1 $(-)$ C D $(+)$ E G O Lepore	Most frequently used	Simple, fast Requires specialized equipment
2. Electrophoresis (acid)	Electrophoretic separation of hemoglobin fractions on agarose gel at pH 6.0 F A_1 S C $(-)$ E $(+)$ D G Lepore	Used for follow-up confirmation of results of alkaline hemoglobin electrophoresis	Simple, fast Requires specialized equipment
3. Solubility (sickling test)	HbS is reduced by dithionite or metabisulfite resulting in formation of denatured hemoglobin. Denatured hemoglobin results in increased turbidity of solution.	Often used as screen for HbS	Subject to interferences (see text)

titate the specific hemoglobin fractions S, A_2, or F. These methods are based upon differences in solubility, charge, or stability in alkaline solution of the various hemoglobin fractions.

The procedure for HbS is based upon the solubility of this hemoglobin (Table 36-8, method 3). Deoxyhemoglobin S is less soluble than deoxy-HbA_1, and treated red blood cells containing elevated levels of HbS assume a sickled appearance. The hemoglobins, including HbS, in a sample are treated with reducing agents, such as sodium dithionite or sodium metabisulfite in a phosphate buffer solution. The solubility, or sickling, test may give erroneous results if the concentration of HbS is less than approximately 25%.[52] In addition, high concentration of HbF can inhibit the ability of these reducing agents to induce sickling. This test has also been found to be unreliable in individuals with low blood hemoglobin concentrations (that is, ≤ 2 g/dL) or with polycythemia. Drugs such as phenothiazines in high concentrations (>128 µg/mL) can also inhibit sickling or reverse the sickling induced by sodium metabisulfite.[53]

Quantitation of HbA_2 is best achieved by column chromatography (Table 36-7, method 4). This technique is based on differences in charge of the various hemoglobin fractions and their affinity for adsorption onto an anion-exchange column containing diethylaminoethyl-cellulose. Under the conditions employed in the procedure, HbA_2 is not absorbed onto the column and is the first fraction eluted from the column. Elution of the remaining hemoglobin fraction or fractions is accomplished by use of buffers of increasing ionic strength. The percentage of Hb present in the eluates is determined by measurement of the absorbance of the eluates at 415 nm. Measurement of HbA_2 by column chromatography is simple, accurate, and precise.[54] However, quantitation of HbA_2 by chromatography in the presence of HbS, HbC, or several other variants can result in error. Accurate quantitation of HbA_2 by densitometry after electrophoretic separation is possible if careful attention to technique is exercised and properly calibrated instruments are used.[55]

The rapid identification of HbF is most frequently performed by use of alkali denaturation methods. Fetal hemoglobin is more resistant to denaturation by strong alkali than other hemoglobins are. The addition of a strong alkali, such as KOH or NaOH, to a hemolysate results in denaturation of hemoglobins other than HbF. After denaturation, an ammonium sulfate solution is added to precipitate the denatured hemoglobins, and centrifugation removes the denatured hemoglobin. The amount of hemoglobin remaining in the supernatant is measured spectrophotometrically at 415 nm and is expressed as alkali-resistant, fetal hemoglobin.

Specimen The type of specimen required, whole blood or hemolysate, is dependent on the type of procedure used. For electrophoretic separation of hemoglobins, column chromatography, and alkali denaturation, whole blood that has been prepared as a hemolysate is required. Whole blood is collected in EDTA, heparin, or other suitable anticoagulant. After centrifugation of the sample, plasma from the separated cells is discarded. One can prepare the hemolysate by lysing the cells with a hemolyzing reagent such as saponin, or by mixing an aliquot of whole blood with distilled water. Whole blood specimens (not hemolysate) for electrophoresis are stable for up to 2 weeks if kept at 4° C; whole blood for determination of HbA_2 by column chromatography is stable for 1 week at 4° C. The required specimen for determination of HbS by solubility is anticoagulated whole blood.

Reference interval Normal healthy adult erythrocytes contain HbA_1, HbA_2, and HbF. HbA_2 usually constitutes approximately 1.5% to 3.5% of the total adult hemoglobin, whereas HbF usually constitutes less than 1% of the total adult hemoglobin. The remainder is composed of HbA_1. In certain hemoglobinopathies, the relative percentages of each fraction may become increased or decreased. There are several texts and a recent review available that offer a more comprehensive overview of expected values seen in patients with hemoglobin disorders.[55,56,57]

ACKNOWLEDGMENTS

The editors wish to acknowledge the author of the previous versions of the Haptoglobin and the Hemoglobin F methods, Robert S. Franco.

REFERENCES

1. Bunn HF, Forget BG: *Hemoglobin: molecular, genetic and clinical aspects,* Philadelphia, 1986, Saunders.
2. Summers RN, Yerlley JC, Hyland VJ, et al: Mapping the human α-globin gene complex to 16p13.2 → pter, *J Med Genet* 4:761, 1987.
3. Shaeffer JR: Evidence for a difference in affinities of human hemoglobin $β^A$ and $β^S$ chains for α chains, *J Biol Chem* 255:2322, 1980.
4. Urbanetti JS: Carbon monoxide poisoning. In Wallach DFH, editor: *The function of the red blood cells: erythrocyte pathobiology,* New York, 1981, Alan R Liss.
5. Schumacher HR: Methemoglobinemia, sulfhemoglobinemia, and carboxy-hemoglobinemia. In Schumacher HR, Garvin DF, Triplett DA, editors, *Introduction to laboratory hematology and hematopathology,* New York, 1984, Alan R Liss.
6. Zijlstra WG, Buursma A, Meewisen van der Roest WP: Absorption of human fetal and adult oxyhemoglobin, deoxyhemoglobin, carboxyhemoglobin, and methemoglobin, *Clin Chem* 37:1633, 1991.
7. Carrell RW, Winterbourn CC, Rachmilewitz EA: Recommended methods for surface counting to determine sites of red cell destruction, *Br J Haematol* 30:250, 1975.
8. Finch CA: Methemoglobinemia and sulfhemoglobinemia, *N Engl J Med* 239:470, 1948.
9. Weatherall DJ, Clegg JB: *The thalassemia syndrome,* Oxford, England, 1981, Blackwell Scientific Publications.
10. Fairbanks VF: Nomenclature and taxonomy of hemoglobin variants. In Fairbanks VF, editor: *Hemoglobinopathies and thalassemias,* New York, 1980, Brian C Decker, Publisher.
11. Westhall DJ: Abnormal hemoglobins and thalassemias. In Hoffbrand AV, Brain MC, Hirsh J, editors: *Recent advances in hematology,* London, 1977, Churchill Livingstone.
12. Lubin BH, Witkowska HE, Kleman K: Laboratory diagnosis of hemoglobinopathies, *Clin Biochem* 24:363-374, 1991.
13. Buihl RW: Physical chemical properties of sickle cell hemoglobin. In Wallach DPH, editor: *The function of red blood cells: erythrocyte pathobiology,* New York, 1981, Alan R. Liss.
14. Ranney HM: The spectrum of sickle cell disease, *Hosp Pract* (off Ed) 27: pp 133-137, 141-144, 149-150 passim, Jan 15, 1992.
15. Bunn HF: Hemoglobin II, sickle cell anemia and other hemoglobinopathies. In Beck WS, editor: *Hematology,* Cambridge, Mass., 1981, MIT Press.
16. Nagel RL, Bookchin RM: Oxygen transport and the sickle cell. In Wallach DFH, editor: *The function of red blood cells: erythrocyte pathobiology,* New York, 1981, Alan R. Liss.
17. Kark JA, Posey DM, Schumacher HR, et al: Sickle cell trait as a risk factor for sudden death in basic training, *N Engl J Med* 317:781, 1987.
18. Charache S: Fetal hemoglobin, sickling and sickle cell disease, *Adv Pediatr* 37:1, 1990.
19. Testa V, Dubait A, Hinard N, et al: Beta⁰-thalassemia/HbE association, *Acta Haematol* 64:42, 1980.
20. Ohba Y: Unstable hemoglobins, *Hemoglobin* 14:353, 1990.
21. Kreimer-Birnbaum M, Pinkerton PH, Bannerman RM, et al: Dipyrrolic urinary pigments in congenital Heinz-body anemia due to Hb Koln and in thalassemia, *Br J Med* 2:396, 1966.
22. Fairbanks VF: Thalassemias and hereditary persistence of fetal hemoglobins (HPFH). In Fairbanks VF, editor: *Hemoglobinopathies and thalassemias, laboratory methods and case studies,* New York, 1980, Brian C Decker, Publisher.
23. Okene-Frempong K, Schwartz E: Clinical features of thalassemia, *Pediatr Clin North Am* 27:403, 1980.
24. Charache S, Clegg JB, Weatherall DJ: The Negro variety of hereditary persistence of fetal haemoglobin in a mild form of thalassemia, *Br J Haematol* 34:527, 1976.
25. Weatherall DJ, Clegg JB: Hereditary persistence of fetal haemoglobin, *Br J Haematol* 29:191, 1975.
26. Jaffe ER: Methemoglobinemia, *Clin Hematol* 10:99, 1981, specific p 103.
27. Jaffe ER: Methemoglobinemia, *Clin Hematol* 10:99, 1981, specific p 117.
28. Dover GJ, Boyer SH, Zinkhorn WH: Production of erythrocytes that contain fetal hemoglobin in anemia, *J Clin Invest* 63:173, 1979.
29. Hardisty RM, Speed DE, Till M: Granulocytic leukemia in childhood, *Br J Haematol* 10:551, 1964.
30. Weatherall DJ, Pembrey ME, Pritchard J: Fetal hemoglobin, *Clin Hematol* 3:467, 1974.
31. Bunn HF, Haney DN, Kain S, et al: The biosynthesis of human hemoglobin A_{1c}, *J Clin Invest* 57:1652, 1978.
32. Landau SA, Winchell HS: Endogenous production of ¹⁴CO: a method for calculation of RBC life-span in vivo, *Blood* 36:642, 1970.
33. Astrup P: Carbon monoxide inhalation-time for clearance from blood in reversible coma, *JAMA* 230:1064, 1974.
34. Smith JR, Landau SA: Smoker's polycythemia, *N Engl J Med* 298:6, 1978.
35. van Lente F, Marchand A, Galen RS: Evaluation of a nephelometric assay for haptoglobin and its clinical usefulness, *Clin Chem* 25:2007, 1979.
36. Sternberg JC: A rate nephelometer for measuring specific proteins by immunoprecipitin reactions, *Clin Chem* 23:1456, 1977.
37. Mancini G, Carbonara AO, Heremans JF: Immunochemical

quantitations of antigens by single radial immunodiffusion, *Immunochemistry* 2:235-254, 1965.

38. Fahey JL, McKelvey EM: Quantitative determinations of serum immunoglobulins in antibody-agar plates, *J Immunol* 94:84-90, 1965.

39. Schrijver J, van Rijn H, Schreurs W: Re-evaluation of the haptoglobin reference values with the radial immunodiffusion technique, *Clin Biochem* 17:258, 1984.

40. Wood WG, Stamatoyannopoulos G, Lim G, Nute PE: F-cells in the adult: normal values and levels in individuals with hereditary and acquired elevations of HbF, *Blood* 46:671-682, 1975.

41. Apt L, Downey WS Jr: "Melena" neonatorum: the swallowed blood syndrome, *J Pediatr* 47:6-12, 1955.

42. Liu N, Wu AB, Wong SS: Improved quantitative Apt test for detecting fetal hemoglobin in bloody stools of newborns, *Clin Chem* 39:2326-2329, 1993.

43. Garver FA, Jones CS, Baker MM, et al: Specific radioimmunochemical identification and quantitation of hemoglobins A_2 and F, *Am J Hematol* 1:459-469, 1976.

44. Chudwin DS, Rucknagel DL: Immunological quantification of hemoglobins F and A_2, *Clin Chim Acta* 50:413-418, 1974.

45. Makler MT, Pesce AJ: ELISA assay for measurement of human hemoglobin A and hemoglobin F, *Am J Clin Pathol* 74:673-676, 1980.

46. Turpeinen U, Stenman U-H: Determination of fetal hemoglobin by time-resolved immunofluorometric assay, *Clin Chem* 38:2013-2018, 1992.

47. Brunnekreeft JW, Eidhof HH: Improved rapid procedure for simultaneous determinations of hemoglobins A1a, A1b, A1c, F, C, and S, with indication for acetylation or carbamylation by cation-exchange liquid chromatography, *Clin Chem* 39:2514-2518, 1993.

48. Tan GB, Aw TC, Dunstan RA, Lee SH: Evaluation of high performance liquid chromatography for routine estimation of hemoglobins A_2 and F, *J Clin Pathol* 46:852-856, 1993.

49. Garver FA, Jones CS, Baker MM, et al: Specific radiochemical identification and quantitation of hemoglobins A_2 and F, *Am J Hematol* 1:459-469, 1976.

50. Nalbandian RM, Nichols BM, Camp FR Jr, et al: Dithionite tube test—a rapid inexpensive technique for the detection of hemoglobins S and non-S sickling hemoglobin, *Clin Chem* 17:1028-1032, 1971.

51. National Committee for Clinical Laboratory Standards: Standard for abnormal hemoglobin detection by cellulose acetate electrophoresis, NCCLS Tentative Standard: TSH-8, Villanova, Penn., 1980, NCCLS.

52. Gottfried EI, Wall B, Robertson NA: Reliable estimation of hemoglobin A_2 concentration by electrophoresis with densitometry, *Am J Clin Pathol* 72:415-420, 1979.

53. Huntsman RG: Sickling tests—microscopic and non-microscopic. In Schmidt RM, Husman THJ, Lehmann H, et al, editors: *The detection of hemoglobinopathies,* Cleveland, 1988, CRC Press.

54. McFadzean JA: The effect of phenothiazines on the sickling phenomenon in vitro, *Br J Haematol* 16:173, 1969.

55. Sonnenwirth AC, Jarett L: *Gradwohl's clinical laboratory methods and diagnosis,* ed 8, vol 1, St. Louis, 1980, Mosby.

56. Miale JB: *Laboratory medicine hematology,* ed 5, St. Louis, 1982, Mosby.

57. Lubin BH, Witkowska HE, Kleman K: Laboratory diagnosis of hemoglobinopathies, *Clin Biochem* 24:363-374, 1991 (review).

BIBLIOGRAPHY

Bick RL, Bennett JM, Brynes RK, et al: *Hematology: clinical and laboratory practice,* St. Louis, 1993, Mosby.

Bunn HF, Forget BG: *Hemoglobin: molecular, genetic and clinical aspects,* Philadelphia, 1986, Saunders.

Hoffbrand AV, Brenner MK: *Recent advances in haematology,* London, 1992, Churchill Livingstone.

Hoffman R, Benz EJ, Shattil SJ, et al: *Hematology: basic principles and practice,* New York, London, 1991, Churchill Livingstone.

Jandl JH: *Blood: textbook of hematology,* Boston, 1987, Little, Brown & Co.

Lee GR, Bithell TC, Foerster J, et al: *Wintrobe's clinical hematology,* ed 9, Philadelphia, 1993, Lea & Febiger.

Rappaport SI: *Introduction to hematology,* ed 2, Philadelphia, 1987.

Schumacher HR: *Introduction to laboratory hematology and hematopathology,* New York, 1984, Alan R. Liss.

Stamatoyannopoulos G, Nieuhaus AW, Leder P, Majerus PW: *The molecular basis of blood diseases,* ed 2, Philadelphia, 1994, Saunders.

Weatherall DJ, Clegg JB: *The thalassemia syndrome,* Oxford, 1981, Blackwell Scientific Publications.

Williams WJ, Beutler E, Eislev E, Lichtman MA: *Hematology,* ed 4, New York, 1990, McGraw-Hill.

Human nutrition

Nancy W. Alcock

■

■

OBJECTIVES

■ Discuss the contribution of individual nutrient classes to human metabolism.

■ Discuss the importance of nutrition in health and disease.

■ Discuss therapeutic nutrition support by enteral and parenteral routes.

■ Discuss the role of the laboratory for the support of nutrition programs and support of patients with inborn errors of metabolism.

■ List the biochemical parameters used to monitor nutritional status.

KEY WORDS

anabolism Biochemical pathways that synthesize macromolecules, such as proteins and nucleic acids.

basal metabolic rate (BMR) The energy expended to maintain the basic physiologic functions.

bioavailability Amount (usually expressed as a percentage) of dietary components that are able to be absorbed from the gastrointestinal tract, either intact or after degradation.

catabolism Metabolic processes that degrade or breakdown macromolecules.

diet The food that is ingested orally.

dysphagia Difficulty in swallowing.

enteral feeding Provision of synthetic nutrients to the gastrointestinal tract through a tube.

essential nutrients Nutrients that are required for normal growth and development and for maintaining the adult body in equilibrium, which cannot be synthesized at all or cannot be synthesized in sufficient amounts. These include vitamins, minerals, trace elements, certain amino acids, and at least one fatty acid.

kilocalorie (kcal) The amount of energy producing food equivalent to the energy required to raise the temperature of 1 kg of water from 15° to 16° C.

kilojoule (kJ) A unit of heat; 1 kJ is equivalent to approximately 0.24 kcal.

kwashiorkor Malnutrition caused by a diet deficient in protein.

malnutrition Suboptimum nutrition arising from inadequate or unbalanced intake, bioavailability, or utilization of nutrients.

marasmus A protein-calorie malnutrition arising from inadequate food intake as the result of partial or complete starvation.

nitrogen balance The difference between total nitrogen intake and the sum of fecal and urinary nitrogen excretion. An estimate of net synthesis of body proteins.

nutrient A dietary component that is utilized by the body in any metabolic pathway.

nutrition The science that studies the processes of requirement, intake, bioavailability, absorption, utilization, and excretion of nutrients.

parenteral nutrition Nutrition administered by a route other than the gastrointestinal tract.

peripheral parenteral nutrition (PPN) Parenteral nutrition introduced through a peripheral vein.

Recommended Dietary Allowance (RDA) Suggested daily requirements for some essential nutrients for healthy subjects of various ages as published by the Food and Nutrition Board of the National Research Council.

resting energy expenditure (REE) Energy expended at resting state, that is, at a basal metabolic rate.

total parenteral nutrition (TPN) Parenteral nutrition administered as the sole source of nutrition.

The science of nutrition is concerned with the qualitative and quantitative aspects of the diet and utilization of the dietary components that are required to sustain health. The major component groups required for human nutrition—carbohydrates, proteins, lipids, minerals, trace elements, vitamins, and fiber—are biochemically well defined. Some nutrients can be synthesized by metabolic processes, but others cannot be synthesized and therefore must be specifically provided in the diet. These nutrients are termed *essential* and include the essential amino acids and fatty acids (see below). All the water-soluble vitamins and fat-soluble vitamins, A, E, and K, are essential. Vitamin D, the fourth fat-soluble vitamin, is required for growing children, but adequate supplies are usually formed from its endogenous precursor, 7-dehydrocholesterol, in the adult human. Dietary fat and its absorption are prerequisites for absorption of the fat-soluble vitamins (see Chapter 30).

The variation in requirement of nutrients depends on the age and sex of the individual, on reproductive status, and on the altered nutritional demands associated with disease, injury, and therapeutic interventions. The Food and Nutrition Board of the Commission on Life Sciences, National Research Council, estimates the levels of dietary essential nutrients that should be adequate to meet the known nutrient needs of practically all healthy persons. These estimates are reported as Recommended Dietary Allowances and are revised from time to time. The latest revision was published in 1989.[1]

Various estimates indicate that at least 40% of hospitalized patients are malnourished. The Joint Commission on Accreditation for Healthcare Organizations has stressed the importance of a nutrition care plan that addresses detection of malnutrition, monitoring the intake of nutrition by the patient, and the route of nutrition delivery. Goals and the means to achieve these goals must be defined for patients at nutritional risk. Although anthropometric measurements are first-tier indicators of suboptimal nutrition, nutritional assessment using biochemical parameters can help to alert the physician to deficiencies. Biochemical measurements are of great importance in the monitoring of the patient's response to nutritional supplementation.

Biochemical and clinical aspects of the essential minerals, electrolytes, trace metals, and vitamins and their function are discussed in detail in the relevant chapters (see Table 37-1). References 2 and 3 provide additional details. Discussion here is limited to the objectives stated above.

NUTRIENT CLASSES
Energy requirements[4,5]

The World Health Organization defines the energy requirement of an individual as follows: "The level of energy intake that will balance energy expenditure when the individual has a body size and composition, and a level of physical activity, consistent with long-term good health.

Table 37-1 Basic classes of nutrients

Nutrient	Chapter discussed
Carbohydrate	Diabetes, 32
Lipids	Lipid, 33
Proteins	Liver, 27
Inorganic elements	
Na, K, Cl	Electrolytes and water balance, 24
Ca, Mg, inorganic phosphorus	Bone, 28
Fe^{++} (Fe^{+++})	Iron, porphyrins, bilirubin, 35
Trace minerals	Trace elements, 38
Vitamins	Vitamins, 39
Water	Renal, 26
	Electrolytes and water balance, 24

The energy requirement should also allow the maintenance of economically necessary and socially desirable physical activity. In children and pregnant or lactating women, the energy requirement includes the energy requirements associated with the deposition of tissues or the secretion of milk at rates consistent with good health."[4]

The body is in energy balance when the metabolizable energy intake is equal to the sum of energy expenditure and changes in stored energy. Energy expenditure can be determined by direct calorimetry (heat generated), indirect calorimetry (from measurement of oxygen consumption and carbon dioxide production), and by isotope-dilution methods using doubly labeled water. An estimate of the expenditure of endogenous energy stores can be quantitated from measurement of the nitrogen balance. A positive nitrogen balance is essential for growth of the fetus, placenta, and other associated changes during pregnancy and lactation. Extra energy is required during periods of growth and during physiologically stressful pathological states. Hormones and cytokines, such as tumor necrosis factor, may initiate a heightened metabolic response to injury and infection. The increased metabolism associated with physiological stress is termed the *hypermetabolic state.*

Patients suffering from trauma and sepsis are often in a hypermetabolic state. The increased metabolic rate, which is proportional to the severity of the condition, results in insulin insensitivity and hyperglycemia. In addition, stored triglycerides are mobilized and oxidized, and, if the patient is not fed, stores of fat and protein may be depleted. The loss of adipose tissue (fat) and muscle tissue (protein) results in the wasted appearance of individuals suffering from protein-calorie malnutrition. In these cases, nutritional support should be given minimally at first and then increased gradually to maintain body cell mass. Biochemical parameters useful in monitoring the patient are discussed below. The use of glutamine, a gut-specific nutrient, in critically ill patients has been shown to be beneficial for the production of ammonia in the kidney. This is a precursor for the synthesis of nucleotides and hence in the regulation of protein synthesis.

Energy intake at birth is approximately 120 kcal/kg/day for both males and females. During the first 2 years of life there is a gradual drop to 90 to 100 kcal/kg/day. From 2 to 14 years of age their energy requirement decreases gradually to approximately 40 kcal/kg/day, with males requiring 5 kcal/kg/day more than females.

Carbohydrates

Carbohydrates are the principal source of energy for the body, contributing 50% to 60% of the total calories.[6] Complex carbohydrates, such as starches and sugars, found in fruits and vegetables are a better source of energy than simple refined sugars and may lower the incidence of hypertension, maturity onset diabetes, and cardiovascular disease. Excessive carbohydrate intake leads to an increase in body weight, whereas insufficient intake stimulates mobilization of lipid stores with associated ketosis, loss of electrolytes, and dehydration. In a healthy adult, carbohydrate is stored as glycogen, principally in muscle (about 150 g) and in the liver (about 90 g). One gram of carbohydrate provides 4 kcal of energy.

Proteins

Requirements. Dietary proteins are the source of amino acids, the building blocks for synthesis and maintenance of tissue proteins.[7] Some amino acids cannot be synthesized either at all or in sufficient amounts to satisfy requirements, and therefore are "essential" in the diet. The essential amino acids are listed in the following box. The quality of dietary protein is determined from its content of all essential amino acids. For infants, children 10 to 12 years of age, and adults, 43%, 36%, and 10% respectively of the total amino acid intake should comprise essential amino acids. Good-quality protein is required to replace losses during the acute phase of physiological stress associated with fevers, burns, surgical trauma, fractures, and other pathological states. On the other hand, protein restriction is required to manage acute liver failure and uremia.

Nitrogen balance. Nitrogen balance studies are used to assess utilization of dietary amino acids for protein synthesis and the balance between anabolic and catabolic processes. An accurate diet record is used to calculate dietary

---

Essential Amino Acids		
Isoleucine	Phenylalanine	Histidine*
Leucine	Threonine	Arginine*
Lysine	Tryptophan	Taurine†
Methionine	Valine	

*Indicated to be unnecessary for maintenance of nitrogen equilibrium in adults in short-term studies but probably necessary for normal growth of children.
†Required in infants.

---

intake of protein nitrogen. Accurate assessment of nitrogen output requires the measurement of both fecal and urinary nitrogen and a correction for nitrogen losses through sweat, hair, nails, and sloughed cells from the skin. The most accurate quantitative assessment of nitrogen excretion measures total nitrogen excretion. This can be achieved by use of instruments that directly measure total nitrogenous compounds in urine or feces by chemiluminescence after pyrolysis of the sample. Because this technique is not in widespread use, an approximate estimate of nitrogen excretion can be obtained from measurement of urine urea nitrogen (UUN). The UUN must be adjusted by a factor that is intended to account for any other body losses. In an adult, a positive nitrogen balance is associated with general good health. A positive nitrogen balance during periods of growth and development and in pregnancy is mandatory. A negative nitrogen balance during periods of starvation, in cachexia, and in many hypermetabolic disease states should alert the physician to consider appropriate nutritional support. The frequency of quantitative measurements is dictated by the patient's response to therapy, but it has been recommended that several assessments a week may be necessary during the most catabolic state of an acute illness.[8]

Protein-deficiency states, such as the disease *kwashiorkor*, occur in underdeveloped countries when breast-fed infants are transferred to a high carbohydrate diet. Kwashiorkor is characterized by edema, rashes and skin lesions, and diarrhea and is often fatal.

An overall nutritional deficiency occurs in marasmus (wasting away) and appears in children with classic signs of starvation, including loss of adipose and muscle tissues, which produces a wasted appearance. There is an overlap between kwashiorkor and marasmus conditions, and the two are often not distinct. Marasmus subjects do not have the severe edema present in kwashiorkor and, by contrast, usually retain their mental alertness.

The Recommended Dietary Allowances (RDA) for protein for various ages and conditions is shown in Table 37-2. One gram of protein provides 4 kcal of energy.

Lipids

Lipids are the most energy dense of the macronutrients, providing 9 kcal/g of fat.[9] Although a typical American diet contains 35% to 45% of calories as fat, the American Heart Association and the Food and Nutrition Board of the National Research Council recommend that fat consumption be reduced to as low as 30% of total calories.

In view of the association of saturated fats from animal sources with heart disease, it is recommended that at least 10% of the fat ingested be polyunsaturated. Some fatty acids found in the structural lipids of cells and the mitochondrial membranes cannot be synthesized in sufficient quantity, and their supply is essential. The essential fatty acids are linoleic acid, linolenic acid, and arachidonic acid,

Table 37-2   Recommended Dietary Allowances for protein for various ages

Category	Age (years) or condition	Weight (kg)	Weight (lb)	Height (cm)	Height (in)	Protein (g)
Infants	0.0-0.5	6	13	60	24	13
	0.5-1.0	9	20	71	28	14
Children	1-3	13	29	90	35	16
	4-6	20	44	112	44	24
	7-10	28	62	132	52	28
Males	11-14	45	99	157	62	45
	15-18	66	145	176	69	59
	19-24	72	160	177	70	58
	25-50	79	174	176	79	63
	51+	77	170	173	68	63
Females	11-14	46	101	157	62	46
	15-18	55	120	163	64	44
	19-24	58	128	164	65	46
	25-50	63	138	163	64	50
	51+	65	143	160	63	50
Pregnant						60
Lactating	1st 6 mo					65
	2nd 6 mo					62

From Food and Nutrition Board, National Academy of Sciences, National Research Council: *Recommended Dietary Allowances,* revised 1989, Washington, D.C.

though there is some question that linolenic acid is essential. Arachidonic acid accounts for 5% to 10% of the fatty acids in phospholipids of the cell membrane. Approximately 2.7 g/day of the essential fatty acids, linoleic, linolenic, and arachidonic acids, are required for normal health.

Lipids are stored as triglycerides, mainly in adipose tissue. Lipid metabolism and associated diseases are discussed in Chapter 33.

Macrominerals

The Recommended Dietary Allowances for the major inorganic components, the macrominerals, of the diet are shown in Table 37-3. The role of each of these is discussed in detail in the relevant chapters listed in Table 37-1. Important aspects of the biological roles and symptoms of deficiency or excess of the individual minerals are shown in Table 37-4.[10,11] A discussion of the biological role of trace elements is found in Chapter 38.

Fiber

Fiber is an important component of the diet. Fiber comprises plant cell components that cannot be digested by enzymes found in the gut. The more insoluble fibers, such as cellulose and lignin found in wheat bran, are beneficial with regard to colonic function, whereas the more soluble gums and pectins found in fruits and vegetables have been associated with the lowering of blood cholesterol.[12] High-fiber diets are associated with reduced incidence of cancer of the colon, cardiovascular disease, and diabetes mellitus.[12] However, high-fiber diets and their phytate content provide binding sites for the divalent metals calcium, iron, and zinc, making these metals less bioavailable. Hence, a requirement for increased intake of these metals should be addressed when high-fiber diets are consumed.

NUTRITION IN HEALTH AND DISEASE[13-16]
General populations

An increased emphasis on wellness has led to suggested improvements in the composition of the American diet to maintain good health and prolong life. The recommendations of the American Heart Association for a decrease in total fat consumption was described above. The increased

Table 37-3   Recommended Dietary Allowances for some minerals and trace elements

Category	Age (years) or condition	Ca (mg)	P (mg)	Mg (mg)	Fe (mg)	Zn (mg)	I (μg)	Se (μg)
Infants	0.0-0.5	400	300	40	6	5	40	10
	0.5-1.0	600	500	60	10	5	50	15
Children	1-3	800	800	80	10	10	70	20
	4-6	800	800	120	10	10	90	20
Males	11-14	1200	1200	270	12	15	150	40
	15-18	1200	1200	400	12	15	150	50
	19-24	1200	1200	350	10	15	150	70
	25-50	800	800	350	10	15	150	70
	51+	800	800	350	10	15	150	70
Females	11-14	1200	1200	280	15	12	150	45
	15-18	1200	1200	300	15	12	150	50
	19-24	1200	1200	280	15	12	150	55
	25-50	800	800	280	15	12	150	55
	51+	800	800	280	10	12	150	55
Pregnant		1200	1200	300	30	15	175	65
Lactating	1st 6 mo	1200	1200	355	15	19	200	75
	2nd 6 mo	1200	1200	340	15	16	200	75

From Food and Nutrition Board, National Academy of Sciences, National Research Council: *Recommended Dietary Allowances,* revised 1989, Washington, D.C.

consumption of fruits and vegetables, especially citrus fruits, leafy vegetables, tomatoes, and orange-colored vegetables, is recommended because these foods are good sources of vitamins. Although a reduction in caloric intake has been demonstrated to be beneficial, excessive caloric intake leads to obesity and its accompanying health problems. Populations requiring special consideration of nutritional requirements are shown in Table 37-5. It is important to note that many of these populations include ambulatory individuals who are not acutely ill and may even be totally healthy (such as pregnant women).

Dietary treatment regimes for individuals with hyperlipidemias or coronary heart disease include a restriction of calories, total fat, saturated fat, and animal protein and an increase in consumption of complex carbohydrates, fiber, vegetable proteins and in the proportion of polyunsaturated and monounsaturated fats. Omega-3 fatty acids are effective in lowering plasma triglyceride levels.[13] The intake of cholesterol should be less than 100 mg/1000 kcal.

Nutrition plans for diabetics who are at risk for development of atherosclerosis recommend that at least 55% to 60% of calories are supplied by carbohydrates.[14] Complex carbohydrates should provide at least two thirds of the total. Protein intake should provide 12% to 16% of calories. Fat intake should be reduced to 20% to 25% of calories, no more than 10% of which should be saturated fats. A high-fiber intake that includes as much as 30 to 50 g/day is usually well tolerated and beneficial.

Drug-nutrient interactions

A comprehensive coverage of the nature of interactions between drugs and nutrients and their consequences is given by Roe.[15] Physicochemical interaction may occur in the gastrointestinal tract and may impair absorption of drug or nutrient, or both. Factors involved may include solubility properties, pH of the milieu, adsorptivity, chelation, gel formation, and ion exchange. Physiological interactions in which gastrointestinal function is altered may alter transit time and hence absorption rate, produce electrolyte imbalance or vasodilatation, or have a modifying effect on appetite resulting in excessive or inadequate food intake. A third category of interaction occurs when pathological changes result from drug toxicity. These may impair the gastrointestinal tract or other organs (such as liver, kidney, brain, blood system, or the fetus) and have a pronounced effect on metabolism in general. Roe lists 59 specific drugs the absorption of which may be reduced or retarded by food or food supplements, and 24 the absorption of which may be increased by food or by enteral formulas. Although the effects of diet composition on drug metabolism and toxicity have been documented extensively in animal experiments, few studies have been reported in humans. As pointed out by Roe, this is an area in which research is wanting, especially in aging populations where the high prevalence of drug reactions, combined with the frequency of multiple drug prescriptions may involve a diet-related explanation.

Low-protein diets reduce renal plasma flow, creatinine clearance, and renal clearance of drugs such as the antiuricemic drug allopurinol, which inhibits xanthine oxidase.

Table 37-4   Major role of macrominerals and associated abnormalities

Element	Major role	Associated abnormality	Comments
Calcium	Major component with phosphorus of skeletal and dental tissues	Deficiency: rickets in children; osteomalacia in adults; contributes to osteoporosis	Hormonal regulation: parathyroid hormone, vitamin D, calcitonin
Chloride	Important in fluid and electrolyte balance; major extracellular fluid anion; contributes to osmolality	Deficiency may occur as result of vomiting, diarrhea, diuretics, renal disease	
Magnesium	Major pools intracellular, bone; cofactor for many enzymes	Deficiency may occur because of malabsorption, diarrhea, alcoholism	Symptom of deficiency: muscle weakness
Phosphorus	Major component with calcium in skeletal and dental tissue; energy source from ATP Phosphorylated intermediate in metabolic pathways; component of nucleic acids	Deficiency: in children, rickets; in adults, osteomalacia	Parathyroid hormone and vitamin D regulatory mechanisms
Potassium	Major intracellular cation; important in muscle and nerve functions Na^+,K^+-ATPase	Muscle weakness, confusion, paralysis	Hormonal regulation of potassium excretion by aldosterone; urine loss increased by diuretics
Sodium	Major extracellular fluid cation contributes to osmolality Important in acid-base balance Na^+,K^+-ATPase	Excess may cause hypertension in some individuals	Hormonal regulation of sodium reabsorption by aldosterone

Table 37-5 Conditions requiring special nutrition considerations

Aging	Immunoincompetence
Alcoholism	Kwashiorkor disease
Cancer	Lactation
Coronary heart disease	Low birth weight infant
Diabetes	Malabsorption
Growth	Marasmus
Hyperlipidemia	Pregnancy
Injury	Sepsis

Basic drugs such as gentamicin are affected by the alkalinizing effect of low-protein diets, presenting a less ionized form of the drug to the kidney and resulting in increased reabsorption. An area requiring further study is the effect of obesity on drug distribution: Should lyophilic drugs be given according to ideal body weight or to the subject's weight?

Amphetamines are known to decrease appetite. Likewise, digitalis given for long periods at a high level causes nausea and cachexia. Many cancer chemotherapeutic drugs also decrease appetite; in some cases this may be attributable to gastrointestinal ulceration.

The mechanism of action of many drugs appears to be as a vitamin antagonist. Although evidence of this has been provided by in vitro studies and observed in animal experiments for many drugs, confirmation in vivo in humans is often lacking. Table 37-6 lists some drugs that are vitamin antagonists.

The effect of drugs on retention or loss of major minerals in humans is well established and is summarized in Table 37-7.

Hospitalized populations

Malnutrition in chronic and acute care institutions can be a major problem.[8] The estimated 40% of hospitalized patients who show signs of malnutrition includes individuals who enter the hospital with preexisting chronic conditions (such as individuals with acquired immunodeficiency syndrome [AIDS], or cancer) as well as those who may become acutely ill as the result of their hospital stay (such as trauma patients, surgery and burn patients, and very low-birth-weight babies). Individuals in chronic care facilities, such as the elderly, may not eat properly and become chronically malnourished.

Cancer patients with cachexia or who have had prior surgery or radiation therapy that interferes with gastrointestinal function will benefit from nutrition support.[16] Progressive weight loss before surgery is an indication for nutrition support before surgery can proceed.

In all these cases, nutritional intervention will be needed to treat the malnourished patient. The nutritional therapy must be tailored to the needs of the individual patient. In all cases, the route of administration depends on the ability of the gut to function effectively.

THERAPEUTIC NUTRITION SUPPORT[17,18]
Enteral feeding

Enteral feeding refers to the introduction of nutrients into the gastrointestinal tract through a tube.[17] This method is

Table 37-6 Examples of drugs that are vitamin antagonists*

Drug	Use/effect	Vitamin affected
Adriamycin	Cancer chemotherapy; dose-dependent cardiomyopathy, if accumulation >500 mg/m² Histologic pattern resembles that of vitamin E deficiency	Incidence, severity of damage reduced by vitamin E supplementation in animals, not in man
Alcohol	Impaired utilization of B vitamins	Thiamine administration improves, as in Wernicke-Korsakoff syndrome
Coumarin drugs Warfarin Dicumerol	Anticoagulants	Vitamin K antagonists; high vitamin K intake decreases anticoagulant effects
Hydralazine	Antihypertensive drug	B_6 antagonist; inhibits nicotinamide synthesis
Isoniazid	Antituberculosis drug	B_6 antagonist; inhibits nicotinamide synthesis
Methotrexate	Cancer chemotherapeutic drug	Folate antagonist
Moxalactam	Antibiotic	Decreases vitamin K–dependent clotting factors
Nitrous oxide	Anesthetic; recently important in cardiac bypass surgery	B_{12} antagonist
Pentamidine	*Pneumocystis carinii* pneumonia therapy	Folate antagonist
Pyrimethamine	Antimalarial agent	Folate antagonist
Sulfasalazine	Anti-inflammatory drug	Folate antagonist
Tramterine	Diuretic	Folate antagonist
Trimethroprim	Antibiotic	Folate antagonist

*From Roe DA: Diet, nutrition, and drug interactions. In Shils ME, Olson JA, Shike M, editors: *Modern nutrition in health and disease,* ed 8, Philadelphia, 1993, Lea & Febinger, with extensive bibliography. It should be noted that demonstration of vitamin antagonism by a drug in vitro in animal models often lacks confirmation in humans.

Table 37-7 Some classes or individual drugs that influence mineral status

Mineral	Mineral status	
	Overload	Depletion
Potassium	Succinylcholine increases serum potassium; potassium-sparing diuretics	Laxatives; potassium-losing diuretics; nephrotoxic antibiotics
Sodium	Antacids containing $NaHCO_3$; diazoxide, an antihypertensive, may increase serum sodium	Sodium-losing diuretics
Calcium	Thiazide diuretics—calcium retention; etidronate, a biphosphonate, increases bone mass; pharmacologic doses of vitamin D and metabolites—hypercalcemia and soft-tissue calcification potential	Aluminum-containing antacids or parenteral fluids— osteomalacia may occur; corticosteroids; phenobarbital; phenytoin
Magnesium	Magnesium-containing antacids	Nephrotic antibiotics; diuretics; cisplatin
Iron		Aspirin; indomethacin
Zinc		Penicillamine; nephrotic antibiotics

necessary when patients are unable to consume sufficient food normally. A brief list of conditions where enteral feeding may be indicated is given in Table 37-8. The availability of a variety of commercial enteral formulas tailored to meet specific circumstances has made this an increasingly practical route for maintaining adequate nutrition. Percutaneous endoscopic gastrostomy and jejunoscopy procedures have simplified the procedures used for guiding placement of the tubes. The placement of the tube is determined by the particular problem; that is, in the presence of recurrent aspiration, the tube must not be placed in the stomach but in the jejunum. Some of the indications for enteral nutrition include burn patients who require increased nutritional support, coma states, partial obstruction of the stomach or small bowel, fistulas of the small bowel or colon, persistent anorexia, and disorders that have specific requirements that can be met by the introduction of tailored solutions. A more detailed discussion of enteral feeding is given in reference 17. Whenever possible, enteral feeding is preferred to total parenteral nutrition (TPN), since it enables the patient to maintain a functioning gut, with its contribution to normal metabolic processes. In addition, enteral formulas are simpler to manage and preferable to intravenous administration, parenteral nutrition. When enteral feeding is not possible, nutrients must be administered intravenously.

Parenteral nutrition (PN)[18]

Parenteral nutrition aims to maintain or improve the nutritional status of patients who are unable to obtain the necessary nutrients from normal feeding or from enteral formulas. Parenteral nutrient solutions are intravenously administered either by peripheral vein (peripheral parenteral nutrition, PPN) or through a central vein where a central catheter has been maintained (TPN). Isotonic lipid emulsions in 5% or 10% glucose, 5% amino acids, electrolytes, and micronutrients supplying up to 2500 kcal in 3 liters can be administered peripherally.[18] When a critically ill patient

is unstable, continued access to a vein is required; hence a central catheter is essential and readily available. Total parenteral nutrition allows larger volumes and therefore more nutrients to be administered than can be delivered by the PPN route. Conditions in which patients may benefit from TPN are summarized in Table 37-9. Nutritional support by TPN has been demonstrated to be advantageous for patients receiving chemotherapy where cachexia is a problem. However, although TPN used preoperatively in patients with gastrointestinal tumors improved the postoperative outcome, there has been no evidence that TPN improved treatment tolerance or outcome in patients receiving chemotherapy. The evidence for a beneficial effect of TPN given preoperatively to malnourished patients is equivocal. Nutritional support by TPN has been demonstrated to be advantageous for patients receiving chemotherapy where cachexia is a problem.

NUTRITION AND INBORN ERRORS OF METABOLISM

Inherited metabolic diseases are the result of "inborn errors" in genes that result in alterations in the structure and function of enzymes or protein molecules (see Chapter 47). Elas and Costa[19] indicate that over 250 genetic disorders have been reported where accumulation, deficiency, or overproduction of substrates or products involved in normal metabolic pathways occurs. They review some 100 of these disorders in which nutritional therapy is an integral component of the treatment of these diseases. Intervention in the first few weeks of life is mandatory for phenylketonuria, galactosemia, isovaleric acidemia, homocystinuria, maple syrup urine disease, arginosuccinic aciduria, and citrullinemia. A description of chemically defined formulas, medications, and dietary guides for many classes of inherited metabolic disorders is included in this reference, as well as a comprehensive discussion of the biochemistry, screening procedures, diagnosis, and treatment for many of these diseases.

Table 37-8 Conditions where enteral nutrition
is indicated

Severe dysphagia
Persistent anorexia
Coma
Short bowel syndrome
Inflammatory bowel disease
Partial obstruction
Nausea, vomiting except with intestinal obstruction
Need for excessive nutritional requirements, as in burn patients
Fistula of small bowel or colon
Requirement for specific nutrient(s)
Persistent aspiration via a jejunostomy

From Shike M: Enteral feeding. In Shils ME, Olson JA, Shike M, editors: *Modern nutrition in health and disease*, ed 8, Philadelphia, 1993, Lea & Febiger.

BIOCHEMICAL PARAMETERS USED TO MONITOR NUTRITIONAL STATUS
General monitoring[8]

Careful assessment of the nutritional status of patients and the monitoring of nutritional therapies includes both anthropometric and laboratory measurements. The properties of an ideal marker for monitoring nutritional status in biological fluids are summarized in Table 37-10. Although these properties cannot all be met for all clinical situations, when used along with considerations of a patient's condition, they enable interpretation of the patient's nutritional status. Routine biochemical screening panels provide data on the patient's status and requirements for carbohydrates and the macrominerals.

Refeeding syndrome

In addition to providing information on specific nutrients, these routine biochemical tests can also be useful for assessment of the general response of patients to nutrition therapy. Specifically, by careful biochemical monitoring physicians can avoid a negative aspect to nutritional treatment called the *refeeding syndrome*.

Table 37-9 Clinical states of patients likely to benefit from parenteral nutrition

Inability to digest food
Persistent vomiting (such as that secondary to obstruction, increased pressure, or medications given intracranially)
Intestinal motility disorders (such as severe pseudointestinal obstruction)
Massive bowel resection
Severe inflammatory bowel disease
Small bowel fistula unable to be bypassed by tube feedings
Immune disease with intestinal villous atrophy
Support for the underweight premature infant
Persistent hypermetabolic states where enteral feeding is contraindicated or inadequate (such as severe burns with trauma or sepsis)

From Shils ME: Parenteral nutrition. In Shils ME, Olson JA, Shike M, editors: *Modern nutrition in health and disease*, ed 8, Philadelphia, 1993, Lea & Febiger.

Table 37-10 Properties of an ideal nutritional marker

Is specific for analyte to be measured
Has a high degree of sensitivity
Indicative of status of a particular analyte
Biological half-life is very short
Response to supplementation is rapid
Indicates onset and degree of deficiency early

The refeeding syndrome describes the negative sequelae that can result when patients who have been chronically starved and severely malnourished receive aggressive nutritional support. This syndrome may begin when the starved individual receives more glucose than can be physiologically processed. Under normal conditions, the maximal rate at which glucose can be metabolized is 2 to 4 mg/kg/min. Under stress, this metabolic rate can increase to 3 to 5 mg/kg/min. If these rates are exceeded, there may be an exaggerated insulin response. In addition to its hypoglycemic effect (see Chapter 32), insulin has strong antidiuretic properties. Thus, in an exaggerated insulin response, which can occur if a malnourished patient is treated with excessive glucose, there will be water and salt retention, increasing the vascular space, leading to fluid overload and stress to the heart.

Other biochemical sequelae to the insulin include decreases in serum phosphate, magnesium, and potassium, as the insulin drives these analytes into peripheral cells, primarily muscle cells. In a body that might already be deficient in these nutrients, hypophosphatemia, hypokalemia, and hypomagnesemia may result.

- A deficiency in serum magnesium may reduce the activity of key enzymes in tissue, especially cardiac tissue.
- The hypophosphatemia can lead to decreased cellular levels of ATP and, in red blood cells, of 2,3-

Table 37-11 Laboratory tests to monitor response to nutrient supplements

Parameter	Rationale/comments
Urine urea nitrogen	*Approximates* nitrogen balance in anabolic and catabolic states
Total urine nitrogen	Direct measure of excreted nitrogen
Plasma albumin	Low in malnutrition, affected by redistribution with fluid shifts or retention
Plasma transthyretin (prealbumin)	Low in malnutrition; half-life of 2 days; reflects hepatic protein synthesis
Plasma transferrin*	Low in malnutrition; half-life of 8 days
Plasma retinol binding protein*	Low in malnutrition; half-life of 10 hours
Plasma zinc	Low levels (500 µg/L) with skin lesions indicate immunoincompetence
Plasma triglycerides	Essential to monitor hypertriglyceridemia in peripheral parenteral nutrition

*Acute phase reactants, see text.

Table 37-12   Proteins used in nutrition assessment

Protein	Half-life	Normal values	Suggested medical decision point
Albumin	21 days	35-55 g/L	30 g/L
Transferrin	8 days	2000-4000 mg/L	1500 mg/L
Prealbumin	2 days	160-350 mg/L	110 mg/L
Retinol binding protein	10 hours	26-76 mg/L	16 mg/L

From Kaplan LA, general editor: *Laboratory support in assessing and monitoring nutritional status,* National Academy of Clinical Biochemistry's "Standards of Laboratory Practice" series.

diphosphoglycerate (2,3-DPG). The decreased 2,3-DPG alters the shape of red blood cells, decreases the half-life of red blood cells, and alters the binding of oxygen to hemoglobin (see Chapters 25 and 36). This results in a diminished delivery of oxygen to peripheral cells and tissue hypoxia.

- The hypokalemia results in an increased irritability of cardiac tissue and reduced ability of cells to take up glucose.

In a severely protein-malnourished individual, muscles have already been weakened because muscle proteins have been catabolized to amino acids that are consumed in the gluconeogenic pathway to increase the availability of blood glucose for the brain. In this weakened condition, the biochemical stresses listed above act to further reduce the capability of muscles to function, leading to respiratory failure and tissue hypoxia, which in turn leads to congestive heart failure and cardiac arrest. These sequelae of aggressive nutrition therapy can be avoided by careful monitoring of the serum levels of these analytes and a cooperative relationship between the physician, laboratory, and pharmacist.

Nitrogen balance

Tests that may be used to monitor nitrogen balance and provide some estimates of the liver's protein synthesis capabilities are shown in Table 37-11. Nitrogen balance may be estimated from calculated dietary intake and determination of 24-hour excretion of urine urea. An adjustment factor for estimated fecal and other nitrogen losses, such as creatinine, uric acid, ammonia, and losses to hair, nails, and sweat, is determined from an individual patient's condition. Limitations of this method in the critically ill patient using the factor urine urea × 1.25 grams to estimate total nitrogen have been discussed.[8,20] A more accurate measure of nitrogen excretion can be made by direct analysis of total nitrogen (see above and reference 8).

Protein synthesis

Interpretation of results of plasma albumin and of specific proteins must take into account the individual patient's condition. Alterations in fluid volume status and fluid shifts into or out of the vascular system produce changes in the concentration of plasma albumin and transferrin. Conditions initiating the acute-phase response, including trauma, infec-tion, malignancy, and myocardial infarction, can affect the levels of specific hepatic proteins. Of the commonly measured specific proteins, ceruloplasmin is a positive acute-phase reactant, and serum levels will be increased because of increased synthesis at the site of injury. At the same time the serum levels of negative-phase reactants are decreased because of enhanced catabolism and decreased synthesis. Hence, a decrease in plasma transthyretin (prealbumin), transferrin, retinol binding protein, and albumin may result, at least in part, in conditions other than malnutrition. Nevertheless, analysis of specific proteins of short biological half-lives are useful in monitoring the response to nutritional supplementation. The half-life of some of the specific proteins and suggested levels where supplementation is indicated are shown in Table 37-12.

Response to protein supplementation is reflected most rapidly by an increase in retinol binding protein, but prealbumin has been found to be more predictive of improved status.

REFERENCES

1. *Recommended Dietary Allowances, 10th edition,* Subcommittee on the 10th Edition of the RDAs, Food and Nutrition Board, Commission on Life Sciences, National Research Council, National Academy Press, Washington, D.C., 1989.
2. Shils ME, Olson JA, Shike M, editors: *Modern nutrition in health and disease,* ed 8, Philadelphia, 1993, Lea & Febiger.
3. Murray RK, Granner DK, Mayes PA, Rodwell VW, editors: *Harper's biochemistry,* ed 23, Norwalk, Conn., 1993, Appleton & Lange.
4. World Health Organization: *Energy and protein requirements,* report of a joint FAO/WHO/UNU expert consultation technical report, series 724, Geneva, 1985, WHO.
5. Sóuba WW, Wilmore DW: Diet and nutrition in the care of the patient with surgery trauma and sepsis. In Shils, ME, Olson JA, Shike M, editors: *Modern nutrition in health and disease,* ed 8, Philadelphia, 1993, Lea & Febiger.
6. MacDonald I: Carbohydrates. In Shils ME, Olson JA, Shike M, editors: *Modern nutrition in health and disease,* ed 8, Philadelphia, 1993, Lea & Febiger.
7. Crim MC, Munro HN: Proteins and amino acids. In Shils ME, Olson JA, Shike M, editors: *Modern nutrition in health and disease,* ed 8, Philadelphia, 1993, Lea & Febiger.
8. Kaplan LA, general editor: *Laboratory support in assessing and monitoring nutritional status,* National Academy of Clinical Biochemistry's "Standards of Laboratory Practice" series, pp 12-13.
9. Linscheer WG, Vergroesen AJ: Lipids. In Shils ME, Olson JA, Shike M, editors: *Modern nutrition in health and disease,* ed 8, Philadelphia, 1993, Lea & Febiger.
10. Nordin BEC, editor: *Calcium in human biology,* London, 1988, Springer-Verlag.
11. Shils ME: Magnesium. In Shils ME, Olson JA, Shike M, editors:

Modern nutrition in health and disease, ed 8, Philadelphia, 1993, Lea & Febiger.

12. Schneeman BO, Tietyen J: Dietary fiber. In Shils ME, Olson JA, Shike M, editors: *Modern nutrition in health and disease,* ed 8, Philadelphia, 1993, Lea & Febiger.

13. Report of National Cholesterol Education Program Expert Panel on Diet, Evaluation and Treatment of High Blood Cholesterol in Adults, *Arch Intern Med* 48:36-69, 1988.

14. Anderson JW, Geil PB: Diabetes, *Am J Med* 85(suppl 5A):1259-1286, 1988.

15. Roe DA: Diet, nutrition, and drug interactions. In Shils ME, Olson JA, Shike M, editors: *Modern nutrition in health and disease,* ed 8, Philadelphia, 1993, Lea & Febiger.

16. Shils ME: Nutrition and diet in cancer management. In Shils ME, Olson JA, Shike M, editors: *Modern nutrition in health and disease,* ed 8, Philadelphia, 1993, Lea & Febiger.

17. Shike M: Enteral feeding. In Shils ME, Olson JA, Shike M, editors: *Modern nutrition in health and disease,* ed 8, Philadelphia, 1993, Lea & Febiger.

18. Shils ME: Parenteral nutrition. In Shils ME, Olson JA, Shike M, editors: *Modern nutrition in health and disease,* ed 8, Philadelphia, 1993, Lea & Febiger.

19. Elsas LJ, Acosta PB: Nutrition support of inherited metabolic disease. In Shils ME, Olson JA, Shike M, editors: *Modern nutrition in health and disease,* ed 8, Philadelphia, 1993, Lea & Febiger.

20. Konstantinides FN, Konstantinides NN, Lin JC, et al: Urine urea nitrogen: too insensitive for calculating nitrogen balance in clinical nutrition, *JPEN* 15:189-195, 1991.

21. Herbert V: Aseptic addition method for *Lactobacillus casei* assay of folate activity in human serum, *J Clin Pathol* 19:212-16, 1966.

CHAPTER 38

Trace elements

Nancy W. Alcock

Classification
Essential trace elements
    Chromium
    Copper
    Fluorine
    Iodine
    Manganese
    Molybdenum
    Selenium
    Zinc
Toxic trace metals
    Aluminum
    Arsenic
    Cadmium
    Lead
    Mercury
Considerations in assessing trace-element status in humans

OBJECTIVES

- To discuss the primary biochemical role of essential trace elements in humans.

- To present the clinical symptoms associated with a deficiency or an excess of essential trace elements.

- To discuss the biological toxicity of trace levels of some metals.

- To discuss considerations in assessing the status of trace metals in humans.

KEY TERMS

deficiency Status of a nutrient in which an abnormal symptom or biochemical function is reversed by supplementation with the nutrient.

dental caries A condition in which the calcified dentin or enamel, or both, of a tooth is destroyed by the action of microorganisms on carbohydrates.

essential trace element An element that, if removed from the diet, produces a biochemical abnormality that is reversed by supplementation with the element.

metallothionein A 6200-dalton protein, with approximately

30% of its amino acid residue content composed of cysteine, which firmly binds Cd>Cu>Zn ions. Metallothionein plays an important role in zinc-copper interactions, and its synthesis is readily induced by zinc.

micronutrients Essential food components that are required or present in the body in very small amounts. Includes vitamins and some metals.

RDA Recommended daily allowance of a micronutrient.

toxic trace elements Those elements found in the environment in abnormal amounts that are antagonistic to biochemical processes. When present in tissues in elevated levels, they can be toxic and may eventually be fatal.

trace elements Elements present in the body in very low amounts (micrograms/gram or less). Some are essential; others may be toxic, even at relatively low levels. Most trace elements are metals, exceptions being the halogens iodine and fluorine.

zinc fingers Specific zinc binding (by histidine and cysteine residues) regions that occur at defined intervals of regulatory proteins. These proteins bind to deoxyribonucleic acid (DNA) and regulate gene expression by controlling DNA transcription.

CLASSIFICATION[1]

Trace elements can be subdivided into four major groupings based on their physiological function.

1. Essential trace elements for which a recommended daily allowance (RDA) has been established. These elements have been shown to be essential for normal growth, development, and maintenance, and a specific biological role has been identified. The elements in this group that are considered in this chapter are zinc, iodine, and selenium. The RDAs for these elements are listed in Table 38-1. Iron, the most abundant of the essential trace metals, is discussed in Chapter 35. Iron and zinc are transition elements in Mendeleef's original classification of the elements, whereas selenium and iodine are members of the "normal" series in group VI and group VII respectively.

2. Trace elements for which there is definite evidence of an essential role in human metabolism but for which an RDA has not yet been established. These include the transition metals copper, manganese, chromium, cobalt, and molybdenum and the group VII halogen fluorine. The estimated safe but adequate dietary intakes for these elements

Table 38-1   Recommended Dietary Allowances established for zinc, iodine, and selenium
The RDA for iron is included for comparison.

Category	Age (years) or condition	Weight kg	Weight lb	Height cm	Height in	Iron (mg)	Zinc (mg)	Iodine (μg)	Selenium (μg)
Infants	0.1-0.5	6	13	60	24	6	5	40	10
	0.5-1.0	9	20	71	28	10	5	50	15
Children	1-3	13	29	90	35	10	10	70	20
	4-6	20	44	112	44	10	10	90	20
	7-10	28	62	132	52	10	10	120	30
Males	11-14	45	99	157	62	12	15	150	40
	15-18	66	145	176	69	12	15	150	50
	19-24	72	169	177	70	10	15	150	70
	25-50	79	174	176	70	10	15	150	70
	51+	77	170	173	68	10	15	150	70
Females	11-14	46	101	157	62	15	12	150	45
	15-18	55	120	163	64	15	12	150	50
	19-24	58	128	164	65	15	12	150	55
	25-50	63	138	163	64	15	12	150	55
	51+	65	143	160	63	10	12	150	55
Pregnant						30	15	175	65
Lactating	1st 6 mo					15	19	200	75
	2nd 6 mo					15	16	200	75

From *Recommended Dietary Allowances,* ed 10, National Research Council, Washington, D.C., 1989, National Academy Press.

are shown in Table 38-2. The only known requirement for cobalt in humans is as a component of the B_{12} molecule, which is discussed in Chapter 39.

3. Trace elements that are consistently found in tissues or biological fluids in "ultratrace" amounts but that have not yet been shown to be either essential or detrimental at these levels of concentration. These include lithium, nickel, tin, silicon, and vanadium. These are not discussed in this chapter.

4. Trace metals that have no known biological function in humans but that, if present at relatively low levels, cause pathological changes. These toxic elements include aluminum, cadmium, mercury, lead, and arsenic. These are discussed in this chapter. Cadmium, arsenic, and mercury are transition elements, whereas aluminum and lead are members of the normal series in group III and group IV respectively.

ESSENTIAL TRACE ELEMENTS

The biological role of essential trace elements and some abnormalities arising from a deficiency or excess of the respective elements are shown in Table 38-3. Reference intervals, taken from the literature, for essential trace elements are listed in Table 38-4, and those for toxic metals are given in Table 38-5.

Chromium (Cr)[2-8]

Chromium is a transition element in period 4 of the periodic table of the elements, with an atomic weight of 52.

Biochemistry. Chromium has been demonstrated to be essential for normal carbohydrate, lipid, and nucleic acid metabolism. Trivalent chromium is a potentiator of insulin action.[3] It is postulated that chromium, which is found in cell nuclei, binds to DNA, RNA, and nuclear proteins. It appears to be involved in the maintenance of the structural

Table 38-2   Estimated safe and adequate daily dietary intakes of selected trace elements

Category	Age (years)	Copper (mg)	Manganese (mg)	Fluorine (mg)	Chromium (μg)	Molybdenum (μg)
Infants	0-0.5	0.4-0.6	0.3-0.6	0.1-0.5	10-40	15-30
	0.5-1	0.6-0.7	0.6-1.0	0.2-1.0	20-60	20-40
Children and adolescents	1-3	0.7-1.0	1.0-1.5	0.5-1.5	20-80	25-50
	4-6	1.0-1.5	1.5-2.0	1.0-2.5	30-120	30-75
	7-10	1.0-2.0	2.0-3.0	1.5-2.5	50-200	50-150
	11+	1.5-2.5	2.0-5.0	1.5-2.5	50-200	75-250
Adults		1.5-3.0	2.0-5.0	1.5-4.0	50-200	75-250

1. Because there is less information on which to base allowances, these figures are not given in the main table of the RDA and are provided herein the form of ranges of recommended intakes.
2. Since the toxic levels for many trace elements may be only several times the usual intakes, the upper levels for the trace elements given in this table should not be habitually exceeded.
From *Recommended Dietary Allowances,* ed 10, National Research Council, Washington, D.C., 1989, National Academy Press.

Table 38-3   Biological role of essential trace elements and associated abnormalities

Element	Biological role	Comments	Deficiency/abnormality/toxicity
Chromium	Metabolism of glucose	Potentiates insulin action	Glucose intolerance in deficiency
Cobalt	Component of vitamin B_{12}	No other function known in man	Vitamin B_{12} deficiency; anemia
Copper	Cofactor for oxidase enzymes	90% to 95% plasma copper bound to ceruloplasmin	Inherited diseases: Wilson's, Menke's
Fluorine	Inhibits dental caries; therapeutically improves quality of hydroxyapatite crystals	Usually supplied as supplement to drinking water	Excessive intake causes fluorosis
Iodine	Component of T_3 and T_4	Concentrated in the thyroid; supplementation by addition to salt common	Iodine deficiency still occurs in various areas
Iron	Component of heme enzymes: hemoglobin, cytochromes	In plasma bound to transferrin; stored as ferritin	Deficiency: hypochromic, microcytic anemia
Manganese	Required for glycoprotein and proteoglycan synthesis	Component of mitochondrial superoxide dismutase	Deficiency not known in man
Molybdenum	Component of sulfite and xanthine oxidases	Essential for production of uric acid	Deficiency reported in TPN patient; inability to metabolize methionine
Selenium	Component of glutathione peroxidase and iodinothyronine-5' deiodinase	Antioxidant properties; selenium and vitamin E act synergistically	Deficiency may occur where soil Se is low and in long-term TPN patients with inadequate supplements
Silicon	Involved in calcification in bone	Role in bone, cartilage, and connective tissue poorly understood	Deficiency: impairment of normal growth in animals; silicosis may occur from industrial exposure
Zinc	Cofactor or component of more than 200 metalloenzymes	Involved in many metabolic processes: protein synthesis; immunological function; growth and development	Deficiency: growth failure, hypogonadism, impaired wound healing; genetic disease: acrodermatitis enteropathica– impaired absorption; toxicity: vomiting, gastrointestinal irritation

TPN, Total parenteral nutrition.

integrity of the nuclear strands and in the regulation of gene expression.[4] The biologically active form is believed to be an organic complex containing trivalent chromium, nicotinic acid, and glutathione or its constituent amino acids. However, the exact structure of the complex has not been elucidated as yet. In humans, several signs and symptoms are indicative of chromium deficiency. These include impaired glucose tolerance, elevated circulating insulin, glucosuria, elevated fasting blood glucose, elevated serum triglycerides and cholesterol, encephalopathy, and neuropathy. Brewer's yeast is a good source of the glucose tolerance factor, but only 5% of its total chromium was found to be associated with the insulin-potentiating activity. It is not known exactly how chromium potentiates the action of insulin in vivo. It may bind directly to insulin, or it may act by increasing receptor number or affinity.

Clinical significance.[5] The status of chromium in the body has not been successfully characterized from its concentration in urine or serum. One reason for this is the difficulty associated with its accurate measurement in biological fluids because of contamination. Stainless steel, which contains chromium, is a common source for gross contamination. Anderson suggests that even when chromium analysis is carefully performed, the levels of chromium in serum

or urine may not be indicative of the body status.[2] Demonstration of a deficiency of chromium has been successful when improvement in glucose or lipid metabolism resulted from the administration of 200 μg of chromium per day to adults over a period of months. Patients receiving long-term total parenteral nutrition (TPN) are at risk for chromium deficiency if their TPN fluids are not supplemented. In the first reported case of chromium deficiency, the patient showed impaired glucose tolerance with normal insulin levels and had elevated fatty acid levels, low respiratory quotient, abnormalities of nitrogen metabolism, and neuropathy. Insulin infusion failed to improve glucose tolerance or respiratory quotient, but these parameters returned to normal after chromium supplementation.

The safe and adequate recommended level of chromium intake is shown in Table 38-2. It is estimated that less than 2% of dietary trivalent chromium is absorbed from the gastrointestinal tract.

Toxicity. Toxicity from trivalent sources of chromium has not been reported in humans. Hexavalent chromium toxicity from industrial exposure through inhalation has been associated with increased incidence of lung cancer.[6] In experimental animals, ingestion as chromate resulted in liver and kidney damage. Chromium in detergents and

Table 38-4 Reference intervals for essential trace elements

Element	Specimen type	Reference interval	
		Concentration	IU
Cr	S	0.12-2.1 μg/L	2.3-40.3 nmol/L
	RBC	20-36 μg/L	384-692 nmol/L
	U	0.1-2.0 μg/L	1.9-38.4 nmol/day
Co	S	0.11-0.45 μg/L	1.9-7.6 nmol/L
	RBC	16-46 μg/L	272-781 nmol/kg
	U	1-2 μg/L	17-34 nmol/L
Vitamin B$_{12}$	S	100-700 pg/mL	74-516 pmol/L
Cu	S	μg/dL	μmol/L
	birth-6 mo	20-70	3.14-10.99
	6 years	90-190	14.13-29.83
	12 years	80-160	12.56-25.12
	Adult (male)	70-140	10.99-21.98
	Adult (female)	80-155	12.56-24.34
	Term pregnancy	118-302	18.53-47.41
	U	3-35 μg/day	0.047-0.55 μmol/day
F	P	0.01-0.2 μg/mL	0.5-10.5 μmol/L
	U	0.2-1.1 μg/mL	10.5-57.9 μmol/L
	Toxicity		
I	U cord	1.7-4.0 ng/dL	21.9-51.6 pmol/L
T$_4$ free	Newborn	2.6-6.3 ng/dL	33.5-81.3 pmol/L
	Adult	0.8-2.3 ng/dL	10.3-31.0 pmol/L
T$_4$ total	S adult	5-12 μg/dL	65-155 μg/L
T$_3$ free (equilibrium dialysis)	S cord	15-391 pg/dL	0.2-6.0 pmol/L
	Children and adults	260-380 pg/dL	4.0-7.4 pmol/L
Radioimmunoassay	Adult	208-674 pg/dL	3.2-104 pmol/L
T$_3$ total	Adult	100-200 ng/dL	1.54-3.08
Mn	S	0.5-1.5 μg/L	9-27 nmol/L
	B		
	U		
Mo	S	0.1-3.0 μg/L	1.0-31.3 nmol/L
Se	S	124.3-165 μg/L	1.57-2.09 μmol/L
	≥11 years	46-143 μg/L	0.58-1.81 μmol/L
	Adult	85-145 μg/L	1.08-1.84 μmol/L
	Toxicity	>400 μg/L	>5.06 μmol/L
	U	7-60 μg/L	0.09-0.78 μg/L
Zn	S	70-120 μg/dL	10.7-18.3 μmol/L
	U	300-500 μg/day	4.58-7.64 μmol

B, Whole blood; *IU,* standard international units; *P,* plasma; *RBC,* red blood cell; *S,* serum; *U,* urine.

bleaches may be associated with the occurrence of dermatitis.

Food sources. Chromium is found in brewer's yeast, mushrooms, molasses, nuts, wine, beer, asparagus, prunes, meats, cheeses, and whole grains. It is difficult to assess accurately the chromium content of foods, since preparation for analysis usually involves homogenization in equipment with stainless steel parts and some contamination usually occurs.

Method.[7,8] Graphite furnace flameless atomic absorption spectrometry is the preferred method of analysis. Although a tungsten halogen lamp provides adequate background correction, graphite furnace atomic absorption spectrophotometry utilizing Zeeman background correction is the preferred instrumentation.

Reference intervals. Normal, nonsupplemented human adults excrete approximately 0.5 μg of chromium/L of urine and have serum levels <0.5 μg/L.[7,8] Erythrocytes have a concentration of 20 to 36 μg/L.

Copper (Cu)[9-16]

Copper is a transition element in period 4 of the periodic table of the elements, with an atomic weight of 64.

Divalent copper forms complexes with proteins, many of which are enzymes. A group of these constitute copper metalloenzymes with oxidase activity. These include cytochrome oxidase, ferroxidase (ceruloplasmin), superoxidase dismutase, lysine oxidase, dopamine beta-hydroxylase (β-hydroxylase), spermine oxidase, tyrosinase, uricase, benzylamine oxidase, diamine oxidase, and tryptophan 3,3-dioxygenase. In biological systems, copper has the ability to induce the synthesis of metallothionein and is intermediate between cadmium and zinc in this activity. Approximately 50% of dietary copper is absorbed, with the process being

Table 38-5 Acceptable and toxic reference ranges for toxic trace metals

Element	Specimen type	Reference range	
		Concentration	IU
Al	S	<4 µg/L	148 nmol/L
	U	0.120 mg/day	0.4-4 µmol/L
	S toxic	See text	
As	B	2-62 µg/L	26-826 µmol/L
	U	5-50 µg/day	66-660 nmol/day
	B acute toxicity; B chronic toxicity	600-9300 µg/L	8-125 µmol/L
Cd	B	<5 µg/L	<44.6 nmol/L
	U	<3 µg/day	<26 nmol/L
	Toxic	>50 µg/L	>446 nmol/L
Hg	B	<5 µg/L	<24.9 nmol/L
	B dentists	5-15 µg/L	24.9-74.7 nmol/L
	U	<20 µg/day	<99.5 nmol/L
	B toxicity	>50 µg/day	>249 nmol/L
	Hair	<1 µg/g	<4.9 nmol/g
Pb	B (children)	<100 µg/L	<480 nmol/L

B, Whole blood; *IU,* standard international units; *S,* serum; *U,* urine.

facilitated by the complexing of copper with amino acids. In plasma approximately 95% of copper is bound to the alpha$_2$-globulin (α_2-globulin), ceruloplasmin, an oxidase with ferroxidase activity. Copper is also transported in the plasma loosely bound to albumin. A small fraction of plasma copper is complexed with amino acids.

Although 1.5 to 3 mg/day of dietary copper has been determined to be safe and adequate (Table 38-2), it is estimated that 35% of diets in the United States provide less than 1 mg/day. Excretion of copper occurs mainly in the bile, with urinary excretion normally <40 µg/day.

Clinical significance. A relatively high carbohydrate intake in the American diet accompanied by marginal intake of copper possibly potentiates subclinical copper deficiency.[11] There is evidence that marginal copper deficiency is associated with heart disease, bone and joint osteoarthritis, and osteoporosis. Microcytic, hypochromic anemia, neutropenia, hypothermia, and demineralization have also been associated with copper deficiency. Copper deficiency in humans results in hypercholesterolemia[12] and decreased antioxidant protection. In an X-linked genetic defect in infants, Menkes' kinky hair syndrome, absorption of copper from the gastrointestinal tract is impaired, resulting in copper deficiency with resultant cerebellar and cerebral degeneration.[13]

Wilson's disease is an inherited autosomal recessive error in copper metabolism that results in excessive accumulation of copper in liver, brain, cornea, and kidneys. Ceruloplasmin levels are low, with elevated levels of nonceruloplasmin bound copper. Tissue copper deposits may be diminished and then excreted by the intravenous administration of a chelating agent. A more recent effective treatment with negligible side effects is the oral administration of zinc acetate,[14] which inhibits copper absorption.

Marginal copper deficiency, especially in adults, has so far proved to be difficult to detect biochemically. Milne[15] has concluded that diminished cytochrome oxidase activity in leukocytes or diminished superoxide dismutase activity in erythrocytes is likely to be the most reliable index of reduced levels of metabolically active copper.

Plasma copper is not a reliable indicator of copper status. Although long-term copper deprivation, as in treatment by total parenteral nutrition, results in low plasma levels, chronic therapy with corticosteroids and ACTH also reduce copper levels. Factors that are associated with elevated serum copper levels include oral contraceptives, pregnancy, and infectious or inflammatory conditions.

Food sources of copper. Most foods contain appreciable amounts of copper. Those rich in copper include shellfish, liver, kidney, egg yolk, and some legumes.

Methods.[16] Either flame atomic absorption spectrophotometry for serum or plasma, or graphite furnace flameless atomic absorption spectrophotometry for urine, where concentration is usually less than 40 µg/L, are the preferred methods of analysis.

Reference intervals. Serum or plasma levels vary with age and are higher in adult women than in men. These are shown in Table 38-3. Most copper is excreted through the bile, and urine levels are usually <40 µg/day.

Fluorine (F)[17-21]

Fluorine, atomic weight 19, is the first member of period 2 of the group VII halogens of the periodic table of elements.

Biochemistry. The fluoride anion may substitute for the hydroxyl ion in the hydroxyapatite crystal structure in calcified tissues, bone, and teeth. The production of a "harder" crystal is believed to account for the protective effect of fluoride against dental caries.[17] Fluoride has also been used therapeutically, alone or in combination with vitamin D, in the treatment of osteoporosis.

Clinical significance. A direct, inverse association between the incidence of dental caries and the fluoride concentration in drinking water ≤1 mg/L has long been recognized. Less convincing is a reported beneficial effect of sodium fluoride as a therapy for osteoporosis.[18,19]

Requirement. 1 to 2 mg/day. Usually a fluoridated water supply with 1 mg/L of fluoride provides the daily requirement.

Food sources. Traces of fluoride are present in most foods. Fluoride can be present in drinking water, either naturally or because of artificial supplementation.

Toxicity. A high intake of fluoride causes *dental fluorosis* characterized by discolored and mottled teeth. Increased bone density and calcification of muscle insertions evident by radiography occur in areas where 10 to 45 mg/L of fluoride is present in water.

Method. An ion-selective electrode[21] method is the preferred method of analysis.

Reference intervals[21]. *Plasma:* 0.01 to 0.2 µg/mL; 0.5 to 10.5 µmol/L. *Urine:* 0.2 to 1.1 µg/mL; 10.5 to 57.9 µmol/L.

Iodine (I)[22-24]

Iodine, atomic weight 127, is in period 5 of the group VII halogens of the periodic table of elements.

Biochemistry. Although iodine is widely distributed throughout the earth's surface, the sea is the major source of iodine. Iodides, oxidized by sunlight to the volatile elemental iodine, are estimated to provide annually some 400,000 tons of iodine to the atmosphere from seawater. The iodide concentration in seawater, approximately 50 μg/L, is similar to that of human serum.

Iodine is of significance in human biology as a constituent of the thyroid gland's hormones, thyroxine (3,5,3'5'-tetraiodothyronine, (T_4) and 3,5,3'-triiodothyronine (T_3), which are synthesized by the iodination of tyrosine (see Chapter 44 for details). These hormones are essential for healthy growth, differentiation, and development. Iodine deficiency occurs in areas where soil is depleted of iodide when heavy rains and snow leach iodine from the soil. Uptake by crops is directly proportional to soil content. Iodine-deficiency disease is still a frequent occurrence in various underdeveloped countries.

Clinical significance. Both maternal and fetal thyroid hormones contribute to fetal development. Iodine deficiency during pregnancy may result in spontaneous abortions, stillbirths, an increase in infant or perinatal mortality, congenital abnormalities or neurological cretinism, fetal hypothyroidism, and psychomotor defects. In the child and adolescent, goiter, mental retardation, and retarded development are prominent signs of hypothyroidism. Myxedematous, or neurological, cretinism is also seen. In adults endemic goiter results from iodine deficiency. Iodine status may be determined by measurement of either serum thyroid hormone levels or urine iodine excretion.[22]

Requirements. Iodine requirements vary with age (see Table 38-1).

Food sources. Marine fish and seaweed are rich in iodine.

Toxicity. Prolonged excess of iodine intake (>2 mg/day) results in iodide goiter and myxedema.

Methods. Immunoassay[24] for thyroid hormones and ion-selective electrode for methods for iodide are the recommended methods of analysis.

Reference intervals[23]. See Chapter 44 for levels of iodine-containing hormones. Reference intervals for plasma inorganic iodide are 0.8 to 6.0 μg/L. Urine inorganic iodide correlates with plasma level. The lower limit of the reference interval is age dependent: 5 to 10 years, 32.5 μg/g creatinine; adolescents, 50 μg/g creatinine; adults, 75 μg/g creatinine.

Manganese (Mn)[25-29]

Manganese is a transition element in period 4 of the periodic table of the elements with an atomic weight of 55.

Biochemistry. Manganese forms divalent and trivalent salts. It is important for proper metabolism in connective tissue, physical growth and development of reproductive functions, and proper carbohydrate and lipid metabolism. It functions as an enzyme activator, however, and other divalent cations, in particular magnesium, may substitute for manganese. Enzymes that may have high specificity for manganese are glycosyl transferases and mitochondrial pyruvate carboxylase and superoxide dismutase.[25] The total manganese content in adult humans is 12 to 20 mg, of which 25% is in the skeleton. The usual intake ranges from 1.7 to 8.3 mg/day, of which 2% to 15% is absorbed. Absorption is inhibited by the presence of other divalent cations, including Fe, Ca, and Mg, and by phosphate, fiber, and phytate. Manganese is excreted through the bile duct and in urine.

Clinical significance. Manganese deficiency in humans has not been unambiguously demonstrated. An anecdotal report in association with experimental vitamin K deficiency has not been substantiated.[27] A manganese deficiency has been suspected in hip abnormalities, joint disease, congenital skeletal deformities, and childhood epilepsy. Increased levels of erythrocyte manganese may be seen in rheumatoid arthritis. Serum manganese has been reported to be increased in myocardial infarction, in acute hepatitis, and in industrial manganese exposure. Industrial poisoning produces schizophrenia-like psychiatric effects and neurological disorders similar to those of Parkinson's disease. Symptoms arising from a decrease in striatal dopamine present in manganese poisoning can be reversed by administration of L-dopa, the precursor of dopamine.[28]

Requirement. The estimated safe and adequate dietary intake for various ages is shown in Table 38-2.

Food sources. Bran flakes and wheat are rich in manganese. Refined grains and meat contain little manganese.

Toxicity. Manganese toxicity from prolonged industrial exposure results in neurological changes resembling those of Parkinson's disease.[28]

Method. Zeeman graphite furnace atomic absorption spectrophotometry is the preferred analytical procedure. Magnesium nitrate is recommended as matrix modifier.[29]

Reference intervals. Whole blood: ~11 μg/L; ~200 nmol/L. *Serum:* 0.5 to 1.5 μg/L; 9 to 27 nmol/L. *Urine:* 0.2 to 0.5 μg/day; 3.6 to 9.0 nmol/L.

Molybdenum (Mo)[30-34]

Molybdenum is a transition element in period 5 of the periodic table of the elements, with an atomic weight of 96.

Biochemistry. Molybdenum is a cofactor of the metalloenzymes xanthine oxidase, sulfite oxidase, and aldehyde oxidase, and thus plays a role in the metabolism of purines to uric acid, the final stages of oxidation of sulfur-containing amino acids, and the oxidation of aldehydes respectively. Absorption of molybdenum from the gastrointestinal tract may be inhibited by competition from dietary copper if copper intake is high.

Clinical significance. Most of the available evidence on the metabolism of molybdenum results from animal studies. Increased intake of molybdenum inhibits copper utilization; this effect is potentiated by increased sulfate intake. Molybdenum retention is decreased in the presence of excess copper or sulfate.[31] An increase in molybdenum intake is accompanied by increased serum levels of uric acid and the development of gout.

A case of molybdenum deficiency in a patient maintained on total parenteral nutrition was reported.[32] Elevated levels of the amino acid methionine and decreased uric acid excretion and sulfate excretion were corrected by administration of molybdenum, indicating a reduced activity of molybdenum-containing metalloenzymes in the molybdenum-deficient patient.

Requirement. An estimate of the safe and adequate daily intake of molybdenum ranges from 10 μg in infancy to 250 μg in adults.

Food sources. Milk, milk products, organ meats, and dried legumes and cereals contain molybdenum.

Toxicity. A single report from Armenia documented elevated blood levels of molybdenum that were associated with high levels of molybdenum in soil and plants.[33] Symptoms of gout were reported, as well as others that indicated possible involvement of the liver, gastrointestinal tract, and kidney.

Method. Graphite furnace atomic absorption spectrophotometry is the recommended method of analysis for molybdenum.[34]

Reference interval. The reference interval for serum molybdenum is 0.1 to 3.0 μg/L.

Selenium (Se)[35-43]

Selenium is in period 4, group VI, of the periodic table of the elements and has an atomic weight of 79.

Biochemistry.[35] Selenium is a member of the same group of elements as oxygen and sulfur. Although selenium biochemistry has not been completely characterized, it is known that in plants selenium is present predominantly as selenomethionine, whereas in animals selenocysteine is the major form. Four selenium atoms are covalently bound to cysteine residues in the enzyme glutathione peroxidase, which has strong antioxidant properties and, in animal models, acts synergistically with vitamin E. Glutathione peroxidase is present in the cytoplasm and mitochondria of tissues. It is also found in erythrocytes, platelets, and plasma. Recently, a second enzyme, type 1 iodothyronine deiodinase, has been identified, and it contains one selenium atom per molecule. This selenium-metalloenzyme plays a role in the conversion of T_4 to T_3.[35]

Selenium enters the food chain via plants. Because of the wide variability in the concentration range of selenium in various areas throughout the world, low availability of selenium may occur in some areas, whereas in seleniferous areas excessive selenium is taken up by plants.[37] In human studies, the bioavailability of selenium from wheat, tuna, and mushrooms was 83%, 57%, and 5%, respectively, compared with that of sodium selenite. However, the form in which selenium occurs in foods is still unknown.

Clinical significance. Although no single marker for selenium status has been identified, plasma selenium is an indication of recent ingestion. Erythrocyte and platelet glutathione peroxidase activity correlates well with selenium supplementation in patients maintained on home total parenteral nutrition.[41] Urine selenium varies with intake, and, at very high levels of intake, volatile forms of selenium are exhaled. Nails and hair, which can have a high presence of sulfur- or selenium-containing proteins, have both been assessed for measurement of selenium status. In the United States the use of selenium-containing shampoos precludes the use of hair for such measurement.

Low selenium status has been recognized when intake is below the RDA shown in Table 38-1; chronic ingestion of levels above the RDA produce clinical symptoms. Experimentally selenium has been shown to be protective against mercury, cadmium, and silver toxicity, suggesting a preventive role for the element.

Selenium deficiency has been demonstrated in Keshan (pronounced kuh-shahn), a city in Manchuria, China, where soil selenium is very low.[40] Although Keshan disease, often associated with a cardiomyopathy in children and young females, responded to supplementation by selenium, the selenium deficiency is not considered to be the sole cause of this condition, and the implication of a virus or other agent has been considered. In other areas such as New Zealand, Finland, and Sweden, where low selenium status has been demonstrated, serious detrimental effects of the low soil selenium have not been observed. A second disease associated with low selenium intake in China is Kashin-Bek disease, which causes cartilage degeneration and osteoarthritis in adolescents and preadolescents. Patients maintained on long-term total parenteral nutrition are at risk of developing selenium deficiency if fluids are not supplemented. Numerous such cases have been reported, and several deaths associated with cardiomyopathy have occurred.

Requirement. The RDA for selenium is shown in Table 38-1 and ranges from 10 μg in infants to 75 μg in adults.

Food sources. In decreasing order of magnitude, organ meats and seafood, cereals and grains, dairy products, and fruits and vegetables are sources of dietary selenium.

Toxicity. Selenium toxicity is characterized by dermatitis, loose hair, and diseased nails. Selenium poisoning resulting from excessive intake of supplements results in acute toxicity. Symptoms include a metallic taste, odor of garlic, mucosal irritation, gastroenteritis, paronychia, and reddening of nails, hair, and teeth.[43] There is evidence that chronic ingestion of moderately elevated levels of selenium may be carcinogenic. Ironically, the use of oral selenium compounds as cancer-prevention agents is being actively studied. In some tumor models selenomethylselenocysteine had greater antitumor activity than sodium selenite, which was more active than selenomethionine.

Method.[44] Zeeman graphite furnace atomic absorption analysis with nickel nitrate or reduced palladium as matrix modifier is the recommended analysis method.

Reference intervals. Reference intervals in serum[42] vary from region to region depending on the selenium content of the soil of food sources. The mean serum levels (± 1 SEM) for adults in the United States are 1.10 (± 0.10) μmol/L for men and 1.20 (± 0.18) μmol/L for women.

Zinc (Zn)[45-52]

Zinc is a transition element in period 4 of the periodic table of the elements that has an atomic weight of 65.

Biochemistry. Zinc forms stable complexes, called *zinc fingers,* with the histidine and cysteine amino acid residues of proteins, and is a component of over 200 metalloenzymes. Important among the enzymes are those involved in nucleic acid and protein synthesis, including DNA and RNA polymerases, and reverse transcriptase. Regulatory proteins containing zinc fingers are central to gene expression.

Zinc induces the synthesis of metallothionein, which serves an important regulatory function of zinc and copper metabolism. The protein binds copper more firmly than zinc and forms an unabsorbable complex in the gastrointestinal tract, hence reducing copper absorption. In the liver, induction of metallothionein synthesis is significant in cases of stress and infection when zinc is sequestered by this organ. Zinc fingers, defined as domains of zinc-binding proteins that also bind to DNA, are involved in the gene expression of metallothionein.

Zinc is an intracellular cation present in all body tissues and fluids and, next to iron, is the second most abundant of the trace metals in humans. Muscle contains 50% to 60% of the 2 g of total body zinc. Bone contains 28% of body zinc stores, and 0.5% is found in blood. Erythrocytes contain 75% to 88% of blood zinc. In the plasma approximately 18% of zinc (normal range 700 to 1200 μg/L) is tightly bound to an α_2-macroglobulin, 80% is loosely bound to albumin, 2% is bound to transferrin, ceruloplasmin, or the amino acids histidine and cysteine, and a small fraction is present as free zinc.

The RDA of 15 mg of zinc for adult males and 12 mg for females is not likely to be provided by many diets consumed in the United States. Red meat is a prime source of bioavailable zinc. Hence, vegetarians are at risk for zinc insufficiency. In addition, the high fiber content of a vegetarian diet binds zinc and hence diminishes its bioavailability. From a usual nonvegetarian diet approximately 20% of zinc is absorbed. Absorption is enhanced by meats, liver, eggs, and seafood, whereas vegetables, whole grain foods, fiber, phytate, calcium, and iron inhibit absorption.

Clinical significance. Because zinc is required for the activity of enzymes that are critical for nucleic acid replication and protein synthesis, it is a necessary component for cell replication. Adequate supplies of zinc are imperative for healthy development of the fetus, and in early pregnancy plasma zinc falls despite increased intake. During pregnancy there is an increase in the plasma zinc fraction bound to α_2-macroglobulin and a decrease in the zinc bound to albumin. Plasma zinc is elevated during lactation.

Zinc deficiency was first described by Prasad et al. in Iran and Egypt.[47,48] Male adolescents showed retarded development and hypogonadism. Experimental zinc deficiency in animals is characterized by fetal abnormalities, impaired embryogenesis, impaired brain development, and impaired vision. Acute zinc deficiency in humans, especially in growing children, is apparent from skin lesions especially on body extremities or around orifices, diarrhea, irritability, loss of hair, growth retardation, and increased susceptibility to infections. An inherited autosomal recessive abnormality in ability to absorb zinc from the gastrointestinal tract was first described by Moynahan and Barnes.[49] In sickle cell anemia, some cancers, and traumas as in burns, stress, and acute infections, plasma zinc may fall precipitously, probably as the result of its redistribution to other tissues such as liver.

Impaired immunological function is associated with zinc insufficiency. In vitro, stimulation of lymphocytes by phytohemagglutin and concavalin A is enhanced by zinc. In vivo, a delayed hypersensitive response to skin allergens occurs consistent with the degree of zinc deficiency.

Identification of a reliable marker for assessment of zinc status has yet to be realized. Although abnormal plasma zinc levels are associated with many pathological conditions, plasma zinc concentrations are a poor indicator of the body status of zinc. Plasma levels of zinc may be lowered in response to stress and trauma but do not reflect intracellular status. Leukocyte zinc has been suggested as a reliable marker, but consistent findings have yet to be reported. Urinary excretion of zinc in response to a zinc challenge has been explored as a marker of zinc nutriture, as has the level of zinc in hair. Further investigation is required before any of these markers can be recommended. The use of stable isotopes of zinc in a recent study[50] showed that in premenopausal women zinc disappeared more rapidly from the plasma of those women judged to be zinc deficient. In both this and an earlier study, an inverse relationship between serum ferritin and zinc status was suggested. A strong association between zinc and iron nutriture was demonstrated. It is considered that marginal zinc deficiency is common and should be considered a public health problem.[51]

Requirement. The RDA for zinc is shown in Table 38-1. An increase in intake to 30 mg/day is recommended during pregnancy.

Food sources. Seafoods, meat, milk, and eggs are good sources of zinc. Although vegetables contain appreciable amounts of zinc, the presence of high concentrations of fiber and phytate account for zinc's low bioavailability in these food sources.

Toxicity. Epigastric pain, diarrhea, and vomiting have been observed from high zinc intake from food stored in galvanized containers. Supplements of as little as 25 mg of zinc have resulted in diminished absorption of copper, presumably because of competition.

Method.[52] The preferred method for zinc analysis is flame atomic absorption spectrophotometry in serum or plasma, with its erythrocytes, and in urine.

Reference intervals. *Serum:* 700 to 1200 µg/L; 10.7 to 18.3 µmol/L. *Urine:* 300 to 500 µg/day; 4.58 to 7.64 µmol/day.

TOXIC TRACE METALS
Aluminum (Al)[53-59]

Aluminum is classified as a period 3 element with an atomic weight of 27.

Basis for toxicity. Aluminum toxicity can result from exposure to industrial sources of aluminum, but most commonly the cause is iatrogenic. Patients who are experiencing renal failure are at high risk for aluminum toxicity from two sources. First, these patients use antacids containing aluminum hydroxide to decrease phosphate absorption. Second, aluminum may be present in the dialysate used for chronic dialysis of patients with end-stage renal disease. A second group of potentially vulnerable patients are those receiving TPN. Premature infants who receive TPN are particularly at risk for aluminum toxicity because of their reduced renal clearance. Casein hydrolysates were found to contain high concentrations of aluminum,[53-56] and more recently, components such as calcium and phosphate[57] have been shown to contain appreciable aluminum contamination.

In all cases of aluminum toxicity, the brain and the skeleton are the two target organs.[53,54] Although the biochemical basis for the neurotoxic effects of aluminum is uncertain, an association was found between high brain-aluminum concentrations at autopsy and dialysis dementia or dialysis encephalopathy in a large number of patients with renal failure who were undergoing chronic dialysis. By contrast, the finding of elevated brain aluminum in patients with Alzheimer's disease has not been uniformly reported.

Deposition of aluminum along the calcification front in bone has long been recognized. The development of bone pain in dialysis patients can indicate an excessive accumulation of aluminum. Bone morphology in these cases is consistent with osteomalacia (see p 538, Chapter 28). Another major sign of aluminum toxicity is microcytic anemia.

The use of free amino acids instead of casein hydrolysate considerably reduced the aluminum load from artificially prepared nutrients used for enteral and parenteral nutritional supplements. The finding of varying amounts of aluminum in different batches of the same ingredient, from the same and different manufacturers, accents the need for monitoring the aluminum content of TPN solutions. A working group for standards for aluminum content of parenteral nutrition solutions supports the Food and Drug Administration's proposal for setting a limit of 25 µg of aluminum per liter in large-volume parenteral fluids. It has been recommended that many TPN components, including solutions of minerals, trace metals, and vitamins and heparin, should require a statement of the aluminum content on their label. Other intravenous fluids such as immunoglobulins and albumin also contain variable amounts of aluminum.

Serum levels and indications for treatment. Reference intervals for serum aluminum vary among laboratories because of the ease of contamination. An upper limit of 4 µg/L (0.15 µmol/L) is considered to be within the reference interval. Serum aluminum levels do not necessarily reflect the amount of metal deposited in bone, liver, and brain. Bone pain is a useful clinical indicator of the degree of aluminum toxicity. The effectiveness of chelation therapy with desferrioxamine during dialysis can be monitored by measurement of serum aluminum.

Method. Zeeman graphite furnace atomic absorption spectrophotometry using magnesium nitrate as matrix modifier[53] is the recommended method of analysis.

Arsenic (As)[60-66]

Arsenic is a period 4 element with an atomic weight of 75.

Basis for toxicity. There is evidence that a very small amount of arsenic is essential in humans.[60] Arsenic has been shown to give protection against selenosis.[62] In tissues, arsenic is present in both trivalent and pentavalent states. Organic arsenic compounds containing methyl groups are the most important biochemically. Arsenate may be able to replace phosphate in some biological molecules.

The relative toxicity of oral arsenic trioxide is low: A fatal acute dose is estimated to be 10.2 to 26 nmol (0.76 to 1.95 µg) of arsenic per kilogram of body weight. In animal experiments 10 g/kg of body weight of arsenobetaine produced symptoms that disappeared within an hour.

Arsenic is usually found in all tissues, with skin, hair, and nails showing the highest concentrations,[61] because of arsenic binding to sulfhydryl (SH—) groups of proteins. Symptoms of acute toxicity in humans from oral intake of arsenic are nausea, vomiting, diarrhea, burning of the mouth and throat, and severe abdominal pain.[62] Chronic exposure to smaller toxic doses causes weakness, prostration, muscle aches, and, in children, loss of hearing at low frequencies. Headaches, drowsiness, and confusion occur both in acute and chronic toxicity. Although the mechanism for the symptoms is not defined, arsenic probably inhibits enzyme activity.

Both the absorption of organic forms of arsenic from the gastrointestinal tract and its excretion in the urine are highly efficient. Urine excretion is an effective mode of monitoring body status.[63] Refined techniques such as high-performance liquid chromatography are required to characterize the form in which arsenic is excreted.

Treatment.[64-66] Treatment of acute poisoning with D-penicillamine, 2,3-dimercapto-1-propanesulfonate, 2,3-dimercaptosuccinic acid, or 2,3-dimercaptopropanol (BAL) has been successful in humans.

Method. The recommended method of analysis is flameless atomic absorption.

Cadmium (Cd)[67-73]

Cadium is a period 5 element with an atomic weight of 112.4.

Basis for toxicity. The primary organs affected by cadmium toxicity are liver and kidney.[68] Cadmium toxicity may be the result of the formation of cadmium-metallothionein, which prevents the usual binding of zinc and copper to metallothionein, thus preventing the healthy functioning of the target organs.

Clinical significance. Cadmium is present in human infants in very low concentrations, but the metal accumulates rapidly within the first 3 years of life and continues to accumulate up to approximately 50 years of age. The level in blood, which is usually <1 μg/L, is increased about 50% in smokers.[69,70] Urinary excretion is approximately 1 μg/L normally, and higher in smokers.

Only small amounts of cadmium are absorbed from the gut. Absorbed cadmium is stored in the liver and preferentially in the renal cortex. Retention in the liver and kidney is explained by the formation of cadmium-metallothionein in these organs.[71] It is estimated that the biological half-life of cadmium is approximately 30 years. It is postulated that in the kidney low levels of cadmium reduce the number of binding sites in metallothionein for zinc and copper, thus interfering with the usual function of metallothionein in the kidney. Inhalation of cadmium results in renal damage even before impaired lung function is detected, causing a low-molecular-weight proteinuria and a reduced glomerular filtration rate. Osteomalacia (itai-itai disease) in Japanese women has been ascribed to cadmium exposure.[72]

Suggestions that cadmium in drinking water was associated with hypertension have yet to be proved.

Treatment. Chelation therapy has been found to be efficient immediately after toxic exposure to cadmium but less effective later. Diethylenetriaminepentaacetate probably does not effectively chelate the less accessible intracellular cadmium. However, BAL, if continuously administered, has been shown to increase biliary excretion of cadmium.[73]

Method. The recommended method of analysis is flameless atomic absorption.

Lead (Pb)[74-81]

Lead is considered to be a heavy metal and lies in period 6 of the periodic table of elements. It has an atomic weight of 207.

Basis for toxicity. The major source of lead in the environment, apart from industrial waste, is lead-based paint in the interior and exterior of wooden houses. Subsequent removal or decay of the paint leads to soil and water contamination and possible exposure of children to lead contamination. Other potential sources of lead contamination, such as lead pipes that are used for conveying water and lead solder used in food cans, have been largely eliminated.

Several enzymes in the heme synthetic pathway are inhibited, in vitro, by lead (see also p 706). The cytosolic enzymes δ-aminolevulinic acid synthetase and δ-aminolevulinic acid dehydratase are readily inhibited.[74] However, this effect has not been unequivocally demonstrated in vivo. Anemia is usually present in subjects when the blood-lead level exceeds 400 μg/L (1.92 μmol/L). In both iron deficiency and lead poisoning there is decreased incorporation of ferrous iron into protoporphyrin IX, a step needed for the synthesis of heme, and the replacement of iron by zinc to form zinc protoporphyrin occurs. Erythrocyte protoporphyrin begins to rise at a blood-lead level of 200 μg/L.

Lead absorption by the intestines is increased when a deficiency of iron, calcium, magnesium, zinc, phosphate, or vitamin D is present.[74] The use of dietary supplements of one or more of these nutrients is suggested as preventive or remedial treatment for lead toxicity.

Clinical significance of lead toxicity. Lead toxicity produces neurological, gastrointestinal, renal, immunological, endocrinological, and hematopoietic changes in humans. Children 6 months to 6 years of age are most affected, since they are growing rapidly and lead crosses the blood-brain barrier at an age when brain development is critical. Although the detrimental effects of lead have been recognized for many years, it is now believed that these effects occur at lower blood-lead concentrations than was previously believed. The work of Needleman and others[75,76,79] convincingly demonstrated a lowering of IQ in children with blood lead as low as 100 μg/L. At this level the magnitude of the problem, which affects millions of children, was recognized, and widespread efforts were undertaken to prevent or minimize the possibility of increasing exposure. In 1991 the Centers for Disease Control and Prevention (CDC) published a statement on preventing lead poisoning in young children.[77]

Blood-lead levels.[78,79] Although the level of blood lead considered to be safe is currently <100 μg/L, there is evidence that even lower blood-lead concentrations may be detrimental in growing children. Although no specific action level has been suggested, the CDC has suggested diagnostic evaluation and medical management of children at lead levels of >200 μg/L. Adults are less vulnerable to the neurological damage caused by lead than children are, but a blood-lead level of 300 μg/L or higher in an adult requires evaluation.

Treatment. The treatment of lead toxicity with chelating agents has included the use of penicillamine, calcium-ethylenediaminetetraacetic acid (Ca-EDTA), and 2,3-dimercaptopropanol. Dimercaptosuccinic acid (Succimer),[80] which may be administered orally, appears to have the least side effects. Effectiveness of treatment may be monitored by measurement of urine excretion of lead.

Method.[8] Zeeman graphite furnace atomic absorption spectrophotometry is the recommended method of analysis. Matrix modifiers of ammonium dihydrogen phosphate and magnesium nitrate together are effective.

Mercury (Hg)[82-86]

Mercury is a transition element also in period 6 of the periodic table of elements, with an atomic weight of 201.

Biochemistry. Mercury is usually present in all body tissues tested in humans, even in the absence of any identified exposure apart from dental amalgams. In fresh tissue, levels ranged from 0.1 to 0.5 μg/g. The highest levels occur in skin, nails, and hair. The kidneys contain higher mercury concentrations than liver, brain, thyroid, and pituitary do. In populations exposed to industrial mercury, the pituitary and thyroid concentrate mercury to a greater degree than other organs. Elevated tissue levels of mercury are usually associated with an elevation of selenium, with both elements present in a 1:1 molar ratio.

Inorganic mercury is poorly absorbed. However, alkyl derivatives of mercury, especially methyl mercury, formed by the action of microorganisms in sediments in both freshwater and seawater, enter the food chain and are approximately 90% absorbed. Mercury vapor is efficiently absorbed by inhalation, and approximately 80% of inhaled mercury is retained in the body.

The most common food source of mercury is fish, where the element is present as methyl mercury.[83] In the United States and other countries, limits of 0.4 to 1.0 mg Hg/kg of fish have been established. The red blood cell readily takes up methyl mercury, with a blood cell-to-plasma ratio of approximately 20:1. Populations with a heavy fish consumption may have blood-mercury levels as high as 400 μg/L. Methyl mercury crosses the placenta, and the level in cord blood correlates well with that of the mother,[84] though slightly higher. Inhalation of mercury vapor results in a smaller increase in red blood cells than is observed from methyl mercury absorption.

Clinical significance. Mercury poisoning affects the central nervous system (CNS). CNS abnormalities associated with mercury poisoning include tremors, incoordination, irritability, moodiness, and depression.[84] Salivation, diarrhea, stomatitis, and impaired vision accompany the neurological abnormalities. The passage of methyl mercury across the placenta is associated with increases in congenital abnormalities, mental retardation, cerebral palsy, and fetal mortality. All these symptoms were present after an incident termed the *Minamata Bay incident,*[83] in which industrial wastes containing mercury were dumped into the bay. In Minamata disease, increased levels of methyl mercury were found in fetal tissue, most particularly in the brain.

Mercury concentration in hair has been shown to correlate well with blood levels of mercury. The concentration in hair is approximately tenfold higher than the levels seen in blood. Clinical manifestations of mercury intoxication appear at whole blood levels of 200 μg/L, which can result from an exposure of about 0.3 mg of mercury per day as methyl mercury; this is a dosage equivalent to approximately 4 μg of mercury per kilogram of body weight in an adult.

Method.[86] Cold vapor atomic absorption spectrophotometry is the preferred method for analysis of inorganic mercury. Predigestion is required to convert methyl mercury to inorganic mercury.

Critical levels in blood and urine.[85] *Blood:* >20 μg/L; 0.10 μmol/L. RBC >40 μg/L; 0.20 μmol/L. *Urine:* 150 to 300 μg/L; 0.75 μmol/L.

CONSIDERATIONS IN ASSESSING TRACE-ELEMENT STATUS IN HUMANS

The roles of essential trace elements in biology are summarized in Table 38-3. The status of most of the essential trace elements cannot be assessed from their concentration in whole blood or plasma, the most easily accessible body component, and this remains a problem in patient care. Because it is not possible to assign a threshold for plasma or serum zinc, copper, selenium, chromium, or manganese below which supplementation of the respective element is indicated, other biochemical parameters should be considered concomitantly for assessment of trace-metal nutriture. These include dietary availability, existing conditions that may involve redistribution within the body, genetic disorders, hormonal regulation in the case of iodine, and the functional state of excretory organs. In addition, the presence of clinical signs and symptoms that are usually associated with a deficiency of a trace metal is an important diagnostic finding. Hence, a plasma zinc amount less than 500 μg/L associated with dermatological lesions, especially in a rapidly growing child, is suggestive of severe acute zinc deficiency. Investigation would be necessary to determine if the deficiency resulted from an insufficient dietary intake of zinc or from malabsorption of zinc as occurs in the genetic disorder acrodermatitis enteropathica. In cases of trauma such as burns, a similarly low plasma zinc level indicates redistribution of zinc, and the necessity for zinc supplementation is equivocal. Usually, the main route of excretion of endogenous zinc is the gastrointestinal tract, with contributions from pancreatic secretions and bile. The intestinal absorption of trace metals can be reduced as a result of the competition between zinc, iron, copper, manganese, and other divalent minerals in the diet. Trace-metal absorption may also be decreased in high-fiber diets because of the binding of the metals to phytates.

Although very low levels of plasma copper, such as 300 μg/L, and ceruloplasmin (which binds 60% to 95% of the copper) are indicative of frank copper deficiency, the plasma level is generally not a good indicator of copper status. Hence, functional tests, such as response to antigenic challenge for zinc and measurement of a copper-requiring enzyme such as superoxide dismutase or cytochrome oxidase, are considered to be useful in the assessment of the status of these metals. Serum selenium is an acceptable indicator of recent selenium absorption.

Chromium status is currently best assessed by the patient's ability to metabolize glucose. Excretion of glucose in the urine can be monitored for this purpose. Difficulties with obtaining an accurate (contamination-free) measurement of the very low levels of chromium seen in either serum or urine minimizes the value of direct chromium measurements for the assessment of chromium status.

Deficiencies of trace elements in patients maintained on TPN or by enteral feeding are now rare, but consideration must be given to ensure adequate supplementation in these groups of patients, especially when the therapy is over a long term. If periodic estimations of zinc, copper, selenium, or manganese reveal a decrease in the plasma levels of a trace metal when the patient's condition is stable, the possibility of a deficiency should be further explored.

Identification of the biochemical parameters that can be measured to indicate the status of trace elements in the body remains a challenge. Appropriate function tests or tests that measure the activity of an enzyme that has a specific requirement for a particular trace metal that are suitable for routine testing in a clinical chemistry laboratory have yet to be realized.

REFERENCES
Classification of trace elements
1. *Recommended Dietary Allowances,* ed 10, Subcommittee on the Tenth Edition of the RDA's Food and Nutrition Board, Commission on Life Sciences, National Research Council, National Academy Press, Washington, D.C., 1989, p 284.

Essential trace elements
Chromium
2. Anderson RA: Chromium. In Wertz W, editor: *Trace elements in human and animal nutrition,* ed 5, New York, 1987, Academic Press, vol 1.
3. Anderson RA, Polansky MM, Bryden NA, et al: Chromium supplementation of human subjects: effect on glucose, insulin, and lipid variables, *Metabolism* 32:894-899, 1983.
4. Okada S, Tsukada H, Ohba HJ: Enhancement of nucleolar RNA synthesis by chromium (III) in regenerating rat liver, *J Inorg Biochem* 21:113, 1984.
5. Jeejeebhoy KN, Chu RC, Marliss EK, et al: Chromium depletion: glucose intolerance and neuropathy reversed by chromium supplementation in a patient receiving long-term total parenteral nutrition, *Am J Clin Nutr* 30:531-538, 1977.
6. Fishbein L: Perspectives of analysis of carcinogenic and mutagenic metals in biological samples, *Int J Environ Anal* 28:21-69, 1988.
7. Veillon C, Patterson KY, Bryden NA: Determination of chromium in human serum by electrothermal atomic absorption spectrometry, *Anal Chim Acta* 164:67-76, 1984.
8. Veillon C, Patterson KY, Bryden NA: Chromium in urine as measured by atomic absorption spectrometry, *Clin Chem* 28:2309-2311, 1982.

Copper
9. Mason K: A conspectus of research on copper metabolism and requirements of man, *J Nutr* 109:1979-2066, 1979.
10. O'Dell BI: Copper. In Brown ML, editor: *Present knowledge in nutrition,* ed 6, Washington, D.C., 1990, International Life Sciences Institute, Nutrition Foundation.
11. Reiser S, Smith JC, Mertz W, et al: Indices of copper status in humans consuming a typical American diet containing either fructose or starch, *Am J Clin Nutr* 42:242-251, 1985.
12. Klevay LM, Inman L, Johnson LK, et al: Increased cholesterol in plasma in a young man during experimental copper depletion, *Metabolism* 33:1112-1118, 1984.
13. Danks DM, Campbell PE, Stevens BJ, et al: Menkes' kinky hair syndrome: an inherited defect in copper absorption with widespread effects, *Pediatrics* 50:188-201, 1972.
14. Brewer GJ, Hill GM, Dick RD, et al: Treatment of Wilson's disease with zinc. III: Prevention of reaccumulation of hepatic copper, *J Lab Clin Med* 109:526-531, 1987.
15. Milne DB, Johnson PE: Assessment of copper status: effect of age and gender on reference ranges in healthy adults, *Clin Chem* 39:883-887, 1993.
16. Alcock NW: Copper. In Pesce AJ, Kaplan LA, editors: *Methods in clinical chemistry,* St. Louis, 1987, Mosby.

Fluorine
17. Krishnamachari KAVR: Fluorine. In Mertz W, editor: *Trace elements in human and animal nutrition,* ed 5, New York, 1987, Academic Press, vol 1.
18. Department of Health and Human Services, Public Health Service: *Review of fluoride benefits and risks,* report of ad hoc subcommittee on fluoride of the committee to coordinate environmental health and related programs, Washington, D.C., 1991, US Government Printing Office.
19. Riggs BL, Seeman E, Hodgson SF, et al: Effect of fluoride/calcium regimen on vertebral fracture occurrence in postmenopausal osteoporosis: comparison with conventional therapy, *N Engl J Med* 306:446-450, 1982.
20. Riggs BL, Hodgson SF, O'Fallon WM, et al: Effect of fluoride treatment on the fracture rate in postmenopausal women with osteoporosis, *N Engl J Med* 322:802-809, 1994.
21. Blancke RV, Decker WJ: Analysis of toxic substances: determination of fluoride in plasma and urine by ion specific potentiometry. In Tietz NW, editor: *Textbook of clinical chemistry,* New York, 1986, Saunders.

Iodine
22. Hetzel BS, Maberly GF: Iodine. In Mertz W, editor: *Trace elements in human and animal nutrition,* ed 5, New York, 1986, Academic Press, vol 2.
23. Clugston GA, Hetzel BS: Iodine. In Shils ME, Olsen JA, Shike M, editors: *Modern nutrition in health and disease,* ed 8, Philadelphia, 1993, Lea & Febiger.
24. Larson PR, Alexander NM, Chopra IJ, et al: Revised nomenclature for tests of thyroid hormones and thyroid related proteins in serum, *J Clin Endocrinol Metab* 64:1089-1094, 1987.

Manganese
25. Keen CL, Zidenberg-Cherr S: Manganese. In Brown ML, editor: *Newer knowledge in nutrition,* ed 6, Washington, D.C., 1990, International Life Sciences Institute, Nutrition Foundation.
26. Hurley LS, Keen CL: Manganese. In Mertz W, editor: *Trace elements in human and animal nutrition,* ed 5, New York, 1987, Academic Press, vol 1.
27. Doisy EA Jr: Effect of a deficiency in manganese upon plasma levels of clotting proteins in man. In Hoekstra WG, Suttie HE, Ganther HE, Mertz W, editors: *Trace elements in animals,* ed 2, Baltimore, 1974, University Park Press.
28. Cotzias GC, Miller ST, Papavasilion PS, Tang LC: Interactions between manganese and brain dopamine, *Med Clin North Am* 60:729-738, 1976.

29. *Techniques for graphite furnace atomic absorption spectrophotometry,* Norwalk, Conn., 1985, Perkin-Elmer Corp, p 189.

Molybdenum

30. Nielsen FH: Ultratrace minerals. In Shils ME, Olsen JA, Shike M, editors: *Modern nutrition in health and disease,* ed 8, Philadelphia, 1993, Lea & Febiger.
31. Mills CF, Davis GK: Molybdenum. In Mertz W, editor: *Trace elements in humans and animals,* ed 5, New York, 1987, Academic Press, vol 1.
32. Abumrad NN, Schneider AJ, Steel D, Rogers LS: Amino acid intolerance during prolonged TPN reversed by molybdate therapy, *Am J Clin Nutr* 34:2551-2559, 1981.
33. Koval'skii UV, Iarovaia, GA, Shmavonian DM: [Modification of human and animal purine metabolism in conditions of various molybdenum bio-geochemical areas], *Zh Obshch Biol* 22:179-181, 1961.
34. International Union of Pure and Applied Chemistry (IUPAC): Determination of molybdenum in biological materials, *Pure Appl Chem* 63:1627-1630, 1991.

Selenium

35. Lockitch G: Selenium: clinical significance and analytical concepts, *Crit Rev Clin Lab Sci* 27:483-541, 1989.
36. Lavender OA, Burke RF: Selenium. In Shils ME, Olsen JA, Shike M, editors: *Modern nutrition in health and disease,* ed 8, Philadelphia, 1993, Lea & Febiger.
37. Robinson MF: Selenium in human nutrition in New Zealand, *Nutr Rev* 47:99-107, 1989.
38. Ip C: The chemopreventive role of selenium in carcinogenesis, *J Am Coll Toxicol* 5:7-20, 1986.
39. Ip C, Ganther HE: Activity of methylated forms of selenium in cancer prevention, *Cancer Res* 50:1206-1211, 1990.
40. Ip C, Hayes C, Budnick RM, Ganther HE: Chemical form of selenium, critical metabolites and cancer prevention, *Cancer Res* 51:595-600, 1991.
41. Lane HW, Lotspeich CA, Moore CA, et al: The effect of selenium supplementation on selenium status of patients receiving chronic total parenteral nutrition, *JPEN* 11:117-120, 1987.
42. Keshan Disease Research Group: *Chin Med J* 92:477-482, 1979.
43. McLaren CS: Clinical manifestations of human vitamin and mineral disorders. In Shils ME, Olsen JA, Shike M, editors: *Modern nutrition in health and disease,* ed 8, Philadelphia, 1993, Lea & Febiger.
44. Jacobson BE, Lockitch G: Direct determination of selenium in serum by graphite furnace atomic absorption spectrometry with deuterium background correction and a reduced palladium modifier: age specific reference ranges, *Clin Chem* 34:709-714, 1988.

Zinc

45. Hambidge KM, Krebs NF: Zinc. In Mertz W, editor: *Trace elements in humans and animals,* ed 5, New York, 1986, Academic Press, vol 2.
46. Cousins RJ, Hempe JM: Zinc. In Brown ML, editor: *Present knowledge in nutrition,* ed 6, Washington, D.C., 1990, International Life Sciences Institute, Nutrition Foundation.
47. Prasad AS, Miale A Jr, Farid Z, et al: Zinc metabolism in patients with the syndrome of iron deficiency anemia, hepatosplenomegaly, dwarfism, and hypogonadism, *J Lab Clin Med* 1:537-549, 1963.
48. Prasad AS: Discovery and importance of zinc in human nutrition, *Fed Proc* 43:2829-2834, 1984.
49. Moynahan EJ, Barnes PM: Zinc deficiency and a synthetic diet for lactose intolerance, *Lancet* 1:676-677, 1973.
50. Yokoi K, Alcock NW, Sandstead HH: Iron and zinc nutriture of premenopausal women: associations of diet with serum ferritin and plasma zinc disappearance and of serum ferritin with plasma zinc and plasma zinc disappearance, *J Lab Clin Med* 124:852-861, 1994.
51. Sandstead HH: Zinc deficiency: a public health problem, *Am J Dis Child* 145:853-859, 1991.
52. Smith JC Jr, Butrimovitz GP, Purdy WC: Direct measurement of zinc in plasma by atomic absorption spectroscopy, *Clin Chem* 25:1487-1491, 1979.

Toxic trace metals

Aluminum

53. Alfrey AC: Aluminum. In Mertz W, editor: *Trace elements in human and animal nutrition,* ed 5, New York, 1986, Academic Press, vol 2.
54. Ott SM, Malong NA, Klein GL, et al: Aluminum is associated with low bone formation in patients receiving chronic parenteral nutrition, *Ann Intern Med* 98:910-914, 1983.
55. Sedman AB, Klein GL, Merritt RJ, et al: Evidence of aluminum loading in infants receiving intravenous therapy, *N Engl J Med* 312:1337-1343, 1985.
56. Klein GL, Alfrey AC, Miller AL, et al: Aluminum loading during total parenteral nutrition, *Am J Clin Nutr* 35:1425-1429, 1982.
57. Koo WWK, Kaplan LA, Horn J, et al: Aluminum in parenteral nutrition solutions—sources and possible alternatives, *JPEN* 10:591-595, 1986.
58. Klein GL, Alfrey AC, Shike M, et al: Parent drug products containing aluminum as an ingredient or a contaminant: response to FDA notice of intent, *Am J Clin Nutr* 53:399-402, 1991.
59. Alcock NW, Goeger MP: *Determination of aluminum with Zeeman graphite furnace atomic absorption spectrophotometry.* (In press.)

Arsenic

60. Anke M: Arsenic. In Mertz W, editor: *Trace elements in human and animal nutrition,* ed 5, New York, 1986, Academic Press, vol 2.
61. Smith HS: *J Forensic Sci Soc* 7:97-102, 1967.
62. Diplock AT, Mehlert A: Arsenic. In Anke M, Schneider HJ, Bruckner C, editors: *Spurenelement—Symposium,* Geneva, 1980, Wiss Publisher, Friedrich-Schiller University, pp 75-81.
63. Tan GKH, Charbonneau SM, Bryce F, Sandi E: Excretion of a single oral dose of fish-arsenic in man, *Bull Envir Contam Toxicol* 28:669-673, 1982.
64. Peterson RG, Rumack BH: D-Penicillamine therapy of acute arsenic poisoning, *J Pediatr* 91:661-666, 1977.
65. Tadlock CH, Aposhian V: Protection of mice against lethal effects of sodium arsenite by 2,3-dimercapto-1-propane sulfonic acid and dimercaptosuccinic acid, *Biochem Biophys Res Comm* 94:501-507, 1980.
66. Levine WG, Goodman LS, Gilman A, editors: Heavy metals and heavy metal antagonists. In *Pharmacological basis of therapeutics,* ed 5, New York, 1975, MacMillan.

Cadmium

67. Kostial K: Cadmium. In Mertz W, editor: *Trace elements in human and animal nutrition,* ed 5, New York, 1986, Academic Press, vol 2.
68. Kjellström T: Exposure and accumulation of cadmium in populations from Japan, the United States, and Sweden, *Environ Health Perspect* 28:169-176, 1979.
69. Smith TJ, Temple AR, Reading JC, et al: Cadmium, lead, and copper blood levels in normal children, *Clin Toxicol* 9:75-87, 1976.
70. Kowal DE, Johnson DE, Kraemer DF, Pahren HR: Normal levels of cadmium in diet, urine, blood, and tissues of inhabitants of the United States, *J Toxicol Environ Health* 5:995-1014, 1979.
71. Nordberg M: Studies on metallothionein and cadmium, *Environ Res* 15:381-404, 1978.
72. Tohyama C, Shaikh ZA, Nogawa K, et al: Urinary metallothionein as a new index of renal dysfunction in "itai-itai" disease patients and other Japanese women environmentally exposed to cadmium, *Arch Toxicol* 50:159-166, 1982.
73. Klassen CD, Waalkes MP, Cantilena LR: Alteration of tissue disposition of cadmium by chelating agents, *Environ Health Perspect* 54:233-242, 1984.

Lead

74. Centers for Disease Control and Prevention (CDC): *Preventing lead poisoning in young children—a statement by the CDC,* Atlanta, 1991, Department of Health and Human Services, Public Health Service.
75. Quarterman KA: Lead. In Mertz W, editor: *Trace elements in human and animal nutrition,* ed 5, New York, 1986, Academic Press, vol 2.

76. Piomelli S, Graziano J: *Laboratory diagnosis of lead poisoning, Pediatr Clin North Am* 27:843-853, 1980.
77. Mahaffey KR: Environmental lead toxicity: nutrition as a component of intervention, *Environ Health Perspect* 89:75-78, 1990.
78. Bellinger DC, Stiles KM, Needleman HL: Low level lead exposure, intelligence, and academic achievement: a long-term follow up study, *Pediatrics* 90:855-861, 1992.
79. Needleman HL: The current status of low level lead toxicity, *Neurotoxicology* 14:161-166, 1993.
80. Jorgensen FM: Succimer: the first approved oral lead chelator, *Am Fam Physician* 48:1496-1502, 1993.
81. Jacobsen BE, Lockich G, Quigley G: Improved sample preparation for accurate determination of low concentrations of lead in whole blood by graphite furnace analysis, *Clin Chem* 37:515-519, 1991.

Mercury

82. Clarkson TW: Mercury. In Mertz W, editor: *Trace elements in human and animal nutrition,* ed 5, New York, 1987, Academic Press, vol 1.
83. Subaki T, Irukagama K: *Minamata disease: methyl mercury poisoning in Minamata and Niigata, Japan,* Amsterdam, 1977, Elsevier Scientific Publishing Co.
84. Choi BH: The effects of methyl mercury on the developing brain, *Prog Neurobiol* 32:447-470, 1989.
85. Swedish Expert Group: MeHg in fish: a toxicologic-epidemiologic level of risks report from an expert, *Nord Hyg Tidsk* (supp 4), pp 1-364, 1971.
86. Magos L, Clarkson TW: Atomic absorption determination total, inorganic and organic mercury in blood, *J Assoc Office Anal Chem* 55:966-971, 1972.

CHAPTER 39 Vitamins

MARGE A. BREWSTER

OBJECTIVES

- Define vitamin.
- List the fat-soluble vitamins, their functions, and conditions that result from a deficiency.
- List water-soluble vitamins, their functions, and conditions that result from a deficiency.
- Describe the functions of vitamin B_{12} and folic acid and describe disease conditions that are a result of deficiencies of these vitamins.

KEY TERMS

angular stomatitis Inflammation at the corner of the mouth.

anorexia Appetite loss.

antioxidant A substance that protects against oxidation, usually by being readily oxidized itself.

aphonia Loss of voice; motions of crying but little sound.

avidin A glycoprotein in raw egg white with strong affinity for biotin.

Batten's disease A progressive childhood encephalopathy with disturbed metabolism of polyunsaturated fatty acids.

carotenoids Compounds structurally similar to β-carotene (provitamin A) occurring naturally in vegetables and pigmented fruits.

cholelithiasis Presence of gallstones.

CNS Central nervous system.

coagulopathy A disorder of coagulation.

creatinuria Excess excretion of creatine in the urine.

cyanosis Blue skin color caused by lack of oxygen.

dry beriberi Thiamin deficiency resulting in poor appetite, fatigue, and peripheral neuritis.

dyspnea Difficult or painful breathing.

ecchymoses Skin discolorations caused by oozing of blood into tissues.

fibrinolysis The process of dissolution of fibrin clots.

flavins Riboflavin, flavin adenine dinucleotide (FAD), and flavin mononucleotide (FMN).

glossitis Smooth tongue.

hydrolases Enzymes that cleave ester bonds by addition of water.

hyperuricemia Increased concentration of serum uric acid.

ischemia Lack of adequate blood supply to tissues.

megaloblastic anemia Anemia in which marrow and blood cells are large and have multilobed nuclei.

osteoblasts Cells that form bone.

osteoclasts Cells that degrade bone.

ozone O_3; increased in air in areas with heavy automobile traffic.

pancytopenia Decrease in all blood cells and platelets.

paresthesias Abnormal sensations such as burning, prickling, or tingling.

pellagra Niacin deficiency resulting in diarrhea, dementia, and dermatitis.

pernicious anemia Anemia (no longer considered pernicious) caused by antibodies interfering with vitamin B_{12} absorption.

photophobia Abnormal sensitivity to light.

PUFA Polyunsaturated fatty acids.

pyrexia Fever.

pyridine nucleotides NAD, NADH, NADP, NADPH.

RDA Recommended Dietary Allowances, quantity of vitamin recommended for daily ingestion to meet essential needs of a healthy person.

rebound scurvy Symptoms of scurvy occurring on sudden withdrawal of a megadosage of ascorbic acid.

rickets Muscle hypotonia and skeletal deformities in children.

scurvy Ascorbic acid deficiency characterized by swollen gums with loss of teeth, skin lesions, and pain and weakness in the lower extremities.

steatorrhea Excessive lipid in feces.

subclinical vitamin deficiency Chemical indices of vitamin status indicate deficiency, but there is no *apparent* clinical symptom.

thioester Ester bond involving —SH.

vitamins Low-molecular-weight components required for metabolic activity that must be supplied by dietary intake.

Wernicke-Korsakoff syndrome Neurological and behavioral alterations seen in some patients with thiamin deficiency.

wet beriberi Thiamin deficiency resulting in edema and cardiac failure.

xanthomatosis Presence of yellow skin deposits.

The vitamins are a group of low-molecular-weight compounds with diverse functions in biological tissues. Primarily they serve as cofactors of numerous enzymatic reactions. Without these cofactors a wide range of enzymes that play critical roles in cellular metabolism become inactive. The term *vitamin* is derived from early evidence that one such compound, thiamin, was an amine vital for health. These compounds or their biologically inactive precursors must be obtained, at least partially, from food sources or, in some instances, from intestinal bacterial synthesis. Inadequacies in supply (resulting from inadequate diet or inadequate intestinal absorption) are termed *vitamin deficiencies.* Abnormalities of metabolism requiring an abnormally high supply of one of these cofactors may be termed *vitamin insufficiencies,* or *vitamin dependencies,* depending on the level of supply demanded for physiological function. Variabilities in clinical expression of vitamin abnormalities result from differences in specific cause and degree and duration of vitamin inadequacy. Additional factors contributing to this variability include the genetic constitution of the individual, simultaneous presence of multiple nutritional insufficiencies, or increased metabolic demands imposed by conditions such as infection, pregnancy, or cancer. We still have limited knowledge of human mechanisms of absorption, transport, storage, and metabolism of vitamins, and we have much to learn with regard to the effects of diseases, therapies, and exogenous agents on these processes.

Because of the pervasive action of vitamins in metabolic processes, the clinical symptoms of vitamin deficiencies are usually nonspecific and vague, often delaying a definitive diagnosis. This is especially true in the early stages of vitamin deficiency or in mild chronic deficiency states; also vitamin deficiency may be complicated by other simultaneous processes. A combination of dietary history, physical examination, and biochemical measurements is often required to diagnose a vitamin deficiency. In addition, a therapeutic trial may also be required for a definitive diagnosis. Because vitamin metabolism is complex and interactive, vitamin supplementation without proper studies may lead to other nutrient deficiencies, toxicities, or an irreversible state of untreated deficiency with symptoms masked by inappropriate therapy. Vitamin functions and the usual symptoms seen in deficient and toxic states are listed in Table 39-1.

Suspicion of dietary deficiency of a vitamin arises primarily from knowledge of dietary sources and dietary practices likely to provide inadequate intake or absorption. Recommended Dietary Allowances (RDA) are defined by the Food and Nutrition Board[1] as the levels of intake of essential nutrients considered, on the basis of available scientific knowledge, to be adequate to meet the nutritional needs of practically all "healthy persons." These levels are defined from information on the daily intake requirements needed to avoid deficiency symptoms and to maintain specific functions. RDA values are generally set high enough to meet the needs of 97.5% of the population; they are sometimes even higher if the nutrient is poorly absorbed or insufficiently used.

Biochemical indices of vitamin status become abnormal before development of obvious clinical changes, thus allowing detection of a vitamin deficiency at a subclinical or nonclassical stage. Chemical determination of human vitamin status has been approached in the following ways:

1. Measurement of the active cofactor(s) or precursor(s) in biological fluids or blood cells
2. Measurement of urinary metabolite(s) of the vitamin
3. Measurement of a biochemical function requiring the vitamin (such as enzymatic activity) with and without in vitro addition of the cofactor form
4. Measurement of urinary excretion of vitamin or metabolite(s) after a test load of the vitamin
5. Measurement of urinary metabolites of a substance, the metabolism of which requires the vitamin, after administration of a test load of the substance

However, reduced serum concentrations of a vitamin do not always indicate a deficiency that interrupts cellular function; on the other hand, values within the reference interval do not always reflect adequate function. Interpretation of chemical values must be done with caution and with knowledge of the physiological and methodological factors that can confound a diagnosis. Several different measures of a vitamin's status are thus desirable.

Table 39-2 lists representative biochemical data that are usually associated with classical deficiency symptoms. These values are, of course, somewhat affected by the age of the patient and by laboratory methodology. A bibliography of articles regarding methodologies and vitamin functions is provided.

FAT-SOLUBLE VITAMINS

Because the fat-soluble vitamins (A, E, K, and D) are absorbed as part of the chylomicron complex (see Chapter 33),

Table 39-1   Vitamin functions and symptoms of deficiency or toxicity

Vitamin	Function	Clinical deficiency	Toxicity
A	Vision, growth, reproduction, mucus secretion, immune responses, cancer prevention (?)	Night blindness, growth retardation, appetite loss, reduced taste, recurrent infections, dermatitis, dry mucous membranes *Late:* bone growth failure, aspermatogenesis, xerophthalmia (dry, thickened, lusterless eyeballs), blindness	*Acute:* raised intracranial pressure and skin desquamation; teratogen *Chronic:* liver damage, skin changes, and exostoses
E	Antioxidant (membrane stability), neurologic function, cardiovascular disease prevention	Mild hemolytic anemia, ataxia, loss of tendon reflexes, pigmentary retinopathy	Creatinuria, decreased platelet aggregation, impaired wound healing, anti-inflammatory activity, hepatomegaly, impaired fibrinolysis, potentiation of vitamin K deficiency, coagulopathy
K	Coagulation (gamma-carboxylation of inactive clotting factors—prothrombin, factors II, IX, and X)	Hemorrhage (ranging from easy bruising to massive ecchymoses, mucous membrane hemorrhage, or posttraumatic bleeding)	*Adults:* cardiac and pulmonary signs *Newborns:* hemolytic anemia
D	Bone calcification	*Children:* rickets *Adults:* osteomalacia	Anorexia, vomiting, headache, drowsiness, and diarrhea
C	Collagen formation, catecholamine synthesis, cholesterol catabolism, antioxidant	*Early:* weakness, lassitude, irritability, vague aches and pains *Late:* scurvy (hemorrhages into skin, alimentary and urinary tracts, other tissues; osteoporotic bones, defective tooth formation, anemia, pyrexia, delayed wound healing)	Increased excretion of oxalate and urate, diarrhea, dyspepsia
Riboflavin	Oxidative enzymatic reactions	Angular stomatitis (mouth lesions), glossitis (smooth tongue), photophobia, blepharospasm (eyelid spasm), conjunctival congestion and other ocular changes, dermatological changes, neurological alterations (behavior changes, decreased hand grip strength, burning feet in adults, retarded intellectual development and EEG changes in children), and hematological dyscrasia (anemia and reticulocytopenia)	Low toxicity
Pyridoxine	Enzyme systems involving amino acid transaminases, phosphorylases, racemases, decarboxylases, deaminases	*Infants:* irritability, seizures, anemia, vomiting, weakness, ataxia, abdominal pain *Adults:* facial seborrhea	Usually low systemic toxicity Reduced milk production? Sensory neuropathy?
Niacin	Oxidation-reduction (as pyridine nucleotides NAD and NADP)	*Early:* lassitude, anorexia, weakness, digestive disturbances, anxiety, irritability, and depression *Late:* pellagra (dermatitis, mucous membrane inflammation, weight loss, disorientation, delirium, dementia)	Cutaneous flushing, gastric irritation, mild liver dysfunction, jaundice, hyperuricemia, impaired glucose tolerance
Thiamine	Decarboxylations, ketol formation	*Infants:* dyspnea and cyanosis, diarrhea, vomiting, wasting, aphonia *Adults:* "dry beriberi" (poor appetite, fatigue, peripheral neuritis) or "wet beriberi" (edema and cardiac failure), Wernicke-Korsakoff syndrome (intelligence disturbance, apathy, ataxia, double vision, nystagmus, drooping eyelids, loss of recent memory)	Anxiety, headache, convulsions, weakness, trembling, neuromuscular collapse

Table 39-1   Vitamin functions and symptoms of deficiency or toxicity—cont'd

Vitamin	Function	Clinical deficiency	Toxicity
Biotin	Coenzyme for CO_2 carboxylation reactions and for carboxyl group exchange	Dermatitis progressing to mental and neurological changes, nausea, anorexia, peripheral vasoconstriction, or coronary ischemia in some cases	None described
Pantothenate	Acyl-group transfer reactions (as part of coenzyme A and acyl carrier protein)	Never spontaneously seen—with chemical agonist: apathy, depression, increased infection, paresthesias (burning sensations), muscle weakness	None described
B_{12}	Myelin formation, methionine synthesis, folate interconversions, and DNA synthesis	*Early:* cognitive impairment? *Late:* megaloblastic anemias, neurological abnormalities (paresthesias progressing to spastic ataxia)	Infrequent adverse reactions are mostly allergic (possibly related to contaminants or preservatives)
Folate	One-carbon transfers	Megaloblastic anemia; organic mental changes?	Few reports—mostly allergic reactions
Carnitine	Energy metabolism and acyl-group transport	Muscle weakness, fatigue	None known

their absorption depends on the presence of adequate bile and pancreatic secretions and on healthy bowel mucosa as well. Therefore chronic malabsorptive states are often associated with a deficiency of one or more of these vitamins (see Chapters 29 and 30). The malabsorptive states include biliary tract disease, pancreatic disease, fistula, small bowel obstruction, and alcoholic liver disease (see Chapter 34). Deficiency of this class of vitamins generally develops slowly as stored supplies of vitamins are depleted. Vitamin A can be stored in liver parenchymal cells for a year or longer, and vitamin E can be stored in body fat for several months. Paradoxically, although they are fat soluble, vitamins K and D appear to be stored only for days or weeks.

Vitamin A

First described in 1909 and found to prevent night blindness in 1925, vitamin A is now known to be made up of three biologically active forms: retinol, retinal, and retinoic acid. These major vitamin A compounds all contain a trimethylcyclohexenyl group and an all-*trans* polyene chain with four double bonds (Fig. 39-1). These compounds are derived directly from dietary sources, primarily as retinyl esters, or from metabolism of dietary carotenoids (provitamin A), primarily β-carotene. Major dietary sources of these compounds include animal products (vitamin A) and pigmented fruits and vegetables (carotenoids). Each of these compounds is soluble in organic solvents, with retinoic acid being more polar than the others. Oxidation of retinol or retinal by peripheral cells is irreversible; thus neither retinoic acid nor retinal is metabolically converted to retinol.

Metabolism. Enzymes of the small intestinal mucosa convert dietary β-carotene and retinal to the predominant form of vitamin A, retinol (Fig. 39-2). The retinyl esters of dietary animal products are cleaved to retinol by pancreatic

and mucosal hydrolases (vitamin A esterases). Once in the mucosal cell, retinol is reesterified, forming retinyl esters (primarily retinyl palmitate) that are transported in lymph chylomicrons to the systemic circulation. After the chylomicrons release their triglycerides to adipose tissue, the retinyl esters are transported to the liver where they are stored associated with lipid droplets in hepatocytes. The more polar retinoic acid does not require this lipoprotein transport route but is directly absorbed into the portal circulation. However, this form is not stored in liver but is excreted through bile as a glucuronide conjugate.

When body demands require mobilization of hepatic vitamin A, the stored retinyl palmitate is hydrolyzed and the free retinol combines with retinol-binding protein (RBP). RBP-retinol is then secreted into the circulation, where it complexes with prealbumin. This large complex then circulates to target tissues that have specific receptor sites for RBP, and retinol is transferred intracellularly to another specific binding protein termed *cytosol-retinol–binding protein* (CRBP). CRBP-retinol presumably transports the retinol to its functional site within the cell. Retinol metabolism is shown in Fig. 39-2.

Function (see Table 39-1). The only clearly defined physiological role for retinol is its role in vision. Retinol is oxidized in the rods of the eye to retinal, which, when complexed with opsin, forms rhodopsin, allowing dim-light vision. In vitamin A–deficiency states epithelial cells (cells in the outer skin layers and cells in the lining of the gastrointestinal, respiratory, and urogenital tracts) become dry and keratinized. Thus vitamin A may help to maintain epithelial cells, which provide protection against infectious organisms. Retinoic acid, a quantitatively minor component of vitamin A, is known to function in growth and maintenance of the epithelium but not in vision and reproduction.

Table 39-2 Concentration or excretion rates associated with classical vitamin deficiency symptoms*†

Vitamin	Chemical value
A	<0.1 mg/L of plasma retinol
	>20% relative dose response (RDR) in plasma
E	<5.0 mg/L of plasma α-tocopherol
K	Plasma prothrombin time greater than normal
D	See Chapter 28
Ascorbic acid (C)	<2.4 mg/L of serum ascorbate
	<3 mg/L of whole blood ascorbate
	<80 mg/L of leukocyte ascorbate
Riboflavin (B₂)	>1.4 AC‡ of erythrocytic glutathione reductase
	<0.1 mg of riboflavin per liter of erythrocytes
	<0.12 mg of urinary riboflavin per day
	≥0.08 mg of urinary riboflavin per gram of creatinine
Pyridoxine (B₆)	≥1.5 AC of erythrocytic AST
	≥1.25 AC of erythrocytic ALT
	<0.8 mg of urinary 4-pyridoxic acid per day
	>25 mg of urinary xanthurenic acid per day
	<30 nM plasma pyridoxal phosphate
Thiamine	>1.25 AC of erythrocyte transketolase
	<0.1 mg of urinary thiamine per day
Niacin	≥1 urinary ratio (α-pyridone/N′-methyl-nicotinamide)
Biotin§	<0.7 μg/L of whole blood?
	15 μg of urinary biotin per day?
Pantothenic acid§	<1.0 mg/L of whole blood pantothenate
	<1.0 mg of urinary pantothenate per day
B₁₂	<150 ng/L of serum vitamin B₁₂
	≥24 mg of urinary methylmalonic acid per day
	>0.44 nM serum methylmalonic acid
	>4 mmol/mole of creatinine in urine
	>15 nM serum total homocysteine
Folate	<140 μg/L of erythrocyte folate
	<3.0 μg/L of serum folate
	≥30 mg of urinary N⁵-formiminoglutamic acid (FIGLU) per 8 hours
	>15 nM serum homocysteine
Carnitine	<30 nM plasma total carnitine

*These are general guidelines with reference intervals dependent on age and methodology used.
†Compiled from references 3, 4, and 42.
‡AC, Activity coefficient; ratio of activities with and without added cofactor.
§Deficient values for biotin and pantothenate are not well established.

Clinical and chemical deficiency signs. Clinical signs of vitamin A deficiency can be separated into early and late signs (see Table 39-1). The chemical sign of deficiency is reduction in plasma vitamin A. Generally retinol values below 0.1 mg/L are associated with clinical symptoms, and values above 0.2 mg/L are not.[2,10] Values below 0.29 mg/L may be inadequate for postadolescent persons. Vitamin A itself is not excreted in human urine. Although several metabolites are excreted, they do not seem to reflect the tissue status of vitamin A. A relatively new method for assessment of vitamin A status is the relative dose response (RDR) test and a modified version of it (MRDR); these tests measure the increase in plasma retinol after administration of retinyl palmitate (RDR) or dehydroretinol (MRDR). Another functional measure of vitamin A status

involves evaluation of the morphology of conjunctival epithelial cells, referred to as conjunctival impression cytology (CIC).[13]

Pathophysiology. Because retinol and RBP are secreted from liver as a 1:1 complex, low plasma concentrations of both are seen in vitamin A deficiency. Adequate concentration of plasma retinol usually indicates dietary and tissue adequacy, but low concentrations *do not* always indicate dietary deficiency. Factors that reduce hepatic synthesis of RBP, or secretion of the RBP-retinol complex, lower plasma concentrations of retinol and RBP, even though dietary intake and the hepatic retinol store are adequate. These states are primarily recognized by the absence of an increase in plasma retinol after oral therapy with vitamin A and include protein-calorie malnutrition, liver disease, zinc deficiency, and cystic fibrosis.

Pathophysiological conditions that can result in increased retinol and RBP include chronic renal disease and use of oral contraceptives.

Toxicity and therapeutic uses. Retinoids have been used therapeutically to prevent noise damage to auditory function and to treat a variety of skin disorders. One retinoid, 13-*cis*-retinoic acid (Accutane) has become the therapy of choice for several forms of acne. Accutane, however, must be used with great caution because large doses of retinoid taken during pregnancy can result in congenital malformations. The anticarcinogenic role of high-dosage retinoids has been well established in animals. An inverse correlation has been noted between serum vitamin A and the incidence of lung cancer, indicating that vitamin A may have a role in prevention of this cancer. RBP and retinol assessments may be useful in selecting those at high risk for lung cancer. Such inverse correlation has also been reported among men later developing prostate cancer. Clinical trials to evaluate antitumor activity of vitamin A and related compounds are in progress.[58] Further discussion of vitamin A and carotenes as antioxidants occurs at the end of this chapter.

Vitamin A deficiency is often associated with disorders of fat absorption.[10-12] Premature infants are born with lower serum retinol and RBP levels, as well as low hepatic stores of retinol. Sick newborns are thus treated with vitamin A as a preventive measure. With excess intake of vitamin A, liver storage capacity can be exceeded, resulting in circulation of free retinol and retinyl esters in lipoproteins. In this instance retinyl ester concentration in plasma becomes quite high. A test of fat malabsorption involves an oral loading dose of vitamin A. With adequate absorption, plasma retinol is unchanged and retinyl palmitate is elevated within 4 hours.

Vitamin E

A factor in vegetable oils that restored fertility to rats was isolated in the early 1920s as vitamin E; later it was given the generic name *tocopherol* and was shown to include sev-

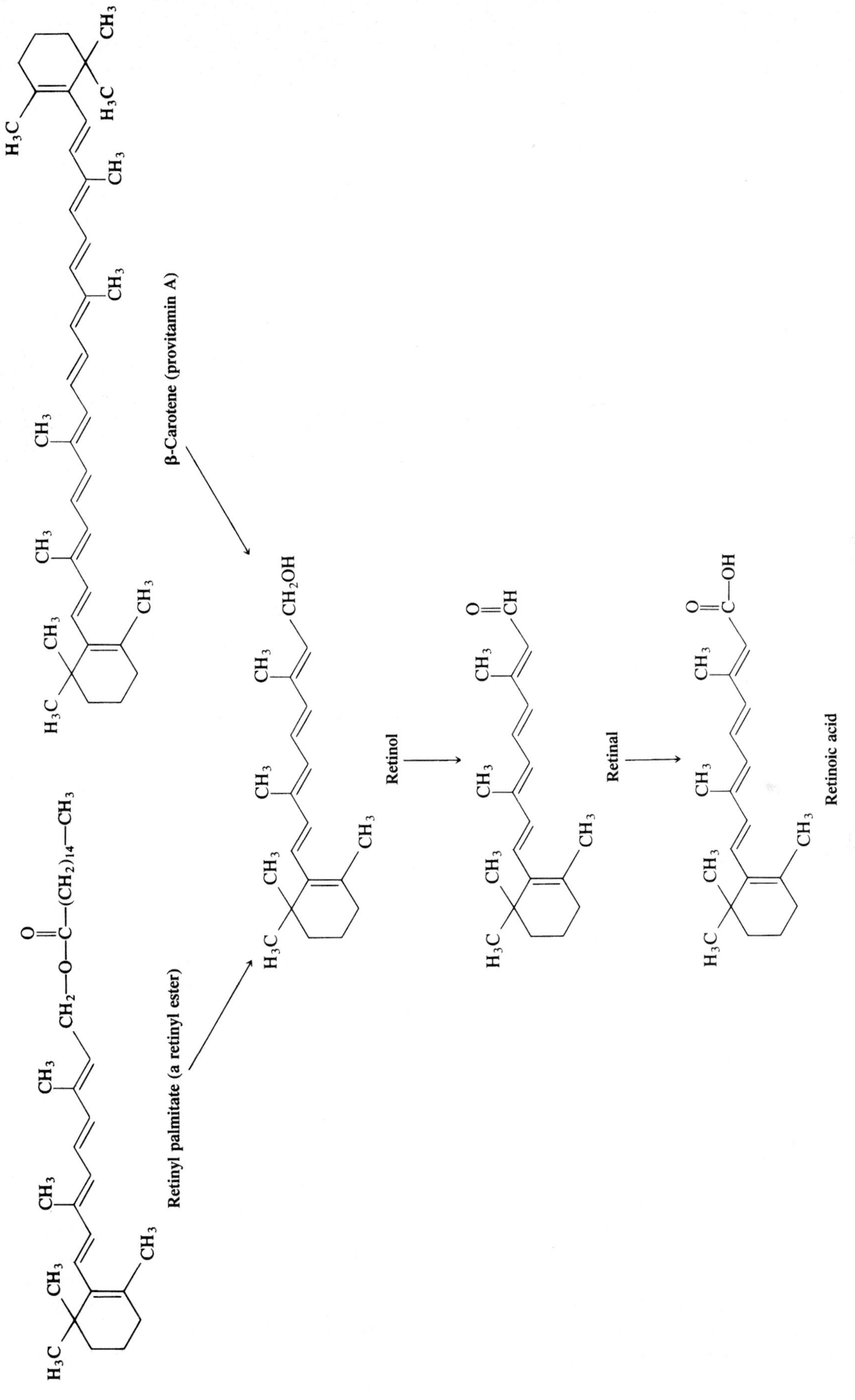

Fig. 39-1 Structures of vitamin A (retinol) with its precursors and metabolites.

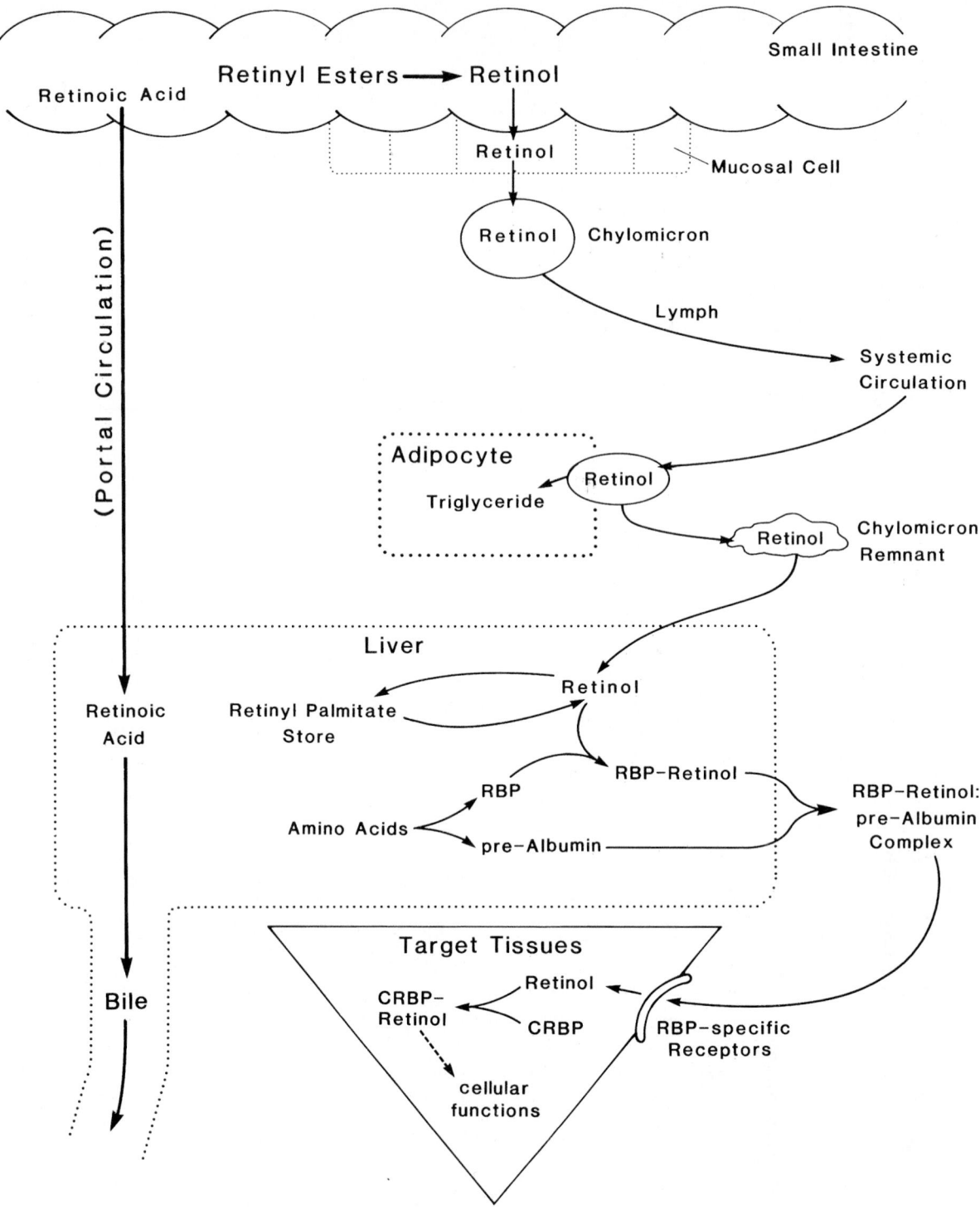

Fig. 39-2   Retinol metabolism. *RBP*, Retinol-binding protein; *CRBP*, cytoplasmic retinol-binding protein.

eral biologically active isomers (Fig. 39-3). The word tocopherol is of Greek derivation, meaning an 'oil that brings forth in childbirth,' but the fertility role of these compounds is still questionable. α-Tocopherol is the predominant isomer in plasma and is the most potent isomer by current biological assays. Whether the tocopherol isomers have separate physiological effects is unknown.

Dietary sources of tocopherols include vegetable oils, fresh leafy vegetables, egg yolk, legumes, peanuts, and margarine. Diets suspect for vitamin E deficiency are those low in vegetable oils or fresh green vegetables or those high in unsaturated fats.

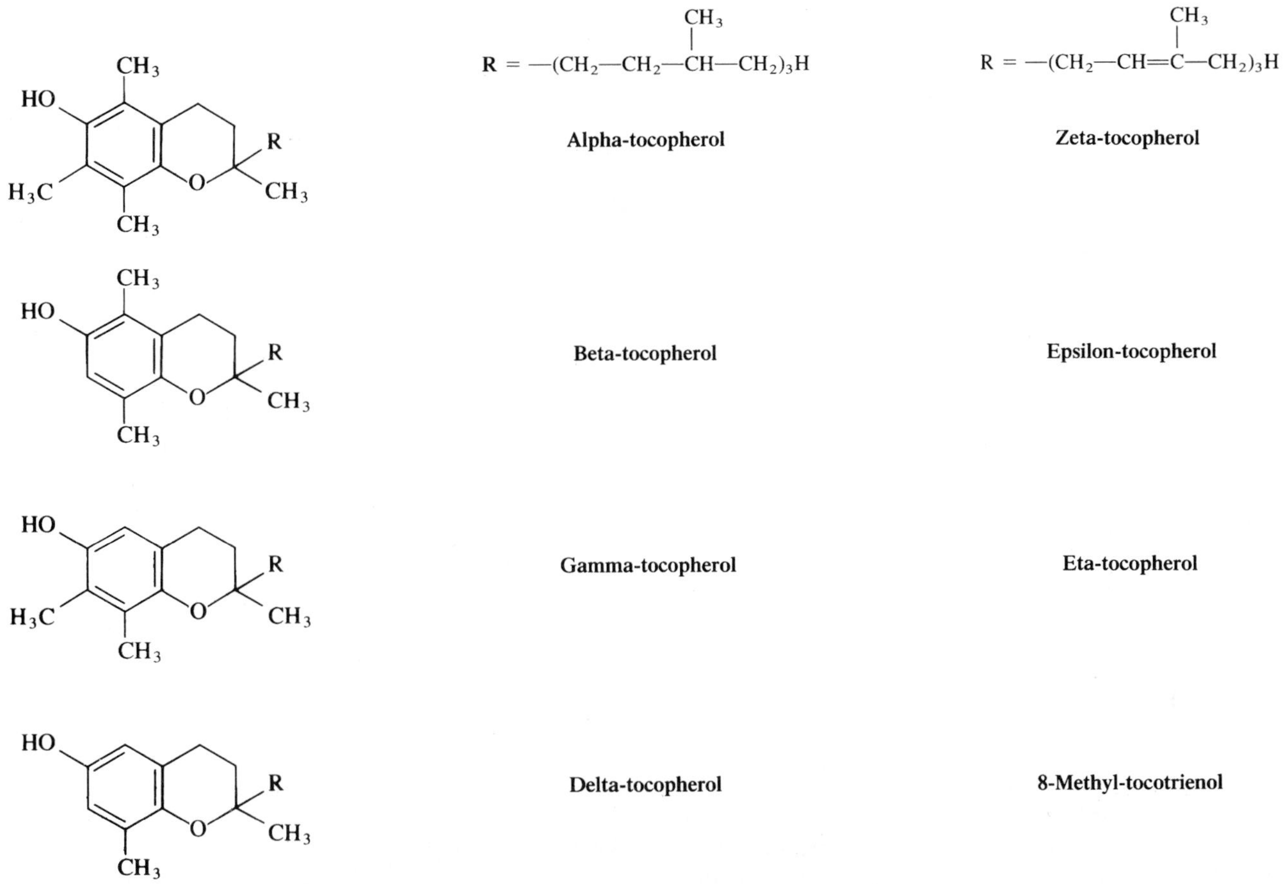

Fig. 39-3 Vitamin E isomers. The structure in the left column is the core ring isomer. The R groups in the second or third columns are the two forms that can be part of the structure. Thus eight forms of the vitamin are described.

Metabolism. The absorption, transport, storage, and metabolism of tocopherols are only partially understood. Absorption is believed to be associated with intestinal fat absorption. Approximately 40% of ingested tocopherol is absorbed; the percentage is affected by the amount and by the degree of unsaturation of dietary fat, as well as by the isomer type. The physiological requirement for vitamin E increases with increasing polyunsaturated fatty acids (PUFA) in the diet. Absorbed vitamin E is first associated with circulating chylomicrons and very-low-density lipoproteins (VLDL) and some is transferred to adipose tissue during triglyceride hydrolysis. The remaining vitamin E in chylomicron remnants is transported to the liver. α-Tocopherol is resecreted as a component of liver-derived VLDLs (and perhaps HDLs).[19] Vitamin E is predominantly found in adipose tissue, though increased dietary α-tocopherol acetate is reflected by increased concentrations in all animal tissues, including plasma, erythrocytes, and platelets. A tocopherol-binding protein (TBP) in the hepatic cell cytosol has been described.[19]

Function. Vitamin E functions as an antioxidant, protecting unsaturated lipids from peroxidation (cleavage of fatty acids at unsaturated sites by oxygen addition across the double bond and formation of free radicals).[14] The role of vitamin E in protecting the erythrocyte membrane from oxidant stress is presently the major documented role of vitamin E in human physiology. There is evidence for preventive roles of vitamin E in retrolental fibroplasia, intraventricular hemorrhage, and mortality of small premature infants.[7] There is now much evidence that vitamin E plays a neurologic role[19] and also may have a preventive role in cardiovascular disease.[59] Further discussion of vitamin E as an antioxidant is presented at the end of this chapter.

Clinical deficiency signs (see Table 39-1). The major symptom of vitamin E deficiency is hemolytic anemia. Although such vitamin E use is still controversial, premature newborns are commonly supplemented with vitamin E to stabilize their red blood cells and prevent hemolytic anemia. Patients with conditions resulting in fat malabsorption, especially cystic fibrosis and abetalipoproteinemia, are very suspect for vitamin E deficiency; a relationship has been recognized between vitamin E deficiency and progressive loss of neurological function in infants and children with chronic cholestasis.[15] Alteration in TBP has been postulated as a cause of vitamin E deficiency without lipid malabsorption.[19]

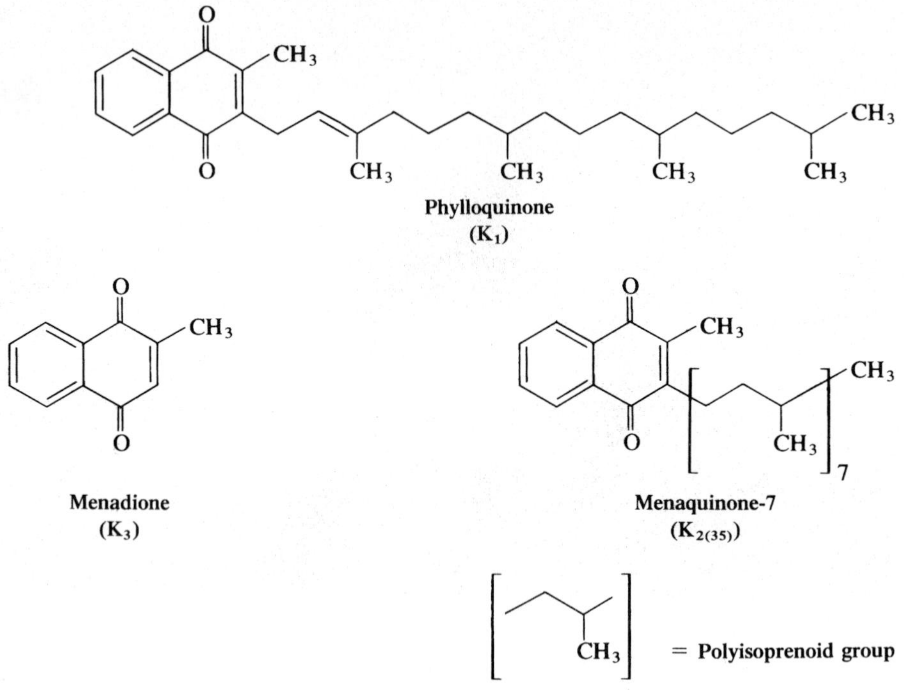

Fig. 39-4 Structures of vitamin K forms.

Chemical deficiency signs. Plasma concentrations of α-tocopherol below 5 mg/L are associated with increased erythrocyte hemolysis in the presence of hydrogen peroxide and are thus designated "deficient."[7,10] There is a strong correlation between plasma α-tocopherol and plasma lipids, indicating that plasma concentrations should be interpreted relative to plasma lipid levels; 0.8 mg of α-tocopherol per gram of total plasma lipids appears to indicate adequate levels of vitamin E in infants. Elevation of plasma total lipids above 15 g/L can apparently shift erythrocyte α-tocopherol to plasma, potentially altering erythrocyte susceptibility despite "adequate" plasma concentrations of α-tocopherol in hyperlipidemic states.[16,17] Breath ethane has been measured as a marker of deficiency.

Pathophysiology. At the present time assessment of vitamin E status is primarily indicated in newborns, in persons with fat-malabsorption states, and in persons receiving synthetic diets. Dietary insufficiency rarely causes vitamin E deficiency.

Elevated values of serum vitamin E have been reported during pregnancy and in patients with Batten's disease (a progressive childhood encephalopathy with disturbed PUFA metabolism). Decreased serum values have been reported in patients with grand mal seizures[4,18] and in persons exposed to nonsymptomatic doses of organophosphates.[5]

Toxicity. Toxicity may result from chronic voluntary overdoses. Premature infants receiving vitamin E sufficient to sustain serum levels above 30 mg/L have an increased incidence of sepsis and necrotizing enterocolitis. Patients receiving synthetic diets should be monitored to avoid vitamin E toxicity (see Table 39-1).

Vitamin K

Experiments in the mid-1930s led to the discovery of the antihemorrhagic factor later called *vitamin K* (from German *Koagulationsvitamin*). Purification efforts revealed several quinone-containing compounds possessing this antihemorrhagic activity, and the term *vitamin K* is now used as a generic descriptor for menadione and derivatives exhibiting this activity. There are a large number of these compounds that are related to those shown in Fig. 39-4 by number and substituents of polyisoprenoid side chains and degree of saturation.

The K vitamins are unstable in acidic or alkaline conditions and are readily oxidized. Major dietary sources are cabbage, cauliflower, spinach and other leafy vegetables, pork, liver, soybeans, and vegetable oils. Uncomplicated dietary deficiency is considered rare in healthy children and adults, but a study of elderly persons revealed deficiencies in a large percentage that were correctable by oral administration of vitamin K.[21]

Metabolism. In infants vitamin K is absorbed in the colon, where bacterial synthesis is the major source of this vitamin. Older children and adults absorb dietary vitamin K in the upper small intestine, where the contribution of intestinal bacteria is insignificant. Absorption of vitamin K in the intestines is chylomicron mediated, and vitamin K malabsorption states include cystic fibrosis, biliary atresia, cholelithiasis and obstructive jaundice resulting from hemo-

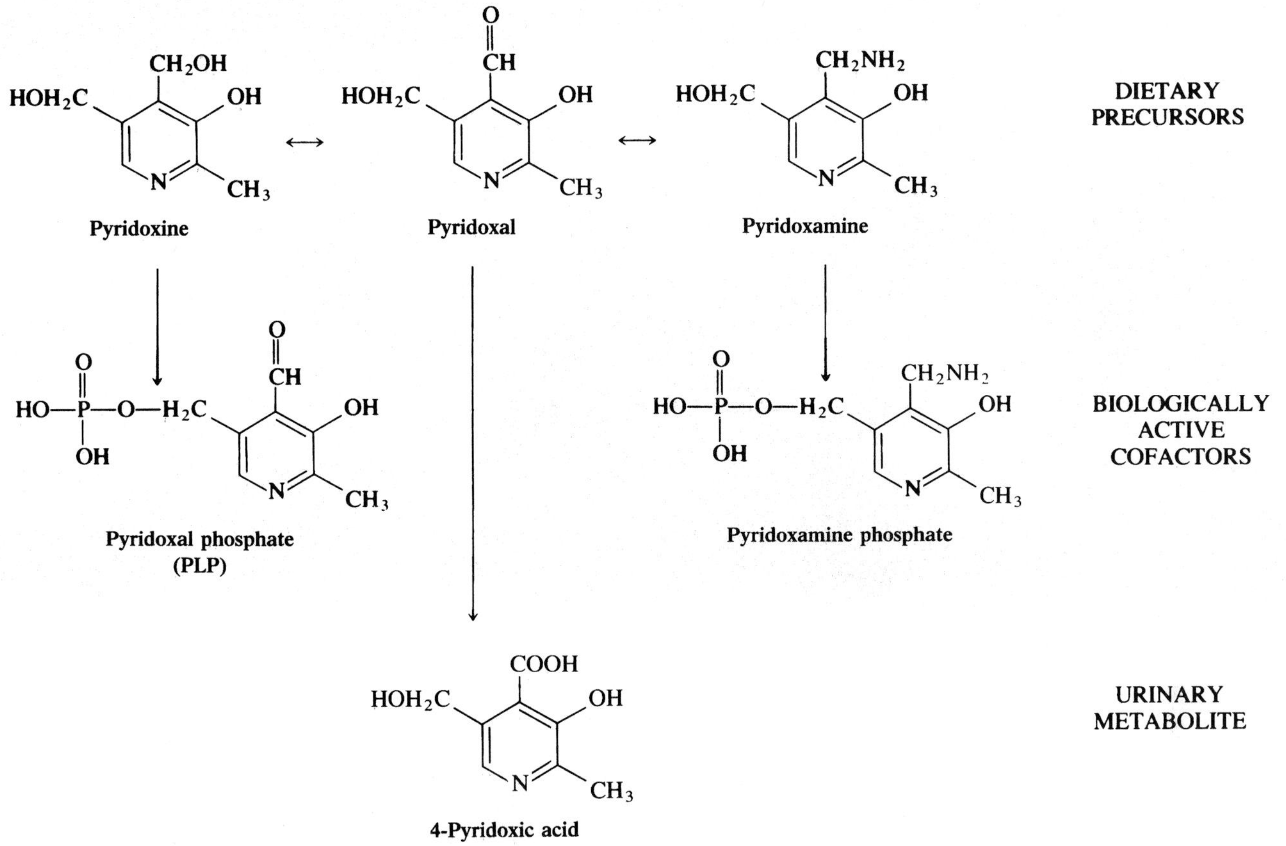

Fig. 39-7 Vitamin B_6 forms and major metabolites.

Function. Almost all pyridoxal phosphate–catalyzed reactions involve transformations of amino acids; the major exception is provided by the phosphorylases. The pyridoxine cofactor forms act in over 60 different enzyme systems catalyzing a variety of reaction types, including the transaminases AST and ALT. The best-known functions of the pyridoxine cofactors are their roles in the conversion of tryptophan to 5-hydroxytryptamine (serotonin) and in the separate pathway of tryptophan to nicotinic acid ribonucleotide (the "niacin pathway"), both shown in Fig. 39-8.

Clinical and chemical deficiency signs. Clinical signs of pyridoxine deficiency for infants and adults are listed in Table 39-1. Chemical indices of pyridoxine depletion include reduction in plasma and erythrocyte concentrations of pyridoxine or pyridoxal phosphate. Urinary pyridoxine (usually representing less than 10% of the pyridoxine intake) and pyridoxic acid, the major urinary metabolite, are also reduced. An oral tryptophan load given to persons suspected of being deficient in pyridoxine results in excretion of several tryptophan metabolites in higher amounts than usual, xanthurenic acid being the one most commonly measured (Fig. 39-8). The involvement of other metabolic and hormonal factors in this pathway necessitates cautious interpretation of the tryptophan challenge test. The

tissue status of pyridoxal phosphate can be assessed by measurement of the increment of erythrocytic aspartate (or alanine) aminotransferase (AST or ALT respectively) after in vitro addition of the pyridoxal phosphate cofactor. Elevation in the ratio of activity plus or minus pyridoxal phosphate (the EAST index) is suggestive of inadequate tissue stores. Pyridoxine-depleted subjects may require several months of repletion to increase enzymatic activity and reduce the stimulation index. Plasmas from normal subjects primarily contain pyridoxal phosphate and 4-pyridoxic acid with lesser amounts of pyridoxal. All the known B_6 vitamins can be measured simultaneously by HPLC. Of the direct measures of B_6 status, plasma pyridoxal phosphate is currently considered most reflective of tissue status. Measurement of plasma pyridoxal phosphate, urinary 4-pyridoxic acid, and an indirect measure (the EAST index or urinary xanthurenic acid) are all recommended to evaluate B_6 status.[35]

Pathophysiology. Conditions associated with low pyridoxine indices include celiac disease, acute alcoholism, psychoses such as paranoia and schizophrenia, epilepsy, ulcerative colitis, renal calculi, and lactation. Although low plasma pyridoxal-5-phosphate levels are seen during the acute phase of myocardial infarction, B_6 deficiency does not

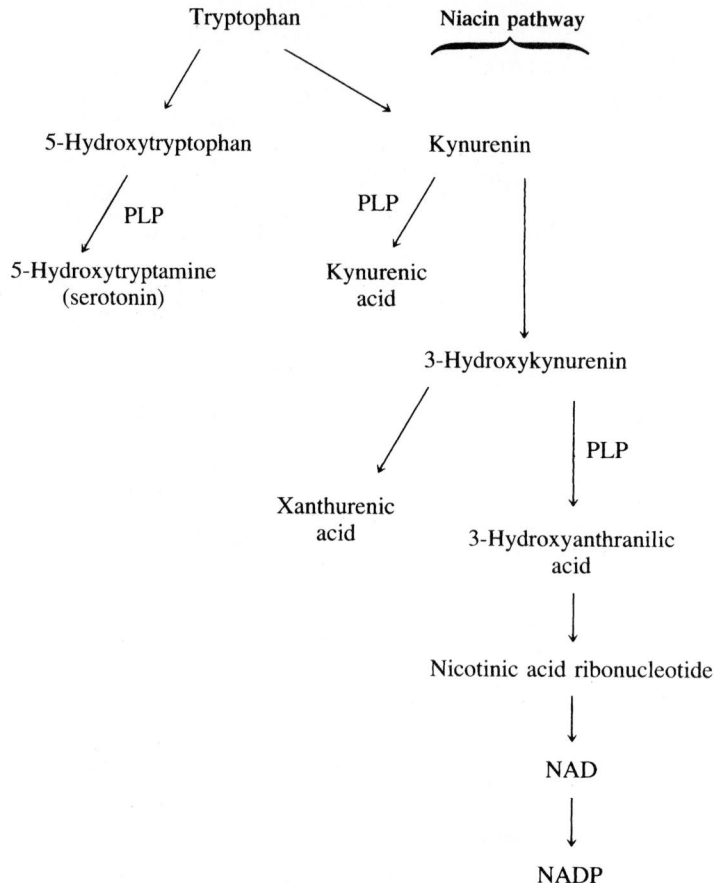

Fig. 39-8 Role of vitamin B_6 in tryptophan metabolism. *NAD,* Nicotinamide adenine dinucleotide; *NADP,* nicotinamide adenine dinucleotide phosphate; *PLP,* pyridoxal phosphate.

appear to be a risk factor for ischemic heart disease.[33] Pyridoxine requirements increase during pregnancy as a result of fetal demand and hormonal induction of maternal enzymes, which increases maternal requirements. Pyridoxine inadequacy during pregnancy has been linked to suboptimal birth outcomes (infants with low Apgar scores and low birth weight).[34] A novel vitamin B_6 compound (adenosine-N_6-diethylthioether-N_1-pyridoxamine-5α-phosphate) is synthesized by tumor cells; higher concentrations of this B_6 relative in sera from patients with different malignancies indicate that it may be a biomarker of tumor presence or metastasis.[35]

Drugs known to antagonize pyridoxine include isonicotinic acid hydrazide (isoniazid, INH), steroids, and penicillamine. Oral contraceptives lower indices of pyridoxine status; depressive mood changes in patients receiving these agents may relate to the role of pyridoxine in serotonin synthesis. Pyridoxine deficiency enhances susceptibility to carbon disulfide toxicity. The vitamin B_6 compounds are of low systemic toxicity, and no teratogenic effect has been detected.

Niacin

Over 200 years ago pellagra (from the Italian, meaning 'rough skin'), which is associated with diarrhea, dementia, dermatitis, and death (the "four *D*'s"), was attributed to poor diet. From 1910 to 1935 pellagra was the worst nutritional disease outbreak in U.S. history, with over 150,000 cases reported annually, most of whom were poor persons in the South. In 1912 nicotinic acid was extracted from rice polishings and was claimed to have vitamin-like effects, but it was not until 1935 that nicotinic acid (also called *niacin*) was shown to cure blacktongue in dogs (a disease similar to pellagra in humans). Thus the responsible nutrient was identified as niacin, and its deficiency was associated with diets high in corn.

Niacin is a simple derivative of pyridine and is extremely stable. Moderately resistant to heat, acid, and alkali, niacin is related chemically to nicotine but has very different physiological properties. The active cofactor forms of NAD and NADP (Fig. 39-9) derived from niacin can also be synthesized from liver tryptophan (Fig. 39-8), and so sufficient dietary tryptophan can abolish the requirement for niacin.

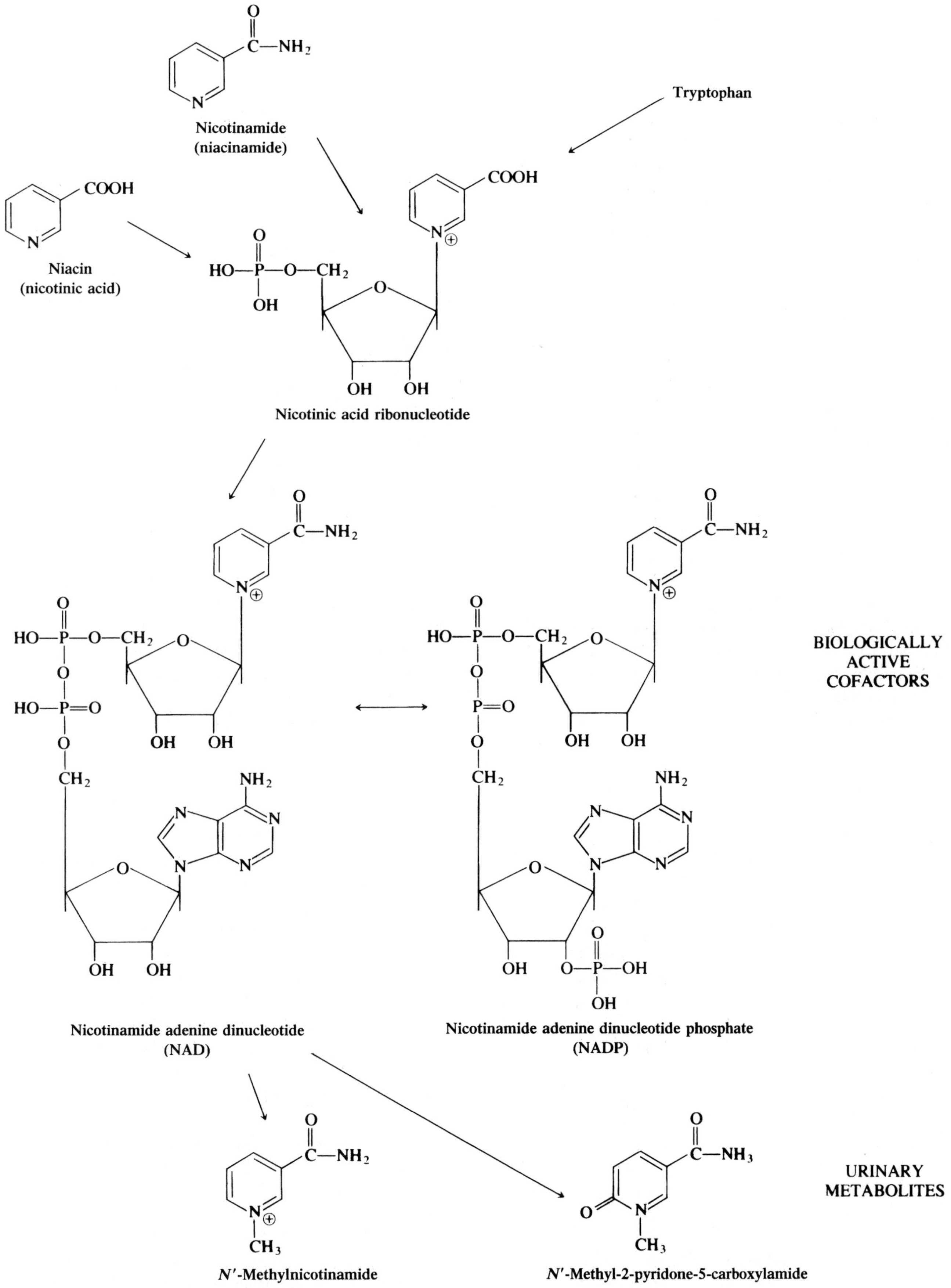

Fig. 39-9 Cofactor forms and metabolites derived from niacin or tryptophan.

Meats and grains are major sources of niacin, and many manufactured food products are supplemented with this vitamin, especially those made from cereals. Dietary deficiency is most likely in persons with diets consisting primarily of corn (such as a diet of pork fat and hominy grits or sorghum). Corn is especially poor in tryptophan, and part of the niacin in corn is not absorbed. The high concentrations of leucine in cereals somehow interfere with the niacin pathway and with conversion of niacin to its cofactor forms. The niacin equivalent of tryptophan is approximately 60 mg of tryptophan, equaling 1 mg of niacin. Most diets have ≥600 mg of tryptophan, but diets low in protein have much less.

Metabolism. Both niacin and nicotinamide are readily absorbed in the gut. Niacin is transported in blood mainly in erythrocytes. There is little storage of niacin in the body, and urine contains nicotinamide and other metabolites of niacin (Fig. 39-9). Plasma nicotinamide readily enters the CSF, whereas niacin does not. Brain tissue does not express the niacin pathway of tryptophan and so must use plasma nicotinamide from the diet or dephosphorylated forms of the cofactors.

Function. NAD and NADP are involved in a large number of oxidation-reduction reactions catalyzed by dehydrogenases including alcohol, glutamate, glucose-6-phosphate, and glycerol-3-phosphate dehydrogenases. Reduction yields dihydronicotinamide (NADH or NADPH), which has a strong absorption at 340 nm, a feature widely used in assays of pyridine nucleotide–dependent enzymes (see Chapter 54).

Clinical and chemical deficiency signs. Clinical signs of niacin deficiency are listed in Table 39-1. Chemical measures of niacin status primarily involve the two major urinary metabolites N'-methylnicotinamide and N'-methyl-2-pyridone-5-carboxylamide. Ratio of 2-pyridone compound to N'-methylnicotinamide is reduced in niacin deficiency; reduction in the individual metabolites is also seen. These metabolites are usually present in plasma also. Only a small percentage of administered niacin is excreted as niacin or as nicotinamide. Measurement of niacin or its nucleotides in blood is generally not considered a reliable index of niacin status, though erythrocytes of deficient persons have lower levels of NAD and NADP and higher amounts of nicotinamide ribonucleotide.

As in the case of pyridoxine, niacin deficiency results in greater susceptibility to toxicity of carbon disulfide. Oral contraceptives stimulate the niacin pathway of tryptophan. Niacin and nicotinamide are widely used in megadoses in the treatment of sprue, psychiatric conditions such as schizophrenia, and a wide range of circulatory disorders including hypertension, cerebral thrombosis, and intermittent claudication (limping). Niacin and its analogs are used in treatment of some hyperlipidemic states to reduce heart and vascular effects.[36] Nicotinic acid is one of several agents known to elevate HDL cholesterol; whether this therapy can retard or reverse the progression of atherosclerosis is not yet clear.[37] Nicotinic acid–induced hyperbilirubinemia response is of diagnostic value in patients with Gilbert's syndrome.[38]

Thiamin

Beriberi, a polyneuritis disease, was first believed to be caused by a toxin that was neutralized by rice husks. This disease was later shown to be a nutrient deficiency caused by removal of an essential factor from rice as it was polished. This antiberiberi factor was finally isolated and crystallized in 1925; then its structure was shown to be a substituted pyrimidine linked by a methylene group to a substituted thiazole (Fig. 39-10). Thus the name reflects its components of amine and sulfur *(thia-)* groups.

Thiamin is easily destroyed in alkaline media. It resists temperatures up to 100° C but is destroyed at greater temperatures, a fact significant for fried foods or those cooked under pressure. Highly water soluble, thiamine is easily leached out of foodstuffs being washed or boiled.

Sources of thiamin include yeast, wheat, whole grain, and enriched breads and cereals, nuts, peas, potatoes, and most vegetables. Dietary deficiency is suspect in persons with a diet primarily consisting of polished rice; alcoholics; persons with anorexia, vomiting, or diarrhea; and postoperative patients. Deficiency of thiamin is common in the elderly.[39]

Metabolism. Dietary thiamin is absorbed in the intestine by a carrier-mediated process that is saturated at an oral intake of about 10 mg. Blood thiamin appears in the CSF and brain to a small degree; the phosphorylated forms are found even less commonly. Thiamin is excreted unchanged or after cleavage between the ring systems by intestinal microorganisms. Thiamin pyrophosphate (TPP) is the predominant moiety in tissues, whereas the major form in plasma is thiamin. Erythrocytes contain TPP at concentrations about fivefold higher than those found in plasma. Liver, heart, and brain have higher concentrations than muscle and other organs have.

Function. In its TPP cofactor form, thiamin catalyzes the decarboxylation of α-keto acids (pyruvate and α-ketoglutarate), the oxidative decarboxylation by α-keto acid dehydrogenases, and the formation of ketols. Thiamin pyrophosphate functions in major carbohydrate pathways and also functions in the metabolism of branched-chain amino acids. Thiamin triphosphate (TTP) may be the thiamin derivative released from nerves after electrical stimulation and as such may play a role in sodium-ion conductance. There is some evidence for decreased brain TTP and an inhibitor of its synthesis (demonstrable in tissues and urine) in patients with Leigh's encephalopathy.

Clinical deficiency signs. Table 39-1 lists the major clinical signs of thiamin deficiency. The Wernicke-Korsakoff syndrome responds to thiamin therapy, and there is evidence for an abnormality of neurotransmitter metabo-

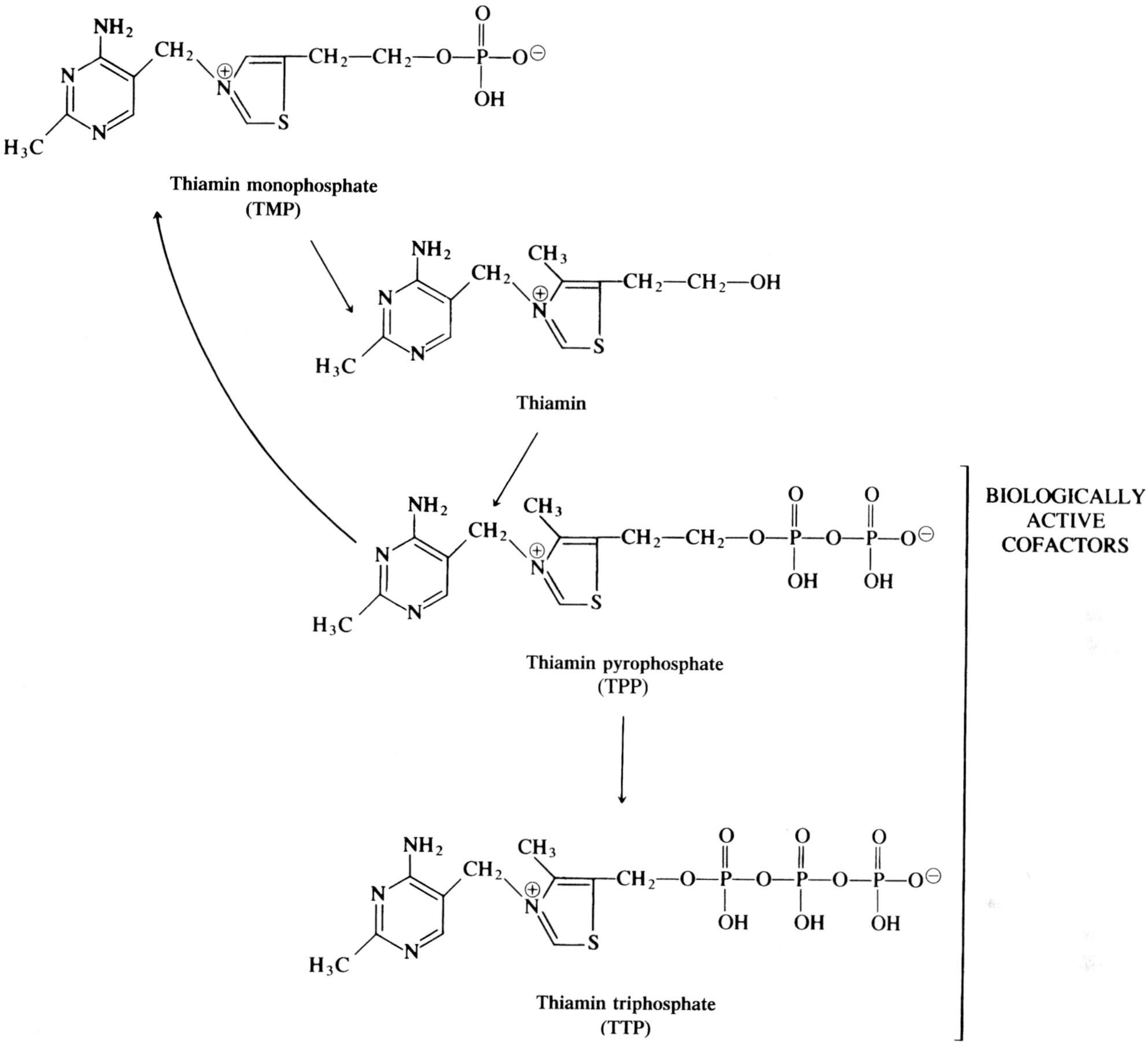

Fig. 39-10   Thiamin and its cofactor forms.

lism, perhaps involving TTP. These patients typically accumulate excessive amounts of pyruvate and lactate in physiological fluids.[40]

Genetic variations in TPP-dependent enzymes modify the effect of dietary thiamin deficiency. Although most patients with thiamin deficiency do not develop Wernicke-Korsakoff syndrome, mild deficiency leads to impairments in higher integrative functions (including memory). More severe deficiency leads either to "dry" or "wet" beriberi, but seldom do both occur together.

Chemical deficiency signs. Chemical indices of thiamin deficiency commonly used are reduction in urinary thiamin, reduction in erythrocyte transketolase (ETK) activity, and stimulation of ETK by in vitro TPP. Prolonged deficiency results in decreased synthesis of the ETK apoenzyme, and so the ETK stimulation test may underestimate

the magnitude of deficiency. There is also evidence of reduction of ETK in undernutrition, diabetes, and liver disease without a TPP stimulation effect. As is possible with all proteins, genetic heterogeneity of ETK has been demonstrated in humans. Correlation between ETK stimulation and dietary thiamin or clinical signs is not always seen. There are conflicting reports as to the usefulness of blood thiamin levels; this is possibly related to low concentrations and measurement difficulties. HPLC separates thiamin and its three phosphate esters.

Pathophysiology. Populations of Southeast Asia who eat foods rich in antithiamin substances commonly develop beriberi. Milder forms of thiamin deficiency are common among pregnant women, elderly persons, and alcoholics. Magnesium deficiency (common in alcoholics) impairs thiamin use. Oral contraceptive use may induce deficiency.

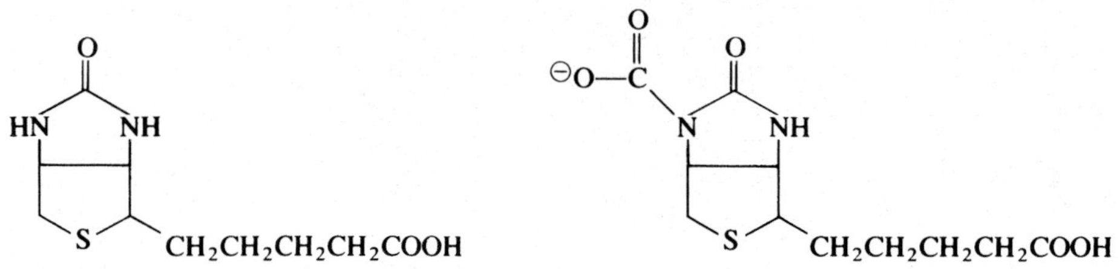

Fig. 39-11 Biotin and its active form.

The total body store of thiamin is only 30 mg, that is, 30 times the daily requirement. Thiamin deficiency symptoms can occur after about 1 month of a thiamin-deficient diet. Thiamin replacement is often warranted in persons with persistent vomiting or prolonged gastric aspiration and in those who go on long fasts. Patients with typical sporadic amyotrophic lateral sclerosis (ALS) reportedly have a very high incidence of decreased CSF thiamine monophosphate with inversion of the thiamin/TMP ratio.[41] There is some evidence for unrecognized thiamine deficiency in chronically ill children (those receiving nasogastric feeding or intensive chemotherapy, or receiving intensive care for a period of weeks).

Biotin

Growth factors separately discovered under the names of bios II, coenzyme R, and biotin were noted to be similar; other research demonstrated the symptom complex produced in rats by feeding them raw egg white was corrected by cooking the eggs or by addition of other foods presumably containing "vitamin H," or "protective factor X." The linkage between vitamin H and biotin was made and the clinical role of biotin was established when human volunteers ingested large amounts of raw egg white and confirmed the "egg white injury" of animals that is correctable with biotin (structure in Fig. 39-11).

Numerous foods contain biotin, though no one food is especially rich (up to 2 mg/100 g). Dietary intake is low in the neonatal period despite the fact that concentrations increase as newborns switch from colostrum to mature breast milk. Enteric bacteria are known to synthesize biotin, though the relative contribution of this source is unclear.

Metabolism. Biotin is absorbed in the proximal half of the small intestine and circulates in blood largely bound to plasma proteins. Avidin, a glycoprotein of egg albumin, has very high affinity for biotin, thus explaining the biotin deficiency resulting from raw egg white ingestion.

Function. Biotin is a coenzyme for carboxylation and carboxyl exchange reactions. Important enzymes include acetyl CoA, propionyl CoA, and pyruvate carboxylases, as well as methylmalonyl-oxaloacetic transcarboxylase.

Clinical deficiency signs. Reported dietary deficiency cases are rare, but each has a history of raw eggs as a large

dietary component for months to years. Table 39-1 lists the major signs of biotin deficiency.

Chemical deficiency signs. Dietary deficiency is accompanied by decreased urinary and plasma[42] biotin and increased urinary organic acids, indicating functional deficiency of β-methylcrotonyl CoA carboxylase and propionyl CoA carboxylase. Genetic alterations in these carboxylases may result in biotin-dependent states that cause metabolic acidosis and require pharmacological biotin doses; these enzyme deficiencies are confirmed in leukocytes. Genetic deficiency of biotinidase, which can be detected by a blood spot assay, is treated with biotin.[43]

Pathophysiology. With proper modern nutrition biotin deficiencies are extremely rare. However, biotin deficiency might be suspected in patients receiving long-term total parenteral nutrition.[16,40] No biotin toxicity has been described,[44] though biotin administration to nondeficient animals influences gene expression and alters astrocyte glucose utilization.

Pantothenic acid

A growth factor occurring in all types of animal and plant tissue was first designated *vitamin B_3* and later named pantothenic acid (from Greek, meaning 'from everywhere'). This factor was chemically identified in 1938, and its deficiency was linked to the "burning feet syndrome" in 1949.

Dietary sources include liver and other organ meats, milk, eggs, peanuts, legumes, mushrooms, salmon, and whole grains. Approximately 50% of pantothenate in food is available for absorption. Pantothenate is unstable to acid, alkali, heat, and some salts. Intestinal microorganisms are a source of B_3 for animals, possibly including humans.

Metabolism. As shown in Fig. 39-12, pantothenate is metabolically converted to 4'-phosphopantothenine, which becomes covalently bound to either serum acyl carrier protein (ACP) or to coenzyme A. Little is known of pantothenate metabolism. Urinary excretion of pantothenate correlates well with intake; no saturation is seen with intakes of 10 mg/day. Free pantothenate is the major form in both urine and serum, whereas coenzyme A is the major erythrocytic form. In contrast to other B vitamins, pantothenate tissue repletion is gradual. Tissues known to contain pantothenate are liver, adrenal glands, brain, kidneys, and heart.

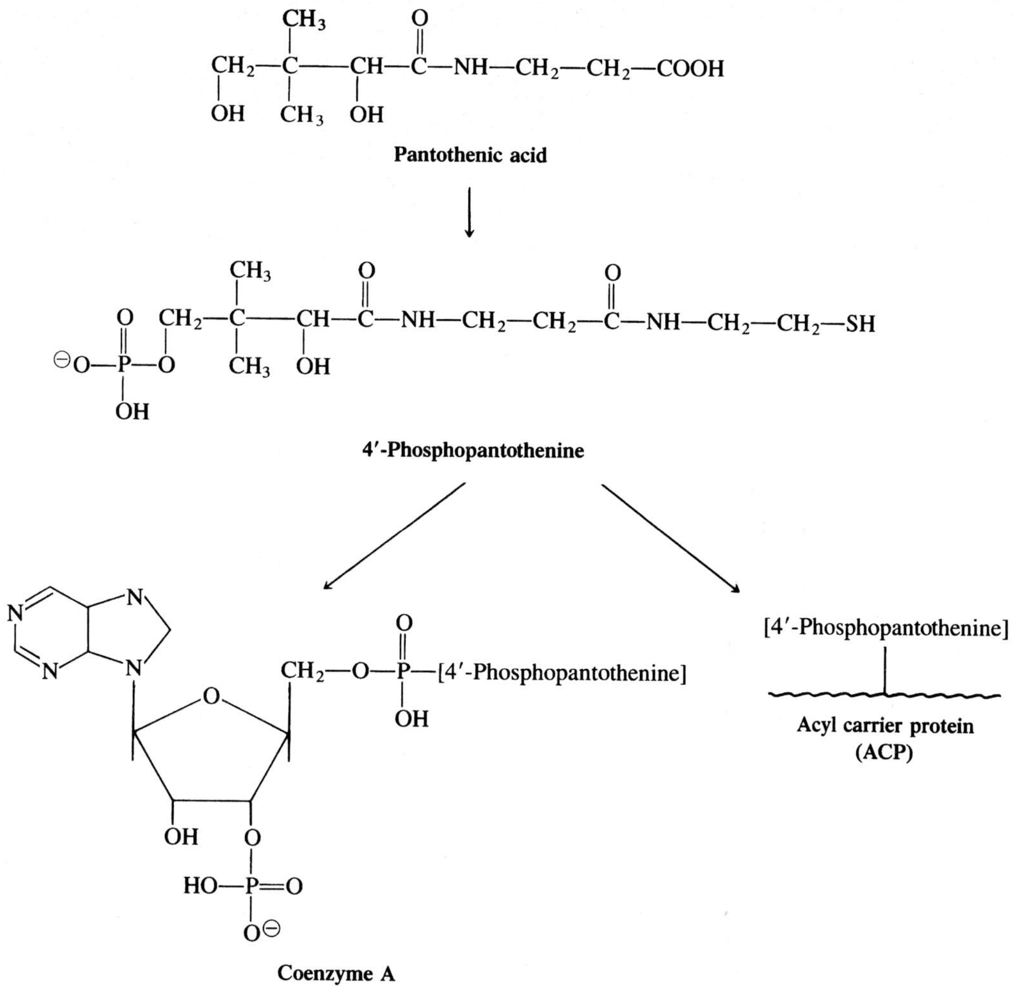

Fig. 39-12 Pantothenic acid and its active cofactors.

Function. Coenzyme A is a highly important acyl-group transfer coenzyme that is involved in a large number of reactions of a great variety of reaction types. Acyl derivatives of coenzyme A are first formed (by thioester linkage), followed by transfer of the acyl group to an acceptor molecule.

Clinical and chemical deficiency signs. No clear-cut case of a pantothenate deficiency has been reported; Table 39-1 lists clinical signs observed in experimentally induced deficiencies. Whole blood pantothenate of less than 1000 mg/L and urinary excretion of less than 10 mg/day are regarded as indicative of deficiency. Most past measurements have used biological assays for free pantothenate, releasing pantothenate from coenzyme A by multiple enzymatic treatments.

Pathophysiology. Low urinary excretion and reduced blood levels of pantothenate have been reported in patients with chronic malnutrition, acute alcoholism, and acute rheumatism. Patients with circulatory and cardiovascular diseases and those with peptic ulcers have reduced circulating pantothenic acid; chronic alcoholics have increased excretion, an indication of impaired use. There is evidence that

the increased occurrence of hypertension in some Japanese populations may be related to pantothenate deficiency.[45] Pantothenate has been given postoperatively to stimulate the gastrointestinal tract and also to treat streptomycin-induced neuropathy. No toxicity is known.

Vitamin B_{12}

Pernicious anemia was described over 100 years ago and was recognized as a disease amenable to liver extract therapy. The antipernicious anemia factor (extrinsic factor), finally isolated, crystallized, and characterized between 1948 and 1956, is now known as *vitamin B_{12}*. In the early 1930s a similar entity, *pernicious anemia of pregnancy,* was shown to be different in that it did not respond to liver extract therapy but did respond to an autolyzed yeast substance. Purification of this substance led to its identification as pteroylglutamic acid, more commonly known as *folic acid.* Thus similar clinical symptoms were found to result from deficiencies of two totally different structures (Figs. 39-13 and 39-14), neither of which could replace the other. The clinical similarities and the metabolic interactions

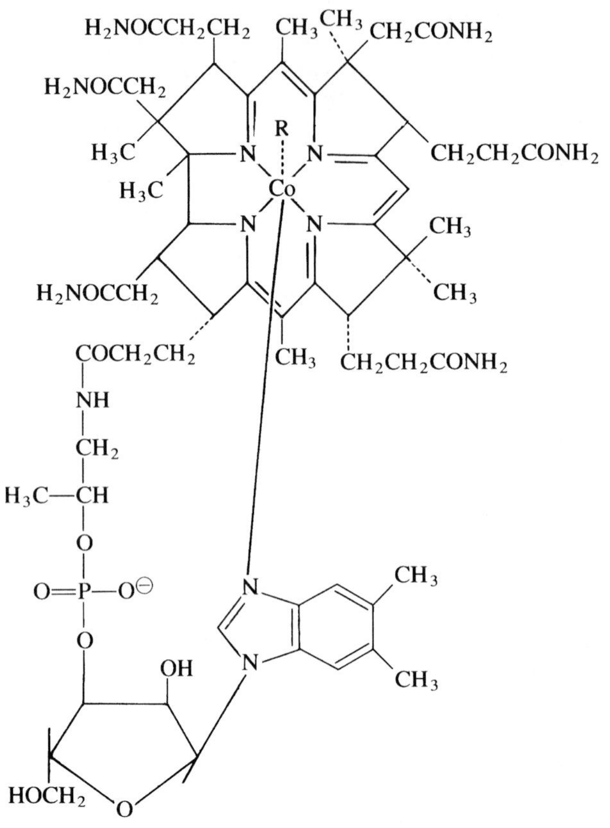

	R		
(Me-B_{12})	CH_3	**Methylcobalamin**	ACTIVE COFACTOR FORMS
(Ado-B_{12})	5′-Deoxy-adenosine	**Deoxyadenosyl-cobalamin**	
(OH-B_{12})	OH	**Hydroxocobalamin**	DIETARY FORMS AND THERAPY
(CN-B_{12})	CN	**Cyanocobalamin**	

Fig. 39-13 Vitamin B_{12} forms.

of vitamin B_{12} and folic acid usually dictate their simultaneous assessment.[46]

Vitamin B_{12} bears a corrin ring (containing pyrroles similar to porphyrin) linked to a central cobalt atom. The pyrroles are almost saturated with side chains (methyl, acetamide, or propionamide groups). Different corrinoid compounds, or cobalamins, are distinguished by the substituent linked to the cobalt with methylcobalamin and 5′-deoxyadenosylcobalamin being the two known coenzyme forms.

Dietary sources of vitamin B_{12} are of animal origin (meat, eggs, milk) except for the plant comfrey. Total vegetarian diets are therefore likely settings for deficiency. Animals derive their vitamin B_{12} from intestinal microbial synthesis. The average daily diet contains 3 to 30 μg of vitamin B_{12}, of which 1 to 5 μg is absorbed. The frequency of dietary deficiency increases with age, occurring in over 0.5% of persons over 60 years of age.

Metabolism. Most vitamin B_{12} absorption is through a complex with intrinsic factor (IF), a protein secreted by gastric parietal cells (Fig. 39-15). This IF-B_{12} complex binds with specific ileal receptors. "Blocking" IF-antibodies prevent binding of vitamin B_{12} to IF, and "binding" antibodies can combine with either free IF or the IF-B_{12} complex, thus preventing attachment of the complex to ileal receptors and intestinal uptake of the vitamin. Parietal cell antibodies have also been identified as a cause of pernicious anemia.

Released from the IF complex within the mucosal cell, vitamin B_{12} circulates in plasma bound to specific transport proteins and is deposited in liver, bone marrow, and other tissues. There is a significant enterohepatic circulation of vitamin B_{12}. As a result of this biliary reabsorption, 10 to 12 years are required for a strict vegetarian to become clinically deficient. A person with normal B_{12} stores but lacking IF requires less time (1 to 4 years) for deficiency to become evident.

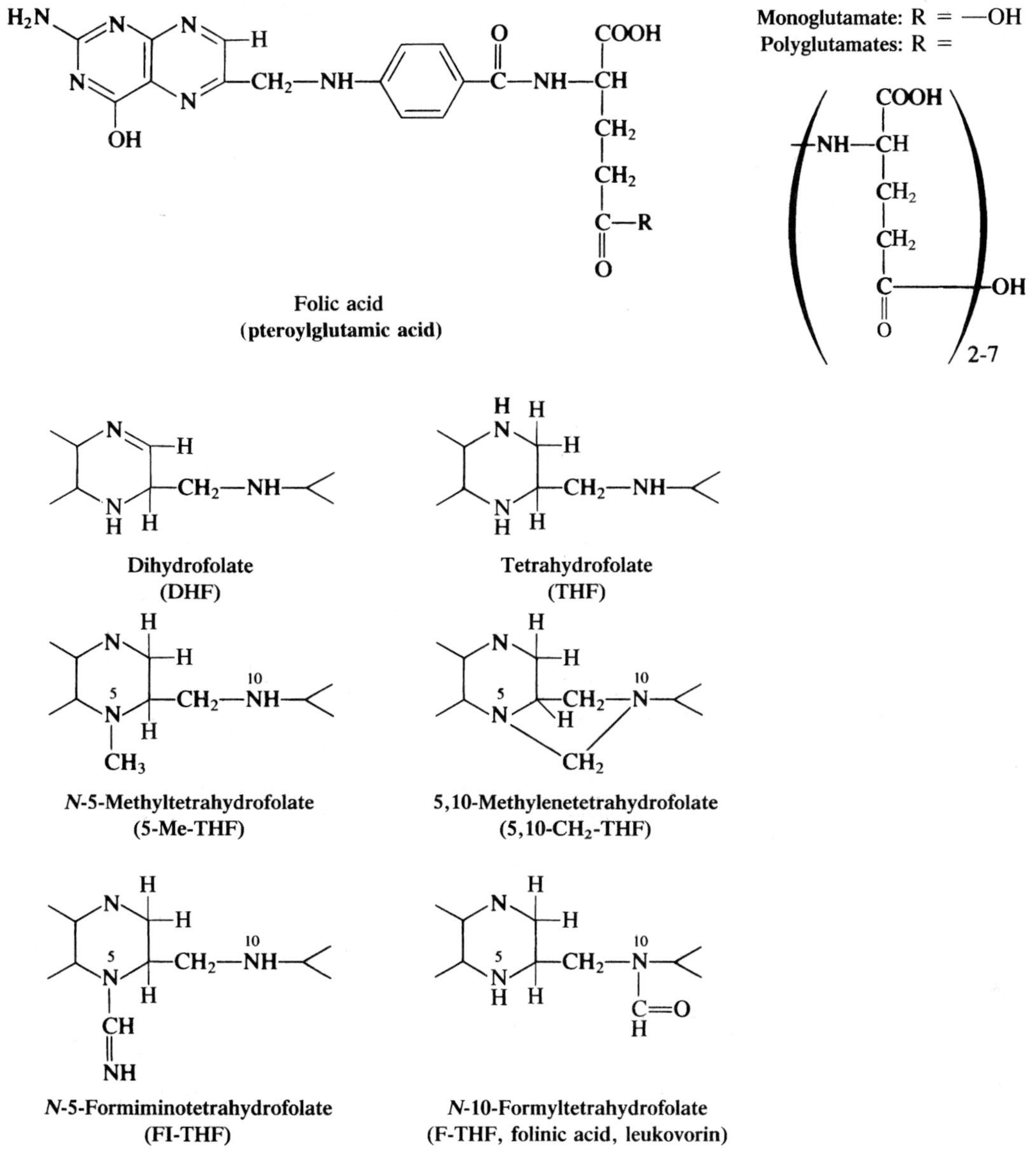

Fig. 39-14   Structures of folic acid forms.

Transcobalamin II (TC II) appears to be the major serum protein transporting exogenous vitamin B_{12} to tissues. Cobalophilin (previously R, or rapidly migrating, binding protein, or TC I) transports endogenous B_{12} and is the binder of food cobalamins. Saliva, breast milk, and granulocytes contain large amounts of this binding protein compared with relatively small amounts of cobalamin. Plasma contains both types of transport proteins and the three forms of vitamin B_{12} (hydroxycobalamin, methylcobalamin, and deoxyadenosylcobalamin). Absorption and transport of this vitamin are illustrated in Fig. 39-15.

Functions. The deoxyadenosylcobalamin form (AdoCbl) is a cofactor for odd-numbered chain fatty acid metabolism (myelin sheath formation); deficiency results in accumulation of the intermediate methylmalonyl CoA and excretion in urine of methylmalonic acid. The methylcobal-

amin form (MeCbl) is required for methyl group transfer reactions; lack of it results in blockage of DNA synthesis, megaloblastic anemia, and elevation in homocysteine. Dietary deficiency of the precursor of these two coenzyme forms results in deficiencies of both active cobalamins. Genetic deficiencies of enzymes in either pathway are known. In the few case reports of inherited deficiency of TC II, symptoms of pancytopenia and failure to thrive develop within a few months of birth. Several large studies have shown a racial difference in serum vitamin B_{12} levels, with blacks maintaining higher B_{12} levels than whites.[47]

Clinical and chemical deficiency signs. Table 39-1 lists signs of vitamin B_{12} deficiency. Diagnostic tests for vitamin B_{12} deficiency include measurement of serum B_{12} by microbiologic or radioligand assay methods, measure-

Dietary OH-cbl : cblin

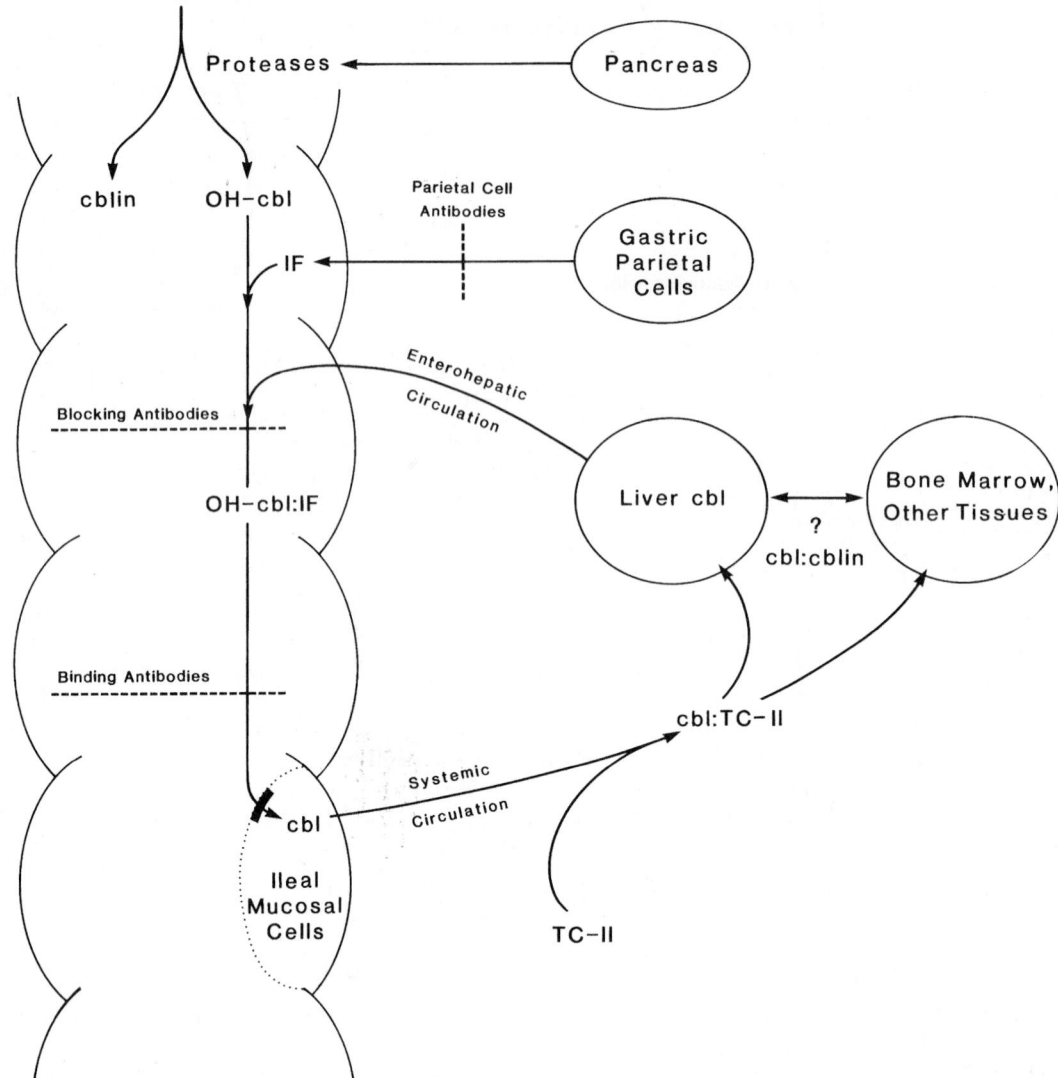

Fig. 39-15 Absorption of dietary vitamin B_{12} and its transport to storage sites. *cblin,* Cobalophilin; *cbl,* cobalamin; *IF,* intrinsic factor; *OH-cbl,* hydroxycobalamin; *TC II,* transcobalamin II.

ment of urinary or serum methylmalonic acid or total homocysteine, and the Schilling test (see pp. 590 and 788).

Early serum B_{12} competitive-binding methods used B_{12} binders with variable purity and binding specificity, yielding unreliable results; there are numerous reports of cobalamin deficiency in patients with normal serum cobalamin concentrations. Analysis of serum methylmalonic acid concentration, by gas chromatography–mass spectrometry, appears to be a more sensitive and specific indicator of cobalamin deficiency than direct measures of serum cobalamin. Urinary methylmalonic acid excretion has been recommended as a sensitive screening test for undetected cobalamin deficiency among the elderly and the newborn. Uremic patients show elevated serum methylmalonic acid

apparently unrelated to cobalamin status; CSF concentrations may be normal in these patients. Hepatic diseases do not appear to affect serum methylmalonic values but may elevate serum cobalamins. The heterozygous methylmalonic acidemia state (2% of the general population) reportedly does not elevate serum methylmalonic acid. Hyperhomocysteinemia is seen in deficiency of B_{12}, folate, or vitamin B_6. It is not an early indicator of B_6 status and does not appear to be superior to serum methylmalonic acid as an index of B_{12} deficiency. Plasma homocysteine has been used to monitor nitrous oxide–induced cobalamin inactivation.[51]

Definition of the cause of vitamin B_{12} deficiency may require additional assays including tests for specific antibodies, the deoxyuridine suppression test, and assessment of the transport proteins.

The deoxyuridine suppression test is based on the fact that preincubation of normal bone marrow with an appropriate concentration of deoxyuridine severely suppresses the subsequent incorporation of tritiated thymidine into DNA. This suppression is subnormal with bone marrow from patients deficient in either vitamin B_{12} or folate and is correctable in vitro by addition of the appropriate deficient vitamin. This test will also show abnormal results in patients with megaloblastic changes resulting from neoplastic, chemotherapeutic, or other agents interfering with DNA synthesis.

Pathophysiology. Inadequate secretion of intrinsic factor may accompany lesions of the gastric mucosa, gastric atrophy, gastrectomy, iron deficiency, and some endocrine disorders. The IF-B_{12} complex may be inadequately formed in pancreatic insufficiency because there is insufficient pancreatic protease activity to split the dietary vitamin B_{12} from cobalophilin in the duodenum. The IF-B_{12} complex may be inadequately absorbed in ileal malfunction (sprue, enteritis, ileal resection, neoplasias, granulomas, and so on). The term *pernicious anemia* is now most commonly applied to vitamin B_{12} deficiency resulting from lack of IF. Antibodies to IF and to parietal cells are common in pernicious anemia patients, in their healthy relatives, and in patients with other autoimmune disorders. Blocking antibodies can result in normal or high serum B_{12} levels in patients with pernicious anemia. Numerous drugs induce vitamin B_{12} malabsorption, and excessive ascorbate intake may convert vitamin B_{12} to analog, blocking forms. Cobalophilin is elevated in patients with chronic myeloproliferative disorders, polycythemia vera, and various neoplasms. There is evidence for B_{12} deficiency in some patients with late-onset dementia. Hyperhomocysteinemia is an independent risk factor for premature vascular disease and is associated with suboptimal status of B_6, B_{12}, or folate. Plasma homocysteinemia correctable by methylcobalamin has been linked to diabetic macroangiopathy.[51]

Folic acid

Structural relatives of pteroylglutamic acid (folic acid) are the metabolically active compounds usually referred to as *folates* (see Fig. 39-14). Up to eight glutamate residues may be found in these naturally occurring compounds.

Food folates are primarily found in green and leafy vegetables, fruits, organ meats, and yeast. Excessive boiling of foods and use of large quantities of water result in folate destruction. The average American diet may be inadequate in folate for adolescents and for pregnant or lactating females.

Metabolism. The naturally occurring folate polyglutamates are hydrolyzed to monoglutamate forms before absorption (which occurs primarily in the proximal jejunum) by the intestinal mucosal cells. After this, folate enters the liver through the portal circulation. The liver converts some of these folate monoglutamates to polyglutamates, which are presumably then stored; another fraction of the folate is excreted in bile as N^5-methyltetrahydrofolate (MeTHF), which is reabsorbed and is the major circulating form of folate. Serum folate (MeTHF), in the monoglutamate form, readily enters the choroid plexus and the CSF. Folic acid, on the other hand, is readily transported from CSF to plasma. A folate-binding protein has been identified in the choroid plexus, probably accounting for the high CSF/plasma ratio. The CSF form is mainly MeTHF; brain folates are predominantly polyglutamate forms of dihydrofolate (DHF). Folate catabolism involves cleavage of the pterin ring, followed by acetylation to form the excreted product, *p*-acetamidobenzoylglutamic acid.

Function. Folate (MeTHF) is a cofactor for enzymatic reactions involving one-carbon transfers. After cellular uptake, the MeTHF is converted to THF while transferring a carbon to homocysteine to yield methionine. As mentioned previously, this reaction requires vitamin B_{12}. In the absence of vitamin B_{12}, the folate is essentially trapped in the MeTHF form, making it unavailable for other reactions, including the synthesis of thymine for DNA (Fig. 39-16).

Clinical and chemical deficiency signs. The major clinical symptom of folate deficiency is megaloblastic anemia. Chemical indices of deficiency are, in order of occurrence, low serum folate (see Table 39-2), hypersegmentation of neutrophils, high urinary FIGLU (a histidine metabolite accumulating in absence of folate), low erythrocyte folate, macro-ovalocytosis, megaloblastic marrow, and finally anemia. The deoxyuridine suppression test, discussed with vitamin B_{12}, is also an index of folate status. Serum folate, although an early index of deficiency, can frequently be low despite normal tissue stores. Hypersegmentation of neutrophils may not be seen in folate deficiency of pregnant women. The urinary FIGLU test requires ingestion of an oral load of histidine, followed by a timed urine collection, and can be abnormally high in deficiencies of either folate or vitamin B_{12}. Because most folate storage occurs after the vitamin B_{12}-dependent step, erythrocyte folate can also be reduced in deficiency of either B_{12} or folate. Despite this overlap, erythrocyte folate concentration is currently accepted as the best laboratory index of folate deficiency. As indicated in the discussion of vitamin B_{12}, homocysteine elevation in serum or urine occurs in folate deficiency. Total homocysteine is generally measured, which is the sum of all homocysteine species, both free and protein-bound forms. The diagnostic utility of this measure of folate deficiency relative to direct folate measures is currently uncertain.[51]

Pathophysiology. Folate requirement is increased during pregnancy and especially during lactation. The increase during lactation partially results from the presence in milk of high-affinity folate binders. Other instances of increased folate requirement include hemolytic anemias, iron defi-

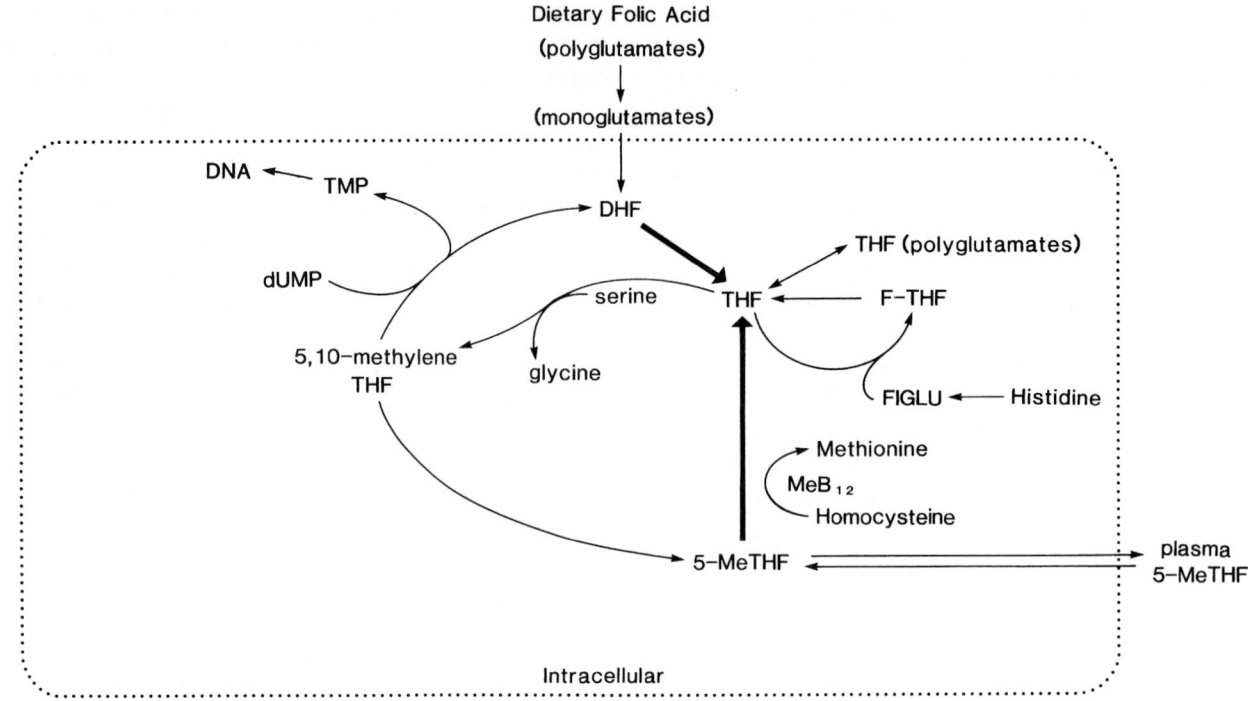

Fig. 39-16 One-carbon transfer using folic acid forms as cofactors. *DHF,* Dihydrofolate; *DNA,* deoxyribonucleic acid; *dUMP,* deoxyuridine monophosphate; *FIGLU,* formimino-L-glutaric acid; *F-THF,* folinic acid; *MeB₁₂,* methylcobalamin; *5-MeTH, N⁵-*methyltetrahydrofolate; *THF,* tetrahydrofolate; *TMP,* thymidine monophosphate.

ciency, prematurity, and multiple myeloma. Patients receiving dialysis treatment rapidly lose folate. Folate deficiency as a result of malabsorption can occur in sprue, celiac disease, inflammatory bowel diseases, cardiac failure, and systemic bacterial infections. Both acidic and alkaline conditions can interfere with intestinal transport; the organic anions that accumulate in uremia also impair folate use. Genetic alterations in most of the folate-interconverting enzymes have been reported. Several mentally retarded children who are unable to transfer folates from blood into CSF have been described; this is probably a result of abnormal folate transport-binding systems in the central nervous system. Folate deficiency of dietary origin commonly occurs in the elderly.[49]

Phenytoin (Dilantin) therapy accelerates folate excretion and interferes with folate absorption and metabolism. Alcohol interferes with folate's enterohepatic circulation, whereas the chemotherapeutic agent methotrexate inhibits the enzyme dihydrofolate reductase. Although decreased serum folate can occur with use of oral contraceptives (cycle-day dependent), this is not believed to cause a functional deficit unless some other problem is also present. There has, however, been concern expressed that there may be a relationship between oral contraceptive–induced cervical folate deficiency and cervical carcinoma. A specific folate-binding protein, possibly of granulocytic source, has been reported

in the serum of some women who were receiving oral contraceptives or who were pregnant.

The therapeutic form of folate is 5-formyl-THF (also known as leucovorin, citrovorum factor, or folinic acid). This form of folate can bypass MeTHF and enter the cycles of folate's one-carbon transfer reactions (see Fig. 39-16). This feature is useful in the "leucovorin rescue" of cancer patients given high-dose methotrexate therapy with toxic levels of methotrexate. The use of folate supplements during conception and early pregnancy is now recommended to reduce the occurrence of neural tube defects.[50]

Carnitine

Carnitine, including L-carnitine and its fatty acid esters (acylcarnitines) (Fig. 39-17), is described as a "conditionally essential" nutrient.

Major dietary sources are meat, poultry, fish, and dairy products. Foods of plant origin generally contain very little carnitine (exceptions being peanut butter, asparagus, and avocados). Average diets provide more than half the human requirement; strict vegetarian diets provide only 10% of the total available carnitine. Most of the dietary carnitine is absorbed.

Metabolism. Endogenous synthesis involves *N*-trimethyllysine residues of proteins; the biosynthetic rate is determined by the available supply of these *N*-tri-methyl-

CH₃   O
| ||
CH₃ — N — CH₂ — CH — CH₂ — C — OH
| |
CH₃   OH

L-Carnitine

CH₃   O
| ||
CH₃ — N — CH₂ — CH — CH₂ — C — OH
| |
CH₃   O
               |
               C = O
               |
               (CH₂)ₙ — CH₃

Acylcarnitine

Fig. 39-17 ʟ-Carnitine and fatty acid esters.

lysine residues. Synthesis occurs in liver, brain, and kidney, with storage primarily in muscle. Carnitine is not degraded but is excreted mainly in the urine both as free and esterified forms.

Function. ʟ-carnitine facilitates entry of long-chain fatty acids into mitochondria for oxidation and energy production. As shown in Fig. 39-18, coenzyme A esters of the long-chain fatty acids (acyl-*S*-CoA) are transesterified to ʟ-carnitine by means of catalysis by an enzyme of the mitochondrial outer membrane, CPT I (carnitine palmitoyltransferase I). Once inside the inner membrane, the long-chain fatty acid is once again transesterified (by CPT II) yielding the CoA ester, which can enter the beta-oxidation pathway for energy production. The carnitine "transporter"

can then leave the mitochondria to be reutilized or it can serve its other known role and carry out short- and medium-chain fatty acids that accumulate in normal or abnormal metabolism. The carnitine esters may be excreted in urine or distributed in tissues; some may be utilized for specific purposes.

Chemical deficiency signs. The major signs of carnitine deficiency are muscle weakness and fatigue. Chemical indices of deficiency include decreased total or free carnitine in serum, urine, or tissues; measurements are generally radioenzymatic. Total carnitine is measured after hydrolysis of ester forms to free carnitine; acylcarnitines represent the difference between these two measures. Short- and long-chain esters can be distinguished by solubilities. Characterization of individual esters is helpful in recognizing disorders of fatty acid metabolism; techniques include gas chromatography–mass spectrometry and fast atom bombardment mass spectrometry.[55] Abnormally high ratios of acylcarnitines to free carnitine are seen in disorders of fatty acid oxidation and also in ketosis (excess acetylcarnitine).

Pathophysiology. Human deficiency can be either hereditary (systemic carnitine deficiency, myopathic carnitine deficiency) or acquired. Acquired deficiency can be caused by inadequate intake, increased requirement (pregnancy and breast feeding), or increased urinary loss (valproic acid therapy). Infants, patients following a course of long-term parenteral nutrition, and perhaps children are groups most vulnerable to deficiency as judged by decreased circulating levels and altered indicators of energy metabolism. Patients receiving hemodialysis may lose carnitine in the dialysis fluid. Excessive loss is also seen in the Fanconi syndrome. Excess production of acids (Reye's syndrome, organic acidemias, and chronic valproic acid therapy) is also accompanied by an excessive conversion of carnitine to ester

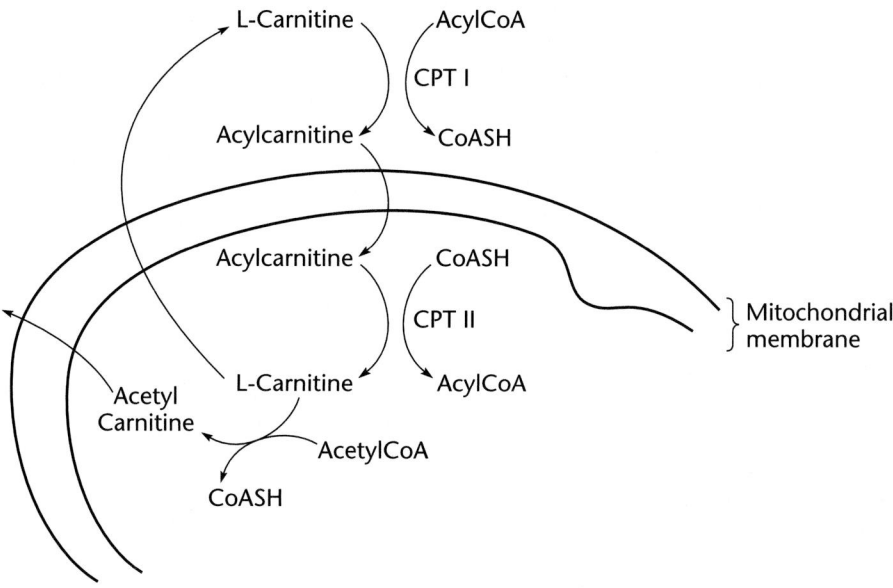

Fig. 39-18 Carnitine transport of acyl groups.

forms. These secondary deficiencies may result in muscular dysfunction. Primary deficiencies show muscle weakness and fatigue and may also have cardiac and hepatic involvement. Carnitine therapies are being evaluated for these circumstances and also in patients with disorders of ammonia metabolism. The three-carbon ester propionyl-L-carnitine has been shown to protect the ischemic heart from reperfusion injury. Function of patients with Alzheimer's disease has been reportedly improved by treatment with acetyl-L-carnitine. Mechanisms for these processes are not yet clear.[54]

VITAMINS AS ANTIOXIDANTS[55-60]

Free radicals are highly reactant molecules generated during ordinary metabolism and from certain drugs or xenobiotics (foreign chemicals). Exposure to ultraviolet radiation, cigarette smoke, and other environmental pollutants increases the body's burden of free radicals. These short-lived free radicals can damage membranes, enzymes, and DNA. An array of antioxidant defenses exist in cells and tissues to prevent formation or limit the effects of free radicals. Free radicals have been implicated as a possible cause of cancer and cardiovascular disease. Vitamins C and E and β-carotene protect against cancer of the lung and other epithelial tissues through a variety of mechanisms. Human intervention trials testing the efficacy of these compounds as anticancer agents are ongoing. Recent evidence indicates that low-density lipoprotein (LDL) apoprotein may be modified by a free radical–driven lipid peroxidation process. The resultant modified ApoB protein has altered receptor affinity leading to macrophage scavenging and initiation of the atherosclerotic lesion. This peroxidation may be prevented by the endogenous vitamin E carried in LDL lipid. Consumption of antioxidants is associated with delayed development of various forms of cataracts. Clinical trials indicate improved immune responses in the elderly upon supplementation with vitamins C, E, and A or β-carotene. Vitamin A supplementation decreases the morbidity and mortality associated with measles infection in children. In addition to specific antioxidant compound assessments, measures of overall oxidant status include breath pentane, electron spin resonance, and measures of base damage to DNA. Exploration of the roles of oxidant damage and of the protective and perhaps therapeutic effects of antioxidants has just begun.

METHODS OF ANALYSIS
Ascorbic acid (vitamin C)
STEVEN C. KAZMIERCZAK

Principles of analysis and current usage Ascorbic acid (AA) is a physiologic reducing agent and many methods are based on the oxidation of ascorbic acid to dehydroascorbic acid or on its reducing properties. Examples of such assays based on an indicator dye are the 2,6-dichlorophenol-indophenol and ferrous chromogenic complex methods. In the 2,6-dichlorophenol-indophenol method, ascorbic acid reduces the dye, resulting in decreased absorbance at 520 nm.[61] Disadvantages of this technique include its poor sensitivity and nonspecificity; a variety of other compounds can reduce the dye.[62]

In the ferrous chromogenic complex method, ascorbic acid reduces ferric ion to ferrous iron.[63] The ferrous iron then reacts with a chelating agent, such as 2,2'-dipyridyl or FerroZine Iron Reagent, to form a colored complex that can be detected spectrophotometrically. This method also suffers from lack of sensitivity and interference from a variety of substances. Modifications introduced to reduce the effects of interfering compounds on this assay as well as the 2,6-dichlorophenol-indophenol assay make these assays tedious to perform. Because of these and other drawbacks, neither of these ascorbic acid reduction assays are used today to any appreciable extent.

The most widely used assay for ascorbic acid is the 2,4-dinitrophenylhydrazine method (Table 39-3, method 1). In this procedure, ascorbic acid is first oxidized to dehydroascorbic acid and 2,3-diketogulonic acid. Copper is the most common agent chosen for oxidation; however, activated charcoal, bromine, 2,6-dichlorophenol-indophenol, and benzoquinone may also be used.[62] After the initial step of oxidizing ascorbic acid, 2,4-dinitrophenylhydrazine is added forming bis-2,4-dinitrophenylhydrazone. Treatment with sulfuric acid results in the formation of a colored product that absorbs at 520 nm. This method measures the total vitamin C content of the sample, since ascorbic acid, dehydroascorbic acid, and diketogulonic acid are also measured. This assay is subject to interference from sugars and amino acids, thiosulfates, and glucuronic acid.[62]

Fluorometric determinations of ascorbic acid have been developed though they are rarely used. Ascorbic acid is first oxidized to dehydroascorbic acid and then reacted with o-phenylenediamine to form a quinoxaline derivative that is a fluorophor.[64] This method measures both ascorbic acid and dehydroascorbic acid.

Enzymatic assays for ascorbic acid that use ascorbic acid oxidase have been developed (Table 39-3, method 2). Ascorbic acid oxidase is highly specific for oxidizing ascorbic acid to dehydroascorbic acid.[65] Specimens are incubated with and without ascorbic acid oxidase and then reacted with ferric iron and a complex-forming reagent 2,4,6-tris(2-pyridyl)-S-triazine. The absorbance of the complex is monitored at 593 nm. The difference in absorbance between the samples with and without ascorbic acid oxidase is proportional to ascorbic acid concentrations.

High-performance liquid chromatography (HPLC) has been developed as a means of bypassing the poor sensitivity and specificity of some of the methods previously described (Table 39-3, method 3). HPLC methods can measure ascorbic acid, dehydroascorbic acid, and the stereoisomer of ascorbic acid, isoascorbic acid. These HPLC methods utilize either ultraviolet detection or electrochemical detection schemes. Ultraviolet detection makes use of the vitamin's peak absorbance at 265-266 nm, whereas electrochemical detection of ascorbic acid utilizes the ease by which the vitamin is oxidized to become electrochemically active. Advantages of HPLC measurements of ascorbic acid include en-

Table 39-3 Methods of ascorbic acid analysis

Method	Principle	Usage	Comments
1. Spectrophotometric (2,4-dinitrophenylhydrazine)	Ascorbic acid is oxidized by copper to dehydroascorbic acid and 2,3-diketogulonic acid Addition of 2,4-dinitrophenyl-hydrazine followed by sulfuric acid results in formation of colored phenylhydrazone	Most common method in use	Subject to interference from sugars, amino acids, thiosulfates, and glucuronic acid
2. Enzymatic	Ascorbic acid is oxidized to dehydroascorbic acid by ascorbic acid oxidase. Addition of ferric ion and 2,4,6-tris(2-pyridyl-*S*-triazine) results in formation of colored complex measured at 593 nm	Not commonly used	More specific than method 1
3. High-performance liquid chromatography (HPLC)	Separation of ascorbic acid and dehydroascorbic acid using octadecylsilyl (C_{18}) columns with ultraviolet or electrochemical detection	Used with increasing frequency	More sensitive and specific than other methods

hanced sensitivity and specificity as a result of decreased substance interference. Because of these advantages, HPLC measurement of ascorbic acid is the preferred technique.

Specimen Serum or plasma collected in tubes containing EDTA, oxalate, or heparin may be used for most assays. The stability of ascorbic acid in biologic samples has not been adequately addressed.[62] Losses of 6% to 12% of ascorbic acid from baseline concentrations have been described for plasma samples that have not been refrigerated or deproteinized.[66] The preparation of metaphosphoric acid or perchloric acid supernates of serum or plasma samples that are not to be immediately analyzed may help prevent loss of ascorbic acid if these protein-free samples are stored at −20° C for 2 weeks or less. The addition of dithiothreitol (1 mg/mL) to samples has also been reported to stabilize specimens against loss of ascorbic acid. However, this and other thiol-reducing compounds can interfere in the popular 2,4-dinitrophenyl-hydrazine procedure.

The presence of any hemolysis is cause for the rejection of samples for ascorbic acid measurements. Hemoglobin causes a very rapid oxidation of ascorbic acid. Since some hemoglobin can be released from red blood cells during the clotting process, plasma specimens may be optimal.

Reference interval Individuals on a normal diet have been reported to have ascorbic acid concentrations from 6.0 to 20.0 mg/L (0.034 to 0.110 mmol/L). Ascorbic acid concentrations less than 2.0 mg/L are associated with a high risk for development of scurvy. Saturation of tissues with ascorbic acid results in plasma ascorbic acid concentrations of 10 to 15 mg/L (0.057 to 0.085 mmol/L).

Folic acid
STEVEN C. KAZMIERCZAK

Principles of analysis Techniques used to measure folate include microbiologic assays and competitive-binding immunoassays that employ radioisotopic, fluorescent, chemiluminescent, and enzyme labels. The microbiological assays were the first to be developed for folate measurement (Table 39-4, method 1). This assay is based upon measurement of the growth of the organism *Lactobacillus casei*, which requires methyltetrahydrofolic acid for growth; the growth of the or-

Table 39-4 Methods for folate analysis

Method	Principle	Usage	Comments
1. Microbiological	Growth of folate-requiring organism proportional to amount of folate present in patient specimen Growth monitored turbidimetrically	Rarely used	Reference method
2. Radiometric	Folate in sample competes with radiolabeled folate for binding sites on milk protein	Most frequently used	Endogenous folate binders must be destroyed
3. Nonradioisotopic	Folate in sample competes with labeled folate for binding to folate-binding protein Amount of folate-label conjugates bound to binding protein inversely related to folate in patient specimen	Increasingly used	Endogenous folate binders must be destroyed Automated

Nonisotropic labels include chemiluminescent, fluorescent, and enzyme labels.

ganism is directly related to the folate concentration in the patient's sample.

Organism growth is monitored by measurement of the turbidity of the growth solution. Microbiological assays for folate are no longer used routinely in the clinical laboratory because of their labor-intensive nature. There has been a recent report of a microbiological assay that measured folate using a 96-well microtiter plate.[67] This procedure was found to be less time-consuming than the traditional microbiological assays and was extremely economical when compared to the competitive protein-binding methods.

The most common methods in use for folate analysis are the radiometric competitive protein-binding techniques (Table 39-4, method 2). These methods are based on competitive binding between folate present in the patient sample and radiolabeled folate for a limited number of sites on a binding agent. Binding agents that are most commonly used are derived from milk,[68] whose varying affinities for the different forms of folate are pH dependent.[69]

The protein-binding assay may be performed as a single-stage or two-stage assay. The single-stage assay is the simplest to perform and involves combining the sample, the binding protein, and the tracer reagent all at once.

The two-stage assay is more sensitive than the former and involves a noncompetitive sequential incubation. In the first step of the procedure, the patient sample is incubated with the protein binder. After an incubation step, the temperature is decreased to 4° C to minimize dissociation of folate from the protein binder, and then radiolabeled folate is added to occupy any remaining binding sites. Separation of bound and unbound radiolabeled folate is usually performed with dextran-coated charcoal at 4° C.

Nonradioisotopic competitive protein-binding methods have been developed to permit automated analysis of folate in serum (Table 39-4, method 3). An example is a competitive radial partition assay (Baxter Diagnostics, Miami, Florida) in which folate present in patient sample is first reduced and then extracted from endogenous binding proteins. In the next stage of the assay, the solution containing the reduced and unbound folate is added to a fiber matrix that contains a folate-binding protein linked to the fiber matrix with an anti–folate binding protein antibody. Next, a folate-enzyme (alkaline phosphatase) conjugate is added so that it will combine with any remaining folate-binding sites. In the last step of the assay, unbound folate-enzyme conjugate is eluted from the reaction area of the fiber matrix, and enzyme substrate is added. The amount of product formed is inversely related to folate concentrations in the patient sample.

Most of the nonisotopic folate assays are hetergeneous assays similar to the one described above. However, the Abbott fluorescence polarization procedure is a homogeneous assay.

Serum contains endogenous binding proteins that can bind folate and result in falsely low serum folate concentrations being measured. These endogenous binding proteins may be inactivated by chemicals or by boiling at a high pH with 2-mercaptoethanol. Care must be taken, however, so that endogenous folate is not destroyed in these extraction steps.

In addition to serum or plasma folate determinations, red blood cell folate determinations may also be performed.

Studies have shown that measurement of red blood cell folate concentrations are of greater clinical utility than serum folate concentrations for the diagnosis of megaloblastic anemia.[70] However, many laboratories perform assays for serum folate only. The reason may be the convenience of dual isotope kits for simultaneous determination of serum folate and vitamin B_{12},[71] or the increased variability and inaccuracy associated with analysis of folate in red blood cells. These analytical problems may result from the various forms of folate in erythrocytes and the problem of adequately converting all the forms to the reduced monoglutamate, methyltetrahydrofolate, during analysis.[71] Folate in serum is almost exclusively present in the monoglutamate form. However, in red blood cells it is present as the polyglutamate form and as high-molecular-weight complexes.[72]

Specimen Samples for serum or plasma folate analysis should be collected from fasting individuals because folate levels can vary with intake of foods containing this vitamin. Plasma samples may be collected into tubes containing EDTA or heparin, however, if the specimen is to be used for simultaneous determination of B_{12}, heparin should be avoided because it can complex with vitamin B_{12}. Serum or plasma may be maintained for 24 hours at 4° C without appreciable loss of folate. For longer term storage, these specimens should be frozen at −10° C. Hemolyzed samples are unsuitable for analysis because of the very high folate concentrations found in red blood cells.

Whole blood for erythrocyte folate analysis may be collected using oxalate or heparin as the anticoagulant. The hematocrit of the sample should also be determined so that results can be expressed as a function of red blood cell mass. Folate within the cells may be liberated by freezing and thawing the specimen or by incubation of the sample with ascorbic acid. Folate in the erythrocyte lysate is stable for up to 4 days at 4° C if ascorbic acid (5 mg/mL) is added to the lysate.[71]

Reference interval The reference interval for folate in serum or plasma is often stated as 1.9 to 14 ng/mL (4.3 to 31.7 pmol/mL). Folate is higher in children. For children 1 to 12 years of age the serum folate was found to be 2.0 to 11.9 ng/mL (4.5 to 27.0 pmol/L for males and 2.5 to 13.8 pmol/L for females).[73] For persons 13 to 18 years of age, a significant decline in folate concentrations has been reported, with an upper reference limit of 8.8 ng/mL (19.9 pmol/L) in males and 7.3 ng/mL (16.5 pmol/L) for females.

Vitamin B_{12}

I-WEN CHEN
MATTHEW I. SPERLING
LINDA A. HEMINGER

Principles of analysis Methods of measurement of vitamin B_{12} have included microbiological assays and radioisotopic/nonradioisotopic competitive-binding immunoassays. Unfortunately, the current assays for quantitating vitamin B_{12} often encounter problems of poor precision and a failure to measure vitamin B_{12} directly.[74]

Microbiological assays (Table 39-5, method 1) were the first procedures established for measurement of vitamin B_{12}. Although no longer in routine use, this assay may be considered the reference method because it measures biologically active vitamin only. The microbiological assays are

Table 39-5   Methods of analysis of vitamin B$_{12}$

Method	Principle of analysis	Usage	Comments
1. Microbiological	Growth of microorganism in solution depends on amount of vitamin B$_{12}$ present in serum sample; Growth monitored by turbidimetry	Not in routine use Used as reference	Tedious Not very sensitive
2. Radioimmunoassay	Competition occurs between radiolabeled B$_{12}$ and nonlabeled B$_{12}$ from patient's sera for limited number of sites on a vitamin B$_{12}$ protein binder	Most common, currently in use Will most likely be replaced by nonradioisotopic assays	Sensitive and precise Often performed with analysis of folic acid
3. Competitive magnetic-separation immunoassay	Enzyme-labeled (ALP) vitamin B$_{12}$ competes with vitamin B$_{12}$ from patients sera for a limited number of binding sites on a vitamin B$_{12}$ protein binder Addition of magnetic monoclonal particle allows separation of bound and unbound enzyme-labeled B$_{12}$	Frequently used	Recently introduced method
4. Microparticle intrinsic factor assay	B$_{12}$ from patient sample binds to solid-phase microparticles B$_{12}$ from sera competes with enzyme-labeled B$_{12}$ for binding to microparticle Amount of enzyme activity is measured and is inversely proportional to serum vitamin B$_{12}$ concentrations	Frequently used	Recently introduced method
5. Cloned enzyme donor immunoassay (CEDIA)	Endogenous B$_{12}$ competes with B$_{12}$ linked to enzyme acceptor molecule for limited number of intrinsic factor–binding sites Endogenous B$_{12}$ allows a greater number of enzyme donor and enzyme receptor molecules to associate to form active enzyme	Frequently used	Recently introduced method

ALP, Alkaline phosphatase.

based on the requirement of certain microorganisms for vitamin B$_{12}$ as a growth factor. The amount of bacterial growth is directly proportional to the B$_{12}$ available in the sample.[75] A standard curve is prepared by measurement of the bacterial growth in standards with known amounts of the vitamin. The bacterial growth is typically measured turbidimetrically. A wide variety of bacteria have been utilized in the microbiological assays; the first to be used was *Lactobacillus lactis*.[76] Further refinements of this technique led to the use of *Euglena gracilis*[77] or *Ochromonas malhamensis*.[78] These latter two microorganisms are considered to be the most sensitive and most specific organisms for vitamin B$_{12}$ assays. Although the microbiological assays are specific for B$_{12}$, they suffer from technical and logistical limitations. High concentrations of folate can inhibit bacterial growth, and deoxyribonucleoside can partially replace the vitamin.[78] The sensitivity of the assay is relatively poor, making it difficult to detect the low concentrations of vitamin found in certain body fluids. The microbiological assays require sterile techniques and therefore cannot be used for samples containing certain antibiotics.

The most common methods currently in use for determination of vitamin B$_{12}$ are the competitive protein-binding radioimmunoassays (Table 39-5, method 2). These assays are based on the principle that vitamin B$_{12}$, which has been released from endogenous binding proteins, can be measured by its competition with ^{57}Co-labeled B$_{12}$ for a limited amount of a specific binding protein. The binding protein typically used is porcine intrinsic factor. Special measures must be taken to eliminate the interference caused by other, nonspecific protein binders of vitamin B$_{12}$. These nonspecific protein binders are commonly referred to as *R-proteins*, or *R-binders*. They exhibit rapid (denoted by *R*) mobility on electrophoresis. These proteins are found in human gastric juice and have a high binding affinity for vitamin B$_{12}$.

The commercially available radioisotopic assays typically use one of two techniques for addressing the issue of B$_{12}$-binding proteins. Some assays employ vitamin B$_{12}$ analogs as R-protein blockers, whereas others use heat denaturation in boiling water to remove interfering compounds.[78] Some assays utilize chemical denaturation of interfering compounds and thus eliminate the boiling step. It has been found that the latter "no-boil" procedures do not completely denature anti-intrinsic factor antibodies.[79] Some assay procedures may exhibit a high degree of nonspecific protein binding as a result of incomplete inactivation of endogenous binding proteins in serum, inadequate separation of free and bound radioisotopes, or the use of nonspecific binders of vitamin B_{12}.[80]

Several nonradioisotopic assays for vitamin B_{12} have been developed for routine laboratory use. One procedure utilizes a competitive magnetic-separation immunoassay (Table 39-5, method 3). This assay has been automated (Miles Inc., Tarrytown, NY 10591) and is based on competitive protein binding. In the first phase of the assay, vitamin B_{12} is released from endogenous binding proteins using a pretreatment reagent containing dithiothreitol, NaOH, and KCN. After this, the released vitamin B_{12} is reacted with reagent containing intrinsic factor. After an incubation step, vitamin B_{12} that is conjugated to the enzyme alkaline phosphatase (ALP) is introduced into the system. This B_{12}-enzyme conjugate competes with vitamin B_{12} from the sample for protein-binding sites on the intrinsic factor. Separation of bound and free labeled vitamin B_{12} is accomplished with use of monoclonal antibodies bound to a magnetic particle. The monoclonal-magnetic particles bind to the intrinsic factor–vitamin B_{12} complexes. In the final step of the assay, substrate for the enzyme label (*para-* or *p*-nitrophenyl phosphate) is added. The substrate is cleaved producing *p*-nitrophenoxide, which can be monitored spectrophotometrically at 405 nm. Samples containing no vitamin B_{12} will have maximum binding of enzyme-labeled vitamin B_{12} to intrinsic factor and thus exhibit maximum absorbance readings, whereas samples with increased B_{12} concentrations will have minimum bound label.

An assay based on very similar principles is the chemiluminescence assay available from Ciba Corning. This procedure, automated on the ACS-180, employs a chemiluminescence label.

Another nonradioisotopic vitamin B_{12} procedure is the microparticle intrinsic factor assay (Table 39-5, method 4).[81] This automated procedure utilizes a two-step competitive assay (Abbott Diagnostics, Abbott Park, IL 60064). In this procedure, a sample is combined with an extractant that serves to free vitamin B_{12} from serum binding proteins. Next, a solid-phase vitamin B_{12} binder (intrinsic factor) is added to bind free B_{12} in the solution. After an incubation period, an aliquot of the solution is deposited onto a reaction cell matrix. Any vitamin B_{12}–bound microparticles are captured by the fibers of the matrix. After a wash step, a tracer reagent consisting of ALP conjugated to vitamin B_{12} is added and allowed to incubate. The final step is the addition of an excess amount of 4-methylumbelliferyl phosphate substrate solution. The reaction product, methylumbelliferone, is produced in inverse proportion to the amount of vitamin B_{12} in the sample.[83]

Another nonradioisotopic assay used in some laboratories is the cloned enzyme donor immunoassay (CEDIA) (Table 39-5, method 5).[84] This assay utilizes the enzyme β-galactosidase, which has been prepared as two separate enzyme fragments using recombinant DNA techniques. Active enzyme is obtained only when these two enzyme fragments are mixed together. One enzyme fragment is prepared as the enzyme acceptor, and the other is prepared as the enzyme donor. The enzyme acceptor molecule is conjugated to vitamin B_{12}. Vitamin B_{12} in the patient sample competes with the enzyme donor–vitamin B_{12} conjugate for a limited number of protein-binding sites (porcine intrinsic factor). The binding of vitamin B_{12} in the sample to the intrinsic factor–binding protein enables more enzyme acceptor/enzyme donorvitamin B_{12} complexes to be formed. The concentration of vitamin B_{12} in the patient sample is directly proportional to the amount of enzyme formed. Enzyme activity is measured by monitoring the hydrolysis of chlorophenol-β-galactopyranoside at 550 nm.

Specimen Serum or plasma are acceptable specimens; however, plasma anticoagulated with heparin is unsuitable for use because of its ability to bind vitamin B_{12}. High concentration of fluoride or ascorbate can destroy vitamin B_{12} and should be avoided. Specimens should be collected from fasting individuals because food intake may increase vitamin B_{12} concentrations in blood.

Vitamin B_{12} is degraded after exposure to light for greater than 24 hours.[85] If analysis is delayed, specimens may be stored at 4° C for several days or frozen at −20° C for several months without appreciable loss. Samples should not be repeatedly frozen and thawed.

Reference interval Reference intervals for vitamin B_{12} are dependent on the assay technique used for its measurement and the type of intrinsic factor preparation employed.[86] The reference interval given for a microbiological assay using *Euglena gracilis* as the organism has been reported as 160 to 950 pg/mL (118 to 700 pmol/L).[87] The reference interval for vitamin B_{12} measured using a competitive magnetic separation immunoassay is 199 to 732 pg/mL (147 to 542 pmol/L). Vitamin B_{12} is higher in newborns when compared to adults and has also been found to be higher in black individuals when compared to whites.[88]

Patients taking certain drugs or medications may show decreased vitamin B_{12} concentrations in serum because of interference with absorption of the vitamin. Compounds exhibiting this effect include methotrexate, phenytoin, barbiturates, and oral contraceptives.

ACKNOWLEDGMENTS

The editors wish to acknowledge the previous version of the Folic Acid method written by Michael D. D. McNeely.

REFERENCES

1. Food and Nutrition Board: *Recommended Dietary Allowances,* ed 10, Washington, D.C., 1989, National Academy of Science.
2. Pesce AJ, Kaplan LA: *Methods in clinical chemistry,* St. Louis, 1987, Mosby.
3. Labbe RF, editor: *Clinics in laboratory medicine,* vol 1, *Laboratory assessment of nutritional status,* Philadelphia, 1981, Saunders.
4. Briggs MH, editor: *Vitamins in human biology and medicine,* Boca Raton, Fla., 1981, CRC Press.
5. Calabrese EJ: *Nutrition and environmental health,* vol 1, *The vitamins,* New York, 1980, Wiley & Sons.
6. Brewster MA, Naito HK, editors: *Nutritional elements and clinical biochemistry,* New York, 1980, Plenum Publishing.
7. Pereira GR, Zucker A: Nutritional deficiencies in the neonate, *Clin Perinatol* 13:175-189, 1986.
8. Rosenthal MJ, Goodwin JS: Cognitive effects of nutritional deficiency, *Adv Nutr Res* 7:71-100, 1985.
9. Snodgrass GR: Vitamin neurotoxicity, *Molec Neurobiol* 6:41-73, 1992.

Vitamin A

10. Garry PJ: Vitamin A. In Labbe RF, editor: *Clinics in laboratory medicine,* vol 1, *Laboratory assessment of nutritional status,* Philadelphia, 1981, Saunders.

11. Shamberger RJ: Vitamin A alterations in disease. In Brewster MA, Naito HK, editors: *Nutritional elements and clinical biochemistry,* New York, 1980, Plenum Publishing, pp 117-130.
12. Sklan D: Vitamin A in human nutrition, *Prog Food Nutr Sci* 11:39-55, 1987.
13. Underwood BA: Methods for assessment of vitamin A status, *J Nutr* 120(suppl 11):1459-1463, 1990.

Vitamin E
14. Bland J: Lipid antioxidant nutrition. In Brewster MA, Naito HK, editors: *Nutritional elements and clinical biochemistry,* New York, 1980, Plenum Publishing.
15. Sokol RJ, Guggenheim MA, Henbi JE, et al: Frequency and clinical progression of the vitamin E deficiency neurologic disorder in children with prolonged neonatal cholestasis, *Am J Dis Child* 139:1211-1215, 1985.
16. Farrell PM, Bieri JG: Megavitamin E supplementation in man, *Am J Clin Nutr* 28:1381, 1975.
17. Bieri JG, Evarts RP, Thorp S: Factors affecting the exchange of tocopherol between red cells and plasma, *Am J Clin Nutr* 30:686, 1977.
18. Ogumekan AO: Vitamin E deficiency and seizures in animals and man, *Can J Neurol Sci* 6:43-45, 1979.
19. Sokol RJ: Vitamin E and neurological deficits, *Adv Pediatr* 37:119-148, 1990.

Vitamin K
20. Suttie JW: Role of vitamin K in the synthesis of clotting factors. In Draper HH, editor: *Advances in nutritional research,* vol 1, New York, 1977, Plenum Publishing.
21. Hazell K, Baloch KH: Vitamin K deficiency in the elderly, *Gerontol Clin* 12:10-17, 1970.
22. Motohara K, Endo F, Matsuda I: Screening for late neonatal vitamin K deficiency by acarboxyprothrombin in dried blood spots, *Arch Dis Child* 62:370-375, 1987.

Vitamin D
23. Taylor CB, Peng S: Vitamin D—its excessive use in the U.S.A. In Brewster MA, Naito HK, editors: *Nutritional elements and clinical biochemistry,* New York, 1980, Plenum Publishing.
24. Holick MF: The use and interpretation of assays for vitamin D and its metabolites, *J Nutr* 120(suppl 11):1464-1469, 1990.

Ascorbic acid
25. Sauberlich HE: Ascorbic acid. In Labbe RF, editor: *Clinics in laboratory medicine,* vol 1, *Laboratory assessment of nutritional status,* Philadelphia, 1981, Saunders.
26. Englard S, Seifter S: The biochemical functions of ascorbic acid, *Annu Rev Nutr* 6:265-304, 1986.
27. Mirvish SS: Effects of vitamins C and E on N-nitroso compound formation, carcinogenesis and cancer, *Cancer* 58:1842-1850, 1986.
28. Jacob RA: Assessment of human vitamin C status, *J Nutr* 120(suppl 11):1480-1485, 1990.
29. Washko PW, Welch RW, Dhariwal KR, et al: Ascorbic acid and dehydroascorbic acid analyses in biological samples, *Anal Biochem* 204:1-14, 1992.

Riboflavin
30. Komindr S, Michaels GE: Clinical significance of riboflavin deficiency. In Brewster MA, Naito HK, editors: *Nutritional elements and clinical biochemistry,* New York, 1980, Plenum Publishing.
31. Bates CJ: Human riboflavin requirements and metabolic consequences of deficiency in men and animals, *World Rev Nutr Diet* 50:215-266, 1987.
32. Pinto J, Raiczyk GB, Huang YP, Rivlin RS: New approaches to the possible prevention of side effects of chemotherapy by nutrition, *Cancer* 58:1911-1924, 1986.

Pyridoxin
33. Vermaak WJ, Bernard HC, Potgieter GM, Theran HD: Vitamin B_6 and coronary artery disease: epidemiological observations and case studies, *Atherosclerosis* 63:235-238, 1987.
34. Shuster K, Bailey LB, Madan CS: Vitamin B_6 status of low-income adolescent and adult pregnant women and the condition of their infants at birth, *Am J Clin Nutr* 34:1731, 1981.
35. Leklem JE: Vitamin B_6: a status report, *J Nutr* 120(suppl 11):1503-1507, 1990.

Niacin
36. Wahlqvist ML: Effects on plasma cholesterol of nicotinic acid and its analogues. In Briggs MH, editor: *Vitamins in human biology and medicine,* Boca Raton, Fla., 1981, CRC Press.
37. Glueck CJ: Nonpharmacologic and pharmacologic alteration of high-density lipoprotein cholesterol: therapeutic approaches to prevention of atherosclerosis, *Am Heart J* 110:1107-1115, 1985.
38. Gentile S, Orzes N, Persico M, et al: Comparison of nicotinic acid- and caloric restriction-induced hyperbilirubinaemia in the diagnosis of Gilbert's syndrome, *J Hepatol* 1:537-543, 1985.

Thiamin
39. Flint DM, Prinsley DM: Vitamin status of the elderly. In Briggs MH, editor: *Vitamins in human biology and medicine,* Boca Raton, Fla., 1981, CRC Press.
40. Blass JP: Thiamin and the Wernicke-Korsakoff syndrome. In Briggs MH, editor: *Vitamins in human biology and medicine,* Boca Raton, Fla., 1981, CRC Press.
41. Poloni M, Mazzarello P, Patrini C, and Pinelli P: Inversion of T/TMP ratio in ALS: a specific finding? *Ital J Neurol Sci* 7:333-335, 1986.

Biotin
42. Roth KS, Allen L, Yang W, et al: Serum and urinary biotin levels during treatment of holocarboxylase synthetase deficiency, *Clin Chim Acta* 109:337, 1981.
43. Wolf B, Heard GS, Weissbecker KA, et al: Biotinidase deficiency: initial clinical features and rapid diagnosis, *Ann Neurol* 18:614-617, 1985.
44. Roth KS: Biotin in clinical medicine: a review, *Am J Clin Nutr* 34:1967, 1981.

Pantothenic acid
45. Schwabedal PE, Pietrzik K, Wittkowski W: Pantothenic acid deficiency as a factor contributing to the development of hypertension, *Cardiology* 71(suppl 1):187-189, 1985.

Vitamin B_{12} and folic acid
46. Steinkamp RC: Vitamin B_{12} and folic acid: clinical and pathophysiological considerations. In Brewster MA, Naito HK, editors: *Nutritional elements and clinical biochemistry,* New York, 1980, Plenum Publishing.
47. Saxena S, Carmel R: Racial differences in vitamin B_{12} levels in the United States, *Am J Clin Pathol* 88:85-87, 1987.
48. Ho CH, Chang HC, Yeh SF: Quantitation of urinary methylmalonic acid by gas chromatography mass spectrometry and its clinical applications, *Eur J Hematol* 38:80-84, 1987.
49. Infante-Rivard C, Krieger M, Bascon-Barre M, Rivard SE: Folate deficiency among institutionalized elderly: public health impact, *J Am Geriatr Soc* 34:211-214, 1986.
50. Bailey LB: Folate status assessment, *J Nutr* 120(suppl 11):1508-1511, 1990.
51. Ueland PM, Refsum H, Stabler SP, et al: Total homocysteine in plasma or serum: methods and clinical applications, *Clin Chem* 39:1764-1779, 1993.

Carnitine
52. Rebouche CJ: Carnitine function and requirements during the life cycle, *FASEB J* 6:3379-3386, 1992.
53. Marzo A, Cardace G, Monti N, et al: Chromatographic and non-chromatographic assay of L-carnitine family components, *J Chromatogr* 527:247-258, 1990.
54. Tanphaichitr V, Leelahagul P: Carnitine metabolism and human carnitine deficiency, *Nutrition* 9:246-254, 1993.

Vitamins as antioxidants
55. Roe CR, Millington DS, Kahler SG, et al: Carnitine homeostasis in the organic acidurias, *Prog Clin Biol Res* 321:383-402, 1990.

56. Bendich A: Physiological role of antioxidants in the immune system, *J Dairy Sci* 76:2789-2794, 1993.

57. Cheeseman KH, Slater TF: An introduction to free radical biochemistry, *Br Med Bull* 49:481-493, 1993.

58. Perera FP, Tang D, Grinberg-Funes RA, et al: Molecular epidemiology of lung cancer and the modulation of markers of chronic carcinogen exposure by chemopreventive agents, *J Cell Biochem,* suppl 17F:119-128, 1993.

59. Manson JE, Gaziano JM, Jonas MA, Hennekens CH: Antioxidants and cardiovascular disease: a review, *J Am Coll Nutr* 12:426-432, 1993.

60. Taylor A: Cataract: relationship between nutrition and oxidation, *J Am Coll Nutr* 12:138-146, 1993.

61. Farmer CJ, Abt AF: Determination of reduced ascorbic acid in small amounts of blood, *Proc Soc Exp Biol Med* 34:146-150, 1936.

62. Washko PW, Welch RW, Dhariwal KR, et al: Ascorbic acid and dehydroascorbic acid analyses in biological samples, *Anal Biochem* 204:1-14, 1992.

63. Zannoni V, Lynch M, Goldstein S, Sato P: A rapid micromethod for the determination of ascorbic acid in plasma and tissues, *Biochem Med* 11:41-48, 1974.

64. Omaye ST, Turnbull JD, Sauberlich HE: In: McCormick DB, Wright LD, editors: *Methods in enzymology,* New York, 1979, Academic Press, vol 62, pp 3-11.

65. Liu TZ, Chin N, Kiser MD, Bigler WN: Specific spectrophotometry of ascorbic acid in serum or plasma by use of ascorbate oxidase, *Clin Chem* 28:2225-2228, 1982.

66. Garry PJ, Owen GM, Lashley DW, Ford PC: Automated analysis of plasma and whole blood ascorbic acid, *Clin Biochem* 7:131-145, 1974.

Folic acid

67. O'Broin S, Kelleher B: Microbiological assay on microtitre plates of folate in serum and red cells, *J Clin Pathol* 45(4):344-347, 1992.

68. Chitis J: The folate binding in milk, *Am J Clin Nutr* 20:1-4, 1967.

69. Givas JK, Gutcho S: pH dependence of the binding of folates to milk binder in radioassay of folates, *Clin Chem* 21:427-428, 1975.

70. Hoffbrand AV, Newcombe BFA, Mollin DL: Method of assay of red cell folate activity and the value of the assay as a test for folate deficiency, *J Clin Pathol* 19:17-28, 1966.

71. Brown RD, Jun R, Hughes W, et al: Red cell folate assays: some answers to current problems with radioassay variability, *Pathology* 22:82-87, 1990.

72. Scott JM, Weir DG: Folate composition, synthesis and function in materials, *Clin Haematol* 5:547-568, 1976.

73. Hicks JM, Cook J, Godwin ID, Soldin SJ: Vitamin B_{12} and folate: pediatric reference ranges, *Arch Pathol Lab Med* 117(7):704-706, 1993.

Vitamin B_{12}

74. Lee DSC, Griffiths BW: Human serum vitamin B_{12} assay methods: a review, *Clin Biochem* 18:261-264, 1985.

75. Ross GIM: Vitamin B_{12} assay in body fluids using *Euglena gracilis,* *J Clin Pathol* 5:250-256, 1952.

76. Shorb MS: Activity of vitamin B_{12} for the growth of *Lactobacillus lactis,* *Science* 107:397-398, 1948.

77. Unavailable.

78. Unavailable.

79. Hunter SH, Provasoli L, Stokstad ELR, et al.: Assay of antipernicious anemia factor with *Euglena,* *Proc Soc Exp Biol Med* 70:118-120, 1949.

80. Hunter SH, Provasoli L, Filfus J: Nutrition of some phagotropic fresh-water chrysomonads, *Ann NY Acad Sci* 56:852-862, 1953.

81. Allen RH: More on no-boil assay, *The Ligand Quarterly* 5:48-49, 1982.

82. Allen RH: *Current status of serum cobalamin (vitamin B_{12}) assays,* syllabus, seventh annual meeting, Clinical Radioassay Society, pp 85-109, Apr 27–May 1, 1981.

83. Kuemmerle SC, Boltinghous GL, Delby SM, et al: Automated assay of vitamin B_{12} by the Abbott IMX Analyzer, *Clin Chem* 38(10):2073-2077, 1992.

84. van der Weide J, Homan HC, Cozijnsen-van Rheenen E, et al: Nonisotopic binding assay for measuring vitamin B_{12} and folate in serum, *Clin Chem* 38(5):766-768, 1992.

85. Mastropaolo W, Wilson MA: Effect of light on serum B_{12} and folate stability, *Clin Chem* 39(5):913, 1993.

86. Chen I-W, Silberstein EB, Maxon HR, et al: Clinical significance of serum vitamin B_{12} measured by radioassay using pure intrinsic factor, *J Nucl Med* 22:447-451, 1981.

87. Reynoso G, Fontelo P, Konopka S, et al: Ligand assay methods for serum cobalamin, *The Ligand Quarterly* 3:34-40, 1980.

88. Chen I-W, Silberstein EB, Heninger LA, et al: Comparison of serum vitamin B_{12} (B_{12}), unsaturated B_{12} binding capacity (UBBC), and folate levels in white and black subjects, *Clin Chem* 32:1186, 1986.

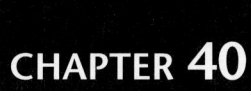

Pregnancy and fetal development

John F. Chapman
Gregory J. Tsongalis

OBJECTIVES

- Describe amniotic fluid including its formation, functions, and normal constituents.
- Describe the usual healthy and pathological maternal biochemical changes that occur during pregnancy.
- Describe fetal biochemical changes that occur during prenatal development.
- Describe pathological conditions associated with pregnancy or the perinatal period and list expected levels of significant laboratory analytes.

KEY TERMS

anencephaly A defective development of the brain wherein the cerebral and cerebellar hemispheres are absent.

blastocyst An early stage in embryonic development characterized by a fluid-filled cavity within the cell mass covered by the trophoblast.

ectopic pregnancy Pregnancy occurring outside the uterine cavity, most commonly in the fallopian tubes.

hemopoietic Related to the process of formation and development of the various types of blood cells.

keratinization The process in skin development and differentiation whereby keratin, a proteinaceous substance, is produced.

lamellar bodies The physical form of pulmonary surfactant extruded from type II pneumocytes.

meningomyelocele A protrusion of the membranes and spinal cord resulting from a defect in the vertebral column.

oligohydramnios The presence of less amniotic fluid than is usual for a given gestational age.

polyhydramnios The accumulation of an excessive amount of amniotic fluid.

spina bifida A developmental abnormality characterized by defective closure of the spinal cord.

transudation The passage of a substance through a membrane as a result of a difference in hydrostatic pressure.

trophoblast The cell layer covering the blastocyst, which erodes

793

the inner lining of the uterus during the process of implantation. Trophoblastic cells do not become part of the embryo itself but contribute to the formation of the placenta.

ANATOMICAL AND PHYSIOLOGICAL INTERACTION OF MOTHER AND FETUS
Fertilization and implantation of the ovum

Chapter 45 reviews the biochemical changes required for the successful development and release of an ovum. After ovulation, the ovum is expelled into the peritoneal cavity where it is moved into either of the two fallopian tubes by the action of the ciliated epithelial cells of the fimbriated tentacles. Fertilization normally occurs either before the ovum enters the tube or shortly thereafter. Approximately 3 days are required for transport of the fertilized ovum through the tube and into the cavity of the uterus. An additional 2 to 5 days are required for implantation of the ovum in the endometrium of the uterus. Thus, implantation of the developing ovum, the *blastocyst,* typically occurs 5 to 8 days after fertilization. Implantation results from the proteolytic digestion of the endometrium by the trophoblasts covering the surface of the blastocyst (Fig. 40-1). Once implantation is complete, both trophoblastic and endometrial cells proliferate rapidly in a coordinated fashion, forming the placenta and its membranes. The placenta serves both to separate the foreign body, the *fetus,* from the maternal host, and to provide an interface between the fetal and maternal circulatory systems. Through this interface, nutrients from maternal blood are delivered to the fetus, and fetal wastes are delivered to the mother for eventual disposal.

As the demands for nourishment and oxygen by the rapidly growing embryo increase, the trophoblast increases its surface area by forming villi. The surface area of these villi is enormous, and from the villi the fetal circulation of the placenta is established. The innermost membrane, the amnion, immediately surrounds the embryo and is filled with fluid. This fluid, referred to as the *liquor amnii,* or *amniotic fluid,* bathes the fetus, thereby preventing desiccation, and buffers the fetus against physical shocks. The blood in the placenta is derived from the fetal circulation.

Fetal growth and nutrition

The fetus grows and develops, using the nutrients provided by maternal blood. To maintain an adequate and continuous supply of necessary substrates for fetal development, continual maternal metabolic adjustments are required. Unlike the *infant* whose diet is a complex mixture of carbohydrates, fats, and proteins, the *fetus* has a diet consisting largely of glucose and sufficient quantities of amino acids to satisfy the nitrogen requirements of protein synthesis. Also included are small amounts of materials such as fatty acids, ketones, vitamins, and minerals that are essential to healthy growth and function. Although glucose provides most of the energy needed for the formation of tissues, amino acids can serve as an alternative source of oxidizable fuel. Ketones may also serve as alternative fetal energy sources and as precursors for proteins and lipids during periods of maternal fasting.

The amount of glucose available to the fetus depends on the concentration of glucose in maternal blood, which is regulated by the action of numerous hormones, including insulin and the placental hormone, human chorionic somatomammotropin (also called *human placental lactogen,* or HPL).

Glucose passes readily from the maternal to the fetal circulation by means of "facilitated diffusion," crossing the placenta at a faster rate than would be expected on physiological grounds alone. A rise in the glucose concentration in maternal blood is followed rapidly by a comparable increase in its concentration in fetal blood. The two levels do not become equal, however, and a concentration gradient from mother to fetus is always present. In addition, a sig-

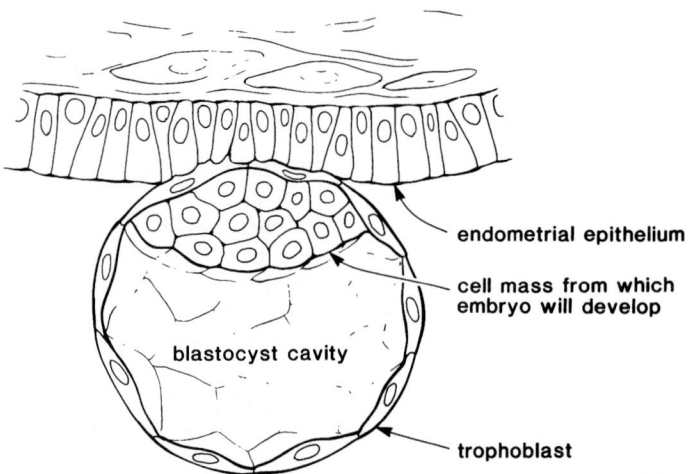

Fig. 40-1 Attachment of blastocyst to endometrial wall.

nificant proportion of glucose is consumed by the placenta to meet its own energy requirements.

Since glucose levels in the fetus mirror those in the mother, there is usually little need for the fetus to regulate its own blood glucose concentrations. Mechanisms for doing so do develop during the fetal period, but, except in infants of hyperglycemic diabetic mothers, these mechanisms are largely dormant until birth, when the supply of glucose through the placenta ends abruptly. Nevertheless, two important processes are active from an early stage. The first is the storage of glucose as glycogen or fat to provide for the metabolic needs of the newborn until feeding begins. The second is the control of the rate at which glucose is used by the growing tissues, and this is attributable primarily to the action of insulin secreted by the fetal pancreas beginning at 8 to 9 weeks of gestational age.

Role of placenta in gas exchange

To meet its metabolic needs the fetus is completely dependent on a continuous delivery of oxygen across the placenta. Transplacental exchanges, including those of gases, depend on both perfusion and permeability. Placental perfusion is a composite of uterine and umbilical blood flows, whereas permeability is a characteristic of the placental membrane. Under healthy conditions with well-oxygenated maternal blood, oxygen transport across the placenta is primarily regulated by blood flow. To meet the increasing demands of the growing fetus, uterine blood flow and placental membrane permeability increase during gestation. In the presence of maternal hypoxia, oxygen transport across the placenta becomes limited primarily by the permeability of the placental membrane.

Carbon dioxide rapidly diffuses across the placenta in either direction. This allows the fetus to maintain a normal P_{CO_2} and the mother to eliminate carbon dioxide. The placenta has limited permeability to bicarbonate ions. The placenta therefore allows the fetus to dispose of carbon dioxide while protecting it from maternal metabolic acidosis.

Formation of amniotic fluid

The volume of blood in the amniotic sac, which surrounds the developing embryo, increases throughout pregnancy until it reaches a maximum volume at about 36 weeks of gestation (Table 40-1). Many maternal and fetal abnormalities can produce oligohydramnios or polyhydramnios states. Amniotic fluid volume at any point in time is the result of a dynamic balance between production and removal. Amniotic fluid originates from multiple sources, and the relative contribution of each source varies depending on the stage of fetal development. The multiple sources include the placenta, fetal kidneys, skin, membranes, lungs, and intestine. In the first half of pregnancy, amniotic fluid forms as a transudate from the skin surface of the fetus. The composition of amniotic fluid is similar to that of extracellular fluid, and the amniotic fluid should be considered as an ex-

tension of the fetal extracellular fluid space. Later in pregnancy, fetal kidneys and lungs assume the major role in the formation of amniotic fluid, and its volume now depends on a balance between fetal urination and volume of amniotic fluid that is swallowed.[1]

Fluid moving from the trachea and pharynx into the esophagus can enter the amniotic cavity. This provides an explanation for the appearance of pulmonary surfactant in amniotic fluid. Respiratory movements by the fetus readily mix fluid with surfactant because the movements produce a tidal volume exchange (in and out) of about 600 to 800 mL/day[2] through the fetal lungs throughout the third trimester.

Amniotic fluid disappearance is in part affected by fetal swallowing. It is estimated that between 200 and 450 mL of amniotic fluid per day flows out from the amniotic cavity by this route, accounting for about half of the daily urine production of the fetus. Since the amniotic cavity gains a fluid volume of no more than 10 mL/day in the third trimester (the total solute concentration always remains in the normal range), a sizable quantity of urine must be reabsorbed by other pathways.[3]

BIOCHEMISTRY OF AMNIOTIC FLUID

Excellent monographs on the subject of amniotic fluid that contain compendia of the biochemical constituents of amniotic fluid are available.[4,5]

Water, electrolytes, and nitrogenous products

Because of the shift in the source of amniotic fluid that occurs about midway through pregnancy, constituents of amniotic fluid also change during gestation. Before keratinization of the skin, amniotic fluid can result as a transudation from the surface of the fetus. After keratinization and with progressive development of the renal system, fetal urine makes a more prominent contribution to the amniotic

Table 40-1   Amniotic fluid volume in normal pregnancy

Gestational age (weeks)	Volume of fluid (mL)
12	5-200
14	50-200
16	150-300
18	200-400
20	225-775
22	300-500
24	500-675
26	500-700
28	500-875
30	400-1300
32	400-1375
34	500-1350
36	525-1500
38	300-1525
40	325-1450
42	600

fluid compartment. The biochemical composition of amniotic fluid therefore reflects the routes of formation of the fluid and is related to the developmental stage of the fetus.

Amniotic fluid is isotonic during early pregnancy but by term becomes moderately hypotonic (mean total solute concentration, 255 mOsm/kg of water) compared with fetal and maternal plasma. This changing concentration of amniotic fluid reflects the maturation of fetal renal function. The osmotic and oncotic pressures in fetal and maternal tissues cause the transfer of water from mother to fetus to amniotic fluid and then back to the mother. It has been calculated that the net transfer of water from mother to fetus reaches 20 to 25 mL/day in late pregnancy.[6]

Amniotic fluid concentrations of nitrogenous products of metabolism, creatinine, urea, and uric acid increase toward the end of the term (see below) but are manyfold lower than concentrations found in maternal urine. The composition difference between amniotic fluid and maternal urine is readily measurable and can be used to determine whether a sample obtained from vaginal leakage or an errant amniocentesis is amniotic fluid.

Proteins

Proteins derived from many sources have been identified in amniotic fluid. Under healthy conditions, amniotic fluid proteins of fetal origin come from the skin, the urinary and gastrointestinal tracts (urine and meconium respectively), and the respiratory tract. Proteins from the respiratory tract are part of the proteolipid product secreted by type II epithelial cells of the fetal lung. These products function as components of the lung surfactant system.[7] At least four surfactant protein (SP) species have been described: SP-A, B, C, and D. These differ in molecular weight and charge and possibly function. Proteins of maternal origin can enter amniotic fluid by transudation across the amnion. Under abnormal circumstances, unusual avenues for protein exchange can occur, such as central neural tube development defects, which increase the α-fetoprotein levels in amniotic fluid (see below).

Over 50 enzymes have been identified in amniotic fluid,[4,5] but the origin of many of these enzymes and their significance in the fluid are not understood. The enzymes fall into two categories: those having an activity greatest early in pregnancy (12 to 20 weeks) and those active at the later stage of pregnancy (35 to 40 weeks). Some enzymes of fetal origin, such as alkaline phosphatase and γ-glutamyltransferase, are used in the diagnosis of particular inborn errors of metabolism.

Hormones

Examples of the hormones that have been identified in amniotic fluid are listed in the box above right. This list includes hormones (such as the catecholamines) derived from steroids, peptides, and amino acids. Although many of these hormones are products of urinary or biliary excretion from

---

Hormones Identified in Amniotic Fluid

Protein and polypeptide
Adrenocorticotropic hormone
Angiotensin
Endorphin
Follicle-stimulating hormone
Growth hormone
Human chorionic gonadotropin
Human placental lactogen
Insulin
Luteinizing hormone
Oxytocin
Prolactin
Relaxin
Renin
Somatomedin
Somatostatin
Thyrotropin
Thyroxine

Steroids
Estradiol
Estriol
Estrone

Prostaglandins
E_2
$F_{2\alpha}$

---

the fetus, a few have clinical usefulness and are discussed later. A more extensive list is available.[4,5]

MATERNAL BIOCHEMICAL CHANGES DURING PREGNANCY
Human chorionic gonadotropin

The urine and serum of pregnant women contain high concentrations of human chorionic gonadotropin (HCG), produced by the trophoblast, and provide the basis of tests for the diagnosis of pregnancy. Specific and sensitive analytical methods for the β-chain subunit of HCG permit the detection of pregnancy as early as 8 days after ovulation (1 day after implantation). Human chorionic gonadotropin concentrations climb early in pregnancy, reaching a maximum by 8 to 10 weeks of gestation (Fig. 40-2).

Human chorionic gonadotropin is one of a family of closely related glycoprotein hormones that regulates reproductive and metabolic functions. This family includes follicle-stimulating hormone (FSH), luteinizing hormone (LH), and thyroid-stimulating hormone (TSH). These hormones are composed of two polypeptide subunits referred to as alpha (α) and beta (β) chains, and each contains carbohydrate; thus the term *glycoprotein* is used. The α chains of HCG, LH, FSH, and TSH are similar in their amino acid sequences, a finding that accounts for the immunological similarity of these protein hormones.[8]

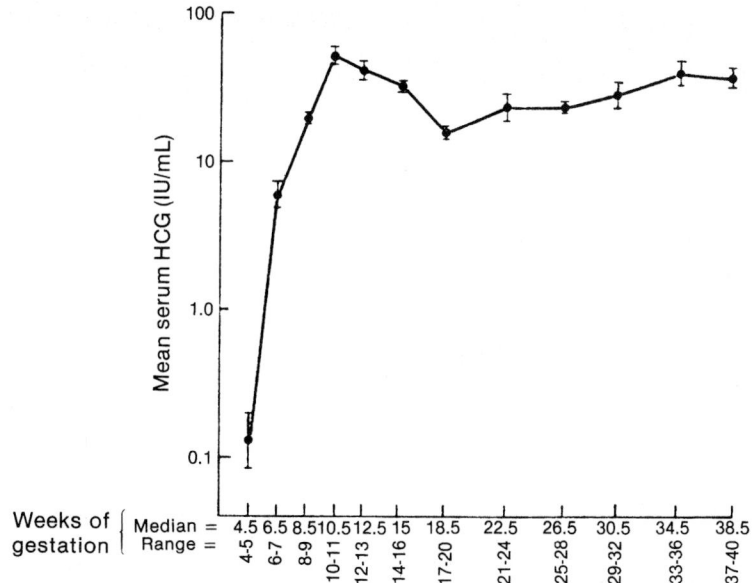

Fig. 40-2 Serum chorionic gonadotropin (HCG) concentrations during pregnancy. (From Goldstein DP, Aon T, Taymor MT, et al: *Am J Obstet Gynecol* 102:110-114, 1968.)

The β chains of the glycoprotein hormones each have a unique amino acid sequence, which gives these hormones their biological specificity. HCG has amino acid sequences in both the α and β chains that are virtually identical to those in LH, differing to a significant degree only in carbohydrate content, with HCG containing about 30% carbohydrate by weight and LH approximately half that amount. This similarity allows HCG to be used instead of LH for such purposes as ovulation induction. The carbohydrate-content difference perceptibly influences the metabolic patterns of these hormones; thus the biological half-life of HCG is about 6 hours, whereas the biological half-life of plasma LH is 12 to 45 minutes. These differences in metabolic clearance correlate well with our understanding of the functions of these hormones, with LH regulating the complicated process of ovulation and subsequent formation of the corpus luteum and HCG providing continued stimulation of the corpus luteum to ensure uninterrupted progesterone production until the placenta can provide sufficient progesterone to maintain the pregnancy (see Chapter 40 for details).

Estrogens

Nearly a half century ago it was recognized that a substantial increase in estrogen excretion accompanied pregnancy. The predominant estrogen was identified as estriol, not the usual ovarian estrogens—estradiol or estrone (Fig. 40-3). It was not until many years later that the unique relationships that described the pathway for estriol formation were elucidated. Estriol formation during pregnancy occurs only in the higher primates, and the obligatory interaction of fetus and placenta required for the formation of this "estrogen of

pregnancy" provides the basis for one of the few biochemical tests available to monitor fetal well-being.

Estrogen formation proceeds in an obligatory sequence of reactions that converts cholesterol to progestin, then to androgens, and then to estrogens (refer to Chapter 45). In the ovary, this sequence occurs solely within that organ. In pregnancy, for this sequence to lead to estriol formation, a complementary relationship is needed between the placenta, the fetal adrenal cortex, and the fetal liver. This unique interrelationship is referred to as the *fetoplacental unit*[9] (Fig. 40-4).

The fetal adrenal gland synthesizes dehydroepiandrosterone (DHEA), which is converted to 16α-hydroxy-DHEA by the fetal liver. The 16α-hydroxy-DHEA is converted to

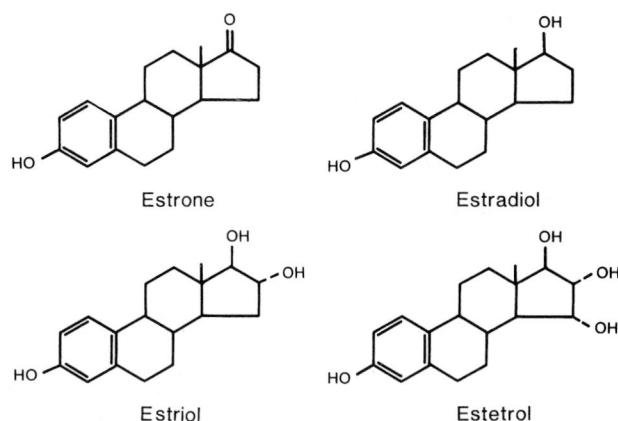

Fig. 40-3 Structures of estrogens. *Dashed lines,* α-stereoconfigurations; *solid lines,* β-stereoconfigurations of hydroxyl groups.

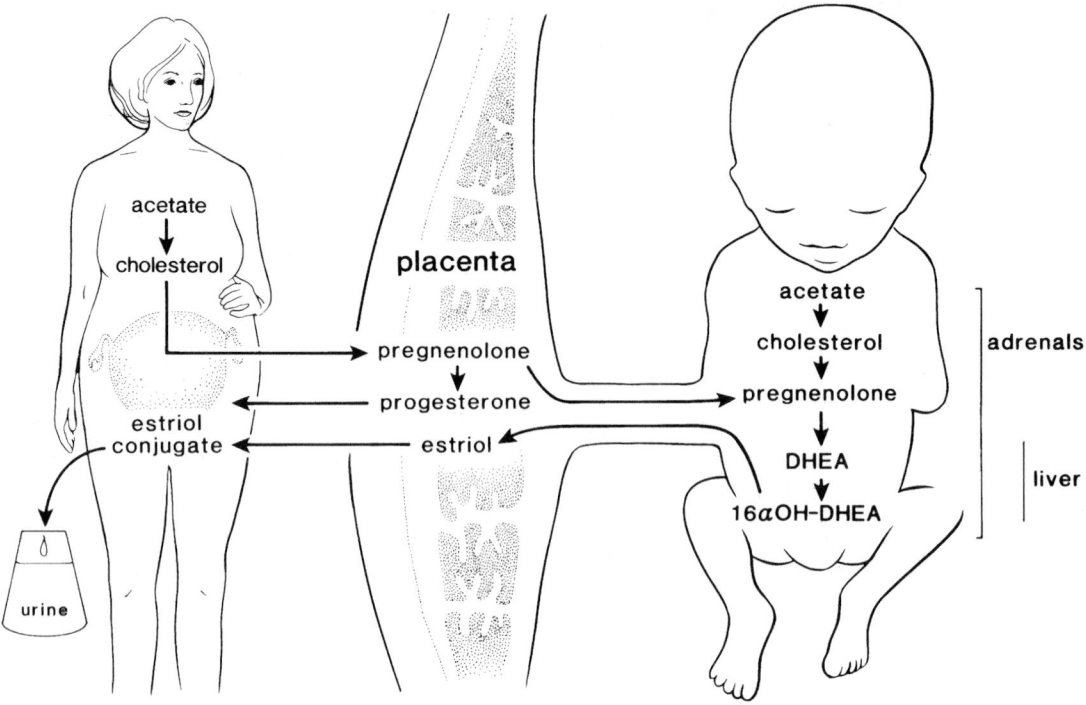

Fig. 40-4 Scheme of fetoplacental unit. *DHEA,* Dehydroepiandrosterone; *16α-OH-DHEA,* 16α-hydroxydehydroepiandrosterone.

estriol by placental aromatizing enzymes. In addition, the placenta possesses a very active sulfatase. Sulfation/desulfation of estriol appears to be integrally involved in the transfer of steroids from the placenta, since, in conditions where the placental sulfatase is absent, low maternal estriol levels are characteristically observed.[10]

Estriol constitutes over 90% of the known maternal estrogens of pregnancy. It is metabolized to both sulfate and glucuronide conjugated forms by maternal liver. These con-jugates are the primary excretory forms of estriol. Concentrations in maternal serum increase with advancing gestation and reach nearly 40 ng/mL at the end of the term. In Fig. 40-5, the patterns of a normal increase in plasma estriol and the patterns seen with a diabetic patient, with fetal death, and with growth retardation are shown. Estriol is also found in amniotic fluid.[11]

The functional role for estriol in pregnancy has prompted much speculation. In many biological test systems, estriol

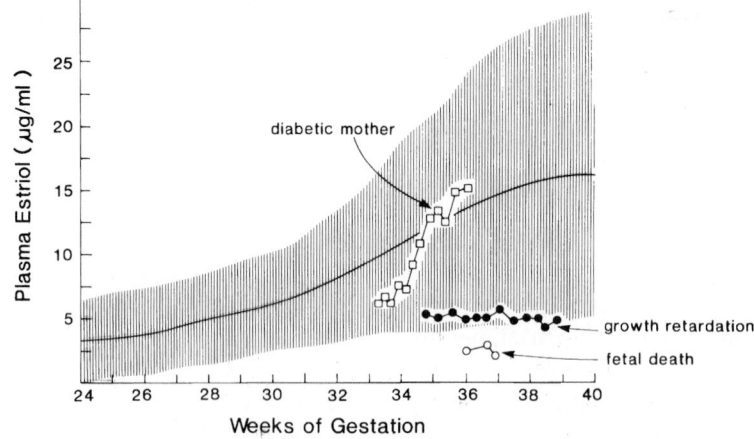

Fig. 40-5 Mean *(solid line)* and estimated 5th and 95th percentiles *(shaded area)* for plasma unconjugated estriol during normal pregnancy. Estriol patterns from three actual pregnancy conditions are shown.

is a weak estrogen, demonstrating only a hundredth of the potency of estradiol and one tenth of the potency of estrone per unit weight. However, estriol can be demonstrated to be equipotent to estradiol in its ability to promote uteroplacental blood flow. For this reason, its role in pregnancy may be to ensure optimum blood flow in the gravid uterus.

It has been suggested that levels of the estrogen *estetrol* (Fig. 40-3) offer more information than estriol levels about the status of the fetus in utero.[12] Estetrol (E_4) is not metabolized further as estriol is in the maternal liver. In addition, E_4 levels specifically reflect fetal liver activity, whereas estriol (E_3) levels depend on the fetal adrenal glands. Once E_4 is formed by fetal liver, it enters the maternal circulation and is excreted in urine as E_4-glucuronide. The presumed advantage of E_4 measurement is based on the belief that this estrogen reflects fetal activity more directly. Clinical evaluations of fetal well-being have not shown a clear advantage of estetrol over estriol, however.[13]

Thyroid

The concentration of thyroxin-binding globulin (TBG) is doubled by the end of the first trimester, and it remains elevated throughout the rest of pregnancy. Because of the increased number of binding sites available for thyroid hormones, the total amount of both thyroxine (T_4) and triiodothyronine (T_3) is increased in the blood; this increase is greater for T_4 than for T_3, which is generally only raised in the last trimester. Pregnant women are generally euthyroid, though hyperthyroxinemic. Although maternal thyroid physiology is clearly altered during pregnancy, the mechanisms by which this occurs are unclear. In response to increased estrogen production during pregnancy, the maternal liver synthesizes increased amounts of TBG.[14] The concentration of TBG is doubled by the end of the first trimester and remains elevated throughout the remainder of the pregnancy. This increase in serum TBG induces an adjustment of thyroid activity by increasing the levels of thyroid hormones in the circulation. However, the degree to which the levels of these hormones change during pregnancy remains controversial, in part because of both methodological and technical analytical flaws in the thyroid hormone analyses.

The maternal thyroid gland enlarges during pregnancy because of glandular hyperplasia and an increased vascularity.[14,15] Although no apparent mechanism has been defined, there is considerable evidence that indicates a possible association between thyroid stimulation and increased levels of HCG.[14,16] Human chorionic gonadotropin and TSH have nearly identical α subunits and similar β chains; thus, HCG may have a TSH-like stimulatory effect on the thyroid. Increased HCG levels have been shown to occur during the first half of gestation, whereas TSH levels increase during the second half of gestation.[14] Numerous studies have shown that the increased levels of HCG associated with trophoblastic disease are accompanied by hyperthyroidism and thyrotoxicosis,[17] and thyroid cells grown in culture have been shown to be stimulated by HCG.[16] The thyroid hormones and TSH do not pass across the placenta. Additional discussion of all facets of thyroid and parathyroid function in pregnancy can be found in Chapter 44. Lowe and Cunningham provide a review of the pathophysiologic mechanisms of thyroid disease during pregnancy.[15]

Serum lipids

Hyperlipidemia develops during a healthy pregnancy and may be the result of alterations in hormone levels. Pregnant women have greatly increased total serum lipid concentrations that increase progressively throughout pregnancy, with highest levels in the second and third trimesters.[18] Interestingly, these levels stabilize to prepregnancy levels after pregnancy, thus lending further support for the role of pregnancy-related hormones in regulating serum lipid levels. All components of the serum lipids are increased, but the triglyceride fraction shows the largest proportionate rise. High-density lipoprotein/low-density lipoprotein (HDL/LDL) ratios decrease with increasing duration of pregnancy, and HDL levels remain decreased 1 year after pregnancy.[18] Oral contraceptives may have some effect on HDL levels, but more thorough studies are needed.

Serum proteins and liver function

The total concentration of serum proteins decreases by about 1 g/L during pregnancy. Most of the decrease occurs during the first trimester. The decrease is mainly in serum albumin. α_1-, α_2-, and β-globulins rise slowly and progressively during pregnancy. γ-Globulin probably decreases slightly. The maternal antibody (IgG) component, which is the major immunoglobulin transferred to the fetus, falls progressively. Throughout pregnancy fibrinogen increases progressively, and values at term are 30% to 50% above nonpregnant levels. Clotting factors VII, VIII, IX, and X are also increased, whereas prothrombin and factors V and XII are reduced. Alterations that occur in the levels of clotting factors and plasminogen are probably brought about by estrogen action on the liver.

Under the influence of increased estrogens, the maternal liver increases the synthesis of transcortin (corticoid-binding globulin). This results in total cortisol levels increasing during pregnancy, almost doubling by late pregnancy. However, the levels of free, active cortisol are normal.

Several liver function tests change as a consequence of healthy pregnancy. For example, nonspecific alkaline phosphatase activity in serum nearly doubles during a pregnancy with a healthy mother and fetus and can reach levels that would be considered abnormal in the nonpregnant woman. Much of this increase is attributable to isoenzymes of this enzyme originating from the placenta.[19]

Glucosuria

Glucosuria is common in healthy, pregnant women. Glucose excretion rises very early in pregnancy, reaching a peak between 8 and 11 weeks of gestation. The degree of glucosuria varies thereafter. The cardinal feature of the glucosuria of pregnancy is a conspicuous variability both from day to day and during the course of a day. The cause of glucosuria in pregnancy appears to be the reduced efficiency of the kidneys to reabsorb glucose.[20]

From these comments it can be seen that pregnancy is potentially diabetogenic. Diabetes mellitus may be aggravated by pregnancy, and clinical diabetes may appear in some women only during pregnancy. The renal processing of glucose during pregnancy is of particular interest because of the frequent appearance of clinical glycosuria and the necessity to differentiate this "renal glycosuria" from that of pregnancy-aggravated diabetes mellitus. Because of the many variables associated with an altered renal physiology in pregnancy, pregnant diabetic women should be monitored by blood glucose levels because urine testing can yield misleading values. Screening for gestational diabetes by a glucose challenge test has become routine. It is important to maintain blood glucose within the reference interval to prevent perinatal morbidity associated with gestational hyperglycemia.

FETAL BIOCHEMICAL CHANGES DURING PRENATAL DEVELOPMENT
Liver function

Fetal liver contains a large number of hematopoietic cells that disappear after birth. In very early fetal life, the liver is the major blood-forming organ, but by 22 to 24 weeks of gestation the bone marrow has assumed the major responsibility for the formation of blood. Because of widely varying amounts of the different cell types in the newborn liver, enzyme-activity patterns are considerably different from the adult.

The fetal yolk sac and later the fetal liver produce α-fetoprotein (AFP), which is released into the fetal circulation. It passes from the bloodstream by way of the urine to amniotic fluid. It is usually removed from amniotic fluid by fetal swallowing. α-Fetoprotein appears in maternal serum throughout gestation (Fig. 40-6), where it can be easily measured to screen for neural tube defects.

The fetus's need for increased quantities of amino acids for protein synthesis is satisfied by placental transport. This is an active process against a concentration gradient that depends on placental blood flow and, to a lesser degree, on the concentration of amino acids in the maternal plasma.

Because maturation of the fetal liver is not complete by the time of birth, some jaundice regularly occurs in virtually every newborn during the first week of life. This is known as *physiological jaundice.* The yellow pigmentation, or jaundice, is caused by bilirubin that comes from the normal destruction of red blood cells. However, since the immature fetal liver has not developed its full capability to clear bilirubin from the blood, jaundice occurs (see pp. 803 and 804 for details).

Renal function

The primary function of the mammalian kidney is to maintain water and electrolyte homeostasis. This is accomplished by selective excretion or retention of water and solutes as

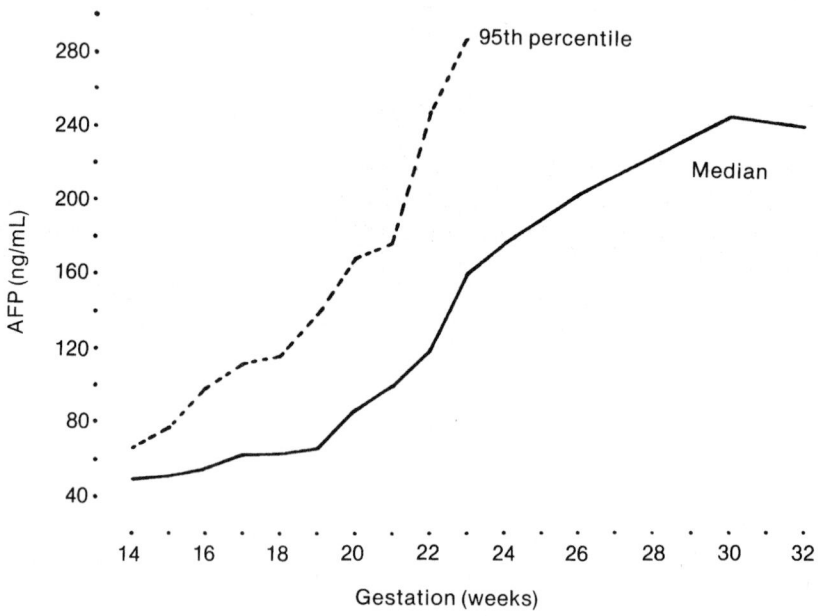

Fig. 40-6 Median and 95th percentile of α-fetoprotein, *AFP,* in maternal serum. (From Crandall BF: In Kirkpatrick AM, Nakamura RM, editors: *Alpha-fetoprotein: laboratory procedures and clinical applications,* New York, 1981, Masson.)

conditions dictate. In the fetus, body water and electrolyte balance are maintained largely by the placenta. For this reason fetuses without functional kidneys often show no water or electrolyte abnormalities. Thus, the full development of mature renal function occurs when it is needed—after birth.

Organic nitrogenous compounds such as urea, uric acid, and creatinine (Fig. 40-7) gradually increase in amniotic fluid as the renal system of the fetus matures. In early pregnancy these compounds are present in amniotic fluid in concentrations similar to concentrations in maternal and fetal blood. Concentrations increased gradually to become significantly higher than levels in maternal or fetal blood. A sharp rise in creatinine at about the thirty-seventh week of gestation elevates the amniotic fluid concentrations of urea and creatinine to levels two to three times higher than those of the reference interval of serum in healthy persons.[21]

Lung development

At birth there is an abrupt physiological transition that requires the newborn infant to assume vital functions that were previously handled by the maternal circulation. The lung is shifted from a fluid-filled organ to a gas-exchange system in a few brief minutes. This functional transition is possible only if sufficient maturation of the fetal lung has occurred during development. The fetal lung maturation process appears to consist of two distinct components: (1) the morphologic development of fetal lungs and (2) the synthesis, storage, and release of pulmonary surfactant. In the latter process, the control mechanisms for synthesis and storage of pulmonary surfactant appear to be distinct from those responsible for surfactant release.[22] Thus, functional

lungs should have developed alveoli with adequate surface area and vascularization for gas exchange, and sufficient surfactant must be available to sustain the ventilatory movements needed for pulmonary function. These processes are highly organized and are coordinated by the timing of anatomical and biochemical events.

Surfactant facilitates pulmonary function in at least two ways: It maintains alveolar stability by preventing collapse of the terminal respiratory tree, and it reduces the pressure that is needed to distend the lungs in the initial phase of inspiration. Infants who develop the respiratory distress syndrome have a higher surface tension at the alveolar air-liquid interface as a result of a pulmonary surfactant deficiency.

Human surfactant is composed principally of phospholipid that contains highly saturated fatty acid moieties.[23] The major constituents and their relative concentrations are shown in Figs. 40-8 and 40-9. In addition to the highly unusual saturated lecithins, other important constituents of the surface-active system include phosphatidylglycerol and the SPs mentioned previously. These proteins may serve a key role in enabling surfactant function by enhancing the rapidity with which surfactant can spread to form a monolayer along the air-water interface of the alveolus. Although functional differences between the individual SPs are incompletely described, recent evidence indicates that surfactant protein B (SP-B) may be the most important of the proteins in pulmonary surfactant.[24] This is believed to be the result of the unique interaction of this protein with phospholipid moities in surfactant. This interaction adds stability to the surfactant monolayer, thus increasing the ability of this layer to resist surface tension and prevent alveolar collapse. Detailed accounts of the function and biochemi-

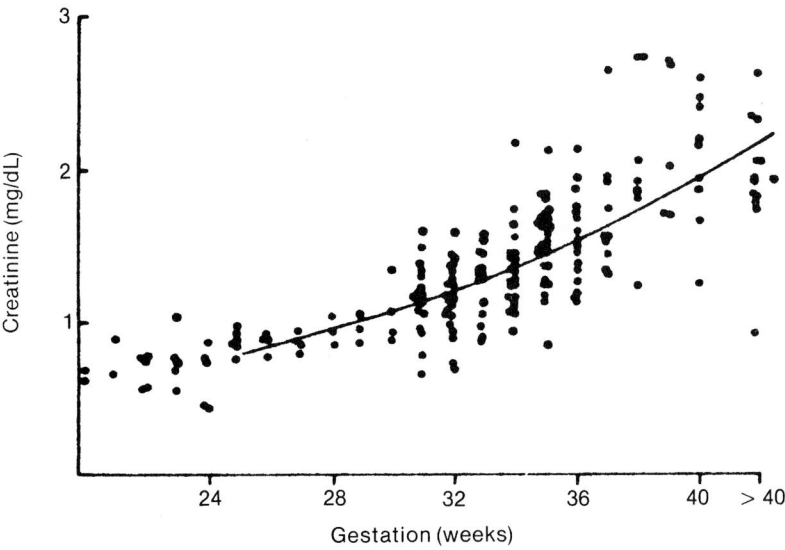

Fig. 40-7 Distribution and regression curve of amniotic fluid creatinine concentration in milligrams per deciliter. (From Lind T: In Fairweather DVI, Eskes TKAB, editors: *Amniotic fluid: research and clinical application,* ed 2, Amsterdam, 1978, Excerpta Medica.)

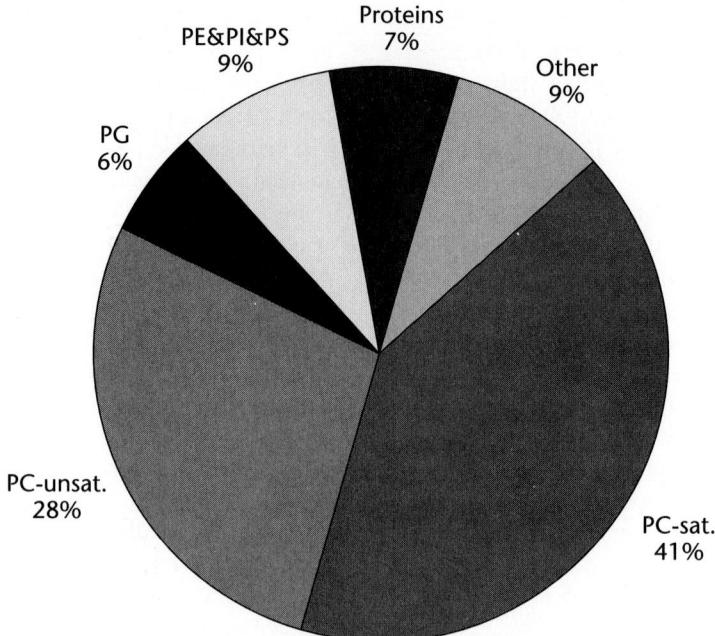

Fig. 40-8 Composition (by weight percent) of human surfactant. *PC-sat.,* Saturated phosphatidylcholine; *PC-unsat.,* unsaturated phosphatidylcholine; *PE,* phosphatidylethanolamine; *PG,* phosphatidylglycerol; *PI,* phosphatidylinositol; *PS,* phosphatidylserine. Proteins include 3.8% SP-A (SP-B and SP-C detected but not quantified). (From Hallman M: *Rev Perinatal Med* 6:197-226, 1989.)

cal composition of pulmonary surfactant have been published.[25,26]

Surfactant is formed in the large alveolar epithelial cells known as type II pneumocytes, which compose about 10% of the cells of the lung. Although the biosynthetic pathways for the individual phospholipids are well described, much remains to be learned about the factors responsible for their regulation. Synthesis and storage begin between 24 and 28 weeks of gestational age.[27] Beginning at about 32 weeks,

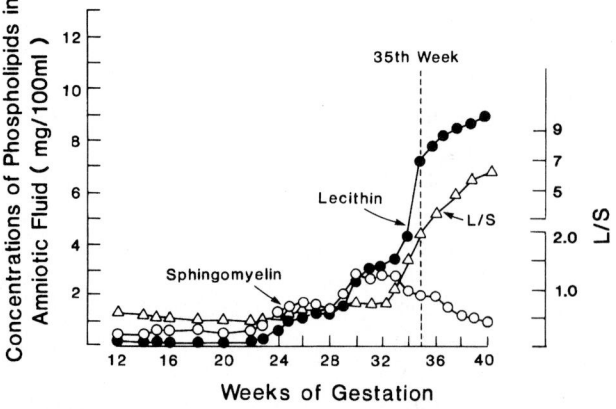

Fig. 40-9 Lecithin, sphingomyelin, and lecithin/sphingomyelin ratios in amniotic fluid during normal pregnancy. (Adapted from Gluck L, Kulovich MV: *Am J Obstet Gynecol* 115:539-546, 1973.)

this material is released from the type II pneumocytes in the form of specialized unique structures called *lamellar bodies* (LB). This term describes the concentrically wound, or "onionlike", structure of these particles when viewed with the electron microscope. Once in the alveolar air space, LBs unravel to form tubular myelin. Tubular myelin then remains in the alveolar space where it eventually spreads into a surfactant monolayer at the air-liquid interface with the alveoli. During normal respiration up to 50% of the surface-active material is reabsorbed and subsequently re-released by the type II pneumocytes.[28]

Hemoglobin

Embryos have a hemoglobin that is unique to the embryonic stage of development. This is replaced during fetal life by "fetal hemoglobin" (HbF) and finally by adult hemoglobin (HbA).[29] The pattern of hemoglobins formed during development is presented in Fig. 40-10. Fetal hemoglobin has been found to constitute 34% of the total in an embryo just less than 7 weeks of age.[30] By approximately 10 weeks of gestation, the embryonic hemoglobins decrease to 10% of the total hemoglobin present. Before the end of the first trimester (less than 12 weeks) the HbF has increased to approximately 90% of the total, with the remaining percentage constituted by HbA. From this point, the percentage of HbF remains constant until about the thirty-sixth week of gestation, when there is a decline. The decline is primarily caused by an increase in HbA synthesis rather than by a

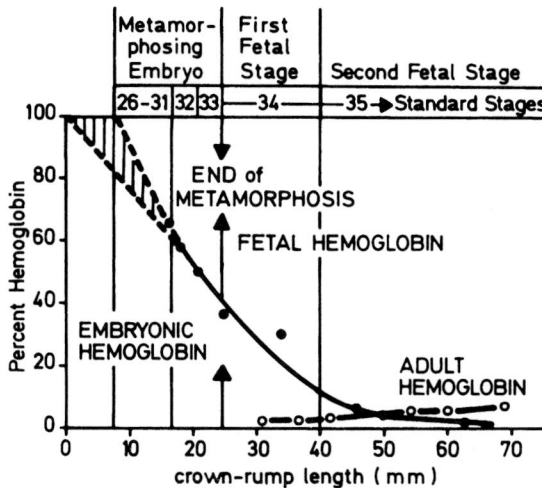

Fig. 40-10 Relationship between hemoglobin types and developmental stages in early human life. *Dashed lines and hatched area,* Expected development. (From Kleihauer E: In Stave U, editor: *Perinatal physiology,* New York, 1978, Plenum Publishing Corp.)

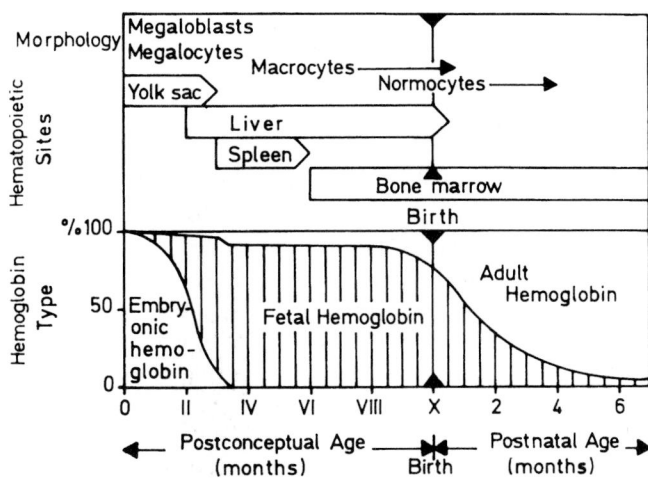

Fig. 40-11 Developmental changes in hematopoietic sites, red blood cell morphology, and hemoglobin types. (From Kleihauer E: In Stave U, editor: *Perinatal physiology,* New York, 1978, Plenum Publishing Corp.)

decrease in HbF. Sharp increases in HbA are seen in reticulocytes and erythrocytes by birth. The developmental changes in hematopoietic sites, the red cell morphology, and the hemoglobin types are shown in Fig. 40-11.

The physiological differences in the hemoglobins are summarized by Kleihauer[29] and include differences in affinities for oxygen; resistance to acid, base, and heat denaturation; and electrophoretic and chromatographic properties. The higher affinity that fetal hemoglobin has for oxygen is reflected in the fetal oxyhemoglobin saturation curve, which lies to the left of the maternal oxyhemoglobin curves under standard conditions. In fact, when oxygen is diffusing from maternal blood with a Pco_2 of about 34 mm Hg to fetal blood at a Pco_2 of about 30 mm Hg, the oxygen is actually moving against a concentration gradient.

Bilirubin

Erythrocyte destruction precedes the formation of bilirubin. Biliverdin is the principal and initial degradation product of hemoglobin and an important intermediate pigment in the formation of bilirubin (see Chapter 27 for details). These relationships are presented in simplified terms:

$$\text{Hemoglobin} \longrightarrow \text{Biliverdin} \xrightarrow{\text{Biliverdin reductase}} \text{Bilirubin}$$
$$\searrow \text{Globin}$$

Plasma concentrations of bilirubin are usually low in the fetal circulation except in unusual circumstances, as in severe *erythroblastosis fetalis* (see p. 804). Even in circumstances where the rapid breakdown of erythrocytes leads to accelerated bilirubin production, as in severe maternal-fetal blood group incompatibility, cord blood bilirubin rarely exceeds 50 mg/L. This fact attests to the rapid, efficient transfer of this pigment across the placenta and the equally efficient disposal of fetal bilirubin by the mother.

After birth, the newborn loses the placental mechanism for bilirubin removal. As a result, there is a modest accumulation of unconjugated bilirubin in the plasma. The jaundice resulting from this change in physiological circumstance is related to the limited uptake, conjugation, and excretion of bilirubin by the immature liver. The degree of neonatal jaundice occurring at birth depends on the maturity and health of the fetal liver at birth. A discussion of the transport and liver metabolism of bilirubin can be found in Chapter 35.

PATHOLOGICAL CONDITIONS ASSOCIATED WITH PREGNANCY AND PERINATAL PERIOD
Placental disorders

Adequate exchange across the placenta between the maternal and fetal circulations is essential for normal fetal growth and metabolism. Less than optimum quantities of nutrients result in small-for-gestational-age fetuses, whereas excessive quantities of nutrients, as with maternal diabetes, result in large-for-gestational-age infants.

Few pathological conditions involving the placenta exist where the monitoring of chemicals by the laboratory is useful. One such example is the hydatidiform mole. Molar tissue is a developmental anomaly of the placenta that has the potential for malignant growth. It is the most common lesion antecedent to choriocarcinoma. Since the mole is trophoblastic tissue, HCG is produced, resulting in a positive pregnancy test result. If serum or urinary HCG levels exceed values typical of specific times in pregnancy, a mole may be suspected. However, because of the variations in gonadotropin values possible for normal pregnancy, no single value can be established as the borderline between normal and abnormal. Because highly sensitive and specific methods are available for monitoring serum HCG, this hormone is useful in monitoring the response of hydatidiform moles to therapy.

Fetal lung immaturity

The last of the organ systems to mature sufficiently to support extrauterine life is the lungs. Fetal lung immaturity, or the respiratory distress syndrome (RDS), occurs most often when insufficient lung surfactant is present.[31] Infants with RDS require increased respiratory effort. The tremendous effort needed to inflate uncooperative lungs often results in the grunting, nasal flaring, and substernal retractions that are characteristic physical signs in these infants. The greater expenditure of energy that is required in order to breathe can result in the death of weak, premature neonates.

Therapy for newborns who have RDS is basically supportive. Clinical management is aimed at thermoregulation, maintaining the infant in an oxygen-rich environment, and keeping the alveoli open artificially during spontaneous or mechanically assisted breathing until such time as surfactant synthesis is adequate for unassisted respiration.[53] Inadequate ventilation can result in acid-base disturbances, which are monitored by use of pH, P_{CO_2}, and bicarbonate values. It is also customary to maintain a venous hematocrit of 40% to 45% during the acute phase of the respiratory distress syndrome to support an adequate oxygen-carrying capacity.

The effect of administration of pulmonary surfactant from exogenous sources (human, mammalian, and artificially synthesized) has been investigated in infants with RDS. Although several studies have demonstrated some reduction in mortality, others have not. In addition, no significant reduction in the development of delayed sequelae such as bronchopulmonary dysplasia have been found.[27,28]

Cortisol stimulates the process of pulmonary maturation, and exogenously administered synthetic corticoids have been used clinically to hasten pulmonary maturation when delivery of a preterm infant was imminent.[32]

No ideal treatment has yet been developed for infants with RDS. Thus, obstetrical management efforts are directed toward prevention of the syndrome in premature infants through antenatal assessment of lung maturation. Because the status of fetal surfactant synthesis and release correlates so well with the probability of lung maturity at delivery, amniotic fluid tests that assess the quantity or quality of pulmonary surfactant present before delivery are used widely for obstetrical management. These are discussed in detail in the next section.

Fetal hemolytic disorders (Rh problems)

Hepatic excretory capacity does not become fully mature until nearly 4 weeks post partum in full-term human infants. The hepatic processing of bilirubin therefore falls short of the maximum before that time. When uptake and conjugation of bilirubin are forced to operate at rates exceeding the capacity of the liver to excrete the quantity formed, as in infants with severe hemolytic disease, unconjugated bilirubin accumulates in liver and serum.

Erythroblastosis fetalis, caused by the Rh-antigen incompatibility of an Rh-negative mother and an Rh-positive father, is a common cause of rapid red blood cell destruction. If the fetus is also Rh-positive, fetal cells entering the maternal circulation may elicit an antibody response to the Rh blood factor. The IgGs cross the placenta into the fetus where they destroy fetal red blood cells.

The healthy fetus generates approximately 35 mg of bilirubin from the catabolism of 1 g of hemoglobin. The high maternal-to-fetal plasma protein gradient facilitates rapid transplacental extraction of unconjugated fetal bilirubin and at the same time suppresses glucuronide conjugation by the fetal liver. The transferred bilirubin is so efficiently conjugated and excreted by the mother that it is uncommon for the neonate to have an elevated cord blood bilirubin level. However, in severe erythroblastosis, particularly if coupled with placental deterioration, unconjugated bilirubin levels can run as high as 80 mg/L. Fetuses receiving intrauterine transfusions are often born with high levels of conjugated bilirubin, probably arising from stimulation of fetal glucuronide formation coupled with decreased placental permeability to the bilirubin glucuronide.

Also unique to the newborn and related to developmental immaturity is the tissue toxicity of unconjugated bilirubin, especially to the brain. In the adult, serum bilirubin elevations are viewed as an important clinical or laboratory sign of disease or altered physiological state. In the neonate, hyperbilirubinemia has a dual significance as a clinical sign and also as a toxin.

Conjugated bilirubin is highly water soluble and is therefore readily excreted in fluids. Unconjugated or indirect bilirubin, on the other hand, is insoluble in aqueous solution but highly soluble in lipids. Under healthy circumstances, unconjugated bilirubin is bound to plasma albumin, and this binding prevents the entrance of free or unbound indirect bilirubin into the lipid-rich central nervous system. When the albumin-binding capacity is exceeded, unbound, unconjugated bilirubin readily passes into the central nervous system cells. Unconjugated bilirubin is toxic to the central nervous system and causes necrosis, a pathological process referred to as "kernicterus." Surviving infants may have mental retardation, hearing deficits, or cerebral palsy. Many affected infants, particularly those of low birth weight, may have no neonatal symptoms but later in childhood can develop hearing deficits, perceptual handicaps, and hyperkinesis.

Usually there is no detectable bilirubin in amniotic fluid when fetus and mother are healthy.[33] However, a neonate who demonstrates significant elevations of unconjugated bilirubin in serum frequently also passes bilirubin into its amniotic fluid. The route by which bilirubin is transferred into amniotic fluid from the fetus is unclear.

Maternal diabetes

There is an increased association of intrauterine deaths, congenital malformations, and perinatal mortality and morbidity in fetuses of diabetic women. For this reason, the pregnant diabetic woman is monitored closely throughout the course of her pregnancy. Monitoring is especially critical in the month immediately after conception, since maintaining a euglycemic state in diabetic women at the time of conception greatly reduces fetal morbidity and mortality (see p. 626). The fetal pancreas does not ameliorate maternal diabetes, since insulin does not cross the placenta.[34] Exogenous insulin therapy and diet are therefore necessary for management of the diabetic mother's insulin-deficient state.

As placental size increases, increasing amounts of HPL and other factors that modify or oppose the action of insulin are produced. Human placental lactogen may be the cause of the increased insulin requirements of pregnancy.[35] Opposing the effect of HPL, maternal pancreatic-cell hyperplasia frequently occurs with pregnancy, increasing the production of maternal insulin. Thus, normal insulin-glucose homeostasis is maintained when there is an increased glucose demand by the fetus.

When insufficient insulin is available to maintain normal glucose homeostasis, maternal hyperglycemia results. This in turn increases the blood glucose of the fetus, which produces a fetal hyperinsulinemia. At delivery, when the fetus is deprived of the maternal glucose source, the excess insulin in the newborn rapidly decreases the blood glucose levels so that the newborn becomes hypoglycemic. Life-threatening hypoglycemic crises are frequently encountered in untreated infants of diabetic mothers. When this happens, glucose must be administered to the newborn until a proper glucose-insulin balance can be achieved.

In pregnancies complicated by diabetes, a significant increase in the incidence of the RDS has been noted, though this is by no means a universal finding.

Toxemia (hypertensive disease of pregnancy)

Toxemia of pregnancy is characterized by hypertension (blood pressure over 140/90 mm Hg), edema, and proteinuria beginning after 20 weeks of gestation. Toxemia is subdivided into *preeclampsia* and *eclampsia*. Eclampsia is characterized by convulsions and is believed to be the sequela of the preeclamptic state.[36] Hypertension of pregnancy affects approximately 0.35 to 0.42 million pregnancies in the United States each year, making this one of the most common medical conditions associated with pregnancy. Preeclampsia tends to occur mostly (85%) in nulliparous women (those having first pregnancies), though women with hypertension predating a pregnancy have a 25% risk of developing preeclampsia.

It is believed that the precipitating cause of pregnancy hypertension is a compromised uteroplacental blood flow.[36] Management includes bed rest, dietary restriction of salt, and the carefully controlled use of magnesium sulfate to prevent eclamptic convulsions. Since the hypertension is a problem associated with implantation, the only satisfactory "cure" for toxemia is delivery, and for this reason information about the pulmonary status of the fetus is of considerable importance. The frequent association of toxemia with diabetes and with vascular disease provides a basis for the correlation of this condition with small-for-gestational-age fetuses. Routine tests for serum uric acid, creatinine, and urine protein are the most common laboratory means of monitoring the toxemic pregnancy. Important adjunct tests are magnesium, levels to monitor magnesium sulfate therapy, and the test of fetal lung maturity.

Spina bifida and anencephaly

Spina bifida and anencephaly are relatively common neural tube defects (NTD) that constitute a large portion of the serious congenital malformations in man. In spina bifida there is a midline defect of the spine that results in a protrusion of the meninges or spinal cord or other neural elements. In anencephaly the brain is a disorganized mass of neural tissues, and the forebrain, overlying meninges, cranial vault, and skin are all absent. Most anencephalic infants are stillborn, and those born alive survive for only several hours.

It is possible to identify women who are at increased risk for carrying fetuses with NTD by measurement of maternal serum AFP levels.[37] Population *screening* for NTD has become widely accepted in the United States. Prenatal *diagnosis* of NTDs by measurement of α-fetoprotein and fetal-specific acetylcholinesterase levels in amniotic fluid has become routine in recent years. Approximately 80% of open spina bifida cases and 95% of anencephaly cases are detectable by measurement of maternal serum α-fetoprotein during 16 to 18 weeks of gestation. In addition, anencephaly specifically affects estriol formation. The absence of fetal pituitary function and fetal adrenal hypoactivity and reduced ACTH levels result in very low rates of production of DHEA from the fetal adrenal glands. Since this androgen is a precursor to estriol, estriol levels are characteristically low.

Down syndrome

Down syndrome, trisomy 21, is the single most common genetic cause of mental retardation with an incidence of 1 in 800 live births. In 1984 Merkatz et al. reported an association of low maternal serum α-fetoprotein with trisomy 21.[38] When the risk for Down syndrome is calculated based on maternal age and maternal serum α-fetoprotein levels, approximately 25% to 33% of Down syndrome cases can be detected. Elevated maternal serum HCG and decreased unconjugated E_3 levels have also been associated with an

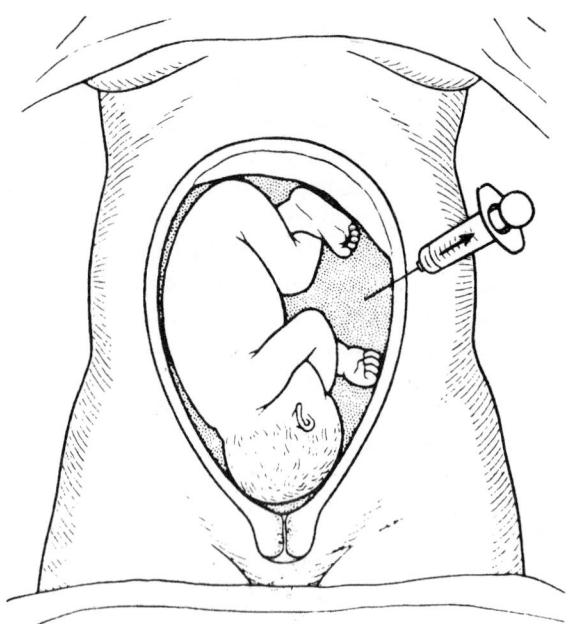

Fig. 40-12 Diagram demonstrating amniocentesis. (From Queenan JT: *Clin Obstet Gynecol* 9:491-507, 1966.)

increased risk for Down syndrome.[39,40] Measurement of these three analytes and maternal age are used in a screening protocol that increases the detection rate for Down syndrome to approximately 67%.

Tubal pregnancy

Usually fertilization occurs in the fallopian tubes. Under usual circumstances, the fertilized egg migrates down the tube and enters and implants in the uterus. Occasionally implantation takes place outside the uterus, most commonly in the fallopian tube itself. Any implantation outside the uterus is called an *ectopic pregnancy,* and an implantation that occurs in the tube is called a *tubal pregnancy.* An ectopic pregnancy can be caused by endocrine imbalances, residual effects stemming from tubal infections, or retrograde movement of the embryo from the uterus to the fallopian tube.[41]

Clinical symptoms include lower abdominal pain and vaginal bleeding. Amenorrhea is not a characteristic feature. Before rupture of the fallopian tube occurs, tubal pregnancies usually give a positive pregnancy test. However, since compromised placentas (that is, those in the process of abruption, degeneration, or penetration of the tubal wall) cannot produce chorionic gonadotropin in usual quantities, the tests may turn negative and become misleading. The recommended procedure for diagnosis of an ectopic pregnancy includes a qualitative pregnancy test (to detect trophoblastic tissues and a conception), followed by serial quantitative serum HCG levels, a serum progesterone level, and visualization of the conception by transvaginal ultrasound. Since serum HCG levels usually double every 2 days, a

longer doubling time can increase the likelihood of an ectopic pregnancy. Serum progesterone levels reflect the activity of the corpus luteum, and high levels can be used to exclude an ectopic pregnancy, whereas very low levels can identify nonviable pregnancies. Since an ectopic pregnancy can be life threatening, these laboratory tests should be routinely available in areas with a high incidence of ectopic pregnancies.[42]

CHANGE OF ANALYTE IN DISEASE

Over the past two decades significant advances elucidating the course of growth and development of the fetus have been made. Part of this new-found knowledge has been possible through the development and application of improved analytical techniques and the improved safety of amniocentesis through ultrasound visualization. Application of much of this knowledge has dramatically altered the course of management of problem or "high-risk" pregnancies. Fig. 40-12 presents a representation of the technique of amniocentesis, and Fig. 40-13 indicates the multifaceted array of its applications.

Three clinical problem areas have been the primary beneficiaries of amniocentesis: (1) the management of Rh-antigen incompatibility of mother and fetus, (2) the identification of the earliest possible time in pregnancy that delivery can be performed with minimal risk of lung immaturity, and (3) the identification of developmental or genetic disorders. Genetic disorders are discussed in Chapter 47.

Human chorionic gonadotropin

Human chorionic gonadotropin is used to identify and follow both trophoblastic disease and the course of normal pregnancy. In a healthy pregnancy, urinary levels of HCG rise to a range of 20,000 to 100,000 U/day and then decrease to a range of 4000 to 11,000 U/day later in the pregnancy. Pregnancy can be detected by analysis of urinary HCG about a week after a missed menses. By using assays of serum HCG, particularly with sensitive and specific methods for the HCG β chains, pregnancy can be detected as early as a few days after conception. In cases of hydatidiform mole, urinary HCG titers rise to over 300,000 U/day. After molar evacuation, these values drop within 1 month, and in about 90% of cases HCG is not detectable by urinary assay after 3 months. In cases where trophoblastic tissue remains, such as retained choriocarcinoma, values remain elevated, and serial assays of urine or serum HCG are of great value in determining the results of treatment, usually chemotherapy.

On a molecular basis, HCG shows about 1/4000 the thyrotropic activity of pituitary TSH. If HCG levels are very high, thyroid-stimulating activity is possible. For this reason, the levels of HCG attained in molar pregnancies are believed to be the reason hyperthyroidism is often associated with molar pregnancies. If HCG values exceed 100,000 U/day in urine or 300 U/mL in serum, the presence of hy-

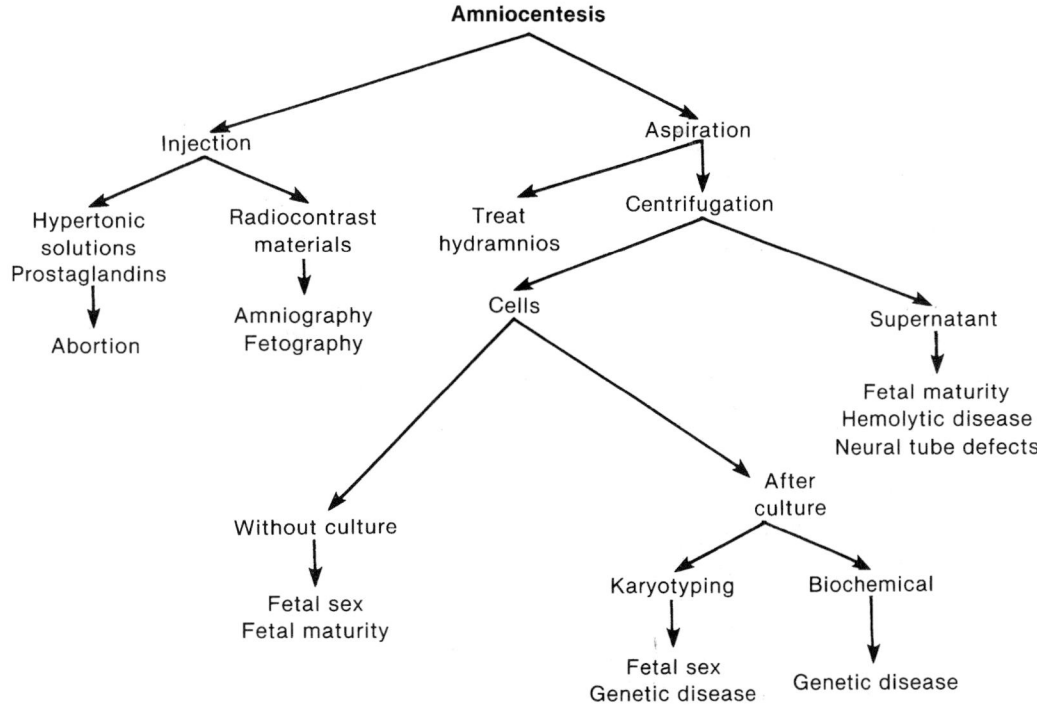

Fig. 40-13 Clinical applications of amniocentesis. (From Pritchard JA, MacDonald PC: In Pritchard JA, MacDonald PC, editors: *Williams obstetrics,* ed 16, New York, 1990, Appleton-Century-Crofts.)

perthyroidism and hydatidiform mole should be suspected.

Human chorionic gonadotropin levels are often low for gestational age with ectopic pregnancies. Positive pregnancy tests have been obtained in only 50% of ectopic pregnancies. A negative test result therefore does not exclude ectopic pregnancy. Newer, more sensitive immunoassays may improve the diagnosis of ectopic pregnancies. Serial, quantitative HCG levels that show a doubling time significantly less than 48 hours are strongly suggestive of an ectopic pregnancy.[42] Low levels of maternal serum HCG have also been associated with fetal trisomy 18, a lethal condition in which 75% of affected fetuses are spontaneously lost in the third trimester.[43] Unlike in trisomy 18, maternal serum HCG levels have been shown to increase in trisomy 21 (Down syndrome).[40,44] Newer, more sensitive immunoassays may improve the diagnosis of ectopic pregnancies. In addition, women with a diagnosis of threatened abortion who have low HCG levels for the estimated time of gestation have been shown to have complete abortions.

Human placental lactogen

Fetal growth is closely associated with placental growth and thus with HPL, which is synthesized by placental syncytiotrophoblasts. Serum HPL levels are related to placental mass (Fig. 40-14), but HPL is not entirely satisfactory as a clinical measure of healthy placental function because there is a wide range of values as gestation advances. Human placental lactogen is not used to follow metastatic tropho-

blastic disease because there is little HPL in comparison to the larger concentrations of HCG. Human placental lactogen, however, can contribute to the identification of a population at risk for perinatal mortality. Carl et al. have proposed a mathematical model based on a modified Gompertz equation to forecast HPL levels in healthy pregnancies, taking into account such factors as maternal height, hemoglobin concentrations, and smoking.[45]

Estriol

Low serum or urinary estriol levels, or, more importantly, declining estriol levels, carry an unfavorable prognostic significance[46] (see Fig. 40-5, showing serial estriol values during various pregnancies). As a rough guideline, a decline of 30% to 50% from the mean of 3 previous days indicates probable impending danger to the fetus. Because of the pronounced diurnal variation in estrogen formation, maintaining a consistent time of day for sampling (particularly when one is measuring estrogen levels in urine) is important. Since the precursors of estriol are androgens produced by the fetal adrenal gland, drugs such as synthetic corticoids that can cross the placenta and suppress ACTH secretion depress maternal estriol levels in both blood and urine.

Serum or urinary estriol levels that are greater than the 95th percentile should be suggestive of the possibility of twins. Estriol values are good predictors of impending fetal death in hypertensive disease, renal disease, and diabetes. Conditions associated with chronically low serum estriol

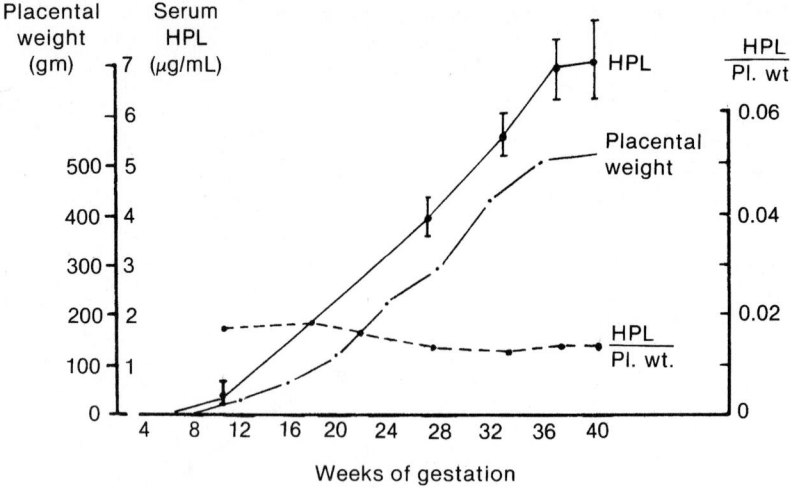

Fig. 40-14 Concentrations of human placental lactogen, *HPL,* during normal pregnancy. (From Selenkow HA, Saxena SM, Dana CL, Emerson K Jr.: In Pecile A, Fenzi P, editors: *The foeto-placental unit,* Amsterdam, 1969, Excerpta Medica.)

levels include toxemia, anencephaly, placental sulfatase deficiency, Down syndrome, and trisomy 18.[44,45] Estriols are not helpful in monitoring erythroblastosis fetalis.

Tests of fetal lung maturation

Antenatal laboratory tests for fetal lung maturity (FLM) are used by the obstetrician to predict the likelihood of RDS subsequent to delivery. Typically, these tests include biochemical or biophysical evaluations of amniotic fluid for the presence of surfactant components derived from maturing fetal lungs. These tests have been designed either to quantify specific surfactant-associated phospholipids (biochemical approach) or to measure the surface-active effects of these pulmonary surfactant components in the amniotic fluid sample (biophysical approach). Other methods that do not seem to fit neatly into either group have been developed. Over the years an enormous number of FLM methods have been developed, though most of these have never gained widespread acceptance for routine use. Some of the more popular, or promising, FLM methods are described below.

Biochemical assays

The lecithin-to-sphingomyelin ratio (LSR) test. Gluck and Kulovich[47] were the first to correlate the relative concentrations of lecithin and sphingomyelin in amniotic fluid to the functional status of the fetal lung, and the lecithin/sphingomyelin ratio (LSR) they described was the first laboratory test for fetal lung maturity to be widely accepted. Rather than quantifying lecithin and sphingomyelin directly, the test is used to determine the ratio of these compounds after thin-layer chromatography (TLC). This semiquantitative approach was designed to provide faster analysis times than quantitative TLC, to be relatively independent of usual

and sometimes significant variations in the volume of amniotic fluid during pregnancy, and to diminish the effects of variations in the extraction recovery of lipids. Using TLC methods of the type originally proposed by Gluck, LSR values of 2 or greater have been found to correlate with fetal lung maturity. Before 34 weeks of gestation, lecithin and sphingomyelin are present in amniotic fluid in approximately equal amounts, but at about 34 weeks the concentration of lecithin begins to rise rapidly compared to sphingomyelin. When the concentration of lecithin in amniotic fluid becomes at least twice that of the sphingomyelin, the likelihood of respiratory distress after delivery is minimal. Because early reports suggested that a greater risk of RDS is associated with the diabetic pregnancy, values of 2.5 or greater have often been used for these pregnancies. The validity of this approach has been questioned by some, however, as no consistent gestationally age-matched differences in LSR results have been observed between diabetic and nondiabetic pregnancies in many recent studies.[22] The clinical predictability of the LSR, like most FLM tests, varies widely. Reported sensitivities and specificities for this test range between 80% and 85%.[80] This variability is likely to be the result of poor analytical standardization, differences in study populations, inherent lack of consistency in the diagnosis of RDS, and the use of different reference values.

Gluck and Kulovich[47] and others have reported that in certain pathological pregnancy conditions pulmonary maturation appears to be accelerated, whereas in others it is delayed. Diseases in which fetal lung maturation may be delayed include diabetes mellitus and hemolytic disease in the fetus. Maternal hypertension and premature rupture of the membranes with delayed delivery have been reported to hasten maturation through increased surfactant production by the fetal lung. However, the exact nature and extent of the effects of these and other maternal and fetal complications on the results obtained for the LSR and most other FLM tests remains largely speculative.

Pathophysiologic factors that alter the overall rate of lung maturation might be expected to affect these processes individually and to differing extents. This proposed effect has been termed the "uncoupling phenomenon" by some[22] and refers to the apparent uncoupling of phospholipid synthesis from clinical outcome. An emerging concept is that FLM tests measure surfactant, *but* lung maturation requires (1) surfactant production and release *and* (2) morphologic development of lung tissue (differentiation, such as production of lung connective tissue and vascularization). Processes (1) and (2) are usually synchronized; however, some disease states may cause morphologic development to occur faster or slower than surfactant development. In these cases, FLM tests, which measure only one component of this process (surfactant release), may not correctly reflect fetal pulmonary status. As an example, β-methasone administration at 30 to 32 weeks of gestational age will promote lung maturation as evidenced by decreased incidence of RDS. However, standard FLM tests do not typically reflect any change from pretreatment levels. β-Methasone effect is believed to be mostly on morphologic development and secondarily on increased surfactant synthesis. This concept is important because it makes the point that lung maturation is a very complicated process with many interrelated factors and is not just surfactant related. In situations where alterations in morphologic factors were predominant in the lung-maturation process, the relationship between FLM test results and the status of fetal lung development could be altered such that the surfactant-based tests lose their usual significance. If this should indeed be the case, the use of altered FLM reference values, as has been the practice for diabetes and other maternal or fetal diseases, would seem to be without foundation unless the nature and extent of specific surfactant-related alterations can be determined.

Contamination of samples with blood tends to produce falsely elevated values for very immature samples and falsely lowered values for very mature samples. Meconium, vaginal secretion, and maternal urine contamination can also produce false results. Also RDS can develop in an asphyxiated neonate, despite a mature LSR.

The LSR was the first laboratory procedure designed to assess fetal lung maturity directly, and largely because of this historical fact, it has come to be considered by many as the "standard" test for fetal lung maturity. Over the years, however, numerous modifications of the original procedure have been proposed in an effort to overcome many perceived practical and analytical deficiencies. Unfortunately, this activity has led to the development of many unique TLC methods for determining the ratio of lecithin to sphingomyelin in amniotic fluid, each of which may produce substantially different LSR values. Up to now, there is no standard method for the LSR, and many problems persist, including poor interlaboratory and intralaboratory reproducibility and excessive analysis time. In addition, there are still many unresolved questions about specific components of the general procedure such as phospholipid extraction, TLC solvent systems, TLC plates, and detecting systems (see below).

Because the LSR method is believed to be less successful in predicting fetal lung maturity in diabetic pregnancies, tests for other surface-active lipids or surfactant proteins have been developed for use either with the LSR or solely as independent tests. These efforts to improve on the clinical reliability of the LSR have led to the development of the "lung profile,"[48,49] which consists of the two-dimensional TLC determination and combined interpretation of the LSR, phosphatidylglycerol (PG), phosphatidylinositol, and the percentage of acetone-precipitable lecithin. Unfortunately, the marginal improvements in clinical reliability associated with this method may be offset by extremely long analysis times and the requirement for high levels of technical expertise.

Phosphatidylglycerol. Because PG does contribute to the functional properties of surfactant, tests for this phospholipid came to be popular as an adjunct to the LSR. Functional lung maturity is clearly associated with measurable quantities of PG;[50] however, the absence of PG does not necessarily mean that RDS is inevitable. Collective experience with the PG test indicates that, whereas the predictive value of the presence of PG is nearly 100% for lung maturity, the predictive value of the absence of PG in predicting RDS may be so low as to be virtually uninformative. Since PG appears to be but a very small constituent of blood, the measurement of PG is especially valuable at times when fetal lung status must be predicted from blood- or meconium-contaminated amniotic fluid samples. The measurement of PG is also considered important when one is evaluating the maturity of fetuses of diabetic mothers, since the LSR and other FLM tests may be less reliable in these cases. When amniotic fluid obtained from leakage into the vagina is the most readily accessible sample, PG is the only phospholipid that should be measured. If a proper vaginal pool sample is obtained, false-positive results are rare, though there have been rare reports of local PG production by vaginal flora. Creatinine or urea values should be obtained on vaginal pool samples suspected of being heavily contaminated with maternal urine to help determine the nature of the sample. Phosphatidylglycerol has been measured by one- or two-dimensional TLC procedures, though both are time-consuming and some TLC methods may be subject to comigration of other phospholipids or interfering substances with the PG spot.[51] More recently, a slide agglutination assay for PG (AmnioStat-FLM, Irvine Scientific, Irvine, California) has become popular. This test employs antiserum specific for PG, can be applied to vaginally collected samples, and is rapid and relatively simple to perform.

Biophysical assays. The methods in this group were originally so classified because they were designed to measure some specific biophysical property of pulmonary surfactant in the amniotic fluid sample. As mentioned recently by Dubin,[52] however, this classification has, over time, come to include a group of fundamentally dissimilar assays that have in common the primary property of not fitting into the biochemical category. They are generally easier, faster, and cheaper to perform than traditional TLC techniques.

Foam-stability assays. The shake test and foam stability index (FSI) test are based on the observation that ethanol acts as a competitive antifoaming surfactant that overcomes the foam-stability effects of most nonpulmonary surfactants in amniotic fluid. Pulmonary phospholipid surfactants, however, are capable of producing a surface tension lower than 29 dynes/cm, thus allowing stable foam formation in ethanolic solutions after vigorous shaking. This is the basis for the semiquantitative shake test developed by Clements and co-workers[53] for assessing fetal lung maturity. The end point of this test is the formation of a continuous ring of bubbles at the meniscus of a tube that was shaken vigorously and that contained equal volumes of 95% (v/v) ethanol and amniotic fluid. This value was roughly equivalent to over 30 mg of dipalmitoyl phosphatidylcholine per liter, and was found to be highly predictive of FLM. In 1978, Sher et al.[54] reported a modification of the original "shake test," named the "foam stability index" (FSI), that allowed the semiquantitative measurement of varying amounts of surfactant, primarily dipalmitoyl phosphatidylcholine, in concentrations ranging from 15 to 30 mg/L. The reported clinical performance of this test is generally quite good. The FSI, which is simple and rapid to perform, is commercially available in the form of the Lumadex-FSI test (Beckman Instruments, Inc., Brea, CA 92621). Drawbacks of this test include the subjective nature of the foam reading and the test's susceptibility to a wide variety of foam-producing contaminants. Because of this, particular care must be taken to ensure that sample containers and glassware for the test are clean and that the reagents and amniotic fluid samples are not contaminated with blood, meconium, excessive numbers of leukocytes, or vaginal secretions.

Fluorescence polarization assays. The assessment of FLM using the fluorescence polarization microviscosity method was first described by Shinitzky et al.[55] The actual analysis is conducted by use of a microviscosimeter called the Fetal Lung Maturity Analyzer (FELMA) (Elscint, Inc., Hackensack, NJ 07602) designed specifically for this test. Although first described in 1976, high instrument cost and practical problems with this particular assay have resulted in its achieving only limited popularity as a routine test for fetal lung maturity.

The TDx Fetal Lung Maturity Assay (TDx-FLM) test is a fluorescence polarization assay designed for use on the Abbott TDx Analyzer (Abbott Laboratories Diagnostics Division, Irving, TX 75015). This test employs a unique fluorescent probe (PC16)[56] that, when added to amniotic fluid, partitions between endogenous albumin (high fluorescence polarization) and phospholipid surfactant (low fluorescence polarization). The overall polarization measured by the analyzer reflects the ratio of surfactant to albumin in the sample, and this value is highly correlated with lung maturity. Recent clinical evaluation demonstrated sensitivity and specificity for this test equal to or exceeding that of the LSR.[57] The test is precise and quantitative, employs standardized reagents and calibrators, requires minimal sample preparation and volume, and can be performed in less than 30 minutes.

Lamellar bodies. Because the lamellar bodies (LBs) are the structural form of pulmonary surfactant extruded by the type II pneumocytes, the concentration of lamellar bodies in amniotic fluid has been evaluated for use in FLM assessment. Early approaches were generally based on ultracentrifugation to separate the LB fraction of the sample followed by quantitation of the phospholipid content of this fraction.[58] Although the clinical performance of this approach was generally quite good, the hardware requirements and procedural complexity exceeded the capabilities of most clinical laboratories.

More recently, Dubin has reported on the measurement of LBs by refractive index–matched anomalous diffraction (RIMAD)[59] and resistive-pulse counting[60] techniques. The RIMAD technique consists in the measurement of the difference in the optical density of amniotic fluid diluted 1:2 in glycerol (reference cuvette) and in saline (test cuvette). Light scattering caused by the lamellar bodies occurs in the test cuvette but not in the glycerol blank because the refractive index of glycerol very closely matches that of the lamellar bodies. Since the light absorbance of common chromogens, such as methene pigments, is independent of the refractive index, any interference should be the same in both the reference and the test cuvettes and should thus be corrected for in a dual-beam spectrophotometer. The net effect is an increase in measured absorbance at 650 nm resulting from the light scattering alone. Using the absorbance (A) difference criterion of A = 0.056, this test has been shown to correlate well with the lamellar body number density (LBND) and fetal lung maturation.[59] Quantitation of LBND by resistive-pulse counting techniques using the platelet channel of commercial cell counters also represents a promising new approach to FLM testing. Lamellar body number density values of 40,000/μL and 26,000/μL, in uncentrifuged and centrifuged specimens respectively, demonstrate strong predictive concordance with other accepted measures of FLM.[60] This method possesses the advantages of little or no sample preparation, relative freedom from common interfering substances, and rapid, semiautomated performance. Because of their procedural simplicity and rapid turnaround times, both of the LB procedures described here appear to be useful tests in the initial screening for FLM.

FLM testing strategies. Although biochemical or biophysical procedures for FLM can provide reliable clinical information if the procedures are properly performed, because of the low prevalence of RDS, there is a high proportion of false-positive predictions of immaturity throughout gestation for all FLM tests. Given this reality, testing strategies for the purpose of enhancing the predictive value of test results that are positive for respiratory immaturity have been developed.[57,61,62] Such strategies rely heavily on the availability of rapid methods for FLM that can be performed in a sequential, or cascade, fashion without substantially lengthening the total turnaround time for results. Typically the easiest and fastest tests are performed first, followed by additional tests until the first mature result is obtained or all tests in the cascade indicate immaturity. Occasionally there is a clinical need to be relatively certain that RDS will not occur after delivery that could be delayed if necessary. In these cases, the requirement for multiple mature test results that indicate fetal maturity, higher reference values, or results from markers that are positive only after fetal maturity is well established, such as PG, are sometimes employed to enhance the predictive value of test results.

Bilirubin (ΔA_{450})

A maternal anti-Rh antibody titer (indirect Coombs' test) of 1 to 16 or more in most cases warrants amniocentesis and appropriately timed measurements of bilirubin pigment in amniotic fluid. The absorbance of bilirubin, when measured in a continuously recording spectrophotometer, is demonstrable as a "hump" or inflection with maximum absorbance at 450 nm (Fig. 40-15). The magnitude of the increase in absorbance above the baseline value (ΔA_{450}) usually but not always correlates well for any gestational age with the intensity of the hemolytic disease.

Liley[63] developed a graph that reasonably allows one to predict the severity of hemolytic disease and to recommend clinical management (Fig. 40-16). The higher the ΔA_{450}, the more severe is the hemolytic disease relative to the gestational age of the pregnancy. In general, a decreasing amniotic fluid bilirubin trend is a good prognostic indicator that a fetus will survive, whereas a horizontal or rising bilirubin level indicates that there is severe erythroblastosis fetalis. The main source of error is the fetus with polyhydramnios because it can cause a false-low bilirubin determination. In addition, maternal hyperbilirubinemia or sickle cell disease may result in elevations of bilirubin in amniotic fluid in the absence of fetal hemolytic disease.

In severe erythroblastotic disease, bilirubin levels of 45 to 60 mg/L and occasionally as high as 80 mg/L are seen. These levels are important in deciding whether to use immediate or delayed exchange transfusions. In neonates receiving intrauterine transfusions, it is not uncommon to see significantly elevated levels of direct bilirubin.

Glucose (see also pp. 626)

After delivery, the glucose concentration in offspring of diabetic mothers declines rapidly below that observed in healthy infants. Blood glucose levels of these infants must be carefully monitored to see if life-threatening hypoglycemia occurs. Approximately 60% of babies from insulin-dependent mothers have glucose concentrations below 300 mg/L in the first 6 hours of life.[64]

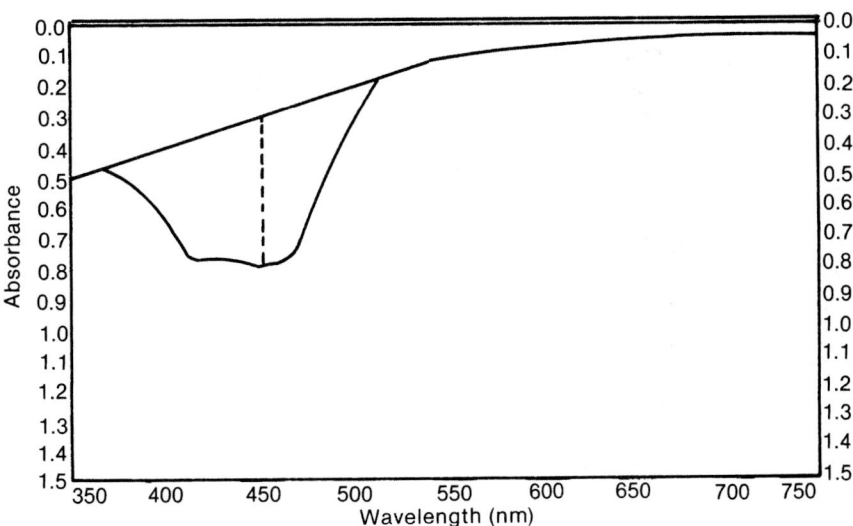

Fig. 40-15 Spectrum of bilirubin. *Dashed line,* Absorbance at 450 nm. (From Queenan JT: *Clin Obstet Gynecol* 14:505-536, 1971.)

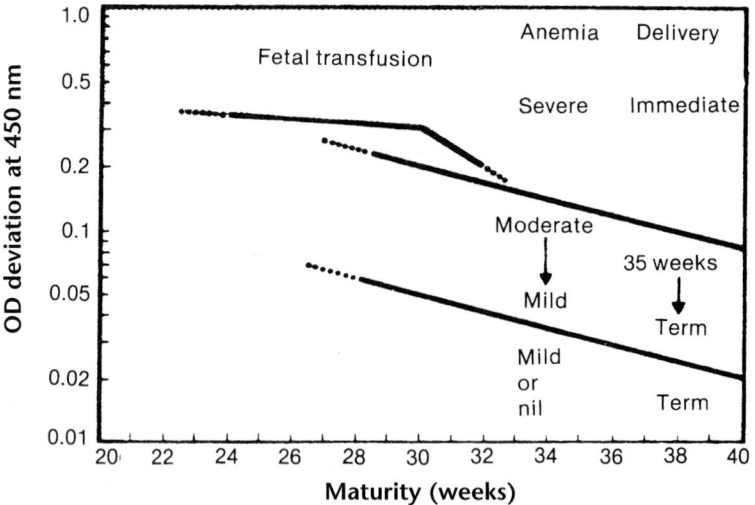

Fig. 40-16 Relationship of absorbance at 450 nm, gestational age of amniotic fluid associated with fetal anemia, and suggested clinical management. *OD,* Optical density (absorbance). (From Liley AW: *Am J Obstet Gynecol* 86:485-494, 1963.)

Renal function tests (see also pp. 493)

During a healthy pregnancy, renal blood flow and the glomerular filtration rate are significantly increased above nonpregnant levels. With the development of pregnancy-induced hypertension, renal perfusion and glomerular filtration are reduced. Most often, therefore, the creatinine or urea concentration in plasma is not appreciably elevated. The plasma uric acid concentration is much more commonly elevated, especially in women with more severe renal disease. The elevation is a result primarily of decreased renal clearance of uric acid by the kidney, a decrease that exceeds the reduction in glomerular filtration rate and creatinine clearance.

α-Fetoprotein

α-Fetoprotein (AFP) is a glycoprotein with molecular weight of approximately 68,000 daltons and physicochemical properties similar to albumin. Several AFP isoforms have been identified, yet their clinical relevance has not been elucidated. It has been speculated that individual isoforms may be associated with phases of development, neoplastic disease, congenital disease, and a variety of biochemical processes. Unlike other analytes, elevations or decreases in AFP levels do not directly confirm a pathologic process. However, this analyte is unique as an identifier of patients at risk for having fetuses with a variety of birth defects, as well as malignant disease in men and nonpregnant women.[37]

Elevated maternal serum AFP levels are associated with an increased risk for NTDs, whereas decreased levels are associated with an increased risk for Down syndrome. However, because maternal AFP levels are dependent on numerous factors, including gestational age, maternal weight and age, race, insulin-dependent diabetes, multiple pregnancies, and drug ingestion, the results are not diagnostic. Thus, maternal serum AFP levels are most useful in identifying those pregnant women who require additional testing (such as ultrasonography and amniocentesis) to exclude the possibility of an affected fetus.

α-Fetoprotein results are routinely reported as a multiple of the normal median (MoM) for the relative gestational week once the value has been normalized for the factors mentioned above. Spina bifida, anencephaly, gastroschisis, and omphalocele are among the differential diagnoses at 15 to 20 weeks of gestation when both the maternal and amniotic fluid AFP levels are above 2.0 MoM and the amniotic fluid acetylcholinesterase levels are increased. When there is increased risk because of maternal age and the maternal serum AFP levels are below 0.4 MoM, Down syndrome is suspected. Decreased maternal serum levels of unconjugated estriol and increased levels of human chorionic gonadotropin have also been associated with Down syndrome. Multiple marker screening, including maternal serum AFP, HCG, and unconjugated estriol, has been shown to be superior in screening for Down syndrome when compared with the use of maternal serum AFP levels only.[40]

Magnesium

Women with toxemia of pregnancy or premature labor are often treated with high levels of magnesium sulfate ($MgSO_4$). These women, usually under hospital care, must be closely monitored for excessive hypermagnesemia (>80 mg/L).

METHODS OF ANALYSIS
Amniotic fluid bilirubin
STEVEN C. KAZMIERCZAK

Principles of analysis The concentration of unconjugated bilirubin in amniotic fluid is relatively low in healthy preg-

Table 40-2   Methods of amniotic fluid bilirubin analysis

Method	Type of analysis	Principle	Usage	Comments
1. Spectrophotometry	Differential absorbance	Bilirubin absorbs at 450 nm; background absorption is corrected by extrapolation.	Common	Accurate except in cases of hemolysis
2. Spectrophotometry with extraction of bilirubin	Differential absorbance	Bilirubin is extracted with chloroform; absorbance at 450 nm is measured as in method 1 above.	Less common	Minimizes effects of interferences

nancies.[65] However, bilirubin concentrations in amniotic fluid may increase significantly in cases of material alloimmunization syndrome. The maximum absorbance of bilirubin occurs at approximately 450 nm, and the magnitude of this peak in an absorbance scan of amniotic fluid has been shown to be predictive of erythroblastosis fetalis.[66,67] The clinical application of the severity of the difference in absorption of amniotic fluid at 450 nm for the evaluation of Rh-immunized patients was popularized by Liley[67] (Table 40-2, method 1).

Because the concentration of bilirubin in normal pregnancies is extremely low, an absorbance spectrum of amniotic fluid obtained from a healthy pregnancy will yield an approximate straight line when scanned between the wavelengths of 365 and 550 nm. If equipment is unavailable for performing a continuous scan between these wavelengths, absorbance readings can instead be taken at 365, 415, 450, and 515 nm. A straight line is then constructed when the points at 365 and 550 nm are connected. As the concentration of bilirubin in the amniotic fluid increases, a peak in the absorbance spectrum occurs at 450 nm, with the height of the peak being proportional to the bilirubin present. Liley[67] developed a chart whereby gestational age is plotted against the net absorbance of amniotic fluid obtained at 450 nm. Determining the location of the intersection of gestational age and net absorbance at 450 nm (expressed as ΔOD at 450 nm) can be used to assess the severity, if any, of hemolytic disease.

Interference in the direct spectrophotometric method can occur if hemoglobin or meconium are present in the sample. Contamination with oxyhemoglobin causes absorbance peaks at 412, 540, and 575 nm, whereas the presence of meconium in the amniotic fluid will result in an increase in absorbance in the region of 350 to 400 nm and decreasing absorbance at higher wavelengths. The interference attributable to the presence of meconium can result in an inaccurate low bilirubin value. If the sample contains intact red blood cells, it should be centrifuged as soon as possible to remove the cells before they hemolyze. In vivo, hemoglobin and its degradation products methemoglobin and methemalbumin as well as meconium take approximately 2 to 3 weeks to clear from amniotic fluid.[68] Biliverdin, which is the oxidation product of bilirubin produced in the intestine, can also stain the amniotic fluid if meconium is excreted into the amniotic fluid. The interference of biliverdin can be overcome by the use of chloroform extraction. The concentration of biliverdin in amniotic fluid can also be estimated by measurement of the difference in absorption at 480 and 500 nm.[69]

To avoid the interference resulting from the presence of blood or meconium in the amniotic fluid, modifications of direct spectrophotometry have been introduced whereby contaminated samples are extracted by chloroform (Table 40-2, method 2).[70-72] The use of an organic solvent such as chloroform allows bilirubin to be separated from other interfering pigments. Bilirubin is readily soluble in chloroform, whereas contaminants such as meconium and blood are more water soluble and therefore remain in the aqueous fluid. A single extraction with an organic solvent such as chloroform can recover up to 90% of the bilirubin present in the sample.

Specimen Because exposure to light can cause a decrease in bilirubin, samples of amniotic fluid should be protected from light before analysis. Amniotic fluid is normally turbid. The turbidity is the result of cellular material and other debris. Turbidity can be reduced by centrifugation of the sample before analysis. If the fluid still remains turbid after centrifugation, filtration of the sample through Whatman No. 42 filter paper can be helpful in the further clarification of the sample.

Amniotic fluid is stable at refrigerated temperatures for up to 24 hours. If analysis is to be delayed for longer than 24 hours, the sample should be frozen. Frozen specimens, if centrifuged before freezing, can be stored for months.[73]

Reference interval The absorbance change at 450 nm (ΔOD 450) caused by the presence of bilirubin is dependent on gestational age. A chart developed by Liley[67] plots gestational age against the change in absorbance at 450 nm caused by the presence of bilirubin and enables the severity, if any, of hemolytic disease to be evaluated.

Fetal lung maturity assessment: amniotic fluid analysis, lecithin-to-sphingomyelin ratio, phosphatidyl glycerol
STEVEN C. KAZMIERCZAK

Principles of analysis Measurement of pulmonary surfactant for the assessment of FLM may be categorized according to what parameter of the surfactant is being assessed. Tests that measure the chemical constituent of surfactant include the L/S ratio, the phospholipid profile, and the fatty acid composition of amniotic fluid lecithin.[74-76] Methods that measure the physical properties of lung surfactant, which reflect amniotic fluid chemical composition, include analysis of surface tension, foam stability, and microviscosity.[77,78]

Measurement of the LSR in amniotic fluid has been the accepted standard indicator of FLM. However, because this approach was believed to be associated with an unacceptably high incidence of false indications of maturity in certain clinical situations (such as diabetes), measurement of

PG was also added to eliminate the high rate of falsely elevated L/S results.

The most common technique used to measure the LSR is TLC (Table 40-3, method 1).[79] The phospholipids of interest in the amniotic fluid are purified before analysis by TLC, usually by multiple organic solvent extractions. Separation of the phospholipids is most frequently carried out using a silica-gel stationary phase and a mobile phase consisting of either chloroform-methanol-water or chloroform–methanol–ammonium hydroxide.[78] The separation of phospholipids may be carried out in one or two dimensions. Once the phospholipids of interest have been separated, visualization of the separated fractions followed by measurement of the LSR can be performed. One can visualize the separated phospholipids by spraying the TLC plates with sulfuric or phosphoric acids and then heating the plates to char the organic phospholipids, spraying the plates with rhodamine B or dichlorofluorescein and visualizing the fluorescent spots under ultraviolet rays, or reacting the fatty acid double bonds with cupric acetate or sulfuric acid (with or without dichromate) to produce a colored product. Quantitation of the individual spots and calculation of the LSR can be performed by several techniques; however, transmission or reflection densitometry are most frequently employed.

Enzymatic methods for determination of lecithin and sphingomyelin have also been developed,[84] though rarely used.

Determination of the LSR by TLC requires a very high degree of skill and is fairly labor intensive, requiring approximately 4 to 5 hours to complete. The technique is also not very reproducible, especially between laboratories. Using an LSR cutoff value of 2.0 to indicate FLM, one can find that the cited values for sensitivity and specificity range from 70% to 90%.[80] As discussed previously, differences in opinion exist regarding the reliability of the L/S in pregnancies complicated by diabetes mellitus.[22] Some studies have failed to demonstrate any significant differences in lung maturation, or L/S predictability, for fetuses of diabetic women when subjects are matched for gestational age, sex, or race.[81] Studies also suggest that clinical interpretation of LSRs may be different between different racial groups.[81] Diabetic patients

often have LSRs in excess of 2.0 even though respiratory distress syndrome still develops in the newborn.

Lipids other than lecithin and sphingomyelin have been shown to have prognostic significance in the evaluation of FLM. Hallman et al.[82] showed that when PG represented 3% or more of the total phospholipids the fetal lungs were mature. Because PG rapidly increases in concentration from the time it first becomes detectable, the presence of any PG on a TLC plate is usually indicative of FLM. Determination of PG may be performed in concordance with measurement of the L/S ratio by TLC. If only the LSR ratio is being determined, one-dimensional chromatography is usually adequate. However, if PG is also to be determined, two-dimensional chromatography is usually indicated to minimize the presence of interfering substances.

Phosphatidylglycerol can be determined by methods other than TLC. Probably the most common of these alternative procedures are the latex agglutination methods. These procedures have adequate analytical sensitivity for detecting PG (0.5 μg/mL). Contamination of the specimen with blood or meconium does not interfere with the assay. Other advantages include the ability to perform the test in a short period of time and the lack of need for specialized equipment. The biggest drawbacks to this procedure is subjectivity of the approach, since the presence or absence of agglutination is visually determined. Enzymatic methods for PG determinations that can be performed rapidly (<1 hour) and are cost effective have also been described.[83] Although endogenous glycerol can produce falsely increased results, contamination of the specimen with glycerol is unlikely.

The major drawback of PG determinations for FLM assessment is the poor clinical specificity.

One of the commonly used biophysical indicators for the assessment of FLM is the foam stability, or shake test (Table 40-3, method 2).[85] In this procedure, serial dilutions of amniotic fluid are mixed with equal volumes of 95% ethanol. The samples are then shaken and inspected for bubbles around the meniscus. If adequate amounts of pulmonary surfactant are present, the bubbles formed as a result of shaking the sample will persist. The final percentage of ethanol used in the test (47.5% after dilution with equal parts of am-

Table 40-3   Methods for assessment of fetal lung maturity

Method	Principle	Comments	Usage
1. Thin-layer chromatography	Chromatographic separation of phospholipids using silica gel solid support is followed by visualization of phospholipids by charring or color formation using various chemical sprays.	Semiquantitative Determination of L/S ratio and PG. Not a stat. type of procedure	Frequently used
2. Foam stability (shake test and foam stability index [FSI])	Presence of adequate surfactant in specimen is measured by its ability to support foam bubbles after shaking of an amniotic fluid/ethanol mixture.	Qualitative Common as stat. procedure	Frequently used
3. Fluorescence polarization	Ratio of surfactant to albumin is determined by use of fluorescent dye that has different levels of fluorescence polarization depending on its association with either surfactant or albumin.	Quantitative Common as stat. procedure	Frequently used

niotic fluid) is optimal to prevent the formation of bubbles because of the presence of proteins, bile acids, or salts of free fatty acids in the amniotic fluid. Drawbacks to the shake test include the lack of complete objectivity in deciding what is meant by foam "stability" and the problem of ascertaining the degree of immaturity if a specimen fails the shake test.[80]

The FSI, a modification of the shake test, was developed in response to the problems associated with the shake test.[86] In this procedure, amniotic fluid is added to a series of tubes with varying quantities of ethanol so that the final ethanol concentrations vary from 44% to 50%. All the tubes are then shaken, and each tube is inspected for the presence of a complete stable ring of foam. The FSI is defined as the tube with the highest ethanol volume fraction that will result in a stable ring of bubbles at the meniscus after shaking. A blue dye added to the solution permits better visualization. An FSI of 0.48 (48% ethanol) is comparable to an LSR of 2.0.[87] Interference in the test can result from amniotic fluid contaminated with blood, meconium, debris found in vaginal pool material, and neutrophil debris not completely removed by centrifugation. The use of siliconized collection tubes can cause false-positive test results, though usually silicon contamination can be inferred from the presence of equally large quantities of foam at every concentration of ethanol.

Another popular biophysical measurement to assess functional lung surfactant is the use of the fluorescence polarization procedure (Table 40-3, method 3).[88] In this procedure, a fluorescent dye added to the specimen partitions between albumin and surfactant present in the specimen. Dye molecules that are associated with albumin are restricted in rotation, which results in a high degree of polarization of the emitted fluorescent light. Those dye molecules that are associated with surfactant are in a much less polar environment, compared to the albumin-bound dye molecules and have a greater ability to rotate. Thus, little of the fluorescent light emitted from dye associated with surfactant will be plane polarized. The amount of polarized fluorescent light measured in an amniotic fluid specimen reflects the distribution of dye between the protein and surfactant components of the amniotic fluid specimen, allowing the ratio of surfactant to albumin present in the specimen to be determined.

Specimen Amniotic fluid collected by means of amniocentesis or from a free-flowing vaginal sample should be transported to the laboratory on ice and processed as soon as possible. If pooled vaginal fluid is the sample, care should be taken to ensure that there is no contamination of the specimen with maternal urine. Specimens to be analyzed by the fluorescence polarization procedure should not be centrifuged because centrifugation falsely decreases the results.[89] These specimens are stable if kept refrigerated (2° to 8° C) or frozen at −10° C for up to 72 hours before testing.

Specimens for other types of analyses should be centrifuged at ≤ 500 *g* for 5 minutes. Centrifuged samples can be stored at −20° C for prolonged periods without significant changes in the L/S ratio.

Reference interval An LSR of greater than 2.0 is usually considered indicative of FLM. The presence of PG is also considered positive for FLM. For the fluorescence polariza-

tion procedure, specimens with surfactant/albumin concentrations of 55 milligrams of surfactant per gram of albumin (55 mg/g) and above are considered mature, with values less than or equal to 39 mg/g being considered immature. Results between 40 and 54 mg/g are considered to be indeterminate.

β-**Human chorionic gonadotropin (β-HCG)**

STEVEN C. KAZMIERCZAK

Principles of analysis Human chorionic gonadotropin is one of the family of dipeptide (α- and β-subunits) glycoprotein hormones, the members of which share a common α-subunit. The β-subunits of each protein hormone determine the specificity of that hormone. The other glycoprotein hormones that share the same α-subunits are LH, FSH, and TSH. Although these three hormones are produced in the pituitary, HCG is secreted by the trophoblast.

In the circulation, HCG is present predominantly in the form of the intact hormone dimer (α-β). Only small amounts are present as free α- or free β-subunits. In the urine, a significant portion of HCG is present as a metabolic fragment commonly referred to as the "β-core."[90] The β-core fragment consists of two polypeptide chains derived from the β-subunit of HCG and joined by disulfide bridges. This fragment still retains the unique immunological determinants found in both the intact HCG and the β-subunit. Urine of pregnant women contains large quantities of β-core, whereas in serum it is essentially undetectable.

Measurements for HCG for the determination of the presence or absence of pregnancy is widely used by both the general public and healthcare professionals. Using a test procedure for HCG that has a sensitivity of 25 mIU/mL, urine may reveal positive results within 3 to 4 days after implantation of the blastocyst. The development of monoclonal antibodies specific for the β-subunit of HCG has essentially eliminated the problems of cross reactivity with LH, FSH, and TSH. Measurement of HCG in urine and serum is almost exclusively by use of immunoassays that utilize nonisotopic markers or, to a much lesser extent, radioisotopes, as labels. Nonisotopic labels in current use include enzymes and fluorescent and chemiluminescent compounds.

The first assays used to measure HCG detected its biological activity and thus measured the intact, heterodimeric molecule only.[93] The biological assays have been totally replaced by immunoassays, which can measure the parent molecule as well as the free subunits of HCG fragments. Immunoassay methods for detection of HCG in the urine and serum are available as both qualitative and quantitative procedures. The major differences in these procedures are the type of label employed and the specificity of the antibody used.

The original qualitative immunoassay procedures used particles (latex or sheep red blood cells) coated with HCG molecules as the label (Table 40-4, method 1). These methods are commonly referred to as agglutination-inhibition procedures (see Chapter 11). Because of their poor sensitivities, approximately 200 to 500 mIU/mL, these tests are no longer used.[92]

The newer qualitative assays (Table 40-4, method 2) for

Table 40-4 Methods of analysis for hCG

Method	Principle	Usage	Comments
1. Agglutination-inhibition (slide or tube tests)	Latex particles or sheep red blood cells coated with HCG mixed with patient specimen reacts with HCG antibody causing inhibition of agglutination of particles. If HCG is absent from patient specimen, HCG antibody will cross-link particles or cells causing agglutination.	Infrequently used	Not very sensitive Detection limit of 200-500 mIU/mL Quantitative assay
2. Immunoenzymatic concentration assay	Sandwich type of assay. HCG in specimen "captured" by first antibody is linked to solid-phase support. Addition of detector antibody results in "sandwich." Detector antibody covalently linked to enzyme label or chromatogenic substance.	Frequently used	Qualitative and semiquantitative Sensitive to approximately 25 mIU/mL
3. Radioimmunoassay (RIA)	Competitive inhibition–based assay. HCG inpatient specimen competes with ^{125}I-labeled HCG for binding to anti-HCG.	Frequently used though decreasing in popularity	Very sensitive
4. Immunoenzymometric (ELISA)	Sandwich type of assay. HCG in patient sample captured by HCG antibody is linked to solid-phase support. Enzyme-labeled anti-HCG detector antibody binds to captured patient HCG forming sandwich. Enzyme substrate is added. Amount of bound enzyme activity is directly proportional to HCG concentration in sample.	Frequently used	Suitable for stat. analysis

HCG have detection limits of approximately 15 to 25 mIU/mL. These immunoenzymatic concentration tests employ either goat polyclonal or mouse monoclonal antibody directed against the HCG α- or β-subunit as the capture antibody. Detection of the captured HCG β-subunit may be performed using a variety of immunological techniques, including mouse monoclonal anti–HCG α-subunit colloid complex, an enzyme-linked anti–HCG β-subunit antibody, or enzyme-linked monoclonal antibody targeted against the intact HCG molecule.[94] These procedures typically do not react with the β-core fragment or free β-subunit of HCG. Although these assays are qualitative in nature, it has been shown that with serum as specimen an approximation of the HCG concentration can be obtained (up to 100 mIU/mL) by measurement of the time (in seconds) from sample or reagent addition to the appearance of a positive test result.[94]

The most frequently employed quantitative assays for HCG in urine and serum include enzyme, chemiluminescent, and radioimmunoassay (RIA) procedures. The RIA procedure (Table 40-4, method 3) utilizes a competitive-binding format whereby HCG in the patient's sample competes with ^{125}I-labeled HCG for binding sites on an HCG antibody.

The development of sensitive and rapid immunoenzymometric assays (Table 40-4, method 4) for HCG have become the most popular methods. A wide variety of enzyme immunoassay systems have been developed for HCG determinations. Variations in the type of solid-phase support that is used, the source and specificity of antibody, and the method of development of the indicator reaction have been described. The capture and detection antibodies used in a particular assay may be monoclonal, polyclonal, or a combination of the two and may be directed toward the α-subunit, β-subunit, or the intact HCG molecule. The detection antibody is usually conjugated to horseradish peroxidase or alkaline phosphatase. Immunometric assays that employ a chemiluminescent label are also widely used. The sensitivity for HCG of all these assays is approximately 2 mIU/mL, which is similar to that achieved with RIA. The assay range of immunoassay procedures typically ranges up to 500 to 1000 mIU/mL, though some procedures have dynamic working ranges of up to 50,000 mIU/mL.[95]

The accuracy of measurement of HCG is dependent on the quality and purity of the reference preparation used to standardize the assay as well as the use of these standards by manufacturers of reagent systems for HCG measurement. International Reference Preparations (IRP) composed of highly purified HCG are provided by the World Health Organization for standardization of these assays. A widely used standard is the first IRP that still contains small quantities of subunit impurities. The first IRP succeeded the Second International Standard (IS), which consisted of a mixture of HCG and subunits. One unit of the second IS is equal to approximately 2 units of the first IRP.[96]

The use of purified HCG for standardizing these assays can lead to significant problems. For example, an assay for HCG that is specific for free β-subunit and reacts only slightly with intact HCG will show very little activity with the first IRP standard. On the other hand, a second assay that reacts predominantly with intact HCG and shows little reactivity with free β-subunit will exhibit high activity with the first IRP standard. More importantly, however, is the difference in results that may be observed with patient specimens measured by two different assays. For example, a urine specimen from a pregnant woman, which contains predomi-

Table 40-5   Serum HCG levels with gestational age

Gestational age	Serum HCG (mIU/mL)
0.2-1 week	5-50
1-2 weeks	50-500
2-3 weeks	100-5000
3-4 weeks	500-10,000
4-5 weeks	1000-50,000
5-6 weeks	10,000-100,000
6-8 weeks	15,000-200,000
2-3 months	10,000-100,000

nantly β-core, will show high concentrations when measured by use of the first assay and low concentrations when measured by use of the second assay. This illustrates how different assays can give different results on the same clinical specimen.

Specimen   Urine or serum can be used as specimens. If urine is used, the specimen should be centrifuged to remove any particulate material. *HCG concentrations in serum are very similar to those found in urine.*[97] *Urinary HCG does not show any consistent variation over a 24-hour period.*[98] *Thus, it is not necessary to perform HCG measurements using the first morning specimen of urine.*

Human chorionic gonadotropin in urine should be frozen, not refrigerated if analysis is delayed. Urine HCG is stable when stored frozen at $-20°$ C. Human chorionic gonadotropin and its free α-subunit are stable in serum stored at $4°$ C for up to 6 days. When stored at $-20°$ C, HCG and the α-subunit are stable for at least 6 months.[99] Specimens for analysis of β-HCG are more labile because of nicking and degradation of the β-subunit peptide chain. Serum or urine for analysis of β-HCG should be immediately frozen if analysis is delayed.[100]

Reference interval   Healthy nonpregnant, premenopausal females and healthy males have low circulating concentrations of HCG of 0.2 to 0.80 mIU/mL.

Postmenopausal females may show values much higher than this.[101] During pregnancy, the concentration of HCG varies greatly with gestational age (Table 40-5). During this time, HCG doubles in concentration approximately every 2 days.[102] A slower rate of increase may indicate a higher risk of abortion.

ACKNOWLEDGMENTS

The editors wish to acknowledge Paul T. Russell, who is the author of the previous versions of the methods Amniotic fluid bilirubin, and Fetal lung maturity assessment: amniotic fluid analysis lecithin-to-sphingomyelin ratio phosphatidyl glycerol.

REFERENCES

1. Abramovich DR: The volume of amniotic fluid and its regulating factors. In Fairweather DVI, Eskes TKAB, editors: *Amniotic fluid: research and clinical application,* ed 2, Amsterdam, 1978, Excerpta Medica.
2. Duenhoelter JH, Pritchard JA: Fetal respiration: quantitative measurements of amniotic fluid inspired near-term by human and rhesus fetuses, *Am J Obstet Gynecol* 125:306-309, 1976.
3. Seeds AE: Current concepts of amniotic fluid dynamics, *Am J Obstet Gynecol* 138:575-586, 1980.
4. Sandler M, editor: *Amniotic fluid and its clinical significance,* New York, 1981, Marcel Dekker.
5. Fairweather DVI, Eskes TKAB, editors: *Amniotic fluid: research and clinical applications,* Amsterdam, 1978, Excerpta Medica.
6. Hytten FE: Water transfer. In Chamberlain GVP, Wilkinson AW, editors: *Placental transfer,* Tunbridge Wells, 1979, Pitman Medica.
7. Weaver TE: Pulmonary surfactant-associated proteins, *Gen Pharmacol* 18:1-8, 1987.
8. Pierce JG, Parsons TF: Glycoprotein hormones: structure and function, *Annu Rev Biochem* 50:465-495, 1980.
9. Eberlein WR: The fetal adrenal cortex. In Christy NP, editor: *The human adrenal cortex,* New York, 1971, Harper & Row.
10. France JT, Seddon RJ, Liggins GC: A study of a pregnancy with low estrogen production due to placental sulfatase deficiency, *J Clin Endocrinol Metab* 36:1-9, 1973.
11. Schindler AE, Siiteri PK: Isolation and quantitation of steroids from normal human amniotic fluids, *J Clin Endocrinol Metab* 28:1189-1198, 1968.
12. Kundu N, Carmody PJ, Didolkar SM, Petersen LP: Sequential determination of serum human placental lactogen, estriol, and esterol for assessment of fetal morbidity, *Obstet Gynecol* 52:513-520, 1978.
13. Notation AD, Tagatz GE: Unconjugated estriol and 15α-hydroxyestriol in complicated pregnancies, *Am J Obstet Gynecol* 128:747-756, 1977.
14. Glinoer D, de Nayer P, Bourdoux P, et al.: Regulation of maternal thyroid during pregnancy, *J Clin Endocrinol Metab* 71:276-287, 1990.
15. Lowe TW, Cunningham FG: Pregnancy and thyroid disease, *Clin Obstet Gynecol* 34:72-80, 1991.
16. Kennedy RL, Darne J, Griffiths H, et al: Thyroid-stimulatory effects of human chorionic gonadotropin in early pregnancy, *Horm Res* 33:177-183, 1990.
17. Desai RK, Norman RJ, Jialal I, et al: Spectrum of thyroid function abnormalities in gestational trophoblastic neoplasia, *Clin Endocrinol (Oxf)* 29:583-592, 1988.
18. van Stiphout WAHJ, Hofman A, de Bruijn AM: Serum lipids in young women before, during, and after pregnancy, *Am J Epidemiol* 126:922-928, 1987.
19. Studd JW, Wood S: Serum and urinary proteins in pregnancy. In Wynn RM, editor: *Obstetrics and gynecology annual,* New York, 1976, Appleton-Century-Crofts.
20. Davison JM: The urinary system. In Hytten F, Chamberlain G, editors: *Clinical physiology in obstetrics,* Oxford, 1980, Blackwell Scientific Publications.
21. van Geuns HJ, van Kessel H: Creatinine in amniotic fluid and fetal renal function. In Fairweather DVI, Eskes TKAB, editors: *Amniotic fluid: research and clinical application,* ed 2, Amsterdam, 1978, Excerpta Medica.
22. Spillman T, Cotton DB: Current perspectives in the assessment of fetal pulmonary surfactant status with amniotic fluid, *CRC Rev Clin Lab Sci* 27:341-389, 1989.
23. Hallman M: Recycling surfactant: a review of human amniotic fluid as a source of surfactant for treatment of respiratory distress syndrome, *Rev Perinatal Med* 6:197-226, 1989.
24. Cochrane CG, Revak SD: Pulmonary surfactant protein B (SP-B): structure-function relationships, *Science* 254:566-568, 1991.
25. Martin RJ, Fanaroff AA, Skalina MEL: The respiratory system. In Fanaroff AA, Martin RJ, editors: *Behrman's neonatal/perinatal medicine,* St. Louis, 1983, Mosby.
26. Reynolds MS, Wallander KA: Use of surfactant in the prevention and treatment of neonatal respiratory distress syndrome, *Clin Pharmacol* 8:559-576, 1989.
27. Shapiro DL: The development of surfactant replacement therapy and the various types of replacement surfactants, *Semin Perinatol* 12:174-179, 1988.
28. Jobe A: Metabolism of endogenous surfactant and exogenous surfactants for replacement therapy, *Semin Perinatol* 12:231-244, 1988.
29. Kleihauer E: The hemoglobins. In Stave U, editor: *Perinatal physiology,* New York, 1978, Plenum Publishing.
30. Hecht F, Jones RT, Koler RD: Newborn infants with Hb Portland 1, an indicator of α-chain deficiency, *Ann Hum Genet* 31:215-218, 1967.
31. Avery ME, Mead J: Surface properties in relation to atelectasis and hyaline membrane disease, *Am J Dis Child* 97:517-523, 1959.

32. Robertson B: Corticosteroids and surfactant for prevention of neonatal RDS, *Ann Med* 25:285-288, 1993.

33. Liley AW: The administration of blood transfusions to the foetus in utero, *Triangle* 7:184-189, 1966.

34. Posner BI: Insulin metabolizing enzyme activities in human placental tissue, *Diabetes* 22:552-563, 1973.

35. Klopper A: Placental metabolism. In Hytten F, Chamberlain G, editors: *Clinical physiology in obstetrics,* Oxford, 1980, Blackwell Scientific Publications.

36. Cunningham FG, Lindheimer MD: Hypertension in pregnancy, *N Engl J Med* 326:927-932, 1992.

37. Sundaram SG, Goldstein PJ, Manimekalai S, et al: Alpha-fetoprotein and screening markers of congenital disease, *Reprod Med* 12:481-492, 1992.

38. Merkatz IR, Nitowsky AM, Macri JN, et al: An association between low maternal serum alpha-fetoprotein and fetal chromosome abnormalities, *Am J Obstet Gynecol* 148:886-894, 1984.

39. Cheng EY, Luthy DA, Zebelman AM, et al: A prospective evaluation of a second trimester screening test for fetal Down syndrome using maternal serum alpha-fetoprotein, HCG, and unconjugated estriol, *Obstet Gynecol* 81:72-76, 1993.

40. Haddow JE, Palomaki GE, Knight GJ, et al: Prenatal screening for Down's syndrome with use of maternal serum markers, *N Engl J Med* 327:588-593, 1992.

41. Martinez F, Trounson, A: An analysis of factors associated with ectopic pregnancy in a human in vitro fertilization program, *Fertil Steril* 45:79-87, 1986.

42. Carson SA, Buster JE: Ectopic pregnancy, *N Engl J Med* 329:1174-1180, 1993.

43. Palomaki GE, Knight GJ, Haddow JE, et al: Prospective intervention trial of a screening protocol to identify fetal trisomy 18 using maternal serum alpha-fetoprotein, unconjugated oestriol, and human chorionic gonadotropin, *Prenatal Diagn* 12:925-930, 1992.

44. Mancini G, Peronam M, Dall'Amico CD, et al: HCG, AFP, and uE3 patterns in the 14-20th weeks of Down syndrome pregnancies, *Prenatal Diagn* 12:619-624, 1992.

45. Carl J, Christensen M, Mathiesen O: Human placental lactogen (HPL) model for the normal pregnancy, *Placenta* 12:289-298, 1991.

46. Little B, Billar RB: Endocrine disorders. In Romney SL, Gray MJ, Little AB, et al, editors: *Gynecology and obstetrics: the health care of women,* New York, 1975, McGraw-Hill.

47. Gluck L, Kulovich MV: Lecithin/sphingomyelin ratios in amniotic fluid in normal and abnormal pregnancies, *Am J Obstet Gynecol* 115:539-546, 1973.

48. Kulovich MV, Hallman MB, Gluck L: The lung profile I: Normal pregnancy, *Am J Obstet Gynecol* 135:57-63, 1979.

49. Kulovich MV, Gluck L: The lung profile II: Complicated pregnancy, *Am J Obstet Gynecol* 135:64-70, 1979.

50. Bent AE, Gray JH, Luther ER, et al: Assessment of fetal lung maturity: relationship of gestational age and pregnancy complications to phosphatidylglycerol levels, *Am J Obstet Gynecol* 139:664-669, 1981.

51. Spillman T, Cotton DB, Lynn SC Jr, Bretaudiere JP: Removal of a component interfering with phosphatidylglycerol estimation in the "Helena" system for amniotic fluid phospholipids, *Clin Chem,* 30:737-740, 1984.

52. Dubin SB: The laboratory assessment of fetal lung maturity, *Am J Clin Pathol* 97:836-848, 1992.

53. Clements JA, Platzker ACG, Tierney DF, et al: Assessment of the risk of respiratory distress syndrome by a rapid test for surfactant in amniotic fluid, *N Engl J Med* 286:1077-1081, 1972.

54. Sher G, Statland BE, Freer DE, et al: Assessing fetal lung maturation by the foam stability index assay, *Obstet Gynecol* 52:673-677, 1978.

55. Shinitzky M, Goldfisher A, Bruck A: A new method for assessment of fetal lung maturity, *Br J Obstet Gynecol* 83:833-844, 1976.

56. Russell JC: A calibrated fluorescence polarization assay for assessment of fetal lung maturity, *Clin Chem* 33:1177-1184, 1987.

57. Herbert WNP, Chapman JF, Schnoor MM: Role of the TDx FLM assay in fetal lung maturity, *Am J Obstet Gynecol* 168:808-812, 1993.

58. Duck-Chong, CG: Lamellar body phospholipid content of amniotic fluid: a possible index of fetal lung maturity, *Am J Obstet Gynecol* 136:191-196, 1979.

59. Dubin S: Determination of lamellar body size, number density and concentration by differential light scattering from amniotic fluid: physical significance of A_{650}, *Clin Chem* 34:938-943, 1988.

60. Dubin S: Characterization of amniotic fluid lamellar bodies by resistive-pulse counting: relationship to measures of fetal lung maturity, *Clin Chem* 35:612-616, 1989.

61. Garite TJ, Freeman RK, Nageotte MP: Fetal maturity cascade: a rapid and cost effective method for fetal maturity testing, *Obstet Gynecol* 67:619-622, 1986.

62. Herbert WNP, Chapman JF: Clinical and economic considerations associated with testing for fetal lung maturity, *Am J Obstet Gynecol* 155:820-823, 1986.

63. Liley AW: Amniocentesis and amniography in hemolytic disease. In Greenhill JP, editor: *Yearbook of obstetrics and gynecology,* 1964-1965 series, St. Louis, 1964, Mosby.

64. Pennoyer MM, Hartman AF Sr: Management of infants born of diabetic mothers, *Postgrad Med* 18:199-206, 1955.

65. Benzie RJ, Doran TA, Harkins JL, et al: Composition of the amniotic fluid and material serum in pregnancy, *Am J Obstet Gynecol* 119:798-810, 1982.

66. Bevis DCA: Blood pigments in haemolytic disease of the newborn, *J Obstet Gynaecol Br Emp* 63:68-75;1956.

67. Liley AW: Liquor amnii analysis in the management of the pregnancy complicated by rhesus sensitization, *Am J Obstet Gynecol* 82:1359-1370;1961.

68. Greene MF, Fenci M deM, Tulchinsky D: Biochemical aspects of pregnancy. In Tietz N, editor: *Textbook of clinical chemistry,* Philadelphia, Penn., 1986, Saunders.

69. van Kessel H: Spectrophotometry of amniotic fluid. In Sandler M, editor: *Amniotic fluid and its clinical significance,* New York, 1981, Marcel Dekker.

70. Brazie JV, Bowes WA, Ibbott FA: An improved, rapid procedure for the determination of amniotic fluid bilirubin and its use in the prediction of the course of Rh-sensitized pregnancies, *Am J Obstet Gynecol* 104:80-86, 1969.

71. Mallikarjuneswara VR, Clemetson CAB, Carr JJ. Determination of bilirubin in amniotic fluid, *Clin Chem* 16:180-184, 1970.

72. Hochberg CJ, Witheiler AP, Cook H: Accurate amniotic fluid bilirubin analysis from the bloody tap, *Am J Obstet Gynceol* 126:531-534, 1976.

73. Queenan JT: Amniotic fluid analysis, *Clin Obstet Gynecol* 14:505-536, 1971.

74. Freer DE, Statland BE: Measurement of amniotic fluid surfactant, *Clin Chem* 27:1629-1641, 1981.

75. Tsao FH, Zachman RD: Prenatal assessment of fetal lung maturations: a critical review of amniotic fluid phospholipid tests. In Farrell PM, editor: *Lung development: biological and clinical perspectives,* vol 2, *Neonatal respiratory distress,* New York, 1982, Academic Press.

76. Chapman JF, Herbert WNP: Current methods for evaluating fetal lung maturity, *Lab Med* 17:597-602, 1986.

77. Clark HW, Jacobson W: Detection of pulmonary surfactant in human amniotic fluid by polarized light microscopy, *J Physiol* 418:139P, 1989.

78. Clements PA, Platzker ACG, Tierney DF, et al: Assessment of the risk of respiratory distress by a rapid test for surfactant in the amniotic fluid, *N Engl J Med* 286:1077, 1972.

79. Gluck L, Kulovich MV, Borer RC Jr, et al: Phosphatidylinositol and phosphatidylglycerol in amniocentesis, *Am J Obstet Gynecol* 109:440, 1971.

80. Dubin SB: Assessment of fetal lung maturity by laboratory methods, *Clin Lab Med* 12(3):603-620, 1992.

81. Richardson DK, Torday JS: Racial differences in predictive value of the lecithin/spingomyelin ratio, *Am J Obstet Gynecol* 170:1273-1278, 1994.

82. Hallman M, Kulovich M, Kirkpatrick E, et al: Phosphatidylinosi-

tol and phosphatidylglycerol in amniotic fluid: indices in lung maturity, *Am J Obstet Gynecol* 125:613, 1976.

83. Chapman JF, Phillips JC, Rosenthal MA, Herbert WNP: Evaluation of the PG-numeric assay for semi-automated analysis for phosphatidylglycerol in amniotic fluid, *Clin Chem* 36:1974-1977, 1990.

84. Bradley CA, Salhany KE, Entman SS, et al: Automated enzymatic measurement of lecithin, sphingomyelin, and phosphatidylglycerol in amniotic fluid, *Clin Chem* 33:81, 1987.

85. Clements JA, Platzker ACG, Tierney DF: Assessment of risk of respiratory distress syndrome by a rapid test for surfactant in amniotic fluid, *N Engl J Med* 286:1077-1081, 1972.

86. Stratland BE, Freer DE: Evaluation of two assays of functional surfactant in amniotic fluid, surface tension lowering ability, and the foam stability index test, *Clin Chem* 25:1770-1773, 1979.

87. Sher G, Statland BE, Freer DE: Clinical evaluation of the quantitative foam stability index test, *Obstet Gynecol* 55:617-620, 1980.

88. Tait JF, Franklin RW, Simpson JB, et al: Improved fluorescence polarization assay for use in evaluating fetal lung maturity. I. Development of the assay procedure, *Clin Chem* 32:248, 1986.

89. Russell J, Cooper C, et al: Multicenter evaluation of TDx test for assessing fetal lung maturity, *Clin Chem* 15:1005-1010, 1989.

90. Wehmann RE, Blithe DL, Flack MR, Nisula BC: Metabolic clearance rate and urinary clearance of purified beta-core, *J Clin Endocrinol Metab* 69:510-517, 1989.

91. Jeng LL, Moore RM, Kaczmarek RG: How frequently are home pregnancy tests used? Results from the 1988 National Maternal and Infant Health Survey, *Birth* 18:11-13, 1991.

92. Chard T: Pregnancy tests: a review, *Hum Reprod* 7:701-710, 1992.

93. Ascheim S, Zondek B: Die Schwangerschaftsdiagnose aus dem Harn durch Nachweis des Hypophysenvorderlappen-hormone II. Praktische und theoretische Ergebnisse aus den Harnuntersuchungen, *Klin Wochenschr* 7:1453-1457, 1928.

94. Mishalani SH, Seliktar J, Braunstein GD: Four rapid serum-urine combination assays of choriogonadotropin (hCG) compared and assessed for their utility in quantitative determinations of hCG, *Clin Chem* 40:1944-1949, 1994.

95. Vankrieken L, De Hertogh R: Rapid, automated quantification of total human chorionic gonadotropin in serum by a chemiluminescent enzyme immunometric assay, *Clin Chem* 41:36-40, 1995.

96. Ooi DS, Perkins SL, Claman P, Muggah HF: Serum human chorionic gonadotrophin levels in early pregnancy, *Clin Chem Acta* 181:281-292, 1989.

97. Lenton EA, Hooper M, King H, et al: Normal and abnormal implantation in spontaneous in-vivo and in-vitro human pregnancies, *J Reprod Fertil* 92:555-565, 1991.

98. Kent A, Kitau MJ, Chard T: Absence of diurnal variation in urinary chorionic gonadotrophin excretion at 8-13 weeks gestation, *Br J Obstet Gynecol* 69:1180-1181, 1991.

99. Rao CV, Hussa RO, Carmen FR, et al: Stability of human chorionic gonadotropin and its α subunit in human blood, *Am J Obstet Gynecol* 146:65-68, 1983.

100. Cole LA, Kardana A: Discordant results in human chorionic gonadotropin assays, *Clin Chem* 38:263-270, 1992.

101. Lee CL, Hes R, Shephert JH, et al: The purification and development of a radioimmunoassay for beta-core fragment of human chorionic gonadotrophin in urine: applications as a marker of gynecological cancer in premenopausal women, *J Endocrinol* 130:481-489, 1991.

102. Schwarz S, Berger P, Wick G: Epitope-selective monoclonal antibody based immunoradiometric assay of predictable specificity for differential measurement of choriogonadotropin and its subunits, *Clin Chem* 31:1322-1328, 1985.

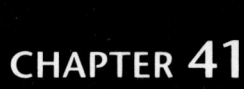

CHAPTER 41

Extravascular biological fluids

Lewis Glasser

Serous fluids
    Formation
    Change of analyte in disease
Synovial fluid (synovia)
    Normal synovial fluid
    Change of analyte in disease

OBJECTIVES

- Define serous fluid and describe the formation of serous fluids.
- Differentiate transudate and exudate based on cause, mode of formation, and protein and enzyme levels.
- List analytes of serous fluids that may be markers of disease conditions.
- Define synovial fluid and describe a normal synovial fluid.
- Describe changes in synovial fluid in pathological conditions.

KEY TERMS

arthritis Inflammation of a joint.
ascites Pathological accumulation of serous fluid in the peritoneal cavity.
chyle Fatty lymph fluid originating from the intestinal lymphatics. It is milky white in appearance.
colloid osmotic pressure of plasma The difference in osmotic pressure between the plasma and interstitial fluid that drives water into the bloodstream from the interstitial spaces.
effusion Pathological accumulation of fluid in a body cavity.
empyema The presence of pus in a body cavity, usually the pleural cavity.
epicardium The visceral layer of pericardium.
exudate A fluid with a high concentration of protein that accumulates in a body cavity when capillary permeability is increased.
gout An inflammatory arthritis of the joint secondary to crystallization of monosodium urate in the joint.
hemothorax Blood in the pleural cavity secondary to rupture of the blood vessels.

hyaluronic acid A high-molecular-weight polymer made up of repeating units of the disaccharide *N*-acetylglucosamine and glucuronic acid.
hydrostatic pressure The lateral pressure of water within a vessel that tends to drive fluid out of the capillaries into the interstitial space.
joint An articulation between bones.
neuroarthropathy Disease of a joint secondary to a disease of the nervous system.
osmotic pressure The force with which a solvent passes through a semipermeable membrane.
osteoarthritis A degenerative form of arthritis that is primarily a disease of the bones with joint involvement.
osteochondromatosis A joint disease characterized by the development of cartilaginous nodules in the synovial tissues.
paracentesis Aspiration of fluid from a body space.
parapneumonic effusion An accumulation of fluid in the pleural space secondary to pneumonia.
parietal membrane The wall of a cavity.
pericardium The sac enclosing the heart.
peritoneum The serous membrane lining the abdominal cavity and the organs of the abdominal cavity.
permeable Allowing the passage of fluid through a membrane.
pigmented villinodular synovitis A disease of the joints of unknown cause characterized by fingerlike proliferative growths of the synovial tissue with hemosiderin deposition within the synovial tissue.
pleura The serous membrane lining the inner surface of the thorax, the diaphragm, and the outer surface of the lungs.
pseudogout An inflammatory arthritis of the joint secondary to crystals of calcium pyrophosphate.
psoriatic arthritis A chronic destructive joint disease that occurs in some patients with the skin disease psoriasis.
Reiter's syndrome A syndrome of unknown cause characterized by inflammation of the joints, urethra, and conjunctivae.
rheumatoid arthritis A chronic progressive inflammatory disease of unknown cause involving multiple joints.
serous fluid Fluid having the characteristics of serum.
synovial fluid Joint fluid.
systemic lupus erythematosus A multisystem disease, caused by an autoimmune reaction, that involves mostly the skin, kidneys, joints, and serosal membranes.
thoracentesis Removal of fluid from the pleural cavity.
transudate Fluid with a low concentration of protein that has accumulated in a body cavity.
visceral membrane The outer wall of an organ.

SEROUS FLUIDS

In this chapter the term *serous fluids* is restricted to pleural, pericardial, or peritoneal fluid. The word *serous* is derived from *serum* and accurately expresses the derivation of the body fluids from plasma. Body fluids are designated by a variety of medical terms. *Pleural fluid* (thoracic or chest fluid) is obtained by surgical puncture of the chest wall *(thoracentesis)*. *Empyema* refers to pus in the pleural cavity. Peritoneal fluid is frequently designated by the nonanatomical term *ascitic fluid*. *Ascites* is derived from the Greek word *askos* (wineskin, belly) and describes the bloated abdomen of the patient afflicted with a massive accumulation of peritoneal fluid. *Paracentesis* means aspiration of fluid from a cavity, and *abdominal paracentesis fluid* is synonymous with *peritoneal fluid*. Whole blood in the body cavities is designated with the prefix *hemo-,* as in *hemothorax*. A *chylous effusion* refers to the accumulation of lymph (chyle) in the body cavity.

Formation

Normal formation. Each body cavity is lined by a thin serosal membrane. The lining of the body wall is the parietal membrane, and the outer lining of the organs is the visceral membrane. The two membranes, which together form the serosal membrane, are continuous, and the space between them is the body cavity (Fig. 41-1). The serosal membrane is composed of a thin layer of connective tissue containing numerous capillaries and lymphatics and a superficial layer of flattened mesothelial cells.

Serous fluid is an ultrafiltrate of plasma derived from the rich capillary network in the serosal membrane. Its formation is similar to the production of extravascular interstitial fluid anywhere in the body. Three factors are important: hydrostatic pressure, colloid osmotic pressure, and capillary permeability. Hydrostatic pressure drives fluid out of the capillaries and, into the body cavities. Impermeable protein molecules in the plasma exert a force that counteracts the hydrostatic pressure and causes capillaries to absorb fluid. This force is called the *colloid osmotic pressure* (COP) and is proportional to the molar concentration of protein. Lymphatics also play an important role in the absorption of water, protein, and particulate matter from the extravascular space. In the thoracic (chest) cavity, fluid is formed at the parietal pleura because the high hydrostatic pressure of the systemic circulation exceeds the colloid osmotic pressure, and fluid is reabsorbed at the visceral pleura, where capillary colloid osmotic pressure exceeds the low hydrostatic pressure of the pulmonary circulation (Fig. 41-2). Normally there is less than 15 mL of fluid in each pleural cavity, 10 to 50 mL in the pericardial sac, and less than 50 mL in the peritoneal cavity.[1]

Abnormal formation. Effusions will form when the normal physiological mechanisms responsible for the formation or absorption of serosal fluid are impaired. Thus, fluid will accumulate if capillary permeability increases, hydrostatic pressure increases, colloid osmotic pressure decreases, or lymphatic drainage is obstructed. Hydrostatic pressure is increased in congestive heart failure, a frequent cause of effusions. Hypoproteinemia decreases the colloid osmotic pressure. A decreased plasma protein can be sec-

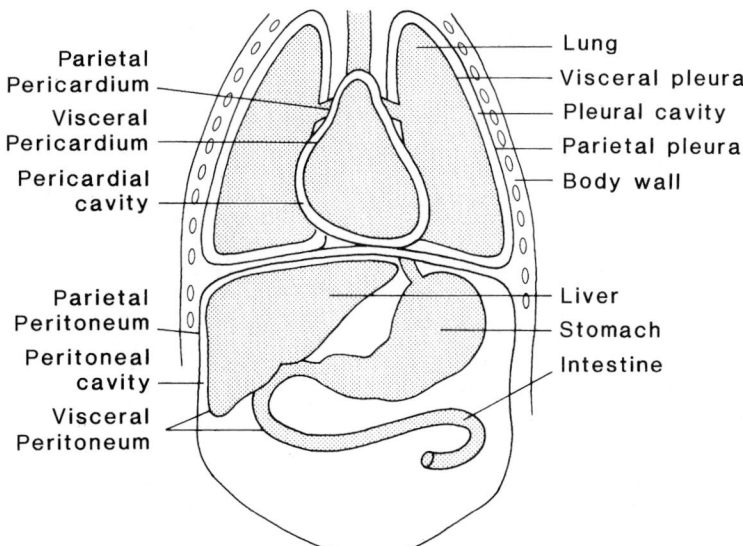

Fig. 41-1   Relationships of serous membranes, body cavities, and viscera. The heart is enclosed in the pericardial sac. The outer layer of pericardium is called "parietal pericardium." Lining the exterior surface of the heart is visceral pericardium, which is also called "epicardium." Parietal peritoneum lines the wall of the abdominal cavity. Visceral peritoneum invests stomach, liver, and intestines. The peritoneal cavity is the space between the two layers of peritoneum.

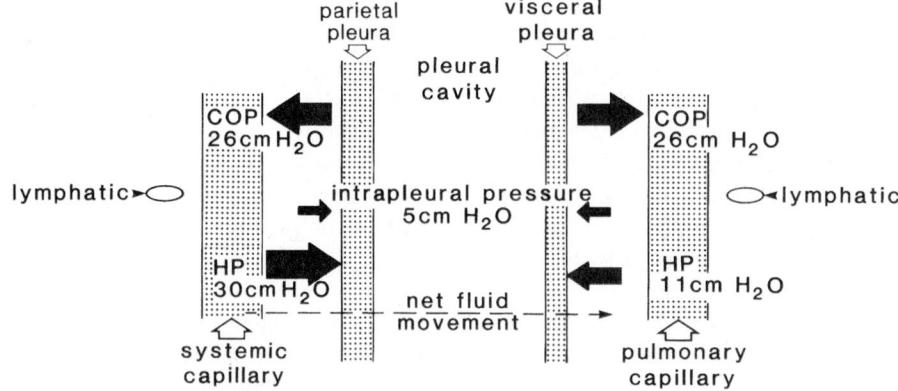

Fig. 41-2 Pleural fluid is formed at the parietal pleura because net forces for flow of fluid out of the systemic capillaries exceed net colloid osmotic pressures. Fluid moves toward the visceral pleura where net colloid osmotic pressure exceeds outward forces because of low hydrostatic pressure in pulmonary capillaries. Lymphatics play a role in absorption of water, protein, and particulate matter. *COP,* Colloid osmotic pressure; *HP,* hydrostatic pressure.

ondary to decreased synthesis or increased loss of protein. Albumin, synthesized in the liver, is the most important protein in the maintenance of colloid osmotic pressure. Diseases of the liver may impair albumin synthesis; the liver disease most frequently associated with hypoproteinemia and effusions is cirrhosis. Hypoalbuminemia is also caused by an increased loss of serum protein, which occurs in the nephrotic syndrome. Capillary permeability increases if the pleural surfaces are inflamed. Increased capillary permeability also results in loss of protein from the vascular space, and so the physical forces that lead to excess fluid formation are accentuated. Conditions causing an increase in capillary permeability include inflammatory diseases, infection, and metastatic tumors. If the lymphatics are obstructed, a protein-rich fluid will accumulate. Neoplasms of the lymph nodes frequently produce pleural effusions. The causes of effusions and the underlying pathogeneses are listed in Table 41-1.

Change of analyte in disease

Transudates and exudates. Serous effusions are designated as transudates or exudates, depending on the protein content of the fluid. The distinction is important because transudates are not caused by inflammations but by disturbances of hydrostatic or colloid osmotic pressure, whereas exudates are caused by increased capillary permeability secondary to diseases that directly involve inflammation of the surfaces of body cavities. Distinguishing between transudates and exudates involves the use of arbitrary medical decision levels that have been empirically determined. The higher the protein content, the more likely it is that the fluid is caused by a process that alters the capillary permeability and involves the surfaces of the body cavity. Measuring the specific gravity will indirectly measure the protein concentration. Pleural fluids are classified as exu-

Table 41-1 Causes of effusions

Cause	Finding	Pathogenesis
Transudates		
Congestive heart failure	↑ HP	Systemtic and pulmonary venous hypertension
Hepatic cirrhosis	↑ HP	Portal and inferior vena cava hypertension
	↓ COP	Hypoalbuminemia
Nephrotic syndrome	↓ COP	Hypoalbuminemia
Exudates		
Pancreatitis	↑ CP	Inflammation secondary to chemical injury
Bile peritonitis	↑ CP	Inflammation secondary to chemical injury
Rheumatoid disease	↑ CP	Inflammation of serosa
Systemic lupus erythematosus	↑ CP	Inflammation of serosa
Infections (bacterial, tuberculosis, fungal, viral)	↑ CP	Inflammation secondary to microorganisms
Infarction (myocardial, pulmonary)	↑ CP	Inflammation secondary to extension of process to serosal surface
Neoplasms	↑ CP	Increased permeability of capillaries supplying tumor implants; pleuritis secondary to obstructive pneumonitis
	↓ LyD	Lymphatic obstruction secondary to lymph node infiltration
Chyle		
Trauma		Disruption of lymphatic ducts
Surgery	↓ LyD	
Neoplasms		
Idiopathic		

COP, Colloid osmotic pressure; *CP,* capillary permeability; *HP,* hydrostatic pressure; *LyD,* lymphatic drainage.

dates if the specific gravity is greater than 1.015 g/mL or the total protein is 30 g/L or greater. Measurement of total protein is preferable to measurement of specific gravity. The distinction between exudates and transudates in pleural fluids is even more precise if the fluid protein is compared to the serum total protein. Dividing the concentration of the protein in the fluid by the concentration of the protein in the serum gives a ratio. A ratio of 0.5 or greater is indicative of an exudate.[2] The distinction is further improved if a large protein molecule such as lactate dehydrogenase (LD) is used as a marker of capillary permeability. Pleural fluid-to-serum LD ratios of 0.6 or greater are diagnostic of exudates.[2] The differences between transudates and exudates in pleural effusions are summarized in Table 41-2. Different cutoff values are used for peritoneal fluid. Protein levels greater than 25 g/L classify the fluid as an exudate.[1] Use of the difference between the serum and peritoneal fluid albumin concentrations provides significantly better discrimination between transudative and exudative ascites than use of the total protein levels; differences less than 11 g/L correlate with malignant effusions.[3,4]

Glucose. Pleural fluid glucose concentrations are similar to plasma glucose levels in normal fluids and transudates. Glucose is decreased in exudates such as those seen with bacterial infection, tuberculosis, neoplasia, and rheumatoid disease.[5,6] A pleural fluid glucose concentration less than 600 mg/L or a difference between the plasma and fluid glucose concentrations of more than 300 mg/L is clinically significant. Only low glucose levels are diagnostically useful, and the various diseases associated with low glucose levels are also associated with normal values. Any etiological diagnosis on the basis of a low glucose level alone is unreliable. Two mechanisms are operative in producing low values. One is increased glucose use, and the second is a relative block in the transport of glucose from the blood to the fluid. The latter occurs in rheumatoid effusions.[7] Interpretation of low glucose concentrations in peritoneal and pericardial fluid is similar to that in pleural fluid.

pH. Measurement of pleural fluid pH is clinically useful in the management of patients with parapneumonic effusions. Patients with pneumonia develop effusions because the infectious process extends to the visceral pleura, causing exudation of fluid into the pleural space. Complications of parapneumonic effusions include loculation and pus in the pleural cavity. Fluids are divided into potentially benign and complicated effusions on the basis of the pH. Fluids with a pH greater than 7.30 resolve spontaneously, whereas a pH less than 7.20 indicates a need for tube drainage.[8] A cautionary note: the specimen must be collected anaerobically in a heparinized syringe, stored on ice, and measured at 37° C. There is a significant relationship between pleural fluid pH and glucose concentration.[9]

Lipid. Chyle is a milky-white emulsion of fatty lymph fluid originating from the intestinal lymphatics. The accumulation of chyle in the pleural space is rare. Even less frequent is chyle accumulation in the peritoneal or pericardial cavities. Chylous fluid accumulates because of the disruption of the thoracic duct. Chylomicrons found on lipoprotein analysis are the best evidence for a chylous effusion. Triglyceride values above 1100 mg/L are highly suggestive of chylous effusion.[10] Cholesterol values do not distinguish between chylous and nonchylous effusions.

Analytes as markers for organs. Chemical substances can serve as markers for the specific organ involved in the pathogenesis of the effusion. The rationale for these tests is easily understood when one considers the anatomical location of the viscera and normal biochemistry (Fig. 41-3). Analytes that have been used as markers include amylase, pH, alkaline phosphatase, urea nitrogen, and creatinine. Pleural effusions accompany most cases of esophageal rupture. The perforation allows secretions from both the oral cavity and stomach to contaminate the effusion fluid. Pleural fluid amylase levels can be elevated, and the levels are higher than the serum amylase. Electrophoretic studies indicate that the amylase is from the saliva.[11] Another indicator of esophageal perforation is the pH of the pleural fluid. Normal gastric juice has a pH below 3.5. Leakage of gastric contents through the esophageal tear will acidify the pleural fluid.[12,13] A pH below 6.0 is clinically significant. The measurement may be performed at the bedside by use of pH reagent paper.

Amylase is a well-accepted marker of pancreatic disease. In acute pancreatitis, amylase-rich fluid seeps into the peripancreatic tissue and causes a chemical peritonitis, with the formation of small amounts of peritoneal fluid in most cases. One study reports fluid amylase levels of 27,800 ±7560 U/L (15,030 ±4086 Somogyi units/dL).[14] The fluid levels are higher and persist longer than the corresponding blood amylase levels.[15] *Pancreatic ascites* is the chronic accumulation of massive amounts of fluid in association with pancreatitis. It is not certain whether the fluid represents leakage of pancreatic secretions from ruptured ducts or exudation of fluid from the serosal surfaces secondary to chemical irritation.[16] In pancreatic ascites, peritoneal fluid amylase concentrations range from 680 to 129,500 U/L (370 to 70,000 Somogyi units/dL).[17] Pleural effusions are present in 15% of cases of pancreatitis. Increased amylase

Table 41-2 Diagnostic criteria of transudates and exudates in pleural fluid

Test	Transudate	Exudate
Appearance	Clear	Cloudy
Fibrinogen	No clot	Clots
Specific gravity	<1.015	≥1.015
Total protein	<30 g/L	≥30 g/L
Total protein (fluid/serum)	<0.5	≥0.5
Lactate dehydrogenase (fluid/serum)	<0.6	≥0.6
Glucose	~ serum	Often <600 mg/L

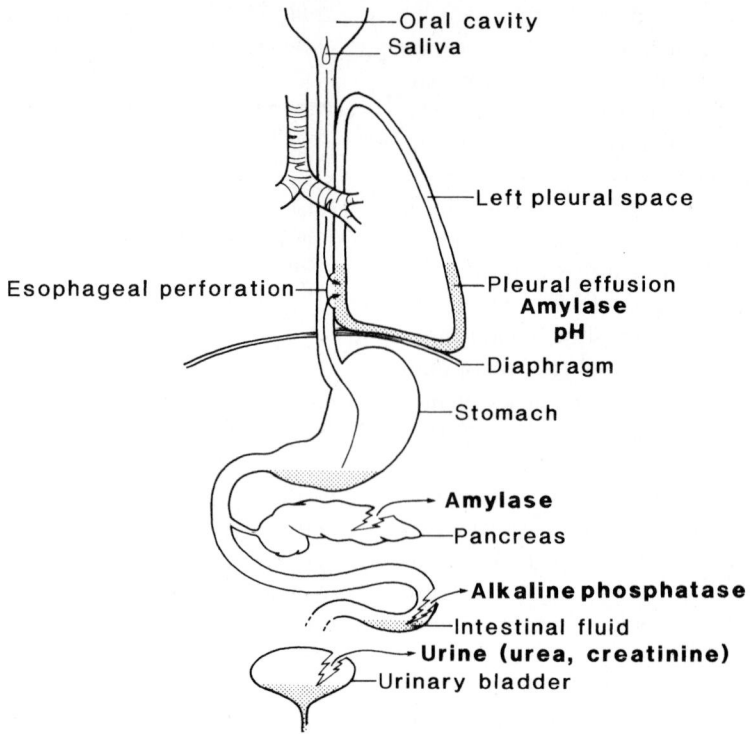

Fig. 41-3 Chemical determinations of body fluids as markers for specific organ involvement.

levels are caused by transdiaphragmatic lymphatic drainage or seepage of the enzyme across the diaphragm.[17] In a rare case pleural fluid is present because of a direct communication between the pleural and peritoneal cavities.[18]

Alkaline phosphatase has been shown to be a marker enzyme for pathological processes of the small intestine. The source of the enzyme can be leakage of alkaline phosphatase–rich fluid from the intestinal contents or extravasation from the wall of the intestine.[19] The enzyme is elevated in peritoneal serous effusions in association with intestinal perforation and infarctions of the small bowel and in peritoneal blood in patients with physically induced injuries of the small intestine.[20] The values are higher than corresponding peripheral blood levels.

Both urea nitrogen and creatinine are helpful in the differential diagnosis of a ruptured urinary bladder after abdominal trauma. Extravasated urine will have high levels of both urea nitrogen and creatinine. The former is freely diffusible and will also elevate the blood urea nitrogen; however, the peritoneum is relatively impermeable to creatinine, and blood levels of creatinine will not increase. In uncomplicated serous effusions, the fluid urea nitrogen and creatinine are low. If the physician inadvertently aspirates urine from the bladder, both urea nitrogen and creatinine will be high, but their concentrations in the blood will be within the reference interval.

SYNOVIAL FLUID (SYNOVIA)

Joints are articulations between bones. Freely movable joints are composed of hyaline articular cartilage and a fibrous capsule lined on its inner surface by a membrane (Fig. 41-4). Synovial fluid fills the joint cavity and acts as a lubricant, keeping to a minimum the friction between bones during movement or weight bearing. The fluid also provides the sole nutrition for cartilage. Synovial fluid enters the cartilage by diffusion and by a spongelike effect when the cartilage is compressed and relaxed. The term *synovia,* coined by Paracelsus, is derived from the Greek *syn* ('with') and *ōon* (Latin *ovum*) ('egg') and *-ia* (probably 'condition'), suggesting the fluid's resemblance to raw egg white.

Synovial fluid is a dialysate of plasma mixed with hyaluronic acid. Ultrafiltration in the rich vascular network in the synovial tissue produces this fluid, whereas hyaluronic acid, a mucoprotein, is secreted into the dialysate by synovial cells.

Normal synovial fluid

The fluid volume in the normal joint depends on the size of the structure. The knee joint usually contains 0.1 to 3.5 mL of fluid.[21] Normal synovial fluid is rarely obtained. If it is obtained, the fluid is clear or pale yellow with a specific gravity close to that of plasma. The viscosity is high relative to that of water because of the protein-

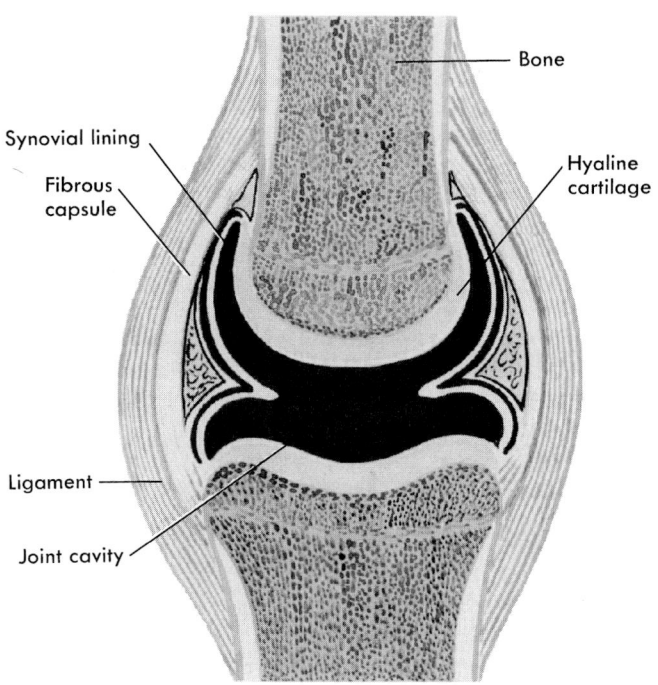

Fig. 41-4 Diagram of normal synovial joint. (From Beck EW: *Mosby's atlas of functional human anatomy,* St. Louis, 1982, Mosby.)

Table 41-3 Physical and chemical characteristics of normal synovia

	Mean	Range
Volume (mL)*	1.1	0.13-3.5
Relative viscosity at 38° C	235	5.7-1160
Hyaluronic acid (g/L)	3600	1700-4050
Total protein (g/L)	17.2	10.7-21.3
Immunoglobulins (mg/L)		
IgG	4530	330-8500
IgA	740	270-1770
IgM	370	0-840
Fibrinogen (mg/L)	0	0
Complement (CH_{50} U/mL)	20†	16-25
Glucose (mg/L)	‡	650-1200
Uric acid (mg/L)	‡	25-72

*Knee.
†Values are approximately 10% of plasma values.
‡Fasting values are similar to plasma values.

polysaccharide complex, hyaluronic acid, which constitutes 99% of the mucoproteins present in the fluid. Hyaluronic acid, a long-chain, high-molecular-weight polymer made up of repeating units of acetylglucosamine and glucuronic acid, is destroyed in inflammatory states by hyaluronidase, an enzyme contained in the neutrophils. When this occurs, the fluid viscosity decreases significantly, giving the clinician a bedside test for the presence of inflammatory fluid.

Synovial protein concentrations are related to the molecular weight of each protein because of the dialytic effect in the synovia. Thus, albumin is present in relatively higher concentrations than the higher-molecular-weight globulins are. Fibrinogen is not present because of its high molecular weight, and so normal synovia does not coagulate. Glucose and uric acid diffuse freely into the synovia and in the fasting state are as concentrated in synovia as in plasma.

The characteristics of normal synovia are summarized in Table 41-3.[22-25]

Change of analyte in disease

Physical and chemical changes that occur in the synovia during disease reflect basic pathological processes occurring in the joint. A pathological classification of synovial fluids and the diseases associated with each category is summarized in Table 41-4. The laboratory tests discussed in this section include viscosity, fibrinogen, total protein, complement, glucose, and uric acid.

Clinically there is no need for a sophisticated measurement of viscosity. Instead, one measures it at the time of aspiration by placing a finger at the tip of the syringe and stringing out the fluid. Noninflammatory fluids will "string out" longer than 4 cm. One can also drip fluid off the needle and syringe, observing it string out if it is a noninflammatory fluid and drip like water if it is the result of inflammation. The depolymerization of the hyaluronic acid by neutrophil hyaluronidase decreases the viscosity in inflammatory disease.

The mucin clot test *(Ropes's test)* is seldom advocated but is frequently described in the literature. This test reflects the degree of hyaluronate polymerization. One performs it by dropping fluid into a dilute acid solution and determining the quality of the clot. Although the test is often mentioned without critical comment in discussions of synovia, the quality of the information obtained by use of this test is inferior to that obtained by use of other procedures, and the test should be considered obsolete.

Normal synovia contains no fibrinogen, but because inflammatory synovitis permits the passage of high-molecular-weight proteins into the fluid, fibrinogen can be present and spontaneous clotting can occur. Thus, anticoagulants are necessary when specimens are collected for microscopic and bacteriological examination.

In synovia, unlike in serous fluids, total protein concentration is not used to distinguish noninflammatory from inflammatory fluids because the leukocyte count is used to make that distinction. Thus, total protein is not included in the routine examination of synovial fluids; however, its measurement can be helpful in interpreting complement levels.[26] Complement proteins are usually present at lower concentrations in synovial fluid than in serum. In systemic inflammatory conditions, complement behaves as an acute-phase reactant, and there is hypercomplementemia. In some conditions, such as Reiter's disease, the joint fluid complement concentration has been reported to be even higher than that of the serum.

In systemic immune complex diseases such as systemic

Table 41-4   Pathological classification of synovial fluids

Test	Noninflammatory	Inflammatory	Septic	Hemorrhagic
Volume (mL)	>3.5	>3.5	>3.5	>3.5
Color	Yellow	Yellow-white	Yellow-green	Red-brown
Viscosity	High	Low	Low	Low
Leukocytes (cells/μL)	200-2000	2000-100,000	10,000->100,000	>500
Neutrophils (%)	<25	>50	>75	>25
Glucose (mg/L)	~ serum	>250 mg/L lower than serum	>250 mg/L lower than serum	~ serum
Culture	Negative	Negative	Positive	Negative
Diseases	Osteoarthritis	Gout	Bacterial infection	Hemophilia
	Osteochondritis dissecans	Pseudogout	Fungal infection	Trauma
	Osteochondromatosis	Psoriatic arthritis	Tuberculous infection	Pigmented villonodular synovitis
	Traumatic arthritis	Reiter's syndrome		
	Neuroarthropathy	Rheumatoid arthritis		
		Systemic lupus erythematosus		

lupus erythematosus (SLE), complement is consumed widely and can be low in both the serum and synovial fluid. In other diseases, such as rheumatoid arthritis and viral synovitis, complement is consumed locally in the synovia while serum levels are usually normal or high.

Measurement of C_3 and C_4 by precipitation methods is preferable to measuring CH_{50}, which will be falsely low if the fluid sits out at room temperature. A decreased C_4 level is suggestive of a classical pathway activation by immune complexes and is more sensitive than C_3 or CH_{50}. The latter two are low in both classical or alternative pathway activation of complement and, if low, are suggestive of more profound systemic activity. The proper approach to interpreting complement levels in synovia is controversial. For practical purposes compare synovia and serum complement levels and consider synovia complement low if it is less than 30% of serum levels. However, in SLE and other severe immune complex diseases both levels may be low. In such a situation one can compare the synovia and serum complement levels with total protein in each fluid.

Interpretation of synovial glucose levels requires knowledge of the patient's simultaneous serum glucose. This is best done in the fasting state, but such preparation is not always clinically feasible. In the ideal situation after an 8-hour fast, the difference between serum and synovia is less than 100 mg/L; levels 250 mg/L or more below the serum level are suggestive of inflammation, and differences greater than 400 mg/L are suggestive of sepsis. In the nonfasting state, synovial glucose levels less than half of serum levels should definitely arouse suspicion of a septic process. Rarely, such findings are noted also in rheumatoid arthritis effusions. Lactic acid and succinic acid have been advocated for use in the diagnosis of septic arthritis; however, these tests have not gained general acceptance.[27]

Serum uric acid levels are important in the diagnosis of gout. The synovial fluid uric acid concentration is similar to that of serum and measurement of uric acid in synovial fluid is of no diagnostic value[28]; however, formation of monosodium urate crystals and their identification by polarized light microscopy in synovia is central to the diagnosis of gouty arthritis.

REFERENCES

1. Krieg AF, Kjeldsberg CR: Cerebrospinal fluid and other body fluids. In Henry JB, editor: *Clinical diagnosis and management by laboratory methods,* Philadelphia, 1991, Saunders.
2. Light RW, MacGregor MI, Luchsinger PC, Ball WC Jr: Pleural effusions: the diagnostic separation of transudates and exudates, *Ann Intern Med* 77:507-513, 1972.
3. Pare P, Talbot J, Hoefs JC: Serum-ascites albumin concentration gradient: a physiologic approach to the differential diagnosis of ascites, *Gastroenterology* 85:240-244, 1983.
4. Rector WG Jr, Reynolds TB: Superiority of the serum-ascites albumin difference over the ascites total protein concentration in the separation of "transudative" and "exudative" ascites, *Am J Med* 77:83-85, 1984.
5. Light RW, Ball WC Jr: Glucose and amylase in pleural effusions, *JAMA* 225:257-260, 1973.
6. Carr DT, Mayne JG: Pleurisy with effusion in rheumatoid arthritis, with reference to the low concentration of glucose in pleural fluid, *Am Rev Respir Dis* 85:345-350, 1962.
7. Dodson WH, Hollingsworth JW: Pleural effusion in rheumatoid arthritis: impaired transport of glucose, *N Engl J Med* 275:1337-1342, 1966.
8. Sokolowski JW Jr, Burgher LW, Jones FL Jr, et al: Guidelines for thoracentesis and needle biopsy of the pleura, *Am Rev Resp Dis* 140:257-258, 1989.
9. Sahn SA, Good JT: Pleural fluid pH in malignant effusions, *Ann Intern Med* 108:345-349, 1988.
10. Staats BA, Ellefson RD, Budahn LL, et al: The lipoprotein profile of chylous and nonchylous pleural effusions, *Mayo Clin Proc* 55:700-704, 1980.
11. Sherr HP, Light RW, Merson MH, et al: Origin of pleural fluid amylase in esophageal rupture, *Ann Intern Med* 76:985-986, 1972.
12. Dye RA, Lafaret EG: Esophageal rupture: diagnosis by pleural fluid pH, *Chest* 66:454-456, 1974.
13. Abbott OA, Mansor KA, Logan WD: Atraumatic so-called spontaneous rupture of the esophagus, *J Thorac Cardiovasc Surg* 59:67-82, 1970.
14. Geokas MC, Olsen H, Carmack C, Rinderknecht H: Studies on the ascites and pleural effusion in acute pancreatitis, *Gastroenterology* 58:950, 1970.
15. Keith LM, Zollinger RM, McCleery RS: Peritoneal fluid amylase determinations as an aid in diagnosis of acute pancreatitis, *Arch Surg* 61:930-936, 1950.
16. Donowitz M, Kerstein MD, Spiro HM: Pancreatic ascites, *Medicine* 53:183-195, 1974.

17. Salt WB, Schenker S: Amylase—its clinical significance: a review of the literature, *Medicine* 55:269-289, 1976.

18. Goldman M, Goldman G, Fleischner FG: Pleural fluid amylase in acute pancreatitis, *N Engl J Med* 266:715-718, 1962.

19. Lee YN: Alkaline phosphatase in intestinal perforation, *JAMA* 208:361, 1969.

20. Delany HM, Moss CM, Carnevale N: The use of enzyme analysis of peritoneal blood in the clinical assessment of abdominal organ injury, *Surg Gynecol Obstet* 42:161-167, 1976.

21. Ropes MW, Rossmeisl EC, Bauer W: The origin and nature of normal human synovial fluid, *J Clin Invest* 19:795-799, 1940.

22. Hamerman D, Schuster H: Hyaluronate in normal synovial fluid, *J Clin Invest* 37:57-64, 1958.

23. Hoeprich PD, Ward JR: *The fluids of the parenteral body cavities*, New York, 1959, Grune & Stratton.

24. Pekin TJ, Zvaifler NJ: Hemolytic complement in synovial fluid, *J Clin Invest* 43:1372-1382, 1964.

25. Pruzanski W, Russell ML, Gordon DA, Ofryzlo MA: Serum and synovial fluid proteins in rheumatoid arthritis and degenerative joint diseases, *Am J Med Sci* 265:483-490, 1973.

26. McCarty DJ: Synovial fluid. In McCarty DJ, Koopman WJ, editors: *Arthritis and allied conditions, a textbook of rheumatology*, ed 12, Philadelphia, 1993, Lea & Febiger.

27. Borenstein DG, Gibbs CA, Jacobs RP: Gas-liquid chromatographic analysis of synovial fluid: succinic acid and lactic acid as markers of septic arthritis, *Arthritis Rheum* 25:947-953, 1982.

28. Baker DG: Chemistry, serology, and immunology. In Gatter RA, Schumacher HR: *A practical handbook of joint fluid analysis*, ed 2, Philadelphia, 1991, Lea & Febiger.

CHAPTER 42

Nervous system

Michael D. Privitera
Christian Kohler

OBJECTIVES

- Define the blood-brain barrier and its physiological function.
- Describe the function and composition of cerebrospinal fluid (CSF) and list the major changes to CSF that are seen in disease states.
- List the major neurotransmitters and define their function.
- List the major causes of coma or altered metal status.
- Name six commonly used classes of antiseizure drugs and describe the most common methods used to measure one of the classes.

KEY TERMS

affective disorder A disorder of mood regulation manifested clinically by episodes or sustained periods of depression or mania or both.

antiepileptic drugs Medications given therapeutically to prevent seizures of various types.

antipsychotic drugs Drugs that are used for the reversal or attenuation of psychotic symptoms (hallucinations, delusions, and disorders of cognition).

anxiety disorders Chronic disorder characterized by inappropriate, pervasive, continuous or paroxysmal feelings of worries or fear.

bipolar affective disease Affective disorder in which episodes of depression and mania are episodically present in the same patient.

blood-brain barrier The barrier between the brain and the blood that allows the brain to maintain a cerebrospinal fluid composition different from that of blood.

cerebrospinal fluid (CSF) Clear, colorless fluid contained within the four ventricles of the brain, the subarachnoid space, and the spinal cord.

coma A state of unconsciousness from which patients cannot be aroused, even by the strongest stimuli.

depression A mood disturbance often described as being sad, blue, hopeless, low, "down in the dumps," or irritable, accompanied by pervasive loss of interest or pleasure in almost all usual activities or pastimes.

epilepsy A disorder characterized by a tendency to have seizures.

IgG index The ratio (CSF IgG × Serum albumin)/(Serum IgG × CSF albumin) used as an indicator of the source of elevated cerebrospinal fluid protein.

mania A periodic disturbance of mood in which the mood is elevated, expansive, or irritable, accompanied by hyperactivity, pressure of speech, flight of ideas, inflated self-esteem, and decreased need for sleep.

meninges The three membranes covering the brain and spinal cord: the dura, arachnoid, and pia.

meningitis Inflammation of the meninges, often caused by viral or bacterial infections.

nerve receptor A protein complex embedded in the cell membrane that binds to a particular neurotransmitter and initiates a series of events that alter the membrane's physiologic functioning.

neurotransmitter A chemical substance released by one neuron onto a specific receptor on an adjacent cell and alters the physiologic functioning of the cell.

reuptake A process by which neurons conserve their own neurotransmitter by recovering it from the synaptic cleft for storage and subsequent rerelease.

schizophrenia A deteriorating psychotic illness with delusions, hallucinations, and disorders of cognition that has lasted more than 6 months and from which full recovery is not expected.

seizure A sudden and transient disturbance of mental function or body movements that results from an excessive electrical discharge of a group of brain cells.

stroke Sudden onset of symptoms caused by acute ischemia in the brain resulting from hemorrhage, embolism, or thrombosis, and is evidenced by loss of neurological functions.

subarachnoid space The space between the arachnoid and pia membranes.

synapse The structural junction of two neurons where chemical messages are carried from the presynaptic neuron to the postsynaptic receptor by neurotransmitters.

unipolar affective disease Affective disorder in which episodes of depression alone occur without episodes of mania.

ventricles Four cavities within the brain filled with cerebrospinal fluid and lined by the pia and the choroid plexus.

xanthochromia A yellow coloring to the cerebrospinal fluid caused by the presence of breakdown products of hemoglobin.

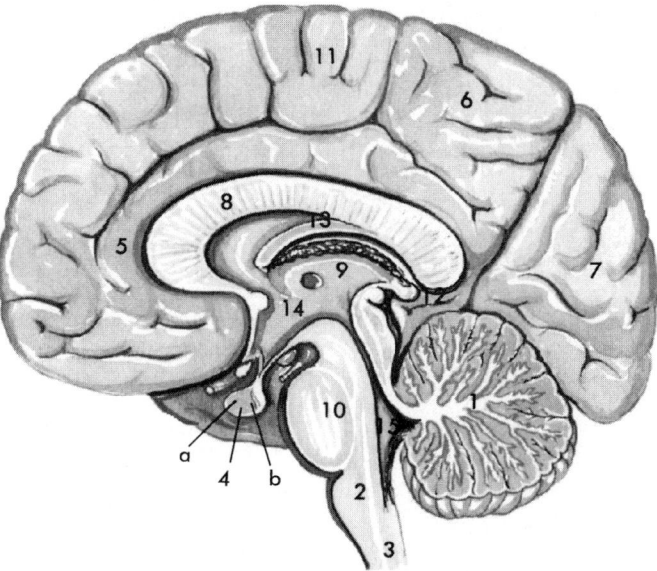

Fig. 42-1 Scheme of functional or motor-control areas of brain (right hemisphere, medial view). *1,* Cerebellum; *2,* medulla oblongata; *3,* spinal cord; *4,* pituitary gland: *a,* anterior lobe, *b,* posterior lobe; *5,* frontal lobe; *6,* parietal lobe; *7,* occipital lobe; *8,* corpus callosum; *9,* thalamus; *10,* pons; *11,* cerebrum; *12,* pineal body; *13,* fornix; *14,* third ventricle; *15,* fourth ventricle. (From Beck EQ: *Mosby's atlas of functional human anatomy,* St. Louis, 1982, Mosby.)

The two cerebral hemispheres are built around a connecting system of hollow spaces called the *ventricular system.* The *ventricles* are filled with cerebrospinal fluid (CSF) (Fig. 42-2).

The brain and spinal cord are both covered by a double membrane called the *meninges* (Fig. 42-3). Its inner mem-

BASIC NEUROANATOMY

The central nervous system (CNS) consists of the brain and spinal cord. The brain includes the two cerebral hemispheres, which are roughly mirror images of one another, the brainstem, a narrow structure through which all the pathways entering and leaving the two hemispheres must pass and that contains the centers that control breathing, heart rate, eye movements, and many other critical functions; and the cerebellum, a rounded structure about the size of a baseball that helps control movement and balance (Fig. 42-1). The lower brainstem flows into the spinal cord. The spinal cord is the point of exit for nerves on their way out to the muscles they control and the point of entry for sensory fibers returning from the body's sensory organs. All the nerves outside the CNS are collectively called the *peripheral nervous system.*

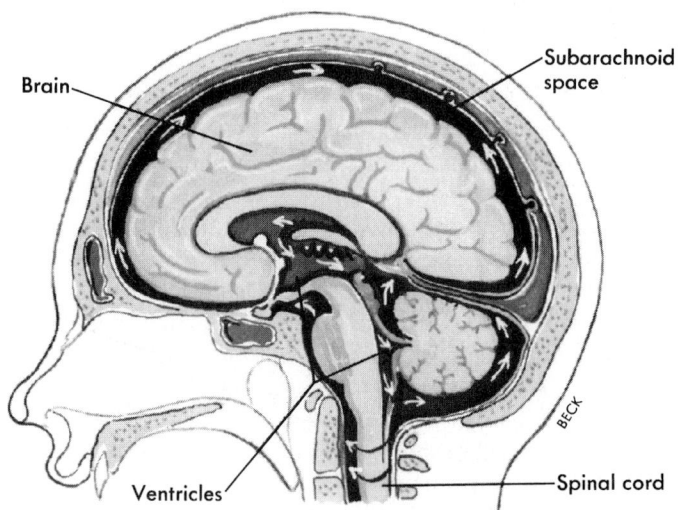

Fig. 42-2 Scheme of brain showing relationships of ventricles and subarachnoid space with rest of brain. (From Beck EW: *Mosby's atlas of functional human anatomy,* St. Louis, 1982, Mosby.)

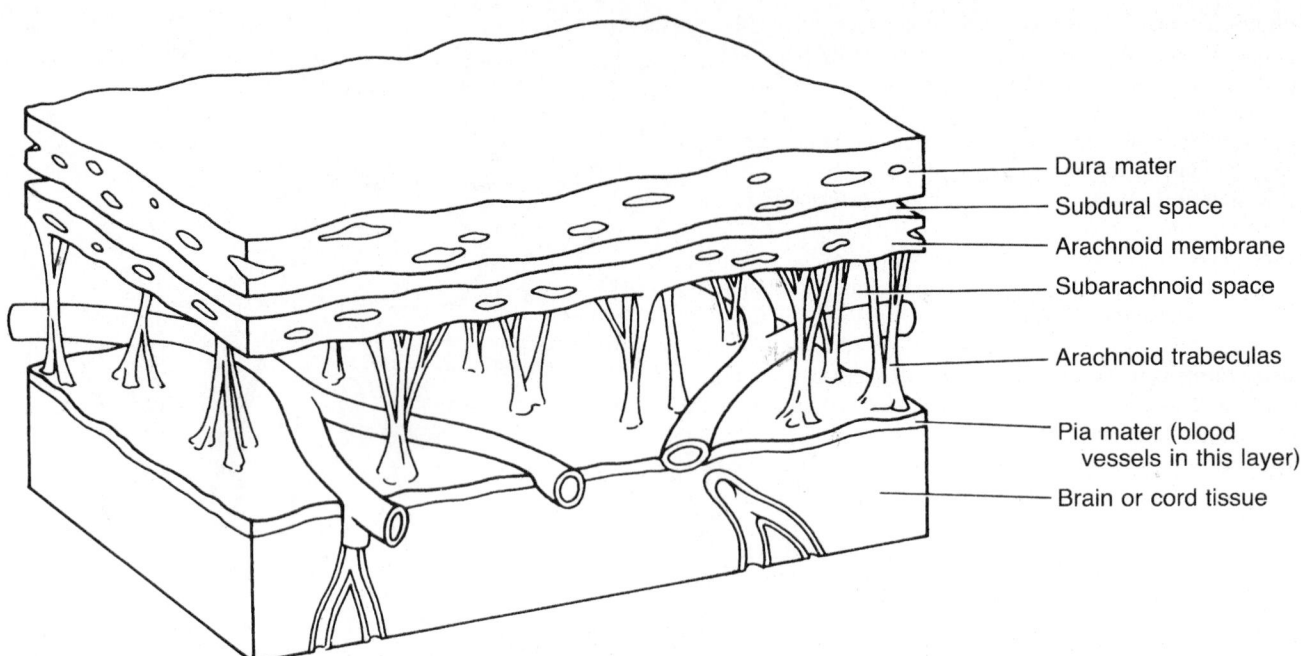

Fig. 42-3 Scheme of meninges. Arrangement may be compared with an underground parking garage. Dura and arachnoid form roof with pia membrane as floor. CSF flows in subarachnoid space. (From Prezbindowski KS: *Guide to learning anatomy and physiology,* St. Louis, 1982, Mosby.)

brane, the *arachnoid,* lies next to the outermost covering of the brain and spinal cord, the *dura.* The dura is a tough, nonelastic membrane that essentially wraps the brain and spinal cord in a nondistensible sac. The brain, blood, and CSF are thus sealed within a space the volume of which is fixed. The space between the pia and the arachnoid is called the *subarachnoid space* and communicates directly with the ventricular system.

PHYSIOLOGY AND BIOCHEMISTRY
Formation of cerebrospinal fluid

The ventricular system and the subarachnoid space are filled with CSF. The total volume of CSF in adults is about 150 mL. CSF is constantly produced and reabsorbed at a rate of approximately 500 mL/day (0.35 mL/min). This means the total amount of CSF is replaced every 6 to 8 hours.

CSF is produced in the ventricles by a specialized sponge-like structure called the *choroid plexus.* Beginning in the lateral ventricles, where it is formed, CSF circulates into the third ventricle and then into the fourth ventricle. It leaves the fourth ventricle by three small openings, or foramina, to circulate through the intracranial and spinal subarachnoid spaces. Circulation may be blocked in any of the ventricles or at the foramina between them, leading to an *obstructive hydrocephalus* (accumulation of fluid in the brain).

New CSF is constantly produced and is *absorbed* at the arachnoid villi and *granulations* to keep volume constant.

These arachnoid villi and granulations are scattered along the entire inner table of the skull and down the spinal canal to the points at which the spinal nerves exit the dura. Thus CSF reabsorption can occur along the entire neuraxis. If absorption is impaired (as after meningeal inflammation, bacterial meningitis, or subarachnoid hemorrhage), CNS pressure and CSF volume both rise; this is called a *communicating hydrocephalus.*

Factors that determine the rate at which CSF is formed and absorbed are complex and not completely understood. Any increase in the size of one component (that is, brain, CSF, or blood) leads to a sharp increase in pressure within the system unless there is a corresponding decrease in the volume of one of the other two components. With increased CSF pressure the brain may suffer from direct effects of the abnormally high pressure or from having its blood flow decreased.

Blood-brain barrier

The term *blood-brain barrier* refers to a physiological barrier separating the brain and CSF from substances borne in the blood. The blood-brain barrier allows brain and CSF composition to be maintained at levels quite different from those of blood with respect to proteins, ions, and other molecular elements. The blood-brain barrier is extremely important in clinical practice. It determines the access of antibiotics to the brain and meninges and contributes to the exquisite control exercised over the brain's chemical milieu despite simultaneous changes occurring in the peripheral blood.

The extracellular fluid (ECF) compartment of the brain is in relatively free communication with the CSF, whereas a barrier exists between capillary blood and the ECF compartment–CSF combination.

Factors that significantly influence the access of substances to brain and CSF include molecular weight, protein binding, and lipid solubility. With molecular weight, entry is inversely related to size, hence the $1:200$ CSF-to-plasma ratio of albumin (molecular weight, 69,000 daltons). Drugs that are highly protein bound enter the CSF much less readily than unbound smaller molecular weight substances. For example, phenytoin is 90% protein bound and 10% free in blood. Only 10% of the total measured blood phenytoin level is easily able to enter the CNS, and only that 10% is "active." Calcium, magnesium, and metabolites such as bilirubin are also highly protein bound and thus relatively restricted from CSF. Highly lipid-soluble substances such as carbon monoxide, neuroactive drugs, and alcohol readily enter the CNS. Substances that are high ionized at physiological pH are relatively excluded. Highly polar substances, such as some amino acids, enter slowly and require an active-transport mechanism.

The blood-brain barrier is readily permeable to water but not to electrolytes. The major cations, sodium and potassium, require hours to reach equilibrium with CSF after changes in peripheral blood. Changes in blood osmolality are followed by parallel CSF changes after a lag time of a few hours.

In the case of drugs, their pK_a, or *ionic dissociation constant,* is important in determining how readily they cross the blood-brain barrier. pK_a refers to the pH at which 50% of a compound is ionized. A nonionized drug is relatively lipid soluble and so more freely enters the CNS. The polarionized fraction is relatively excluded.

Finally, the characteristics of the blood-brain barrier can be dramatically altered by disease states. Penicillin, an acidic substance, is normally excluded from the CNS after parenteral injection, and yet it is an effective agent for treating meningitis. The reason is that meningeal inflammation alters (damages) the blood-brain barrier, allowing greater access of drugs, such as penicillin, that normally would not reach infected tissue.

Some specific factors that alter permeability of the blood-brain barrier are as follows:

1. Inflammation can increase the ease of entry into the nervous system of macromolecules such as albumin and penicillin.
2. Neovascularity, in association, for example, with tumor, trauma, or ischemia, alters the blood-brain barrier. This may be caused by defects in the new vessels or by their immaturity.
3. Toxins can change blood-brain barrier characteristics, and some agents used in radiographic studies increase

the permeability of the barrier by direct toxic effects. When they are injected in hyperosmolar concentrations, the effect is greater.
4. Finally, the blood-brain barrier of the immature nervous system is more permeable to a variety of substances. For infants below 6 months of age, CSF protein is normally as high as 100 mg/L.

Functions of cerebrospinal fluid

Why should the brain be suspended in and bathed by this distinctive fluid? First, CSF provides mechanical support to the brain. Second, CSF probably functions to help remove metabolic products from the brain, a function that is poorly understood but probably important in both healthy and diseased states. Third, there is some evidence that CSF transports biologically active compounds that may function as chemical messengers. Finally, it plays an important role in maintaining the chemical environment of the brain. Although its communication with the plasma compartment is tightly regulated, CSF seems to be in relatively free communication with the brain's extracellular fluid compartment, which aids brain cells themselves. The following section examines the composition of CSF more closely.

Composition of cerebrospinal fluid

The ionic and molecular composition of CSF differs from that of plasma for some components and is the same for others (see box on following page). Changes in serum sodium are followed by corresponding changes in CSF sodium so that after a lag time of about 1 hour sodium values are nearly the same. However, CSF potassium is lower than plasma potassium, and furthermore potassium is maintained within a very narrow concentration range in CSF despite wide fluctuations in plasma values. Active transport in and out of the CSF space appears to be largely responsible for maintaining these differences. Chloride and magnesium are somewhat higher in CSF than in plasma, and bicarbonate is somewhat lower.

CSF glucose normally ranges from 450 to 800 mg/L (2.5 to 4.44 mmol/L), that is, between 60% and 80% of the blood glucose concentration after equilibration. Blood and CSF glucose equilibrate only after a lag period of about 4 hours, and so CSF glucose at any given time reflects blood glucose levels during the past 4 hours. When a lumbar spinal puncture (LP) is performed and CSF glucose is to be determined, a simultaneous sample of peripheral blood must also be drawn. CSF glucose is altered by certain disease processes, as is discussed later. Equilibrated CSF glucose is definitely abnormal when it is less than 40% of the simultaneous blood glucose value; values less than 400 to 450 mg/L are almost always abnormal.

One should also be aware that the expected percentage of CSF glucose to blood glucose (60% to 80%) falls as blood glucose rises. That is, one would expect a CSF-to-blood ratio of 0.5 when blood glucose values reach 5000

Characteristics of Normal Spinal Fluid

Total volume: 150 mL
Color: colorless, like water
Transparency: clear, like water
Osmolarity at 37° C: 281 mOsm/L
Specific gravity: 1.006 to 1.008
Acid-base balance:

pH	7.31
Pco_2	47.9 mm Hg
HCO_3^-	22.9 mEq/L

Sodium: 138 to 150 mEq/L
Potassium: 2.7 to 3.9 mEq/L
Chloride: 116 to 127 mEq/L
Calcium: 2.0 to 2.5 mEq/L (40 to 50 mg/L)
Magnesium: 2.0 to 2.5 mEq/L (24.4 to 30.5 mg/L)
Lactic acid: 1.1 to 2.8 mmol/L
Lactate dehydrogenase: Absolute activity depends on method; approximately 10% of serum value
Glucose: 450 to 800 mg/L
Proteins: 200 to 400 mg/L

At different levels of spinal tap:

Lumbar	200 to 400 mg/L
Cisternal	150 to 250 mg/L
Ventricular	150 to 100 mg/L

Normal values in children:

Up to 6 days of age	700 mg/L
Up to 4 years of age	244 mg/L

Electrophoretic separation of spinal fluid proteins (% of total protein concentration):

Prealbumin	2% to 7%
Albumin	56% to 76%
α_1-globulin	2% to 7%
α_2-globulin	3.5% to 12%
β- and γ-globulin	8% to 18%
γ-globulin	7% to 12%
IgG	10 to 40 mg/L
IgA	0 to 0.2 mg/L
IgM	0 to 0.6 mg/L
κ/λ ratio	1

Erythrocyte count:

Newborn	0 to 675/mm³
Adult	0 to 10/mm³

Leukocyte count:

<1 year of age	0 to 30/mm³
1 to 4 years of age	0 to 20/mm³
5 years of age to puberty	0 to 10/mm³
Adult	0 to 5/mm³

---

mg/L and a ratio of 0.4 if blood glucose reaches 7000 mg/L.

Proteins found in the CSF ordinarily originate from serum and reach the CSF space by pinocytosis across the capillary endothelium. The normal ratio of serum to CSF protein is 200:1 (with serum equal to 70 g/L and CSF equal to 350 mg/L).

Brain metabolism

The brain's metabolic rate is one of the highest of any of the body's organs, whether one is awake or asleep. But unlike most other organs, which store and reserve some supplies of energy to sustain themselves, the brain has almost no energy reserve. It depends entirely on an uninterrupted supply of glucose and oxygen delivered by peripheral blood. The brain uses glucose almost exclusively to supply its energy needs (see Chapter 32). To get an idea of just how hungry the brain is and how dependent it is on a constant, swift flow of blood, consider that under resting conditions total cerebral blood flow equals 15% to 20% of cardiac output (or about 500 mL per 100 g of brain per minute). Although *total* cerebral blood flow remains remarkably constant, discrete areas within the brain show striking variability; gray matter receives three to four times the blood flow compared to white matter. Moreover, *regional* blood flow is known to vary during performance of certain tasks, with regional flow increasing in the appropriate areas during tasks such as hand movement, speaking, or mental problem solving. Blood flow is also altered in response to disease states, as in stroke.

Neurotransmitter systems

Neurons (nerve cells) within the central nervous system process information arriving from multiple internal and external sources. To maintain physiological and psychobiological homeostasis, CNS neurons communicate both with one another and eventually with effectors outside the central nervous system by means of neurotransmitters released by each neuron on to specific receptors. Neurons are characterized by the anatomical distribution, by the path of projection to their areas of innervation, and by the nature of the neurochemical hormone or transmitter that they synthesize and release (Fig. 42-4).

The function of the neurotransmitter is to propagate an electrical impulse from one neuron to another. The electrical impulse travels down a neuron causing the release of a neurotransmitter from presynaptic vesicles in which the neurotransmitter is synthesized and stored. Subsequently several thousand molecules of neurotransmitter are released into the synaptic cleft, the space between the presynaptic and postsynaptic neurons. There they bind to transmitter-specific receptors of the presynaptic neurons and produce either an excitatory or inhibitory impulse. Neurotransmitters are broken down by enzymes in the synaptic cleft. Both the metabolites and the parent compounds bind to receptors on the presynaptic membrane, where they are again taken back into the presynaptic neuron (reuptake) for formation of new neurotransmitter.

Norepinephrine. Norepinephrine is formed in presynaptic noradrogenic neurons from the substrate tyrosine by means of the intermediary products of dopa and dopamine (Fig. 42-5). Norepinephrine produces an excitatory response at postsynaptic receptors. It is either broken down in the cleft to 3-methoxy-4-hydroxyphenylglycol (MHPG) or taken up into the presynaptic neuron where it is metabolized by a cytoplasmic enzyme called *monoamine oxidase,*

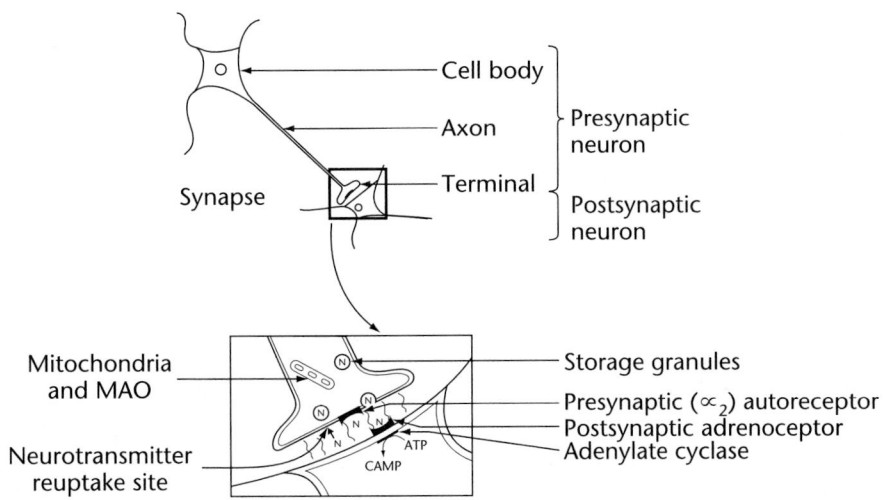

Fig. 42-4 Norepinephrine neuron, synapse, and postsynaptic connections.

and the breakdown product is resynthesized to norepinephrine. By this mechanism most of the norepinephrine released into the synaptic cleft is recovered by the noradrenergic neuron. MHPG also crosses the blood brain barrier, enters the circulatory system, and is excreted into urine; approximately 50% of urinary MHPG is derived from the CNS.

Dopamine. Dopamine is formed by the same metabolic pathway as shown in Fig. 42-5 in dopaminagenic neurons that lack the enzymes for further metabolism of dopamine into norepinephrine. These neurons project from the brainstem to the limbic system and frontal cortex. Dopamine appears to be mainly inhibitory in action. There now appear to be five to seven different types of dopamine receptors; these subtypes may have significance in pharmacological treatment of mental disorders. Dopamine is metabolized to homovanillic acid and is excreted into urine.

Acetylcholine. Acetylcholine, the first demonstrated neurotransmitter, is formed in presynaptic cholinergic neurons from acetyl CoA, a ubiquitous metabolite, and choline, which is derived from lipid metabolism. The essential enzyme for this reaction is choline acetyltransferase.

Once released from presynaptic vesicles into the synaptic cleft acetylcholine binds to postsynaptic receptors and acts as an excitatory neurotransmitter. It is broken down by the enzyme acetylcholinesterase in the synaptic cleft. Ten percent of all synapses in the central and peripheral nervous system use acetylcholine. The synapses are located in all the neuromuscular junctions, the major portion of the autonomic nervous system, and in brain areas such as motor pathways, the hippocampus, which is part of the limbic system, and the basal ganglia.

Serotonin (5-hydroxytryptamine, 5-HT). Serotonin is formed in presynaptic serotoninergic neurons from the

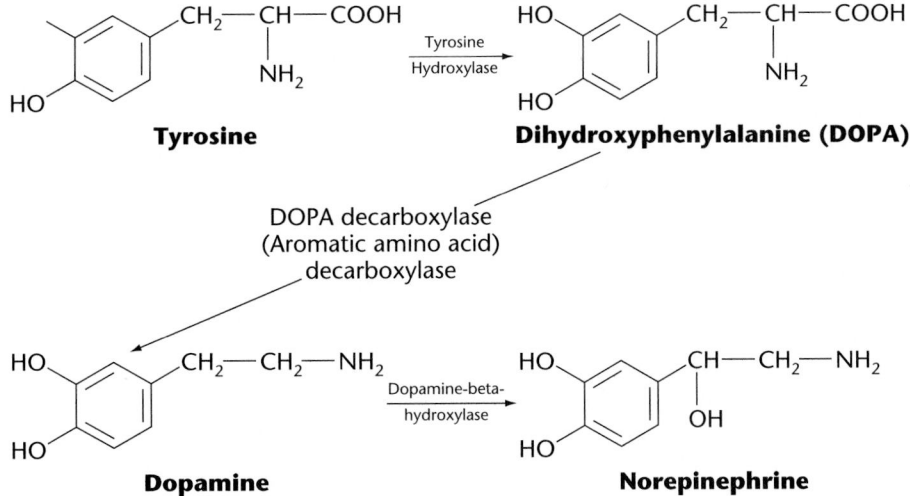

Fig. 42-5 Enzymatic pathway for synthesis of dopamine and norepinephrine. (From Kaplan H, Sadock B: *Clinical psychiatry,* Baltimore, 1988, Williams & Wilkins.)

amino acid tryptophan, by means of hydroxytryptophan. Most serotoninergic neurons originate in the raphe nuclei in the pons from where projections run diffusely throughout the brain and spinal cord. The raphe nuclei are part of the reticular formation, which regulates general arousal. Serotonin binds to the postsynaptic hydroxytryptamine receptor, where it produces an excitatory response. Both serotonin and its metabolite 5-hydroxyindoleacetic acid (5-HIAA) are taken up into the presynaptic neuron.

GABA (gamma-aminobutyric acid). GABA is formed from the amino acid glutamic acid by decarboxylation. GABA is used as a neurotransmitter by 30% to 40% of all synapses in the brain and is diffusely located throughout the brain, brainstem, and spinal cord. It acts as an inhibitory neurotransmitter. The postsynaptic GABA receptor complexes also bind drugs like phenobarbital, valproate and benzodiazepines.

Other neurotransmitters. A variety of other substances make up the majority of neurotransmitters in the central nervous system, but their clinical significance is poorly understood at the present time. Such substances are glutamate, an amino acid that has excitatory function in synapses in the brain; glycine, another amino acid that has inhibitory function in the spinal cord; endogenous opioids, such as endorphine and enkephalin; and substance P, which is found in neuronal pathways transmitting pain. Most recently, two gases, nitric oxide and carbon monoxide have been shown to act as neurotransmitters.

PATHOLOGICAL CONDITIONS: NEUROLOGICAL

Loss of neural function with resulting disease states is caused by abnormalities of the neurotransmitter biochemical pathways. For example, in the early stages of Alzheimer's disease there is a large decrease in choline acetyltransferase activity along with degeneration of neurons utilizing acetylcholine. Loss of acetylcholine activity in the hippocampus may explain the hallmark symptom of early memory loss in Alzheimer's disease, since the hippocampus is involved in acquisition of memory. In Huntington's disease there is degeneration of cholinergic neurons in the basal ganglia, contributing to the movement disorder and dementia seen in Huntington's disease. Dysfunction of GABA-ergic systems is postulated in idiopathic generalized epilepsy, Huntington's disease, and anxiety disorders. Clinical disease states attributable to dopaminergic neuron dysfunction vary according to the anatomic location of the dysfunctional neurons. Dopaminergic neuron dysfunction in pathways from the brainstem to the frontal cortex and limbic system may contribute to clinical symptoms of schizophrenia, whereas dysfunction of dopaminergic neurons that project from the brainstem to the corpus striatum is important in movement disorders such as Parkinson's disease.

Damage to *discrete* (focal) areas of the brain or spinal cord produces predictable circumscribed signs and symp-toms, such as paralysis of an arm, leg, or side of the body, loss of ability to speak or comprehend spoken language, incoordination, visual or sensory loss. *Diffuse* impairment of cerebral tissue, on the other hand, leads to a different characteristic clinical picture. Failure of various intellectual functions such as attention, concentration, judgment, memory, problem-solving ability, and insight are early findings with mild diffuse disease. Other symptoms include changes in alertness beginning with clouding of consciousness and proceeding to drowsiness, stupor, and coma. Excessive synchronized nerve transmission can cause sudden transient abnormalities of mental function or body movement, called *seizures*. Seizures can accompany both diffuse and focal brain damage.

Various disease states tend to produce either focal or diffuse brain damage, and so the pattern of deficits described above is often helpful to the clinician in working backward toward a specific diagnosis. Some examples of conditions that cause focal damage are stroke caused by arterial occlusion or hemorrhage; trauma; cerebral abscess; and tumors. Many of these conditions also cause changes in the CSF by damaging the blood-brain barrier (elevating CSF protein) and stimulating inflammatory changes (with leukocytosis), tissue necrosis (elevating CSF protein and cell count), or shedding of tumor cells (observed in cytological specimens).

Examples of conditions associated with diffuse cerebral dysfunction (encephalopathic states) are anoxia, generalized ischemia, hypoglycemia, sepsis, thyroid abnormalities, disseminated intravascular coagulation, and the entire group of toxic and metabolic derangements. The diagnosis of these states often rests on laboratory findings.

A summary of some of the clinical and pathological changes commonly found in many conditions are briefly discussed.

Coma

Coma is a state of unconsciousness from which the patient cannot be aroused. A coma is but one aspect of altered states of consciousness that can be present in patients. *Confusion* is the least altered state, in which there is disorientation with respect to time, associated drowsiness, and altered attention span. *Stupor* is a state in which the patient is unresponsive but can be aroused back to a near-normal state with appropriate stimuli.

A patient with an altered mental state, as seen in an emergency department, must first be given any life support, such as ventilation, necessary to maintain vital functions. The next step is to determine the underlying cause of the altered mental status. Readily treatable causes can be corrected by procedures, such as administration of dextrose to relieve coma caused by severe hypoglycemia. Table 42-1 lists the most important causes of coma and altered mental states, which include metabolic, structural, or infectious causes. Many of these causes are described in detail below.

Table 42-1   Some causes of coma and altered mental states

Type	Cause	Laboratory findings
Metabolic	Alcoholism	Increased blood ethanol, metabolic acidosis, and ketosis
	Hyperosmolar coma	Blood glucose ≥5000 mg/L, no ketosis, dehydration
	Diabetic ketoacidosis	Increased blood glucose, ketosis, acidosis, dehydration
	Metabolic acidosis of other origin	Decreased pH, increased lactic acid
	Hypoglycemia	Decreased blood glucose (<500 mg/L)
	Hypercalcemia or hypocalcemia	Changes in calcium levels; hypomagnesemia can be found with hypocalcemia
	Drugs	Presence of any of many drugs on serum or urine toxicology screen, often at very high levels
Systemic metabolic diseases	Hepatic coma	Increase in blood ammonia, increased liver function tests
	Uremic coma	Increased serum urea, creatinine with metabolic acidosis
	Ischemia; cardiac, pulmonary	Lactic acidosis
	Hypothyroidism or hyperthyroidism	Abnormal thyroid function tests
Encephalopathy	Intracranial hemorrhage	Blood in CSF
Trauma	—	None, or blood in CSF if traumatic hemorrhage is present
Infectious	Bacterial, viral	Decreased CSF glucose, increased protein
Psychiatric	—	None

Intracranial bleeding

Bleeding from a vessel on the surface of the brain, such as an arterial aneurysm, pours blood between the brain's surface and the pia and arachnoid layers and is called a *subarachnoid hemorrhage*. Blood thus mingles with CSF, and red blood cells appear on examination of the CSF. Furthermore, because blood is an extremely irritating substance when it escapes from its usual vascular channels, it may provoke an inflammatory response in the meninges, called a *chemical meningitis,* and leukocytes will be shed into the CSF by the irritated meninges. Since meninges are pain sensitive, a subarachnoid hemorrhage typically causes acute, severe headache.

Infectious diseases

Both the type of invading bacterial or viral organism and the intracranial structures they invade help determine CSF changes seen in the infectious process. The CSF parameters that reflect CNS invasion by an infectious agent are white cell count and differential, glucose, and to a lesser extent protein concentration.

Meningitis is an inflammation of the meninges leading to several clinical patterns. Bacterial, or *purulent,* meningitis is associated with a CSF polymorphonuclear (PMN) leukocytosis, with cell counts ranging from a very few to many thousands of PMNs. The CSF glucose levels may be depressed to strikingly low values, and CSF protein concentrations may be elevated. Later in the course of illness lymphocytes can become prominent or dominant, especially if the infection has been partially treated with antibiotics. Partial treatment of bacterial meningitis that fails to eradicate the infection can produce confusing findings and may make diagnosis difficult.

Viral meningitis causes a predominantly or exclusively lymphocytic leukocytosis. Red blood cells may be seen with herpes simplex encephalitis. CSF glucose levels usually remain within the healthy reference interval but may be decreased in mumps, herpes simplex or herpes zoster encephalitis. Protein is usually within the healthy reference interval or slightly elevated in these diseases.

Fungi also invade the CNS and may cause no change in CSF other than a lymphocytosis and increased protein concentration. Glucose levels usually remain within the healthy reference interval.

The presence of bacteria should be determined by Gram stain and culture of CSF. Viruses can be sought with appropriate serological tests or culture, and fungi can be found with culture or immunological procedures as well as with appropriate staining. For example, carefully performed india ink staining may reveal *Cryptococcus* species.

The CSF findings in syphilis depend on the stage of illness, disease activity, and whether previous treatment was given in adequate amounts. Pleocytosis is lymphotic or mononuclear in character, with white cell counts in the range of 100 to 1000/microliter. CSF protein levels may be elevated. CSF VDRL (Venereal Disease Research Laboratory) and serum FTA (fluorescent treponemal antibody) tests are usually positive, and oligoclonal bands may be present.

Organisms can invade the brain substance, in which case the term *encephalitis* is used. CSF findings are comparable to findings in meningitis or may be quite minimal.

Abscess formation in the brain may produce no CSF changes even though a potentially deadly infection is present.

Finally, any of the above conditions can and frequently do lead to increased CSF pressure. This is especially true of meningitis, which obstructs the usual flow of CSF, causing an obstructive hydrocephalus. Meningitis can also impair CSF absorption, causing a communicating hydrocephalus.

A variety of organisms that do not usually cause serious

infections in healthy individuals may produce life-threatening infections in patients whose immune system is compromised. Patients at risk for these "opportunistic" infections include those with acquired immunodeficiency syndrome (AIDS), cancer, or those taking immunosuppressant drugs for other reasons (for example, to treat an immune-mediated disease like myasthenia gravis).

AIDS is caused by the human immunodeficiency virus (HIV) and is invariably fatal. Direct HIV invasion of the nervous system may produce neurologic manifestations but AIDS also predisposes affected individuals to opportunistic infections and unusual malignant tumors that can involve the nervous system. Opportunistic infections, AIDS related neoplasms, or HIV can affect the brain, spinal cord or peripheral nerves; usually multiple sites are affected by multiple causes. With direct HIV infection of the CNS, oligoclonal bands and elevated protein concentrations are usually present in the CSF. The most common CNS tumors are lymphoma and metastatic Kaposi sarcoma. Common infections are toxoplasmosis, progressive multifocal leukoencephalopathy, fungal and mycobacterial granulomas, and herpes simplex virus encephalitis.

Lyme disease, first identified in 1975 by a cluster of cases in Old Lyme, Connecticut, is caused by a spirochete *(Borrelia burgdorferi)* and is spread through tick bites. Clinical symptoms include arthritis, meningitis, radiculitis, neuropathy, and in late stages, concentration, memory and sleep disorders. The diagnosis is made by organism specific IgG or IgM in the serum, but CSF typically shows elevated white blood cells and protein levels, and the measure of oligoclonal bands.

Inflammatory diseases

Multiple sclerosis and sarcoidosis are inflammatory CNS diseases of unknown cause. *Multiple sclerosis (MS)* is a disorder of unknown cause usually affecting young adults. MS produces numerous areas of demyelination in the CNS and is characterized by a waxing and waning but usually progressive course. The diagnosis of MS is best made by magnetic resonance imaging (MRI) by which approximately 90% of patients show white matter lesions. Examination of CSF, however, can clarify the diagnosis in many cases. Five major CSF abnormalities are seen in MS: (1) an elevation of up to 40 cells/mm^3 of white blood cells, (2) an elevation of protein up to 1000 mg/L, (3) elevation in IgG, (4) presence of oligoclonal bands, (5) elevation in myelin basic protein. However, none of these CSF abnormalities are specific for multiple sclerosis.

Sarcoidosis is a generalized disease of unknown cause that may affect the nervous system. Serum angiotensin-converting enzyme (ACE) is usually elevated and CSF shows elevations in protein concentration, cells, and occasionally decreased glucose levels.

Further information regarding infectious disorders of the nervous system can be found in general textbooks of neurology or infectious disease (see the bibliography).

Ischemia

Although immensely dependent on glucose for its energy source, the brain's own glucose reserves are small. With *oxygen* being available and the brain's metabolic needs being supplied by respiration using only glucose stored in the brain itself, those stores could supply the brain's needs for only 2 to 3 minutes. If *both* glucose and oxygen are cut off (as in ischemia) glycolysis becomes the dominant source of energy, and glucose stores in the brain can support its energy metabolism for only about 14 seconds. When energy metabolism ceases, the integrity of cellular membranes fails, potassium begins leaking from the cells, osmotic balance is lost, fluid rushes into the damaged cells, and within seconds cells begin to die.

The term *ischemia* can be defined as inadequate blood flow to a tissue. In the brain, ischemia can be present for many reasons. For example, if the heart stops, total cerebral blood flow ceases; if the blood pressure drops low enough, the flow of blood becomes inadequate; and if a single large vessel such as the carotid artery becomes narrowed, too little blood passes through. If a cerebral blood vessel becomes occluded by an embolus or an atherosclerotic plaque, the tissue that it irrigates becomes ischemic. Other blood vessels usually try to supply the area and make up the difference, but if the area of brain supplied by an occluded vessel cannot be supplied with blood from surrounding vessels, the cells in that area die. This is called a cerebral *infarction,* or a *stroke.*

Stroke

When a stroke occurs, the functions served by the infarcted region are damaged. For example, if the area controlling strength and movement in one extremity or one side of the body is infarcted, that extremity or side becomes weak or paralyzed. If the area subserving speech is damaged, the patient may lose the ability to talk or to comprehend what is heard. The dying or dead area of brain may release protein into the CSF. Because blood vessels in the area are also damaged by ischemia, some bleeding may occur. Only a few cells may appear in the CSF, if only a little blood has escaped from the area, or the CSF may become frankly bloody if an actual hemorrhage occurs in the damaged area. Finally, as the brain begins to clear away the damaged tissue, some white blood cells may appear in the CSF. In summary, then, after a stroke that has not involved significant hemorrhage, one can expect to find the CSF either normal or more likely containing an elevated protein level, a few red blood cells, and possibly some white blood cells.

Diffuse cerebral ischemia and hypoxia

If total cerebral circulation stops, as in cardiac arrest, consciousness is lost within 6 to 8 seconds. On the other hand, if oxygen supply becomes inadequate but circulation continues, the clinical result is usually a feeling of light-headedness followed by mental confusion in mild cases, proceeding to loss of consciousness, seizures, and coma with moderate to severe hypoxia. Precipitating events include pulmonary edema, carbon monoxide poisoning, pulmonary embolism, strangulation, respiratory failure during mechanical ventilation and exposure to ambient air at high altitudes. Failure to restore cerebral circulation and oxygenation within 4 to 5 minutes after their total cessation may result in cell death and irreversible damage.

Neuromuscular diseases (see also Chapter 31).

The term *neuromuscular disease* refers to disorders that affect peripheral nerves, neuromuscular junctions, or muscle cells, typically causing weakness, sensory loss, or loss of autonomic function. A detailed discussion of these disorders is beyond the scope of this chapter, but we will attempt to focus on laboratory aids in their diagnosis.

Peripheral nerve disorders are either hereditary or acquired. The diagnosis of hereditary *neuropathies* usually requires nerve biopsy for histologic evaluation of the nerve; however, neuropathy resulting from porphyria is frequently associated with elevated levels of delta-aminolevulinic acid and porphobilinogen in urine. Guillain-Barré syndrome (acute idiopathic demyelinating polyneuropathy) and its chronic form cause weakness and loss of reflexes, and have a characteristic CSF finding of elevated protein levels without elevated cell counts. Other causes of neuropathy where laboratory diagnosis is essential include diabetes (see Chapter 32), hypothyroidism (see below), vasculitis, uremia (see Chapter 26), hepatic dysfunction (see Chapter 27), or heavy metal (arsenic, lead, mercury, and thallium) poisoning. Infectious causes of neuropathy include AIDS, Lyme disease, herpes zoster, diphtheria and leprosy. Amyloidosis causing neuropathy can be secondary to a plasma cell dyscrasia or because of hereditary amyloidosis.

Myasthenia gravis is a disorder of the neuromuscular junction where antibodies are directed against the acetylcholine receptor. Patients have fluctuating weakness typically affecting the face, limbs, and eye movements. Approximately 85% of patients with active myasthenia will show elevated acetylcholine receptor antibody titers.

Muscle disorders can be hereditary or acquired. Hereditary forms of muscular dystrophy typically show elevated serum creatine kinase, aldolase, and lactate dehydrogenase. Recently a defect in the gene coding for a muscle protein called *dystrophin* has been found in the Duchenne and Becker forms of muscular dystrophies and may prove to be an important diagnostic test in these disorders. Periodic paralysis refers to a group of familial diseases of unknown cause characterized by attacks of generalized weakness with either high or low serum potassium concentrations. Myoglobinuria occurs when necrosis of muscle is acute and myoglobin from muscle escapes into the blood and then into the urine. Myoglobinuria can be caused by hereditary muscle disorders, seizures, trauma, ischemia, and toxic or metabolic disorders. Dermatomyositis and polymyositis are termed "inflammatory myopathies" and are associated with elevated erythrocyte sedimentation rate and elevated creatine kinase.

Neoplastic and paraneoplastic syndromes

Neoplasms affecting the CNS can be present in neural tissue (brain, cranial nerves, spinal cord or peripheral nerves) or related structures (skull, meninges, blood vessels, pituitary or pineal glands). Carcinomatous meningitis refers to invasion of the CSF and meninges by neoplastic cells. If the neoplasm arises directly from these structures, it is termed *primary;* it is termed *metastatic* if it has spread from a neoplasm elsewhere in the body. The symptoms that develop with various types of nervous system tumors are related to the nature of the tumor, its size, and its location. Approximately one third of patients with cerebral tumors will develop seizures.

Neoplasms outside the nervous system can produce paraneoplastic syndromes where nervous system function is affected without direct invasion. The most common neurologic paraneoplastic syndromes affect the cerebellum, peripheral nerves, or neuromuscular junction.

Modern imaging techniques such as MRI and computerized tomography (CT) can identify nervous system neoplasms with extraordinary accuracy. Laboratory diagnosis, however, can still be useful for certain neoplasms. The diagnosis of carcinomatous meningitis is made by examination of the CSF for neoplastic cells. Elevated CSF beta-glucuronidase and carcinoembryonic antigen (CEA) are also found in some cases.

Epilepsy

A seizure is a sudden and transient disturbance of mental function or body movements that results from an excessive electrical discharge by a group of brain cells. There are two main types of seizures: *focal onset* and *generalized onset.* Focal onset seizures begin in a discrete region of the brain and then have varying degrees and patterns of spread. Generalized onset seizures begin throughout the brain at once. The clinical manifestations of the seizure depend on the areas of the brain involved. For example, a focal onset seizure involving the motor cortex may manifest as twitching of one hand, whereas a seizure involving the temporal lobe may show alteration in consciousness with staring and memory loss (known as a *complex partial seizure*). Staring spells of generalized onset are known as *absence* or *petit mal seizures.* Either focal onset or generalized-onset seizures may spread to involve the entire brain and cause a *generalized tonic clonic seizure* with generalized motor activity, sometimes called a *convulsion* or *grand mal seizure.*

Focal-onset seizures are usually caused by some localized abnormality of the brain that can sometimes be identified by using brain-imaging procedures such as CT or MRI. Frequent causes of focal onset seizures include: stroke, brain tumors, birth injuries, or severe head injury. Generalized seizures can be idiopathic (no obvious cause) or symptomatic resulting from a generalized insult to the brain such as drug overdose, renal failure, encephalitis, or illicit drugs. The type and duration of treatment are determined by the seizure type and presumed cause. Each person who has seizures needs a careful evaluation by a physician searching for an underlying cause that can be corrected.

Persons with seizures are usually placed on antiepileptic drugs (AEDs) for months or even for the rest of their lives in an attempt to stop or at least reduce the frequency of seizures. Once treated most persons with seizures obtain excellent control and can live normal lives, and often the medication can be stopped after some period of time. However, about 30% to 40% of persons with seizures will obtain inadequate seizure control or have unacceptable side effects from AEDs.

Intoxication with drugs and poisons

Many drugs and poisons affect the nervous system directly, producing confusion, drowsiness, stupor, coma, seizures, or psychotic states. Drugs may also cause respiratory depression, alter the systemic metabolic balance, or otherwise indirectly damage the nervous system. In many cases, the differential diagnosis of these states requires laboratory confirmation of the presence of an offending drug or toxin. When specific drugs are known or suspected to be available to the patient, the search is simplified.

Physical findings may raise suspicion of a certain class of drugs; for example, small pupils are suggestive of the presence of opiates, and widely dilated pupils are suggestive of drugs with atropine-like effects such as tricyclic antidepressants or amphetamines with adrenergic actions. Unfortunately, many cases of intoxication involve multiple substances, whether "street" drugs or medications. For these cases or because the circumstances surrounding an ingestion are unclear, a *toxic screen* for common substances is necessary.

Metabolic diseases

A variety of metabolic disorders can affect the nervous system and usually present with episodic confusion, stupor or coma. Metabolic diseases affecting mental status include respiratory acidosis, hypoglycemia, ketoacidosis, nonketotic hyperosmolar coma, hepatic failure, renal failure, renal dialysis, and electrolyte disturbances. *Anoxic encephalopathy* occurs when there is a lack of oxygen delivery to the brain, caused by failure of respiration, circulation, or both. Mild degrees of hypoxia may produce only transient confusion, whereas severe degrees may cause coma sometimes with permanent brain injury. *Hypercapnia* (elevated pressure of CO_2 in the blood) can produce alterations in level of con-

sciousness. *Hypoglycemia* is an infrequent cause of CNS symptoms unless it is severe (plasma glucose below 250 to 300 mg/L (1.4 to 1.7 mmol/L) as may occur with insulin overdose, acute severe alcohol intoxication, or various conditions in children and neonates. Hyperglycemia uncommonly causes stupor or coma except when severe ketoacidosis or hyperosmolar nonketotic hyperglycemia occurs (see Chapter 32). Hepatic failure can cause impaired consciousness by elevating serum ammonia. Altered consciousness in patients with renal insufficiency can be attributable to uremia or to a "disequilibrium syndrome" associated with dialysis. Altered consciousness sometimes accompanied by seizures may result from a variety of electrolyte disturbances including (but not limited to) metabolic acidosis, hypernatremia and hyponatremia, hypokalemia and hypocalcemia.

Endocrine diseases

Adrenal disease. Inadequate release of cortisol affects the brain in ways that are complex and not well understood. In chronic untreated hypoadrenalism, apathy, depression, fatigue, and even mild delirium are common. Stupor and coma usually occur only when there is an abrupt severe worsening of chronic illness, the so-called *addisonian crisis*. Other metabolic derangements secondary to the hypoadrenalism such as hyponatremia, hyperkalemia, hypoglycemia, and hypotension may occur and produce additional CNS dysfunction.

Excess glucocorticoid products and the administration of steroid medications are associated in some patients with disturbances of mood (depression, elevation, or hypomania), mild confusion, delusion, hallucinations, impaired insight, and grossly inappropriate behavior.

Hypothyroidism. In the fetus and during infancy can cause irreversible brain damage and profound mental retardation (cretinism) unless the condition is corrected without delay. Chronic hypothyroidism is associated with depression or lability of mood, listlessness, confusion, and sometimes delusions and hallucinations (see Chapter 44). Peripheral neuropathy and unsteady gait related to impaired cerebellar functions also occur together with abnormal deep tendon reflexes. For obscure reasons, elevated CSF protein is a common finding in hypothyroidism. Severe hypothyroidism (myxedema coma) may cause decreased body temperature, slowed respiration, and hypometabolism, usually occurring in a setting of chronic hypothyroidism on which some acute event is superimposed, such as infection, surgery, trauma, or congestive heart failure. Because myxedema coma is rapidly fatal, correct diagnosis and prompt treatment are essential.

Signs of thyroid hypermetabolism (thyrotoxicosis) distinguish the state of thyroid excess that is associated with disturbances in thinking and emotion. Because the clinical appearance of thyroid disease can mimic psychiatric disease or CNS dysfunction, thyroid function tests are frequently ordered from psychiatric and emergency areas of the hospital.

PATHOLOGICAL CONDITIONS: PSYCHIATRIC
Schizophrenia

Description. Approximately 1% of the population is afflicted with the mixed group of chronic reoccuring disorders termed *schizophrenia* that usually start in young adulthood and persist throughout life. Schizophrenia disease patterns include active phases in which illogical thinking, delusions (fixed false beliefs), and auditory hallucinations with frequently threatening content and bizarre behavior may be prominent. Because of its chronic relapsing nature and the frequent gradual decline of the patient to function in a socially rational manner, the cost of care to society is tremendous. In the current classification of psychiatric disorders (DSM III-R) several subtypes, that is, disorganized, paranoid, undifferentiated, catatonic and residual type, are described.

Pathophysiology. The cause of this disorder remains unknown, and theories include developmental abnormalities and aberrant neurotransmitter function. Increased production of neurotransmitters in the mesolimbic dopaminergic pathway appears to be correlated with hallucinations and delusions, whereas decreased production in the mesocortical dopaminergic pathway is postulated to be associated with the autistic, withdrawn behavior and gradual decline in function in chronic schizophrenic patients (Davis 1991). Supporting this concept is the observation that at postmortem examination, the neurons of substantial numbers of chronic schizophrenic patients have an increased number of dopamine-related postsynaptic receptors.

Treatment. Antipsychotic medication ameliorates and stabilizes schizophrenic disorder; however, these medications seem to provide no cure. The mechanism by which these medications act on schizophrenic symptoms is poorly understood but they all share the blockade and antagonism of dopamine receptors to a variable extent. The most important side effects manifest as extrapyramidal syndromes such as dystonia; rigidity; the extreme form of neuroleptic malignant syndrome, that, if untreated can be lethal; sedation; orthostatic hypotension; dry mouth; urinary retention; and constipation caused by adrenergic and cholinergic blockade.

Affective disorders

Description. The affective disorders are diseases of mood regulation. Clinical symptoms may be *depression, mania* (abnormally elevated mood), or *bipolar disorder* (mood alternating between depression and mania). The manifestation of affective disorder, ranges from major depression and bipolar disorder where the episodic mood disorder is accompanied by changes in *neurovegetative* functions such as sleep, appetite, and energy and possibly including psychotic symptoms such as hallucinations and de-

lusions, to *dysthymic disorder* and *cyclothymia* in which the mood disorder appears long standing and less severe without prominent neurovegetative or psychotic symptoms.

The cause of major depression and bipolar disorder is more closely linked to a genetic and biological basis, whereas dysthymia and cyclothymia are more the result of life events and maladaptive behavior. Bipolar disorder appears to have a stronger genetic link than major depression because patients with bipolar disorder have an approximate 30% to 35% chance of another family member being afflicted with the disorder. In one genetic study of a familiar bipolar disorder a mutation was found on chromosome 11. This gene appears to be involved in the regulation of tyrosine hydroxylase, the rate-limiting enzyme for synthesis of norepinephrine and dopamine (Kaplan 1988).

Pathophysiology. In the past and at present, much effort has been invested in the search for a neurotransmitter disturbance as the underlying biochemical component for affective disorders. Some investigators characterize depression into serotonin-related and norepinephrine-related depressions.

Evidence for the role of serotonin in depressive disease comes from numerous reports of diminished quantities of its metabolite, 5-HIAA, in the cerebrospinal fluid of depressed patients; furthermore 5-hydroxytryptophan (5-HT), a precursor of serotonin, is an effective antidepressant only in depressed patients with decreased cerebrospinal fluid 5-HIAA. However, only patients with a recent suicide attempt consistently have decreased cerebrospinal 5-HIAA.

Norepinephrine appears critically important in affective disorders. The presence of large norepinephrine-containing cells in specific areas of the brain is suggestive of the possibility of a critical regulating role of norepinephrine in a variety of neurovegetative changes that are important in depression: appetite, sexual function, sleep, and cognition. Depressed patients have been shown to have abnormally low levels of CSF norepinephrine and urinary MHPG, half of which has its origin from central nervous system norepinephrine metabolism. Patients with decreased urinary MHPG excretion often respond to antidepressants that selectively inhibit the reuptake of norepinephrine into the presynaptic neuron. As a consequence of this reuptake inhibition more norepinephrine is available in the synaptic cleft to act on the postsynaptic receptor, correcting the central norepinephrine deficiency.

Treatment. The primary treatment of depression has been the tricyclic antidepressants, which to a variable degree bind to both presynaptic and postsynaptic noradrenergic and serotoninergic receptors in the synaptic cleft. The mechanism of action of these medications appears to be a competitive blockade of these receptors, which become unavailable for norepinephrine and serotonin to bind to, resulting in increased availability of neurotransmitter. Antidepressant drugs that are relatively selective in inhibition of neuronal reuptake of norepinephrine include desipramine, protriptyline and maprotiline (see Table 42-2). Pharmacological agents such as amitriptyline, trazodone and fluoxetine, which are effective in the treatment of depression, have been shown to inhibit selectively the neuronal reuptake of 5-HT from the synapse, though this is not their only pharmacologic effect. Most other antidepressants, except bupropion, are believed to act by increasing the availability of these neurotransmitters. On the other hand, the monoamine oxidase inhibiters work by irreversibly inhibiting cytoplasmic monoamine oxidase A and B in the presynaptic neuron and thus inhibiting the break down norepinephrine, serotonin, and dopamine. This inhibition takes place within 5-10 days after start of medication and makes more neurotransmitter available for neuronal transmission. Apart from treating episodes of depression with antidepressants and manic episodes with sedating medication such as benzodiazepines and antipsychotics, the main treatment for bipolar disorder is with lithium which has nonspecific membrane-stabilizing properties. Carbamazepine and valproate are medications introduced as antiepileptic drugs, but both have been shown to have some effect in bipolar disorder.

Anxiety disorders

Anxiety disorders have as their hallmark pervasive chronic or paroxysmal feelings of apprehension that are often accompanied by physical signs such as sweating, shortness of breath, increased heart rate, and restlessness.

The range of anxiety disorders includes generalized *anxiety disorder* with chronic fears, anxiety, and physical symptoms; *panic disorder*, with well-circumscribed anxiety attacks provoked by situations such as open spaces or certain objects; and *obsessive compulsive disorder*, with pervasive or repetitive worries (obsessions) and repetitive actions (compulsions), both beyond the person's ability to control.

The pathophysiologic characteristics of anxiety disorders is poorly understood at the present time, and a variety of biological, genetic, and behavioral theories exist. Research into neurotransmitter systems is focused on the noradrener-

gic and GABA-ergic systems. Drugs such as benzodiazepines increase the affinity of GABA for the receptor complex.

Treatment. Pharmacological treatment of generalized anxiety disorder and panic disorder is by drugs that affect the noradrenergic system and probably downregulate its activity. Such drugs are beta-adrenergic receptor blockers, tricyclic antidepressants, monoamine oxidase inhibitors, and benzodiazepines. Benzodiazepines bind to specific receptor sites throughout the brain and spinal cord. These binding sites are coupled to a GABA-receptor complex that mediates the anxiolytic, sedative, and antiepileptic action for which there might be specific receptors on the complex.

Obsessive compulsive disorder, which was long believed to respond best to psychotherapy, shows impressive improvement on administration of drugs such as clomipramine and fluoxetine affecting mostly serotonin pathways but to a small and essential extent norepinephric pathways.

FUNCTION TEST
Dexamethasone suppression test

Cortisol, the major corticosteroid hormone, is secreted by the adrenal glands in a circadian rhythm, with a peak occurring in the early morning hours. Production of this hormone is regulated by the release of pituitary ACTH, which in turn is under the control of CRH (corticotropin-releasing hormone) that is produced by the hypothalamus (see pp. 918 and 919 for details). Under physiologic conditions cortisol production is suppressed by the presence of even small amounts of exogenous corticosteroids such as dexamethasone.

The dexamethasone suppression test was originally used for the evaluation of the hypothalamic pituitary axis in Cushing's syndrome (see p. 925). It was subsequently shown that a subgroup of depressed patients who mainly displayed features of unipolar depression or psychoses had an abnormal response to the dexamethasone depression test; that is, unsuppressed cortisol levels after dexamethasone administration. Since then it has been postulated that depressed patients with abnormal dexamethasone suppression tests respond to standard antidepressant medication better than those patients with a normal dexamethasone suppression test response. It has further been shown that the normalization of the dexamethasone suppression test after treatment of depression correlates with the degree of clinical response. On the other hand, depression in the absence of dexamethasone suppression normalization carries with it the risk of early relapse, should antidepressant medication be discontinued.

Description of test. In the dexamethasone suppression test 1 mg of dexamethasone (a synthetic corticosteroid) is administered orally around bedtime and plasma cortisol levels are measured at 4 and 11 P.M. the following day (see p. 925). Plasma cortisol levels of over 50 µg/liter are abnormal and are suggestive that depression will respond to an

Table 42-2   Site of action of some antidepressants

	Reuptake blockade		Receptor blockade		
	NE	5-HT	Muscarinic ACh	H₁	H₂
Imipramine	+	+	++	±	±
Desipramine	+++	±	±	−	−
Trimipramine	±	±	++	++	?
Amitriptyline	±	++	+++	++	++
Nortriptyline	++	±	+	±	±
Protriptyline	+++	±	+	+++	−
Amoxapine	++	±	+	±	?
Doxepin	+	±	++	+++	+
Maprotiline	+++	−	+	±	?

From Kaplan H, Sadock B: *Clinical psychiatry,* Baltimore, 1988, Williams & Wilkins.
ACh, Acetylcholine; *H,* histamine; *5-HT,* 5-hydroxytryptophan; *NE,* norepinephrine.

tidepressant medications. The best predictive value of this test appears to be in the setting of patients who suffer from unipolar depression with psychotic or melancholic features. The test is not used routinely but may be helpful in selected cases.

CHANGE OF ANALYTE IN DISEASE: NONDRUG ANALYTES (Table 42-3)
Appearance of cerebrospinal fluid

CSF is normally crystal clear and free from all pigmentation, that is, "clear and colorless." One should examine it in a glass tube while comparing it with a tube of water while both are held in white light against a pure white background. It is best to look down the long axis of the tube. At least 1 mL of fluid should be observed.

A red blood cell count of 500/mm^3 gives a pink or yellow tinge to the fluid. White counts of 200/mm^3 will give a slightly cloudy appearance. Xanthochromia (a yellow tinge) will appear when blood has been mixed with CSF. This yellowing does not occur immediately but requires from 2 to 4 hours. A "traumatic" lumbar puncture occurs when the lumbar puncture needle pierces small blood vessels near the spinal cord coverings and blood enters the CSF collection tubes. Since blood in the CSF may represent subarachnoid bleeding or may be simply the result of a traumatic lumbar puncture (a common occurrence), the CSF sample should be centrifuged immediately. If this is done promptly, bleeding that is caused by a traumatic lumbar puncture should produce no xanthochromia. Xanthochromia indicates that the bleeding may have occurred at least 2 to 4 hours before observation of the sample. As many as 10% of patients with subarachnoid hemorrhage actually have clear CSF at 12 hours, but beyond that time 100% will show xanthochromia if the sample is examined carefully. A more sensitive technique, such as second deviative spectrophotometry, can increase the ability to detect low levels of xanthochromia.

Protein concentrations greater than 1500 mg/L will also give a slightly xanthochromic appearance to CSF. Hemoglobin from hemolyzed red blood cells will appear in CSF after about 10 hours. When a patient is jaundiced (that is, when serum bilirubin is elevated, as it may be in liver failure), bilirubin may enter the CSF. However, this requires serum bilirubin levels of at least 100 to 150 mg/L before CSF xanthochromia is found.

Proteins of cerebrospinal fluid

In disease states the local production or modification of proteins within the CNS may lead to diagnostically useful changes in CSF protein patterns. In general, diseases that interrupt the integrity of the capillary endothelial barrier lead to an increase in total CSF protein. Examples are brain tumor, purulent (bacterial) meningitis, cerebral infarction, and trauma.

Immunoelectrophoresis allows further fractionation of CSF protein constituents. The major *immunoglobulins* in CSF are IgG, IgA, and IgM (with only trace amounts of IgD and IgE). Of all these, IgG is quantitatively the most important. It is often useful to know whether an elevated IgG value is caused by local production of that immunoglobulin within the CNS (as may be the case in some demyelinating diseases such as multiple sclerosis) or by the leakage of IgG across a damaged blood-brain barrier (as in some infections). Since the normal serum IgG is 15% to 18% of total serum protein and normal CSF IgG is 5% to 12%, the ratio of IgG to total protein is sometimes used to estimate the source of IgG elevation. That is, if the ratio in a sample more nearly approximates the ratio ordinarily found in serum, one tends to suspect that the IgG has been somehow transferred into the CSF from serum. But this is a crude and not especially reliable estimate. A more widely used measure currently is the IgG-albumin index. The formula for determining it is as follows:

$$\text{IgG index} = \frac{\text{IgG (CSF)} \times \text{Albumin (serum)}}{\text{IgG (serum)} \times \text{Albumin (CSF)}}$$

Table 42-3 Change of analyte in CNS disease

Disease	Analyte in CNS					
	Glucose	Total protein	IgG	IgG index	Xanthochromia	Lactic acid
Stroke (cerebral infarction)	N	↑	N	↓	N, ↑	N, ↑
Hemorrhage	N	N, ↑↑	N	N	↑↑	N
Epilepsy	N	N	N	N	N	N
CNS tumor	N, ↓	↑	N, ↑	↓	N, ↑	N, ↑
Infection						
Fungal, bacterial	↓	↑	↑	↑	N	↑
Viral	N	N	↑	↑	N	N
Coma	↑↑ hyperosmolar ↓ hypoglycemia	↑ (trauma)	N	N	N, ↑ (trauma) N	N
Meningitis, viral	N	N, ↑	N, ↑	↑	N	N

N, Little or no change; ↑, increase; ↑↑, large increase; ↓, decrease.

The upper reference interval for this index must be determined for each laboratory, but generally it ranges between 0.25 and 0.85. The IgG index is elevated in diseases in which there is increased CNS IgG production and an intact blood-brain barrier (as in multiple sclerosis). The IgG index is decreased when the blood-brain barrier is compromised, allowing serum proteins to cross into the CSF (as in strokes, tumors, and some forms of meningitis).

Myelin basic protein (MBP) concentration increase in serum is a potential indicator of demyelination. Myelin is a complex substance that surrounds many CNS axons like the insulation on a wire cable and is necessary for normal conduction of nerve impulses down the axon. *Demyelinating diseases* are a group of disorders in which the primary insult is some form of damage to the myelin coating of CNS axons. MBP is a constituent of normal myelin, and has been found to be elevated in a variety of conditions involving myelin damage. Initially it was believed that MBP was specific for multiple sclerosis, but it is now known to be elevated in many CNS disorders.

Gamma globulin synthesis

Elevations of CSF gamma globulin may be caused by changes in serum proteins, such as the small-molecular-weight Bence Jones proteins seen in multiple myeloma, which cross the blood-brain barrier and appear in the gamma fraction of CSF proteins. However, there is evidence that local CNS immunoglobulin production occurs in many diseases. Examples include multiple sclerosis, subacute sclerosing panencephalitis (a rare devastating process of myelin damage that occurs in children and young adults in association with greatly elevated CSF measles titers), many chronic and acute infections (neurosyphilis, tuberculous meningitis, abscess, viral meningoencephalitis, and sarcoidosis), and some brain tumors. As a practical point, in those settings in which CSF total protein rises as a result of increased permeability of the blood-brain barrier, the addition of serum protein (which normally contains 15% to 18% gamma globulin) raises the CSF gamma fraction. It thus becomes difficult to estimate the upper reference interval for gamma globulin as a percentage of total protein when total protein is significantly elevated. In any case, when CSF gamma globulin is elevated, a clinician may order a simultaneous serum protein electrophoresis to help determine the source of the increased CSF gamma fraction.

Oligoclonal bands

The gamma fraction of CSF is composed of a variety of immunoglobulins. Agarose gel electrophoresis performed on concentrated CSF can demonstrate elevation of a population of proteins within the gamma range. When these proteins all share the same electrophoretic mobility they are called *oligoclonal bands*. The population of gamma proteins that separates as oligoclonal bands is believed to derive from a few clones of immunocompetent cells. The appearance of oligoclonal bands has been reported in 79% to 90% of patients with multiple sclerosis and in a variety of CNS inflammatory conditions. Interestingly, this change in the composition of the gamma fraction may occur without any increase in the total gamma globulin concentration.

A final practical point should be made about protein determinations in CSF. When there is blood in the CSF from a traumatic lumbar puncture or bleeding within the nervous system, one expects that the blood will elevate the CSF protein value. One can still determine the CSF protein level by correcting for the amount of blood present. Simply allow 10 mg/L of protein for every 1000 red blood cells/mm^3. For example, if the red cell count is 10,000 in the CSF sample and its total protein is 1000 mg/L, the corrected total protein equals 900 mg/L. The cell count should be performed as rapidly as possible after lumbar puncture, preferably in the first half hour and certainly not later than 2 hours, since hemolysis will occur after that time.

Glucose in cerebrospinal fluid (see the methods, p. 635, Chapter 32)

Determination of CSF glucose helps distinguish bacterial from viral meningitis; the glucose value is often quite *low* (less than 40% to 45% of simultaneously analyzed serum glucose) in bacterial meningitis and tuberculous meningitis and is generally normal in viral disease. Carcinomatous meningitis (widespread infiltration of the meninges by tumor cells) also drives CSF glucose values below the normal range.

Thyroid function tests (see the methods, p. 886)

Diseases of the thyroid gland can result in changes of mood that are difficult to distinguish from psychiatric illnesses. Therefore, as part of the diagnostic evaluation of patients newly admitted to psychiatric wards, thyroid tests are ordered to rule out thyroid imbalance as a cause (see p. 886 for recommended thyroid testing).

Toxicology screen (see the methods, p. 1026)

One of the causes of abnormal behavior is the presence of drugs or toxins in the afflicted patient. A urine drug screen is frequently ordered by emergency unit physicians to establish drugs as a cause of acute psychoses. These are usually focused to search for a limited number of abused stimulant drugs, such as amphetamines, cocaine and phencyclidine. Less frequent causes of abnormal behavior or neurologic symptoms are the result of heavy metal poisoning. In these cases, analyses of blood lead and urine mercury may be requested.

3-Methoxy-4-hydroxyphenylglycol (MHPG). The amount of MHPG excreted in 24-hour urine collections is believed to reflect noradrenergic activity in the brain. MHPG excretion of less than 1400 ng in males and less than 1200 ng in females in 24 hours is suggestive of depression caused by noradrenergic deficiency (Beckman

1975). Thus, in theory, depressed patients with low 24-hour MHPG excretion respond best to antidepressant medications, such as desipramine, nortriptyline, and protriptyline, that increase the availability of norepinephrine as a neurotransmitter in the brain. However, in clinical practice the use of urinary MHPG is limited because the patient must be kept drug-free from psychotropic medication for a 2-week period before MHPG measurements can be obtained.

5-Hydroxyindoleacetic acid (5-HIAA). 5-HIAA can be measured in the cerebrospinal fluid typically by a lumbar puncture performed in the morning hours. Levels of less than 15 ng/mL are suggestive of depressive disorder caused by a deficiency of the neurotransmitter serotonin. Depressive disorders can be subtyped into those with low, medium, and high MHPG levels (Schildkraut 1982). If both MHPG and 5-HIAA are evaluated two subgroups of depressive disorders emerge: (1) one group with low levels of norepinephrine but high serotonin metabolites and that show a favorable response to drugs increasing noradrenergic activity, and (2) a second group with high levels of norepinephrine but low serotonin metabolites and that show a favorable response to drugs increasing serotonin activity (Goodwin 1978). Urinary MHPG and cerebrospinal 5-HIAA levels remain an intriguing research tool to identify depression subtypes and treatment response but are not routinely used in clinical practice.

CHANGE OF ANALYTE IN DISEASE: THERAPEUTIC DRUG MONITORING

Therapeutic drug monitoring (TDM) is essential in optimally managing many neurologic and psychiatric disorders. The clinician can more readily assess efficacy, toxicity, drug interactions, or the effect of generic substitution when the plasma concentration of the drug is known (see Chapter 56). More advanced tests, such as unbound plasma concentra-

tion or measurement of active metabolites, can further refine patient management.

Antiepileptic drugs (see pp. 605-615 in Pesce AJ, Kaplan LA: *Methods in clinical chemistry*)

Among neurologists, measurement of plasma concentrations of antiepileptic drugs (AEDs) is probably the most widely used laboratory test. Table 42-4 presents pharmacokinetic data on the most commonly used AEDs. The "therapeutic range" is an important concept but should be used only as a general guide in patient management. The goal of treatment is control of seizures without toxic side effects, and many patients achieve this goal with plasma concentrations of AEDs either below or above the "therapeutic range." Furthermore, several recent studies show that most patients taking a single AED can tolerate plasma concentrations above the "therapeutic range" and obtain improved seizure control (Lesser 1984). Thus, AED plasma concentrations can be quite useful to the clinician; however, decisions about patient management should always combine information about the patient's clinical state with plasma-concentration data.

Plasma concentrations of AEDs should always be interpreted with knowledge of whether the patient has taken the drug over a long enough period of time to have reached a steady-state concentration, especially with AEDs that have a longer half-life (Table 42-4). This is even more important in the case of phenytoin, which shows saturable metabolism and can have a half-life that ranges from a few days to several weeks, depending on the plasma concentration. AEDs with a shorter half-life (valproate or carbamazepine) may show substantial variation between peak and trough concentrations. Carbamazepine plasma concentrations may fall after the first 2 to 3 weeks of use because of the drug's induction of liver enzymes that speed its metabolism. Plasma concentrations of AEDs that

Table 42-4 Commonly used antiepileptic drugs

Antiepileptic drug	Common trade name	"Recommended" therapeutic range* (μg/mL)	Approximate time to steady state (days)	Other features
Phenytoin	Dilantin	10-20	3-21†	Highly protein bound
Carbamazepine	Tegretol	4-12	3-5	Active metabolite
Primidone	Mysoline	5-12	1-2	Active metabolite
Phenobarbital	—	10-40	15-25	—
Valproate/divalproex	Depakene/Depakote	50-100	2-5	Active metabolites; saturable protein binding
Ethosuximide	Zarontin	40-100	7-13	—
Clonazepam	Klonopin	13-72 (ng/mL)	4-8	—
Felbamate	Felbatol	Not established	4-5	Acts as hepatic enzyme inhibitor, increasing concentrations of most other AED; associated with aplastic anemia
Gabapentin	Neurontin	Not established	1-2	Renal elimination; no metabolism

*See text.
†Exhibits saturable metabolism, and so time to steady state increases as plasma concentration increases.

Table 42-5   Commonly used antidepressant drugs

Antidepressant drug	Common trade name	Therapeutic plasma level (μg/mL)	Half-life (hours)	Other features
Tricyclic antidepressants				
Amitriptyline	Elavil	150-500*	24	Highly anticholinergic
Nortriptyline	Pamelor	50-150	24	
Doxepin	Sinequan	150-500	24	High antihistaminic
Imipramine	Tofranil	150-500†	24	
Desipramine	Norpramin	150-500	24	Low anticholinergic activity
Amoxapine	Asendin	150-250	24	Loxapine (neuroleptic metabolite)
Monoamine oxidase inhibitors				
Isocarboxazid	Marplan	N/A	8-10	
Phenelzine	Nardil	N/A	8-10	
Tranylcypromine	Parnate	N/A	8-10	Stimulatory effect
Atypical antidepressants				
Trazodone	Desyrel	N/A	8-10	Potential priapism
Fluoxetine	Prozac	N/A	48-72	Metabolite with long half-life
Sertraline	Zoloft	N/A	—	

*Measurement includes amitriptyline and its metabolite, nortriptyline.
†Measurement includes imipramine and its metabolite, desipramine.

cause toxicity are generally close to concentrations that are needed for seizure control; thus, frequent plasma AED determinations may be necessary when generic AED substitutions are used.

Measurement of non–protein bound (free) AED plasma concentrations are useful when patients receive phenytoin or valproate in combination with other drugs, in patients with renal or hepatic failure, or in patients with hypoalbuminemia. In these instances the free plasma drug concentration may increase and produce toxic symptoms while the total plasma concentration remains unchanged. Active metabolites of primidone, carbamazepine (especially carbamazepine 10,11-epoxide), and possibly valproate can produce toxicity, and measurement of these metabolites may improve patient management in selected cases.

Antipsychotic medication

Antipsychotics, also known as *neuroleptics,* are a heterogeneous group of medications used to treat psychotic disorders such as schizophrenia, depression, dementia, and nonspecific agitation. They may also be useful in a variety of movement disorders such as Huntington's Disease and Gilles de la Tourette's syndrome.

Neuroleptics include the drug class phenothiazines, all of which share the three-ring phenothiazine structure but differ in the side-chain varieties (see Table 42-5).

Clozapine is the only dibenzodiazepine in use in the United States, and patients receiving clozapine are followed with bimonthly white blood cell counts.

Another major group of neuroleptics are the butyrophenones such as droperidol, haloperidol and pimozide, which have structures dissimilar to those of the phenothiazines. At present haloperidol is the most widely prescribed neuroleptic in the United States.

In contrast to antidepressant and antiepileptic medications, an efficacious response to most neuroleptic medication is not linked to a certain blood concentration of the drug.

It has been suggested that a plasma level of 5 to 20 ng/mL is the optimal therapeutic window for haloperidol treatment of psychotic symptoms and schizophrenia. Haloperidol levels above 20 ng/mL are linked to subjective and objective medication side effects such as dysphoria, hypotension and parkinsonian effects (extrapyramidal), which may interfere with a therapeutic response.

Antidepressant medications

Tricyclic antidepressants (pp. 667 to 677 in Pesce AJ, Kaplan LA: *Methods in clinical chemistry*). Apart from reuptake blockade of serotonin and norepinephrine, the tricyclic antidepressant medications block alpha-adrenergic, muscarinic, and histaminic receptors to a variable degree resulting in the medication side effects such as orthostatic hypotension, dry mouth, constipation, and sedation (see Table 42-5).

The dosage range for most tricyclic antidepressants usually lies between 75 and 300 mg/day, depending on age, body weight, liver, and renal function. The notable exceptions are nortriptyline and protriptyline, both of which have dosage requirements between 50 and 150 mg/day. The linkage between plasma levels of tricyclics and their clinical response appears clearest in patients with major depression. For most tricyclic antidepressants, the relationship between response and plasma level appears sigmoidal (Fig. 42-6). Yet, for nortriptyline and to a lesser extent protriptyline, the

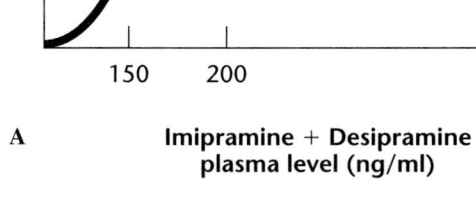

A   **Imipramine + Desipramine**
     plasma level (ng/ml)

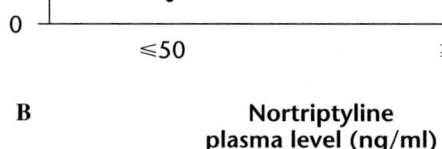

B   **Nortriptyline**
     plasma level (ng/ml)

Fig. 42-6 **A,** Sigmoidal relationships between clinical response and imipramine plus desipramine plasma levels. **B,** Curvilinear relationship between clinical response and nortriptyline plasma levels. (From Schatzberg AF, Cole JO: *Manual of clinical psychopharmacology,* Washington, D.C., 1986, American Psychiatric Press.)

relationship is curvilinear, and when plasma levels are above the therapeutic range the clinical response falls dramatically and side effects are more prominent.

Monoamine oxidase inhibitors. There are two classes of monoamine oxidase inhibitors: the *hydrazine class,* which includes isocarboxazid and phenelzine, and the *nonhydrazine class,* which includes tranylcypromine. The clinical effects of these and other antidepressant medications take 2 to 3 weeks to develop for reasons that are not understood. The side effects and dietary restrictions required for patients receiving the monoamine oxidase inhibitors has limited use of this class of drug. Tyramine, which is usually broken down in the gastrointestinal tract by monoamine oxidase A, must be eliminated from the diet, otherwise rapid and dangerous elevation of blood pressure can occur. Tyramine is found in large quantities in cured foods such as beer, wine, cheese and sausage. Other side effects include orthostatic hypotension, muscle pain attributable to vitamin B_6 deficiency, and agitation or insomnia. There is no relationship between medication plasma level and response rate.

Atypical antidepressants

This group includes *trazodone,* which is a potent serotonin reuptake inhibitor; *bupropion,* which is a dopamine blocker; *fluoxetine,* which has mostly serotonin but also some norepinephrine reuptake blockade; and *sertraline,* which is a pure serotonin reuptake blocker. Since the introduction of fluoxetine on the United States market in 1988, it has become the most widely prescribed antidepressant. These medications differ from other antidepressants in that they lack a ring structure and have fewer side effects. Trazodone

is noted for its potential side effect of priapism, which occurs in one of 10,000 males treated and may require emergency treatment.

Anxiolytics

Anxiolytics are a group of medications used for treatment of anxiety disorders. The medications included in this group are *benzodiazepines* and *buspirone.* All benzodiazepines share the same three-ring structure, but differ mainly in substitutions on the heptagonal ring. There are three established subgroups: (1) the 2-ketobenzodiazepines including chlordiazepoxide, diazepam, and prazepam, which are oxidized in the liver to desmethyldiazepam (active metabolite) with a half-life of 60 hours, (2) the 3-hydroxybenzodiazepines (oxazepam, lorazepam and temazepam), metabolized in the liver with a half-life of 9 to 15 hours, and (3) the triazolobenzodiazepines (alprazolam and triazolam), metabolized in the liver with a 3- to 8-hour half-life.

The most common side effects include sedation at low doses, ataxia at higher doses, and respiratory suppression at toxic doses. Generally, it is believed that these drugs have a wide safety margin and overdose only rarely leads to lethal outcome. An important recent development is the availability of a benzodiazepine antagonist, flumazenil, which can be used acutely in benzodiazepine overdose.

Dosage for the individual benzodiazepines differs widely, from 6 mg/day for alprazolam to 200 mg/day for chlordiazepoxide. Unlike other psychiatric medications discussed in this section, benzodiazepines have potentially strong addictive properties causing psychological and physical drug dependence and possible withdrawal upon cessation of the drug. Therapeutic plasma concentrations of benzodiazepines have not been established, except for clonazepam, which is also used as an antiepileptic.

Apart from the benzodiazepines, buspirone is the other commonly used class of anxiolytics. It is a nonbenzodiazepine, nonsedating anxiolytic. This drug probably does not act directly through the GABA receptor complex. It is believed that its anxiolytic effects might be mediated by dopaminergic pathways. The daily dosage ranges from 5 to 40 mg. Side effects upon use include nausea and headaches. Plasma levels are not in use at the present time.

Mood stabilizers

This group of drugs includes lithium carbonate, carbamazepine, valproate, and clonazepam. Their therapeutic use in psychiatry is for treatment of bipolar disorder, schizoaffective disorder, explosive disorders, and unstable behavior related to personality disorders.

Physiologically *lithium* ions (see the methods, p. 1107 are indistinguishable from sodium and replaces sodium along cell membranes. The exact mode of lithium action is unknown. Because lithium replaces sodium throughout the whole body, its side effects may involve most organ systems. Neurological effects such as tremor, ataxia, confusion, sedation at higher and toxic levels, and encephalopathy in conjunction with haloperidol administration have been described. Long-term lithium treatment can result in hyperthyroidism from a nontoxic goiter. Renal effects such as polyuria with secondary polydipsia, renal diabetes insipidus, and interstitial nephritis are also occasionally seen.

Dosage range is 600 to 2100 mg/day in two or three divided doses. Plasma levels should be measured approximately 12 hours after the previous dose to obtain a trough value. Plasma levels from 0.8 to 1.5 mEq/L have been shown to produce a therapeutic response in the treatment of acute mania. Slightly lower lithium levels have been recommended for maintenance treatment of bipolar disorders and treatment of other conditions. The plasma level of lithium which can be achieved and maintained is often limited by subjective side effects and by development of thyroid or renal impairment.

Carbamazepine, valproate, and *clonazepam* are used as antiepileptics but recently have found increasing use in psychiatry for disorders such as rapid cycling bipolar disorder and explosive disorder. They are generally used as an alternative to lithium, but recent studies suggest that they can be used as first-line medication.

The dosage and plasma level ranges, particularly for valproate and carbamazepine, are similar to their use as antiepileptics.

Tricyclic antidepressants are absorbed from the gastrointestinal tract to a variable and incomplete degree. Protein binding appears to be 75%, and the medications are highly lipid soluble. In the liver, tertiary amines (amitriptyline and imipramine) are desmethylated to secondary amines (nor-

triptyline and desipramine) which are active metabolites. Half-life lies between 10 hours and 70 hours and can be even longer as with nortriptyline and protriptyline. Steady-state plasma levels are achieved within 5 to 7 days, and once-a-day dosage is possible.

Monoamine oxidase inhibitors are completely absorbed in the gastrointestinal tract. Metabolism occurs in the liver by acetylation. The half-life is extremely variable because up to 50% of whites and more than 50% of people of Asian descent are slow acetylators. Dosage range is from 30 to 50 mg for isocarboxazide and tranylcypromine to 45 to 90 mg for phenelzine per day.

Fluoxetine has a half-life of 24 to 72 hours and is broken down into a desmethylated metabolite with a half-life of 7 to 15 days. Trazodone and bupropion have a much shorter half-life of 8 to 12 hours and, unlike most other antidepressants, have to be given either two or three times per day.

METHODS OF ANALYSIS
Barbiturates
MARK W. LINDER

Principles of analysis and current usage Barbiturates are hypnotic drugs that act as sedatives or analgesics (painkillers) and are also used to help control seizure disorders. Phenobarbital, one member of this class of drugs, is frequently prescribed for the control of epilepsy. Quantitation of this compound is probably the most frequently performed analysis in the clinical laboratory for this group of drugs. In addition to their legitimate use in the treatment of various medical conditions, barbiturates are also abused substances.

Both qualitative and quantitative assays may be performed for barbiturate determinations. The type of assay that is performed is determined by the medical condition that is being evaluated. Qualitative tests, typically performed in patients with suspected drug overdose, are useful because of their rapid performance and their ability to react with any drug of the barbiturate class. Quantitative barbiturate analyses are performed to establish proper therapeutic levels. The quantitative analyses utilize blood as specimen, since blood concentrations correspond most closely with pharmacologic effect, whereas qualitative analyses typically employ urine or gastric contents as specimen.

Some qualitative procedures for barbiturate require extraction of the drug followed by analysis by colorimetric or ultraviolet spectroscopy and chromatographic techniques, such as thin-layer chromatography (TLC), gas chromatography (GC), and high-performance liquid chromatography (HPLC).

The most common qualitative procedures in use today are the immunoassay methods and chromatographic procedures such as TLC and HPLC. The immunoassay of urine by EMIT (Table 42-6, method 1) is currently the most widely used procedure to screen for barbiturates. The EMIT assay is described on p. 262. The amount of enzyme activity in the EMIT assay is directly related to the amount of drug present in the specimen.

Table 42-6 Methods for barbiturate analysis

Method	Principle	Usage	Comments
1. EMIT (enzyme multiplied immunoassay technique)	Antibody competes for unbound and enzyme labeled drug. Binding of antibody to enzyme-labeled drug causes drug loss of functional enzyme activity. Loss of enzyme activity is monitored through reduction in formation of measurable product (i.e., NADH).	Serum, urine	Most widely used Both qualitative and quantitative procedures
2. HPLC (high-performance liquid chromatography)	Barbiturates are identified by retention time and ultraviolet absorption characteristics.	Blood, plasma, serum, urine, gastric contents	Both qualitative and quantitative analyses Can be used to quantitate several antiepileptic drugs simultaneously.
3. FPIA (fluorescence polarization immunoassay)	Competition between labeled and unlabeled drug for antibody. Bound labeled drug has higher polarized fluorescence than free. Amount of polarized fluorescence inversely proportional to specimen drug concentration.	Serum, plasma	Frequently used Precise
4. Nephelometric inhibition	Competitive inhibition of precipitation	Serum	Requires specialized instrumentation
5. Turbidimetric inhibition	Competitive inhibition of insoluble particle–phenobarbital–antibody aggregates. Rate of particle aggregation is inversely proportional to sample phenobarbital concentration.	Serum, plasma	

Devices developed for point of care testing allow for visual detection of barbiturates and other abused drugs (Triage, Biosite Diagnostics, San Diego, California).[1] This device utilizes colloid gold particles conjugated to the drug or drugs of interest and monoclonal antibodies directed toward these drugs. Addition of a specimen containing a drug(s) allows competition between drugs in urine and the drug bound to gold colloid for binding sites on the antibody. If the specimen contains a drug above a set concentration limit of the system, some of the drug bound to the gold colloid will not be covered with antibody. Colloid-bound drug will remain covered with antibody in the presence of specimens with little or no drug. The reaction mixture is transferred to a nylon membrane with additional bound antibody. Specimens with drug present will have the antibody gold-colloid complex pass through the membrane whereas specimens with no drug will have the gold-colloid pass through the membrane. Binding of the gold colloid to the nylon membrane results in the appearance of a colored bar that appears in the area containing antibody directed toward the drug of interest.

Chromatographic procedures using TLC were once widely used to detect barbiturates as well as other drugs. Both serum and urine may be used as specimen. Although this method is relatively inexpensive to perform, it is very labor intensive and requires a high degree of skill to interpret. The presence of the drug of interest is detected by its characteristic extent of migration on the chromatographic strip, along with its characteristic color under white light and ultraviolet radiation after the reaction of the drug with various reagents (see p. 618 in Pesce AJ, Kaplan LA: *Methods in clinical chemistry*).

The development of a dedicated HPLC system for drug detection (REMEDi System, Bio-Rad Laboratories Inc., Hercules, California) has enabled this type of chromatographic separation of drugs to be carried out more readily in clinical laboratories (Table 42-6, method 2). Both serum and urine can be analyzed with minimal sample preparation. Unfortunately the sensitivity of the system for detecting barbiturates in urine is unacceptable. Also the system is subject to interference and misidentification of drugs caused by coeluting compounds.[2]

Quantitative tests for barbiturates typically include a variety of immunoassay techniques. The quantitative immunoassay procedures are normally employed for measurement of a specific barbiturate (such as phenobarbital). Quantitative assays currently used include EMIT, fluorescence polarization (Table 42-6, method 3), nephelometric inhibition (Table 42-6, method 4), and turbidimetric inhibition (Table 42-6, method 5).

If the specimen to be analyzed contains a mixture of barbiturates, gas or liquid chromatography or HPLC procedures are best used because they allow separation of barbiturates before quantitation.

Specimens Specimens for barbiturate analysis include blood, plasma, serum, or urine. Refrigeration or freezing of the sample until analysis will help maintain the stability of the drug.

Therapeutic range The therapeutic concentrations for barbiturates measured in serum are as follows:

Amobarbital	Up to 8 μg/mL	(< 35 μmol/L)
Butabarbital	Up to 8 μg/mL	(< 34 μmol/L)
Pentobarbital	Up to 4 μg/mL	(< 16 μmol/L)
Phenobarbital	15 to 40 μg/mL	(64-172 μmol/L)
Secobarbital	Up to 6 μg/mL	(< 23 μmol/L)

REFERENCES

Wu AHB, Wong SS, Johnson KG, et al: Evaluation of the triage system for emergency drugs-of-abuse testing in urine, *J Anal Toxicol* 17:241-245, 1993.

Binder SR, Adams AK, Regalia M, et al: Standardization of multiwavelength UV detector for liquid chromatography–based toxicological analysis, *J Chromatogr* 550:449-459, 1991.

BIBLIOGRAPHY

Beckman H, Goodman FK: Antidepressant response to tricyclics and urinary MHPG in unipolar patients, *Arch Gen Psychiatry* 32:17-21, 1975.

Davis K, Kahn R, Ko G, Davidson M: Dopamine in schizophrenia, *Am J Psychiatry* 148:1474-1486, 1991.

Fishman RA: *Cerebrospinal fluid in diseases of the nervous system,* Philadelphia, 1980, Saunders.

Garvey M, Rubeis R, Hollon S, et al: Response of depression to very high plasma levels of imipramine plus desipramine, *Biol Psychiatry* 30:57-62, 1991.

Goodwin FK, Cowdry RW, Webster MH: Predictors of drug response in the affective disorders. In Lipton MA, Maschio A, Killam KF, editors: *Psychopharmacology: a generation of progress,* New York, 1978, Raven Press.

Kaplan H, Sadock B: *Clinical psychiatry,* Baltimore, 1988, Williams & Wilkins.

Lesser RP, Pippenger CE, Lueders H, Dinner DS: High-dose monotherapy in treatment of intractable seizures, *Neurology* 34:707-711, 1984.

Pesce AJ, Kaplan LA: *Methods in clinical chemistry,* St. Louis, 1987, Mosby.

Peter JG: *Use and interpretation of tests in neuroimmunology,* Santa Monica, Calif., 1991, Specialty Laboratories.

Plum F, Posner JB: *The diagnosis of stupor and coma,* ed 3, Philadelphia, 1980, FA Davis.

Rowland LP, editor: *Merritt's textbook of neurology,* ed 8, Philadelphia, 1989, Lea & Febiger.

Schildkraut JJ, Orsulak PJ, Schatzberg AF, et al: Biochemical discrimination of subgroups of depressive disorders based on differences in catecholamine metabolism. In Usdin E, Hanin I, editors: *Biological markers in psychiatry and neurology,* New York, 1982, Pergamon Press.

van Putten T, Marder S, Mintz J, Poland R: Haloperidol plasma levels and clinical response, *Am J Psychiatry* 149:500-505, 1992.

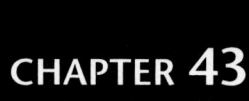

CHAPTER 43 *General endocrinology*

Laurence M. Demers

OBJECTIVES

- Describe the mechanism of action of steroid and peptide hormones.

- Describe the regulatory control of hormone biosynthesis and release.

- List the hypothalamic factors and the pituitary hormones they control.

- Describe the pathological conditions of pituitary deficiency and excess.

- List the major hormones that provide an assessment of pituitary function.

KEY TERMS

acromegaly A pathological state in adults that is associated with hypersecretion of growth hormone.

adenohypophysis The anterior lobe of the pituitary gland, which secretes trophic hormones.

amenorrhea The absence of a menstrual cycle and menstrual period.

autocrine factor A cellular factor that interacts with receptors that are found on the same cell that released the factor.

bioavailable hormone Hormone in the circulation, whether free or weakly bound to plasma proteins, that is available for tissue receptor binding and cell uptake.

cytokines Peptides synthesized and released by white blood cells and tissue macrophages that stimulate or suppress the functional activity of lymphocytes, monocytes, neutrophils, fibroblast cells, and endothelial cells.

diabetes insipidus A pathological state associated with inappropriately low secretion of antidiuretic hormone and excessive water excretion.

endocrine gland A specialized gland that releases hormones into the circulation affecting a tissue or organ at a distal site.

feedback loop A loop integrating two endocrine glands by means of a positive or negative hormone signal.

galactorrhea An uncontrolled secretion of fluid from the breast.

G-protein A regulatory protein found in the membrane of all mammalian cells that acts to transmit an extracellular hormone signal to inner membrane factors as part of a cell-membrane transduction signaling system.

hormone A chemical substance released by an endocrine gland into the circulation.

hormone transport The mechanism by which hormones are carried in the bloodstream, bound to protein carriers.

hypothalamus The portion of the brain that possesses both endocrine and neurotransmitter functions.

intracrine factor A cytosolic factor made by a cell that travels to the nucleus and binds to a specific receptor on DNA to regulate gene activity.

juxtacrine factor A membrane bound growth factor that interacts with the membrane receptor of a neighboring cell by direct cell-to-cell contact.

neurohypophysis The posterior part of the pituitary gland that is an extension of the central nervous system.

paracrine factor A factor that is released by one cell in a tissue and binds to receptors of a different cell in that same tissue.

peptide hormones Hormones made from amino acids by specialized endocrine glands, and are released into the circulation to interact with membrane bound receptors of other tissues and organs.

pituitary portal circulation The vascular channel connecting the hypothalamus with the anterior pituitary.

pituitary adenoma A tumor of the pituitary that produces excess amounts of a particular pituitary hormone.

pulsatile release The release of hypothalamic and pituitary hormones in short bursts, or pulses, during the course of a 24-hour day. The amplitude and frequency of the pulse is unique to each hormone.

receptor Specific cytosolic and membrane proteins that bind a hormone or growth factor with high specificity and affinity.

releasing factors Peptides synthesized by the hypothalamus and released into the portal circulation to affect pituitary hormone synthesis and secretion.

steroids Hormones made by endocrine glands from cholesterol that have as a basic structure the cyclopentanophenanthrene nucleus.

FUNDAMENTALS OF ENDOCRINOLOGY

The endocrine system comprises part of the extracellular communication system within the body that links the brain to organs and functions to control body metabolism, growth and development, and reproduction. The other two major components of this communication system, the central nervous system and the immune system, are also linked to the endocrine system as part of the overall control of bodily function. The endocrine system itself functions through an elaborate network of chemical messengers called hormones that are produced by highly specialized endocrine organs. The location of the endocrine glands is shown in Fig. 43-1. The hormones enter the circulation to effect their action at a site usually distant from their site of production. Hormones interact with specific receptors on the target cell, conferring the selectivity of hormone action. The traditional definition of endocrinology, that is, the study of hormone action distal to the site of hormone production, has become obscured in recent years because we now recognize the important local effects of hormone metabolism and action within a given endocrine gland or tissue. In addition, many growth factors produced locally by specific cells elicit a network of cellular communication akin to the hormone receptor interactive event. Many of the biological effects of hormones are produced at the target site through local metabolism of hormone precursor substances. The local biosynthesis of estrogen from steroid precursor substrates like androstenedione and the formation of triiodothyronine from T_4 are examples of local hormone synthesis at the target cell.

Control of the endocrine system is affected primarily by its linkage to the central nervous system through the hypothalamus and pituitary glands. This aspect of the endocrine system is referred to as the neuroendocrine system and involves an intimate relationship between neurosecretory chemicals formed in the brain and hormonal factors produced by the master endocrine organs located within the brain. It is now evident that the immune system also acts at nerve centers of the brain to facilitate the orchestration of hormone signals, both positive and negative, by the elaboration of a network of cytokine factors produced both by endocrine tissues and immunocompetent cells residing in the brain.

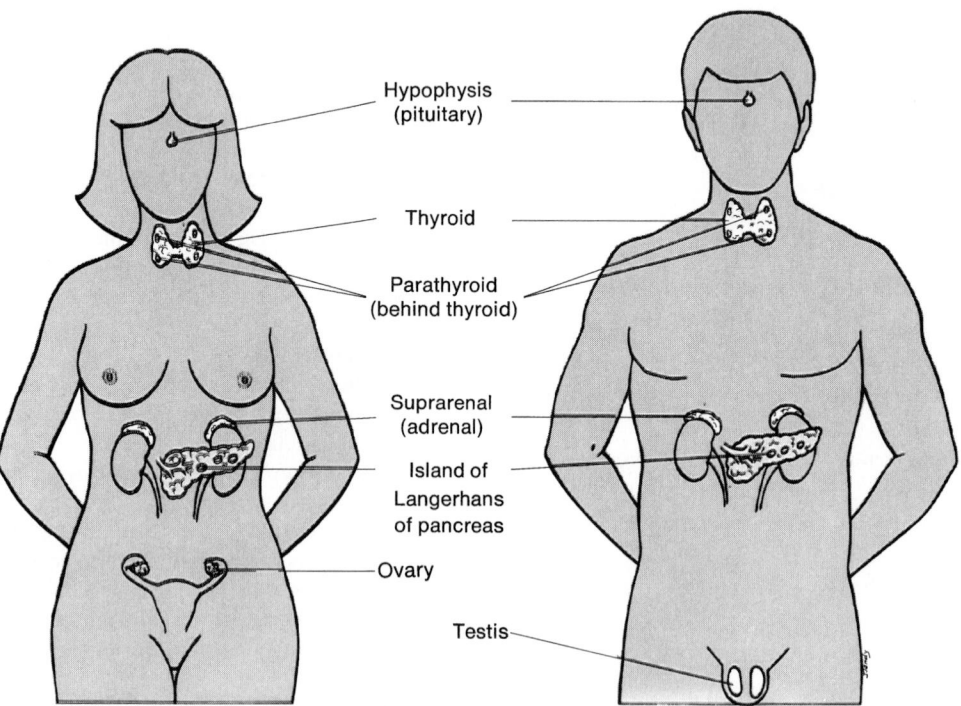

Fig. 43-1   Location of endocrine glands. (From Toporek M: *Basic chemistry of life,* St. Louis, 1980, Mosby.)

The chemical nature of hormones

Hormones are divided into basically two broad classes, peptides and steroids. Most hormones are amino acid and peptide in nature, ranging from complex carbohydrate-polypeptide molecules such as human chorionic gonadotropin to single amino acid moieties such as the catecholamines. Steroids are all derived from cholesterol and are subdivided into two types, those containing an intact cyclopentanophenanthrene nucleus, such as adrenal and gonadal steroids, and those like vitamin D that have an alteration in the B ring of the basic phenanthrene nucleus. It is the chemical makeup of the hormone that is integral to its ability to interact with a specific tissue-based receptor to bring about hormone action. For example, the simple lack of a methyl group between the A and B rings of a steroid molecule along with a saturated A ring determine the difference between a female steroid hormone such as estradiol and the male hormone testosterone. It is this subtle chemical difference and the presence of highly specific protein receptors in tissues that allow the hormone to recognize a particular tissue or organ and invoke its biological effect. A list of the major peptide and steroid hormones and their primary sites of action is shown in Table 43-1.

Mechanisms of hormone action

All hormones act on their respective target glands and tissues through highly specific binding proteins, called *receptors,* that are located either on the surface of the membrane or within the cytosol of the target cell. The binding of a hormone to its specific receptor serves as an initial signal to a cell. An amplification of the signal then ensues, involving many intermediate messenger signals. These signals ultimately impact on the nucleus of the target cell to elicit an alteration in gene expression, resulting in the synthesis of a specific mRNA message and new protein synthesis. Figs. 43-2 and 43-3 provide examples of hormone binding and the mechanism of hormone action as they are currently understood.

Steroid hormones. All steroid hormones interact with their target cells by binding to specific protein receptors located in both the cytoplasmic and nuclear fractions of the cells (Fig. 43-2). Each steroid responsive tissue contains a

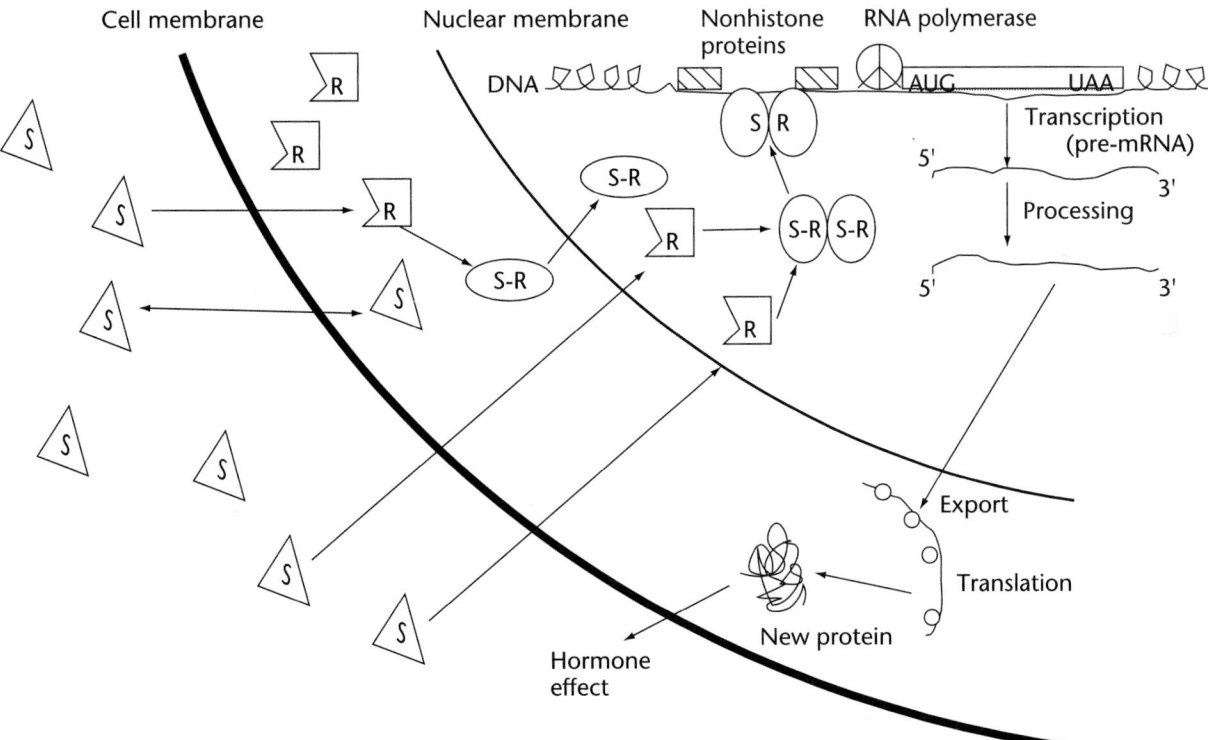

Fig. 43-2 Current proposed mechanism of action of steroid hormones (estrogens, androgens, progesterone, glucocorticoids, aldosterone). Steroids, *S,* diffuse across the plasma membrane and bind to a cytosolic protein receptor, *R.* Steroid binding activates the receptor complex, which then translocates to the nucleus of the cell where it interacts with chromatin at a specific binding site on DNA called the *steroid-response element.* This binding activates the transcription of specific genes involved in steroid hormone action. Transcription of messenger RNA then takes place with the eventual synthesis of specific proteins by the cells that are linked to steroid hormone action.

Table 43-1   Steroid and peptide hormones

Hormone	Source	Target organ	Circulating level	Biological effect
Steroid hormones				
Androgens				
Testosterone (dihydrotestosterone)	Testis	Accessory sex glands	3.0-10.0 ng/mL	Male, secondary sex characteristics, protein anabolism
DHEAS (dehydroepiandrosterone sulfate)	Adrenal	Liver, fat tissue	1500-4000 ng/mL	Androgen substrate
Estrogens				
Estradiol	Ovary	Accessory sex glands, liver, brain	50-300 pg/mL	Female, secondary sex characteristics
Estrone	Ovary, fat tissue	Accessory sex glands	50-200 pg/mL	Estradiol substrate
Progesterone	Ovary	Uterus, breast, brain	5-20 ng/mL	Pregnancy hormone
Adrenal steroids				
Cortisol	Adrenal	Liver, muscle, brain, fat tissue	50-250 µg/L	Gluconeogenesis, immune system control
Aldosterone	Adrenal	Kidney	50-300 ng/L	Salt homeostasis
Peptide hormones				
Anterior pituitary				
TSH (thyroid-stimulating hormone)	Anterior pituitary	Thyroid gland	0.4-4.0 µU/mL	Biosynthesis of thyroid hormones
ACTH (adrenocorticotropic hormone)	Anterior pituitary	Adrenal	25-80 pg/mL	Biosynthesis of adrenocortical hormones
FSH (follicle-stimulating hormone)	Anterior pituitary	Ovary/testis	5-20 mIU/mL	Follicular development, ovary and sperm formation, testis
LH (luteinizing hormone)	Anterior pituitary	Ovary/testis	5-25 mIU/mL	Corpus luteum, ovary Leydig cell, testis
Prolactin	Anterior pituitary	Mammary gland, uterus, ovary, testis	5-20 ng/mL	Mammary gland development, ovary and testis steroid production
GH (growth hormone)	Anterior pituitary	All tissues	2-5 ng/mL	Tissue growth, fat and CHO metabolism
Posterior pituitary				
AVP (arginine vasopressin)	Posterior pituitary	Kidney	2-8 pg/mL	Water homeostasis
Oxytocin	Posterior pituitary	Breast, uterus	1-5 pg/mL	Milk secretion, uterine contractility
Calcitropic hormones				
PTH (parathyroid hormone)	Parathyroid	Bone, kidney, intestine	10-55 pg/mL	Calcium homeostasis
Calcitonin	Thyroid	Bone	0-50 pg/mL	Calcium regulation
Pancreatic hormones				
Insulin	Pancreas	Most tissues	6-25 µU/mL	Carbohydrate metabolism
Glucagon	Pancreas	Liver	50-100 pg/mL	Glycogenolysis
Gastrointestinal hormones				
Gastrin	Stomach	Stomach	30-150 pg/mL	Acid secretion
Secretin	Small intestine	Stomach, pancreas	0-50 pg/mL	Stomach and pancreatic fluid secretion
Thyroid hormones				
T_4 (thyroxine)	Thyroid	All tissues	40-120 µg/L	Basal metabolism
T_3 (triiodothyronine)	Thyroid	All tissues	800-2200 ng/L	Basal metabolism

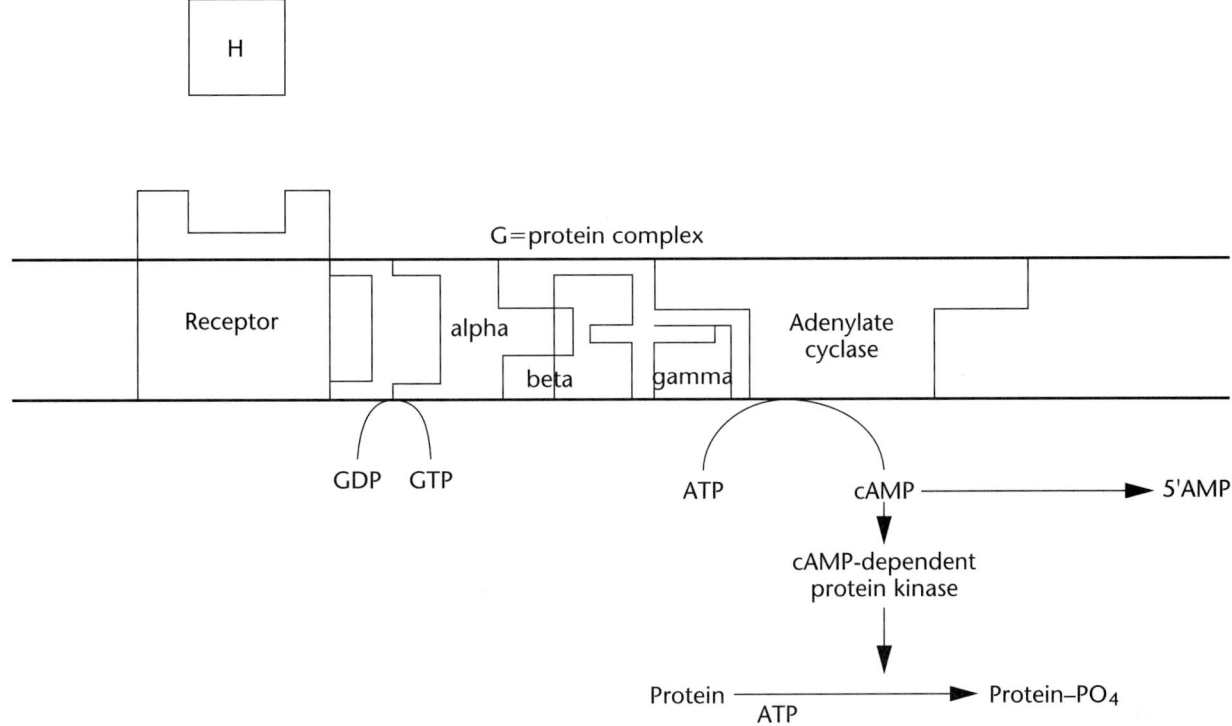

Fig. 43-3 Current proposed mechanism of action of peptide hormones. Peptide hormones bind to a specific receptor on the external domain of the plasma membrane. Hormone binding causes activation of a G-protein complex in the cell membrane that is coupled to and activates the enzyme adenylate cyclase. When the catalytic component of adenylate cyclase is activated, ATP is converted into cyclic AMP, which in turn activates cAMP-dependent protein kinase, resulting in protein phosphorylation and expression of the peptide hormone effect.

finite concentration of receptor protein with an affinity constant that is greater than that of other steroid binders, such as the transport proteins. Transport proteins, which are found in the circulation, carry steroids from the organ of synthesis to the target organ or tissue. The higher affinity of the receptor protein enables the tissue to sequestrate a specific steroid from the hormone's specific carrier protein as the tissue is perfused with blood containing the circulating steroid.

Steroids enter the cell primarily through diffusion, bind to the receptor molecule, and produce a conformational change in the receptor structure. This conformational change in the receptor activates the receptor complex, forming a *transformed receptor–steroid activated complex*. This complex has a high affinity for nuclear binding sites on chromatin and binds to both regulatory and nonregulatory DNA sequences in the 5' end of the responsive gene element. Binding of the transformed receptor–steroid complex to the regulatory elements of the gene results in gene activation and subsequently the synthesis of specific proteins. The net result is altered cell metabolism, which can lead to cell growth and differentiation and the secretion of specific cell products. All steroid hormones interact with their re-

ceptor complexes in a similar fashion. Thus the interaction is much the same for a cortisol-activated event and for estrogen acting on uterine cell growth.

Although we speak of cytosol receptors for steroids, it is important to understand that thyroid hormone also exerts its biologic effect through a cytosol-receptor complex with translocation of the complex to the nucleus in a fashion quite similar to that of the steroid hormones. Under certain circumstances, the measurement of tissue steroid receptor levels is used for determining the course of treatment for certain malignancies. In the case of breast cancer, estrogen and progesterone tissue receptor levels are important prognostically and allow one to categorize the subtype of breast cancer. Normal breast tissue contains very small amounts of estrogen and progesterone–receptor proteins. Certain forms of breast cancer demonstrate an increase in the level of breast tissue steroid–receptor protein. These breast cancers are termed *hormone dependent*. They require a particular modality of antihormonal therapy for the patient. Hormone ablative therapy (reduction of hormone levels) thus becomes an alternative means of chemotherapy for the patient. This therapy is based on the use of drugs that either inhibit the binding of estrogen to its receptor, or inhibit the biosynthesis of estrogenic hormones. Thus the measurement of breast tissue steroid–receptor protein content has proved to be an important clinical tool that categorizes the subtype of hormone–dependent breast cancer and helps select appropriate antihormonal therapy for these patients.

Peptide hormones. Peptide hormones interact with cellular receptors located on the surface of the cell membrane, in contrast to the intracellular cytoplasmic receptors that bind steroid and thyroid hormones. The receptor protein comprises three areas, or domains—an extracellular hormone-binding domain, a transmembrane spanning domain, and the intracellular kinase domain. The receptor mechanism located in the cell membrane appears to be much more complex than the cytosolic-based receptor mechanism. The signaling mechanism involved with peptide hormone–receptor interaction includes postreceptor

cascade events that involve multiple effector systems such as the cyclic nucleotides, arachidonic acid metabolites, G-proteins, and inositol phospholipids. These signaling systems act as secondary messengers that transmit the signal of the initial receptor-hormone interaction to other areas of the cell. In many cases, when the hormone binds to the extracellular domain of the membrane-bound receptor, there is activated a membrane-bound intermediate signal that translates the signal to an intracellular event. This membrane-bound signal transducer is often a guanine nucleotide–binding regulatory protein (G-protein). The G-protein is coupled to the adenylate cyclase and phospholipase enzyme systems that activate subsequent intracellular protein kinases to transmit the biologic response. Some receptor systems contain the effector component as part of the intrinsic structure of the receptor. Most of the growth factors,

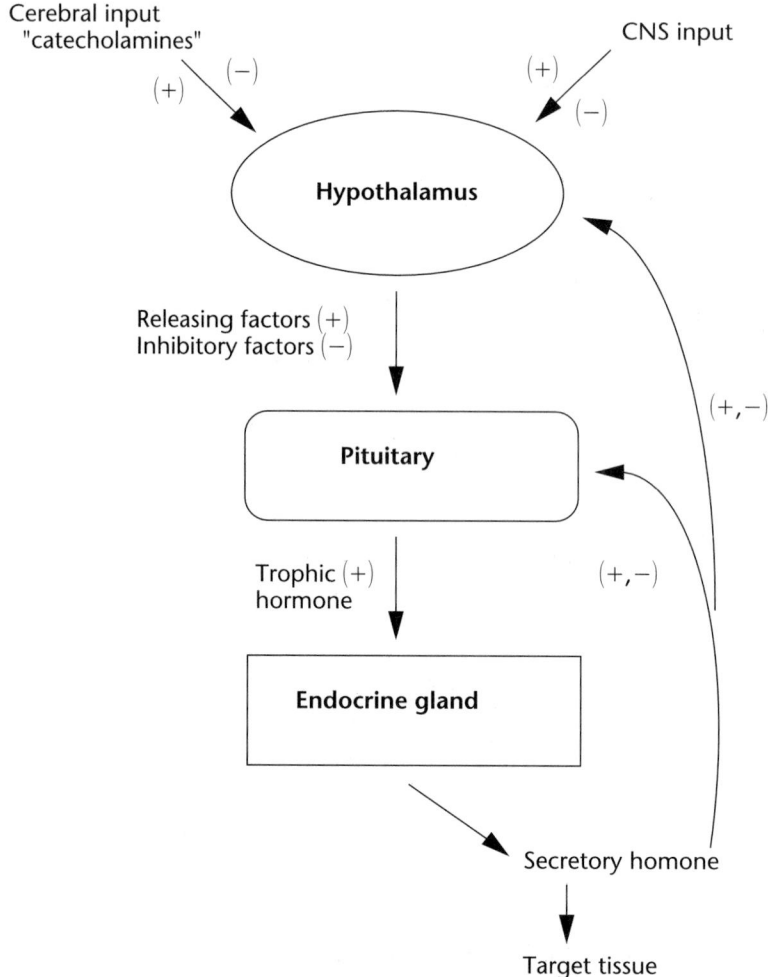

Fig. 43-4 Regulatory feedback loops of the hypothalamic-pituitary-target organ axis. The hypothalamus receives neural and sensory input to produce pituitary hormone–releasing and inhibitory peptides and factors. The pituitary responds by releasing trophic hormones that act on specific endocrine glands or tissues to promote primary gland hormone synthesis and release. The secretory hormone from the endocrine organ negatively feeds back to the higher centers of control to maintain a homeostatic balance of hormone in the circulation.

such as insulin, insulin-like growth factor, and epidermal growth factor, interact with a surface receptor that has inherent protein tyrosine kinase enzyme activity within the intracellular domain of the receptor. An example of the G-protein–membrane receptor complex and the activation sequence by a peptide hormone is shown in Fig. 43-3.

Regulatory control of hormone synthesis and release

Feedback control mechanism. A unique feature of the endocrine system is its ability to regulate itself by providing negative or positive feedback stimuli to each gland that produces a secretory hormone. All hormone production comes under some form of feedback control. A "feedback" control system requires two production units, in which the product of one unit directly affects the production of the other unit. The products of the two units compose the two halves of a continuous loop. The product of one unit usually causes the second unit to increase the production of its

product. The second unit's product "feeds back" to the original unit to control the output of that unit. Most often, the feedback is negative; that is, the product of the second unit causes a decrease in the first unit's production. This negative-feedback loop, in turn, results in a diminished stimulation of the second unit. Under normal physiological conditions, the overall effect of the two parts of the feedback loops in the endocrine system is to maintain relatively constant levels of circulating hormones.

Hormone feedback to the hypothalamus-pituitary axis from endocrine glands is the most well-known feedback loop; however, other feedback loops exist in endocrinology, for example, calcium feedback to the parathyroid glands to reduce PTH secretion, and glucose feedback control of pancreatic insulin secretion. When studying endocrine feedback control, however, the paradigm is usually the hypothalamic-pituitary-endocrine gland axis (Fig. 43-4). Hormone output from the target endocrine gland, such as the thyroid gland, adrenal gland, or the gonads, is controlled primarily by

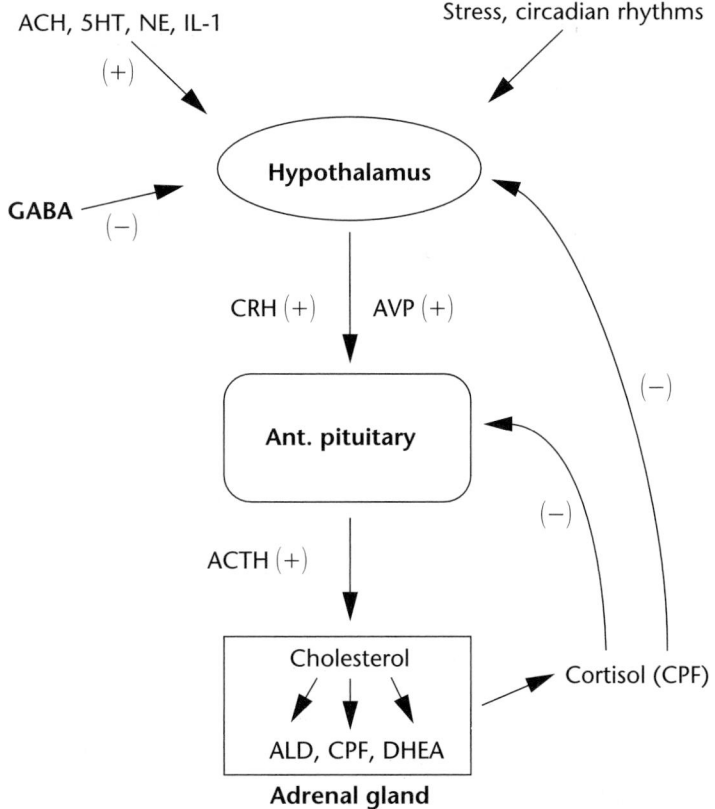

Fig. 43-5 The regulatory feedback loop of the hypothalamic-pituitary-adrenal axis. Several neurotransmitters including acetylcholinesterase (ACH), 5-hydroxytryptamine (5-HT), norepinephrine (NE), and the cytokine interleukin-1 (IL-1) have a positive effect on the release of corticotropin-releasing factor (CRH) from the hypothalamus. Gamma-aminobutyric acid (GABA) has a negative influence. Stress and circadian rhythm also influence the release of CRH from the hypothalamus. Both CRH and arginine vasopressin (AVP) stimulate the pituitary to release adrenocorticotropin (ACTH), which in turn stimulates the adrenal gland to synthesize and release three major classes of hormones (aldosterone, ALD; cortisol, CPF; and dehydroepiandrosterone, DHEA). Cortisol is the only adrenal steroid to feed back negatively to the hypothalamic-pituitary axis to control its own biosynthetic rate.

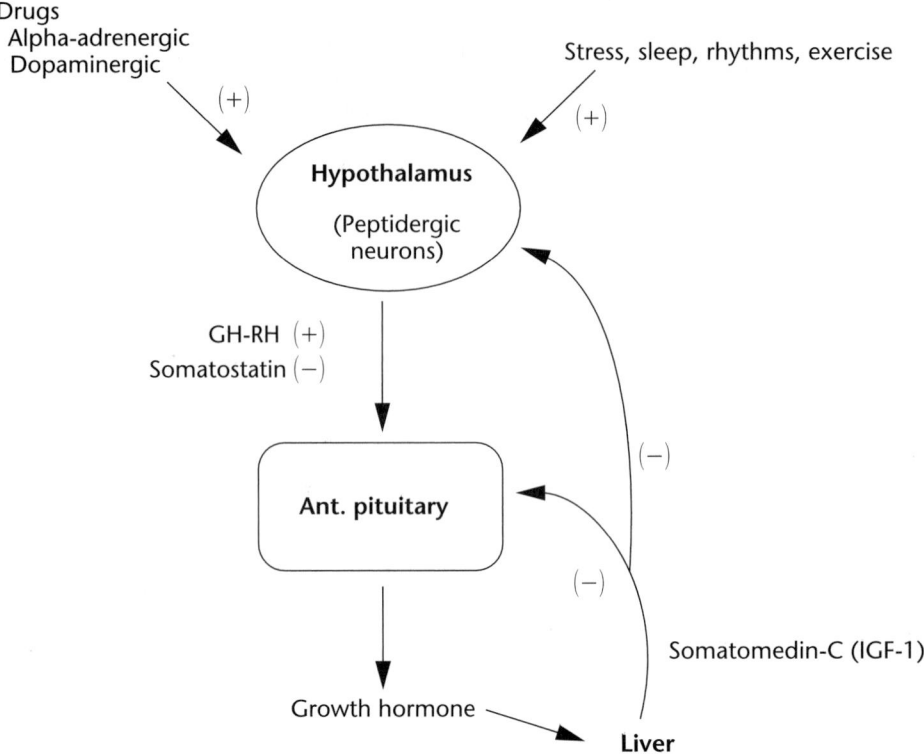

Fig. 43-6   The regulatory feedback loop of the hypothalamic–pituitary–growth hormone axis. Growth hormone release from the pituitary is driven primarily by growth hormone–releasing hormone (GH-RH) from the hypothalamus. GH-RH release from the hypothalamus is positively influenced by alpha-adrenergic and dopaminergic drugs and by stress, sleep patterns, and exercise. Growth hormone acts on the liver to produce somatomedin-C, or insulin-like growth factor–1 (IGF-1). This factor in turn negatively feeds back to the hypothalamic-pituitary axis to maintain homeostatic control over growth hormone secretion.

negative feedback to the hypothalamus and the pituitary, which maintain central nervous system (CNS) control over the circulating level of each gland's hormone. When circulating hormone levels decline, the hypothalamus rapidly senses the decline in hormone output and increases its production of hypothalamus-based releasing factors that enter the portal circulation in the brain to stimulate pituitary hormone synthesis and secretion and reestablish normal hormone output. This stimulus is termed *a positive-feedback loop*. Conversely, when the hormone output from the endocrine gland becomes excessive, the high levels of circulating hormone feedback negatively to the hypothalamic-pituitary axis, reducing the synthesis of the hypothalamic releasing factors and hence pituitary hormone secretion. The reduced pituitary secretion in turn reduces the original stimulation of the target glands to maintain hormone levels.

Negative-feedback control predominates in endocrinology, though positive feedback is also important. An example of positive feedback is the ovarian estrogen–pituitary positive-feedback event, occurring at the midpoint of the monthly menstrual cycle, in which estradiol stimulates the

ovulatory surge of pituitary gonadotropin release. Each target organ controls its own biosynthetic rate and increases the synthesis of hormone when needed through attenuation of the negative-feedback loop that decreases hypothalamic-pituitary secretions. Examples of the feedback and stimulus loops that tie the hypothalamic pituitary axis to the primary endocrine organ or tissue are shown in Figs. 43-5 through 43-9.

The hypothalamic and pituitary hormones are secreted in cyclic patterns that vary in duration. Studies in recent years have focused on the *pulsatile* and *circadian* release of the pituitary hormones. It is now evident that virtually all hypothalamic and pituitary hormones are synthesized and released in a minute-to-minute pulsatile fashion. For example, in both men and women, pituitary FSH and LH release occurs every 30 to 40 minutes as a consequence of the pulsatile release of gonadotropin-releasing hormone (GnRH) from the hypothalamus. Overlaying this shorter, pulsatile cycle, pituitary hormone secretion also exhibits a cyclic change in secretion rates that occurs over a 24-hour period, termed a *circadian rhythm*. The frequency and magnitude

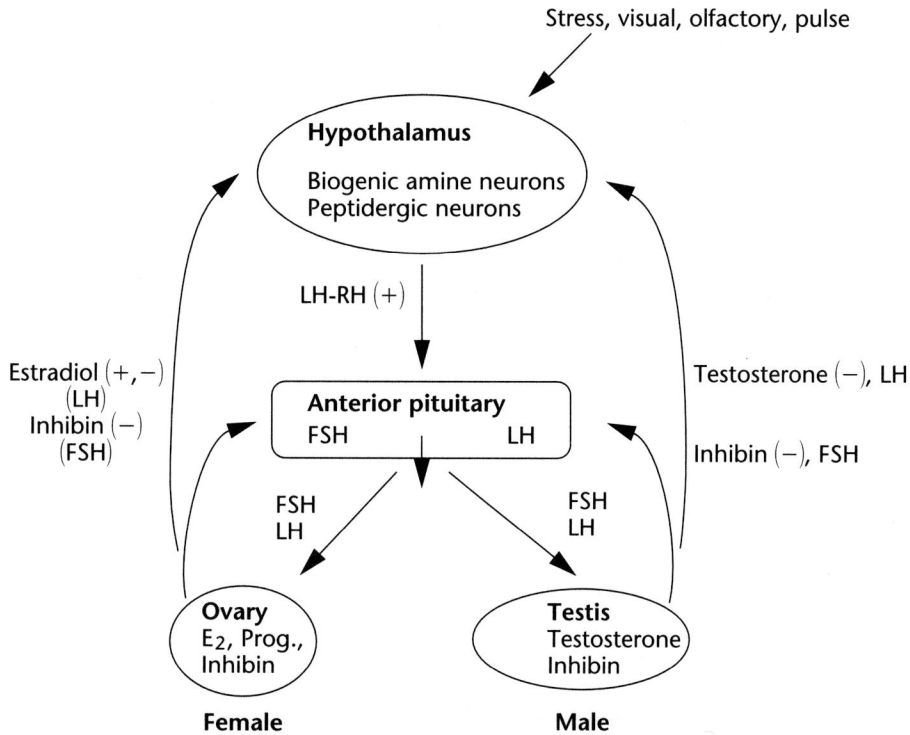

Fig. 43-7 The regulatory feedback loop of the hypothalamic-pituitary-gonadal axis. Biogenic amine and peptidergic neurons in the hypothalamus respond to neural and sensory input from the brain to elicit the release of gonadotropin hormone–releasing hormone (LH-RH). This input can be visual and olfactory in origin and occurs in a pulsatile fashion. Stress can override these inputs in a negative fashion. LH-RH in turn acts on the pituitary to synthesize and release the gonadotropins FSH and LH. In the female, FSH causes ovarian follicular development and the production of estradiol, whereas LH causes corpus luteum development and the secretion of progesterone. Estradiol feeds back both negatively and positively to the hypothalamic-pituitary axis to control the menstrual cycle and LH secretion. FSH-release feedback control is orchestrated by an ovarian peptide called *inhibin*. In the male, FSH causes testicular spermatogenesis, whereas LH stimulates testosterone production by the testes. Testosterone negatively feeds back to the hypothalamic-pituitary axis to control LH release, whereas a testicular peptide, inhibin, feeds back to control FSH release.

of the pulsatile release is different for the individual pituitary hormones. For example, in the case of pituitary ACTH secretion, there is a characteristic circadian rhythm during the course of the 24-hour day, with a much higher output in the early morning hours and a nadir around midnight. Growth hormone output exhibits increased amplitude and frequency during periods of REM sleep, a period from about midnight to 4:00 in the morning. In women, there is the added factor of menstrual cyclicity of the pituitary reproductive hormones LH and FSH, which occurs over the course of a 30-day menstrual cycle (see Chapter 45). Pulsatility and variable hormone secretory behavior are important considerations when one is interpreting the circulating levels of hormones within the context of the normal biological rhythms.

Control of hormone availability. Hormones are potent, biologically active compounds. The physiological activity of hormones is controlled by changing their rates of synthesis and release. In addition, however, two other mechanisms act by limiting the hormones' availability after they have been released into the circulation. These mechanisms are rapid catabolism (breakdown) and sequestration.

Catabolism—peptide hormones. Except for the thyroid hormones, peptide and amino acid–derived hormones are water soluble and are found free in plasma. However, rapid catabolism of these hormones to inactive compounds by tissue and plasma enzymes reduces the availability of the original intact hormone and gives it a relatively short half-life. For example, PTH is released from parathyroid glands as an 84–amino acid, intact peptide. Within a few minutes, it is acted upon by proteolytic enzymes in the circulation to reduce this hormone to inactive fragments. Thus control of plasma circulatory levels of active hormone becomes a balance between new hormone synthesis and release from tissues and the metabolic inactivation of existing hormone.

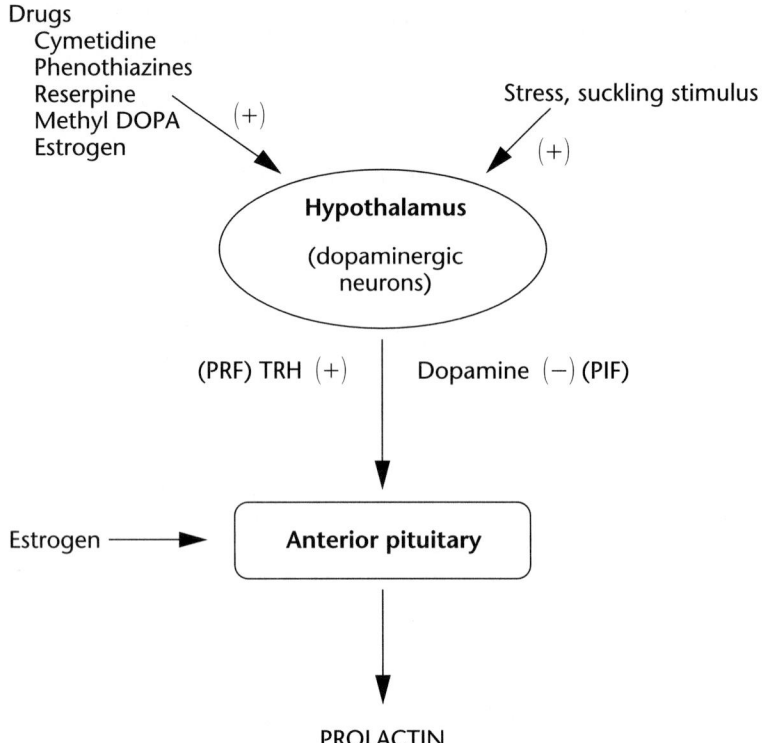

Fig. 43-8 The regulatory feedback loop for prolactin secretion. Prolactin release from the pituitary is under tonic inhibitory control from hypothalamus-derived dopamine, or prolactin inhibitory factor (PIF). Thyrotropin-releasing factor (TRH) in turn is stimulatory to prolactin release. Prolactin release is affected by many factors that influence dopamine release. Drugs, estrogen, and stress are overriding factors that can produce an augmentation in prolactin release from the pituitary. Estrogen can directly sensitize the pituitary to release prolactin.

Sequestration—free and bound transport of steroid and thyroid hormones. Immediate control of the activity of steroid and thyroid hormones in plasma is exercised by sequestration of most of the hormone into a protein-bound, inactive form. Since steroid hormones are themselves water insoluble, plasma proteins also serve as the transport medium for these hormones. The transport/binding proteins, which are synthesized in the liver, are listed in Table 43-2. There are generally three pools of hormones that are, in order of increasing bioavailability, bound to specific proteins with high affinity for the hormone; bound to proteins with low affinity for the hormone; and totally free in the plasma. An example of the binding of testosterone to its respective carrier proteins is shown in Fig. 43-10. In the case of thyroid hormone, three different proteins, each with different binding affinities, participate in the transport of T_4 and T_3 in the circulation: thyroxine-binding globulin, thyroxine-binding prealbumin, and albumin (see Chapter 44). There is speculation that hormones bound to proteins with high affinity represent a circulating storage form of the hormone that is not immediately bioavailable to the target organ. When hormone is transferred from the free or weakly bound form to its tissue receptor, the hormone equilibrium shifts

from the storage form to the more weakly bound form to maintain appropriate availability of free hormone within the circulation (see below).

Free and protein-bound hormone transport

Several proteins serve as carriers of hormones in plasma and also serve as a form of hormone storage within the circulation (see above). Albumin and prealbumin serve as general transport proteins for the steroid hormones and thyroid hormones. Binding of thyroid hormones and steroid hormones to albumin and prealbumin is weak, however, with an affinity constant that is much lower than that of the tissue receptor. Thus the hormones bound to albumin and pre-

Table 43-2 Hormone transport proteins

	Protein	Hormone
CBG	(cortisol-binding globulin)	Cortisol
SHBG	(sex hormone–binding globulin)	Estradiol, testosterone
TBG	(thyroid-binding globulin)	T_3, T_4
TBPA	(thyroxine-binding prealbumin)	T_4
VDBG	(vitamin D–binding globulin)	Vitamin D
ALB	(albumin)	All hormones

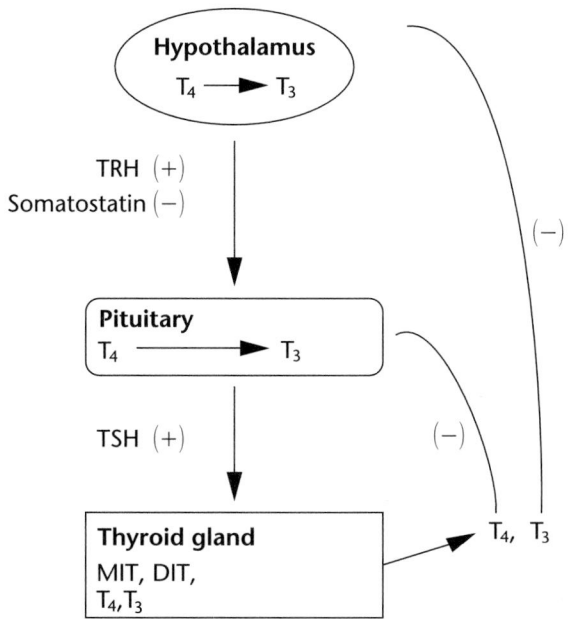

Fig. 43-9 The regulatory feedback loop of the hypothalamic-pituitary-thyroid axis. The hypothalamus secretes thyrotropin-releasing factor (TRH) to stimulate the synthesis and release of TSH from the pituitary. TSH in turn stimulates the thyroid gland to grow, vascularize, and produce the thyroid hormones tetraiodothyronine (T_4) and triiodothyronine (T_3). T_3 is primarily formed from T_4 outside the thyroid gland. T_4, through hypothalamic and pituitary conversion to T_3, and T_3, directly, feed back to the hypothalamic-pituitary axis to maintain a homeostatic balance of circulating thyroid hormone.

albumin are a weakly bound form of free hormones and are considered to be readily bioavailable to tissues. This is in contrast to previous thinking that only hormones absolutely free of carrier proteins could gain access to tissue receptors. This new concept has led to the description of free hormone as inclusive of free and weakly bound hormone.

In addition to general, low-affinity, transport proteins like albumin, there exist specific transport proteins. These specific transport proteins have a high affinity for the hormones they carry, which closely parallels the binding and specificity characteristics of intracellular receptors; thus they significantly influence the metabolic clearance rate for hormones. Several important considerations underscore the role of all the transport proteins that carry hormones in the circulation. The high-affinity binding proteins act as reservoirs for the storage and transport of hormones in the circulation. Once free or weakly bound hormone enters the tissue rapid circulatory adjustments are made in the free hormone level through an exchange and reequilibration between specific transport protein-bound hormone and weakly bound transport protein-bound hormone. The overall decline in circulatory hormone is then eventually compensated for through activation of positive feedback to higher cen-

ters of control, like the hypothalamic-pituitary axis. This keeps a sufficient amount of life-sustaining hormones like thyroxine and cortisol available continuously with a significant circulating reservoir available as soon as it is needed.

Many laboratories now measure bioavailable (that is, free and albumin- or prealbumin-bound) hormone, in contrast to previous measurements, which included only the free concentration of hormone. An example of the utility of measuring both the free and weakly bound hormone can be seen in the measurement of free and weakly bound testosterone (see Fig. 43-10). Testosterone is carried in the circulation bound tightly to its specific carrier protein, sex hormone-binding globulin (SHBG), and bound weakly to albumin. Only a small (<10%) fraction of the testosterone in the circulation is actually free. When blood perfuses an organ containing testosterone receptors, both the free and albumin-bound fractions of testosterone are available for immediate binding to an available receptor. Hence the term *bioavailable testosterone* is used to describe the free and albumin-bound fraction of total hormone in the circulation.

Some steroid hormones, like dehydroepiandrosterone (DHEA), a major androgenic steroid produced by the adrenal gland, lack a specific transport protein. To compensate for the lack of a specific carrier protein for this steroid, DHEA is sulfated at the 3-hydroxyl position of the basic steroid molecule. This step increases the solubility of this steroid for general transport in the circulation. Thus DHEA circulates primarily as DHEA-S in the blood.

Local hormone and growth factor action

Our classical understanding of endocrinology and hormones is that a hormone is produced by a specialized gland in one part of the body and travels through the bloodstream to a distant site to elicit a biological effect. The recent discovery of a family of peptide growth factors, however, has challenged our current perception of classical endocrinology. Like hormones, these growth factors can be extracellular regulators of cell growth and function. The major difference is that growth factors' actions are local and rely on cell-to-cell communication within the tissue and cellular environment.

Terms like *autocrine* and *paracrine* action have been coined to describe the local synthesis and release of growth factors that interact with receptors on neighboring cells within the same tissue (paracrine action) or with receptors from the same cell that release the growth factor (autocrine action) (Fig. 43-11).

The gastrointestinal tract is a prime example of local regulatory interaction between hormones, growth factors, and neurotransmitters that influence cell function through cell-to-cell communication (see Chapter 30). An analogy to this system of communication is the cytokine network of communication that exists between the lymphoid cells of the immune system and the cells of a particular tissue, such as the tissue macrophage and an epithelial cell.

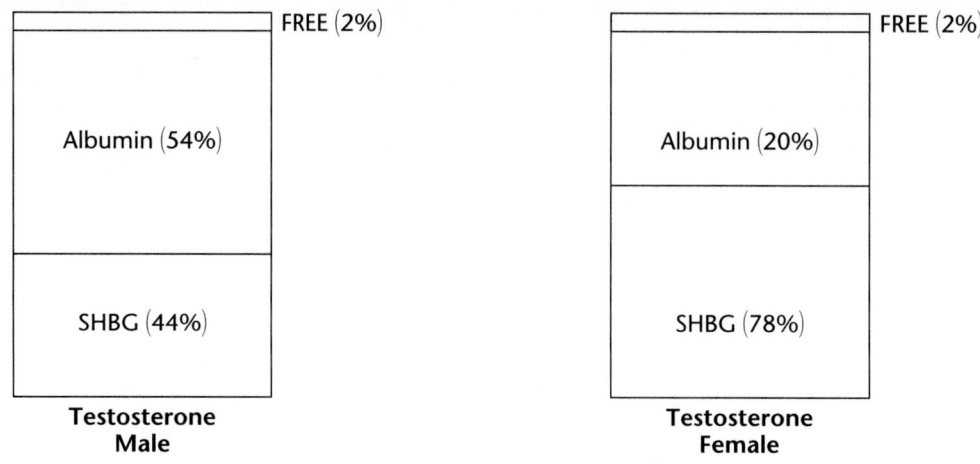

Male: Total testosterone	250-900 ng/dL
Bioavailable T	140-504 ng/dL
Female: Total testosterone	20-80 ng/dL
Bioavailable T	5-18 ng/dL

Fig. 43-10 Free and weakly bound testosterone. Testosterone circulates bound to two proteins—a specific binding protein, sex hormone–binding globulin (SHBG), and albumin. Only a small fraction of testosterone circulates in a free state. Total testosterone levels are a combination of SHBG-bound, albumin-bound, and free testosterone. The bioavailable form of circulating testosterone, the form that "sees" the tissue receptor, is composed of the free fraction and that bound to albumin. Thus bioavailable testosterone is the biologically active form of the hormone found in the circulation.

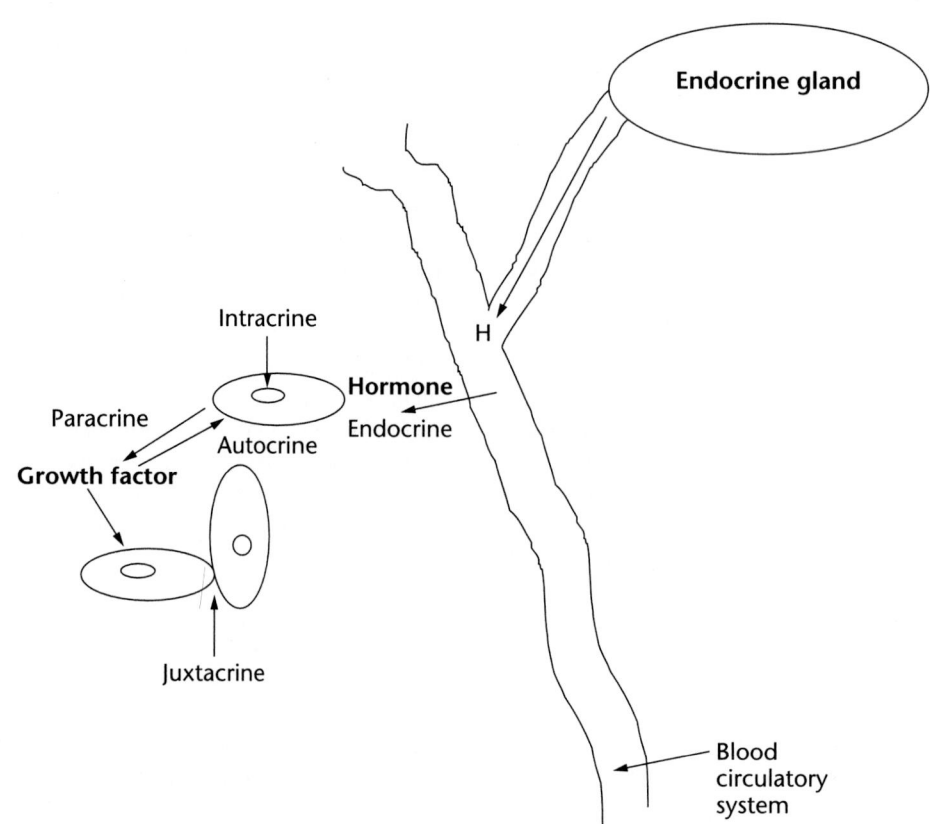

Fig. 43-11 Local and systemic modalities of hormone and growth factor action. Hormones, *H,* are the chemical messengers released into the circulation by endocrine glands to effect a response.

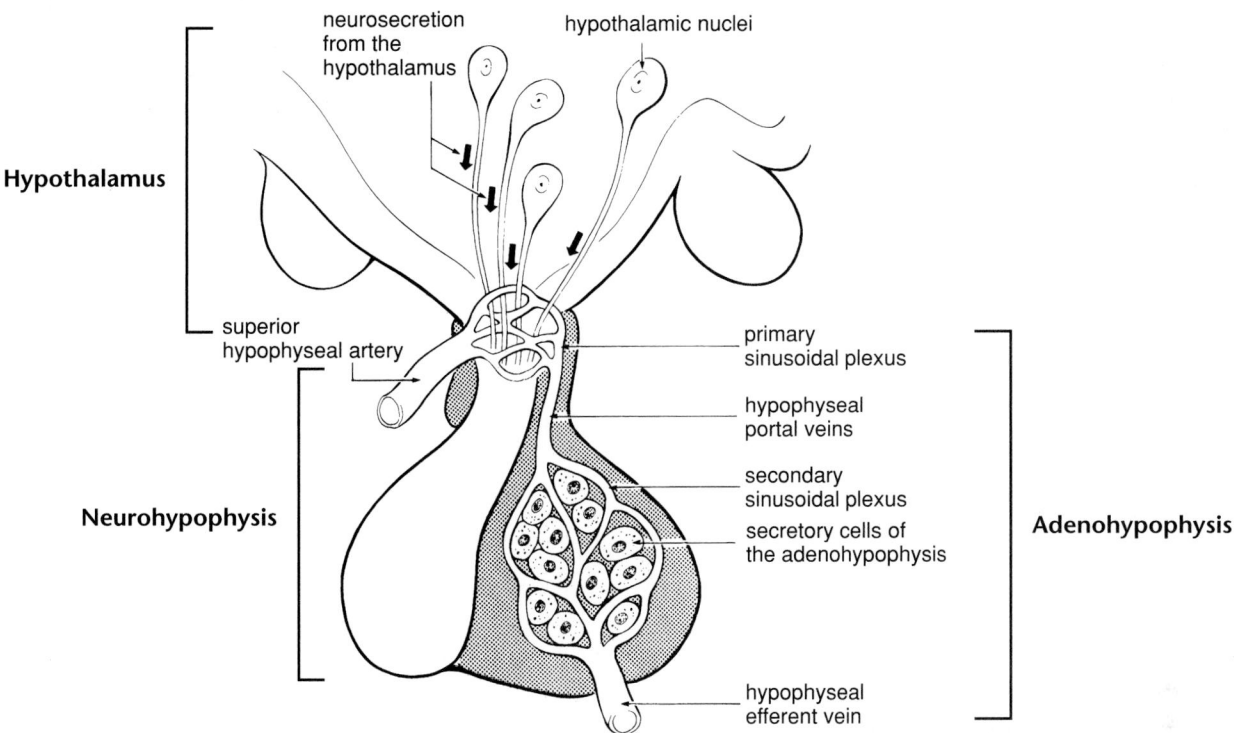

Fig. 43-12 Sinusoidal portal system of pituitary gland.

Two additional terms have been used to describe growth factor communication within the local cellular environment. *Intracrine* is a term used to describe an intracellular cytosolic factor that travels to the nucleus in the same cell to bind to a specific receptor within the DNA-binding region of chromatin. The term *juxtacrine* describes direct cell-to-cell communication elicited by growth factors that are still anchored to each cell's membrane. When the cells come into contact with each other, this membrane-bound growth factor directly influences its neighboring cell. As the family of growth factors continues to expand, a reclassification of the nomenclature will be needed to assign hormones, growth factors, and neural peptides to their proper location and function.

THE HYPOTHALAMIC-PITUITARY AXIS
Hypothalamus

The hypothalamus exerts control over pituitary function by both direct neurostimulation and neurosecretion events of the hypothalamus. The anatomic positioning of the hypothalamus at the base of the brain with both neural and anatomic connection to the pituitary through the pituitary stalk and the portal circulation ensures the close interdependence of these two important organs. The pituitary is anatomically configured with a posterior and an anterior lobe (Fig. 43-12). The hypothalamus directly innervates the posterior lobe (neurohypophysis), and hypothalamic stimulation causes the posterior pituitary to release stored peptide hor-

mones like arginine vasopressin (AVP) and oxytocin. These two hormones are synthesized by the neurosecretory cells of the hypothalamus and are stored in the neurohypophysis. In contrast, the anterior lobe (adenohypophysis) responds to hypothalamus-derived neuropeptides, which, when released directly into the portal circulation, cause the release of the corresponding pituitary hormones (see Table 43-1).

In addition to the classical hypothalamic releasing factors, there exists a hypothalamic peptide, *somatostatin,* that exerts a negative influence on TSH, GH, and several other hormone secretions, including gastrointestinal and pancreatic hormones. Somatostatin is a peptide synthesized not only by the hypothalamus but also within the lumen of the gastrointestinal tract and the pancreas. Different isoforms are synthesized in the brain and gastrointestinal tract. This neurohormone exerts a profound inhibitory effect on both the synthesis of GH and TSH and the secretion of these hormones from the pituitary. Somatostatin inhibits virtually all endocrine secretions, including gastrin, insulin, glucagon, and secretin, of the gastrointestinal tract, pancreas, and gallbladder. Its primary role is to attenuate hypersecretion of these hormones in pathologic states, such as endocrine-secreting tumors like insulinomas and carcinomas. Somatostatin analogs have been used as effective therapeutic agents to treat endocrine-secreting pituitary tumors like acromegaly and pancreatic tumors like insulinomas.

Neurohypophysis

The neurosecretions of vasopressin and oxytocin have specialized roles in mammalian physiology that involve water-conserving (antidiuretic) and nonvascular smooth muscle contracting properties respectively. Arginine vasopressin (AVP) is the major homeostatic factor that maintains normal water concentration in the blood, keeping plasma volume and blood osmolality tightly controlled. Control of blood volume plays an important role in the maintenance of normal blood pressure (see p 933). The release of AVP occurs immediately in response to increases in plasma osmolality, and AVP acts in the kidney to increase water reabsorption by the distal kidney tubules and the collecting ducts. AVP also participates in volume regulation. A sudden reduction in blood volume of greater than 10%, as occurs with a massive hemorrhage, can evoke a rapid release of AVP. Volume receptors for AVP are located in the heart and carotid sinus. Under normal conditions, AVP is released in response to changes in plasma osmolality. Severe volume depletion, however, can override the influence of osmolality on AVP release.

Oxytocin appears to have a role in mammalian physiology that transcends reproductive behavior. Release of oxytocin is generally brought about through a neurogenic reflex transmitted primarily from nerve endings in the nipple of the breast. The stimulus is transmitted through the spinal cord, midbrain, and ultimately to the hypothalamus. Suckling of the breast induces the release of oxytocin, which causes contraction of epithelial cells that encircle mammary acini. This produces expulsion of milk from the milk ducts of the breast, termed *milk letdown,* which is a key event in breast feeding. Oxytocin also plays a role in the induction of labor in pregnancy by stimulating the nonvascular smooth muscle of the uterus to contract. Although the exact signal precipitating the onset of human labor has not yet been identified, oxytocin receptors in the uterus translate the oxytocin signal to produce rhythmic myometrial contractile changes and the physical events of labor. The secretion of oxytocin from the posterior pituitary occurs independent of AVP secretion; thus it is believed that both fall under independent control mechanisms.

Adenohypophysis

The anterior lobe of the pituitary is responsible for the secretion of trophic hormones that govern virtually the entire endocrine system. As noted previously, pituitary cell differentiation, proliferation, and hormone synthesis are controlled by neurosecretory factors of hypothalamic origin. All the releasing factors are peptides except dopamine (Table 43-3). Dopamine, a neurotransmitter, is also synthesized and released from the hypothalamus and plays an important regulatory role over pituitary hormone secretion. Dopamine is believed to be the major regulator of prolactin secretion, exerting a continuous and sustained inhibition on its release from the pituitary. In addition to its effect on pro-

Table 43-3 Human hypothalamic neurosecretory factors

Vasopressin	cys-tyr-phe-gln-asn-cys-pro-arg-gly-NH$_2$ (1084.38 daltons)
Oxytocin	cys-tyr-ile-gln-asn-cys-pro-leu-gly-NH$_2$ (1007.35 daltons)
CRH	ser-glu-glu-pro-pro-ile-ser-leu-asp-leu-thr-phe-his-leu-leu-arg-glu-val-leu-glu-met-ala-arg-ala-glu-gln-leu-ala-gln-gln-ala-his-ser-asn-arg-lys-leu-met-glu-ile-ile-NH$_2$ (4758.14 daltons)
GH-RH	tyr-ala-asp-ala-ile-phe-thr-asn-ser-tyr-arg-lys-val-leu-gly-gln-leu-ser-ala-arg-lys-leu-leu-gln-asp-ile-met-ser-arg-gln-gln-gly-glu-ser-asn-gln-glu-arg-gly-ala-arg-ala-arg-leu-NH$_2$ (5040.40 daltons)
LH-RH	pglu-his-trp-ser-tyr-gly-leu-arg-pro-gly-NH$_2$ (1182.39 daltons)
TRH	pglu-his-pro-NH$_2$ (362.42 daltons)
Somatostatin	ala-gly-cys-lys-asn-phe-phe-trp-lys-thr-phe-thr-ser-cys (1638.12 daltons)
Dopamine	3,4-dihydroxyphenylmethylamine

CRH, Corticotropin-releasing factor; *GH-RH,* growth hormone–releasing hormone; *LH-RH,* luteinizing hormone–releasing hormone; *p-,* pyrido-; *TRH,* thyrotropin-releasing hormone.

lactin, dopamine also inhibits the secretion of TSH, FSH, LH, and GH.

Although each hypothalamic releasing factor has a targeted hormone, some integration of hormone release does occur. For example, TRH causes synthesis and release of not only TSH but prolactin as well. Similarly, LH-RH stimulates the release of both FSH and LH. Only CRH and GH-RH act through a single pituitary hormone release mechanism. All releasing factors interact with the pituitary through the same receptor mechanism used by other peptide hormones. Although they are generally restricted to the portal circulation, several releasing factors have been measured in blood and urine. Direct target organ effects have been described for LH-RH in the ovary and testis. The exact physiological meaning of this interaction is still unclear.

PATHOLOGICAL CONDITIONS

Diseases and disorders of the hypothalamic-pituitary axis can strike at any age and can produce a myriad of symptoms that are often subtle in presentation. Many early forms of endocrine disease are detected only with provocative testing. Bacterial infections, tumors, and head trauma are the most usual causes of alterations in central hormone regulation in the young. In the elderly, vascular disease, inflammatory diseases, and nutritional deficiencies are additional causes of neuroendocrine disorders (Table 43-4). Associated with these diseases are deficits in the autoregulatory feedback loop from the target organs. The loss of circadian rhythm, for example, of ACTH secretion with bacterial infection brings about subsequent compromise in pituitary-adrenal function. This effect can be subtle but nevertheless

Table 43-4   Disorders of the hypothalamic-pituitary axis

Hypopituitarism
  Congenital
    Gene deletions
    Aplasia, hypoplasia
    Disconnection of pituitary stalk
    Septo-optic dysplasia
    Hypoxia
  Acquired
    Infections
    Trauma
    Radiation
    Neoplasms
    Drugs
    Surgery
  Functional defects
    Isolated hormone deficiency
    Severe illness
    Multiple hormone defects
  Secondary hypothyroidism
  Secondary hypoadrenalism
  Hyposomatotropism
  Hypogonadotropic hypogonadism

Hyperpituitarism
  Hypothalamic
    Irradiation
    Infection
    Tumor
  Primary pituitary
    Hyperplasia or adenoma
  Hypersomatotropism
    Acromegaly
    Starvation
    Infection
  Adrenocorticotropin
    Pituitary adenoma
    Addison's disease
  Thyrotropin
    Primary hypothyroidism
  Hypergonadotropism
    Primary organ failure
  Hyperprolactinemia
    Pituitary stalk section
    Pregnancy
    Pituitary adenoma
    Hypothyroidism

important, since cortisol production is a key factor in the control of immune cell function. Because we cannot easily determine the local hormone environment of the portal circulation, we rely on the measurement of pituitary hormones in the systemic circulation to provide a clinical picture of events at the hypothalamic level in health and disease.

Abnormalities of hormone secretion are usually defined in terms of the serum levels of the hormone, that is, high or low levels, and the endocrine gland directly demonstrating the abnormality. In addition, the disease is defined by whether the hormone abnormality is the result of the endocrine gland producing the hormone (primary disease), a disease of the pituitary gland controlling the primary gland (secondary disease), a disease of the hypothalamus controlling the pituitary (tertiary disease), or an inability of the hormone's target tissue to respond to the hormone (end-organ, or quaternary, disease). For example, secondary hyperthyroidism is defined by increased levels of thyroxine resulting from a pituitary gland producing excessive TSH.

Pituitary hormone deficiency

Deficiencies in a specific pituitary cell type can result in primary pituitary failure. A list of primary causes of hypopituitarism can be found in Table 43-4.

Secondary pituitary failure can occur as a result of a deficiency or excess in one or more hypothalamic releasing factors brought on by infection, tumors, or a congenital defect. Hypothalamic tumors, such as a craniopharyngioma, or inflammatory events of the brain, such as meningitis, can result in inadequate synthesis of certain releasing factors that leads to eventual compromise in pituitary hormone synthesis. Hypothalamic hypothyroidism, for example, is a deficiency syndrome of TRH secretion that is initially diagnosed by observation of a suppressed circulating level of TSH. Provocative testing in the form of the intravenous TRH stimulation test can help sort out the hypothalamic origin of TRH deficiency.

An isolated LH-RH deficiency is the most common form of hypothalamic hormone deficiency and can be caused by a congenital defect in the development of LH-RH–containing neurons in embryological life. A deficiency in the release of growth hormone–releasing hormone (GH-RH) is yet another hypothalamic disorder; this disorder results in idiopathic dwarfism. This disorder is diagnosed by documentation of inappropriate levels of circulating growth hormone before and after provocative stimulation. Deficiencies of TRH, LH-RH, GH-RH, and CRH have all been described and are categorized as tertiary endocrine hypofunction.

Pituitary hormone excess

Primary hyperpituitarism. Pituitary hypersecretion is most commonly caused by the presence of a pituitary adenoma or benign tumor of pituitary origin. Prolactin-secreting pituitary adenoma is by far the most common form of pituitary disease. Prolactin, the secretion of which is usually under continuous negative control by the neurosecretory factor dopamine, is produced and secreted uncontrollably in large amounts by pituitary prolactinomas. Prolactin-secreting tumors are diagnosed more readily in women, since disruption of the normal menstrual cycle and amenorrhea usually herald a potential problem early in the manifestation of the disease. Women with prolactinomas can also manifest *galactorrhea,* that is, an abnormal secretion of fluid from the nipple of the breast. Males who develop a prolactinoma, in contrast, are less fortunate and usually do not present at a microadenoma stage as females do. Growth of the prolactin-secreting pituitary tumor usually continues in the male without overt symptoms, and the tumor eventually reaches the size of a macroadenoma before symptoms appear. Headache, impotence, and visual-field disturbances as a consequence of tumor extension that compresses the optic nerve are the classical symptoms that result from a pituitary macroadenoma. The diagnosis of a prolactinoma is usually confirmed by the appearance of blood levels of prolactin in excess of 200 ng/mL.

Growth hormone- and ACTH-producing pituitary tumors are also relatively common pituitary disorders, though of lower prevalence than prolactin-secreting tumors. Growth hormone excess is characterized by the development of acromegalic features, including soft tissue and cartilaginous growth, that result in characteristic facial features of *gigantism*. This growth hormone–excess disease entity is called *acromegaly*. The major effect of growth hormone is to induce the synthesis of an insulin-like growth factor (IGF-1) by the liver. In patients with acromegaly, IGF-1 levels are raised to a greater extent than those of growth hormone itself. The recent availability of commercial immunoassays for IGF-1 has allowed for the routine measurement of this circulating growth factor for the diagnosis and monitoring of acromegaly.

Pituitary adenomas hypersecreting ACTH are also common and lead to the condition known as Cushing's syndrome (see Chapter 46). This syndrome is associated with bilateral adrenal hyperplasia and clinical manifestations of cortisol overproduction as a consequence of excessive ACTH. TSH-producing pituitary adenomas leading to thyroid gland hyperstimulation have also been described but are much less common than the previously mentioned pituitary adenomas.

Secondary hyperpituitarism. Pituitary hypersecretion can be induced by numerous factors including neurogenic tumors of the hypothalamus. Overproduction of releasing factors will hyperstimulate the pituitary, leading to an excessive pituitary hormone release that overrides the usual negative-feedback mechanisms. LH-RH hypersecretion associated with precocious puberty, GH-RH–secreting gangliocytomas causing acromegaly, and CRH-secreting tumors producing Cushing's disease are examples of releasing factor hypersecretion and secondary causes of hyperpituitarism. Hypothalamus-based disorders are relatively rare, however, compared to the hypersecretion that occurs with primary pituitary disease.

Inappropriate release (hypersecretion) of AVP can bring about excessive water retention and a dangerous expansion of plasma volume. Brain injury resulting from physical trauma, infection, or tumors in the brain can bring about excessive AVP release, leading to the clinical condition known as *SIADH* (syndrome of inappropriate secretion of antidiuretic hormone). The ectopic production of AVP by certain tumors can also lead to inappropriate water retention. The thirst mechanism in the brain is also linked to AVP secretion from the neurohypophysis. Both drinking behavior and AVP release are believed to be activated by similar hyperosmotic stimuli resulting in repletion of plasma water in states of dehydration. SIADH is associated with hyponatremia and the production of urine that is hypertonic relative to plasma, despite normal renal and adrenal function. Clinically, SIADH is associated with symptoms of muscle weakness, malaise, and poor mental status, ultimately progressing to convulsions.

TESTS OF HYPOTHALAMIC AND PITUITARY FUNCTION

Evaluation of pituitary disease is very often difficult because of subtle disease presentation. The diagnosis usually requires some form of provocative testing of gland function either by suppressing or stimulating the pituitary gland through exogenous hormone treatment, or provocation of symptoms with stress or exercise. These challenge tests are then followed by measurement of specific pituitary hormones. For each suspected pituitary adenoma a specific testing protocol is usually employed to confirm the clinical suspicion. Many factors, however, must be considered when one is interpreting these functional tests. The pulsatile nature of pituitary hormone secretion, the time of day the test is performed, whether stress or infection might be present, and the concentration of circulating hormone are all factors that affect the interpretation of pituitary function tests. In addition, clinical laboratories have access to a wide variety of immunoassays with differing specificities and sensitivities that affect interpretability of provocative hormone testing.

ACTH EXCESS

Dexamethasone suppression tests (see p. 925) The existence of a tumor secreting ACTH is usually suspected when an abnormal elevation in urine or blood cortisol levels is observed. In these patients, cortisol determinations are made after a low-dose dexamethasone suppression test. A lack of cortisol suppression is suggestive of a pituitary tumor. One then gives a higher dose of dexamethasone that will elicit a modest but still incomplete suppression of cortisol output in the patient with a functional pituitary adenoma. Cortisol output in patients with ACTH from an ectopic source will not be suppressed by either low or high dose dexamethasone.

GH DEFICIENCY

Insulin challenge test. The most commonly performed challenge test for a growth hormone problem is the challenge test used to determine the presence of a GH deficiency in young children. Most pediatric endocrinologists use a combination of insulin-induced hypoglycemia, which produces a form of stress through carbohydrate sensing, and the drug levodopa (L-dopa), which acts in the CNS to induce pituitary release of GH. Insulin is usually administered first, and blood is collected for the assessment of GH at 30-minute intervals for 90 minutes. This is followed by the administration of L-dopa over the subsequent 120 minutes with the additional collection of blood for GH measurement every 30 minutes. Because of the influence of stress, baseline levels can be slightly raised because of the venipuncture and can sometimes cause misinterpretation of the results. The recent availability of the releasing factor GH-RH for clinical use has allowed for a better clinical work-up of patients with a subtle manifestation of pituitary growth hormone deficiency. Administration of GH-RH and the measurement of GH are useful in discerning growth deficiencies that are of hypothalamic origin.

SECONDARY HYPOGONADISM

LH-RH challenge. LH-RH is usually given intravenously to stimulate pituitary secretion of FSH and LH; low FSH and LH levels after this challenge are suggestive of hypopituitary function. LH-RH analogs are available for use in provocative testing and in the treatment of a variety of reproductive disorders and malignancies, such as endometriosis and prostate cancer.

CHANGE OF ANALYTE IN DISEASE
Prolactin

The pulsatile secretion of prolactin has little effect on its measurement or interpretation for the diagnosis of a prolactinoma because of the high levels of prolactin that are usually achieved in this disease. Prolactin hypersecretion is usually established simply by the observation of an elevated basal level. A prolactin level above 200 ng/mL is virtually diagnostic of a prolactinoma. Mild elevations of prolactin (25 to 50 ng/mL), however, can easily be achieved in response to the stress of venipuncture or simply after physical examination and examination of the breasts, but one must obtain repeated measurements after mild elevations to confirm the presence of a prolactinoma. Levels up to 150 ng/mL, which are elevated approximately tenfold, can be achieved in normal individuals who are receiving certain medications. The phenothiazines and antiulcer medications, such as Tagamet, can produce a significant increase in prolactin secretion, and so a careful drug history is important when one is assessing the patient with raised levels of prolactin. A CAT scan of the pituitary of a patient with raised prolactin levels is usually required to confirm the presence of a pituitary tumor.

ACTH

Patients with an ACTH-producing pituitary adenoma are usually diagnosed through an elevation in basal blood cortisol levels; ACTH measurements are not routinely needed in these cases. ACTH measurements are more commonly used for patients requiring *localization* of the tumor within the pituitary before surgical removal of the pituitary adenoma. In these cases, blood samples are collected from the petrosal sinus. Occasionally patients with a suspected ectopic source of ACTH, from an ACTH-producing tumor, are candidates for blood ACTH measurements. The highest values for ACTH are usually found in patients producing this peptide from a tumor source. The dexamethasone suppression test is used for this diagnosis (see above). Sustained high levels of ACTH can be helpful in establishing the presence of a nonpituitary source for ACTH. Tumors of the lung, particularly oat cell carcinoma, are commonly associated with nonpituitary sources of ACTH. Blood levels of ACTH in a patient with a pituitary adenoma rarely exceed 1000 pg/mL; however, with an ectopic source the levels are frequently in excess of this concentration. Pancreatic tumors are also commonly associated with ectopic ACTH release.

ACTH measurements are not routinely used. The short half-life of ACTH, stringent collection requirements because of the lability of this peptide (antiproteases are required in the collection vial), and the need for immediate sample storage at $-20°$ C are factors that impede the routine use and the interpretation of an ACTH result.

Growth hormone

Growth hormone is secreted in healthy individuals in a pulsatile fashion, with the greatest amounts produced during rapid-eye-movement sleep. During the day, blood levels of GH can range from undetectable to 5 ng/mL. However, GH levels can be greatly influenced by stress and also by the recent ingestion of food, with carbohydrates suppressing and proteins stimulating GH secretion. Thus a single determination of GH is not particularly useful in establishing either inadequate or excessive release of GH from the pituitary. When a GH deficiency is suspected, provocative testing is usually required to confirm this suspicion (see above).

To evaluate the possibility of pituitary hypersecretion of growth hormone in a patient suspected of having acromegaly one can measure the concentration of somatomedin C, or IGF-1. The concentration of this liver factor, which mediates the effects of growth hormone, is raised in the circulation in patients with acromegaly, and its measurement can be useful to confirm the diagnosis in borderline cases. IGF-1 measurements are also helpful in monitoring therapy of patients treated for acromegaly.

TSH

The availability of ultrasensitive TSH assays has greatly enhanced the usefulness of TSH measurements for the diagnoses of hypofunction and hyperfunction of the pituitary-thyroid axis. Before the advent of these highly sensitive tests, TRH stimulation tests were important provocative tests that helped distinguish hypothalamic from pituitary disease as the cause of the thyroid dysfunction. This was particularly important when hyperthyroidism from euthyroidism are being distinguished. The newer highly sensitive TSH assays can reasonably be expected to distinguish between depressed and normal TSH secretion, thus obviating, in most patients, the need to carry out TRH provocative testing. Basal TSH level becomes the important parameter to determine when the adequacy of pituitary TSH release is being assessed. A basal serum TSH level of less than 0.05 μU/mL, for example, indicates with virtual certainty that primary hyperthyroidism exists for whatever clinical reason. TRH testing has been quietly abandoned for the most part and has been reserved for establishing the differential diagnosis of suspected hypothalamus-based thyroid disease in patients who have a complex disease presentation (see p. 881). Patients who have a TSH level in excess of 10 μU/mL are strongly suspected of having hypothyroidism, and when the TSH level exceeds 25 μU/mL, the diagnosis is usually established as primary hypothyroidism.

FSH/LH

Of all the pituitary hormones influenced by pulsatile release, the gonadotropins are the most affected. In males, this pulsatility doesn't interfere with the clinical utility of gonadotropin measurements, since the assessment of primary gonadal disease is the usual reason for determining gonadotropin levels in the male. Testosterone measurements provide the initial biochemical indication for the diagnostic work-up of the hypogonadal male. Measurement of the gonadotropins with LH-RH provocative testing can be useful in the diagnosis of males with hypogonadatropic hypogonadism (secondary hypogonadism) (see above).

In women, the situation is more complex because menstrual cyclicity, menopause, and the pulsatility and frequency of hypothalamic LH-RH secretion all affect the interpretation of serum FSH and LH levels. A single gonadotropin measurement is of little practical use in the female unless one simply wants to determine the probability of menopause. In this case, use of FSH is a better test to confirm menopause than LH. In dealing with the more intricate cases of infertility, amenorrhea, and the many disorders that influence the hypothalamic-pituitary-ovarian axis, multiple blood measurements of the gonadotropins are necessary to pinpoint the disorder (see p. 902). An alternative to this is the use of timed urine gonadotropin measurements, which can effectively integrate the pulsatile secretion and concentrate the gonadotropins for use in the different clinical diagnoses. Pediatric endocrinologists routinely use urinary gonadotropin measurements to diagnose delayed puberty, precocious puberty, and functional disorders of the pituitary-ovarian and pituitary-testicular axis in young girls and boys.

In general, dynamic testing of pituitary function takes on the uniqueness of the specific disorder. With the current clinical availability of the four hypothalamic releasing factors, GH-RH, CRH, LH-RH, and TRH, direct pituitary responses can now be monitored by the measurement of the corresponding pituitary peptide. This allows the clinician to distinguish between hypothalamic and pituitary disease and determine adequacy of the hypothalamic-pituitary-endocrine axis.

BIBLIOGRAPHY

Wilson JD, Foster DW: *Williams' textbook of endocrinology,* ed 8, Philadelphia, 1992, Saunders.
DeGroot LJ: *Endocrinology,* Philadelphia, 1989, Saunders.
Besser GM: *Clinical endocrinology,* ed 2, St. Louis, 1994, Mosby.
Hall R: *Color atlas of endocrinology,* ed 2, St. Louis, 1990, Mosby.

CHAPTER 44

Thyroid

Marvin H. Lucas
Mariano Fernández-Ulloa

OBJECTIVES

- Describe the synthesis, transport, function, and regulation of thyroid hormones.
- Describe pathological conditions resulting in hyperthyroidism or hypothyroidism.
- State the importance of the analysis of the free hormone levels of T$_4$ and T$_3$ and the meaning of the free thyroxine measured.
- Describe the thyroid function tests and which analytes are used.
- State the diagnostic value of the following laboratory tests in assessing thyroid conditions: T$_4$, T$_3$, FT$_4$, T$_3$RU, FTI, and TSH.

KEY TERMS

acromegaly Enlargement of the extremities (especially hands and feet) caused by an increased secretion of pituitary growth hormone.

adrenergic activity Pharmacologic and metabolic effects caused by the hormone epinephrine (adrenaline) or norepinephrine (noradrenaline).

anabolic agents Compounds (usually androgens) that promote synthesis of new tissue.

androgen Natural or synthetic substance (usually a hormone) that produces masculinizing effects.

antimicrosomal antibody An antibody against thyroid peroxidase, the principal antigen in thyroid microsomes.

aplasia Lack of development of any organ.

C-cells Calcitonin-secreting cells of the thyroid.

calorigenesis Production of heat and energy.

cretinism Hypothyroid condition caused by congenital lack of thyroid hormone secretion and characterized by impaired physical and mental development.

DIT Diiodotyrosine.

dysgenesis Abnormal or defective development.

dysplasia Abnormal development of an organ resulting in alteration of configuration, size, or cell organization.

endocytosis The uptake by a cell of material from the environment by invagination of its plasma membrane.

factitial Produced by artificial means; unintentionally produced.

follicular cells Thyroid hormone–producing cells arranged in units of spherical vesicles.

goiter Enlargement of the thyroid gland.

Graves' disease Immune disorder caused by the binding of antibodies to thyroid-stimulating hormone (TSH) receptors, resulting in an unregulated increase in thyroid hormone production and release.

Hashimoto's thyroiditis Inflammatory process of the thyroid caused by a derangement of the immune system, which may or may not lead to abnormal thyroid function.

hyperthyroidism Metabolic and clinical state caused by an increase in circulating active thyroid hormone.

hypothyroidism Metabolic and clinical state caused by decreased levels of circulating active thyroid hormone or increased tissue resistance; primary—decreased thyroid function caused by disease of the thyroid gland; secondary—decreased thyroid function caused by disease of the pituitary gland; tertiary—decreased thyroid function caused by disease of the hypothalamus.

iatrogenic Any adverse condition resulting from the actions of a physician.

interstitium Pertaining to the intercellular spaces of a tissue.

iodine trapping The ability of the thyroid gland to sequester iodine against a concentration gradient.

medullary carcinoma (thyroid) Cancer of the C-cells.

MIT Monoiodotyrosine.

monodeiodination Loss or removal of a single iodine atom.

multinodular goiter Enlarged thyroid containing numerous superficial and deep indurations.

myxedema Advanced hypothyroid state characterized clinically by distinctive external appearance: pallor, skin edema (swelling) of face and hands, apathy, and so on.

organification Incorporation of ionic form of iodine into the molecular structure of tyrosine.

parafollicular C-cells Calcitonin-secreting cells located between follicles.

parenchyma A group of basic morphological and functional cellular units that constitute any organ.

prohormone A compound requiring chemical transformation to become an active hormone.

protein-bound iodine (PBI) The total amount of iodine bound to proteins in the plasma.

radioiodine thyroid uptake Measurement of thyroid functions based upon percentage of ^{123}I or ^{131}I accumulation after a known dose is administered orally.

resin-uptake test Measurement of the number of available binding sites of plasma thyroid hormone–transporting proteins.

solitary nodule Localized enlargement of a portion of the thyroid gland.

struma ovarii Rare teratoid tumor of the ovary composed almost entirely of thyroid tissue.

T_3 Thyroid hormone with iodine atoms in positions 3, 5, and 3′ (triiodothyronine).

T_4 Thyroxine, a thyroid hormone with iodine atoms in positions 3, 5, 3′, and 5′ (tetraiodothyronine).

rT_3 Reverse T_3, triiodothyronine with iodine in positions 3, 3′, and 5′.

thyroglobulin A glycoprotein of molecular weight 660,000 daltons produced by the follicular cells and containing the precursors of T_3 and T_4.

thyroid colloid The material found within the follicles of the thyroid and containing thyroglobulin and thyroid hormone.

thyroid hormone–binding ratio (THBR) Current terminology for the T_3 or T_4 resin-uptake tests.

thyroiditis A general term for inflammation of the thyroid gland.

thyrotoxicosis Condition caused by excess thyroid hormone secretion; often used as synonym for hyperthyroidism.

thyrotropin A synonym for thyroid-stimulating hormone (TSH).

thyroxine-binding globulin (TBG) A glycoprotein of alpha-mobility that transports thyroid hormone in the blood.

transthyretin Thyroxine-binding prealbumin, a protein that transports thyroid hormone in the blood.

TRH (thyrotropin-releasing hormone) A hypothalamic tripeptide that promotes release of TSH.

trophic action Stimulation of cell reproduction and enlargement.

trophoblastic tumor Tumor originating from extraembryonal cells of ectodermic nature located in the blastocyst.

TSH (thyroid-stimulating hormone, thyrotropin) A glycoprotein composed of alpha and beta subunits that is released from the pituitary. TSH promotes thyroid hormone production and release.

TSI Thyroid-stimulating immunoglobulin.

Wolff-Chaikoff effect Decreased formation and release of thyroid hormone in the presence of excess iodine.

ANATOMY

The thyroid is usually formed of two lobes, one on either side of the neck. The thyroid gland consists of two types of cells, follicular and parafollicular (Fig. 44-1). Follicular cells are arranged spherically in a single layer with an apical end facing the center of the follicle and a basal end facing the interstitium. Follicular cells produce thyroid hormone, which is then stored in the central portion of the spherical follicle in a material called "colloid." The interstitium contains the blood supply and parafollicular cells. Parafollicular cells secrete the hormone calcitonin. For this reason they are called *C*-cells.

THYROID PHYSIOLOGY

The thyroid gland has as its main function the production and secretion of metabolically active hormones that are essential for the regulation of various metabolic processes. Thyroid hormones are produced within the cells of the follicles from the amino acid tyrosine and the halogen element iodine. The two most important thyroid hormones are thyroxine (T_4), which contains four iodine atoms, and triiodothyronine (T_3), which contains three iodine atoms (Fig. 44-2).

Thyroid hormones are released from the colloid and secreted into circulation in response to stimulation of the thyroid gland by the pituitary hormone called *thyroid-stimulating hormone* (TSH).

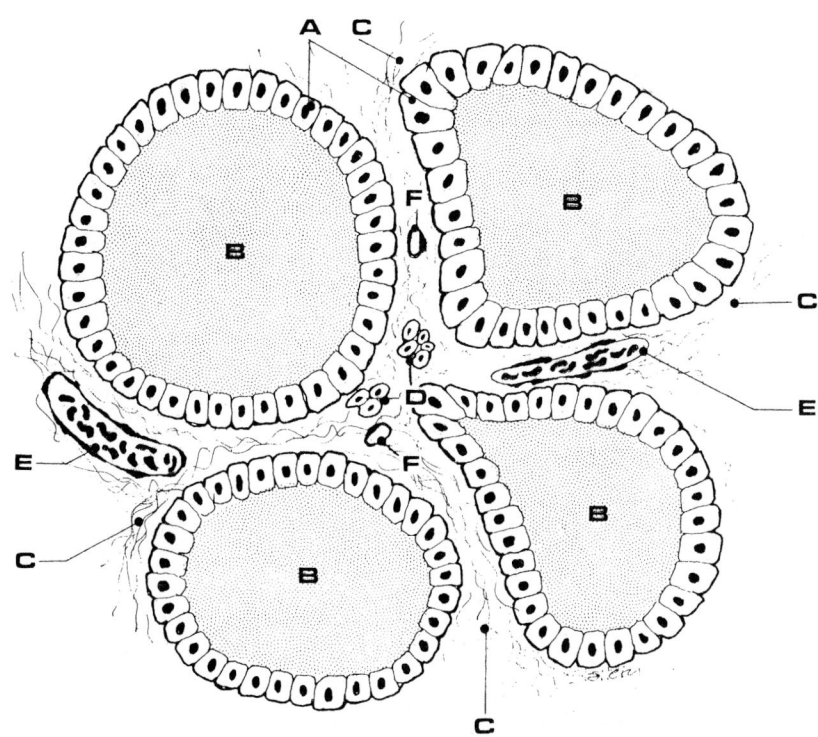

Fig. 44-1 Thyroid gland structure consists of follicular cells, *A;* enclosing colloid, *B;* and parafollicular "C" cells, *D,* in the interstitium, *C. E,* Venule; *F,* capillary.

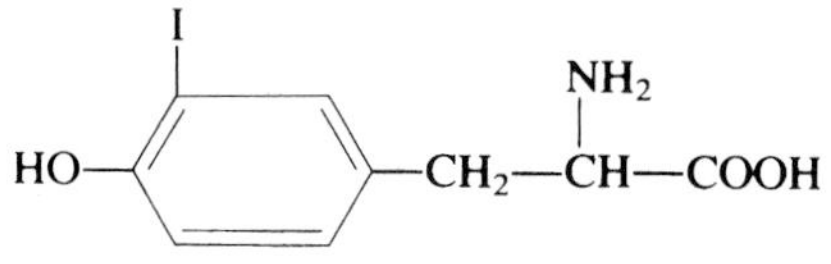

MIT
(Monoiodotyrosine)

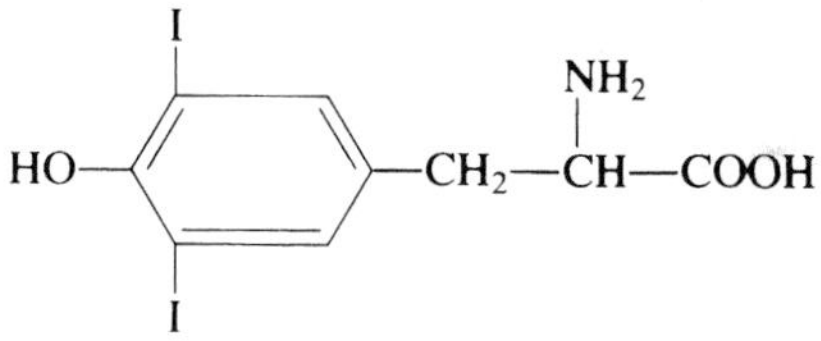

DIT
(Diiodotyrosine)

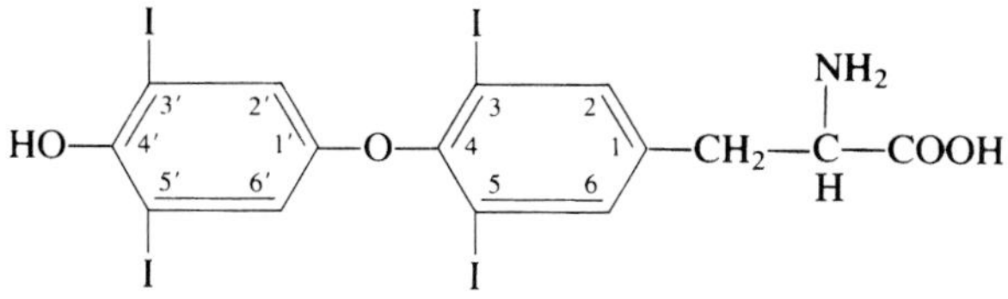

T₄
(3,5,3′,5′-Thyroxine)

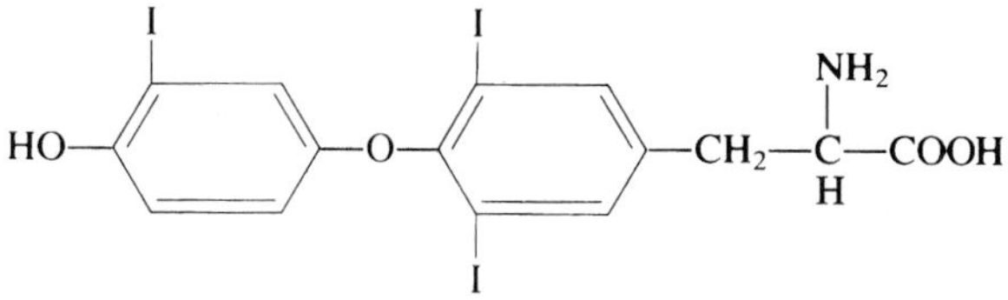

T₃
(3,5,3′-Triiodothyronine)

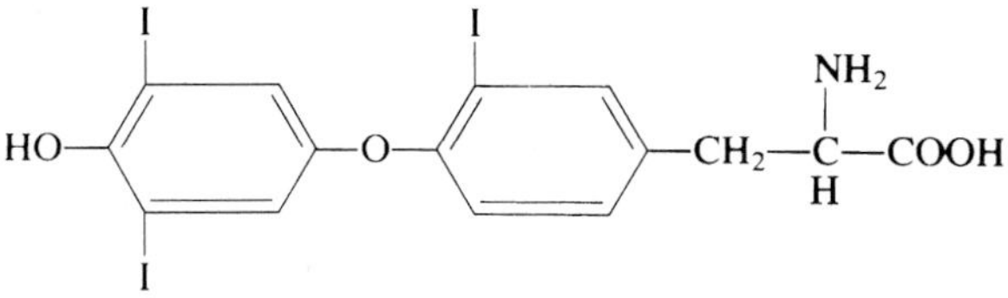

rT₃
(3,3′,5′-Triiodothyronine)

Fig. 44-2 Chemical structure of thyroid hormones and iodinated precursors and metabolites.

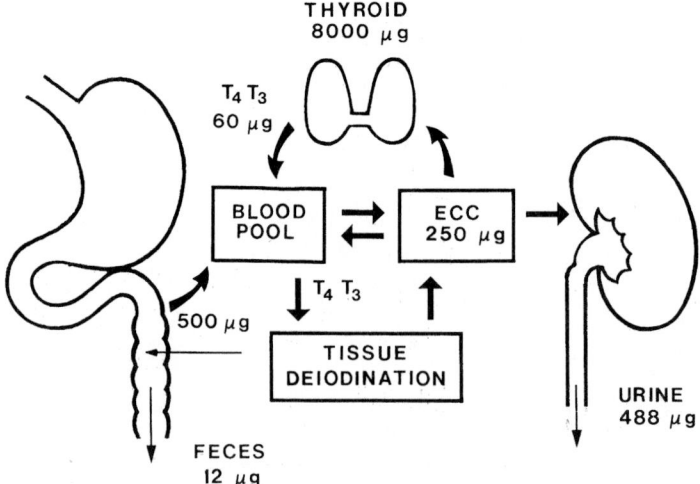

THYROID
8000 μg

T₄ T₃
60 μg

BLOOD POOL ⇌ ECC 250 μg

500 μg

T₄ T₃

TISSUE DEIODINATION

URINE 488 μg

FECES 12 μg

Fig. 44-3   Iodine metabolic pathway in a 24-hour period. *ECC,* Extracellular compartment.

Metabolism of iodine and thyroid hormone synthesis

Iodine is a natural component of many foods, and in the United States it is provided in adequate amounts by a well-balanced diet. Extra amounts of iodine are currently provided by the ingestion of iodine-enriched foods and numerous "vitamin pills." The daily intake of iodine varies widely in different parts of the world. In the United States iodine intake ranges from 250 to 700 μg or more daily. In countries such as Japan, intake may reach several milligrams per day, whereas in some areas of Africa, South America, Asia, and Europe daily intake may be as low as 50 μg.

Under physiological conditions, iodine, which is reduced to iodide (I⁻) in the gastrointestinal tract, is absorbed in the small bowel and then enters either the excretory or metabolic pathways (Fig. 44-3). Between 60% and 80% of the ingested iodine is excreted by the kidneys. Small amounts are excreted through the intestinal route. Fecal excretion is derived mostly from hormones degraded by the liver and excreted into the bowel by the biliary tract. The remainder of the iodine is distributed into the extracellular and thyroid compartments. The intrathyroid iodine compartment contains about 90% of the total body iodine and can amount to as much as 6000 to 12,000 μg. The extracellular compartment contains most other iodine, except for a small but important amount that is found in cells. The metabolism of iodine is closely related to the process of thyroid hormonogenesis.

Classically, intrathyroidal iodine metabolism has been divided into the following stages: (1) iodine trapping or uptake of iodine by the follicular cells, (2) organification, (3) coupling, (4) storage, and (5) secretion (Fig. 44-4). During trapping, thyroid cells concentrate iodine against high chemical and electrical gradients, which requires an active energy-dependent mechanism at the level of the cell membrane.[1]

This trapping mechanism for iodine has been exploited for many years in clinical tests to assess thyroid function. Radioactive iodine is given orally to patients, and its degree of concentration in the thyroid is subsequently measured. Various physiological and pharmacological factors influence trapping. The most important factor is thyroid-stimulating hormone (TSH), which stimulates trapping of iodine. Iodine excess inhibits the transport of iodine; iodine deficiency stimulates it.

The second step of intrathyroidal iodine metabolism is organification by means of which iodine is incorporated into thyroid hormone.[2] The iodine used comes from trapping and from the intrathyroid deiodination of stored thyroid hormone precursors. Iodine in the thyroid is oxidized in the presence of a peroxidase enzyme into a reactive form that combines with the protein thyroglobulin.[2]

Thyroglobulin is a glycoprotein with a molecular weight of about 660,000 daltons. Thyroglobulin serves as a preformed matrix containing 140 tyrosine residues to which reactive iodine is attached to form monoiodotyrosine (MIT) and diiodotyrosine (DIT). After their formation, enzymatic coupling of MIT and DIT takes place to form intrathyroglobulin triiodothyronine (T₃), and thyroxine (T₄). The thyroglobulin is then released from the cells into the colloid of the follicle where it is stored. The function of iodinated thyroglobulin is to serve as a storage pool of thyroid hormone.

When TSH stimulates the thyroid, a series of cellular and biochemical changes takes place in the gland, all directed toward the synthesis and release of thyroid hormone.[3] Initially, droplets of colloid are engulfed by the follicular cells and digested by proteases, releasing MIT, DIT, T₃, and T₄ from the thyroglobulin matrix. Intracellular MIT and DIT are immediately deiodinated, and their iodine is reused in subsequent thyroid hormone synthesis, whereas the T₃ and T₄ are resistant to intrathyroid deiodination and are imme-

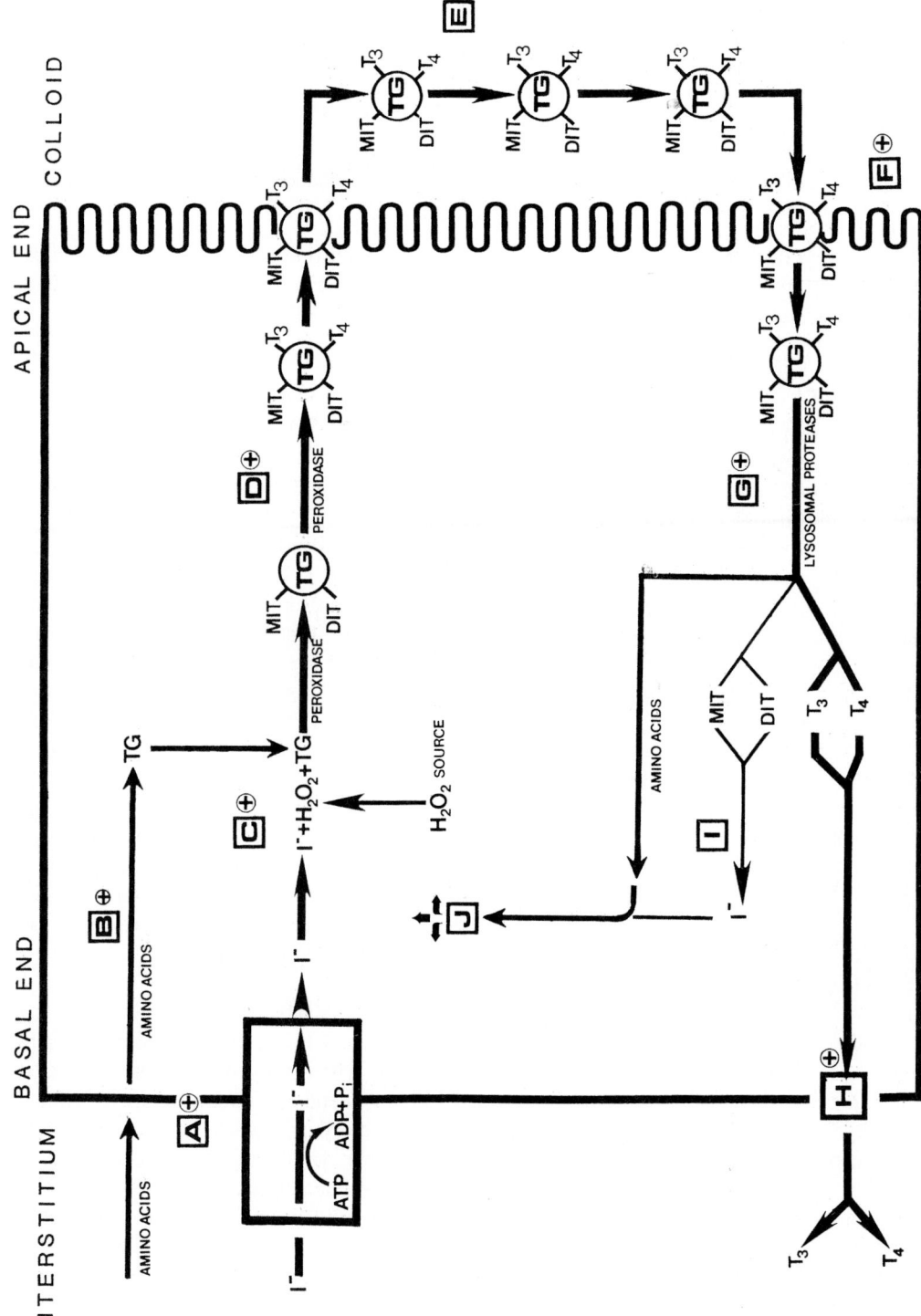

Fig. 44-4 Thyroid cell. Schema depicting stages of thyroid hormonogenesis and intrathyroidal iodine metabolism. *A*, Iodine transport; *B*, thyroglobulin (TG) synthesis; *C*, iodide organification; *D*, intrathyroglobulin oxidative coupling; *E*, storage; *F*, endocytosis; *G*, hydrolysis; *H*, hormone secretion; *I*, intrathyroidal deiodination; *J*, recycling. Steps influenced by the thyroid-stimulating hormone (TSH) are indicated by the symbol ⊕.

Table 44-1 Physiological relationship between thyroxine-binding globulin (TBG) and serum thyroid hormone concentrations

Biological modulators	Initial biochemical changes	Intermediate biological response	Final equilibrium conditions
Increased TBG Pregnancy Oral contraceptives	Increased TBG levels, decreased saturation Augmented binding of hormone (T_4, T_3) Decreased free T_4, T_3	Decreased negative-feedback mechanism Increased serum TSH Increased T_4 and T_3 production	Increased TBG Elevated serum T_4 and T_3 levels Normal TBG saturation Normal free T_4 and T_3
Decreased TBG Androgens Malnutrition Liver disease	Decreased TBG, increased saturation Diminished binding of hormone (T_4, T_3) Increased free T_4 and T_3	Increased negative-feedback mechanism Decreased serum TSH Decreased T_4 and T_3 production	Decreased TBG Decreased T_4 and T_3 Normal TBG saturation Normal free T_4 and T_3 serum

diately secreted. The daily secretion of thyroid hormone includes about 80 to 100 µg of T_4 and about 7 µg of T_3.[4] Small amounts of reverse T_3 (rT_3) are also secreted by the thyroid.

Transport of thyroid hormones

After they are released into the bloodstream, the thyroid hormones are transported in two forms, protein bound and free. The free hormone, which is most readily available for cellular uptake and is thus the physiologically active fraction, represents only a small fraction (less than 0.1%) of the total plasma thyroid hormone content. The bound hormone is metabolically inactive and serves as a large, stable reservoir of hormone, and thus a constant supply of hormone is available to tissues.

Thyroid hormones are bound to three plasma proteins.[5] The most important of these is the thyroxine-binding globulin (TBG), which is a 55,000-dalton glycoprotein synthesized in the liver. The second most important is thyroxine-binding prealbumin (TBPA), also called *transthyretin*, which has a molecular weight of 50,000 daltons. The third transporting protein is albumin. The role of each of these binding proteins in the transport of T_3 and T_4 is related to their relative affinities for each of the thyroid hormones and on their relative concentrations in plasma. Almost all the circulating T_4 (99.98%) is bound to these plasma proteins. Under physiological circumstances, TBG transports 70% to 75% of total T_4. TBPA and albumin transport 15% to 20% and 10% of T_4 respectively. As is true for T_4, most (99.7%) plasma T_3 circulates in the bound form. The affinity of TBG for T_3 is lower than its affinity for T_4, and binding of T_3 to TBPA is negligible. T_3 is mostly bound to TBG and to a lesser extent to albumin.

T_4 has different affinities for each of its binding proteins, which must be compared to its affinity to the intracellular T_4 receptor (see below). T_4's affinity for TBG is greater than its affinity for the T_4 receptor. T_4's affinity for albumin, however, is weaker than its affinity for the T_4 receptor. Thus there are three pools of protein-bound T_4 in decreasing order of amount of T_4 bound: high-affinity, low-availability (TBG); medium-affinity, medium-availability (TBPA); and low-affinity, high-availability (albumin). This

allows a rapid shifting of T_4 among all pools as described in the following equation and ensures a constant availability of T_4 to target cells:

$$\overbrace{\text{TBG-}T_4 \rightleftharpoons \text{TBPA-}T_4 \rightleftharpoons \text{Albumin-}T_4}^{\textbf{Protein bound } T_4} \rightleftharpoons \text{Free } T_4 \rightleftharpoons \text{Intracellular receptor-}T_4$$

Abnormalities of the binding proteins may result in abnormal total (bound) hormone concentrations in the blood even when normal amounts of free hormone are present. Since both T_4 and T_3 are bound to TBG, changes of TBG levels affect total serum T_4 and T_3 levels. Changes in TBG concentrations in blood have an indirect effect on the negative-feedback mechanisms of thyroid hormone regulation (Table 44-1). An increase in levels of TBG binding will result in an immediate increase in the amount of thyroid hormone that is protein bound, with a subsequent decrease in circulating free hormone. The decrease in thyroid hormone immediately triggers the secretion of TSH, which results in increased thyroid hormone production and release. All of these changes are transient, and a new equilibrium with preservation of the normal thyroid status is quickly reached. Decreases of TBG serum levels will cause the opposite biological changes.

Metabolism of thyroid hormones

Circulating T_3 and T_4 are either incorporated into the intracellular pool, where they undergo partial transformations and exert their metabolic effects, or are degraded and eliminated by excretory organs.

Although all circulating T_4 originates in the thyroid gland, the more metabolically important T_3 originates from both direct thyroid secretion (about 20%) and peripheral conversion of T_4 to T_3 by monodeiodination (about 80%).[4] The total daily production of T_3 from all sources ranges from 22 to 47 µg. T_3 has been established as the main active hormone at the tissue level. The role of T_4 as a hormone with direct biological activity has been questioned, and some workers consider T_4 to be a prohormone. However, T_4 is believed to have some direct biological activity, albeit much less than T_3.

THYROID   BLOOD   CELLS

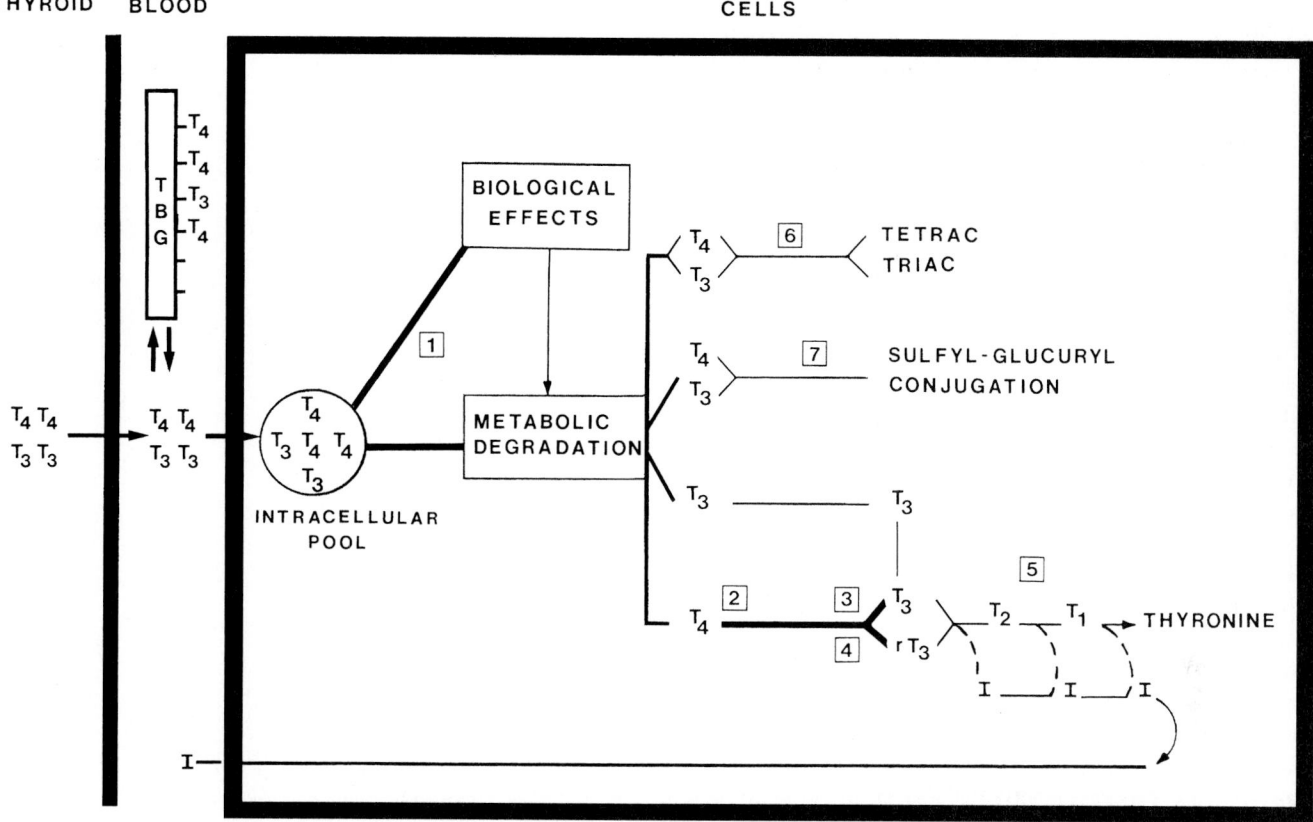

Fig. 44-5   Metabolic pathways of thyroid hormone. *1,* Biological effects through binding to intracellular receptors; *2,* main deiodinative pathway for T_4; *3,* conversion of T_4 into T_3; *4,* conversion of T_4 into rT_3; *5,* serial deiodinations of T_3 and rT_3; *6,* deamination and decarboxylation pathway; *7,* conjugative pathway.

The thyroid hormones are metabolized through deiodinative and nondeiodinative mechanisms. The following are some of the most important metabolic steps (Fig. 44-5):

1. Both T_4 and T_3 exert their biological effects by binding to specific intracellular receptors and are subsequently degraded through successive deiodinations.

2. Deiodination accounts for 80% to 85% of the metabolism of T_4 and T_3.[6]

3. About 35% to 50% of the T_4 undergoing deiodination is converted to T_3.[6,7]

4. About 50% to 65% of the deiodinated T_4 is converted into rT_3.[7]

5. Most of the T_4, T_3, and rT_3 are metabolized through a chain of successive deiodinations, resulting in the formation of iodinated intermediary metabolites and ultimately thyronine.

6. Both T_4 and T_3 undergo oxidative deamination and decarboxylation of the alanine side chains to form the acetic acid analogs tetrac and triac.[4]

7. Small amounts of free T_4 are eliminated in the bile and urine.

8. Small amounts of T_3, rT_3, and indirectly T_4 are me-

tabolized through processes of conjugation with glucuronic acid and sulfate.

Conversion of T_4 to active T_3 by monodeiodination of the outer ring is one of the most important metabolic pathways of T_4. In T_3, iodine atoms are located at positions 3 and 5 of the inner (nonphenolic) ring and at position 3' of the outer (phenolic) ring (Fig. 44-2). Two types of 5'-deiodinases have been identified. Type 1, 5'-deiodinase, maintains the plasma T_3 concentration and is found in the liver and kidney. Its activity increases in hyperthyroidism and decreases in hypothyroidism. There is a reduced amount of type 1 5'-deiodinase activity in severe illness, fasting states, and significant hepatic disease. Reduced activity is also seen in the fetus and secondary to certain medications, including propylthiouracil (PTU), propranolol, and excess glucocorticoids. Type 2, 5'-deiodinase, maintains the local T_3 concentrations in the tissue in which it is present. It predominates in the brain, pituitary, placenta, and brown fat and is under noradrenergic control. Its activity increases in hypothyroidism, maintaining the constant intracellular T_3 levels, and decreases in hyperthyroidism as a compensatory mechanism. Decreased amounts of both types of 5'-

deiodinases may be caused by the administration of iodinated radiographic contrast material or by the administration of amiodarone, an antiarrhythmic drug that causes inhibition of T_4 monodeiodination.

If the inner ring of T_4 undergoes monodeiodination, the product is *reverse T_3* (rT_3), which is metabolically inactive. In rT_3, the iodine atoms are found in position 3 of the inner ring and positions 3' and 5' of the outer ring. Almost all rT_3 derives from inner ring monodeiodination of T_4.

Mechanisms of action

Mechanisms of action of the thyroid hormones at the cellular level have been the focus of intensive research. Initially the thyroid hormone appears both to bind to cell membrane receptors and to cross the cell membrane by direct diffusion. Once inside the cell, the thyroid hormone binds to cytosol and nuclear receptor sites. The T_3 nuclear receptors are the gene products of the c-*erb* A proto-oncogene. Mutations of these sites are believed to be the cause for familial thyroid hormone resistance. Once the T_3 binds to the nuclear receptor sites, messenger ribonucleic acid (mRNA) is formed and directs the synthesis of proteins and enzymes responsible for metabolic functions.[8] Other postulated mechanisms of action at the cellular level are (1) mitochondrial activation, (2) stimulation of Na^+,K^+-adenosine-triphosphatase (ATPase) activity,[9] (3) stimulation of cell membrane functions, probably through a specific receptor, and (4) interaction with the adrenergic system.

Control and regulation of thyroid function

Hypothalamic-pituitary-thyroid axis (HPTA). The HPTA is a group of physiologically interrelated neuroendocrine and endocrine organs that regulate and control the secretion of thyroid hormone (Fig. 44-6). The ultimate effector in this axis is the thyroid gland, which produces, stores, and secretes the hormones thyroxine and triiodothyronine. The hypothalamus, located in the brain, acts as a crucial regulating organ (see also Chapter 43).

Thyrotropin-releasing hormone (TRH) is a tripeptide produced in the hypothalamus and secreted into the venous system, which then drains into the pituitary. The TRH attaches to receptor sites in the pituitary, where it causes increased production and secretion of thyroid-stimulating hormone (TSH). TSH is a glycopeptide structurally composed of two subunits, alpha and beta. The β subunit confers on TSH the specific physiological properties that differentiate it from other pituitary glycopeptides. TSH is released from the pituitary into the bloodstream. At the thyroid, TSH attaches to specific cell membrane receptors thereby activating adenylate cyclase and increasing intracellular levels of cyclic AMP (cAMP). The increased levels of cAMP have two main actions. The first action is the stimulation of cell reproduction and hypertrophy. The second effect is the stimulation of production and secretion of thyroid hormone by the thyroid cell.

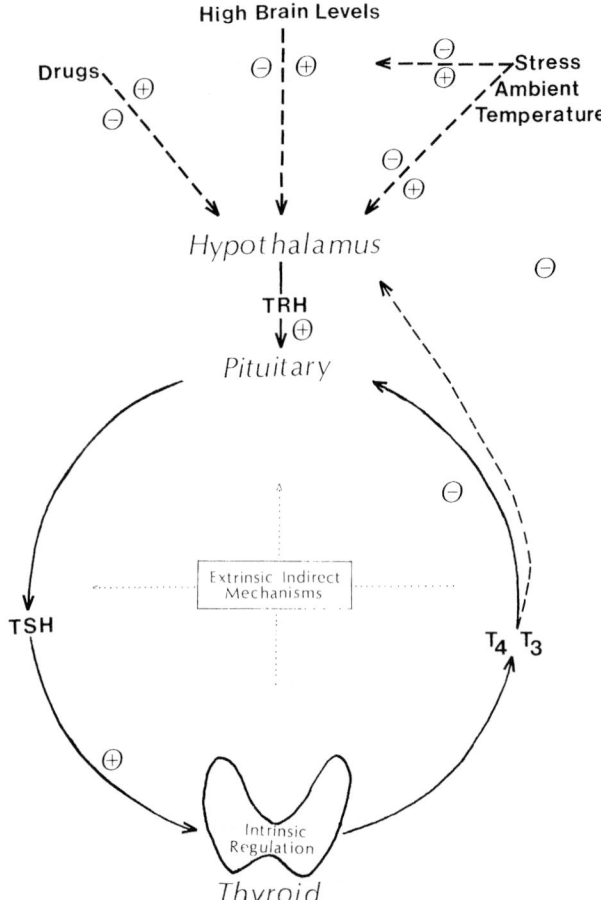

Fig. 44-6 Hypothalamic-pituitary-thyroid axis (HPTA). Stimulatory, ⊕, or inhibitory, ⊖, effect of agent.

In healthy persons an increase in blood TRH levels will affect the blood levels of TSH and thyroid hormone (Fig. 44-7). After the intravenous administration of synthetic TRH, blood levels of TSH begin to increase within 10 minutes, reach a maximum at 15 to 45 minutes, and return to normal base levels in 1 to 4 hours.[10] Elevations of TSH after the administration of TRH result in increases in serum T_4 and T_3. The initial increases in T_3 are higher (75% increase over basal levels) than those in T_4 (15% to 50% over basal levels). The T_3 and T_4 levels subsequently drop slowly. The TSH (and occasionally T_3 and T_4) responses to intravenous administrations of synthetic TRH are occasionally used for diagnostic purposes (see p. 881).

Negative-feedback system on pituitary secretion of TSH. Increased levels of thyroid hormones in blood inhibit TSH secretion by the pituitary (negative feedback). The mechanism of this inhibitory effect appears to involve circulating free T_3 and T_4. The pituitary and hypothalamus glands are also able to convert T_4 directly to T_3. This locally generated T_3 then acts with circulating T_3 on the pituitary gland cells to inhibit the secretion of TSH in response to TRH and on the hypothalamus to reduce TRH

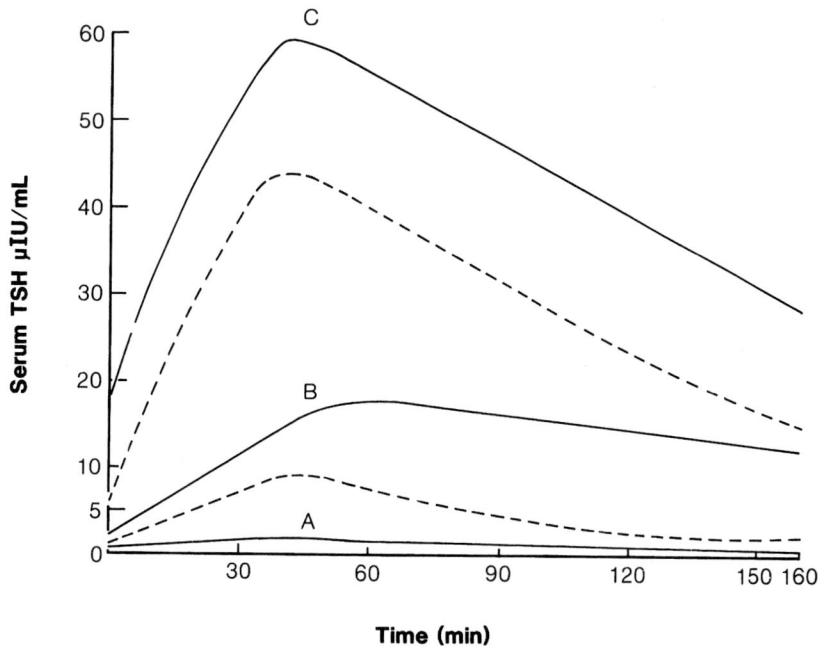

Fig. 44-7 Changes in serum TSH levels in response to TRH (given at 0 min). The upper and lower ranges of normal responses are shown by the dashed lines. Serum TSH changes after TRH challenge in pituitary, *A;* hypothalamic, *B;* and primary hypothyroid, *C,* disease are also shown.

output. Conversely, decreased levels of thyroid hormone result in increased secretion of TRH and TSH.

Other factors affecting thyroid function. Thyroid function is finely regulated by both extrinsic and intrinsic mechanisms. The extrinsic direct mechanism is referred to as the HPTA (hypothalamic-pituitary-thyroid axis). The extrinsic indirect mechanisms, which include neurogenic, metabolic, and pharmacological mechanisms, exert inhibitory and stimulatory effects centrally at all levels of the HPTA and peripherally on the metabolism of the thyroid hormones (see below). The intrinsic mechanisms are those that act within the thyroid cells, ensuring that adequate amounts of intrathyroid hormone are produced. These mechanisms are closely dependent on the availability and effects of iodine.

When the thyroid gland is exposed to rapid and large increases of iodine, there is an inhibition of the formation and release of thyroid hormone. This inhibition is known as the "Wolff-Chaikoff effect."[11] If the thyroid continues to be exposed to increased concentrations of iodine, the inhibitory effects of excess iodine on hormone formation and release decrease and eventually cease.[11]

Effects of drugs and other compounds on thyroid function. Various drugs and substances may interfere with thyroid function. Their pharmacological effects may take place at one or several levels (Table 44-2). For example, the drug amiodarone causes elevations of free and total T_4, decreased T_3, and increased rT_3.[12] Various other drugs affect TBG levels and hormone binding and thus total T_3 and T_4 determinations (see box, p. 877).

Interrelationships between thyroid gland and other functions

Various physiological factors indirectly influence thyroid function and the effects of thyroid hormones. The effects of sex hormones and sex type on thyroid function are variable. Thyroid disease is known to predominate in females. Estrogens cause an increase in TBG and therefore total serum T_3 and T_4 content, whereas androgenic hormones have the opposite effect. On the other hand, states of decreased (hypothyroidism) and increased (hyperthyroidism) thyroid function are associated with alterations of the reproductive system, abnormalities of the menstrual cycle, delayed or precocious puberty, infertility, and growth retardation.

The newborn has lower levels of total T_3 and higher levels of total T_4 and rT_3 than adults have.[13] Immediately after birth there is an increase of TSH, with corresponding elevations of total T_3 and total T_4 that reach their zenith the second day after birth and then gradually decrease toward normal adult levels by the end of the first year of life. There is also a slow progressive decrease of T_3 levels in adults during the aging process.

Striking changes in thyroid function occur during pregnancy (see also Chapter 40). The normal placenta produces significant amounts of nonthyroid hormones (especially estrogens), which stimulate the synthesis of TBG, increasing

Table 44-2 Effects of various drugs on thyroid function

Mechanism of action	Drug	Effects
Hypothalamic stimulation	Amphetamine	Increased T_4, T_3, and free T_4
Inhibition of TSH secretion	Dopamine Levodopa Glucocorticoids Bromocriptine	Decreased TSH Blunted TSH response to TRH
Enhanced TSH secretion	Metoclopramide	Increased TSH response to TRH
Blocking of iodine trapping	Perchlorate Thiocyanates Nitroprusside	Block production of T_4 and T_3
Inhibition of organification	Propylthiouracil Methimazole Sulfonylureas 6-Mercaptopurine	Decreased T_4 and T_3 production
Inhibition of release of T_4 and T_3	Lithium	Mild transient decrease of T_4, T_3 Induction of goiter
Decreased conversion of T_4 and T_3 Decreased type I 5'-deiodinase	Propylthiouracil Propanolol Glucocorticoid excess	Decreased T_3
Decreased type I and II 5'-deiodinase	Amiodarone Telepaque (iopanoic acid) Oragrafin (ipodic acid sodium calcium salt)	Decreased T_3
Increased degradation	Phenobarbital	Slight decrease of T_4 and T_3 and increase in TSH
Modulation of excess of β-adrenergic receptors	β-Adrenergic blockers	Blunted adrenergic-related effects of T_3 and T_4
Decreased hormone protein-binding to TBG	Salicylates Phenytoin Fenclofenac Furosemide	Decreased T_3 and T_4 Increased T_3RU

From Kaplan MM: *Med Clin North Am* 69:863-880, 1985; Oppenheimer JH, Schwartz HL, Surks MI: *J Clin Invest* 51:2493-2497, 1972; Singer I, Rotenberg D: *N Engl J Med* 289:254-260, 1973; Cavalieri RR, Gavin LA, Wallace A, et al: *Metabolism* 29:1161-1165, 1979.

serum TBG levels. Both total T_4 and, to a lesser extent, total T_3 levels in serum increase during pregnancy because of these increases in TBG concentration.[14] Levels of free hormone remain normal.

In fasting states, changes in levels of thyroid hormone in serum occur within 24 to 48 hours. Initially serum T_3 decreases rapidly. If fasting is maintained, the decrease slows, becoming more gradual. The decrease in T_3 levels is caused by decreased peripheral conversion of T_4 to T_3. Concomitantly there is an increase in rT_3 levels. Chronic decreased caloric intake also results in a decline in thyroxine-binding prealbumin (TBPA), probably caused by decreased hepatic production.

General metabolic and physiological effects of thyroid hormone

Increases and decreases in hormone production will result in states of hyperfunction (hyperthyroidism) and hypofunction (hypothyroidism) respectively. The clinical presentation of hyperthyroidism or hypothyroidism reflects the ba-

sic effects of thyroid hormone on various organs and metabolic systems.

Table 44-3 depicts some general effects that thyroid hormone has on various metabolic functions and systems. The effects of thyroid hormone can be classified according to their clinical expression into (1) general metabolic effects, (2) growth and maturation effects, and (3) organ-specific effects. Generally speaking, both intermediary metabolic pathways and specific metabolic pathways are stimulated by the thyroid hormone resulting in increased oxygen consumption and calorigenesis. Thyroid hormone has important actions as a promoter of cell differentiation, growth, and maturation. Deficiency of thyroid hormone in early life results in severe impairment of physical growth, maturation, and brain development. The third class of thyroid hormonal effects represents many direct effects exerted on specific organs and systems, such as the brain and heart. Finally, increased thyroid function is associated with an elevated catecholamine (hyperadrenergic) state important in the genesis of some symptoms of hyperthyroidism.

Causes of Abnormalities in Thyroxine-Binding Globulin (TBG)

Quantitative

Increased TBG serum levels
  Pregnancy
  Estrogen therapy
  Clofibrate treatment
  Oral contraceptives
  Perphenazine
  Abuse of heroin or methadone
  Acute hepatitis
  Hypothyroidism
  Neonatal period
  Acute intermittent porphyria
  Genetic TBG excess
Decreased TBG serum levels
  Androgens
  Anabolic agents
  Cirrhosis
  Acute illness
  Surgical stress
  Severe chronic illness
  Severe hypoproteinemia
  Protein malnutrition
  Nephrotic syndrome
  Hyperthyroidism
  Corticosteroid therapy
  L-Asparaginase therapy
  Active acromegaly
  Klinefelter's syndrome
  Cushing's syndrome
  Down's syndrome
  Type III hyperlipidemia
  Chronic metabolic acidosis
  Genetic deficiency (usually x-linked)

Qualitative

Genetic
  Genetically determined increase in binding affinity
  Genetically determined decrease in binding affinity
Drugs competing with T_4 and T_3 for TBG-binding sites
  Phenytoin (diphenylhydantoin, Dilantin)
  Dicumarol
  Heparin
  Atromid S
  Aspirin
  Phenylbutazone

Decreased thyroid hormone results in deposition of mucoproteins and mucopolysaccharides in various tissues such as the skin, muscles, and heart. This phenomenon partly explains the thick skin, muscle weakness, enlarged heart, and symptoms of heart failure seen in hypothyroidism.

Thyroid function in nonthyroid disease (NTD)

Certain conditions do not directly alter the output of hormone by the thyroid but rather interfere with the normal transport and metabolism of thyroid hormones. These conditions, including those abnormalities in thyroxine-binding globulin (see box at left). These conditions produce changes in standard blood tests of thyroid function but are generally not accompanied by true thyroid dysfunction. The disorders are of clinical importance because they may mimic true thyroid disease or confound the diagnosis of concomitant thyroid dysfunction.

Malnutrition, renal and hepatic dysfunction are the three most important nonthyroid factors leading to abnormalities of thyroid function tests. States of malnutrition are often seen in chronic and debilitating diseases. The most conspicuous physiological abnormality found in malnourished patients is the impaired peripheral conversion of T_4 to T_3.[15] As a result, serum total and free T_3 concentrations decrease significantly while the serum total T_4 concentration stays relatively stable. The levels of rT_3 may double.

The liver plays an important role in the metabolism of thyroid hormones by its production of thyroxine-binding proteins, conversion of T_4 to T_3 or rT_3, and removal of thyroid hormones. Alterations in these functions can occur in liver disease, resulting in abnormal test results in the absence of thyroid disease.

The kidneys have two main functions in relation to the thyroid: the first concerns iodine metabolism, since the kidneys represent a major pathway of iodine elimination; the second is the prevention of excessive losses of thyroxine-binding globulins in the urine. Kidney disease can result in either decreased iodine clearance and excretion, with the secondary increases in blood and interstitial pools of iodine seen in renal failure, or the augmented loss of thyroxine-binding proteins seen in the nephrotic syndrome. Finally, although it plays a less important role than that of the liver, the kidney has the metabolic function of converting T_4 to T_3. In acutely and severely ill patients, the serum T_3 may be undetectable, the serum T_4 greatly reduced, and the serum TSH normal or mildly increased. As the patient recovers, there is an approximate increase in TSH until free T_4 and free T_3 return to normal.

PATHOLOGICAL CONDITIONS
Hyperthyroidism

Causes. Hyperthyroidism refers to the clinical syndrome caused by an excess of circulating active thyroid hormone. Hyperthyroidism is caused by numerous pathological conditions that have as a common denominator an increase in circulating thyroid hormone (see box on p. 878).

Graves' disease is caused by an immunological disorder in which serum autoantibodies bind to TSH receptors in the thyroid cell and stimulate the production and release of thyroid hormone. These antibodies compose a heterogeneous group of serum immunoglobulins that belong to the IgG fraction and are generically termed *thyroid-stimulating immunoglobulins* (TSI)[16] because of their ability to stimulate function in thyroid cells. The long-acting thyroid stimula-

Table 44-3   Basic physiological effects of thyroid hormone and their relationship with syndromes of thyroid dysfunction

System	Thyroid hormone effects	Usual symptoms	
		Hyperthyroidism	Hypothyroidism
Metabolic	Increased calorigenesis and O_2 consumption Increased heat dissipation Increased protein catabolism Increased glucose absorption and production (gluconeogenesis) Increased glucose use	Heat intolerance Flushed skin Increased perspiration Increased appetite and food ingestion Muscle wasting and proximal weakness Weight loss Onycholysis (nail disease) Lid lag Proptosis (exophthalmos)	Cold intolerance Dry and pale skin Coarse skin Lethargy Generalized weakness Weight gain Voice coarsening, slow speech Myxedema
Cardiovascular	Increased adrenergic activity and sensitivity Increased heart rate Increased myocardial contractility (inotropy) Increased cardiac output Increased blood volume Decreased peripheral vascular resistance	Palpitations Fast heart rate (tachycardia) Bouncy, hyperdynamic arterial pulses Shortness of breath Atrial fibrillation Widened pulse pressure ($\uparrow$ systolic BP, $\downarrow$ diastolic BP)	Slow heart rate (bradycardia) Low blood pressure Heart failure Heart enlargement
Central nervous	Increased adrenergic activity and sensitivity	Restlessness, hypermotility Nervousness Emotional lability Fatigue Exaggerated reflexes Tremor	Apathy Mental sluggishness Depressed reflexes Mental retardation
Gastrointestinal (GI)	Increased motility	Hyperdefecation	Constipation

BP, Blood pressure.

Causes of Hyperthyroidism

Primary hyperthyroidism

Primary thyroid abnormalities
   Toxic multinodular goiter (Plummer's disease)
   Thyroid adenoma
   Thyroid carcinoma
   Struma ovarii (ovarian teratoma with thyroid elements)

Secondary hyperthyroidism

Endogenous: increased serum levels of TSH (thyroid-stimulating substances), resulting in thyroid hyperactivity:
   Graves' disease
   Neonatal hyperthyroidism
   Pituitary tumors (TSH-secreting)
   Trophoblastic tumors
      Hydatiform mole
      Choriocarcinoma
      Embryonal carcinoma of testes
Exogenous:
   Iatrogenic
   Factitious hyperthyroidism (Jod-Basedow phenomenon)

Thyroiditis

Subacute thyroiditis (early phase)
Lymphocytic (Hashimoto's) thyroiditis
Radiation
Postpartum thyroiditis (early phase)

---

tor (LATS) antibody was the first TSI described and is present in about 60% of patients with Graves' disease.

Graves' disease is characterized clinically by the presence of diffuse goiter (enlarged thyroid gland), symptoms and signs of hyperthyroidism (Table 44-3), ophthalmopathy, and, occasionally, pretibial (swelling of the shins) edema. Graves' ophthalmopathy is characterized by a myxedematous (swelling observable by pressing on the tissue) infiltration of the tissues and muscles of the orbit, resulting in protrusion of the eyes and ocular muscle dysfunction. The ophthalmopathy may exist without accompanying thyroid hyperfunction.

Toxic multinodular goiter is a frequent cause of hyperthyroidism and usually appears in patients with preexisting nodular goiters. Nodular goiters are discrete portions of the thyroid gland that are no longer under normal feedback control and secrete excess amounts of thyroid hormone. This condition occurs more frequently in elderly patients and is not accompanied by ophthalmopathy or pretibial edema.

Thyroid adenomas are benign tumors that do not respond to the normal control mechanism and can occasionally produce excess thyroid hormone. Patients with adenomas have thyroid nodules that concentrate radioactive iodine avidly (hot nodules). It should be emphasized that most adenomas do not cause thyroid hyperfunction. Thyroid cancer is a rare cause of hyperthyroidism.

Table 44-4 Hyperthyroidism: laboratory findings in various clinical conditions

Clinical entity	T_4	T_3	FT_4	T_3RU	FT_4I	TSH	TRH stimulation	TSI	Thyroid ^{123}I uptake
Graves' disease	↑	↑	↑	↑	↑	↓, U	Blunted	↑	
Euthyroid Graves' disease	N	N	N	N	N	N	Blunted, N	+	N
Toxic multinodular goiter	↑	↑	↑	↑	↑	↓, U	Blunted	−	↑, N
Toxic adenoma	↑	↑	↑	↑	↑	↓, U	Blunted	−	↑, N
T_3 toxicosis	N	↑	N	N, ↑	N	↓, U	Blunted	+, −	N, ↑
Hyperthyroidism in pregnancy	↑	↑	↑	N, ↓	↑	↓, U	Blunted	+, −	*
Neonatal hyperthyroidism	↑	↑	↑	↑	↑	↓,N	Blunted	+	*
Subacute thyroiditis	↑, N	↑, N	↑, N	↑, N	↑, N	N,↓, U	Blunted, N	−	↓, N
Exogenous hyperthyroidism with T_4	↑	↑	↑	↑	↑	↓, U	Blunted	−	↓
Trophoblastic tumors	↑	↑	↑	↑	↑	↑, N, ↓	Blunted	−	↓, N, ↑
Pituitary TSH-secreting tumors	↑	↑	↑	↑	↑	↑	N, ↑	−	↑
Pseudohyperthyroidism	↑	↑, N	↑, N	↑, N	↑, N	↑, N	N	−	N or ↑

FT_4, Free thyroxine; FT_4I, free thyroxine index; *N*, normal; *TRH*, thyrotropin-releasing hormone; T_3RU, triiodothyronine resin-uptake test; *TSH*, thyroid-stimulating hormone; *TSI*, thyroid-stimulating immunoglobulins; *U*, undetectable.
↑, Elevated; ↓, decreased; +, present; −, absent; *, test contraindicated or not recommended.

Thyroiditis is a general term used to describe an inflammation of the thyroid gland. All forms of thyroiditis can potentially cause hyperthyroidism because large quantities of hormone can be released from the inflamed and disrupted follicles. *Subacute thyroiditis* and its variant, *painless thyroiditis,* are considered to be caused by a viral infection of the gland and have two phases. The early phase is characterized by active inflammation of the thyroid, which results in enlargement and tenderness of the gland and clinical and laboratory findings of thyroid hyperfunction caused by release of hormones.[17,18] During the late phase, recuperation takes place and function usually returns to normal. Some patients may evolve through an intermediary state of hypothyroidism. *Chronic lymphocytic thyroiditis* (Hashimoto's thyroiditis) is occasionally associated with an overactive thyroid state but more often results in hypothyroidism.

Postpartum thyroiditis occurs in 3.9% to 8.2% of women after delivery.[19,20] Similar to subacute thyroiditis, there may be three phases beginning with a painless thyrotoxicosis with greatly diminished radioactive iodine uptake. This typically occurs 1 to 3 months post partum and lasts for 1 to 2 months.[19] The thyroid gland often becomes enlarged. The patient may then develop hypothyroidism before recovery. Fatigue and depression are common symptoms. Postpartum thyroiditis is believed to be attributable to an autoimmune process and thyroid autoantibodies may be present.[21]

A sudden release of hormone may be seen after irradiation of the thyroid gland *(radiation thyroiditis).* Thyroid hyperfunction caused by this radiation thyroiditis as suggested by elevations of serum T_3 and T_4 is usually mild and self-limited.

Exogenous hyperthyroidism is caused by the administration of excessive thyroid hormone by the physician (iatrogenic) or as a result of surreptitious intake of thyroid hormone by patients (factitious).

Tumors originating from the trophoblast, or outer cellular layer of the forming embryo, can secrete large amounts of human chorionic gonadotropin (hCG). This hormone has been found to have a weak thyroid-stimulating action. As a result, such tumors may cause an increased secretion of thyroid hormones. Secondary hyperthyroidism caused by pituitary tumors that secrete high levels of TSH is a rare occurrence.

Some iodine-deficient patients develop hyperthyroidism after replacement of iodine either through diet or after the administration of radiographic iodine contrast material. This condition, known as the Jod-Basedow phenomenon, is postulated to occur in patients with occult Graves' disease or multinodular goiter.

Laboratory findings. Graves' disease is the classic example of hyperthyroidism. It occurs in 0.4% of the United States population. Its laboratory abnormalities (Table 44-4) include (1) elevation of thyroid hormones in serum, (2) decreased serum levels of TSH, and (3) blunted responses to TRH (see p. 881). In addition, patients with Graves' disease may have elevated serum levels of thyroglobulin and thyroid-stimulating immunoglobulin. In general there is a disproportionately higher rate of production of T_3 in Graves' disease.

As many as 5% of people with thyroid disease have been described with symptoms of hyperthyroidism and normal total T_4 and free T_4 concentrations, normal or mildly elevated thyroidal radioactive iodine uptake, and elevated T_3 levels in blood (T_3 thyrotoxicosis). This syndrome, which may be present in patients with Graves' disease, has also been observed in 5% of patients with toxic nodular goiter, in patients with previous iodine deficiency after iodine ingestion, and in patients with recurrent hyperthyroidism after treatment with radioactive iodine, thyroid-blocking agents, or surgery.

A less frequently found entity, T_4 *toxicosis,* refers to a condition in which the T_3 is normal or only mildly elevated and T_4 is quite elevated. This condition is seen most often in patients with an alteration in conversion of T_4 to T_3 as a result of chronic debilitating diseases or in patients acutely exposed to large amounts of iodine (such as x-ray contrast media).

Neonatal hyperthyroidism refers to a state of increased thyroid function seen in newborn infants of mothers whose serum may contain thyroid-stimulating immunoglobulins (TSI). This condition is postulated to be caused by transplacental transfer of maternal TSI.[22] Its course is benign with spontaneous remission.

Treatment. The treatment of hyperthyroidism can be aimed at eliminating excess functioning thyroid tissue (surgery or radioiodine), inhibiting the production of thyroid hormone by thyroid-blocking drugs such as propylthiouracil (PTU), methimazole, SSKI (saturated solution of potassium iodide), or Lugol's solution, inhibiting thyroid hormone release from the thyroid (SSKI, Lugol's solution), or suppressing the symptoms of hyperthyroidism (beta-adrenergic receptor blockers). All these methods are currently used, and the choice depends on the cause of the hyperthyroidism, special clinical situations, and the physician's personal preferences.

Hypothyroidism

Causes. A clinical state of hypothyroidism develops whenever insufficient amounts of thyroid hormone are available to tissues. By and large the most common group of entities causing hypothyroidism are those that involve the thyroid gland itself (see accompanying box).

Hashimoto's thyroiditis is probably the single most common cause of hypothyroidism. It is believed to result from a derangement of cellular and humoral components of the immune system.[23] The most important characteristic of Hashimoto's thyroiditis is the presence of a defect in organification, accompanied by lymphocytic infiltration of the gland with concomitant loss of thyroid tissue. These elements of the disease are reflected clinically by the presence of an enlarged thyroid gland, thyroid hypofunction, and presence in serum of antithyroid antibodies. The antimicrosomal (peroxidase) antibody is found in 90% to 95% of patients with Hashimoto's thyroiditis.

Hypothyroidism can result from various other conditions. It often follows surgical thyroidectomy or therapy with radioiodine for treatment of Graves' disease. Developmental abnormalities and tumors and other infiltrative disorders that displace and destroy thyroid tissue can occasionally cause hypothyroidism. Congenital defects in hormonogenesis and the effect of drugs can also result in hypothyroidism. Pituitary and hypothalamic disease are rare conditions that occasionally lead to hypothyroidism caused by inadequate TRH or TSH secretion.

Laboratory findings. Regardless of the cause, the laboratory findings in hypothyroidism are characterized by

Causes of Hypothyroidism
Primary thyroid dysfunction
Parenchymal damage
Thyroiditis
Chronic lymphocytic (Hashimoto's) thyroiditis
Subacute thyroiditis
Therapeutic ablation
After ^{131}I therapy
After surgery
Thyroid dysgenesis
Aplasia
Dysplasia
Thyroid infiltration
Tumors
Iodine deficiency (endemic goiter)
Iodine excess (>6 mg/day)
Thyroid-blocking drugs (lithium, sulfonamides, etc.)
Congenital and acquired defects of hormone synthesis and thyroglobulin metabolism defects
Abnormal hormonogenesis
Pituitary hypothyroidism (TSH deficiency)
Hypothalamic hypothyroidism (TRH deficiency)
Reduced peripheral response to thyroid hormone

decreased total serum T_4, T_3, FT_4, FT_4I, and T_3RU. The degree of abnormality of these tests varies widely, depending on the cause of hypothyroidism and stage of the disease.

Some distinctive laboratory findings can be found in Table 44-5. For example, hypothyroidism caused by intrinsic thyroid disease (primary hypothyroidism) will be characterized by elevated TSH levels and exaggerated TSH response to TRH stimulation. Hypothyroidism caused by pituitary (secondary) and hypothalamic (tertiary) disease will be characterized by low or borderline normal levels of TSH and TRH test responses as noted earlier.

Hypothyroidism in the neonatal period can lead to severe retardation of the growth and maturation of the central ner-

Table 44-5   Laboratory findings in hypothyroidism

Type	T_4	T_3	T_3RU	FT_4I	TSH	TRH stimulation*	Ab
Primary	↓	↓, N	↓, N	↓	↑	↑	†
Secondary	↓	↓	↓	↓	↓, N	↓	—
Tertiary	↓	↓	↓	↓	↓, N	N	—
Peripheral unresponsiveness	↑	↑	N	↑ or N	↑ or N	N or ↑	

*Assessed by response of serum TSH to TRH administration.
†10% of normal population has acute antiperoxidase antibody, with females more than males.
Ab, Antibodies to thyroid microsomal peroxidase; *N,* Normal; ↑, elevated; ↓, decreased. See Table 44-4 for abbreviations.

vous system (cretinism). Routine screening of neonates for hypothyroidism is an important tool for the early diagnosis of hypothyroidism.[24] TSH-blocking antibody, which has been found in the serum of patients with atrophic thyroiditis, may be transmitted across the placenta and cause temporary hypothyroidism in the newborn. Disappearance of the antibody is associated with remission of the hypothyroid state.

Treatment. The treatment of hypothyroidism consists in thyroid hormone replacement given orally, which reverses the abnormal laboratory findings and clinical symptoms and signs, provided that there are no abnormalities in the transport and peripheral use of thyroid hormones. The most common agent used is levothyroxine (T_4), which is converted peripherally to T_3. The average replacement dose in most adults is 1.6 μg/kg body weight.

Goiter

Goiter is a generic reference to an enlargement of the thyroid gland. It may be associated with a hyperthyroid, hypothyroid, or euthyroid state. Diffuse goiter is characterized by uniform enlargement of the thyroid gland. In multinodular goiter the thyroid gland is enlarged in a nonuniform fashion, resulting in nodules located both superficially and deep within the gland.

Solitary nodule

A solitary nodule refers to the presence of a solitary localized enlargement of a portion of the thyroid gland. Although most of these nodules represent benign conditions, such as cysts, localized hemorrhages, focal thyroiditis, and adenomas, they may also represent malignant tumors of the thyroid. External radiation therapy used in the past for acne and enlarged tonsils and other conditions of the head, neck, and chest has been associated with an increased risk for the development of both thyroid cancer and benign thyroid neoplasms.[25]

Thyroid cancer

The most common primary malignant thyroid tumors originate from the epithelial cells of the follicles. Patients with thyroid cancer usually do not display significant abnormalities of thyroid function. These tumors often release thyroglobulin into the circulation, where it may be followed as a tumor marker. Rarely, a patient may have an antithyroglobulin antibody, which invalidates the use of the thyroglobulin assay. Since other thyroid diseases can also result in increased levels of thyroglobulin, this parameter is most useful for following the activity of thyroid cancer once a specific diagnosis has been made.

A different type of thyroid cancer originates from the parafollicular C-cells of the thyroid and is termed *medullary carcinoma*. These tumors secrete calcitonin, a hormone that lowers blood calcium, which is a useful tumor marker for diagnosing and following these patients.

Peripheral resistance to thyroid hormone

Cases of abnormally high T_4 and T_3 hormone levels have been described in patients with otherwise normal baseline TSH concentrations and a normal or increased response to TRH stimulation. Clinical features of this disease vary. They range from euthyroid to an expression of thyroid deficiency.

TESTS OF THYROID FUNCTION

The iodine-concentrating property of the thyroid is used to estimate thyroid function and to obtain functional anatomical images of the gland. For these studies tracer amounts of a radioiodine (^{123}I or ^{131}I) are administered to the patient. Gamma rays emitted by the radioiodine concentrated in the thyroid are detected by specially designed imaging and counting devices and transformed into thyroid radioiodine-uptake percentages and images of the gland. ^{123}I is the preferred radioisotope because it produces better images and delivers lower radiation doses to the patient's thyroid. Serum samples for hormone radioassays that are obtained after the administration of radioactive materials to the patient must be checked for residual radioactivity before the assay is started or spurious results may be obtained.

Thyroid iodine uptake

The thyroid iodine-uptake test measures the percentage of an administered dose of radioiodine that is concentrated in the thyroid by the trapping and organification mechanisms. This measurement may be obtained at various intervals after radioiodine administration. Imaging and counting of the radioiodine can be performed 4 to 24 hours after the radioisotope dose. For ^{123}I the dose is approximately 200 μCi. Theoretically the amount of radioiodine in the thyroid at a given time reflects thyroid hormone synthesis and secretion and therefore reflects the functional status of the thyroid. Graves' disease is characterized by an elevated radioactive-iodine uptake. Low thyroid uptakes are found not only in hypothyroidism but also in certain conditions actually associated with thyroid hyperfunction, including (1) thyrotoxicosis factitia caused by exogenous thyroid hormone, (2) subacute thyroiditis, (3) iodine-induced hyperthyroidism, (4) chronic lymphocytic thyroiditis, and (5) ectopic thyroid tissue.

TRH stimulation test

The TRH stimulation test takes advantage of the interrelationship between the TRH and TSH secretions. Normally, after the intravenous administration of TRH, there is an increase of TSH levels in blood, which in turn elicits an elevation of T_3 and T_4 serum levels.[11,26] Various factors influence the TSH response to TRH stimulation. Abnormal responses to TRH stimulation are of two types. The first type is characterized by lower-than-normal responses of serum TSH to TRH stimulation. In these cases the TSH response to TRH is said to be blunted. A blunted response is usually associated with pituitary dysfunction. The second type of abnormal response mainfests as higher-than-normal increments of serum TSH after TRH stimulation and is associated with primary hypothyroidism. Responses of TSH to TRH in various clinical conditions are depicted in Fig. 44-7. Falsely low TSH responses may be associated with depression, with excessive use of glucocorticoids, and serious illnesses.

The main clinical applications of the TRH stimulation test are (1) diagnosis of subclinical and early biochemical hyperthyroidism, (2) evaluation of patients with ophthalmopathy without overt hyperthyroidism, and (3) diagnosis of hypothalamic and pituitary hypothyroidism. A significant increment in TSH eliminates the diagnosis of hyperthyroidism except in the extremely rare patient with the TSH-induced form of this disease.

TSH stimulation test

Administration of exogenous TSH will stimulate all phases of thyroid function, which will be reflected by increases in the uptake of radioiodine by the thyroid and increases in blood levels of thyroid hormone. The TSH stimulation test is performed by monitoring of the thyroidal radioiodine uptake before (baseline value) and after the administration of bovine TSH for 3 consecutive days. Normally there is an increase of serum T_4 and radioiodine uptake to more than 1.5 times the baseline value in response to TSH administration. The chief use of this test has been to differentiate primary hypothyroidism (increase of serum T_4 and decrease in radioiodine uptake) from secondary or tertiary hypothyroidism. The TSH stimulation test has been replaced largely by TSH determinations in serum and by the TRH stimulation test.

Triiodothyronine (T_3) or Cytomel suppression test

This test is performed by a determination of 24-hour thyroid radioiodine uptake before (baseline value) and then after the oral administration of T_3 for 7 to 10 days.[27] Images of the thyroid gland and thyroid radioisotope uptake determinations are obtained simultaneously. The purpose of this test is to establish the presence of thyroid tissue that has become autonomous and unresponsive to TSH changes. Normally the administration of thyroid hormone (T_3 or T_4)

will shut off the secretion of TSH by the pituitary gland. The subsequent absence of TSH results in diminished thyroid concentration of radioiodine. A thyroid gland that is overactive is often autonomous, and so suppression of TSH production by administration of exogenous thyroid hormone will not be followed by corresponding declines of thyroid radioiodine uptake. Normally a drop in thyroid uptake (suppression) to 30% to 50% of the baseline value occurs after T_3 administration.

Perchlorate-discharge test

The perchlorate-discharge test detects defects of iodine organification present in conditions such as Hashimoto's thyroiditis and congenital goiters. It is also used to determine the degree of organification defect caused by certain thyroid-blocking drugs used for treatment of hyperthyroidism to assess their therapeutic effects.

CHANGE OF ANALYTE IN DISEASE

Thyroid function can be assessed by determination of various analytes in blood. Tables 44-4 to 44-6 summarize the changes of some analytes in various disease states.

Protein-bound iodine (PBI)

Historically protein-bound iodine (PBI) was used to assess indirectly the concentration of thyroid hormone in the blood. This test measured iodine contained in thyroid hormones, as well as iodine of nonhormonal origin, which is bound to proteins. This test has been replaced by more accurate ones

Serum T_4 (see method, p. 888)

Elevations in total serum T_4 can occur as a result of increased hormone synthesis, increased hormone release from the thyroid cells, or increased binding capacity of plasma proteins, especially TBG. Increased hormone secretion is most frequently seen in states of hyperthyroidism. Causes of hyperthyroidism are listed in the box on p. 878.

Increased T_4 release also occurs in subacute thyroiditis and Hashimoto's thyroiditis and after radiation. Increased levels of serum TBG from various causes (see box, p. 877) produce elevations of total serum T_4. These conditions are not accompanied by hyperthyroidism.

Table 44-6 Thyroid-function tests in nonthyroid diseases (NTD)

	T_4	T_3RU	FT_4I	Free T_4	Free T_3	T_3	rT_3	TSH	TBG
General NTD*	N, ↓	↑, N	↓, N	N, ↑	↓, N	↓, N	↑, N	N	↓, N
Acute hepatitis	N, ↑	↓	N, ↓	N, ↑	N, ↓	↓, N	↑	N	↑
Chronic active hepatitis	N, ↑	↓	N, ↓	N, ↑	N	N	↑	N	↑
Alcoholic cirrhosis	N, ↓	N, ↑	N, ↑	N, ↑	↓	↓	↑	N	↓, N
Renal failure	N, ↓	N	N, ↓	N, ↓	↓	↓	N	N	N
Acute psychiatric illness	N, ↑	—	N, ↑	N, ↑	N	N	—	N	—

Normal thyroid function in patients with very complex problems; findings in individual patients may vary widely.
N, Normal; ↑, augmented; ↓, diminished.
*Includes all patients with NTD.

Serum T₃

In general, elevations of serum T_3 are proportionally greater than the increases of T_4 found in most states of hyperthyroidism. Thus routine measurements of total serum T_3 are not necessary. In approximately 5% of cases, elevations of T_3 occur while serum T_4 levels remain normal. This condition is termed T_3 thyrotoxicosis. Total T_3 measurements will be needed to monitor the treatment of thyroid disease in these cases.

Free hormone levels: estimates or direct measurements

Thyroid hormones in the blood are distributed into two compartments: protein-bound and unbound, or free, compartments (Fig. 44-8). Variations in total thyroid hormone in blood can result from changes in the concentration of binding protein. Hypothyroidism and hyperthyroidism will occur only if a net persistent decrease of free unbound thyroid hormone exists in the blood. Because of the limited utility of total thyroid hormone measurements, in 1990, the American Thyroid Association had recommended that free thyroid hormones be either measured directly or estimated indirectly.[28] Blood level determinations of total T_4 and T_3 are clinically meaningful only if the functional levels of thyroid hormone-binding protein in blood are known. This is achieved by use of the resin-uptake test, which does not measure a specific analyte per se but measures the functional state (ability to bind hormone) of the hormone-binding proteins (such as TBG).

Resin-uptake test (T₃RU or T₄RU)

The resin-uptake test is an estimate of the number of available binding sites on the plasma thyroid hormone–transporting proteins, especially TBG, which is the most important transporter of thyroid hormones. Samples of patient serum are mixed with labeled thyroid hormone (T_3 or T_4). The amount of labeled hormone that remains unbound in the mixture is inversely proportional to the number of available binding sites (Fig. 44-8). This unbound hormone is separated from the mixture when one adds a relatively low-affinity binder, such as a resin, to the system (Fig. 44-8). The resin is then separated from the serum, and the amount of labeled hormone bound to the resin (resin uptake) is determined. In the classic uptake procedure, the amount of resin uptake is directly proportional to the degree of saturation of T_4-binding sites on carrier proteins (see discussion at right).

In cases of increased TBG in plasma, although free thyroid hormone levels are normal, the total T_4 is increased, since the total number of binding sites in TBG is increased. Labeled T_4 or T_3 will find an increased pool of TBG (available binding sites), and less labeled hormone will remain free to bind to resin. Therefore the resin uptake is low. The opposite changes occur in states of decreased TBG. Conditions that cause abnormalities of the binding sites (TBG) are listed in Table 44-4. Certain drugs (salicylates, phenytoin, furosemide, and fenclofenac) compete with thyroid hormone for the TBG-binding sites. This phenomenon is reflected by normal free T_4, low total T_4, and high resin-uptake values.

In hyperthyroidism, free thyroid hormone in plasma increases. This results in complete or almost complete saturation of binding sites in TBG, which in turn will result in fewer molecules of labeled hormone bound to TBG and increased amounts of free labeled hormone. This results in an increased resin uptake.

Recently, there has been an attempt to change the nomenclature from T_3 (T_4) resin-uptake test to thyroid hormone–binding ratio (THBR) to avoid confusion with direct measurements of serum T_3 (T_4).[29]

Free thyroxine hormone index (FT₄I)

It is the free hormone that induces metabolic and biological effects in target cells. The free T_4 index (FT_4I) indirectly estimates the level of free T_4 in blood and adjusts for most interferences caused by binding-protein abnormalities.[30] The FT_4I is determined from total T_4 and resin-uptake values obtained on the sample. The FT_4I is calculated as follows:

$$FT_4I = \frac{\text{Total serum } T_4 \times \% \text{ T uptake of patient serum}}{\% \text{ T uptake of pooled reference serum}}$$

As expected, most alterations of binding proteins produce reciprocal changes in resin uptake and total serum T_4 or T_3, resulting in normal values of the FT_4I, whereas true alterations of free thyroid hormone content cause concordant, unidirectional changes of the FT_4I. The FT_4I is elevated in hyperthyroidism (see Table 44-4) and is decreased in states of hypothyroidism (see Table 44-5).

The calculation of the free T_3 index is similar to that used for the FT_4I, except that total serum T_3 is used.[31] It has similar applications and significance as the FT_4I. The FT_3I may be helpful to exclude T_3 toxicosis in some patients taking oral contraceptives in whom isolated serum T_3 increases are found without corresponding elevations of T_4. In general, the FT_3I offers no advantages to the FT_4I and is used less frequently in clinical practice.

Free T₄ (FT₄) and free T₃ (FT₃)

Serum FT_4 correlates very well with secretion and metabolism rates of T_4. FT_4 and FT_3 levels tend to parallel changes in total T_4 and total T_3 concentrations. Measurement of the free hormone levels is useful in routine clinical practice and in instances in which other test results are borderline or conflicting. Elevations and decreases of free T_4 and free T_3 theoretically are true reflections of hyperthyroidism and hypothyroidism. However, the results are very dependent on the analytical method used to measure "free" hormone and clinically have been less useful than originally hoped.

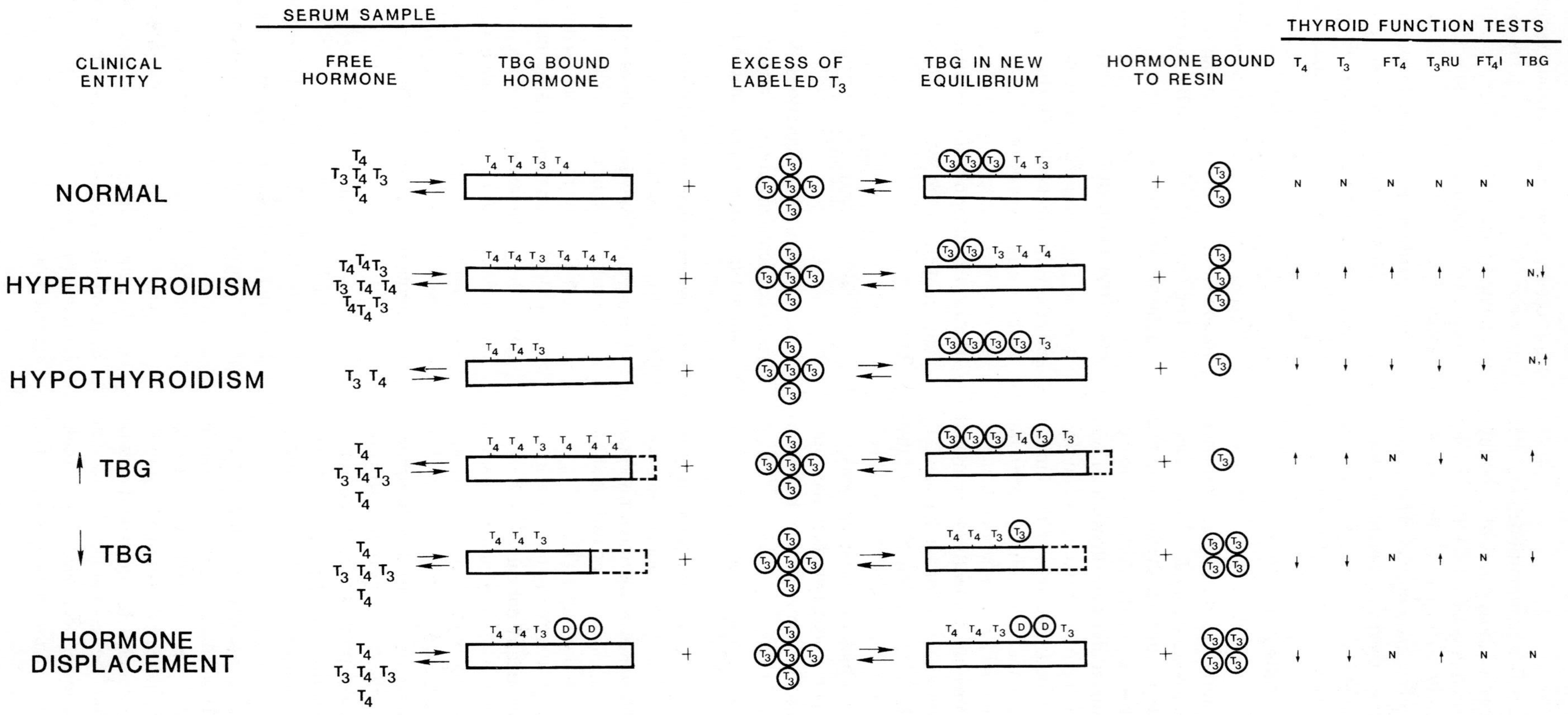

Fig. 44-8 Interrelationships between serum TBG (thyroxine-binding globulin), the T_3RU, and other thyroid function tests. *D*, Drugs occupying binding sites on TBG; FT_4I, free thyroxine hormone index.

Thyroxine-binding globulin (TBG)

Many diseases produce alterations of TBG (see box, p. 877) and other thyroid hormone–transporting proteins in plasma. Changes in concentrations of such proteins affect the total plasma concentrations of T_4 and T_3 (Fig. 44-8). Since most of the T_4 and T_3 is bound to TBG, changes in this protein level are clinically important. Quantitative abnormalities are those characterized by absolute increases or decreases of TBG levels in plasma. Consequently, the total amount of thyroid hormone transported in plasma will increase (increased TBG) or decrease (decreased TBG).

Qualitative abnormalities of TBG refer to those stemming from alterations of the hormone-binding affinity rather than from absolute changes of TBG amounts in plasma. The binding affinity of the TBG may be increased or decreased in intrinsic TBG defects. Various compounds and drugs may strongly bind to TBG and result in displacement of thyroid hormone from binding sites. The result is decreased total serum T_4 and T_3 (Fig. 44-8) and increased free T_4 and free T_3.

Serum thyroid-stimulating hormone (TSH) (see method, p. 886)

A principal use of thyroid-stimulating hormone (TSH) determinations in serum is the diagnosis of hypothyroidism. Patients with untreated hypothyroidism stemming from intrinsic thyroid defects (primary hypothyroidism), regardless of the cause, have elevated serum levels of TSH. Patients with hypothyroidism caused by pituitary lesions (secondary) or hypothalamic (tertiary) lesions have normal or low TSH levels. Differentiation between secondary and tertiary hypothyroidism is accomplished by use of the TRH stimulation test.

Most patients with hyperthyroidism have low or undetectable TSH levels in serum, reflecting the inhibitory effects of high levels of circulating thyroid hormone on the hypothalamic-pituitary axis.

Recent advances have dramatically enhanced the clinical utility of TSH determinations. Immunometric assays (IMAs) for TSH measurement are much more sensitive than the radioimmunoassay (RIA) method. Clinicians often refer to the updated techniques as either second-generation (functional sensitivity approximately 0.1 μIU/mL) or third-generation (functional sensitivity approximately 0.01 μIU/mL) assays. Because of the increased sensitivity of second- and third-generation TSH assays, the very low TSH levels encountered in patients with hyperthyroidism can be discriminated from those levels found in euthyroid states.[32] The diagnosis of hypothyroidism can also be made earlier and with more certainty by finding an elevated TSH by an IMA method. The specificity of TSH-IMA is also greater than TSH-RIA because the former employs antibodies to the β subunit of TSH, resulting in less cross-reactivity with LH, FSH, and hCG, which have α subunits that are similar to those of TSH. With the availability of the third-generation

TSH assays, TSH levels can now be used as accurate indicators of thyroid suppression in patients with thyroid carcinoma or thyroid nodules.[33]

Immunoglobulins

It has been suggested that immunological abnormalities play an important role in thyroid pathologic conditions.[16] Antibodies against components of thyroid cells are found in many patients with thyroid disease. High levels of antibodies against thyroglobulin or thyroid peroxidase frequently are found in patients with Hashimoto's thyroiditis. High titers of thyroid-stimulating immunoglobulins may be found in Graves' disease.

TSH-blocking antibody may be transmitted across the placenta in patients with atrophic thyroiditis and cause temporary hypothyroidism in the newborn. TSH-receptor antibodies may differ in their actions. They may (1) displace TSH without activating the receptor, (2) activate the receptor and mimic TSH, (3) block the action of TSH and cause atrophy of the gland, or (4) stimulate growth of the thyroid gland without increasing secretion of thyroid hormone. The presence of antithyroglobulin antibody interferes with the measurement of serum thyroglobulin.

Laboratory findings in nonthyroid disease (NTD)

The abnormal changes in thyroid test results that may be seen in patients with NTD are listed in Table 44-6. These changes can mimic thyroid disease or modify and confound laboratory findings in patients with thyroid disease. Chronic diseases that alter laboratory tests of thyroid function are more frequent than thyroid disease. NTD includes patients with general chronic debilitating conditions and patients with specific conditions, namely, alcoholic cirrhosis, hepatitis, renal failure, and acute psychiatric illness.

As a group, euthyroid patients with NTD have either normal or low total T_4, normal or low FT_4I, normal or low total T_3 and free T_3, normal or high rT_3, normal or high T_3RU, and low or slightly high TSH levels in serum.[28,34-36] The free T_4 index (FT_4I), which is often a reliable indicator of thyroid function, is usually normal but may also be low in patients with NTD.

Low total T_4, low FT_4I, and low or subnormal T_3 levels indicate the possible presence of hypothyroidism in patients with NTD. The presence of high serum levels of rT_3 is useful in excluding hypothyroidism in this circumstance.[34] However, it would be more cost effective to measure the TSH by immunometric assay to assess the possibility of underlying hypothyroidism.

Liver disease is characterized by abnormalities of protein synthesis, including the thyroid-binding proteins, and by alterations of T_4 metabolism. Alcoholic liver cirrhosis is accompanied by decreased binding capacity of thyroid hormones, resulting in high T_3RU[37] (Table 44-6). Total T_4 is usually normal or low,[36] and free T_4 is slightly elevated.

There is depressed conversion of T_4 to T_3 with decreased serum levels of T_3 and occasionally free T_3.

Acute hepatitis is characterized by an increase of the serum TBG[38] (see Table 44-6), which results in increased levels of T_4 and decreased T_3RU. In general, chronic active hepatitis also produces the same changes in blood as those seen in acute hepatitis. These include (1) lower than expected T_4, (2) low free T_4 index, (3) decreased free T_4, (4) normal serum TSH, and (5) abnormally increased TSH response to TRH.[39]

In patients with renal failure the most common findings are decreased total and free T_3 in the serum,[40] caused by diminished peripheral conversion of T_4 to T_3. Serum thyroxine-binding protein, T_3RU, and total T_4 usually are normal. However, the total T_4 and free T_4 may be slightly low.[41] Diminished total T_4 can result from renal failure with severe catabolic states, probably caused by decreased thyroxine-binding proteins in serum. Concentration of TSH in serum is normal.

There is a selective increase in T_4 in patients with an acute psychiatric illness. The reason for the increase is not known, but it is postulated that there is an acute redistribution of T_4 out of the liver, which contains one third of the total body pool of T_4 outside of the thyroid. T_4 levels typically normalize in 1 to 2 weeks after the acute psychiatric event.[42]

Association of NTD with hyperthyroidism is found occasionally. In these situations there is a disproportionate increase of T_4 in serum with only modestly elevated or normal T_3 levels. This is caused by a decreased peripheral conversion of T_4 to T_3 concomitant with the increased T_4 production.

Laboratory findings after therapeutic interventions for thyroid disease

The two most frequently found clinical situations that require closely monitored treatment are hyperthyroidism and hypothyroidism.

Graves' disease, when successfully treated surgically, results in normalization of T_4, T_3, T_3RU, FT_4I, and TSH. In patients treated with antithyroid drugs, such as propylthiouracil (PTU), improvement of thyroid function tests may be occasionally seen as soon as 2 weeks after initiation of treatment. Because of the blocking effect of PTU on conversion of T_4 to T_3, a disproportionately rapid decrease in T_3 may be seen in some cases.

Therapy with ^{131}I is now used more frequently to treat hyperthyroidism. After this treatment, laboratory tests show a decrease of T_4, T_3, T_3RU, and FT_4I in approximately 6 to 10 weeks. Residual radioactivity in the serum must be considered when one is using radioassay methods within 90 days of therapy.

Patients treated for thyrotoxicosis by any of the methods may follow one of three courses. Ideally normal thyroid function ensues and is reflected by normal laboratory val-ues. Occasionally patients remain hyperthyroid, and abnormal laboratory tests persist. More often patients become hypothyroid with low T_4, T_3RU, and FT_4I values. The earliest indication of the ensuing hypothyroidism is a depressed T_4 followed by an elevation of TSH levels as the hypothalamic-pituitary axis recovers. The TSH may remain elevated with normal T_4 levels, a condition known as *biochemical hypothyroidism*. Patients with treated Graves' disease may develop a hyperthyroid status with normal or subnormal T_4 values but elevated T_3 levels.

The treatment for hypothyroidism is thyroid hormone replacement. During the monitoring of thyroid hormone replacement, it is very important to keep in mind the effect that changes in TBG levels produce on thyroid hormone levels. Laboratory tests should therefore include those that indirectly or directly assess TBG levels, such as the T_3RU, FT_4I, and TBG determinations. With the development of the sensitive TSH-IMAs, it is most practical to diagnose hypothyroidism by detection of an elevated serum TSH. After thyroid hormone replacement therapy for hypothyroidism, it is necessary to wait at least 6 weeks before reevaluating the TSH response to therapy. When preparations containing T_4 and T_3 are used, normalization of both T_3 and T_4 values is expected. When preparations containing only T_3, such as Cytomel, are used, T_3 values become normal or slightly elevated, but the T_4 values may remain mildly depressed. Normalization of T_4 and T_3 values is accompanied by a corresponding decline in TSH levels. When one is monitoring patients on T_4 replacement, it is important to take into consideration the fluctuation of serum levels caused by the oral administration of the preparation. Increases of T_4 from baseline levels can be observed 2 to 10 hours after ingestion of T_4-containing medications.[43] More accurate interpretation of serum T_4 levels is accomplished by measurement of serum T_4 levels after this peak absorption period, that is, at least 10 hours after dosage.

METHODS OF ANALYSIS

Thyroid-stimulating hormone (thyrotropin)
I.-WEN CHEN

Principles of analysis   Thyrotropin is composed of two subunits, alpha and beta. The α subunit is identical to the α subunit of human LH and differs only slightly from the α subunits of human FSH and hCG. The β subunit of thyrotropin has a primary amino acid structure that is significantly different from those of LH, FSH, and hCG.

Historically, measurement of TSH in serum was performed using radioimmunoassay (RIA) to diagnose primary hypothyroidism, a condition characterized by an increased TSH concentration. The development of more sensitive immunoassay methods have enabled the clinical role of TSH measurements to include the assessment of thyrotoxicosis, a condition associated with subnormal circulating concentrations of TSH. Although all immunoassay procedures can detect increased serum TSH concentrations, only the newer immunoassay methods can readily detect the very low, suppressed serum TSH concentrations of <0.1 mIU/L.[44]

The RIA procedure for TSH is commonly referred to as a first-generation procedure. The development of more sensitive immunoassay procedures with lower limits of detection have led to the use of terms such as "sensitive," "supersensitive," and "ultrasensitive" for describing the performance characteristics of each particular assay. These designations have been replaced by the use of terminology such as second, third, and fourth generations to describe limits of detection of 0.1, 0.01, and 0.001 mIU/L respectively.[45] These limits are defined by their "functional sensitivity," that is, by their ability to achieve a long-range precision of ≤20% CV at these TSH concentrations. All second- and third-generation assays can readily distinguish between the euthyroid range and untreated hypothyroid and most hyperthyroid individuals.

The majority of initially available commercial TSH immunoassays were capable of distinguishing normal TSH levels from hyperthyroid values but could not reliably differentiate between mildly subnormal values (0.01 to 0.1 mIU/L) and the profoundly low values (<0.01 mIU/L) typical of thyrotoxicosis.[44]

The RIA procedure for TSH (Table 44-7, method 1) is based on competitive binding between a fixed amount of radiolabeled TSH and TSH from the patient's serum, for a fixed and limited number of TSH-antibody binding sites. The amount of radiolabeled TSH that binds to antibody is inversely related to TSH levels present in the patient's sample.

Two-site immunoradiometric assay has also been developed (Table 44-7, method 2).[46] These newer "sandwich" assays make use of two or more antibodies directed against different portions of the TSH molecules, which results in TSH becoming "sandwiched" between the antibodies. The second anti-TSH antibody may also employ various labels including radioisotopes, enzymes, fluorophors, or chemiluminescent molecules (see below). In this procedure, TSH is first reacted with an excess of radiolabeled antibody directed toward a unique site on the TSH molecule so that all TSH present in the patients become bound by antibody. In the second phase of the assay, labeled antibody-TSH complexes react with a second antibody attached to a solid-phase support. This second antibody is directed against a site on the TSH molecule different from the first antibody. The radiolabeled antibody/TSH/solid-phase antibody complex is then separated from the reaction mixture, washed to remove any remaining unbound labeled antibody, and the bound label is counted. The amount of label is directly related to TSH concentrations present in the patient's serum.

The use of enzyme labels for immunometric measurement of TSH has supplanted RIA in terms of overall use. Enzyme immunoassays typically use horseradish peroxidase or alkaline phosphatase as enzyme labels. More sensitive TSH assays, based on chemiluminescence and time-resolved fluorescence, have been introduced.[45,47] Chemiluminescent labels include acridinium esters, luminol (3-aminophthalhydrazide), and dioxitane phosphates, whereas the immunofluorometric assays employ europium labels.

A variety of separation systems have been developed for use with these newly developed immunoassay systems. Separation may be performed by immobilization of the capture antibody on a solid phase such as a plastic bead, glass fiber paper, or test tube so that bound and free analyte are separated by washing or decanting. Other systems utilize ferromagnetic particles attached to antibody to allow separation to be accomplished with magnets. Another variation is to attach biotin, a high-affinity binder of avidin, to the antibody.

Table 44-7 Methods for TSH analysis

Method	Principle	Usage	Comments
1. Radioimmunoassay (RIA)	Competition occurs between radiolabeled TSH and TSH in patient serum for limited number of antibody-binding sites.	Currently used Uses ^{125}I label	Lacks sensitivity for subnormal TSH concentrations
2. Immunoradiometric assay (IRMA)	TSH is first reacted with excess of radiolabeled antibody. In second step, labeled antibody-TSH complex binds to second antibody attached to solid-phase support.	Currently used Uses ^{125}I label	Better sensitivity compared with conventional RIA procedure Nonradioactive labels also used
3. Immunochemiluminometric assay (ICMA)	TSH reacts with antibody coated onto solid phase. Detector antibody conjugated to alkaline phosphatase binds to second antigenic site on TSH forming antibody-TSH-antibody enzyme sandwich complex. After wash step to remove unbound antibody, substrate for ALP is added.	Currently used	Good sensitivity
4. Time-resolved immunofluorometric assay (TR-IFMA)	TSH first reacts with capture antibody conjugated to solid-phase support. Addition of europium-labeled antibody forms TSH-antibody sandwich complex. In final step, europium ions are dissociated from labeled antibodies and form fluorescent chelates.	Currently used	Good sensitivity

Separation of the TSH sandwich complexes is accomplished by the use of avidin that is linked to a solid phase.[44]

An immunochemiluminometric method (ICMA; Table 44-7, method 3) utilizes mouse monoclonal antibody directed toward whole TSH, which is coated onto a solid phase. The detector antibody, polyclonal goat antibody to TSH, is conjugated to alkaline phosphatase. After an incubation period, any unbound conjugated is removed, and a chemiluminescent substrate is added. In the presence of ALP this substrate undergoes hydrolysis to form an unstable intermediate compound with the production of light. The light production is detected by use of a luminometer and is proportional to the TSH concentration within the sample.

Measurement of TSH based on a time-resolved immunofluorometric assay (TR-IFMA) (Table 44-7, method 4) (such as Delphia; Wallae, Turku, Finland) uses a two-site solid phase involving three monoclonal antibodies directed against TSH.[48] The capture antibody is coated onto a microtiter well, and two other antibodies, labeled with europium, are directed against different antigenic sites on the β subunit of TSH. After an incubation period and wash step to remove any unbound labeled antibody, an enhancement solution is added to dissociate europium ions from the labeled antibodies into solution. The dissociated europium ions form fluorescent chelates with the components of the enhancement solution. Fluorescence intensity is measured with a time-resolved fluorometer.

A major source of interference in some immunoassay procedures for TSH has been attributed to the presence of heterophilic antibodies in the patient's serum. These antispecies immunoglobulins act like TSH to "crosslink" the capture labeled monoclonal antibody. The presence of these antibodies has been attributed to exposure to animal proteins by individuals treated with vaccines prepared in tissue culture, by animal handlers, and by individuals exposed to radiolabeled mouse monoclonal antitumor antibodies for imaging or therapy. Mouse sera can be added to the reagent or patient sample to eliminate this problem for assays using mouse monoclonal antibodies.[49] However, it should be noted that some interference in TSH assays may be the result of other, nonspecific effects on the solid-phase assay and are not corrected by the addition of mouse serum.

Specimen Serum or plasma are acceptable specimens, though some TSH methods recommend use of serum only. There is a small but significant circadian rhythm of TSH secretion. Peak values occur in late evening and near midnight.[44] However, this does not influence the clinical utility of the measurement, and useful clinical information can be obtained from samples collected at any convenient time. TSH is stable in serum for up to 5 days at 4° C. However, samples that have testing delayed for more than 24 hours should be frozen at −20° C for best results. Previously frozen samples should be thoroughly mixed before analysis to ensure homogeneity. Grossly hemolyzed or lipemic specimens should not be used.

Reference interval The reference interval for TSH is dependent on the assay used and the reference population that has been tested. The approximate reference interval is 0.5 to 5.75 milli-International U/L.[50] Concentrations of TSH are similar for both sexes up to approximately 60 years of age. Women older than 60 years show higher mean TSH concentrations compared to younger women.[51] Newborns show increased TSH concentrations that decline to reach adult levels within the first week of life.

Thyroxine
I.-WEN CHEN

Principles of analysis Modern methods for measuring serum levels of thyroid hormones began with the development of competitive protein-binding assays for measuring total T_4, first described by Ekins in 1960.[52] This procedure utilized the specific binding characteristics of thyroxine-binding globulin (TBG) for T_4. Purified TBG was linked to a solid support and incubated with patient sample and a fixed amount of radiolabeled T_4. The patient T_4 and radiolabeled T_4 competed for a limited number of binding sites on TBG. A wash step removed any unbound T_4, and the radioactivity remaining in the column was then counted.

The TBG binding assay for T_4 had several inherent analytical problems. The presence of endogenous binding proteins in the patient's serum can interfere with binding of T_4 to the TBG. In addition, since more than 99.9% of T_4 in serum is bound to TBG or other thyroxine-binding proteins, it was necessary to extract T_4 from endogenous TBG and then to remove the endogenous TBG so that it did not interfere with the binding of T_4 by TBG linked to the solid phase. Extraction of T_4 from TBG can be accomplished by incubation of the serum with ethanol or by use of 8-anilino-1-naphthalenesulfonic acid (ANS). Dilution of the sample with barbital buffer prevents binding of T_4 to other T_4-binding proteins, such as prealbumin or albumin.

The development and application of techniques for producing antibodies directed against T_4 led to the use of radioimmunoassay (RIA) (Table 44-8, method 1) for measurement of T_4. The basic principles of RIA and the competitive protein-binding thyroxine assays are the same, except that in RIA the binding protein is an antibody. Differences between the various commercially available RIA procedures are in the techniques used for separation of antibody-bound and free radioligands. The most commonly used techniques employ a solid-phase separation procedure. T_4 antibody is chemically or physically bound to a solid-phase support, such as a glass bead, plastic tube, or magnetic particle. The labeled and unlabeled T_4 compete for binding to this bound antibody; unbound T_4 is removed from the bound T_4-antibody complex by a wash step. Separation of the T_4-antibody complex can also be accomplished with use of a second antibody or polyethylene glycol.

The use of immunoassay methods that employ nonradioisotopic labels have gained widespread acceptance. Many of the original nonradioisotopic assays were, like RIA, heterogeneous assays where a separation step was required to remove any unbound labeled ligand from the reaction mixture (see below). To avoid the separation steps of the heterogeneous immunoassays, immunoassays methods that do not require separation of bound and unbound label have been developed. These homogeneous assays (no separation step required) utilize a label that has some changed physicochemi-

Table 44-8 Methods for thyroxine analysis

Method	Principle	Usage	Comments
1. Radioimmunoassay (RIA)	Competition occurs between radiolabeled T_4 and patient T_4 for a limited number of antibody binding sites.	Currently used Uses ^{125}I label	Requires separation step
2. Enzyme-multiplied immunoassay (EMIT)	T_4 and T_4 labeled with enzyme glucose-6-phosphate dehydrogenase compete for antibody binding sites. Binding of enzyme-labeled T_4 to antibody results in decrease in activity of G-6-PD.	Frequently used	Automated homogeneous assay
3. Fluorescence polarization immunoassay (FPIA)	T_4 competes with fluorescein-labeled T_4 for antibody-binding sites. Binding of fluorescein-labeled T_4 to antibody results in an increase in polarized fluorescent light.	Frequently used	Automated homogeneous assay
4. Cloned enzyme-donor immunoassay (CEDIA)	The enzyme β-galactosidase is cloned as two separate inactive fragments. One fragment is labeled with T_4. Patient T_4 and T_4-enzyme fragment complex compete for antibody-binding sites. Binding of T_4-enzyme fragment to antibody results in inability of both fragments combining to form active enzyme.	Frequently used	Automated homogeneous assay
5. Fluorometric enzyme immunoassay	Patient T_4 and enzyme-labeled T_4 compete for binding to antibody immobilized in glass fiber matrix. Unbound enzyme-labeled T_4 is washed from fiber by the process of radial elution before enzyme substrate is added.	Frequently used	Automated heterogeneous assay

cal characteristic when the labeled T_4 is bound to the antibody.

One of the first homogeneous immunoassays to be developed was the enzyme-multiplied immunoassay technique (EMIT, Syva Inc., Palo Alto, Calif.). In this assay system (Table 44-8, method 2), T_4 is labeled with the enzyme glucose-6-phosphate dehydrogenase (G-6-PD). When the enzyme-labeled T_4 binds to anti-T_4 antibody, the active site of the enzyme is blocked, resulting in decreased G-6-PD activity. The presence of patient T_4 prevents binding of the labeled T_4, resulting in higher enzyme activity. The concentration of serum T_4 is directly proportional to the enzyme activity in this EMIT assay.

Another homogeneous immunoassay technique in wide use is the fluorescence polarization immunoassay (FPIA) (Table 44-8, method 3). In this assay, T_4 in the specimen competes with fluorescein-labeled T_4 for a limited number of antibody-binding sites. Absorption of polarized light by the fluorescein-labeled T_4 results in the reemission of polarized fluorescent light only if the fluorescein-labeled T_4 is bound to antibody; the rapidly moving unbound fluorescein-labeled T_4 emits depolarized light (see Chapters 4 and 13).

Another homogeneous immunoassay technique for measuring T_4 is the cloned enzyme-donor immunoassay assay (CEDIA) (Table 44-8, method 4). This procedure utilizes the enzyme β-galactosidase, which has been cloned as two inactive fragments. One fragment is used as the label for T_4. Addition of anti-T_4 antibody results in the binding of enzyme fragment-T_4 complexes to the antibody thus preventing reassociation of the inactive enzyme fragments and the formation of active enzyme. However, the presence of patient T_4

results in some of the enzyme fragment-T_4 complexes being displaced from the antibody, allowing association of the enzyme fragments to produce active enzyme. Serum T_4 levels are directly related to the enzyme activity in the CEDIA assay.

The development of instrumentation for performing the separation step required in heterogeneous assays has resulted in a variety of analytical systems that can perform automated heterogeneous assays. One example of these systems is the fluorometric enzyme immunoassay technique (Baxter Stratus; Dade Division, Miami, Florida) (Table 44-8, method 5). The specimen is applied to the center portion of a glass fiber membrane containing immobilized T_4 antibody. Thyroxine in the sample binds to T_4 antibody. Next, enzyme-labeled T_4 is added so that it will bind to any unoccupied antibody-binding sites. Unbound enzyme-labeled T_4 is removed by application of a wash solution to the center of the reaction zone to elute this unbound fraction. The enzymatic activity of the bound fraction is then measured with use of a suitable fluorescence substrate.

Other automated heterogeneous assay techniques employ centrifugation to wash and remove any unbound reagents and wash solution from antibody-coated beads (Diagnostic Products Corp., Los Angeles, Calif.) or magnetic particles, which can be separated with magnets (Tosoh, San Francisco, Calif.). Ciba Corning uses magnetic particles and a bioluminescence label.

Specimen Serum is the specimen of choice for T_4 analysis. Plasma is also acceptable, though care must be taken to avoid fibrin in samples that have been previously frozen. Thyroxine is stable in serum for up to 14 days even if stored at room temperature. However, it is recommended that samples be stored frozen if not analyzed within 24 hours of collection.

Reference intervals Thyroxine concentrations vary significantly among euthyroid individuals because of the high degree of protein binding of T_4 and the great variability in serum protein concentrations. Reference intervals for total T_4 are approximately 40 to 120 mg/L (51 to 154 nmol/L). Premenopausal women have T_4 concentrations that are approximately 5 to 10 mg/L (6 to 13 nmol/L) higher than those in men and postmenopausal women as the result of the effect of estrogen on increased TBG concentrations.[53]

REFERENCES

1. Wolff J: Transport of iodide and other anions in the thyroid gland, *Physiol Rev* 44:45-79, 1964.
2. DeGroot LJ, Niepomniszcze H: Biosynthesis of thyroid hormone: basic and clinical aspects, *Metabolism* 26:665-718, 1977.
3. Dumont JE: The action of thyrotropin on thyroid metabolism, *Vitam Horm* 29:287-412, 1971.
4. Chopra IJ, Solomon DH, Chopra U, et al: Pathways of metabolism of thyroid hormones, *Recent Prog Horm Res* 34:521-567, 1978.
5. Woeber KA, Ingbar SH: The interactions of the thyroid hormones with binding protein. In Greer MA, Solomon DH, editors: *Thyroid, American handbook of physiology,* vol 3, Washington, D.C., 1973, American Physiological Society.
6. Chopra IJ: An assessment of daily production and significance of thyroidal 3,3'5'-triiodothyronine (reverse T_3) in man, *J Clin Invest* 58:32-40, 1976.
7. Schimmel M, Utiger RD: Thyroidal and peripheral production of thyroid hormones, *Ann Intern Med* 87:760-768, 1977.
8. Oppenheimer JH, Samuels HH, editors: *Molecular basis of thyroid hormone action,* New York, 1983, Academic Press.
9. Edelman IS, Ismail-Beigi F: Thyroid thermogenesis and active sodium transport, *Recent Prog Horm Res* 30:235-257, 1974.
10. Erfurth EM, Nordén NE, Hedner P, et al: Normal reference interval for thyrotropin response to thyroliberin: dependence on age, sex, free thyroxine index and basal concentrations of thyrotropin, *Clin Chem* 30:196-199, 1984.
11. Wolff J: Iodide goiter and pharmacologic effects of excess iodide, *Am J Med* 47:101-124, 1969.
12. Mason JW: Amiodarone, *N Engl J Med* 316:455-466, 1987.
13. Abuid J, Stinson DA, Larsen PR: Serum triiodothyronine and thyroxine in the neonate and the acute increases in these hormones following delivery, *J Clin Invest* 52:1195-1199, 1973.
14. Selenkow HA, Birnbaum MD, Hollander CS: Thyroid function and dysfunction during pregnancy, *Clin Obstet Gynecol* 16:66-68, 1973.
15. Portnay GI, O'Brian JT, Bush J, et al: The effect of starvation on the concentration and binding of thyroxine and triiodothyronine in serum and on the response to TRH, *J Clin Endocrinol Metab* 39:191-194, 1974.
16. McKenzie JM, Zakarija M, Sato A: Humoral immunity in Graves' disease, *Clin Endocrinol Metab* 7:31-45, 1978.
17. Christiansen NJB, Sierboek-Nielson K, Hansen JEM, Christiansen LK: Serum thyroxine in the early phase of subacute thyroiditis, *Acta Endocrinol* 64:359-363, 1970.
18. Dorfman SG, Cooperman MT, Nelson RL, et al: Painless thyroiditis and transient hyperthyroidism without goiter, *Ann Intern Med* 86:24-28, 1977.
19. Roti E, Emerson CH: Clinical review 29: postpartum thyroiditis, *J Clin Endocrinol Metab* 74:3-5, 1992.
20. Gerstein HC: How common is postpartum thyroiditis? *Arch Intern Med* 150:1397-1400, 1990.
21. LiVolsi VA: Postpartum thyroiditis: the pathology slowly unravels [editorial], *Am J Clin Pathol* 100:193-195, 1993.
22. McKenzie JM, Zakarija M: Pathogenesis of neonatal Graves' disease, *J Endocrinol Invest* 2:183-189, 1978.
23. Brown J, Solomon DH, Beall GN, et al: Autoimmune thyroid dis-

ease—Graves' and Hashimoto's, *Ann Intern Med* 88:379-391, 1978.
24. Dussault JH, Coulombe P, Laberge C, et al: Preliminary report on a mass screening program for neonatal hypothyroidism, *J Pediatr* 86:670-674, 1975.
25. Maxon HR III, Saenger EL, Thomas SR, et al: Clinically important radiation-associated thyroid disease: a controlled study, *JAMA* 44:1802-1805, 1980.
26. Snyder PJ, Utiger RD: Response to thyrotropin-releasing hormone (TRH) in normal man, *J Clin Endocrinol Metab* 34:380-385, 1972.
27. Werner SC, Spooner M: A new and simple test for hyperthyroidism employing L-triiodothyronine and the 24 hour ^{131}I uptake method, *Bull NY Acad Med* 31:139-145, 1955.
28. Surks MI, Chopra IJ, Mariash CN: American Thyroid Association guidelines for the use of laboratory tests in thyroid disorders, *JAMA* 263:1529-1532, 1990.
29. Larsen PR, Alexander NM, Chopra IJ, et al: Committee on Nomenclature, American Thyroid Association: Revised nomenclature for tests of thyroid hormones and thyroid-related proteins in serum [letter to the editor], *J Clin Endocrinol Metab* 64:1089-1094, 1986.
30. Stein RB, Price L: Evaluation of adjusted total thyroxine (free thyroxine index) as a measure of thyroid function, *J Clin Endocrinol Metab* 34:225-228, 1972.
31. Sawin CT, Chopra D, and Albano J: The free triiodothyronine (T_3) index, *Ann Intern Med* 88:474-477, 1978.
32. Toft AD: Use of sensitive immunoradiometric assay for thyrotropin in clinical practice, *Mayo Clin Proc* 63:1035-1042, 1988.
33. Schlumberger M, De Vathaire F, Wu-Ahouju G, et al: Postoperative surveillance of differentiated thyroid carcinoma: contributions of the ultra-sensitive TSH assay, *Presse Méd* 16:1791-1793, 1987.
34. Chopra IJ, Solomon DH, Hepner GW, et al: Misleadingly low free thyroxine index and usefulness of reverse triiodothyronine measurement in nonthyroidal illnesses, *Ann Intern Med* 90:905-912, 1979.
35. Chopra IJ, Solomon DH, Chopra U, et al: Alterations in circulating thyroid hormones and thyrotropin in hepatic cirrhosis: evidence for euthyroidism despite subnormal serum triiodothyronine, *J Clin Endocrinol Metab* 39:501-511, 1974.
36. Grenn JRB: Thyroid function and thyroid regulation in euthyroid men with chronic liver disease: evidence of multiple abnormalities, *Clin Endocrinol* 7:453-461, 1977.
37. Inada M, Sterling K: Thyroxine turnover and transport in Laënnec's cirrhosis of the liver, *J Clin Invest* 46:1275-1282, 1967.
38. Tabei A, Shimoda S: Increased TBG-T_4-binding capacity in acute hepatitis, *Folia Endocrinol* 49:1025-1033, 1973.
39. Schussler GC, Schaffner F, Korn F: Increased serum thyroid hormone binding and decreased free hormone in chronic active liver disease, *N Engl J Med* 299:510-515, 1978.
40. Spector DA, Davis PJ, Helderman JH, et al: Thyroid function and metabolic state in chronic renal failure, *Ann Intern Med* 85:724-730, 1976.
41. Lim VS, Fang VS, Katz A, et al: Thyroid dysfunction in chronic renal failure, *J Clin Invest* 60:522-523, 1977.
42. Cavalieri RR: The effects of nonthyroid disease and drugs on thyroid function tests, *Med Clin North Am* 75:27-39, 1991.
43. Maxon H, Volle C, Hertzberg V, et al: Variation in serum thyroxine concentrations with time after oral replacement dose, *Clin Nucl Med* 12:369-370, 1987.
44. Hay ID, Bayer MF, Kaplan MM, et al: American Thyroid Association assessment of current free thyroid hormone and thyrotropin measurements and guidelines for future clinical assays, *Clin Chem* 37:2002-2008, 1991.
45. Spencer CA, Presti JSL, Patel A, et al: Applications of a new chemiluminometric thyrotropin assay to subnormal measurement, *J Clin Endocrinol Metab* 70:453-460, 1990.
46. Miles LEM, Hales CN: Labeled antibodies and immunological assay systems, *Nature* 219:186-189, 1968.
47. Taimela E, Aalto M, Koshinen P, Irjala K: Clinical and laboratory studies of time-resolved fluorescence immunoassays of thyrotropin and free triiodothyronine, *Clin Chem* 39:679-682, 1993.

48. Taimela E, Tähtelä R, Koskinen P, et al: Ability of two new thyrotropin (TSH) assays to separate hyperthyroid patients from euthyroid patients with low TSH, *Clin Chem* 40:101-105, 1994.

49. Marstein S: Caution against spuriously increased thyrotropin values as determined by two-site immunoradiometric assays, *Clin Chem* 33:1290-1291, 1987.

50. Chen I-W, Heminger LA, Barnes EL, et al: A sensitive radioimmunoassay (RIA) for detection of serum thyrotropin (TSH) in healthy subjects and patients with suppressed pituitary function, *J Nucl Med* 24:114, 1983.

51. Lipson A, Nickoloff EL, Hsu TH, et al: A study of age-dependent changes in thyroid function tests in adults, *J Nucl Med* 20:1124-1130, 1979.

52. Ekins R: The estimation of thyroxine in human plasma by an electrophoretic technique, *Clin Chim Acta* 5:453-459, 1960.

53. Libson A, Nickoloff EL, Hsu TH, et al: A study of age-dependent changes in thyroid function tests in adults, *J Nucl Med* 20:1124-1130, 1979.

CHAPTER 45

The gonads

Karen L. Nickel

(With acknowledgment to the previous authors
Elizabeth J. Kicklighter *and* **Robert J. Norman***)*

Anatomy
   Male: the testes
   Female: the ovaries
Normal physiology
   Male
   Female
Biosynthesis of steroid hormones
   Testicular steroid hormones
   Ovarian steroid hormones
Transport and metabolism
   Transport
   Catabolism and excretion
Pathological conditions
   Abnormalities of ovarian function
   Abnormalities of testicular function
   Premenstrual syndrome (PMS)
   Dysmenorrhea
   Other disorders causing infertility
   Disorders of sexual differentiation
   Amenorrhea
Fertility and infertility
   Disorders leading to infertility in women
   Disorders leading to infertility in men
Evaluation of the infertile couple
   Induction of ovulation
   Assisted reproduction
Contraception through endocrine intervention
Function tests
   Male dynamic tests
   Male physical tests
   Female dynamic tests
   Female physical tests
Changes of analyte in disease
   Gonadotropins (FSH and LH)
   Androgens
   Estrogens
   Progesterone

OBJECTIVES

- Describe the hypothalamus-pituitary-gonadal axis and its regulation.
- Discuss the menstrual cycle and dysfunction leading to infertility.
- Outline the pathways of biosynthesis, transport, and excretion of sex hormones.
- Discuss disorders leading to infertility.
- Describe disorders of sexual differentiation.
- Discuss evaluation of the infertile couple.
- List function tests in evaluating infertility.
- Describe change of analyte with gonadal disease.

KEY TERMS

amenorrhea Absence or abnormal cessation of menstruation.
androgens Sex steroid hormones responsible for the development of the male secondary sex characteristics.
anovulation Inability of the ovary to produce ova.
anorchia Congenital absence of the testis.
cryptorchidism Failure of the testes to descend into the scrotum.
dysmenorrhea Cramping and pain associated with menstruation.
endometrium Inner layer of the uterus.
epididymis Elongated, cordlike structure of the testis that contains ducts capable of storing spermatozoa.
estrogens Sex steroid hormones responsible for the development of the female secondary sex characteristics. Most bioactive is estradiol.
fallopian tube Long, slender tube that extends from the ovary to the uterus.
fecundability Rate of conception in a population.
gametogenesis The development of male and female sex cells, called *gametes*.
gonadotropins Protein hormones (FSH and LH) secreted by the pituitary that stimulate the gonads.
gonadotropin-releasing hormone Decapeptide hormone produced by the hypothalamus, which stimulates the anterior pituitary to produce gonadotropins.
gynecomastia Benign glandular enlargement of the mammary glands in males.
hirsutism An undesirable increase in body hair in women.
hypogonadism Abnormally low activity of the gonads.
infertility Failure to conceive during 1 or more years of unprotected intercourse.

in vitro fertilization (IVF) Assisted reproduction in which the ova are harvested, conception is promoted outside the womb, and then embryos are returned to the fallopian tube. Also, GIFT (genetic intrafallopian tube transfer) and ZIFT (zygote intrafallopian tube transfer).

Klinefelter's syndrome Sexual abnormality in a man characterized by presence of a female chromatin pattern (XXY) with male morphology.

Leydig cells Interstitial cells of the testes that produce the male sex steroids.

luteal phase defects Abnormalities of the corpus luteum of the ovary characterized by insufficient progesterone production.

menarche Beginning of menstruation.

menopause (climacteric) Cessation of the reproductive period in adult women.

menstruation Cyclical uterine bleeding that occurs at about every 28 days during the reproductive period of women.

oral contraceptives Female contraceptives that prevent ovulation by hormone (usually estrogen-progestin) therapy.

ovum Female reproductive cell produced by the ovary.

polycystic ovary syndrome (Stein-Levanthal syndrome) Condition characterized by bilateral polycystic ovaries, amenorrhea, and anovulation.

premenstrual syndrome (PMS) Behavioral changes associated with the menstrual cycle.

pseudohermaphroditism Condition in which the gonads are of one sex, but the other morphology is of the other sex.

sex hormone–binding globulin A liver protein that binds testosterone and estradiol in the circulation.

spermatozoa Male reproductive cell produced in the testes.

testosterone Most important male hormone

virilism Development of male secondary sex characteristics in a female.

ANATOMY
Male: the testes

The normal mature testis (Fig. 45-1) contains approximately 250 pyramidal lobules of seminiferous tubules, which are separated by the fibrous septa. The tubules compose over 85% of the volume of the testis. Surrounding the central lumen of the seminiferous tubule is a structured epithelium containing Sertoli cells and spermatogenic cells. The interstitial tissue between the tubules contains Leydig cells, which are responsible for the production of testicular androgens.

The adult testes (Fig. 45-1) are spheroids located within the scrotum. The scrotum not only serves as a protective envelope, but also helps to maintain the testicular temperature about 2 Celsius degrees below abdominal temperature. Within each testis are about 250 pyramidal lobules that contain coiled seminiferous tubules accounting for 80% to 90% of the testicular mass. The approximately 350 million androgen-producing Leydig, or interstitial, cells, as well as

blood and lymphatic vessels, nerves, and fibroblasts, are interspersed between the seminiferous tubules. The Leydig cells constitute the major endocrine component of the testes. The primary secretory product of these cells, *testosterone,* is responsible for embryonic differentiation of male traits, male secondary sexual development at puberty, and maintenance of libido and potency in the adult male. The seminiferous tubules are responsible for production of approximately 30 million spermatozoa per day during the male's reproductive life. Both these components are related, and both require an intact hypothalamic-pituitary axis for initiation and maintenance of function (see Chapter 43). In addition, several accessory genital structures, discussed below, are required for functional maturation and transport of spermatozoa.

The seminiferous tubules are lined with Sertoli cells and germinal cells. Germinal cell production occurs after about 74 days of orderly development, yielding mature spermatozoa. The seminiferous tubules empty into a highly convoluted network of ducts called the *rete testis.* Spermatozoa are then transported into a single duct, the *epididymis.* During their 12-day transit time, they undergo morphologic and functional changes essential for fertilization. The epididymis also serves as a reservoir for sperm, which then enter the vas deferens and are propelled into the ejaculatory duct.

In addition to the spermatozoa and secretory products of the testes, the *ejaculatory ducts* receive fluid from the *seminal vesicles.* These glands are the source of seminal *fructose,* which serves as an energy source for spermatazoa as well as *phosphorylcholine, ascorbic acid,* and *prostaglandins.* About 60% of the seminal fluid volume derives from the seminal vesicles. The ejaculatory ducts terminate in the prostatic urethra. There about 20% of the seminal fluid is added by the *prostate gland.* Constituents of prostatic fluid include *spermine, citric acid, fibrinolysin, prostate specific antigen,* and *acid phosphatase.* Fluid is also added to the seminal plasma by the Cowper glands and the urethral glands during its transit through the penile urethra.

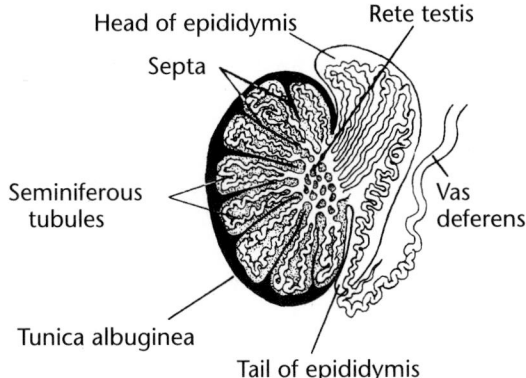

Fig. 45-1 Anatomy of testis. (From Ganong WF: *Review of medical physiology,* ed 2, Los Altos, Calif., 1983, Lange Medical Publications.)

Female: the ovaries

The mature ovaries are paired, nodular organs weighing from 4 to 8 g each, varying during the menstrual cycle. The ovaries are attached to the uterus by the ovarian ligament and lie in proximity to the uterine tubes (oviducts, fallopian tubes).

The ovaries serve a twofold purpose: (1) *production of ova* and (2) *secretion of female sex hormones estrogen and progesterone.* The oocyte, the germ cell of the ovary, is the largest cell in the body with a diameter of about 100 μm at ovulation. Unlike the testis, which continues to produce spermatozoa throughout the entire lifetime of the male, the ovary contains its full supply of oocytes at the time of birth. However, only about 400 oocytes complete the complex process of maturation and ovulation, leaving most of the 400,000 immature oocytes, or follicles, unused. Over the reproductive lifetime of a woman there is gradual degeneration and depletion of oocytes until menopause, when the supply is essentially exhausted.

The mature follicle is composed of three layers of cells—the *theca externa,* the *theca interna,* and the *granulosa cells* (Fig. 43-2). The cells of the theca interna are the primary source of estrogens. After rupture of the follicle and release of the ovum (ovulation), clotting leads to the formation of the *corpus hemorrhagicum.* The granulosa and theca externa cells of the follicle start to proliferate at that site, forming the *corpus luteum.* The luteal cells secrete the estrogens, estrone and estradiol, and progesterone. If there is no pregnancy, the luteum begins to degenerate about 4 days before the next menses and is eventually replaced by scar tissue called the *corpus albicans.* Fertilization of the released oocyte may then take place within the ampullary portion of the fallopian tube. The fertilized ovum would then continue to the endometrium of the uterus, where it would be implanted for the term of the pregnancy.

NORMAL PHYSIOLOGY
Male

In both the male and female, all reproductive function is dependent on a complicated interrelationship of the hypothalamus, the pituitary gland, and the gonads. The hypothalamus synthesizes a decapeptide, gonadotrophin-releasing hormone (GnRH), and secretes it in pulses every 2 minutes. After reaching the anterior pituitary, GnRH stimulates the release of both luteinizing hormone (LH) and, to a lesser extent in the male, follicle-stimulating hormone (FSH) into the general circulation.

In males, LH is bound to specific cellular membrane receptors of the Leydig cells. This leads to generation of cAMP and other messengers that ultimately result in secretion of androgens, male hormones. The primary endocrine product of these cells is testosterone, the male sex hormone. Elevation of androgens, in turn, inhibits secretion of LH from the pituitary by a negative feedback mechanism on both the pituitary and hypothalamus. Both the pituitary and hypothalamus have androgen receptors. Leydig cells also produce small amounts of other bioactive substances, such as *oxytocin, prostaglandins and endorphins,* which may be important in regulation of testicular function. The testosterone released by the Leydig cells is responsible for embryonic differentiation of male traits, male secondary sexual development at puberty, and maintenance of libido and potency in the adult male.

Pituitary FSH binds to specific cell membrane receptors

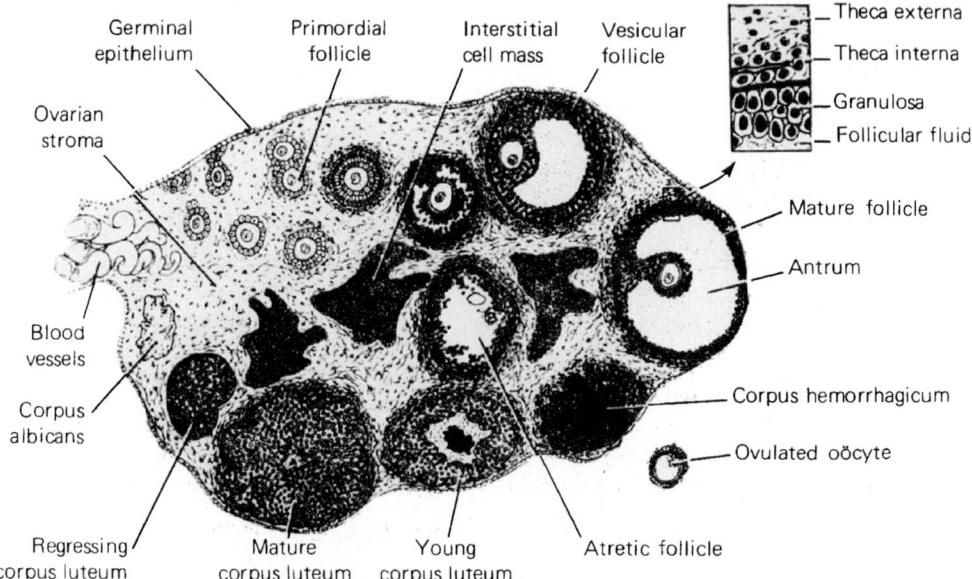

Fig. 45-2 Diagram of ovary, showing sequential development of a follicle and formation of corpus luteum. Section of wall of a mature follicle is enlarged at upper right. (From Gorbman A, Bern HA: *A textbook of comparative endocrinology,* New York, 1962, Wiley & Sons.)

of the Sertoli cells, stimulating production of androgen-binding protein (ABP). FSH is necessary for the initiation of spermatogenesis; however, full maturation of spermatozoa also requires testosterone. The major action of FSH on spermatogenesis may be its role in stimulating ABP production, which in turn maintains the needed level of testosterone.

The Sertoli cells produce a number of other substances besides ABP, such as transferrin, inhibin, ceruloplasmin, and H-Y antigen. Two forms of *inhibin* have been found, both of which have the same alpha subunit cross-linked to different beta subunits. Both inhibins selectively inhibit FSH release from the pituitary without affecting LH release. Since FSH directly stimulates the Sertoli cells to secrete *inhibin*, inhibins (and possibly the gonadal steroids) are probably the physiological regulators of pituitary FSH secretion.

Female

Throughout the reproductive years in a woman, the structural composition and hormonal activity of the ovary are continually changing. These changes are responsible for many of the physiological events of the normal menstrual cycle. The two major functions of the adult ovary are the synthesis and secretion of sex hormones and the release of a mature ovum every 28 to 30 days. These two functions are closely related and interdependent and are part of the menstrual cycle described below.

The ovary. The basic reproductive unit of the ovary is the primordial follicle consisting of a small oocyte arrested in the diplotene stage of meiotic prophase. These follicles are the resting pool from which all ovulatory follicles will eventually develop. Each month after puberty, a follicle leaves the pool of resting follicles and begins to enlarge. Unknown local factors must play a role in its selection as dominant preovulatory follicle. This oocyte starts a process of growth, leading to development of a fully grown ovum that is released at ovulation. This process is dependent on the interaction of pituitary gonadotropins, ovarian steroids, and other local factors within the follicle. Binding of FSH to its ovarian receptor stimulates conversion of androgen precursors to estrogens. Estradiol, in turn, plays a critical role in follicular growth by a direct effect on the ovary and by positive- and negative-feedback regulation of FSH and LH secretion (see below).

Immediately after ovulation there are remarkable changes in cellular organization of the rupture area of the follicle that go beyond normal tissue repair and lead to the formation of the corpus luteum. The corpus luteum lasts for about 14 days, during the low levels of LH available during the luteal phase of the menstrual cycle. If LH were to be replaced by human chorionic gonadotrophin (hCG) produced by the trophoblast after a successful implantation, the corpus luteum would be maintained. However, if no pregnancy occurs, the corpus luteum rapidly ages and menses occurs (see p. 896).

Ovarian hormones. The mature ovary actively synthesizes and secretes estrogens (estradiol and estrone), progesterone, androgens, and their precursors. The most biologically active ovarian estrogen is estradiol. The ovary also produces *relaxin, inhibin, prostaglandins,* and other substances. The ovary is normally the major source of estrogens, though conversion of androgens and their precursors in other tissues may be clinically important after menopause or in ovarian dysfunction. *Progesterone* is produced in large amounts during the luteal phase of the menstrual cycle. The ovary also produces small amounts of testosterone and other androgens that act peripherally and also serve as precursors for the synthesis of estrogens. *Estrone,* another important estrogen, is the product of both ovarian secretion and peripheral conversion of prohormones of adrenal and ovarian origin.

Menstrual cycle. Cyclic ovarian function depends on appropriately timed secretions of both FSH and LH by the anterior pituitary in response to hypothalamic GnRH. Release of GnRH by the hypothalamus and, in turn, FSH and LH secretion by the pituitary in response to GnRH are modulated by the estrogen and progesterone reaching these glands. Both negative and positive feedback are essential for appropriate coordination of endocrine and morphological events in the adult female reproductive cycle (Fig. 45-3). Negative feedback is seen in suppression of FSH and LH secretion in response to increased levels of estradiol and progesterone. Estradiol appears to inhibit mainly FSH secretion, whereas progesterone, in combination with estradiol, seems to reduce both LH and FSH secretion. Positive feedback is characterized by estradiol stimulation of the synthesis or release of LH from the pituitary.

The normal ovarian, or menstrual, cycle is regulated by the hypothalamic-pituitary-ovarian feedback mechanism, which may be divided into four phases: *early follicular, late follicular, midcycle,* and *luteal.*

Estradiol seems to be the most effective agent in eliciting a negative-feedback response to inhibit FSH release. If circulating estradiol levels fall, FSH secretion rises promptly. This is seen at the onset of menstruation when the corpus luteum ceases to secrete estradiol and progesterone. Conversely, FSH levels fall during the second half of the follicular phase when the maturing follicle secretes increasing amounts of estradiol and inhibin and during the luteal phase. The effect of estradiol on LH production is not so straightforward, since there may be a pronounced concentration-dependent effect.

Hypothalamic-pituitary regulation of ovarian function is governed not only by steroid and peptide hormones, but also by neural stimuli from the central nervous system. The hypothalamus receives both neural as well as hormonal signals, which are translated into GnRH secretions and can affect the menstrual cycle. This is seen in cases of stress or profound weight loss, which may lead to amenorrhea.

The physiology of reproduction in the female is domi-

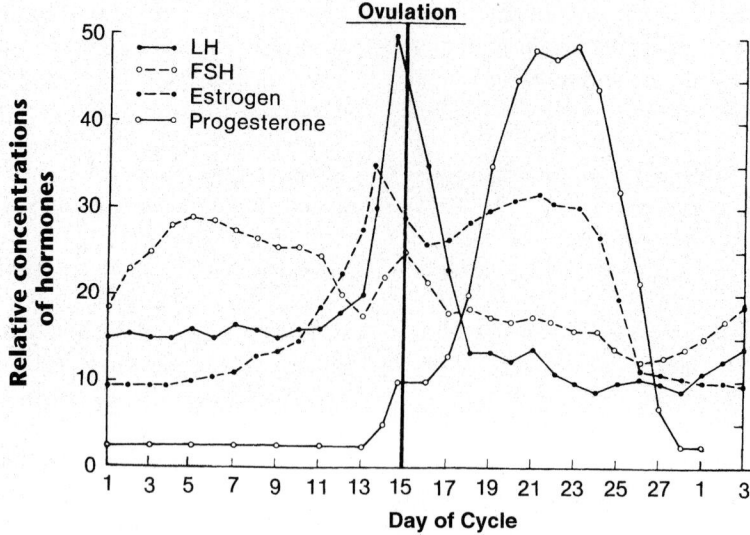

Fig. 45-3 Changes in blood levels of various hormones throughout menstrual cycle. (Modified from Taymor ML, Berger MJ, Thompson IE, Karamo KS: *Am J Obstet Gynecol* 114:445, 1972.)

nated by the events of the menstrual cycle. *Menstruation* is the regular cyclic shedding of the surface layer of the endometrium along with blood. This cyclic phenomenon is the result of interaction of its hormone effectors, as described above.

In the beginning of the menstrual cycle, in the follicular phase, several follicles begin to develop, but only one will mature in about 10 to 12 days. In the early follicular phase, when the preceding month's corpus luteum ceases to function, the levels of estradiol and progesterone are relatively constant and low, the FSH levels are rising, and the LH levels are also low (see Fig. 45-3). These high levels of FSH stimulate follicular growth and release of estradiol. By days 7 to 8, the estradiol level is rising at a rapid rate, reaching its first peak before ovulation. The rising levels of estradiol result in negative feedback on the hypothalamus and pituitary, causing a fall in FSH levels. At the same time, the rise in estradiol triggers a rapid rise in LH through positive feedback. Estradiol reaches a maximum on the day before the LH peak.

During the midcycle there is a peak rise in LH, which leads to final maturation and rupture of the ovum at ovulation, usually 16 to 24 hours after the LH peak. This usually occurs at day 14 of the 28-day cycle. Before the LH surge and before ovulation, the estradiol level drops considerably and then rises again after ovulation.

The ruptured follicle becomes the site of corpus luteum formation, and the ovary is said to be in the *luteal phase*. Progesterone produced by the corpus luteum begins to increase 3 days after ovulation, and the rising progesterone levels cause an inhibition of the secretion of LH. A sharp increase in progesterone follows and reaches a maximum in about 8 or 9 days after the LH peak (days 23 to 25 of

the cycle). As estradiol and progesterone increase, FSH and LH decline throughout the luteal phase, and the decreasing FSH causes regression of the corpus luteum. As the corpus luteum regresses, the levels of both estradiol and progesterone begin to diminish. Removal of the inhibitory effect of these two compounds results in an increase of FSH, which stimulates the growth of a new crop of follicles in the ovary. During the menstruation phase, estradiol, progesterone, and LH are at relatively constant low levels, whereas FSH is the only hormone present at elevated and rising levels.

Effect of ovarian hormones on uterus (endometrium). As a physiological result of the ovarian hormones estradiol and progesterone, definite changes occur in the endometrium in preparation to receive and implant a fertilized ovum. The rising levels of estradiol stimulate the reconstruction of the endometrium, blood vessels, and secretory glands of the uterus. This change in the endometrial growth is called the *proliferative phase* and corresponds with the follicular phase of the ovary. The newly formed glands begin to release glandular substances. Hence the phase is called the *secretory phase* of the endometrium, and it corresponds to the luteal phase of the ovary. During days 1 to 5 of the cycle, enough estrogen is secreted by the follicles to start the deep layer of the endometrium growing, but it is not enough to support the thickened secretory endometrium of the previous cycle. As a result, this well-developed surface of the endometrium sloughs off as the estradiol levels decrease. This is menstruation. Thus menstruation occurs during the later stages of the proliferative phase of the endometrium because of withdrawal of hormonal support. If a fertilized egg is successfully implanted in the enriched endometrium, the implantation causes additional estrogen to be produced; thus menstruation is prevented and the development of a pregnancy is begun (see Chapter 40).

Menopause. Cyclic changes of hormones of the hypothalamic-pituitary-ovarian axis (Fig. 45-4) occur usually 30 to 35 years after menarche. As a woman approaches the age of menopause the remaining follicles begin to perform less well. During this "perimenopausal" period, called the *climacteric,* women can have lower estradiol levels and higher FSH levels even though their periods are regular. LH levels, on the other hand, are largely unchanged. This plateau is probably caused by the declining negative effect of inhibin on FSH production by the pituitary. Major characteristics seen during this time are disturbances in menstrual pattern, including anovulation and reduced fertility, decreased (or increased) flow, and irregular frequency of menses. Occasionally corpus luteum formation and function occur during this time, and the perimenopausal woman is not safe from unexpected pregnancy until elevated levels of both LH and FSH can be demonstrated.

After menopause, usually between 48 to 55 years of age for American women, there are no remaining follicles, inadequate estrogen production, and no menses. There is a tenfold to twentyfold increase in FSH and about a threefold increase in LH, peaking about 3 years after menopause. FSH levels are higher than LH because LH is cleared from the blood much faster than FSH (serum half-lives are 4 hours for FSH and 30 minutes for LH). Estradiol production does not continue after menopause; however, estrogen levels may be significant because of peripheral conversion of androgens to estrogen. The major estrogen in menopausal women is estrone, not estradiol.

BIOSYNTHESIS OF STEROID HORMONES
Testicular steroid hormones

The ultimate precursor of all steroid hormones is acetate, from which cholesterol is synthesized. Cholesterol can be made anew from acetate in the gonads, or it can be derived from systemic circulation. The conversion of cholesterol (a C27 steroid) to both androgens (C19) and estrogens (C18) is shown in Fig. 45-5. These metabolic pathways are similar in the testis, ovary, and adrenal glands. The first step is cleavage of the cholesterol side chain, resulting in formation of pregnenolone, a C21 steroid. Pregnenolone is then converted through a series of intermediates to testosterone or estradiol. The pathway through progesterone is called the Δ^4 pathway, and the one through DHEA the Δ^5 pathway. In the male, testosterone is further reduced to DHT, androstanolone, and androstanediol in target tissues such as the prostate.

The testis is the primary site of androgen production in the male, and the major circulating androgen is testosterone. By definition, androgens are steroid hormones capable of stimulating the development and maintaining the normal function of male sex organs. There are several androgens

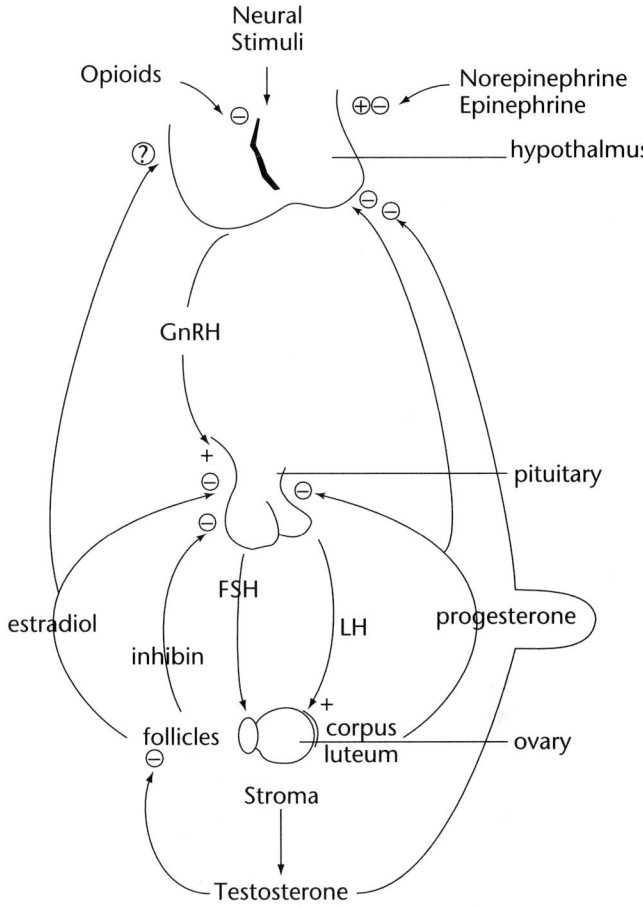

Fig. 45-4 Diagram of hypothalamic-pituitary-ovarian axis. *FSH,* Follicle-stimulating hormone; E_2, estradiol; *GnRH,* gonadotropin-releasing hormone; *LH,* luteinizing hormone; +, positive effect; −, negative effect. (After Greenspan FS: *Basic and clinical endocrinology,* East Norwalk, Conn., 1991, Appleton & Lange.)

besides testosterone, such as androstenedione and dehydroepiandrosterone (DHEA), which are weak androgens, and 5α-dihydrotestosterone (DHT), which is a potent androgen. 5α-reductase is a key enzyme for converting testosterone into the more potent DHT. Specific pharmicological inhibitors of 5α-reductase (such as Proscar) are used to treat benign prostatic hypertrophy and prostatic cancer, both of which are stimulated by testosterone and DHT. The testis also secretes other steroids such as estradiol and 17-hydroxyprogesterone, the latter being the second major hormone product of the testes. Secretion of testosterone by the testes is episodic; a circadian pattern can be demonstrated, with a maximum in the early morning (about 7 A.M.) and a minimum about 13 hours later.

Ovarian steroid hormones

The ovary is the major source of estrogen and progesterone in the female, as described previously. Estradiol, the most active estrogen produced, is synthesized from andro-

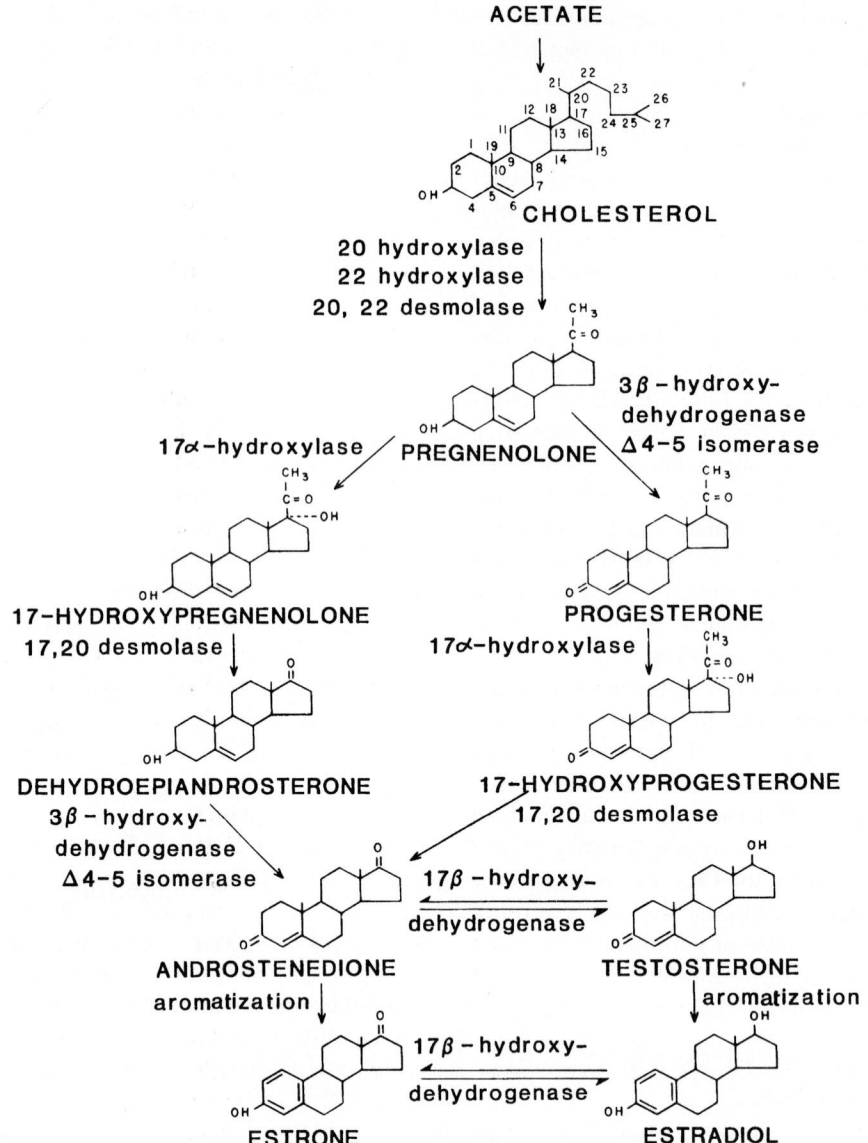

ACETATE

CHOLESTEROL

20 hydroxylase
22 hydroxylase
20, 22 desmolase

PREGNENOLONE

3β − hydroxy-
dehydrogenase
Δ4−5 isomerase

17α−hydroxylase

17-HYDROXYPREGNENOLONE

17,20 desmolase

PROGESTERONE

17α−hydroxylase

DEHYDROEPIANDROSTERONE

3β − hydroxy-
dehydrogenase
Δ4−5 isomerase

17-HYDROXYPROGESTERONE

17,20 desmolase

ANDROSTENEDIONE

17β −hydroxy-
dehydrogenase

TESTOSTERONE

aromatization

aromatization

17β −hydroxy-
dehydrogenase

ESTRONE

ESTRADIOL

Fig. 45-5 Pathways of sex steroidogenesis. *Capitals,* Metabolic products; *lower-case lettering,* enzymes in metabolic pathway. (From Felig P et al: *Endocrinology and metabolism,* New York, 1981, McGraw-Hill.)

gens by a group of microsomal enzymes known as the *aromatase system.* Progesterone serves as a precursor for androgen and estrogen, depending on cleavage of the two-carbon (C20-C21) side chain. Little hormone is stored in the ovary, and so secretory activity is closely related to biosynthetic activity. During pregnancy the fetoplacental unit produces large amounts of steroid hormone, such as progesterone, pregnenolone, and estriol (see Chapter 40).

TRANSPORT AND METABOLISM
Transport

When secreted into the circulation, the gonadal steroids exist either in a free (unbound) state or weakly or strongly bound to plasma transport proteins. Only the free and the

weakly bound hormones are biologically active. The major steroid binders in plasma are albumin and a beta globulin, called *sex hormone–binding globulin* (SHBG). SHBG binds approximately 97% of estradiol and 60% of testosterone; albumin binds 38% of testosterone. Thus only 3% of estradiol and 2% of testosterone remain in the free, active form in plasma. SHBG, synthesized by the liver, is under hormone regulation and is distinct from androgen-binding protein (ABP), which is produced by the Sertoli cells in the testes. Progesterone binds strongly to corticosteroid-binding globulin (CBG) and only weakly to albumin. The concentration of these binding proteins is increased by estrogen and thyroxine and decreased by androgens and progestins. Binding by transport protein is a way of exerting control over the biological availability of active hormones, since only free hormone can enter a cell (see p. 858). Disturbances in hormone binding may have clinical importance after menopause or in women with abnormal ovarian function associated with excess androgens.

Catabolism and excretion

Although testosterone is converted to DHT within specific androgen target tissues, the liver is the key organ for the catabolism of sex hormones. Plasma testosterone is converted by the liver into various metabolites such as androsterone and etiocholanolone, which, after conjugation with glucuronic or sulfuric acid, are excreted in the urine as 17-ketosteroids. It is important to note, however, that only about 25% of urinary ketosteroids are derived from testosterone. Most, such as DHEAS, originate from adrenal steroid metabolism. Circulating estradiol is rapidly converted in the liver to estrone, some of which reenters the circulation. However, most is further metabolized to estriol or 2-hydroxyestrone, a catechol estrogen, conjugated, and excreted by the kidney. Progesterone is rapidly cleared, having a half-life of about 5 minutes. It is converted in the liver to pregnanediol, conjugated to glucuronic acid, and excreted by the kidneys.

PATHOLOGICAL CONDITIONS

Abnormalities of gonadal function can be expressed in a variety of pathological conditions. Some of these conditions can result in death, whereas others, such as hirsutism, are not life threatening. One of the most important clinical manifestations of many gonadal abnormalities is infertility. This clinical problem is discussed in a separate section below.

Abnormalities of ovarian function

Endocrine disorders of the ovary may be classified as "hypo-" or "hyper-"; primary ovarian in origin or secondary to disturbances of hypothalamic-pituitary function; and congenital or acquired. The clinical manifestations of ovarian function may be very subtle because the ovary is mainly an organ of reproduction. Thus its disturbances may be picked up only in a work-up for infertility or for precocious or delayed puberty (see the discussion of fertility and infertility, pp. 901 and 904).

Ovarian hypofunction. Symptoms of gonadal hypofunction depend on whether the condition manifests itself before or after puberty. Ovarian hypofunction that develops in the prepubertal period will manifest itself clinically as delayed or absent menarche or primary amenorrhea. Ovarian hypofunction developing after puberty may manifest itself as secondary amenorrhea.

Primary ovarian hypofunction. The causes of primary ovarian disorders may be caused by functional or developmental dysfunction of the gland. Premature ovarian failure, resistant ovary syndrome, and ovarian tumors can result in loss of ovarian function. Disturbance of development is seen in gonadal agenesis, Turner's syndrome, and 17α-hydroxylase deficiency. Because of the lack of estrogenic feedback on the hypothalamic-pituitary axis, primary ovarian hypofunction is characterized by increased levels of gonadotropins in association with decreased estrogen levels.

A normal pattern of ovarian hypofunction is female climacteric, or menarche, resulting in *menopause.* The climacteric normally begins to occur in women in their late forties to early fifties and, within a few years, results in complete cessation of the menstrual cycle (menopause). The climacteric is the result of primary ovarian hypofunction despite the very high elevation in LH. Physical and psychological discomfort accompanies the withdrawal of estradiol during the climacteric. The long-term lack of estradiol also places women at increased risk for osteoporosis and heart disease, and the decreased progesterone increases the risk of breast cancer. For this reason, most American women are prescribed estrogen replacement therapy during menarche, continuing this therapy for decades afterwards.

Secondary ovarian hypofunction. Secondary ovarian hypofunction is characterized by decreased estrogen and progesterone levels in association with decreased gonadotropin levels. It may be attributable to hypothalamic, pituitary, or constitutional disturbances.

Secondary ovarian failure occurs when the pituitary does not produce FSH and LH in response to GnRH stimulation or to decreasing estrogen levels. The most common cause of abnormal pituitary hypofunction is pituitary trauma (accidental injury, surgery), in which gonadotrophin production is usually the first function to be lost. Space-filling pituitary tumors and necrosis resulting from postpartum hemorrhages also result in loss of pituitary function.

Functional abnormalities in the neural mechanisms that regulate the pulsatile secretion of GnRH can lead to hypothalamic amenorrhea *(tertiary amenorrhea).* In such cases, pituitary and ovarian function may be normal, but conditions such as emotional stress or physical illness may disrupt LHRH secretion and normal ovulation. Amenorrhea may also be seen in athletes and patients suffering from anorexia.

Clinical laboratory tests can be used to help differentiate ovarian (primary), pituitary (secondary), or hypothalamic (tertiary) causes of amenorrhea in women (see below). One can show the presence of endogenous estrogen by attempting to induce withdrawal uterine bleeding by administering progesterone. The presence of vaginal bleeding within 7 days after the end of progesterone treatment indicates the patient is capable of producing sufficient estrogen to stimulate endometrial growth. The patient may still be anovulatory, and the method of treatment depends on her objectives. Failure to induce bleeding by progesterone indicates insufficient estrogen production secondary to hypothalamic-pituitary-ovarian dysfunction. Analysis of FSH and LH levels and a GnRH challenge will help differentiate secondary and tertiary causes of amenorrhea. Prolactin (PRL) is the first test of choice to rule out a pituitary tumor as the cause of amenorrhea.

Ovarian hyperfunction

Primary ovarian hyperfunction. The main cause of primary ovarian hyperfunction is estrogen-secreting tumors; granulosa and thecal cell tumors are the most common. Approximately 5% arise before puberty, 55% during the period of reproductive life, and 40% after menopause. Precocious puberty and intermittent uterine bleeding result from tumors during the premenarchal years. Irregular uterine bleeding frequently alternating with periods of amenorrhea is common during the active reproductive life. Uterine bleeding is the characteristic manifestation of tumors during the postmenopausal years. Primary ovarian hyperfunction results in decreased levels of FSH and LH because of increased negative feedback on the hypothalamic-pituitary axis.

Secondary ovarian hyperfunction. Secondary ovarian hyperfunction is characterized by increased levels of gonadotropins resulting in increased estrogen secretion. Sexual precocity results from pituitary stimulation of ovarian function.

An unusual form of precocious puberty is associated with hypothyroidism, where the ovary has increased sensitivity to endogenous gonadotropins. The precocity can be reversed by treatment of the hypothyroidism. These observations contrast with the effects of hypothyroidism on adult women who commonly experience a failure of ovulation.

Abnormalities of testicular function

As in women, male gonadal dysfunction can be divided into two categories: those resulting in decreased androgen production, or hypogonadism, and those resulting in excessive androgen production, or hypergonadism (Table 45-1). Either disorder may be attributable to a primary dysfunction of the testes, or may be secondary to a derangement of the pituitary-hypothalamic axis and may result in infertility.

Hypogonadism

The clinical picture of hypogonadism is directly related to the time of development of androgen deficiency. Androgen deficiency during the second to third months of fetal development can cause sexual ambiguity and pseudohermaphroditism. In prepubertal hypogonadism, absence of androgen production by the testis is associated with persistent infantile genitalia, a barely palpable prostate, poor secondary sexual development and lack of normal secondary sexual characteristics, and eunuchoid characteristics. Prepubertal hypogonadism is usually inapparent until the adolescent period, when normal adolescent development, including genital and secondary sexual changes, does not occur.

Postpubertal hypogonadism results in minimal changes. In young males, there is usually diminished beard growth

Table 45-1   Causes of male hypogonadism

Primary hypogonadism

Klinefelter's syndrome
Other chromosomal defects (that is, XX male, XY/XXY, XX/XXY, etc.)
Leydig cell aplasia
Cryptorchidism
Adult seminiferous tubule or Leydig cell failure
Testicular trauma

Secondary hypogonadism

Panhypopituitarism
Isolated LH deficiency
LH and FSH deficiency

Defects in androgen action

Complete androgen insensitivity (testicular feminization)
Incomplete androgen insensitivity (such as 5α-reductase deficiency)

---

and thinning of body hair. The prostate atrophies, and sexual desire and performance decrease. The genitalia may decrease somewhat in size. In older men, none of these changes may be noted.

Primary hypogonadism. Because of the lack of androgenic feedback on the pituitary-hypothalamic axis, primary hypogonadism is manifested by increased serum and urine gonadotropins and by decreased serum androgen levels and decreased urinary 17-ketosteroid levels (see p. 904). The testicular abnormality may be secondary to a developmental abnormality, such as a genetic or embryological defect, or it may occur at any time later in life. Developmental abnormalities account for most prepubertal cases of hypogonadism.

The majority of cases of primary hypogonadism manifesting themselves after puberty are the result of testicular infections, trauma, irradiation, a tumor that has replaced the testicular parenchyma, or surgical or accidental castration. Other rare congenital disorders may be manifested as a primary hypogonadal state after puberty. These include such conditions as myotonia dystrophica and cystic fibrosis.

Secondary hypogonadism. Secondary hypogonadism results from failure of the pituitary to produce LH and FSH. This is usually the result of primary hypopituitarism, though rarely this condition may be secondary to a failure of the hypothalamus to release LHRH. This results in inadequate synthesis of FSH and LH by the pituitary.

In most cases of primary hypopituitarism there is a loss of pituitary hormones, resulting in decreased thyroid, adrenal, and gonadal function at all ages. This *panhypopituitarism* may be idiopathic, part of a congenital disorder, or secondary to a neurohypophysial lesion such as a neoplasm, cyst, or granulomatous process. When there is a progressive loss of the pituitary function because of a neurohypophysial lesion, a decrease in gonadotropins is at times the first deficiency observed, and the patient may present with isolated hypogonadism.

The absence of serum and urinary gonadotropins after the age of adolescence in patients with diminished gonadal function is diagnostic of secondary hypogonadism. Studies of growth, thyroid, adrenal, and antidiuretic hormones may reveal clinically unsuspected deficiencies in other pituitary hormones.

Hypergonadism

Hypergonadism may occur as a primary process because of excessive androgen production from a testicular tumor (Leydig cell or interstitial cell carcinoma). Hypergonadism may also occur secondary to altered pituitary-hypothalamic axis function with increased LH/FSH secretion. Primary hypergonadism is noted for high serum androgen levels, high urinary 17-ketosteroids, and low serum gonadotropins. Secondary hypergonadism is differentiated by elevated androgens and their urinary metabolites and elevated gonadotropins.

The production of excessive quantities of androgenic hormones in adult males results in little if any morphological change. However, excessive production in children results in precocious puberty. When precocious puberty occurs in males without a family history, it is almost always associated with a space-occupying lesion in the region of the third ventricle of the brain.

Premature puberty in the male may also result from excessive adrenal androgens. The pattern of growth and development is similar to that produced by increased testicular steroids; however, the testes remain prepubertal in size.

Premenstrual syndrome (PMS)

The premenstrual syndrome (PMS) is commonly recognized by behavioral changes associated with the menstrual cycle. PMS appears as a variety of psychological and physiological manifestations triggered by normal, physiologic hormonal changes. The most frequently encountered symptoms include abdominal bloating, anxiety, breast tenderness, crying spells, depression, fatigue, irritability, thirst, and appetite changes, all occurring during the last 7 to 10 days of the menstrual period. There seems to be no single cause of PMS, and various treatments have been used, such as oral contraceptives, vitamin B$_6$, bromocriptine, and synthetic progesterone agents. The physician needs to modify the treatment of his patient to alleviate her specific symptoms.

Dysmenorrhea

Dysmenorrhea is a condition of cramping and pain that affects over half the menstruating women and is associated with ovulatory cycles. Primary dysmenorrhea is caused by myometrial contractions induced by prostaglandins, especially prostaglandin F$_{2\alpha}$ (PGF$_{2\alpha}$) originating in secretory endometrium. Other symptoms include headache, nausea and vomiting, backache, and diarrhea. Drugs that act as prostaglandin synthetase inhibitors effectively relieve the pain of dysmenorrhea in about 80% of women with the problem. These drugs include ibuprofen, naproxen, flufenamic acid, and indomethacin. Another benefit of prostaglandin inhibition is the reduction in the amount of blood lost with menstrual flow. Indeed these agents may also be used to treat idiopathic menorrhagia and excess flow associated with an intrauterine device (IUD).

Other disorders causing infertility

Infertility may be defined as a failure to conceive during 1 or more years of unprotected intercourse. Eighty percent of couples attempting a pregnancy achieve a conception within 1 year with regular intercourse, with an additional 10% by the end of the second year. Ten percent will remain infertile after 2 years. Fertility problems generally involve one of the following areas in either the male or female: defects of the hypothalamic-pituitary-gonadal axis, congenital disorders, chromosomal abnormalities, infections, autoimmune reactions, or physical dysfunction.

Female factors usually account for about 40% to 50% of an infertility problem and include problems related to ovulation, anovulation (no ovulation), or oligo-ovulation (little ovulation).

Anovulation is the inability of the ovary to produce ova. Abnormal ovarian function may result from primary disorders of the ovary itself or disorders of the controlling mechanisms (see above). Ovarian failure occasionally occurs in women under 35 years of age after spontaneous sexual maturation. In some patients, it is associated with ovarian autoantibodies and is probably the result of autoimmune destruction of the ovary. In other patients, the ovaries show a few primordial follicles, and in some they resemble menopausal ovaries. The presence of excessive amounts of androgen is also associated with oligomenorrhea or amenorrhea. Evaluation of FSH, LH, and estrogen levels in the patient will help diagnose the cause of anovulation. Female infertility can also result from luteal phase defects.

Luteal phase defects are defined as abnormalities of corpus luteum function in the ovary characterized by insufficient progesterone production. Inadequate production of progesterone may prevent implantation (infertility) or may lead to inability to maintain the early embryo (spontaneous abortion). Unless hCG is produced by the trophoblast to continue stimulation, the corpus luteum degenerates, progesterone level falls, and menses occurs. In patients with luteal phase defect, the amount or duration of progesterone secretion may be deficient, whereas the production of estrogen usually remains normal. Classification of luteal defect may be performed by carefully timed analysis of serum progesterone (specifically 7 days after ovulation), endometrial biopsy (5 days later), and perhaps ultrasonographic examination of the ovaries.

Other causes of female infertility can include poor tubal patency and antibodies against sperm. Tubal closure can result from scarring after pelvic inflammatory disease (PID);

about 20% of infertility in women is caused by tubal disease.

Male infertility occurs in about 40% to 50% of couples. An additional 10% to 20% of cases of infertility result from problems in both partners.

Disorders of sexual differentiation

There are seven characteristics that can be used to determine a person's sex: (1) sex chromosomes, (2) gonadal histological appearance, (3) morphology of external genitalia, (4) morphology of internal genitalia, (5) hormonal status, (6) sex of rearing, and (7) sex role of individual. The sex chromosomes of the zygote determine the type of gonad that will be developed. Differentiation begins during the fourth to sixth week of gestation. Testicular development occurs as directed by genes in the Y chromosome, including the testis-determining factor (TDF) and HY antigen genes. Ovarian development occurs in the absence of the Y chromosome, and the importance of the X chromosome appears to be for oocyte maintenance. Various deletions along the X chromosome have been identified to cause ovarian and menstrual disorders.

Sexual ambiguity is said to occur if the above classifications do not clearly describe a person's sex. For example, if the gonads are masculine but the other morphogenetic sexual characteristics are mixed, the person is said to be a male pseudohermaphrodite, or similarly for a person with female genitalia.

There are two basic causes for physiological disorders of sexual ambiguity: (1) defects in gonadal development because of a chromosome aberration, or (2) disorders in development because of a hereditary defect despite normal chromosomes. The chromosomal defects that cause abnormal gonadal development are attributable to errors in meiosis or mitosis. They occur by chance and are not hereditary or more likely to occur in siblings. The normal female has 44 autosomes and two X sex chromosomes, whereas the normal male has 44 autosomes and one X and one Y sex chromosome. Several errors of meiotic division can cause euploidy, an abnormal number of sex chromosomes (either extra or absent), as well as structurally abnormal sex chromosomes. When an ovum with extra or absent sex chromosomes is fertilized by normal sperm, for example, various forms of sexual abnormalities occur, such as Klinefelter's syndrome (47,XXY) or Turner's syndrome (45,X).

Klinefelter's syndrome is the most common disorder (1 in 4000 live male births) that is characterized by small testes, gynecomastia, azoospermia, and infertility. This is a disorder of intersexuality, since there is a female chromatin pattern with a completely male sexual morphology.

Turner's syndrome is also quite common (1 in 7000 live female births). Turner's syndrome is characterized by short stature, webbing of the neck, and heart malformations.

These patients have immature internal and external genitalia and no sexual development.

True hermaphroditism occurs when both male and female gonadal tissue is present. A uterus is nearly always present, and at puberty most hermaphrodites develop breasts and menstruate. The most common karyotype is 46,XX.

Diagnosis of abnormalities of sexual differentiation is best done soon after birth. Early sex identification will often determine the success of the final outcome for both the child and the family. Sex assignment is based on appearance of external genitalia and ultrasound appearance of internal organs (uterus and cervix). Karyotyping is used only to confirm the anatomic findings.

Amenorrhea

Biochemical disorders with androgen excess. Excessive androgen (male hormone) in women usually leads to menstrual disorders, including amenorrhea. The major androgens in women are testosterone, dihydrotestosterone, DHEA, and DHEA sulfate, with free testosterone being the bioactive form of testosterone. Androgens can arise from ovarian or adrenal sources. Testosterone is derived from both the ovary and adrenal glands, whereas DHEA and its sulfate are derived from adrenal glands only.

The most common causes of androgen excess are listed in Table 45-2. One of the most frequent symptoms of hyperandronism in women is hirsutism. *Hirsutism* is defined as an abnormal increase in body hair in women. Although approximately 5% of women have hirsutism, only 40% to 60% of these women will have elevated levels of serum androgens. Over 95% of hirsute women will have the more benign conditions of idiopathic hirsutism (the most common disorder) or the polycystic ovary syndrome. The remaining women must be investigated for the presence of other, more life-threatening causes of their hirsutism, including congenital adrenal hyperplasia and Cushing's syndrome (see Chapter 46) and tumors (benign or malignant) of the adrenal gland or ovaries.

Approximately 20% of women with androgen excess have polycystic ovaries. The polycystic ovary syndrome (PCO, Stein-Leventhal) is characterized by anovulation in association with continuous stimulation of the ovary by high

Table 45-2 Causes of androgen excess in women

Ovarian causes
  Polycystic ovary syndrome
  Hyperthecosis
  Androgen-producing tumors
Adrenal causes
  Congenital or adult-onset hyperplasia
  Androgen-producing tumors
  Cushing's syndrome
Obesity
Postmenopausal state
Drug induced (as phenytoin, danazol, minoxidil)
Idiopathic or familial

---

levels of LH. This causes increased ovarian androgen production usually, testosterone and androstenedione, and characteristic morphologic changes in the ovaries. The hyperandrogenemia leads to amenorrhea, hirsutism, acne, and, if uncorrected, male pattern balding, clitoral hypertrophy, and voice changes. These unwanted changes are most frequently the complaints leading to a work-up of hyperandrogenemia. As in the case of hirsutism, most cases of androgen excess in the PCO syndrome are caused by ovarian failure rather than adrenal dysfunction. The exact cause needs to be determined to rule out ovarian or adrenal tumors, Cushing's syndrome, and mild forms of congenital adrenal hyperplasia.

Clinical laboratory tests are available to evaluate a hirsute woman with suspected androgen excess, and a guide to their use is given in Figs. 45-6 and 45-7 and Table 45-3. The rate of ovarian and adrenal androgen secretion can be

evaluated initially by measurement of the testosterone (total and free, plus weakly bound), androstenedione, and DHEA sulfate. If the DHEA sulfate is normal, adrenal androgen excess can usually be eliminated. If the other hormones are elevated, the patient can be treated with a combination oral contraceptive to suppress pituitary LH and FSH secretion. If the excess androgen is gonadotrophin dependent and of ovarian origin (as in PCO syndrome), serum androgen levels will be suppressed after a 1-month trial of oral contraceptives. Failure to suppress indicates that excessive production is either of adrenal origin (as by a tumor or because of an enzyme defect) or is the result of an ovarian tumor. If the patient's DHEAS level is elevated, a 5-day, low-dose dexamethasone suppression test will indicate whether the adrenal gland's production of hormone can be suppressed, differentiating adrenal hyperplasia or adenoma (suppression) from an adrenal or pituitary tumor (no-

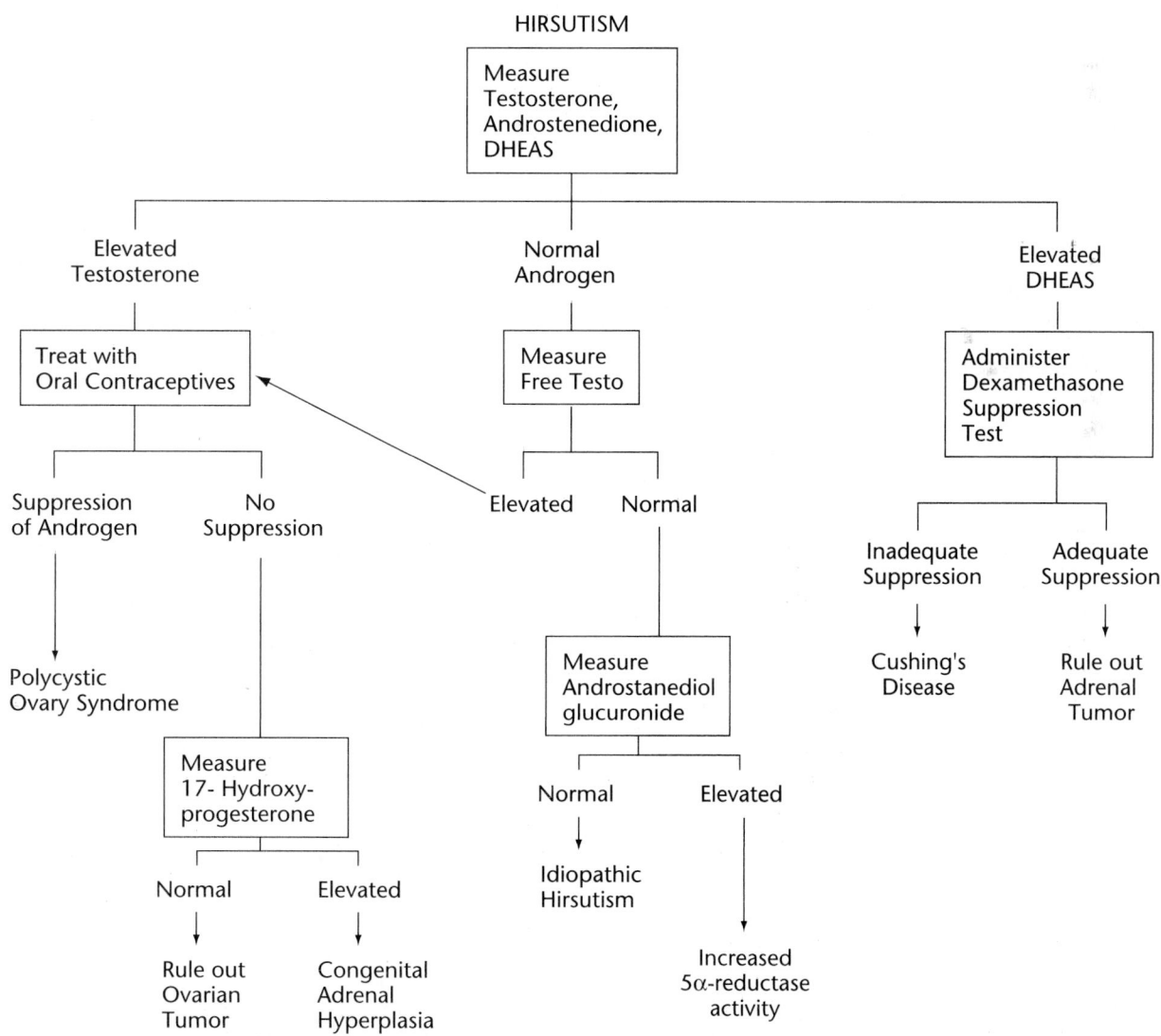

Fig 45-6 Clinical evaluation of hirsutism.

Table 45-3 Laboratory findings in hirsutism

Condition	Total testosterone	Free testosterone	DHEAS
		Analyte	
Idiopathic hirsutism	↑	↑↑↑	↑
Polycystic ovary syndrome	↑	↑↑	↑
Congenital adrenal hyperplasia	↑↑	↑↑	↑↑↑
Virilizing tumors			
Ovarian	↑↑↑	↑↑↑	↑
Adrenal	↑↑	↑↑	↑↑↑

Modified from Demers LM: *Hirsutism and virilization, News and Views,* in-service training material produced by the American Association for Clinical Chemistry, Inc, Washington, D.C., April 1989.
DHEAS, Dehydroepiandrosterone sulfate.

suppression). Women with adult-onset adrenal hyperplasia with a 21-hydroxylase deficiency will have elevated levels of 17-hydroxyprogesterone that are readily suppressed by dexamethasone.

Women with normal levels of total testosterone and androstenedione and apparent hirsutism can be evaluated further with free testosterone measurement. If free testosterone is also normal, 5α-reductase activity in the hair follicles can be estimated by measurement of serum levels of androstenediol glucuronide. If this is also within normal limits, the woman is said to have idiopathic hirsutism.

FERTILITY AND INFERTILITY
Disorders leading to infertility in women

There are several disorders that lead to infertility in women, such as primary ovarian disorders, central nervous system disease, pituitary disorders, androgen excess, and physical disorders (Table 45-4). The endocrine and biochemical bases for these disorders have been discussed above. Evaluation for female infertility will occur as part of the work-up for hirsutism and amenorrhea (Fig. 45-6 and 45-7).

Physical disorders. Patients with amenorrhea who appear to be normally sexually mature may have abnormalities of the outflow tract. These patients cannot be induced to bleed after treatment with a progestational agent and do not respond to mixed estrogen-progestational agents. The presence or absence of ovulation in these patients can be followed by basal body temperature or by measurement of serum progesterone levels once a week for several weeks. A number of müllerian defects can cause amenorrhea, such as imperforate hymen, abnormal cervix, interruptions of the vaginal canal, or absence of the vagina. The menstruum collects at the point of obstruction, causing pain, distension, and accumulation of blood in the peritoneal cavity. Destruction of the endometrium, as in tuberculosis or by improper curettage, can also lead to amenorrhea.

Table 45-4 Causes of female infertility

Primary hypogonadism
Secondary (pituitary) and tertiary (hypothalamic) hypogonadism
Primary hypergonadism
Genetic abnormalities resulting in abnormal sexual differentiation
Amenorrhea with androgen excess
  Luteal phase defect of insufficient progesterone production
Physical disorders
  Blocked fallopian tubes
  Abnormal cervix or vagina

Disorders leading to infertility in men

As in women, male infertility can be caused by disorders in the gonads themselves, the pituitary, or the hypothalamus. These general disorders have been discussed above. There are several other causes of male infertility, as shown in Table 45-5. Idiopathic infertility, in which no cause can be identified, is most common (about 35%). Sex chromosomal abnormalities, cryptorchidism, adult seminiferous tubule failure, and other forms of primary testicular failure are the most common identifiable causes (15% of infertile males). Physical factors, such as ductal problems, and ejaculatory disturbances, such as retrograde or absent ejaculation, are found in about 10% of the cases, whereas endocrine-caused infertility is found in about 4% of infertile men. Poor ejaculation may be associated with chronic diabetes. Autoimmune disturbances cause infertility in only a small fraction of patients. Long-term abuse of alcohol and marijuana can adversely affect spermatogenesis.

Evaluation of adult male hypogonadism (see Table 45-1) as a cause of infertility involves semen analysis and measurements of basal and challenged levels of testosterone, FSH, and LH. Several drugs are used to evaluate functional hormone level and to elucidate the cause of dysfunction. Human chorionic gonadotrophin (hCG) is a glycoprotein hormone similar to LH. On administration it stimulates Leydig cells to produce testosterone, thereby allowing assess-

Table 45-5 Causes of male infertility

Endocrine
  Hypothalamic-pituitary disorders
  Gonadal disorders
  Defects of androgen action
  Thyroid disorders
  Adrenal disorders
Defects in spermatogenesis
Systemic illness and general state of health
Gonadal and urological infections (prostatitis, orchitis); testicular infection (mumps)
Ductal obstruction
Varicocele
Retrograde ejaculation
Antibodies to sperm or fluid
Anatomic defects
Idiopathic

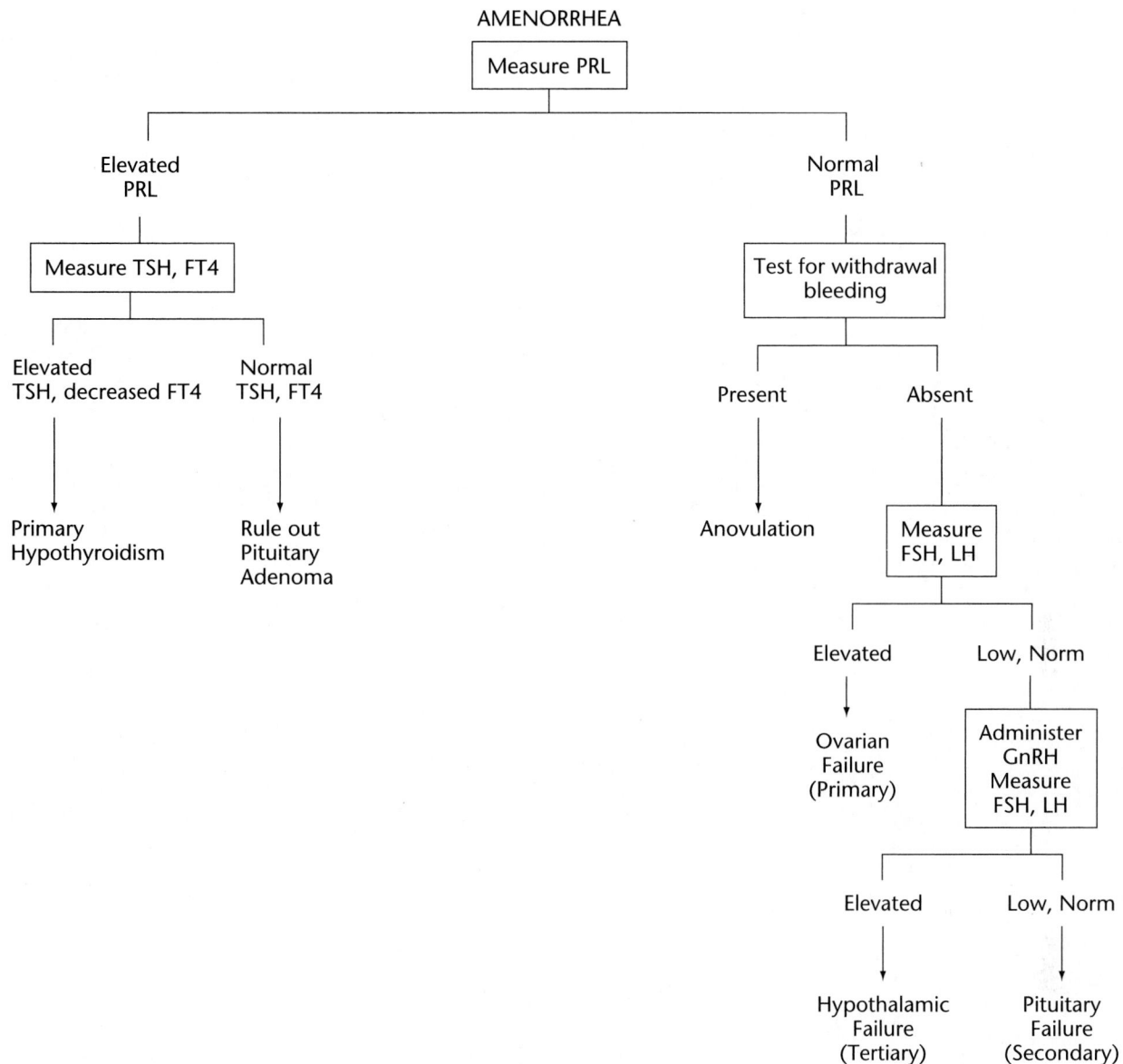

Fig. 45-7 Clinical diagnostic evaluation of amenorrhea. *PRL,* prolactin.

ment of testicular func tion. Clomiphene citrate (Clomid) stimulates production of GnRH and, ultimately, LH and FSH. Clomid would be expected to cause an increase in testosterone, LH, and FSH in the normal male with no pituitary or hypothalamic disease. GnRH can be used to distinguish between hypothalamic and pituitary disorders by measurement of the response of LH and FSH levels after administration. These challenge tests are discussed on p. 909.

A diagnostic scheme for evaluating male hypogonadism is shown in Fig 45-8. A patient with primary gonadal failure has poor semen characteristics, low or normal testosterone, and elevated FSH and LH. Secondary gonadal failure is characterized by low or inappropriately normal FSH and LH levels and must be evaluated by

function tests as described below. Oligospermia or azoospermia in the presence of normal hormone levels may indicate tubule or ductal failure, or inappropriate spermatogenesis.

Klinefelter's syndrome is the most common cause of male infertility resulting from abnormal sexual differentiation. It is present in about 0.2% of live-born males and is caused by an extra X chromosome. The XXY genotype patient is characterized by delayed puberty, hypogonadism, gynecomastia, intellectual impairment, dystocia, dissocial behavior, and infertility. The resulting gonadal phenotype can vary from obviously feminized males to normally virilized males with only microscopic physical defects and minor biochemical deficits. Adult seminiferous tubule failure is found in about half the infertile males. Adult Leydig cell

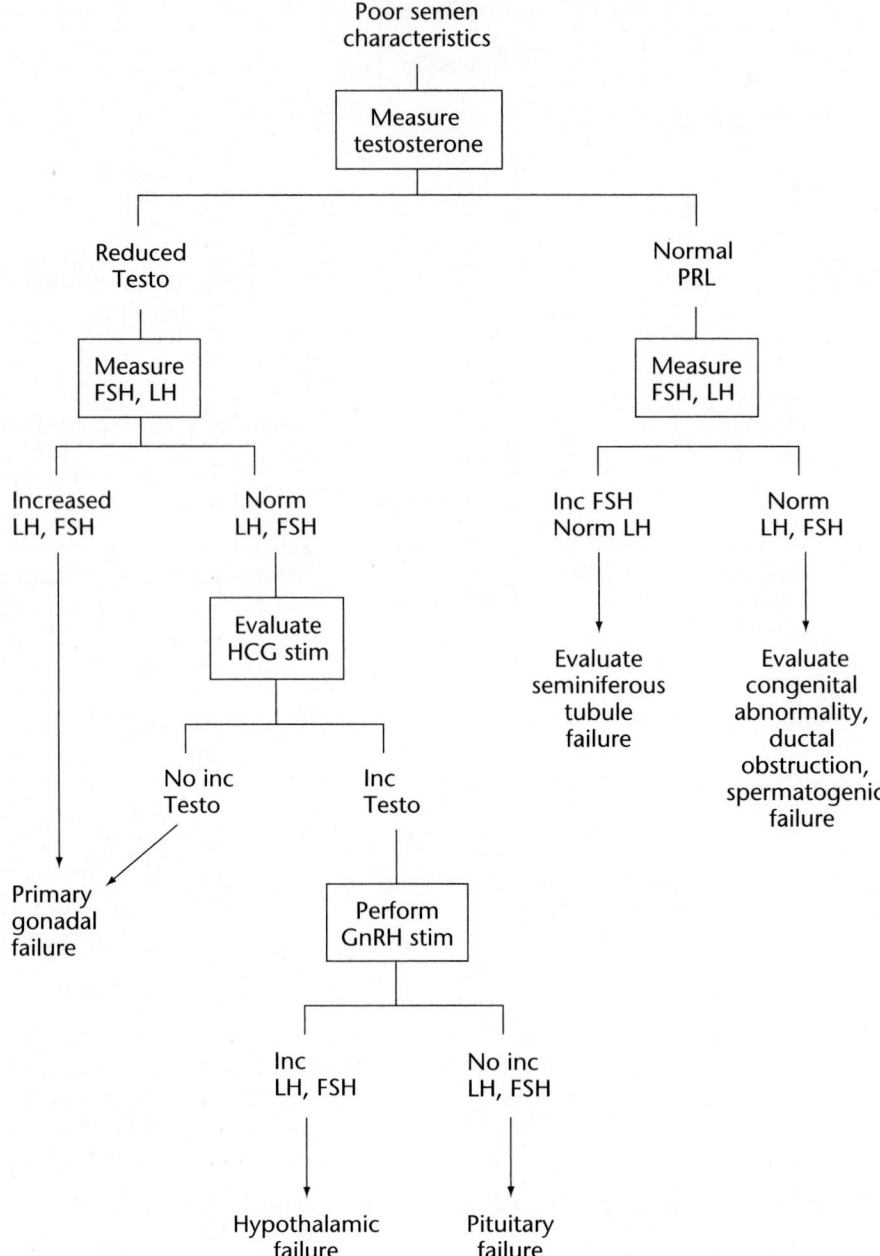

Fig. 45-8 Clinical diagnostic evaluation of male hypogonadism.

failure, with reduced levels of testosterone, is also called the *male climacteric syndrome,* since it mimics menopause seen in women.

To ensure fertility in a man, spermatogenesis must be normal, the sperm must be nourished with seminal plasma of adequate volume and with proper nutrient elements, must appear structurally normal, must have motility and fertilizing capacity, and must be depositable near the female's cervix. Any defect in this complex pathway can result in infertility attributable to a male factor problem.

EVALUATION OF THE INFERTILE COUPLE

Infertility, as defined above, is the inability of a couple to conceive after 1 year of unprotected intercourse (Table 45-6). In the medical sense, infertility is reduced ability to conceive when compared to the general population. *Fecundability* is the rate of conception occurring in a population in a given time period, usually a month. In normal fertile couples, the typical fecundity is about 20%. Of those couples with infertility, some are merely *hypofertile* and may conceive with treatment, whereas others are *sterile,* or unable to conceive in any event.

Table 45-6   Causes of infertility

Target	Result	Cause
Female		
Hypothalamus	Decreased gonadotropin-releasing hormone	Drugs Increased stress Diet
Pituitary	Decreased FSH, LH	Destructive tumor or vesicular lesion
Ovaries	Decreased estradiol or progesterone	Organ failure Organ dysgenesis Organ tumors Antiovarian antibodies Malnourishment, very low weight, metabolic disease
Fallopian tubes and uterus	Inadequate endometrium Tubal scarring and closure Decreased cervical mucus	Low progesterone output Pelvic inflammatory disease Cervical infections
Conception	Immobilization and destruction of sperm	Antisperm antibodies
Male		
Hypothalamus and pituitary	Azoospermia (no sperm) to oligospermia	Primary defects in hypothalamic or pituitary glands Exogenous androgens Testicular dysfunction with decreased testicular production
Testes	Azoospermia (no sperm) to oligospermia	Orchitis, testicular infections, such as mumps Alcoholism and substance abuse
	Delayed or deficient sexual maturity; decreased testosterone	Chromosomal defects
Prostate	Decreased seminal fluid	Infections of prostate or seminal vesicles
Urethrogenital tract	Retrograde or absent ejaculation	Physical abnormalities; chronic diabetes

According to the National Center for Health Statistics, in 1982 about 8.5% of all United States couples with wives 15 to 44 years of age were infertile. Of these, about 40% had no children (primary infertility), and 60% had at least one child (secondary infertility). Between 1965 and 1982 the incidence of primary infertility had increased, probably because of increased incidence of pelvic inflammatory disease caused by genital infection with gonorrhea and chlamydia (see above).

Age of the couple has a definite bearing on fertility. The incidence of infertility increases with increasing age of the female partner. Delayed marriages increase infertility from the baseline 9% in women 20 to 24 years to 15% at 30 to 35, and 64% between 40 and 44. The probability of conception is significantly reduced by delaying childbirth until later in life. The fecundity is significant in evaluating infertile couples using unprotected intercourse. If the mean fecundability of their population is 20%, it would be expected that 14% of the couples would not have conceived after 1 year, still 4% after 2 years, 2% after 3 years, and 1% after 4 to 6 years. Since infertility is defined as inability to conceive in 1 year, it should be noted that many hypofertile couples would eventually conceive without therapy. Often therapy is used to hasten conception that likely would have happened normally.

Diagnostic evaluation of an infertile couple involves laboratory tests, physical examinations, and perhaps some invasive diagnostic procedures (see the discussion of function tests, p. 909). All patients need to have a complete history taken, including a sexual history and physical examination. Initial laboratory tests usually done are the complete blood count and urinalysis on both, a Pap smear and fasting blood glucose on the woman, and a semen analysis on the man. Further laboratory tests may be warranted later as the evaluation continues (see earlier discussions on infertility and hypogonadism).

Documentation of ovulation by measurement of daily basal body temperature (BBT) is routinely done. Ovulation usually occurs 1 to 3 days after BBT nadir. The couple is counseled to have daily intercourse for 3 consecutive days at midcycle, starting the day before ovulation. The analysis of serum progesterone 7 to 8 days after BBT shift indicates not only whether ovulation has occurred but also if the corpus luteum is producing sufficient progesterone to support implantation.

Semen analysis provides one of the most important objective means of evaluating male fertility. Collection and analysis of the sample are equally important. Abnormally low volume indicates disturbances in secretory function of the seminal vesicles. Absence of fructose is suggestive of a disorder of the ejaculatory duct, whereas leukocytes or pus cells may indicate prostatitis. Severe oligospermia, low motility, or irregular sperm morphology may be associated with testicular disease, partial obstruction of the epididymal duct, or an endocrine disorder. Azoospermia is suggestive of a complete block of the testicular ejaculatory system. The presence of antibodies to sperm or constituents of the seminal plasma may lead to nonviable sperm. The *sperm penetration assay (SPA)* uses hamster eggs to assess fertilizing capacity of the sperm.

Any abnormality found in these preliminary procedures should be treated. For example, if the woman has oligomenorrhea and does not ovulate each month, ovulation may be induced with clomiphene citrate before other diagnostic measures are performed. A higher incidence of multiple gestations occur with this treatment, however. If no abnormality in these procedures is found, a hysterosalpingography or a laparoscopy, or both should be performed during the follicular phase of the woman. If all the tests are normal, additional tests are used by some to assess the cause of infertility. These include immunologic tests, cultures of cervical mucus and semen, measurement of thyroid-stimulating hormone (to rule out hypothyroidism) and prolactin (to rule out a hyperprolactinemia), luteal phase biopsy, and a hamster-egg penetration test.

Couples should be advised as to the prognosis for curing their particular cause of infertility. The highest chance of conception is among those couples for whom anovulation is the only abnormality. In couples with unexplained infertility, more than half eventually conceive within 1 year after completion of infertility evaluation. Aggressive treatment of infertility may only hasten a conception that would happen inevitably.

Induction of ovulation

Clomiphene citrate (Clomid) and gonadotropin-releasing hormone *(GnRH, Factrel)* may be administered to induce ovulation by mechanisms that have been discussed before. Clomid is given for 5 days in 50 mg doses, and if no ovulation occurs, the dose is doubled to 100 mg for 5 days. About 80% of anovulatory patients respond to this treatment, and about half will become pregnant. There is increased incidence of multiple births after Clomid therapy. GnRH is used in patients with amenorrhea resulting from hypothalamic dysfunction associated with decreased secretion of endogenous GnRH. In this case GnRH, in pulsatile doses of 1 to 10 μg per pulse at 60- to 120-minute intervals, may induce ovulation.

Human menopausal gonadotropin (Pergonal), used with hCG, can stimulate ovulation in anovulatory patients who have potentially functional ovarian tissue. For various reasons this procedure is generally used only after failure with Clomid. Pergonal administration is potentially dangerous and is complicated, time consuming, and expensive. Also there are increased incidences of multiple births and abortions with Pergonal. Typically one or more ampules of Pergonal (containing 75 units each of FSH and LH) are injected intramuscularly daily until estrogen production is optimal (600 to 1000 pg/mL). hCG in doses of 5000 to 10,000 units is then given intramuscularly to induce ovulation from the mature follicle and then several times after ovulation to support corpus luteum function.

Bromocriptine is occasionally used to induce ovulation in patients who have excessive serum levels of prolactin with or without galactorrhea. This will suppress prolactin secretion and allow normal cycling.

Assisted reproduction

Assisted reproductive technologies can be used to treat couples with prolonged unexplained infertility. These include *in vitro fertilization and embryo transfer (IVF), gamete intrafallopian tube transfer (GIFT),* and *zygote intrafallopian tube transfer (ZIFT).* IVF, first successfully done in 1978, involves follicle stimulation and monitoring, ova retrieval, gamete maintenance, and return of embryo to the female reproductive tract. Clomiphene citrate or menopausal gonadotropins are given to induce multiple follicular maturation, and then hCG is given to provide an identifiable preovulatory stimulus. GIFT is a similar procedure, except that the ovum is deposited into the fallopian tube with a quantity of freshly collected sperm, and conception takes place "normally." In the ZIFT procedure, the ovum is harvested, conception takes place in vitro, and then the zygote is transferred 24 hours later to the fallopian tube. With these procedures, the fecundities approach normal, but the methods are invasive, time consuming, costly, and uncomfortable.

CONTRACEPTION THROUGH ENDOCRINE INTERVENTION

Oral contraceptives (OCs) have been marketed in the United States since 1960. Because of their high rate of effectiveness, ease of administration, and low cost, they have become the most widely used method of reversible contraception. The dosages of estrogen and progestin in OCs have decreased over the years, as have side effects of the drug. The combination formulations consist of tablets containing synthetic estrogen and progestin, given continuously for 3 weeks with the fourth week off. These hormones inhibit midcycle FSH and LH surge, preventing ovulation, by interfering with the release of GnRH from the hypothalamus. They also have other physiological effects that alter fertility.

Small doses of progestins administered orally can be used for contraception. They are particularly suited for patients who cannot take estrogens. Although there is a high incidence of abnormal bleeding, they are about as effective as intrauterine devices in preventing pregnancy. Postcoital pregnancy can also be prevented by administration of estrogens alone or in combination with progestins.

A synthetic antiprogestin agent, mifepristone, commonly called RU-486, has received much attention because of its ability to induce menstruation in women even days after fertilization has occurred. It is being evaluated for use as a contraceptive and as a "morning-after" pill to terminate possible early pregnancies.

FUNCTION TESTS

The gonad is part of a complex system involving the hypothalamus, pituitary, gonad, and target tissue. Sometimes dynamic testing is necessary to ascertain dysfunction of a particular member of this network. Measurement of FSH, LH, prolactin, and estradiol in the female patient, and testosterone in the male, before and after stimulation or suppression can be invaluable in establishing proper diagnosis of hormone disorder. The following are provocative tests of gonad function.

Male dynamic tests

Human chorionic gonadotrophin (hCG) is a hormone with biological actions similar to LH. Leydig cell function may be directly assessed by intramuscular injection of 4000 IU of hCG for 4 days. In a normal response, the Leydig cells are stimulated to synthesize and secrete testicular steroids; the serum testosterone level doubles after the fourth injection. Patients with primary gonadal disease will have diminished response, whereas patients with secondary gonadal failure caused by pituitary or hypothalamic disease will have a qualitatively normal response.

Clomiphene citrate (Clomid) is a nonsteroidal compound with weak estrogenic activity. It causes the hypothalamus to increase GnRH release, which in turn stimulates the pituitary to produce LH and FSH and the Leydig cells to produce testosterone. The test is performed by the administration of clomiphene citrate, 100 mg orally twice a day for 10 days. Baseline samples are drawn before drug administration and then again after days 9 and 10. Healthy men show a 50% to 250% increase in LH, a 30% to 200% increase in FSH, and a 30% to 220% increase in testosterone by day 10 of the test. Patients with primary disease show no response in testosterone, whereas those with secondary or tertiary dysfunction show abnormal response of gonadotropins.

GnRH (Gonadorelin) directly stimulates pituitary production of FSH and LH and may be used to assess pituitary gonadotrophic function. A rapid, intravenous bolus of 100 μg of GnRH is administered, and blood is drawn at intervals from starting time to 180 minutes. Normal males show a twofold to fivefold increase in LH and a twofold rise in FSH over the baseline value. Patients with primary testicular disease may respond with exaggerated increases, whereas those with pituitary dysfunction will show no increase.

Male physical tests

Semen analysis is usually an evaluation of sperm density, motility, and morphology.

The *sperm penetration assay* is a functional test that measures the ability of a sperm population to penetrate (fertilize) oocytes. The assay commonly uses hamster oocytes that have been treated to remove the outer layers of the ova that would normally prevent cross-species fertilization. Each egg is then incubated with sperm, and their penetration ability is evaluated. This test is controversial because it is performed under artificial conditions and a nonviable product is formed. It is believed to be useful, however, especially for couples desiring in vitro fertilization.

Sperm antibody testing measures antibodies directed against sperm. These antibodies may arise from the male whose self-directed antibodies may be found in the seminal plasma or serum or from the female's cervical mucus or serum. In any case, these antibodies interfere with fertilization in several different ways. If the antibody is directed toward the tail of the sperm, motility will be affected. The presence of head-directed antibody interferes with sperm-egg binding. Most procedures in current use employ a sperm sample that has been incubated with the test fluid of interest, followed by separation by anti-immunoglobulin-coated beads and microscopic visualization.

Female dynamic tests

The *GnRH test* may be used in women to permit assessment of pituitary response and the ability to produce FSH and LH. A 100 μg bolus is given, followed by collection of blood samples for up to 180 minutes afterwards. In healthy patients there is a doubling of both LH and FSH within 30 to 45 minutes after injection. A reduced or absent response to GnRH indicates pituitary hypofunction. The possibility of hypothalamic abnormality is confirmed with the clomiphene citrate test.

Clomiphene citrate normally stimulates hypothalamic release of GnRH, resulting in increased secretion of FSH and LH. The female patient is given 50 or 100 mg of the drug for 5 days (days 2 to 6 of her menstrual cycle). A healthy response is a doubling of LH concentration over the next 10 days. A diminished response indicates hypothalamic hypofunction.

Dexamethasone suppression of adrenal androgens can be used to evaluate the cause of hirsutism. A short course of suppression uses 1 mg of dexamethasone overnight, whereas longer protocols of 2 to 14 days use 0.5 mg of the drug hourly. The test helps discriminate Cushing's disease from an adrenal tumor (see previous discussion).

The *progestogen withdrawal test* is used as an indirect measure of endogenous estradiol levels. The principle of this test is that uterine bleeding will occur after treatment with progesterone only if there has been prior priming of the uterine endometrium by estrogen. Progestogen is given orally daily for 5 days, after which uterine bleeding should occur.

Female physical tests

Tubal patency should be assessed when there is a history of pelvic inflammation or pelvic surgery. Hysterosalpingography or diagnostic laparoscopy can detect the presence and indicate the extent of any intrapelvic disease.

Cervical factors are a cause of about 5% of infertility and may create a hostile environment for conception. Cervical mucus can be evaluated for stretchability (*"Spinnbarkeit"*), appearance on slide after drying ("ferning"), thickness, and clarity, as well as the presence of live spermatozoa after intercourse.

CHANGES OF ANALYTE IN DISEASE (Table 45-7)
Gonadotropins (FSH and LH)

Measurement of serum FSH and LH levels provides input on hypothalamic-pituitary axis function and helps distinguish between primary and secondary gonadal dysfunction. Since pulsatile and cyclic changes occur throughout the menstrual cycle, it is common practice to draw a woman's blood during the follicular phase and to obtain 2 to 3 samples several minutes apart. A pooled serum sample will yield a more accurate estimation of hormone level.

Increased levels of FSH and LH are seen in primary gonadal failure. Examples of this are, in women, Turner's syndrome or menopause and, in men, Klinefelter's syndrome or cryptorchidism in men (see Table 45-1). In polycystic ovary syndrome, LH levels may be elevated, with normal or low levels of FSH. A ratio of LH to FSH greater than 2:1 would support the diagnosis of this disorder.

Decreased levels of FSH and LH are significant in the presence of low sex hormones, since this would indicate a defect of the pituitary-hypothalamus axis. Further testing would be required (see previous discussion) to determine the cause of low levels of gonadotropin.

Androgens

The clinically significant androgens (male hormones) are testosterone, androstenedione, DHEA sulfate, and dihydrotestosterone. Upsets in natural balance of androgens can lead to virilization in women and feminization in men.

Increased levels of androgen (>2000 ng/L of total testosterone and >8000 µg/L of DHEAS) are seen in women with virilizing tumors, whereas slightly increased levels are found in polycystic ovary syndrome (see Table 45-3 and Fig. 45-6). Increased androgen levels in men are generally not clinically significant but will cause precocious puberty in prepubertal boys.

Decreased androgen is found in men with testicular hypofunction and Klinefelter's syndrome. Low androgen may arise from failure at any site along the gonad-pituitary-hypothalamus axis. Generally, low levels of androgen are not significant in women.

Estrogens

Estrogens are found in the circulation as estrone, estradiol, or estriol, and at different conditions one or another may be significant. The estrogen usually tested, however, is estradiol, since it is present in the highest level and is the most biologically active.

Increased levels of estrogen result from ovarian hyperfunction in a woman, whether from a feminizing tumor (pseudoprecocious puberty) or from a switched-on hypothalamic-pituitary axis. Very high levels are found during induction of ovulation and in pregnancy. In pregnancy, the primary estrogen is estriol (see p. 797). In the male, increased levels of circulating estradiol and estrone may reflect not only increased aromatization and secretion by the

---

Table 45-7   Change of analyte in disease

Disease	Analyte			
	FSH	LH	Estradiol	Testosterone
Female				
Primary ovarian failure (including menopause)	↑	↑	↓	—
Secondary ovarian failure	↓	↓	↓	—
Feminizing tumors	↓	↓	↑	
Masculinizing tumors	↓	↓	—	↑
Exogenous gonadotropins or gonadotropin-producing tumor (rare)	↑	↑	↑	—
Polycystic ovary syndrome	N to ↓	↑	—	↑
Male				
Primary testicular failure	↑	↑	—	↓
Secondary testicular failure	↓	↓	—	↓
Primary testicular overactivity (e.g., because of a tumor, testotoxicosis)	↓	↓	—	↑
Secondary testicular overactivity (e.g., because of a precocious puberty)	↑	↑	—	↑

↑, Increased; ↓, decreased; *N*, normal.

testis and adrenal, but also altered aromatization activity in other organs, as seen in liver disease. Increased estrogen levels in males manifest as gynecomastia.

Decreased levels of estrogen are clinically significant in women, for whom ovarian hypofunction is indicated. Low levels of estrogen are not significant in men.

Progesterone

Progesterone levels in women vary throughout their menstrual cycles, with the highest levels occurring during the luteal phase. A single progesterone level of 4 to 10 ng/mL obtained between 4 and 10 days after ovulation is presumptive evidence of luteinization. A value greater than 10 ng/mL is excellent evidence of good ovulation.

Increased levels of progesterone are seen in pregnancy or in the luteal phase of the menstrual cycle.

Decreased progesterone is observed in infertility or threatened abortion.

BIBLIOGRAPHY

Alsever RN: Hormone assays in endocrine systems. In Gold JJ, Josimovich JB, editors: *Gynecologic endocrinology,* New York, 1987, Plenum Medical Book Co.

Andrews WC: Investigation of the infertile couple. In Gold JJ, Josimovich JB: *Gynecologic endocrinology,* New York, 1987, Plenum Medical Book Co.

Bernstein GS, Siegel MS: Male factor in infertility. In Mishell D, Davajan V, Lobo RA, editors: *Infertility, contraception, and reproductive endocrinology,* Boston, 1991, Blackwell Scientific Publications.

Braunstein GD: Testes. In Greenspan FS, editor: *Basic and clinical endocrinology,* Norwalk, Conn., 1991, Appleton & Lange.

Gibbons WE, Battin DA, diZerega GS: Mechanism of action of reproductive hormones. In Mishell D, Davajan V, editors: *Infertility, contraception, and reproductive endocrinology,* Oradell, N.J., 1986, Medical Economics Books.

Goebelsmann U: Steroid hormones. In Mishell D, Davajan V, editors: *Infertility, contraception, and reproductive endocrinology,* Oradell, N.J., 1986, Medical Economics Books.

Goldfien A, Monroe SE: Ovaries. In Greenspan FS: *Basic and clinical endocrinology,* Norwalk, Conn., 1991, Appleton & Lange.

Hylka VW, DiZerega GS: Reproductive hormones and their mechanism of action. In Mishell DR, Davajan V, Lobo RA, editors: *Infertility, contraception, and reproductive endocrinology,* Boston, 1991, Blackwell Scientific Publications.

Lobo RA: The menstrual cycle. In Mishell DR, Davajan V, Lobo RA, editors: *Infertility, contraception, and reproductive endocrinology,* Boston, 1991, Blackwell Scientific Publications.

Lobo RA, Kletzky OA: Dynamics of hormone testing. In Mishell DR, Davajan V, Lobo RA, editors: *Infertility, contraception, and reproductive endocrinology,* Boston, 1991, Blackwell Scientific Publications.

Lipsett MG: Steroid hormones. In Yen SSC, Jaffe RB: *Reproductive endocrinology: physiology, pathophysiology, and clinical management,* Philadelphia, 1986, Saunders.

March CM, Mishell DR: Induction of ovulation. In Mishell DR, Davajan V, Lobo RA, editors: *Infertility, contraception, and reproductive endocrinology,* Boston, 1991, Blackwell Scientific Publications.

March CM, Shoupe D: Luteal-phase defects. In Mishell DR, Davajan V, Lobo RA, editors: *Infertility, contraception, and reproductive endocrinology,* Boston, 1991, Blackwell Scientific Publications.

Mishell DR: Oral steroid contraceptives. In Mishell DR, Davajan V, Lobo RA, editors: *Infertility, contraception, and reproductive endocrinology,* Boston, 1991, Blackwell Scientific Publications.

Mishell DR, Davajan V: Evaluation of the infertile couple. In Mishell DR, Davajan V, Lobo RA, editors: *Infertility, contraception, and reproductive endocrinology,* Boston, 1991, Blackwell Scientific Publications.

Mishell DR, Lobo RA: Disorders of sexual differentiation. In Mishell DR, Davajan V, Lobo RA, editors: *Infertility, contraception, and reproductive endocrinology,* Boston, 1991, Blackwell Scientific Publications.

Mooradian AP, Morley JE, Korenman, SG: Biological action of androgens, *Endocr Rev* 8:1, 1987.

Ross GT, Schreiber JR: The ovary. In Yen SSC, Jaffe RB: *Reproductive endocrinology: physiology, pathophysiology, and clinical management,* Philadelphia, 1986, Saunders.

Speroff L, Glass RH, Kase NG: The ovary from conception to senescence. In *Clinical gynecologic endocrinology and infertility,* Baltimore, 1989, Williams & Wilkins.

Steinberger E: Male infertility. In Gold JJ, Josimovich JB: *Gynecologic endocrinology,* New York, 1987, Plenum Medical Book Co.

Swerdloff RS: Infertility in the male, *Ann Intern Med* 103:906, 1985.

CHAPTER 46

Adrenal hormones and hypertension

Morris R. Pudek

OBJECTIVES

■ List the principal glucocorticoids, mineralocorticoids, adrenal androgens, and medullary hormones and state their physiological effects.

■ Describe the synthesis, transport, catabolism, and regulation of glucocorticoids, mineralocorticoids, adrenal androgens, and medullary hormones.

■ Describe each of the following pathological conditions, including diagnostic laboratory results: Cushing's syndrome, hyperaldosteronism, congenital adrenal hyperplasia, Addison's disease, and pheochromocytoma.

■ Describe each of the following adrenal function tests and the interpretation of results: clonidine suppression test, overnight and 2-day dexamethasone suppression tests, ACTH stimulation test, CRH stimulation test *and* bilateral petrosal sinus sampling, captopril suppression test, and metyrapone test.

■ Describe some of the factors regulating blood pressure and list the major causes and complications of hypertension.

■ Describe the minimum laboratory evaluation for the initial work-up of a patient with hypertension and the indications for testing for secondary hypertension.

■ List some of the most important metabolic complications associated with antihypertensive therapy.

KEY TERMS

Addison's disease Primary adrenal insufficiency, most commonly the result of an autoimmune adrenalitis.

adrenal cortex The outer portion of the adrenal gland, which produces various steroid hormones.

adrenal medulla The inner portion of both adrenal glands, which produces catecholamines.

adrenocorticosteroids Refers to all steroids secreted by the adrenal cortex.

adrenocorticotropic hormone (ACTH) A polypeptide hormone secreted by the anterior pituitary gland, that primarily stimulates the synthesis and release of glucocorticoids from the adrenal cortex.

adrenocorticotropic hormone (ACTH) stimulation test An initial screening test used in the assessment of adrenal insufficiency.

adrenoleukodystrophy An inherited X-linked disorder in the metabolism of very long chain fatty acids that can lead to severe neurological problems and primary adrenal insufficiency.

captopril suppression test A test that is useful in the investigation of Conn's syndrome. Captopril is an angiotensin-converting enzyme inhibitor and blocks the formation of angiotensin II, which normally will result in a fall in aldosterone.

catecholamines Epinephrine and norepinephrine, which are produced in the adrenal medulla and are responsible for maintenance of blood pressure.

chromaffin cells Cells found in the adrenal medulla and other sites throughout the body that produce catecholamines.

clonidine suppression test A function test used in the diagnosis of pheochromocytoma.

congenital adrenal hyperplasia Also known as *adrenogenital syndrome*. A group of hereditary diseases that result from enzyme deficiencies in the steroid hormone production pathways.

Conn's syndrome Another name used to denote primary hyperaldosteronism.

corticosteroid-binding globulin Also known as *transcortin*. A protein that binds and transports the majority of cortisol in the circulation.

corticotropin-releasing hormone (CRH) A hypothalamic polypeptide that stimulates ACTH secretion.

Cushing's disease A form of Cushing's syndrome specifically attributable to an ACTH-secreting pituitary adenoma.

Cushing's syndrome A range of specific symptoms resulting from the elevation of blood glucocorticoid levels from primary or secondary causes.

dexamethasone suppression test A function test that is used in the diagnosis and differentiation of various causes of Cushing's syndrome.

glucocorticoids A group of steroid hormones secreted by the adrenal cortex that have multiple physiological effects including regulation of carbohydrate metabolism. Cortisol is the major glucocorticoid in man.

hyperaldosteronism Increased secretion of aldosterone from the adrenal cortex either because of elevated blood renin levels or autonomous adrenocortical secretion (Conn's syndrome).

hypoadrenalism Adrenal insufficiency resulting in decreased output of steroid hormones from the adrenal cortex.

metyrapone test An adrenal function test that can be used in the assessment of both hyperadrenal and hypoadrenal function. Metyrapone blocks 11-hydroxylase activity, and the response is usually determined by measurement of the 11-deoxycortisol in blood.

mineralocorticoids Steroid hormones secreted by the adrenal cortex that stimulate the resorption of sodium and the excretion of potassium in the distal tubules of the kidneys. Aldosterone is the major mineralocorticoid in man.

pheochromocytoma A tumor of the chromaffin cells, usually located in the adrenal medulla, that results in hypersecretion of epinephrine and norepinephrine.

primary hypertension Also called *essential hypertension*. It is an elevated systemic arterial pressure for which no cause can be found and that is often the only significant clinical finding.

renin-angiotensin system This system is responsible for the regulation of aldosterone secretion from the adrenal cortex.

secondary hypertension Elevated blood pressure associated with several primary diseases, such as renal, endocrine, and vascular diseases.

zona fasciculata The middle portion of the adrenal cortex in which glucocorticoids and various sex hormones are produced.

zona glomerulosa The outer portion of the adrenal cortex in which the mineralocorticoids are produced.

zona reticularis The innermost portion of the adrenal cortex, next to the adrenal medulla, that acts in concert with the zona fasciculata.

Part I: The adrenal hormones
ANATOMY

The adrenal glands are situated at the upper pole of each kidney (Fig. 46-1). In the adult the adrenal cortex, which constitutes 90% of the gland volume, is made up of three distinct layers. The outer layer is called the *zona glomerulosa*. The wide middle layer and the inner layer are called the *zona fasciculata* and the *zona reticularis* respectively. These three layers secrete steroid hormones that may have mineralocorticoid, glucocorticoid, or androgen functions. The gland is highly vascular with a complex venous circu-

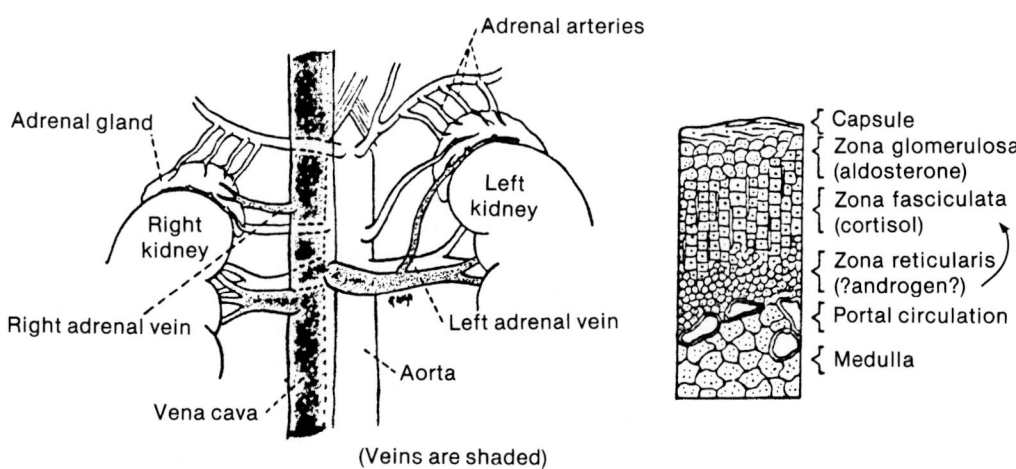

(Veins are shaded)

Fig. 46-1 Adrenal gland anatomy and histology. (From Ryan W: *Endocrine disorders,* St. Louis, 1980, Mosby.)

lation that is believed to play a role in regulating steroid hormone synthesis.

The adrenal medulla consists of sheets of irregular cells with small nuclei called *chromaffin cells*. These cells synthesize and secrete the catecholamines.

PHYSIOLOGY OF ADRENAL HORMONES

All adrenal steroids secreted by the adrenal cortex (adrenocorticosteroids) have the same basic cyclopentanoperhydrophenanthrane nucleus consisting of three 6-carbon hexane rings and one 5-carbon ring. The numbering of the carbon atoms is indicated in Fig. 46-2. The steroid molecules with 21 carbon atoms and a hydroxyl group at the carbon-17 position are termed *17-hydroxysteroids*. The steroid structures with 19 carbon atoms with a ketone group at C-17 are termed *ketosteroids*.

There are three major functional groups of steroids secreted by the adrenal cortex. These are the *mineralocorticoids* secreted by the zona glomerulosa and the *glucocorticoids* and *androgens* secreted by the zona reticularis and

zona fasciculata. Relatively minor differences in the chemical structure result in major differences in the physiological function of these steroid molecules.

The adrenal medulla secretes the catecholamines. These molecules are not related in structure to the adrenal steroids and have very different physiological functions.

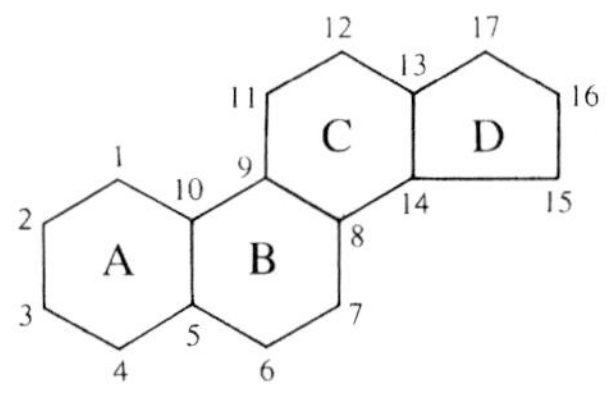

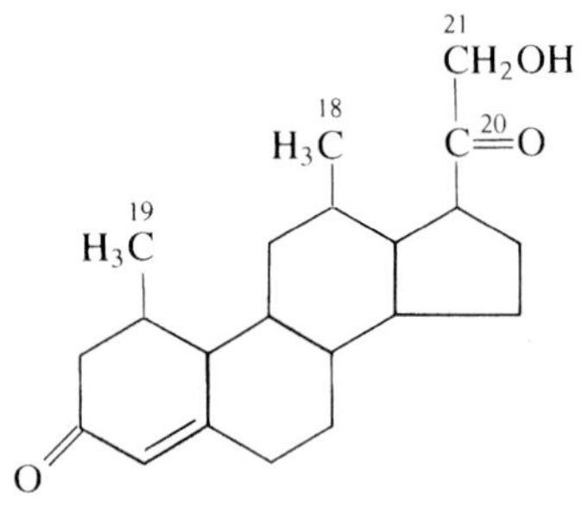

Glucocorticoids

The glucocorticoids (primarily cortisol in humans) are synthesized and secreted by the zona fasciculata and the zona reticularis. These steroid molecules are involved in the regulation of carbohydrate, protein, and lipid metabolism. Cortisol at high concentrations also demonstrates mineralocorticoid activity. Some of the more important physiological effects of the glucocorticoids are summarized in the box. These hormones are essential for life, especially when the human body is subjected to a stress such as surgery, major illness, or severe trauma. Cortisol concentrations increase greatly during these stresses, with the output of cortisol from the adrenal glands increasing from 25 mg/day to as high as 300 mg/day. Stress induces the release of numerous mediator substances such as catecholamines and kinins that can affect cardiovascular function, and, if unchecked, can lead to cardiovascular collapse. The glucocorticoids block mediator production and action and prevent them from becoming life threatening.

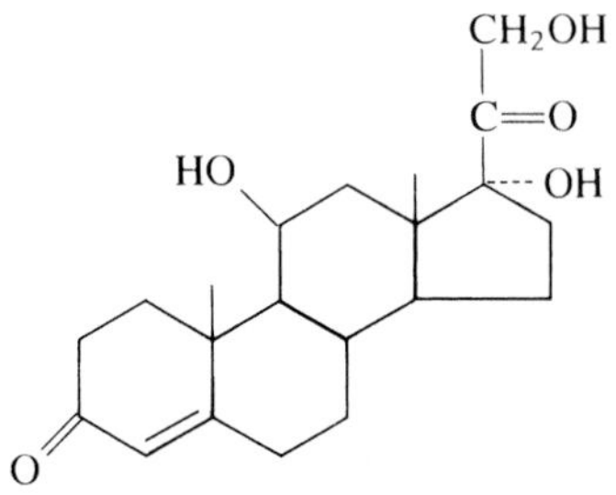

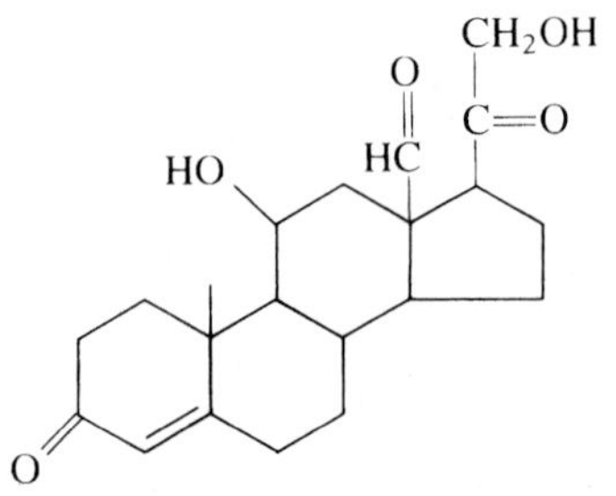

The overall metabolic action of glucocorticoids is catabolic, promoting protein and lipid breakdown and inhibiting protein synthesis in muscle, connective tissue, adipose tissue, and lymphoid cells. Wound healing is inhibited, and osteoporosis is promoted. Glucocorticoids, however, have an anabolic effect on liver metabolism. The effects of cor-

Fig. 46-2   Structures of adrenocortical hormones.

Physiological Functions of Cortisol
Effects on intermediary metabolism
Increases gluconeogenesis
Increases glycogen synthesis
Increases lipolysis
Increases blood glucose levels
Decreases glucose utilization
Effects on protein metabolism
Increases protein catabolism
Decreases protein synthesis
Effects on immunologic and inflammatory responses
Decreases antibody formation
Decreases circulating lymphocytes, eosinophils, and monocytes
Decreases production and inhibits actions of interleukins and interferons
Stabilizes lysosomes
Inhibits leukocyte migration
Inhibits phagocytosis

tisol are antagonistic to those of insulin, increasing the concentration of glucose by stimulating gluconeogenesis. The amino acids and glycerol released by the catabolic action of cortisol on protein and fat are used as gluconeogenic substrates. Cortisol increases the synthesis and activity of numerous enzymes in the liver that are involved in amino acid and glucose metabolism. The net effect is increased production and conservation of glucose for use by essential tissues, such as the brain and red blood cells, at the expense of "less essential" tissues during times of stress or starvation.

Cortisol also contributes to the maintenance of normal blood pressure through unknown mechanisms. Cortisol increases urine flow by stimulating glomerular filtration rate and decreasing water resorption. At high concentrations, however, cortisol can act like a mineralocorticoid promoting sodium and water retention and causing hypokalemia. Cortisol interacts avidly with the mineralocorticoid receptor. In fact, free serum cortisol levels are 150-fold higher than free serum aldosterone levels; therefore the mineralocorticoid receptor is saturated by cortisol in most tissues except the kidney. Renal cells rapidly convert cortisol to cortisone, allowing aldosterone to be the predominant regulator of renal sodium resorption and potassium excretion.

The hematologic effects of cortisol are multiple, stimulating erythropoiesis and causing leukocytosis, neutrophilia, lymphocytopenia, monocytopenia, and eosinopenia. Glucocorticoids also suppress the inflammatory and immune response by stabilizing lysosomes, interfering with leukocyte migration, and inhibiting phagocytosis. Some of the glucocorticoid action is mediated through its effects on the production and actions of mediators such as the interleukins and interferons.

The molecular basis for steroid hormone actions is described in Chapter 43.

Mineralocorticoids

Aldosterone is the primary product of the zona glomerulosa with approximately 200 μg produced per day, roughly one hundredth the amount of cortisol synthesized daily. The major physiological functions of aldosterone are (1) regulation of extracellular fluid volume and (2) regulation of potassium metabolism. Its actions are mediated through a high-affinity mineralocorticoid receptor found in a variety of tissues. Its most important action is in the cells of the renal distal convoluted tubule where it promotes sodium resorption in exchange for excretion of potassium. Water passively follows the transported sodium (see Chapter 24).

Cortisol and other corticosteroids such as corticosterone and deoxycorticosterone have some mineralocorticoid activity that can become clinically significant when serum levels of these compounds are elevated. This can occur with the high cortisol levels seen in Cushing's syndrome. Aldosterone in turn has weak glucocorticoid activity, but its concentration is too low to have any physiological effect.

Adrenal androgens

The predominant androgens secreted by the adrenal cortex are dehydroepiandrosterone sulfate (DHEA-S), dehydroepiandrosterone (DHEA), and androstenedione. Small amounts of testosterone (T) and dihydrotestosterone (DHT) are also secreted. The average daily production rate of DHEA-S is approximately 30 mg in young men and 20 mg in young women. The half-life of DHEA-S is between 8 and 11 hours, whereas it is only 30 to 60 minutes for the unconjugated androgens. Adrenal androgen production reaches a peak between 20 and 30 years of age and then gradually falls with age to about 20% of peak levels after 70 years. This is in contrast to cortisol production, which does not change with age.

The biological effects of the adrenal androgens are either direct or indirect. These steroids can be converted by peripheral tissues to the primary sex hormones testosterone, DHT, and estradiol. Adrenal androgens are the major source of testosterone in females. Some direct effects of DHEA have been determined. It can inhibit the enzyme glucose-6-phosphate dehydrogenase, an important factor controlling the synthesis of NADPH, which is required for many important biological reactions including lipogenesis. DHEA may also have important effects on immune regulation.

Catecholamines

The naturally occurring catecholamines are norepinephrine (NE, noradrenaline), epinephrine (E, adrenaline), and dopamine. The main secretory products of the adrenal medulla are epinephrine and norepinephrine. Production of catecholamines is not restricted to the adrenal medulla, however, and synthesis of these hormones also occurs in the neurons of the sympathetic and central nervous systems (CNS) and in scattered groups of chromaffin cells found in other regions of the abdomen and neck. Norepinephrine is the principal product synthesized in the CNS, and epinephrine is the principal catecholamine produced by the adrenal glands.

Physiological actions of the catecholamines are diverse. Norepinephrine functions primarily as a neurotransmitter. Both norepinephrine and epinephrine influence the vascular system, whereas epinephrine affects metabolic processes such as carbohydrate metabolism. The biological actions of the catecholamines are initiated through their interaction with two different types of specific cell membrane receptors, the alpha-adrenergic and beta-adrenergic receptors. These receptors have different affinities for norepinephrine and epinephrine and cause opposing physiological effects. Norepinephrine primarily interacts with alpha-adrenergic receptors, whereas epinephrine interacts with both alpha- and beta-receptors.

Stimulation of alpha-adrenergic receptors results in vasoconstriction, decrease in insulin secretion, sweating, piloerection (hair standing on end), and stimulation of glycogenolysis in the liver and skeletal muscle leading to an

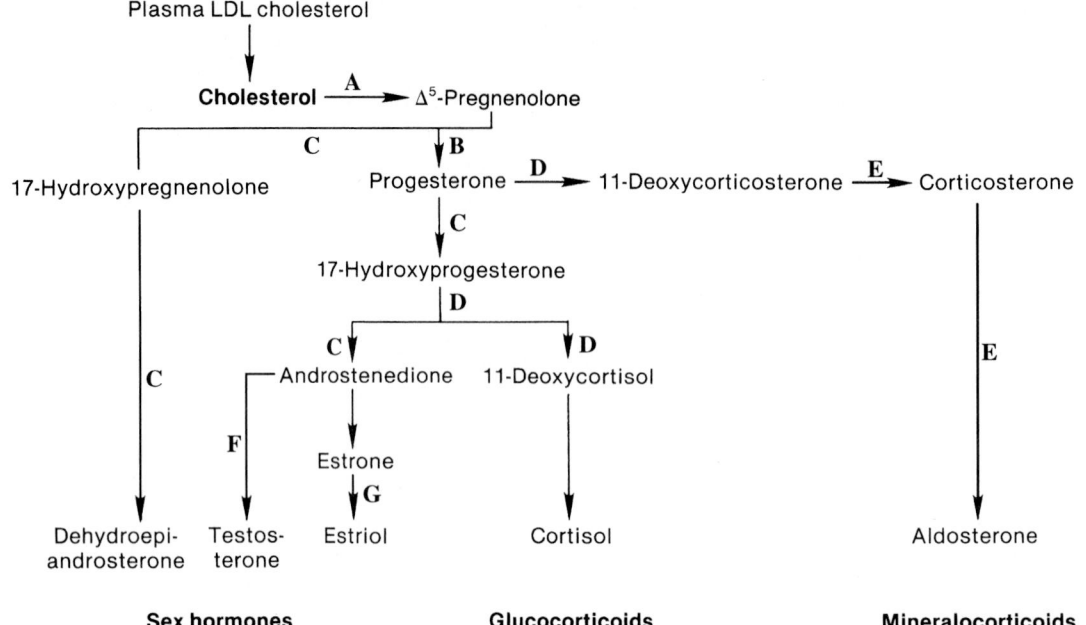

Fig. 46-3 Principle pathways of adrenal steroidogenesis. The letters represent the different enzymes responsible for catalysis of each of the biochemical transformations. Notice that the same enzyme may be responsible for more than one type of reaction. *A,* Mitochondrial cytochrome P-450scc catalyzes the side chain cleavage of cholesterol. *B,* 3β-hydroxysteroid dehydrogenase bound to the endoplasmic reticulum also catalyzes Δ^5-Δ^4 isomerase activity. *C,* P-450c17 is responsible for both 17-hydroxylase activity and 17,20-lyase activity, which cleaves off the remaining side chain at C-17 position. *D,* P-450c21 catalyzes 21-hydroxylation of progesterone and 17-hydroxyprogesterone. *E,* Mitochondrial P-450c11 catalyzes three different reactions: 11-hydroxylation, 18-hydroxylation, and 18-methyloxidase. *F,* 17-Ketosteroid reductase is found mainly in the testes and ovaries. *G,* P-450aro mediates the aromatization of ring A and is located mainly in the ovaries.

increase in blood glucose concentration. Stimulation of beta-receptors, however, leads to vasodilatation; stimulation of insulin release; increased cardiac contraction rate; relaxation of smooth muscle in the intestinal tract; bronchodilatation by relaxation of smooth muscles in bronchi; stimulation of renin release, which enhances sodium resorption from the kidney; and enhanced lipolysis.

BIOSYNTHESIS
Adrenocorticosteroids

All adrenal steroid synthesis begins with cholesterol. Cholesterol in the adrenal tissue may be synthesized in situ from acetate or may come from cholesterol made in the liver and transported to the adrenal glands by low-density lipoprotein.

The biosynthetic pathway leading to the three major groups of adrenal steroids is outlined in Fig. 46-3. Several of the reactions in steroidogenesis involve cytochrome P-450 enzymes. The rate-limiting step in the synthesis of all steroids is the conversion of cholesterol to pregnenolone. This step is stimulated by ACTH in the zona fasciculata and zona reticularis and by angiotensin II and III in the zona glomerulosa. The pathway leading to progesterone is common to both aldosterone and cortisol synthesis. In the zona reticularis and zona fasciculata, progesterone is hydroxylated at the 17, 21, and 11 positions to form cortisol. Under normal circumstances, 10 to 30 mg of cortisol is synthesized per day. The zona glomerulosa does not contain 17-hydroxylase activity. Instead, hydroxylation occurs at positions 21, 11, and 18; finally a dehydrogenase reaction forms aldosterone.

The androgens are derived from the major pathway of steroid biosynthesis after cleavage of the side chain attached to carbon 17 in ring D. See Chapter 45 for a description of the synthesis of androgens. The adrenal gland production of androgens is significant, indirectly generating 60% of the circulating testosterone in females, mainly through peripheral tissue conversion of testosterone precursors.

Catecholamines

The biochemical pathway leading to the synthesis of the catecholamines is outlined in Fig. 46-4. The rate-limiting step is the hydroxylation of the amino acid tyrosine leading to the formation of dihydroxyphenylalanine (dopa). This step

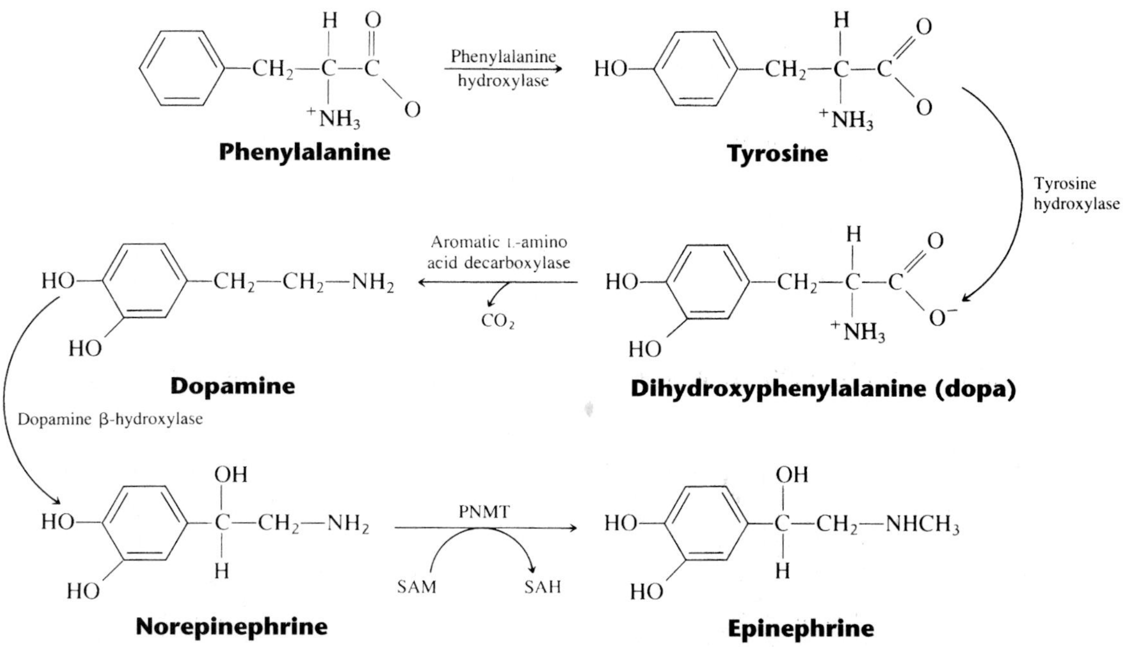

Fig. 46-4 Synthesis of medullary hormones. *PNMT*, Phenylethanolamine *N*-methyltransferase; *SAH*, S-adenosyl homocysteine; *SAM*, S-adenosylmethionine. (From Orten JM, Neuhaus OW: *Human biochemistry*, St. Louis, 1982, Mosby.)

is inhibited by both epinephrine and norepinephrine. Tyrosine comes from the diet or from hydroxylation of phenylalanine. Dopa is decarboxylated to form dopamine, which is a major end product in the central nervous system where it functions as a neurotransmitter. Dopamine is stored in granules that are present in both neurons and the adrenal medulla. Within the granules, dopamine β-hydroxylase converts dopamine to norepinephrine. Finally, the norepinephrine is released from the storage granules, and phenylethanolamine *N*-methyltransferase (PNMT) methylates the norepinephrine to form epinephrine. PNMT, which is found only in the adrenal medulla, is induced by glucocorticoids (cortisol). The hormones of the adrenal medulla are stored complexed with proteins (chromogranin A, dopamine-β-hydroxylase) and adenosine-5'-triphosphate (ATP) in chromaffin granules. Nerve stimulation results in release of the stored catecholamines from these vesicles by the process of exocytosis.

TRANSPORT AND CATABOLISM
Adrenocorticosteroids

In plasma, aldosterone and cortisol are bound to plasma proteins to different degrees. Aldosterone exists approximately 40% in the free state, whereas 4% of cortisol is free in solution. Albumin and corticosteroid-binding globulin (CBG, transcortin, cortisol-binding globulin) account for most of the binding of these two steroids. CBG is a high-affinity, low-capacity steroid binder, binding 90% of the cortisol under normal circumstances, whereas albumin is a low-affinity, high-capacity binding protein. The proportion of

cortisol in the free state greatly increases as the concentration of cortisol exceeds the binding capacity of CBG (approximately 550 nmol/L). The binding affinity of CBG for cortisol is reduced in areas of inflammation. This increases the concentration of free cortisol, therefore increasing its effectiveness at that site. CBG levels are increased in hyperestrogenic states such as those found in pregnant women and in women taking estrogen-containing birth control pills. The free cortisol levels remain normal under these circumstances because of a compensatory increase in total cortisol. Aldosterone is much less affected by these hormonally induced changes.

Steroid catabolism is quite complex, and only a brief discussion of it is necessary for the understanding of the pathogenesis and laboratory investigation of adrenal disorders. Most steroids are catabolized by the liver and the kidneys. Examples of the types of reactions that are carried out include further hydroxylation of the steroid nucleus, conjugation with glucuronic acid, and reduction of the double bond in ring A. These transformations increase the water solubility of the steroids, allowing for their excretion into the urine. Only a small portion of aldosterone and cortisol is excreted unmetabolized into the urine.

The amount of cortisol directly secreted into the urine is related to the proportion of cortisol that circulates in the free form. CBG is saturated at high physiological concentrations of cortisol. Therefore any increase in cortisol above this level will result in a pronounced increase in the amount of cortisol excreted into the urine, making urinary free corti-

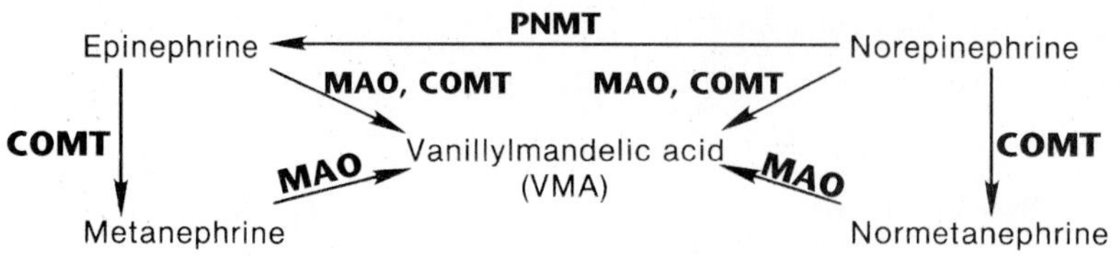

Fig. 46-5 Metabolism of medullary hormones (see text for description of abbreviations).

sol a valuable test in the investigation of Cushing's syndrome, as is discussed later.

Catecholamines

The catecholamines are stable within the storage granules of the adrenal medullary cells. However, when they are released they are rapidly degraded by two enzymes: catechol-*O*-methyltransferase (COMT) and monoamine oxidase (MAO) (Fig. 46-5). Only a small fraction of catecholamine output (2%) is excreted unmetabolized as free catecholamines into the urine. COMT is present in many tissues, especially liver and kidney, and in erythrocytes. This enzyme methylates the C-3 hydroxyl group of norepinephrine and epinephrine, resulting in normetanephrine and metanephrine respectively. Approximately 20% of catecholamines are excreted into the urine as metanephrines. Most catecholamines, however, are further converted to vanillylmandelic acid (VMA) by the combined action of COMT and MAO; the latter is a ubiquitous enzyme that deaminates these amines. The measurement of free catecholamines, metanephrines, and VMA in the urine may be useful in the diagnosis of adrenal medullary disease.

CONTROL AND REGULATION
Glucocorticoids

Cortisol released from the adrenal cortex is regulated by the hypothalamic-pituitary-adrenal axis (Fig. 46-6 and Chapter 43). The hypothalamus synthesizes a 41–amino acid polypeptide, corticotropin-releasing hormone (CRH), which is carried by the circulation to the anterior pituitary gland. There it causes the release of adrenocorticotropic hormone (ACTH), a 39–amino acid polypeptide. The first 18 amino acids are essential for biological activity. The ACTH molecule interacts with membrane receptors of the cells of the adrenal cortex and through its second messenger, cyclic AMP, stimulates the rate-limiting step in steroidogenesis (the conversion of cholesterol to pregnenolone) leading to cortisol secretion. The free circulating cortisol acts in a negative-feedback manner to control the release of ACTH from the pituitary gland. Overriding this system of negative-feedback control are the higher centers of the brain, which establish the normal diurnal variation of cortisol (Fig. 46-7). Serum cortisol levels are normally highest in the morning on waking and lowest in the late evening. This pattern is mainly affected by the sleep-wake cycle of the individual. If the sleep-wake cycle is altered, several days are required for the pattern to change. The circadian pattern of

ACTH release is controlled by means of CRH secretion from the hypothalamus. Short-term release of cortisol is episodic, following the pattern of ACTH pulses by about 2 to 3 minutes. Stress is another factor that can override the negative feedback of cortisol on ACTH release. Stress stimulates release of neurogenic amines, which in turn stimulates the release of CRH. The inflammatory cytokines, tumor necrosis factor α, interleukin-1, and interleukin-6, also stimulate the release of ACTH. ACTH levels can increase up to tenfold in times of stress, resulting in high levels of cortisol. Hypoglycemia, which is a form of chemical stress, can also increase CRH release, ultimately leading to an increase in cortisol. This effect is mediated by glucose receptors in the hypothalamus.

Mineralocorticoids

In normal individuals three main factors control the secretion of aldosterone from the zona glomerulosa: (1) the renin-angiotensin system, (2) potassium, and (3) ACTH. Under normal circumstances, the renin-angiotensin system predominates. Fig. 46-8 outlines the normal regulation of aldosterone secretion. A more detailed description is found in Chapter 24.

Renin is a proteolytic enzyme stored by specialized cells in the wall of the afferent arteriole of the glomerulus. These cells are associated with the *macula densa,* which is part of the juxtaglomerular apparatus. A drop in blood pressure or serum sodium concentration will result in the release of renin. Renin cleaves a peptide bond in circulating angiotensinogen, a protein secreted by the liver, releasing a decapeptide called *angiotensin I.* Angiotensin I in turn is cleaved by angiotensin-converting enzyme (ACE), forming an octapeptide called *angiotensin II.* Angiotensin II is a potent vasoconstrictor that increases blood pressure directly. This peptide also stimulates aldosterone release, which causes sodium retention and potassium loss. Finally, angiotensin II is converted to a heptapeptide, *angiotensin III,* by a carboxypeptidase. Angiotensin III still retains the capacity to stimulate aldosterone release but has little pressor activity.

Potassium stimulates aldosterone secretion directly at the adrenal level. Hyperkalemia stimulates and hypokalemia inhibits renin release. ACTH can also stimulate aldosterone secretion directly; however, this is only an acute phenomenon that is short lived. There is normally a circadian rhythm in plasma aldosterone concentration with highest values occurring in the morning. In addition, there are al-

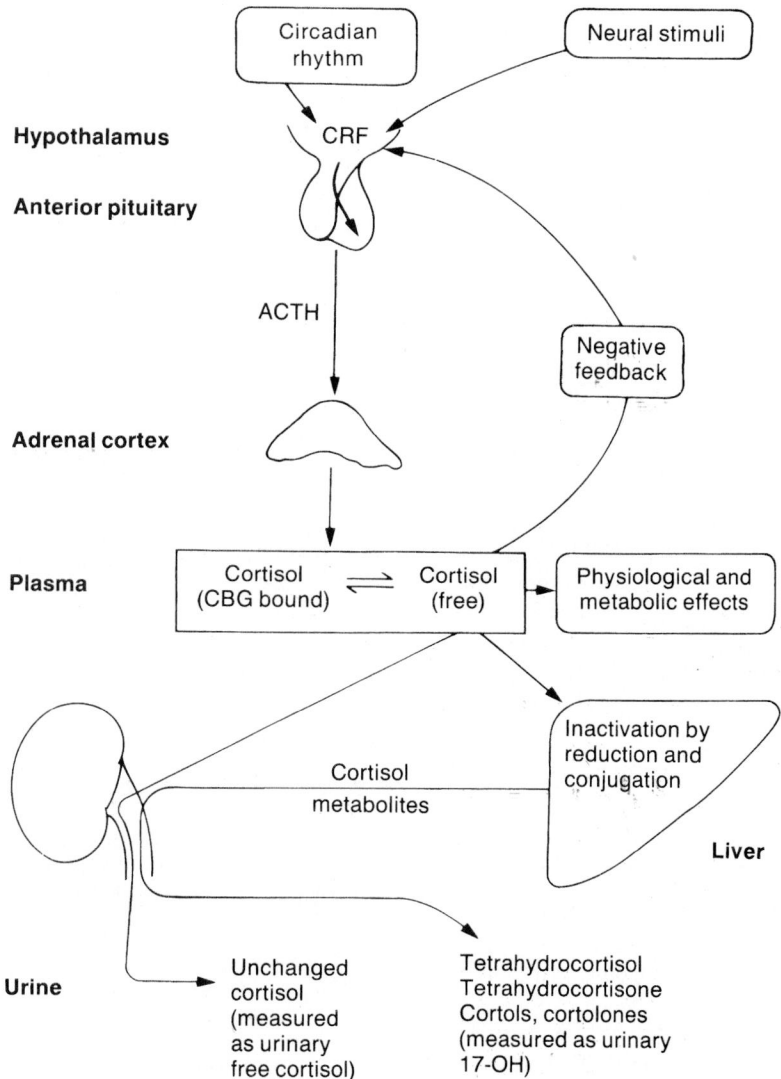

Fig. 46-6 Control and metabolism of glucocorticoids. (From Toft A: *Diagnosis and management of endocrine diseases,* St. Louis, 1981, Blackwell Scientific Publications.)

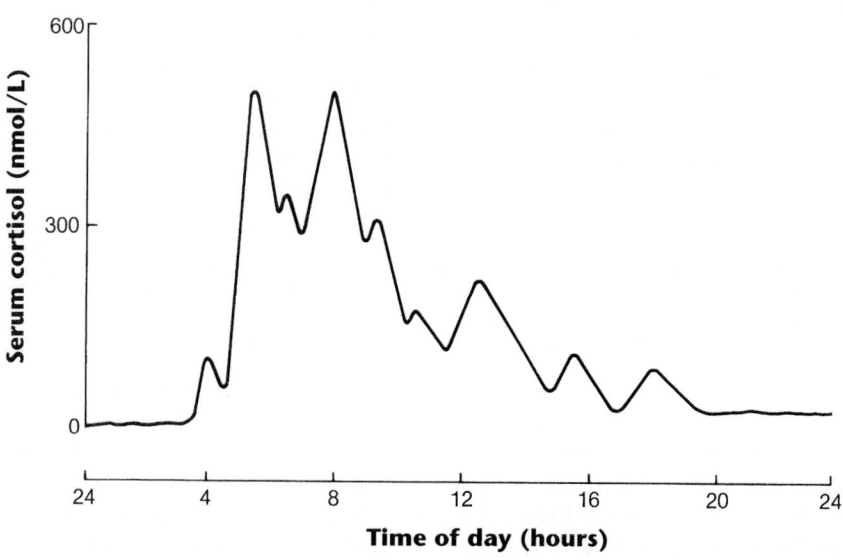

Fig. 46-7 Variation of serum cortisol concentration during 24-hour period in normal individual.

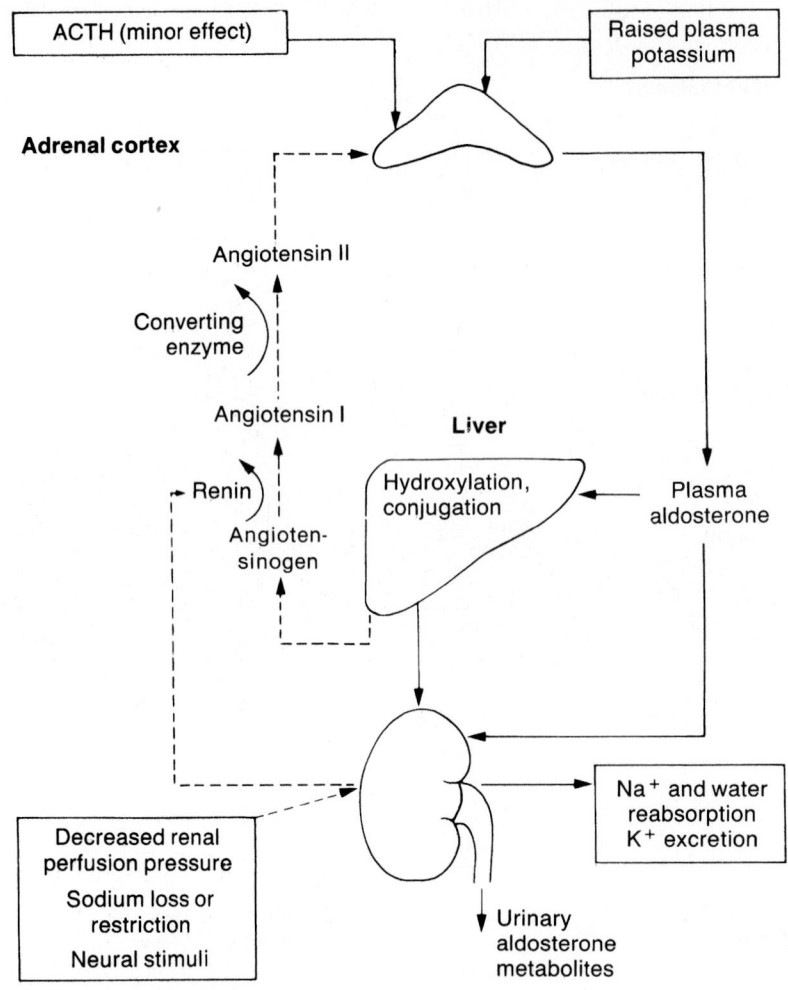

Fig. 46-8 Control and metabolism of aldosterone. (From Toft A: *Diagnosis and management of endocrine diseases,* St. Louis, 1981, Blackwell Scientific Publications.)

terations in aldosterone levels with postural changes. Plasma levels range from 50 to 150 ng/L (140 to 420 pmol/L) in healthy individuals when recumbent and from 150 to 300 ng/L (420 to 840 pmol/L) when upright. Approximately 150 to 200 μg of aldosterone is secreted per day under normal circumstances. Dopamine, serotonin, γ-MSH, beta-endorphin, and an unidentified pituitary aldosterone-stimulating factor also participate in aldosterone regulation.

Adrenal androgens

Androgen secretion is partially regulated by ACTH but not by gonadotropins. ACTH stimulation is variable, and dexamethasone (a synthetic corticosteroid) administration decreases adrenal androgen production to a dissimilar degree when compared to cortisol. In other instances, as at adrenarche or puberty, or with aging or severe illness, cortisol and androgen production diverge, and such divergence indicates that other factors are playing a role in the regulation of adrenal androgen secretion. These factors may in-

clude the arrangement of the blood supply to the adrenal cortex, intrinsic properties of the adrenocortical cells, and other unknown factors exogenous to the adrenal, such as factors from the pituitary.

Catecholamines

The synthesis of epinephrine and norepinephrine is regulated by the intracellular concentrations of these hormones by negative-feedback inhibition, as stated previously. The catecholamines are released from the adrenal medulla in response to hypotension, hypoxia, exposure to cold, muscular exertion, pain, and emotional disturbances.

PATHOLOGICAL CONDITIONS

In this section the causes and clinical features associated with the disorders of the adrenal cortex and the adrenal medulla are discussed. In general, the gland may hyperfunction and produce excess quantities of bioactive molecules, or the gland may hypofunction and secrete too little of certain important molecules that may be essential for the normal maintenance of life. The pathological cause of these disorders may be neoplastic, hyperplastic, vascular, inflammatory, autoimmune, infectious, hereditary, or idiopathic.

Disorders of the adrenal cortex

Hyperadrenalism. There are three basic conditions associated with hyperadrenalism, each of which may have more than one cause. These are Cushing's syndrome, resulting from excess cortisol production; primary hyperaldosteronism, or Conn's syndrome; and congenital adrenal hyperplasia caused by an enzymatic block in the steroid synthetic pathway.

Cushing's syndrome. *Cushing's syndrome* is the term used to describe any condition resulting from an increased concentration of circulating glucocorticoid, usually cortisol. The most common cause of excess cortisol is iatrogenic, resulting from high doses of cortisol or other glucocorticoids used in the management of a wide variety of clinical problems. The most common noniatrogenic causes are, in order, pituitary tumors (60%), ectopic ACTH (20%), and adrenal adenoma and adrenal carcinoma (combined 20%). The estimated prevalence of Cushing's syndrome is approximately 1:10,000 women and 1:30,000 men. The most common cause of Cushing's syndrome in children is adrenal carcinoma.

Cushing's syndrome may be divided into two broad categories: ACTH dependent and ACTH independent. ACTH-dependent Cushing's syndrome is caused by excess ACTH and results in bilateral adrenal hyperplasia. This is most commonly caused by autonomous ACTH secretion by a benign pituitary adenoma, also called *Cushing's disease.* This condition is much more common in women than in men (F:M ratio 7:1 or 8:1). Ectopic sources of ACTH include carcinoma of the lung (oat cell or small cell) (50%), thymic cancer (10%), pancreatic cancer (10%), neural crest tumors (5%), bronchial carcinoid (2%), medullary carcinoma of the thyroid (5%), and miscellaneous tumors (18%). It is now known that many nonendocrine tissues of the body can synthesize small amounts of proopiomelanocortin (POMC), the precursor to ACTH. Very few tissues can actually metabolize POMC and release bioactive ACTH. Most lung tumors produce POMC, but only 3% of these have the right proteolytic enzymes to release active ACTH, thus causing Cushing's syndrome.

In ACTH-independent Cushing's syndrome, serum ACTH levels are low because of the negative inhibition that results from the increased cortisol production of adrenal adenomas and carcinomas. Adrenal carcinoma has a particularly bad prognosis, with most patients dying within 3 years despite surgical intervention. Adrenal neoplasms are usually unilateral. In adults, about half of these are malignant, whereas in children neoplasms of the adrenal are more often malignant.

Rare causes of Cushing's syndrome include ectopic CRH secretion, macronodular adrenal hyperplasia (elevated

---

Major Causes and Clinical Features of Cushing's Syndrome

Causes
ACTH independent
 Adrenal adenoma
 Adrenal carcinoma
ACTH dependent
 Pituitary adenoma secreting ACTH (Cushing's syndrome)
 Ectopic ACTH
 Ectopic corticotropin-releasing hormone
Nodular hyperplasia
 Macronodular hyperplasia
 Primary pigmented nodular hyperplasia
 Gastric inhibitory polypeptide–dependent Cushing's
  syndrome
Iatrogenic
 Glucocorticoid therapy
 ACTH therapy

Clinical features
Central obesity
Hypertension
Glucose intolerance
Plethoric facies
Purple striae
Menstrual dysfunction
Muscle weakness
Hirsutism
Bruising
Osteoporosis
Psychiatric problems

ACTH and elevated cortisol), primary pigmented nodular hyperplasia (a familial autoimmune disorder analogous to Graves' disease), and gastric inhibitory polypeptide (GIP)–dependent cortisol hypersecretion (food-dependent Cushing's syndrome).

Cushing's syndrome in advanced stages may be easy to recognize (see the box). In early stages of the disease, however, patients can have a wide variety of clinical symptoms that may be confused with other common problems such as idiopathic hypertension, glucose intolerance, depression, and obesity. The laboratory plays a major role in sorting out the diagnosis. Central obesity is a characteristic redistribution of adipose tissue with increased deposition around the face (moon facies), in the supraclavicular region, in the interscapular region (buffalo hump), and in the mesenteric bed (truncal obesity). The reason for this is not known. Less common findings include neuropsychiatric dysfunction, pigmentation, acne, and hypokalemic alkalosis. Polyuria may be seen because cortisol in high concentrations may suppress antidiuretic hormone (ADH) release. The neuropsychiatric problems include depression, manic behavior, psychoses, and attempts at suicide.

The catabolic effect of glucocorticoids on protein metabolism can account for the bruising, striae (stretch marks), osteoporosis, and muscle weakness. Hypertension and hypokalemia can be explained by the mineralocorticoid actions of excess cortisol. Hirsutism, acne, and menstrual dysfunction, a result of excess androgen production, may most dramatically be seen in some cases of adrenal carcinoma. Hyperpigmentation sometimes occurs in association with ectopic ACTH where the high levels of ACTH release may be associated with increased release of melanocyte-stimulating activity causing generalized hyperproduction of melanin. Some patients may also suffer from impotence, decreased libido, and infertility.

Hyperaldosteronism. Primary autonomous hypersecretion of aldosterone by the zona glomerulosa is mainly caused by two disorders: (1) an adrenal adenoma–producing aldosterone (APA), or Conn's syndrome (approximately 70% of cases), and (2) idiopathic hyperaldosteronism (IHA) caused by bilateral hyperplasia (approximately 30% of cases). Primary adrenal hyperplasia, which is indistinguishable biochemically from APA, may account for 1% to 2% of patients with this problem. Carcinomas secreting aldosterone are even more rare (<1%). A rare form of primary hyperaldosteronism, glucocorticoid-remediable aldosteronism (GRA), has clinical features of Conn's syndrome but results from an ectopic expression of aldosterone synthase (AS). GRA, with a characteristic overproduction of 18-hydroxycortisol, is caused by chimeric duplication of two linked genes, 11-β-hydroxylase and AS on chromosome 8.

The major clinical feature of hyperaldosteronism is hypertension. The estimated prevalence of this disorder in the hypertensive population varies from 0.05% to as high as 2.0%. The hypertension associated with primary hyperaldosteronism can be explained by the actions of aldosterone that result in retention of sodium and water and decreased plasma potassium levels (see Chapter 24). The most consistent laboratory finding in patients with primary aldosteronism is hypokalemia. Spontaneous hypokalemia is found in 80% to 90% of patients. Administration of sodium chloride for several days will provoke hypokalemia in the remainder. The prevalence of primary hyperaldosteronism in patients with hypertension and spontaneous hypokalemia is more than 50%. The degree of hypokalemia is affected partly by the sodium intake. Many patients with hypokalemia will not experience symptoms (see the box). Abnormal glucose tolerance can be observed in more than half the patients. Hypokalemia impairs insulin release from the beta cells of the pancreas. The hallmark of primary hyperaldosteronism is inappropriately elevated aldosterone in the presence of suppressed plasma renin activity.

Hyperaldosteronism may also result from secondary causes. In these situations the adrenal gland is not autonomously secreting aldosterone but is responding to enhanced production and release of renin from the kidney, which may be triggered by sodium loss, decreased renal perfusion, renal artery stenosis, or vascular volume depletion. Rarely the

---

Major Causes and Clinical Features of Primary Hyperaldosteronism (Conn's Syndrome)
Causes
Adrenal aldosterone-producing adenoma, APA (70% of cases)
Idiopathic hyperaldosteronism, IHA (30% of cases)
Clinical features
Hypertension
Symptoms resulting from hypokalemia
Muscle weakness
Polyuria and polydipsia
ECG changes
Glucose intolerance

---

hypersecretion of renin may be inappropriate, as in *Bartter's syndrome,* a kidney defect in chloride resorption, or in patients with renin-secreting tumors. In contrast to primary aldosteronism where renin is decreased, plasma renin is elevated in secondary aldosteronism.

Congenital adrenal hyperplasia. Congenital adrenal hyperplasia, or adrenogenital syndrome, describes a group of inborn errors of metabolism that are caused by deficiencies of enzymes in the biosynthetic pathways leading to cortisol and aldosterone production. There are at least six distinct inheritable defects in this pathway, the most common of which is a 21-hydroxylase deficiency, which accounts for 95% of all cases of congenital adrenal hyperplasia. These enzyme defects lead to diminished production of cortisol, which results in increased levels of ACTH. This in turn stimulates adrenal hyperplasia and steroid production as the body attempts to overcome the enzyme deficiency. The block is usually partial, and the patient may be capable of maintaining normal levels of cortisol and aldosterone under normal circumstances at the expense of the accumulation of steroid precursors that are diverted down other metabolic pathways. Commonly there is hypersecretion of various androgens including DHEA and androstenedione, which after peripheral conversion to testosterone, may lead to precocious puberty in males and varying degrees of masculinization and sexual dysfunction in females.

Symptoms in congenital adrenal hyperplasia are related to both the decrease in the final product of metabolism and the accumulation of its precursors. In the case of 21-hydroxylase deficiency, the accumulation of 17-hydroxyprogesterone results in a salt-wasting tendency. Plasma renin levels increase in response, triggering greater demand for aldosterone synthesis, which also requires 21-hydroxylase activity. If the deficiency is partial, the salt-losing tendency is compensated. If it is more complete, more severe salt wasting will occur and an addisonian crisis (see p. 923) is more likely. The non–salt wasting variant of this condition, seen in two thirds of patients with this disorder, is primarily characterized by the problems associated with increased androgens. More severe deficiencies may be manifested in childhood. The less severe deficiencies may not become clinically apparent until after puberty. Without treatment the excess androgen results in precocious development in both males and females with rapid growth, pubic hair, and acne at an early age. There is also premature epiphyseal closure. Additional problems for females include clitoromegaly, deepening voice, increased muscle mass, failure of breast development, primary amenorrhea, and facial hair.

The 21-hydroxylase deficiency is inherited through an autosomal recessive trait with an estimated heterozygote frequency of approximately 1 in 50 of the population. The approximate frequency of homozygous 21-hydroxylase deficiency causing congenital adrenal hyperplasia is 1 in 10,000 births (M:F ratio 1:1). Mild, nonclassic 21-hydroxylase deficiency is much more common, with a prevalence of 1 in 1000 in the general population. The prevalence is much higher in some populations; for example, among Ashkenazi Jews it may be as high as 1 in 30. Because of the high incidence of nonclassic congenital adrenal hyperplasia, some have questioned whether it is a disease.

A deficiency of 11-hydroxylase is the second most common cause of congenital adrenal hyperplasia. Again, depending on the severity of the deficiency, cortisol production may or may not be adequate. A unique feature of this enzyme deficiency is the accumulation of 11-deoxycorticosterone, a precursor in the aldosterone pathway. This steroid promotes sodium resorption and therefore can cause hypertension. Excess androgen production is also a problem.

Treatment for both of the above forms of congenital adrenal hyperplasia is simply glucocorticoid replacement therapy. Female patients in addition require surgical correction for ambiguous genitalia. Male patients tend to respond well to therapy, whereas female patients, despite adequate therapy, have a high incidence of sexual identity disorders, infertility, hirsutism, and virilization.

Hypoadrenalism. Adrenal hypofunction or insufficiency can be caused by (1) primary adrenal disease, involving the entire adrenal cortex; (2) secondary adrenal insufficiency caused by decreased levels of CRH or ACTH, as a result of pituitary or hypothalamic disease; or (3) long-term suppression of the hypothalamic-pituitary-adrenal axis by glucocorticoids, which leads to adrenal atrophy. Secondary adrenal insufficiency resulting from decreased ACTH or CRH is discussed further in Chapter 43.

Addison's disease. Primary adrenal hypofunction or insufficiency, also known as *Addison's disease,* is relatively rare (estimated prevalence 1 in 50,000). A major cause of Addison's disease today, accounting for 70% of all cases, is autoimmune adrenalitis with circulating adrenal antibodies. This disorder, accounting for 70% of Addison's disease,

---

Major Causes and Clinical Features of Primary Adrenal Insufficiency

Causes
Autoimmune adrenalitis
Granulomatous disease
   Tuberculosis
   Histoplasmosis
   Sarcoidosis
Neoplastic infiltration
Hemochromatosis
Amyloidosis
Bilateral adrenalectomy
Infarction
Infectious disease
Drugs (metyrapone, ketoconazole, o,p'-DDD)
Adrenoleukodystrophy
Congenital adrenal hyperplasia

Clinical features
Muscle weakness
Fatigue
Weight loss
Orthostatic hypotension
Pigmentation
Anorexia
Addisonian crisis
   Fever
   Dehydration
   Nausea
   Hypotension
   Shock
   Abdominal pain

---

may be associated with other autoimmune disorders such as Hashimoto's thyroiditis, hypoparathyroidism, diabetes mellitus, pernicious anemia, vitiligo, and primary ovarian failure. Other causes of primary adrenal failure are listed in the box. Tuberculosis was the leading cause of adrenal failure in the first half of this century.

Symptoms of Addison's disease begin to appear after about 90% of the adrenal cortex has been destroyed (see box). The disease usually develops slowly with progressive loss of cortisol and increasing ACTH levels, resulting in hyperpigmentation of the patient because of the melanocyte-stimulating hormone properties of ACTH. Because of coincident aldosterone deficiency, there is sodium loss and potassium retention. Hypoglycemia may be present because of cortisol deficiency. These symptoms may be vague and nonspecific. However, some patients may be seen with an acute life-threatening disease that is termed an *addisonian crisis* after stress caused by illness, surgery, or trauma. An *addisonian crisis* is a result of an acute deficiency of both mineralocorticoids and glucocorticoids. An *addisonian crisis,* the signs of which are listed in the box, can rapidly evolve into circulatory shock. Hyperkalemia and hyponatremia are common laboratory findings along with hemoconcentration and elevated urea levels resulting from fluid loss. The hyperkalemia may be severe enough to induce cardiac arrhythmias and cardiac arrest.

Congenital adrenal hyperplasia, discussed in the previous section, can result in primary adrenal insufficiency. Certain drugs, such as metyrapone used in the treatment of Cushing's syndrome, *o,p'*-DDD (mitotane) used in the treatment of adrenal cancer, and other therapeutic agents such as ketoconazole and etomidate, which interfere with steroid synthetic pathways, all have the potential to cause primary adrenal insufficiency.

The X-linked form of adrenoleukodystrophy (ALD) should also be considered in the differential diagnosis of primary adrenal insufficiency in the male patient. It occurs more frequently than recognized, with up to 40% of males with Addison's disease having this problem. The defect is caused by a deficiency of a peroxisomal enzyme (lignoceroyl CoA ligase), which results in decreased oxidation and therefore accumulation of very long chain fatty acids (VLCFAs). Pathological changes are found in the adrenal cortex, testes, CNS white matter, and the peripheral nervous system. The cells of the adrenal gland in the zona fasciculata and zona reticularis tissues become swollen with lamellar inclusions consisting of cholesterol esters of VLCFAs and eventually atrophy and die. Patients with ALD may present with adrenal insufficiency alone, both neurological and adrenal problems, or neurological problems alone. The neurological problems include emotional lability, failure at school, and hyperactivity that progresses to visual impairment, diffuse cerebral demyelination, seizures, mental deterioration, and death.

The primary adrenal insufficiency in ALD is mainly the result of diminished cortisol reserve. Primary gonadal insufficiency is a problem in 20% of patients with decreased testosterone and increased gonadotropins.

Patients with secondary adrenal insufficiency do not usually experience symptoms related to hypoaldosteronism because aldosterone synthesis and secretion depend on the renin-angiotensin system rather than on ACTH. Hyperpigmentation is also not a feature of this disorder. However, patients with secondary adrenal insufficiency may show other signs of hypothalamic or pituitary disease including concomitant hypogonadism and hypothyroidism. Symptoms common to both primary and secondary disease of the adrenal cortex include weakness, hypoglycemia, weight loss, and gastrointestinal discomfort.

Disorder of the adrenal medulla: pheochromocytoma

Pheochromocytoma, a relatively rare, usually benign tumor arising from chromaffin cells, results in hypersecretion of the catecholamines epinephrine and norepinephrine. It is estimated that at least 0.1% of patients with persistent diastolic hypertension may have this tumor. Although it is a rare cause of hypertension, it is important to diagnose because it is surgically curable, and, even more significantly, it can cause death from acute hypertensive attacks. This tumor can present as an isolated problem at any age; for example, 10% of pheochromocytomas are reported in children. Overall incidence is estimated at 1 to 2 per 100,000. The autopsy incidence is considerably higher at 0.3%. Pheochromocytomas are most commonly discovered in the third to fifth decades of life.

Approximately 90% of pheochromocytomas occur in the adrenal glands, with the remainder occurring in extra-adrenal chromaffin cells, anywhere from the base of the brain to the lower abdomen. Approximately 10% of pheochromocytomas are bilateral or multiple, and approximately 10% are malignant. Pheochromocytomas also occur as an inheritable disorder. In this case they may be associated with multiple endocrine neoplasia (MEN) type II syndrome, which manifests as pheochromocytoma, hyperparathyroidism, and medullary carcinoma of the thyroid, or MEN type III, which manifests as multiple mucosal neuromas, medullary carcinoma of the thyroid, and pheochromocytoma. There is also a significant association with neurofibromatosis (von Recklinghausen's disease) and with von Hippel-Lindau disease.

Pheochromocytomas may release their hormones in a sustained or episodic fashion. Clinically the most significant finding is persistent or paroxysmal hypertension; other common findings are summarized in the box. Many of the symptoms may be persistent or episodic. Episodes can be as infrequent as once every few weeks or as frequent as 20 to 30 times daily, with attacks persisting for less than a minute or for as long as a week. The symptom pattern de-

---

Major Causes and Clinical Features of Pheochromocytoma

Causes
Benign adrenal chromaffin cell tumor (80%)
Malignant adrenal chromaffin cell tumor (10%)
Extra-adrenal chromaffin cell tumor (10%)

Clinical features
Episodic or sustained hypertension
Headache
Sweating
Palpitations with or without tachycardia
Nervousness
Weight loss
Nausea
Weakness or fatigue
Less common:
   Flushing
   Dyspnea
   Dizziness

pends on the specific catecholamine secreted by the tumor. Rarely hypotension may be the clinical problem. This is the case if the tumor primarily secretes epinephrine, dopa, or dopamine. Some patients may first present with cardiac hypertrophy or cardiac failure. It must be emphasized that the clinical symptoms are often subtle. A high degree of clinical alertness is required by the physician. The associated symptoms when they do occur are not specific for pheochromocytoma. A common cause of death in patients with unsuspected pheochromocytoma is hypertensive or hypotensive crisis precipitated by surgery. Paroxysmal attacks may be precipitated by palpation of the tumor, postural changes, emotional trauma, and even rarely micturition (in the case of a rare bladder tumor).

CHANGE OF ANALYTE IN DISEASE (Table 46-1)
Hyperadrenalism

Cushing's syndrome. In the laboratory investigation of Cushing's syndrome, the first step is to establish that the patient actually has autonomous cortisol production, or Cushing's syndrome. Once this is established, the next step is to differentiate the cause of the Cushing's syndrome.

One of the simplest and most important tests to perform initially is the overnight dexamethasone suppression test. Dexamethasone is a synthetic glucocorticoid that is 30 times as potent as cortisol. The patient is given a tablet containing 1 mg of dexamethasone and instructed to take this at 11 P.M. and come to the laboratory for plasma cortisol determination at 8:00 the following morning. A morning cortisol level less than 140 nmol/L (50 µg/L) usually excludes any cause of hypercortisolism. This is a normal response. Levels greater than 280 nmol/L (100 µg/L) indicate hypercortisolism. This test has a reported sensitivity of 98% for Cushing's syndrome. The specificity is not so good, and false positive results can be seen in patients with some forms of mental depression, stress-induced hypercortisolism, pseudo–Cushing's syndrome resulting from chronic alcoholism, and increased levels of cortisol-binding globulin associated with pregnancy or the use of birth control pills. False-positive results are also seen in patients receiving drugs, such as phenytoin or rifampin, that increase the rate of clearance of dexamethasone. However, the dexamethasone suppression test remains an ideal screening test for Cushing's syndrome, since false-negative results are a more serious problem than false-positive results in screening procedures. To minimize false-negative results some centers lower the expected cortisol suppression to below 85 nmol/L (30 µg/L).

Another useful initial investigative test is the estimation of a 24-hour urine free cortisol level. This is in essence a direct measure of the amount of cortisol that is not bound to plasma protein and is thus excreted unmetabolized in the urine over a 24-hour period. This test also has good sensitivity (95%) for Cushing's syndrome. A 24-hour urine cortisol determination is required along with a urine creatinine determination to ensure the adequacy of collection. The measurement of other steroid metabolites in urine that reflect glucocorticoid output, such as 17-hydroxycorticosteroids and 17-ketogenic steroids, is not considered reliable.

A traditional test that is no longer part of the standard work-up for Cushing's syndrome is the morning and afternoon serum cortisol determination. Plasma cortisol values usually display diurnal variation, with the highest levels occurring in the morning and the lowest levels in the early evening. Evening values are usually less than 50% of the

Table 46-1   Change of analyte with disease

Disease	24-hour urinary free cortisol	17-OHCS	Plasma ACTH	Urinary aldosterone	Plasma aldosterone	Plasma cortisol	Plasma renin activity	Urine or plasma catecholamines	Urine vanillylmandelic acid and metanephrine
Hypercortical disease									
Primary Cushing's syndrome	↑	↑	↓			±			
Cushing's disease (secondary)	↑	↑	±			±			
Ectopic ACTH	↑	↑	↑			±			
Primary hyperaldosteronism				↑	↑		↓		
Secondary hyperaldosteronism				↑	↑		↑		
Hypocortical disease									
Primary	±	↓	↑			↓			
Secondary	±	↓	↓			↓			
Pheochromocytoma								↑	↑

↑, Elevated; ±, variable response; ↓, diminished.
ACTH, Adrenocorticotropic hormone; *17-OHCS*, 17-hydroxycorticosteroid.

early morning concentrations. Classically, samples are drawn at 8 A.M. reference interval 140 to 660 nmol/L, 50 to 239 μg/L) and 4 P.M. (reference interval 50 to 330 nmol/L, 18 to 119 μg/L). Many patients with Cushing's syndrome will not show this diurnal variation and will have elevated concentrations at both times. However, the release of cortisol is episodic, and there is considerable overlap between healthy patients and patients with Cushing's syndrome. To differentiate patients with Cushing's syndrome from healthy patients it is best to take the sample at the time when cortisol is usually at its lowest concentration in the circulation. This time happens to be at midnight, and because it is not always practical to draw blood at this time, the more practical time of 4 P.M. is often chosen. Plasma cortisol levels greater than 420 nmol/L (152 μg/L) at this time are highly suggestive of hypercortisolism. Loss of diurnal variation can also occur with stress, anorexia, obesity, and emotional disturbances, or it may be secondary to sedatives, stimulants, or psychotropic or antiepileptic drugs.

Another variation of the overnight dexamethasone suppression test is the low-dose dexamethasone suppression test, which can also be used to confirm that the patient has Cushing's syndrome. This test is more time consuming and is not included in some of the recent protocols for this disorder. Some now suggest that one should go straight to the high-dose dexamethasone suppression test, which is discussed below. In the classic low-dose dexamethasone suppression test the patient is given a total dose of 2 mg of dexamethasone per day for 2 days in 0.5 mg doses every 6 hours. This dose is equivalent to about four times the usual adrenal output. During the second day a 24-hour urine specimen is collected for urine free cortisol. Plasma cortisol measurements may also be performed. Patients with Cushing's syndrome generally will not show significant suppression of cortisol output with this dose of dexamethasone. Normal patients should show greater than 50% suppression of the urine cortisol output present before the test. Urine cortisol usually falls to less than 50 nmol/L (18 μg/L) and morning serum cortisol to less than 140 nmol/L (50 μg/L).

There are several possible approaches that can be used to determine the cause of Cushing's syndrome. One can perform a high-dose dexamethasone suppression test. This can be done as an overnight procedure using 8 mg of dexamethasone, or it can be carried out over 2 days, giving a total of 8 mg of dexamethasone per day divided into four aliquots of 2 mg every 6 hours. The response can be determined by measurements of plasma cortisol or 24-hour urine free cortisol. Patients who have pituitary tumors secreting excess ACTH (Cushing's disease) will show greater than 50% suppression of the glucocorticoid output after the high-dose dexamethasone suppression test because pituitary tumors remain responsive to negative feedback though requiring higher levels of corticosteroid than normal. Patients with adrenal tumors or ectopic sources of ACTH will fail to show

suppression of glucocorticoids. Anomalous responses, however, do occur.

Plasma ACTH levels, which can be measured by radioimmunoassay, are essential in determining the specific cause of Cushing's syndrome. ACTH is a labile polypeptide hormone, and special precautions are required in its handling. Plasma samples should be collected on ice, and the plasma should be separated in a refrigerated centrifuge and stored frozen. ACTH can now be measured by a two-site immunoradiometric assay that has better precision, specificity, and sensitivity than a traditional competitive radioimmunoassay. The new assays do not measure fragments of ACTH and do not react well with "big" ACTH, a precursor to ACTH that is produced by some tumors. ACTH levels in the upper limit of the reference interval (<11.4 pmol/L) and up to twice the upper limit of normal are consistent with a pituitary cause of Cushing's syndrome. Nondetectable levels of ACTH (less than 2 pmol/L) are suggestive of an adrenal tumor. Very high levels of ACTH (greater than 50 pmol/L) are suggestive of an ectopic source, such as a malignant tumor. There is some overlap in the plasma concentrations of ACTH associated with ectopic and pituitary causes of Cushing's syndrome.

The metyrapone stimulation test has also been used to delineate the cause of Cushing's syndrome. Metyrapone acts by inhibiting the enzyme 11-hydroxylase and therefore blocking the synthesis of cortisol. In healthy patients, the cortisol level drops, and ACTH levels will increase because of loss of negative-feedback inhibition from cortisol. The response to metyrapone can be determined by measurement of either serum or plasma 11-deoxycortisol or urine 17-hydroxycorticosteroids. The following protocol is recommended: First measure the baseline serum cortisol and 11-deoxycortisol values in serum at 8 A.M. Give the patient 750 mg of metyrapone every 4 hours for 24 hours, and then repeat the measurement of serum cortisol and 11-deoxycortisol. In Cushing's syndrome caused by a pituitary tumor the ACTH response remains intact, and 11-deoxycortisol levels increase to levels greater than 200 nmol/L. Levels of 11-deoxycortisol that are less than this are consistent with an adrenal tumor or ectopic ACTH. Some investigators have suggested that this test may be better than the high-dose dexamethasone suppression test in determining the cause of Cushing's syndrome; however, most laboratories do not perform this protocol.

If ACTH is suppressed in a patient with Cushing's syndrome, a CT scan is usually successful in identifying the adrenal lesion. Adrenal adenomas are usually obvious because the adjacent normal adrenal tissue and the contralateral adrenal have become atrophic. With adrenal carcinoma the gland is usually very large, with dimensions that exceed 6 cm. Other features that help distinguish between adrenal adenoma and carcinoma include increased androgen production associated with adrenal carcinoma; benign tumors may respond to ACTH and malignant tumors are usually pleomorphic and invasive.

The most difficult causes of Cushing's to differentiate are ectopic ACTH production and a pituitary adenoma. This differentiation was not necessary until the 1970s because bilateral adrenalectomy was standard treatment for both. Starting in the late 1970s transsphenoidal surgery became the treatment of choice for pituitary adenoma. It subsequently became clear that not all patients with an apparent pituitary adenoma had this problem. Patients with bronchial carcinoids most often had biochemical parameters, including ACTH and high-dose dexamethasone suppression test results, that were similar to those patients with Cushing's disease. These slow-growing tumors were not radiologically apparent for years in some cases. Pituitary imaging techniques may give high rates of false-positive and false-negative results. False-negative results are usually a problem with small pituitary tumors. The false-positive results occur because of the high incidence of nonfunctional pituitary tumors. There was some hope that the corticotropin-releasing hormone (CRH) stimulation test would be more helpful. In principle, ACTH-secreting tumors usually retain CRH receptors and after the administration of 100 μg of CRH, will respond with a brisk increase in ACTH release. Patients with other causes of Cushing's syndrome should theoretically show no response. Unfortunately, as with the previously discussed tests, false-positive and false-negative results do occur. The overall diagnostic accuracy of the CRH stimulation test is approximately 90%, which is only marginally better than that of the high-dose dexamethasone suppression test.

The test that is now considered definitive in the differentiation of pituitary causes of Cushing's syndrome from other causes is bilateral inferior petrosal sinus sampling after CRH administration. In this test a radiologist inserts catheters into both inferior petrosal sinuses, which drain from the anterior pituitary. Venous samples are drawn before and 2, 5, and 10 minutes after 100 μg of CRH has been administered intravenously. The ACTH gradient between the inferior petrosal sinus and peripheral venous sites after CRH stimulation is greater than 2 or 3 if the patient has a pituitary tumor. The average gradient seen in patients with a pituitary tumor secreting ACTH is about 50. A gradient of less than 2 indicates a nonpituitary source of ACTH. Since samples are taken simultaneously from the right and left sinuses, it is possible to localize the tumor to the right or left side of the anterior pituitary in about 80% of cases. This is useful information for subsequent surgical procedures. If there is no identifiable lesion, the surgeon may remove only the left or right side of the pituitary, thereby lessening the risk of panhypopituitarism.

The petrosal sinus sampling procedure is demanding and requires a skilled radiologist. Therefore not everyone agrees that this test should be performed routinely in all patients who are suspected of having pituitary tumors. Data from the National Institutes of Health indicate that a 50% suppression of cortisol output by high-dose dexamethasone may be inadequate to confirmation that the patient has a pituitary tumor. They recommend confirm that the patient has the diagnosis of a pituitary tumor only when the urine free cortisol has decreased by 90% from baseline value. In their experience, no patient with ectopic ACTH experienced cortisol suppression to this degree. The more invasive petrosal sampling protocol described above may then be reserved for those patients who show only partial suppression of urine cortisol excretion.

Pituitary Cushing's syndrome is much more common in women than in men, with a female-to-male ratio of 7 or 8 to 1, whereas with ectopic ACTH the ratio is approximately equal. Forty percent of men with Cushing's syndrome may have an ectopic source of ACTH. As mentioned earlier, the presence of bronchial carcinoids can cause confusion in the diagnostic protocol. Petrosal vein sampling for ACTH helps to resolve this confusion. Localizing bronchial carcinoids remains a problem because they are small and slow growing. These tumors are benign but have malignant potential and must eventually be found.

In summary, if a patient is suspected of having Cushing's syndrome, begin with an overnight dexamethasone suppression test. Confirm a positive result with a 24-hour urine free cortisol with or without a subsequent low-dose dexamethasone suppression test. To determine the cause of Cushing's syndrome, ACTH measurements and the urine and serum cortisol responses to high-dose dexamethasone are useful. In centers where CRH is available, measurement of the ACTH response to CRH administration can be used in determining the cause of the excess cortisol. Finally, if the results of the investigation are not definitive, bilateral petrosal sinus sampling for ACTH after CRH administration should provide a definitive diagnosis. See Fig. 46-9 for an outline of the diagnostic protocol.

Primary hyperaldosteronism. Conn's syndrome, or primary hyperaldosteronism, is a rare cause of hypertension. The investigation process leading to a diagnosis for this disorder is costly and time consuming, and therefore patients with hypertension should be investigated for this disorder only when indicated. A scheme for the investigation of primary hyperaldosteronism is outlined in Fig. 46-10. The laboratory should play a major part in advising on the collection and handling of the specimens required for these expensive investigations to ensure a successful outcome. The simplest method for screening for this disorder is the measurement of serum and urine potassium when the patient is not receiving diuretics. Primary aldosteronism should be suspected in all patients with spontaneous hypokalemia. It should also be suspected in those who become hypokalemic on a high-salt diet or in those who develop hypokalemia very quickly when placed on diuretics. If the potassium is low, the next step in the investigation is to determine 24-hour urine potassium and sodium values. Values of serum

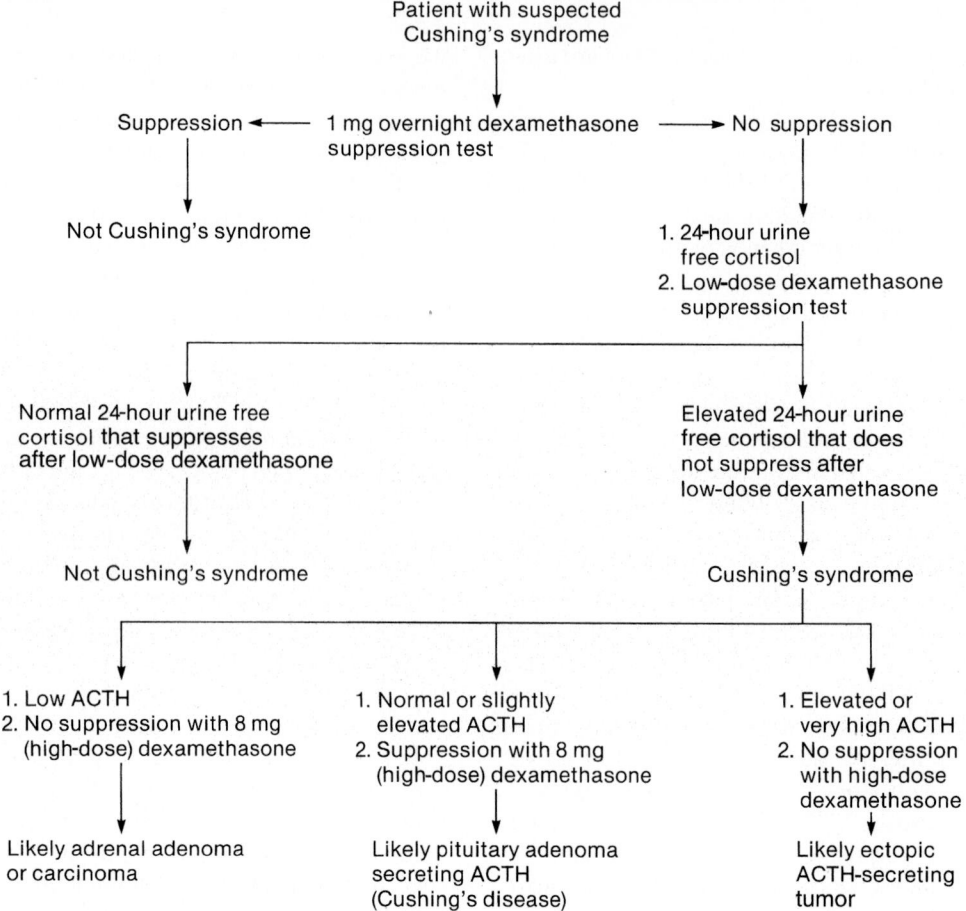

Fig. 46-9   Laboratory protocol for the investigation of Cushing's syndrome.

potassium of less than 3.5 mmol/L along with a urine potassium excretion rate of greater than 30 mmol/24 hours are not usually seen with essential hypertension but are commonly seen with primary hyperaldosteronism. The 24-hour urine sodium should be ≥100 mmol/L in order for the urine potassium result to be valid; a low sodium intake may decrease potassium excretion and yield a false-negative result. This screen is not entirely reliable because a serum potassium within the reference interval may be seen in some patients with primary hyperaldosteronism. The test may have to be repeated on two or three occasions.

The confirmation of the diagnosis of primary aldosteronism is dependent on the demonstration in serum of both a suppressed renin concentration and an increased aldosterone. Diuretics and spironolactone should be discontinued for at least 4 weeks before assessment of the patient.

Aldosterone is generally measured under conditions that will ordinarily suppress its secretion. One can most simply carry this out by prescribing for the patient a regimen that entails a moderately large sodium intake for 1 week (>100 mmol/day). Plasma aldosterone is then measured in the morning with the patient in a supine position. A second specimen, drawn 4 hours after the patient assumes an upright position, is used for measurement of plasma aldosterone and renin activity. The diagnosis of primary aldosteronism is confirmed if the supine plasma aldosterone is

>150 ng/L (420 pmol/L) and the upright renin activity is <1 ng/mL/hour. A simultaneous measurement of aldosterone in a 24-hour urine collection should be >65 μg/day in a patient with Conn's syndrome.

Another approach is to measure supine plasma aldosterone before and after infusion of 2 liters of normal saline over a 4-hour time span. Normal patients and patients with essential hypertension will suppress their plasma aldosterone to <50 ng/L (140 pmol/L). This test is not advised in patients with evidence of heart failure. Since the patient must be carefully monitored, this is an expensive test to perform.

Plasma renin activity may also be measured after challenge with a low-salt diet (<20 mmol/day) for 3 days, or after a 1-day low-salt diet followed by ingestion of 40 mg of furosemide taken three times during the day. A plasma sample is taken the following day after 4 hours in the upright position. This procedure causes salt and water depletion. Normal patients and patients with essential hypertension will respond with an increase in renin activity, whereas patients with primary hyperaldosteronism will not respond, and renin activity will remain low.

Low plasma renin activity may also be seen with congenital adrenal hyperplasia caused by 11-hydroxylase deficiency, excessive licorice ingestion, and low-renin essential hypertension.

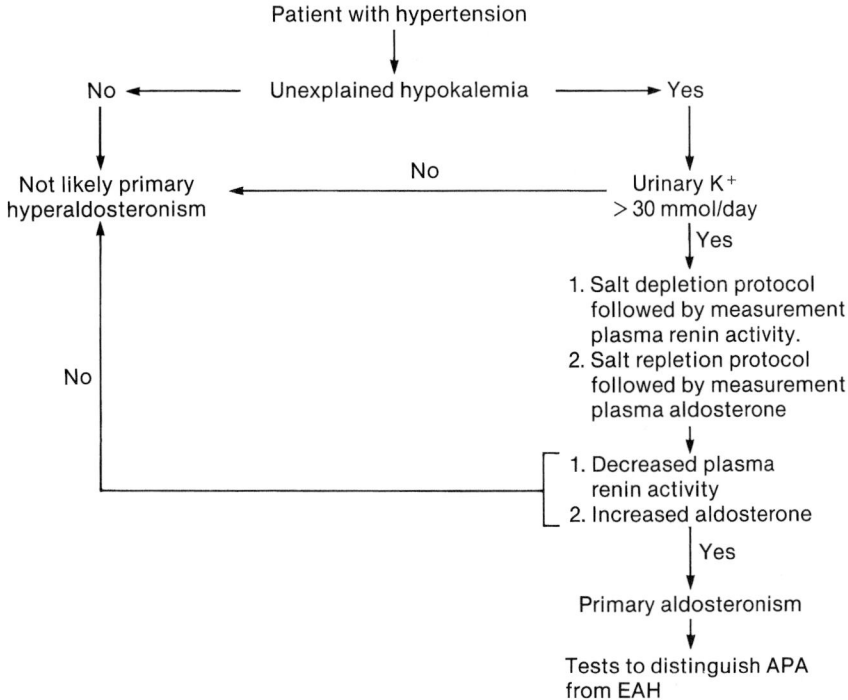

Fig. 46-10   Laboratory protocol for the investigation of a patient with suspected primary hyperaldosteronism (Conn's syndrome). Alternative approaches may be used (see text).

If the results are ambiguous, the "captopril test" may be useful. Captopril is a drug used to treat some patients with hypertension. Its primary mechanism of action is inhibition of angiotensin-converting enzyme, which converts angiotensin I to angiotensin II. Patients without Conn's syndrome will respond with a drop in plasma aldosterone, but patients with Conn's syndrome will not suppress the aldosterone levels. Aldosterone is usually measured 2 to 3 hours after a 25 mg oral dose of captopril. The expected response is that plasma aldosterone should decrease to <100 ng/L (<280 pmol/L).

Once the diagnosis of primary aldosteronism has been established, the cause of the disorder must be determined so that the proper course of treatment can be chosen. Surgical adrenalectomy is indicated for aldosterone-producing adenoma (APA), whereas medical therapy is required for idiopathic hyperaldosteronism (IHA). Several tests can be used to accomplish this task. The availability and accuracy of these tests vary, and a direct approach employing radiological imaging is limited because lesions associated with primary aldosteronism may be small (<2 cm). Also, nonfunctioning adrenal masses are quite common and may give false-positive results. The overall accuracy of imaging is only 75%. Slightly better results are seen when biochemical responses to posture change are used. In patients with APA, aldosterone levels may drop after assumption of an upright posture, whereas in patients with IHA, aldosterone usually rises. This indicates that plasma renin activity (PRA) may still be involved in aldosterone regulation in pa-

tients with IHA despite the low PRA levels. Another biochemical difference that can be measured involves 18-hydroxycorticosterone. This substance is higher in patients with APA than in patients with IHA. This test has limited availability.

Adrenal imaging with radioactively labeled iodocholesterol can accurately locate the tumor in 90% of patients with APA. The ^{131}I-labeled cholesterol should be administered after dexamethasone treatment to reduce uptake by healthy adrenal tissue.

The best procedure for localizing the lesion is bilateral adrenal venous sampling. The ratio of the ipsilateral to contralateral concentration of serum aldosterone is usually greater than 10:1. The success of this procedure is dependent on the ability of the radiologist to place the catheter accurately. The results can be improved by simultaneous determination of ACTH-stimulated cortisol from both adrenal veins, which should be symmetrical. Although this test is considered the standard, it is usually reserved for those cases where the simpler tests are inconclusive.

After adrenalectomy for APA, 70% of patients are normotensive 1 year later. Drugs such as amiloride and spironolactone have been used to treat IHA. Surprisingly, some patients respond to angiotensin-converting enzyme inhibitors. Such a response again indicates that angiotensin II may be playing a role in IHA.

Congenital adrenal hyperplasia. The reported incidence of congenital adrenal hyperplasia (CAH) ranges from 1:5000 to 1:62,000 births. The most common cause is a

21-hydroxylase deficiency, accounting for 95% of all cases. A child with this disorder may have evidence of adrenal insufficiency, as discussed earlier, and may be investigated from this point of view, as outlined in the next section of this chapter. However, the child may also suffer the biochemical consequences of excess androgen, with females showing signs of virilization and males demonstrating precocious puberty. The definitive test for this condition is the finding in the serum of an elevated serum level of 17-hydroxyprogesterone, the immediate precursor to the metabolic block. Measurements of testosterone in serum and pregnanetriol, a metabolite of 17-hydroxyprogesterone, in urine may also be useful. Measurement of serum 17-hydroxyprogesterone is also useful in following the adequacy of glucocorticoid replacement therapy in patients with 21-hydroxylase deficiency. The healthy reference interval for 17-hydroxyprogesterone is 0.5 to 3 nmol/L. Levels may be higher in normal maternal and fetal blood but drop dramatically after birth and reach normal adult levels by 2 to 7 days. Homozygotes for the 21-hydroxylase deficiency have 17-hydroxyprogesterone levels in the 300 to 3000 nmol/L range, whereas heterozygotes have levels between 3 and 30 nmol/L. An 11-hydroxylase deficiency may also lead to virilization or precocious puberty but is most frequently associated with hypertension and can best be diagnosed by measurement of serum or plasma deoxycortisol. Diagnostic tests for the other forms of congenital adrenal hyperplasia are not discussed because of the rarity of these disorders.

Hypoadrenalism, or primary adrenal insufficiency (Addison's disease)

When a patient has orthostatic (postural) hypotension, low serum sodium, and increased serum potassium, the possibility of primary adrenal insufficiency, or Addison's disease, should be considered. Samples should be drawn immediately for ACTH and baseline cortisol determinations. Aldosterone determinations may also be useful but are not usually performed. Patients with hypoadrenalism may have cortisol levels within the reference interval if they have inadequate adrenal reserves. In these cases an ACTH-stimulation test must be performed. A synthetic form of ACTH (cosyntropin, Cortrosyn), consisting of the first 24 amino acids of ACTH, can be injected intravenously or intramuscularly. Blood samples for serum cortisol should then be drawn at 30 to 60 minutes after injection. A normal response to this cosyntropin (ACTH) stimulation test manifests as a rise in the serum cortisol of at least 280 nmol/L (100 μg/L) to a level greater than 550 nmol/L (200 μg/L), unless the baseline value is already above 550 nmol/L. A low baseline cortisol result with a failure to respond to ACTH may be suggestive of primary adrenal failure or may be a result of atrophy caused by long-term steroid therapy or pituitary insufficiency. In primary adrenal insufficiency the ACTH levels will be greatly elevated (greater than 50 pmol/L) and in fact may be clinically apparent because of hyperpigmentation of the patient. In secondary adrenal insufficiency or atrophy resulting from exogenous steroids, the ACTH levels will be suppressed (less than 10 pmol/L).

If the response to the Cortrosyn stimulation test is abnormal and secondary adrenal insufficiency is suspected, a prolonged (3- to 5-day) ACTH stimulation test or an insulin-induced hypoglycemia stress test should be performed. Intravenous administration of ACTH over several days generally results in a gradual increase in cortisol output if the adrenal insufficiency is a result of long-term deficiency of ACTH from the pituitary. Hypoglycemia ordinarily stimulates release of ACTH from the pituitary. A failure to show increased ACTH or increased cortisol in response to hypoglycemia is suggestive of pituitary or hypothalamic disease. A CRH stimulation test could also be used and would give results comparable to the insulin hypoglycemia test. This test would be much safer, though CRH is not yet generally available at all diagnostic centers.

The metyrapone stimulation test is also sometimes used in the investigation of adrenal insufficiency. A protocol similar to that outlined earlier can be followed. A normal response usually results in increased levels of 11-deoxycortisol in the serum or increased output of 17-hydroxycorticosteroids in the urine. There is no response or an inadequate response in the case of both primary and secondary adrenal insufficiency. A simplified scheme for the investigation of adrenal insufficiency is shown in Fig. 46-11.

Transient adrenal insufficiency can result from long-term use of glucocorticoids, which inhibit ACTH and CRH release causing adrenal cortex atrophy. Short-term glucocorticoid therapy is rapidly reversible, but high-dose long-term therapy may result in adrenal insufficiency for as long as 2 years after the steroid medication is discontinued, and patients are at risk of cardiovascular collapse when severely stressed. It is impossible to predict which patients will have a problem, and therefore a laboratory assessment of adrenal reserve should be routinely performed. If a random cortisol is greater than 400 nmol/L (145 μg/L), there is little likelihood of a problem. However, the best assessment for reserve capacity is the rapid ACTH-stimulation test discussed above.

Adrenoleukodystrophy, which may also be a cause of adrenal insufficiency in males, is diagnosed by measurement of increased levels of very long chain saturated fatty acids ($C_{26:0}$, $C_{25:0}$, $C_{24:0}$) in plasma, red blood cells, white blood cells, or cultured fibroblasts. This assay is available in very few centers. Magnetic resonance imaging may also show characteristic white matter lesions.

Pheochromocytoma

There are many possible ways to investigate pheochromocytoma. One can measure urinary vanillylmandelic acid (VMA), metanephrines, total catecholamines, or fraction-

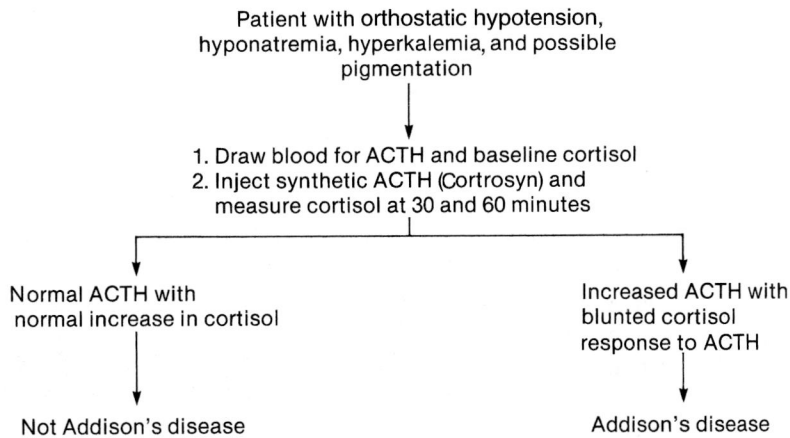

Fig. 46-11 Laboratory protocol for investigation of Addison's disease.

ated catecholamines. In addition, one can measure plasma epinephrine and norepinephrine. Most methods used to measure these analytes are analytically specific, but many drugs such as monoamine oxidase inhibitors and reserpine can alter catecholamine metabolism and may interfere with the interpretation of the results. The patient should not receive any medication, if possible, before the laboratory investigation is begun. Ideally a 24-hour urine sample should be collected when the patient is not receiving any drugs or under any stress and is medically stable. With the newer more specific methods available today, dietary restrictions are not required. Nevertheless, many drugs can either affect catecholamine metabolism directly or may interfere with their measurement. This is especially true for spectrophotometric and fluorometric methods. Increased catecholamine concentrations may be associated with administration of exogenous catecholamines (found in nose drops and appetite suppressants), amphetamines, vasodilators, alpha-adrenergic receptor antagonists (prazosin and phentolamine), diuretics with hyponatremia, caffeine, cigarette and marijuana smoking, beta-blockers, and tricyclic antidepressants. There are other drugs that may decrease catecholamine levels, including clonidine, bromocriptine, dexamethasone, and monoamine oxidase inhibitors.

Most of the literature indicates that a 24-hour urine metanephrine (reference interval, less than 5 μmol/day) determination may be the best screening test for pheochromocytoma, with a sensitivity of 98% to 99%. HPLC methods for VMA analysis (reference interval, 10 to 35 μmol/day) are not so sensitive, with a reported sensitivity of 90% for pheochromocytoma. The more recent literature indicates that quantitation of fractionated urine free catecholamines may be the most sensitive and specific test to order in the investigation of pheochromocytoma (sensitivity >95%). One continuing problem is that patients with hypertension from other causes may have borderline deviations of catecholamines and their metabolites. In patients with pheochromocytoma, the most common finding obtained after

fractionation of urine catecholamines is an increased norepinephrine level with smaller increases or normal levels of epinephrine and dopamine. A less common pattern is a pronounced increase in both norepinephrine and epinephrine with a smaller increase in dopamine. A rare pattern is a pronounced increase in epinephrine with smaller increases or normal levels of norepinephrine and dopamine. This last pattern is seen only in association with adrenal tumors. Some malignant pheochromocytomas may secrete large amounts of dopamine primarily. This is the result of a deficiency of dopamine-β-hydroxylase in malignant cells. The reference intervals for urine norepinephrine, epinephrine, and dopamine are up to 470, 160, and 3300 nmol/day respectively. An increase in urine norepinephrine is one of the more specific findings associated with pheochromocytoma when a value greater than 900 nmol/day (approximately 2 $\times$ the upper reference level) is used as the decision level. At this concentration, specificity of the assay is greatly improved without loss of sensitivity. Urine norepinephrine measurements are especially useful when the patient has episodic hypertension of short duration. A random urine collected shortly after the attack may indicate abnormal catecholamine excretion, whereas the metabolite concentrations may be normal.

There has been considerable interest in plasma catecholamine measurements, especially in combination with the clonidine suppression test. The analysis of plasma catecholamines is very difficult because the concentrations are very low and the compounds very labile. Many conditions can cause elevations of plasma catecholamines into the range seen in patients with pheochromocytoma, including volume depletion, anxiety, exercise, anorexia, smoking, renal failure, obesity, and several drugs such as L-dopa and methyldopa. Sensitivity of plasma catecholamine measurements for the diagnosis of pheochromocytoma may be as high as 95%, but the specificity is suboptimal. Using higher, more specific decision levels results in a drop in sensitivity. With plasma catecholamines, despite precautions to minimize stress during the evaluation period, a significant portion of patients with essential hypertension may have plasma norepinephrine concentrations in the equivocal range that could be the result of increased activity of the sympathetic nervous system (SNS).

The measurement of catecholamines in a 24-hour urine sample has several advantages. Urine collections induce minimal stress in the patient, and integration of production of catecholamines over 24 hours minimizes fluctuations in SNS activity. In addition, the considerably higher concentrations of analyte in a urine sample make the procedure less technically demanding.

The clonidine suppression test may be of some use in difficult diagnoses. Plasma catecholamines are measured before and 3 hours after the administration of 0.3 mg of clonidine. Patients with pheochromocytoma show no suppression, whereas patients with essential hypertension suppress their catecholamine levels into the reference interval. Best results are obtained with methods that are specific for free catecholamines. If conjugated catecholamines, which have longer half-lives, are included, false-positive results may occur. A recent modification of this protocol involves measurement of urine catecholamines in a timed urine specimen after administration of clonidine.

To localize the tumor before surgery, CT scans, venous sampling for catecholamines, radioisotope imaging with metaiodo[^{131}I]benzylguanidine, and MRI, are all useful techniques.

It is important to diagnose pheochromocytomas early because of the potential for a life-threatening hypertensive crisis, which may be triggered by a surgical procedure, major trauma, or certain drugs used in the treatment of depression or hypertension. The indications for testing for pheochromocytoma include the list of signs and symptoms described in the previous section. An adrenal mass, which may be an incidental finding on an abdominal CT scan, must be considered a potential pheochromocytoma, and this diagnosis must be ruled out before any surgical procedure is performed. Pheochromocytoma should also be considered in any patient with a history of hypertension after general anaesthesia or trauma. Finally, monitoring for pheochromocytoma should be initiated in patients with medullary carcinoma of the thyroid or a family history of MEN type II or type III.

To summarize, no single test or 24-hour urine sample is sufficient to define the diagnosis. If clinical suspicion is high, it is justifiable to analyze more than one urine sample and to order determinations of free catecholamines and the metabolites. Appropriate patients should be screened with 24-hour urinary fractionated free catecholamine analysis, preferably analyzed by HPLC methods combined with electrochemical detection or other specific methods. Equivocal results should be confirmed by the analysis of 24-hour urine VMA or metanephrines. There has been recent interest in the determination of fractionated metanephrines by HPLC. The analytical procedure is more complicated than that for

fractionated catecholamines but may prove to be more sensitive as a screen. These tests may have to be performed on more than one occasion. In patients with episodic hypertension, an analysis of a random urine sample for fractionated free catecholamines may be useful. In very difficult cases, a clonidine suppression test combined with plasma catecholamine measurements may be useful.

Part II: Hypertension
DEFINITION AND CRITERIA

Chronic hypertension is a common health problem in industrialized countries, with approximately 25% of the adult population affected. The higher the individual's blood pressure the greater the risk is for developing heart disease, stroke, renal failure, and peripheral vascular disease. The risk for development of these complications extends down to blood pressure values below the population mean. Therefore, any definition of hypertension is purely arbitrary. Other factors such as cigarette smoking and hyperlipidemia increase the risk for hypertension-associated complications.

The criteria for hypertension defined by the World Health Organization (WHO) are a systolic blood pressure greater than 160 mm Hg or a diastolic blood pressure of greater than 90 mm Hg (Table 46-2). It is important not to make the diagnosis of hypertension on the basis of a single measurement, since the stress of visiting a physician may be sufficient to elevate blood pressure in some persons.

It is important to recognize hypertension, since it is treatable, and treatment reduces the incidence of complications. Laboratory testing can be used to monitor the course of some of the complications of hypertension and also, importantly, to screen patients for potentially curable secondary hypertension. This may save the hypertensive patient from life-long expensive medical therapy; the extensiveness and expense of medical therapy may themselves be associated with complications.

Table 46-2   Clinical classification of blood pressure

	Blood pressure (mm Hg)	Category
Diastolic	<85	Normal
	85-89	High normal
	90-104	Mild hypertension
	105-114	Moderate hypertension
	≥115	Severe hypertension
Systolic (Diastolic <90)	<140	Normal
	140-159	Borderline isolated systolic hypertension
	≥160	Isolated systolic hypertension

FACTORS REGULATING NORMAL BLOOD PRESSURE

To better understand the pathophysiology of hypertension, it is necessary briefly to review factors responsible for normal blood pressure regulation. Cardiac output and peripheral vascular resistance are the primary determinants of systemic blood pressure. Cardiac output is determined by plasma volume, cardiac stroke volume (the volume of blood expelled from the heart with each contraction), heart rate, and myocardial contractility. Peripheral vascular resistance is a function of the balance of humoral vasoconstriction (to increase blood pressure) and vasodilatation (to decrease blood pressure), adrenergic activity, and arteriole smooth muscle tone. Ordinarily blood pressure is adjusted to maintain sufficient organ perfusion without producing organ or vascular damage. Several systems play a role in modulating cardiac output and peripheral vascular resistance. These are the arterial baroreceptor reflex, the body fluid or plasma volume regulatory system, and vascular autoregulation.

Baroreceptors in the aortic arch and carotid arteries sense the perfusion pressure and wall tension. Through the afferent autonomic nervous system, these then signal the brainstem to modulate efferent adrenergic and vagal nerve activity, which in turn regulates myocardial contractility, heart rate, and peripheral vascular resistance. The release of antidiuretic hormone from the hypothalamus is regulated by plasma osmolality and blood pressure. This hormone enhances water resorption by the kidney. The renin-angiotensin system stimulates aldosterone release when blood pressure or sodium concentration drops and leads to sodium and water conservation. Angiotensin II generated by this cascade is also a potent vasoconstrictor. This system has been described in greater detail earlier in this chapter.

The arterioles have the intrinsic capability to alter muscular tone in response to local perfusion pressures. With this vascular autoregulatory system, when cardiac output rises, the arterioles constrict to protect capillaries and tissues from hyperperfusion.

All these systems work together when there is a change in blood pressure. Table 46-3 summarizes some of the factors that play a role in regulating blood pressure. Through our understanding of the physiology of blood pressure control, newer specific therapeutic agents have evolved for treating hypertension.

PATHOLOGICAL CONDITIONS

In the majority of patients the cause of the hypertension is unknown. Definable causes such as renal vascular disease, chronic renal failure, and endocrine abnormalities are uncommon and account for 5% to 10% of cases at most. Unknown genetic and environmental factors may play a role in the approximately 95% of patients with "essential," or "primary," hypertension. There is some evidence that salt intake, alcohol intake, and obesity may have important influences.

It is beyond the scope of this chapter to delve into the many theories behind the mechanisms leading to primary hypertension. It can be most simply stated that the final common pathway is increased peripheral arteriolar vasoconstriction. The initiating factor is not known.

Primary hypertension

The two broad categories in hypertension are primary, or "essential," hypertension and secondary hypertension. The cause of primary hypertension is unknown, and it is improbable that there is a single cause to explain the diversity of hemodynamic pathophysiologic derangements in this condition. Hereditary and environmental factors (salt intake, stress, obesity, and alcohol) may play a role. The sympathetic nervous system and the renin-angiotensin system have been most often implicated as the source of the problem. A high resting pulse rate is sometimes an early predictor of subsequent hypertension. Some but not all hypertensive individuals have higher than normal catecholamine output. Plasma renin activity is usually normal in hypertensives, but it may be suppressed in some (approximately 25%) and elevated in others (approximately 15%). The ma-

---

Table 46-3   Factors that regulate blood pressure

Factor	Site of synthesis	Mechanism and sites of action
Arterial baroreflex activators		
Epinephrine	Adrenal medulla	Vasodilatation of arterioles of skeletal muscle; vasoconstriction of arterioles of skin, mucous membranes, and viscera; increases in rate and force of cardiac contraction
Norepinephrine	Terminals of sympathetic nervous system	General vasoconstriction
Body fluid volume regulators		
Antidiuretic hormone (ADH)	Neurohypophysis	Enhanced water reabsorption; increased plasma volume
Aldosterone	Adrenal cortex	Renal tubular sodium reabsorption; increased plasma volume
Renin	Juxtaglomerular cells of kidney	Converts angiotensinogen to angiotensin I
Angiotensin-converting enzyme	Lung	Converts angiotensin I to angiotensin II (potent vasoconstrictor, stimulates aldosterone production)
Vascular autoregulation	Tissue/organ specific	Local mechanisms to maintain constant tissue perfusion

lignant (accelerating) phase of hypertension is nearly always accompanied by increased renin.

Initially there may be a single derangement, but hypertension appears to beget hypertension, and other mechanisms become involved as the hypertension continues over time. This may explain why secondary hypertension is not always cured when the primary defect has been corrected.

Many other factors have been implicated. Whether these are causative or simply epiphenomenal is not known. There are reported defects in sodium transport across cell walls either attributable to Na^+, K^+-ATPase dysfunction or because of increased sodium permeability. It is also speculated that hypertension may result from a deficiency of vasodilators rather than an excess of vasoconstrictors. At this point there is no single unifying hypothesis.

Secondary hypertension

Although secondary causes of hypertension account for only 5% to 10% of all cases, they are important to recognize because of the possibility of a more specific medical therapy or surgical cure. Table 46-4 summarizes the major causes of hypertension.

Renal disease. A leading cause of secondary hypertension is renal disease. Glomerulonephritis, pyelonephritis, polycystic renal disease, renin-secreting tumors, and chronic renal failure are all associated with hypertension.

Renovascular hypertension. Stenosis, or occlusion of one or both main renal arteries or branches, can cause hypertension by stimulating release of renin from the juxtaglomerular cells of the affected kidney. Greater than 60% occlusion is required to have a significant hemodynamic effect. In patients who are older than 50 years of age, atherosclerosis is the most important cause. In younger patients

Table 46-4 Principle causes of hypertension

	Cause	Relative incidence (%)
I	Primary hypertension	90-95
II	Renal disease	4-5
III	Renovascular hypertension	2-5
IV	Drug- or exogenous agent–induced hypertension	<2
	Oral contraceptives	
	Sympathetic amines (decongestants)	
	Licorice	
	High-dose corticosteroids	
V	Endocrine	<2
	Conn's syndrome	
	Cushing's syndrome	
	Pheochromocytoma	
	Primary hyperparathyroidism	
	Hypothyroidism	
	Hyperthyroidism	
	Acromegaly	
	Congenital adrenal hyperplasia (17-hydroxylase and 11-hydroxylase deficiencies)	
VI	Coarctation of the aorta	<1

fibromuscular dysplasia is the leading cause. Renovascular hypertension, or renal artery stenosis, is the most frequent cause of curable secondary hypertension, but it is discovered in only about 2% of hypertensive patients. Renovascular hypertension should be suspected when hypertension develops rapidly in those less than 30 or more than 55 years of age, or when there is sudden worsening of previously stable hypertension. The most important physical finding is a systolic-diastolic bruit in the epigastrium, but this sign is present in only 50% of patients.

Drug-induced hypertension. Many drugs may cause hypertension. Oral contraceptives may cause a mild degree of hypertension through an increase in the liver production of angiotensinogen (renin substrate). Oral contraceptives may also cause, directly, some degree of sodium retention. Licorice and carbenoxolone, by enhancing mineralocorticoid activity, also causes sodium and water retention. Nasal decongestants can cause hypertension through vasoconstriction. Administered glucocorticoids given in excess will also increase mineralocorticoid activity. The above are just a few examples of drug-induced causes of hypertension.

Coarctation of the aorta. Coarctation of the aorta is usually first identified in childhood. In this condition there is an arterial defect with a fibrous aortic stricture reducing blood flow to the lower body and extremities. The result is restricted blood flow to the kidneys and, as a consequence, activation of the renin-angiotensin system. These patients will then have upper extremity hypertension relative to the lower extremities. A soft bruit, louder in the back, is often heard over the coarctation site. Femoral pulses are diminished and delayed when compared to the brachial pulses.

Endocrine causes of hypertension. Several adrenal disorders are associated with hypertension. These include Cushing's syndrome, pheochromocytoma, and Conn's syndrome. The causes, clinical features, and laboratory investigation of these problems are summarized in the first section of this chapter. Other endocrine disorders that may be associated with hypertension are acromegaly, primary hyperparathyroidism (50% are hypertensive), hypothyroidism (rarely hypertensive), and thyrotoxicosis (high systolic blood pressure).

COMPLICATIONS OF HYPERTENSION

Blood pressure may gradually rise over many years, and the patient may remain asymptomatic for a long time. Hypertension is usually discovered during a routine physical examination. Unfortunately it is too often discovered after vital organ injury has already occurred, such as ischemic injury to the brain after a stroke or cardiac injury after a myocardial infarct. Headache and light-headedness, symptoms sometimes associated with hypertension, are seen in less than 25% of patients, and the physical examination is usually unremarkable. Years of uncontrolled hypertension may produce damage to several vital organs, in particular the eyes, the brain, the heart, the kidneys, and the aorta.

In the eyes, retinal hemorrhages, exudates, and papilledema may occur. Hypertension is a very important risk factor for stroke. Peripheral resistance in hypertension is high, a condition that increases afterload on the left ventricle, causing left ventricular hypertrophy. Hypertension also accelerates atherogenesis. Long-standing hypertension induces both vascular and glomerular damage in kidneys, causing nephrosclerosis. The renal blood vessels show fibrous atherosclerotic thickening and narrowing of the lumen. The kidneys' ability to regulate blood flow becomes impaired. Glomerulosclerosis also is initiated with resulting increase in proteinuria. This will eventually lead to the loss of the glomerular filtration rate and end-stage renal disease. Large-vessel atherosclerosis, including that of the aorta, is accelerated by hypertension. Aortic aneurysm and intramural dissection may occur. Aneurysms evolve slowly and may be asymptomatic, whereas a dissection is always a painful episode often accompanied by shock.

CHANGE OF ANALYTE WITH DISEASE

Once hypertension has been identified in a patient through multiple determinations of blood pressure, a simple minimum evaluation should be initiated. See the box for a summary. This evaluation serves three main purposes: (1) to exclude treatable causes of secondary hypertension, (2) to detect evidence of organ damage, (3) to identify other risk factors that may accelerate cardiovascular disease. This evaluation mainly involves inexpensive, high-volume laboratory tests. The choice of these tests is justified below.

Urinalysis. Routine urinalysis can detect proteinuria, hematuria, and glycosuria. Proteinuria and hematuria may be attributable to hypertensive nephrosclerosis or to intrinsic renal disease, which may in fact be the cause of the hypertension. A renal biopsy is required to distinguish the cause if an abnormality is observed. The presence of proteinuria in a hypertensive patient may be suggestive of a bad prognosis. There has been some interest in diagnosing this problem earlier using sensitive assays for albumin (microalbuminuria) analogous to diabetic nephropathy. It may be possible to reverse the process, for example, by the use of angiotensin-converting enzyme inhibitors. The presence of glycosuria, which is suggestive of diabetes mellitus, will affect the choice of antihypertensive therapy. For example,

thiazide diuretics are contraindicated in diabetes because they can exacerbate glucose intolerance. It is also possible that the glucose intolerance may be secondary to other endocrine causes of hypertension such as pheochromocytoma, Cushing's syndrome, or acromegaly.

Sodium. An elevated sodium is not a sensitive or specific test, but it may be elevated in some patients with primary hyperaldosteronism. Another consideration is that serum sodium may be decreased in hypertensive patients receiving thiazide or loop diuretics. This test is therefore also important for monitoring patients undergoing diuretic therapy.

Potassium. The finding of a low potassium value is a very important clue in a hypertensive patient not receiving medication, suggestive of the possibility of either primary (Conn's syndrome) or secondary (that is, renal artery stenosis) hyperaldosteronism. Also, serum potassium levels may be raised in patients with acute or chronic renal failure and lowered in patients receiving diuretics.

Creatinine. Creatinine is a specific screen for renal impairment that may be caused by hypertension or be the cause of hypertension. Creatinine should be assessed on presentation and on an annual basis in all hypertensives.

Calcium. The serum calcium level is elevated in primary hyperparathyroidism, which is one of the causes of hypertension. About 50% of patients with this problem will be hypertensive. It is of interest that despite this connection the blood pressure most often does not normalize after surgical cure. Another consideration is that thiazide diuretics can rarely cause hypercalcemia and thus should be excluded before one pursues the diagnosis of primary hyperparathyroidism.

Uric acid. Uric acid is elevated in about 40% of patients with essential hypertension. The connection is unclear but is more common in patients with renal failure. Uric acid levels may also be elevated by thiazide diuretics, in some cases leading to gout.

Glucose. An elevated fasting plasma glucose greater than 1400 mg/L on two or more occasions is sufficient to allow one to diagnose diabetes mellitus. About 50% of diabetics have hypertension, and up to 10% of hypertensive patients are diabetic. Calcium-channel blockers and angiotensin-converting enzyme inhibitors are the preferred antihypertensive drugs in diabetics. Thiazide diuretics and beta-blockers should be avoided.

Cholesterol. The presence of hyperlipidemia is an important risk factor for atherosclerosis along with hypertension. The presence of hyperlipidemia is a contraindication for the use of some antihypertensive medications, such as beta-blockers and thiazide diuretics, which may exacerbate the lipid problem.

Electrocardiogram. An electrocardiogram should be obtained in all cases to assess cardiac status as a baseline parameter and to determine if left ventricular hypertrophy is present.

Minimum Evaluation of the Hypertensive Individual

Complete history and physical examination
Serum creatinine, sodium, potassium, glucose, uric acid, cholesterol, and triglyceride concentrations
Hemoglobin
Urinalysis
Electrocardiogram

Chest x-ray film. A chest x-ray film may identify aortic dilatation or elongation and rib notching, which may occur in coarctation of the aorta.

Gamma-glutamyltranspeptidase. This is an optional test that serves as a screen for alcohol abuse. Alcohol consumption may elevate blood pressure acutely and chemically. One ounce of alcohol per day, equivalent to about two drinks, will raise the systolic blood pressure by an average of 2 to 6 mm Hg.

SECONDARY STUDIES

Clues from the history, physical examination, and the basic laboratory studies may indicate a possible secondary cause for the hypertension. Some of these clues include:

1. Abrupt onset of severe hypertension, or onset before 25 years of age or after 50 may be suggestive of pheochromocytoma or renovascular disease.
2. A history of palpitations, anxiety attacks, sweating, hyperglycemia and weight loss may be suggestive of pheochromocytoma.
3. An abdominal bruit may be suggestive of renovascular disease.
4. Bilateral upper abdominal mass on physical examination may imply polycystic kidney disease.
5. Abnormal renal function test results may be suggestive of renal insufficiency.
6. Hypokalemia in an untreated hypertensive or easily provoked hypokalemia should be a trigger to look for hyperaldosteronism, or Conn's syndrome.

The investigation of adrenal disorders with associated hypertension is discussed earlier in this chapter. Other endocrine causes of hypertension are suspected on clinical grounds, and laboratory investigations for these disorders are reviewed in other chapters. The focus at this point will be on the investigation of renovascular hypertension.

Renovascular hypertension. The standard screening test for renal vascular hypertension has been the rapid-sequence intravenous pyelogram (IVP). Abnormalities of contrast excretion and kidney shape and size may be suggestive of this disorder. The definitive test for surgically correctable renal artery stenosis until recently has been the combination of a renal angiogram and renal-vein renin determinations. The angiogram can identify the stenotic lesion, whereas the bilateral renal vein catheterization and subsequent measurement of renin activity confirm the functional significance of the observed lesion. The narrow renal artery supplies less blood to the affected kidney, and renin secretion will be higher on this side. A renal-vein renin ratio of greater than 1.5:1 is associated with cure or amelioration of hypertension after angioplasty or surgical intervention in 80% of cases. Before performance of this test the patient must not be receiving beta-blockers, which may suppress renin, and should be on a low-salt diet for 4 days.

Another screening procedure is the captopril renogram, which provides an indirect measure of the glomerular filtration rate and its dependence on angiotensin II. In this test renal uptake of radiolabeled diethylenetriaminepentaacetic acid (DTPA) or *o*-iodohippurate sodium (Hippuran) is measured before and after ACE inhibition with captopril. An abnormal result indicates that the stenosis is functionally significant and will respond to revascularization. This test has replaced renal-vein renin assessment in some centers. Pharmacologic screening with an ACE inhibitor is another sensitive but not highly specific means of assessing patients suspected of having renovascular hypertension. Administration of the ACE inhibitor (that is, captopril) normally leads to an increase in plasma renin activity and a drop in blood pressure. This response is exaggerated in patients with renovascular hypertension. The problem is that there are false-positive results.

Angioplasty is the initial treatment of choice for renal artery stenosis. It works best in younger patients with fibromuscular dysplasia. If angioplasty is unsuccessful or if restenosis occurs, the angioplasty procedure may be repeated. If this fails, surgical revascularization should be attempted.

DRUG THERAPY

Although medical therapy is beyond the scope of this chapter, it is of value to summarize briefly the major classes of drugs used in the initial treatment of hypertension, primarily focusing on the metabolic complications that may result from their use. Some patients will be receiving several of these drugs. In recent years there has been a gradual shift from dependence on diuretics and beta-blockers to use of ACE inhibitors and calcium-channel blockers to control blood pressure because of the lower incidence of side effects. Effectiveness of drug therapy is best assessed by routine monitoring of blood pressure and patient history.

Diuretics. The group of approximately 50 different drugs called diuretics promotes the formation and excretion of urine with the intent in hypertension to reduce extracellular fluid volume. In large doses they can cause hypovolemia, electrolyte imbalance, and prerenal failure. Diuretics can also be associated with sexual dysfunction in males. Metabolic side effects include hypokalemia, hypomagnesemia, hyperuricemia, hyperglycemia, and hyperlipidemia. Despite these disadvantages, diuretics are effective and inexpensive, and most of the side effects are minimal if the patient is properly managed and monitored.

Beta-adrenergic receptor blockers. Drugs that block beta-adrenergic receptors decrease the rate and force of cardiac contractions, among other effects. If the patient has diabetes mellitus, chronic occlusive peripheral arterial disease, or chronic obstructive pulmonary disease, cardioselective beta-blockers should be used. These do not completely eliminate complications in the above patients, however. Like diuretics, beta-blockers can cause sexual dysfunction and some metabolic disturbances such as impaired glucose tolerance or decreased high-density-lipoprotein cholesterol and increases in serum total cholesterol and triglycerides.

Angiotensin-converting enzyme (ACE) inhibitors. ACE inhibitors block the conversion of angiotensin I to angiotensin II, which is a stimulator of aldosterone release and a potent vasoconstrictor. This group of drugs has a low reported incidence of side effects. ACE inhibitors neither cause sexual dysfunction in males nor adversely affect lipids, glucose, or uric acid, though they tend to increase potassium. ACE inhibitors reduce proteinuria in patients with diabetic nephropathy and may retard glomerulosclerosis by selectively dilating the efferent arteriole, reducing glomerular capillary pressure without compromising blood flow. ACE inhibitors can cause acute renal failure in patients with severe renal artery stenosis and, in large doses, can cause nephrotic syndrome, nephritis, and leukopenia.

Calcium antagonists. Calcium antagonists are potent peripheral vasodilators and reduce blood pressure by decreasing peripheral resistance. Verapamil has a direct effect on the myocardium. Calcium antagonists do not have adverse metabolic side effects but are as expensive as ACE inhibitors.

BIBLIOGRAPHY
General

Baxter J, Tyrell JB: The adrenal cortex. In Felig P et al, editors: *Endocrinology and metabolism,* ed 2, New York, 1987, McGraw-Hill.

Besser GM, Cudworth AG, editors: *Clinical endocrinology: an illustrated text,* Philadelphia, 1987, Lippincott.

Howanitz PJ, Howanitz JH: Hormones. In Howanitz PJ, Howanitz JH, editors: *Laboratory medicine,* New York, 1991, Churchill Livingstone.

Orth DN, Kovacs WJ, DeBold CR: The adrenal cortex. In Wilson JD, Foster DW, editors: *Williams' textbook of endocrinology,* ed 8, Philadelphia, 1992, Saunders.

Williams GH, Dluhy RG: Diseases of the adrenal cortex. In Wilson JD et al, editors: *Harrison's principles of internal medicine,* ed 12, New York, 1991, McGraw-Hill.

Mineralocorticoids

Bravo EL, Tarazi RC, Dustan HP, et al: The changing clinical spectrum of primary aldosteronism, *Am J Med* 74:64-651, 1983.

Lyons DF, Kem DC, Brown RD, et al: Single dose captopril as a diagnostic test for primary aldosteronism, *J Clin Endocrinol Metab* 57:892-896, 1983.

Melby J: Diagnosis of hyperaldosteronism, *Endocrinol Metab Clin North Am* 20(2):247-255, 1991.

Scully RE, Marj EJ, McNeely WF, McNeely BV: Case records of the Massachusetts General Hospital, *N Engl J Med* 326:1617-1623, 1992.

Short F, James VHT: Primary hyperaldosteronism in England and Wales: a review of the use of a supraregional assay service laboratory for the measurement of aldosterone and plasma renin activity, *Ann Clin Biochem* 28:218-225, 1991.

Steigerwalt SP: Unraveling the causes of hypertension and hypokalemia, *Hosp Pract* 30(7):67-79, 1995.

Ulick S: Two uncommon causes of mineralocorticoid excess, *Endocrinol Metab Clin North Am* 20(2):269-276, 1991.

Glucocorticoids

Baxter JD: The effects of glucocorticoid therapy, *Hosp Pract* (Off Ed) 27(9):111-114, 115-118, 123, passim, 1992.

Chrousos GP: The hypothalamic-pituitary-adrenal axis and immune-mediated inflammation, *N Engl J Med* 332:1351-1362, 1995.

Findling J: Cushing's syndrome—an etiological work-up, *Hosp Pract* 27(10):107-122, 1992.

Freeman DA: Steroid hormone–producing tumors of the adrenal, ovary and testes, *Endocrinol Metab Clin North Am* 20(4):751-766, 1991.

Godl PW, Loriaux DL, Roy A, et al: Responses to CRH in hypercortisolism of depression and Cushing's disease, *N Engl J Med* 314:1329-1335, 1986.

Grua JR, Nelson DH: ACTH producing pituitary tumors, *Endocrinol Metab Clin North Am* 20(2):319-362, 1991.

Hermus AR, Pesmon GJ, Benraad TJ, et al: The CRH test versus the high-dose dexamethasone test in the differential diagnosis of Cushing's syndrome, *Lancet* 2:540-544, 1986.

Kaye TB, Crapo L: The Cushing syndrome: an update on diagnostic tests, *Ann Intern Med* 112:434-444, 1990.

Lacroix A, Bolte D, Tremblay J: Gastric inhibitory polypeptide–dependent cortisol hypersecretion, a new cause of Cushing's syndrome, *N Engl J Med* 327:914-980, 1992.

Loriaux DL: The treatment of Cushing's syndrome and adrenal cancer, *Endocrinol Metab Clin North Am* 20(4):767-771, 1991.

Loriaux DL, Nieman L: Corticotrophin-releasing hormone testing in pituitary disease, *Endocrinol Metab Clin North Am* 29(2):363-369, 1991.

Oldfield EH, Doppman JL, Lynette KN, et al: Petrosal sinus sampling with and without corticotrophin-releasing hormone for the differential diagnosis of Cushing's syndrome, *N Engl J Med* 325:897-905, 1991.

Orth DN: Differential diagnosis of Cushing's syndrome, *N Engl J Med* 325:957-959, 1991.

Adrenal androgens

Parker LN: Control of adrenal androgen secretion, *Endocrinol Metab Clin North Am* 290(2):401-421, 1991.

Meikle WA, Dagnes RA, Aranco BA: Adrenal androgen secretion and biologic effects, *Endocrinol Metab Clin North Am* 29(2):381-400, 1991.

Catecholamines

Bravo EL, Tarazi RC, Fouad RM, et al: Clonidine-suppression test: a useful aid in the diagnosis of pheochromocytoma, *N Engl J Med* 305:623, 1981.

Bravo EL, Tarazi RC: Plasma catecholamines in clinical investigation: a useful index or a meaningless number? *J Lab Clin Med* 100:155-162, 1982.

Bravo EL, Gifford RW: Pheochromocytoma: diagnosis, localization and management, *N Engl J Med* 311:1298-1303, 1984.

Cryer PE: Diagnosis of the sympathochromaffin system. In Felig P et al, editors: *Endocrinology and metabolism,* ed 2, New York, 1987, McGraw-Hill.

Landsberg L, Young JB: Pheochromocytoma. In Wilson JD et al, editors: *Harrison's principles of internal medicine,* ed 12, New York, 1991, McGraw-Hill.

Landsberg L, Young JB: Catecholamines and the adrenal medulla. In Wilson JD, Foster DW, editors: *William's textbook of endocrinology,* ed 8, Philadelphia, 1992, Saunders.

Ross GA, Newbould EC, Thomas J, et al: Plasma and 24-hour urinary catecholamine concentrations in normal and patient populations, *Ann Clin Biochem* 3990:38-44, 1993.

Shepps SG, Jiang N, Klee GC: Diagnostic evaluation of pheochromocytoma, *Endocrinol Metab Clin North Am* 17(2):397-414, 1988.

Shepps SG, Jiang N, Klee GC, Heerden JA: Recent developments in the diagnosis and treatment of pheochromocytoma, *Mayo Clin Proc* 65:88-95, 1991.

Smythe GA, Edwards G, Graham P, Lazarus L: Biochemical diagnosis of pheochromocytoma by simultaneous measurement of urinary excretion of epinephrine and norepinephrine, *Clin Chem* 38:486-492, 1992.

Stenström G, Sjögren B, Waldenström J: Excretion of adrenalin, noradrenaline, vanilmandelic acid and metanephrines in 64 patients with pheochromocytoma, *Acta Med Scand* 214:145-152, 1983.

Hypertension

Harvey JM, Beevers DG: Biochemical investigation of hypertension, *Ann Clin Biochem* 27:287-296, 1990.

Mahrensmith RL: Hypertension. In Abuelo JG, editor: Renal pathophysiology—the essentials, Baltimore, 1989, Williams & Wilkins.

Oparil S: Arterial hypertension. In Wyngaarden JB et al, editors: *Cecil textbook of medicine,* ed 19, Philadelphia, 1992, Saunders.

Williams GH: Hypertensive vascular disease. In Wilson JD, et al, editors: *Harrison's principles of internal medicine,* ed 12, New York, 1991, McGraw-Hill.

The 1988 report on the Joint National Committee on Detection, Evaluation and Treatment of High Blood Pressure, *Arch Intern Med* 148:1023-1038, 1988.

Miscellaneous

Migeon CJ, Donohue PA: Congenital adrenal hyperplasia caused by 21-hydroxylase deficiency, *Endocrinol Metab Clin North Am* 29(2):277-206, 1991.

Miller WL: Congenital adrenal hyperplasias, *Endocrinol Metab Clin North Am* 20(4):721-749, 1991.

Moser HW, Bergin A, Naida S, Ladenson PW: Adrenoleukodystrophy, *Endocrinol Metab Clin North Am* 29(2):297-318, 1991.

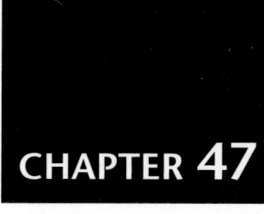

CHAPTER 47

Diseases of genetic origin

Thaddeus E. Kelly
Revised by Donald L. Rucknagel

———————————■———————————

———————————■———————————

OBJECTIVES

■ Briefly describe the chromosome abnormality associated with the following pathological disorders: Down's syndrome, Turner's syndrome, Klinefelter's syndrome, chronic myelogenous leukemia, Fanconi anemia, and fragile X syndrome.

■ Briefly describe the metabolic disorder in each of the following and state the primary abnormal clinical chemistry results:

Gaucher's disease
Niemann-Pick disease
Tay-Sachs disease
Hurler's syndrome
Phenylketonuria
Maple-syrup urine disease
Galactosemia
Fanconi syndrome
von Gierke's disease
Vitamin D–resistant rickets
Wilson's disease
Familial hypercholesterolemia
Lesch-Nyhan syndrome
Leber's optic atrophy and myopathies caused by mitochondrial mutations
Zellweger's cerebrohepatorenal syndrome

■ Describe the role of genetic screening in the diagnosis of genetic disease.

KEY TERMS

allele One of various forms of a gene that may appear at a specific locus.

amniocentesis A transabdominal aspiration of the uterus by syringe to obtain amniotic fluid.

aneuploidy A chromosomal abnormality caused by the addition or absence of an entire chromosome.

autosomal Pertaining to any of the 22 chromosomes except the X and Y chromosomes.

Barr body The condensation of nuclear (genetic) material of the inactivated X chromosome.

chromosome Nuclear structure containing a linear array of genes. Humans have 23 pairs of chromosomes.

diploid The duplicate representation of each gene and chromosome.

dominant trait A trait that is expressed or determined by the heterozygous presence of an allele at the locus on the chromosome.

Down's syndrome A condition characterized by mental retardation and physical abnormalities caused by trisomy of chromosome 21.

dysmorphogenesis Physical defects caused by intrinsically altered embryonic development.

exon The portion of a gene that codes for the amino acid sequence of a protein.

galactosemia A toxicity syndrome associated with intolerance to dietary galactose and characterized by deficiency of the enzyme galactose-1-phosphate uridyl transferase.

gene The smallest biological unit of heredity, located on specific sites of specific chromosomes. A gene contains the encoding for one specific protein.

gene clones Colonies of bacteria derived from a single progenitor bacterium containing plasmids into which a human gene or DNA fragment has been spliced.

Guthrie test A microbiologic assay for serum phenylalanine; used to screen for phenylketonuria.

haplotype The alleles of linked genes contributed by either of the biological parents.

heteroplasmic Pertaining to presence of both abnormal and normal mitochondria in cells.

heteronuclear RNA The initial RNA transcription product of a gene containing both coding sequences (exons) and noncoding sequences (introns).

heterozygous Pertaining to a state in which a pair of alleles are dissimilar at both positions of the same locus.

homozygous Pertaining to a state in which a pair of alleles are the same at both positions of the same locus.

intron (intervening sequence) A sequence composed of a few or several thousands of base pairs interposed in structural genes.

karyotype The chromosomal makeup of a nucleated cell.

Lesch-Nyhan syndrome A rare X-linked error of purine metabolism characterized by mental retardation and self-mutilation. There is a deficiency of the enzyme hypoxanthine-guanine phosphoribosyl transferase.

locus The particular location on a given chromosome occupied by a structural gene.

lyonization A process of random inactivation of an X chromosome to compensate for the double-gene dosage of two X chromosomes in females.

meiosis Segregation of genes and chromosomes with reduction from a diploid to a haploid number in sperm and egg formation.

mitogen A chemical substance that induces cells in culture to divide.

monosomy Absence of one chromosome from an otherwise diploid cell. Only known disorder is absence of Y or X chromosome in Turner's syndrome.

phenylketonuria (PKU) An autosomal, recessively inherited disorder resulting from a defect in conversion of phenylalanine to tyrosine because of a phenylalanine hydroxylase deficiency.

polymerase chain reaction An analytic method whereby repeated replication of a restricted sequence of DNA or RNA is mediated in vitro by DNA polymerase or reverse transcriptase resulting in a manyfold amplification of the region of interest.

promotor A small DNA sequence at the 5′ end of structural genes; binding of specific proteins to promotors regulates transcription of the structural gene.

recessive trait The expression of a trait that requires that both alleles at a locus are mutated.

restriction endonuclease Enzymes that cleave DNA wherever specific sequences of four to nine base pairs occur.

Tay-Sachs disease Infantile form of a recessive hereditary disorder caused by a defect in lipid metabolism in which sphingolipids accumulate in the brain, resulting in progressive mental and physical degeneration. The disease occurs primarily in children of Jewish ancestry.

trait An observable feature of an organism that is visually apparent or laboratory derived.

translocation A term used in genetics to describe the movement of a portion of one chromosome into the structure of another.

trisomy Presence of one additional chromosome of a specific pair in an otherwise diploid cell ($2n + 1$ chromosomes). See *Down's syndrome*.

Turner's syndrome A condition consisting of absent ovarian function, short stature, and physical anomalies; most commonly caused by a 45,X karyotype.

X-linked Pertaining to a trait carried on the X chromosome.

GENETIC BASIS OF INHERITANCE

In the 1860s, after a series of simple experiments, Gregor Mendel proposed two laws regarding the transmission of traits across generations. In the first law Mendel stated that the segregation of factors determining a trait followed predictable patterns and that one could anticipate the proportion of offspring expressing various forms of a given trait. The second law, the law of independent assortment, stated that the inheritance of one trait had no effect on the inheritance of a second trait. Approximately 40 years later, with the capability of observing cellular division under the microscope, it was recognized that the behavior of chromosomes during cellular division was consistent with the predictions made by Mendel regarding the segregation of traits. We now recognize that the factors described by Mendel are genes and that these are carried by chromosomes the segregation of which can be observed in cellular division.

A large number of inherited diseases have been shown to be caused by the structural abnormality of a protein that is the product of a defective gene. The genes responsible for most of the major inherited diseases have now been cloned and their DNA sequenced, some without the protein involved being identified first. The following is not a comprehensive review but, rather, uses specific examples to illustrate the current state of our knowledge of inherited diseases.

Chemical basis

Genes are composed of DNA and, occasionally (in viruses), RNA. DNA and RNA are made up of nucleotide sequences. A triplet code of nucleic acid pairs encodes the sequence of amino acids in polypeptide chains. A gene might be defined as the amount of DNA equivalent to a polypeptide chain. *Eukaryotic genes* are more complex than those of bacterial or viral genes, however, and contain blocks of nucleotides, composed of several hundred to many thousands of base pairs, inserted into the coding sequence. These inserted sequences, called *intervening sequences,* or *introns,* are transcribed along with the coding sequences to form *het-*

eronuclear RNA (hnRNA) in the nucleus of the cell. To convert hnRNA to messenger RNA, the hnRNA must be processed, whereby a cap is applied to the 5′ end, the intron (noncoding sequences) transcripts are spliced out of the hnRNA, and a polyadenylate tail is attached to the 3′ end. The resulting RNA, *messenger RNA,* serves as a template for polypeptide chain synthesis. Genes of higher organisms occupy specific locations on chromosomes and code for polypeptides that have specific physiological functions. Each polypeptide may function as a single protein or combine with other polypeptides to form a heteropolymeric functional unit. However, the basic premise remains that one structural gene encodes a unique polypeptide with a specific function (Fig. 47-1). A change in the DNA sequence of an exon of a structural gene, a mutation, will result in a structurally altered polypeptide.

Most mutational changes are single base-pair substitutions that produce single amino acid substitutions in the resultant protein or polypeptide chain. Depending on its location in the molecule an amino acid substitution may profoundly affect function or may be silent. Other mutational changes that have been documented are insertions or deletions of blocks of DNA, *frameshift mutations* caused by insertions or deletions of multiples of one or two base pairs, formation of nonsense chain-terminating codons, and base substitutions that interfere with heteronuclear RNA processing to produce complex insertions or deletions in the amino acid sequence of the gene product. Finally, some mutational changes interfere with the regulatory DNA sequences on either side of a gene to alter the rate at which ordinarily normal gene sequences are transcribed. The prototype for such changes is the β-thalassemia mutation of the hemoglobin β-chain loci. The kind of disease that results from such a mutation depends on the function of the polypeptide. Examples are illustrated in Table 47-1. The specific methods employed to detect mutations are discussed below (p. 945) and more fully in Chapter 48.

The genetic material of human cells is diploid in that each gene is represented twice, one of each pair occupying a specific location, or a locus, on each of a pair of similar, or homologous, chromosomes. The chromosomes segregate during meiosis, reducing the chromosome number from a diploid to haploid number. Humans have a chromosomal or modal number of 46 in somatic cells and 23 in gametes. Virtually every structural gene locus has a series of alleles that may occur. In most instances these alleles were created by mutations consisting of a single nucleotide change in the structure of the gene and thus a single amino acid substitution in the gene product. Many of these gene products are equally functional but may be recognized by different electrophoretic or immunological properties of the gene product. On the long arm of chromosome 1 is the locus for the Duffy blood group. At that locus, various alternative forms of the gene, or alleles, may occur giving rise to different Duffy blood types. The two most common al-

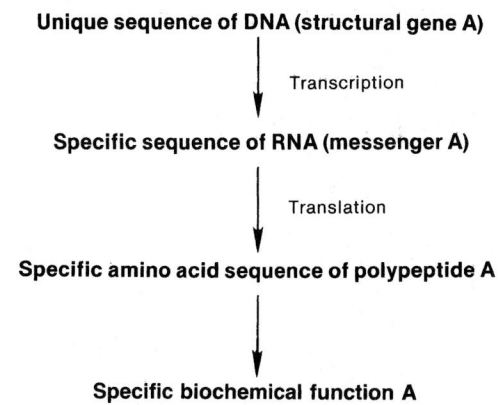

Unique sequence of DNA (structural gene A)

↓ Transcription

Specific sequence of RNA (messenger A)

↓ Translation

Specific amino acid sequence of polypeptide A

↓

Specific biochemical function A

Fig. 47-1   Sequence of events from a structural gene leading to a specific, normal biochemical function.

leles at the Duffy blood group locus are designated **a** and **b** (that is, Fy^a and Fy^b respectively). The gene products for the **a** and **b** alleles of the Duffy blood group are recognized by standard blood-typing techniques. When the pair of alleles at a given locus are the same, the person is said to be homozygous at that locus. Thus a person with the **a** allele at both positions on the pair of 1 chromosomes for the Duffy blood group is homozygous **a.** When the pair of alleles are dissimilar, such as the Duffy allele **a** and **b,** the person is a heterozygote.

A series of allelic mutations may impart a range of functional consequences on the polypeptide gene product. For example, many different mutations occur in the structural gene for the β chain of hemoglobin. This series of alleles results in functional changes in β-hemoglobin chains that range from insignificant, no disease, to lack of the gene product and severe disease, β-thalassemia.

Table 47-1   Diseases caused by various genetic mutations

Protein type	Consequences of mutation	Example
Enzyme	Loss of enzyme activity	Phenylketonuria
Hemoglobin	Altered protein aggregation	Sickle cell disease
Structural protein (cartilage collagen)	Defective bone matrix	Osteogenesis imperfecta
Receptor	Altered metabolic regulation	Familial hypercholesterolemia
Membrane protein	Altered membrane transport	Cystinuria
Coagulation protein	Defective coagulation	Hemophilia
Carrier protein	Inability to transport compound	Hemochromatosis

Single gene patterns of inheritance

The chromosomes in the pairs numbered 1 to 22 are called *autosomes,* and the chromosomes in the remaining pair are called the *sex chromosomes* (X and Y). When a trait is determined by the presence of one mutant allele at the locus on an autosome, that trait is inherited as an *autosomal dominant trait.* A person exhibiting that trait can be either homozygous (two mutant alleles) or heterozygous (one mutant allele) for that trait. When the expression of the trait requires that both genes consist of the same mutant allele, the trait is said to be an *autosomal recessive trait.* The terms *dominant* and *recessive* refer to the trait in question and not to the genes determining that trait. Whether a trait is classified as dominant or recessive can depend on the definition of what constitutes presence of the disease. For example, if one studies families with the sickle cell gene only by detecting morphologic sickling, the disease would be classed as dominantly inherited because only one gene would be sufficient to cause the trait. If, on the other hand, one uses only measurement of the total hemoglobin concentration, the disease is classed as an autosomal recessive disorder because heterozygotes and homozygotes for the normal allele would be indistinguishable. When one uses electrophoresis, all three genotypes are definable, and the trait is classified as codominantly inherited. One parent may transmit an autosomal dominant disorder to his or her offspring since a dominant disorder is determined by the presence of a single allele, but an autosomal recessively inherited disorder requires the inheritance of mutant alleles from both parents. It can be seen from Fig. 47-2 that one may inherit the carrier state for sickle cell disease from a single parent, but sickle cell disease itself must be inherited from both parents. In general, the disorders that are characterized by altered biochemical metabolism and are diagnosable through biochemical means are conditions that are autosomal recessively inherited.

The two sex chromosomes of the human male consist of an X chromosome and a Y chromosome. The human female has two X chromosomes. The enzyme glucose-6-phosphate dehydrogenase (G-6-PD) is coded for by a gene on the X chromosome. Because a female has two X chromosomes and a male has one X chromosome, it might be expected that a female would make twice as much G-6-PD as a male does. On the average, however, females and males make equal amounts of G-6-PD. There is gene dosage compensation that occurs by a mechanism called *lyonization,* or random inactivation of the X chromosome. During early embryonic development of the 46,XX female, one of the two X chromosomes is randomly inactivated; it no longer produces gene products. Because this is a random process, each female is a mosaic, or mixture, of cells in which one or the other, but not both, X chromosomes is functioning (Fig. 47-3). The presence of a Y chromosome is associated with maleness, and its absence is associated with femaleness. The Y chromosome carries a factor, called the *testis determining factor* (TDF), that induces the embryonic gonad to develop into a testis; in its absence the gonad develops as an ovary. There are no other genes residing on the Y chromosome that have been shown to code for proteins. The X chromosome carries many structural genes and codes for proteins similar to those coded for by autosomes.

The difference in the sex chromosome constitution of

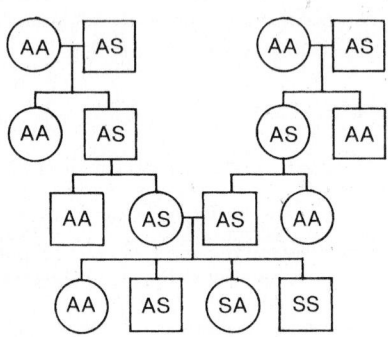

AA, Homozygous for normal hemoglobin A
AS, Heterozygous for hemoglobins A and S (sickle cell carrier)
SS, Homozygous for mutant hemoglobin S (sickle cell disease)

Fig. 47-2 Pedigree that demonstrates segregation of single-gene mutations. Heterozygous state (carrier for sickle-cell disease in this example) is inherited from a single parent, whereas homozygous state (a person affected with sickle cell disease in this example) requires inheritance of a mutant gene from each parent.

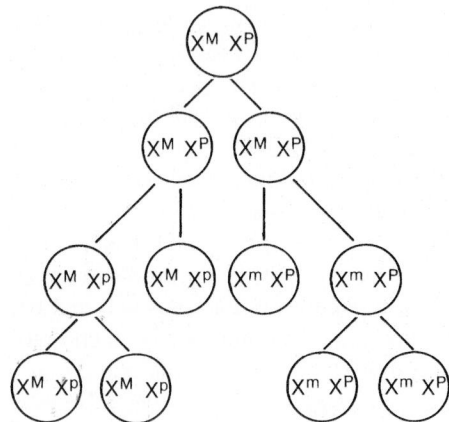

X^M, Active maternally derived X chromosome
X^P, Active paternally derived X chromosome
X^m, Inactive maternally derived X chromosome
X^P, Inactive paternally derived X chromosome

Fig. 47-3 Random inactivation of the X chromosome in the 46,XX female. Once an X chromosome is inactivated, that particular X is inactivated in all subsequent progeny of that cell.

males and females is the basis for the particular pattern of inheritance that is known as *X-linked*. If there is a mutation on the single X chromosome of a male, that male will always transmit that mutant gene to all of his daughters and to none of his sons. A heterozygous female may give either of her X chromosomes, one of which has the normal gene and one of which has the mutant gene, to a son or daughter. If the mutation on the X chromosome results in a disease when present in the heterozygous state of the female, the trait is known as an X-linked dominant disorder and will be observed in both males and females. Because the single X of the male carries a mutation, the disease is usually more severe in the male than in the female who has a mutant gene and a normal gene. If the mutation is not expressed as a recognizable trait in the heterozygous state of the female, the disorder is X-linked recessively inherited. Males will manifest the disorder and females will carry but not manifest the gene for the disorder. Females are carriers for hemophilia and Duchenne muscular dystrophy, but the disease occurs among males who have a single copy of the mutant gene. There are tests that will identify the carrier female for most X-linked recessive diseases. In general these tests demonstrate a partial expression in females of the defect seen in affected males.

Many traits such as height and intelligence and isolated birth defects such as cleft lip and congenital heart disease are determined by the joint action of many genes and the environment. This mode of inheritance is called *multifactorial causation*. Such traits are familial and have a major genetic input but do not segregate in families in a manner similar to that seen for autosomal dominant and recessive traits. An expressed trait is the consequence of numerous genes received from each parent and a variable environmental influence that determines the expression of the trait. In addition to isolated birth defects seen in infants, multifactorial causation is responsible for many common diseases of adults. Examples include insulin-independent diabetes mellitus, osteoarthritis, gout, and certain forms of hypertension and coronary artery disease.

PATHOLOGICAL DISORDERS ASSOCIATED WITH ABNORMAL CHROMOSOMES
Aneuploidy

Disorders that occur as the result of a chromosome abnormality involve a change in the gene dosage for a large number of genes rather than a change in the gene structure. This produces a change in the blueprint for the structural development of the embryo. Such an abnormality can come about in two ways. First, there is the presence or absence of an entire chromosome, an aneuploidy. This is exemplified by the presence of an extra 21 chromosome in trisomy 21, which causes Down's syndrome, and by the presence of a single X chromosome resulting in monosomy, which occurs in Turner's syndrome. Trisomy means the presence of three copies of a chromosome rather than the normal two, and

monosomy means the presence of single copy. Second, there are structural alterations in chromosomes that result in the loss or addition of part but not all of a chromosome. A variety of structural abnormalities of chromosomes can lead to such a deviation from the normal amount of chromosomal material.

Chromosomal abnormalities involving the autosomes, whether they involve a partial or a complete loss or addition of a chromosome, always result in altered morphogenesis expressed as major and minor birth defects and altered mental development in the form of mental retardation. The altered physical development in a chromosomally abnormal embryo is called *dysmorphogenesis;* the individual physical abnormalities are called *dysmorphic features*. In Down's syndrome this consists of such features as small ears, unusual creases on the palms, upward slant of the eyes, small head size, congenital heart disease, and short stature.

Down's syndrome is an easily recognized combination of major and minor physical abnormalities associated with mental retardation. It occurs as the specific result of the presence of a triple dose of chromosome 21 material. This occurs most commonly as trisomy 21, the presence of three separate 21 chromosomes as the result of meiotic nondisjunction. Meiosis is the special form of cell division that occurs in germ cells that produce ova or sperm. This division reduces the chromosome number from 46 to 23, with one member of each pair of chromosomes being represented. Nondisjunction is the failure of one of a pair of chromosomes to go to each daughter cell during division; instead both go to one daughter cell (Fig. 47-4). The frequency of nondisjunction increases with maternal age. For that reason, prenatal diagnosis through amniocentesis with cytogenetic study is recommended for women 35 years of age or older. This form of Down's syndrome does not occur with an increased familial incidence.

Structural abnormalities of chromosomes

A familial form of Down's syndrome occurs with a structural abnormality known as a *Robertsonian translocation*. This translocation is formed by the fusion of the centromeres, most commonly of chromosomes 14 and 21. A carrier of a 14/21 translocation will have a total chromosomal number of 45. However, the translocation chromosome contains the normal amount of chromosomal material of two separate chromosomes and the carrier is phenotypically normal. Meiosis in a translocation carrier can result in a variety of different gametes. Among the offspring of carriers of a 14/21 translocation, one may observe normal infants with 46 normal chromosomes, phenotypically normal infants with 45 chromosomes and a translocation similar to the parent, and infants with 46 chromosomes of which there are two normal 21 chromosomes and the material of a third 21 present in the translocation (Fig. 47-5). Such children have typical Down's syndrome. The translocation may occur in multiple members of a family, each of whom is a carrier at

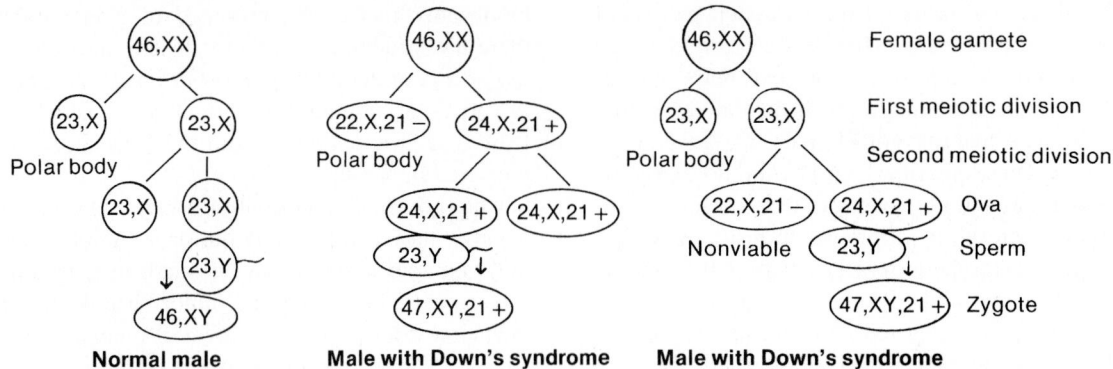

Normal male   **Male with Down's syndrome**   **Male with Down's syndrome**

Fig. 47-4   Meiotic nondysjunction. *Left,* Normal meiosis of an ovum fertilized by a normal sperm yielding a normal zygote. *Center,* Error in first cell division of meiosis results in an aneuploid ovum that when fertilized yields a 47,XY,21+ male with Down's syndrome. *Right,* Error has occurred in second cell division of meiosis with same result.

increased risk of having a child with Down's syndrome. One can differentiate the familial and sporadic forms of Down's syndrome by chromosomal studies. For that reason it is advisable that each person with Down's syndrome undergo chromosomal analysis to determine whether there is an increased risk for other family members of having children with Down's syndrome.

Sex chromosome abnormalities

Alterations in the number of sex chromosomes are common, and several types of aneuploidy can occur. These conditions were originally recognized through the use of buccal smear for Barr body analysis. Each X chromosome in excess of 1 in the cell nucleus is inactivated and is seen microscopically as the Barr body. The Barr body, named for its discoverer, is the nuclear condensation of the inactivated X chromosome and appears as a clump inside and adjacent to

the nuclear membrane (Fig. 47-6). The cells of a normal male contain only one X chromosome; thus no Barr body is present. Cells of a normal female contain two X chromosomes and demonstrate a single Barr body.

Abnormalities of sex chromosomes in females occur most commonly as a 45,X and a 47,XXX karyotype. The former is the most common chromosomal finding in Turner's syndrome. This disorder has three major features: short stature, minor dysmorphic abnormalities and congenital malformations, and sexual infantilism. The sexual infantilism occurs as a result of fibrosis of the infantile ovary, and so at the time of puberty there are neither follicles nor hormone-producing cells present. In its classic form this syndrome is diagnosed by buccal smear, which will show the absence of Barr bodies. However, a variety of X-chromosome abnormalities may result in Turner's syndrome; for that reason a full lymphocyte karyotype should

		14, 21	45,XX,t14/21	Carrier
		t14/21		
Gametes			**Zygotes**	**Phenotype**
Ovum	14, 21		46,XX	Normal
Sperm	14, 21			
Ovum	t14/21		45,XX,t14/21	Normal (carrier)
Sperm	14, 21			
Ovum	t14/21,21		46,XX,t14/21	Down's syndrome
Sperm	14, 21			

Fig. 47-5   Translocation 14/21. Carrier has 45 chromosomes with one normal 14, one 21, and genetic content of a 14 and 21 contained in translocation. A person with Down's syndrome as a result of such a translocation has two separate 21s and a third 21 as part of translocation. Such a person has a total of 46 chromosomes but genetic content of three number 21s, that is, trisomy 21.

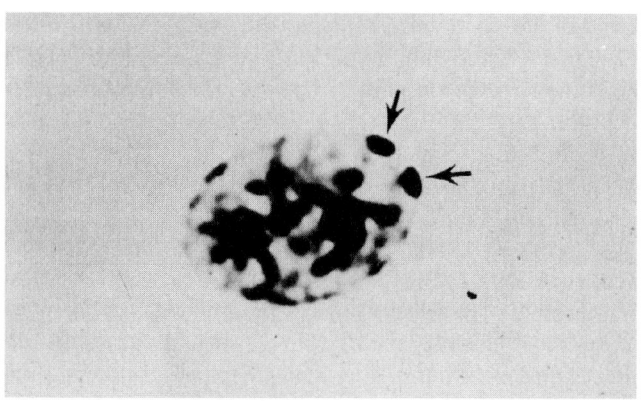

Fig. 47-6 Barr body. This cell has two Barr bodies seen as nuclear condensations just inside nuclear membrane at 3-o'clock position *(arrow)*. Two Barr bodies would be seen in a male with 48,XXXY and a female with 47,XXX.

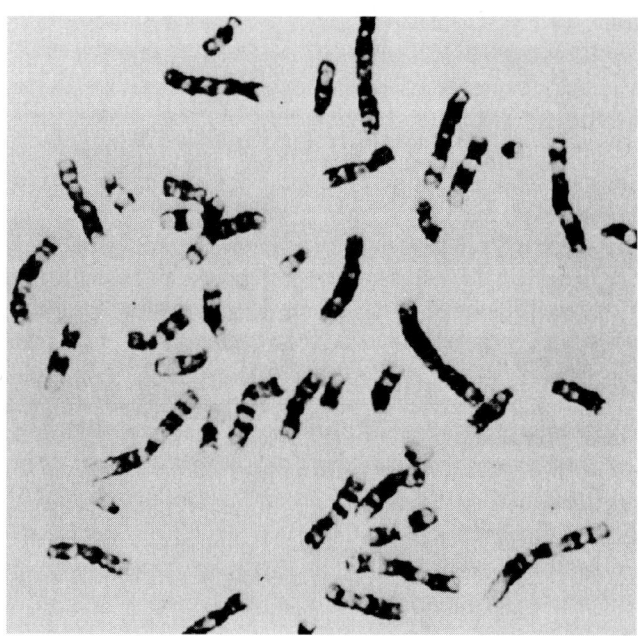

Fig. 47-7 Metaphase spread. Chromosomes as seen through microscope in a spread stained by G-banding technique.

always be done regardless of the findings on buccal smear. The 47,XXX karyotype is not associated with significant clinical abnormalities.

The most common abnormalities of sex chromosomes in males include the 47,XXY and 47,XYY karyotypes. Klinefelter's syndrome (47,XXY) has three major clinical findings: minor to no dysmorphic abnormalities, normal to mild retardation in cognitive function, and failure of testicular development with secondary sexual infantilism and a eunuchoid body habitus. Because of the lack of testosterone production at the age of puberty, such males may respond to ovarian estrogens with breast enlargement or gynecomastia. Surgical correction of gynecomastia and testosterone replacement therapy will correct most of the problems associated with this disorder. There is considerable controversy regarding the type and frequency of clinical manifestations associated with the 47,XYY karyotype. Males with the 47,XYY karyotype are physically and sexually normal, but some studies have suggested that an increased proportion of men with this karyotype exhibit sociopathic behavior.

Cytogenetic methods

The most common method of chromosome analysis involves the culture of peripheral lymphocytes. These are mature cells circulating in the peripheral blood that are not actively undergoing cell division. Such cells can be stimulated to divide by the addition of a mitogen to the culture medium. The most commonly used mitogen in human cytogenetics is phytohemagglutinin (PHA). Lymphocytes in the presence of PHA are commonly cultured for 72 hours. Toward the end of the culture period, colchicine is added to the culture. This agent acts as a microtubular poison and thereby disrupts the mitotic spindle during cell division. Thus cells can be arrested in metaphase, the only time during cell division when chromosomes can be easily visualized and studied (Fig. 47-7). At the end of the culture period the cells can be harvested, spread on a slide, and stained with a number of fluorogens or chromagens. When special fixative techniques are used, the chromosomes take on a banded appearance. These bands are specific for each chromosome and allow detailed analysis of the structure of each chromosome.

The normal Y chromosome contains a large fluorescent segment in the long arm. If a buccal smear from a 46,XY male is stained with a fluorescent dye, a bright fluorescent spot called the *F body,* or *Y body,* will be revealed. The use of Giemsa staining for Barr bodies and fluorescent staining for Y bodies allows determination of the sex-chromosome constitution from a buccal smear. The recognition of both Barr bodies and Y bodies is sufficiently subjective that an experienced technician, using control cells from a normal male and female, is necessary for an accurate determination. The expected findings of Barr body and Y body determination on a buccal smear for normal and abnormal sex chromosomal constitutions are shown in Table 47-2.

Recently techniques have been developed for hybridizing RNA or DNA (see Chapter 48) labeled with chromogenic enzymes or fluorochromes to chromosome preparations that have been fixed during metaphase. Labeling the molecular probes with different colored fluorochromes allows complex karyotypic abnormalities, including single-copy genes, to be defined. Fusion genes hybridized with probes for the constituent genes labeled with fluorochromes of complementary colors will appear as a third color. The use of fluorescent in situ hybridization (called FISH) has added another dimension to karyotypic analysis.

Table 47-2 Buccal smear findings in sex chromosome abnormalities

Karyotype	Sex	Barr body	Y body
46,XX	F	+	0
46,XY	M	0	+
45,X	F	0	0
47,XXX	F	++	0
48,XXXX	F	+++	0
49,XXXXX	F	++++	0
47,XXY	M	+	+
47,XYY	M	0	++
48,XXYY	M	+	++
49,XXXXY	M	+++	+

Chromosomal markers of disease

The analysis of the chromosomes in dividing cells may reveal abnormalities of three types: first, a change in the amount of chromosomal material present as in aneuploidy or partial duplication or deletion; second, no alteration in the amount of chromosomal material but chromosomal changes that are diagnostic of specific disease states; third, nonspecific changes in chromosomal structure or number that reflect the consequences of environmental influences such as drugs or radiation or the abnormal chromosomal behavior seen in malignant cells.

Improvements in culture techniques and staining of chromosomes have revealed that malignant cells often demonstrate a consistent and specific chromosomal abnormality that is of major diagnostic assistance. Such an abnormality is best exemplified by the Philadelphia chromosome (Ph[1])

found in the majority of persons with chronic myelogenous leukemia (CML). The Philadelphia chromosome represents a deletion in chromosome 22, which renders it a small acrocentric chromosome (Fig. 47-8). The deleted material is most often translocated to a 9 chromosome. Thus there is no loss or gain of chromosomal material, but there is a structural rearrangement. The Philadelphia chromosome is confined to the malignant cells of the bone marrow, and analysis for the Philadelphia chromosome is done on bone marrow aspirate. The breakpoints of these chromosomes have been cloned into bacteria using recombinant DNA technology. The translocation creates a fusion gene, the 5' portion of which is derived from the c-*Abelson* oncogene that is usually present in the long arm of chromosome 9; the 3' end is derived from a gene in the break-cluster region on chromosome 22. The resulting fusion protein is a truncated protein kinase. The clinical expression of the associated malignancy is correlated with the precise location of the translocation. The translocations accompanying many malignancies transect oncogenes, immunoglobulins, and various cell receptors.

A second type of chromosomal marker used diagnostically is that of chromosomal breakage. This is most dramatically illustrated in the Fanconi anemia. Persons with this form of autosomal, recessively inherited, aplastic anemia demonstrate a pronounced increase in the frequency of spontaneous chromosomal breaks and gaps in cultured peripheral lymphocytes. Aplastic anemia occurs as a result of failure of the bone marrow to produce blood cells. Studies of cultured somatic cells from persons with Fanconi's ane-

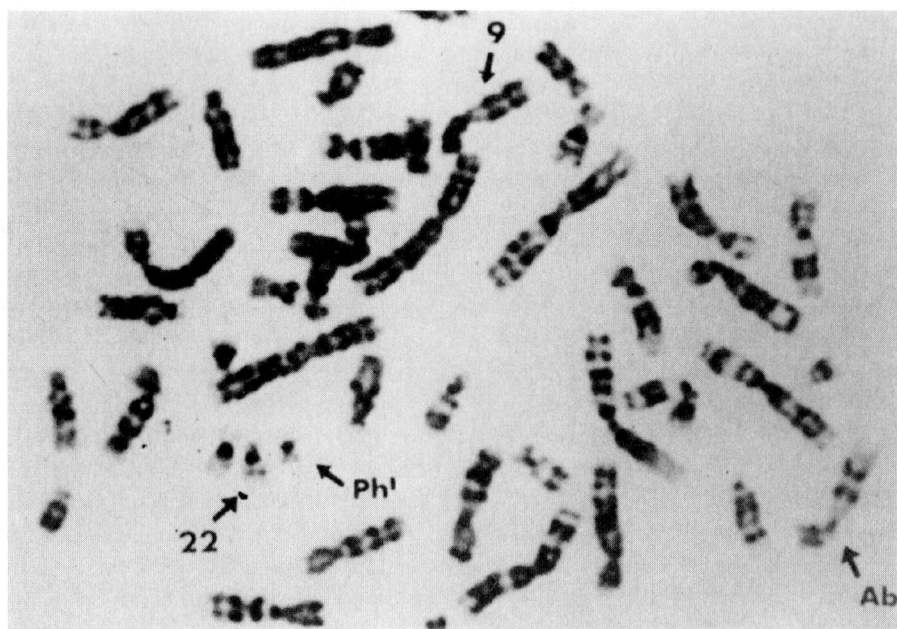

Fig. 47-8 Philadelphia chromosome. A metaphase spread with banded chromosomes shows small number 22, or Ph[1] chromosome, and normal 22 + normal chromosome 9 and chromosome 9(Ab) involved in 9/22 translocation producing Ph[1] chromosome.

mia imply four different genetic mechanisms that are believed to affect DNA repair proteins. Thus the various dysmorphic features are believed to be the result of multiple somatic mutations resulting from defective repair of DNA.

The autosomal recessively inherited disorder Bloom's syndrome is also characterized by a sharp increase in the frequency of sister chromatid exchanges in cultured lymphocytes. Bloom's syndrome is typically characterized by intrauterine growth retardation and short stature thereafter. Such patients have increased sensitivity of skin to ultraviolet rays and a significant risk of malignancies including leukemia during late childhood and early adult years.

A fourth type of specific chromosomal marker is the fragile X chromosome recognized in one X-linked form of mental retardation. The characteristic findings in this disorder include postpubertal enlargement of the testes, large, simply formed ears, a jovial personality, and moderate to severe mental retardation. Approximately 10% of carrier females for this form of X-linked mental retardation show a mild form of mental retardation. The culture of lymphocytes with the standard growth media used for cytogenetic studies will not demonstrate the fragile X chromosome. However, the use of media that are deficient in folic acid will show a *fragile X* chromosome in a significant percentage of cells from an affected male. The designation fragile X is used because the X chromosome in these males appears to have a break at the end of the long arm.

The mode of inheritance of the fragile X syndrome has several unusual features. Carrier females have only mild mental retardation, never severe mental impairment. In affected males, the defect appears to be progressively more severe in subsequent generations of the same family, and the age of onset is progressively earlier. The fragile X site has now been cloned, and the basic defect has been shown to be a defect of amplification of DNA. In the normal population, a highly polymorphic sequence of 5 to 54 CGG triplet repeats is found between the 5′ end of the chromosome and the fragile X gene (called the *FMR-1 gene*). Carriers in affected families have an abnormally increased number of triplets. The threshold for clinical expression of the gene defect is approximately 80 triplets. The offspring of individuals with more than 50 repeats are at increased risk of larger amplifications. Severely affected individuals may have up to 4000 tandem copies of the CGG triplets, with severity being proportional to the number of repeats. The number of triplets transmitted by males to their daughters is stable. A manyfold amplification can occur during a single meiosis in a female carrier. Although the FMR-1 protein is expressed in brain and testicle, its function is still not known.

Similar defects in amplification are found in spinal and bulbar muscular atrophy, or Kennedy disease, in which the 11 to 31 CAG repeats normally present in the first exon of the gene for the androgen receptor are represented by a polyglutamine stretch in the protein. In myotonic dystrophy

5 to 30 copies of a GCT repeat are normally present in the untranslated region between the 3′ end of the chromosome and the termination codon of a gene designated the myotonin protein kinase (MT-PK) gene on chromosome 19. Huntington's disease is also caused by perturbed amplification of sequences found between the 5′ end of the chromosome and the Huntington gene on chromosome 7. Additional information on the effect of amplification of repeat sequences can be found in Chapter 48.

PATHOLOGICAL DISORDERS ASSOCIATED WITH BIOCHEMICAL CHANGES
Lysosomal storage diseases

Lysosomal storage diseases are recessively inherited disorders, each of which is the result of a deficiency of a specific acid hydrolase. These acid hydrolases are located within membrane-bound cytoplasmic organelles called *lysosomes*. If there is a complete or nearly complete deficiency of a specific hydrolase, the macromolecular compound that it normally degrades will accumulate within tissue. The primary organs affected will depend on the tissue distribution of the macromolecular compound. These organs include (1) the reticuloendothelial system, (2) the central nervous system (CNS), and (3) the skeleton and connective tissues and other somatic tissues. In a given disorder the clinical manifestations may be apparent in only one or in any combination of these three organ systems. The box lists a classification scheme for lysosomal storage diseases.

Classification of Lysosomal Storage Disease

Mucopolysaccharidoses
Mucolipidoses (ML)
   ML I (now called "salidosis")
   ML II or I-cell disease
   ML III or pseudo-Hurler polydystrophy
   ML IV
Gangliosidoses
   G_{M1} gangliosidosis, or generalized gangliosidosis
   G_{M2} gangliosidosis
      Tay-Sachs disease
      Sandhoff's disease
Leukodystrophies
   Metachromatic leukodystrophy
   Krabbe's disease
   Adrenoleukodystrophy
Glycoproteinosis
   Mannosidosis
   Fucosidosis
   Sialidosis
   Aspartylglucosaminuria
Others
   Ceramidosis
   Cholesterol ester storage disease
   Pompe's disease, or glycogen-storage disease II

Varying degrees of deficiency or altered activity of a hydrolase may result in several different clinical syndromes occurring as a result of the same enzyme deficiency. This is demonstrated by deficiency of the hydrolase α-L-iduronidase. Deficiency of this enzyme results in the accumulation of the glycosaminoglycans, dermatan sulfate, and heparan sulfate. In its most severe form with the greatest degree of enzyme deficiency, Hurler's syndrome occurs with severe skeletal, somatic, and central nervous system manifestations and death by 5 to 8 years of age. In its mildest form, deficiency of this enzyme results in the Scheie syndrome with normal height, life expectancy, and intelligence but with skeletal, ocular, and cardiac abnormalities. An intermediate form, known as the *Hurler-Scheie syndrome,* is intermediate in its clinical manifestations.

Reticuloendothelial system involvement

The two disorders in which involvement of the liver and spleen is most prominent and may represent the major manifestation are Gaucher's and Niemann-Pick diseases. Gaucher's disease occurs as a result of the deficiency of the acid hydrolase β-glucosidase.

$$\text{Ceramide-}\beta\text{-glucose} \xrightarrow{\text{β-Glucosidase + H}_2\text{O}} \text{Ceramide + Glucose}$$

Deficiency of this enzyme results in the lysosomal accumulation of the phospholipid glucosylceramide. This disorder occurs in several forms. The most severe form is known as neuronopathic Gaucher's disease (type 2) in which, although liver and spleen enlargement occur, massive accumulation of phospholipids within the central nervous system predominates and affected infants die within the first year of life. The other extreme is illustrated by the adult form of Gaucher's disease (type 1) recognized by hepatosplenomegaly, in which good general health and normal life expectancy occur. Before the use of enzyme assays for specific diagnoses, Gaucher's disease was most often recognized by the demonstration of Gaucher cells (large macrophages) in a bone marrow aspirate. Because the gene for ceramide glucosidase has been cloned, diagnosis with an accuracy heretofore impossible is allowed. Gaucher's disease is prevalent in Ashkenazi Jews. A mutation at nucleotide 1226 accounts for 73% of the mutant alleles (gene frequency, 0.035) in this population. Additional alleles account for a total-population heterozygote frequency of 8.9% and a disease incidence at birth of 1:450. The enzyme, ceramide glucosidase, is now available commercially, though at great cost. Use of this enzyme as a therapeutic agent can allow mobilization of the accumulated ganglioside from bone and liver. Reversal of the neurological disease is still not possible. The second disorder in this group, Niemann-Pick disease, also occurs in several forms ranging from a severe infantile to a mild adult disease. This disorder occurs as a result of a deficiency of sphingomyelinase.

$$\text{Sphingomyelin} \xrightarrow{\text{Sphingomyelinase + H}_2\text{O}} \text{Ceramide + Phosphorylcholine}$$

Niemann-Pick disease is also associated with enlargement of the liver and spleen. Niemann-Pick disease can be diagnosed by the demonstration of storage cells on bone marrow aspirate that represent macrophages with lysosomes engorged with sphingomyelin. The acid sphingomyelinase gene has been cloned and mapped to chromosome 11p15; numerous mutations have been defined at the molecular level.

DISORDERS OF INTERMEDIARY METABOLISM
CNS predominance

The lysosomal storage diseases that affect primarily the CNS clinically involve gray matter or white matter initially. When the initial accumulation is within white matter, the disorder is known as a leukodystrophy, and motor abnormalities are seen early in the course of the disease. The most commonly recognized leukodystrophy is metachromatic leukodystrophy, in which neural tissue demonstrates a particular metachromatic staining property resulting from the lysosomal accumulation of sulfated galactosylceramide. The deficient enzyme is called arylsulfatase A, or cerebroside sulfate sulfatase. Several screening tests are available for this disorder and include the examination of urine for metachromatic granules.

$$\text{Ceramide-}\beta\text{-galactose-3 sulfate} \xrightarrow{\text{Sulfate acrylsulfatase A + H}_2\text{O}} \text{Ceramide-}\beta\text{-galactose + Sulfate}$$

In normal urine adequate amounts of this enzyme are present for a simple colorimetric assay of arylsulfatase activity. The presence of an adequate amount of enzyme activity will exclude this diagnosis, but lack of enzyme activity is not diagnostic and indicates that more specific assay systems should be used. The specific diagnosis of metachromatic leukodystrophy requires the demonstration of arylsulfatase A deficiency in homogenized peripheral leukocytes or cultured skin fibroblasts. Arylsulfatase occurs in two lysosomal forms known as A and B. The use of cellulose acetate electrophoresis is a second diagnostic method. In metachromatic leukodystrophy a normal arylsulfatase B band will be observed, and no A band will be recognized.

The best known lysosomal storage disease that results in macromolecular compound accumulation initially within gray matter is Tay-Sachs disease. This disorder occurs as a result of the accumulation of G_{M2} ganglioside (Fig. 47-9) within the CNS. In the classical form it results in early regression of CNS function, and so by 1 year of age children with this disease have delayed cognitive development, impaired hearing and sight, and a characteristic cherry-red spot found on funduscopic examination. The accumulation of G_{M2} ganglioside within the CNS occurs as a result of deficiency of the acid hydrolase *N*-acetyl-β-D-galactosaminidase. Many variant juvenile and adult-onset

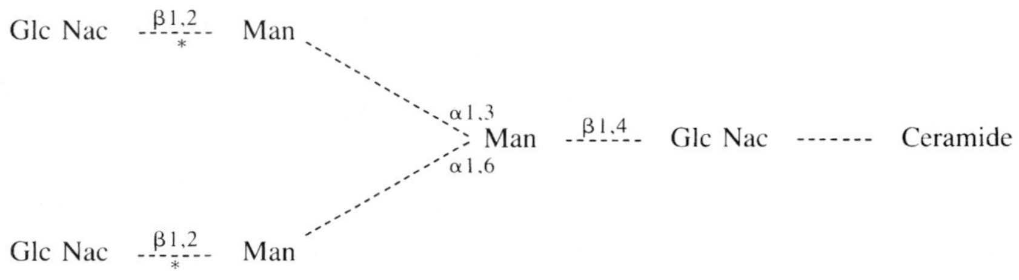

Fig. 47-9 Tay-Sachs disease. G_{M2} ganglioside accumulates in the gray matter of brain because of deficiency of N-acetyl-β-1,2-glucosaminidase (hexosaminidase A). *Glc Nac,* N-Acetylglucosamine; *Man,* mannose.

forms have been defined, often appearing as the late onset of cerebellar ataxia or convulsions. The activity of N-acetyl-β-D-galactosaminidase is assayed with an artificial substrate, either a glucosamine or a galactosamine. Therefore the enzyme activity so measured is based on *hexosaminidase*. Hexosaminidase occurs as a heat-labile form, hexosaminidase A, a heteropolymer of α and β subunits, and a heat-stabile form, hexosaminidase B, a homopolymer of β subunits. Tay-Sachs disease is usually characterized by the specific deficiency of hexosaminidase A. Sandhoff's disease is associated with numerous mutations of the β gene. Measurement of enzyme activity with and without heat inactivation gives levels of hexosaminidase B and total hexosaminidase respectively. The difference between the two determinations is thus the calculated level of hexosaminidase A, or the heat-labile form. A so-called associated activation protein has been found to be a small protein that forms a complex with G_{M2} ganglioside making it accessible to the hexosaminidase. Mutations of the gene coding for this protein may impair the functional activity of both the A and B enzymes and also affect the disease.

Because Tay-Sachs disease occurs most commonly among Ashkenazi Jewish infants, this target population can be screened for carrier detection. Determination of the percentage of hexosaminidase A present as a function of total hexosaminidase activity represents the most accurate screening method for detecting carriers of Tay-Sachs disease. In the establishment of a screening assay system for Tay-Sachs disease carriers, it is necessary that each laboratory determine its reference values and values for Tay-Sachs disease carriers. Confirmation of the carrier state requires study of hexosaminidase A activity in peripheral leukocytes and additional family studies if necessary to resolve questionable results. The use of such carrier tests among Ashkenazi Jews and subsequent use of prenatal diagnosis has significantly reduced the incidence of Tay-Sachs disease in the United States.

Application of recombinant DNA technology to the study of Tay-Sachs disease has greatly expanded understanding of the clinical heterogeneity of the disease that has been evi-

dent. The structural genes for the α and β subunits of hexosamidase and the activator proteins are on chromosomes 15, 5, and 5 respectively. Of the 3% of Ashkenazi Jews who are heterozygotes for this disease, approximately 73% have an insertion of 4 nucleotide base pairs in exon 11 to create a frameshift mutation; 15% have a G to C substitution in the first nucleotide of intron 12 to create a splicing abnormality; 4% have a glycine 269 substitution by serine at the 3' end of exon 7, which is responsible for adult-onset disease, and 8% have either false-positive results or have a heterogeneous group of other mutations. The presence of multiple mutations, all of eastern European Ashkenazic origin, argues for some selective advantage for heterozygote formation rather than a "founder effect" (passing on original mutations) as the explanation for the high frequency. Eighty percent of non-Jewish heterozygotes have other mutations.

Connective tissue and skeletal predominance

Lysosomal storage diseases in which involvement of connective tissue, especially the skeletal system, predominates are referred to as *Hurler-like disorders*. With skeletal system involvement there may also be CNS or reticuloendothelial involvement. Table 47-3 lists a classification of lysosomal disorders that are seen with this phenotype.

Hurler's syndrome represents the prototype of diseases involving glycosaminoglycan metabolism and resulting in a connective tissue disorder. This form of α-L-iduronidase deficiency is characterized by multisystem involvement that

Table 47-3 Hurler-like disorders

Disorders	Screening test
Mucopolysaccharidoses	Urinary screening for mucopolysacchariduria
Mucolipidoses ML II and ML III	Serum levels of acid hydrolases Urinary bound sialic acid
Glycoproteinosis	Urinary oligosaccharide TLC Urinary bound sialic acid

IA—Glc Nac—GA—Glc Nac—IA—Glc Nac
  *   *

Dermatan sulfate

IA—Gal Nac—GA—Gal Nac—IA—Gal Nac
  *   *

Heparan sulfate

*Site of hydrolysis by α-L-iduronidase in oligosaccharide chain of dermatan and heparan sulfate

Fig. 47-10   Hurler's syndrome. Deficiency of lysosomal hydrolase α-L-iduronidase results in widespread accumulation of both heparan and dermatan sulfate. *GA,* Glucosamine; *Gal Nac,* N-acetylgalactose; *Glc Nac,* N-acetylglucosamine; *IA,* iduronic acid.

is usually apparent by 6 months of age (Fig. 47-10). It follows a rapidly progressive course thereafter with all organ systems involved and mental deterioration predominating late in the disorder, with death ultimately occurring between 5 and 8 years of age. These diseases were classified initially on the basis of the urinary pattern of mucopolysaccharide or glycosaminoglycan excretion. In Hurler's syndrome massive amounts of dermatan sulfate and heparan sulfate are excreted in the urine. Mucopolysacchariduria is detected by a variety of screening tests including a urine spot test, the toluidine blue test.

Recognition of the clinical phenotype and the presence of a positive urine screening test are followed by the study of mucopolysaccharide metabolism in cultured fibroblasts and the assay of specific hydrolases that can cause the mucopolysaccharidoses. Inorganic sulfate added to tissue culture media is exclusively incorporated into cultured fibroblasts as sulfated glycosaminoglycans. The use of radioactive sulfate allows the recognition of accumulation of these sulfated compounds within cultured fibroblasts and therefore provides direct evidence for tissue accumulation of glycosaminoglycans. A specific diagnosis can be pursued by the assay of the individual hydrolases that, when deficient, result in a mucopolysaccharidosis. The pattern of mucopolysacchariduria and the specific acid hydrolase deficient in the mucopolysaccharidoses are shown in Table 47-4.

Another disorder that results in a Hurler-like clinical picture is *mucolipidosis II,* or I-cell disease. Children with this disease are similar clinically to those with Hurler's syndrome but are diagnosed at an earlier age and follow a more rapid downhill course with death by 3 to 5 years of age. There is no mucopolysacchariduria. When cultured skin fibroblasts from affected children were first analyzed under phase microscopy, a sharp increase in cytoplasmic inclusions was noted, hence the name *I-cell,* or *inclusion cell disease.* Lysosomal hydrolases are glycoproteins. Each lysosomal enzyme has a unique structural gene that codes for the protein component of the glycoprotein. There is, however, commonality in the posttranslational modification of these proteins to form the oligosaccharide component of the glycoproteins. It has been recognized that mannose-6-phosphate sugars in the oligosaccharide chain of the glycoprotein structure of acid hydrolases are required for their appropriate intracellular localization. This is accomplished through several posttranslational enzymatic steps in the modification of the oligosaccharide chain. Deficiency of a transferase involved in such posttranslational modifications represents the primary molecular defect in I-cell disease. Cultured skin fibroblasts from affected children show deficient levels of numerous acid hydrolases in cultured cells. The ultimate defect resides in the abnormal intracellular localization of these hydrolases. The urine of patients with I-cell disease shows increased levels of lysosomal hydrolases and an increase in the amount of sialic acid oligosaccharides. The measurement of bound sialic acid in urine is a relatively simple procedure and represents an excellent screening test for a large number of lysosomal storage diseases.

Disorders of intermediary metabolism

Disorders of intermediary metabolism occur as a result of three basic mechanisms: an enzyme deficiency with defective substrate conversion, a membrane transport defect resulting in failure of absorption or excessive excretion of a compound, and defects in receptors involved in mediating metabolism. The biochemical basis for the resulting disease occurs as a result of (1) accumulation of a substrate to levels that become toxic, (2) deficiency through lack of production or excessive loss of a needed compound, and (3) conversion of an elevated compound to an altered metabolite that itself is a toxic material (Fig. 47-11). In general, defects in intermediary metabolism result in alterations of compounds with a molecular weight lower than those seen in lysosomal storage diseases. As a result, they are more likely to result in more acute manifestations and are less likely to be associated with the striking physical features that dominate the lysosomal storage disorders. Defects in intermediary metabolism result in a disruption of a normal metabolic process and often produce an elevated urinary excretion of a normal metabolite or the urinary excretion of an abnormal metabolite. Therefore urine screening tests are the principal means of recognizing the presence of such a disorder, prompting more specific diagnostic assays.

Aminoacidopathies.   Table 47-5 is a list of the more common amino acid disorders and their clinical chemical characterizations. *Phenylketonuria* (PKU) is the best known and best understood of the amino acid disorders. This autosomal recessively inherited disorder occurs as a defect in phenylalanine conversion to tyrosine because of a deficiency of the enzyme phenylalanine hydroxylase (PAH).

Phenylalanine   ———Defective phenylalanine hydroxylase———→   Tyrosine

Alternative metabolic pathway

↘ Phenylpyruvic acid

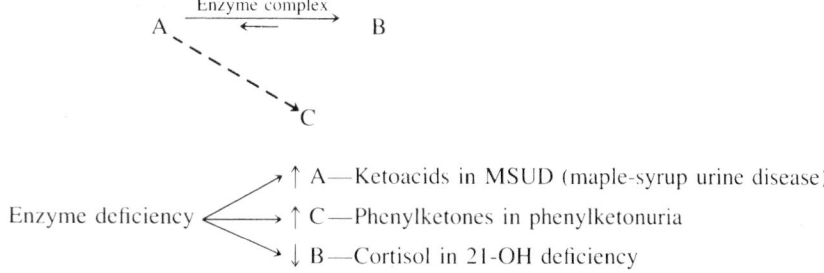

Fig. 47-11 Enzyme deficiency. Deficiency of enzyme in metabolic pathway may produce clinical symptoms because of accumulation of substrate, *A;* lack of production of product, *B;* or shunting of substrate to alternative pathway with production of a toxic compound, *C.*

The deficiency of phenylalanine hydroxylase results in a shunting of phenylalanine metabolism to several ketoacids, the principal one being phenylpyruvic acid. This disease occurs in approximately 1 in 15,000 live-born infants. The enzymatic activity is restricted to the liver, and therefore diagnosis is accomplished through demonstration of alterations in phenylalanine metabolism.

Ferric chloride screening of the urine in the newborn had been used both for diagnosis and dietary management from early infancy; for the former it has been supplanted by the Guthrie test, in which a bacterial inhibition assay is used to detect an elevated level of phenylalanine. In newborn screening a Guthrie test is considered positive when the phenylalanine level exceeds 60 mg/L. Given a positive result, approximately 1 in 10 to 1 in 20 infants will in fact have phenylketonuria. The specific diagnosis of phenylketonuria after a positive screening test requires the demonstration of plasma levels of phenylalanine greater than 200 mg/L on 2 consecutive days while normal feedings are given. After institution of dietary restriction in phenylalanine intake, urine screening tests will revert to normal. Subsequent monitoring of children on dietary management requires quantitative plasma determinations of phenylalanine levels.

The gene for phenylalanine hydroxylase (PAH) has been mapped to chromosome 12q22-q24.1. Approximately 50 haplotypes have been defined on the basis of seven restriction fragment length polymorphisms (RFLP; see p. 975). The most prevalent base mutation among whites is a G to A substitution in intron 12; this mutation is on haplotype 3 and the combination is widely distributed throughout Europe. The PAH mutations seen in African-Americans are distributed among five haplotypes, one common and one rare in whites, the other three unique to African-Americans. Some mutations are found on more than one haplotype, reflecting either a new mutation or a chromosomal cross-over.

Maple-syrup urine disease was so named because of the obvious odor of urine in affected infants. This disease occurs in roughly one in 250,000 live-born infants. Many disorders of amino acid metabolism are characterized by unusual odors. The odor is usually the result of the excessive urinary excretion of an organic acid that imparts a specific odor. The three branched-chain amino acids, leucine, isoleucine, and valine, undergo transamination, transketolation, and decarboxylation through a common pathway (Fig. 47-12). Maple-syrup urine disease occurs as a result of a deficiency in the multicomponent enzyme branched-chain ketoacid decarboxylase. This enzyme activity resides in two proteins, E1 composed of subunits E1α and E1β, and E2. The gene for E1α has been cloned and assigned to chromosome 19; E2 is on chromosome 1. Mutants of all three loci have been defined.

Table 47-4 Mucopolysaccharidoses

Eponym	Number	Mucopolysacchariduria	Enzyme deficiency
Hurler	HPS I-H	DS, HS	α-L-Iduronidase
Scheie	MPS I-S	DS, HS	α-L-Iduronidase
Hurler-Scheie	MPS I-H/S	DS, HS	α-L-Iduronidase
Hunger	MPS II	DS, HS	Iduronide sulfate sulfatase
Sanfilippo	MSP III-A	HS	Heparan-*N*-sulfate sulfatase
Sanfilippo	MPS III-B	HS	α-Glucosaminidase
Sanfilippo	MPS III-C	HS	Acetyl-CoA:α-glucosaminide *N*-acetyltransferase
Morquino A	MPS IV-A	KS	Galactosaminyl-6-sulfate sulfatase
Morquino B	MPS IV-B	KS	α-Galactosidase
Maroteaux-Lamy	MPS VI	DS	Galactosaminyl-4-sulfate sulfatase (arylsulfatase B)
Sly	MPS VII	DS or HS or DS, HS	β-Glucuronidase

DS, Dermatan sulfate; *HS,* heparan sulfate; *KS,* keratan sulfate.

Table 47-5 Inborn errors of intermediary metabolism of amino acids

Condition	Defective enzyme	Biochemical features	Clinical features	Treatment
Alkaptonuria*	Homogentisate oxygenase	Urinary excretion of homogenetisic acid.	Urine darkens; ochronosis; arthritis in later life.	Not known
Phenylketonuria†	Phenylalanine 4-hydroxylase	Phenylalanine accumulates in blood, CSF, etc.; urinary excretion of phenylpyruvic acid and related compounds.	Severe mental deficiency, epilepsy, abnormal EEG, eczema, behavioral disorders.	Diet low in phenylalanine beginning at early age
Albinism‡	o-Diphenol oxidase (tyrosinase)	Lack of melanin in skin, hair, and eyes.	Photophobia, nystagmus, carcinomas of the skin.	None known
Goitrous cretinism (several types)	(1) Tyrosine iodinase (2) Coupling enzyme (3) Deiodinase	Lack of thyroid hormone.	Cretinism, goiter.	Thyroid, thyroxine, or triiodothyronine
Maple-syrup urine disease (leucinosis)	Enzyme responsible for oxidative decarboxylation of α-ketoisocaproic, α-keto-β-methyl-*n*-valeric and α-ketoisovaleric acids	Leucine, isoleucine, and valine accumulate in blood, CSF, etc.; urinary excretion of the 3 keto acids and related compounds.	Cerebral degeneration; usually early death, milder form with partial enzyme deficiency, symptomless except during infections, etc.	Diet low in leucine, isoleucine, and valine
Cystinosis	Cystine reductase (?)	Cystine is deposited in reticuloendothelial system; aminoaciduria, glucosuria, proteinuria, phosphaturia, dilute urine.	Dwarfism, photophobia, renal acidosis, hypokalemia, vitamin-resistant rickets; death before puberty. A benign (nonrenal?) variant occurs in adults.	Palliative: potassium salts, alkalis, vitamin D; diet low in cystine and methionine (efficacy doubtful)
Homocystinuria	L-Serine dehydratase	Urinary excretion of homocystine.	Mental retardation, retinal defects, dislocated lenses, malar flush, thromboses.	Diet low in methionine, high in cystine; pyridoxine
Hyperglycemia (several types)	(Uncertain, depends on type)	Glycine accumulates in blood, etc.; urinary excretion of glycine and, in one type, methylmalonic acid.	Neonatal lethargy and ketosis, neutropenia, hypo-γ-globulinemia; mental retardation.	Diet low in protein
Oxalosis	Excessive conversion of glycine to oxalic acid	Calcium oxalate accumulates in kidneys, heart, bone marrow and cartilages.	Nephrocalcinosis leading to progressive renal failure.	None known
Histidinemia	Histidine ammonialyase	Urinary excretion of β-imidazolylpyruvic acid and related compounds	Speech defects; mental retardation in some.	Diet low in histidine
Familial tyrosinemia	Fumarylacetoacetase	Tyrosine levels in blood and urine raised; urinary excretion of phenolic acids related to tyrosine; generalized aminoaciduria; glucosuria; fructosuria.	Rapidly enlarging liver; jaundice; hypoprothrombinemia; death common in infancy; survivors may have vitamin D–resistant rickets and acidosis.	Diet low in tyrosine and phenylalanine (efficacy doubtful)
Hyperprolinemia Type I	Pyrroline-5-carboxylate reductase	Hyperprolinemia; urinary excretion of proline, glycine, and hydroxyproline.	Mental retardation, convulsions, renal disease, deafness.	None known
Type II	Pyrroline-5-carboxylate dehydrogenase			
Hydroxyprolinemia	3-Hydroxypyrroline-5-carboxylate reductase (?)	High levels of hydroxyproline in blood and urine.	Mental retardation (?).	None known
Citrullinemia	Argininosuccinate synthetase	High blood and urinary levels of citrulline; blood ammonia increased; urea excretion normal.	Mental retardation, epilepsy, vomiting, ammonia intoxication.	Diet low in protein
Argininosuccinic-aciduria	Argininosuccinate lyase	Urinary excretion of argininosuccinic acid; high blood and CSF ammonia levels; urea excretion normal.	Mental retardation, convulsions, hair abnormalities, ammonia intoxication.	Diet low in protein
Hyperammonemia Type I	Ornithine carbamolytransferase	Blood ammonia about 10 mg/L; urea excretion normal.	Mental retardation, ammonia intoxication.	Diet low in protein(?)
Type II	Carbamolyl-phosphate synthase			

From *Geigy scientific tables,* ed 7, 1970, Ciba-Geigy Corp, Summit, N.J.
*Incidence 1 in 100,000.
†Incidence varies from 1 to 3200 to 1 in 10^7 according to locality.
‡Incidence 1 in 13,000.

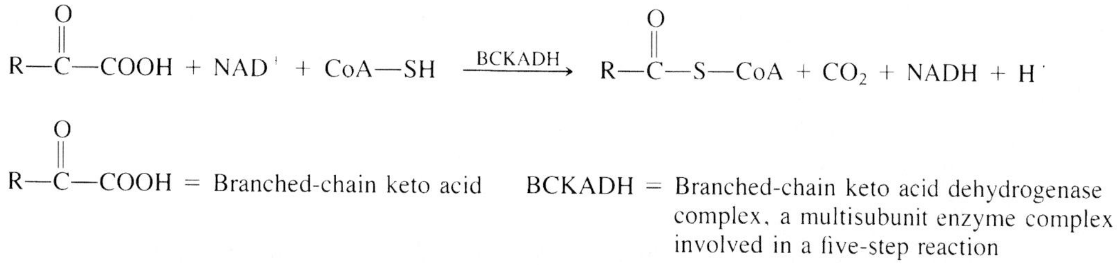

$$R\!-\!\overset{\displaystyle O}{\overset{\|}{C}}\!-\!COOH + NAD^{+} + CoA\!-\!SH \xrightarrow{\text{BCKADH}} R\!-\!\overset{\displaystyle O}{\overset{\|}{C}}\!-\!S\!-\!CoA + CO_{2} + NADH + H^{+}$$

$$R\!-\!\overset{\displaystyle O}{\overset{\|}{C}}\!-\!COOH = \text{Branched-chain keto acid}$$

BCKADH = Branched-chain keto acid dehydrogenase complex, a multisubunit enzyme complex involved in a five-step reaction

Fig. 47-12 Maple-syrup urine disease. Branched-chain keto acid decarboxylase enzyme complex when deficient results in elevation of branched-chain amino acids valine, isoleucine, and leucine, as well as their keto acid analogs.

Deficiency of this enzyme results in the elevated urinary excretion of the ketoacid analogs of these three branch-chained amino acids and gives positive ferric chloride and dinitrophenol hydrazine screening tests. The plasma is characterized by elevations in the levels of leucine, isoleucine, and valine. This disorder is screened for in the newborn using a bacterial-inhibition assay system, similar to the Guthrie test, that detects elevated levels of plasma leucine in the newborn. After the diagnosis, special diets that restrict the intake of isoleucine, leucine, and valine combined with careful monitoring can provide adequate control of this disease. Affected children who are not detected by newborn screening within the first month of life generally become acutely ill with hypoglycemia and ketoacidosis. Without early recognition and treatment death, most commonly occurs, and in those in whom diet is instituted late, significant mental retardation results.

Homocystinuria is generally recognized in late childhood because of physical abnormalities with or without mental retardation. Homocystine is an intermediate amino acid in the metabolism of methionine to cystine. The most common form of homocystinuria occurs because of a deficiency of the enzyme cystathionine synthetase, which results in elevated plasma and urinary levels of homocystine. The elevation in plasma levels of homocystine results in conversion of most of this substance to methionine. Thus one can screen for homocystinuria in newborn blood by analyzing plasma levels of methionine. This condition results in clinical manifestations through two mechanisms: (1) the elevated levels of homocystine have been shown to be toxic to vascular endothelium and account for the thromboembolic phenomenon (plugging of brain or lung blood vessels by blood clots) of this disease, and (2) the failure of production of cystine results in a deficiency of this essential amino acid in connective tissue, specifically collagen, metabolism. The enzymatic activity of cystathionine synthetase requires as its cofactor the B vitamin pyridoxine. Different mutations in the gene locus for cystathionine synthetase result in two distinct forms of homocystinuria. In approximately half the patients with cystathionine synthetase deficiency, a sufficient enhancement of residual enzyme activity can be achieved by the addition of therapeutic doses of pyridoxine to the diet essentially to cure the disease.

Cyanide-nitroprusside is used as a urine-screening test for this disease. Nitroprusside combines with sulfhydryl-containing amino acids to produce a red color. The cyanide reduces disulfide bonds and gives a positive screening result. Homocystinuria and cystinuria give a positive cyanide-nitroprusside reaction, whereas silver nitroprusside, which does not reduce the disulfide bond of homocystine, gives a positive result only when cystinuria is present.

Organic acidurias

The metabolism of amino acids involves several intermediate steps. During each step organic acids are produced. A defect in the subsequent metabolism of these compounds results in disorders that are characterized by a severe metabolic acidosis. Among this group of disorders, the ketotic hyperglycinemia syndrome is composed of several defects in propionic acid and methylmalonic acid metabolism. The amino acids leucine, isoleucine, valine, threonine, and methionine and odd-numbered fatty acids lead to the production of propionyl CoA, which is converted to methylmalonyl CoA. Methylmalonyl CoA is converted into succinyl CoA, which can then enter the tricarboxylic acid cycle (Fig. 47-13). Infants with these disorders usually are seen within the first few weeks of life with severe ketoacidosis, which may be accompanied by hypoglycemia. The urine yields a strongly positive dinitrophenyl hydrazine reaction and by amino acid analysis shows striking elevations in glycine. If methylmalonic acid is not found in the urine, one can make a presumptive diagnosis of propionicaciduria. A definitive diagnosis of this disorder can then be further pursued through the demonstration of the presence of methylcitrate in the urine, the gas-liquid chromatographic analysis of organic acids in the urine, or the assay of propionyl CoA carboxylase in cultured cells. The conversion of propionyl CoA to methylmalonyl CoA uses biotin as a cofactor, which may in therapeutic doses enhance residual enzyme activity. The conversion of methylmalonyl CoA to succinyl CoA involves the metabolism of B_{12}, which in therapeutic doses can also result in significant biochemical improvement. In those instances in which vitamin therapy

$$\text{Propionyl CoA} + \text{HCO}_3^- \xleftrightarrow{1} \text{D-Methylmalonyl CoA} \xleftrightarrow{2} \text{L-Methylmalonyl CoA} \xleftrightarrow{3} \text{Succinyl CoA}$$

If enzyme 1 is missing → Propionic acid

If enzyme 2 is missing → Methylmalonic acid

1 = Propionyl/CoA carboxylase (biotin, ATP, Mg^{++})
2 = Methylmalonyl-CoA racemase
3 = Methylmalonyl-CoA mutase

Fig. 47-13 Propionic aciduria and methylmalonic aciduria. This sequence of metabolism of organic acids can be interrupted at several points, each of which results in a specific organic aciduria.

does not result in a significant therapeutic response, a low-protein diet is used.

Defects in carbohydrate metabolism

Galactosemia is a toxicity syndrome associated with an intolerance to dietary galactose. This recessively inherited disorder occurs as a result of a deficiency of the enzyme galactose-1-phosphate uridyltransferase.

$$\text{Galactose-1-phosphate} + \text{UDP-glucose} \xrightarrow{\text{Gal-1-P uridyltransferase}}$$
$$\text{UDP-galactose} + \text{Glucose-1-phosphate}$$

Lactose, composed of galactose and glucose, is the major disaccharide in mammalian milk. Hydrolysis of lactose by the intestine results in the release of the monosaccharides glucose and galactose. The main pathway of galactose metabolism in humans involves the conversion of galactose to glucose by epimerization of the hydroxyl group at the carbon-4 position. The reaction catalyzed by galactose-1-phosphate uridyltransferase involves galactose-1-phosphate with UDP-glucose, yielding UDP-galactose and glucose-1-phosphate. The UDP-galactose can by further conversion yield UDP and glucose-1-phosphate. Humans are thus capable of metabolizing large amounts of galactose. However, with deficiency of the transferase enzyme, galactose is reduced to galactitol and oxidized to galactonate. It is the presence of these two intermediate products of galactose metabolism that has direct toxic effects and results in the clinical manifestations of galactosemia. The classic clinical presentation of galactosemia is one of failure to thrive in early infancy complicated by vomiting and diarrhea. In addition, these infants show deranged hepatic function with jaundice and hepatomegaly. Severe hemolysis can also occur, and cataracts may be noted shortly after birth. Without dietary therapy, retarded mental development can be apparent in the newborn after only a few months of age. Many states have instituted newborn screening for galactosemia using the disk of blood collected for the Guthrie test to assay for galactose-1-phosphate uridyltransferase. Metabolic screening tests of the urine from acutely ill infants should include a test for reducing substances in the urine. Urine dipsticks impregnated with glucose oxidase are specific for glucose. Such a urine screening would be negative in most infants with galactosemia. An infant with the clinical manifestations described above who has a negative dipstick urine

test result for glucose but a positive copper sulfate test result (such as Clinitest) for reducing substances in the urine has strong presumptive evidence for galactosemia. Dietary control of the disease in the first few years of life can result in normal growth and development.

A second defect in galactose metabolism occurs as a result of deficiency of the enzyme galactokinase:

$$\text{Galactose} + \text{ATP} \xrightarrow{\text{Galactokinase}} \text{Galactose-1-phosphate} + \text{ADP}$$

This disorder is recognized most commonly after a screening of urine metabolites of patients with cataracts. Deficiency of galactokinase results in the accumulation of galactitol as an end product in galactose metabolism. This compound accumulates within the lenses and is responsible for the cataracts. There are no hepatic or other systemic manifestations of this defect. One can assay the enzyme in red blood cells, and the excretion of galactose and galactitol in urine will give a positive reducing substance reaction. Early recognition of this disorder and the elimination of galactose from the diet will prevent the development of cataracts.

Lactic acidosis is a commonly observed complication of many diseases that result in increased anaerobic metabolism. Primary abnormalities in carbohydrate metabolism leading to lactic acidosis are rare. Anaerobic metabolism and defective carbohydrate metabolism may give rise to elevations in both pyruvic and lactic acid. However, because pyruvate is shunted rapidly to lactate and most clinical laboratories perform lactate assays but not pyruvate assays, lactic acidosis rather than pyruvic acidosis is more commonly recognized and referred to. A primary abnormality in pyruvate metabolism or in muscle mitochondrial metabolism of glucose will result in an increased pyruvate and lactate level after a glucose load. Patients with lactic acidosis in whom no abnormality in tissue blood perfusion or oxygenation is apparent may require additional tests to rule out a primary abnormality in carbohydrate or pyruvate metabolism.

Glycogen-storage diseases (see Chapter 31). The glycogen-storage diseases combine two different types of metabolic defects. First, because of the alterations in glycogen metabolism, inadequate glucose stores are available for metabolic needs, and symptoms of acute hypoglycemia occur. Second, the accumulation of glycogen results in the

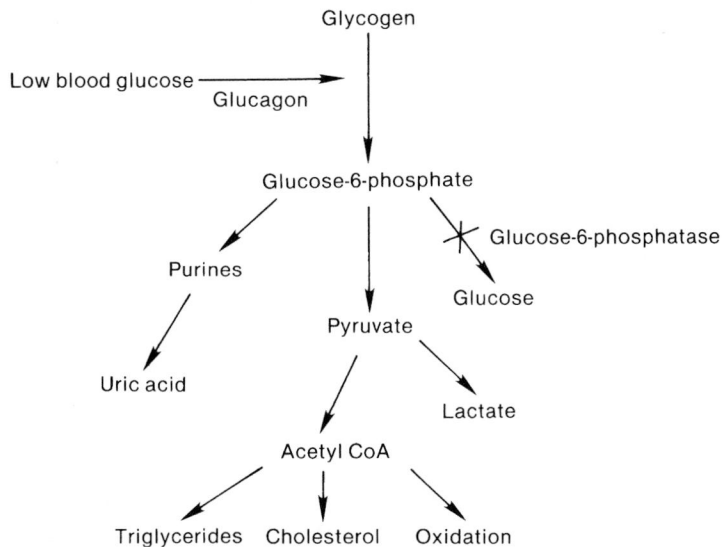

Fig. 47-14   Glycogen-stored disease type 1 (von Gierke's disease). Use of glycogen to form free glucose requires hepatic action of glucose-6-phosphatase to transport glucose extracellularly.

long-term, chronic effects of a storage disease. Table 47-6 lists a classification scheme of the glycogen-storage diseases.

The classic form of glycogen-storage disease is von Gierke's disease, which occurs as a result of a deficiency of glucose-6-phosphatase. All metabolic sources of blood glucose are channeled through the intrahepatic formation of glucose-6-phosphate (see Chapter 32). Glucose in this form cannot be transported outside the liver cell. Thus the for-

mation of glucose from amino acids through gluconeogenesis or the conversion of other carbohydrates into glucose uses the intermediate of glucose-6-phosphate. With a deficiency of glucose-6-phosphatase, the only carbohydrate available to maintain blood glucose is the glucose metabolite glucose-1-phosphate. A simplified scheme of glycogen metabolism and the consequences of glucose-6-phosphatase deficiency are shown in Fig. 47-14. Infants with type 1 glycogen-storage disease, glucose-6-phosphatase defi-

Table 47-6   Inborn errors of glycogen deposition or utilization

Condition	Cori type	Biochemical features	Clinical features
Glucose-6-phosphatase deficiency (von Gierke's disease)	1	Normal glycogen accumulates in liver and kidney	Hepatomegaly, hypoglycemia; stunted growth with retarded bone age, etc.
Idiopathic generalized glycogenosis (Pompe's disease)	2	Normal glycogen accumulates in all organs	Cardiac failure, muscle hypotonia, neurological disorders, death in infancy
Dextrin-1,6-glucosidase (debrancher) deficiency (limit dextrinosis; Forbes' disease)	3	Abnormal glycogen with short branches deposited in liver and sometimes skeletal and cardiac muscle	Hepatomegaly, hypoglycemia; less severe than von Gierke's disease
α-Glucan-branching glycosyltransferase (brancher) deficiency (amylopectinosis; Andersen's disease)	4	Abnormal carbohydrate with long inner and outer branches deposited in liver, spleen, and lymph nodes	Hepatic cirrhosis; death within 2 years of birth
Glycogen phosphorylase (glycogen phosphorylase of the muscle deficiency (McArdle's syndrome)	5	Moderate accumulation of normal glycogen in skeletal muscles; lactate and pyruvate levels in blood fall during exercise	Generalized muscular fatigability and pain
Glycogen phosphorylase (hepatic glycogen phosphorylase) deficiency (Hers' disease)	6	Normal glycogen accumulates in liver; phosphorylase content of liver and leukocytes reduced	Hepatomegaly; relatively benign
Deficiency of UDP glucose glycogen glycosyltransferase (glycogen synthetase)	7	Liver glycogen almost completely absent	Severe fasting hypoglycemia

From *Geigy's scientific tables,* ed 7, 1970, Ciba-Geigy Corp, Summit, N.J. From Field RA. In Stanbury JB et al, editors: *The metabolic basis of inherited disease,* ed 2, New York, 1966, McGraw-Hill, p 141; Hers HG: *Adv Metab Disord* 1:1, 1964; *Control of glycogen metabolism,* Ciba Foundation symposium, London, 1964, Churchill.

ciency, usually have recurring episodes of hypoglycemia within the first few days of life that are often accompanied by ketoacidosis and lactic acidosis. If there is no elevation in blood glucose after administration of glucagon, a defect in glycogen metabolism must be assumed. Specific diagnosis of type 1 glycogen-storage disease requires a liver biopsy for the demonstration of glucose-6-phosphatase deficiency. Children with type 1 glycogen-storage disease are unable to maintain an adequate blood glucose for more than 2 to 2½ hours after a normal feeding. The management of infants with this disorder cannot be satisfactorily accomplished through the use of frequent oral feedings. For that reason, nasogastric tubes and feeding gastrostomies have been used to improve the management of this disease during the first few years of life.

Pompe's disease, or type I glycogen-storage disease, is a condition that is entirely different from the remainder of the glycogen-storage diseases. This disorder is the result of a defect in lysosomal degradation of glycogen. The deficient enzyme is α-glucosidase, an acid hydrolase similar to the deficient enzyme of other lysosomal storage diseases. Deficiency of this enzyme results in widespread systematic lysosomal storage of glycogen and is seen in infancy with hepatomegaly, cardiomegaly, and central hypotonia. The disease follows a rapidly downhill course, with death by 1 to 2 years of age. This alteration of glycogen metabolism does not affect normal glucose homeostasis. Diagnosis of this form of glycogen-storage disease is indicated by lysosomal accumulation of glycogen demonstrated on muscle or liver biopsy. The enzyme α-glucosidase can be assayed in peripheral lymphocytes or in cultured skin fibroblasts to make a specific diagnosis. Because this enzyme is present in cultured cells, prenatal diagnosis exists for this form of glycogen-storage disease.

Transport defects. There are many conditions that lead to altered metabolic states as a result of a defect in membrane transport of metabolites rather than as a result of an enzyme deficiency in a metabolic pathway. After glomerular filtration of plasma, there is the selective reabsorption of metabolites through the renal tubules so that urine ultimately contains only waste products and nonwaste products

are conserved. Single gene-determined components of the plasma membrane of the renal tubule are responsible for the selective reabsorption of individual compounds. One selective renal tubular reabsorption mechanism exists for the four amino acids cystine, lysine, ornithine, and arginine. Homozygotes for a mutation involving this reabsorptive system have a pronounced renal loss of these four amino acids. The condition is known as *cystinuria* because it is the renal loss of cystine that contributes to the clinical disorder. Cystine is less soluble in an acid urine than in an alkaline urine. With an increased renal loss of cystine this amino acid precipitates out to form stones in renal papillae and the collecting system. Cystinuria is seen in early childhood as a form of chronic renal insufficiency usually first manifest as growth retardation. Metabolic screening of urine because of failure to thrive or short stature will detect cystinuria through a positive cyanide-nitroprusside reaction.

There are several conditions in which there is defective renal transport of amino acids; these are shown in Table 47-7.

Vitamin D–resistant rickets, or hypophosphatemic rickets, represents a defect in renal tubular reabsorption of phosphate. This condition is inherited as an X-linked dominant disorder. As a result, its effect is quite variable in heterozygous females who may show no clinical manifestations or who may exhibit moderate short stature and evidence of rickets. In affected males there is hypophosphatemia and hyperphosphaturia with short stature and bowing of the legs accompanying the roentgenographic evidence of rickets. Definitive diagnosis is made by demonstration of a greatly elevated 24-hour urine phosphate excretion. This disorder is called vitamin D–resistant rickets because massive doses of vitamin D will not correct the altered plasma and urine levels of calcium and phosphate. With regular intake of the maximum gastrointestinal tolerance of phosphate, males with this condition can have significant improvement of rickets and enhancement of their adult height. Phosphate is rapidly cleared from plasma when taken orally, and replacement therapy must include ingestion of phosphate every 4 hours. This disease is the first to be found that is a mutant

Table 47-7   Errors in renal amino acid transport

Disorder	Urine analysis	Findings
Cystinuria	Urine cyanide-nitroprusside	Renal failure resulting from cystine stones
Hyperdibasic aminoaciduria	Elevated urinary lysine, ornithine, arginine	Autosomal dominant asymptomatic
Fanconi syndrome	Elevated urinary amino acids, bicarbonate, phosphate, glucose, potassium, uric acid	Growth failure in primary form, occurs secondarily in Wilson's disease and galactosemia
Glucoglycinuria	Glucosuria, glycinuria	Autosomal dominant asymptomatic
Hartnup's disease	Elevated neutral and ring amino acids	Asymptomatic with good nutrition, especially nicotinic acid
Familial renal iminoglycinuria	Elevated urine proline, hydroxyproline, glycine	Autosomal recessive asymptomatic
Lowe's (oculocerebrorenal) syndrome	Renal aminoaciduria, proteinuria, aciduria, phosphaturia	X-linked recessive cataracts, mental retardation, and hypotonia

of a hormone receptor; it is a vitamin D_3 intracellular receptor.

Disorders of mineral metabolism. The most common and best-known disorder involving mineral metabolism is *Wilson's disease,* or *hepatolenticular degeneration.* Copper is accumulated in pathological quantities. This autosomal, recessively inherited disorder involving copper metabolism is often observed symptomatically as cirrhosis in adolescents or as a psychiatric disorder in older teenagers or young adults. The gene responsible for Wilson's disease has not been cloned but is closely linked to a marker on chromosome 13. Although the exact genetic basis of the specific abnormality in copper metabolism remains unknown, derangements in tissue and urinary levels of copper are diagnostic for the disease. Clinically this disorder is characterized by a triad of findings: a peculiar neurological syndrome, cirrhosis of the liver, and Kayser-Fleischer rings of the cornea. The neurological abnormalities take two forms: the first is lenticular degeneration (loss of cerebellar function), which is also known as the dystonic form (abnormal movement and tone of muscles) of the disease. The second neurological form is pseudosclerosis. This involves flapping tremors of the wrist and shoulders associated with rigidity and spasticity. The hepatic involvement of this disease is first manifest as an enlarged liver with associated splenomegaly. Thereafter the course is one similar to that of chronic hepatitis. Ultimately the disease progresses to the full-blown picture of cirrhosis. The Kayser-Fleischer ring is still considered as the single most important clinical diagnostic finding of this disease. It is a ring of a golden-brown or greenish discoloration that appears at the margin of the cornea near the limbus.

There are several laboratory approaches to the diagnosis of Wilson's disease. Most but not all patients with this disorder will have a depressed plasma level of ceruloplasmin. Ceruloplasmin is a metalloglycoprotein containing copper. It acts as an oxidase in the enzymatic oxidation of iron from the ferrous to the ferric state. Early in the course of the disease the 24-hour urine level of copper may be within the reference interval to slightly increased but is uniformly strikingly elevated in advanced stages of the disorder. Given a clinical suspicion of this disorder, one diagnostic approach is the 24-hour urine measurement of copper followed by a 24-hour urine measurement of copper during administration of penicillamine. With increased tissue levels of copper the chelating agent penicillamine will result in a striking increase in copper excretion. The most definitive and in some cases the only assured way of making a diagnosis is by liver biopsy and tissue analysis of copper content. Wilson's disease can be essentially controlled by the long-term administration of penicillamine. Patients who have serious side reactions to penicillamine can be treated with zinc sulfate, which blocks metallothionine receptors in the gut, preventing reabsorption of copper excreted in the bile.

A second disorder of copper metabolism is known as *Menkes' syndrome,* or *kinky-hair disease.* This disorder is an X-linked recessive neurological disease that is seen in early infancy with failure to thrive, lethargy, hypothermia, and myoclonic seizure activity. Affected male infants have pallid skin and a characteristic facial appearance. The hair may appear normal at birth, but thereafter a characteristic pattern develops. The hair lacks luster and is somewhat depigmented; it also has a steely feel. Children with Menkes' syndrome have low serum levels of copper and ceruloplasmin. However, attempts at treatment through copper administration have been unsuccessful. A defect in copper transport is demonstrated through the study of radioactive copper metabolism in cultured skin fibroblasts. This approach has also been successfully used in the prenatal diagnosis of this disease.

Disorders of urea cycle and hyperammonemias. The principal end product of nitrogen metabolism in humans is urea. Protein metabolism results in the production of ammonia, which enters the urea cycle (Fig. 47-15) in the synthesis of carbamyl phosphate and leaves through the urea in the conversion of arginine to ornithine. Within this cycle there have been recognized five distinct enzymatic deficiencies, each of which results in hyperammonemia. Disruption of the urea cycle does not produce acidosis, ketosis, or hypoglycemia but manifests itself clinically as the direct toxic effect of ammonia on the CNS. The clinical diagnosis should be suspected in infants with CNS depression after protein intake, a condition that should prompt an analysis of a blood ammonia level. The degree of hyperammonemia is massive and in itself does not indicate a particular disorder but rather an interruption in the urea cycle. Quantitative determination of plasma and urine amino acids may show elevations in amino acids suggestive of defects in earlier steps in the urea cycle or demonstrate the specific compound elevated in the latter steps of the urea cycle. Carbamyl phosphate synthetase and ornithine transcarbamylase deficiencies require liver biopsy for specific diagnosis using an enzymatic analysis. Citrullinemia, argininosuccinicaciduria, and argininemia are diagnosed by demonstration of an elevation of these substrates through two-dimensional paper chromatography of urine or by column chromatography for amino acid analysis. The enzyme defect in these latter three conditions is demonstrated in cultured skin fibroblasts.

Receptor defects. Receptors are discrete gene products that function as membrane-bound or cytoplasmic agents required for the transport of specific compounds across membranes or as the intracellular regulators of metabolic activity. Knowledge about receptor function has been greatly enhanced through the study of single gene disorders that result in specific receptor defects. Such genetic disorders are illustrated by the conditions familial hypercholesterolemia and testosterone-resistant syndromes (testicular feminization syndrome).

Familial hypercholesterolemia is a dominantly inherited

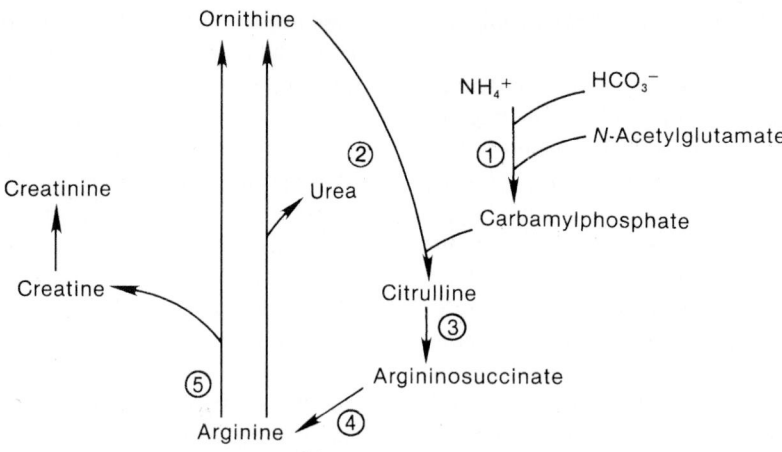

Fig. 47-15 Urea cycle defects. Five primary hyperammonemias include type 1, or carbamyl phosphate synthetase deficiency; type 2, or ornithine transcarbamyltransferase deficiency; type 3, or citrullinemia caused by argininosuccinate synthetase deficiency; type 4, or argininosuccinicaciduria caused by argininosuccinase deficiency; type 5, or hyperargininemia caused by arginase deficiency.

disorder that is the most common single gene cause of coronary artery disease and myocardial infarction in young adults. In humans, low-density lipoprotein (LDL) is the carrier for most of the cholesterol in plasma. After cholesterol is synthesized within the liver, it is transported within LDL particles to cells, where it is internalized through the binding of the LDL molecules to a specific cell surface receptor. After binding of LDL molecules to the cell surface receptors, an endocytotic vesicle is formed, which fuses with lysosomes. Within the lysosome the LDL molecules are degraded to free amino acids, eventually unesterified free cholesterol. As adequate amounts of cholesterol are internalized, there is suppression of 3-hydroxy-3-methylglutaryl coenzyme A reductase (HMG-CoA reductase), which causes a reduction in cellular cholesterol synthesis. Conversely, an intracellular requirement for cholesterol stimulates HMG-CoA reductase activity. The familial hypercholesterolemia disorder results from a mutation affecting the LDL receptor. With a reduced number of cell surface receptors for LDL cholesterol and thus reduced uptake of cholesterol, there is inadequate suppression of HMG-CoA reductase activity. This results in stimulation of further cholesterol synthesis. The net result is familial, or type IIa, hypercholesterolemia. There are rare persons who are homozygous for a defect in the LDL receptor. During early childhood such persons have greatly elevated levels of plasma cholesterol and severe coronary artery disease, usually leading to death at adolescence. Study of cultured skin fibroblasts from homozygously affected persons allowed elucidation of the defect in LDL receptors and the concomitant effect on the regulation of HMG-CoA reductase activity. As a result of this work, it was possible to show that the more common heterozygous form of autosomal dominant hypercholester-

olemia represented a partial defect in LDL receptors and regulation of HMG-CoA reductase activity.

The term *testicular feminization syndrome* is an older designation for a disorder involving an abnormality in testosterone metabolism. Affected individuals are phenotypic females who develop female secondary sexual characteristics at puberty but fail to undergo menarche. A laparotomy in such a person will show absence of a uterus and the presence of intra-abdominal testes. Chromosome analysis reveals a normal male 46,XY karyotype. These chromosomal males embryologically develop the external genitalia of a female because of a cellular resistance to the action of testosterone. There is normal testosterone generation by the testes, but there is an unresponsiveness of target tissues to testosterone. The action of testosterone (androgens) on target cells is mediated by specific cytoplasmic receptors. Dihydrotestosterone combines with a cytosol-binding protein (the receptor) to form a hormone-protein complex that is transported into the cell nucleus, where it exerts its action on chromatin. A defect in the receptor results in an inability of target cells to respond to the testosterone.

Disorders of purine metabolism. The best known disorder involving a defect in purine metabolism is the *Lesch-Nyhan syndrome*. Affected males are seen with a disorder of self-mutilation, mental retardation, and cerebellar dysfunction. Their urine contains excessive amounts of uric acid crystals. The hyperuricemia characteristic of this X-linked recessively inherited disorder is the result of a deficiency of hypoxanthine-guanine phosphoribosyltransferase (HGPRT). This enzyme is involved in the metabolism of the purine nucleotides guanylic acid (GMP) and inosinic acid (IMP). These two purines regulate the activity of several enzymes in purine metabolism including HGPRT.

The deficiency of this enzyme results in an accelerated rate of purine biosynthesis, and because of the block, increased amounts of hypoxanthine and xanthine are synthesized, which are readily converted in the liver by xanthine oxidase to massive amounts of uric acid. Allopurinol is used to lower the serum and urinary levels of uric acid in these patients, but this does not alter the CNS abnormalities that are part of the disorder.

When cells deficient in HGPRT are cultured, they are resistant to the effects of purine analogs such as 8-azaguanine and 6-mercaptopurine, which inhibit the growth of normal cells. Because the female carrier for this X-linked condition by lyonization has cells with HGPRT and cells without HGPRT, fibroblasts will grow in both normal media and media with one of these purine analogs. Cells from a noncarrier female will grow in the normal media but not in media with the analog. This selective medium system has proved to be a powerful tool in the detection of carriers for the Lesch-Nyhan syndrome. As prenatal diagnosis is available, study of females in a family in which this condition has occurred is important for genetic counseling. The gene for HGPRT seems to be susceptible to a large number of mutations, ones that may be seen on a single individual or family ("private" mutations). This makes the diagnosis of this disorder by molecular means more difficult.

Mitochondrial disorders. Each cell contains hundreds of mitochondria, which are subcellular organelles responsible for a large number of metabolic functions, including most oxidative processes. Many of the proteins and enzymes contained within the mitochondria are coded by the mitochondrial genome, a double-stranded circle of DNA, 16.6 kilobases (kb) in length. Since mitochondria also have their own protein synthesis machinery and a genetic code slightly different from the one used by the nuclear genes, it is appropriate that the translation apparatus (including 22 transfer RNAs and two ribosomal RNAs) also be encoded in the mitochondrial DNA. Thirteen subunits of the respiratory chain, which is responsible for producing ATP, are encoded in the mitochondrial DNA, including the proteins composing the NADH-coenzyme Q reductase (complex I), the cytochrome-*b* subunit of coenzyme Q–cytochrome-*c* (complex III), three subunits of cytochrome-*c* oxidase, and two subunits of ATPase (complex IV). The remaining subunits of these complexes are encoded by nuclear genes. Numerous diseases, which have been recognized to be consistent with a sex-limited, or maternal, mode of inheritance, have been found to be caused by mutations in genes encoded by the mitochondrial DNA.

A classic example of a maternally inherited mitochondrial disorder is *Leber's optic atrophy.* Because mitochondria are inherited only from the mother, females transmit the disease to sons and daughters; more males are affected than females, but males never transmit the disease to their offspring. One seventh of the mothers of affected males are themselves affected. In 1988, Wallace et al. demonstrated that this disease was caused by an error in the mitochondrial gene encoding the NADH-dehydrogenase subunit 4. Other point mutations underlie mitochondrial myopathies (muscle disorders). These are characterized by syndromes given the acronyms "MELAS" (myopathy, encephalopathy, lactic acidosis, and stroke-like episodes) and "MERRF" (myoclonus, ataxia, seizures, dementia, and ragged red fibers). In these cases mutations occur in genes coding for tRNAs. Mutational changes may also consist of large deletions or duplications of the same genes, such as in the *Kearns-Sayre syndrome* (progressive ophthalmoplegia, ptosis, proximal myopathy, pigmentary retinopathy, ataxia, and heart block) in which a deletion of 4.9 kb of DNA removes several tRNA genes from mitochondria, primarily in muscles, or the Pearson syndrome (sideroblastic anemia, exocrine pancreatic dysfunction, lactic acidosis) in which large insertions or deletions are found in mitochondria in all tissues. The mutant phenotype is found in both normal and abnormal mitochondria in heteroplasmic individuals. The clinical manifestations are influenced by the proportion of mutant mitochondria in relevant tissues in heteroplasmic individuals. The proportion can vary from cell type to cell type and with age of the individual in ways that are not yet clear (Johns DR: Mitochondrial DNA in disease, *N Engl J Med* 333: Sept. 1995). Although disease severity appears correlated with proportion of affected mitochondria in specific tissues, sufficient exceptions have been observed to indicate that much remains to be learned about the biology of mitochondria.

Peroxisomal disorders. Peroxisomes are subcellular organelles that contain oxidizing enzymes called *peroxidases.* The *Zellweger cerebral hepatorenal syndrome* (craniofacial dysmorphology, abnormalities of the hands and feet, polycystic kidneys, and intrahepatic dysgenesis) is the prototypic peroxisomal abnormality. Elevated pipecolic acid, abnormalities in very-long-chain fatty acid metabolism (impaired beta-oxidation), and absence of peroxisomes all indicate that the fundamental defect may be a structural abnormality of this organelle. Indeed, a gene for a peroxisomal assembly factor–1 (PAF1) has been cloned and found to contain a point mutation in a Japanese family with a child with CHR syndrome. *Neonatal adrenoleukodystrophy* and *infantile Refsum's disease* may be additional examples of this class of defect. Inasmuch as peroxisomes contain over 40 enzymes and up to eight complementation groups have been identified in the CHR syndrome, additional genes may also be implicated in defective peroxisome biogenesis.

GENETIC SCREENING
Role of mass screening

Screening tests play a major role in the diagnosis and population study of genetic disease (Table 47-8). A screening test is not designed as a primary diagnostic tool. Rather, its pur-

Table 47-8 Genetic screening tests

Nature of screening test	Condition(s) screened for	Definitive diagnostic test
Buccal smear for Barr bodies	Numerical abnormalities of the X chromosome	Peripheral blood lymphocyte karyotype
Serum assay for percent hexosaminidase A	Carriers for Tay-Sachs disease	Hexosaminidase A in peripheral leukocytes
Guthrie test for semiquantitative blood phenylalanine level	Phenylketonuria among newborn infants	Quantitative plasma level of phenylalanine
Maternal serum alpha-fetoprotein determination	In utero detection of neural tube defects and Down's syndrome	Amniocentesis for chromosomes, alpha-fetoprotein, and acetylcholinesterase
RBC mean corpuscular volume	Carriers for thalassemia	Hemoglobin electrophoresis or chromatography
Stool for trypsin activity	Cystic fibrosis among newborns	Sweat test for 1 month of age
Serum CK levels in males with delayed walking	Duchenne muscular dystrophy	Restriction analysis
Fasting blood sugar or 2-hour postprandial blood glucose	Diabetes mellitus	Glucose tolerance test
Urine for reducing substances	Newborn with jaundice	Galactosemia
Hematocrit and RBC morphology among black infants	Sickle cell disease	Hemoglobin electrophoresis
Urine nitroprusside test among people with dislocated lenses	Homocystinuria	Quantitative plasma amino acids
Bleeding and clotting times in preoperative evaluation	Hemophilia A	Plasma factor VIII levels

pose is to identify a subpopulation of persons on whom definitive diagnostic testing would be cost beneficial. In general, the more specific a particular screening test, the greater is its cost, thus reducing its utility for screening large populations. A definitive diagnostic test for a given entity is one that has a sensitivity and specificity of close to 100%. The sensitivity of a test is a measure of how frequently a test will detect a disorder under question. The specificity of a test is a measure of how well a test discriminates one disorder from other disorders (see Chapter 20 for details). The sensitivity and specificity that are required of a screening test depend on the population to be studied and the purpose for which the screening test is undertaken. This is best illustrated when one considers the purposes for screening tests: (1) screening tests for the early detection of disease in the presymptomatic state when effective therapy exists (phenylketonuria or penicillin prophylaxis for sickle cell anemia), (2) carrier detection for inherited disease, especially in the context of prenatal diagnosis (Tay-Sachs disease), and (3) epidemiological studies of the frequency of a given disorder within the population (47,XXY or 47,XYY karyotype). If a disease can be effectively treated when detected early and if the consequences of nondetection are unacceptable, it is desirable to have a test with maximum sensitivity in order to detect all possibly affected persons. Those persons identified through a positive screening test can undergo additional testing with more specific assays that will establish a specific diagnosis. For a disease in which successful treatment is not readily available for the clinical manifestations, less-sensitive screening tests may be used. By lowering the sensitivity one can improve the specificity of the test. The few persons with the disease who are missed by the screening test will not be unduly compromised. Universal screening of newborns for sickle cell he-

moglobinopathies is an example of a situation where priorities are not easily set. Cellulose acetate electrophoresis is sensitive enough to detect the gene for HbS. Isoelectric focusing is a very sensitive but expensive technique for differentiating sickle cell trait from sickle cell–β^+-thalassemia. Sickle cell trait is sufficiently common, however, that locating all heterozygotes with β^+-thalassemia also is more would be very expensive. Thus, for screening purposes the use of less expensive techniques such as cellulose acetate electrophoresis followed by confirmatory isoelectric focusing with densitometry or HPLC that can be used on a large population may be the best approach. The cost of locating children for repeated testing may dictate a more definitive initial analysis.

Detection of heterozygote carriers

During the past 20 years considerable information about the specific molecular abnormalities underlying many genetically determined disorders has been amassed. In recessively inherited disorders, knowledge of the molecular defect can be used for the detection of carriers through demonstration of a partial expression of the molecular defect in heterozygous individuals. The accuracy of these carrier detection tests generally is directly proportional to the accuracy of the assay system that measures the specific molecular defect of the disorder under question. Some assay systems used for the detection of carriers of recessively inherited disorders are listed in Table 47-9. Some biochemical abnormalities have been noted in cystic fibrosis (CF), most notably an elevation in the chloride content of sweat. The gene for CF is genetically linked to that for the enzyme paroxonase and has been cloned by positional cloning and mapped to chromosome 7. The cystic fibrosis transmembrane conductance regulator (CFTR), as the gene is called,

Table 47-9 Carrier detection for genetic diseases

Disease	Carrier test	Findings
Sickle cell disease	Hemoglobin electrophoresis	S and A hemoglobin bands
Tay-Sachs disease	Serum hexosaminidase (Hex) A and total assay	% Hex A <45%
Hurler's syndrome	α-L-Iduronidase assay	Level <50% control
Duchenne muscular dystrophy	Serum CK assay	Elevated levels
Hemophilia A	Factor VIII assay	Low level
	DNA genotyping	Genotype of carriers in family
Phenylketonuria	Phenylalanine (phe) tolerance test	Higher than normal phe level after load
	DNA genotyping	Genotype of one carrier patient

CK, Creatine kinase.

is large, encoding a protein of 1480 amino acid residues (see below and Chapter 48). Its structure indicates that it is a membrane chloride-transport regulator, defects of which allow water and chloride to leak from the cells involved, resulting in the viscous secretions associated with the disease. The most severe mutation, dF508, is characterized by deletion of a phenylalanine codon at that amino acid position 508 of the gene. This allele accounts for 70% of the mutations at this locus, and homozygotes constitute approximately 57% of persons with CF. The majority of the remainder of CF patients are compound heterozygotes with mutations that can involve a large number of additional alleles.

This creates a substantial public health dilemma. Population mass screening using allele-specific oligonucleotide hybridization that will detect a high proportion of heterozygotes will be very expensive. Use of a smaller number of oligonucleotides will decrease sensitivity.

Prenatal diagnosis

Once the prevalence of a disease is shown to be high enough to justify the investment involved in establishing a method to detect that disease, there are several criteria that a diagnostic method must meet if it is to be used successfully in prenatal diagnosis. First, there must be a means of identifying couples at sufficient risk for a particular condition to warrant incurring the risks and costs of amniocentesis and other diagnostic procedures. Parents may be determined to be at risk for producing an offspring with genetic disease because they have at least one child with a genetic birth defect that has a significant recurrence risk, because they are determined by previous carrier detection, guided perhaps by knowledge of their racial or ethnic origin, to be carriers for an autosomal, recessively inherited disorder, or because of the age of the mother.

Second, the disorder under question should by its nature warrant prenatal diagnosis. At present this is generally true, since almost all conditions for which a prenatal diagnosis

is available are severe disorders for which there is no effective therapy for affected infants.

Third, the accuracy of the diagnostic method used should be well established because there is little margin for error with these studies. For diagnoses of many cytogenetic disorders and biochemical disorders using cultured amniotic fluid cells, the laboratory receives a 20 to 30 mL sample for a one-time opportunity of establishing a culture and performing a limited number of assays. The results of these assays will be used to determine whether the pregnancy will be continued. One wants to have supreme confidence in the systems used under these circumstances.

The recombinant DNA techniques that have proved so useful in the study of gene structure and function have provided the means for accurate prenatal diagnosis of several conditions. The best known example is the test for the prenatal diagnosis of sickle cell disease. With sickle cell disease it has been possible to combine the use of restriction endonucleases that recognize the specific nucleotide change of the mutant sickle cell gene with probes that bind to that portion of the hemoglobin gene that codes for the beta-globin chain. Use of the polymerase chain reaction is more sensitive and faster and does not require use of radioisotopes. The allele specific oligonucleotide (ASO) hybridization allows detection of base-pair abnormalities that are not detectable by use of restriction endonuclease analysis. The reverse ASO employs multiple DNA fragments (oligonucleotides) for various thalassemic base substitutions that are bound to a single membrane and then hybridized by labeled genomic DNA. The reverse ASO technique allows testing for multiple mutations simultaneously. All these techniques require neither the culturing of amniotic fluid cells nor special studies on the parents, provided that they are known carriers for sickle cell disease. It is possible to imagine a time when probes and restriction endonucleases will exist for the diagnosis of all genetic disorders. See Chapter 48 for a more detailed description of these techniques.

The box on p. 962 lists the various diagnostic modalities used in prenatal diagnoses, with an example of each.

ALPHA-FETOPROTEIN TESTING
Maternal serum alpha-fetoprotein screening

Alpha-fetoprotein (AFP) is a plasma protein made by the fetal liver. The plasma of a nonpregnant woman contains virtually no detectable AFP. During pregnancy, the maternal serum AFP level is related to the level of AFP in the amniotic fluid. Any fetal condition that results in increased passage of fetal plasma into amniotic fluid will increase the maternal serum level of AFP. Such conditions include open neural tube defects, such as anencephaly or meningomyelocele; abdominal wall defects, such as gastroschisis or omphalocele; and renal loss of plasma proteins from congenital nephrotic syndrome. These disorders can be screened for by the measurement of the AFP concentration in maternal serum. However, elevated levels of maternal se-

METHODS OF PRENATAL DIAGNOSIS

Cultured amniotic fluid cells
  Cytogenetic
    Advanced maternal age for Down's syndrome
  Biochemical
    Hexosaminidase assays for Tay-Sachs disease
  Morphological analysis
    Electron microscopy for mucolipidosis IV
  Substrate analysis
    Radioactive copper in Menkes' syndrome
Uncultured amniotic fluid cells
  Restrictive endonuclease analysis
    Beta-hemoglobin gene study in sickle cell disease
  Genetic polymorphisms for linkage diagnosis
    HLA determination and 21-hydroxylase deficiency
Amniotic fluid analysis
  Quantification of marker components
    Alpha-fetoprotein for open neural tube defects
  Analysis of abnormal metabolites
    Methylmalonate in methylmalonicaciduria
  Genetic polymorphisms for linkage diagnosis
    Secretory status and myotonic dystrophy
Imaging techniques
  Ultrasonography
    Autosomal recessive polycystic kidneys
  Roentgenography
    Skeletal dysplasia—achondrogenesis
  Fetoscopy
    Polydactyly in Ellis–van Creveld syndrome
Fetal sampling
  Fetal blood sampling
    Factor VIII antigen assay in hemophilia A
  Skin biopsy
    Histological appearance in epidermolysis bullosa
      dystrophica

rum AFP are also indicative of pregnancy complications in the absence of a fetal malformation; such complications include fetomaternal transfusion, increased risk of premature delivery, increased risk of fetal death, and the presence of twins.

From empirical experience it has been found that expression of the level of AFP in multiples of the median (MoM) lead to a better correlation with infant risk than use of standard deviations of the mean does. Most screening programs use 2.5 MoM as the upper limit of the reference interval for maternal serum; this is roughly equivalent to 5 SD above the mean. The amount of AFP produced by the fetus is relatively consistent from pregnancy to pregnancy, but the level of maternal serum AFP will vary with the maternal blood volume. It is necessary to adjust for this by correcting for maternal weight. Other factors that affect the maternal serum level are diabetes and race. The level of maternal serum AFP varies with gestational age, increasing gradually during the time appropriate for screening, 14 to 24 weeks of pregnancy. The maternal serum level in MoM is based on the median determination for each gestational week of

pregnancy, and interpretation requires accurate dating of the pregnancy.

Retrospective analysis of maternal serum screening for elevated AFP levels showed a correlation between low levels of AFP and the presence of a fetus with Down's syndrome. This correlation was subsequently confirmed in a series of prospective studies so that, currently, low levels of maternal serum AFP are considered an indication for amniocentesis and determination of the fetal karyotype. An independent correlation also exists between maternal age and the risk for a fetus with Down's syndrome; a maternal age of 35 years or older is the most common indication for prenatal diagnostic testing by amniocentesis or chorionic villus sampling. Levels of maternal serum AFP can be expressed as a risk for Down's syndrome for specific maternal ages. Thus, if a woman's age and her low level of AFP combine to generate a risk equivalent to that of a 35-year-old woman, she is offered prenatal diagnosis.

Amniotic fluid determination of alpha-fetoprotein

Maternal serum AFP determination is a screening test considered applicable to all pregnancies. Given an abnormal result, further testing in the form of ultrasonography and amniocentesis is offered. Normally, AFP determinations are done any time amniotic fluid samples are taken as with amniocentesis for advanced maternal age. A close correlation exists between the level of amniotic fluid AFP and the fetal conditions cited above; additionally, these structural defects can often be visualized by ultrasonography. If AFP is elevated in maternal serum and, upon amniocentesis, in amniotic fluid but no fetal defect is seen upon ultrasonography, electrophoresis of amniotic fluid acetylcholinesterase will reveal a specific band if an open neural tube defect is present. Amniotic fluid levels of AFP also vary with gestational age; levels are expressed as MoM with the median established for each gestational week of pregnancy between 16 and 26 weeks.

METHODS OF ANALYSIS

Each disease caused by an inborn genetic error results in a unique defect in a protein or enzyme function, or both. The consequence of this defect is a singular pattern of analyte change in biological fluids. Tables 47-4 to 47-11 list the pathognomonic analyte changes for many of these genetic defects. In addition, the major clinical findings for each disease are also given.

Alpha₁-antitrypsin

STEVEN C. KAZMIERCZAK

Principles of analysis and current usage Alpha₁-antitrypsin (AAT) is a glycoprotein with a molecular weight of approximately 55,000 daltons that is found in serum and other body fluids. AAT migrates in the alpha₁ region on agarose gel electrophoresis at pH 8.6. Major sites of synthesis of AAT are hepatocytes and alveolar macrophages. In serum AAT is responsible for about 90% of total antitrypsin activity, inhibiting a variety of proteolytic enzymes including trypsin, chy-

Table 47-10 Inborn errors of purine and pyrimidine metabolism

Condition	Defective enzyme or system	Biochemical features	Clinical features	Incidence and genetics
Gout (hyperuricemia)	Excessive synthesis of uric acid from precursors	Concentration of uric acid is increased in serum and often in urine.	Acute arthritic attacks, chronic arthritis with urate deposition in tissues; urinary urate calculi causing kidney damage; asymptomatic in 80% of cases	Hyperuricemia in 1% to 2%, clinical gout in 2 to 4/1000; probably autosomal dominant with variable and sex modified expression
Xanthinuria	Deficiency of xanthine oxidase and defective renal tubular reabsorption of xanthine	Xanthine is excreted in large amounts.	Xanthine calculi in urinary tract	Rare recessive
Oroticaciduria	Absence of orotidine-5'-phosphate pyrophosphorylase or decarboxylase, or of both	Orotic acid accumulates and is excreted in urine.	Severe megaloblastic anemia, orotic acid crystalluria	Very rare; recessive
β-Aminoisobutyricaciduria	Deficiency of a catabolic enzyme	High urinary excretion of β-aminoisobutyric acid.	Harmless	0 to 46%, depending on ethnic group; recessive

From Scientific tables, ed 7, 1970, Ciba-Geigy Corp, Summit, N.J.

motrypsin, elastase, collagenase, and plasmin.[1] AAT is an acute-phase reactant protein that may increase in concentration in serum by twofold to threefold in conditions such as inflammation, neoplastic disease, pregnancy and after the administration of estrogens.[2] Deficiency of AAT is strongly associated with early obstructive lung disease, whereas severe deficiency is associated with a high risk of developing pulmonary emphysema.[3] Because AAT inhibits a wide range of proteolytic enzymes in addition to antitrypsin, *alpha₁-protease inhibitor* is a more appropriate name for AAT.

AAT concentrations in serum can be approximated by use of electrophoretic separation of serum proteins (Table 47-12, method 1). Since AAT constitutes approximately 90% of the alpha₁-globulin band, deficiency of the enzyme results in virtual absence of this protein fraction.

Measurement of AAT can be performed by use of immunochemical or functional methods. The former measure the concentration of protein present, whereas the latter indicate the functional activity, or ability, of AAT to inhibit protease activity.

Measurement of the capacity of AAT to inhibit trypsin can be performed by measurement of the percentage of known trypsin activity that is inhibited by serum (Table 47-12, method 2).[4] In addition to inhibition of trypsin by AAT, elastase has also been used to evaluate the protease inhibitory capacity of AAT.[5] Although some have questioned the utility of assays for determining the functional activity of AAT, studies have found that in cigarette smokers, the functional activity of AAT is diminished even though the immunochemical concentration may be normal or increased.[6]

Most of AAT determinations performed in clinical laboratories measure the concentration of AAT in serum by use of immunochemical techniques. The most common immunochemical method in use for measurement of AAT in serum is immunonephelometry (Table 47-12, method 3). This technique measures the increase in light scattered as a result of AAT–anti-AAT antibody complex formation. Samples containing increased quantities of AAT will produce more antigen-antibody complexes resulting in a greater rate of in-

crease in light scatter when compared to samples with low concentrations of AAT.

A small percentage of laboratories measure AAT concentrations by use of immunodiffusion techniques such as radial immunodiffusion (Table 47-12, method 4). In this procedure, serum containing AAT is applied onto agarose gel containing anti-AAT antibody. The serum containing AAT diffuses into the gel where the diameter of the AAT–anti-AAT antibody precipitate is related to AAT concentrations in the sample.

Measurement of AAT activity in stool samples is performed for assessment of protein-losing enteropathy in patients with Crohn's disease, ulcerative colitis, or inflammation caused by enteric pathogens.[7] AAT is resistant to proteolytic digestion within the intestinal tract, and such a property makes it a useful marker for disease activity. The technique most commonly used for measuring AAT in stool specimens is radial immunodiffusion.[8] Immunonephelometric methods for measurement of AAT in stool samples have also been developed. However, studies comparing the immunonephelometric methods versus radial immunodiffusion for AAT in stool reveal radial immunodiffusion to have better sensitivity and a greater positive predictive value than immunonephelometric techniques.[9]

Individuals who are suspected of having AAT deficiency may be further characterized according to their AAT genotype. Various genotypes of AAT deficiency have been described, some of which are associated with low activities of AAT. The most common allele of the AAT gene is designated as PiM. The Z mutation results from a single-base substitution of the normal M allele. Individuals with the ZZ AAT phenotype have an associated severe deficiency of AAT. The method most commonly performed for evaluating a patient's AAT phenotype is electrophoretic separation using acid-starch gel followed by crossed antigen-antibody electrophoresis (Table 47-12, method 5). The first electrophoretic separation resolves AAT into several protein fractions labeled Z, S, M, and F from cathode to anode, respectively.[10] Charge differences causing the different rates of migration

Table 47-11   Lipidoses

Condition	Lipid accumulating	Site	Clinical features	Age at which symptoms appear	Genetics
Gaucher's disease (a) 'Adult' (b) Acute infantile (c) Juvenile and adult neurological	Glucocerebroside	Spleen, liver, bone marrow, leukocytes Brain in (b) and (c); lung in (b)	Splenomegaly, often gross; hepatomegaly; anemia; bone disorder; purpura; cerebral degeneration in (b) and (c).	(a) 1-60 years (b) 1st or 2nd half-year of life (c) 6-20 years	(a), (b), and (c) in different families, all recessive
Tay-Sachs disease (infantile amaurotic familial idiocy)	Ganglioside G_{M2} (G_0), amino glycolipid	White and gray matter of the brain	Cherry-red spot, retina of eye; progressive cerebral degeneration; death at age 1-5 years.	Usually 4-6 months, sometimes earlier	Recessive
Juvenile and adult amaurotic familial idiocy	Ganglioside G_{M1} (G_1)	Brain (moderate increased)	Progressive loss of vision and cerebral degeneration.	From 5 years onward	Probably recessive
Neimann-Pick disease (a) Acute infantile (b) Cerebral juvenile (c) Noncerebral	Mainly sphingomyelin	Spleen, bone marrow, liver; usually also brain and retina	Often cherry-red spot, retina of eye; hepatosplenomegaly; hepatic cirrhosis; usually cerebral degeneration and death in first 2½ years. Some adult cases are without neurological involvement.	(a) From birth (b) Childhood (c) Up to 30 years or later	(a) Recessive (b) Recessive (c) Uncertain
Metachromatic leukodystrophy (a) Infantile (b) Adult	Sulfatides	Brain, kidney, urine, gallbladder	(a) Cerebral and cerebellar degeneration; spasticity; dementia; death after 1-6 years. (b) Psychotic changes; blindness; aphasia; tetraplegia. Death after 3-12 years.	(a) 1-2 years (b) Late childhood or adulthood	(a) Recessive (b) Uncertain
Essential familial hyperlipemia	Triglycerides, lipoproteins	Blood plasma (chylomicrons)	Hepatosplenomegaly; sometimes xanthomas. Relatively benign.	Usually early childhood	Complex
Hypercholesterolemia	Cholesterol (free and esterified), phosphatides, sometimes triglycerides	Blood plasma (lipoproteins), tendons, skin, blood vessels	Cutaneous and tendinous xanthomas; atheroma of endocardium, coronary arteries, or great vessels.	From childhood onward	Usually dominant

*From *Scientific tables,* ed 7, 1970, Ciba-Geigy Corp, Summit, N.J.

are caused by amino acid substitutions in various fractions. The second step used in this procedure for determining AAT phenotypes consists in performing electrophoresis perpendicular to the first separation so that the AAT fractions migrate into agarose containing antibody directed against AAT. Precipitin bands occur wherever AAT and antibody react within the gel. The procedure requires technical expertise and takes approximately 1½ days to complete.

Another common method in use for evaluation of an individual's AAT phenotype is isoelectric focusing in polyacrylamide gel (Table 47-12, method 6).[11] This assay is performed with use of acrylamide gel with 3% cross-linking, which creates a slight molecular sieving effect. A pH gradient is produced in the gel by use of ampholine compounds composed of polyamino-polycarboxylic acids. Ampholines with a pH range of 3 to 6 are used. After electrophoretic separation, Coomassie Blue R-250 dye is used to stain the bands.

Current methods for phenotyping AAT such as acid starch gel electrophoresis and isoelectric focusing require technical skills and expertise not easily maintained in most laboratories because of the infrequent performance of this test. Alternative methods that have been devised include the use of monoclonal antibodies specific for either Z or non-Z AAT[11] and a colorimetric solid-phase minisequencing assay for the detection of the Z mutation of the AAT gene.[12]

Specimen   Serum is the specimen of choice for analysis for AAT by use of radial immunodiffusion or immunonephelometry. Samples may be kept refrigerated at 4° C for up to 5 days; however, storage at −20° C is optimal.

Phenotyping studies may be performed with use of serum or plasma. Specimens may be stored for up to 2 weeks at −20° C; for longer periods of storage, freezing at −70° C is preferable. Specimens that are stored improperly or have

Table 47-12   Methods for alpha₁-antitrypsin analysis

Method	Type of analysis	Principle	Sample	Comments
1. Electrophoresis	Estimation of alpha₁-globulins by electrophoretic separation	Proteins are separated based on migration in charged electrical field.	Serum	Useful as screen for severe alpha₁-antitrypsin deficiency
2. Trypsin-inhibitory capacity	Enzyme inhibition measured spectrophotometrically	Trypsin-inhibitory capacity of alpha₁-antitrypsin is determined by measurement of the esterolytic activity of trypsin and its inhibition spectrophotometrically.	Serum	Infrequently used
3. Nephelometry	Quantitation by immunoprecipitate in solution	Reaction of alpha₁-antitrypsin with its specific antibody results in immunoprecipitate, which has light-scattering properties; amount of light scatter is proportional to alpha₁-antitrypsin concentration.	Serum	Most common method in use
4. Radial immunodiffusion	Quantitation by immunoprecipitate in gel	Alpha₁-antitrypsin diffuses into gel containing antibody. Ring-shaped immunoprecipitate forms; diameter of ring is proportional to concentration.	Serum	Infrequently used
5. Electrophoresis of serum on acid starch gel followed by antigen-antibody crossed electrophoresis	Physical separation of alpha₁-antitrypsin variants followed by immunoprecipitating reaction in agarose	Two-step procedure: 1. Separation of alpha₁-antitrypsin variants on acid-starch gel by electrophoresis. 2. Second electrophoresis causes the separated variants to migrate perpendicularly to the first separation into agarose containing antibody to alpha₁-antitrypsin; precipitin peak forms.	Serum	Time consuming (1½ days) and technically difficult
6. Isoelectric focusing	Separation of alpha₁-antitrypsin variants on polyacrylamide gel based on surface-property charge	Alpha₁-antitrypsin variants are electrophoresed on polyacrylamide gel with a pH gradient ranging from 3.5 to 5 or 3 to 6.	Serum	Faster procedure—4 hours; produces band patterns similar to electrophoresis on acid-starch gel followed by antigen-antibody crossed electrophoresis

bacterial contamination may show altered rates of migration of AAT bands.[13]

Stool specimens obtained for analysis for AAT may be stored at 4° C for up to 3 days. Specimens may be stored frozen at −20° C until analysis.

Reference interval   Reference intervals for quantitation of AAT by use of rate nephelometry are approximately 0.9 to 2.1 g/L.[14] No significant age- or sex-related differences in AAT concentrations exist, though newborns may have slightly higher concentrations, which decline to adult ranges within approximately 60 days.[15]

Carbohydrate screen
STEVEN C. KAZMIERCZAK

Principles of analysis and current usage   The detection of carbohydrates in urine is clinically important in the evaluation of certain inborn errors of metabolism and for the evalu-

ation of other conditions resulting in excretion of carbohydrates into the urine. The carbohydrate most frequently assayed for in urine is glucose. Both quantitative and semiquantitative procedures have been developed for glucose determinations. Semiquantitative screening test for glucose, as well as other reducing carbohydrates, is a modification of the Benedict test (Table 47-13, method 1; see also p. 634). The sensitivity of this assay for detecting glucose is approximately 3500 mg/L when the two-drop method is used and 2500 mg/L using the five-drop procedure. Although this procedure suffers from a lack of sensitivity, its nonspecificity for glucose makes it useful for screening for other reducing sugars including galactose, fructose, lactose, mannose, and xylulose. Noncarbohydrate compounds, which can interfere with this assay producing a positive reaction, include sialic acid and homogentisic acid. Glucose in urine can be determined by use of quantitative enzymatic procedures that em-

Table 47-13   Tests for common carbohydrates

Method	Type of analysis	Principle	Usage	Comment
1. Modified Benedict test	Semiquantitative	Color is produced because of reaction of reducing substances with reagent containing copper sulfate, sodium hydroxide, sodium carbonate, and citric acid.	Commonly used	Detects reducing carbohydrates
2. Glucose oxidase	Semiquantitative	H_2O_2 is liberated from oxidation of glucose by glucose oxidase. H_2O_2 reacts with chromogen to form a colored dye.	Commonly used	Specific for glucose
3. Paper chromatography	Semiquantitative	Ascending or descending chromatography; sugars are located after color development with dinitrosalicylic acid or aniline-diphenylamine reagent.	Infrequently used	Good sensitivity and specificity
4. Thin-layer chromatography	Semiquantitative	Single-dimensional color development with aniline–phthalic acid reagent.	Infrequently used	Good sensitivity and specificity

ploy glucose oxidase or hexokinase (Table 47-13, method 2; see also Chapter 32). A positive test result obtained by use of the nonspecific Clinitest reagent coupled with a negative test result obtained by use of the glucose-specific enzymatic method is strongly suggestive of the presence of nonreducing sugars other than glucose. Unfortunately, this technique does not detect the presence of sucrose or other nonreducing carbohydrates.

The identification of carbohydrates in urine other than glucose requires more elaborate schemes to separate the various carbohydrates that may be present. Paper chromatography (Table 47-13, method 3) and thin-layer chromatography (Table 47-13, method 4) are the techniques most often employed for the detection of urinary carbohydrates. Thin-layer chromatography is more sensitive and specific and gives more accurate information when compared to paper chromatography.[16] Various solvent systems have been described for use with both paper chromatography and thin-layer chromatography.[16,17] A variety of support media have also been used with thin-layer chromatography.

Chemical detection stains vary in their abilities to detect carbohydrates separated by thin-layer or paper chromatography. General-purpose reagents include aniline phthalate and aniline phosphate. These stains readily detect most carbohydrates except for fructose and other ketones, which stain poorly, and sucrose, which does not react at all. Other chemical stains that may help in detecting these carbohydrates include aniline-diphenylamine phosphate reagent, which detects sucrose, and naphthoresorcinol, which reacts with ketose sugars.

Specimen   A random urine specimen is suitable for screening of urinary carbohydrates. Samples should be frozen as soon as possible after collection to prevent bacterial degradation of carbohydrates. Samples are stable for 12 months when frozen at $-20°$ C.

Reference interval   Healthy individuals have no carbohydrates detectable in urine. Premature infants and, to a lesser extent, term infants may excrete small amounts of glucose during the first few weeks of life. In addition to glucose, galactose may also be seen in the urine during this time. Beyond 1 month of age, however, the presence of carbohydrates in urine should be regarded as an abnormal finding.

Ceruloplasmin

STEVEN C. KAZMIERCZAK

Principles of analysis and current usage   Ceruloplasmin, the primary copper-containing protein in plasma, is also a late acute-phase reactant synthesized by the liver. During protein electrophoresis on agarose or cellulose acetate gel, it migrates in the α_2 region of the electrophoretogram. Ceruloplasmin normally does not make any visible contribution to the α_2 band except in instances where the concentration of the protein is greatly increased.

One function of ceruloplasmin is the oxidation of Fe^{2+} to Fe^{3+} as a preliminary step for the binding of iron to transferrin. Ceruloplasmin may also help prevent copper toxicity. A final role of ceruloplasmin may be that of an antioxidant, by preventing lipid peroxidation and mediating free-radical production in inflammatory states.

A wide variety of techniques have been employed for measurement of ceruloplasmin. Early methods that were developed were based on measurement of the oxidase activity of the enzyme. (Table 47-14, method 1). In these methods, ceruloplasmin reacts with a substrate to form a colored product.[18,19] The substrates most common in use are *p*-phenylenediamine and *o*-dianisidine dihydrochloride. These methods are subject to interference from certain anions and organic compounds.[20] Free metal ions such as cupric and ferrous ions can oxidize the substrate causing falsely increased results. Inhibition of the reaction can occur with samples containing increased concentrations of blood urea nitrogen (BUN >1 g/L), bilirubin (>163 mg/L), and uric acid (>200 mg/L).[19] The use of *o*-dianisidine is preferred over *p*-phenylenediamine as a substrate because the latter is not specific for ceruloplasmin, and both phenylalanine and its product are not so stable as *o*-dianisidine and its product.

The most common methods in use today for determination of ceruloplasmin concentrations are immunochemical procedures including radial immunodiffusion (Table 47-14, method 2) and immunonephelometry (Table 47-14, method 3). The immunochemical methods are more specific for ceruloplasmin and less subject to chemical interferences when compared to the enzymatic procedures.

Specimen   Serum is the specimen of choice for ceruloplasmin determinations. Plasma anticoagulated with

Table 47-14   Methods of ceruloplasmin analysis

Method	Principle	Usage	Comment
1. Colorimetric	Ceruloplasmin oxidizes substrate in the presence of oxygen to form a colored product.	Infrequently used Serum	Subject to variety of interferences
2. Radial immunodiffusion	Antibody to ceruloplasmin forms precipitin ring in agarose gel.	Frequently used Serum	Simple, specific method
3. Immunonephelometry	Antibody to ceruloplasmin forms antigen-antibody complexes, which scatter light.	Frequently used Serum	Requires specialized instrumentation

EDTA or citrate is unsuitable for use with the enzyme methods and is also not recommended for use with the immunochemical procedures. Freshly drawn serum is preferred, but samples stored at 4° C are stable for up to 3 days. Specimens frozen at −20° C are stable for up to 4 weeks.[21]

Reference interval When one is using an immunonephelometric procedure, the normal reference interval for ceruloplasmin in adults is 250 to 630 mg/L. Factors such as age, sex, and hormone use can affect ceruloplasmin concentrations. Neonates have lower concentrations of ceruloplasmin, which do not reach adult levels until 3 to 6 months of age. Females taking oral contraceptives show higher concentrations of ceruloplasmin when compared with age-matched females.[22]

Cholinesterase
STEVEN C. KAZMIERCZAK

Principles of analysis and current usage Cholinesterase (ChE) is a generic term used to describe a group of related enzymes that hydrolyze choline esters. Two types of cholinesterases are present in blood: acetylcholinesterase (AChE), also called RBC, or erythrocyte cholinesterase; and pseudocholinesterase (BuChE), also called plasma or serum cholinesterase.[23] The substrates utilized by AChE include acetylcholine and acetyl-β-methylcholine; BuChE can utilize butyrylcholine, propionylcholine, and benzoylcholine. Both AChE and BuChE hydrolyze acetylcholine. AChE can hydrolyze acetylcholine and propionylcholine at essentially the same rate, whereas it hydrolyzes butyrylcholine very slowly. In contrast BuChE hydrolyzes butyrylcholine at a faster rate than propionylcholine, whereas acetylcholine is hydrolyzed slowly. This difference in substrate specificity allows for the determination of both AChE and BuChE activities within the same sample.

Measurement of ChE is usually performed for the evaluation of organophosphorus poisoning, for the identification of the presence of abnormal genetic variants of ChE, and in amniotic fluid as a marker for the presence of neural tube defects.

The earliest chemical methods for measurement of ChE were titrimetric,[24] manometric,[25] and electrometric[26] methods based on the measurement of acid formed. These historical methods are no longer used.

Spectrophotometric methods are the most common methods in use today (see the method in Table 47-15). The substrate typically used is acetylcholine that is hydrolyzed by ChE to form thiocholine. The thiocholine formed in this reaction reacts with 5,5′-dithiobis(2-nitrobenzoic acid) (DTNB) to form a yellow-colored product, the formation of which is monitored at 412 nm.[27] Modifications to this procedure have been proposed including the use of 6,6′-dithiodinicotinic acid (DTNA) instead of DTNB[28] as the coupling reagent and the use of acetylcholine instead of acetylthiocholine as substrate with subsequent formation of hydrogen peroxide after the reaction of choline oxidase with choline.[29]

A variety of miscellaneous procedures for ChE have also been described. These include radiometric techniques that use acetylcholine labeled with ^{14}C or ^3H in its acetate moiety,[30] fluorometric procedures,[31] ion-selective electrode techniques,[32] and enzyme-linked immunosorbent assay (ELISA) procedures.[33]

Specimen Both serum and heparin or EDTA plasma are acceptable specimens. Serum should be separated as soon as possible because up to 25% increases in BuChE activity can occur in serum left in contact with the clot for 24 hours.[23] Samples may be stored for up to a year at −20° C. However, samples kept at room temperature for several hours can show loss in enzyme activity.

Reference interval Individuals up to 6 months of age have ChE activities that are 40% to 50% of adult levels.[34] ChE activities in young adult females (<35 years) are approximately 64% to 74% of those found in adult males. Pregnant females show decreased ChE activities compared to nonpregnant females.[35]

Table 47-15   Method for quantitative cholinesterase (ChE) analysis

Method	Type of analysis	Principle	Usage	Comments
Colorimetric	Spectrophotometric, kinetic end point	1. Acetylthiocholine + H_2O $\xrightarrow{AChE}$ Thiocholine + Acetate 2. Thiocholine + DTNB $\rightarrow$ Mixed disulfide + 5,5′-dithiobis(2-nitrobenzoic acid) *(yellow)*	Serum or plasma; most commonly used method	Preferred method sensitive

AChE activities in neonates are approximately 65% of those found in adults and reach adult values by 1 year of age.[36] No sex-related differences in AChE activities have been noted.

ACKNOWLEDGMENTS

The editors wish to acknowledge the previous authors of the following methods: Alpha$_1$-antitrypsin and ceruloplasmin, Gayle Jackson; Carbohydrate screen, Helen Berry; Cholinesterase, Mary Ellen King.

REFERENCES

1. Prinsen JH, Schweisfurth H, Rasche B, Breuer J: Comparison of three methods for the determination of serum alpha-antitrypsin in patients with pulmonary diseases, *Clin Physiol Biochem* 7:198-202, 1989.
2. Viedma JA, de la Iglesia, Parera M, López MT: A new automated turbidimetric immunoassay for quantifying α_1-antitrypsin in serum, *Clin Chem* 32:1020-1022, 1986.
3. Carrell RW, Owen MC: Alpha$_1$-antitrypsin: structure, variation and disease, *Essays Med Biochem* 4:83-119, 1978.
4. Cooper GR, editor: *Selected methods of clinical chemistry,* 8:149-153, Washington, D.C., 1977, American Association for Clinical Chemistry.
5. Nethercott SE, Kalsheker NA: Kinetic fluorimetric assay for alpha$_1$-antitrypsin elastase-inhibitory capacity in serum, *Clin Chem* 34:178-179, 1988.
6. Cox DW, Billingsley GD: Oxidation of plasma alpha$_1$-antitrypsin in smokers and nonsmokers and by an oxidizing agent, *Am Rev Resp Dis* 130:594-9, 1984.
7. Brouwer J, Smekens F: Determination of α_1-antitrypsin in fecal extracts by enzyme immunoassay, *Clin Chim Acta* 189:173-180, 1990.
8. Wilson CM, McGilligan K, Thomas DW: Determination of fecal α_1-antitrypsin concentration by radial immunodiffusion: two systems compared, *Clin Chem* 34:372-376, 1988.
9. Buffone GJ, Shulman RJ: Characterization and evaluation of immunochemical methods for the measurement of fecal α_1-antitrypsin, *Am J Clin Pathol* 83:326-330, 1985.
10. Morse JO: Alpha-1-antitrypsin deficiency. Part 1, *N Engl J Med* 299:1045-1048, 1978.
11. Zegers ND, Classen E, Gerritse K, et al: Detection of genetic variants of α_1-antitrypsin with site-specific monoclonal antibodies, *Clin Chem* 37:1606-1611, 1991.
12. Harju L, Weber T, Alexandrova L, et al: Colorimetric solid-phase minisequencing assay illustrated by detection of α_1-antitrypsin Z mutation, *Clin Chem* 39:2282-2287, 1993.
13. Ritchie RF, Smith R: Immunofixation II: application to typing of alpha-1-antitrypsin at acid pH, *Clin Chem* 22:1735-1737, 1976.
14. Gaidulis L, Muensch HA, Maslow WC, Borer WZ: Optimizing reference values for the measurement of alpha-1-antitrypsin in serum: comparison of three methods, *Clin Chem* 29:1838-1840, 1983.
15. Tietz NW: *Clinical guide to laboratory tests,* Philadelphia, 1983, Saunders.
16. Young DS, Jackson AJ: Thin-layer chromatography of urinary carbohydrates: a comparative evaluation of procedures, *Clin Chem* 16:954-959, 1970.
17. Szustkiewicz C, Demetriou J: Detection of some clinically important carbohydrates in plasma and urine by means of thin-layer chromatography, *Clin Chim Acta* 32:355, 1971.
18. Mukerjee H: A kinetic method for determination of serum ceruloplasmin, *Clin Chem* 36:391-392, 1990.
19. Schosinsky KH, Lehmann HP, Beeler MF: Measurement of ceruloplasmin from its oxidase activity in serum by use of o-dianisidine dihydrochloride, *Clin Chem* 20:1556-1563, 1974.
20. Curzone G, Spezler BE: Inhibitors of ceruloplasmin, *Biochem J* 105:243-250, 1967.
21. Tietz NW: *Clinical guide to laboratory tests,* Phildelphia, 1983, Saunders, p 108.
22. Milne DB, Johnson PE: Assessment of copper status: effect of age and gender on reference ranges in healthy adults, *Clin Chem* 39:883-887, 1993.
23. Dass P, Mejia M, Landes M, et al: Check sample, *Clin Chem* 34:135-158, 1994.
24. Crane CR, Sanders DC, Abbot JN: Cholinesterase use and interpretation of cholinesterase measurements. In Sunshine I, editor: *Methodology for analytical toxicology,* Cleveland, 1975, CRC Press.
25. Ammon R: Die fermentative Spaltung des Acetylcholine, *Pflugers Arch* Ges Physiol 233:486-491, 1933.
26. Ravin HA, Tsou KC, Seligman AM: Colorimetric estimation and histochemical demonstration of serum cholinesterase, *J Biol Chem* 191:843-857, 1951.
27. Ellman GL, Courtney KD, Andres V Jr, Featherstone RM: A new and rapid colorimetric determination of acetylcholinesterase activity, *Biochem Pharmacol* 7:88-95, 1961.
28. Brownson C, Watts DC: The modification of cholinesterase activity by 5,5'-dithiobis(2-nitrobenzoic acid) included in the coupled spectrophotometric assay, *Biochem J* 131:369-374, 1973.
29. Abernethy MH, Fitzgerald HP, Ahern KM: An enzymatic method for erythrocyte acetylcholinesterase, *Clin Chem* 34:1055-1057, 1988.
30. Johnson CD, Russel RL: A rapid, simple radiometric assay for cholinesterase, suitable for multiple determinations, *Anal Biochem* 64:229-238, 1975.
31. Parvari R, Pecht I, Soreq H: A microfluorometric assay for cholinesterase, suitable for multiple kinetic determinations of picomoles of released thiocholine, *Anal Biochem* 133:450-456, 1983.
32. Baum G, Ward FB: General enzyme studies with a substrate-selective electrode: characterization of cholinesterase, *Anal Biochem* 42:487-493, 1971.
33. Brock A: Inter and intraindividual variations in plasma cholinesterase activity and substance concentration in employees of an organophosphorous insecticide factory, *Br J Ind Med* 48:562-567, 1991.
34. Zsigmond EK, Downs JR: Plasma cholinesterase activity in newborns and infants, *Can Anaesth Soc* 18:278-283, 1971.
35. Howard J, East N, Chaney J: Plasma cholinesterase activity in early pregnancy, *Arch Environ Health* 33:277-279, 1978.
36. Kaplan E, Tildon JT: Changes in red cell enzyme activity in relation to red cell survival in infancy, *Pediatrics* 32:371-375, 1963.

BIBLIOGRAPHY

Caskey CT, Pizzuti A, Fu YH, et al: Triplet repeat mutations in human disease, *Science* 256:784-789, 1992.

de Grouchy J, Turleau C: *Clinical atlas of human chromosomes,* New York, 1977, Wiley & Sons.

Kelly TE: Clinical genetics and genetic counseling, ed 2, St. Louis, 1986, Mosby.

King RA, Rotter JI, Motulski AG: *The genetic basis of common diseases,* New York, 1992, Oxford University Press.

McKusick VA: Mendelian inheritance in man, ed 10, Baltimore, 1992, Johns Hopkins University Press.

Neufeld EF: Natural history and inherited disorders of a lysosomal enzyme, beta hexosaminidase, *J Biol Chem* 264:10927-10930, 1989.

Poulton J: Mitochondrial DNA and genetic disease, *Dev Med Child Neurol* 35:833-840, 1993.

Scriver CR, Rosenberg LB: *Amino acid metabolism and its disorders,* Philadelphia, 1973, Saunders.

Shimozawa N, Tsukamoto T, Suzuki Y et al: A human gene responsible for Zellweger syndrome that affects peroxisome assembly, *Science* 255:1132-1134, 1992.

Simpson JL: *Disorders of sexual differentiation,* New York, 1976, Academic Press.

Stanbury JB, Wyngaarden JB, Fredrickson DS, et al, editors: *Metabolic basis of inherited disease,* ed 5, New York, 1983, McGraw-Hill.

Thomas GH, Howell RR: *Selected screening tests for genetic metabolic diseases,* St. Louis, 1973, Mosby.

CHAPTER 48

Molecular biology in the clinical laboratory

W. Edward Highsmith, Jr.

Jay Stoerker

Lawrence M. Silverman

OBJECTIVES

■ Review the structure of DNA, and describe how its properties of complementary base pairing and digestion by specific nucleases can be used to identify specific sequences of DNA.

■ List the major clinical uses of techniques to identify specific DNA sequences.

■ Describe restriction fragment length polymorphisms and variable numbers of tandem repeats, and explain how they can be used to detect the presence of specific genes.

■ Describe the Southern blot technique.

■ Describe the polymerase chain reaction.

KEY TERMS

base pairing The process by which purine and pyrimidine bases bind through hydrogen bonds. The bases pair in a specific complementary fashion: adenine with thymine (or uracil) and guanine with cytosine.

base sequence The exact order of purine bases (guanine and adenine) and pyrimidine bases (cytosine and thymine or uracil) found in nucleic acids. The order defines the primary amino acid sequence of the gene products, which are proteins.

complementary DNA (c-DNA) A DNA copy of an mRNA molecule. Prepared by the reverse transcriptase using the mRNA as the template.

denaturation The process by which double-stranded nucleic acid separates to form single strands. Denaturation can be accomplished by heat, salts, or chemicals. *Also termed melting.*

double-stranded DNA Two complementary strands of DNA that are bound together through base pairing.

gene The smallest biological unit of heredity, located on specific sites on specific chromosomes. A gene contains the encoding for one specific protein.

hybridization The process by which complementary single strands of nucleic acid form double-stranded complexes of nucleic acid through base pairing.

linkage A term defining the association of genes on a chromosome to specific sequences of DNA.

melting temperature The temperature at which one half a population of identical DNA species exists in double-stranded form and one half exists in the single-stranded (denatured) form. The melting temperature is dependent on the ionic strength of the solution, the length of the DNA strands, and the %[G+C] content of the DNA.

northern blot A process similar to the Southern blot, except RNA is the molecule transferred and analyzed.

polymerase chain reaction An oligonucleotide directed, *in vitro* method for the rapid amplification of specific DNA sequences.

probe A sequence of complementary DNA or RNA that is labeled with a radioisotope, enzyme, or other marker. Probes are used to detect specific sequences of nucleic acid by hybridization.

restriction endonucleases Class of nucleases (usually bacterial) that act within a strand of DNA at specific base sequences to cleave the DNA.

restriction fragment length polymorphism (RFLP) The heritable differences in restriction digest patterns seen when a

DNA sequence polymorphism creates or destroys a restriction enzyme recognition site. RFLPs can be observed with either Southern or PCR analysis.

restriction site The base sequence that a particular restriction endonuclease recognizes and cleaves.

single-stranded DNA A length of DNA that is not paired to its complementary strand.

Southern transfer A process by which electrophoretically separated, denatured DNA is transferred from the electrophoretic gel (usually agarose) onto a nitrocellulose filter or membrane for subsequent hybridization analysis.

stringency The conditions under which a hybridization experiment is conducted. High-stringency conditions (low ionic strength, temperature at about DNA melting temperature) allow the hybridization of only perfectly base-paired strands. Low-stringency conditions (high ionic strength, temperature less than DNA melting temperature) allows hybridization of homologous but not perfectly base-paired strands.

The smallest unit of inheritance, the *gene,* codes for specific protein chains, each with a specific function in cell physiology. Chemically, genes are usually composed of deoxyribonucleic acid (DNA, see below). The base sequences are grouped into informational units of three bases, called *codons.* Each triplet sequence composing a codon either codes for a specific amino acid or serves a regulatory function, such as stopping or starting protein chain synthesis. Structurally, the base sequence that composes a gene is linked to other genes, to regulatory sequences, and to (apparently) functionless DNA sequences. DNA is associated with a large number of proteins that serve regulatory functions and also to package the genetic material into larger units called *chromosomes.*

As the number of genes identified and implicated in a variety of human diseases grows, the clinical laboratory faces new challenges. We know that disease or abnormal states can occur when genes are damaged and that this damage usually results from chemical changes to the genes, called *mutations* (see below). The laboratory now utilizes the techniques and technology of molecular biology to identify and characterize specific gene mutations associated both with single-gene disorders, such as cystic fibrosis or Duchenne muscular dystrophy, and polygenic disorders, such as cancer or atherosclerosis. Additionally, molecular techniques receive wide use for the detection of infectious agents, including organisms that are difficult to culture or are present in low numbers.

This chapter introduces the use of these techniques in the clinical laboratory for the detection and characterization of single-gene disorders. Also, the applicability of these techniques for detecting infectious diseases and cancer are discussed.

GENETIC MATERIAL
Chemical composition and structure of DNA

Fig. 48-1 shows the unique arrangement of sugar, phosphate, and the purine and pyrimidine bases that form the double-helical structure known as DNA. DNA usually consists of two strands of base sequences that are bound to each other by hydrogen bonding between the bases of each single strand of DNA (Fig. 48-1). The bases bind to each other in a specific, or *complementary,* fashion. Adenine binds only to thymine, whereas guanine binds only to cytosine. Thus one chain of double-stranded DNA has a base sequence that is complementary to the other strand. A single strand of DNA will bind to another single DNA strand if the strands contain a high proportion of complementary sequences. For example, if a mixture consists of single strands of DNA-A and its complementary strand and an excess of other non-complementary DNA strands, strand A will form only double-stranded complexes with its complementary strand and none other. In the laboratory the process of allowing complementary single strands of DNA to form double-stranded DNA is called *hybridization.* Hybridization can also be performed between single strands of DNA and

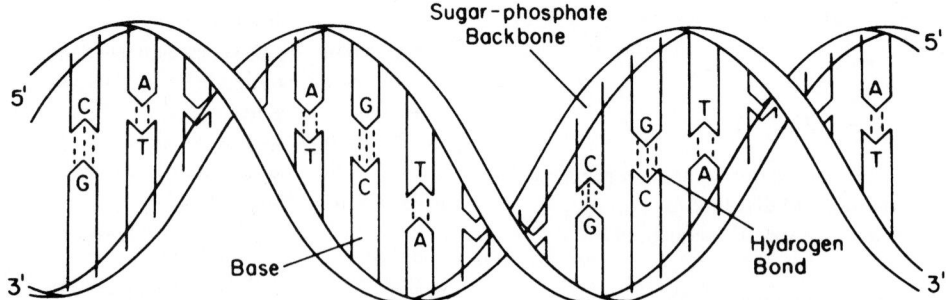

Fig. 48-1   Structure of DNA. DNA molecule is a double helix that consists of two sugar-phosphate backbones with four bases: cytosine (C), guanine (G), adenine (A), and thymine (T) attached. *C* and *G* residues and *A* and *T* residues on opposite strands pair through hydrogen bonding. (From LeGrys V, Leinbach SS, Silverman L: *CRC Crit Rev Clin Lab Sci* 25:255, 1987.)

complementary strands of ribonucleic acid (RNA). For measurement of a specific DNA base sequence, a known copy of that base sequence is prepared. This copy of complementary DNA (c-DNA), known as a DNA *probe,* is labeled in some fashion to allow monitoring of the hybridization reaction. The basis of the techniques described later in the chapter hinge on the hybridization properties of a specific sequence of bases that make up a single strand of the double-stranded helix of DNA.

Mutations and gene expression

A genetic mutation is a stable change in the DNA structure that usually is caused by a change in the base sequence that composes a codon. The base change usually results in a change in the code and the information residing in that code. A mutation occurring in the portion of DNA that codes for a protein usually results in a change in the amino acid structure of that protein. This change can result in no change in the function of the protein, a total loss of function, or a partial loss of function. It is the partial or total loss of function that usually results in a pathological state. The effect of a loss of function can be direct, such as the conformation dysfunction of hemoglobin that results in the disease sickle cell anemia (see Chapter 36), or indirect, such as the loss of function of regulators of gene expression that can result in cancers (see p. 976 and Chapter 49).

Mutations can occur by a wide variety of mechanisms. For the purposes of the discussion of cancer and inherited disease, mutations can be divided into germline and somatic events. A germline mutation is one that is present in all cells of the body and is passed from generation to generation by meiosis (creation of germ cells—sperm and egg) and sexual reproduction. Somatic cells are those mutations that arise in tissue cells, generally as a result of some environmental insult or DNA replication error. For additional information on genetic inheritance, see Chapter 47.

Abnormal expression of genes can also result from inheritable changes to the chemical structure of genes that are not a result of a change of a base in a codon triplet. Methylation of the nucleotide bases is a postsynthetic modification to DNA that affects the expression of genes. Abnormal patterns of DNA methylation can cause abnormal gene expression (transcription) and disease states. Repeat base sequences that have no apparent informational content regarding protein structure exist throughout the DNA. The expansion of the number of repeats in a gene has been associated with specific diseases, and this change in the gene structure is inheritable (see p. 975).

TECHNIQUES OF DNA ANALYSIS

Several core technologies are central to the modern practice of molecular biology. The first takes advantage of the ability of complementary strands of DNA to find each other in solutions containing a complex mixture of DNA and bind together to form the familiar DNA double helix. This spe-

cific binding technique is termed *hybridization* and forms the basis for almost all types of DNA detection methods. The second set of techniques that are crucial for manipulation and detection of specific nucleotide sequences involve a large number of enzymes that are commercially available. These restriction endonucleases, which in vivo are involved in DNA metabolism and repair or in bacterial host defense, provide the molecular tools with which nucleic acids can be manipulated with extraordinary specificity.

The third set of core techniques of modern molecular biology are the detection methods. These methods possess extreme specificity, not for the chemical structure of DNA, which is identical for all genes, but for the sequence of the bases, which determines the information that a particular piece of DNA is carrying. Further, because specific gene sequences form only a tiny fraction of the whole human genome and because DNA is typically available only in microgram amounts, these methods must possess extreme sensitivity. The first of these methods to be described and widely adopted is the Southern transfer. The second is the polymerase chain reaction (PCR).

General techniques

Restriction digestion and gel electrophoresis. A specific property of DNA (and RNA) is its susceptibility to enzymes called *nucleases.* Nucleases hydrolyze the phosphodiester bonds that connect bases within a nucleic acid strand, resulting in cleavage of the strand. Certain nucleases have a very high substrate specificity and will cleave a DNA strand only at specific base sequences, often as small as 4 to 8 bases in length. Because these nucleases are employed by bacteria to restrict entry of foreign DNA into their cells, they are called *restriction endonucleases.* The sequences that the enzymes recognize and cleave are referred to as *restriction sites.* These enzymes require Mg^{++} ion for activity. Over 400 enzymes recognizing different restriction sites have been identified. Most of these are commercially available.

Restriction endonucleases are critical reagents in laboratories investigating DNA base sequences because they cleave the double-stranded nucleic acid only at specific points. After these endonucleases degrade DNA into a series of many smaller fragments, specific sequences can be more readily identified by the hybridization technique. To aid in the identification of a specific base sequence, the fragments can be first separated into molecules of differing molecular size. This is accomplished by either agarose or polyacrylamide (or their derivatives) gel electrophoresis.

The most common method for the visualization of DNA after electrophoretic size separation is by staining with the intercalating agent ethidium bromide. When this compound is in solution, it is free to lose energy, acquired from incident radiation, by increased rotation and collision with solvent molecules. However, when a molecule of ethidium bromide is intercalated into the DNA double helix, these motions are lost, and the molecule rids itself of excess energy by fluorescence. The fragments of DNA generated by restriction enzyme digestion are at equal molar concentrations with respect to each other, giving an easy method for determining the completeness of a given restriction digestion reaction. The hybridization of the separated fragments is then achieved by the Southern transfer techniques.

Southern transfer. Blood samples for linkage analysis are collected into acid-citrate-dextrose (AC) anticoagulant tubes, and the white cells are then isolated from each sample. DNA is extracted from the white cells and incubated with a restriction endonuclease to cleave the DNA into smaller fragments. The digested DNA sample is applied to an agarose gel and electrophoresed to separate the fragments according to size. The fragments are then treated by either chemicals or high temperatures to separate the double-stranded DNA into single strands; this process is termed *denaturation*. The separated, denatured fragments are then transferred (either by blotting or by electrophoresis) from the gel onto another support medium, such as a nitrocellulose or nylon membrane (the *Southern* blot procedure). The fragment or fragments containing the DNA sequence of interest are identified by incubation of the membrane with a labeled DNA probe that contains sequences complimentary to the sequence of interest. The label can be a radioisotope, an enzyme, or a fluorescent dye. The complementary sequence of the probe permits it to hybridize to the sample DNA containing the desired sequences. In the case of radiolabeled c-DNA, the membrane is then incubated with x-ray film to expose areas *(bands)* on the film where the probe has bound to the sample DNA, resulting in an *autoradiogram* (Fig. 48-2).

The procedure described requires 7 to 10 days from DNA extraction from whole blood to development of the autoradiogram. Usually DNA is extracted on the first day, digested with restriction endonucleases on day 2, electrophoresed overnight on day 3, and hybridized on days 4 and 5. The membrane is then placed in an x-ray cassette with x-ray film for 1 to 4 days and then developed. Alternative, nonisotopic detection methods that utilize colorimetric or luminescent detection are gaining in popularity because they reduce the time required for band visualization and technologist exposure to ionizing radiation. These methods employ a second incubation step using an enzyme-coupled antibody to a hapten that has been incorporated into the probe DNA instead of ^{32}P. The action of the enzyme then generates the colored or chemiluminescent material from a colorless or inactive substrate. Several nonisotopic detection systems for use with Southern transfer are commercially available—examples are the GENIUS kit from Boehringer-Mannheim (colorimetric) and the ECL system from Amersham (chemiluminescent).

Polymerase chain reaction (PCR). Although the Southern procedure combines reasonable sensitivity with excellent specificity, it is technically demanding, typically

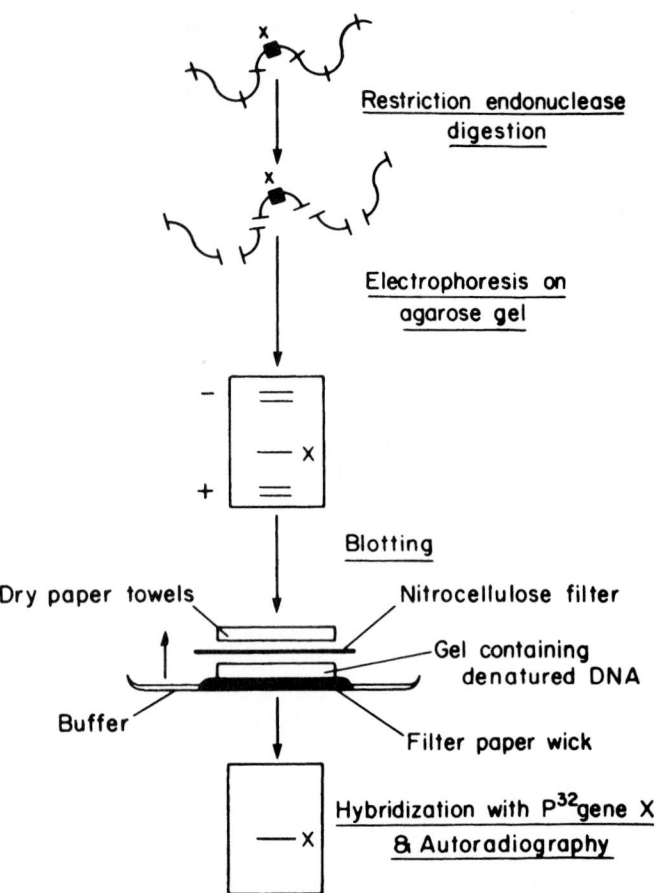

Fig. 48-2 Identification by Southern blot hybridization of DNA fragment–containing gene X. DNA was digested with restriction endonuclease, and resulting fragments were fractionated according to size by electrophoresis in agarose gel. DNA fragments in gel were denatured and blotted to nitrocellulose filter as a result of flow of buffer through gel and nitrocellulose filter to dry paper towels. Subsequent hybridization of DNA on the filter to a ^{32}P-labeled gene X probe and autoradiography revealed single DNA fragment–containing gene X. (From LeGrys V, Leinbach SS, Silverman L: *CRC Crit Rev Clin Lab Sci* 25:255, 1987.)

requires the use of hazardous, high-energy beta-particle emitters, such as ^{32}P, and has a long turnaround time. Several of the objections to the Southern procedure can be eliminated by use of the polymerase chain reaction (PCR). PCR is a technique developed for the rapid in vitro amplification of specific DNA sequences.

Knowledge of the sequence of the region of DNA flanking the area of interest is required for PCR. Two synthetic oligodeoxynucleotides (primers), typically 20 to 30 bases in length, are prepared (or purchased) such that one of the primers is complementary to an area on one strand of the target DNA that is 5′ (see Fig. 48-1 for description of the 5′ and 3′ ends of the DNA strand) to the sequences to be amplified, and the other primer is complementary to the op-

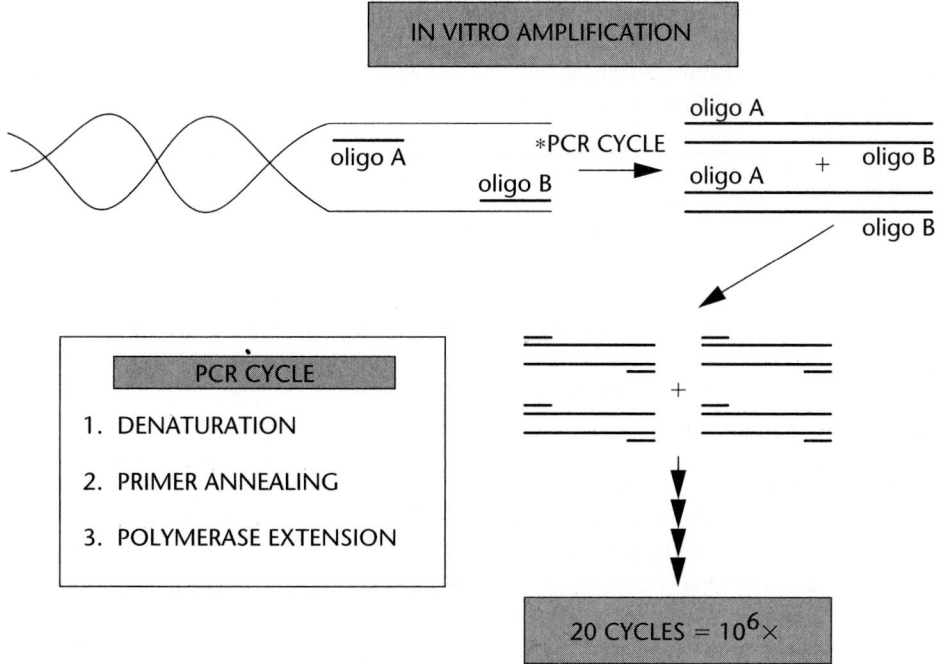

Fig. 48-3 Schema of the first cycle of a PCR reaction. (From Highsmith WE, Silverman LM: *Lab Med Bull* 104:1-4, 1989.)

posite strand of the target DNA, again 5′ to the region to be amplified. A schema is shown in Fig. 48-3.

To perform the amplification, one places the sample DNA in a tube along with a large molar excess of the two primers, all four deoxynucleotide triphosphates (dNTPs), buffer, magnesium ion, and a thermostable DNA polymerase. The most commonly used polymerase is isolated from the thermophilic organism *Thermus aquaticus*. This enzyme, termed *Taq*. polymerase, has its optimal activity at 72° C but can survive for short periods at temperatures up to 95° C without being irreversibly denatured. The reaction is first heated to 95° C to denature, or *melt,* the test DNA from its double-stranded to its single-stranded form. The temperature is then decreased, typically to 50° to 60° C, to allow annealing, or hybridization, of the primers to their complementary sites on the single-stranded sample DNA. It should be noted that the vast molar excess of the primers, as well as their small size, will ensure that the hybridization is between the sample DNA and the primers and not between the two strands of the test DNA. The temperature is then increased to 72° C, the temperature optimum for *Taq*. polymerase. The polymerase extends the primers in the 5′ to 3′ direction by incorporating the dNTPs into the growing complementary DNA strands. It is crucial that the polymerase extends far enough along each strand to create a new binding site for the opposite primer. After holding the temperature at 72° C for a period of time sufficient to synthesize a new DNA strand from one primer to the binding site of the other primer (typically 15 to 60 seconds), the process of temperature cycling is repeated. After heating to de-

nature the newly formed DNA, the temperature is again decreased to allow annealing of the primers, this time to the newly synthesized binding sites as well as those on the original template DNA. The temperature is again increased to 72° C to extend the four bound primers (Fig. 48-3). As the temperature changes are repeated, the DNA between the two primers is synthesized. The amount of DNA produced is exponential with respect to cycle number. After 20 cycles of annealing, extension, and denaturation, 2^{20}, or approximately 10^6, copies will have been generated.

In a typical experiment starting with 100 to 1000 ng of human DNA, 30 cycles of amplification will produce enough specific DNA to be visualized on an ethidium bromide–stained gel. Because each cycle takes 2 to 5 minutes, amplification of a specific sequence can easily be accomplished in several hours. After amplification, the DNA can be analyzed by one of several techniques, depending on the specific problem.

Techniques for genetic disorders

Direct analysis. Many laboratory tests used in the diagnosis of genetic disorders give results that may be characteristic of a disorder but are not entirely specific. These tests are generally *phenotypic* tests; that is, they reflect how a particular gene is expressed rather than the exact DNA sequence, or *genotype*. Therefore, phenotypic tests can be misleading, particularly in the absence of complete clinical data and family history. *Direct,* or *genotypic,* tests could avoid these problems by detecting the specific alterations in DNA that result in the disorder. Several techniques, principally based on PCR, have been developed for the direct detection of known mutations. The following is a brief explanation of some of the most frequently used techniques.

Allele-specific oligonucleotide hybridization (ASO, or dot blot). DNA is amplified by PCR and spotted onto two nylon membranes. Each membrane is then hybridized with one of two synthetic, radiolabeled oligonucleotides *(oligo)* that span the region of DNA containing a specific mutation. One oligo has the sequence complementary to the *wild type,* or normal DNA sequence, whereas the other is perfectly complementary to the mutant allele. Under appropriate conditions of temperature and salt concentration (stringency), hybridization will occur only when the probe and the target DNA are perfectly base paired. Thus, the normal oligo will bind only the normal amplified target, but the mutant oligo will hybridize only with the mutant allele. Detection is usually by autoradiography. Variants of this procedure include nonisotopic detection and hybridization in microtiter trays instead of on a membrane.

Reverse dot-blot. The reverse dot-blot is a variant on the ASO technique in which the allele-specific oligonucleotides (normal and mutant) are bound to a nylon membrane. Amplification of the sample DNA is preformed as usual but with one of the PCR primers labeled at the 5′ end with a biotin molecule. The amplified DNA is hybridized with the ASOs on the membrane under the appropriately stringent conditions for allele specific hybridization. After the hybridization and washing steps, avidin conjugated to alkaline phosphatase is bound to the biotin. Detection of the hybrids is by monitoring action of the enzyme on a substrate to produce a colored, insoluble product. This system is commercially available for HLA genotyping.

Allele-specific PCR (AS-PCR). In this allele-specific PCR, also called *amplification-resistant mutation scanning* (ARMS), three PCR primers are prepared. One of them, the constant primer, is 100 to 200 bases away from the site of the mutation. Two of the primers overlap the site of the mutation by one base at the 3′ end of the primer. The normal oligo is complementary to the normal sequence, and the mutant oligo is complementary to the mutant sequence. Two amplification reactions are performed, one with each of the normal or mutant primers and the constant primer. Only when the primers are perfectly base paired at the 3′ end will amplification occur.

Restriction analysis. Occasionally, a disease-causing mutation will create or destroy a restriction enzyme recognition site. The classic example is sickle cell anemia. In this case, the mutation replacing A by T eliminates a restriction site for the enzyme *Mst II.* Thus, detection consists in PCR amplification of a region of the beta-globin gene that contains codon 6, digestion with Mst II, and determination of the PCR fragment sizes after gel electrophoresis. In the presence of adequate controls, failure of the enzyme to cleave the PCR-applied DNA into two smaller pieces indicates the presence of this specific mutation.

PCR-mediated, site-directed mutagenesis (PSM). When a disease-causing mutation does not create or destroy a restriction site, one can often be created that is specific for either the wild type or the mutant allele by using a primer that is 100 to 200 bases away from the mutation site and that abuts but does not overlap the mutation site. By introducing a mismatch into the abutting primer, the sequence of the amplified material after PCR will be altered to contain the base that was present in the primer rather than the one in the corresponding position in the target (that is, site-directed mutagenesis). By introducing a point mutation within several bases of the mutation, it is often possible to introduce a restriction site that is associated with either the wild type or the mutant sequence, but not both. After PCR and restriction digestion, the alleles are identified by their different lengths on gel electrophoresis.

Limitations of direct analysis. The number of diseases for which mutations in single genes have been identified in the past 5 years is impressive. Theoretically, direct tests could be developed for all these disorders. Although tests are available for many of them, *genetic heterogeneity* prevents the use of a few simple tests for diagnosis of disease states or carrier detection in all patients or families. Genetic heterogeneity refers to the observation that although a clinical disorder is typically caused by mutations in a single gene, the range of mutations in that gene that can cause disease is very large. This genetic heterogeneity is reflected by a phenotypic heterogeneity, that is, a wide degree of severity of the same disease entity. The exception to this rule is sickle cell anemia. Every case of sickle cell anemia is caused by the same mutation, an A-to-T mutation in codon 6 of the beta-globin gene. More typical are the mutational profiles of cystic fibrosis (CF) and Duchenne muscular dystrophy (DMD). There is one mutation (termed ΔF508) in the cystic fibrosis transmembrane conductance regulator (CFTR) gene that accounts for approximately 70% of disease alleles in populations derived from northern Europe. However, over 300 different mutations have been described on the CF gene that do not carry the most common mutation. In the case of DMD, large deletions in the dystrophin gene account for approximately 60% of cases of DMD. These deletions, although clustered in two hot spots, are heterogeneous, with few affected boys sharing the same deletion. The nondeletion cases are heterogeneous as well, with only a single report of two apparently unrelated boys sharing the same point mutation. Thus, even after a disease gene has been identified, it still may not be possible to provide a direct test. In these cases, an *indirect genotypic* approach is necessary. This indirect approach, called *linkage analysis,* is discussed below and a case study of the clinical application of linkage analysis is described for cystic fibrosis.

Indirect analysis

Linkage analysis: restriction fragment length polymorphisms.

Linkage analysis can be used in following the inheritance of single-gene disorders within a family. For example, color blindness is a phenotypic marker that can be followed within families. The most common form of color blindness is manifested only in males; this is an example of a genetic linkage. In this case the gene of interest is linked to the X chromosome.

This type of linkage analysis is at the level of the phenotypic expression of a specific gene on a specific chromosome. Monitoring the expression of abnormal genes at the molecular level is more difficult, especially when the gene product and specific DNA sequence may not be known. In the laboratory, the mutation-bearing chromosome is identified by linkage to *restriction fragment length polymorphisms* (RFLPs, pronounced "riflips"). It has been estimated that, between any two human genomes, DNA-sequence differences exist every 100 to 300 bases. Because most of these differences occur in noncoding sequences, these changes are silent and have no phenotypic effect on the individual. Occasionally, one of these single base changes will alter a small region of DNA sequence that defines a specific restriction enzyme recognition site. In these cases, if samples of DNA that differ at a restriction site are treated with that enzyme and subjected to Southern transfer with an appropriate probe, the difference will be detected by the difference in length of the restriction fragments in the two samples. Similarly, if PCR amplification is performed with primers that flank the polymorphic restriction site, restriction enzyme digestion will either cut the amplified DNA (if the DNA contains the restriction site) or not (if the restriction site is not present). Again, the presence or absence of a restriction site is revealed by size differences of the alleles on gel electrophoresis. If a polymorphic restriction site happens to lie near the target disease gene on the chromosome, it will likely be coinherited with the disease gene. When this is the case, the polymorphism and the disease gene are said to be *linked*. There is an error rate associated with linkage analysis determined by the physical distance (in base pairs) between the polymorphism affecting the restriction site and the disease gene. If the distance is large, there is a high probability that a chromosomal crossover event in meiosis will separate the two. On the other hand, if the distance between the two loci is small, there is a low probability of a crossover between them. To be useful in a clinical setting, it must be demonstrated that a particular RFLP and the disease locus are tightly linked enough that crossovers rarely occur between them. A crossover rate of <1% (1 centimorgan) is generally required before a given RFLP is considered useful for prenatal diagnosis.

Linkage analysis: microsatellite sequences.

After the demonstration that human DNA contained restriction fragment length polymorphisms, Botstein et al. (1980) suggested that these polymorphisms could be used to map disease genes to specific areas of specific chromosomes. This suggestion and the identification of RFLPs from many laboratories worldwide began the era of gene mapping and positional cloning. This era is culminating in the Human Genome initiative. One of the priorities of the Human Genome Project is to construct physical and genetic maps of the human genome. The first polymorphisms to be extensively used were the RFLPs. This type of polymorphism was used in the positional cloning of several important disease genes, including the cystic fibrosis and Duchenne muscular dystrophy genes. Although RFLPs have proved to be very useful tools for gene mapping, they are limited in their information content. Since a RFLP can have only two alleles, the presence or absence of a restriction site, the maximum heterozygosity for that polymorphism is 50%; furthermore, most RFLPs have heterozygosities far less than the theoretical maximum. The consequence of this limited information content is that it is likely that useful information will not be produced for many families in a given linkage study.

Beginning with the observations of Jeffries, multiallelic polymorphisms have become more widely used. These multiallelic polymorphisms are the result not of single base changes as in RFLP's but of variable numbers of repeated base sequences. Thus these types of polymorphisms are called *VNTRs* (variable number of tandem repeats). A particular type of VNTR in which the locus containing the repeated sequence is small enough to be amplified by PCR is termed a *microsatellite*. In these cases, the repeats consist of very short, simple sequence motifs. The most common repeated sequence observed up to now is the $(CA)_n$, but other dinucleotide, trinucleotide, tetranucleotide, and even larger repeats have been observed. The expansion in the number of repeated sequences of the trinucleotide CAG in the gene on chromosome 4p16.3 associated with Huntington's disease has been shown to be the molecular defect causing the disease. The greater the number of repeats, the earlier the onset of the disease (see Kremer et al in the bibliography). Because of their higher heterozygosity and informativity, the use of PCR-based analysis of microsatellite DNA has all but supplanted the use of RFLPs for linkage studies. Indeed, in ongoing searches for disease genes, a large percentage of the research efforts are focused on the identification of CA repeats near the gene of interest. In addition to their use in gene mapping and clinical genetics, the use of VNTRs have been shown to be extremely useful in forensic analysis of biological evidence (such as blood or semen stains) and paternity determination.

To use linkage analysis, it is necessary to trace the coinheritance of the polymorphic marker and the disease allele through the entire family; thus, key family members' DNA must be available. An important point to remember is that the differences in the DNA sequences detected by analysis of polymorphic sites do not cause the disorder; they merely allow one to follow the inheritance of a closely linked mutant gene throughout a family.

CLINICAL APPLICATIONS OF MOLECULAR TECHNIQUES

The nucleic acid probe technology can be used to detect specific DNA or RNA sequences in human samples. DNA sequences of interest to the clinician include normal gene sequences, abnormal gene sequences associated with specific disease states, abnormal gene sequences associated with cancer, and exogenous base sequences associated with infectious organisms, such as bacteria and viruses.

Cancer

Cancer is defined as an autonomous proliferation of cells with metastatic potential. It is fulfillment of the metastatic potential that differentiates a rapidly growing, life-threatening neoplasm from slow-growing, local cancers and benign (non–life threatening) neoplasms, such as adenomas. Using the tools of molecular biology, a picture of the exquisite interplay of genes and gene products that serve to regulate the cell cycle and cell proliferation has emerged. When one or more of these gene products fails to fulfill its intercellular task, uncontrolled growth can result. The mechanism that brings about failure (inactivity or inappropriate high activity) of these protein growth regulators is the occurrence of a mutation in the DNA coding for that particular protein.

Although certain rarer types of cancer are associated with germline transmission of mutant genes, most cancers are the result of somatic mutations. Among the hundreds of thousands of genes in the human genome, mutation of only a few of them is necessary or sufficient to cause the deregulation of cell growth. According to our present understanding, there exist two broad classes of genes with these properties—the oncogenes and the tumor-suppressor genes.

Oncogenes (see also Chapter 49). The oncogenes were the first class of genes shown to be involved n the transition from normal, well-regulated cells to the cell mass whose uncontrolled proliferation characterizes cancers. An *oncogene* is defined as a gene that, when activated inappropriately, results in uncontrolled cell division and tissue growth. Because only one copy of the gene needs to be mutated for the genotype to affect the phenotype (malignant versus normal), oncogenes are said to act in a dominant fashion. Although the first oncogenes discovered were of viral origin, it is now clear that the majority of oncogenes are the result of mutations of the normal cell's regulatory genes. These normal genes are referred to as *proto-oncogenes*. The biochemical activities of proto-oncogenes generally fall into one of three categories: (1) protein kinases and phosphorylases, (2) GTP binding proteins (G-proteins) and signal transduction proteins, and (3) transcription factors. When activated inappropriately, protein kinases

and phosphorylases initiate phosphorylation cascades, with the result often being cell division. Examples include the *erbB* oncogene, which is a mutant form of the epidermal growth factor receptor, and the *raf1* gene, a serine kinase that is believed to transmit signals generated at the cell membrane to nuclear proteins that regulate cell division.

The G-proteins are part of signal transduction pathways. These pathways connect events at the cell surface, such as the binding of a hormone to its receptor, to the nucleus. The G-proteins are activated by the binding of GTP and inactivated by the GTPase-catalyzed hydrolysis of GTP to GDP. The activated G-proteins interact with second-messenger systems, such as adenyl cyclase and cyclic AMP, to stimulate RNA transcription in the nucleus. The best known example is the *ras* family of oncogenes. Although normal G-proteins possess a GTPase activity that serves to terminate the signal transduction, these mutant genes are incapable of hydrolyzing GTP and are thus inappropriately maintained in an active state. Several proto-oncogenes code for transcription factors and thus directly modulate gene expression. The *myc* family of oncogenes is perhaps the most well-studied system. *Myc* is overexpressed in several different types of tumors and serves to deregulate the production of cellular growth factors.

There are several mechanisms for mutations that result in activation of proto-oncogenes. The common mechanisms are (1) overproduction of the proto-oncogene by loss of the ability to regulate that gene, (2) increased concentration of the proto-oncogene by amplification of the number of genomic copies of that gene, and (3) activation of a proto-oncogene by chromosomal translocation in which the promotor region for a constitutively regulated gene (one that is normally "on" during most of the cell cycle) is brought into position to regulate a proto-oncogene. Although several of these mechanisms have been studied and some are common for particular types of cancer, the most common alteration of function or stability of a proto-oncogene is by means of a small mutation in the DNA coding for that gene.

Detection of activated forms of several oncogenes has been associated with poor clinical prognosis, such as the amplification of N-*myc* in neuroblastoma or the activation of *ras* genes in a variety of tumors. There is a compelling need to determine the relationship between genotype and phenotype and the clinical utility of detecting mutant oncogenes in particular tumors.

Tumor-suppressor genes. The existence of a class of genes that restricts cell division and thus could act as tumor suppressors was postulated before they were actually shown to exist. After observing familial cases of bilateral retinoblastoma (RB) and comparing those cases with sporadic (nonfamilial) cases of unilateral RB, Knudson proposed that two "hits," or mutational events, were needed for the initiation of tumor growth. In the cases of familial RB, a germline mutation in one tumor-suppressor allele was postulated. In familial RB, there was a much higher probability of tumor initiation because the individual is born with one "hit." Therefore, somatic mutations that "hit," or render nonfunctional, the remaining normal allele would be tumorigenic. In contrast, that same somatic event in a normal individual (one not carrying a mutant RB gene) would not lead to the initiation of a tumor because one functional allele would still be retained. Tumor initiation would take place in a normal individual only if two somatic events occurred at the same locus. Because tumor initiation is not observed with a single abnormal allele, it is said that tumor-suppressor genes act as recessive alleles.

Since the cloning of the RB gene and the proof of the two-hit hypothesis, several recessively acting tumor-suppressor genes have been identified. These include the Wilms' tumor gene (WT), p53, the neurofibromatosis type 1 and type 2 genes (NF1 and NF2), the adenomatous polyposis coli gene (APC), and the deleted colon cancer gene (DCC). As a rule, these genes have been identified when genes were searched for in chromosomal locations that are commonly deleted in cancers.

Because tumor-suppressor genes are activated only by mutations that destroy the function of the gene, it seems reasonable that mutations that give rise to premature "stop" codons (those that instruct translation of the RNA messages) appearing in the reading frame of the gene would be over-represented. This has been observed and will influence methodologic choices in the clinical analysis for the inactivation of these genes in clinical samples.

Familial cancer syndromes. Extensive epidemiologic evidence demonstrates that many cancers have a higher incidence in relatives of patients than in the general population. Many but not all of these cancers follow straightforward mendelian inheritance patterns (generally autosomal dominant with reduced penetrance or, rarely, autosomal recessive) (see Chapter 47). These genes are believed to involve germline defects in single genes. On the other hand, familial cancers in which mendelian inheritance patterns cannot be demonstrated (that is, relatives with risk levels that are elevated relative to the general population but far less than the risk predicted for single-gene disorders) are most likely the result of multiple factors. It is difficult to separate the increased risk in these families into genetic and environmental factors; undoubtedly, both are important.

Together there are over 50 recognized mendelian disorders in which the risk of cancer is very high, sometimes approaching 100%. A particularly striking aspect of the inherited cancer syndromes is that multiple primary tumors often occur, whereas more than one tumor in a sporadic case is rare. The genes responsible for some of the cancer syndromes have been recently identified, including those responsible for adenomatous polyposis coli (colon cancer), neurofibromatosis type 1 (neurofibromas) and type 2 (acoustic neuroma), and the Li-Fraumani syndrome (cancer of multiple tissues). Not surprisingly, these genes belong to the class of tumor-suppressor genes. Although as previously discussed tumor-suppressor genes act in a recessive manner (the phenotype of a cell with one or two normal copies of a tumor-suppressor gene are indistinguishable, that is, normal), the inheritance pattern is dominant with reduced penetrance. Reduced gene penetrance refers to the fact that not all patients who receive a mutated gene at birth will go on to express the phenotype of that gene or, in this case, to develop cancer. The resolution of this apparent paradox is the realization that the inherited trait is the increased probability of developing a cancer as the result of having inherited one mutated gene.

Although the numbers of individuals affected by specific mendelian familial cancers is small, in aggregate the number of cancer types is significant, totaling approximately 5% of total cancers. The ability to detect germline tumor-suppressor gene mutations will be of extreme importance to families who are shown to be transmitting a cancer of this type. For these families, it will be crucial to identify the causative mutation in the relevant gene and then trace that mutation through the family. Individuals who are found not to carry the mutation do not have to fear the likelihood of cancer. Individuals who are found to carry the mutation before the onset of symptoms will benefit from increased surveillance in order to identify tumors while they are small and can be treated effectively.

Sporadic cancers. Most (95%) cancers arise without the inheritance of a mutant tumor-suppressor gene. Rather, they arise as a result of mutations in somatic (nongermline) cells. In contrast to the linear view of carcinogenesis, that is, first a mutation occurs in gene A, followed by a mutation in gene B, followed by a mutation in gene C, and so forth, current theory suggests a stochastic, or web-of-causation, model. In this theory, the order of gene mutation is not important; the mutation of any proto-oncogene or tumor-suppressor gene can serve as a first hit. It is not necessary for the first mutational event to be followed by a mutation of a specific gene. Rather, the cumulative mutation of some number of genes (a number unknown at the present time) will be necessary for the development of a malignant phenotype. Further, the identity of those genes is not fixed. There are a large number of genes that can, in theory, act in concert when mutated to allow the cell to divide in an uncontrollable fashion.

Because tumors vary widely in their characteristics, such as aggressiveness or response to a given therapeutic modality, it is not unreasonable to search for correlations between the genotype of the tumor (the set of genes that are mutated and the types of mutations that they harbor) and the tumor's phenotype (the observed behavior of the tumor). Although the ability to make genotype/phenotype correlations is in its infancy, the identification of cancer-associated mutations and their correlation with clinical phenotype will yield important insights into the functional characteristics of both oncogene and tumor-suppressor proteins. Ultimately, these structure/function relationships will contribute to understanding these proteins' roles in cell growth and development and assist in the development of therapeutic strategies for modifying or bypassing abnormal function.

Among the first genes for which genotype/phenotype correlations has begun to emerge is p53. This protein has multiple roles in the normal cell. It is associated with both the transcriptional activation of cellular growth factors and the downregulation of growth-suppressor genes. Further, p53 has been recently shown to mediate the apoptotic (programmed cell death) pathway that is activated in response to severe cellular damage. p53 was originally classified as an oncogene. The first mutations discovered for p53 met the standard criteria for an oncogene; that is, its effect was manifest in a dominant fashion. It was shown that the majority of missense mutations of p53 had essentially the same effect on the p53 protein, that is, to increase its half-life. Missense mutations result in an incorrect amino acid replacing the normal amino acid, whereas nonsense mutations result in the deletion of an amino acid in the peptide chain. Thus, the degradation-resistant mutant p53 continues to stimulate cell growth even when growth is an inappropriate response to external or internal stimuli. However, it was soon noted that many (approximately one half) of mutant p53 genes characterized were nonsense mutations with an inability to produce p53 protein. Further, it was shown that many tumors had nonsense mutations on both p53 alleles. Thus, not only could the gene function as an oncogene, but as a tumor-suppressor gene as well.

The identity of specific p53 mutations has implications for therapy. In the case of a long-lived p53, the apoptotic pathway is still viable; therefore, therapeutic maneuvers such as radiation therapy aimed at causing enough cellular damage for the cells to undergo programmed death are effective. On the other hand, in the complete absence of p53, the apoptotic pathway cannot be engaged, resulting in a radiation-resistant phenotype. Recently, it has been shown that p53 plays a central role in the angiogenesis (production of a blood-supplying network) of metastatic tumors. Knowledge of p53 mutations will be critical in the proper application of emerging therapies in these cases.

Infectious disease

Nowhere has the revolution of DNA diagnostics had more profound effects than in the detection of infectious agents. It is likely that, in a few short years, PCR-based techniques will probably supplant even routine cultures for the detection of common bacterial pathogens like *Escherichia coli*. Economic considerations already point the way to PCR-based drug-resistance testing. Just as important is the ability of molecular techniques to identify the presence of infectious organisms in situ, that is, directly in the pathological processes. This can be accomplished by extraction of nucleic acids directly from thin sections of biopsied tissue, or by in situ hybridization or amplification techniques.

Currently the clinical use of molecular methods extends only into the detection of organisms that are difficult or impossible to culture, such as *Mycobacterium* species, fungi, and viruses. In these cases the economic advantages already outweigh classical approaches. In addition, molecular diagnostics provide superior information in terms of sensitivity and even specificity. Most compelling, molecular diagnostics can provide results in a same-day or overnight turnaround time frame for diagnoses that previously required weeks.

Detection of infectious agents by molecular methods presents different problems from the analysis of endogenous cellular DNA sequences. The nucleic acid sequences of infectious agents tend to be novel and provide clean signals so that detection methods relying on hybridization by probes or amplification of the target can be used. However, samples needed for analysis may be much more difficult to obtain than by a simple venipuncture. For example, the branched-chain amplification method for the diagnosis of *Mycobacterium* species (Chiron, Alameda, California) must contend with nonuniform materials such as sputum, which contains wax-coated pathogens in irregular clusters. Other useful samples may be feces, urine, or tissue. The opportunity for sampling error is large, and sample preparation protocols are key. Even though the sequences of infectious agents are novel with regard to human DNA, contamination can be a particular problem when one is detecting organisms that survive in the environment. Greater than 50% of house dust, for example, is composed of desquamated human skin. Assays for nonculturable dermatophytes such as human papillomaviruses (HPV) are highly susceptible to contamination from such sources.

Although unique concerns exist for the use of molecular methods in the detection of infectious agents, some of the earliest clinical tests using DNA technology were developed in this area. A list of infectious agents and suppliers of kit materials is given in Table 48-1. Since the primary consideration for microbiological tests is often sensitivity, and the novel sequences of the organisms usually allow very clean amplifications using PCR, several methods have been developed to enhance signal transmission even further. These methods generally employ immobilization of PCR products or viral DNAs by antibody or avidin capture molecules, followed by signal generation by an appropriate complex of

Table 48-1 Some representative nucleic acid probes commercially available for diagnosis of infectious diseases (not an inclusive list of agents or suppliers)

Infectious agent	Supplier
Chlamydia trachomatis	Gen Probe (San Diego, Calif.)
Salmonella	Gen Probe (San Diego, Calif.)
Human immunodeficiency virus	Gen Probe (San Diego, Calif.)
Human papillomavirus	Digene (Silver Springs, Md.)
Hepatitis B virus	Enzo Diagnostics (Syosset, N.Y.)
Mycobacterium sp.	Chiron (Alameda, Calif.)

second capture molecule and enzyme. Examples of this type of assay are the SHARP (Sandwich Hybridization Assay for PCR Products, Digene Diagnostics, Silver Springs, Maryland) and the EMHA (Enhanced Microplate Hybridization Assay, ENZO Diagnostics, Syosset, New York). The assay signal can be colorimetric or luminometric, employing common clinical chemistry instruments. Another promising approach is the direct measurement of PCR product by electrochemical luminescence (ECL), which may be detected manually or with specific instrumentation, such as the PCR 5000 (Perkin Elmer, Foster City, California).

Many methods other than PCR are important for the diagnosis of infectious disease. Very often the important question is not the presence of an organism but the activities going on in the infectious process. For example, HPV and the herpes viruses are ubiquitous. Positive findings of HPV in the genital tract or EBV in the lymphocyte population of a given patient are of very limited value indeed. However, information regarding the transcriptional activity of these agents can be important for the management of the patient. One important technique used to gain this kind of information is in situ hybridization. In this method, a thin section of tissue from fresh or fixed samples can be probed for viral DNA and RNA sequences. This information is a powerful adjunct to classical cytology. Recently, in situ PCR has been described, and manufacturers of PCR instrumentation have begun to develop instruments for this purpose. It is important to remember that the biggest single problem with using these methods on fixed and embedded materials is the quality of the fixation process. Neutral formalin-buffered saline is preferred, since many other fixatives have detrimental effects on DNA and RNA in tissue sections.

Genetic disorders

Abnormal variants of normal DNA sequences are associated with diseases of genetic origin (see Chapter 47). Molecular techniques can be used to make prenatal diagnoses of these diseases, giving prospective parents the opportunity to seek genetic counseling. The box below lists genetic disorders for which DNA probe analysis is currently avail-

able. As the Human Genome Project continues, this list should rapidly expand.

In general, genetic disorders can be grouped into the following categories: chromosomal abnormalities, multifactorial disorders, and single-gene disorders. The discussion in this chapter centers on single-gene disorders.

Single-gene disorders are inherited in one of the following patterns: autosomal dominant, autosomal recessive, or X-linked. The terms *autosomal* and X-linked refer to the chromosomal location of the disease-causing, or mutant, gene. Generally, in X-linked disorders, males with the mutant gene express the disorder, whereas females with the same gene are *carriers* and are usually disease free. Examples of X-linked disorders include Duchenne's muscular dystrophy and hemophilia. *Dominant* disorders are expressed whether an individual is heterozygous or homozygous; *recessive* disorders are expressed only when an individual is homozygous for a mutant gene and carries two copies of the defective gene. Examples of the former are the autosomal dominant disorders achondroplasia and Huntington's disease; examples of the latter are the autosomal recessive disorders cystic fibrosis, sickle cell anemia, and phenylketonuria. Individuals who are heterozygous for these recessive disorders are carriers.

Prenatal diagnosis. Nucleic acid probes and linkage analysis have been used successfully for the prenatal or presymptomatic diagnosis of genetic disorders. To perform prenatal tests, one must obtain DNA from the fetus either by *amniocentesis,* in which fetal cells are obtained by removal of amniotic fluid (see Chapter 40), or by *chorionic villus sampling,* in which fetal cells are obtained from the chorionic villus membrane when a fetus is about 9 weeks old.

The use of linkage analysis to detect genetic disorders begins when an interested family seeks genetic counseling. The genetic counselor explains the procedures and limitations to the family (that is, amniocentesis versus chorionic villus sampling), obtains a *pedigree* (detailed family history), completes the appropriate consent forms, and answers any questions that the family may have. Peripheral blood samples are obtained from the *proband* (the family member affected with the disorder), the natural parents, and any interested family members. If a prenatal diagnosis is requested, a fetal sample is obtained by either chorionic villus sampling (at 9 to 11 weeks of gestation) or amniocentesis (15 to 17 weeks). Direct mutation detection or linkage analysis with appropriate RFLPs is carried out. If the results can clearly determine the genetic status of all family members, the family is informed and counseled appropriately. If the status cannot be unequivocally determined, the previous procedure is repeated with additional probes and restriction endonucleases. As a result, the entire process may require 2 to 3 weeks. In addition, DNA samples obtained by chorionic villus sampling and amniocentesis for prenatal diagnosis often require cell culturing to yield ad-

---

Common Clinical Applications of DNA Linkage Analysis

Cystic fibrosis
Duchenne's muscular dystrophy
Hemophilia A and B
Alpha$_1$-antitrypsin deficiency
Sickle cell anemia
Thalassemia
Phenylketonuria
Adult polycystic kidney disease
Huntington's disease

equate amounts of DNA, which further lengthens the total turnaround time. Ideally, prenatal diagnosis should follow preconception family studies that have determined the appropriate DNA probes and restriction endonucleases to be used on the fetal sample.

Factors affecting gene testing for genetic disorders. The following are factors that can decrease test accuracy:

1. Recombination (crossovers) that occurs between the DNA sequence recognized by the probe and the gene of interest. This problem can be minimized by employing probes that are tightly linked (very close) to the gene of interest.
2. Incorrect identification of paternal relationships can cause misinterpretation of the results, since the procedure is based on comparing inheritance patterns from generation to generation.
3. Erroneous diagnosis of the proband will invalidate the results, since the basis of linkage analysis depends on comparing the restriction fragment patterns of the affected individual to those with a specific disease.
4. Genetic heterogeneity or disorders can be the result of more than one gene defect, sometimes on different chromosomes.
5. Laboratory errors can include specimen mislabeling, probe contamination, incomplete DNA digestion by the restriction endonuclease, or misinterpretation of the autoradiogram.

In addition, not all families can benefit from the application of linkage analysis to their genetic disorder for the following reasons:

1. Linkage analysis is an indirect test that requires comparing patterns of restriction fragments of the affected individual's DNA to those of other family members. The test cannot be done without a DNA sample from the affected individual and his or her natural parents. For this reason, the test cannot be used to screen the general population.
2. The DNA of some families may not yield informative RFLP patterns using the existing probes and restriction enzyme combinations.

CASE EXAMPLE: CYSTIC FIBROSIS
Clinical background (see also Chapters 29 and 47)

Both direct mutation analysis and linkage analysis are used for the prenatal diagnosis and detection of carrier status of cystic fibrosis (CF). CF is inherited as an autosomal recessive disorder and is caused by mutations in the CFTR gene on chromosome 7. CF is characterized by thick secretions obstructing the exocrine glands and leading to chronic pulmonary disease, pancreatic insufficiency, and abnormal sweat electrolytes. CF is diagnosed on the basis of clinical manifestations, a positive family history for the disease, and elevated sweat chloride concentration (see p. 566). Other laboratory tests that may be useful in document-

ing pancreatic insufficiency include the *p*-aminobenzoic acid (PABA) test and the pancreatic stimulation test (see p. 562). Pilot programs screen newborns for CF on the basis of elevated immunoreactive trypsin (IRT) activity in blood spots collected shortly after birth. Decreased activity of microvillar enzymes (the intestinal isoenzyme of alkaline phosphatases, leukocyte alkaline phosphatases, and gamma-glutamyltransferase) is seen in amniotic fluid from fetuses with CF and can be used as the basis for a prenatal diagnosis when DNA testing is not available or useful.

Genetic testing options

In 1989, the gene coding for the protein that is defective in CF, termed the *Cystic Fibrosis Transmembrane Conductance Regulator,* or CFTR, was identified by a new approach to the cloning of disease genes termed *positional cloning.* This approach depends not on classical biochemical techniques but on finding ever more closely linked polymorphisms. Before the actual identification of the gene itself, several RFLPs that were useful clinically in determining family members' carrier status and in prenatal diagnosis were identified. It was hoped that the identification of the gene would allow the replacement of all indirect DNA laboratory procedures by direct tests. However, this has not proved to be possible in all cases. The reason for the continued reliance on indirect testing is genetic heterogeneity. Although a single mutation, a three-base deletion resulting in the deletion of a single phenylalanine residue from position 508 of the mature CFTR protein (ΔF508), is observed on approximately 70% of CF chromosomes worldwide, the remaining mutations are extremely heterogeneous. Up to now over 400 different CF-causing mutations have been identified. In addition to the ΔF508 mutation, several other mutations are present on greater than 0.1% of CF chromosomes. Thus, current familial carrier identification and prenatal diagnosis strategies consist in performing 6 to 30 direct tests for specific mutations, optimally on the proband, followed by linkage analysis using closely linked and intragenic polymorphisms if necessary. This combination testing is informative in virtually all CF families.

Case report

Mr. and Mrs. K have one child, a 3-year-old girl with CF. The child was diagnosed at 18 months of age on the basis of recurrent pulmonary infections and elevated sweat chloride concentrations of 100 to 105 mEq/L. When Mrs. K was 16 weeks pregnant with another child, the K family spoke to their physician about prenatal diagnosis. Their physician referred them to a genetic counselor for information. After genetic counseling, blood was obtained on Mr. and Mrs. K and their affected child, and amniocentesis was performed to obtain fetal DNA. The DNA from the proband was first screened using a 12-mutation panel, which identifies approximately 85% of CF alleles in the North American population. The genotype of the affected girl was ΔF508/Unk

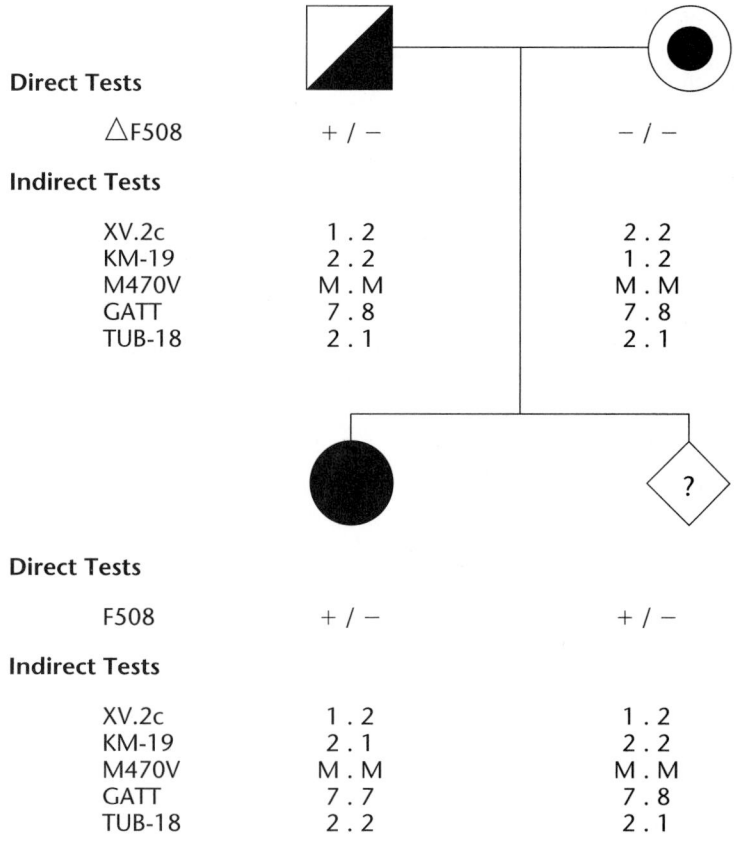

Direct Tests

△F508	+ / −	− / −

Indirect Tests

XV.2c	1 . 2	2 . 2
KM-19	2 . 2	1 . 2
M470V	M . M	M . M
GATT	7 . 8	7 . 8
TUB-18	2 . 1	2 . 1

Direct Tests

F508	+ / −	+ / −

Indirect Tests

XV.2c	1 . 2	1 . 2
KM-19	2 . 1	2 . 2
M470V	M . M	M . M
GATT	7 . 7	7 . 8
TUB-18	2 . 2	2 . 1

Fig. 48-4 Pedigree of the K family with results from a panel of both direct and indirect test procedures.

(unknown mutation). The fetal DNA was then tested and found to have one copy of the △F508 mutation. The parents were given the option of having a 50-mutation test panel performed in the hopes of identifying the unknown CF mutation, or to proceed with linkage analysis. The parents had another meeting with the genetic counselor, who informed them that the extra mutation panel identifies a further 1% to 2% of CF alleles, and informed them of the potential mechanisms of error in linkage analysis. After consideration, this family elected to proceed with linkage analysis. RFLPs at two extragenic but closely linked loci (XV.2c and KM-19) and three intragenic loci (M470V, GATT, and TUB-18) were analyzed by use of PCR-based methods. The family's pedigree and results are shown in Fig. 48-4. The fetus received the CF-bearing chromosome from the father; that chromosome bears the △F508 mutation and the haplotype (or series of polymorphism), resulting in 1,2,M,7,2. This indicates that the fetus is at least a carrier of CF. However, the affected girl received the haplotype 2,1,M,7,2 from the mother, an indication that the unknown CF mutation from the mother is coinherited with this haplotype. The fetus received the opposite maternal chromosome, that bearing the haplotype 2,2,M,8,1. Thus the combination of direct and linkage analysis in this family indicates that the fetus is a carrier but is not affected with CF. Because of the

extremely tight linkage, with two informative loci being inside the gene itself (note that the M470V locus is not informative in this family), the estimated risk of error caused by recombination is extremely small. Mr. and Mrs. K were informed of the results by the genetic counselor and decided to continue the pregnancy, with plans to employ the sweat test for the baby a few months after birth. When the infant was 3 months old, sweat testing was performed with normal results.

BIBLIOGRAPHY
General

Dracopoli NC, Haines JL, Kork BR, et al, editors: *Current protocols in human genetics,* New York, 1994, Wiley & Sons.

Farkas D, editor: *Molecular biology and pathology: a guidebook for quality control,* New York, 1993, Academic Press.

Silverman LM, Hine R, editors: *Molecular pathology,* Durham, N.C., 1994, Carolina Academic Press.

Cancer Genetics

Cho Y, Gorina S, Jeffrey PD, Pavletich NP: Crystal structure of a p53 tumor suppressor–DNA complex: understanding tumorigenic mutations, *Science* 265:346-355, 1994.

Dean M, Vande Woude GF: Introduction to methods in molecular biology. In DeVita VT, Hellman S, Rosenberg SA, editors: *Cancer: principles and practice of oncology,* ed 3, Philadelphia, 1989, Lippincott.

Friend S: p53: a glimpse at the puppet behind the shadow play, *Science* 265:334-335, 1994.

Hodgson SV, Maher ER: *A practical guide to human cancer genetics,* New York, 1993, Cambridge University Press.

Knudson AG: Mutation and cancer: statistical study of retinoblastoma, *Proc Nat Acad Sci USA* 68:820-824, 1971.

Levine AJ: The tumor suppressor genes, *Annu Rev Biochem* 62:623-51, 1993.

Lemoine NR, Wright NA, editors: *The molecular pathology of cancer,* Plainview, N.Y., 1993, Cold Spring Harbor Press.

Special Cancer Issue, *Science* 254:1131-1177, 1991.

Infectious Disease

Greer CE, Peterson HT, Kiviat NB, Manos MM: PCR amplification from paraffin embedded tissues, *Am J Clin Pathol* 95:117, 1991.

Naber SP: Molecular pathology: diagnosis of infectious disease, *N Engl J Med* 331:1212-1215, 1994.

Nuovo JN, Gallery F, MacConnell P, et al: An improved technique for the *in situ* detection of DNA after polymerase chain reaction amplification, *Am J Pathol* 139:1239, 1991.

Rersing DH, Smith TF, Tenover FC, White TJ, editors: Diagnostic molecular microbiology: principles and applications, Washington, D.C., 1993, American Society for Microbiology.

Terry G, Ho L, Szarewski A, Cuzick J: Semi-automated detection of human papillomavirus DNA of high and low oncogenic potential in cervical smears, *Clin Chem* 40:1890-1892, 1994.

Tsongalis GJ, McPhail AH, Daniel R, et al: Localized in situ amplification (LISA): a novel approach to in situ PCR, *Clin Chem* 40:381-384, 1994.

Genetics

Botstein D, White R, Scolnick M, Davis R: Construction of a genetic linkage map in man using restriction fragment length polymorphisms, *Am J Hum Genet* 32:314, 1980.

Buffone GJ, Spence JE, Fernbach SD, et al: Prenatal diagnosis of cystic fibrosis: microvillar enzymes and DNA analysis compared, *Clin Chem* 34(5):933, 1988.

Kerem B-S, Rommens JR, Buchanan JA, et al: Identification of the cystic fibrosis gene: genetic analysis, *Science* 245:1073-1087, 1989.

Kremer B, Goldberg P, Andrew SE, et al: A worldwide study of the Huntington's disease mutation: the sensitivity and specificity of measuring CAG repeats, *N Engl J Med* 330:1401-1406, 1994.

LeGrys V, Leinbach SS, Silverman L: Clinical applications of DNA probes in the diagnosis of genetic diseases, *CRC Crit Rev Clin Lab Sci* 25:255, 1987.

Pearson PL: Restriction fragment length polymorphisms and their use in mapping the human genome. In Kare B, editor: *Progress in clinical biology research,* New York, 1985, Alan R Liss.

Pena SDJ, Chakraborty R, Epplen JT, Jeffreys AJ, editors: *DNA fingerprinting: the state of the science,* Boston, 1993, Birkhäuser Verlag.

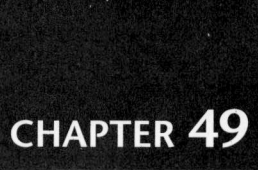

CHAPTER **49**

Neoplasia

Bernard E. Statland
Per Winkel

OBJECTIVES

■ Briefly describe the biological factors that can result in cancer.

■ List the roles of laboratory tests in the assessment of cancers.

■ Define and describe an ideal tumor marker.

■ List commonly used chemical and cellular markers and state their clinical significance in relation to cancers.

KEY TERMS

carcinoembryonic antigen A glycoprotein produced by or associated with cancer cells, which is also expressed by fetal cells.

Small levels are detected in healthy individuals. Detection is by immunochemical analysis.

carcinogen An agent, usually a chemical, that transforms a cell from a normal to a cancerous state.

cocarcinogen An agent that by itself does not transform a normal cell into a cancerous state but in concert with another agent can effect the transformation.

confirmation Use of a second test with very high specificity to verify the observation of a less specific test (such as a biopsy to verify a mass as a tumor).

dedifferentiation The process by which cells go from the more specific to the more general in nature. Usually such cells lose their morphological architecture and ability to synthesize specific cell components (such as estrogen receptors).

dissemination The phase of cancer in which the cells spread to various parts of the body distant from the site of origin.

ectopic hormones Hormones that are produced in tissues that do not normally do so (such as hormones produced by cancers).

estriol receptor The specific tissue membrane receptor in breast that binds the hormone estriol. Its presence in breast cancer signifies a differentiated tumor.

heterogeneity Variation in gene expression among cancer cells. Differences between cells exist, and not all cells within a tumor are positive for the same antigen or respond to the same drug.

induction phase The period during which a normal cell becomes transformed into a cancerous cell.

in situ A term used to show that cancer cells are localized at their place of origin.

invasion The process by which malignant cells move into deeper tissue and through the basement membrane and gain access to blood vessels and lymphatic channels.

metastases Cancer cells that have spread to other organs and have formed colonies that are growing and often invading the organ.

monitoring Measurement of a biochemical marker of cancer after a confirmed diagnosis (such as the use of carcinoembryonic antigen to monitor colorectal cancer) *to evaluate* the presence or growth of the cancer.

neoplasia 'New growth', the unrestricted growth of cells resulting in cancer.

oncogene A gene whose protein product can cause the development of a cancer when the protein is present (or absent) in abnormal amounts.

oncofetal protein A protein produced by or associated with cancer cells that is made by the fetus; however, it is usually produced in the child or adult at very low levels.

Pap (Papanicolaou) smear A common screening test for cancer in which cells from the cervix are examined for cytological abnormalities consistent with cancer.

staging A process of diagnosis in which the pathologist determines the position of cancer in the progressive cycle of phases: induction, in situ, invasion, and dissemination.

transformation In oncology, the process by which a normal cell becomes malignant, that is, cancerous.

tumor marker A misused term applied to molecules that can be used to diagnose or monitor the presence or growth of a cancer. Usually such markers are not specific for cancer.

CANCER INCIDENCE IN THE UNITED STATES

Changes in longevity, introduction of carcinogens into the environment, and other factors have changed the incidence of cancer in the United States. Table 49-1 presents percentages of cancer deaths by organ site and sex as tabulated in 1987 in the United States. The sites associated most strongly with cancer deaths in males of all ages are, in descending order, lung, colorectal area, prostate, pancreas, and stomach. Carcinogens in tobacco are believed to be responsible for the alterations in cellular genetic material (deoxyribonucleic acid, DNA) that lead to lung cancer, whereas ingested carcinogens cause similar DNA lesions that lead to colorectal cancer. In females of all ages the most common cancer sites are breast, colorectal area, lung, uterus, and ovary. The incidence of smoking in men and women is directly related to the incidence of lung cancer. The distribution of deaths by organ site is affected by geographical factors as well. For example, in Japan, unlike in the United States, esophageal and stomach cancers are the most common types of malignancy. In Western countries cancer is the second greatest cause of death. Approximately one in five persons in the United States will die of cancer.

CANCER: NATURE OF THE DISEASE

The clonal theory of carcinogenesis states that cancers derive from an original, transformed cell. This transformed cell, or clone, is a normal cell whose genetic material has been altered such that the cell and its progeny lose those regulatory functions that govern cell replication and cell death. By an evolutionary, multistep process, cells derived from the initially modified cell begin to multiply, uncontrolled by the usual local inhibitory systems, often invading other parts of the body. This last phase, called *metastases,* is usually the cause of deaths by cancer.

Several points of evidence have led scientists to believe that more than one gene must be altered before a malignant cell is formed. First, the relationship between cancer and age is an experiential one; that is, as an individual ages the likelihood of cancer increases. Time is needed to allow the accumulation of genetic damage, which can lead to the transformed state (see below). Second, cancer cells can be

Table 49-1 Estimated new cancer cases and deaths in 1995 in the United States by site and sex*

Site	Sex	
	Male (%)	Female (%)
Breast	—	32
Colon and rectum	10	12
Blood and lymphoid tissue (leukemia and lymphomas)	8	7
Lung	14	13
Oral cavity	3	2
Ovary	—	5
Pancreas	2	2
Prostate gland	36	—
Skin	3	3
Urinary tract	8	4
Uterus	—	8
Other	16	13

*Data supplied by the American Cancer Society.

shown to have multiple genetic lesions. Third, cancer is more likely to occur in cells that proliferate. Thus cancer of the heart is very rare, but cancers of the white blood cell are very common. Because white blood cells proliferate, there is far greater potential for the expression of genetic lesions and for the process of cell division to become unregulated.

Etiology

Sager[1] has described the cause of cancer as a multistage genetic process. The stages include

1. Initial DNA damage
2. Chromosome breakdown and rearrangement; gene replication
3. Selection of successfully growing mutant cells

The initial changes in cellular DNA can be caused by a variety of carcinogens, including radiation, chemicals, viruses, and unknown agents. This leads to faulty growth control and loss of chromosome stability. The chromosome breakage and rearrangement occur in several continuous phases after the initiation of cell division. This is later manifested in terms of aberrant chromosomal transpositions, which lead to genomic rearrangements (see Chapter 47).

The changes in the DNA and chromosomes result in a new pattern of gene expression, creating a new phenotype, in which previously quiescent genes are now expressed, previously expressed genes are now quiescent, or there is overexpression of certain key genes. It is now believed that the earliest changes in gene expression that can lead to a transformed cell occur in genes that normally regulate cell growth and cell death.[2] These newly expressed or suppressed regulatory genes are known as *oncogenes.*[3] A list of the cell-derived oncogene products by class is presented in Table 49-2. Assays that detect oncogenes in human cancer tissues are rapidly becoming available (see Chapter 47). These assays may be potentially useful for the prediction

Table 49-2   Classes of oncogenes and their derived protein products

Class of factor	Factor	Gene product
Growth factors	*sis*	PDGF B, chain growth factor
Protein tyrosine kinase	*sic*	Membrane associated, receptor protein tyrosine kinase
Receptors lacking protein kinase activity	*mas*	Angiotensin receptor
Membrane-associated G-proteins	H-*ras*	Membrane-associated GTP-binding/GTPase
Cytoplasmic protein kinase	*rat/mil*	Cytoplasmic protein kinases
Cytoplasmic regulators	*crk*	SH-23 protein
Nuclear transcription cofactors	*myc*	Sequence-specific, DNA-binding protein

of the development of oncogene-associated cancers in high-risk groups.[4]

A cell that has been transformed has only the potential for developing into a cancer. The expression of the cancer phenotype requires cell division, which can be induced by additional genetic damage or can result from a natural induction of cell division. This can be seen in the inverse relationship between the development of breast cancer and the age at which a woman first carries a pregnancy to near term. This relationship is likely the result of the one-time induction of breast epithelial cell hyperplasia that occurs in a first pregnancy. The later in life that the first pregnancy occurs, the greater the likelihood of the accumulation of a cancer phenotype in breast epithelium.

As cancer cells multiply, there may be additional phenotypic changes in the now unstable genetic material. As a result, a process of natural selection allows the most "successful" cancer cell to proliferate the most and to dominate the cancer mass. As the environment surrounding the cancer changes, such as that from therapy, the selection process continues.

Diversity of cancer cells

Variation of gene expression. There is a broad range of possible combinations of gene expression in the human cell. It varies from normal cells to the most atypical cancer cells. As a result of the genetic changes described above, cancer cells develop new combinations of gene expression and therefore new phenotypes. The phenotypic variation occurs not only from cancer cells to normal cells, or from cancer type to cancer type, but also within particular cancer types and even within a single tumor. For example, in patients with cancer of the breast there is a heterogeneity of genes expressed by various cells; that is, not all cells express the same genes. An example is the heterogeneous expression in breast tumors of the gene for the estrogen receptor (see below).

Variable gene expression and its manifestations. Variable gene expression leads to biological and biochemical diversity of cancer cells; consequently various tumor-specific markers are not necessarily elaborated by all cancer cells of the same type or even by a single cancer over time. This is very important clinically when one is trying to determine which analyte to follow in monitoring patients with known malignancy. The cellular diversity within a single tumor also means that a cancer's clinical manifestation, such as a tumor's response to therapy, may change with time.

Clinical manifestations. The clinical manifestations of cancer vary widely, depending on the type of tumor, the tissue affected, and the stage of tumor development. For example, cancer of the gastrointestinal tract is manifested by obstruction, hemoptysis, and bloody stools. Cancer of the lung is manifested by hypoxia, chest pain, and often various neurological symptoms. The clinical manifestations are related to the physiological function of the organ with the primary cancer and the effect of the cancer on other organs as well. For example, cancer of an endocrine gland can result in production of excess hormone with many systemic hormonal effects. New symptoms are evidenced with the spread (metastasis) of the cancer cells to other organs. Cancer spreads through the lymphatic system and the bloodstream, resulting in liver, bone, and pulmonary metastases.

Time as a factor

Cancer as a long-term process. Cancer is a long-term process and progresses through four obligatory phases: an induction phase, an in situ phase, an invasion phase, and a dissemination phase. During the *induction phase,* which can last up to 30 years or more, the cells are exposed to one or more carcinogens. These environmental carcinogens may include radiation or various toxins. It has been estimated that approximately three fourths of all human cancers may be caused by these environmental factors.

It is now believed that a period of many years after exposure may be necessary before a carcinogen is able to have its effect on the host. The histological changes begin with severe dysplasia, eventually leading to cancer. It should be obvious that not everyone who is exposed to the same carcinogen will develop cancer. Additional factors that play a role in deciding which individual may get cancer include individual (genetic) or tissue susceptibility, the presence of other carcinogens or cocarcinogens, the site at which the carcinogen may act, the duration of exposure (see above), and obviously the nature, amount, and concentration of the carcinogen under question. Often the time between the induction phase and the clinically apparent cancer can be as long as 20 years.

After induction there is the *in situ phase.* The in situ phase represents that time during which the transformed cell actually develops into a cancer, but the cancer remains localized in the original site and does not invade other tissues. Clonal selection (see above) for those cancer cells that grow most successfuly occurs during this phase.

The third phase is called the *invasion phase*. During the invasion phase the malignant cells multiply and invade into the deeper tissues through the basement membrane, thereby gaining access to blood vessels and lymphatic channels.

The fourth stage is that of dissemination. During the *dissemination phase*, which lasts 1 to 5 years, the invading cancer spreads to various parts of the body distant from the site of origin, often through the blood and lymphatic systems. For the tumor to grow during this phase it must form a new blood supply, using a process that is termed *angiogenesis*.

It is critical to detect cancer early, before metastatic spread. Ideally it should be detected during the induction phase. However, this is impossible because before the in situ phase one is *not* certain if cancer will actually develop in the individual. The next approach is to detect the cancer in the in situ phase. This has been done with great success in patients with cancer of the cervix. Here the Pap (Papanicolaou) smear technique has been of great benefit. When in situ cancer of the cervix is detected, the prognosis is excellent. Most cancers are detected during the invasion phase. If dissemination has not yet occurred, the prognosis is reasonable. Detection of local spreading with or without involvement of the lymph nodes often leads to a cure. However, if dissemination has already occurred, the prognosis is very poor.

Invasion by cancer cells of surrounding tissue. Several factors play a role in determining the cancer's ability to invade the surrounding tissue. Such factors include increased motility of the cells, increased pressure within the tumor caused by active multiplication of the cells, elaboration by the cancer of lytic substances, lack of intercellular bridges found between all normal cells, decreased cohesiveness between cells, and eventual spread of the tumor cells to the regional lymph nodes. However, when the metastases are still microscopic (micrometastases), the clinician's ability to detect them is very poor. It has been estimated that approximately half the patients who appear to be clinically free of metastases do in fact have unrecognized distant micrometastases at the time of initial diagnosis and treatment.

Change in cell division. Cancer is often manifested by a change in cellular division rate. Although most cancers are associated with an increased rate of cell division, there are examples in which this is not always the case, such as nephroma.

Dedifferentiation of cells. A common phenomenon of cancer is dedifferentiation, in which cells go from a more specific cell type to a more general cell type by the process of clonal selection. Thus it is not uncommon for cancer cells to synthesize various compounds that are normally present only in the embryonic or fetal stage. On the other hand, as cells dedifferentiate, they may lose certain specific cellular

properties such as receptor activity or an enzyme activity. These phenotypic changes can be used as prognostic indicators.

Chromosomal changes in cancer. Chromosomal changes in cancer have been extensively studied in patients with leukemia, and various types of leukemia are often confirmed on the basis of these chromosomal changes.

OVERVIEW OF ROLES OF LABORATORY TESTS
Detection (screening)

There are four major functions that laboratory tests can serve in the field of neoplasia. They are detection or screening, confirmation, classification (staging), and monitoring.

Table 49-3 lists several screening tests for early detection of cancer.[5] The quality of a screening test is usually expressed by its clinical sensitivity and specificity (see p. 375). The observations from the screening tests are divided into negative and positive results. Each person examined is classified as either a diseased or a nondiseased person.

A rigid classification of test results into positive and negative results may sometimes be too simplistic. Outcomes of screening tests can usually be ordered from very negative to very positive. The latter approach allows for a more sophisticated test interpretation in actual screening programs. For example, patients whose results are not negative but also are not alarming enough to justify immediate diagnostic action can be scheduled for earlier repeat screenings.[6] Another example is a stepwise screening policy in which only individuals with positive results at the first screening test are subject to further diagnostic testing.[7]

Sometimes the use of more than one screening test may seem advantageous. However, assessment of the sensitivity and specificity of a combination of screening tests based on data available for the individual tests is complicated by the fact that usually the tests are not independent in a sta-

Table 49-3   Screening tests for early detection of cancer

Site	Test
Bladder	Cytological analysis of urine
Breast	Mammography, physical examination, self-examination
Cervix	Papanicolaou smear, pelvic examination
Colon and rectum	Testing stool for occult blood, sigmoidoscopy
Hodgkin's disease	Physical examination and roentgenography
Lung	X-ray, cytological analysis of sputum
Oral cavity	Visual examination
Prostate	Digital palpation per rectum, prostatic massage and cytological examination
Skin	Visual inspection
Stomach	Photofluorography, saline wash and cytological examination of gastric contents, examination of stool for occult blood

From Habbema JDF, van Oortmarssen GJ, van der Maas, PJ. In Statland BE, Winkel P, editors: *Laboratory measurements in malignant disease*, vol 2, Philadelphia, 1982, Saunders.

tistical sense. In general, it is more effective to combine two tests that are complementary (that is, directed at different anatomical or biochemical features of the tumor) than to combine tests directed at the same types of features.

Complementary tests include sputum cytological examination and chest x-ray examination for lung cancer screening.[8] Palpation and mammography in breast cancer screening are examples of two related tests. They both detect tumors largely on the basis of size. One study[9] showed that when mammography was performed, the physical examination proved to be almost completely redundant.

Confirmation

Additional tests are used to confirm the suspicion of cancer based on clinical symptoms or signs. Tests that tend to confirm the presence of a cancer include, for example, bone marrow examination for leukemia, urinary catecholamines for pheochromocytoma, and alpha-fetoprotein for testicular cancer. The confirmatory results must be above a certain decision level.[10] For a laboratory test result to be confirmatory, it should possess 100% diagnostic specificity, that is, contain no false-positive results. For example, all cases in which the catecholamine level is above a certain value should be associated with pheochromocytoma.

Classification and staging

Classification of tumors is used to describe the degree of tumor differentiation. Tumors are classified as well differentiated, moderately well differentiated, and poorly differentiated. Poorly differentiated tumors are more aggressive and have a poorer prognosis. Surgical pathologists have developed various staging approaches based on the size and extent of invasion of surrounding tissues by the tumor, the number of cancer cell–positive lymph nodes, and the presence or absence of metastases. This has been called the TNM (tumor, nodes, metastases) system.[11] The purpose of such staging is to give reasonable estimates of prognosis (that is, recurrence of cancer), appropriate response to therapy, or the likely course of the disease. In addition to staging based on gross or microscopic pathological data, it would be of great value to have biochemical tests that could classify cancers appropriately. It has been suggested that an elevated serum prostatic acid phosphatase level, if measured by an enzymatic procedure, can indicate the presence of metastatic prostate cancer.

Monitoring

The most important function of laboratory tests in cancer is that of monitoring the course of the disease or its response to therapy. Winkel et al.[12] have developed various strategies to monitor patients known to have breast cancer. The problem addressed was that of predicting on the basis of sequential values whether a patient would have recurrence of this disease. Other approaches have been used to monitor patients on the basis of carcinoembryonic antigen (CEA)

in colon cancer,[13] prostate-specific antigen (PSA) for prostate cancer,[14] and others. An increased CEA or PSA value is a signal to explore the patient surgically again to remove additional cancer or change the course of chemotherapy. It is assumed that the CEA- or PSA-producing tumor has reached clinical proportions when the serum values for PSA or CEA reach a certain threshold.

All four major functions—screening, confirming, classifying, and monitoring—are possible roles for laboratory tests for neoplasia.

DEFINITION OF IDEAL TUMOR MARKER

Coombes and Neville[15] have suggested that the *ideal* tumor marker should fulfill the following criteria:

1. Be easy and inexpensive to measure in readily available body fluids.
2. Be specific to the tumor studied and commonly associated with it.
3. Have a stoichiometric relationship between plasma level of the marker and tumor mass.
4. Have an abnormal plasma level, urine level, or both, in the presence of micrometastases, that is, at a stage at which no clinical or presently available diagnostic methods reveal their presence.
5. Have plasma levels, urine levels, or both, that are stable and not subject to wild fluctuations.
6. If present in the plasma of healthy individuals, exist at a much lower concentration than that found in association with all stages of cancer.

Obviously much additional research must be done before such ideal tumor markers will be found. However, it is important to recognize that the evaluation of an ideal tumor marker should relate to the clinical setting. To do so, it has been suggested that all tumor markers should also comply with the following major criteria[16]:

1. They should prognosticate a higher or lower risk for eventual development of recurrence.
2. They should change as the current status of the tumor changes over time.
3. They should precede and predict recurrences before they are clinically detectable.

In addition, if a tumor marker is to be used to detect very early stages of cancer, a treatment for that cancer must be available. It might be unethical to detect cancers for which no effective treatment is available (see below).

All tumor markers should be analyzed both according to the criteria that Coombes and Neville have presented and according to the considerations just mentioned. For a tumor marker to be of some value, it must give information beyond that readily seen on the basis of physical examination or history, and it must give this information with a reasonably long lead time to allow appropriate therapy to be given in a timely manner. Lead time is the time elapsed between the time a test result will be positive and the time that the disease will be clinically evident or advanced.

ETHICS OF TESTING

Even when a tumor marker can be used to detect the presence of disease, it may not always be beneficial to use it. Prostate cancer, for example, is present in about 40% of males 50 to 70 years of age, but only about 4% of these men will die from this disease itself. The reason is that prostate cancer is usually slow growing and in most cases it is more likely that a patient will die from some other cause, rather than from the prostate cancer. The standard treatments for prostate cancer, surgical intervention, chemotherapy, and radiation, can result in unwanted side effects, including impotence, incontinence, and the need for colostomy. In addition, a significant number of patients can die from the treatments themselves. Thus the ethical question arises: should PSA be used to detect prostate cancer when the therapy is not without a great cost in unnecessary morbidity and its effect on the longevity of patients unproved?

CHANGE OF ANALYTE IN DISEASE

Classes of biochemicals used as tumor markers
(Table 49-4)

This section is a review of several biochemical tests that have been used either as primary tumor markers or as secondary tests to note invasion or dissemination of cancer. The types of analytes are listed in the box and are discussed in terms of their clinical usefulness and applications. This chapter is a discussion of assays that are commonly in use or that seem to have potential value. The Food and Drug

---

Examples of Tumor Markers

Oncofetal proteins
Carcinoembryonic antigen (CEA)
Alpha-fetoprotein (AFP)
Human chorionic gonadotropin (hCG)
SCC (squamous cell carcinoma) antigen

Mucin glycoproteins (carbohydrate antigen)
CA-125
CA-19-9

Enzymes
Prostatic acid phosphatase (PAP)
Prostate-specific antigen (PSA)

Hormones and hormone receptors
ACTH and all other endocrine hormones
Breast estrogen and progesterone receptors

Cell surface proteins (other than receptors)
Beta$_2$-microglobulin

Cellular markers
Oncogenes, such as N-*ras*
Suppressor genes, such as p53

Administration regulates which tumor markers can be used. The current FDA-approved list of protein tumor markers includes CEA, AFP, PSA, PAP, and CA-125. As large clinical trials are completed, other such markers will be approved. Reviews that cover some of these assays in greater depth are recommended for further reading (such as references 16 and 17).

Oncofetal antigens

Many of the oncofetal antigens are measured in the laboratory by use of immunoassays; either competitive-binding radioimmunoassays or solid-phase immunometric assays, employing either second antibodies labeled with ^{125}I, enzymes, fluorescent, or chemiluminescent compounds. These proteins are NOT recommended for cancer screening.

Carcinoembryonic antigen. CEA is a glycoprotein present in colonic adenocarcinoma and fetal gut; it was first described by Gold and Freedman.[18] The detection of CEA in various tissues or serum is complicated by the presence in these tissues of CEA cross-reacting antigens.

In general, CEA plasma levels increase with increasing age and smoking. This has prevented the use of CEA levels for the purpose of general screening.[19] The results of screening programs confined to subpopulations with higher-than-average risk of developing cancer have been equally discouraging.[20] Thus, neither the sensitivity nor the specificity of CEA justifies its use for the definitive diagnosis of cancer.[21]

In specific situations, however, CEA has proved of diagnostic value. CEA is useful, for example, for the detection of primary colorectal cancer[22] when used in combination with a barium enema and with radioiodide imaging for the detection of carcinoma metastatic to the liver. According to the consensus statement of the National Cancer Institute,[19] only values five to ten times the upper normal reference limit in patients with symptoms should be considered strongly suggestive of the presence of cancer. In some can-

Table 49-4 Classes of biochemicals used as tumor markers

Class of biochemical	Examples	Use
Increased production of endogenous biochemicals	Hormones, enzymes, polyamines, and so on	Confirmation, diagnosis, monitoring
Synthesis of biochemicals of previously quiescent genes	Oncofetal proteins, cell surface antigens, enzymes	Monitoring, prognosis
Receptors	Estriol receptor (breast cancer), androgen receptor (prostate cancer)	Prognosis, treatment
Modification of usual cell or organ function	Gamma-glutamyltransferase (GGT) or 5'-nucleotidase	Diagnosis

cers, including colorectal and breast cancer, the plasma level of CEA and the frequency of elevated values are positively correlated with the severity of the disease as assessed by clinical staging. Currently, CEA is approved only for monitoring of colorectal cancer.

Postoperative monitoring of plasma CEA levels for the detection of recurrence or metastases has proved valuable in colorectal cancer. Most clinicians now respond to consecutively increasing serum CEA values with second-look operations in patients with surgically treated colorectal cancer. A significant number of patients do benefit from a second surgery.[23]

CEA is not approved for breast cancer because postoperative CEA levels are less frequently elevated in patients with breast cancer who eventually develop overt metastatic disease than in corresponding patients operated on for colorectal cancer. In only 10% to 15% of patients with breast cancer does the plasma CEA level rise to values above 10 μg/L.[24]

Alpha-fetoprotein and human chorionic gonadotropin.

Alpha-fetoprotein (AFP) is an oncofetal glycoprotein. In early embryonic life it is a predominant component of the serum proteins. It is first synthesized by the yolk sac and later by the fetal liver. Later in life it is mainly produced in the liver. AFP was first recognized as a tumor marker by Abele in 1963.[25]

Serum AFP values should be less than 10 μg/L in healthy subjects. In benign hepatic disorders, moderate (40 μg/L) elevations may be seen. Values above 400 μg/L are almost always associated with hepatocellular carcinoma, germ cell carcinoma (such as testicular carcinoma), chronic aggressive hepatitis, or subacute hepatic necrosis. Currently, AFP is approved only for use with testicular carcinoma.

Human chorionic gonadotropin (HCG) is a glycoprotein hormone that shares indistinguishable biological activity and extensive structural homology with its pituitary counterpart, human luteinizing hormone (HLH).[26] Although the α subunits of HLH and HCG are essentially identical, the β subunits can be differentiated on the basis of specific immunoassay techniques (see Chapter 40). Tumors of the placenta and the testes that contain trophoblastic tissue secrete excessive amounts of HCG. Specific and sensitive assays have revealed that many cancers also secrete HCG. However, available data[27] clearly show that HCG determinations are of no value in screening for cancer.

The main clinical use of AFP and HCG is related to the diagnosis, therapy, and follow-up study of germ cell tumors.[28] Table 49-5 presents the World Health Organization (WHO) classification of germ cell tumors and associated markers in tissue and serum. In general, AFP and HCG provide the most information about tumor status when they are persistently elevated. The absence of a marker does not preclude the presence of germ cell tumors.

Carbohydrate antigen-19-9.

Carbohydrate antigen-19-9 (CA-19-9) occurs in tissue as a monosialoganglioside and in serum as mucin, a high-molecular-weight, carbohydrate-rich glycoprotein. Results of clinical studies indicate that the CA-19-9 level in serum or plasma of patients with an intra-abdominal carcinoma frequently is increased. It is correlated most strikingly with cancer of the pancreas, for which early studies have shown a sensitivity of 90% and a specificity of 85%. CA-19-9 also may be increased with other adenocarcinomas such as lung, gastric, biliary, and colonic.

Carbohydrate antigen-125.

Serum carbohydrate antigen-125 (CA-125), a glycoprotein antigen, is elevated in the serum of patients with ovarian cancer. Increased concentrations of CA-125 were found in many patients with epithelial ovarian cancer and in ovarian teratoma. Changes in CA-125 concentrations in serum during chemotherapy mirrored the progress of the disease as assessed by clinical and radiological evidence. It should be noted that CA-125 provides no real assistance for diagnosis; however, it does have value as a marker for monitoring responsiveness to chemotherapy.

Enzymes

Schwartz[30] reviewed the use of enzyme tests in the management of patients with cancer. The box presents various enzymes that have been used for this purpose. As with many putative tumor markers discussed in this chapter, the use of enzyme markers is fraught with difficulties. Not all patients

Table 49-5   WHO classification of germ cell tumors and associated tumor markers

WHO classification	Immunohistochemistry		Serology		Comments
	AFP	HCG	AFP	HCG	
Seminoma (S)	−	±	No	± Yes	HCG in giant cells
Embryonal carcinoma (EC)	+	+	± Yes	± Yes	HCG in giant cells AFP controversial, may occur in undiagnosed yolk sac elements
Yolk sac tumor (YST)	+	−	± Yes	No	
Choriocarcinoma (CC)	−	+	No		
Teratoma (TT)	−	−	No?	No?	

From Norgaard-Pedersen B, Hangaard J: In Statland BE, Winkel P, editors: *Laboratory measurements in malignant disease*, Philadelphia, 1982, Saunders.
AFP, alpha-fetoprotein; *HCG*, human chorionic gonadotropin.

Enzymes Useful in Cancer Detection

Acid phosphatase (ACP)
Alkaline phosphatase (ALP)
Creatine kinase BB (CK-BB)
Gamma-glutamyltransferase (GGT)
Glycosyltransferases
Lactate dehydrogenase (LD)
Lysozyme (muramidase)
5'-Nucleotidase
Pancreatic enzymes (amylase, lipase, ribonuclease, trypsin)
Phosphohexose isomerase (PHI)
Prostate specific antigen (PSA)
Terminal deoxynucleotidyltransferase (TDT)

Table 49-6 Diagnostic sensitivities (percent positive) of several PAP assays for prostatic carcinoma*

Stage	Chemical†	Radioimmunoassay			
		†	‡	§	‖
A	12	33	13	0	8
B	15	79	26	20	21
C	29	71	30	33	40
D	60	92	94	79	86

*Sensitivities were calculated from data presented in the reference listed for each assay.
†Foti AG, Cooper JF, Herschman H, et al: *N Engl J Med* 297:1357-1361, 1977.
‡Mahan DE, Doctor BP: *Clin Biochem* 12:10-17, 1979.
§Chu TM, Wang MC, Scott WW, et al: *Invest Urol* 15:319-323, 1978.
‖New England Nuclear, April 1979, Study Report, Boston.

---

with a particular cancer type have elevations in an enzyme (poor sensitivity), and many noncancer diseases are associated with elevations of many of these enzymes. An exception to this is PSA, which is an extracellular protease (see above). Thus the most frequent uses of these enzymes are as objective markers to give semiquantitative estimates of response to therapy or as prognostic indicators.

Acid phosphatase. There are two isoenzymes of the 13 known for acid phosphatase (ACP) that appear to have important roles in managing patients with cancer. The first is the prostatic isoenzyme, and the second is the bone isoenzyme. The former is inhibited by tartrate, whereas the bone isoenzyme is tartrate resistant.

The prostatic acid phosphatase (PAP) isoenzyme has not proved useful for diagnostic purposes.[31] Most assays investigated have low sensitivities in the early, more treatable stages of prostatic carcinoma (A and B) (Table 49-6). The use of many of these assays to confirm the presence of prostatic carcinoma in men with urological complaints has also been limited.[32] The primary use of PAP is to help determine the likelihood of metastatic prostate cancer.

Pancreatic enzymes (amylase, lipase, ribonuclease, and trypsin). Serum amylase elevations have been found in approximately 25% of patients with pancreatic cancer. Unfortunately lipase assays are not more useful than amylase assays are. Various workers have examined ribonuclease as a marker of pancreatic cancer. Reddi and Holland[33] observed that this enzyme was elevated in 90% of patients with pancreatic cancer and in only 10% of patients with pancreatitis. Fitzgerald et al.[34] repeated these studies and found that 50% of patients with pancreatic cancer and, unfortunately, 35% of patients with noncancerous pancreatic disease had elevated ribonuclease values.

Immunoreactive trypsin has been used to study patients with pancreatic cancer. In one study all 17 patients with pancreatic cancer had elevated renal clearance of immunoreactive trypsin, whereas 67% of patients with acute pancreatitis had elevated values. This should be compared with the fact that all patients with chronic pancreatitis had values within the control range.[35]

Prostate-specific antigen. Prostate-specific antigen (PSA) is a glycoprotein protease found in the epithelial cells of the prostatic duct and acini. PSA is elevated in all four stages of prostate cancer as well as in benign prostatic hypertrophy (BPH). It is a much more sensitive assay for a prostate cancer than prostatic acid phosphatase is.[13] However, because serum PSA levels are elevated in BPH, PSA has a relatively poor clinical specificity and *cannot* be used as the sole test for the diagnosis of prostate cancer. It has been recommended that PSA be used in combination with a direct rectal examination to screen for prostate cancer. However, the utility of *any* screening for prostate cancer has become controversial, since the proper treatment for this disease has not been determined. Although some argue that "watchful" waiting is sufficient for most prostate cancers, others see immediate intervention, especially for small, early prostate cancers, as a cure. This ethical question will be resolved with ongoing clinical trials.[29]

Terminal deoxynucleotidyltransferase. Terminal deoxynucleotidyltransferase (TdT) is a polymerase that is found in high concentrations in normal thymus and in T and non-T, non-B acute lymphoblastic leukemia cells. High TdT activity in peripheral blood lymphocytes and in bone marrow is observed in most patients at initial diagnosis of acute lymphoblastic leukemia (see below).

Other enzymes (Table 49-7)

Additional enzyme tests that may be of value in patients with cancer include alkaline phosphatase, which is elevated in the presence of bone or liver metastases; creatine kinase BB elevations in a small percentage of patients with lung cancer; gamma-glutamyltransferase and 5'-nucleotidase elevations in patients with liver metastases; galactosyltransferase II elevations in patients with pancreatic cancer; lactate dehydrogenase (LD) elevations as the LD_5 isoenzyme in patients with liver metastases and as the LD_2 or LD_3

Table 49-7   Liver metastasis and serum enzyme activity in 95 patients

Enzyme	Patients with metastasis		Patients without metastasis		Number of patients*
	Normal	Abnormal	Normal	Abnormal	
Alkaline phosphatase (ALP)	9	31	36	18	94
5'-Nucleotidase (5'-NT)	13	24	50	4	91
Gamma-glutamyltransferase (GGT)	1	35	30	25	91
Glutamate dehydrogenase (GD)	11	26	36	19	92

From Kim NK, Yasmineh WG, Freier EF, et al: *Clin Chem* 23:2034-2038, 1977.
*The total is less than 95 because some enzyme determinations were omitted.

isoenzyme in patients with lymphoma; and lysozyme (muramidase) elevations in patients with various types of leukemia.

Collagen-breakdown products

In patients with bone metastases of an osteolytic nature there is an increase in urinary excretion of both hydroxyproline and hydroxylysine. In fact, hydroxyproline excretion in urine is often the first sign of bony metastases in certain malignancies.

Cellular markers

Several markers associated with the plasma membrane, cytoplasm, or nuclei of the lymphoid cell have been identified. Various techniques have been used. These techniques, which tend to be immunological in nature, include rosetting, immunofluorescence, and immunoenzymatic testing. The rosetting technique is based on a reaction between an indicator cell (usually an erythrocyte) and the lymphoid cell to form rosettes in cases in which the lymphoid cell carries a particular membrane marker. By such techniques the cells may be mixed directly, or the indicator cell may first be coded with antibody or complement to demonstrate receptors for the Fc part of immunoglobulin or complement components. The use of flow cytometry in combination with immunofluorescence has proved to be a powerful technique for detecting cell markers.

It appears that the various antigens demonstrated by these techniques are not tumor-specific antigens but rather are tumor-associated differentiation antigens that represent the expression of oncofetal antigens not normally expressed by differentiated cells.

Lymphocytic leukemias and non-Hodgkin lymphomas have been subdivided into clinically usable subgroups on the basis of biochemical cell markers. The most striking evidence of the value of typing lymphocytes with a panel of markers comes from studies of acute lymphocytic leukemia (ALL). Table 49-8 gives the five prognostically distinct groups of ALL and the relevant markers for each. The groups are ordered according to prognosis. The cells of the B-cell type are characterized by the presence of surface membrane immunoglobulin (SmIg), as are normal mature B-cells. The cells of the T-cell type are characterized by the

presence of sheep erythrocyte receptors and human thymocyte antigen, as are mature T-cells. The cells of the pre-B-cell type are characterized by a cytoplasmic IgM heavy chain but no SmIg, which corresponds to the characteristics of an early stage during the B-cell differentiation.

The terminal deoxynucleotidyltransferase and the common ALL antigen are of value not only for the classification of ALL (Table 49-8), but also because they are very useful in distinguishing between acute lymphoblastic and myeloblastic leukemia.

ALL may be classified into B-cell leukemia (95%), which is characterized by low-density monoclonal surface membrane immunoglobulins, usually IgM or IgM and IgD with one light chain, and the more rare, but also more aggressive, T-ALL (5%). The cells of the last type form E rosettes and have T antigens but lack SmIg.

Steroid receptor analysis

Both estrogen and progesterone receptor assays are useful in the assessment of the prognosis of patients with breast cancer.[36] These procedures evaluate the relative concentration of receptors for estrogen and progesterones in breast tumor excised during surgery. Individuals who are positive both for estrogen and progesterone receptors tend to have a longer survival time and thus a better prognosis than individuals who are deficient in these receptors. Of the two, estrogen receptor appears to be the most important of the two factors. The presence or absence of steroid receptors can

Table 49-8   Phenotypic heterogeneity of ALL

ALL	E	HTA	SmIg	Cyμ	CALLA	HLA-DR	TdT
Common ALL	−	−	−	−	+	+	+
Pre-B ALL	−	−	−	+	+	+	+
Null-ALL	−	−	−	−	−	+	+
T-ALL	+	+	−	−	−	−	+
B-ALL	−	−	+	−	−	+	−

From Plesner T, Wilken M, Avenstrøm S: In Statland BE, Winkel P, editors: *Laboratory measurements in malignant disease,* Philadelphia, 1982, Saunders. *ALL,* Acute lymphocytic leukemia; *B-ALL,* B-cell type of acute lymphoblastic leukemia; *CALLA,* common ALL antigen; *Cyμ,* cytoplasmic IgM heavy chain; *E,* sheep erythrocyte receptor; *HLA-DR,* human Ia-like antigen; *HTA,* human thyrocyte antigen or antigens; *SmIg,* surface membrane immunoglobin; *T-ALL,* T-cell type of acute lymphoblastic leukemia; *TdT,* terminal deoxynucleotidyltransferase.

help determine the type of therapy. For those women devoid of receptors, a more aggressive therapy may be used, whereas women with the estrogen receptors can be treated with antiestrogen therapy with great success.

Hemostasis-related factors

Plasma fibrinogen levels are generally elevated in patients with cancer. However, in patients with disseminated intravascular coagulation (DIC) hypofibrinogenemia has also been noted. As expected, DIC is also associated with decreased values for antithrombin III (AT III). Consequently, in patients with DIC associated with cancer, AT III values will be decreased.

Increased fibrinolytic or fibrinogenolytic activity has been reported in patients with cancer. Consequently the fibrinogen-degradation products are often elevated in the plasma or urine in patients with cancer. It is interesting that plasminogen activators are often elevated in patients with cancer.

CONCLUSIONS

The scope of the problem is too large to be covered in one chapter in a textbook of clinical chemistry. More important than merely enumerating all the assays available is the fact that there is a challenge that must be presented for any candidate tumor marker. The challenge is that it be useful clinically in the management of patients with the disease or suspected of having the disease. Unfortunately the present scene is a very pessimistic one. It is hoped that with further research and clear thinking additional strategies and new markers will be made available.

METHODS OF ANALYSIS

Acid phosphatase

STEVEN A. NOEL
JOHN A. LOTT

Principles of analysis Phosphatases that catalyze the hydrolysis of a variety of phosphate esters at an acid pH are collectively called *acid phosphatase* (ACP). ACP enzymes are widely distributed in human tissues, with the greatest concentrations occurring in liver, spleen, erythrocytes, platelets, bone marrow, and the prostate gland. At least four separate genetic loci encode for the different ACP isoenzymes.

The most widely studied ACP isoenzyme is prostatic acid phosphatase (PAP). PAP has long been used as a test for the detection or monitoring of carcinoma of the prostate. In addition, because PAP is present in very high concentrations in semen, measurement of this isoenzyme is used in the investigation of rape. Other ACP isoenzymes that have been utilized for clinical diagnosis or monitoring purposes include erythrocytic ACP and bone ACP. Erythrocytic ACP is used in genetic and familial studies, whereas interest in the bone isoenzymes is attributable to increased ACP activities found in Gaucher's disease,[37] in hairy cell leukemia,[38] and in patients with increased osteoclastic activity and bone resorption.[39,40]

A multitude of assays have been developed for measure-

ment of ACP activity. The natural substrate for ACP is unknown, and the variety of substrates that have been used in various methods for ACP show differing specificities for the ACP isoenzymes. The methods that have been developed for ACP are the result of attempts to maximize the sensitivity and specificity of the assay for a particular ACP isoenzyme. Unfortunately, no substrate reacts specifically with a particular isoenzyme.[41,42]

Historically, measurement of ACP activity was performed using modifications to assays that had been previously developed for measurement of ALP activity. Changing the buffer to an acidic pH was often the only modification performed. One early method employed phenyl phosphate as substrate in a citrate buffer at pH 4.8 (Table 49-9, method 1). This procedure required a 3-hour incubation, after which time the reaction was stopped by the addition of alkali, and the phenol liberated from the substrate by the action of ACP was measured colorimetrically using the Folin-Ciocalteu reagent.

Other substrates that have been used include β-glycerophosphate, *p*-nitrophenyl phosphate, phenolphthalein phosphate, β-naphthyl phosphate, and α-naphthyl phosphate. None of these substrates are specific for any one particular ACP isoenzyme, except α-naphthyl phosphate, which exhibits fairly good specificity for PAP. All the above-mentioned substrates, with the exception of α-naphthyl phosphate, find limited use today. The use of kinetic methods employing substrates that are more specific for PAP have supplanted these methods.

The most popular substrates for measurement of ACP that are in use today include thymolphthalein monophosphate, α-naphthyl phosphate, and methylumbelliferone phosphate.

Thymolphthalein monophosphate (Table 49-9, method 2) exhibits greater specificity for PAP when compared to the other ACP isoenzymes. PAP hydrolyzes the monophosphate from thymolphthalein and the released thymolphthalein produces a color when NaOH is added to the reaction mixture.[43] The intensity of the color that is produced is directly proportional to ACP activity and can be measured colorimetrically at 590 nm.

Methods for ACP which use α-naphthol phosphate (Table 49-9, method 3) as substrate make use of the reaction of α-naphthol, released from its phosphate ester, with 2-amino-5-chlorotoluene-1,5-naphthalene disulfonate (Fast Red TR) to form a colored product. Fluorometric methods for ACP utilize 4-methylumbelliferone phosphate as substrate (Table 49-9, method 4). The rate at which methylumbelliferone is liberated by the action of ACP is measured in a fluorometer with an excitation wavelength of 365 nm and an emission wavelength of 455 nm.

The substrates that are currently used are hydrolyzed less readily by nonprostatic ACP isoenzymes when compared to PAP. In addition to the use of these substrates, specificity for PAP can be enhanced to an even greater degree by the use of certain enzyme inhibitors. One commonly used inhibitor is L-tartrate, which inhibits the prostatic ACP fraction. One can determine the prostatic ACP fraction by measuring total ACP activity and then repeating the assay with tartrate included in the reaction mixture. The activity of tartrate-inhibitable PAP is calculated as the difference between the two measurements. It must be noted, however, that measure-

Table 49-9   Methods of measurement of total and prostatic acid phosphatase (PAP)

Method	Type of analysis	Principle	Usage	Comments
1	End-point spectrophotometric	Phenol liberated from monophenyl phosphate substrate is measured with Folin-Ciocalteu reagent.	Serum Manual	Historical interest only
2	Kinetic spectrophotometric	Thymolphthalein released from thymolphthalein monophosphate substrate is measured colorimetrically after addition of base.	Commonly used All body fluids and tissues Manual or automated	High specificity for PAP sensitive, self-indicating substrate
3	End-point or kinetic spectrophotometric	α-Naphthol liberated from α-naphthyl phosphate reacts with Fast Red TR to form colored product.	Commonly used Serum Manual or automated	Not specific for PAP
4	Fluorometric kinetic	Rate of appearance of fluorescent 4-methylumbelliferone liberated from 4-methylumbelliferone phosphate by ACP is measured.	All body fluids Manual or automated Infrequently used	Sensitive substrate; requires specialized instrument
5	Radioimmunoassay	Antibody is directed against PAP coated onto solid support.	All body fluids Infrequently used	Specific for PAP
6	Enzyme immunometric assay	Monoclonal antibody linked to solid support binds PAP. Second antibody conjugated to enzyme (ALP or peroxidase) binds to bound PAP; amount of bound enzyme activity is proportional to PAP concentrations.	Frequently used Automated, rapid analysis time	Specific for PAP

ACP, Acid phosphatase; *PAP*, prosthetic acid phosphatase.

ment of tartrate-inhibited ACP is not entirely specific for PAP because other ACP isoenzymes show varying degrees of inhibition by tartrate.[44]

Immunologic methods for determination of PAP are seeing increased use. Radioimmunoassays (Table 49-9, method 5) have been developed to make use of monospecific antibodies directed against PAP that has been coated onto a solid support such as a bead or a polypropylene tube. Both fluorometric and colorimetric immunoassay procedures (Table 49-9, method 6) have gained widespread acceptance because of their specificity for PAP and ease of use as a result of automation. One procedure employs a dual monoclonal "sandwich" enzyme immunoassay whereby PAP in the specimen binds to an antibody coated onto a solid phase. This is followed by addition of a second antibody that has been conjugated to alkaline phosphatase. After a wash step to remove any unbound antibody, methylumbelliferyl phosphate substrate is added. Similar immunological "sandwich" type of assays employ peroxidase-linked anti-PAP as the second antibody to form the "sandwich." The peroxidase is used to form a chromophore, and the amount of color formation is proportional to PAP concentrations.

Specimen Both serum and heparinized plasma are acceptable specimens, though plasma results are usually lower than serum because of the release of ACP from platelets. Plasma obtained from tubes containing EDTA is acceptable; however, oxalate has been found to inhibit ACP activity.[45] Other compounds that inhibit ACP activity include fluoride, phosphate in high concentrations, ethanol, and tartrate. Hemolysis in trace amounts is tolerable; however, moderate to gross hemolysis causes significant overestimation of ACP because of the release of the enzyme from erythrocytes.

The stability of ACP is dependent on maintenance of an acidic pH. ACP is irreversibly inactivated when kept at room temperature and at a pH of greater than 6.0 for several hours or longer. Once separated from blood cells, serum or plasma should be treated by the addition of citric acid tablets or acetic acid (5 mol/L) to maintain a pH of approximately 5.4, at which the enzyme is stable.

Reference interval The reference interval for ACP activity in healthy men and women is 0.5 to 1.9 U/L when determined using methods employing thymolphthalein monophosphate as substrate. Biological factors influencing total and tartrate-resistant ACP activities include age, sex, sexual maturity, and hormonal status in women, that is, puberty and menopause. Reference intervals based on these various factors have been proposed and are described elsewhere.[46]

Beta₂-microglobulin

DONALD T. FORMAN

Principles of analysis   Beta₂-microglobulin (β_2M) is a protein with a molecular mass of approximately 11,800 daltons.[47] β_2M composes the light chain of the class I antigen of the major histocompatibility complex (HLA) and is noncovalently linked to the HLA heavy chain; it is present on the surface of all nucleated cells.[48] Small amounts of β_2M occur in various biologic fluids after its dissociation from the HLA heavy chain.[49,50] Concentrations in β_2M in serum are influenced by the turnover of nucleated cells, renal function, and immune activation.[51] Increased concentrations of β_2M in serum are found in patients with malignancies, renal diseases characterized by reduced glomerular filtration, and several infectious conditions, including human immunodeficiency virus (HIV) infection.[52,53] In patients with multiple myeloma, serum β_2M had been found to be the single most powerful prognostic indicator.[54]

Current methods for measurement of β_2M are all immunochemical procedures (see Chapters 11-13); radial immunodiffusion (RID), radioimmunoassay (RIA), immunonephelometric and turbidimetric assays, enzyme immunoassays, and fluoroimmunoassays have all been described. Most of these methods make use of polyclonal antisera; however, use of monoclonal antibodies has also been described.[55] Although the amino acid sequence of β_2M has a considerable degree of homology with the constant region (C_{H3}) of immunoglobulin G, β_2M is immunologically unrelated to the immunoglobulins, and antisera (monoclonal or polyclonal) prepared to β_2M do not cross-react with the immunoglobulins.

Historically, measurement of β_2M was performed by RID (Table 49-10, method 1).[56] The RID assay is the least sensitive of the assays developed for β_2M, and, in addition, it requires very long incubation times.

Immunoturbidimetric[57] procedures for β_2M have been described. These assays can be adapted to a variety of automated instruments. Pretreatment of sample with polyethylene glycol may be required to remove lipoproteins, immunoglobulins, and other proteins that may be precipitated and interfere with β_2M measurements during the assay.[58]

Immunonephelometric[59] assays for β_2M, based upon the amount of light-scattering, have been automated. The sensi-

Table 49-10   Methods for measurement of serum and urine beta₂-microglobulin (β_2M)

Method	Type of analysis	Principle	Usage	Assayable concentration range (mg/L)	Comments
1. Single radial immunodiffusion (RID)	Quantitative	Diffusion of protein is through medium containing specific antibody.	Serum, urine Manual	5-75	Requires preconcentration of sample, very long incubation time
2. Latex immunoassay	Quantitative	Direct agglutination is by β_2M of latex particles on which β_2M is absorbed.	Serum, urine Automated	0.25-16	Requires particle counter or turbidimeter
3. Radioimmunoassay (RIA), solid phase, double antibody, and monoclonal antibody procedures	Quantitative	See text.	Serum, urine Semiautomated	0.15-20.0	Adequate precision and sensitivity, can be completed within 1 working day
4. Fluoroimmunoassay (FIA), solid phase	Quantitative	Dissociation of fluorescent europium ion from labeled β_2M, which competes with β_2M in sample for binding to monoclonal anti-β_2M antibodies.	Serum, CSF Automated Commercially available	0.2-32	Accurate, small sample volume required, long shelf life, nonradioactive available europium label
5. Enzyme immunoassay (EIA), solid phase	Quantitative	Competitive enzyme immunoassay, β_2M competes with a fixed amount of enzyme-labeled β_2M for binding sites on anti-β_2M. Bound enzyme is measured by specific substrate hydrolysis. Absorbance produced is inversely proportional to concentration of β_2M.	Serum, urine Semiautomated Commercially available for clinical use	0.2-10.5	Reproducible and sensitive, correlates with RIA, stable reagents Convenient incubation and separation steps; assay can be completed within 4 hours

CSF, Cerebrospinal fluid.

tivity of these assays has been increased by the use of latex microparticles (diameter 0.1 μm) coated with antibody directed against β_2M (Table 49-10, method 2). Strongly turbid lipemic samples must be clarified before analysis. Immunoturbidimetric and immunonephelometric methods are rapid, precise, and accurate for measuring β_2M in serum. However, these methods are relatively insensitive for detecting β_2M in urine from healthy persons without a preliminary concentration step.

β_2M is frequently measured by RIA methods (Table 49-10, method 3).[59] RIA methods can accurately measure nanogram quantities of β_2M in serum and urine without preconcentration of the sample. The types of RIA procedures that have been developed include the use of a solid-phase support, where, for example, β_2M in the patient's sera competes with a fixed amount of labeled β_2M for binding to anti-β_2M antibodies that have been linked to Sephadex particles.[60] Traditional RIAs for β_2M have also been devised whereby β_2M and labeled β_2M compete for a limited amount of antibody.[61] The resulting antigen-antibody complexes are then precipitated by a second antibody, and the radioactivity of the precipitant is measured. The amount of radioactivity is inversely related to serum or urine β_2M concentration.

An immunofluorometric method for β_2M has been developed and is commercially available (Table 49-10, method 4).[62] This assay is based upon the competition between europium-labeled β_2M and β_2M in the sample for binding to specific monoclonal antibodies. The monoclonal antibody-β_2M complexes are detected by a second antibody coated onto a solid-phase support. Addition of an enhancement solution to the reaction system causes dissociation of europium ions from the labeled immune complex. The dissociated europium ions form highly fluorescent chelates; the degree of fluorescence is inversely proportional to β_2M concentrations in the sample.

Highly sensitive and accurate enzyme immunoassay (EIA) procedures (Table 49-10, method 5) have been developed and are commercially available.[63] Sample containing β_2M competes with β_2M conjugated to an enzyme (β-galactosidase or horseradish peroxidase) and covalently bound to a solid support, such as Sephadex particles or a microtiter plate well. After an incubation period, any unbound enzyme-β_2M complexes are removed by washing, and a suitable enzyme substrate is added to the system. The bound enzyme tracer is assayed by monitoring of the amount of substrate that is converted to a product that can be measured spectrophotometrically. The enzyme activity is inversely proportional to the concentration of β_2M in the sample.

An automated ELISA assay based on the fluorescence of the hydrolized substrate umbelliferone galactose with the enzyme label β-galactosidase is also available.

Specimen Serum and plasma collected in sodium heparinate yield comparable results.[64] Samples can be stored for 1 week at 2° to 8° C or for up to 1 year at −20° C. β_2M in CSF may also be measured and is useful for monitoring patients with malignancy or HIV infection.

Analysis of β_2M in urine samples is problematic. β_2M is known to be unstable in urine, and the degree of instability depends on factors such as the urine pH and temperature.[65]

For best results, urine should be refrigerated and alkalinized as soon as possible following collection. Properly collected and alkalinized urine specimens can be stored for 2 days at 2° to 8° C or for up to 2 months at −20° C.

Reference interval β_2M concentrations in serum and plasma are reported to be independent of body mass and sex but are slightly higher in the elderly.[66] The reference interval for β_2M in the serum of healthy individuals varies slightly depending on the type of method used for its measurement. A 95% reference interval of 0.95 to 2.78 mg/L has been reported by use of an immunofluorometric assay,[55] whereas nephelometric measurement of β_2M yields a 95% reference interval of 0.87 to 2.42 mg/L.[57] The reference interval of β_2M in CSF obtained from healthy individuals is identical for that obtained in serum.[67] Concentrations of β_2M in urine from healthy individuals has been found to average 98 μg/L with an upper limit (+2 SD) of 320 μg/L.[68]

Carcinoembryonic antigens (CEA)

GREGORY A. HOBBS

Principles of analysis and current usage Measurement of carcinoembryonic antigen (CEA) is commonly employed for use as a tumor marker for monitoring patients with colorectal cancer. Increased serum concentrations of CEA are also found in patients with other types of cancer, in patients with benign hepatobiliary and some inflammatory diseases, and in smokers.[69] CEA is a collective term used to describe a family of cancer-associated molecules. The molecule is not homogeneous in terms of its antigenic epitopes[70] and measurement of CEA by different immunoassay techniques involving different antibody reagents often yield discrepant CEA values.[71]

The earliest technique for measuring CEA was by radioimmunoassay (RIA), which is still in use today (Table 49-11, method 1). RIAs for CEA may employ an extraction step that extracts glycoproteins, such as CEA, into the fluid phase, while precipitating most of other serum proteins that might cause nonspecific protein binding. Assays employing an extraction step are also termed *indirect* assays. *Direct* assay of CEA (no extraction step employed) is typically not required for specimens containing greater than 20 ng/mL of CEA where assay sensitivity is not critical.

Extraction of CEA may be performed by use of perchloric acid, heat, or both. These techniques do result in the loss of some immunoreactive CEA. Perchloric acid, but not heat extraction, also releases CEA from immune complexes, allowing for a more sensitive assay. Although the use of perchloric acid allows for a more sensitive assay, it requires the removal of the acid before assay of CEA can occur. Methods of acid removal include dialysis, gel exclusion chromatography, or ultrafiltration.

Immunochemical methods for CEA that employ antibodies directed toward CEA that are irreversibly bound to a solid phase support are the most common assays in use (Table 49-11, method 2). CEA is bound by a capture antibody followed by the addition of a second anti-CEA antibody containing an enzyme label to form a "sandwich" complex. Nonspecific protein binding is eliminated by use of a

Table 49-11   Methods of CEA analysis

Method	Principle	Usage	Comments
1. Radioimmunoassay (RIA)	Plasma may be extracted (indirect assay) with acid or heat to remove proteins, or plasma may be used without first performing an extraction step (direct assay). Plasma is reacted with antibody for 30 minutes at 45° C followed by addition of ^{125}I-CEA for 30 minutes at 45° C.	Plasma or serum Declining usage	Extraction step allows for increased assay sensitivity. Direct assay is used to monitor patients with ≥20 ng/mL of CEA.
2. Enzyme immunoassay (EIA)	"Sandwich" type of immunoassay employs anti-CEA antibody bound to solid phase followed by addition of second antibody with enzyme label. Addition of enzyme substrate results in formation of product that can be detected spectrophotometrically.	Plasma or serum Most common method in use	

series of wash steps performed before the addition of the second antibody. Addition of substrate that can react with the enzyme label to produce a product capable of being measured by spectrophotometric means completes the assay.

The various assay kits that are commercially available may employ antibodies with differing degrees of specificity. This fact makes it difficult for laboratories to change from one CEA method to another without making interpretation of results by physicians difficult. In addition, differences in the form of extraction (heat versus acid) used in indirect methods, as well as the differences in CEA values measured by means of direct versus indirect methods, contribute to differences in quantitative results obtained with the various available assays.

Specimen   EDTA plasma is the preferred specimen for CEA analysis. Serum contains the proteolytic enzyme plasmin, which can inactivate CEA. Plasma requires calcium as cofactor for activity. Thus plasma anticoagulated with EDTA to remove calcium is required. Specimens should be centrifuged and immediately frozen at −20° C to pre-

vent proteolytic degradation of CEA. If serum has been collected, any remaining specimen should be kept at 0° to 4° C during analysis in the event that the assay needs to be repeated.

Reference interval   The reference interval for CEA in healthy individuals is influenced by the method used for measurement and the smoking status of the patient. An upper reference interval of 2.5 ng/mL has previously been established for CEA when measured by RIA.[72] In smokers who are otherwise healthy, values up to 5.0 ng/mL may be seen. When CEA is measured by enzyme immunoassay, an upper reference of approximately 4.0 ng/mL may be appropriate.[73]

Immunoelectrophoresis
STEVEN C. KAZMIERCZAK

Principles of analysis   Immunoelectrophoresis (Table 49-12, method 1) is a very common type of technique in use in clinical laboratories today for the identification of proteins, especially *monoclonal gammopathies*. This method is usually performed with an agarose gel solid sup-

Table 49-12   Immunoelectrophoretic methods

Method	Principle	Usage	Comments
1. Immunoelectrophoresis (IEP)	Proteins are first separated in agarose by zone electrophoresis. Antiserum is next placed in trough horizontal to separated proteins. Precipitin bands appear in areas where antigen and antibody meet.	Serum, urine, other body fluids	Used as confirmatory test for identification of monoclonal proteins.
2. Immunofixation	Proteins are separated by zone electrophoresis followed by application of monospecific antisera to area containing protein to be identified.	Serum, urine, other body fluids	More sensitive than IEP for identification of monoclonal proteins

Table 49-13   Method for immunoglobulin quantitation

Method	Principle	Usage	Comments
1. Radial immunodiffusion (RID)	Immunoglobulin diffuses into gel containing antibody resulting in formation of immunoprecipitate. Diameter of precipitin ring is proportional to concentration of immunoglobulin.	Serum, CSF, other body fluids Frequently used	Slow and labor intensive Accurate
2. Nephelometry	Reaction of immunoglobulin with antibody results in formation of immunoprecipitate, which scatters light. Amount of light scatter is proportional to immunoglobulin concentration.	Serum, CSF, other body fluids Most commonly used	Automated Requires specialized instrumentation Accurate
3. Turbidimetry	Reaction of immunoglobulin with antibody results in formation of immunoprecipitate, which increases turbidity of sample and scatters light.	Serum Commonly used	Automated Requires specialized instrumentation

CSF, Cerebrospinal fluid.

port medium. Patient samples are separated by zonal electrophoresis into their usual protein fractions. Antiserum of the appropriate specificity is then placed in a trough that runs parallel to the separated proteins. Diffusion of antigen and antibody toward each other results in the formation of precipitin arcs. The shape of the arc and the migration position of the arc from the origin can be compared to a control sera allowing for identification of the protein of interest. See Chapter 12 for additional details on this method, and Fig. 12-2 for an example of the technique.

Immunofixation electrophoresis (Table 49-12, method 2) eliminates the long diffusion time required for antigen-antibody reactions inherent to the immunoelectrophoresis method of protein identification. This procedure, like immunoelectrophoresis, first requires the separation of proteins by zone electrophoresis. After this, monospecific antiserum is overlaid on the zone occupied by the protein of interest. After an incubation period, excess antiserum is removed from the gel by washing, and the remaining antigen-antibody precipitation band is stained. This technique is more sensitive than immunoelectrophoresis for the detection of monoclonal proteins. Protein identification by use of western blot analysis is one type of immunofixation procedure.

Specimen Serum, urine, or other body fluids are acceptable specimens for performing immunoelectrophoresis. If plasma is used, the fibrinogen present in the sample may be misinterpreted as a monoclonal band. If analysis is delayed more than 48 hours, samples should be frozen. Specimens that normally contain low concentrations of protein, such as urine or cerebrospinal fluid, may need to be concentrated before analysis.

Immunoglobulin quantitation

GAYLE JACKSON

Principles of analysis Immunoglobulins in serum, urine, and other body fluids can be measured by a variety of semiquantitative or quantitative techniques. Semiquantitative methods measure immunoglobulins as the fraction of the to-

tal globulins present in the specimen, whereas quantitative methods determine the concentrations of each of the individual immunoglobulin classes.

Semiquantitative assessment of immunoglobulins in serum is most frequently performed using electrophoretic separation of total globulins into alpha, beta, and gamma globulin components. Since the gamma fraction consists almost entirely of immunoglobulins, this technique allows for fairly good assessment of the total immunoglobulin concentration. This method also serves as a good screening method for the detection of monoclonal immunoglobulins.

Quantitative measurement of each of the immunoglobulin (Ig) classes has been made possible by the development of antibodies directed toward each class (IgG, IgM, IgA, IgD, and IgE). A variety of immunochemical procedures have been developed for quantitation of these Ig classes because of the vast differences in concentration between each class of immunoglobulin. For example, up to a millionfold difference may exist between the serum concentrations of IgG and IgE.

The technique of radial immunodiffusion (Table 49-13, method 1) is commonly used in clinical laboratories for measurement of IgG, IgM, or IgA concentrations. This method is described in depth on p. 236. The sensitivity of this method for the different immunoglobulin fractions is dependent on the concentration of antibody incorporated into the gel. Standard-level immunodiffusion plates have sensitivities for IgG, IgM, and IgA of approximately 4 g/L, 300 mg/L, and 600 mg/L respectively, whereas low-level immunodiffusion plates have sensitivities for IgG, IgM, and IgA of approximately 20, 25, and 20 mg/L respectively. The radial immunodiffusion methods are accurate but suffer from the drawback of being slow and labor intensive. Thus they are best suited for use where a limited number of samples need to be assayed.

The most common method in use for quantitation of immunoglobulins IgG, IgM, and IgA is immunonephelometry (Table 49-13, method 2). In this procedure immunoglobulin reacts with its specific antibody to form an immunoprecipitate complex that results in an increase in light scatter. The amount of light scatter is proportional to the concentration of immunoglobulin within the specimen. Samples that are turbid may need to be filtered to remove the turbidity before analysis. Another common procedure used for immunoglobulin determinations is turbidimetry (Table 49-13, method 3). This method is similar to immunonephelometry except that the increase in absorbance is used to calculate the immunoglobulin concentration. Absorbance measurements can be taken after completion of the reaction or at selected time intervals during the assay.[74] See Chapter 12 for details on both methods.

The usual serum concentrations of IgD (300 μg/mL) and IgE (2 to 2000 ng/mL) are below the limits of detection for the assay techniques described above. The measurement of IgD is generally not indicated except in cases where production of monoclonal IgD by plasma cell malignancy is suspected.

Measurement of IgE concentrations is frequently performed for the work-up of allergy. A modification of the immunonephelometric technique of particle-enhanced turbidimetry (PET) does permit measurement of IgE. This modification employs anti-IgE antibody covalently bound to small latex particles. These uniformly sized particles scatter light better than the immunocomplexes do and thus provide the sensitivity needed to measure IgE.

The techniques most frequently used to measure the relatively low concentrations of IgE are radioimmunometric assay (RIA) and enzyme immunoassay. The RIA technique commonly used to measure IgE is a paper-radioimmunosorbent test (PRIST). This technique employs anti-IgE immobilized on paper, which reacts with IgE

present in the specimen. After an incubation period followed by a wash step to remove excess serum, ^{125}I-anti-IgE is added forming a "sandwich" with the IgE/anti-IgE complexes.

Enzyme immunoassay methods used to measure IgE include ELISA. In this technique, specimen is incubated in tubes coated with anti-IgE followed by addition of peroxidase-labeled anti-IgE. Addition of enzyme substrate results in color formation, which can be measured in a spectrophotometer.

Specimen Serum is most frequently used for immunoglobulin quantitation. However, cerebrospinal fluid and urine are also frequently analyzed. Urine specimens must be concentrated approximately 20 to 50 times before being evaluated by electrophoresis or immunoelectrophoresis.

Samples are stable for up to 5 days at 2° to 8° C. For longer periods of storage, freezing at lower than −20° C is recommended. Refreezing of thawed samples is not recommended because of the increased risk of protein denaturation.

Reference interval The normal reference intervals for immunoglobulins in serum stratified by age are as shown in Table 49-14.

Prostate-specific antigen

WILLIAM R. JOHNSON
JOHN A. LOTT

Principles of analysis Prostate-specific antigen (PSA) is a glycoprotein produced by the epithelial cells of the prostate gland as well as the periurethral and perirectal glands.[75,76] Because PSA is a serine protease, PSA in serum binds to protease inhibitors such as α_2-macroglobulin and α_1-antichymotrypsin. Binding of PSA to α_2-macroglobulin renders the PSA undetectable by current immunoassay pro-

Table 49-14 Physical properties of human immunoglobulins

Immunoglobulin class	IgG	IgM	IgA	IgD	IgE
Molecular weight (daltons)	150,000	900,000	160,000 (monomer) 320,000 (dimer)	185,000	200,000
Sedimentation coefficient, S	6.6	18.0-19.0	6.25-10.9	6.2-7.0	7.86-7.92
Heavy chains	γ	μ	α	δ	ϵ
Heavy-chain subclasses	$\gamma_1, \gamma_2, \gamma_3, \gamma_4$	μ_1, μ_2	α_1, α_2	—	—
Light chains	κ or λ	κ or λ	κ or λ	κ or λ	κ or λ
Molecular formula	IgG(κ)2γ2κ IgG(λ)2γ2γ	IgM(κ)(2μ2κ)$_5$ IgM(γ)(2μ2λ)$_5$	IgA(κ)(2α2κ)$_{1-3}$ IgA(λ)(2α2λ)$_{1-3}$	IgD(κ)2δ2κ IgD(λ)2δ2λ	IgE(κ)2ε2κ IgE(λ)2ε2λ
Reference interval serum concentrations (mg/mL) (by age)					
Cord specimen	7.66-16.93	0.04-0.26	0.0004-0.09		
0.5-3 months	2.99-8.52	0.15-1.49	0.03-0.66		
3-6 months	1.42-9.88	0.18-1.18	0.04-0.90		
6-12 months	4.18-11.42	0.43-2.23	0.014-0.95		
1-2 years	3.56-12.04	0.37-2.39	0.13-1.18		116-122 ng/mL
2-3 years	4.92-12.69	0.49-2.04	0.23-1.37		80-122 ng/mL
3-6 years	5.64-13.81	0.51-2.14	0.35-2.09		
4-7 years					140-442 ng/mL
6-9 years	6.58-15.35	0.50-2.28	0.29-3.84		
10-14 years					374-674 ng/mL
12-16 years	6.80-15.48	0.45-2.56	0.81-2.52		
Adult	8.00-16.00	0.50-2.00	1.40-3.50	0-0.14	2-2000 ng/mL

Data from Seligson O, editor: *Handbook series in clinical laboratory science.* Section F. *Immunology,* vol 1, part 1, Boca Raton, Fla., 1978, CRC Press; and Meites S, editor: *Pediatric clinical chemistry,* ed 2, Chicago, 1981, American Association for Clinical Chemistry.

cedures. However, binding of PSA to α_1-antichymotrypsin results in the formation of a complex that is detectable by current PSA immunoassays. In addition to these PSA-protease inhibitor complexes, serum also contains unbound PSA, which is also detectable by PSA immunoassays. The current difficulty for PSA methods is reconciling the standardization of different methods, using antibodies that recognize the various PSA forms to different degrees and therefore do not produce similar results on all samples.

Techniques for measurement of PSA may be described as standard methods and ultrasensitive methods.[77] The standard methods were the first immunoassay procedures to be developed for PSA measurement. Using these assays, detection of PSA above the biological detection limit often corresponded to the presence of residual tumor after surgical intervention.[78] The biological detection limit is defined as the lower limit of detection of the assay plus two standard deviations from the interassay precision data.[77] Using this cutoff point, which was typically set at <0.4 µg/L for the standard assays, approximately 40% to 60% of patients who underwent "curative" radical prostatectomy and whose serum PSA levels were below the cutoff value of the standard assays at 6 months eventually showed evidence of residual progressive disease.

The development of ultrasensitive PSA procedures capable of accurately measuring less than 0.1 µg/L provide advantages over the standard PSA assays, including (1) the early identification of residual disease in patients undergoing radical prostatectomy, (2) evaluation of the virulence of residual disease by the assessment of PSA doubling times within the ultrasensitive range, and (3) assurance that patients with PSA concentrations below a certain concentration for an extended period of time would have low probability of developing progressive disease.[77]

The earliest commercial assays for PSA were radioimmunoassays (RIA) and immunoradiometric assays (IRMA).[79] The RIA procedure (Table 49-15, method 1) utilized a polyclonal antibody in a traditional competitive-binding assay format. The IRMA procedure (Table 49-15, method 2) has been replaced with immunometric assays employing nonisotopic labels.[80]

The most common procedure currently in use for PSA is based on a microparticle capture, enzyme immunoassay (MEIA) (Table 49-15, method 3). In this procedure, monoclonal antibody directed toward PSA is coated onto inert microparticles. PSA present in the specimen binds to the microparticles. The microparticles are next trapped on a glass-fiber matrix where a second antibody labeled with enzyme binds to the PSA forming a sandwich complex. Enzyme substrate is added, and it reacts with the bound enzyme. The product, which is directly related to PSA concentrations, is measured.

Another popular immunoassay procedure is an enzyme immunoassay version of the IRMA procedure previously described as method 2 in Table 49-11 (Table 49-15, method 4). In this EIA procedure, the label is alkaline phosphatase (ALP) instead of ^{125}I. The reaction of *p*-nitrophenyl phosphate with ALP results in the production of *p*-nitrophenol, which is monitored bichromatically at 405 and 450 nm.

Other nonradioisotope immunometric procedures for PSA include fluorescence enzyme immunoassays that use enzyme-labeled antibody directed against PSA linked to glass-fiber paper (Baxter-Dade, Miami, Florida) or magnetic beads (Tosoh, San Francisco, California), and a bioluminescence assay (Ciba-Corning).

Specimen Serum is the specimen of choice for measurement of PSA. In addition to serum, PSA has also been measured in urine.[81] Urine PSA concentrations reflect residual

Table 49-15 Methods for analysis of PSA

Method	Principle	Usage	Comments
1. Radioimmunoassay (RIA)	Competitive binding between PSA and ^{125}I-PSA for antibody-binding sites.	Decreasing usage	Requires separation step
2. Immunoradiometric assay (IRMA)	PSA in patient sample binds to antibody linked to solid phase. Second antibody labeled with ^{125}I binds to solid-phase antibody–PSA complex to form a sandwich.	Decreasing usage	Requires separation
3. Microparticle-based enzyme immunoassay (MEIA)	PSA in sample binds to antibody-microparticle complex, which is then trapped on a glass-fiber matrix. Second antibody labeled with ALP is added, and it binds to PSA on microparticles. Substrate containing 4-methyl-umbelliferyl phosphate is added, and fluorescence of the product 4-methylumbelliferone is measured.	Most frequently used	Automated Good sensitivity
4. Enzyme immunoassay (EIA)	Similar to method 2 described above except label used is ALP instead of ^{125}I. Absorbance of *p*-nitrophenol formed from reaction of ALP and *p*-nitrophenyl phosphate is directly related to PSA concentration in patient sample.	Frequently used	Automated

prostatic tissue in prostatectomy patients. The stability of PSA has been found to be up to 4 days at room temperature[82] and at least 6 months at $-20°$ C.[83] The effect of freezing and thawing on PSA concentrations is controversial. Increases, decreases, and no effect of freeze-thaw cycles have been reported.[84,85] At present, avoidance of repeated freezing and thawing of specimens is indicated.

Reference interval PSA is present in low concentrations in the sera of healthy men. When used as a screening tool, a PSA value of >4.0 µg/L but <10 µg/L is suggestive more of benign prostatic hypertrophy than of a significant risk for prostate cancer. Patients with PSA levels between 10 and <20 µg/L have an even greater risk for prostatic cancer, and this interval identifies those patients who may require further evaluation and possible biopsy.[86] PSA levels >20 µg/L are usually associated with prostatic cancer. When PSA is used for assessment of disease recurrence after radical prostatectomy, 0.5 µg/L has been suggested as a medical decision value.[87]

Serum protein electrophoresis

DAVID A. SMITH
JOHN A. LOTT

Principles of analysis and current usage Human serum contains a myriad of proteins ranging from simple polypeptide hormones to large and complex proteins such as immunoglobulins. A variety of techniques can be employed for differentiating the large number of proteins present in serum. Highly sensitive methods such as two-dimensional electrophoresis coupled with improved staining methods can distinguish more than 500 different serum proteins. However, in the typical clinical laboratory the term "serum protein" usually refers to the dozen or so proteins that are in great enough concentrations to be detected by the commonly used method of electrophoresis for protein separation and dye-binding methods for visualization of the individual protein fractions.

Historically the differentiation of proteins in serum was based upon their characterization into one of two broad categories termed *albumin* and *globulins*. This classification was based upon the finding that the addition of salts to serum resulted in the preferential precipitation of globulins. Removal of the salt by dialysis followed by evaporation of the supernatant resulted in the formation of a white residue termed *albumin*.

The most common technique for separating proteins in serum is electrophoresis. This method is based on the principle that when an electric current is applied to a medium containing charged particles those particles with a negative charge will migrate toward the positive electrode and those particles with a positive charge will migrate toward the negative electrode.

The support matrix is the medium through which proteins migrate during the electrophoretic process. Supporting media can be of various types. Media that are used can separate proteins based on either molecular charge alone, or on the basis of both molecular charge and size. Commonly used support media that separate proteins on the basis of molecular charge include both agarose and cellulose acetate. Support media used to separate proteins on the basis of both size

and charge include starch and polyacrylamide gel; these media are porous and thus impede the migration of larger protein molecules, whereas smaller protein molecules migrate without hindrance. This allows for the separation of molecules with different size but identical charge-to-mass ratios.

Proteins can carry a positive or negative charge, or be uncharged, depending on the pH of their environment. For electrophoretic separation of proteins, a buffer is used to impart a charge to serum proteins. The pH and ionic strength of the buffer are important factors affecting the separation of proteins. Typical buffers that are used include barbital, tris-barbital, and a borate buffer composed of boric acid, tris, and EDTA. These buffers are ordinarily used at a pH of 8.6, which imparts a negative charge to most plasma proteins. The concentration of the buffer usually ranges from 0.05 to 0.15 mol/L. If the buffer concentration is too high, the migration of proteins through the support media is slowed because the ions within the buffer compete with the proteins for current.

Another factor affecting the separation of proteins is the phenomenon called *electroendosmosis*. Electroendosmosis describes the flow of buffer toward the cathode as a consequence of the negative surface charge present on certain types of support media. The negative surface charge attracts a layer of positively charged solute ions. When current is applied, a thin zone of mobile positive ions will migrate toward the cathode. The migrating ions are associated with buffer solvent. Proteins that do not possess a sufficient charge-to-mass ratio to overcome this flow of buffer solvent will be swept backwards from their point of application toward the cathode. Gamma globulins, which have an isoelectric point (pI) close to pH of the buffer, are one group of proteins affected by electroendosmosis.

Once separated, the individual protein bands are visualized by use of a dye that stains the various protein fractions. Dyes that are used include amido black, ponceau S, bromphenol blue, and Coomassie brilliant blue. The dyes have differing affinities for the various protein fractions and behave differently with respect to the support medium that has been used for protein separation. Amido black is commonly used for staining agarose gels; however, the dye has a slightly greater affinity for albumin and transferrin than for globulin fractions. Ponceau S works best with cellulose acetate. One drawback of ponceau S is that it stains albumin with greater intensity than it does the globulins. Bromphenol blue is useful for staining of proteins on agarose support media. However, like ponceau S, it gives more color with albumin than with the globulins.[90] Coomassie bue dye has approximately an order of magnitude greater analytical sensitivity than the other dyes making it suitable for use after electrophoresis of specimens such as urine and CSF, which usually have protein concentrations much less than those found in serum.[91]

Individual protein bands may also be detected immunlogically by use of specific antisera. The advantage of performing immunoelectrophoresis or immunofixation electrophoresis in conjunction with serum protein electrophoresis (SPE) is in the identification of abnormal monoclonal immunoglobulins, which do not migrate with the other gamma globu-

Table 49-16 Approximate reference intervals for serum protein fractions

	Total	Albumin	Alpha₁	Alpha₂	Beta	Gamma
Quantity (%)	50	5	10	15	20
Interval, g/dL*		3.2-5.5	0.1-0.3	0.6-1.0	0.7-1.1	0.8-1.6

*If one assumes a usual total protein reference interval of 6.0 to 8.3 g/dL

lins and might be mistaken for another protein (that is, fibrinogen, hemoglobin, or transferrin).

Common methods in use today for electrophoretic separation of serum proteins include zone electrophoresis and high-resolution electrophoresis. Zone electrophoresis[88,89] uses an inert supporting medium such as agarose gel.

The use of high-resolution electrophoresis (HRE) is preferred over the less-sensitive zone electrophoresis.[92] This technique enables the separation of additional proteins that are not usually detected by SPE. Either agarose gel or cellulose acetate can be used as the support medium. With polyacrylamide as the supporting medium, over 100 serum protein bands may be observed.

Other, more elaborate techniques used to separate proteins, which are used primarily in research and critical analytical settings, include isoelectric focusing (IEF) and two-dimensional electrophoresis. IEF separates proteins on the basis of their individual isoelectric points. A pH gradient is created within the gel by the use of a mixture of ampholytes, which quickly migrate to their individual isoelectric points during electrophoresis. Proteins will migrate in the gel until they reach a position within the gel where the gel pH is the same as their isoelectric pH. At their isoelectric pH, or pI, the proteins no longer carry a charge and thus stop migrating. IEF can be used to detect the presence of paraproteins in serum[92] and oligoclonal bands in CSF.[93] It has also been particularly useful in delineating fetal hemoglobin from glycosylated hemoglobin and for identifying alpha₁-antitrypsin phenotypes.[91]

The most powerful technique available today for protein separation is two-dimensional electrophoresis. This method separates proteins first by IEF in one dimension and then by molecular weight in a second dimension. More than 1000 proteins can be separated and identified when this method is used with computer analysis. The relatively high cost and difficulties in interpreting the results of two-dimensional electrophoresis limits its use to special clinical circumstances.[95,96]

Specimen Serum is the specimen of choice for protein electrophoresis. Plasma can be used; however, the fibrinogen present in plasma will migrate between the beta globulins and the application point and give rise to an additional protein band. Protein present in urine and cerebrospinal fluid can be analyzed if the concentration of protein present in these specimens is increased. Ultracentrifugation and dialysis are two common techniques used to concentrate protein in urine and CSF.

Reference interval Reference intervals for each of the five commonly measured serum protein fractions should be individually established by each laboratory performing serum protein electrophoresis. The various dyes that are available for staining the various protein fractions give different reference intervals because each of the individual protein fractions bind these dyes with differing affinities. Approximate reference intervals for the five commonly measured protein fractions in serum are given in Table 49-16.[91]

REFERENCES

1. Sager R: Explorations on the origin of cancer, *Focus* 2/3:1-3, 1983.
2. Aaronson SA: Growth factors and cancer, *Science* 254:1146-1153, 1991.
3. Cantley LC, Auger KR, Carpenter C, et al: Oncogenes and signal transduction, *Cell* 64:281-302, 1991.
4. Niman HL: Detection of oncogene-related proteins with site-directed monoclonal antibody probes, *J Clin Lab Anal* 1:28-41, 1987.
5. Habbema JDF, van Oortmarssen GJ: Performance characteristics of screening tests. In Statland BE, Winkel P, editors: Laboratory measurements in malignant disease, vol 2, Philadelphia, 1982, Saunders.
6. EVAC: *Rapport eerste screeningsronde,* Leidschendam, 1980, Ministerie van Volksgezondheid en Milieuhygiene.
7. Tabar L, Gad A: Screening for breast cancer: the Swedish trial, *Radiology* 138:219-222, 1981.
8. Woolner LB, Fontant RS, Sanderson DR, et al: Mayo Lung Project: evaluation of lung cancer screening through December 1979, *Mayo Clin Proc* 56:544-555, 1981.
9. Shapiro S: Evidence on screening for breast cancer from a randomized trial, *Cancer* 39:2772-2782, 1977.
10. Statland BE: *Clinical decision levels for lab tests,* Oradell, N.J., 1983, Medical Economics Co.
11. Rubin P: Clinical oncology for medical students and physicians, ed 5, New York, 1978, American Cancer Society.
12. Winkel P, Bentzon MW, Statland BE, et al: Predicting recurrence in patients with breast cancer from cumulative laboratory results: a new technique for the application of time series analysis, *Clin Chem* 28:2057-2067, 1982.
13. Ravry M, Moertel CG, Schutt AJ, et al: Usefulness of serial serum carcinoembryonic antigen (CEA) determinations during anticancer therapy or long-term follow-up of gastrointestinal carcinoma, *Cancer* 34:1230-1234, 1974.
14. Chan DW: PSA as a marker for prostatic cancer, *Clin Chem* 33:1916-1920, 1987.
15. Coombes RC, Neville AM: Significance of tumor-index substances in management. In Stoll BA, editor: *Secondary spread in breast cancer,* Chicago, 1978, William Heinemann Medical Books.
16. Rej R, et al: Clinical laboratory testing in cancer patient diagnosis and management, *Clin Chem* 39:2359-2452, 1993.
17. Sell S, editor: *Serological cancer markers,* Totowa, N.J., 1992, Humana Press.
18. Gold P, Freedman SO: Demonstration of tumor-specific antigens in human colonic carcinomata by immunological tolerance and absorption techniques, *J Exp Med* 121:439-462, 1965.
19. *CEA as a cancer marker,* vol 3, no 7, Bethesda, Md., 1981, National Institutes of Health, Consensus Development Conference Summary.
20. Holyoke ED, Chu TM, Murphy GP: CEA as a monitor of gastrointestinal malignancy, *Cancer* 35:830-836, 1975.
21. Costanza ME, Das S, Nathanson L, et al: Proceedings: carcinoembryonic antigen: report of a screening study, *Cancer* 33:583-590, 1974.
22. McCartney WH, Hoffer PB: The value of carcinoembryonic antigen (CEA) as an adjunct to the radiological colon examination in the diagnosis of malignancy, *Radiology* 110:325-328, 1974.
23. Wanebo HJ, Rao B, Pinsky CM, et al: Preoperative carcinoembryonic antigen level as a prognostic indicator in colorectal cancer, *N Engl J Med* 299:448-452, 1978.
24. Statland BE, Winkel P: Usefulness of clinical chemistry measurements in classifying patients with breast cancer, *CRC Crit Rev Clin Lab Sci* 26:255-290, 1982.

25. Sell S, Becker FF: Alpha-fetoprotein, *J Natl Cancer Inst* 60:19-26, 1978.

26. Vaitukaitis JL: Secretion of human chorionic gonadotrophin by tumors. In *Carcino-embryonic proteins,* vol 1, New York, 1979, Elsevier/North Holland, pp 447-455.

27. Braunstein GD: Human chorionic gonadotropin in nontrophoblastic tumors and tissues. In Talwar GP, editor: Recent advances in reproduction and regulation of fertility, Amsterdam, 1979, Elsevier/North Holland Biomedical Press.

28. Anderson CK, Jones WG, Ward A: *Germ cell tumors,* London, 1981, Taylor and Francis.

29. Carter HB, Pearson JD, Metter EJ, et al: Longitudinal evaluation of prostate specific antigen levels in men with and without prostate disease, *JAMA* 267:2215-2220, 1992.

30. Schwartz MK: Enzyme tests in cancer. In Statland BE, Winkel P, editors: *Laboratory measurements in malignant disease,* Philadelphia, 1982, Saunders.

31. Chu TM, Wang MC, Scott WW, et al: Immunological detection of serum prostatic acid phosphatase: methodology and clinical evaluation, *Invest Urol* 15:319-323, 1978.

32. Watson RA, Tang DB: The predictive value of prostatic acid phosphatase as a screening test for prostatic cancer, *N Engl J Med* 303:497-499, 1980.

33. Reddi K, Holland JF: Elevated serum ribonuclease in patients with pancreatic cancer, *Proc Natl Acad Sci* 73:2308, 1976.

34. Fitzgerald PJ, Fortner JG, Watson RC, et al: The value of diagnostic aids in detecting pancreas cancer, *Cancer* 41:868- 879, 1979.

35. Lake-Bakaar G, McKavanaugh S, Summerfield JA: Urinary immunoreactive trypsin excretion: a non-invasive screening test for pancreatic cancer, *Lancet* 2:878-880, 1979.

36. Pertschuk LP, Eisenberg KB, Carter AC, Feldmann JG: Immunohistologic localization of estrogen receptors in breast cancer with monoclonal antibodies, *Cancer* 55:1513-1520, 1985.

37. Robinson DB, Glew RH: Acid phosphatase in Gaucher's disease, *Clin Chem* 26:371-382, 1980.

38. Yam LT, Li CY, Finkel HE: Leukemic reticuloendotheliosis: the role of tartrate-resistant acid phosphatase in the diagnosis and splenectomy in treatment, *Arch Intern Med* 130:248-256, 1972.

39. Deftos LJ, Glowacki J: Mechanisms of bone metabolism. In Kem DC, Frohlich E, editors: *Pathophysiology,* ed 3, Philadelphia, 1984, Lippincott.

40. Lau KH, Onishi T, Wergedal JE, et al: Characterization and assay of tartrate-resistant acid phosphatase activity in serum: potential use to assess bone resorption, *Clin Chem* 33:458-462, 1987.

41. Teshima S, Hayashi Y, Ando M: Determination of acid phosphatase in biological fluids using a new substrate, 2,6-dichloro-4-nitrophenyl phosphate, *Clin Chim Acta* 168:231-238, 1987.

42. Gavella M: Simple, rapid determination of zinc and acid phosphatase in seminal plasma with an ABA-100 bichromatic analyzer, *Clin Chem* 34:1605-1607, 1988.

43. Ewen LM: Acid phosphatase activity (thymolphthalein monophosphate substrate). In Faulkner WH, Meites S, editors: *Selected methods for the small clinical laboratory,* Philadelphia, 1982, Saunders.

44. Townsend RM: Enzyme tests in diseases of the prostate, *Ann Clin Lab Sci* 7:254-261, 1977.

45. Young DS: *Effects of drugs on clinical laboratory tests,* Washington, D.C., 1990, American Association for Clinical Chemistry Press, pp 3-4 and 3-5.

46. Schiele F, Artur Y, Floch AY, Siest G: Total, tartrate-resistant, and tartrate-inhibited acid phosphatase in serum: biological variations and reference limits, *Clin Chem* 34:685-690, 1988.

47. Berggård I, Bearn AG: Isolation and properties of a low molecular weight β_2-globulin occurring in human biological fluids, *J Biol Chem* 243:4095-4103, 1968.

48. Bjorkman PJ, Saper MA, Samraoui B, et al: Structure of the human class I histocompatibility antigen, HLA-A$_2$, *Nature* 329:506-512, 1987.

49. Plesner T, Bjerrum OJ: Distribution of "free" and HLA-associated human β_2-microglobulin in some plasma membranes and biological fluids, *Scand J Immunol* 11:341-351, 1980.

50. Nilsson K, Ervin P-E, Welsh KI: Production of β_2-microglobulin by normal and malignant human cell lines and peripheral lymphocytes [Review], *Transplant Rev* 21:53-84, 1974.

51. Fuchs D, Hausen A, Reibnegger G, et al: β_2-Microglobulin and immune activation [Letter], *Clin Chem* 35:2158-2159, 1989.

52. Bhalla RB, Safai B, Pahwa S, Schwartz MK: β_2-Microglobulin as a prognostic marker for development of AIDS, *Clin Chem* 31:1411-1412, 1985.

53. Wibell L, Ervin PE, Berggård I: Serum beta-2-microglobulin in renal disease, *Nephron* 10:320-331, 1973.

54. Durie BGM, Stock-Novack D, Salmon SE, et al: Prognostic value of pretreatment serum β_2 microglobulin in myeloma: a Southwest Oncology Group study, *Blood* 75:823-830, 1990.

55. Tienhaara A, Eskola JU, Näntö: Double monoclonal time-resolved immunofluorometric assay of β_2-microglobulin in serum, *Clin Chem* 36:1961-1964, 1990.

56. Peterson PA, Ervin PE, Berggård I: Differentiation of glomerular, tubular, and normal proteinuria: determinations of urinary excretion of β_2-microglobulin, albumin, and total protein, *J Clin Invest* 48:1189-1198, 1969.

57. Rifai N, Morales A: Immunoturbidimetry of β_2-microglobulin in serum, *Clin Chem* 35:1996-1997, 1989.

58. Desjarlais F, Daigneault R: Limitations of conventional laser nephelometry for the measurement of β_2-microglobulin, lysozyme, α_1-fetoprotein and myoglobin in serum and urine, *Clin Biochem* 14:146-149, 1981.

59. Viedma JA, Pacheco S, Albaladejo MD: Determination of β_2-microglobulin in serum by a microparticle-enhanced nephelometric immunoassay, *Clin Chem* 38:2464-2468, 1992.

60. Ervin PE, Peterson PA, Wide L, Berggård I: Radioimmunoassay of β_2-microglobulin in human biological fluids, *Scand J Clin Lab Invest* 28:439-443, 1971.

61. Shuster J, Gold P, Poulik MO: β_2M levels in cancerous and other disease states, *Clin Chim Acta* 67:307-313, 1976.

62. Meillet D, Bélec L, Schuller E, Delattre J: Time-resolved fluoro-immunoassay of β_2-microglobulin in serum and cerebrospinal fluid, *Clin Chem* 39:552-553, 1993.

63. Bjerrum OW, Birgens HS: Measurement of beta-2-microglobulin in serum and plasma by an enzyme-linked immunosorbent assay (ELISA), *Clin Chim Acta* 155:69-76, 1986.

64. Swanson RA, Tracy RP, Katzman JA, et al: β_2-microglobulin determined by radioimmunoassay with monoclonal antibody, *Clin Chem* 28:2033-2039, 1982.

65. Bastable MD: β_2-microglobulin in urine: not suitable for assessing renal tubular function, *Clin Chem* 29:996-997, 1983.

66. Forman DT: Serum beta-2-microglobulin as an indicator of neoplasia, *J Clin Immunoassay* 6:228-233, 1983.

67. Lutz CT, Cornell SH, Goeken JA: Establishment of reference interval for β_2-microglobulin in cerebrospinal fluid with use of two commercial assays, *Clin Chem* 37:104-107, 1991.

68. Forman DT, Finn W, Mandel S: Comparison of an enzyme immunoassay for serum beta-2-microglobulin (β_2M) with a radioimmunoassay technique, *Clin Chem* 29:1245, 1983.

69. Turpeinen U, Haglund C, Roberts P, Stenman U-H: Comparability of three assays for carcinoembryonic antigen, *Clin Chem* 38(8):1506, 1992.

70. Hammarstrom S, Shively JE, Paxton RJ, et al: Antigenic sites is carcinoembryonic antigen, *Cancer Res* 49:4852-4858, 1989.

71. Börmer O: Standardization, specificity, and diagnostic sensitivity of four immunoassays for carcinoembryonic antigen, *Clin Chem* 37(2):231-236, 1991.

72. Hansen H, Snyder J, Miller E, et al: Carcinoembryonic antigen (CEA) assay: a laboratory adjunct in the diagnosis and management of cancer, *Hum Pathol* 5:139, 1974.

73. Rule A: Carcinoembryonic antigens (CEA). In Kaplan LA, Pesce AJ, editors: *Clinical chemistry theory: analysis and correlation,* Philadelphia, 1989, Mosby.

74. Finley PR, Williams RJ, Lichti DA, et al: Immunochemical determination of human immunoglobulins: use of kinetic turbidimetry and a 36-place centrifugal analyzer, *Clin Chem* 25:526-530, 1979.

75. Papsidero L, Kuriyama M, Wang M, et al: Prostate antigen: a marker for human prostatic epithelial cells, *J Natl Cancer Inst* 66:37-41, 1981.

76. Iwakiri J, Grandbois K, Graves HCB, Stamey T: An analysis of urinary prostate-specific antigen before and after radical prostatectomy: evidence for secretion of prostate-specific antigen by the periurethal glands, *J Urol* 149:783-786, 1993.

77. Vessella KL: Trends in immunoassays of prostate-specific antigen: serum complexes and ultrasensitivity, *Clin Chem* 39(10):2035-2039, 1993.

78. Lange PH, Ercole CJ, Lightner DJ, et al: The value of serum prostate-specific antigen determinations before and after radical prostatectomy, *J Urol* 141:873-879, 1989.

79. Oesterling JE: Prostate specific antigen: a critical assessment of the most useful tumor marker for adenocarcinoma of the prostate, *J Urol* 145:907-923, 1991.

80. Armbruster DA: Prostate-specific antigen: biochemistry, analytical methods, and clinical application, *Clin Chem* 39(2):181-195, 1993.

81. White RW, Meyers FJ, Soares SE, et al: Urinary prostate specific antigen levels: role in monitoring the response of prostate cancer to therapy, *J Urol* 147:947-951, 1992.

82. Brawer MK: Laboratory studies for the detection of carcinoma of the prostate, *Urol Clin North Am* 17:759-768, 1990.

83. Killian CS, Chu TM: Prostate-specific antigen: questions often asked, *Cancer Invest* 8:27-37, 1990.

84. Simm B, Gleeson M: Storage conditions for serum for estimating prostate-specific antigen, *Clin Chem* 37:113-114, 1991.

85. van Dieijen-Visser MP, Delaere KPJ, Gijzen AHJ, Brombacher PJ: A comparative study on the diagnostic value of prostatic acid phosphatase (PAP) and prostatic-specific antigen (PSA) in patients with carcinoma of the prostate gland, *Clin Chem Acta* 174:131-140, 1988.

86. Babaian R, Camps J: The role of prostate-specific antigen as part of the diagnostic triad and as a guide when to perform a biopsy, *Cancer* 68:2060-2063, 1991.

87. Fritsche HA, Babaian RJ: Analytical performance goals for measuring prostate-specific antigen, *Clin Chem* 39(7):1525-1529, 1993.

88. Rosenfield L: Serum protein electrophoresis: a comparison of the use of thin-layer agarose gel and cellulose acetate, *Am J Clin Pathol* 62:702-706, 1974.

89. Jeppsson JO, Laurell CB, Franzen B: Agarose gel electrophoresis, *Clin Chem* 25:629-638, 1979.

90. Ojala K, Weber TH: Some alternatives to the proposed selected method for "agar gel electrophoresis," *Clin Chem* 26:1754-1755, 1980.

91. Harrison HH, Levitt MH, Bedford K: *Serum protein electrophoresis: basic principles, interpretations, practical considerations, and new techniques.* ASCP Check Sample Core Analyte No. PTS93-8 (PTS-74), Chicago, American Society of Clinical Pathologists, pp 1-10.

92. Whicher JT, Spence CE: Serum protein zone electrophoresis—an outmoded test? *Ann Clin Biochem* 24:133-139, 1987.

93. Sinclair D, Kumeraratre DS, Forrester JB, et al: The application of isoelectric focusing to routine screening for paraproteins, *J Immunol Methods* 64:147-156, 1983.

94. Roos RP, Lichter M: Silver staining of cerebrospinal fluid IgG in isoelectric focusing gels, *J Neurosci Methods* 8:375-380, 1983.

95. Harrison HH, Miller KL, Dickinson C, Daufeldt JA: Quality assurance and reproducibility of high-resolution two-dimensional electrophoresis and silver staining in polyacrylamide gels, *Am J Clin Pathol* 97:97-105, 1992.

96. Janson RW, Verstosick FT Jr, Kelly RH: A method for recovery of active, clonally-restricted immunoglobulins from agarose gels, *Electrophoresis* 10:11-15, 1989.

CHAPTER 50

Laboratory evaluation of the transplant recipient and donor

Timothy J. Schroeder
Stephen J. Rossi
Kevin T. Schlueter
M. Roy First

OBJECTIVES

- Outline the laboratory testing performed before transplantation in potential living related and cadaver kidney donors, liver donors, heart donors, and pancreas donors as well as potential transplant recipients.

- Define the different types of rejection seen in transplant patients with regard to timing, organ involvement, and diagnosis.

- List the most important components of the laboratory evaluation of the following transplant types:
Kidney
Pancreas
Liver
Heart

- List the immunosuppressive agents that are assessed by therapeutic drug monitoring.

- Define the pretransplant immunological assays utilized to predict the compatibility of a donor with a potential recipient.

KEY TERMS

allogeneic Refers to organs or cells from another person, which may or may not have the same histocompatibility antigens as the recipient.

antibody A class of serum proteins induced after contact with antigen. An antibody binds specifically to the antigen that induced its formation. Most antibodies are present in the gamma globulin fraction of serum.

antigen Any molecule that can be recognized by the immune system. In general, immunoglobulins recognize and bind to intact antigens.

azathioprine and 6-mercaptopurine These are purine analogs that act on small lymphocytes and dividing cells, thereby blocking development of organ-rejecting T-cells.

B-cells Lymphocytes that develop in the fetal liver and subsequently in the bone marrow. They respond to antigenic stimuli by dividing and differentiating into plasma cells under the control of cytokines released by T-cells.

CD markers This system of nomenclature is used for leukocyte surface molecules as identified by monoclonal antibodies. More than 80 individual molecules are recognized by this series, and some of them are found on cells other than leukocytes.

corticosteroids Agents that have numerous immunosuppressive and anti-inflammatory effects. They interfere with antigen presentation, inhibit the primary antibody response, and reduce the number of circulating T-cells.

cyclophosphamide A drug that prevents DNA replication by covalently adding to the DNA through an alkylation reaction. It acts primarily on lymphocytes and strongly inhibits antibody responses.

cyclosporin A A drug that is obtained from a fungus and interferes with early events in lymphocyte activation and transformation. It acts primarily on T-cells and has become the main immunosuppressive agent used after transplantation.

cytokines Substances released by leukocytes and other cells that control the development of the immune response. Often termed the "hormones of the immune system," they modulate the differentiation and division of hematopoietic stem cells and activation of lymphocytes and phagocytes.

cytotoxicity A general term for the ways in which lymphocytes, mononuclear phagocytes, and granulocytes can kill target cells.

histocompatibility complex The complex of glycoproteins on the surface of cells that is used by the immune system to define self and nonself.

human leukocyte antigen (HLA) The major histocompatibility complex. It is divided into seven main groups: A, B, C, Class III, DR, DQ, and DP.

immunosuppression Measures used to reduce immune responses after transplantation to prevent graft rejection. Most are not specific for the transplant antigens.

interleukin-2 A cytokine that is an essential T-cell growth factor required for division of antigen-activated T-cells.

major histocompatibility complex (MHC) A large group of genes including those encoding the class I and II MHC molecules that are involved in presentation of antigen to T-cells.

OKT3 A murine monoclonal antibody directed against the CD3 receptor on human T-cells. It is used to prevent and treat acute rejection after transplantation.

polyclonal antilymphocyte agents Immunosuppressive antibodies made by injecting human lymphoid material (spleen, thymus, lymph node) into an animal (horse, goat, sheep, rabbit) that makes an antibody response against the human tissue. The animal immune globulin is purified and used to prevent or treat rejection in human transplant patients.

rejection A reaction induced by recipient T-cells that recognize allogeneic MHC molecules. The T-cells can activate graft-infiltrating mononuclear cells, damaging the graft.

T-cells Lymphocytes that develop in the thymus and whose role is to recognize antigens originating from within cells of the host as self and foreign antigen as nonself.

tacrolimus (FK506) A fungal compound that prevents T-cell activation by inhibiting early calcium-signaling events. It is approximately 100 times more potent than cyclosporin A and has recently been approved by the Food and Drug Administration.

tissue typing The technique used to determine the major histocompatibility specificities carried on an individual's cells.

tolerance The acquisition of nonresponsiveness to a molecule that is normally recognized by the immune system.

Solid-organ transplantation has become the therapy of choice for end-stage diseases of the kidney, liver, and heart. Advances in surgical techniques and diagnostic capabilities, progress in immunology and histocompatibility analysis, development of more specific and potent immunosuppressive agents, improvements in donor management and organ preservation, and new antimicrobial agents have all contributed to the success of transplanting solid organs. Reflecting these improvements, the total number of each type of transplants tripled in the United States over the past decade (Table 50-1).

The term *graft* is used to describe a transplanted organ. *Allografts* refer to tissue that is taken from one individual and used for a second individual. An allograft from a relative is termed a *living related donor graft* (LRD). Allografts from individuals who have been declared legally dead ("brain dead") are termed *cadaver allografts.* Transplants are high-risk medical procedures.

The major factor limiting transplantation is the shortage of organs. By the end of 1994, the waiting list for solid-organ transplants in the United States exceeded 35,000. This represented more than a 100% increase since 1988. In cases of heart and liver disease, failure to receive a timely transplant results in death. The overall percentage of registrants who died while waiting for a transplant in 1993 was 5.8%. The highest death rates were for heart and heart-lung recipients at 13.1% and 16.2% respectively.

As transplantation has progressed, the role of the clinical laboratory has become more clearly defined. This chapter is a description of the utility of monitoring both transplant donors and recipients of solid organs.

PRETRANSPLANT EVALUATION

No transplant is performed without a thorough clinical investigation of both the donor and the recipient. Each organ has specific criteria that must be reviewed before the transplant is performed.

Live donor (kidney)

Allograft survival rates are greater when the graft is obtained from a LRD rather than from a cadaver donor. A second important advantage of live donor transplants is the

Table 50-1 Transplants performed in the United States in 1994

	1994
Kidney	11,104
(LRD)	(2,730)
(Cadaver)	(8,374)
Liver	3,590
Heart	2,334
Pancreas	841
Lung	703
Heart-lung	70
Total	18,642

Table 50-2 Medical evaluation of the potential live kidney donor

Complete history and physical examination

Laboratory studies*
  Complete blood count
  Serum urea and creatinine, sodium, potassium, chloride,
    bicarbonate
  Fasting blood glucose (glucose tolerance if family history of
    diabetes)
  Serum calcium, phosphorus, uric acid
  Liver function tests including bilirubin, alkaline phosphatase,
    transaminases
  Fasting lipids including cholesterol, triglycerides, high-density
    lipoproteins, low-density lipoproteins
  Prothrombin time, partial thromboplastin time
  Antibodies to cytomegalovirus (CMV), Epstein-Barr virus (EBV),
    human immunodeficiency virus (HIV), *Treponema pallidum*
  Hepatitis B antigen and antibody, hepatitis C antibody
  Urine analysis and microscopy
  Urine culture
  24-hour urine for creatinine, protein, calcium, uric acid

Electrocardiogram

X-ray studies
  Chest x-ray film
  Intravenous pyelography
  Renal arteriogram

*There are no absolute acceptable ranges for these lab tests. The aim is to
ensure that the potential donor is in excellent general health with no contraindication to the removal of one kidney and no potential infections or
malignancies to transmit to the recipient.

Table 50-3 United Network for Organ Sharing: mandatory laboratory testing of the potential cadaver donor

Complete blood count
Electrolytes
Blood gases
ABO typing
Hepatitis screen
Syphilis screen (VDRL or RPR)
Screen for antibodies to:
  HIV
  HTLV-1
  Cytomegalovirus
Blood and urine cultures if hospitalized more than 72 hours

Renal specific*
  Serum creatinine and urea
  Urinalysis

Liver specific*
  Liver enzymes: transaminases and alkaline phosphatase
  Total and direct bilirubin
  Prothrombin time and partial thromboplastin time

Heart specific*
  12-lead electrocardiogram
  Consultation with cardiologist
  Chest x-ray film

Pancreas specific*
  Serum amylase
  Serum lipase
  Glucose

*There are no absolute acceptable ranges for these lab tests. The aim is to
ensure that organs function after transplant and no infections or malignancies are passed from donor to recipient.

elective nature of the procedure, sparing the recipient the long waiting period on dialysis that frequently occurs when one is waiting for a suitable cadaveric transplantation. A third reason for the continued use of related donors is the shortage of cadaver donors.

The potential donor and recipient must be tested to demonstrate ABO blood type compatibility. Another immunocompatibility test, termed a *cytotoxic T-cell crossmatch*, must be performed between the donor and the recipient. This ensures that the recipient has no preformed antibodies against the donor. All potential donors must be emotionally stable and must fully understand the process of donating a kidney. Potential donors are meticulously evaluated to ensure that they are in excellent general health and that there are no contraindications to the removal of one kidney (Table 50-2). One goal of this evaluation is the detection of unsuspected disease in the donor, such as diabetes, hypertension, anemia, renal calculi, or malignancy. Another goal is to detect infections that may be transmitted to the recipient. The goal of the remainder of the studies is to assess whether the renal function and structure of the potential renal allograft are completely normal. The age of the potential living related donor is obviously important. Minors are not eligible for kidney donation, but older donors, up to 70 years of age, may be used if in excellent health. Kidney donors who have been monitored for up to 20 years after donation exhibit a slight reduction in glomerular filtration

rate and a mild increase in urine protein excretion without an increase in hypertension.

Cadaver donor

Cadaver donors are previously healthy individuals who suffer irreversible brain death. Once they are declared legally dead, to sustain cardiovascular function, they are maintained on a ventilator and clinically managed with appropriate fluids and medications until the organs are removed. Each donor undergoes an extensive history and physical as well as rigorous laboratory testing to assure optimal organ function. The laboratory studies obtained upon admission are important and establish baseline values of the individual organ systems. The United Network for Organ Sharing (UNOS) has established mandatory laboratory tests (Table 50-3), though additional tests may occasionally be requested. For example, if the donor's heart or lungs are being considered for transplantation, an echocardiogram, ECG, chest x-ray film, and measurement of creatine kinase-MB levels may be ordered at the time of the evaluation.

Kidney. Most cadaver kidney donors are between 2 and 70 years of age. However, kidneys from neonates and donors more than 70 years of age have been successfully transplanted. A thorough past and present medical history of the donor is necessary. The laboratory studies should include those listed in Table 50-3, with specific attention placed on the results of serum creatinine and urea levels and on urinalysis. Only patients with laboratory values that are within the reference intervals, or patients with laboratory values or clinical findings that are returning to normal after management, are usually accepted as cadaveric kidney donors.

Liver. Donor livers from individuals up to 70 years of age can safely be used. Older donors who are healthy enough to remain hemodynamically stable after brain death can become acceptable donors. Social history and the cause of death are often valuable pieces of information for potential liver donors. Laboratory testing includes those tests listed in Table 50-3 with particular attention to bilirubin, AST, ALT, and alkaline phosphatase. Moderate elevations in liver function studies are acceptable, especially if the trend is toward the reference range.

Pancreas. In general, donors who are acceptable for renal or liver transplants are also acceptable as pancreas donors. The primary contraindications for the acceptance of a donor for pancreas transplantation is a history of diabetes and acute or chronic pancreatitis. Hyperglycemia is frequently seen in individuals after severe head trauma or as a result of the administration of glucose-containing solutions. These factors are not a contraindication for pancreas retrieval if the patient has no history of diabetes. In questionable cases, the measurement of glycosylated hemoglobin levels may demonstrate that long-term pancreas function has been normal. An elevated serum amylase is not necessarily indicative of pancreatic trauma. Direct visualization of the pancreas is the best way to assess pancreatic injury in trauma cases. Evidence of pancreatic trauma precludes retrieval. The age of the potential donor is generally not a factor for pancreatic transplants, though age criteria are slightly more restrictive than for kidney transplants.

Heart. The donor's cardiac assessment combines the history, physical examination, and diagnostic tests. Contraindicating problems include prominent blunt chest trauma, prolonged hypotension, cardiac arrest, and premorbid cardiac symptoms. If blunt trauma or cardiac arrest occurred, the measurement of serum lactate dehydrogenase and creatine kinase isoenzyme levels, in addition to a chest x-ray film and ECG, may help in judging the severity of myocardial damage. Generally, individuals older than 50 years of age are not considered as cardiac donors.

Recipient

A detailed medical and psychologic evaluation of all potential transplant recipients is essential. Patients must be sufficiently healthy and motivated to undergo the surgical procedure, to withstand the potential problems of immunosuppressive agents, and to comply with a complex and demanding medical regimen.

Renal. The pretransplantation evaluation of the recipient of a kidney is listed in Table 50-4. The purpose of this evaluation is to detect any problem that may reduce the chance of success of the procedure and to take corrective

---

Table 50-4 Pretransplantation evaluation of the renal recipient

Complete history and physical examination

Dental evaluation

Gynecologic evaluation

Laboratory studies*
  Serum creatinine, urea, AST, ALT, bilirubin, and alkaline phosphatase
  Hepatitis B antigen and antibody, hepatitis C antibody
  Antibodies to CMV, HIV, and EBV
  Urine culture

X-ray studies
  Chest x-ray film
  Upper gastrointestinal series
  Barium enema (age >40 years)
  Gallbladder ultrasound scan
  Voiding cystourethrogram
  Mammography (female >40 years)

*There are no absolute acceptable ranges for these lab tests. The aim is to ensure that the potential recipient is sufficiently motivated to undergo the surgical procedure and to withstand the potential problems of immunosuppressive agents.

---

measures when necessary. Not all patients with end-stage renal disease are candidates for transplantation. Patients of advanced age or with prominent systemic illness are generally not acceptable candidates. The American Society of Transplant Physicians has published a list of absolute contraindications to renal transplantation. They include active infection, advanced cardiovascular disease, advanced pulmonary disease, severe chronic liver disease, malignancy, acute vasculitis or glomerulonephritis, uncorrectable lower urinary tract disease, primary oxalosis, age greater than 70 years, morbid obesity, severe psychosocial problems, drug or alcohol abuse, and positive current T-cell crossmatch.

Other recipients. Similar laboratory evaluations are used to assess potential liver, heart, pancreas, and lung transplant recipients. The primary goal is to be assured that the patient is healthy enough to survive the surgery and posttransplantation complications associated with life-long immunosuppression. Obviously, advanced cardiac disease would not be a contraindication to heart transplantation but would be a contraindication to liver transplantation. Active infection, malignancy, severe psychosocial problems, and any active drug or alcohol abuse are contraindications to all transplants.

CLINICAL AND PATHOLOGICAL DIAGNOSIS OF TRANSPLANT REJECTION

Allograft rejection is the destruction of a transplanted organ resulting from an immune attack mounted by the recipient's body. The rejected organ loses function. The process of monitoring the health of a transplanted organ includes a large component of laboratory testing.

The diagnosis of transplant rejection is often an exclusionary process by which the clinician rules out other posttransplantation complications. For example, kidney rejection must be differentiated from the nephrotoxic effects of the drug cyclosporin A, which is used to suppress the recipient's immune response. Liver allograft rejection must be differentiated from drug-induced hepatic injury, surgical complications, and hepatitis. Although biochemical and immunological testing and clinical symptoms may be strongly suggestive of organ rejection, a definitive diagnosis is made through histological examination of the transplanted organ. This is an invasive procedure that requires a core of tissue to be biopsied from the allograft for microscopic examination.

Allograft rejection can be caused by T-cells of the immune system, the antibodies produced by B-cells, or both. The differentiation between these processes is based on clinical presentation, timing of the event, and histological examination. *Hyperacute rejection,* defined as organ rejection beginning within minutes of transplantation, occurs because antibodies against the donor tissue are already present in the recipient. Clinical manifestations are noted immediately after the blood supply of the graft is restored. *Acute cellular rejection* is a T-cell–mediated process and is the most common form of rejection. It can occur at any time after transplantation but is most common in the first 6 months after transplantation. *Chronic rejection* is a slow, progressive loss of organ function that generally follows episodes of acute cellular rejection. The course of chronic rejection is generally months to years.

Kidney

Hyperacute rejection of the kidney is a rare occurrence with current cross-matching techniques. Clots form in the renal arteries, followed by necrosis of the renal cortex. Acute cellular rejection ranges from mild to severe forms, depending on the degree of renal damage (Table 50-5). Chronic rejection results in a progressive, irreversible deterioration of renal function.

Table 50-5   Banff grading scale of acute renal allograft rejection*

Classifications	Description
Borderline changes	Mild lymphocytic invasion of tubules (tubulitis)
Mild acute rejection (grade I)	Interstitial infiltrates with moderate tubulitis
Moderate acute rejection (grade II)	Interstitial infiltrates with severe tubulitis and/or mild to moderate intimal arteritis
Severe acute rejection (grade III)	Severe intimal and/or transmural arteritis, fibrinoid changes, medial smooth muscle cell necrosis often with patchy infarction and interstitial hemorrhage

International standardization of criteria for the histologic diagnosis of renal allograft rejection developed by a group of renal pathologists, nephrologists, and transplant surgeons meeting in Banff, Canada, August 2-4, 1991.
*Histological grading may or may not correlate with biochemical indices such as serum creatinine.

Table 50-6   Grading of acute cellular liver allograft rejection*

Grade	Description
Consistent with rejection	Lymphocytic or mixed portal infiltrate with minimal bile duct damage (<50%) and no endothelialitis
Mild rejection	Mild portal infiltrates with endothelial and biliary epithelial hypertrophy and damage
Moderate rejection	Lymphocytic or mixed portal infiltrate with significant bile duct damage (>50%), with or without endothelialitis
Severe rejection	Lymphocytic or mixed portal infiltrates, arteritis, paucity of bile ducts, central hepatocellular ballooning with confluent dropout of hepatocytes

*Histological grading may or may not correlate with biochemical indices such as AST, ALT, and bilirubin.

Liver

Hyperacute rejection of liver allografts rarely occurs in ABO-compatible donors. However, the paucity of donors has made ABO-incompatible liver transplantation more common, thus increasing the risk for this type of rejection. Acute cellular rejection of liver allografts is characterized by portal inflammation with a predominant lymphocytic infiltrate. The severity of rejection (Table 50-6) will determine the therapy implemented. Hepatic chronic rejection, or "vanishing bile duct syndrome," is characterized by progressive cholestasis and deteriorating liver function. Bile duct injury is the result of a vascular arteriopathy that diminishes the blood supply to the biliary tree.

Heart

Hyperacute rejection in cardiac allografts is extremely rare but has been noted in both ABO compatible and incompatible transplants. Because of the rapidity of this process, patient and graft survival is generally poor. Acute cellular re-

Table 50-7   International Society for Heart Transplantation standard cardiac biopsy grading*

Grade	Description
0	No rejection
1A	Focal perivascular or interstitial infiltrate without myocyte damage
1B	Diffuse but sparse perivascular and/or interstitial infiltrate without myocyte damage
2	One focus only with aggressive infiltration and/or focal myocyte damage
3A	Multifocal infiltrates and/or myocyte damage
3B	Diffuse inflammatory process with myocyte damage
4	Diffuse aggressive polymorphous infiltrate ± edema ± hemorrhage ± vasculitis with necrosis

*Histological grading does not correlate with biochemical indices such as creatine phosphokinase and lactate dehydrogenase.

jection is detected by serial endomyocardial biopsies. The grade of the severity of acute cellular rejection is based on the criteria established by the International Society of Heart and Lung Transplantation (Table 50-7). Chronic rejection generally manifests itself as accelerated arteriosclerosis.

Pancreas

Routine biopsy of the pancreas to diagnose rejection is infrequently performed because of the high morbidity associated with this procedure. Hyperacute rejection has not been clearly described in the pancreatic allograft. In acute cellular rejection, a lymphocytic infiltrate of the small vessels of the allograft results in damage to the surrounding acini and small ductule arteries. Chronic rejection results in eventual loss of both exocrine and endocrine pancreatic function.

LABORATORY MONITORING OF THE TRANSPLANT RECIPIENT

The clinical development of acute rejection of a transplanted organ generally results in progressive allograft destruction with accompanying organ dysfunction. Histopathologic examination of transplanted tissue remains the standard for the determination of rejection after it has become clinically apparent. However, the continued success

of organ transplantation is largely the result of the use of laboratory tests to detect early signs of rejection and to monitor treatment. These tests measure biochemical markers that reflect organ allograft damage and organ function.

Kidney

The laboratory evaluation of posttransplantation renal function employs the same tests routinely used to monitor glomerular and tubular function. Rejection remains an important cause of renal dysfunction after kidney transplant, but cyclosporin A nephrotoxicity, recurrent disease, infection, and vascular complications can cause renal dysfunction in these patients. Routine analysis of serum creatinine and urea remains the most practical clinical measure of renal function. Elevations in serum creatinine are often the initial presentation of posttransplantation renal complications. Both the degree of creatinine elevation and the rate of rise are important in the diagnosis. The rate of increase in serum creatinine, in combination with other clinical and histopathologic findings (Table 50-8), can be used to differentiate acute rejection from cyclosporin A nephrotoxicity. Other serum chemistry results may have some utility in this differential diagnosis.

Cyclosporin A–induced tubular dysfunction can cause el-

Table 50-8 Comparison of acute rejection versus cyclosporin A (CYA) nephrotoxicity

Parameter	Acute rejection	CYA nephrotoxicity
Clinical		
Onset	<60 days	Variable
Fever >37.5° C	+	−
Weight gain >0.5 kg	+	±
Oliguria	++	±
Biochemical		
Creatinine	Rapid rise (>3 mg/L/day)	Gradual rise (1-2 mg/L/day)
BUN:creatinine	<20:1	>20:1
Potassium (serum)	Increased	Increased ++
Bicarbonate (serum)	Decreased +	Decreased ++
Uric acid (serum)	No change	Increased +
Magnesium (serum)	No change	Decreased +
Sodium (urine)	Decreased ±	Decreased ++
Cyclosporin A* trough level	Low, <150 ng/mL	High, >400 ng/mL ·
Lymphocytes (urine)	++	−
Pathological		
Biopsy	Endovasculitis	Arteriolopathy
	Tubulitis	Tubular vacuolation and mitochondria
	Interstitial edema	Minimal edema
	Glomerulitis	Interstitial fibrosis
	Diffuse infiltrates	Focal infiltrates
Diagnostic tests		
Ultrasonography	Increased graft cross-sectional area	Normal graft cross-sectional area
Magnetic resonance imaging	Swelling	Normal
Radionucleotide	Decreased perfusion	Decreased tubular function
	Patchy arterial flow	Normal or decreased perfusion

+ indicates a positive response, and a − indicates no response.
*TDx whole blood, monoclonal assay.

evations in serum potassium, bicarbonate, and uric acid while causing a decrease in serum magnesium. Alterations in the urinary excretion of sodium and potassium are consistent with cyclosporin A nephrotoxicity. Functional tests such as renal manometry, ultrasonography, magnetic resonance imaging, and radionuclide scans may further delineate the cause of renal allograft dysfunction.

Pancreas

Since the pancreas is usually transplanted in combination with the kidney, biochemical markers of renal function are often utilized as early indicators of the status of the pancreatic transplant. Increases in serum amylase and glucose occur very late in the process of pancreas rejection and remain largely unreliable as indicators of early allograft rejection. The majority of pancreas transplants are performed so that the pancreatic enzymes drain into the bladder. Consequently, falling urinary amylase levels have been shown to correlate with early pancreatic transplant dysfunction. The frequency of this testing is a prominent factor in its sensitivity for detecting allograft rejection. Most centers initially monitor urinary amylase levels daily or at least three times per week. Other pancreatic enzymes such as trypsinogen may also be of value. Pancreatic fluid cytological findings may also be of diagnostic value; an increase in lymphocytes and blast cells is indicative of rejection, whereas a predominance of neutrophils is more characteristic of infection. Functional tests that evaluate insulin response to a glucose load may also be useful in the assessment of pancreatic reserve.

Liver

Biochemical markers are routinely used in monitoring liver allograft function. The various tests used to evaluate liver function can be divided into two categories: (1) *static tests,* which allow one to assess liver function indirectly by measuring substances produced by the liver, and (2) *dynamic tests,* which directly measure the metabolic and clearance capacities of the liver.

Static tests. In general, the serum levels of bilirubin, alkaline phosphatase, aspartate aminotransferase (AST), and alanine aminotransferase (ALT) are routinely used liver function tests. These tests are evaluated daily during the first few weeks of the posttransplantation period. Testing frequency decreases as stable graft function is demonstrated and increases when liver dysfunction occurs. Other tests of serum analytes, such as lactate dehydrogenase (LD), 5'-nucleotidase (5-NT), and gamma-glutamyltransferase (GGT) are considered secondary tests and may not be part of standard post–liver transplantation monitoring. Small incremental increases in standard liver tests do not necessarily indicate liver allograft rejection. However, serial increases of ≥25% over several days are considered a reliable indicator of liver allograft dysfunction.

The results of the liver function tests, such as bilirubin,

Table 50-9 Relative changes in laboratory values after liver transplantation

Clinical condition	Bilirubin	Alkaline phosphatase	AST	ALT
Rejection				
Mild	++	++	+	+
Moderate	++	++	++	++
Severe	+++	+++	+++	+++
Other conditions				
Cholestasis	++	++	±	±
Ischemic necrosis	++	++	+++	+++
Hepatitis	+	+	++	++

ALT, Alanine aminotransferase; *AST,* aspartate aminotransferase.

alkaline phosphatase, AST, and ALT, do not always indicate transplant rejection, since evaluations in test results are also associated with other clinical conditions (Table 50-9). For example, although serum bilirubin and alkaline phosphatase are progressively elevated with development of acute cellular rejection, both are also elevated during cholestasis secondary to biliary obstruction, drug toxicity, injury resulting from the process of preserving an organ before transplantation, and infection. Early elevations in serum aminotransferases may occur with rejection but elevations become progressively higher ($>2\times$ the upper limit of normal) in severe cases. Acute elevations in AST and ALT are also reflective of ischemic hepatocellular injury, necrosis, and hepatitis. Serum markers of hepatic synthetic function (serum proteins, serum ammonia, and coagulation factors) generally become abnormal as the result of longstanding progressive liver disease or severe fulminant hepatic failure. In general, static tests are sensitive early indicators of liver allograft dysfunction but are not specific for rejection.

Dynamic tests. Dynamic tests of liver function have been developed in an attempt to measure the functional status of the liver. Dynamic tests assess the liver's ability to clear or metabolize various substrates. Several of these tests have been extensively evaluated as part of the clinical assessment of liver transplant donors and recipients (Table 50-10).

The state of hepatocellular oxygenation is reflected by the ratio of serum acetoacetate (AcAc) to 3-hydroxybutyrate (HB), known as the ketone body ratio (KBR). As the oxygenation state of the liver decreases and the NAD/NADH ratio decreases, more HB is formed from AcAc. Clinically, a KBR of <0.7 is associated with diminished hepatocellular function in both liver allograft donors and recipients.

The hepatic clearance of exogenous substances has also been evaluated for assessing liver status. Indocyanine green (ICG) is removed from blood by the liver and is excreted unchanged into the bile. Its removal from blood is primarily reflective of hepatic blood flow. Another measure of hepatocellular metabolism is galactose-elimination capacity

Table 50-10   Dynamic liver function tests

Test	Functional assessment	Utility
Lidocaine metabolism/ monoethylglycinexylidide formation	Cytochrome P-450 activity, liver blood flow	Assessment of potential donor and recipient before transplantation and assessment of recipient after transplantation
Indocyanine green clearance	Liver blood flow	Assessment of potential recipient before transplantation
Galactose elimination	Hepatocellular function by means of enzymatic saturation capacity	Assessment of potential donor before transplantation
Acetoacetate/3-hydroxybutyrate ratio (ketone body ratio)	Reduction/oxidation function, hepatocellular respiration	Assessment of potential donor before transplantation and recipient after transplantation

(GEC), which is the saturation of the enzyme responsible for galactose elimination from blood. Lidocaine metabolism and the formation of its primary oxidative metabolite monoethylglycinexylidide (MEGX) reflect both hepatic cytochrome P-450 activity and hepatic blood flow. MEGX formation has been clinically correlated with varying degrees of liver function in both donors and recipients. Other exogenous agents that have been evaluated as potential dynamic markers of liver function include antipyrine, caffeine, lorazepam, and debrisoquine. A limitation of these dynamic tests is that they appear to be a sensitive indicator of liver injury but not of liver regeneration after transplantation. The role of dynamic monitoring of the posttransplantation liver recipient requires further clinical evaluation.

Heart

The use of biochemical markers for the evaluation of cardiac allograft complications is limited by the mechanism of rejection of this organ. In noncardiac allografts, injury to epithelial cells is the cause of the observed biochemical alterations. Unlike the kidney, liver, or pancreas, the heart lacks epithelial cells as a primary target for rejection. Thus, in cardiac allograft recipients, changes in levels of analytes used to measure cardiac function, such as creatine kinase, myoglobin, LD, and AST, have no clinical correlation with rejection. Electrocardiography, echocardiography, and radionuclide scanning are only of value in determining functional status late in rejection and are not reliable indicators of early allograft rejection. Because of the lack of sensitive and specific markers of rejection, routine serial endomyocardial biopsies are the standard for posttransplantation cardiac allograft monitoring.

PHARMACOLOGICAL MONITORING

The continued improvement of immunosuppressive therapies for transplant recipients depends on appropriate monitoring of these therapies and optimal adjustment of the multiple immunosuppressive drug regimens. The available choices for immunosuppressive therapy have expanded and now include not only irradiation, steroids, and antimetabolites, but also cyclosporin A, tacrolimus, and the polyclonal and monoclonal antilymphocyte agents (Table 50-11).

Immunosuppressive protocols vary with organ type, patient status, and the treatment philosophies of the physician and transplant center. Posttransplantation immunosuppressive therapy can involve single, double, triple, or even quadruple drug therapy (Table 50-11).

Corticosteroids

Corticosteroids were among the earliest compounds found to have immunosuppressive activity. The binding of the glucocorticoids to their receptors blocks the synthesis or release of lymphokines and cytokines. This results in an inhibition of T-cell response to stimulation, a redistribution of lymphocytes from the vascular to the lymphatic system, and a decrease in the number of circulating T-cells and B-cells. The cellular immune response is blunted, but almost no immunosuppressive effect is seen in the humoral response (antibody production).

Total steroid dosing is generally quite high (100 to 500 mg/day) in the immediate posttransplantation period but is reduced to 10 to 20 mg daily within 2 weeks after transplantation. Often additional doses of intravenous or oral corticosteroids are used to treat acute rejection episodes. Since the liver and kidney are the major organs that metabolize

Table 50-11   Common immunosuppressive protocols

Monotherapy
Cyclosporin A
Tacrolimus

Double therapy
Cyclosporin A + Prednisone
Tacrolimus + Prednisone
Prednisone + Azathioprine

Triple therapy
Cyclosporin A + Prednisone + Azathioprine
Tacrolimus + Prednisone + Azathioprine

Quadruple therapy
Antilymphocyte therapy (OKT3 or ATG) + Cyclosporin A + Prednisone + Azathioprine
Antilymphocyte therapy (OKT3 or ATG) + Tacrolimus + Prednisone + Azathioprine

glucocorticoids, dysfunction of these organs may require modification of the dosage.

The acute adverse effects associated with corticosteroids include hypertension, glucose intolerance, hyperlipidemia caused by altered lipid metabolism, negative calcium balance and bone disease, growth retardation in children, weight gain, psychological changes, reduced wound healing, and cataracts. These acute adverse effects may be new symptoms or seen as an aggravation of preexisting conditions. The acute effects are most often dose-related and diminish as the patient progresses to lower doses. Adverse effects associated with long-term glucocorticoid therapy lead to cushingoid appearance, osteoporosis or avascular bone necrosis, and cardiovascular disease secondary to hypertension and hyperlipidemia.

The hepatic metabolism of corticosteroids can be affected by multiple drug interactions. Inducers of cytochrome enzymes can increase the oxidative capacity of the liver and cause decreased levels of steroids for a given dose, whereas inhibitors of cytochrome enzymes tend to spare the circulating steroids from degradation and elimination. No specific monitoring of corticosteroids is routinely performed. Dosing is typically driven by protocols, to minimize side effects, and by the immune response of the patient.

Azathioprine and cyclophosphamide

Azathioprine is a prodrug for 6-mercaptopurine, which is a potent inhibitor of cellular proliferation. It inhibits purine metabolism and thus interferes in nucleic acid replication. Azathioprine diminishes the clonal expansion of lymphocytes, resulting in suppression of bone marrow function and the cellular immune response. Azathioprine is administered orally once a day. Standard dosages are in the range of 1 to 2 mg/kg/day. Dosages may need to be reduced if myelosuppression occurs. If significant leukopenia (reduced white blood cell levels) occurs, azathioprine therapy may be temporarily or permanently discontinued. Azathioprine therapy is monitored primarily by following the white blood count (WBC). Generally, full doses of azathioprine are maintained while the WBC count remains above 5000/mm³. Dosages are reduced by half if the WBC count decreases into the 3000 to 5000/mm³ range and discontinued when the WBC count falls below 3000 WBC/mm³, at least until the leukopenia is resolved. Acute administration of granulocyte colony–stimulating factor (G-CSF) may be used to alleviate the myelosuppression.

Cyclophosphamide is a nitrogen mustard precursor, which is activated in the liver. It acts as an alkylating agent and disrupts cell division, having the greatest effect on rapidly dividing cells such as lymphocytes. It is more toxic and less well tolerated than azathioprine. Its use as an immunosuppressant is generally limited to cases of azathioprine intolerance, usually resulting from hepatotoxicity.

Cyclosporin A

Cyclosporin A transformed the practice of transplantation from an experimental procedure to the treatment of choice for end-organ failure. It is an 11-residue cyclic peptide that is chemically neutral and mostly hydrophobic. Cyclosporin A is formulated for oral administration in an olive oil solution or gel capsule and for intravenous (IV) administration as a surfactant dispersant. The avidity of cyclosporin A for hydrophobic surfaces has caused concern. Dosage can be dangerously reduced because of its adsorption to plastic drinkware, nasogastric feeding tubes, and IV lines. Cyclosporin A is believed to cause immunosuppression by inhibiting the synthesis and release of interleukin-2 (IL-2) and other lymphokines. Cyclosporin A accomplishes this by inhibiting early calcium-dependent events in signal transduction during T-cell activation.

Pharmacokinetics. Absorption of cyclosporin A after oral dosing is quite variable. Approximately one third of the dose is absorbed, but its bioavailability can range from 5% to 90%. The absorption in the gut is aided by dietary fat and excretion of bile fluids. Patients with diarrhea, nausea, vomiting, or reduced bile secretion may have a significantly reduced bioavailability of orally administered cyclosporin A. Peak blood levels occur 2 to 6 hours after oral dosing.

Cyclosporin A is widely distributed in tissues. Because of its hydrophobic nature it is tightly bound and can be detected in tissue as long as 2 weeks after discontinuation of therapy. Approximately 10% of cyclosporin A in the blood is carried in leukocytes, whereas 40% to 60% is carried in the red blood cells; the balance is carried in the plasma bound to lipoproteins.

Binding to erythrocytes is nonlinear temperature dependent and may change with hematocrit. This variability in distribution within blood fractions has necessitated that whole blood anticoagulated with EDTA be the specimen customarily used for clinical analysis.

Cyclosporin A undergoes extensive hepatic metabolism. Many changes occur at the extended side chains, but little or no modification occurs on the cyclic core configuration. The microsomal oxidases, especially the cytochrome P-450IIIA4 isoenzyme, are responsible for metabolism. These oxidases are present in intestinal mucosa and play a significant role in gut metabolism of cyclosporin A. Most metabolites identified have undergone oxidation or N-demethylation.

Elimination of cyclosporin A is primarily through hepatobiliary excretion with elimination in the feces. Urinary concentrations of cyclosporin A and metabolites account for less than 10% of the administered dose.

Adverse effects. Serious adverse effects related to cyclosporin A treatment are dose-related nephrotoxicity, hypertension, neurotoxicity, gingival hyperplasia, hirsutism, hyperlipidemia, and glucose intolerance. Many of these side effects are similar to side effects of corticosteroid treatment,

Table 50-12   Cyclosporin A drug interactions

Decreased cyclosporin A levels	Increased cyclosporin A levels	Nephrotoxic synergy
Carbamazepine	Diltiazem	Acyclovir
Isoniazid	Erythromycin	Aminoglycosides
Phenobarbital	Fluconazole	Amphotericin B
Phenytoin	Itraconazole	Cotrimoxazole
Rifampicin	Ketoconazole	Furosemide
Nafcillin	Metoclopramide	Ganciclovir
	Methylprednisolone	H_2-antagonists
	Nicardipine	Melphalan
	Verapamil	Nonsteroidal anti-inflammatory agents
		Vancomycin

adding to their severity. There are general risks of overimmunosuppression as well, with an increased risk of chronic viral infections, which, although mostly innocuous in the general population, can be a threat to the transplant patient. Both acute and chronic nephrotoxicity can occur. In the early posttransplantation time when the cyclosporin A dosage and levels are highest, the probability of occurrence of acute cyclosporin A–induced nephrotoxicity is greatest. This toxicity manifests as a reduction in renal blood flow, glomerular filtration rate, and urine output. It may be difficult to distinguish this nephrotoxicity from acute rejection in renal transplants (see Table 50-8). These short-term effects can usually be reversed when one decreases the cyclosporin A dose. Long-term administration of cyclosporin A and the associated renal vasoconstriction can lead to a nephropathy characterized by interstitial fibrosis. Secondary to the chronic nephropathy are hypertension and hyperuricemia. Decreasing the cyclosporin A dose or switching

to alternative therapies are the most commonly used strategies for dealing with these chronic side effects.

Drug interactions. The pharmacokinetic and pharmacodynamic properties of cyclosporin A may be affected by many drugs commonly used to treat transplant recipients (Table 50-12). Drug interactions with cyclosporin A may occur as a result of an alteration of the pharmacokinetic parameters, an alteration of the physiological or pharmacological effect, or a combination of these effects. The most common mechanisms for these drug interactions are induction or inhibition of the cytochrome P-450 system, which results in a reduction or an increase in blood cyclosporin A levels respectively. Close monitoring of the patient is suggested when the administration of drugs known to interact with cyclosporin A is initiated or stopped. This monitoring includes the assessment of organ function and known adverse effects of cyclosporin A, and the measurement of cyclosporin A blood concentrations.

Monitoring. Since its introduction, monitoring of cyclosporin A has been used by most transplant centers to optimize immunosuppression while minimizing toxicity. Evolving technology for monitoring cyclosporin A, as well as changes in immunosuppressive protocols, has made it difficult to establish appropriate therapeutic ranges (Table 50-13). Therapeutic ranges are often specific to each institution with different ranges developed for each organ type and for various times after transplantation (Table 50-14). Clinical response does not correlate with dose as a result of the variability in cyclosporin A pharmacokinetics and pharmacodynamics. Frequent monitoring of cyclosporin A levels is particularly valuable when one is following the progress of individual patients. The assay techniques vary from institution to institution, but assays specific for the parent drug are recommended. Whole blood is the matrix of

Table 50-13   Summary of assay parameters for monitoring cyclosporin A

Assay	Type of antibody, automated	Sample matrix, automated	Linearity	% CV	Turnaround (20 samples) Estimated time	Turnaround (20 samples) Specific or nonspecific
³H Sandoz	Polyclonal, No	Plasma	50-1000	4-12	8 hours	Nonspecific
		Whole blood	62.5-2000			
HPLC	Not applicable	Whole blood	50-1000	7-10	8 hours	Specific
TDx	Polyclonal, Yes	Plasma	10-1000	3-4	45 min	Nonspecific
		Whole blood	25-2000	2-6	45 min	
INCstar	Polyclonal, No	Plasma			3 hours	Nonspecific
		Whole blood	50-1000	5-10		
³H Sandoz	Monoclonal, No	Plasma	10-500	3-6	8 hours	Specific or nonspecific
		Whole blood				
INCstar	Monoclonal, No	Plasma				Specific or nonspecific
		Whole blood	50-1000	5-10	3 hours	
TDx	Monoclonal, Yes					
		Whole blood	25-1500	5-7	45 min	Specific
Du Pont	Monoclonal, Yes	Whole blood	25-350	2-8	30 min	Specific
Syva	Monoclonal, Yes	Whole blood	50-500	5-8	120 min	Specific

Table 50-14 Cyclosporin A whole blood TDx monoclonal assay therapeutic ranges at the University of Cincinnati

Kidney and kidney-pancreas transplants
<6 months   (250-375 ng/mL)
>6 months   (100-250 ng/mL)

Liver transplants
≤1 month   (350-450 ng/mL)
2-6 months (250-350 ng/mL)
>6 months   (170-240 ng/mL)

Cardiac transplants
<6 weeks   (300-420 ng/mL)
6-12 weeks (180-300 ng/mL)
>12 weeks   (120-180 ng/mL)

choice and trough level monitoring is the standard of practice. Frequent inpatient monitoring early after transplantation is performed in many centers with daily monitoring preferred. The frequency of monitoring decreases after discharge and generally occurs whenever the patient is evaluated in the outpatient clinic. Early after transplantation this may occur as often as three times per week, but much later it may only occur three or four times per year. The amount of monitoring generally increases when physiologic changes occur in the transplant recipient (rejection, infection, drug toxicity, and so forth).

Tacrolimus

Tacrolimus (FK506), a novel macrolide immunosuppressant, is a powerful and selective anti–T cell agent that has a similar mode of action to cyclosporin A. It has been approved by the FDA for use in liver transplant recipients, and many studies are in progress, evaluating its use in other transplant types. Tacrolimus is approximately 100 times more potent than cyclosporin A and has been particularly impressive in treating previously uncontrollable rejection.

The pharmacokinetics of tacrolimus exhibit many of the same features that cyclosporin A exhibits. It is poorly, erratically, and incompletely absorbed in the gut, though its absorption appears to be less dependent on the availability of bile than is that of cyclosporin A. In plasma, the drug binds primarily to α_1-acid glycoprotein, whereas in whole blood it is mainly found in erythrocytes. Tacrolimus is metabolized by the microsomal cytochrome P-450 system of the liver and the small intestine. After hepatic metabolism, more than 95% of the drug is eliminated by the biliary route. Drug interactions with tacrolimus are probably very similar to cyclosporin A, although this is not so well studied.

Variability in blood concentrations because of erratic pharmacokinetics and drug interactions together with the dose-dependent immunosuppressive effects and toxicities justify careful monitoring of this drug. The correlation between tacrolimus concentrations and efficacy or toxicity is

still unclear. Many transplant centers are targeting whole blood levels from 5 to 20 ng/mL.

Polyclonal antilymphocyte preparations

Polyclonal antilymphocyte agents were first used in clinical transplantation in 1967. An antihuman immunoglobulin is prepared from the serum of horses, rabbits, or goats immunized with human lymph nodes, thymus, or spleen. The effect of these agents is dependent on timing and dose. A transient but significant immunosuppression is gained by removal of lymphocytes from circulation. This therapy is utilized most often to reduce the activity of the highly stimulated immune system during the first few days after transplantation and during serious rejection episodes. Antilymphocyte agents are generally administered intravenously. One can assess the progress and effectiveness of antilymphocyte therapy by monitoring lymphocyte counts, total T-cell counts, or T-cell subsets such as CD2+ or CD3+ cells. Lower T-cell counts are a general indication of immunosuppression through lymphocyte elimination. Efficacy of treatment with polyclonal antilymphocyte preparations may be compromised by the patient's development of antibodies to the animal source of the antisera.

OKT3

Monoclonal antilymphocyte antibodies have better specificity than polyclonal preparations. Instead of targeting all lymphocytes or thymocytes, a specific subset of cells can be chosen for suppression. The mouse monoclonal antibody, OKT3, is used widely to prevent and treat acute rejection. OKT3 is usually administered intravenously (5 mg/day) for 7 to 14 days. Its most noted adverse effect has been termed the *cytokine release syndrome.* Symptoms include fever, pulmonary edema, dyspnea, and progressive hypotension. A further consideration in the use of OKT3 is that the patient may develop antibodies to the mouse protein (human antimouse antibody, HAMA). This response may occur as early as 3 to 10 days after the patient's first exposure to OKT3, but it generally does not appear until after cessation of therapy. The elicited antibodies may be isotypic, in which case there is no therapeutic interference; or they may be idiotypic, in which case they neutralize the OKT3 activity.

OKT3 therapy can be monitored by several means. Measurement of lymphocyte subsets, specifically CD3+ cells, is the primary monitor of OKT3 efficacy. CD3+ counts below a range of 10 to 50/mm³ are considered indicative of effective immunosuppression. The serum concentration of OKT3 can be measured by various immunoassays and by flow cytometry. A trough OKT3 serum level of 500 to 1200 ng/mL is usually considered to be therapeutic. The presence of a high-titer HAMA response will lead to reduced efficacy and is a contraindication to possible OKT3 retreatment. The HAMA titer is assessed by ELISA technology during and after treatment.

IMMUNOLOGICAL MONITORING
Human leukocyte antigen testing

The host immune system discriminates self from nonself by recognizing the human leukocyte antigens (HLA) on the major histocompatibility complex. HLA matching, or histocompatibility testing, is utilized to help predict the compatibility of donor tissue with a potential recipient. The HLAs, which mediate transplant rejection, are divided into two molecular groups: class I HLA molecules and class II HLA molecules. Class I HLA comprises two antigenic loci, HLA-A, and HLA-B, which are found on the surface of most cells. Similarly, class II HLA has three primary antigenic loci: HLA-DR, HLA-DQ, and HLA-DP, but these antigens are found primarily on B-lymphocytes and macrophages. Each antigenic locus has two antigenic haplotypes, which are identified for typing.

In general, a complement-dependent lymphocytoxicity test is used for tissue typing. The unknown tissue, a lymphocyte, is exposed to a broad panel of standardized antisera of known HLA specificity. If the antisera bind to the cell, complement is fixed, and the lymphocyte is killed, and such a response indicates that the HLA of the cell is similar to that of the known antisera. Class I HLA are typed as a mixed lymphocyte preparation, whereas Class II antigens generally require a B lymphocyte–enriched preparation for adequate typing. The process of HLA typing generally takes several hours, which may be a rate-limiting step in utilizing this test in the clinical setting.

The clinical implications and utility of HLA typing vary depending on the organ transplanted. In general, HLA typing is used clinically only for the matching of renal allograft donors and recipients. Six antigen matches of a cadaveric donor and a recipient are linked automatically through United Network of Organ Sharing (UNOS); all other matches are based on a combination of HLA match, crossmatch negativity, panel-reactive antibody status (see below), medical urgency, geographic location, and length of time on the recipient waiting list.

Early data indicated that short-term and long-term kidney allograft survival was strongly influenced by HLA-A, HLA-B, and HLA-DR matching. Although the introduction of cyclosporin A has reduced the effect of HLA matching on short-term graft survival, long-term survival still appears to be HLA dependent. It has been estimated that the half-life for HLA-matched kidney transplants from cadaveric donors is twice that for unmatched donors (17.3 years versus 7.8 years; see Takemoto et al. in the bibliography). The use of HLA matching has been demonstrated to improve graft survival in patients with heart transplants. However, the shortage of organs, combined with a minimal preservation time, have made HLA typing impractical in this population. There appears to be a limited benefit to HLA matching in liver allograft recipients, though some evidence indicates a possible detrimental effect on graft survival with no HLA matching. Limited data exist regarding the effects of HLA matching on pancreas and lung allograft survival.

Panel reactive antibody testing

Panel reactive antibody (PRA) testing is performed as frequently as once per month for assessment of anti-HLA antibodies in transplant candidates. The appearance of these antibodies is generally the result of blood transfusions, pregnancy, and previous transplants. PRA testing uses a serological assay of complement-mediated lymphocytotoxicity. Recipient serum is reacted with a reference panel of cells representing known HLA specificities. The result is expressed as a percentage, with 100% representing sensitization against the entire panel of HLA antibodies. Prioritization is given to kidney transplant recipients with a negative T-cell crossmatch who are highly sensitized over those patients with lower sensitization. PRA test results are not usually utilized in heart and liver transplants for assessment of donor and recipient compatibility.

Lymphocyte crossmatch

The lymphocyte crossmatch is used to detect donor-specific cytotoxic antibodies in the recipient. Purified donor lymphocytes are reacted against the sera of recipients. Both a T-cell and a B-cell crossmatch are performed. A positive crossmatch can allow one to predict the likelihood of hyperacute rejection. Renal transplants are not performed when there is a positive crossmatch. The urgency of heart transplants requires that surgery be performed before crossmatch results are usually available. If a positive crossmatch is found in a patient with a heart transplant, increased immunosuppression including plasmapheresis is usually instituted. Crossmatches have little predictive value in liver transplant recipients.

Mixed lymphocyte cultures

Although serologic testing of HLA differences provides an initial indication of donor-recipient compatibility, a more specific test has been developed to assess the degree of antigenic incompatibility. This procedure, known as the *mixed lymphocyte culture (MLC) test,* allows one to evaluate the degree of histocompatibility of the primary activating antigen, the class II HLAs. MLC testing is based on the principle that two cells of different HLA composition will activate and proliferate upon exposure whereas HLA identical cells will remain unstimulated. The greater the degree of antigenic disparity, the greater amount of cellular activity and therefore potential for graft rejection. In general, the two cell types in question are incubated for 5 or 6 days, allowing them to interact and activate each other. The degree of cellular DNA synthesis, as determined by radiolabeling, is equivalent to the relative amount of T-lymphocyte activation. Because of the length of time required to perform the test, the primary clinical use of MLC testing is in the evaluation of potential living related donors.

Soluble interleukin-2-receptor monitoring

The expression and release of the soluble interleukin-2 receptor (sIL-2R) is an indication of T-lymphocyte activation. The use of sIL-2R for immunologic monitoring has been evaluated in the transplant recipient as a predictive, noninvasive parameter of acute allograft rejection. Enzyme immunoassays have been developed for use with various biologic matrixes, with most monitoring performed with serum. Significant elevations in serum sIL-2R levels have been noted during acute cellular rejection in kidney, kidney/pancreas, liver, and heart allograft recipients. Additionally, urine and bile sIL-2R levels correlate with rejection in kidney and liver transplants respectively and sIL-2R levels in serum and urine have been used to distinguish between acute rejection and cyclosporin A nephrotoxicity in renal transplant recipients. In addition, sIL-2R levels have been shown to be useful in the diagnosis and monitoring of infectious complications in transplant patients; sIL-2R levels are elevated in viral infections but not bacterial infections. The levels are elevated as early as 2 weeks before the clinical diagnosis of cytomegalovirus, and such elevation demonstrates that prospective serial monitoring may provide an early indication of host immune response to viral infection.

CONCLUSION

The role of the clinical laboratory in the transplantation process has become well defined. Successful transplantation depends on a multidisciplinary approach including surgery, medicine, nursing, radiology, pathology, pharmacy, nutrition, and psychiatry. The monitoring of transplant donors and recipients crosses and joins these many areas. Although the demands and responsibilities that transplantation puts on the clinical laboratories may be great, the rewards seen in the patient successes are far greater. Future advances in transplant science include new procedures (small bowel transplant, pancreatic islet transplants), new immunosuppressive agents (mycophenolic acid, mofetil, rapamycin, brequinar, leflunomide, deoxyspergualin, and mizorbine), and new solutions to previously unsolvable problems (xenotransplantation and tolerance induction). As the field of transplant science grows, the responsibilities of the laboratory will change to meet each new development.

BIBLIOGRAPHY

1993 Annual Report, U.S. Scientific Registry of Transplant Recipients and the Organ Procurement and Transplantation Network.

Abbas AK, Lichtman AH, Pober JS, editors: *Cellular and molecular immunology,* Philadelphia, 1994, Saunders.

Balistreri WF, A-Kader HH, Setchell KDR, et al: New methods for assessing liver function in infants and children, *Ann Clin Lab Sci* 22:162-174, 1992.

First MR: Pre-transplant evaluation and preparation of donors and recipients. In Jacobson HR, Striker GE, Clark SS, editor: *The principles and Practice of nephrology,* St. Louis, 1995, Mosby.

Flye MW, editor: *Principles of organ transplantation,* Philadelphia, 1989, Saunders.

Klintmalm G: A review of FK506: a new immunosuppressive agent for the prevention and rescue of graft rejection, *Transplant Rev* 8:53-63, 1994.

Phillips MG, editor: *Organ procurement, preservation and distribution in transplantation,* Richmond, Va., 1993, The William Byrd Press Inc.

Rossi SJ, Schroeder TJ, Hariharan S, First MR: Prevention and management of the adverse effects associated with immunosuppressive therapy, *Drug Safety* 9:104-131, 1993.

Schroeder TJ, Pesce AJ, Vine WH, First MR: Cyclosporine monitoring—An update, *American Association for Clinical Chemistry—TDM/Tox* 13:7-22, 1991.

Schroeder TJ, First MR: Monoclonal antibodies, *Am J Kidney Dis* 23:138-147, 1994.

Takemoto S, Terasaki PI, Cecka JM, et al: Survival of nationally shared, HLA-matched kidney transplants from cadaveric donors, *N Engl J Med* 327:834-839, 1992.

Terasaki PI, Cecka JM, editors: *Clinical transplants 1993,* Los Angeles, 1994, UCLA Tissue Typing Laboratory.

Yatscoff RW: Laboratory support for transplantation, *Clin Chem* 40:2166-2173, 1994.

CHAPTER 51

Toxicology

Alphonse Poklis
Steven H.Y. Wong
Amadeo J. Pesce

OBJECTIVES

- Define toxicology, poison, toxicity, and LD_{50}.
- Describe the mechanisms of toxicity and factors that influence toxicity.
- List some general effects of toxic agents.
- List and describe classes of drugs frequently encountered in overdose situations.
- Define drug interaction.

KEY TERMS

abused substances Potentially addictive compounds such as alcohol, cocaine, and marijuana that are taken to induce pleasure. These are often toxicants.

acute toxicity Usually refers to the harmful effect of a toxic agent that manifests itself in seconds, minutes, hours, or days after entering the patient.

analgesics A class of drugs that reduce pain.

antidepressants A class of drugs that alleviate depression.

antidote Any agent that counteracts the effects of a poison.

benzodiazepines A group of antianxiety sedative drugs.

biotransformation The chemical modifications of chemicals as they pass through the body.

chiral drugs Drugs (stereochemical isomers) with four different chemical groups attached to a carbon atom, resulting in nonsuperimposable structures. (*Chiral* is based on Greek 'hand'.)

chronic toxicity Usually refers to the long-term harmful effects of an agent, weeks, months, and years after it first affects the patient.

confirmation The process of verifying the identity of a drug or a drug metabolite by the use of at least two different tests. The initial screening test is followed up by a second confirmatory test, which must employ an analytical principle that is different from that used by the screening test.

designer drugs Analogs of controlled substances whose legal status has not yet been defined by the U.S. Drug Enforcement Agency.

drug interaction The difference that is observed between the independent actions of two or more drugs and their combined actions when administered together.

drug screen A test that qualitatively identifies the presence of one or more drugs or classes of drugs.

enantiomers Stereochemical isomers of a compound that are capable of rotating polarized light clockwise are designated as *d* and those counterclockwise, designated as *l,* or more properly *(R)* and *(S)* respectively.

forensic toxicology A branch of the discipline of toxicology concerned with the medical and legal aspects of the harmful effects of chemicals or poisons.

hypnotics A class of drugs often used as sedatives.

inhalants Volatile chemicals, such as toluene, that are components of household products but can be abused by breathing in of their fumes, leading to neural damage.

LD_{50} The amount of a substance that will cause death in half the test animal population.

lethal dose The amount of a substance that if ingested will cause death.

mixed-function oxidases A group of enzymes present in the microsomes of the liver that add oxygen to a drug.

opiates Drugs with chemical structures similar to those of heroin and morphine. Synthetic opiates include meperidine, oxycodone, and others.

phenothiazines Drugs used to treat psychoses.

therapeutic dose The amount of a substance that will produce a desired pharmacological effect.

toxicant or poison A substance that, when taken in sufficient quantity, will cause sickness or death.

toxicokinetics The quantitative study of a toxicant's disposition in the body of an affected person with time. Similar to pharmacokinetics.

toxicology The study of poisons.

tricyclic antidepressants Mood-elevating drugs.

xenobiotics Compounds, usually drugs, that do not normally occur in the body.

DEFINITIONS

Toxicology is the study of poisons. More specifically, toxicology concerned with the chemical and physical properties of poisons, their physiological or behavioral effects on living organisms, qualitative and quantitative methods for their analysis in biological and nonbiological materials, and the development of procedures for the treatment of poisoning. A poison (or toxicant) is regarded as any substance that, when taken in sufficient quantity, will cause sickness or death. The key phrase in this definition is "sufficient quantity." As the sixteenth-century physician Paracelsus observed, "All substances are poisons; there is none which is not a poison." The right dose often differentiates a poison from a "remedy." For example, minute quantities of cyanide, arsenic, lead, and dichlorodiphenyltrichloroethane (DDT) are regularly ingested from food sources or inhaled as environmental contaminates and retained by the human body. However, the amounts of these toxicants are insufficient to cause obvious deleterious effects. On the other hand, a substance as apparently innocuous as pure water will, if ingested in sufficient quantity, cause incapacitating electrolyte imbalance or even death.

There is often no difference between the mechanism of action of a drug and that of a poison. A drug is administered in doses that alter physiological function to produce a desired therapeutic effect. If administered in greater than therapeutic quantities, a drug may produce toxic (harmful) effects. Thus toxicology is a quantitative discipline that seeks to identify the amount of a substance that, in particular exposure situations, will cause deleterious effects in a particular animal or patient.

Because of a diversity of concerns and applications, modern toxicology has developed into five specialized branches: clinical, therapeutic drug monitoring, forensic, drug control in sports medicine, and environmental testings. Clinical toxicology is concerned with the harmful effects of chemicals on living organisms. Therapeutic drug monitoring is the rational utilization of drug therapy for selected groups of drugs with laboratory monitoring of drug concentration in accordance with the clinical pharmacokinetic principles. Forensic toxicology is the branch of toxicology that is concerned with the medical and legal aspects of the harmful effects of chemicals or poisons. Within the specialized area of forensic drug urine testing, preemployment and for-cause working-place drug testing are used as a means of detering against illicit drug use. Sports medicine toxicology is a newly established specialty concerned with the harmful effects of performance-enhancing drugs such as anabolic steroids and stimulants such as amphetamine and caffeine. Environmental toxicology is concerned primarily with the harmful effects of chemicals that are encountered incidentally because they are in the atmosphere, food chain, or occupational or recreational environments.

DOSAGE RELATIONSHIPS

Toxicity is a relative term used to compare one substance with another. To state that one substance is more toxic than another is to make a quantitative comparison of a dose. Such a comparison is valid only in a specific organism under identical exposure conditions. A toxicity rating of the lethal dose of a substance for a normal man (body weight 150 pounds, or 70 kg) is presented in Table 51-1. In the vernacular, toxic substance refers to substances with a toxicity defined in Table 51-1 as "extremely toxic," or "super toxic" (arsenic, cyanide, strychnine).

Important parameters in toxicology include the amount of an agent introduced into a person (that is, a dose), the route of administration, the number of doses, and the period over which the agent is administered. Time is an essential quantity, since the effect of many agents is time dependent. For convenience, terms such as *acute toxicity* and *chronic toxicity* are used. To some extent, these terms overlap. In general, the toxic reactions observed in the emergency room are caused by the acute ingestion, inhalation, or injection of some agent, whereas the reactions caused by environmentally toxic agents are more often observed in the chronic care setting. Thus toxic agents can have an acute

Table 51-1   Toxicity rating chart

Toxicity rating or class	Probable lethal dose (human)	
	Amount	For 70 kg (150-pound) man
6 Supertoxic	< 5 mg/kg	A taste (<7 drops)
5 Extremely toxic	5-50 mg/kg	Between 7 drops and 1 teaspoonful
4 Very toxic	50-500 mg/kg	Between 1 teaspoonful and 1 ounce
3 Moderately toxic	0.05-5 g/kg	Between 1 ounce and 1 pint (or 1 pound)
2 Slightly toxic	5-15 g/kg	Between 1 pint and 1 quart
1 Practically nontoxic	>15 g/kg	More than 1 quart

effect when the action of the chemical is observed from seconds to days after dosage, or a chronic effect when the time scheme is in weeks, years, or decades.

A dose-response relationship occurs when an increased toxic effect is observed as the dose is increased. However, the increased toxic effect may not be observed in all persons at the same dose. Only a portion of the population may be affected at a given dose, but as increasing amounts of the agent are given, the dose becomes great enough so that the entire population is affected.

Fig. 51-1 illustrates the overlap between therapeutic and toxic effects on a population. The horizontal (logarithmic) axis depicts a drug dosage of 1 to 10 U, while the vertical axis shows the cumulative percentage of treated individuals who have a response, that is, the percentage of the total population that is affected. The curve termed *therapeutic effect* applies to the designated drug effect, such as prevention of seizures in the case of phenytoin. A point on the curve at which 50% of the people are effectively treated is the ED_{50}. The *toxic effect* curve describes an unwanted effect, such as nausea, dizziness, or in extreme cases death. It is important to note that in this example, and indeed in many cases, the therapeutic and toxic dose ranges overlap. In some individuals a large dose is needed for treatment, whereas in other cases this same dosage can result in a toxic effect. Thus the therapeutic range usually describes the range of doses in which the desired effect occurs. However, in this range a few patients will not benefit from the drug, whereas others will have a toxic reaction. The reasons for such individual variability in response are many, including age, sex, race, health status, and genetic factors. All contribute to the distribution of the effect of an agent on a population.

One important quantitative parameter used in toxicology

is the dose necessary to cause the death of an animal. If increasing doses are given, an increasing percentage of animals will die. The lethal dose for 50% of the population, termed the LD_{50}, is an important value that is used for many drugs or agents. Table 51-2 shows the LD_{50} for a selected number of drugs and chemicals.[1] For humans, such values are extrapolated from survivors or deaths reported in the literature. The agent does not have to affect the entire population. If only 1% of the animals died at a given dose, the term would become LD_1, the dose lethal for 1% of the animals. If 99% died, the term would then be LD_{99}.

MECHANISMS OF TOXICITY

There are many ways in which toxic agents can cause their effects. They can be subtle, such as promoter molecules, which affect cells only if a carcinogen has been given, or dramatic, such as that of a caustic agent, which destroys tissue on contact. The examples listed in the box on p. 1020 illustrate only a few of the ways that toxic agents act.

FACTORS THAT INFLUENCE TOXICITY
Nature of toxicant

Solubility properties. One of the most important properties of a toxicant is its solubility in various tissues of the body. For example, toxicants that are water soluble are less likely to penetrate the skin. Those that are lipid soluble tend to be more readily absorbed; however, the ionic form of the chemical and its molecular size are also important chemical properties affecting the solubility.

Physical properties. Another important property of a toxicant is the physical state of the compound, whether gas, liquid, or solid. Gases are readily inhaled and pass immediately into circulation. In addition, they pass through skin. In contrast, liquids are not inhaled unless in a vaporous state or aerosol form. Liquids can, however, pass through the epi-

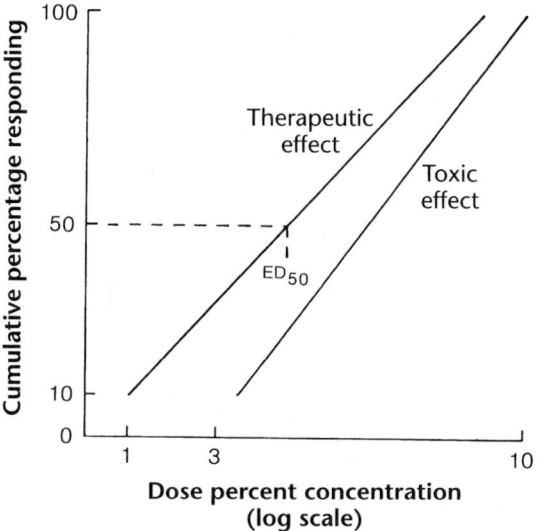

Fig. 51-1 Results of therapeutic and toxic effects on a population. *ED_{50},* Effective dose for 50% of population.

Table 51-2 Approximate LD_{50} of a selected variety of chemical agents

Agent	Animal	Route	LD_{50} (mg/kg)
Ethyl alcohol (ethanol)	Mouse	Oral	10,000
Sodium chloride	Mouse	i.p.	4,000
Ferrous sulfate	Rat	Oral	1,500
Morphine sulfate	Rat	Oral	900
Phenobarbital, sodium	Rat	Oral	150
DDT	Rat	Oral	100
Picrotoxin	Rat	s.c.	5
Strychnine sulfate	Rat	i.p.	2
Nicotine	Rat	i.v.	1
d-Tubocurarine	Rat	i.v.	0.5
Hemicholinium-3	Rat	i.v.	0.2
Tetrodotoxin	Rat	i.v.	0.10
Dioxin	Guinea pig	i.v.	0.001
Botulinus toxin	Rat	i.v.	0.00001

i.p., Intraperitoneal; *i.v.,* intravenous; *s.c.,* subcutaneous
From Loomis TA: *Essentials of toxicology,* ed 3, Philadelphia, 1978, Lea & Febiger.

Molecular Mechanisms of Toxicity*

Interference with enzyme action and systems
  Irreversible enzyme inhibition (organophosphates)
  Reversible enzyme inhibition (atropine)
  Uncoupling of oxidative phosphorylation (dinitrophenol)
  Synthesis of lethal compounds (fluoroacetic acid)
  Chelation of metals required for enzyme activity (dithiocarbamates)

Blockage of oxygen usage and transport
  Inhibition of cytochrome oxidase (cyanide)
  Inhibition of oxygen transport (carbon monoxide)
  Red blood cell lysis (arsine gas)

Interference with cell function
  Interaction with lipid phase of the cell membranes affecting its reaction to a depolarizing pulse (anesthetics)
  Interference with DNA and RNA synthesis (chemotherapeutic agents such as 5-fluorouracil, and many carcinogens)

Hypersensitivity reactions
  Immune reaction to specific chemicals (diisocyanates)

---

*Compounds in parentheses are examples of each class of toxic agent.

dermal barrier. Although particulates can be inhaled, they are not absorbed quickly through the skin. Solids usually must be ingested or dissolved before they have an effect. Compounds (such as mercury) with a liquid form that have a significant gas phase under exposure conditions can have an adequate amount of the compound in the gas phase to induce toxicity by vapor inhalation.

Exposure variables

Dose dependency. For common pharmacological agents or drugs, increased dosage results in an increase in the percentage of a population that will be affected and also an increase in the severity of the toxicological reaction. In contrast, continued exposure in very low concentrations can be noncumulative and relatively innocuous. Such an effect of concentration is observed with the drug acetaminophen. At low concentrations this analgesic is commonly used to treat pain and is metabolized in the liver to nontoxic forms by a pathway involving glutathione. At high concentrations of acetaminophen, this pathway is depleted of glutathione, and free radical damage occurs. This can irreversibly damage liver cells, causing cell death.

Also keep in mind that the symptoms of a toxicological response may not be obviously related to the intended clinical response to the drug. In the case of the tricyclic antidepressants, the desired effect is a mood elevation resulting from drug action on central nervous system receptors. When the drug is present in an overdose, it may affect similar receptors in the heart, causing arrhythmia. As the concentra-

tion of the tricyclic increases, so do the arrhythmias that can cause heart failure and death.

Route, rate, and site of administration. The route of administration can be percutaneous, inhalation, oral, rectal, subcutaneous, or intravenous. Of these routes, the percutaneous route is usually not considered in a hospital environment because most agents are given by the other routes. However, the skin has a very large surface and is permeable to many chemicals. Several new systems that deliver medications using transcutaneous membranes, or *patches,* have resulted in overdoses when the slow-release formulation was incorrectly made and the drug was released in a rapid manner.

Variation in the amounts of an agent causing death based on the route of administration can be quite large. For example, a twentyfold difference between the effect of procainamide given intravenously versus subcutaneously has been demonstrated. For other compounds, such as pentobarbital, there is less than a twofold difference in dosage between these two routes to achieve the same lethal effect. Thus the route of administration can lead to considerable differences in the dose-response curve to a toxic agent.

Duration and frequency of exposure. Duration of exposure is the time in seconds, minutes, hours, days, months, or years that a person is exposed to a toxicant. For some agents, such as carbon monoxide, the duration can be a few seconds or minutes, such as an exposure in a room with a high concentration of carbon monoxide, or chronic as in cigarette smoking. One calculation often used is *exposure time × dosage.* The derived value is used to compare persons with different levels of toxicant, such as the blood-lead levels of workers, and toxicological symptoms, such as renal disease. Frequent exposure in many cases leads to an accumulation of toxic effects, but this will vary, depending on the agent. An unusual case is that of a delayed hypersensitivity reaction, in which a minute amount of a substance can result in a toxic anaphylactic reaction, even though the amount may be subtoxic for the same person under presensitizing conditions.

Biological variables

Age affects the rate of metabolism of compounds. In general, younger subjects will metabolize a drug more rapidly than older ones. Older patients are often given the same dosage as younger ones; however, because their metabolism may be one half to one third as rapid as that of younger patients, the drug may build up to toxic levels. Part of the age difference is attributable to changes in organ function. For example, renal clearance in an aged population is 20% to 50% of that of young medical technology students.

Difference in genetic makeup can be one of the most dramatic factors influencing the toxic effect of an agent. Succinylcholine, a muscle relaxant, is hydrolyzed to succinic acid and choline. However, certain persons (1 in 3000) either do not have the enzyme that will hydrolyze this compound or have a defective form of the enzyme. Thus they have prolonged muscle relaxation and possible apnea (stoppage of breathing) and therefore are at risk when given this drug. It is possible to screen a population for this deficiency by measuring acetylcholinesterase levels in the presence of the inhibitor dibucaine and thus find those persons with this enzyme deficiency.

Another example of genetic differences in drug metabolism involves the ability to *N*-acetylate certain compounds. One drug, procainamide, is *N*-acetylated as part of the normal metabolic detoxification pathway. It has been found that there are two groups of persons, those who are fast acetylators and those who are slow acetylators. This may be characterized by a bimodal distribution (see Chapter 19). The slow acetylators who form *N*-acetylprocainamide at a less rapid rate are more likely to have an immunological reaction to the drug. However, the *N*-acetylated drug is cleared more slowly, thus leading to higher blood levels at a given dosage for fast acetylators. Thus drug levels are dependent on the *N*-acetylation rate.

Chiral pharmacology

Enantiomers of drugs are chiral drugs with four different chemical groups attached to a carbon atom, capable of rotating polarized light to the right or left, and are referred to as *d* or (+), and *l* or (−) respectively.[3,4] The properties of enantiomers may vary from identical to different efficacy and toxicity. To illustrate the difference in toxicology, *(S)*-(+)-methamphetamine has considerable abuse potential whereas *(R)*-(−)-methamphetamine is used as a nasal decongestant. Stereospecific immunoassay is capable of distinguishing these enantiomers in urine.

Toxicokinetics

The principles of toxicokinetics are similar to those of pharmacokinetics discussed in Chapter 56 on therapeutic drug monitoring. Most toxicants, such as gases or drugs, must pass through membranes or be absorbed and then pass through the circulation before they exert their effect on a particular target tissue; thus the first steps of liberation and absorption may be quite different in overdoses. In addition, many toxicants must be transformed by metabolic processes before they can exert action on receptor or cell. Finally, most drugs or compounds must be metabolized before they are excreted. In general one can use the same equations presented for therapeutic monitoring to follow these agents. However, often in overdose situations, as with phenytoin, the pattern of elimination can change from first order to zero order as the elimination pathways are saturated. Other toxicants, such as caustic agents (lye, acid, corrosives), have a direct tissue-damaging effect and thus are not studied in this manner.

Biotransformation of xenobiotics

Most chemicals or agents that enter the body (xenobiotics) undergo a change in structure termed *biotransformation*. There are numerous pathways for this to occur. A list of such reactions is presented in the box. Biotransformed molecules can have properties that make them biologically less active than, more active than, or as reactive as the parent compound. Atropine is hydrolyzed to the inactive moieties tropic acid and tropine. On the other hand, cyclophosphamide, an anticancer alkylating agent, must be activated by liver microsomes to be effective. Finally, the drug amitriptyline is demethylated to form nortriptyline, which is equipotent as a tricyclic antidepressant.

The microsomes of the liver contain a group of enzymes that oxidize various chemicals such as steroids, fatty acids, drugs, pesticides, and carcinogens. These microsomal systems are termed *mixed-function oxidases*. The last oxidase in this chain of oxidases is cytochrome P-450, so termed because of its spectral absorption at 450 nm. Recently, the P-450 superfamily (CYP) has been characterized, consisting of about 16 human genes.[5] Oxidation of a drug occurs by a reaction that involves oxygen, the drug or substrate, and the appropriate cytochrome P-450 enzyme:

$$\text{Substrate} + O_2 + \text{NADPH} + H^+ \xrightarrow{\text{Cytochrome P-450}} \text{Oxidized substrate} + H_2O + \text{NADP}^+$$

Many of the biotransformation reactions listed above are oxidations catalyzed by the microsomal cytochrome *CYP* superfamily; these include epoxidations, hydroxylations of aryl and alkyl hydrocarbons, oxidation of alcohols, removal of the alkyl group from ether type of linkages, *N*-hydroxylation, nitroxidation, *N*-dealkylations, oxidative deamination, sulfoxidation, and dehalogenation. For ex-

---

Biotransformation reactions of xenobiotics*

Azo reduction (azobenzene → aniline)
Nitro reduction (nitrobenzine → aniline)
Hydrolysis of esters (procaine → 2-diethylaminoethanol and *p*-aminobenzoic acid)
Acylation (procainamide → *N*-acetylprocainamide)
Conjugation with glucuronic acid (morphine → morphine glucuronide)
Conjugation with mercaptic acid (dichlorobenzene → dichlorobenzene mercaptic acid)
Oxidative deamination (amphetamine → phenylacetone)
Dealkylation (meperidine → normeperidine)
Aromatic ring oxidation (*n*-butylaniline → *n*-butyl-*p*-aminophenol)
N-oxidation (trimethylamine → trimethylamine oxide)
S-oxidation (chlorpromazine → chlorpromazine sulfoxide)
Oxidation of alcohols (benzyl alcohol → benzoic acid)
Hydroxylation of alkyl side chain (*p*-nitrotoluene → *p*-nitrobenzyl alcohol)

*Examples of each reaction are given in parentheses.

ample, the subfamily of *CYP2D6* catalyzes the hydroxylation of debrisoquin and amitriptyline. These enzyme reactions are induced by some drugs, such as phenobarbital or alcohol, and inhibited by others, such as cimetidine; thus administration of one of these drugs will change the rate of metabolism and effectively alter the steady-state level of the drug. In general, the drugs oxidized by the microsomal enzyme system are lipid soluble. After oxidation, they are more water soluble and thus more likely to be excreted. The P-450 system is under genetic control, and the variation in ability to metabolize drugs is attributable to these genetic differences in the P-450 systems.

DRUGS AND NONTHERAPEUTIC AGENTS ENCOUNTERED IN THE CLINICAL LABORATORY

One role of the clinical toxicology laboratory is to help the clinician determine whether a patient's pathological condition is the result of a toxic agent. Although a great many deaths are the result of poisonings, a far greater number of individuals are brought to the hospital with a diagnosis of potential poisoning. The physician must differentiate between a condition that is the result of poisoning and one that is not. Recent advances in immunoassay methodologies provide rapid point-of-care testings for a selected number of therapeutic and illicit drugs such as cocaine, cannabinoids, phencyclidine, amphetamines, barbiturates, and benzodiazepines. These rapid screening tests may enhance patient management.

Agents used in suicide

Table 51-3 gives the number of deaths from poisoning for the year 1991 by class of agent.[6] Most of these deaths are the result of suicides; the remainder are the result of accidental poisoning. It should be noted that most poisonings

are caused by agents that are easily available as over-the-counter medications or are prescribed for medicinal purposes; these include analgesics, tranquilizers, psychotropic agents, barbiturates, and others. The most frequent problem facing the laboratory is the determination of the agent employed in an attempted suicide. When depressed individuals are given access to potentially lethal agents, they often attempt suicide with these agents.

Drugs in emergency situations

In a hospital, particularly one involved in emergency care, the pattern of toxic drug ingestion or abuse observed in acutely ill patients is somewhat different from that seen in suicide. Table 51-4 lists the number of cases showing the presence of a particular class of drugs.[7] Notice that the major drugs or drug classes observed were cocaine, ethanol, opiates, acetaminophen, cannabinoids, antidepressants, and benzodiazepines. Again, prescription drugs make up a significant portion of the observed toxic agents. Most important is the observation that many patients will have ingested more than one drug. In one study about half the patients seen in an emergency room had ingested two or more drugs.[8] Drug screening tests are ordered for a variety of patients in emergency situations who may appear clinically hyperactive, hallucinating, or in coma. A description of the

Table 51-3 Number of deaths reported by drug category and calculated as a percentage of the number of exposures (potential poisonings)

Category	Number	Percentage of all exposures in category
Analgesics	190	0.104
Antidepressants	188	0.525
Sedative/hypnotics	97	0.166
Stimulants and street drugs	90	0.434
Cardiovascular drugs	87	0.348
Alcohols	72	0.143
Gases and fumes	49	0.188
Asthma therapies	39	0.229
Chemicals	37	0.069
Hydrocarbons	36	0.057
Cleaning substances	26	0.014
Pesticides (including rodenticides)	18	0.026

From Litovitz TL, Schmitz BF, Bailey KM: *Am J Emerg Med* 10:452-505, 1992.

Table 51-4 Drug screen results of the toxicology laboratory at the Johns Hopkins Hospital for the months of October, November, and December 1989

Pharmaceuticals	
Cocaine/metabolite	837
Ethanol	757
Opiates	677
Acetaminophen	373
Cannabinoids	311
Antidepressants	279
Benzodiazepines	218
Diphenhydramine	208
Salicylate	205
Methadone	203
Lidocaine	161
Barbiturates	156
Ephedrine/pseudoephedrine	138
Phenytoin	121
Phenothiazine/metabolites	121
Others	
Amphetamine	2
Carbamazepine	50
Phencyclidine	4
Nonpharmaceuticals	
Nicotine/cotinine	1691
Caffeine	1310
Quinine/quinidine	896
Methanol	5
Total drugs/substance identified	6874

From Wong SHY: *Crit Care Rep* 2:295-306, 1991.

various grades of coma in toxic cases is given by Hanenson as follows[9]:

Coma gradation

Grade 1—Drowsy but responds to verbal commands

Grade 2—Unconscious but responds to mild painful stimulus

Grade 3—Unconscious and responds only to maximum painful stimulus

Grade 4—Unconscious without response to painful stimulus

When a comatose or bizarrely acting patient is seen in an emergency room, the possibility of a drug overdose is one of the diagnoses that must be considered by a physician. For the most efficient use of laboratory facilities, it is important for the physician to try and ascertain the nature or identity of the drug or drugs used. A physician's judgment about the presence of intoxicating or lethal drugs is based on many clinical observations (Table 51-5). A history obtained from an alert patient can be helpful, though in general, patient history is not a reliable index of what drugs may have been taken (less than 50% reliability).

General effects of toxic agents can include symptoms such as respiratory depression, shock, convulsions, hyperthermia, or hypothermia. Some clinical effects and symptoms observed in patients intoxicated with very high doses of these agents are summarized in Table 51-5. The size of pupils, respiration rate, cardiac status, and the condition of other organ systems are all important signs and can provide information about the nature of the toxic substance. An alternative approach is to establish the toxidrome (toxic syndromes). Since drugs and poisons cause autonomic dysfunction with accompanying physical clues, toxidromes are listed in Table 51-6.[10]

If the physician suspects the presence of one or more drugs, laboratory tests may be ordered to confirm the presence of the drug or drugs and to determine the amount present. These data can establish the therapy to be used. If the clinician is not certain if drugs are present, a general drug screen may be ordered. The drug screen will rapidly test for the presence of some of the major drug groups; positive results should be confirmed by an alternative procedure (see p. 1026). Electrolytes, BUN, and glucose may also be ordered to rule out renal or diabetic disease states.

ANTIDOTES AND TREATMENT

The history of poisons is intertwined with that of antidotes. Currently there are only a few antidotes specific for those agents commonly observed in a hospital setting. These are presented in Table 51-7. Usually most therapy is supportive, involving treatment for respiratory depression, aspiration, shock, convulsions, delirium, methemoglobinemia, hyperthermia, and hypothermia. Supportive therapy is used to maintain a patient's vital functions until the body is cleared of the drug.

Removal of the toxic agent can often be effected by emesis (vomiting), gastric lavage, or skin decontamination. Other forms of treatment include agents that help remove the toxicant from the body. Dimercaprol is used to treat arsenic and mercury poisoning, and the salts of the divalent metals (lead, mercury, copper, nickel, zinc, cadmium, cobalt, beryllium, and manganese) are chelated by ethylenediaminetetraacetate (EDTA). The chemical deferoxamine is used to remove excess amounts of iron and aluminum. Charcoal may be swallowed or placed in the stomach to enhance the rate of removal of drug from the body. In the case of childhood lead poisoning specific protocols using BAL (British anti-Lewisite), EDTA, and succimer have been designed by the Centers for Disease Control and Prevention.

Many agents are removed more rapidly if urine flow is increased (forced diuresis). This is often accomplished by the intravenous administration of a diuretic such as mannitol. In addition, because of a lower concentration in the kidney under diuretic conditions, the potential for nephrotoxicity of some agents (such as cisplatin) is diminished. The

---

Table 51-5   Some clinical features of severe drug intoxication encountered in overdose cases

Class	Agent	Pupils	Respiration	Other
Analgesic	Acetaminophen	—	—	Liver toxicity
Hypnotic	Barbiturates	Dilated, light reactive	↓	Flaccid paralysis, hypothermia, hypotension
Minor tranquilizer	Benzodiazepines	—	↓	CNS depression, extrapyramidal system changes, autonomic nervous system changes, hypotension
Depressant	Ethanol	—	↓	CNS depression (in some, grand mal seizures)
Analgesic	Narcotics and propoxyphene	Pinpoint	↓	CNS depression
	Salicylates	—	↓	Metabolic acidosis (later)
Antidepressant	Tricyclics	Constricted	—	Tachycardia, arrhythmia
Stimulant	Cocaine	Dilated	↑	CNS effects, euphoria, agitation, seizures, cardiac effects, tachycardia

CNS, Central nervous system.
From Kulig K: *N Engl J Med* 326:1677-1681, 1992.

Table 51-6 The most common toxic syndromes

Anticholinergic syndromes

Common signs	Delirium with mumbling speech, tachycardia, dry, flushed skin, dilated pupils, myoclonus, slightly elevated temperature, urinary retention, and decreased bowel sounds. Seizures and dysrhythmias may occur in severe cases.
Common causes	Antihistamines, antiparkinsonian medication, atropine, scopolamine, amantadine, antipsychotic agents, antidepressant agents, antispasmodic agents, mydriatic agents, skeletal-muscle relaxants, and many plants (notably jimsonweed and *Amanita muscaria*).

Sympathomimetic syndromes

Common signs	Delusions, paranoia, tachycardia (or bradycardia if the drug is a pure alpha-adrenergic agonist), hypertension, hyperpyrexia, diaphoresis, piloerection, mydriasis, and hyperreflexia. Seizures, hypotension, and dysrhythmias may occur in severe cases.
Common causes	Cocaine, amphetamine, methamphetamine (and its derivatives 3,4-methylenedioxyamphetamine, 3,4-methylenedioxymethamphetamine, 3,4-methylenedioxyethamphetamine, and 2,5-dimethoxy-4-bromoamphetamine), and over-the-counter decongestants (phenylpropanolamine, ephedrine, and pseudoephedrine). In caffeine and theophylline overdoses, similar findings, except for the organic psychiatric signs, result from catecholamine release.

Opiate, sedative, or ethanol intoxication

Common signs	Coma, respiratory depression, miosis, hypotension, bradycardia, hypothermia, pulmonary edema, decreased bowel sounds, hyporeflexia, and needle marks. Seizures may occur after overdoses of some narcotics, notably propoxyphene.
Common causes	Narcotics, barbiturates, benzodiazepines, ethchlorvynol, glutethimide, methyprylon, methaqualone, meprobamate, ethanol, clonidine, and guanabenz.

Cholinergic syndromes

Common signs	Confusion, central nervous system depression, weakness, salivation, lacrimation, urinary and fecal incontinence, gastrointestinal cramping, emesis, diaphoresis, muscle fasciculations, pulmonary edema, miosis, bradycardia or tachycardia, and seizures.
Common causes	Organophosphate and carbamate insecticides, physostigmine, edrophonium, and some mushrooms.

From Kulig K: *N Engl J Med* 326:1677-1681, 1992.

Table 51-7 Specific antagonists and antidotes

Drug or toxin	Antagonist or antidote
Acetaminophen	Methionine, *N*-acetylcysteine
Amphetamines	Chlorpromazine
Anticholinergic drugs (tricyclic antidepressants, atropine, scopolamine)	Physostigmine
Benzodiazepines	Flumazenil
Beta-adrenergic receptor blockers	Glucagon
Calcium-channel blockers, hydrofluoric acid, fluorides	Calcium
Carbon monoxide	Oxygen
Cyanide	Sodium nitrite
Isoniazid, hydrazine, monomethylhydrazine (in *Gyromitra* species of mushrooms)	Pyridoxine
Methanol, ethylene glycol	Ethanol
Nitrates and nitrites	Methylene blue
Opiates	Naloxane
Organophosphates	Atropine and pralidoxime
Tricyclic antidepressants	Bicarbonate

pH of urine is also important. For basic drugs such as the amphetamines, excretion is enhanced by an acid urine, in which the drugs are ionized. Barbiturate excretion is increased by alkaline urine, in which the molecule is ionized and therefore more soluble.

DRUG INTERACTIONS

When two drugs are given to a patient, their actions may not be independent; that is, one drug may affect the pharmacological action of the other. This phenomenon is called *drug interaction*. The effects of drug interactions are not obvious, and much information about these phenomena has been gathered from case reports. Many types of interactions have been noted, and it is not possible to provide a comprehensive list here. Stockley[11] has listed the types of interactions, though he notes that "interactions which occur when drugs are given concurrently are often the result of not a single mechanism, but of two or more mechanisms acting in concert. . . ." Table 51-8 gives this listing with an example of each type of interaction.

Important drug interactions are observed between ethanol and other agents that affect the central nervous system. Ethanol is frequently encountered in drug interactions because of its wide usage and because ethanol has a wide range of depressant effects on the central nervous system. For example, the concomitant use of the barbiturates and alcohol can have deleterious effects. The lethal dose of barbiturates is almost 50% lower when combined with alcohol. This same effect occurs with concomitant use of alcohol and agents such as chloral hydrate, paraldehyde, glutethimide, meprobamate, and other tranquilizers.

Table 51-8 Examples of classes of drug interactions.

Action	Example
Drugs with similar effects	Multiple nephrotoxic drugs such as gentamicin and cephalosporin yield increased nephrotoxicity.
Drugs with opposing effects	Hynotics and caffeine result in antagonism to the hypnotic effect.
Absorption interactions	Tetracycline and iron (Fe^{++}) supplement result in decreased oral uptake of drug.
Drug displaced interactions	Theoretical displacement of bound drug from albumin yields increased free-drug level.
Drug metabolism interactions	
Enzyme induction	Barbiturates stimulate microsomal oxidation of drugs such as dicumarol, resulting in lower plasma levels.
Enzyme inhibition	Cimetidine blocks the P-450 oxidation pathway, slowing theophylline metabolism and resulting in a longer half-life and higher plasma levels.
Altered excretion interactions	
Changes in urine pH	Acid urine enhances basic drug excretion. The reverse is true for acidic drugs.
Competition for active tubular secretion	Probenecid decreases the active secretion of drugs such as penicillin, thus increasing serum levels.
Interactions at adrenergic neurons	Tricyclic antidepressants prevent the uptake of guanethidine into neurons, thus blocking its antihypertensive effect.

MEDICOLEGAL ASPECTS

Technologists in the toxicology laboratory may become involved in the medicolegal system because of their need to document under oath the validity of analytical results. The technologist may also have to document the laboratory's procedures and produce a chain-of-custody document (see Chapter 3) to ensure that the specimen was not tampered with.

For some types of testing, such as screening for the presence of abused drugs, the methods of screening by immunoassay and confirmation by gas chromatography or mass spectroscopy may be specified by a federal agency such as the Substance Abuse Mental Health Service Administration (SAMHSA) (formerly the National Institute for Drug Abuse). The current testing for abused substances (alcohol, marijuana, cocaine, heroin, amphetamines, phencyclidine) is based on the assumption that the use of certain drugs, particularly cocaine and marijuana, may be illegal and that individuals will have impaired performance, affecting their job or resulting in an accident. In either case, litigation involving a civil or a criminal suit may result. The laboratory's role is to supply and document legally admissible and defendable data.

METHODS OF ANALYSIS

Acetaminophen

HELEN M. DODDS
JULIA M. POTTER

Principles of analysis A variety of chromatographic and spectrophotometric methods for both the qualitative and quantitative measurement of acetaminophen have been described. The most commonly performed qualitative test for the detection of acetaminophen in urine is the "spot test" (Table 51-9, method 1). This sensitive and inexpensive method is based upon the reaction of the conjugated metabolites of acetaminophen with *o*-cresol in ammonium hydroxide to produce a blue-indigo color (indophenol blue). The spot test exhibits good sensitivity; a positive spot test result can be obtained in a urine sample collected 24 hours after ingestion of 1 g of acetaminophen. False-positive spot test results can be seen in patients who have taken *p*-aminophenol because both acetaminophen and *p*-aminophenol are metabolized to phenacetin, which produces a positive test result.

Another qualitative method for the detection of acetaminophen is thin-layer chromatography on silica gel (see Chapter 5 for a description of the principles of thin-layer chromatography).

Quantitative analysis of acetaminophen was originally based on spectrophotometric methods but have since been largely replaced by immunoassay procedures. The original spectrophotometric methods were time consuming. The modified spectrophotometric method of Glynn and Kendal[12] (Table 51-9, method 2) exhibits adequate sensitivity and has no known interferences. In this procedure, plasma is deproteinized by trichloroacetic acid followed by centrifugation. An aliquot of the protein-free supernatant is then mixed with 6 M hydrochloric acid and sodium nitrite to form a nitrous acid derivative. In the final step of the assay, sulfamic acid is added followed by the addition of sodium hydroxide, resulting in the production of a yellow color, which is read at 430 nm.

High-performance liquid chromatographic (HPLC) procedures have also been employed for acetaminophen analysis. Approaches used include purification of the analyte using cation exchange and silica absorption. Reversed-phase HPLC has been suggested as a possible reference method for acetaminophen quantitation (Table 51-9, method 3).[13]

The most popular assays currently in use to measure acetaminophen are immunoassays. One frequently used immunoassay procedure (Syva Co., Palo Alto, CA 94303) employs a homogeneous enzyme immunoassay technique (EMIT) (Table 51-9, method 4). In this procedure, acetaminophen in the patient's sample competes with glucose-6-phosphate dehydrogenase–labeled acetaminophen for binding to antibody directed against acetaminophen. Binding of enzyme-labeled acetaminophen to antibody results in inhibition of enzyme activity. Thus, in cases where high concentrations of acet-

Table 51-9   Methods for acetaminophen analysis

Method	Principle	Usage	Comments
1. Spot test	Acetaminophen reacts with o-cresol to produce indophenol blue colored comple.	Urine Screening test	Qualitative Sensitive
2. Spectrophotometric (nitro dye formation)	Absorbance of product is monitored at 430 nm.	Plasma Infrequently used	Linear in range of 100 to 500 μg/mL Specific
3. High-performance liquid chromatography (HPLC) (reversed phase)	Chromatographic separation of acetaminophen utilizing column packed with 10-octadecylsilane-coated silica columns with water/acetic acid/ethyl acetate mobile phase.	Possible reference method	Most sensitive (1 μg/mL)
4. Enzyme-multiplied immunoassay technique (EMIT)	Competitive binding assay. Drug in patient sample competes with drug-enzyme complex for limited number of binding sites on acetaminophen antibody. Binding of drug-enzyme complex to antibody inhibits enzyme activity. Amount of active enzyme is directly related to drug concentration.	Frequently used	Automated Available on stat. basis
5. Fluorescence polarization	Competitive binding assay. Drug in patient sample competes with fluorescein-labeled drug for limited number of antibody-binding sites. Amount of polarized light emitted from reaction vessel is inversely related to drug concentration.	Most frequently used	Automated Available on stat. basis Requires specialized equipment

aminophen are present in the patient's sample, less of the enzyme-labeled acetaminophen will be bound by antibody resulting in greater enzyme activity. The NADH formed as a result of enzyme activity is monitored spectrophotometrically at 340 nm.

Another popular immunoassay procedure for acetaminophen analysis utilizes the principle of fluorescence polarization (Table 51-9, method 5). This assay is based on competitive binding between acetaminophen in the patient's sample and fluorescein-labeled acetaminophen for a limited amount of antibody. Specimens containing high concentrations of acetaminophen will exhibit decreased emission of polarized fluorescent light because few fluorescein-labeled acetaminophen complexes are bound to antibody. Little or no acetaminophen present in patient sample results in more fluorescein-labeled acetaminophen being bound to antibody and in a greater amount of plane-polarized fluorescent light being emitted.

Specimen   Serum or plasma can be used with the quantitative procedures. For the spot test, urine is the specimen employed.

Therapeutic range   Therapeutic concentration of acetaminophen in serum or plasma is 10 to 20 μg/mL (66 to 132 μmol/L). In cases of toxic ingestion of acetaminophen, a concentration of greater than 200 μg/mL 4 hours after ingestion, or a half-life of greater than 4 hours, indicates the potential for serious liver damage by free radicals and other

toxic metabolites that result from hepatic metabolism of acetaminophen. In these situations, treatment with *N*-acetylcysteine (Mucomyst) may provide protection. This compound helps to replenish gluthathione, which is consumed by the liver in the metabolism of acetaminophen and prevents the production of toxic free radicals. Fig. 51-2 shows a nomogram developed for estimating the severity of liver damage as a function of plasma acetaminophen concentrations at various times after ingestion.

Drug screen
F. MICHAEL HASSAN

Principles of analysis   The rapid analysis of urine for drugs of abuse is important for the detection of acute drug overdoses. Drug testing is also now used for preemployment screening, for monitoring compliance of patients enrolled in drug rehabilitation programs, and in the investigation of accident-related injuries.

A two-tiered approach is commonly employed for testing for drugs of abuse, typically screening and confirmation tests. Samples that give a positive test result using a screening procedure may be subject to further testing by use of a different method from that originally used in order to confirm the presence of the drug of interest. Ideally, screening procedures should be simple, rapid, inexpensive, and capable of automation.[14] Screening procedures may be performed for the detection of a particular drug or class of drug, or may

Table 51-10   Spot tests

Drug	Specimen used	Reaction	Test time (min)	Comments	Reference
Acetaminophen	Urine	o-Cresol + Acetaminophen $\xrightarrow{\text{NH}_4\text{OH}}$ *Blue color*	15	Highly sensitive and relatively specific	16
Ethanol	Urine, serum	Microdiffusion into dichromate $2K_2Cr_2O_7 + 10H_2SO_4 + 3C_2H_5OH \rightarrow$ $2Cr_2(SO_4)_4 + 2K_2SO_4 + 3CH_3COOH$ $+ 11H_2O + 4H^+$ *(green to blue color)*	15-30	Good sensitivity Nonspecific for ethanol	17
Salicylate	Urine, serum	Trinder's solution Salicylate + FeCl$_3$ → *Violet-colored complex*	2	Good specificity if serum used Good sensitivity	18
Carbamates (meprobamate)	Urine	Furfural + Meprobamate + Antimony trichloride → *Black color on thin-layer chromatography plate*	5	Not specific for meprobamate Good sensitivity	19
Imipramine/ desipramine	Urine	Forrest reagent K$_2$CrO$_3$ (acidic) + Imipramine → *Green-colored complex*	2	Phenothiazines may interfere	20
Ethchlorvynol	Urine, serum	Diphenylamine + Ethchlorvynol in acid → *Red color*	10	Good sensitivity and specificity	21
Phenothiazines	Urine	FPN reagent (ferric chloride/perchloric acid/nitric acid) + Phenothiazines → *Red- to violet-colored complex*	2	Nonspecific Poor sensitivity for some phenothiazines	22
Iron	Serum	Bathophenanthroline color change with iron *(blue)*	15	Will not react at normal serum concentrations	23

entail the analysis for as many drugs as is technically and economically feasible. When screening for a single particular drug, the screening test that is used should ensure adequate sensitivity and specificity for accurate identification of the compound of interest. When the drug screen entails a comprehensive analysis for a large number of drug compounds, less specific assays that enable the detection of many different compounds may be employed.

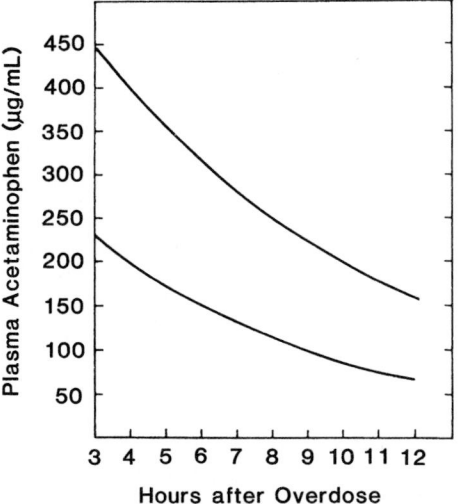

Fig. 51-2   Plasma acetaminophen concentration in relation to time after an acute overdose. Liver damage is likely to be severe above upper line, severe to mild between lines, and clinically insignificant under lower line. (From Prescott LF, Sutherland GR, Park J, et al: *Lancet* 2:109-113, 1976.)

Typically, six or seven different classes of drugs are analyzed in a limited drug screen. Compounds usually screened for, which are listed by the Department of Health and Human Services for workplace drug testing, include cocaine metabolite, benzoylecgonine; opiates; amphetamines; tetrahydrocannabinol; and phencyclidine.[15] Other classes of drugs also included in many comprehensive screening procedures include barbiturate and benzodiazepines.

Methods for analysis of drugs of abuse can be divided into several categories based on the general analytical procedure employed. The major categories include spot tests, immunoassay-based procedures, and chromatographic procedures. The spot tests are the simplest and most rapid of those methods in use for screening. These tests may be used for the detection of a specific drug, such as acetaminophen or salicylate, or for a class of drugs, such as phenothiazines. Spot tests do not usually require any type of specimen pretreatment; unprocessed urine or serum is added directly to the test reagent. Presence of the drug (or drugs) of interest is indicated by the formation of a colored reaction product. Table 51-10 lists spot tests commonly used by laboratories. Although spot tests offer the advantages of simplicity and rapid turnaround time, many suffer from lack of specificity for the drug or class of drug the test is designed to measure. In addition, because the formation of a colored complex resulting from the presence of drug is visually determined, spot tests are very subjective in interpretation, especially when only a faint color change is present.

The development and automation of immunoassay-based procedures have become the most widely used methods for detection of drugs of abuse. Radioimmunoassay (RIA) procedures were the first to be developed; however, these have been replaced by enzyme immunoassays and fluorescence polarization methods. The RIA methods suffer from various practical drawbacks including short reagent shelf-life, special reagent handling and waste disposal requirements, and lack of completely automated analysis.[14]

The homogeneous enzyme immunoassays, such as the EMIT System (Syva Co., Palo Alto, CA 94303) (Table 51-11, method 1) are well established and widely used for screening for drugs of abuse in urine (DAU). This procedure is based on competitive binding between nonlabeled drug present in the patients' sample and enzyme-labeled drug for antibody. These assays may be performed with urine or serum being used as specimen and offer good sensitivity and specificity for a wide variety of drugs. The assays must be performed separately for each individual drug or class of drug being evaluated. Quantitative results may also be obtained.

Fluorescence polarization (Abbott Labs, Chicago, IL 60064) assays are also widely used and provide good sensitivity and specificity for detection of drugs. These assays utilize a six-point calibration curve and also can provide quantitative results.

A second homogeneous immunoassay system, the cloned enzyme donor immunoassay (CEDIA) method[22] (Table 51-11, method 2) is also available for drug analyses. In this procedure, the enzyme β-galactosidase is produced as two inactive enzyme fragments, termed an *enzyme donor* and an *enzyme acceptor fragment*. The enzyme donor fragment is conjugated to the drug of interest to be measured in the pa-

tient's specimen. In the absence of drug in the patient's specimen, antibody directed against the drug of interest binds to a drug–enzyme donor conjugate. This binding of antibody to the enzyme donor–drug conjugate prevents the association of enzyme donor and enzyme acceptor fragments to form active enzyme. On the other hand, if drug is present in the patient's specimen, the drug will compete with the drug–enzyme donor conjugate for antibody-binding sites. The more drug present in the patient specimen, the greater the likelihood that enzyme donor and enzyme acceptor fragments will be able to form active enzyme. The amount of active enzyme formed is directly related to the concentration of drug in the sample. The active enzyme is monitored by the conversion of the enzyme substrate galactopyranoside to a colored product.

Another new immunoassay methodology for drugs of abuse is the kinetic interaction of microparticles in solution, or KIMS (Table 51-11, method 3). In this turbidimetric procedure, the drug of interest to be measured is conjugated to microparticles in the reagent. Binding of specific antidrug antibody to the drug-microparticle conjugates results in the formation of microparticle-antibody lattices, which block transmission of light, resulting in increased absorbance of the reaction solution. Addition of patient specimen containing the drug results in competition between the drug and the drug-microparticle conjugates for binding to antibody present in the reagent. Thus, high concentrations of the drug of interest causes an inhibition of microparticle-lattice formation and increased transmission of light through the re-

Table 51-11   Methods of analysis for drugs of abuse

Method	Principle	Usage	Comments
1. Enzyme immunoassay (EIA)	Competitive binding between drug in patient's urine and enzyme-labeled drug for antibody.	Most frequently used Serum, urine	Good sensitivity and specificity Quantitative results available
2. Cloned enzyme donor immunoassay (CEDIA)	Competitive binding between patient drug and drug conjugated to enzyme-donor fragment. Binding of antibody to drug–enzyme-donor conjugate prevents reassociation of enzyme-donor and enzyme-acceptor fragments to produce active enzyme. Amount of active enzyme is directly proportional to drug concentration in specimen.	Urine	Automated
3. Kinetic interaction of microparticles in solution (KIMS)	Competitive binding between drug in patient specimen and drug conjugated to microparticles. Lack of drug in patient specimen results in antibody binding predominately to microparticles causing formation of microparticle-antibody lattices, which block transmission of light through reagent solution resulting in increased reagent absorbance.	Urine	Automated
4. Thin-layer chromatography (TLC)	Drug is extracted from specimen and subjected to chromatography. Chromatographically-separated drug is identified by its specific chemical reaction and chromatography properties.	Frequently used	Subjective Not automated Limited sensitivity

agent solution with subsequent low measured absorbance. The concentration of drug is inversely related to absorbance of the reaction mixture.

An immunoassay that provides a simultaneous and discrete visual detection of seven drug classes in 10 minutes is available (Triage DOA; Biosite Diagnostics, San Diego, CA 92121).[23] This system uses an immunochemical technique utilizing seven different monoclonal antibodies to analyze multiple analytes simultaneously in a competitive-binding mode. The conjugate-label consists of a representative drug of each class that is conjugated to a colloid gold particle. Urine sample containing one or more drugs results in competition between the free drug and conjugated drug for antibody-binding sites. Competition between the free drug and conjugated drugs results in some of the drug conjugates not being bound to antibody. After a 10-minute incubation period, the reaction mixture is transferred to a detection area consisting of a nylon membrane containing monoclonal antibodies immobilized on the membrane. Urine specimens that contain the drug or drugs being measured will result in some of the drug conjugates not being bound by antibody in the reaction mixture. The drug conjugates that are not bound by antibody in the initial phase of the assay will be captured by the second immobilized antibody resulting in the production of a colored band in the zone corresponding to each positive drug. The presence or absence of the color bands are visually determined.

The use of chromatographic procedures, such as thin-layer chromatography (TLC) (Table 51-11, method 4), has the advantage that no instrumentation is required and the procedure is relatively inexpensive to perform.[24] This procedure also enables the simultaneous detection of a large number of drugs. Although the sensitivity of TLC is not as good as the immunoassay procedures, it is adequate to identify the patient with a drug overdose as well as recreational drug users. TLC does not offer stat. capabilities because the assay may take up to 3 hours to perform. The assay is also labor intensive and subject to interpretive errors. TLC analysis has largely been replaced by immunoassays.

High-performance liquid chromatography (HPLC) and gas chromatography (GC) enables complex mixtures of drugs to be separated and quantitated. Analysis of drugs of abuse by chromatographic techniques has been a multistep procedure requiring sample extraction, elution, and data reduction. As a result of its labor-intensive nature, the use of HPLC and GC for screening for drugs of abuse has been limited. An automated HPLC System (REMEDI; Bio-Rad Laboratories, Hercules, CA 94547) has been introduced; it utilizes a multicolumn approach for drug extraction and separation. Drugs or metabolites are identified by ultraviolet scanning with subsequent identification performed by matching the relative retention time and spectral characteristics with an "on-line" drug library stored within the systems computer. This system has a high degree of automation, ease of operation, and a relatively rapid analysis time of approximately 30 minutes.

Specimen Various biological specimens including urine, gastric lavage or emesis, and serum or plasma may be submitted for screening for drugs of abuse. Urine is generally considered the optimal specimen because it is generally easy to obtain, and most drugs are found in sufficient quantities to be identified. Disadvantages of using urine as specimen include the finding of many metabolic products hampering identification, and the fact that parent drug is often not present. In addition, quantitation of drugs in urine usually does not correlate with the clinical effects of the drug. Analysis of gastric lavage or emesis offers the advantage that the parent drug may be present, though drugs that are quickly absorbed or those drugs not orally ingested will not be detected. In addition, interference from ingested foodstuffs hampers identification. Analysis of serum or plasma enables the identification of the parent drug, and quantitation may aid in patient management. Disadvantages of serum or plasma screening include the limitations of the sample volume available, the low concentration of drug, and the inability to identify certain drugs in patients in a nonoverdose situation.

Lead

M. WILSON TABOR

Principles of analysis One early method developed to measure lead in both biological and environmental samples is the dithizone (diphenylthiocarbazone) compleximetric method (Table 51-12, method 1).[25] In this procedure, samples (blood, urine, or tissue) are ashed by use of acid oxidation with heating to 400° C to remove organic material. After ashing, the sample is redissolved in acidified water and then alkalinized with $KCN-NH_4^+$ to a pH of 9 or 10. Cyanide is next added to prevent side reactions with other metals, and then the sample is reacted with diphenylthiocarbazone to produce a red lead-dithizonate complex. The complex is extracted into chloroform, and its absorbance is measured at 510 nm. This procedure is tedious and time consuming, requires large quantities of clean glassware and reagents, and is subject to interference from tin (II), bismuth, and thallium.

The most frequently used technique to measure lead is by atomic absorption spectroscopy (AAS), usually flameless AA (FAAS). In the classical AAS method (Table 51-12, method 2a) the sample is ashed by use of a procedure similar to that described for the dithizone procedure. After ashing of the sample, the solution containing ionic lead is aspirated into an air-acetylene flame where the lead is reduced to the atomic state P^0. Quantitation of the lead is performed by spectrophotometric measurement of the light absorbed by the lead at its characteristic resonance frequency of 283.3 nm. Numerous variations of this procedure have been described.[26,27]

The Delves microscale technique (Table 51-12, method 2b) is one variation of AAS that is commonly used for measurement of lead in blood or urine.[28] This procedure does not utilize the sample ashing procedure. Instead, the specimen is added to a special nickel cup that contains hydrogen peroxide, which partially oxidizes the sample. The advantages of this technique include the use of a small sample size and improved speed of analysis because of minimal sample pretreatment. However, variations in the quality of sample cups requires careful attention.

The most widely used and recommended procedure for measuring serum lead is the "flameless" or electrothermal AA procedure, also referred to as the graphite furnace[29] and carbon rod techniques[30] (Table 51-12, method 2c). In the electrothermal procedures, sample is applied to a graphite tube or carbon rod. The sample is usually mixed with a "matrix modifier," which places the lead in a constant form and minimizes matrix interferences. The graphite tube is then heated by electrical resistance in a stepwise sequence; a drying temperature of 100° C, a charring temperature of 400° C, and finally an atomization temperature of 2000° to 2500° C. The charring step removes inorganic and organic material that might interfere in the assay. Atomization results in the production of Pb^0 vapor, which absorbs light at 280.2 and 283.3 nm. Because the Pb^0 formed during atomization quickly escapes by diffusion, the signal is generated over only a few seconds. The concentration of lead in the sample is usually calculated from the absorbance peak area.[31]

Another technique of lead analysis is the electrochemical method of anodic stripping voltammetry (ASV) (Table 51-12, method 3). This method is widely used for measurement of lead in biological samples. In this procedure, ionic lead in blood or urine is reduced to elemental lead by the negative potential of a mercury electrode:

$$Pb^{++} + 2e^- \rightarrow Pb^0 \text{ (deposited on mercury electrode)}$$

After a preselected time interval, the potential of the mercury electrode is adjusted to more positive values, resulting in the reoxidation of lead from the electrode. The reoxidation of lead results in the production of an anodic current that is proportional to the concentration of lead in the specimen.

$$Pb^0 \text{ (from mercury electrode)} \rightarrow Pb^{++} + 2e^-$$

The ASV methods have had difficulty reaching the sensitivity to measure blood lead below the required reference interval's upper limit of 100 μg/L, though recent improvements to the method may have resolved this problem. The ASV technique has a wide linear range of approximately 60 to 10,000 μg/L.[32] Disadvantages of this technique are the interference from thallium, which can occur when lead and thallium are present in the specimen at comparable concentrations, and its relatively low throughput.

Specimen For the determination of lead in humans, whole blood is the specimen of choice though urine can also be used. Lead-free vacutainers containing heparin or EDTA may be used. Extreme care must be taken to prevent external contamination of the specimen. Lead-free blood sampling tubes are commercially available (Becton Dickinson, Rutherford, NJ 07070).

Table 51-12 Methods for analysis of lead

Method	Principle	Usage	Comments
1. Spectrophotometric	Sample is ashed, dissolved in acidified water, and then reacted with diphenyl-thiocarbazone to form red complex. Complex is extracted into chloroform, and absorbance is measured at 510 nm.	Rarely used Blood, urine, tissues, environmental	Technically demanding Does not require expensive equipment
2. Atomic absorption spectrometry (AAS) a. Classical	Sample is ashed, and ionized lead is reduced in heat of acetylene flame. Atomic lead absorbs light at 283.3 nm.	Rarely used Blood, urine, environmental	Fairly simple to perform Requires expensive equipment
b. Delves microscale technique	Same procedure as in 2a, except that ashing of sample is not performed. Instead, sample is oxidized in nickel microcup by H_2O_2.	Infrequently used Blood, urine	Same as in 2a Applicable to microsample
c. Graphite furnace or carbon rod (FAAS).	Same procedure as in 2a, except that sample is ashed, dried, and vaporized on a graphite platform in furnace.	Most frequently used Blood, urine	Same as in 2b Semiautomatable Recommended
3. Anodic stripping voltammetry (ASV)	Ionic lead in solution is reduced to elemental lead at negative Hg electrode. Potential is then adjusted to more positive values causing reoxidation of lead from Hg electrode. Resulting anodic current caused by oxidation is measured and is proportional to lead concentration.	Frequently used Blood, urine	Simple to perform Wide analytical range

Lead can be lost during storage by its absorption onto the container used for its storage. Up to 80% of lead can be lost after storage for 1 week.[33] The addition of 1% nitric acid or 3% hydrogen peroxide to the specimen will help preserve samples for up to 5 days.[34] Samples collected in EDTA (1.5 mg/mL of blood) and frozen at $-20°$ C are stable for several months.[35] With EDTA as anticoagulant and with a chemical method of analysis chosen, calcium chloride (1.4 mg/mL of blood) must be added to enhance the recovery of lead from the specimen.[35]

Urine for lead determinations must be collected in lead-free bottles. Thymol (500 mg/L of urine) should be added as preservative. Properly collected and preserved specimens are stable for up to 1 week if kept refrigerated.

Reference interval Exposure of individuals to lead may be classified as either occupational or environmental. Occupational exposure limits for blood lead concentration in workers has been set at 600 μg/L (2.9 μmol/L).[36] At this concentration of lead, effects of lead on good health may be observed. The approximate range for lead in the blood of individuals who are environmentally exposed is 100 to 200 μg/L (483 to 9654 nmol/L). Values in children are lower than those found in adults; values <100 μg/L are considered safe for children.[36] Male children and adults have been reported to have blood and urine lead concentrations up to 20% higher than those concentrations found in female children and adults.[37]

Salicylates

ROSS L. G. NORRIS
DONALD DAVIS
JULIA M. POTTER

Principles of analysis Acetylsalicylic acid (aspirin) is a commonly used analgesic that is responsible for a substantial number of accidental poisonings in children. Acetylsali-

cylic acid is hydrolyzed to salicylic acid and acetic acid within the stomach, allowing the salicylic acid to be readily absorbed into blood.

The most common methods in use for measurement of salicylates are still spectrophotometric. The most frequently used spectrophotometric procedure is based on absorbance changes at 540 nm that occur as a result of the production of a colored complex formed after the reaction of salicylate with ferric ion (Table 51-13, method 1a). A variety of modifications to this procedure have been suggested including extraction of salicylate into acidified ethylene dichloride to eliminate interference from salicylate metabolites[38] and protein precipitation with mercuric chloride and hydrochloric acid.[39] This latter modification, proposed by Trinder,[39] has been automated and is one of the most common procedures in use (ACA Discrete Analyzer, Wilmington, Delaware). This automated procedure utilizes a blank reading to enhance assay specificity.

Another type of spectrophotometric procedure employs a mixture of phosphotungstic acid and phosphomolybdic acid (Folin-Ciocalteu reagent) to reduce salicylates to a blue complex that can be measured at 660 nm (Table 51-13, method 1b).[40] This procedure is subject to interference from endogenous substrates including tryptophan, tyrosine, and uric acid; all react to form blue complexes.

A commonly used procedure for salicylate determination is fluorescence polarization (FPIA) (Table 51-13, method 2). This assay is based on the competitive binding of fluorescein-labeled salicylate and salicylate present in patient sample for a limited number of antibody binding sites. See Chapter 13 for a description of the FPIA technique.

The enzyme-multiplied immunoassay technique (EMIT) (Table 51-13, method 3) is another frequently used competitive immunoassay procedure for measuring salicylate. The

Table 51-13 Methods for salicylate analysis

Method	Principle	Usage	Comments
1. Spectrophotometry			
a. Ferric nitrate complex	Salicylate reacts with Fe^{3+} to form colored complex ($A_{max}=$, 540 nm)	One of most common methods in use	Automated
b. Folin-Ciocalteu reagent reduction	Phosphotungstic acid + phosphomolybolic acid reduces salicylates to form blue complex (A_{max}, 660 nm)	Not commonly used	Subject to tryptophan, tyrosine and uric acid interference
2. Fluorescence polarization (FPIA)	Competition between fluorescein-labeled salicylate and patient salicylate for limited number of antibody-binding sites	One of most common methods in use	Automated, interference from endogenous fluorescence
3. Enzyme-multiplied immunoassay technique (EMIT)	Competition between enzyme-labeled salicylate and salicylate in patient sample for binding to antibody. Binding of antibody to enzyme-labeled salicylate results in inhibition of enzymatic activity	Commonly used	Automated
4. Gas-liquid chromatography	Acetylsalicylate and metabolites extracted with ether	Candidate for reference method For research use	Very sensitive No interfering compounds

general principle of this spectrophotometric assay is described in Chapter 13.

The candidate reference method for salicylate determinations employs a chromatographic separation by gas-liquid chromatography (GLC) with flame ionization detection (Table 51-13, method 4).[41] This procedure allows for quantitation of acetylsalicylate and its metabolites after their extraction from plasma into diethyl ether, along with *p*-toluic acid, an internal standard. The ether is then evaporated and bis(trimethylsilyl)trifluoroacetamide (BSTFA) is added to the residue and heated. An aliquot of this mixture is then analyzed by GLC.

Specimen Serum or plasma may by used. For the automated modified Trinder colorimetric procedure, use of plasma should be restricted to heparinized plasma. In addition, sodium azide at concentrations of 1 mg/mL (15.4 mmol/L) has been shown to increase results significantly.

Therapeutic range Therapeutic ranges for total salicylates in serum need to be interpreted in context to the condition being treated. For use as an analgesic or antipyretic, the therapeutic range is less than 100 μg/mL (<0.72 mmol/L). If used as an anti-inflammatory agent, therapeutic concentrations are from 150 to 300 μg/mL (1.09 to 2.17 mmol/L). Nausea, vomiting, and hyperventilation may be observed at concentrations of 250 to 400 μg/mL (1.81 to 2.90 mmol/L), but concentrations greater than 600 μg/mL (4.34 mmol/L) are often lethal.

REFERENCES

1. Loomis TA: Essentials of toxicology, ed 3, Philadelphia, 1978, Lea & Febiger.
2. Gossel TA, Bricker JD: Principles of clinical toxicology, ed 2, New York, 1990, Raven Press, pp 413.
3. Porter WH: Chiral pharmacology; the left- and right-hand nature of drugs, *Therapeutic Drug Monitoring/Toxicology In-Service Training & Continuing Education* 11(1):7-115, 1989.
4. Wainer IW, Granvil CP: Stereoselective separations of chiral anticancer drugs and their application to pharmacodynamic and pharmacokinetic studies, *Ther Drug Monit* 15:570-575, 1993.
5. Nebert DW, Nelson DR, Coon MJ, et al: The P-450 superfamily: update on new sequences, gene mapping, and recommended nomenclature, *DNA Cell Biol* 10:1-14, 1991.
6. Litovitz TL, Schmitz BF, Bailey KM: 1991 Annual report of the American Association of Poison Control Centers National Data Collection System, *Am J Emerg Med* 10:452-505, 1992.
7. Wong SHY: Rational utilization of the toxicology laboratory, *Crit Care Rep* 2:295-306, 1991.
8. Merigian KS, Schroeder TJ, Tasset JJ, Pesce A: Toxicology screening pattern in Hamilton County, Ohio: review of 1710 comprehensive drug screens in 5 area hospitals, *J Clin Lab Anal* 2:112-116, 1988.
9. Hanenson IB, editor: *Quick reference to clinical toxicology*, Philadelphia, 1980, Lippincott.
10. Kulig K: Initial management of ingestions of toxic substances, *N Engl J Med* 326:1677-1681, 1992.
11. Stockley I: Drug interactions: a source book of adverse interactions, their clinical importance, mechanisms and management, ed 2, Oxford, 1991, Blackwell Scientific Publications.
12. Glynn JP, Kendal SE: Paracetamol measurement, *Lancet* 1:1147-1148, 1975.
13. Howie D, Adriaenssens PI, Prescott LF: Paracetamol metabolism following overdose: application of high performance liquid chromatography, *J Pharm Pharmacol* 29:235-237, 1977.
14. Armbuster DA, Schwarzhoff RH, Hubster EC, Liserio MK: Enzyme immunoassay, kinetic microparticle immunoassay, radioimmunoassay, and fluorescence polarization immunoassay compared
15. Department of Health and Human Services: Mandatory guidelines for federal workplace drug testing programs: final guideline notice, *Fed Reg* 53:11969-11989, 1989.
16. Berry DJ, Grove J: Emergency toxicological screening for drugs commonly taken in overdose, *J Chromatogr* 80:205-220, 1973.
17. Sunshine I, editor: Methodology for analytical toxicology, ed 2, Cleveland, 1975, CRC Press.
18. Natelson S: *Techniques in clinical chemistry*, ed 3, Springfield, Ill., 1971, Charles C Thomas, Publisher.
19. Curry A: *Poison detection in human organs*, ed 4, Springfield, Ill., 1988, Charles C Thomas, Publisher.
20. Selected methods of emergency toxicology. In Frings CS, Faulkner WR, editors: *Selected methods of clinical chemistry*, vol 11, Washington, D.C., 1986, American Association for Clinical Chemistry.
21. Fisher DS: A method for rapid detection of acute iron toxicity, *Clin Chem* 13:6-11, 1967.
22. Wu AHB, Wong SS, Johnson KG, et al: Evaluation of the triage system for emergency drugs-of-abuse testing in urine, *J Anal Toxicol* 17:241, 1993.
23. Armbruster DA, Hubster EC, Kaufman MS, Ramon MK: Cloned enzyme donor immunoassay (CEDIA) for drugs-of-abuse screening, *Clin Chem* 41(1):92-98, 1995.
24. Blass KG: A rapid simple thin-layer chromatography drug screening procedure, *J Chromatogr* 95:75-79, 1974.
25. Cholak J, Hubbard D, Burkey R: Microdetermination of lead in biological material with dithizone at high pH, *Anal Chem* 20:671-672, 1948.
26. Kopito L, Schwachman H: Measurement of lead in blood, urine and scalp hair by atomic absorption spectrometry, *Standard Methods Clin Chem* 7:151-162, 1972.
27. Yeager DW, Cholak J, Henderson EW: Determination of lead in biological and related material by atomic absorption spectrophotometry, *Environ Sci Technol* 5:1020-1022, 1971.
28. Olsen ED, Jatlow PI: An improved Delves cup atomic absorption procedure for determination of lead in blood and urine, *Clin Chem* 18:1312-1317, 1972.
29. Sunderman FW: Electrothermal atomic absorption spectrometry of trace metals in biological fluids. In Forman DT, Matton RW, editors: *Clinical chemistry: ACS Symposium Series 36*, Washington, D.C., 1975, American Chemical Society.
30. Parsons PJ, Slavin W: A rapid zeeman graphite furnace atomic absorption spectrometric method for the determination of lead in blood, *Spectrochimica Acta* 48B: 925-939, 1993.
31. Lead in blood, method no. P&CAM 195. In Taylor DG: *Manual coordination: NIOSH Manual of analytical methods*, ed 2, vol 1, Washington, D.C., 1977, US Government Printing Office, pp 195-1 to 195-7.
32. Meranger JC, Hollebone BR, Blanchette GA: The effects of storage times, temperature and container types on the accuracy of atomic absorption determination of Cd, Cu, Hg, Pb, and Zn in whole heparinized blood, *J Anal Toxicol* 5:33-41, 1981.
33. Unger BC, Green VA: Blood lead analysis: lead loss to storage containers, *Clin Toxicol* 11:237-243, 1977.
34. Critique: Blood lead analysis, 1981, document no. 34Q205158208, Atlanta, Ga., May 1982, Centers for Disease Control, US Department of Health and Human Services.
35. *"Criteria for a recommended standard. Occupational exposure to inorganic lead,"* revised criteria, NIOSH, DHEW Publ no 78-158, Washington, D.C., 1978, Superintendent of Documents, US Government Printing Office.
36. *Airborne lead in perspective*, Report of the Committee on Biological Effects of Atmosphere Pollutants of the National Research Council—National Academy of Sciences, Washington, D.C., 1972, Printing and Publishing Offices.
37. *Airborne lead in perspective*, Report of the Committee on Biological Effects of Atmospheric Pollutants of the National Research Council—National Academy of Sciences, Washington, D.C., 1972, Printing and Publishing Offices.
38. Brodie BB, Udenfriend S, Coburn AF: The determination of salicylic acid in plasma, *J Pharmacol* 80:114-117, 1944.

39. Trinder P: Rapid determination of salicylate in biological fluid, *Biochem J* 57:301-303, 1954.
40. Weichselbaum TE, Shapiro I: A rapid and simple method for the determination of salicylic acid in small amounts in blood plasma, *Am J Clin Pathol* 9:42-44, 1945.
41. Rance ML, Jordan BI, Nichols JD: A simultaneous determination of acetylsalicylic acid, salicylic acid, and salicylamide in plasma by gas-liquid chromatography, *J Pharm Pharmacol* 27:425-429, 1975.

BIBLIOGRAPHY

Bailey DN: Drug use in patients admitted to a university trauma center: results of limited (rather than comprehensive) toxicology screening, *J Anal Toxicol* 14:22-24, 1990.

Baselt RC, Cravey RH: *Disposition of toxic drugs and chemicals in man,* ed 4, Chicago, 1994, Chem Toxicol Inst, p 1000.

Bayer MJ, Rumack BH, Wanke LA: *Toxicologic emergencies,* Bowie, Md., 1984, Prentice-Hall, pp 341.

Bowman WC, Rand MJ: *Textbook of pharmacology,* ed 2, Oxford, England, 1980, Blackwell Scientific Publications.

Brancato DJ, Nelson RC: Poisoning mortality in the United States 1980, *Vet Hum Toxicol* 26:273-275, 1984.

Cravey RH, Baselt RC: *Introduction to forensic toxicology,* Davis, Calif., 1981, Biomedical Publications, pp 299.

Dreisbach RH, Robertson WO: *Handbook of poisoning,* ed 12, Los Altos, Calif., 1987, Appleton & Lange.

Evans WE, Schentag JJ, Jusko WJ, editors: *Applied pharmacokinetics: principles of therapeutic drug monitoring,* ed 3, Spokane, Wash., 1992.

Gerson B: Clinical toxicology I & II, *Clin Lab Med* 10:261-439, 441-647, 1990.

Gibaldi M: *Biopharmaceutics and clinical pharmacokinetics,* ed 4, Philadelphia, 1991, Lea & Febiger, pp 406.

Goodman AG, Goodman LS, Gilman A: *The pharmacological basis of therapeutics,* ed 8, New York, 1990, Macmillan, pp 1840.

Haddad LM, Winchester JF: *Clinical management of poisoning and drug overdose,* ed 2, Philadelphia, 1990, Saunders, pp 1608.

Klaassen CD, Andur MO, Doull J, editors: *Casarett and Doull's toxicology: the basic science of poisons,* ed 5, New York, 1995, Macmillan, p 1056.

Lave LB, Upton AC, editors: *Toxic chemicals, health, and the environment,* Baltimore, 1987, Johns Hopkins University Press.

Merigian KS: *Drug overdose,* parts I and II. Therapeutic Drug Monitoring and Toxicology LIP Program, 13(17)7-13, (18)7-14, Washington, D.C., 1992, American Association for Clinical Chemistry.

Morrow CT, Popper C: The clinical utility of toxicologic testing, *Crit Care Rep* 2:307-317, 1991.

Noji EK, Kelen GD: *Manual of toxicologic emergencies,* St. Louis, 1989, Mosby, p 850.

Poklis A: Toxicology. In Dufour R, Rifai N, editor: *Professional practice in clinical chemistry: a review,* Washington, D.C., 1993, American Association for Clinical Chemistry.

Rumack BH, Peterson RC, Koch GG, Amara IA: Acetaminophen overdoses: 662 cases with evaluation of oral acetylcysteine treatment, *Arch Intern Med* 141:380-385, 1981.

Warner AM, Hohnadel DC, Pesce AJ, editors: *Professional practice in toxicology: a review,* Washington, D.C., 1992, American Association for Clinical Chemistry, pp 598.

Wong SHY: Novel liquid chromatographic techniques for clinical drug analysis, *Therapeutic Drug Monitoring/Toxicology In-Service Training & Continuing Education* 13(16):5-18, 1992.

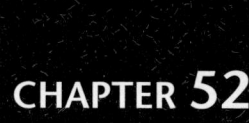

CHAPTER 52

Addiction and substance abuse

R. Jeffrey Goldsmith

OBJECTIVES

- Describe the series of steps resulting in addiction. Differentiate the causes and factors that result in prevalence of addiction in young people.
- Describe the method of diagnosis of addiction
- Describe how drug screens are used to detect drug abuse and monitor rehabilitation.

KEY TERMS

addiction The compulsive use of a pyschoactive chemical, causing problems in the person's life on a physical, psychological, or sociocultural level. Unconscious psychological defenses like denial are a common feature, distorting the addict's self-awareness and confusing the people around him. Addiction is a chronic deteriorating process that leads to death or institutionalization if unchecked. Abstinence allows the mind and body to recover sufficiently to work on the social deficits and deteriorated relationships.

contingency contracts Behavioral plans that engage the addict in a carefully delineated treatment program. The consequences of failure to follow through are clearly spelled out in the hope that this will encourage the addict to remain in treatment.

craving An intense urge to use the drug; it may be short lived or tormentingly chronic. Some addicts have environmental triggers of this craving; others have psychological states that evoke the urge, but many don't have craving at all.

drug screens Qualitative analyses of a body fluid (urine, blood, saliva, and so forth) of a patient in a search for the possible presence of addictive substances. There is usually a brief list of five to 10 drugs that are screened; however, more comprehensive lists are sometimes requested.

recovery The process of growth and development that occurs after sustained abstinence. Spirituality is an important element in recovery because of the need to transcend the intense self-focus or experience of victimization that many addicts exhibit.

rehabilitation A comprehensive, multicomponent treatment for alcoholics and addicts who are abstinent and not in withdrawal. It addresses the consequences of alcohol or drug use, the personal problems that are not directly related to the chemical use, and the necessary skills for ongoing abstinence and recovery.

substance abuse A generic term that covers the pathological use of psychoactive substances. It is not a specific diagnosis and includes both psychological dependence and physiological dependence. For some, this term includes alcohol and drug misuse that would not be covered in DSM-IIIR and therefore would not be a psychiatric diagnosis.

tolerance The behavioral and neurochemical adaptation to the drug effects of a psychoactive substance. It allows the person to experience less toxicity from the substance. Everyone can exhibit some tolerance; however, most addicts exhibit a great deal of tolerance.

withdrawal The central nervous system adjustment to the relatively sudden cessation of a psychoactive substance. There are physical, psychological, and behavioral changes that occur in these states. The symptoms of withdrawal are frequently opposite the acute effects of that substance.

Addiction and abuse of alcohol and drugs affect a significant portion of the population of many countries. Alcohol is the most commonly abused substance in Western civilization, and the patterns of behavior with alcohol are common to other drugs such as marijuana (marihuana), cocaine, opiates, benzodiazepines, and agents, such as glue and petrol (gasoline), that are sniffed. The term *addiction* is defined as the compulsive use of a psychoactive chemical, causing problems in the person's life on a physical, psychological, or sociocultural level. Unconscious psychological defenses against the consequences of addiction, like denial, are a common feature that distort the addict's self-awareness and confuse the people around him. Addiction is a chronic deteriorating process that leads to death or institutionalization if unchecked. Abstinence from the addictive agent allows the mind and body to recover sufficiently to work on the social deficits and deteriorated relationships that may have predated or resulted from the addiction.

THE ADDICTION PROCESS

It is important to understand that alcohol and drug use by itself is not addiction. For example, among teenagers 12 to 17 years of age, roughly 50% have tried alcohol, 15% marijuana, and less than 3% cocaine.[1] If recent drug use by the same age group is examined, percentages decrease considerably; only 25% had used alcohol, 5% marijuana, and 0.6% cocaine in the previous month. Since addiction implies the need to use the drugs frequently, it is clear that not all those who have used the drugs are addicted to them.

The usual history of addiction begins with an early stage in which the patient learns that the drug produces an effect that is desirable.[2] This is often described as *positive reinforcement*. The desirable effects of drugs are more likely related to physiological stimulation of brain receptors. For example, the euphoriant and stimulant effects of cocaine are likely caused by stimulation of specific areas of the brain, areas also affected by opiates. This early stage often occurs during a phase of experimentation and risk-taking in a young person's life in which many new experiences are tried. This is followed by a middle stage where tolerance is manifested. The term *tolerance* is used to describe the requirement for increased amounts of drug to achieve the desired psychological and physiological states. Tolerance implies using a lot of the drug without toxic effects. In this middle stage some negative consequences of drug abuse occur with psychological pain as a secondary phenomenon. Agitation, nervousness, and worry begin as a result of increased usage, intensifying the pain. The late stage of drug addiction begins when the individual uses drugs to feel normal. This occurs because there is tolerance to the positive reinforcement of the drug and increasing negative reinforcement. *Negative reinforcement,* which may include ill health, loss of jobs and friends, as well as pain and discomfort of

the drug withdrawal, encourages the addict to continue abusing the drug. Discontinuance leads to a heightened experience of the pain, and the addict runs back to the drug to feel better. This is the epitome of the addictive cycle. In the last two phases, the addict loses the ability to regulate the amount of drug consumed once the consumption has begun. This is termed *loss of control*. Not only does the drug use get out of control, but the family functioning and the addict's behavior do too.

Part of the addiction is the psychology of denial.[3] Everyone intends to behave in a particular way, and there is a variety of culturally determined intentions that is *behavior*. The chemicals taken by individuals alter their behavior in such a way that some people behave differently from the way they intend to and from what is culturally determined as appropriate. The discrepancy between the intended behavior and what actually occurs may be explained by excuses and alibis. Explaining away these behavioral discrepancies is termed *denial*. The affected individual wants to believe the denial to avoid the pain of acknowledging the unintended behavior. The person becomes progressively more invested in the denial as a way of understanding his world. In other words, since the rest of the world is reacting unfavorably to his or her behavior, the denial becomes a method of rationalizing the behavior. Many modes of treatment involve disrupting the denial so that the person can see his or her actual behavior. This approach leads to a heightened consciousness of pain and a motivation to stop using the agents. It is suggested that it is the pain that is the motivation to stop using a drug. Because the negative consequences of drug abuse appear after a long delay, the individual abusing a drug may already be addicted before these consequences can have an inhibitory effect. Part of the late stage of addiction is the withdrawal syndrome, which reinforces substance abuse. A partial listing of withdrawal symptoms observed with some of the addicting substances is presented in Table 52-1.

Another aspect of addiction is craving. Craving is an intense desire to use a drug. This can occur when the indi-

Table 52-1 Withdrawal symptoms

Alcohol and sedatives	Tobacco	Stimulants and cocaine	Opiates	Caffeine	Marijuana
Tremor	Craving	Sleepiness or hypersomnia	Lacrimation	Craving	Irritability
Nausea	Irritability	Hyperphagia	Rhinorrhea	Headaches	Loss of appetite
Vomiting	Anxiety	Depressed mood	Dilated pupils	Sleepiness	Insomnia
Tachycardia	Difficulty in	(± suicidal)	Piloerection	Irritability	
Sweating	concentrating		Sweating		
High blood pressure	Restlessness		Diarrhea		
Anxiety	Headache		Yawning		
Irritability or depressed	Drowsiness		Mild hypertension		
mood	Gastrointestinal		Tachycardia		
Orthostatic hypotension	disturbances		Fever		
			Insomnia		
			Flu-like syndrome		
			with myalgia		

vidual is placed in situations that remind him of previous drug use or when a particular mood triggers the urge to get high. Some people do not have craving.

THEORIES TO EXPLAIN ADDICTION

A variety of proposed models have been used to explain the addiction process. All the models use the observation of the addict's high affinity for alcohol and drug use as well as the large quantities consumed. The models differ in how they explain the individual's progress down the path to addiction and the addicted state once it has been achieved. Because the theories suggest different cause-and-effect relationships, each theory in turn dictates different types of treatment interventions. The *disease concept* is a proposition that addictions are rooted in a biological vulnerability that predisposes the individual to tolerance and loss of control.[4] This hypothesis suggests that abstinence is the only solution, and treatment is directed toward realization of this loss of control. The *cognitive/behavioral model* of addiction suggests that addicts have different expectancies about their use of alcohol and drugs and get locked into a pattern of use by positive reinforcement (euphoria, being cool socially, feeling less tense), and other negative reinforcements (withdrawal symptoms upon cessation).[4] Treatment is aimed at providing alternative problem-solving skills and coping devices that lead to a sense of self-efficacy. The self-medication hypothesis stresses the psychological motivation to drink alcohol or use drugs in order to alter an unhappy emotional state.[5] Treatment is focused on making the usual state less painful and thereby render the individual less motivated to use alcohol and drugs.

PREVALENCE OF ADDICTION AMONG VARIOUS GROUPS

The prevalence of drug use can be categorized on the basis of age and sex. The onset of use of drugs and alcohol usually occurs between 16 and 20 years of age with a peak usage for alcohol and drugs being the 18- to 25-year-old group.[1] After 25 years of age people begin to decrease their drinking and illegal drug use. However, regular early onset of drinking or drug use is unusual, and these patients may well be in the addiction cycle. In addition, heavy drinking and drug use beyond 25 years of age should also be taken as potential indicators of addiction. There needs to be careful scrutiny of the behavior and other indications of addiction of individuals in the 18- to 25-year-old group to differentiate the potential drug abuser or addict from the other population.

Table 52-2 describes the various types of alcohol and drug abuse among populations. It can be seen that the heaviest alcohol use occurs in the 18- to 25-year-old age group and this decreases in the 26- to 34-year-old group. It is also important to note that males are five times more likely than females to be heavy drinkers. There are also social and cultural differences. This is most striking in the substantial use of tobacco among European Americans, who are more likely to have smoked than African American and Hispanic populations. Although cocaine use in the United States has received a lot of media attention, actual use of cocaine is under 3%. Cocaine use historically has been associated with an older population (25 to 40 years of age) though there is currently a shift toward the younger age groups who are more likely to experiment with drugs. The sequence of alcohol and drug abuse ordinarily follows a particular pattern.[6] Usually a teenager uses alcohol and tobacco before using marijuana. This is especially true for boys, whereas girls sometimes will use one or the other before trying marijuana. Marijuana use often precedes the use of other illegal drugs. Thus highly addictive and illegal drugs are preceded by less addictive and legal substances. The use of legal drugs is a necessary beginning in the addictive process that has something to do with the person's willingness or commitment to use alcohol or drugs. It is possible that these "gateway drugs" sensitize certain parts of the brain. Another hypothesis is that the legal drugs start the individual on the psychological pathway to denial, and this accommodates other drug use.

The abuse and misuse of prescription drugs is a common and complex problem, being involved in nearly 60% of drug-related emergency room visits and 70% of all drug-related deaths.[7] Prescription drug abuse (PDA) covers drugs diverted for addiction purposes (both sale and consumption) by the physician or by the patient, patients inadvertently addicted while taking the medication as prescribed, patients taking medication obtained on the street or from family, as well as overdoses. Alcoholics and the elderly are prone to PDA when suffering from pain, insomnia, anxiety, or depression.

The addict or drug abuser may use more than one drug.[8] About half of the alcoholics are also dependent on other illegal drugs. With alcoholics, 80% to 95% are regular cigarette smokers, which is about triple the national average. In the case of methadone-maintenance patients, at least 50% are also alcohol dependent. In individuals dependent on alcohol or cocaine, very often other drugs will be found; thus the person who is positive for an illegal substance will probably also be positive for alcohol and marijuana.

Table 52-2 Prevalence of drug use (percentage of population)

Males	Alcohol*	Tobacco	Marijuana	Cocaine
12-17	2-3%	12%	?	1%
18-25	11%	30%	13%	2%
26-34	7%	30%	8.6%	1.7%
>34	2-3%	24%	2%	0.2%

*Heavy drinkers use 5 or more drinks per occasion on 5 or more days in the previous 30 days.

PATHOPHYSIOLOGY OF CHRONIC SUBSTANCE ABUSE

The sequelae of chronic use are several diseases with a variety of organ damage.[9] The most commonly known example is that of liver damage and alcoholic cirrhosis, from alcohol dependence. Table 52-3 lists some medical problems associated with chronic abuse.[9-11] In addition, direct damage to the central nervous system is often observed in individuals who sniff petrol (gasoline) or glue. Cocaine and alcohol can also affect the fetus.[10] Infants exposed to cocaine are more often premature and can be fussy, difficult-to-manage babies at first. In utero damage has been reported if the vascular effects of cocaine cause a local loss of blood flow to the placenta. This can cause a stroke or organ damage to a fetus. The long-term effects of in utero exposure to cocaine in terms of intelligence and organ failure are not known at this time. The *fetal alcohol syndrome* is characterized by mental retardation, growth retardation, and a variety of craniofacial anomalies. Such babies also exhibit social-skill deficits and attentional problems when they are older and perform poorly in school without special attention. It is believed that there is a less severe syndrome, called *fetal alcohol effect,* that affects many more children. Because of the subtlety of this neurological deterioration, it is difficult to say how many individuals are affected.

DIAGNOSIS OF ADDICTION AND SUBSTANCE ABUSE

It can be difficult to diagnose addiction because the chronic use of alcohol or drugs often mimics other psychiatric syndromes. A history of alcohol abuse is an important diagnostic finding. However, the presence of denial is common and often thwarts the clinician, and if the history of alcohol or drug use is not elicited, an erroneous diagnosis is frequently made. The coexistence of mental illness with psychoactive substance dependence is considered fairly common, with 30% to 40% of the alcohol/drug-addicted population having a comorbid psychiatric diagnosis.[12] In turn, such psychiatric problems as depression and mania need to be differentiated from medical conditions that may mimic these disorders, such as thyroid disease, Wilson's disease, and others.

Alcoholism is believed to be inherited. Therefore the history of alcoholism in a patient's family establishes that the patient is in a high-risk group for alcohol or drug dependence.[14]

The presence of withdrawal symptoms is important and, when present, is diagnostic. On the other hand, many people are dependent on alcohol and drugs without obvious withdrawal symptoms. They are psychologically dependent and fall into the middle stage of addiction. Blackouts and denial are two other phenomena that are important to understand, but they are not considered diagnostic evidence of addiction. *Blackouts* are true amnestic episodes that are commonly associated with alcoholism and sedative or hypnotic dependence. Although they are not currently diagnostic criteria, they are highly suggestive of dependence. *Denial* is a common psychological defense and is used by the alcoholic or addict to prevent awareness of the addiction, which deflects the fear of losing control. Denial can be recognized only as such after the addiction is identified; therefore it is not a diagnostic criterion.

Diagnosis and treatment of prescription-drug abuse hinges on the recognition of what is happening. Demanding prescriptions or running out of pills before the proper date may be signs of addiction or selling pills on the street. Chronic daily use of a medication that is habituating, predominantly sedatives and narcotics, is a setup for physical dependence and withdrawal symptoms upon sudden discontinuation. Visits to several doctors on a regular basis can be a sign of drug-seeking behavior or an opportunity for inadvertent overmedication. Each one of these situations would be handled differently depending on the patient and the physicians involved. Drug screens can be crucial in the confirmation that a patient is using a drug not prescribed by the physician or is using it beyond the prescribed cutoff date. A quantitative analysis may be useful where the patient is suspected of escalating the dose on his own, or getting prescriptions from other doctors surreptitiously when the drug is known to be present but the amount of drug is in question.

In general, more than 50% of alcoholics give unreliable histories, often because of denial. In part, this unreliable history occurs because alcoholics and addicts are highly stigmatized; people with these disorders are accustomed to considerable negative feedback and disguise their disability until they feel safe to acknowledge it. The criteria listed in Table 52-4 for the diagnosis of substance abuse are primarily subjective ones and therefore more difficult to apply.

Table 52-3 Examples of medical pathophysiology associated with chronic abuse*

Substance	Disease	
Alcohol	Liver cirrhosis	Cardiomyopathy
	Fetal alcohol syndrome	Trauma of all types
	Gastrointestinal cancer	Strokes
		Depression
Cocaine	Nasal septum perforation	Cardiac arrest
	Seizures	Panic attacks
	Paranoia	Premature births
	Neonatal withdrawal	
Opiates	Infections, AIDS	Hepatitis
	Self-poisoning	Neonatal withdrawal
Tobacco	Emphysema	Cancer of various types
	Heart attack	Osteoporosis
	Low birth weight	

* These are in addition to withdrawal symptoms.

Table 52-4 Diagnostic criteria of addiction

Tolerance
Loss of control
Narrowing of life-style
Use despite reasons not to use
Withdrawal symptoms

Many attempts to employ quantitative laboratory data often meet with mixed success. Combination of tests that include gamma-glutamyltransferase, mean corpuscular volume, and aspartate aminotransferase can have a diagnostic sensitivity and specificity for alcoholism in the 70% to 95% range.

The positive drug screen is *not* diagnostic for addiction. The use of alcohol and drugs is a very common phenomenon in the United States in the 1990s. The positive drug screen indicates only that these substances were *used* within a certain time period of the collection of body fluids. A positive drug screen is an important finding. Final diagnosis must be made on clinical grounds by a clinician and physician taking a history and observing the signs and symptoms of addiction. This clinical observation is especially important when serious legal consequences are possible.

THE TREATMENT PROCESS

The major obstacle to the treatment of drug addiction is the patient's continued denial.[3] Even court-enforced monitoring may not remove the denial, and the treatment intervention may fail. A major part of the treatment process is increasing the awareness of the patient's problem to enhance the motivation for treatment and to elicit patient cooperativeness.[16] Families can help increase awareness, and external coercion by courts and other agencies can help improve retention of the patient in treatment. When the addict appreciates that the alcohol or drug use is out of control and that it makes life unmanageable, the addict is more likely to commit to a program of abstinence. With the commitment to abstinence comes a greater cooperation from the patient to reverse the problems of addiction. These rehabilitation programs attempt to rebuild the sectors in the addict's life that have been underdeveloped or undermined by the addiction. One must rally spiritual help and make efforts to prevent relapse by exploring the triggers to relapse and avoiding situations that could precipitate the relapse. Relapse prevention depends on the discovery of alternative, nondrug coping mechanisms for life's problems.

Both inpatient and outpatient programs to stop the addiction cycle have considerable success. Although many return to use their drugs or alcohol, repeated efforts to quit pay off. Over half of the patients completing treatment (50% to 80%) remain abstinent for at least a year.

Strategies of rehabilitation involve the use of *contracts* and drug screens. In this particular circumstance the addict agrees, or contracts, to fulfill a series of rehabilitation steps, which may include attending meetings such as Alcoholics Anonymous. In general, the contract specifies that if the person prematurely leaves treatment or is found to be using drugs by history or by screening he or she will have some consequences, such as violation of probation, the loss of his or her job, or termination from treatment.

Drug screening is a common component of contracts and rehabilitation. They are frequently ordered on a weekly basis, but many may be used more often. Outpatient treatment may require drug screens on an as-needed basis. The screens usually test for a group of the most commonly abused drugs, but less common drugs are added specifically if there is specific concern. Detoxification medication frequently causes a positive screen, as would narcotic analgesics, certain antiseizure medications, and hypnotic drugs used for insomnia. Since addicts often use somatic complaints to obtain these medications from physicians unnecessarily, it is wise to have a physician experienced with the addictions assess positive drug screens and the medication that addicts claim to need. The information is used to confront the addict if surreptitious drug use is suspected. By doing so, the addict has a chance to stop a relapse early, before serious damage occurs.

THE PREEMPLOYMENT OR RANDOM DRUG SCREEN

Many employers use the preemployment drug screen to weed out those potential workers whom they believe will be at risk to their company. This risk may be one of endangering other workers through job-related accidents or placing the employer at risk for the higher health care costs of individuals who have such addictions.[17] Various substances are measured in preemployment screens, depending on the situation. Urinary alcohol is commonly measured in many programs. By law, those individuals employed by the federal government or who are under the aegis of the Department of Transportation will be screened for those drugs specified by the Substance Abuse Mental Health Service Administration, formerly National Institute of Drug Abuse, including opiates, cocaine, barbituates, marijuana, and phencyclidine. Increasingly, many employers also screen for illegal substances in individuals already employed. These screens are performed "for cause," that is, because of actions that raise the suspicion of drug abuse, at prescheduled times or randomly.

The purposes of *intra-employment* drug screens are similar to the preemployment screens. *Random-drug screens* are used to increase the likelihood of detecting individuals who are using illegal drugs. In the case of transportation workers the time and place of the drug screen is usually specified. For other groups such as the military, the screening is often on a random basis.

WHY PATIENTS FAIL DRUG SCREENS

Even individuals who know in advance that they will be tested for drugs of abuse still fail drug screens. There are several explanations. The first is that the person did not understand the physiological aspects of drug testing. Many people are not familiar with the drug half-lives and do not appreciate how long drugs remain detectable in the blood and urine after the time of last use. Secondly, an individual who is tested may be in denial about his own addiction and would not comprehend that the drug testing was in place to pick up drugs in *his* body but only those in someone else's. The rationale is that drug testing is to catch an addict: since I am not an addict, it is not going to catch me. Lastly, the addicted individual may have no intention to use drugs around the time of the announced drug screen; however, loss of control may cause him to use drugs at the inopportune moment.

Loss of control may come about in several different ways. One of which is that drug use may be a mechanism of coping with psychological distress. As the drug screen itself becomes a psychological stressor, a drug is used in an attempt to deal with the added tension of the situation. Drug use may occur impulsively when there is a craving, as at a party just preceding the drug screen.

Individuals may not intend to use the drug but do so because of their inability to refuse the drug when offered in a particular setting. The loss of control also occurs with the experience of withdrawal symptoms. Such an individual will feel compelled to use the drug to reduce those symptoms. Possible psychological reasons why an individual may fail a drug test deal with guilt and the working of the unconscious in certain neurotic individuals.

One important issue regarding individuals testing positive on a drug screen is that some prescription drugs will give an appropriately positive result on the screen. Therefore, every type of drug screen must be reviewed by a *medical review officer* who can interpret the drug screen and take a history of the person who has tested positive. This is particularly important when dealing with positive results in a setting where disciplinary action may take place. The medical review officer can establish if the positive test was the result of prescription drugs, agents such as poppy seeds, or indeed truly illegal drug use.

CHANGE OF ANALYTE IN DISEASE

A drug screen is often used as part of the diagnostic and treatment process. What is meant by a drug screen is referred to in Chapter 51. In general drug screens use untimed urine specimens obtained from the patient at random intervals, or when certain changes in behavior occur, or at specified intervals. There are many different uses for drug screening in drug addiction treatment programs. The identification of drug is an important function of drug screening given the unreliability of the alcohol or drug history given by the patients. The use of drug screens can also be critical in the confrontation of active denial in these patients. Although the purpose is to identify alcohol or drug abuse, the data are also used to confront the person's denial. The

drugs that are screened for, based on the above discussion, include alcohol, marijuana, cocaine, opiates, and so forth. It must be kept in mind that some agents such as LSD cannot be screened using current technology.

Drug screening is a very powerful tool to enforce rehabilitation contracts that explicitly require abstinence from certain drugs. Without drug screening the contracts are often unenforceable. Relapse prevention programs use drug screening to monitor the ongoing abstinence. The patient in the relapse prevention program has made a commitment to abstinence; however, with certain drugs like nicotine and cocaine, this commitment can be shaken by the experience of craving. Finally the drug screening is a legal requirement of the treatment in methadone maintenance clinics. Patients receiving methadone are required by law to get drug screening, and the results are frequently used to determine the future doses of methadone. If the methadone patient is still using opiates in addition to the prescribed methadone, programs will often change the methadone dose to see if that induces the illegal opiates to be discontinued. The drugs to be screened may be only one, such as alcohol, or several depending on the program. It is to be realized that many addicts are multidrug users and this information is important in the use and interpretation of drug screens.

An important component of drug screens may be the need for confirmation of a positive result (see p. 1026). Certainly positive results from employment drug screens *must* be confirmed, and results from rehabilitation clinics may or may not require confirmation.

REFERENCES

1. National Institute on Drug Abuse: *National household survey on drug abuse: main findings 1990*, Rockville, Md., 1991, U.S. Department of Health and Human Services.
2. Johnson VE: Intervention: how to help someone who doesn't want help, Minneapolis, 1986, Johnson Institute Books.
3. Goldsmith RJ, Warner A, Hassan FM: Substance abuse testing, *In-service Training and Continuing Education* 11:7-13, 1989.
4. Meyer RE, Babor TF: Explanatory models of alcoholism. In Tasman A, Hales RE, Frances AJ, editors: *Review of psychiatry*, vol. 8, Washington, D.C., 1989, American Psychiatric Press.
5. Goldsmith RJ. An integrated psychology for the addictions: beyond the self-medication hypothesis, *J Addict Dis* 12:137-152, 1993.
6. Yamaguchi K, Kandel DB: Patterns of drug use from adolescence to young adulthood: II. Sequences of progression, *Am J Public Health* 74:668-672, 1984.
7. Weiss KJ, Greenfield DP: Prescription drug abuse, *Psychiatr Clin North Am* 9:475-490, 1986.
8. Chan AWK: Multiple drug use in drug and alcohol addiction. In Miller NS, editor: *Comprehensive handbook of drug and alcohol addiction*, New York, 1991, Marcel Dekker.
9. Benzer DG: Medical consequences of alcohol addiction. In Miller NS, editor: *Comprehensive handbook of drug and alcohol addiction*, New York, 1991, Marcel Dekker.
10. Engel CJ, Benzer DG: Medical complications of drug addiction. In Miller NS, editor: *Comprehensive handbook of drug and alcohol addiction*, New York, 1991, Marcel Dekker.
11. Geller A: Neurological effects of drug and alcohol addiction. In Miller NS, editor: *Comprehensive handbook of drug and alcohol addiction*, New York, 1991, Marcel Dekker.
12. Regier DA, Farmer ME, Rae DS, et al: Comorbidity of mental dis-

orders with alcohol and other drug abuse, *JAMA* 264:2511-2518, 1990.

13. Kosten TA, Kosten TR: Criteria for diagnosis. In Miller NS, editor: *Comprehensive handbook of drug and alcohol addiction,* New York, 1991, Marcel Dekker.

14. Schuckit MA: Biological vulnerability to alcoholism. In Miller NS, editor: *Comprehensive handbook of drug and alcohol addiction,* New York, 1991, Marcel Dekker.

15. Chan AWK: Biochemical markers for alcoholism. In Miller NS,

editor: *Comprehensive handbook of drug and alcohol addiction,* New York, 1991, Marcel Dekker.

16. Tiebout H: The problem of gaining cooperation from the alcoholic patient. *Q J Study Alcohol* 8:47-54, 1947-1948.

17. Engelhart P, Robinson H, Carpenter HD: The workplace. In Lowinson JH, Ruiz P, Millman RB, Langrod JG, editors: *Substance abuse: a comprehensive textbook,* Baltimore, 1992, Williams & Wilkins.

CHAPTER 53

Classifications and descriptions of proteins, lipids, and carbohydrates

Lawrence A. Kaplan
Herbert K. Naito

OBJECTIVES

- Describe how proteins are classified.
- List the unique chemical properties of proteins.
- Outline some of the biological properties of proteins.
- Describe how lipids are classified.
- Outline some of the biological properties of lipids and their location in specific tissues.
- Describe how carbohydrates are classified.
- Understand how the chemical and physical properties of carbohydrates are related to their biological properties.

KEY TERMS

aldose The chemical form of monosaccharides in which the carbonyl group is an aldehyde.

apoprotein Polypeptide chain not yet complexed to its specific prosthetic group.

carbohydrates Chemicals with the general formula of hydrated carbon, $(CH_2O)_n$, that are an aldehyde or ketone derivative of polyhydric alcohols. Commonly called *sugars.*

compound (conjugated) proteins Polypeptide chain complexed with other chemical classes such as lipids (lipoproteins), carbohydrates (glycoproteins), or nucleic acids (nucleoproteins).

conjugated lipids Esters of fatty acids and alcohols containing additional chemical moieties. Group includes phospholipids, sphingolipids, sterols, bile acids, and so on.

denaturation Unfolding the tertiary structure of a protein that often renders it insoluble, causing it to precipitate out of solution.

derived lipids Lipids derived from the hydrolysis of simple and conjugated fats; these include the fatty acids.

disaccharide Two monosaccharides linked together by a $1{\rightarrow}4$ or $1{\rightarrow}6$ glycosidic linkage, such as sucrose, maltose, or lactose.

furanose Five-membered rings of monosaccharides formed by intramolecular reaction between the carbonyl group and a hydroxyl group; present in alpha or beta stereoisomeric forms.

isoelectric point pH at which a molecule containing many ionizable groups is electrically neutral; that is, the number of positively charged groups equals the number of negatively charged groups.

ketose The chemical form of a monosaccharide in which the carbonyl group is a ketone.

monosaccharide Basic monomeric carbohydrate unit in which n in the formula $(CH_2O)_n$ ranges from 3 to 8.

polypeptide bond The covalent amide bond between a primary amino group of one amino acid and the carboxylic acid group of a second amino acid.

polysaccharide Polymer usually containing more than 10 monosaccharides linked by glycosidic bonds; branched and unbranched chains up to many millions of molecular weight can be formed, as in cellulose, starch, or glycogen.

primary structure The linear sequence of amino acids in a protein, defined by the genetic code resident in DNA.

prosthetic group A nonprotein chemical group that is bound to a protein and is responsible for the biological activity of the protein. The functional complex between protein and a prosthetic group is called a *holoprotein,* and the protein without the prosthetic group is called an *apoprotein.*

pyranose Six-membered rings of monosaccharides formed by intramolecular reaction between a carbonyl group and a hydroxylin group, present in an alpha or beta stereoisomeric form.

quaternary structure The three-dimensional spatial arrangement of polypeptide chains resulting from the combining of more than one polypeptide chain into a larger, stable complex.

Schiff's base Covalent complex between a primary amine and carbonyl function of an aldose.

secondary structure The spatial arrangement of a linear chain of amino acids in a polypeptide; common structures include the beta-plated sheet, alpha-helix, and random coil.

sialic acids N-acetyl derivatives of neuraminic acid that are covalently linked to many proteins.

simple lipids Esters of fatty acids with various alcohols, including the triglycerides and some steroids.

simple proteins Polypeptide chain consisting only of amino acid groups.

steroids Lipids containing four six-membered rings and including many hormones, vitamins, and drugs.

tertiary structure The intramolecular folding of a polypeptide chain on itself resulting from interactions between side-chain groups of individual amino acids.

zwitterion Molecule containing two ionized groups of opposite charge. (Pronounced tsvit′-er-í-on.)

This chapter is not intended to provide a complete biochemical review of the analytes measured in the chemistry laboratory. For this, readers are encouraged to use the excellent biochemistry texts listed in the bibliography. Instead, an emphasis has been placed on those properties of proteins, lipids, and carbohydrates that affect how the analytes may be measured.

Part I: Proteins

LAWRENCE A. KAPLAN

DEFINITION AND CLASSIFICATION

Proteins are linear polymers of alpha-amino acids. There are 20 natural amino acids with the general structure as shown in Fig. 53-1. These exist as the L-stereoisomeric form with the amino group placed on the alpha-carbon atom next to the carboxylic acid group. The pK_a of the carboxylic acid group is approximately 1.8 to 2.4, whereas the pK_a of the alpha-amino group is approximately 8.53 to 10.53. This means that at pH less than 2.53, the carboxylic acid will be in the nonionized form (COOH), whereas the alpha-amino

group will remain ionized at pH values less than 9.53 (Fig. 53-2). At physiological pH (approximately 7.4), both groups are ionized. A compound, such as an amino acid, with two opposite charges is called a *zwitterion* ("hybrid ion," or "hermaphrodite ion").

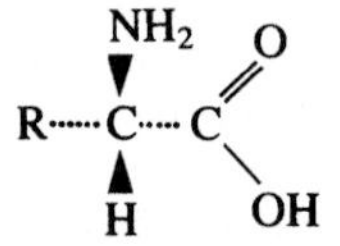

The side chain groups of the 20 amino acids are listed in Table 53-1, along with the pK_a's of all ionizable groups. These side-chain groups can interact with one another to determine the overall chemical, physical, and biological properties of the polypeptide chain.

The amino acids are covalently linked together by the protein-synthesizing machinery of cells. The actual *order* or sequence of amino acids in a protein chain is predetermined by the genetic code within the cell. The sequence of genetic information in DNA is transcribed into messenger RNA, which is translated in the cytoplasm into protein (Fig. 53-3). The specific sequence of amino acids for protein is called its *primary structure*.

The amino acids are linked together by the peptide bond. As shown in Fig. 53-4, this bond has a specific arrangement in three-dimensional space. The linear polypeptide chain can exist in three possible conformations, alpha-helix, beta-plated sheet, and random coil (Fig. 53-5). These conformations are called the *secondary structure* of the protein.

When a polypeptide chain is in solution, it is flexible enough for the molecule to bend, allowing the side chain groups to interact with one another. The types of interactions are listed in Table 53-2. Although the interaction energy of each side group is small, the net energy of all these interactions is great enough to stabilize proteins in a folded, convoluted, three-dimensional spatial arrangement called the *tertiary structure* (Fig. 53-6). Each protein's unique tertiary structure confers on it specific biological properties.

The folded polypeptide chains are often organized as aggregates with identical or different polypeptides. The specific number and type of these polypeptide chains determines the specific properties of the entire complex. The spatial arrangement of these multichain proteins is called the *quaternary structure* of the protein. Usually the biological properties of such quaternary proteins consisting of subunit chains is the sum of each individual chain.

Proteins are generally classified into two major groups, simple and conjugated, with several subdivisions within each group. This classification scheme is based on the

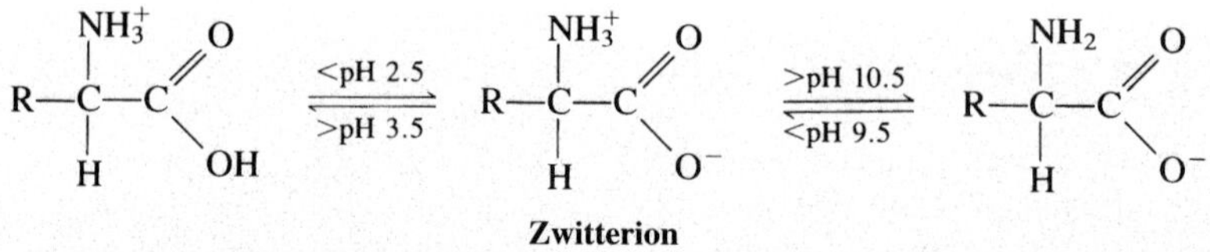

Fig. 53-1 General structure of amino acid of L-stereoisomeric form. *Heavy lines,* Bonds coming out of plane of page; *dotted lines,* bonds extending behind plane of paper.

Zwitterion

Fig. 53-2 Various ionized and nonionized forms of amino acids present at various pH levels. When two opposite charges are present on same molecule, molecule is called a *zwitterion.*

Table 53-1   Classification and properties of side chain (R groups) for naturally occurring amino acids

R group (R—CHCOOH) $\begin{array}{c}NH_2\\|\end{array}$	L-Amino acid (symbol)	Amino acid molecular weight	pK$_a$* (25° C) Primary —COOH	Primary —NH$_2$	Secondary groups
Nonpolar (hydrophobic)					
H—	Glycine (gly), G	75.07	2.34	9.60	—
CH$_3$—	Alanine (ala), A	89.09	2.34	9.69	—
$\begin{array}{c}CH_3\\ \ \ \ \diagdown\\ \ \ \ \ CH—\\ \ \ \diagup\\ CH_3\end{array}$	Valine (val), V	117.15	2.32	9.62	—
$\begin{array}{c}H_3C\\ \ \ \diagdown\\ \ \ \ CH—CH_2—\\ \ \ \diagup\\ H_3C\end{array}$	Leucine (leu), L	131.18	2.36	9.60	—
CH$_3$CH$_2$—CH— $\ \ \ \ \ \ \ \ \ \ \ |$ $\ \ \ \ \ \ \ \ \ \ \ CH_3$	Isoleucine (ile), I	131.18	2.36	9.68	—
—CH$_2$— (benzyl)	Phenylalanine (phe), F	165.19	1.83	9.13	—
H$_2$C—CH$_2$ H$_2$C CH$_2$ \ / N H (proline ring)	Proline (pro), P	115.13	1.99	10.60	—
CH$_3$—S—CH$_2$CH$_2$	Methionine (met), M	149.21	2.28	9.21	—
Neutral polar (hydrophilic)					
OHCH$_2$—	Serine (ser), S	105.09	2.21	9.15	—
CH$_3$CH— $\ \ \ \ |$ $\ \ OH$	Threonine (thr), T	119.12	—	—	—
NH$_2$—CCH$_2$— $\ \ \ \ \ \| \ \ \ \ O$	Asparagine (asp), D	132.12	2.02	8.80	—
NH$_2$—CCH$_2$CH$_2$— $\ \ \ \ \ \| \ \ \ \ O$	Glutamine (gln), Q	146.15	2.17	9.13	—
HSCH$_2$—	Cysteine (cys), C	121.16	1.96 (30°)	10.28	8.18 (SH)
HO—⟨ ⟩—CH$_2$—	Tyrosine (tyr), Y	181.19	2.20	9.11	10.07 (OH)
—C–CH$_2$— ‖ CH (indole) N H	Tryptophan (trp), W	204.23	2.38	9.39	—
Acidic polar (hydrophilic)					
HOOCCH$_2$—	Aspartic acid (asp)	133.10	1.88	9.60	3.65 (COOH)
HOOCCH$_2$CH$_2$—	Glutamic acid (glu)	147.13	2.19	9.67	4.25 (COOH)

Continued.

Table 53-1   Classification and properties of side chain (R groups) for naturally occurring amino acids—cont'd

R group $\underset{\substack{|\\ (\text{R—CHCOOH})}}{\overset{NH_2}{}}$	L-Amino acid (symbol)	Amino acid molecular weight	pK$_a$* (25° C) Primary —COOH	Primary —NH$_2$	Secondary groups
Basic polar (hydrophilic)					
H$_2$NCH$_2$CH$_2$CH$_2$CH$_2$—	Lysine (lys)	146.19	2.18	8.95	(10.53 (E—NH$_3$)
$\underset{H}{\overset{NH}{\overset{\|}{H_2N—C—N}}}$—CH$_2CH_2CH_2$—	Arginine (arg)	174.20	2.17	9.04	12.48(guanidinium)
HC=CH$_2$— (imidazole ring)	Histidine (his)	155.16	1.82	9.17	6.00(imidazolium)

From Cohn EJ, Edsall JT: *Proteins, amino acids and peptides,* New York, 1943, Reinhold Co.
*The pK$_a$ values will be slightly different in a protein molecule.

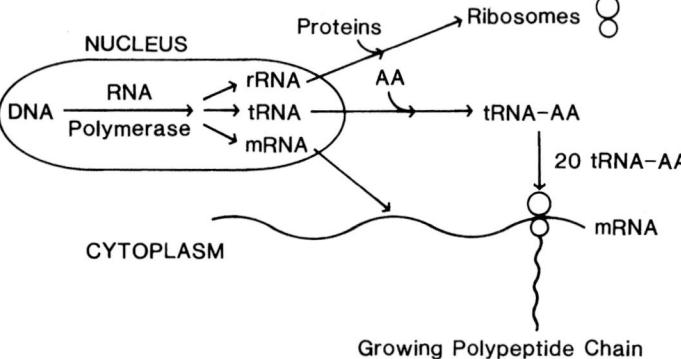

Fig. 53-3   Scheme of synthesis of proteins. *AA,* Amino acid; *DNA,* deoxyribonucleic acid; *tRNA,* transfer ribonucleic acid; *mRNA,* messenger ribonucleic acid; *rRNA,* ribosomal ribonucleic acid (18S and 28S forms); *tRNA-AA,* activated amino acid covalently bound to amino acid-specific tRNA.

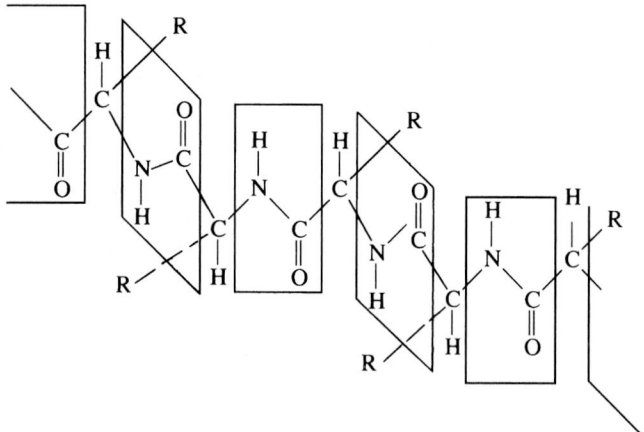

Fig. 53-4   Spatial relationships of a polypeptide bond. *C,* Carbon atom; *N,* nitrogen atom; *H,* hydrogen atom; *O,* oxygen atom. (From Orten JM, Neuhaus OW: *Human biochemistry,* ed 10, St. Louis, 1982, Mosby.)

physical properties and chemical composition of the protein.

I. *Simple proteins*—generally not associated with other major chemical classes
   A. Globular proteins—relatively symmetric, water-soluble or saline-soluble proteins
      1. Albumin—major serum protein
      2. Globulins—most other serum proteins
      3. Histones—basic proteins, found associated with nucleic acids
      4. Protamines—strongly basic proteins found associated with nucleic acids
   B. Fibrous proteins—asymmetric proteins that are insoluble in water or dilute salts; highly resistant to most proteolytic enzymes
      1. Collagens—major proteins of connective tissue, high in hydroxyproline content
      2. Elastins—found in elastic tissue such as tendon and arteries
      3. Keratins—major proteins in animal hair, nails, hooves, and so on
II. *Conjugated proteins*—combined with other non–amino acid biochemicals; considered to consist of two components—the protein, called the *apoprotein,* and the nonprotein *prosthetic* group (The ability of the prosthetic group and apoprotein to dissociate varies from group to group.)
   A. Nucleoproteins—the prosthetic groups are the nucleic acids (DNA or RNA)
   B. Mucoproteins—in which large amounts (more than 4% by weight) of complex carbohydrates are covalently linked to the protein
   C. Glycoproteins—also contain covalently linked carbohydrate residues but usually less than 4% by weight.
   D. Lipoproteins—contain cholesterol, triglycerides,

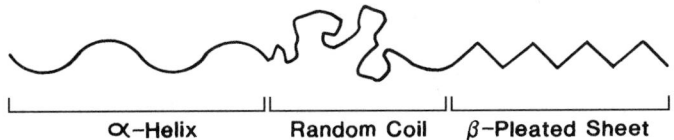

Fig. 53-5 Scheme of three possible polypeptide chain conformations defining secondary structure of proteins.

and phospholipids associated with highly water-insoluble proteins.

E. Metalloproteins—include proteins that contain metals strongly bound to the protein, either as the ion, or as complex metals such as the flavoproteins and hemoproteins

F. Phosphoproteins—contain high concentrations of phosphate groups covalently linked to protein

The biological functions of the proteins are extraordinarily varied, but many functions (see next page) are specific for only one or two of these classes of proteins.

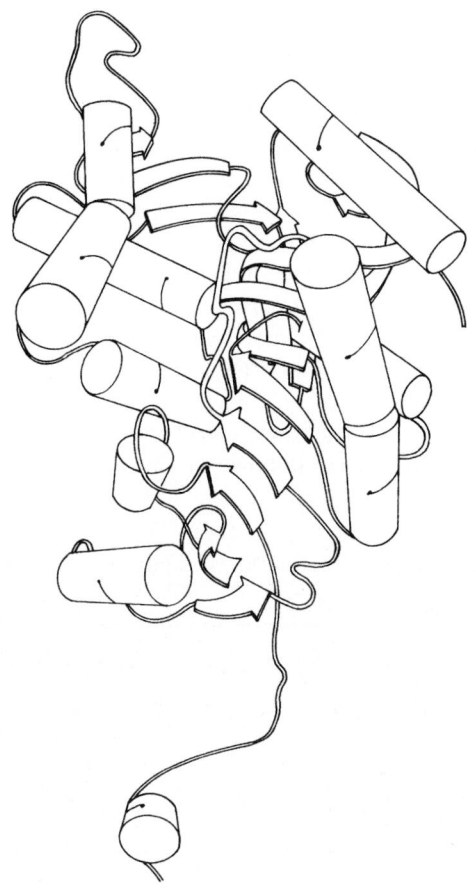

Fig. 53-6 Scheme of tertiary structure of a protein. *Cylinders,* α-helix; *flat arrows,* β-plated sheet; *lines,* random coil secondary structure of lactate dehydrogenase. (From Orten JM, Neuhaus OW: *Human biochemistry,* ed 10, St. Louis, 1982, Mosby.)

CHEMICAL PROPERTIES

The chemical properties of proteins are based on the sum of their parts, that is, the constituent amino acids and prosthetic groups. The peptide bond is chemically reactive and is the basis of the most popular, specific method for quantifying total protein in serum. This is the biuret reaction. The amino acid side-chain groups are also chemically reactive, though only a few of these reactions are used in the chemistry laboratory. The amino groups at the N-terminus of the polypeptide chain and those of lysine and the guanidino groups of arginine can react with several compounds to produce an intense fluorescence. These same groups can react with ninhydrin to give a blue color. Both of these reactions have been used to quantify total protein.

Table 53-2 Types of intramolecular side-chain interactions of protein R-groups

Type of bone	Schematic*
Covalent	
Disulfide (cystine)	$-S-S-$
Lysinonorleucine (in collagen)	$-(CH_2)_3-CH_2-\overset{H}{N}-(CH_2)_4-$
Noncovalent	
Electrostatic	$\overset{C}{\underset{O}{\diagup}}O^{\ominus}$ $^{\oplus}NH_3$
Hydrogen	$O{-}H{\cdots}O{=}C{-}O^-$
Hydrophobic	
Van der Waals	CH_2OH CH_2OH

*Wavy line, Polypeptide chain.

The phenolic group of tyrosine and the indole group of tryptophan react with the oxidizing reagent of the Folin-Wu or Lowry reactions to form a blue color. This method is employed with dilute solutions or microanalysis.

PHYSICAL PROPERTIES

The aromatic amino acids (tryptophan, phenylalanine, and tyrosine) give most proteins an absorption spectrum with the unique absorption maximum at 278 to 280 nm. The absorption at 280 nm is used to estimate the concentration of proteins in solution. In addition, complex proteins such as hemoglobin, which have prosthetic groups with unique absorption properties, can be individually quantitated without extensive purification on the basis of their specific absorption spectra. The Soret absorption band of hemoglobin at 415 nm is used extensively to quantitate the concentration of hemoglobins.

Polypeptide chains vary widely in molecular size. The smallest polypeptides, such as the endorphins or the hypothalamic hormones, contain 5 to 25 amino acids, whereas the largest proteins, containing several subunits, can have molecular weights in the millions of daltons. Although separation of protein on the basis of different molecular weights can be done, it is a method rarely used in the chemistry laboratory.

The density of most proteins falls within a fairly narrow range of about 1.33 g/mL. Lipoproteins represent an important exception because the lipid content of these proteins gives them an unusually low density, allowing the various classes of lipoproteins to be separated from each other and from other proteins on the basis of their density. This technique is used mainly in specialized laboratories.

An important physical property of proteins is the net charge on the protein molecule. The net charge on a protein is the sum of all ionic charges of the amino acids and the carbohydrate and the prosthetic groups of the protein. Since the various chemical groups are ionized at different pH levels, the net charge of a protein varies with pH. The pH at which a protein carries no net charge is called the *pI*, or *isoelectric point*; the isoelectric point of a protein is the point at which the number of positively charged groups equals the number of negatively charged groups. At a pH greater than the pI, the protein will be negatively charged, whereas at a pH less than the pI, it will be more positively charged. At physiological pH most serum proteins are negatively charged.

Since proteins differ in the number and type of constituent amino acids, they also differ in their pIs. Therefore, at different pH levels, proteins will carry different net charges. This difference in net charge is the basis of many procedures for separating and quantifying classes of proteins or individual proteins. The most common procedures are electrophoresis, ion-exchange chromatography, and isoelectric focusing. After separation, individual proteins are detected by use of specific stains.

Proteins found in body fluids are readily water soluble but can become insoluble in the presence of a wide range of denaturing or precipitating agents. These include organic solvents (such as acetone and acetonitrile), heavy metals (such as tungstic acid), certain salts (such as zinc hydroxide and ammonium sulfate), and strong acids (such as sulfosalicylic acid, trichloroacetic acid, and mineral acids). The ability to precipitate proteins from solution by the use of one or more of these chemicals is the basis for a few routine clinical analyses. Cerebrospinal fluid and urine protein measurements are commonly performed by turbidimetric analysis. In addition, protein precipitation steps are often included as part of purification schemes for analytes before analysis.

BIOLOGICAL PROPERTIES

All proteins fulfill some physiological or biological function. The known functions of proteins cover a wide range of activities and are listed in Table 53-3. Often the known biological property of a protein is the basis of a method for its detection and quantification.

Of the important physiological functions of proteins, the most important to the clinical chemistry laboratory are the transport, receptor, and catalytic functions. Many serum proteins function as specific transporters of small molecules. Most transport proteins are globular proteins. Examples are thyroid-binding globulin (TBG), which binds thyroxine; transcortin, which binds cortisol; and albumin, which transports free fatty acids, unconjugated bilirubin, calcium, and many other endogenous and exogenous compounds. The specific binding properties of these transport proteins have been used as the basis for procedures to measure the serum concentrations of cortisol, TBG saturation, and other analytes. The lipoproteins function as transporters of lipids in serum (see Chapter 33).

Many cellular proteins act as intermediary information processors for hormone molecules. Each protein, called a *receptor*, binds a specific hormone and then acts to transmit the hormonal message to the cell. Receptor proteins are

Table 53-3 Biological functions of proteins

Function	Example
Transport of small molecules	Transcortin (cortisol), thyroxine (TBG)
Receptors	Estriol receptors (cytoplasmic), insulin receptors (surface)
Catalytic	All enzymes
Structural	Collagen
Nutritional (source of calories and amino acids)	Albumin
Oncotic pressure	Albumin
Host defense versus foreign antigens	Antibodies (all classes)
Hormonal	Thyroid-stimulating hormone (TSH)
Coagulation	Filminogen

usually glycoproteins. Assays for specific receptors, such as estriol and progesterone receptors, are valuable for the management of certain types of cancers.

An important biological property of some proteins is their ability to catalyze biochemical reactions. The serum concentrations of these proteins, called *enzymes,* are often important in determining the nature of a disease process. Most proteins exhibiting catalytic properties are globular or metalloproteins. An enzyme is most often measured by monitoring the specific biochemical reaction it catalyzes. The conditions of the enzyme assay are carefully defined so as to give maximum enzymatic activity and therefore sensitivity of analysis (see Chapter 54).

One of the most important biological properties of proteins is their ability to act as antigens (see Chapter 11). An antigen inserted into an immunologically competent host will stimulate the synthesis of antibodies by the immune system of the host. Antibodies are also globular proteins. An antibody raised against a specific antigen will be able to bind specifically to that antigen. This antibody-antigen interaction is the basis of many assays for the sensitive and specific measurement of proteins that are not able to be detected by other means, and it is used to increase both the sensitivity and specificity of older assays.

Proteins play a major role both intracellularly and in tissues. For example, connective tissue is composed primarily of collagen and mucoproteins. The proteins forming the cytoplasmic endoskeleton also fall into this group.

Part II: Lipids
HERBERT K. NAITO

DEFINITION AND CLASSIFICATION

Lipids (fats) constitute a wide range of organic compounds that differ greatly in their chemical and physical properties and in their physiological roles. They include a variety of substances, such as fatty acids, sterols, triacylglycerides (more commonly called *triglycerides*), phosphorus-containing compounds (phospholipids), fat-soluble vitamins, bile acids, waxes, and other complex fats. As a consequence, it is difficult to provide a uniform and clear-cut definition of lipids that is broad enough to encompass all these diverse compounds. In general, however, one can say that lipids are substances that are insoluble in water but soluble in organic solvents such as alcohol, chloroform, ether, acetone, hexane, and benzene. Even with this general definition, there are some exceptions, such as phospholipids, which are rather insoluble in acetone. In addition, some phospholipids, such as phosphatidyl serine, phosphatidyl inositol, and phosphatidyl ethanolamine, have a limited but significant ability to dissolve in water.

There is no generally agreed on system for the classification of lipids, but for simplicity, the following commonly used classification of lipids can be used.

Simple lipids

Simple lipids are esters of fatty acids with various alcohols.

Neutral fats. Neutral fats are esters of fatty acids and glycerol (triglycerides). Because they are uncharged, cholesterol and cholesterol esters are also termed *neutral lipids.* However, structurally they are steroids and not neutral fats.

The neutral fats contain mixtures of triglycerides—esters of glycerol and fatty acids (such as stearic, palmitic, or oleic acid). The general formula for such a fat is:

$$
\begin{array}{l}
H_2C-O-C-R_1 \\
\qquad\quad \|\ \\
\qquad\quad O \\
\\
HC-O-C-R_2 \\
\qquad\quad \|\ \\
\qquad\quad O \\
\\
H_2C-O-C-R_3 \\
\qquad\quad \|\ \\
\qquad\quad O
\end{array}
$$

If $R_1 = R_2 = R_3$ (where R = fatty acid), one has a simple triglyceride. If the Rs are not the same, one has a mixed triglyceride. Naturally ocurring fats usually exist as mixtures of mixed triglycerides.

The fats then are triesters of the trihydric alcohol (glycerol) and of certain but not all organic acids. Since all three glycerol alcohol radicals are esterified, they are termed *triacylglycerides,* or more commonly called *triglycerides*. A simple ester would be formed by the combination of an acid and an alcohol:

$$CH_3COOH + C_2H_5OH \rightarrow CH_3COOC_2H_5 + H_2O$$

A fat is formed by the combination of a fatty acid (usually of relatively high molecular weight) with the alcohol glycerol.

Being esters, the fats are readily hydrolyzed:

$$
\begin{array}{l}
H_2C-O-C-C_{15}H_{31} \\
\qquad\quad \|\ \\
\qquad\quad O \\
\\
HC-O-C-C_{15}H_{31} + 3H_2O \rightarrow 3C_{15}H_{31}COOH + \begin{array}{l} CH_2OH \\ CHOH \\ CH_2OH \end{array} \\
\qquad\quad \|\ \\
\qquad\quad O \\
\\
H_2C-O-C-C_{15}H_{31} \\
\qquad\quad \|\ \\
\qquad\quad O
\end{array}
$$

Tripalmitin   **Palmitic acid**   **Glycerol**

This hydrolysis is accomplished by use of acid, alkali, superheated steam, or an appropriate enzyme (such as pancreatic lipase). In acid hydrolysis, the free fatty acid is liberated. When alkali is used, a soap is formed, and the process is called *saponification:*

$$C_3H_5(O\!-\!CO\!-\!C_{17}H_{35})_3 + 3NaOH \rightarrow$$
Stearin

$$3C_{17}H_{35}COONa + C_3H_5(OH)_3$$
Sodium stearate   Glycerol
(a soap)

The fats we eat are mostly triglycerides that contain even-numbered fatty acids because of their mode of biosynthesis. These range from butyric (C_4) to lignoceric (C_{24}) and probably higher fatty acids (see Table 53-5). Odd-numbered fatty acids do occur naturally.

Waxes. Waxes are esters of fatty acids with higher molecular weight alcohols than glycerol. Examples are carnauba wax, wool wax, beeswax, and sperm oil. Industrially, they are used in the manufacture of lubricants (sperm oil), polishes (carnauba wax), ointments (lanolin, which contains wool wax), candles (spermaceti), and so on.

Aside from cholesterol, the common alcohols found in waxes are cetyl alcohol ($C_{16}H_{33}OH$), ceryl alcohol ($C_{26}H_{53}OH$), and myricyl alcohol ($C_{30}H_{61}OH$).

Conjugated lipids

Conjugated lipids are esters of fatty acids containing groups as well as an alcohol and a fatty acid (Table 53-4).

Phospholipids. Phospholipids are lipids having, in addition to fatty acids and glycerol, a phosphoric acid residue, nitrogen-containing bases, and other constituents. These lipids include phosphatidyl choline (lecithin), phosphatidyl ethanolamine, phosphatidyl inositol, phosphatidyl serine, sphingomyelins, and plasmalogens. Phosphatidyl ethanolamine, phosphatidyl serine, and phosphatidyl inositol (lipositol) are also known as cephalins.

This class of complex lipids is also called *glycerophosphatides, phosphoglycerides, glycerol phosphatides,* or more commonly *phospholipids.* Keep in mind that not all phosphorus-containing lipids are phosphoglycerides; that is, sphingomyelin is a phospholipid because it contains phosphorus, but it is better classified as a sphingolipid because of the nature of the backbone structure to which the fatty acid is attached. In phospholipids, one of the primary OH groups of glycerol is esterified to phosphoric acid; the other OH groups are esterified to fatty acids. The parent compound of the phospholipids is phosphatidic acid, which contains no polar alcohol head group. The phospholipids are constituents of all animal and vegetable cells. They are present in abundance in brain, heart, kidney, eggs, soybeans, and so on. The phospholipids have been commonly separated into five distinct groups of compounds: phosphatidic acid, lecithin, cephalin, plasmalogens, and sphingolipids. In addition to carbon, hydrogen, and oxygen, the compounds contain the elements nitrogen and phosphorus. In lecithin and cephalin, the nitrogen-phosphorus ratio is 1:1; in sphingomyelin it is 2:1.

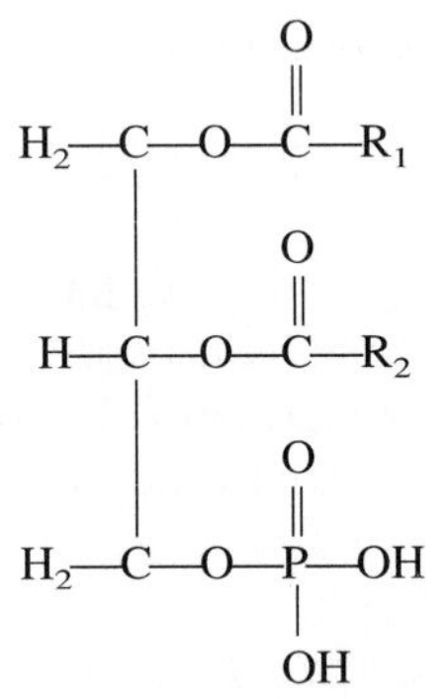

Phosphatidic acid

Phosphatidic acid. Phosphatidic acid is important as an intermediate in the synthesis of triglycerides and phospholipids, but it is not found in any quantity in

---

Table 53-4   Classification of phosphatides and glycolipids

Name	Main alcohol component	Other alcohol components
Glycerophosphatides		
Phosphatidic acid	Diglyceride (= glycerol diester)	
Lecithin	Diglyceride (= glycerol diester)	Choline
Cephalin	Diglyceride (= glycerol diester)	Ethanolamine, serine
Inositide	Diglyceride (= glycerol diester)	Inositol
Plasmalogens (acetal phosphatides)	Glycerol ester and enol ether	Ethanolamine, choline
Sphingolipids		
Sphingomyelins	*N*-Acylsphingosine	Choline
Cerebrosides	*N*-Acylsphingosine	Galactose,* glucose*
Sulfatides	*N*-Acylsphingosine	Galactose*
Gangliosides	*N*-Acylsphingosine	Hexoses,* hexosamine,* neuraminic acid*

*These components are not present as phosphoric esters but rather in glycosidic linkage; for this reason, cerebrosides, sulfatides, and gangliosides are called *glycolipids.*

tissues. Phosphatidic acid is the simplest type of phospholipid. Phosphatidic acid is derived from glycerophosphoric acid by esterification of the two remaining OH groups with fatty acids.

Lecithins. On hydrolysis, a typical lecithin forms glycerol, 2 mol of fatty acids, phosphoric acid, and the nitrogenous base, choline. Most lecithins have a saturated fatty acid in the C-1 position and an unsaturated fatty acid in the C-2 position. The structural formula may be written as follows:

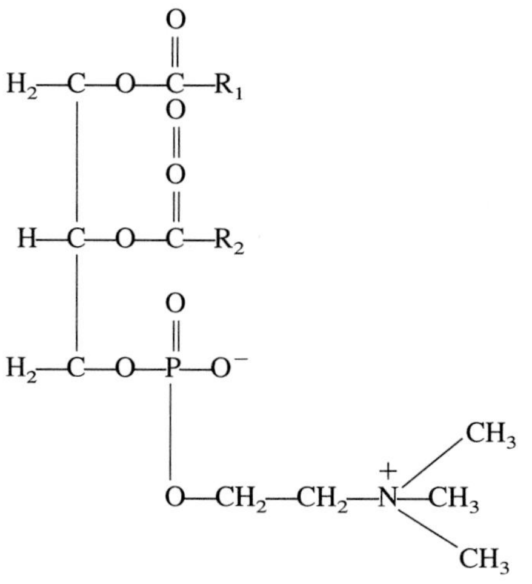

Lecithin
(phosphatidyl choline)

The lecithins, like cholesterol, are common cell constituents that occur principally in animal tissue, having both structural (as part of cell membranes) and metabolic functions. Although not found in depot fat, they make up a considerable proportion of the liver and brain lipids. They also occur in the plasma as part of the lipid-protein complexes called *lipoproteins;* thus they are important for the formation of these macromolecules, which play an important role in fat transport. Lecithins play an important role in the esterification of free cholesterol to form ester cholesterol. Lecithins are an important precursor for the formation of lung surfactant. Lecithins form colloidal solutions with water, but one can prepare an aqueous solution of lecithin by the addition of bile salts. It is believed that a bile salt–lecithin compound is formed that is water soluble. Lecithins are not soluble in acetone; this property is used to separate them from other phospholipids and lipids.

Cephalins. The cephalins resemble the lecithins in structure except for the component corresponding to choline. There are three main fractions: the ethanolamine cephalins, serine cephalins, and inositol cephalins.

The cephalins differ from lecithins in their insolubility in ethanol or methanol.

Phosphatidyl ethanolamine. Phosphatidyl ethanolamine differs from lecithins in that ethanolamine replaces choline.

Both alpha and beta cephalins are known. This is one of the more abundant cephalins found in higher plants and animals.

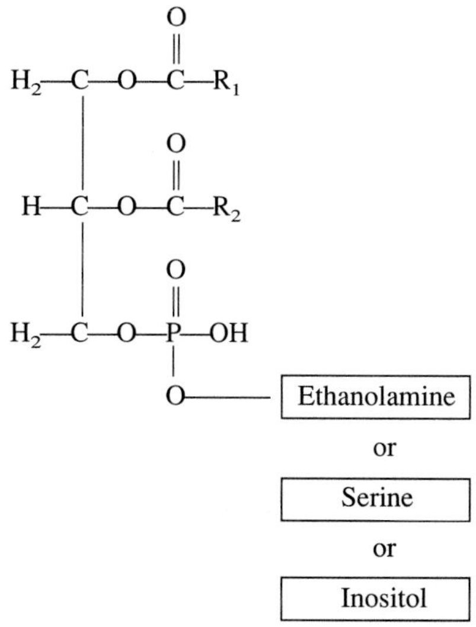

Phosphatidyl serine. Phosphatidyl serine, which contains the amino acid serine rather than ethanolamine, has been found in tissues, like the brain.

Phosphatidyl inositol. Phosphatidyl inositol is found in phospholipids of brain tissue and of soybeans and in other plant phospholipids as well. The inositol is present as the stereoisomer myoinositol.

Plasmalogens. Plasmalogens constitute as much as 10% of the phospholipids of the membranes of nerves and muscles. They are also found in the liver and other organs. Structurally, the plasmalogens resemble lecithins and cephalins but give a positive reaction when tested for aldehydes with Schiff's reagent (fuchsin–sulfurous acid) after pretreatment of the phospholipid with mercuric chloride. These phospholipids contain higher fatty aldehydes in place of fatty acids. Thus the basic units of this class of compounds include glycerol, phosphorus, fatty aldehyde, and ethanolamine.

Sphingolipids. The amino dialcohol group sphingosine characterizes all sphingolipids. It serves as a structural unit for substitution, just as the trihydroxyalcohol glycerol does in glycerides. Sphingosine is a long-chain C_{18} compound that contains a *trans*-double bond, an NH_2 group on C-2, and two OH groups (on C-1 and C-3). Sphingolipids are especially abundant in the brain. Some storage diseases are characterized biochemically by the accumulation of certain sphingolipids. There are four major categories (see Table 53-2): sphingomyelins, cerebrosides, sulfatides, and gangliosides.

Sphingomyelins. Sphingomyelins are found in the brain and other organs. Stearic, lignoceric, and nervonic acid are the sole fatty acids present in brain sphingomyelins, whereas palmitic and lignoceric acids are the fatty acids in lung and spleen sphingomyelins. A typical formula is shown at the top of p. 1050.

Sphingomyelin

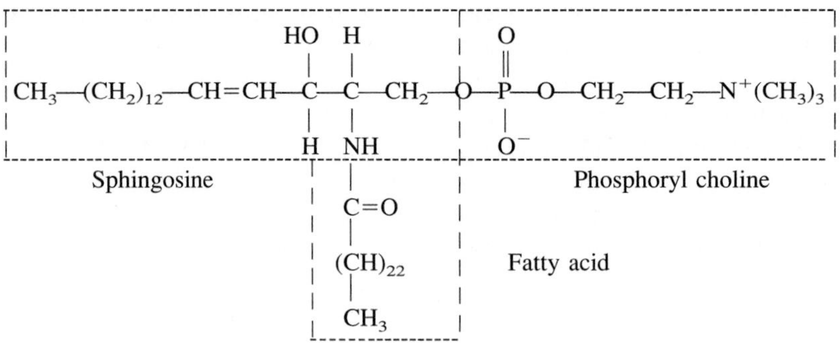

$$CH_3-(CH_2)_{12}-CH=CH-\underset{\underset{H}{|}}{\overset{\overset{HO}{|}}{C}}-\underset{\underset{NH}{|}}{\overset{\overset{H}{|}}{C}}-CH_2-O-\underset{\underset{O^-}{|}}{\overset{\overset{O}{\|}}{P}}-O-CH_2-CH_2-N^+(CH_3)_3$$

Sphingosine

Phosphoryl choline

$$C=O$$
$$(CH)_{22}$$ Fatty acid
$$CH_3$$

and its two important constituents are:

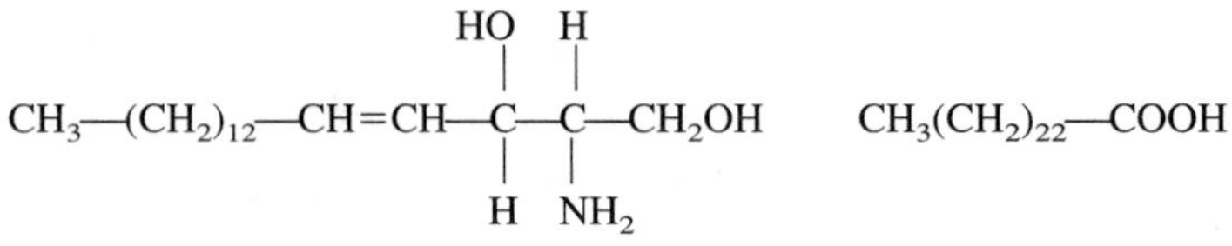

$$CH_3-(CH_2)_{12}-CH=CH-\underset{\underset{H}{|}}{\overset{\overset{HO}{|}}{C}}-\underset{\underset{NH_2}{|}}{\overset{\overset{H}{|}}{C}}-CH_2OH \qquad CH_3(CH_2)_{22}-COOH$$

Sphingosine

Lignoceric acid

Cerebrosides. Cerebrosides contain galactose or glucose, a high-molecular-weight fatty acid, and sphingosine. Thus cerebrosides have the following basic structure:

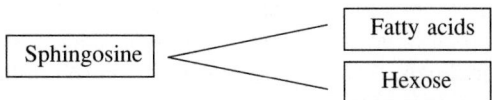

They are structurally similar to sphingomyelins. Cerebrosides may also be classified with the sphingomyelins as sphingolipids. Individual cerebrosides are differentiated by the type of fatty acid in the molecule: *kersins* contain lignoceric acid; *cerebrons* contain a hydroxylignoceric acid (cerebronic acid); *nervons* contain an unsaturated homolog of lignoceric acid called nervonic acid; and *oxynervons* apparently contain the hydroxyl derivative of nervonic acid as a constituent fatty acid.

$$CH_3-(CH_2)_{22}-COOH$$

Lignoceric acid

$$CH_3-(CH_2)_{21}-CH(OH)-COOH$$

Cerebronic acid

$$CH_3-(CH_2)_7-CH=CH-(CH_2)_{13}-COOH$$

Nervonic acid

$$CH_3-(CH_2)_7-CH=CH-(CH_2)_{12}-CH(OH)-COOH$$

Oxynervonic acid

Cerebrosides are found in many tissues besides the brain. In Gaucher's disease, the cerebroside content of the reticuloendothelial cells (as in the spleen) is very high. The cerebrosides are in much higher concentration in myelinated than in nonmyelinated nerve fibers.

Sulfatides. Sulfatides are sulfate derivatives of the galactosyl residue in cerebrosides.

Gangliosides. Gangliosides are glycolipids occurring in the brain (in ganglionic cells). The main components are sphingosine, fatty acids, and branched-chain carbohydrates with as many as seven sugar residues. The construction of gangliosides is similar to that of cerebrosides, but the carbohydrate moiety is far more complex. The various gangliosides are different primarily in the number of sugar residues.

Derived lipids

Derived lipids are compounds derived from the hydrolysis of simple and conjugated fats. These include the compounds described below.

Fatty acids. Fatty acids are straight-chain carboxylic acids (both saturated and unsaturated). More than 100 different kinds of fatty acids have been isolated from various lipids of animals, plants, and microorganisms. All possess a long hydrocarbon chain and a terminal carboxyl group. Fatty acids are obtained from the hydrolysis of fats or can be synthesized from two carbon units (acetyl radicals). Fatty acids that occur in naturally occurring fats usually contain an even number of carbon atoms (because they are synthesized from two carbon units) and are straight-chain derivatives. The chain may be saturated (containing no double bonds) or unsaturated (containing one or more double bonds).

Some generalizations may be made about the fatty acids present in lipids of higher plants and animals. Nearly all have an even number of carbon atoms and have chains that are between 14 and 22 carbon atoms long; those having 16 or 18 carbons are by far the most abundant. In general, unsaturated fatty acids predominate over the saturated type, particularly in the neutral fats and in cells of poikilothermic (cold-blooded) organisms living at lower temperatures. Unsaturated fatty acids have lower melting points than saturated fatty acids. Most neutral fats rich in unsaturated fatty acids are liquid down to 5° C or lower. In most unsaturated fatty acids in higher organisms, there is a double bond between carbon atoms 9 and 10; additional double bonds usually occur between C-10 and the methyl end of the chain.

In fatty acids containing two or more double bonds, the double bonds are never found in conjugation but are separated by one methylene group. The double bonds of nearly all the naturally occurring unsaturated fatty acids are in the *cis* configuration. The most abundant unsaturated fatty acids in higher organisms are oleic, linoleic, linolenic, and arachidonic acids (Table 53-5).

Alcohols. Straight-chain alcohols and cyclic alcohols (such as the sterols) are a subclass of derived lipids.

The steroids may be classified into the following groups:
Sterols
Bile acids
Substances obtained from cardiac glycosides
Substances obtained from saponins
Sex hormones
Adrenocorticosteroids
Vitamin D

These compounds are widely distributed in plant and animal tissues, either in the free state or in the form of esters (in combination with higher fatty acids). Chemically, they are known to be phenanthrene derivatives, or more correctly cyclopentanoperhydrophenanthrene derivatives.

Steroids. The best known steroid is cholesterol. It is present in all animal cells and is particularly abundant in nervous tissue and liver. Varying quantities of this steroid are found admixed in animal fats but not in vegetable fats. The structure of a cholesterol molecule is illustrated in Fig. 53-7.

Cholesterol is the precursor of many other steroids in animal tissues, including the bile acids, detergent-like compounds that aid in emulsification and absorption of lipids in the intestine; the androgens, or male sex hormones; the estrogens, or female sex hormones; the progestational hormones; and the adrenocortical hormones.

Cholesterol is a member of a large subgroup of steroids called the *sterols*. It is a steroid alcohol containing a hydroxyl group at carbon 3 of ring A and a branched aliphatic chain of eight or more carbon atoms at carbon 17. Sterols occur either as free alcohols or as long-chain fatty acid esters of the hydroxyl group at carbon 3; all are solids at room temperature. Cholesterol melts at 150° C and is insoluble in water but readily extracted from tissues with chloroform, ether, or hot alcohol. Cholesterol occurs in the plasma membranes of animal cells and in the lipoproteins of blood. Cholesterol is found only in animal tissues and fluids, never in plants.

Other similar steroids are phytosterols, which are steroids from plants. Among these are stigmasterol, campesterol, and sitosterol.

Fungi and yeasts contain still other types of sterols, the mycosterols. Among these is ergosterol, which is converted to vitamin D.

Bile acids. Bile acids (a C_{24} steroid) are digestion promoting constituents of bile. They are surface-active agents. This means that they lower surface tension and thus can emulsify fats, an important step in the formation of micelles. Bile acids also activate gastrointestinal lipases. For these reasons, bile acids play an important physiological role in the digestion and absorption of fats.

The major primary bile acids are cholic acid and chenodeoxycholic acid, which are made in the liver by the enzymatic cleavage of the terminal three carbons on the cholesterol molecule (a C_{27} hydrocarbon). Thus the bile acids are one of the end products of the metabolism of cholesterol; however, it should be noted that bile acid constitutes the acidic sterol fraction of the bile, which is about 50% to 60% of the total steroid excreted. The remainder of the steroid output in the bile is in the form of neutral steroids, such as cholesterol.

Hydrocarbons. The hydrocarbons are both aliphatic and cyclic compounds.

Vitamins. Vitamins and their structures are presented in Chapter 39. Hormones are presented in Chapter 43.

Other compound lipids. Sulfolipids, aminolipids, and lipoproteins may also be placed in this category.

CHEMICAL AND PHYSICAL PROPERTIES
Melting point

The melting point of fatty acids is influenced by the chain length and degree of chain unsaturation. Increasing the chain length and decreasing the number of unsaturated double bonds will increase the melting point of fatty acids. The melting points of fatty acids and other lipids can be used to identify the compound, but this property is not routinely used in analysis.

Table 53-5 Common unsaturated fatty acids, number of double bonds, and length of carbon chain

Fatty acid	Number of double bonds	Number of carbons
Palmitoleic	1	16
Oleic	1	18
Linoleic	2	18
Linolenic	3	18
Arachidonic	4	20

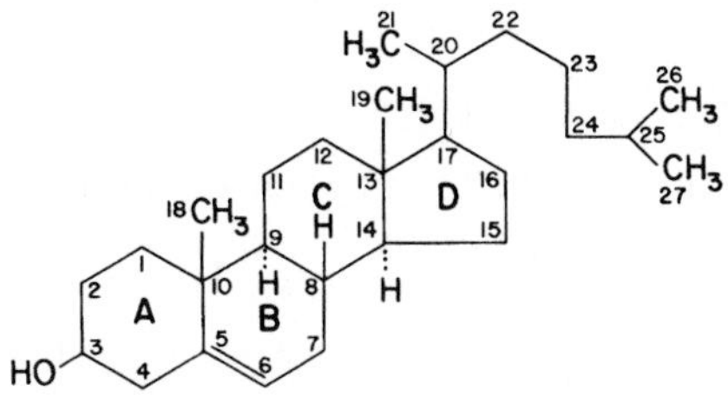

Fig. 53-7 Structure of cholesterol molecule, a C_{27} hydrocarbon sterol.

Solubility

The relative insolubility of lipids in aqueous solutions is an important property of lipids. The major consequence of this insolubility is that analyses of lipids often require a prior treatment of the sample to extract the lipid into a more lipid-soluble medium, such as methanol, chloroform, or ether.

The insolubility of unesterified cholesterol has been used in the past for certain cholesterol assays. Cholesterol can be quantitatively separated from cholesterol esters by precipitation with digitonin as a 1:1 molecular complex of cholesterol digitonide. Measurement, gravimetrically, of the amount of digitonide complex formed has been the basis of cholesterol quantitation in the past.

Specific gravity

The specific gravity of all fat is less than 1 g/mL. Consequently, all fats float in water. This characteristic has enabled lipoproteins to be selectively separated from more dense proteins, and individual lipoproteins to be separated from each other on the basis of varying proportions of lipid content.

Alcohol groups of steroids

The chemically reactive alcohol group of steroids is the basis of many assays for quantitating cholesterol. The group can react with strong mineral acids, such as sulfuric acid, and salts to form a chromogen. The Burchard-Liebermann reaction is the most frequently used example of such a chemical reaction.

The hydroxyl group can be specifically oxidized by the enzyme cholesterol oxidase. Monitoring of this reaction is the basis for enzyme assays for cholesterol.

Triglyceride composition

The chemical composition of triglycerides (that is, the esterification of glycerol by three fatty acids) is the basis of all methods for quantitating triglycerides. These techniques are based on the quantitation of glycerol released from triglycerides after chemical or enzymatic hydrolysis of the fatty acid esters. The glycerol can be chemically or enzymatically oxidized to form measurable chromogens.

Chemical composition

The phospholipids are detectable by specific reactions for phosphorus after chemical reaction.

BIOLOGICAL PROPERTIES

The most important biological properties of lipids are structural, nutritional, and hormonal. Almost all classes of lipids are used as structural components of membranes. The triglycerides are essential components in the formation of the bimolecular protein-lipid–lipid-protein membranes. Cell membranes also contain varying amounts of steroids, phospholipids, and other complex lipids.

Triglycerides also function as an important source of calories and as a source of carbon atoms for the synthesis of other macromolecules.

The role of steroids as hormones has a large influence on a laboratory because the measurement of many of these hormones is required. These hormones were initially measured by some of the chemical techniques discussed above. However, these have been replaced by immunochemical methods.

Part III: Carbohydrates

LAWRENCE A. KAPLAN

DEFINITION AND CLASSIFICATION

The earliest carbohydrates were found to have the empirical formula of $(CH_2O)_n$. Thus these chemicals were simply defined as compounds consisting of hydrated (H_2O) carbon, hence the name *carbohydrate*. Subsequently the existence of complex carbohydrates containing other chemical moieties was noted. Thus carbohydrates can be covalently linked to proteins, lipids, and nucleic acids. The various classes of carbohydrates are discussed below.

Simple monomeric carbohydrates (saccharides)

Saccharides are also known as *sugars,* and their common names all end with the suffix *-ose,* meaning 'sugar.' The smallest sugar units are called *monosaccharides,* in which n in the above formula is from 3 to 8. If $n = 3$, the sugar is a triose; if $n = 4$, a tetrose; and so on. The monosaccharides are straight carbon chains in which each carbon atom except one carries a hydroxyl group (—OH); the one remaining carbon atom has a carbonyl group. If the carbonyl group is on the first or last carbon atom, the carbonyl group is an aldehyde and the monosaccharide is called an *aldose.* If the carbonyl group is on an internal carbon atom, it is a *ketone,* and the monosaccharide is called a *ketose* (Fig. 53-8). Thus a 4-carbon aldose is an *aldotetrose,* a 6-carbon ketose is a *ketohexose,* and so on.

The monosaccharides found in nature are all stereoisomers. Stereoisomerism is physically defined by the ability of a molecule to rotate the plane of incident polarized light. The physical and chemical properties of, for example, all

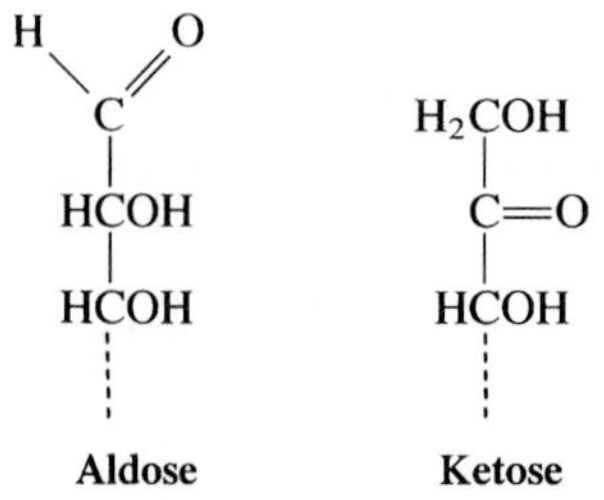

Fig. 53-8   Structural differences between aldoses and ketoses, which are aldehydes and ketones respectively.

the eight aldohexoses (6-carbon chain) are exactly the same except for their different actions on polarized light. All the monosaccharides in human biochemistry are of the dextro-isomeric (D) form. Examples of some monosaccharides are given in Fig. 53-9.

The pentose and hexose monosaccharides also have the ability to form ring structures by intramolecular reaction of the terminal hydroxyl group with the carbonyl function. The six-membered ring forms of the sugars are called *pyrano-ses,* whereas the five-membered rings are called *furanoses.* The aldohexoses, such as D-glucose, form six-membered rings, whereas an aldoketose, such as D-fructose, forms a five-membered ring (Fig. 53-9).

Glucose can form two types of six-membered rings. The rings differ in how the hydroxyl group at the number 1 carbon atom is positioned with respect to the plane of the ring. If the hydroxyl group is on the same side of the molecule as the ring oxygen (Fig. 53-9), the isomer is known as the α-D-glucose isomer, whereas if the hydroxyl group is on the opposite side of the ring oxygen, then this isomer is known as the β-D-glucose. Enzymes acting on carbohydrates usually have a specificity directed toward one of the isomers, usually the most common one found, such as β-D-fructose.

Derived monosaccharides

Derived monosaccharides are formed by reduction or oxidation of the carbonyl groups. The products of reductive reactions are polyols (polyalcohols), such as D-sorbitol or D-mannitol, whereas the products of oxidation are acids, such as D-glucuronic acid (from D-glucose). Many acid forms of monosaccharides are important constituents of more complex carbohydrates, such as mucopolysaccharides.

An important group of derived monosaccharides is the result of the replacement of a hydroxyl group by an amino group. The term *sialic acid* is used to describe the important *N*-acetyl derivatives of neuraminic acid, which are often found covalently linked to proteins (Fig. 53-10).

Complex carbohydrates

These molecules are formed by linking two or more monosaccharides by a glycosidic linkage (Fig. 53-11). The simplest disaccharides, important nutritionally, are maltose (two glucose), lactose (milk sugar, one galactose and one glucose), and sucrose (one fructose and one glucose). Oligosaccharides are often defined as carbohydrates containing two to 10 monosaccharide subunits. Polysaccharides are larger polymers of up to 100 million daltons. All three of the most important polysaccharides contain glucose as the

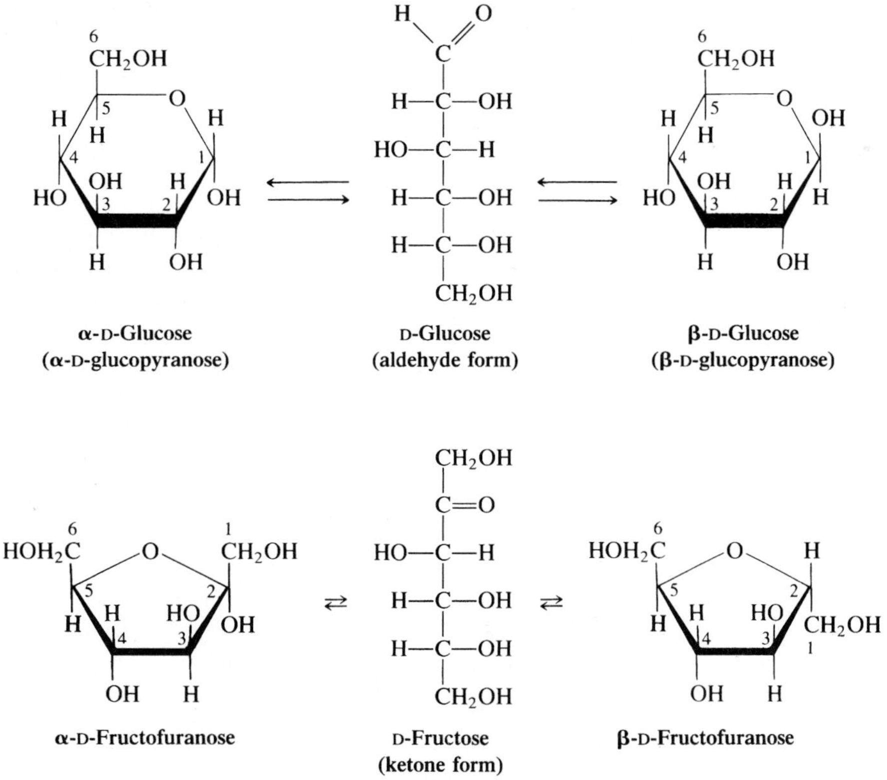

Fig. 53-9 Interrelationships between straight-chain and ring forms of D-glucose and D-fructose, which form pyranose and furanose rings. (From Orten JM, Neuhaus OW: *Human biochemistry,* ed 10, St. Louis, 1982, Mosby.)

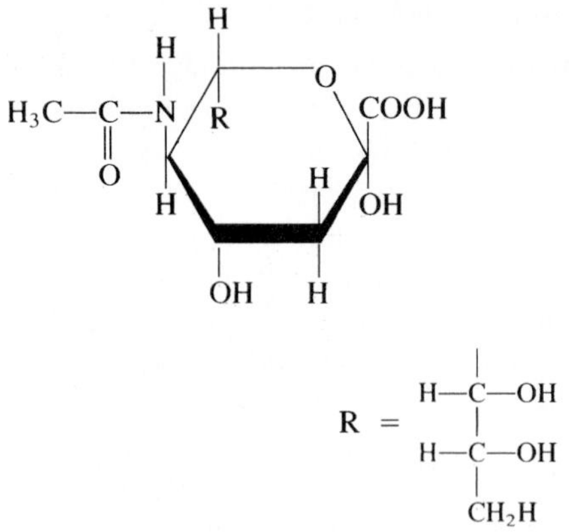

N-Acetylneuraminic acid

Fig. 53-10 Structure of *N*-acetylneuraminic acid ("sialic acid"). (From Orten JM, Neuhaus OW: *Human biochemistry,* ed 10, St. Louis, 1982, Mosby.)

monomeric subunit. Cellulose, a structural component of plant walls, consists of glucose units linked by a β-(1→4) glycosidic bond to form long, unbranched chains. Starch, a storage form of glucose in plants, consists of glucose residues connected by α-(1→4) glycosidic linkages, which, unlike the β-(1→4) linkages of cellulose, are amenable to degradation by human hydrolytic enzymes (such as amylase). Starch also differs from cellulose in that it is a branched molecule. Branching points are scattered throughout the molecule formed by α-(1→6) bonds. The two forms of starch are therefore called *amylose* (the straight-chain fraction) and *amylopectin* (the highly branched fraction). Glycogen is the glucose-storage molecule found in animal cells. Glycogen more closely resembles amylopectin than amylose because of its highly branched nature (see Fig. 32-4).

Complex polysaccharides containing hyaluronic acid, chondroitin-4-sulfate, and keratin sulfates as the repeating subunits are important constituents of synovial fluid and connective tissue. Heparin is a complex polysaccharide containing D-glucuronic acid-2-sulfate–*N*-acetyl-D-glucosamine-6-sulfate as the repeating subunit.

CHEMICAL PROPERTIES

The monosaccharides (pentoses and larger) can undergo dehydration in the presence of hot mineral acids to form the cyclic furfural derivatives. One can dehydrate glucose in this manner to form 3-hydroxymethylfurfural, a reaction that is the basis for a colorimetric assay for glycosylated proteins.

An important chemical property of the monosaccharides is the ability of these compounds to be oxidized or reduced and in turn to reduce or oxidize some other compounds. The ability of reducing aldoses, such as glucose, to be oxidized to the acid form has been the historic basis for chemical assays for glucose. The glucose in turn reduced such compounds as Cu^{++} or $Fe(CN_6)^-$ with the formation of colored complexes of the reduced forms of these compounds (such as Cu^+ and Cu_2O).

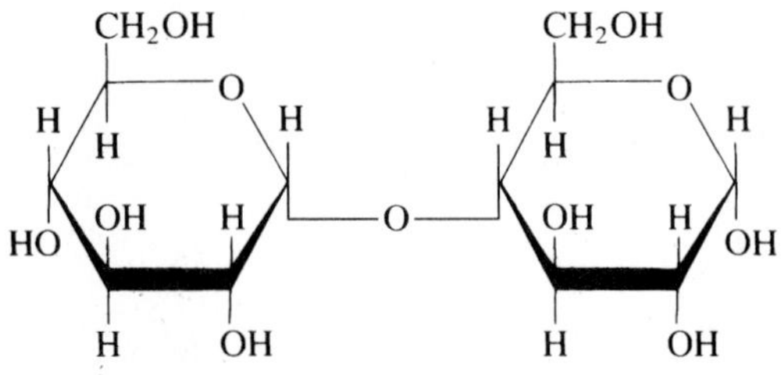

(D-glucose) (D-glucose)
(4-*O*-α-D-glucopyranosyl-D-glucopyranose)
Maltose (α-form)

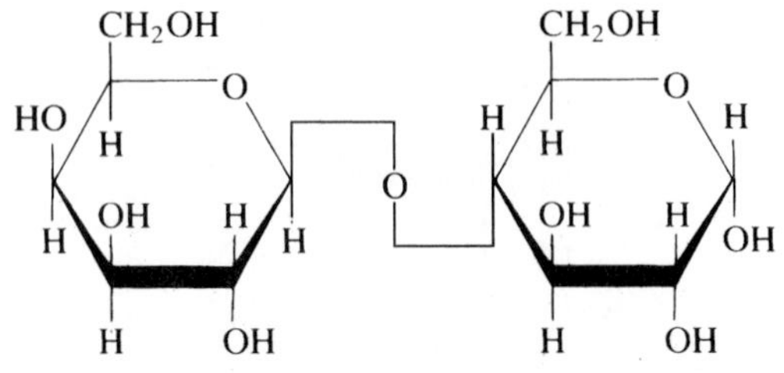

(D-galactose portion) (D-glucose portion)
(4-*O*-β-D-galactopyranosyl-α-D-glucopyranose)
Lactose (α-form)

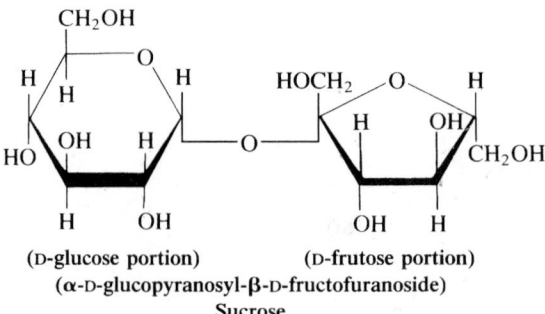

(D-glucose portion) (D-frutose portion)
(α-D-glucopyranosyl-β-D-fructofuranoside)
Sucrose

Fig. 53-11 Common disaccharides linked by β-glycosidic bonds. (From Orten JM, Neuhaus OW: *Human biochemistry,* ed 10, St. Louis, 1982, Mosby.)

The enzymatic oxidation of glucose by glucose oxidase is the basis of many of the current glucose assay procedures, whereas the oxidation of glucose-6-phosphate is the basis of the hexokinase assay for glucose.

Aldoses, such as glucose, can react with primary amines to form a Schiff base. This nonenzymatic condensation is the mechanism for the formation of glycoproteins in blood. In addition, the reaction of glucose with aromatic primary amines, such as *o*-toluidine, is the basis of an important historic method for measuring blood glucose.

PHYSICAL PROPERTIES

The commonly measured monosaccharides and disaccharides are highly water-soluble compounds. Assays for these analytes thus do not require prior extraction or purification. Separation of the monosaccharides by adsorption chromatography is possible, though this is usually performed by specialized metabolic laboratories. The simple monosaccharides, disaccharides, or polysaccharides are not readily distinguished by their spectral or electrophoretic properties.

BIOLOGICAL PROPERTIES

The monosaccharides and disaccharides are the major source of calories for the human body and as such serve as a primary form of nutrition. Polymeric forms of glucose, such as glycogen, serve as a storage for glucose in liver and muscle cells. Complex polysaccharides are found in body fluids and connective tissue.

BIBLIOGRAPHY
General
Friedman PJ: *Biochemistry*, New York, 1995, Little, Brown & Co.
Glick DM: *Biochemistry*, Stamford, Conn., 1995, Appleton & Lange.
Werner R: *Essential biochemistry and molecular biology*, Stamford, CT, 1992, Appleton & Lange.

Proteins and amino acids
Creighton TE: *Proteins: structure*, New York, 1995, WH Freeman.
Kyle J: *Structure in protein chemistry*, New York, 1995, Garland Press.

Lipids
Sebedio JL, Perkins EG, editors: *New trends in lipid and lipoprotein analysis*, Champaign, Ill., 1995, AOCS Press.
Cave G, Paltauf F, editors: *Phospholipids: characterization, metabolism, and novel biological applications*, Champaign, Ill., 1995, AOCS Press.

Carbohydrates
Brinkley RW: *Modern carbohydrates chemistry*, New York, 1988, Marcel Dekker.
Chaplin MF, Kennedy JF, editors: *Carbohydrate analysis*, ed 2, New York, 1994, Oxford University Press.

CHAPTER 54

Clinical enzymology

David C. Hohnadel

OBJECTIVES

- Understand the IUB classification of enzymes and why other names are used.

- Describe the differences between apo enzymes, cofactors, holoenzymes.
- List the major kinetic parameters used to describe enzyme activity.
- Be able to derive the Michaelis Menten equation.
- Understand how pH, buffers, cofactors, and temperature affect assay kinetics.
- List how reference intervals are influenced by preanalytical variables.

KEY TERMS

activation energy The energy required in a chemical reaction to convert reactants to activated or transition-state species that will spontaneously proceed to products.

activators Inorganic ions that are required cofactors for an enzyme reaction.

active sites The specific areas on an enzyme where a substrate binds and catalysis takes place.

activity The amount of substrate for a particular enzymatic reaction that is converted to product per unit time under defined conditions.

allosteric sites, or regulatory sites The sites, other than the active site or sites, of an enzyme that bind regulatory molecules and affect the activity of the enzyme.

apoenzyme An enzyme without any associated cofactors or with less than the entire amount of cofactors or prosthetic groups.

auxiliary enzyme In a coupled assay system, an enzyme that links the enzyme being measured with an indicator enzyme.

binding sites The sites on the surface of the enzyme that serve to bind the substrate or product of the reaction.

bond specificity The nature of enzyme action that causes the disruption of only certain bonds between atoms.

catalyst A substance that increases the rate of a reaction without being changed by the reaction.

catalytic site Another name for active site.

coenzymes Organic cofactor compounds, such as thiamine pyrophosphate and pyridoxyl-5-phosphate.

cofactors Nonprotein substances associated with an enzyme that are needed for catalytic activity.

competitive inhibitor An inhibitor of an enzyme reaction that competes with the substrate by binding at the active site.

constitutive enzymes Enzymes that are always present during the life of a cell.

coupled assays Assays with several enzyme reactions leading to an indicator reaction that has an easily measured substance.

denaturation The loss of the biological properties of a protein, usually as a result of changes in tertiary or quaternary structure.

EC code The four-number Enzyme Commission code for the systematic classification of enzyme reactions.

ELISA Enzyme-linked immunosorbent assay.

EMIT Enzyme-multiplied immunoassay technique.

end-point assays Assays in which a single measurement is made at a fixed time.

endopeptidases Protein-hydrolyzing enzymes that break bonds in the interior of a protein substrate.

enzyme kinetics The study of enzyme reaction rates and the factors that affect them.

enzyme specificity The degree to which an enzyme will catalyze one or more reactions.

enzyme-substrate complex An intermediate active complex formed between the substrate and the enzyme during the reaction.

enzymes Biological materials (proteins) with catalytic properties.

equilibrium constant The ratio of the concentration of product to the concentration of substrate when the reaction is at equilibrium.

exopeptidases Protein-hydrolyzing enzymes that break bonds proceeding from one end of the protein substrate toward the center of the substrate.

first-order kinetics State occurring when the rate of an enzyme reaction is proportional to the concentration of the substrate.

holoenzymes The complete enzyme-cofactor complex that gives full catalytic activity.

hydrophilic amino acids Polar, water-loving amino acids.

hydrophobic amino acids Nonpolar, water-hating amino acids.

inactivation A reversible denaturation of a protein.

indicator enzymes Enzymes that produce (or consume) an easily measured substance.

inducible enzymes Enzymes whose cellular concentrations increase when presented with the appropriate stimulus.

inhibitors Materials that reduce the catalytic activity of an enzyme.

initial rates Enzyme measurements made at the start of a reaction just after the lag phase.

international unit of enzyme activity The amount of enzyme that catalyzes the conversion of one micromole of substrate per minute under defined conditions, $1 \text{ U} = 1.67 \times 10^{-8}$ katal.

in vitro systems Those systems outside of a living organism, that is, in a test tube.

isoenzymes Different forms of an enzyme that catalyze the same reaction.

katal (kat, K) An enzyme unit in moles per second defined by the SI system: $1 \text{ K} = 6.0 \times 10^7 \text{ U}$.

K_m The symbol for the Michaelis-Menten constant.

kinetic assays Assays that form increasing amounts of product with time, usually monitored by multiple datum points.

labile enzymes Unstable or easily denatured proteins.

lag phase The early time in an assay when mixing occurs and temperature and kinetic equilibrium are becoming established.

linear phase Time when an assay is following zero-order kinetics producing a constant amount of product per unit of time.

metalloenzymes Enzymes that contain very tightly bound metal ions.

Michaelis-Menten constant A constant related to the rate constants of an enzyme reaction and equal to the concentration of substrate that gives one half the maximal catalytic velocity.

noncompetitive inhibitor An inhibitor that binds to an allosteric site of an enzyme and does not compete with the substrate by binding at the active site.

optimal assay conditions Conditions for reaction concentrations of substrates, cofactors, activators, and buffer that produce the maximum rate of enzyme catalysis.

primary structure The sequence of amino acids of a protein.

prosthetic groups Cofactors that are so tightly bound that they are considered to be part of the enzyme structure.

quaternary structure The structural relationship of various enzyme subunits to one another.

reactivation The restoration of biological properties of a protein after a temporary loss.

regulatory sites See *allosteric sites*.

secondary structure of an enzyme The twisting of amino acids into a semifixed steric relationship in two dimensions.

specific activity The enzyme activity expressed as units per milligram of protein.

stereoisomeric specificity The specificity of an enzyme for one form of a DL pair of compounds with an asymmetric carbon atom.

substrate-depletion phase The time late in an enzyme assay when the substrate concentration is falling and the assay is not following zero-order kinetics.

substrates The materials enzymes act upon.

subunits Single protein chains from enzymes composed of two or more peptide chains in an active form.

Système International d'Unités An international system of rational and internally consistent units for all types of scientific quantities; SI units.

tertiary structure of an enzyme The folding of amino acid chains into a three-dimensional structure.

uncompetitive inhibitor An inhibitor that appears to bind only to the enzyme-substrate complex and not to the free enzyme.

V_{max} The maximum rate of catalysis obtained from variation of substrate.

zero-order kinetics State occurring when the rate of an enzyme reaction is independent of the concentration of the substrate.

THE NATURE OF ENZYMES

Enzymes are biological materials with catalytic properties; that is, they increase the rate of chemical reactions in cells and in in vitro systems that otherwise proceed very slowly. They are large naturally occurring proteins with molecular weights usually between 13,000 and 500,000 daltons. The study of these molecules and the changes in enzyme activity that occur in body fluids over time has become a valuable diagnostic tool for the elucidation of various disease states and for testing organ function.

Different tissues or cellular materials do not contain the same amounts or types of enzymes. The hundreds of different enzymes in each cell are attached to the cell walls and membranes and are dissolved in the cytoplasm, or sequestered in the nucleus and other specialized subcellular organelles including microsomes, mitochondria, and lysosomes. Often the determination of one or several enzymes in plasma gives a pattern of activities that is indicative of the tissue or cell type from which the enzymes have been derived. Different cells or compartments within a single cell can even contain different forms of an enzyme that catalyses the same chemical reaction. Assays for these different forms can sometimes be performed to determine the tissue or compartment from which an enzyme has come. A few enzymes are found in plasma or other extracellular fluids where they seem to perform a physiological function, but most enzymes catalyze reactions inside cells or in the lumen of various organs.

Composition and structure

All enzymes are proteins; that is, they are complex compounds of high molecular weight; they contain amounts of carbon, hydrogen, oxygen, nitrogen, and sulfur that are similar to amounts found in other protein materials; and hydrolysis with strong acid yields a mixture of amino acids and small peptides. Enzymes are distinguished from other proteins that are not enzymes by their catalytic action.

The catalytic behavior of an enzyme is dependent on the primary, secondary, tertiary, and quaternary structures of the protein molecule, which is discussed on p. 1042. Changes to the primary amino acid sequence will usually result in the differences in the three-dimensional structure because the secondary and tertiary folding will be different. However, changes to any one of these structures can affect the enzymatic activity of the protein, usually reducing or abolishing it.

Apoenzymes and cofactors

An enzyme may have nonprotein substances associated with it that are needed for maximal activity. These other materials, called *cofactors,* may be either loosely or tightly bound to the protein portion of the enzyme. Those that are loosely bound can often be removed by dialysis. These materials may be organic compounds such as the oxidized form of nicotinamide adenine dinucleotide phosphate ($NADP^+$) and pyridoxyl-5-phosphate, which are called *coenzymes,* or inorganic ions like chloride (Cl^-) and magnesium (Mg^{++}), which are called *activators.* Cofactors like the heme portion of peroxidase that are so tightly bound that they are considered to be part of the enzyme structure are termed *prosthetic groups.* Enzymes that have metal ions bound very tightly are called *metalloenzymes.* Two examples of metalloenzymes are ferroxidase, also called *ceruloplasmin,* an enzyme containing a relatively large amount of tightly bound copper, and carbonate dehydratase, also called *carbonic anhydrase,* an enzyme with a large amount of zinc.

The term *coenzyme* is often loosely used when referring to the compound NADH (or NADPH) in a reaction like the lactate dehydrogenase reaction.

$$\text{Pyruvate} + \text{NADH} + \text{H}^+ \overset{\text{LD}}{\rightleftharpoons} \text{L-Lactate} + \text{NAD}^+$$

In a formal kinetic sense, both pyruvate and NADH are substrates for the enzyme reaction, and lactate and NAD^+ are the products. In this case, pyruvate and NADH react with one another on a molar basis. The NADH that reacts is still called a coenzyme, that is, a nonprotein organic material needed for maximal activity, perhaps for historic reasons, even though it should be more correctly called a *second substrate,* or *cosubstrate.*

Since it is possible to dialyze away loosely held cofactors from some enzymes and still retain some activity, an enzyme without the associated cofactors is referred to as an *apoenzyme,* and the complete enzyme-cofactor complex is termed a *holoenzyme.* In the clinical use of enzyme assays, the enzyme assay mixture must contain an excess of all the activators and cofactors to ensure that the holoenzyme is the enzyme form being measured, rather than a mixture of apoenzyme and holoenzyme forms.

Catalysts

Enzymes function as biological catalysts. They are proteins that have the property of accelerating specific chemical reactions toward equilibrium without being consumed in the process. The material the enzyme reacts with is termed the *substrate,* and a simple enzymatic reaction for one substrate and one product is listed below:

$$\text{E} + \text{S} \underset{k_{-1}}{\overset{k_{+1}}{\rightleftharpoons}} \{\text{ES}\} \underset{k_{-2}}{\overset{k_{+2}}{\rightleftharpoons}} \text{P} + \text{E} \qquad \textit{Eq. 54-1}$$

In this case the enzyme is represented by *E,* the substrate on which the enzyme acts by *S,* a postulated enzyme-substrate intermediate complex by *{ES},* and the product of the reaction by *P.* The forward reaction rate constants are represented by k_{+1} and k_{+2}, whereas the reverse reaction rate constants are represented by k_{-1} and k_{-2}. An example of a single substrate enzyme reaction is the action of the enzyme urease on the substrate urea, though in this case two products are produced:

$$\underset{\textbf{Urea}}{\text{H}_2\text{N}\overset{\overset{\displaystyle\text{O}}{\displaystyle\|}}{-}\text{C}-\text{NH}_2} + \text{E} \underset{k_{-1}}{\overset{k_{+1}}{\rightleftharpoons}} \{\text{Urea} - \text{E}\} \underset{k_{-2}}{\overset{k_{+2}}{\rightleftharpoons}} \underset{\textbf{Ammonia}}{2\text{NH}_3} + \underset{\substack{\textbf{Carbon}\\\textbf{dioxide}}}{\text{CO}_2} + \text{E}$$

Water also participates in the reaction but has not been included for clarity. These biological catalysts are like other chemical catalysts in many respects, except that they function in biological systems. Enzyme catalysts, though they are unstable and easily destroyed, have catalytic properties similar to those of other chemical catalysts. These include the following: they are effective in small concentrations; they are unchanged by the reaction; they affect the speed of attaining equilibrium but do *not* change the final concentrations of the substrates and products of the *equilibrium* state; and they demonstrate a much greater degree of specificity than the usual chemical catalysts for the reactions they accelerate.

It is the first property that makes enzymes such a valuable diagnostic tool. Since they are effective in such small amounts, measurement of changes in enzyme concentrations is a very sensitive way to follow changes that have occurred in various types of tissues.

The amount of enzyme involved in an enzyme assay is very much smaller than the amount of glucose present in an assay for glucose. A conventional chemical assay for enzyme material would be very difficult to produce and require large amounts of sample. Of the several thousand enzymes in plasma, the measurement of the concentration of a single enzyme, even if it is present at a very elevated value, is below the limit of detection for most chemical protein assays. What is easier to measure and is biologically related to many clinical conditions is the amount of catalytic activity of the enzyme and how it changes with time.

The *activity* of an enzyme is the amount of substrate for a particular enzyme reaction that is converted to product per unit time under defined conditions (see p. 1067). The assumption that is made for the use of activity as a concentration is that a given weight of enzyme has a fixed number of units of activity. That is, the specific enzyme activity, in units per milligram of protein, remains constant even when the increase in enzyme activity observed during a particular disorder may come from a different tissue. The increased enzyme activity is assumed to occur because of the presence of more enzyme with the same specific activity rather than the presence of another form of the enzyme with a different and perhaps higher specific activity. In practice, activity measurements of enzymes are used as if they were enzyme concentrations.

If the enzyme were acting as a catalyst, it would be unchanged by the reaction, but because of the unstable nature of most enzymes, this property is difficult to demonstrate. It is possible with many current assays to use very short analysis times with sufficient precision to calculate enzyme activity early in an assay period and again after 10 to 15 minutes without showing a decrease in enzyme activity. The amount of substrate converted to product during this time might be 5% to 10% of the initial amount present. Since the enzyme activity determined at both times is unchanged, it is concluded that the enzyme does not participate in the reaction on a molar basis with the substrate and is acting as a catalyst.

Another property of biological catalysts is that they accelerate the attainment of equilibrium but do not shift the final proportions of S and P in the equilibrium state. One way of considering this process is to examine the effect of lactate dehydrogenase on the conversion of pyruvate to lactate. In the presence of the enzyme LD and the coenzyme NADH, the conversion of pyruvate to lactate occurs rapidly, but without the enzyme the process is so slow that it can hardly be demonstrated.

$$\text{Pyruvate} + \text{NADH} + \text{H}^+ \underset{}{\overset{\text{LD}}{\rightleftharpoons}} \text{L-Lactate} + \text{NAD}^+$$

$$\text{Pyruvate} + \text{NADH} + \text{H}^+ \xrightarrow{\text{No enzyme}} \text{No detectable reaction}$$

This is not a one-way process but an approach to the equilibrium concentrations of pyruvate and lactate, since the same enzyme converts lactate to pyruvate with the coenzyme NAD^+. The speed of the reaction and the conditions employed are not the same in both directions, since they are related to the equilibrium constant. It is possible to measure the conversion from either direction, and both methods are widely used to determine LD activity in the clinical laboratory.

Reactive sites

The Gibbs free-energy change $(-\Delta G)$ is the measure of the amount of work a chemical reaction can produce. All reactions that proceed from reactants to products have a net negative free energy $(-\Delta G)$. However, the reactants do not become products directly but must absorb enough energy to pass through an activated, or transition, state.

Enzymes lower the energy required for activation to the transition state. Without the enzyme present, even with a favorable negative free energy, that is, with products having a $-\Delta G$ lower than that of substrates, the reaction may not proceed to any appreciable extent (Fig. 54-1). The reactants must gain the energy to overcome this activation-energy barrier to enter the transition state (activated state) and then pass on to products. Without a catalyst present, the reaction will occur only if enough heat or energy can be added to the reaction system. With an enzyme catalyst, the reaction may easily proceed at normal physiological temperatures. Rewriting Equation 54-1 to account for this transition state in an enzyme-catalyzed reaction, we find that:

$$\text{E} + \text{S} \underset{k_{-1}}{\overset{k_{+1}}{\rightleftharpoons}} \{\text{ES} \rightarrow \text{ES*} \rightarrow \text{EP}\} \underset{k_{-2}}{\overset{k_{+2}}{\rightleftharpoons}} \text{P} + \text{E} \quad \textit{Eq. 54-2}$$

where *ES** is the transition state form of the substrate and *ES* and *EP* are enzyme-substrate and enzyme-product forms with materials bound but not activated. Substantial reduc-

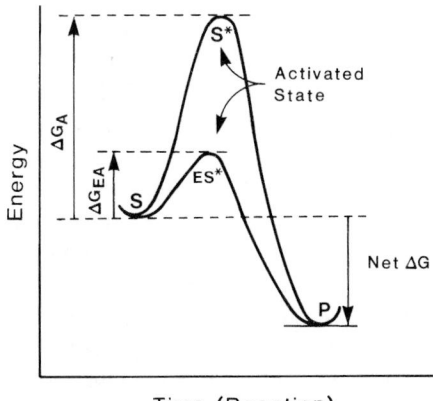

Fig. 54-1 Energy diagram showing reduction in activation energy $\Delta G_{EA} \ll \Delta G_A$ that occurs for same reaction with and without enzyme catalyst. *A,* Activated state (also ***); *EA,* enzyme activation; *ES,* enzyme substrate; *G,* energy; *P,* product; *S,* substrate.

tions in the activation energy requirements are often found when enzymes are used as catalysts for the process. For example, the activation energy necessary for the decomposition of hydrogen peroxide is 18,000 cal/mole, but in the presence of the enzyme catalase the activation energy is less than 2000 cal/mole.

One of the most difficult problems enzyme chemists had faced was to explain how an enzyme can reduce the activation energy and at the same time remain unchanged by the reaction. Equation 54-2 schematically shows one general possibility. To better understand the mechanisms of enzyme catalysis, one needs an examination of the details of enzyme structure.

A wide variety of nonpolar *hydrophobic* and polar *hydrophilic* amino acids are present in enzyme proteins. The external surface of the enzyme for reasons of solubility is believed to be composed of mostly polar but generally unreactive side chains of amino acids. The unreactive amino acid side chains may contain structures like the methyl and isopropyl groups (that is, R—CH_3 and R—CH_3—CH_3), found in alanine and leucine.

Some areas of the enzyme surface contain amino acids with reactive side chains as a part of their structure. The reactive amino acid side chains may contain charged groups like carboxyl and amino groups (that is, $RCOO^-$ and RNH_3^+) found in aspartic and glutamic acids or lysine and arginine. Noncharged moieties like the hydroxyl and sulfhydryl groups (that is, ROH and RSH) found in serine, tyrosine, and cysteine are also reactive. There are other types of reactive groups that are present in amino acids, such as histidine, which has an active nitrogen in a ring structure. The reactive amino acids within an active catalytic site bind portions of the substrates, products, activators, and inhibitors through ionic and hydrogen bonds. These reactive areas of the enzyme may be on the surface or can exist in more hidden clefts or folds in the enzyme surface and can be involved in the catalytic process itself.

There are only a limited number of places on the enzyme where catalysis can take place. These specific areas are called *active sites,* or *active centers,* and may involve only 5 to 10 amino acids out of a total of 200 to 300 in the entire enzyme. The active site, which has catalytic properties, serves to bind the substrate in a specific way so as to facilitate the breaking and forming of new bonds. The substrate is positioned so that other reactive amino acids at the active site cause this conversion from substrate to product.

The sites on the surface of the enzyme that bind the substrate or product of the reaction are termed *binding sites.* Enzymes, particularly those of a complex structure composed of several subunits, often have these sites that are far removed from the primary amino acid sequence at the active site but that affect enzyme activity. These sites are called *allosteric sites,* or *regulatory sites.* Although one would expect great diversity among the types of catalytic

sites to occur for the many kinds of reactions that enzymes catalyze, there are some common features that have been observed.

The substrate of the reaction binds to the active site and is oriented so that a particular bond is subject to attack (Fig. 54-2). The reactive side-chain moieties of the enzyme interact with the group on the substrate so that the covalent bond to be altered becomes weakened. This bond weakening decreases the activation energy needed for chemical reaction. The weakened bond now undergoes a chemical reaction that breaks the covalent bond and allows new ones to form. The product no longer has the same affinity for the active site as the original substrate and will be released from the enzyme.

Changes in the amino acid sequence of a protein could produce different enzymes presumably with different active and binding sites, or even similar proteins without catalytic activity. Such changes, caused by genetic mutations, are often the cause of *inborn errors of metabolism* and other diseases of genetic origin (see Chapter 47).

The chemical reactions in which these reactive amino acids take part not only define the enzyme's specific catalytic activity but also determine the sensitivity of the enzyme to losses of activity by such factors as heavy metals, detergents, or even other reactive parts of the same protein molecule. Metals or detergents may bind to active groups and inactivate them. Changes in surface tension, that is, vigorous shaking, may cause unfolding of the protein or dena-

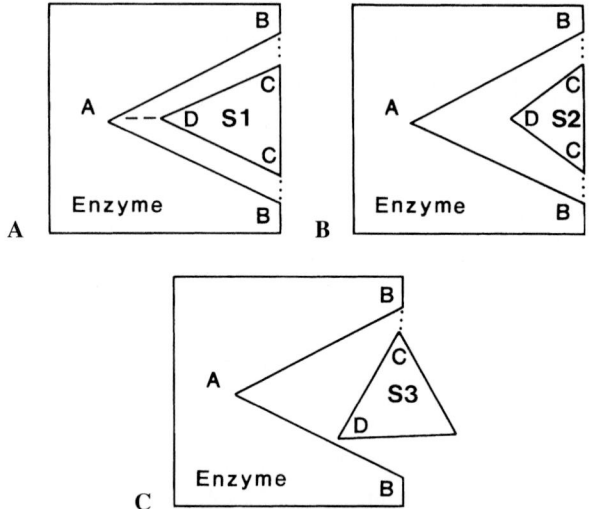

Fig. 54-2 Active site on enzyme is at point *A,* and binding sites are at points *B.* **A,** Correct substrate, *S1,* has complementary binding sites at *C,* and active site can react at point *D* on substrate. **B,** Substrate *S2* has complementary binding sites, but point *D* is too far away for catalysis to take place. If *S2* were present with *S1,* it could act as an inhibitor depending on relative binding constants by preventing *S1* from binding. **C,** Substrate *S3* has only one complementary binding site, *C,* and point *D* is not aligned correctly for catalysis.

turation. As a result, the spatial relationships of these reactive amino acids with each other are disrupted, preventing the usual reaction from taking place.

Specificity of reaction

Differences in enzyme specificity are believed to be related to physical differences at the active site. Some enzymes will react with many related compounds and are said to have a broad specificity. Acid phosphatase is one of the enzymes that exhibits a broad *bond specificity* by hydrolyzing several types of organic phosphate esters, such as β-glycerol phosphate, thymolphthalein phosphate, *para*-nitrophenyl phosphate, α-naphthyl phosphate. At an acid pH, the enzyme-catalyzed reaction

$$R\!-\!O\!-\!P + H_2O \xrightarrow{\text{Acid phosphatase}} R\!-\!O\!-\!H + P_i$$

produces an organic alcohol and an inorganic phosphate.

Many enzymes that hydrolyze proteins also exhibit a broad bond specificity, hydrolyzing a large number and variety of peptide bonds within a protein substrate. If the peptide bonds of the substrate that are hydrolyzed are located on the inside of the protein, the enzyme is called an *endopeptidase,* such as pepsin A. Alternatively, carboxypeptidases are enzymes that act on protein substrates cleaving peptide bonds starting from the outside carboxyl end of the substrate and moving toward the middle of the protein. These enzymes are termed *exopeptidases,* and they also demonstrate a broad substrate specificity.

In contrast to the broad specificity of many peptidases, other enzymes are more specific in their action, in that they will catalyze only a definite reaction with a few substrates. In extreme cases, an almost absolute specificity is demonstrated where only a single compound will serve as a substrate, such as, phospho*enol*pyruvate, for the pyruvate kinase reaction:

Phospho*enol*pyruvate (PEP)		Pyruvate (PYR)
+	$\underset{\rightleftharpoons}{\overset{PK}{}}$	+
Adenosine diphosphate (ADP)		Adenosine triphosphate (ATP)

Enzyme specificity should be described for each substrate involved in a reaction. In contrast to the absolute specificity shown for phospho*enol*pyruvate in the pyruvate kinase reaction, several natural and synthetic nucleoside diphosphates, such as UDP, IDP, GDP, and CDP will also serve as phosphate acceptors in the reaction in place of ADP. Thus, although an absolute specificity is shown for one substrate (PEP), an intermediate degree of specificity is shown for the other substrate (ADP).

An intermediate degree of specificity for each substrate is shown by the hexokinase reaction, in which D-glucose and several other sugars may be phosphorylated, that is, D-mannose, 2-deoxy-D-glucose, and D-glucosamine.' However, D-galactose and 5-carbon sugars like D-xylose are not

substrates. The enzyme can also use a variety of nucleoside triphosphates as phosphate donors, such as ITP and GTP as well as ATP.

D-Glucose + Adenosine triphosphate (ATP)	$\overset{HK}{\rightarrow}$	Glucose-6-phosphate + Adenosine diphosphate (ADP)

Many enzymes demonstrate a *stereoisomeric specificity* for either the L-form or the D-form of a pair of compounds. Hexokinase is absolutely specific for the D-form of glucose; the L-form is not a substrate. Malate dehydrogenase acts only on the L-form of malate, not the D-form. Lactate dehydrogenase acts only on L-lactate, not on D-lactate. However, stereoisomeric specificity does not necessarily mean that the enzyme is absolutely specific, since some forms of lactate dehydrogenase act on hydroxybutyrate as well as lactate, and as mentioned above, hexokinase functions with several D-form substrates.

Subunit structure

Some enzymes occur in nature in several natural forms. That is, there may be several types of enzyme that catalyze the same reaction. These are known as *isoenzymes,* or *isozymes.* In a few well-studied enzymes, it has been found that the different forms of isoenzymes occur because the enzymes are composed of two of more different polypeptide chains or subunits bound into an active form. The subunits alone do not have the catalytic properties of the whole enzyme. The isoenzymes may have different kinetic or other physical properties that allow the different forms to be separated or measured. Many of these features have been used to differentiate and characterize the various enzyme forms as well as to assay for their presence in a sample. Other types or classes of isoenzymes can occur and are considered in the section on isoenzymes (p. 1077), but clinically the most widely used forms are the subunit type of isoenzymes. See Chapter 55 for a longer discussion of isoenzymes.

Anabolism and catabolism

The synthesis of all enzymes is assumed to occur by intracellular protein synthetic pathways within the tissues that contain the enzymes. Extracellular enzymes like those involved in the coagulation process are synthesized in the liver and elaborated into the plasma. In some cases other organs, that is, the kidney, lung, and pancreas, also contribute to the extracellular enzyme pool.

The large size and complexity of structure of enzymes results in molecular forms that are somewhat unstable and are therefore said to be *labile.* Many enzymes in vitro lose their catalytic activity with relatively slight changes in pH, temperature, or even salt concentration of the surrounding medium. It is presumed that similar processes occur intracellularly and that constant, though slight, synthesis of enzymes occurs in a steady-state fashion to maintain the required amounts of intracellular enzymes needed for intermediary metabolism.

A loss of enzyme activity can be either reversible and temporary or irreversible and permanent. *Denaturation* is a process whereby biological properties are lost by a protein; that is, enzyme activity is lost. It has been suggested that the denaturation process is an unfolding or "melting" of tightly coiled peptide chains leading to a more disorganized structure.

There is much experimental support for this idea, including increased reactivity of side chains, changes in viscosity, and changes in the sedimentation behavior, of the "melted" protein solutions. *Irreversible denaturation* can occur when the enzyme protein chains unfold and are unable to refold to their biologically active form, or when a heavy metal ion (such as mercury or lead) or other material binds tightly at or near the active site. Many other factors and events can lead to denaturation and loss of activity including changes in temperature, the addition of strong acids or bases, exposure to high pressure, treatment with ultraviolet rays, repeated freezing, and the addition of detergents, or organic solvents, or the presence of high concentrations of urea or guanidine.

A *reversible denaturation,* or loss of enzyme activity, is called *inactivation.* For example, inactivation can occur if an enzyme solution is allowed to remain for an extended time at room temperature and the enzyme partially loses activity. This temporary activity loss can have several causes including heat instability with the breaking of hydrogen bonds or oxidation of sulfhydryl groups. In both of these cases, there is some loss of the natural structural form. With some enzymes, reducing the temperature of the solution or the addition of a sulfhydryl reducing agent like dithiothreitol may allow the enzyme to refold to the original active form, with reformation of hydrogen bonds or reduction of oxidized sulfhydryl groups, thus producing a *reactivation* of the enzyme and a restoration of lost activity.

Little is known about the mechanism of removal of enzyme proteins from the extracellular fluid compartment. Certainly, extracellular proteases will hydrolyze the protein material thus inactivating enzymes that are lost from cells. The degraded inactive proteins are then removed by one of several excretory routes, that is, excretion in bile, the intestine, liver, kidney, or the reticuloendothelial system. In addition, it is known that various enzymes have different half-lives, an indication that several mechanisms of removal may be present.

ENZYME CLASSIFICATION

Many enzymes were first named for their function (such as lactate dehydrogenase), but some have also been named for the type of substrate on which they act: urease hydrolyzes urea, lipase hydrolyzes lipids, and phosphatases act on organic phosphates. Many of the clinically important enzymes are still known by these trivial names that arose from his-

toric circumstances and will continue to pervade the literature because of their simplicity. A systematic convention for the naming of enzymes was developed by the Enzyme Commission (EC) of the International Union of Biochemistry (IUB) and is widely used.

International Union of Biochemistry (IUB) names and codes

The IUB systematic name describes the reaction catalyzed. The IUB also recognized that trivial names were important and assigned practical names to many enzymes but no abbreviations. For each individual enzyme the system provides a numeric EC code designation consisting of four numbers separated by periods. The first number assigns the enzyme to one of six categories of reaction. The second number denotes the subclass, which is often based on the type of group, such as amino group or hydroxyl group, that takes part in the reaction. The third number indicates the different subsubclass of reaction, often the acceptor group, and the last number is merely the serial number of the particular enzyme in this subsubgroup. For the enzyme lactate dehydrogenase (EC 1.1.1.27), the first number, *1,* indicates that the enzyme is an oxidoreductase; the second number, *1,* indicates that the enzyme acts on the CH—group of donors; the third number, *1,* indicates that the acceptor is NAD^+ or $NADP^+$; and the fourth number, *27,* is merely the serial number of the enzyme in the EC 1.1.1.*x* group.

Enzyme Commission (EC) classification

All enzymes are divided into one of six general classes depending on the type of reaction they catalyze. A few clinically important enzymes are listed in Table 54-1 along with the EC code and systematic names.

The first class includes the *oxidoreductases,* those enzymes that catalyze electron transfer or oxidation-reduction reactions, which can be illustrated schematically as follows:

$$A_{red} + B_{ox} \rightleftharpoons A_{ox} + B_{red}$$

An example of an enzyme in this category is lactic dehydrogenase (EC 1.1.1.27). Some common names of enzymes in this category include dehydrogenases, reductases, oxidases, and peroxidases.

The second group of enzymes contains the *transferases,* those enzymes that catalyze the transfer of a group, such as an amino, carboxyl, glucosyl, methyl, or phosphoryl group, from one molecule to another. These reactions can be listed schematically as:

$$A-X + B \rightleftharpoons A + B-X$$

Alanine aminotransferase (EC 2.6.1.2) is an example of this group. Other common enzymes in this category include kinases and transcarboxylases.

A third group includes the *hydrolases,* which catalyze the cleavage of C—O, C—N, C—C, and some other bonds with

Table 54-1 Examples of enzyme nomenclature

EC code	Recommended name (trivial)	Abbreviation*	Systematic name	Other name or abbreviation
Oxidoreductases				
1.1.1.27	Lactate dehydrogenase	LD	L-Lactate:NAD$^+$ oxidoreductase	LDH
1.1.1.37	Malate dehydrogenase	MD	L-Malate:NAD$^+$ oxidoreductase	MDH
1.1.1.42	Isocitrate dehydrogenase (NADP$^+$)	ICD	*threo*-D$_s$-Isocitrate:NADP$^+$ oxidoreductase (decarboxylating)	
1.1.1.49	Glucose-6-phosphate dehydrogenase	GPD	D-Glucose-6-phosphate:NADP$^+$ 1-oxidoreductase	G6PDH, G-6-PDH
1.4.1.2	Glutamate dehydrogenase	GLD	L-Glutamate:NAD$^+$ oxidoreductase (deaminating)	—
1.16.3.1	Ferroxidase	—	Iron(II):oxygen oxidoreductase	Ceruloplasmin
Transferases				
2.1.3.3	Ornithine carbamoyltransferase	OCT	Carbamoylphosphate:L-ornithine carbamoyltransferase	Ornithine carbamyltransferase
2.3.2.2	γ-Glutamyltransferase	GGT	(5-Glutamyl)-peptide:amino acid 5-glutamyl transferase	—
2.6.1.1	Asparate aminotransferase	AST	L-Aspartate:2-oxoglutarate aminotransferase	Serum glutamic oxaloacetic transaminase, SGOT
2.6.1.2	Alanine aminotransferase	ALT	L-Alanine:2-oxoglutarate aminotransferase	Serum glutamic pyruvic transaminase, SGPT
2.7.1.1	Hexokinase	HK†	ATP:D-hexose-6-phosphotransferase	—
2.7.1.40	Pyruvate kinase	PK	ATP:pyruvate 2-O-phosphotransferase	—
2.7.3.2	Creatine kinase	CK	ATP:creatine *N*-phosphotransferase	CPK
Hydrolases				
3.1.1.3	Triacylglycerol lipase	LPS	Triacylglycerol acyl hydrolase	Lipase
3.1.1.8	Cholinesterase	CHS	Acylcholine acyl hydrolase	Pseudocholinesterase
3.1.3.1	Alkaline phosphatase	ALP	Orthophosphoric-monoester phosphohydrolase (alkaline optimum)	—
3.1.3.2	Acid phosphatase	ACP	Orthophosphoric-monoester phosphohydrolase (acid optimum)	—
3.1.3.5	5'-Nucleotidase	NT	5'-Ribonucleotide phosphohydrolase	—
3.2.1.1	α-Amylase	AMS	1,4-α-D-Glucan glucanohydrolase	Diastase
3.4.11.1	Aminopeptidase (cytosol)	LAS‡	α-Aminoacyl-peptide hydrolase (cytosol)	Arylaminadase, LAP, leucine aminopeptidase
3.4.21.1	Chymotrypsin	—	None (preferred cleavage: Tyr, Trp, Phe, Leu)	Chymotrypsin A and B
3.4.21.4	Trypsin	TPS	None (preferred cleavage: Arg, Lys)	α- and β-trypsin
Lyase				
4.1.2.13	Fructose-bisphosphate aldolase	ALS	D-Fructose-1,6-bisphosphate: D-glyceraldehyde-3-phosphate-lyase	Aldolase
4.2.1.24	Porphobilinogen synthase	—	5-Aminolevulinate hydrolyase	—
Isomerases				
5.3.1.1	Triose phosphate isomerase	TPI	D-Glyceraldehyde-3-phosphate: ketol-isomerase	Triosephosphate mutase
5.3.1.9	Glucose phosphate isomerase	GPI	D-Glucose-6-phosphate: ketol-isomerase	Phosphohexose isomerase
Ligases				
6.3.1.2	Glutamine synthetase	—	L-Glutamate:ammonia ligase (ADP-forming)	—

*Baron DN et al: *J Clin Pathol* 24:656-657, 1971 (ref. 4) and Baron DN et al: *J Clin Pathol* 28:592-593, 1975 (ref. 5) are *not* recommended by the International Union of Biochemistry but are in common use.
†Not listed in references 4 and 5 but in common use in biochemistry laboratories.
‡Reference 5 incorrectly lists (EC 3.4.11.2) the microsomal form of this enzyme as "leucine aminopeptidase."

the addition of water. These hydrolysis reactions can be illustrated as follows:

$$A\!-\!B + H_2O \rightleftharpoons A\!-\!OH + B\!-\!H$$

An example of this group is acid phosphatase (EC 3.1.3.2). Other common enzymes in this category are amylase, urease, pepsin, trypsin, chymotrypsin, and various peptidases and esterases.

A fourth group contains the *lyases,* which hydrolyze C—C, C—O, and C—N bonds by elimination, with the formation of a double bond or catalyze the reverse reaction, the addition of a group to a double bond. In cases where the reverse reaction is important the term *synthase* is used in the name.

This type of reaction is illustrated as follows:

$$A + B \rightleftharpoons AB \text{ (synthase)} \quad \text{or} \quad AB \rightleftharpoons A + B \text{ (lyase)}$$

An examination of the EC listing shows that this and the subsequent groups contain relatively few enzymes that are used in clinical diagnosis.

The fifth group includes the *isomerases,* which catalyze structural or geometric changes in a molecule. They are also called *epimerases, isomerases,* and *mutases* depending on the type of isomerism involved. This reaction can be illustrated as follows:

$$ABC \rightleftharpoons CAB$$

An example of this group is the enzyme glucose phosphate isomerase (EC 5.3.1.9). It is not commonly used diagnostically.

A sixth and last group consists of the *ligases,* or synthetases. In this reaction two molecules are joined, coupled with the hydrolysis of the pyrophosphate in ATP. Many of these enzymes are involved in DNA, RNA, and protein synthesis; none are currently used in clinical diagnosis. The synthetic reaction type is illustrated as follows:

$$A + B + ATP \rightleftharpoons AB + ADP + P_i$$

An example of this reaction is the enzyme glutamine synthetase (EC 6.3.1.2), which is rarely used clinically.

Nonstandard abbreviations

A variety of simple abbreviations containing four or fewer capital letters are also used to represent the enzymes that are routinely measured. These abbreviations are widely used in practice but are *not* part of the IUB system. They are so popular and have become so commonly used that it would be difficult to discard them, and they are listed in Table 54-1.

MEASUREMENT OF ENZYMES

In most enzymatic procedures, the reaction rates are found not to be constant with time. By observing the rate of change of absorbance for a substrate or product at a specific wavelength, one can follow the reaction. Initially,

there is a *lag phase* with little change of absorbance per unit time when the reactants are mixed and reach thermal and kinetic equilibrium, then a *linear phase* of constant absorbance change per unit time, and finally a *substrate-depletion phase* with little change of absorbance per unit time.

Enzyme assays must be performed during the linear phase of absorbance change where a constant amount of activity can be determined for a period of time (Fig. 54-3,*A*). Thus measurements do not start at zero time but begin after the lag phase has occurred. Measurements can be made at any time during the linear phase and can continue up to the substrate-depletion phase.

If the enzyme activity is too great, substrate depletion may occur before the measurements have been completed. Rather than changing the assay time, the most common way to handle samples with high activity is to dilute them twofold or threefold with saline solution or water (Fig. 54-3, *B*). However, not all enzymes demonstrate linearity on dilution, particularly if the enzymes are active at a lipid-water interface, such as lipase (EC 3.1.1.3), or if there are inhibitors present in the sample, such as LD (EC 1.1.1.27) when measured in urine.

One of the more convenient methods of assaying enzyme activity is based on measurement of the absorbance of either the substrates or the products. There are some enzyme systems that involve the conversion of NAD^+ to its reduced form NADH, or vice versa. The reduced form, NADH, has a much greater absorption at 340 nm than the oxidized form does, and consequently, reactions that convert one form to the other may be conveniently followed by measurement of the change in absorption at this wavelength. The difference in the absorption spectrum of the reduced and oxidized compounds is shown in Fig. 54-4.

Enzyme assays

Enzymes currently are measured by either their immunochemical or catalytic properties. The two most commonly employed methods that measure their catalytic properties are the one-point method at a fixed time, sometimes called an *end-point method,* and the multipoint fixed time assay, called the *kinetic method.*

End-point assays are still used in some cases, but in general shorter periods are employed. In these assays a reaction is started and allowed to incubate at a constant temperature for a fixed period, such as 30 minutes. The reaction is then stopped, perhaps by the addition of another reagent, and the amount of product is measured. The assumption in this type of assay is that a constant amount of product is produced throughout the entire assay period.

If the rate of reaction is followed continuously or with many points as a function of time, the assay is termed a *kinetic assay.* Usually the reaction time is short, that is, a

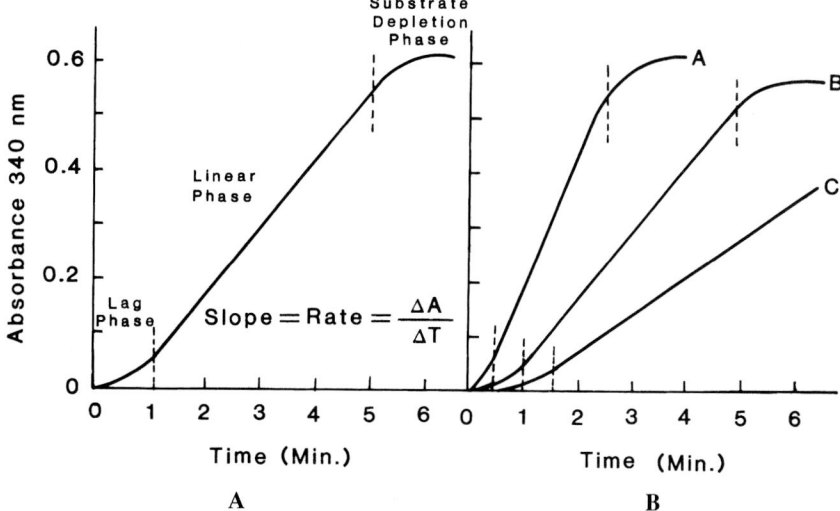

Fig. 54-3 **A,** Typical enzyme reaction with initial lag phase, linear change of absorbance, and final phase of substrate depletion. Enzyme activity is slope of linear phase. **B,** Time course of an enzyme reaction with three different amounts of enzyme present. Curve *A* has a high activity, *B* has a medium activity, and *C* has a low activity. As enzyme activity is increased in an assay system, lag phase decreases, linear phase decreases, and substrate depletion occurs sooner. *ΔA,* Change of absorbance; *ΔT,* change of time.

few seconds to a few minutes, and there is little danger of enzyme degradation. The term *kinetic assay* is also used to describe enzyme reactions that form increasing amounts of product with time; the reactions may be monitored as one-point *end-point assays* or *multiple-point* (continuous-monitoring) *assays.* Although this kinetic method terminology is not strictly correct, the continuous or multiple-point assays are superior to the single-point, fixed time assays, since it is easier to demonstrate approximate linearity of the reaction over the entire measurement period.

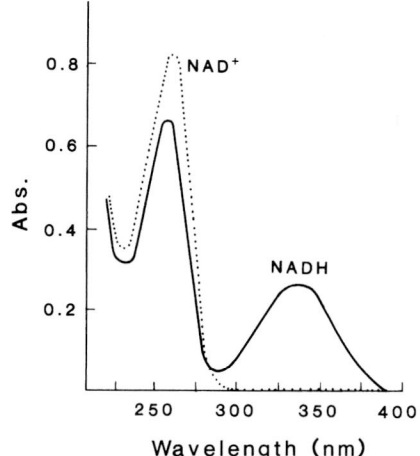

Fig. 54-4 Absorption spectrum, *Abs.,* of 5 × 10^{-5} M NAD$^+$ in 0.1 M Tris buffer, pH 7.5 (dotted line), and absorption spectrum of 4 × 10^{-5} M NADH in 0.1 M Tris buffer, pH 9.5 (solid line).

Principles of kinetic analysis

Enzyme kinetics is the study of enzyme reaction rates and the factors that affect them. Initially, many experiments are performed to examine the effects of different assay conditions on measurements of enzyme activity. Eventually, a series of specific conditions are established that give rise to the maximum rate of enzyme activity.

The general enzyme reaction given previously for a *single substrate reaction* may be rewritten slightly for *initial rates,* as in Equation 54-3. In this case, the amount of product is very small and the reverse reaction of P combining with E and forming {ES} is ignored, since initial rate measurements are to be made. The initial rate is the rate at the start of the reaction, after the lag phase and during the linear phase in Fig. 54-5*A,* but before substantial product formation.

$$E + S \underset{k_{-1}}{\overset{k_{+1}}{\rightleftharpoons}} \{ES\} \overset{k_{+2}}{\rightarrow} P + E \qquad \textit{Eq. 54-3}$$

For a given quantity of enzyme, the rate of activity that is observed increases with increasing amounts of substrate, as is shown in Fig. 54-5. At low substrate concentrations the rate is linearly dependent on the amount of substrate, that is, *first order,* but at high substrate concentrations the rate is essentially independent of substrate concentration, that is, *zero order.* A mathematical description of the reaction must explain how the reaction can be first order at low substrate concentrations and zero order at high substrate concentrations.

If the enzyme has a limited number of active sites, at a low substrate concentration the rate will be dependent on

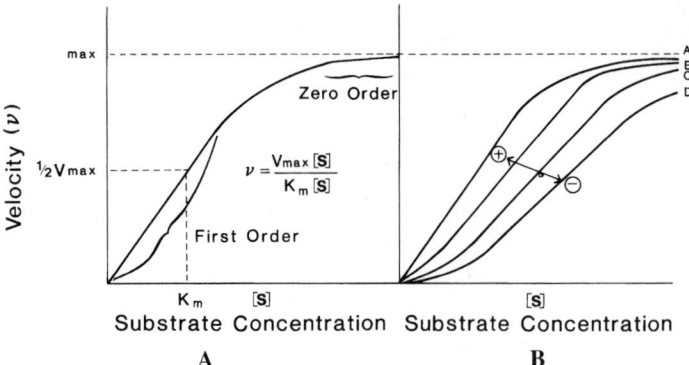

Fig. 54-5 **A,** Relationship of substrate, *S*, to velocity of reaction. At low substrate concentrations, the rate is first order (linearly dependent) with respect to substrate concentration. At high substrate concentrations the rate becomes zero order (independent) with respect to substrate concentration. K_m, Michaelis-Menten constant; V_{max}, maximal rate of reaction. **B,** Relationship between velocity and substrate concentration for an allosteric enzyme. Presence of positive or negative effectors shifts curve toward the + or − side respectively.

the amount of substrate present, since there will be a large effective concentration of unfilled active sites. However, since the total number of sites on the enzyme is limited and the amount of enzyme is constant, then, as the amount of substrate is increased, the sites will become increasingly saturated with substrate until the reaction will appear to be independent of the substrate concentration. At these high substrate concentrations all the enzyme active sites are filled and the reaction proceeds at maximal velocity. Small changes in the substrate concentration after saturation will not affect the enzyme rate.

The second step, product formation, is assumed to be the rate-limiting step or the one that determines the overall activity. The equilibrium for the formation of ES complex can be written as follows with the molar concentrations of all the reacting species expressed in brackets:

$$K_{eq} = \frac{k_{+1}}{k_{-1}} = \frac{[ES]}{[E][S]}$$

The equilibrium constant, K_{eq}, is equal to the ratio of the forward over the reverse rate constants. From Equation 54-3, the rate of formation of the product *P* is the amount of *[ES]* times the rate k_{+2} at which the enzyme complex is converted to *E + P*. Thus the rate of formation of product is:

$$\text{Velocity, or Rate} = [ES] \times k_{+2}$$

Since the rate is the amount of product formed for some period of time:

$$\text{Rate} = \frac{\Delta P}{\Delta T} = [ES] \times k_{+2}$$

and substituting $K_{eq}[E][S]$ for [ES] and rearranging gives:

$$\Delta P = K_{eq} \times [S] \times [E] \times k_{+2} \times \Delta T$$

The amount of product formed is proportional to the amount of enzyme present, the time of the assay, and the amount of substrate present. When a proportionality constant is substituted for the rate constants, the equation becomes:

$$\Delta P = K_1 \times [S] \times [E] \times \Delta T$$

where ΔP is the amount of product formed during the assay time, *[E]* is the amount of enzyme, *[S]* is the amount of substrate, ΔT is the assay time, and K_1 is a proportionality constant. The enzyme activity, or rate of product formation over time, is then given by:

$$\text{Rate} = \frac{\Delta P}{\Delta T} = K_1 \times [S] \times [E]$$

Usually enzyme assays are performed at a high substrate concentration for a short enough period so that the substrate concentration can be assumed to be constant. The value of this constant substrate concentration can be combined with K_1 to produce a second proportionality constant, K_2, which is the product of K_1 times the substrate concentration. The rate can then be expressed so that it is dependent only on the amount of enzyme present, that is, a zero-order reaction, independent of substrate concentration.

$$\text{Rate} = \frac{\Delta P}{\Delta T} = K_2 \times [E]$$

This rate of reaction, or velocity, is often listed as *v*, or V_i, or V_o, in the enzyme kinetic literature.

K_m and V_{max}

The enzyme activity, that is, rate, or velocity, is dependent on the substrate concentration when the amount of substrate is low relative to the amount of enzyme present in an assay. This relationship for a single substrate reaction is shown graphically in Fig. 54-5, with the same enzyme concentration assayed at many different substrate concentrations.

At steady state, before much product is present, the rate of formation of the [ES] complex will equal the rate of breakdown. One can describe this using the following rate equation:

Formation		**Breakdown**
k_{+1} [E][S]	$= k_{-1}$ [ES]	$+ k_{+2}$ [ES]

By collecting terms and rearranging, one can remove the rate constants and a constant, K_m, is defined.

$$\frac{[E][S]}{[ES]} = \frac{k_{-1} + k_{+2}}{k_{+1}} = K_m \qquad \textit{Eq. 54-4}$$

The rate or velocity of product formation, *v*, at any time and the free enzyme concentration, *[E]*, are described by:

$$v = k_{+2}\,[ES] \quad \text{and} \quad [E] = [Et] - [ES]$$

where *[Et]* is the total amount of enzyme and *[ES]* is the amount complexed with substrate. When all the enzyme is present in the form of [ES] (that is, at very high [S] in a zero-order reaction), the maximum rate, V_{max}, is as follows:

$$V_{max} = k_{+2}\,[Et]$$

Combining the above three equations gives:

$$[E] = \frac{V_{max}}{k_{+2}} - \frac{v}{k_{+2}} = \frac{V_{max} - v}{k_{+2}}$$

Since from Equation 54-4:

$$[E] = \frac{K_m\,[ES]}{[S]} \quad \text{and} \quad [ES] = \frac{v}{k_{+2}}$$

then:

$$\frac{K_m\,[ES]}{[S]} = \frac{V_{max} - v}{k_{+2}} \quad \text{or} \quad \frac{K_m \times v}{[S] \times k_{+2}} = \frac{V_{max} - v}{k_{+2}}$$

Rearranging gives:

$$K_m \times v = (V_{max} - v)[S] \quad \text{or} \quad v(K_m + [S]) = V_{max}[S]$$

When this equation is solved for *v*, it gives the *Michaelis-Menten equation*, which is the equation for the rectangular hyperbola shown in Fig. 54-5, *A*.

$$v = \frac{V_{max}\,[S]}{K_m + [S]} \qquad \qquad \textit{Eq. 54-5}$$

[S] is the concentration of substrate, *v* is the velocity, V_{max} is the maximal rate of reaction when the enzyme is saturated with substrate, and K_m, the Michaelis-Menten constant, is that substrate concentration that produces one half the maximal velocity.

At the fixed high substrate concentration found in the usual clinical laboratory assays, the velocity, *v*, approaches V_{max} and is proportional to the amount of enzyme present, since all other factors are constant. The reaction is said to be zero order with respect to substrate, that is, independent of the concentration of substrate. The common condition used for assaying enzyme activity is a high substrate concentration where $[S] \cong 10 \times K_m$ or higher. The rate at a substrate concentration of $10 \times K_m$ is given by the following equation:

$$v = \frac{V_{max}(10 \times K_m)}{K_m + (10 \times K_m)} = V_{max}\,\frac{10 \times K_m}{11 \times K_m} = 0.91\,V_{max}$$

Thus at $[S] = 10 \times K_m$ the rate produced is greater than 90% of V_{max}.

Another way to examine the Michaelis-Menten equation is to see if it is consistent with first-order kinetics at low substrate concentrations and zero-order kinetics at high substrate concentrations.

At low substrate concentrations where $[S] \ll K_m$:

$$v = \frac{V_{max}[S]}{K_m + [S]} \cong \frac{V_{max}[S]}{K_m}$$

and since K_m and V_{max} are constants:

$$v = K_1\,[S]$$

it shows that the rate is dependent only on the first power of the substrate concentration.

At high substrate concentrations where $[S] \gg K_m$,

$$v = \frac{V_{max}[S]}{K_m + [S]} \cong \frac{V_{max}[\cancel{S}]}{[\cancel{S}]} = V_{max}$$

showing that the rate *(v)* does not depend on substrate concentration.

As shown in Fig. 54-5, *A*, the relationship of substrate concentration to enzyme activity is a curve that is often similar to a rectangular hyperbola. For multisubstrate enzyme reactions the kinetics are more complex. The presence of activators and inhibitors acting at allosteric or regulatory sites tends to make the curves less linear because of the complex kinetics.

The accurate determination of K_m and V_{max} for each substrate or activator from Michaelis-Menten curves such as those shown in Fig. 54-5, *A,* is very difficult, even if the curves are fairly linear. However, it is necessary to determine these constants so that assays may be established using optimal conditions to correctly measure enzyme activity. If the curve is transformed into a straight line, the K_m and V_{max} can be determined with greater accuracy. One may transform the Michaelis-Menten equation mathematically and obtain the equation of a straight line in several ways. The K_m and V_{max} can then be graphically determined from the line slopes and intercepts using these transformed equations. Common graphical presentations are shown in Fig. 54-6.

Calculation of enzyme activity

The results of an enzyme determination are expressed as an *activity* unit in terms of the amount of product formed per unit of time under specified conditions for a given volume of sample, which is often serum. Thus one unit of enzyme activity might be the amount of enzyme that would, under certain specified conditions, cause the formation of 1 mg of the product, *P,* per minute when 1 mL of the sample was used. In older procedures arbitrary units like these were often employed.

In 1961 the Enzyme Commission recommended the adoption of an international unit (IU) of enzyme activity. The IU was defined as the amount of enzyme that would convert 1 micromole of substrate per minute under standard conditions.

$$1\ IU = 1\ micromole/minute$$

In those instances where one molecule of substrate is transformed into two or more molecules of a

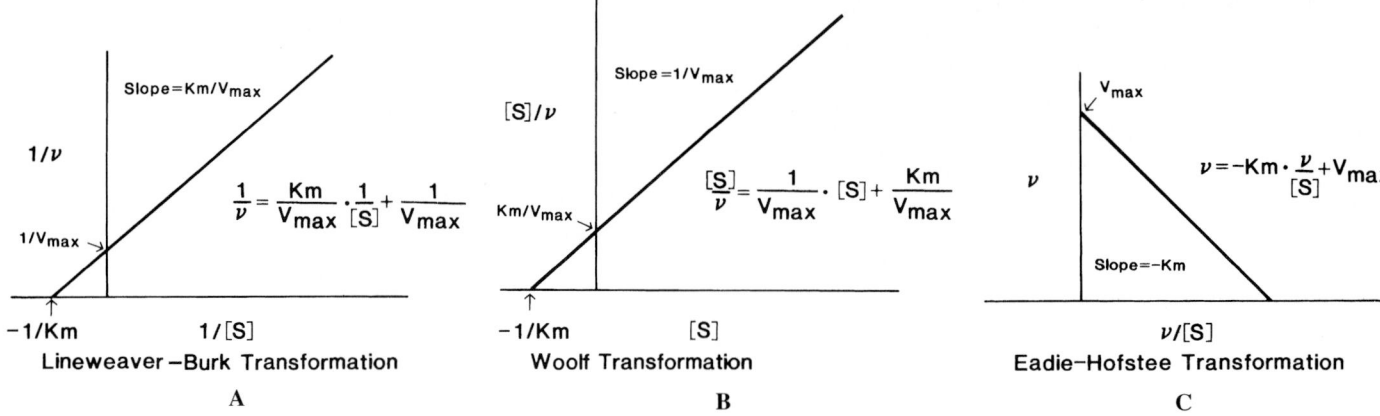

Fig. 54-6 Graphic representations of linear forms of Michaelis-Menten equation.

product, the definition is per micromole of product formed.

This unit has been widely adopted, and in some respects it has standardized assay units. It has not reduced the number of reference intervals because if the standard conditions change the apparent enzyme activity changes. For example, if a new buffer were used in the assay, it may affect the enzyme rate and produce a different reference interval.

The Systmème International d'Unités (SI), as originally adopted by the World Health Organization, established the unit of enzyme activity as the katal (K). This is defined as 1 mole/sec of substrate changed. This unit is too large to be useful clinically, and so it has met with little acceptance in the United States though it was recommended by the EC in 1972.

To convert international units to katals:

$$1 \text{ IU} = \frac{\text{Micromole}}{\text{Minute}} \times \frac{10^{-6} \text{ mole}}{\text{Micromole}} \times \frac{1 \text{ min}}{60 \text{ sec}} = 1.67 \times 10^{-8} \text{ K}$$

Thus, 1.0 IU = 16.7 nK (nanokatals). Only the international units IU have been widely adopted by workers in the field of clinical enzymology. The katal has not gained widespread acceptance.

Pure human enzyme materials are not available, and so enzyme assays cannot be standardized in each laboratory by calibration with pure materials. Other methods of standardization of enzyme assays must be used. The alternative method that is used most widely depends on having an accurately calibrated spectrophotometer. Many enzyme assays are followed by spectrophotometric measurements being made at a specific wavelength. With the spectrophotometric method usually one assumes that at 340 nm, NADH has a molar absorption coefficient, ϵ, of

$$A/(l \times c) = 6.22 \times 10^3 \text{ L} \cdot \text{mol}^{-1} \cdot \text{cm}^{-1}$$

where A is the actual absorbance of a solution, l is the light path in centimeters through the solution, and c is the concentration in moles per liter of the absorbing substance (see Chapter 4). For a 1 cm light path, rearranging for c:

$$c = A \times 10^{-3}/6.22 \text{ mol/L}$$

When the concentration is expressed in micromoles per liter instead of moles per liter, the expression is:

$$c = A \times 10^3/6.22 \text{ } \mu\text{mol/L}$$

From the absorbance change that was measured and the volume of solution used, one can readily calculate the number of micromoles of NADH formed or used up during the enzyme-measurement period.

$$c = \Delta A \times 10^3/6.22 \text{ } \mu\text{mol/L}$$

For example, in the lactate dehydrogenase reaction above, if a change in absorbance of 0.06 per minute was observed at 340 nm in a 1 cm curette and a 0.1 mL sample was used with a total assay volume of 3.0 mL, the calculation of activity would be as follows:

$$\text{International units/L} = \frac{0.06 \times 1000 \text{ } \mu\text{mol/mmol} \times 3.0 \text{ mL}}{6.22 \text{ mmol/L} \times 0.1 \text{ mL}}$$
$$= 289 \text{ IU/L}$$

Both of the enzyme units that have been described express the activity in terms of units per volume of sample. This is a particularly convenient unit of measure in the clinical laboratory when one is assaying enzymes in biological fluids like serum and plasma. If one is measuring an enzyme found in erythrocytes (RBC) or in white blood cells (WBC), another unit of measure is needed. In the case of RBC and WBC enzymes, the enzyme activity can be expressed as units per 10^{10} cells.

In biochemistry laboratories where enzyme purification is important, the activity might be expressed as milligrams of protein or as dry weight of cells or as micrograms of DNA, but these are not convenient units for the clinical laboratory.

Analytical factors affecting enzyme measurement

The rate of reactions involving enzymes is greatly influenced by temperature, pH, concentration of substrate, and several other factors. Accordingly, all the details of a given procedure must be followed exactly to produce precise and accurate results.

Assays of enzyme activity should be performed under optimal conditions of zero-order kinetics, and so the measured rate is dependent only on the amount of enzyme present. To optimize an assay, such as the lactate dehydrogenase reaction given earlier, a series of reaction assays are set up with increasing concentrations of lactate but with a high fixed NAD^+ concentration and a fixed amount of enzyme. The enzyme rates are then measured, and a graph similar to that in Fig. 54-6 is constructed. A second series of assays is then performed with increasing concentrations of NAD^+ but at the fixed high concentration of lactate determined from the first experiment, that is, $[S] \cong 10\ K_m$ for lactate, and the same amount of enzyme present. The enzyme rates are again determined and another graph is created to determine the K_m for NAD^+. This same type of experiment is performed for each item of the assay mixture (such as metal ions, pH, buffer) until all the variables have been evaluated for the production of maximal enzyme activity. The final conditions determined from this set of experiments would be the *optimal assay* conditions. Experiments to determine optimal assay conditions have been performed for the current clinically important enzymes, and diagnostic kits are commercially available with all the materials at usually optimal concentrations.

pH

Changes in pH will considerably affect the enzyme reaction rate. For most enzymes there is a definite pH range where the enzyme is most active. A pH near the center of this range is usually specified for the measurement of that particular enzyme. The optimal pH is different for different enzymes. Reduced activity is observed at pH values greater or less than the optimal.

A typical pH curve of enzyme activity is given in Fig. 54-7. This is a bell-shaped curve showing changes in enzyme activity versus pH.

At pH values other than the optimal pH, the enzyme activity may be affected because of changes in the structure of the enzyme. These changes may occur at the active site, or may result from conformational changes affecting the three-dimensional structure.

Since the active site of an enzyme often contains ionizable side chains of amino acids, such as $RCOO^-$ or RNH_3^+, a significant change in the pH can lead to the gain or loss of a proton. The result will be a substantial change in surface charge at the active site. The active site might, therefore, lose its ability to attract a substrate with an opposing charge. A similar loss of activity would occur if the change in charge were on the substrate molecule rather than on the

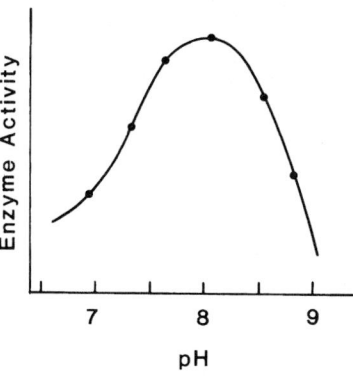

Fig. 54-7 Enzyme activity as a function of pH. Optimal pH range is 7.8 to 8.2; lower activities are observed at pH < 7.8 and pH > 8.2.

enzyme. A change of pH might bring about an unfolding of the enzyme and loss of activity if the effect of pH change was to disrupt hydrogen bonds and other intramolecular forces holding the enzyme in an active conformation.

Buffer

In many cases, as the enzyme reaction proceeds, products that tend to alter the pH are produced. Most assays include a buffer to maintain the assay pH within the optimal pH range. The buffer chosen should have a pK_a within 1 pH unit of the optimal pH of the enzyme to exert effective pH control.

Buffers not only serve to regulate the pH of an assay, but may also take part in the reaction as well. Alkaline phosphatase (ALP, EC 3.1.3.1) assays with *p*-nitrophenyl phosphate as a substrate use the buffer 2-amino-2-methyl-1-propanol (AMP) to maintain the pH at 10.2. The enzyme hydrolyzes the substrate into *p*-nitrophenol and inorganic phosphate in a multistep process, part of which involves a temporary phosphorylation of the enzyme. The final and rate-limiting step includes hydrolysis of the enzyme-phosphate bond to regenerate free enzyme. At similar pH values, buffers that are phosphate acceptors in a transphosphorylation process with the enzyme will produce rates of alkaline phosphatase activity higher than those of buffers that do not act as phosphate acceptors. Thus AMP buffer produces rates of alkaline phosphatase activity at pH 10.2 higher than those of glycylglycine buffer at pH 10.2 because AMP is a phosphate acceptor. In the case of buffers that do not participate in the reaction, the concentration of buffer that gives maximal enzyme activity at the optimal pH must also be experimentally determined.

It has been found that the buffer and certain salts may have an unusual effect on the K_m. When the buffer-to-substrate ratio is very large, the buffer may compete with the substrate for the enzyme and make the enzyme activity appear to be related to substrate concentration in a nonlinear way. This has been observed with NADH in the LD reaction. Here the buffer-to-substrate molar ratio is $10^4:1$ and the rate of reaction is affected by Tris, phosphate, and NH_4HCO_3 buffers and certain salts, such as NaCl and $(NH_4)_2SO_4$, which are often found in the coupling or auxiliary enzymes used to prepare assays. There seems to be no effect at buffer concentrations below 0.05 mol/L, which is consistent with several recommendations for optimal LD assay conditions. It would seem prudent to maintain as low a concentration of buffer as possible without compromising pH stability or enzyme rate.

Cofactors

Many enzymes require a nonprotein, often dialyzable, material for maximal activity. Some of these materials are related to vitamin structures. For example, thiamine or vitamin B_1 can be converted to thiamine pyrophosphate, a cofactor in many decarboxylation reactions. Niacin can be converted to nicotinamide adenine dinucleotide, and vitamin B_2, riboflavin, can be converted to flavin adenine dinucleotide. Both of these compounds are involved in many dehydrogenation reactions. Pyridoxine, vitamin B_6, is modified to pyridoxal phosphate, which is used in many transamination reactions.

In analytical assays of transaminase activity, pyridoxyl-5-phosphate is an example of a tightly bound cofactor that is not a substrate. The optimal concentration of a cofactor is determined in the same way as a substrate so that assay conditions can be established with a cofactor concentration of approximately $10\ K_m$ or higher.

Activators and inhibitors

Many enzymes require specific ions for maximal activity. All phosphate-transferring enzymes, such as hexokinase, require magnesium ions (Mg^{++}). Other common metal ion activators are manganese (Mn^{++}), calcium (Ca^{++}), zinc (Zn^{++}), iron (Fe^{++}), and potassium (K^+). Amylase requires chloride (Cl^-) for maximal activity, and there are enzymes that require several ions for maximal activity; for example, pyruvate kinase requires magnesium (Mg^{++}) and potassium (K^+). In each case, the optimal concentration of the activator must be determined just as the optimal concentration of substrate is determined.

Inhibitors are materials that reduce the catalytic activity of an enzyme. There are many types of inhibitors and several classes of inhibition. Inhibitors may act by removing an activator by chelation; for example, Ca^{++} and Mg^{++} are removed by EDTA or oxalate to cause the inhibition of hexokinase. They may also act by binding to the active site to compete with the substrate or by forming a complex at a different site, that is, an allosteric site, which may affect the enzyme activity.

Inhibitors are classed into three main groups. *Competitive inhibitors* bind at the active site and compete with the substrate for binding sites. These materials demonstrate a reversible inhibition that can often be reduced when one uses a higher substrate concentration.

$$
\begin{array}{ccc}
E & + S \rightleftharpoons \{ES\} & \rightarrow P + E \\
+ & & + \\
I & & I \\
\updownarrow & & \updownarrow \\
\{EI\} & + S \rightleftharpoons \{ESI\} &
\end{array}
$$

The maximum rate of reaction is not affected if enough substrate is present because of the reversibility of the reactions. The binding of the substrate is affected, and thus the apparent K_m will be higher while the V_{max} remains the same.

Noncompetitive inhibitors bind at an allosteric or regulatory site, which may be at or far removed from the active site. These inhibitors cannot be reversed by the addition of more substrate because they bind at a different location on the enzyme surface.

$$
\begin{array}{c}
S \rightleftharpoons \{ES\} \rightarrow P + E \\
+ \\
E \\
+ \\
I \rightleftharpoons \{EI\}
\end{array}
$$

Since the inhibitor does not compete with the substrate, the K_m will be unaffected, but the amount of E or ES that converts substrate to product will be reduced and the V_{max} will be lessened.

Uncompetitive inhibitors, a third group of inhibitors, are believed to bind to the enzyme substrate complex and not to the free enzyme. In this case, at low substrate concentrations, the addition of more substrate increases the inhibition, since it produces more enzyme-substrate complex to react with the inhibitor. The result of this type of inhibition is that the V_{max} is reduced and the K_m is increased.

$$
\begin{array}{c}
E + S \rightleftharpoons \{ES\} \rightarrow P + E \\
+ \\
I \\
\updownarrow \\
\{ESI\}
\end{array}
$$

The type of inhibition a substance exerts can be determined when one examines the results of kinetic studies, with and without inhibitors, using a linear graph of enzyme activity, as is shown in Fig. 54-8. A brief summary of the effects of the types of inhibition is given in Table 54-2. The simple types of inhibition may be classified by examination of the kinetic effect on the K_m and V_{max}.

Coupling enzymes

Some enzyme reactions of interest, such as alanine aminotransferase (ALT) and aspartate aminotransferase (AST), do not have substrates or form products that can be monitored directly. One may couple the initial enzyme reaction to a second *indicating enzyme* reaction that, for example, does contain the $NAD^+/NADH$ conversion to make a convenient assay. The AST enzyme reaction can be coupled to the malate dehydrogenase reaction (MD, EC 1.1.1.37):

$$\text{L-Aspartate} + \alpha\text{-Ketoglutarate} \overset{\text{AST}}{\rightleftharpoons} \text{L-Glutamate} + \text{Oxaloacetate}$$

$$\text{Oxaloacetate} + NADH + H^+ \overset{\text{MD}}{\rightleftharpoons} \text{L-Malate} + NAD^+$$

This gives the following net reaction:

$$\text{L-Aspartate} + \alpha\text{-Ketoglutarate} + NADH + H^+ \rightleftharpoons$$
$$\text{L-Glutamate} + \text{L-Malate} + NAD^+$$

In this case, the substrate for the second reaction, oxaloacetate, is supplied as the product of the first reaction. Oxaloacetate from the AST reaction and the cofactor NADH serve as the substrates for the malate dehydrogenase reaction. This assay would have L-aspartate, α-ketoglutarate,

Table 54-2 Kinetic effects of inhibition

Type of inhibition	Change in K_m	Change in V_{max}
Competitive	Increased	No change
Noncompetitive	No change	Decreased
Uncompetitive	Increased	Decreased

NADH, and the enzyme malate dehydrogenase (MD) present at large excesses so that the rate-limiting item in the assay would be the amount of AST in the sample.

For other enzymes, such as creatine kinase (CK, EC 2.7.3.2), the measurement of the first enzyme requires an intermediate *auxiliary enzyme reaction* and then an *indicator enzyme*. In the measurement of CK, hexokinase (EC 2.7.1.1) is used as an *auxiliary enzyme* and glucose-6-phosphate dehydrogenase (EC 1.1.1.49) is used as an *indicating enzyme*. Both of these additional enzymes would have to be present in large excesses to correctly measure CK. It is difficult to establish optimum assays that have more than two coupled reactions because of the large number of components in the assay system and the problems with maximizing all the components without causing inhibition of the limiting reaction.

Temperature

There is no optimal temperature for enzyme assays. Most enzymes show increasing activity as the temperature is raised over a limited temperature range, such as 10° to 40° C; an example is shown in Fig. 54-9.

To minimize any losses of activity if the enzyme cannot be assayed immediately after collection, one should store samples at refrigerator temperatures, 2° to 6° C, or frozen (Table 54-3). In a few cases, some forms of enzymes, such as LD_4 and LD_5, have been found to be more stable at room temperature than at refrigerator temperatures. The repeated freezing and thawing of a specimen will often cause denaturation and loss of activity. Above 40° C most enzymes are rapidly denatured and lose almost all activity after a

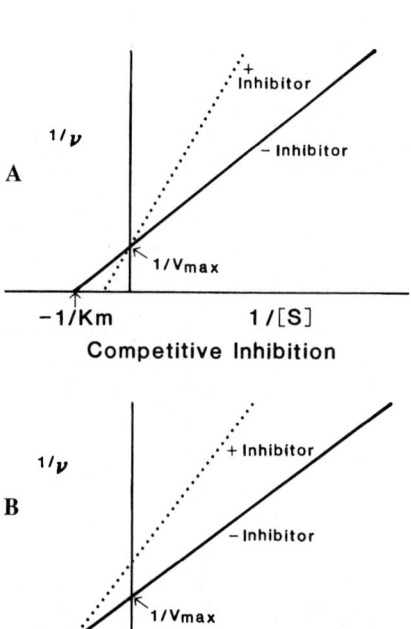

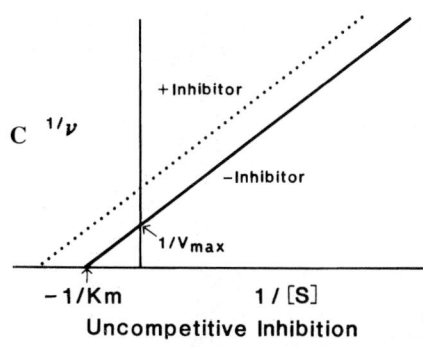

Fig. 54-8 The three types of inhibition are shown by use of Lineweaver-Burk graphic method to demonstrate effect of type of inhibition of K_m and V_{max}.

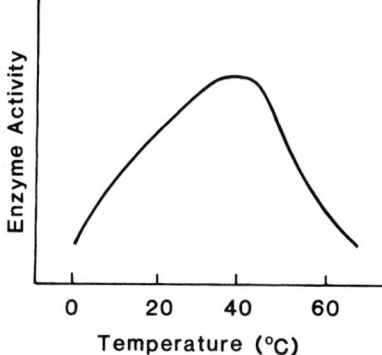

Fig. 54-9 Enzyme activity as a function of temperature of assay. At low temperatures activity decreases. As temperature is raised, activity increases until rate of denaturation is greater than increase in activity.

Table 54-3   Enzyme stability under various storage conditions (less than 10% change in activity)

Enzyme	Room temperature (about 25° C)	Refrigeration (0° to about 4° C)	Frozen (−25° C)
Aldolase (ALS)	2 days	2 days	Unstable*
Alanine aminotransferase (ALT, GPT)	2 days	5 days	Unstable*
α-Amylase (AMS)	1 month	7 months	2 months
Aspartate aminotransferase (AST, GOT)	3 days	1 week	1 month
Ferroxidase I (ceruloplasmin)	1 day	2 weeks	2 weeks
Cholinesterase (CHS)	1 week	1 week	1 week
Creatine kinase (CK)	1 week	1 week	1 month
γ-Glutamyltransferase (GGT)	2 days	1 week	1 month
Isocitrate dehydrogenase (ICD)	1 day	2 days	1 day
Lactate dehydrogenase (LD)	1 week	1 to 3 days†	1 to 3 days†
Leucine aminopeptidase (LAP)	1 week	1 week	1 week
Lipase (LPS)	1 week	3 weeks	3 weeks
Phosphatase, acid (ACP)	4 hours‡	3 days§	3 days§
Phosphatase, alkaline (ALP)	2 to 3 days‖	2 to 3 days	1 month

*Enzyme does not tolerate thawing well.
†Depending on isoenzyme pattern in the serum.
‡Unacidified.
§With added citrate or acetate to pH ~5.
‖Activity may increase.

short time. An exception to this general rule is amylase, which seems to be stable up to about 60° C before significant losses of activity occur.

For many enzymes a 1 Celsius degree change in temperature would produce about a 10% change in activity. A tolerance of ±0.1 Celsius degree for temperature control of an enzyme analyzer is recommended, since this would produce approximately a ±1% change in the activity that was measured. This amount of variation would be small enough to be ignored as an insignificant source of error for most clinical work. A recommendation of ±0.05 Celsius degree for temperature control, which would reduce the change in activity to ±0.5%, has also been suggested.

The apparent increase in activity with increasing temperature means that assays that are performed at higher temperatures, such as 37° C, will be more sensitive to slight changes in the amount of enzyme in a sample. The common enzymes employed for clinical diagnosis are less stable at this temperature than at 25° to 30° C, and therefore assays carried out at 37° C must be performed with relatively short assay times, so that enzyme denaturation is minimized.

Arguments for the use of both higher temperatures, that is, 37° C, and lower temperatures, that is, 25° C, have been presented based primarily on scientific and technical reasoning. A reasonable compromise seems to be measurement at 30° C, which is the recommendation of the International Federation of Clinical Chemistry (IFCC). A very accurate gallium standard melting point cell is now available to all laboratories from the National Institute of Standards and Technology. This material has a melting temperature plateau of 29.772° C and can be used to calibrate or check the assay temperature of a wide variety of instruments.

Defining assay conditions

Although an optimal set of conditions for the assay of an enzyme can be established, it is clear that not all assays are being performed optimally. At times, the differences between assays may not appear to be significant, and yet the results obtained will be substantially divergent. The effect of various components of an assay upon one another, and thus the result, is even more significant when one considers a coupled assay. These assays not only have the concentrations of substrates and activators of the primary reaction to consider, but also must have excesses of the auxiliary and indicating enzymes and their associated activators.

Alanine aminotransferase (ALT) is often measured in an assay that contains an excess of lactate dehydrogenase and NADH, plus L-alanine and α-ketoglutarate and buffer. The usual commercially available kits often specify that about 500 U/L of LD are present as an indicating enzyme and perhaps the animal source of this enzyme. This is not sufficient to define the assay completely, since the K_m of pyruvate varies with the LD isoenzyme type. About four times as many units of M_4-LD_1 would be required than if H_4-LD_5 were used to achieve an equivalent reaction rate. A crude mixture of isoenzymes would be somewhere in between these extremes. Even if the units of LD added to different commercial assays were the same, the measured enzyme rates might vary with each lot of a kit if the indicating enzyme were added without regard to the isoenzyme content. This same kind of variability would occur between manufacturers' kits that contained the same concentrations of substrates, activators, and units of LD if a different source, such as bacterial, of the indicating enzyme were used. It is for this reason that the reference interval for each enzyme assay must be checked by each laboratory, particularly when one is changing reagent manufacturers.

Enzymes as reagents

It is possible to measure the serum levels of the substrate of many enzyme reactions by using many of the principles of enzyme kinetics applied in a slightly different way. The enzyme activity at low substrate concentrations is first order, that is, linear, with respect to substrate concentration. To measure the concentration of pyruvate in a sample, for example, a special assay mixture would be prepared, with only a small amount of the sample being added so that the amount of unknown pyruvate in the assay is low, that is, less than the K_m. One would use an assay mixture that contains an excess of LD, an excess of the coenzyme NADH, the amount of pyruvate present, and a buffer. The reduction in the amount of NADH in this assay is related to the amount of pyruvate present and the millimolar absorption coefficient of NADH at 340 nm. Alternatively a series of pyruvate standards could be used to calibrate the assay. Other enzymatic assays of a similar nature that are commonly used in the clinical laboratory include the determination of glucose, urea, ethanol, cholesterol, triglycerides, and uric acid. Enzymes are also used as indications for immunoassays.

Storage of enzymes

Most of the enzymes that are utilized clinically are stable at refrigerator temperatures for 2 to 3 days to about a week and at room temperature for a shorter time. Table 53-3 summarizes data for three temperatures.

Several enzymes deserve particular comment. Acid phosphatase is unstable at all temperatures unless the pH of the serum is reduced to about 5 to 6 with citrate or acetate. Alkaline phosphatase in human serum demonstrates a linear increase in activity dependent on temperature and time. At 96 hours (4 days) there is a 6% increase at room temperature, a 4% increase at refrigerator temperature, and a 1% increase at $-20°$ C. Enzymes in control materials are usually of nonhuman origin and are much more varied, with some being more stable and some being less stable than human serum.

The observed biological half-lives of several human enzymes in plasma are given in Table 54-4.

CLINICAL ENZYME MEASUREMENTS

A few enzymes have been used since the turn of the century to evaluate chronic diseases, but it wasn't until 1954 that LaDue, Wróblewski, and Karmen found a temporary increase in serum aspartate aminotransferase (EC 2.6.1.1) activity after an acute myocardial infarction. After this time, the measurement of changes in plasma enzyme activity gained importance as a means of following the course of a disease or to improve clinical diagnosis. Many investigators began to look for changes in enzyme activity that were specific for a disease state or reflected damage to a particular tissue.

Table 54-4 Plasma half-lives for clinically important enzymes

Enzymes	Half-life (hours) (mean ± 2 SD)
LD$_1$	53-173
LD$_5$	8-12
CK	15
AST (GOT)	12-22
ALT (GPT)	37-57
AMS	3-6
LPS	3-6
ALP	3-7 days
GGT	3-7 days

Changes in enzyme activity in the plasma or serum are followed, since it is known that enzymes are primarily intracellular constituents that are released after cell damage or cell death has taken place in a specific organ or tissue. The changes that occur with many diseases or in a particular organ can often be understood by examination of the pattern of several enzyme or isoenzyme changes over a period of hours or days.

Extracellular versus cellular enzymes

The enzymes that are found in plasma can be categorized into two major groups. These major subdivisions are the plasma-specific enzymes and the non–plasma specific enzymes.

The plasma-specific enzymes are those enzymes that have a definite and specific function in plasma. Plasma is their normal site of action, and they are present in plasma at higher concentrations than in most tissues. Among these are the enzymes involved in blood coagulation, as well as ferroxidase, pseudocholinesterase, and lipoprotein lipase. These enzymes are synthesized in the liver and are constantly liberated into the plasma to maintain a steady-state concentration. These enzymes are clinically of interest when their concentration decreases in plasma and some have historically been used as estimates of liver function.

The non–plasma specific enzymes are those enzymes with no known function in plasma. Their concentrations in plasma are usually found to be lower than that in most tissues, and there may be a deficiency in plasma of the activators or cofactors that are necessary for maximum enzyme activity. These enzymes can be further divided into the enzymes of secretion, and the enzymes of intermediary metabolism.

The enzymes of secretion are those enzymes secreted from exocrine glands, that is, the pancreas and prostate, and some enzymes from the gastric mucosa and the bones. Enzymes in this group are clinically important when their concentrations are either higher or lower than the reference interval. Elevated values are found when the usual mode of excretion is blocked or when the amount of enzyme produced is increased. Decreases in the amount of enzyme are found when the tissue that ordinarily produces the enzyme is damaged or necrotic. Common examples of this group are amylase, lipase, and acid and alkaline phosphatases.

The other major group of non–plasma specific enzymes are the enzymes of metabolism. The concentrations of these enzymes in tissues are very high, sometimes thousands of times higher than in the plasma. Cellular damage resulting in leakage or necrosis allows a fraction of these proteins to escape into the plasma and causes a sharp rise in the concentration usually observed. Some common examples are creatine kinase (CK), lactate dehydrogenase (LD), alanine aminotransferase (ALT), and aspartate aminotransferase (AST).

Enzymes as tumor markers

Excesses of specific proteins are often elaborated into the plasma during tumor cell growth. In some cases, these specific proteins are enzymes, such as prostatic acid phosphatase (PAP), or creatine kinase (CK), and can be conveniently measured to monitor response to therapy and estimate tumor mass.

FACTORS AFFECTING REFERENCE VALUES

Several important factors affect the reference intervals for enzyme determinations. If these factors are not accounted for in the interpretation of the results, a misdiagnosis is possible. In the following items a brief comment on the problem and an example is given.

Sampling time

Since enzymes do not undergo any significant circadian rhythm, sampling time with respect to time of day is unimportant for the determination of enzyme normal or reference intervals. On the other hand, the sampling time with respect to the onset of a clinical condition may be important for detection of a variety of acute and chronic conditions if the changes observed are sufficiently rapid. The classic average time for maximum elevation for a series of enzymes in patients with a myocardial infarction was reported to be as follows: CK-MB, 6 hours; CK, 18 hours; AST, 24 hours; and LD, 48 hours. Not all patients follow this classical pattern, and a spread of several hours is seen for the rapidly changing analytes and several days for the slower changing analytes if a variety of patients are tested.

Age

There are variations in the amounts of enzymes usually present in serum that are the result of differences in age between various subgroups in the population. There are three principle ages to consider as a factor for determining

a reference interval for an enzyme assay. These are during the first year of life as various organs, such as liver, are becoming functional, during puberty, and in late middle age when hormonal changes occur.

Perhaps some of the most dramatic changes are seen with the enzyme alkaline phosphatase. Using an alkaline phosphatase method with AMP buffer and p-nitrophenyl phosphate substrate at 30° C, one finds the following values: 135 to 270 U/L for children 6 months to 10 years of age, 90 to 320 U/L for children 10 to 18 years of age, and 40 to 100 U/L for adults.

Sex

Differences between the enzyme reference intervals for male and female populations are seen with some enzymes. These differences are most probably related to muscle mass, exercise, or hormone concentration.

An example of these effects is seen with the enzyme creatine kinase, where males are reported to have higher reference intervals than females, which is most likely attributable to increased muscle mass. Alcohol dehydrogenase in gastric mucosa is also reported to be higher in males than in females, allowing males to metabolize ethanol more rapidly. An alcohol load would therefore not adversely affect males as much as females.

Race

Race may also be a factor in a limited number of assays, but data are sparse. Black populations are reported to have higher reference intervals than comparable white populations for creatine kinase, but the effect may be an indirect result of several factors other than race in the two populations.

Exercise

Exercise and ambulation are important variables in the consideration of reference intervals for several enzymes. Patients who have been at complete bed rest for several days are found to have 20% to 30% lower values for creatine kinase than ambulatory patients have. Normal amounts of exercise will also elevate creatine kinase. The additional creatine kinase caused by normal exercise is of the MM type, CK_3. Thus the distinction between these elevations and those that are caused by an acute myocardial infarction, which is the MB type, CK_2, is easily accomplished by determination of the isoenzyme pattern, or direct measurement of CK_2. The increases seen after exercise usually disappear after 12 to 24 hours, unless the exercise is extremely strenuous. In ultralong-distance runners, those that run races longer than 26 miles, the CK_2 can be up to threefold higher than the reference interval and the total CK can be up to fortyfold higher than usual. Even when CK isoenzymes are determined, it may be difficult to distinguish a runner with chest pain from a runner with chest pain and a myocardial infarct.

ISOENZYMES
Nomenclature

The multiple natural forms of an enzyme catalyzing the same reaction in a single species are known as *isoenzymes,* or *isozymes.* The Enzyme Commission of the International Union of Biochemistry has designated that this term is to apply only to those forms of enzymes arising from genetically determined differences in the amino acid structure, though there is not complete agreement on this designation. Isoenzymes are to be distinguished on the basis of electrophoretic mobility and subscripted with the first form having the mobility closest to the anode (+). For example, CK-BB would be subscripted as CK_1, CK-MB as CK_2, and CK-MM as CK_3. Although there exist many reports to the contrary in the literature, isoenzymes should not be labeled on the basis of tissue distribution (that is, heart type, brain type), since some confusion may arise as a result of differences in the predominant form found in various species. Three groups of multiple enzyme forms have been defined as isoenzymes by the IUB. These are grouped as follows: genetically independent proteins, such as mitochondrial and cytosol forms of CK and malate dehydrogenase; heteropolymers of two or more different subunits, such as CK and LD; genetic variants in protein structure, such as glucose-6-phosphate dehydrogenases, with more than 50 varieties known in man.

In a few unusual cases, an enzyme subunit, such as glutamate dehydrogenase, may have catalytic activity by itself. In these cases, the natural enzyme form is made up of several subunits and has a greater activity than the sum of the activities of the separate subunits. In addition, the multiple subunit form of the enzyme often has activators and inhibitors that may more closely control the enzyme activity. A more complex biological structure exists in this case, one whose enzyme activity can be more finely regulated.

The polymeric forms of glutamate dehydrogenase and phosphorylase are not isoenzymes by the IUB definition, since they are polymers of a single subunit and do not differ in amino acid composition. Some additional forms of enzymes that do not fit the strict definition of isoenzymes are those with variations in molecular weight (or length). These forms may occur with the cleavage of different terminal segments of a protein that does not affect the enzyme activity, thus producing various isoenzymes. Hexokinase and carbonate dehydratase are examples of this type of isoenzyme.

Isoforms

The isoenzymes that are released from tissue (CK-MM or CK-MB) are a single unmodified isoenzyme form. As a part of the normal clearance process of the body, carboxypeptidases in serum cleave the terminal lysine from the CK-M subunit and produce other isoforms of the isoenzyme with slightly different charges. High-resolution electrophoresis or isoelectric focusing can be used to demonstrate the presence of three CK-MM isoforms and two CK-MB isoforms, forming and disappearing with time. The CK-MM isoforms differ only in whether none, one, or two lysines have been removed from the CK-M subunits. The two CK-MB isoforms are the intact CK-MB and the CK-MB where the M subunit has had a lysine removed. These are of interest as possible early diagnostic markers of acute myocardial infarction. Examples of the CK isoforms are given in Table 54-5. A more complete description of isoenzymes is given in Chapter 55.

Clinical significance

Creatine kinase. Creatine kinase (CK) is found primarily in muscle tissue. Significant increases of CK occur in serum when either skeletal muscle or cardiac muscle has been damaged. Because the primary isoenzyme in the skeletal muscle is CK-MM, large increases in this isoenzyme occur in serum when damage occurs to the skeletal system (as by auto accidents). In contrast, significant amounts of CK-MB and CK-MM occur in cardiac muscle and are released when the heart is damaged by anoxia, surgery, or myocardial infarction. Isoenzyme analysis is required to differentiate the tissue source of the increase of the CK that is present after injury to either skeletal muscle or myocardium. Large increases of CK may be shown to be from skeletal muscle if CK-MM is the predominant isoenzyme and CK-MB is present at less than 5%. Increases in serum of CK-MM with greater than 5% of CK-MB often occur when the heart has been damaged.

There are some problems of interpretation, since skeletal muscle has the CK-MB isoenzyme as well as myocardial tissue. The simple presence of CK-MB in the serum is not enough to indicate a cardiac problem. For example, certain muscle diseases including Duchenne's muscular dystrophy are associated with muscle regeneration, which increases the amount of CK-MB that is usually present in muscle from less than 5% to between 5% and 15%. Damage to the muscle will therefore produce a pattern in the serum that is consistent with myocardial damage, not skeletal muscle damage.

Sometimes CK-BB isoenzyme is seen in patient samples.

Table 54-5 CK isoforms

Isoform	Subunit	Comment
MM_3	CK-MM	Unchanged isoenzyme
MM_2	CK-MM$_{-L}$	End lysine removed from one M subunit
MM_1	CK-M$_{-L}$M$_{-L}$	End lysine removed from both subunits
MB_2	CK-MB	Unchanged isoenzyme
MB_1	CK-M$_{-L}$B	End lysine removed from M subunit

Isoforms are numbered with the same convention as isoenzymes, with the band with the fastest electrophoretic mobility toward the anode (+) subscripted as the first form.

The presence of this isoenzyme is more rare than the finding of CK-MB.

Lactate dehydrogenase. Lactate dehydrogenase (LD) is widely distributed in many tissues. The heart, however, contains an unusual distribution of LD isoenzymes, with an LD_1 concentration greater than LD_2. This LD result is similar to the finding of an unusual distribution of CK isoenzymes, in this tissue. The combination of both CK and LD isoenzyme analyses is more powerful than either determination alone, since these results tend to support one another but are somewhat independent measures of cardiac damage.

The timing of sampling after an event is important. For acute clinical events such as myocardial infarctions, obtaining several samples spread out in time is diagnostically significant. More information is obtained this way, since the pattern of the appearance of isoenzymes at various times in the serum is important. The average time for maximum elevation for a series of enzymes and isoenzymes in patients with a myocardial infarction has been reported to be: CK-MB, 6-12 hours; total CK, 18-24 hours; and LD, 48-72 hours. LD_1 appears to be less than LD_2 in early samples, when CK-MB is rising, but as the total LD concentration increases, both LD_1 and LD_2 increase in serum. Eventually the LD_1-to-LD_2 ratio flips, and so the LD_1 concentration is greater than the LD_2. As the time after the clinical event increases, the LD_1 concentration eventually returns after several days to normal values, which are lower than that of LD_2. Not all patients follow this classical pattern, and a spread of several hours is seen for the rapidly changing analytes and several days for the slower changing analytes if a variety of patients are tested.

Methods of analysis

Many older methods of analysis took advantage of slight differences in physical properties or of substrate specificity or inhibition patterns of some of the isoenzymes. These methods are only rarely used today. The common methods of analysis either take advantage of differences in migration in electric fields or are based on immunologic differences in the isoenzyme subunits. These methods are reviewed in more detail in Chapter 55.

The reference method for both CK and LD isoenzyme analysis is electrophoresis. This method is somewhat technique dependent but generally is easy to use and is relatively inexpensive. A large variety of different immunologic methods are also available. Because of the ease of use and sensitivity, these methods are gaining popularity. Some of them suffer from poor specificity, and they are all significantly more expensive than electrophoresis is.

BIBLIOGRAPHY

Bakerman P, Strausbauch P: *Bakerman's ABC's of interpretive laboratory data*, ed 3, Myrtle Beach, S.C., 1994, Interpretative Laboratory Data, Inc.

Baron DN, Moss DW, Walker PG, Wilkinson JH: Revised list of abbreviations for names of enzymes of diagnostic importance, *J Clin Pathol* 28:592-593, 1975.

Bowers GN Jr, Inman SR: The gallium melting-point standard: its evaluation for temperature measurements in the clinical laboratory, *Clin Chem* 23:733-737, 1977.

Committee on Standards, Expert Panel on Enzymes: Provisional recommendation (1974) of IFCC methods for the measurement of catalytic concentrations of enzymes, *Clin Chem* 22:384-391, 1976.

Enzyme nomenclature: recommendations on enzyme nomenclature of the Commission on Nomenclature and Classification of the Enzymes of the International Union of Biochemistry, New York, 1979, Academic Press.

Hohnadel DC: Clinical enzymology. In Tilton RC, Balows A, Hohnadel DC, Reiss RF: *Clinical laboratory medicine*, St. Louis, 1992, Mosby.

Kaplan LA, Pesce AJ, editors: *Clinical chemistry: theory, analysis, and correlation*, ed 2, St. Louis, 1989, Mosby, Chapters 52 and 53.

Pappas NJ Jr, editor: Theoretical aspects of enzymes in diagnosis. Why do serum enzymes change in hepatic, myocardial, and other diseases? *Clin Lab Med* 9:595-626, 1989.

Swaroop A: CK isoenzyme variants in electrophoresis, Lab Med, pp 305-310, May 1989.

Wallach JB: *Interpretation of diagnostic tests*, ed 5, Boston, 1992, Little, Brown & Co.

Wu AHB: Creatine kinase isoforms in ischemic heart-disease, *Clin Chem* 35:7-13, 1989.

Zilva JF, Pannall PR, Mayne PD: *Clinical chemistry in diagnosis and treatment*, ed 5, St. Louis, 1988, Mosby, Chapter 15.

CHAPTER 55

Isoenzymes and isoforms

Robert H. Christenson
Kalpana Panigrahi
John F. Chapman
Lawrence M. Silverman

OBJECTIVES

- Define the structural differences of isoenzymes.
- Describe the genetic basis of isoenzymes.
- Show the type of differences between enzymes that make them isoforms.
- Discuss the purpose or functions of isoenzymes.
- Describe the clinical significance of creatine kinase.
- List the ways that isoenzymes are measured.

KEY TERMS

artifactual modification Change in protein structure caused by in vitro manipulation.

dimer A protein composed of two subunits.

heteropolymer A polymeric compound, such as an isoenzyme, that has more than one type of subunit.

homopolymer A polymeric compound, such as an isoenzyme, in which all subunits are identical.

immunoinhibition Inhibition of enzyme activity by reaction with an antibody.

isoenzymes Multiple forms of an enzyme that catalyze the same biochemical reaction; different isoenzymes may exist in different species, within an organism, or in different cellular organelles. Various isoenzymes may differ chemically, physically, or immunologically.

isoforms Multiple forms of serum protein that result from post-translational modifications of the gene product.

macroenvironment On the organ or tissue level, a specific environment that is associated with a specific physiological function.

microenvironment On the cellular level, a specific environment or location that is associated with a specific physiological function.

Regan isoenzyme A specific alkaline phosphatase isoenzyme associated with some cancers.

subunit A polypeptide chain that is an integral part of a protein or enzyme.

tetramer A protein composed of four subunits.

DEFINITIONS
Isoenzyme properties

Isoenzymes, also termed *isozymes,* are multiple forms of an enzyme that catalyze the same biochemical reaction and share the same Enzyme Commission (EC) number. Although isoenzymes of a particular enzyme usually do not differ substantially in molecular size, each isoenzyme has a distinct polypeptide structure and may have a different affinity for substrates and cofactors. Various isoenzymes of an enzyme can differ in three major ways. They may differ in their enzymatic properties, specifically by their ability to be inhibited by specific agents, in their Michaelis-Menten constants (K_m), and their reactivity with different substrates. Second, they may differ in their physical properties, such as heat stability and charge. Last, they may differ in their biochemical properties, such as amino acid composition and immunological reactivities.[1]

Most or all of the above differences have been used for measurement of specific isoenzymes. Assays based on these differences are discussed on p. 1084.

Structural basis

The isoenzymes of greatest interest in clinical chemistry are proteins composed of two or more polypeptide chains or subunits. The global properties of an isoenzyme are dependent on the number and type of polypeptide subunits composing the complete molecule. For example, consider an isoenzyme that is a dimer, that is, composed of two subunits. If the subunits can be either type A or type B, there are three possible combinations: AA, AB, and BB. If there are three subunits (a trimer), each of which can be either A or B, there are four possible isoenzymes: AAA, AAB, ABB, and BBB; with four subunits (a tetramer), there are five possible combinations: AAAA, AAAB, AABB, ABBB, and BBBB. If all subunits are identical in primary, secondary, and tertiary structure, as in AA, BB, AAA, or BBB, the isoenzyme is termed a *homopolymer*. If different subunits are present, as in AB, AAB, or ABBB, the isoenzyme is termed a *heteropolymer*. This concept is illustrated by the dimeric isoenzymes of creatine kinase (CK), which are formed by different paired combinations of two types of subunits, termed *M* (muscle) and *B* (brain), that differ from each other in primary, secondary, and tertiary structure. Both the CK-MM and CK-BB are homopolymers; the hybrid CK-MB isoenzyme is a heteropolymer.

ORIGIN
Genetic basis

The existence of isoenzymes was established in early studies that used electrophoresis and other physical techniques. Much progress has been made in elucidating the chemical basis for the structural diversification of isoenzymes; for example, tryptic digestion and amino acid sequencing of subunit chains led to the discovery that subunits are often the products of two related but separate genes.[2] Many amino acid sequences within each subunit chain are identical, often including the enzymatically active site; however, there are also differences in the amino acid composition and the physical and antigenic properties of different subunit types. The presence of these different but highly homologous amino acid sequences indicates that isoenzyme diversity may have arisen through gene duplication, followed by independent mutations of the two genes, resulting in different subunits. An example of this diversity is lactate dehydrogenase (LD), a tetrameric enzyme the subunits of which may be either of the H or the M type.[3] The amino acid sequences of the subunits of the H and M type are similar, including the active site. However, small differences in the amino acid sequences between the subunits impart a differ-

ent overall charge to the various LD isoenzyme combinations. Cytosolic CK is a dimer consisting of combinations of M and B subunits, each of which is coded by a different gene. These subunits associate to form the three major CK isoenzymes: CK-MM, CK-MB, and CK-BB. A mitochondrial gene codes for the distinct mitochondrial CK.

There are four known distinct structural genes that encode for multiple forms of ALP.[4] These genes have been cloned, sequenced, and mapped to human chromosomes. The tissue nonspecific ALP (TNALP) gene is located on chromosome 1 and determines the ALP activity expressed in bone, liver, and kidney. The remaining three ALP genes, which encode for intestinal, placental, and placenta-like germ cell ALP, are in proximity to each other on chromosome 2, reflecting their close resemblance to each other and their difference from TNALP.[5] Evolutionary selection evidently favors the retention of genes for different isoenzyme forms because they pass on some biological advantage to the organism (see below, p. 1079).

Posttranslational and artifactual modifications

Different subtypes, or *isoforms,* of enzymes may result from posttranslational modifications of the parent enzyme structure by either addition of chemical moieties or partial degradation.[6] These changes can occur intracellularly, as in the addition of carbohydrate side chains, or after the proteins are released from cells into plasma, as in the changes seen with CK isoenzymes.[7,8] Although the term *isoenzyme* is often used to refer to both the gene product and posttranslational modifications, here we will use this term to indicate the gene product only. The term *isoform* will be used to refer to differences based solely on posttranslational modifications.

Associations between different monomer units of an enzyme can result in a variety of enzymatic properties. Oxidation or reduction of functional groups in the enzyme molecule may also result in identifiable isoforms.[6] Modifications of the protein chain, such as the addition of sialic acid, can result in a large number of subtypes with different net charges and physical properties, thus allowing separation and identification of the isoenzyme activities.[6] For example, a comparison of heat stability and catalytic properties of ALP from bone, liver, and kidney indicates that these isoforms result from different posttranslational modifications of a single gene product (TNALP, see above) common to them all.[9] Evidence from selective modifications of enzymes by glycosidases indicates that the differences in the ALP isoforms may be the result of variations in carbohydrate side chains that are enzymatically added to the gene product.[10] The ALP isoforms are difficult to separate by electrophoretic methods because the carbohydrate side chains do not substantially alter the overall electrical charge of the enzyme. It is possible for one to measure such isoforms by immunoassays, by measuring differences in enzyme activity in the presence of different substrates, or by binding a low-molecular-weight substance, such as NAD^+, which will influence the enzyme's electrophoretic mobility.

Isoforms of some enzymes and isoenzymes are formed by degradation of the gene product by serum enzymes called *peptidases*. This degradation occurs after release of the gene product from the intracellular compartment into plasma. A clinically useful example of this process is seen with the dimeric homopolymer CK-MM.[7,8] After release of intracellular CK-MM into plasma, the terminal lysine residue of each M subunit can be successively cleaved by an irreversible enzyme reaction catalyzed by a plasma carboxypeptidase.[11] Because lysine residues impart a positive charge, three CK-MM isoforms can be separated by serum electrophoresis; the three isoforms are named according to their electrophoretic mobility. $CK-MM_3$ migrates closest to the cathode and is the "tissue" isoform that predominates (>95%) within the intracellular compartment; $CK-MM_2$ shows intermediate migration and is formed after $CK-MM_3$ is released from the cell by cleavage of the terminal lysine from one of the $CK-MM_3$'s two M subunits; $CK-MM_1$ migrates closest to the anode and results from cleavage of the remaining intact terminal lysine from the $CK-MM_2$'s unmodified M subunit.[7,8] A similar enzymatic processing of CK-MB occurs to allow the formation of $CK-MB_1$ from the tissue isoform $CK-MB_2$.[11]

PURPOSE OR FUNCTION
Microenvironmental factors

The functional significance of isoenzymes and isoforms remains an intriguing biological question that has been approached by the study of individual cells, by the study of the organization of cells into tissues, and by the study of the developmental processes of the organism as a whole. The finding that isoenzymes and isoforms are compartmentalized within the organelles of cells has led to theories that hypothesize a role for these compounds in subcellular interactions and specific metabolic processes. The different net charges of the isoenzymes may influence their interactions with other charged molecules within the cell. This may result in a logical differential location of specific isoenzymes with respect to the specialized organelles of the cell.

Microenvironmental factors are also important for ALP. All ALP isoenzymes and isoforms are attached to the membranes of cells by a COOH-terminal glycan-phosphatidylinositol "anchor."[12] Although the exact function of ALP is unknown (see ALP assay, p. 521), based on the enzyme's location it is hypothesized that ALP may play a relatively nonspecific role in several transport processes by dephosphorylating metabolites, thereby facilitating their cellular entry through the selectively permeable cell membrane.[4] In addition, because the bone ALP isoforms on the cell membrane of osteoblasts are not specific for any one tissue and because of the association of this ALP with mineralization of bone, it has been suggested that ALP func-

tions to promote bone mineralization by removing inhibitors of crystallization such as inorganic phosphate.[13] Evidence in support of this theory has mainly come from hypophosphatasia, which is characterized by the deficiency of both the enzyme and mineralization.[13]

Macroenvironmental factors

Differential location of isoenzymes and isoforms has also been observed on a larger scale, that is, within different tissues. For example, tissues such as heart, brain, and renal cortex show a predominance of LD_1 and LD_2, whereas other tissues such as skeletal muscle have a high content of LD_5. The tetramer of H chains composing LD_1 has an affinity for pyruvate that is tenfold less than the affinity of LD_5, a tetramer of M chains. Thus LD_1 preferentially catalyzes the conversion of lactate to pyruvate. It has been suggested that because of its kinetic properties the LD_1 isoenzyme predominates in tissues that receive a rich oxygen supply, since these tissues undergo oxidative metabolism and ordinarily do not accumulate lactate (or pyruvate) because they can use lactate as a fuel.[14] The LD_5 isoenzyme is the major LD form in skeletal muscle, which is more dependent on anaerobic glycolysis and accumulates pyruvate under anaerobic conditions. By having the LD_5 isoenzyme, muscle cells are better able to convert pyruvate to lactate and regenerate NAD^+, permitting the energy-producing reactions of the Embden-Meyerhof pathway (see Chapter 32 for further detail). Thus it has been proposed that the isoenzyme and isoform distribution in tissues is based on the particular needs and metabolic demands that have evolved for various tissues.

Developmental factors

Developmental changes in the organism are reflected by a change in the isoenzyme and isoform distribution for many tissues as a result of differential gene activation and repression during ontogeny. These changes in distribution are indicative of the tremendous changes in the interaction of the organism with its environment. During fetal development, the organism must optimize enzymatic reactions to adapt to dramatic changes in intracellular aerobic metabolism. This is accomplished through major shifts in tissue isoenzyme composition by the activation of different genes. This process is very similar to the shift from the fetal form of hemoglobin to the adult form (see Chapter 36). Although the oxygen affinities of purified fetal and adult hemoglobin are very similar, at physiological concentrations of 2,3-diphosphoglycerate in the blood, the adult type of hemoglobin has lower affinity for oxygen than the fetal form has. Fetal hemoglobin's greater oxygen affinity allows the ready transfer of oxygen from maternal hemoglobin to the fetal circulation. Thus different hemoglobins, as with certain isoenzymes and isoforms, serve the different biological needs of the developing organism.

Biochemical evidence indicates that fetal intestinal ALP

may be a heterodimer of the placental ALP and the intestinal subunits that are found in the adult.[15] This pattern of expression presumably results because, during fetal development, the placental gene and the intestinal gene are co-expressed in enterocytes, resulting in the appearance of a hybrid ALP isoenzyme. The amount of this hybrid enzyme is decreased toward term as the result of diminished expression of the placental gene. This pattern is similar to the ontological change in expression of CK subunits in skeletal muscle. During initial fetal development only the B subunit gene is expressed, allowing the CK-BB dimer to form. Later during differentiation, there is a shift to expression of the M subunit gene, resulting first in a transient appearance of the CK-MB heterodimer as both the M and B subunits are expressed and then in the appearance of the CK-MM dimer, which is present almost exclusively at term. The LD isoenzymes also show developmental differences; undifferentiated embryonal tissues have maximal activity in the hybrid isoenzymes LD$_2$, LD$_3$, and LD$_4$.[16] As tissues differentiate, the LD pattern shifts to adapt to the energy production requirements for the tissues' specific functions (see above).

TISSUE DISTRIBUTION OF MAJOR ISOENZYMES

Although many enzymes exist as isoenzymes and isoforms, only a few have proved clinical value. The focus of this section is on the CK, LD, ALP, and acid phosphatase (ACP) isoenzymes and isoforms because they are the enzymes of major clinical interest.

CK-MM is the predominant CK isoenzyme in adult skeletal muscle tissue, with only a small concentration of CK-MB, representing up to 3% of the total CK activity in most skeletal muscle. However, the proportion of CK-MB can reach as high as 10% in some types of noncardiac muscle (see p. 602). Unlike skeletal muscle, adult myocardium contains 14% to 42% of CK-MB, with the remainder of activity contributed by CK-MM. In brain tissue, the CK isoenzyme primarily expressed is the CK-BB isoenzyme (Table 55-1).

The heart is the organ richest in LD$_1$ isoenzyme (H$_4$), whereas LD$_5$ (M$_4$) is found predominately in liver and skeletal muscle.[17] Red blood cells are also rich in LD$_1$. In the lung, the LD$_2$ and LD$_3$ isoenzymes predominate (Table 55-2).

The TNALP form of alkaline phosphatase (liver/bone/kidney) is expressed in virtually all tissues. High activity is particularly noted in mineralizing bone where ALP is located in the plasma membrane of osteoblastic cells. Intestinal ALP is expressed in the intestinal mucosa and is abundant in the brush borders of epithelial cells. Recently, expression of this enzyme has also been observed in kidney where it is mainly localized in the distal (S$_3$) segment of the proximal tubule.[18] Placental ALP becomes detectable in the serum of pregnant women between the sixteenth and twentieth weeks of pregnancy and disappears within 3 to 6

days after delivery. It is also present in relatively small amounts in lung and cervix. Placenta-like germ cell ALP has been found in very small amounts, in the testis and thymus of healthy individuals. At birth, ALP in the serum appears to come almost entirely from bone, differing from the pattern observed in fetuses whose serum contains both bone and fetal intestinal forms. Serum from adults contains many ALP isoenzymes and isoforms (Table 55-3), though the major forms released into serum are bone, liver, kidney, and intestinal.[19] The reasons for characteristic differences in the expression of various isoenzymes and isoforms in different tissues and in different cells within the same tissue are not known.

ACP is a ubiquitous enzyme, located in the lysozomes of all cells. Red blood cells, white blood cells, platelets, and the prostate gland have particularly high concentrations of ACP. Immunologically, ACP isoenzymes from the last three tissues listed are closely related. Most of the ACP activity found in the serum of normal individuals is probably de-

Table 55-1   Creatine kinase activity in various human tissues

Tissue	Isoenzyme distribution in U/g of wet tissue (% of total activity)		
	MM	MB	BB
Skeletal muscle	3281 (100)	0-623 (0-19)	0
Heart	313 (78)	56-169 (14-42)	0
Brain	0	0	157 (100)
Colon	4 (3)	1 (1)	143 (96)
Stomach	4 (3)	2 (2)	114 (95)
Uterus	1 (2)	1 (3)	45 (95)
Thyroid	7 (26)	0.3 (1)	21 (73)
Kidney	2 (8)	0	19 (92)
Lung	5 (35)	0.1 (1)	9 (64)
Prostate	0.3 (3)	0.4 (4)	9.3 (93)
Spleen	5 (74)	0	2 (26)
Liver	3.6 (90)	0.2 (6)	0.2 (4)
Pancreas	0.4 (14)	0 (1)	2.6 (85)
Placenta	1.4 (48)	0.2 (6)	1.4 (46)

From Chapman J, Silverman L: *Bull Lab Med* (National Committee for Mental Health), no 60, pp 1-7, Jan 1982.

Table 55-2   Lactate dehydrogenase activity, expressed as percentage of activity distributing

Organ	Isoenzyme distribution				
	H$_4$	H$_3$M$_1$	H$_2$M$_2$	H$_1$M$_3$	M$_4$
Heart	60	30	5	3	2
Kidney	28	34	21	11	6
Cerebrum	28	32	19	16	5
Liver	0.2	0.8	1	4	94
Skeletal muscle	3	4	8	9	76
Skin	0	0	4	17	79
Lung	10	18	28	23	21
Spleen	5	15	31	31	18

From Pfleiderer G et al: In Schmidt E et al, editors: *Advances in clinical enzymology,* Hannover, West Germany, 1979, S Karger AG.

Table 55-3 Alkaline phosphatase activity in human tissues*

Tissue	Activity (U/g of wet tissue)	
	MAP	DEA
Adrenal	30	66
Placenta	36	—
Liver	12.6	27
Bone	7.5	18
Spleen	7.5	18
Lung	6.6	15
Intestine	4.8	9
Kidney	4.2	11
Prostate	3.3	6.6
Thyroid	2.1	5.1
Heart	1.8	3.6
Erythrocytes	0.02	—

Data calculated from Bowers GN et al: *Clin Chem* 21:1988-1995, 1975.
MAP, 2-Methyl-2-amino-1-propanol buffer.
DEA, Diethylamine buffer.
*Mean activity in two buffer systems of tissue specimens from human autopsies. Notice the greater than twofold activity between the buffer systems.

rived from blood cells, whereas in men only a small fraction is derived from the prostate gland (see also p. 992).

CHANGE IN ISOENZYME PATTERN SECONDARY TO PATHOLOGICAL PROCESSES

Changes in the relative proportion and concentration of each isoenzyme or isoform may occur as a result of a variety of pathological processes. For example, LD activity in normal adult aortic tissue involves primarily the LD_3 fraction[16]; however, in atherosclerotic aortic tissue, maximal LD activity is present as the LD_5 fraction. Likewise, myocardial LD activity shifts from predominantly LD_1 to LD_3 during the progression of ischemic heart disease.[16] There is a greater expression of CK-MB activity in ischemic myocardial tissue compared with normal adult myocardium.

Pathological conditions that result in regeneration of damaged tissue may cause changes in isoenzyme composition that resemble the pattern observed during embryological development. For example, many muscle diseases, such as Duchenne's muscular dystrophy, are characterized by muscle fiber regeneration that results from the destruction of adult muscle fibers. These newly formed, immature muscle fibers may contain isoenzyme distributions that are similar to those seen in early development. Because CK-MB is expressed in fetal skeletal muscle, this hybrid isoenzyme is often identified in blood from patients with muscle diseases in whom there is active skeletal muscle regeneration.

Interpretation of isoenzymes and isoforms must be performed with caution because the fetal isoenzyme from one tissue may represent the adult isoenzyme form from another tissue. For example, the CK-MB isoenzyme represents a significant proportion of the CK activity in both fetal and adult myocardium, whereas in the fetus, CK-MB is also present in large amounts in skeletal muscle. Increased

amounts of CK-MB isoenzyme in the sera of normal adults would probably represent damage to the heart, whereas in children CK-MB increases may be from either heart or skeletal muscle. For a more complete discussion of the interpretational problems associated with the presence of CK-MB in patient sera, refer to Chapter 31.

The cellular dedifferentiation associated with the development of malignancy may also result in altered isoenzyme and isoform patterns. The isoenzymes and isoforms associated with tumors are often referred to as *oncofetal tumor markers* because their expression is similar to that observed during early embryological development. For example, although CK-BB is the predominant isoenzyme in all early embryonic tissue, expression of this isoenzyme in most adult tissues is associated primarily with the brain and some tissues found in the gut (see Table 55-1). In patients without malignancy, detection of CK-BB in the serum is often associated with a pathological condition affecting the nervous, pulmonary, or gastrointestinal systems.[20] However, during the process of cell dedifferentiation, some cells may express significant amounts of CK-BB, which may be detected in the serum.[20] The LD isoenzymes in serum from patients with lymphoid malignancies are predominantly LD_2, LD_3, and LD_4.[21] A shift to this pattern in serum may indicate the presence of increased numbers of lymphoid cells resulting from malignant proliferation. A shift toward LD_5 expression is observed in many solid tumors, especially in carcinomas of the genitalia or the digestive tract, whereas in some tumors, such as those of germ cell origin, there is a shift toward LD_1 expression.

Human tumors are found to produce increased concentrations of the placental (PL-ALP), intestinal (I-ALP), and germ cell (GC-ALP) isoenzymes and isoforms of ALP. It appears that malignant processes either activate or amplify the expression of an ALP gene that is normally either repressed or expressed at a very low level.

In disorders of bone, increased enzyme production results in elevated levels of bone ALP because of increased osteoblastic activity. Increased serum levels of liver ALP in hepatobiliary disease presumably result from injury to hepatocytes as well as from the accumulation of bile acids as a result of cholestasis. An explanation for some of the alternative ALP isoforms detectable in serum, especially in hepatobiliary disease,[22] is provided by the presence of inositol-specific phospholipase D activity in serum and its apparent absence in bile. In hepatobiliary disease, a hydrophilic, nonaggregating ALP is released from hepatocytes into serum by the action of serum phospholipase D. Since this phospholipase D is absent in bile, a higher-molecular-mass aggregate of the ALP is released from hepatocytes forming a so-called fast-liver fraction. This fast-liver fraction enters serum where the presence of this fraction is regarded as valuable evidence of obstructive liver disease, particularly in the extrahepatic circulation.

CLINICAL SIGNIFICANCE OF SPECIFIC ISOENZYMES

For an enzyme, isoenzyme, or isoform to be clinically useful as a marker of disease, several criteria must be met. For example, the marker must have a favorable tissue-to-plasma concentration ratio, and it must have a substantial lifetime in blood. These criteria and others are discussed further in Chapter 54.

For all practical purposes, serum and plasma have been the only clinical specimens examined for isoenzyme and isoform markers of specific tissue abnormalities. Normal cell turnover and characteristic "leakage" from living cells is responsible for the baseline enzyme, isoenzyme, and isoform concentrations in serum. These baseline concentrations define the laboratory reference intervals. Concentrations of enzymes, isoenzymes, and isoforms in excess of these reference intervals are associated with a variety of pathological abnormalities, which result in cellular destruction, thus forming the basis for clinical utility of enzyme determinations. The purpose of the next section is to discuss the major disease states associated with increased levels of isoenzymes and isoforms and to provide a basis for interpretation of abnormal values. Determination of isoenzymes and isoforms in other body fluids is unusual and is discussed briefly at the conclusion of this section. Although isoenzymes and isoforms have been shown to be an important tool for the diagnosis of many conditions, the assumption that abnormal isoenzymes are associated with only one particular tissue must be discouraged.

Creatine kinase

Although the CK-MM, CK-MB, and CK-BB isoenzymes are cytoplasmic, there is creatine kinase (CK) activity in other subcellular locations, particularly in the mitochondrion. The 85,000-dalton molecular weight of CK precludes its passage across the blood-brain barrier except in cases of severe trauma; therefore, significant increases in serum CK levels usually reflect either skeletal or cardiac muscle release. By measurement of the CK isoenzymes, skeletal muscle release can usually be discriminated from cardiac tissue release. As with most laboratory studies, the complexities of enzyme release and the various clearance mechanisms require that the interpretation of serum enzyme or isoenzyme concentrations be made in the context of the clinical situation. Often, combining multiple serum markers yields information that makes interpretation of enzyme concentrations more practical.

In the past, the combined use of the LD and CK isoenzymes was necessary to yield the necessary information for evaluating patients admitted for the diagnosis of myocardial infarction (MI). However, CK-MB has evolved into the standard for diagnosing most cases of MI. LD is a late marker of MI that is not substantially abnormal until 18 to 24 hours after the acute event. LD isoenzyme analysis becomes useful when serum samples are available only after the peak levels of serum CK activity have passed (see p. 600).

A common interpretative problem is encountered when skeletal muscle injury results in significant elevation of CK activity in serum. Because skeletal muscle contains eightfold higher CK concentrations per gram of wet tissue than cardiac tissue does, small areas of skeletal muscle damage or disease can result in serum CK-MB concentrations consistent with substantial damage to the heart. In uncomplicated cases, the use of isoenzyme fractionation can usually differentiate the source of the elevated CK serum activity because skeletal muscle usually consists of greater than 97% CK-MM isoenzyme. Calculation of a relative index, in which CK-MB concentration is the numerator and total CK is the denominator, can help elucidate the source of CK-MB. For cases in which both cardiac and muscle damage is suspected, as in cases of trauma or surgery (see below), interpretation of CK-MB levels is more difficult (see below and p. 602).

It is important to note that an increased proportion of CK-MB content is frequently associated with muscle fiber regeneration. For this reason, certain diseases of skeletal muscle, such as Duchenne's muscular dystrophy or polymyositis, often result in serum elevations of total CK and an abnormal increase in serum CK-MB concentrations often to 5% to 15% of the total CK activity. Because the majority of patients with these muscle diseases are not being evaluated for myocardial infarction (MI), misinterpretation of these CK-MB elevations is infrequent. However, this situation underscores the importance of obtaining appropriate clinical information for proper interpretation of isoenzyme results.

Further difficulty in CK isoenzyme and isoform interpretation may be encountered when one is evaluating patients undergoing thoracic and other surgery, particularly coronary artery bypass graft surgery. Surgical procedures involving the heart can be expected to cause the release of myocardial enzymes and isoenzymes with isoenzyme concentrations reaching levels consistent with MI. In such patients the clinician is frequently concerned about perioperative MI either during surgery or during recovery. In these cases, CK isoenzyme results are extremely difficult to interpret. Experience has led many laboratories to require multiple serum samples for CK isoenzymes during the recovery period (4, 12, 24, and 48 hours and 3, 5, and 7 days postoperatively). In an uncomplicated recovery the CK-MB levels return to normal within 24 hours or decrease to levels approaching normal. With serious complications involving extension of myocardial necrosis or reinfarction, CK-MB levels continue to rise during the recovery period or rise after an initial diminution. More specific markers of myocardial injury, such as troponin-I or troponin-T, show great promise for improving the ability to diagnose perioperative MI.[23,24] Additional information on this subject is found in Chapter 31.

With high-voltage electrophoresis, the CK-MM and CK-MB isoenzymes can each be fractionated into subtypes, or isoforms, which differ in their isoelectric points. Isoform formation appears to play a role in normal clearance of the CK-MM and CK-MB isoenzymes from plasma. Of the five collective CK-MM and CK-MB isoforms, only MM_3 and MB_2 are found within tissue; upon release into circulation, they are irreversibly converted to their isoforms (see p. 1079).

CK-MM isoforms have been used for the early diagnosis of acute myocardial infarction (MI) and for monitoring the success of thrombolytic therapy, which can dissolve the clots that cause MI.[7,8,25] The pattern of CK-MM isoforms can indicate how recently enzymatic release from tissue has occurred. Shortly after release, the $CK-MM_3$ isoform predominates in serum; later, after enzymatic cleavage of both terminal lysines, the $CK-MM_1$ isoform is most prevalent. An increased ratio of MM_3/MM_1 concentrations indicates either recent release of $CK-MM_3$ from tissue or its recent entry into systemic circulation; a lower MM_3/MM_1 concentration ratio indicates either that release has not occurred or has occurred much earlier (see Chapter 31 for detail).

Occasionally CK isoenzymes are used to evaluate tissues other than the heart or muscle. For example, CK-BB concentrations can be elevated in the sera of patients with various conditions, including malignancy and prostatic, pulmonary, and neurological disorders. However, it must be noted that although elevations of serum CK-BB can be associated with these disease states CK-BB levels have poor sensitivity and specificity for these diseases, making such measurements only rarely useful.

Acid phosphatase

Although acid phosphatase (ACP) isoenzymes are found in a variety of cells including red blood cells, white blood cells, and platelets, the most common isoenzyme measured in the clinical laboratory is the fraction denoted as prostatic acid phosphatase (PAP). The method of measurement of PAP affects the clinical usefulness of the results and is discussed in Chapter 49 on p. 992.

For nearly 40 years PAP has been shown to be frequently elevated in patients with advanced stages of prostatic cancer. However, PAP is rarely useful for diagnosis of early stages of prostate cancer because the clinical sensitivity of PAP is low and concentrations of the isoenzyme are often normal when a patient has prostate cancer. False-positive ACP results are associated with benign prostatic hypertrophy in which there is increased growth of noncancerous prostate tissue, leading to various urological problems. Unfortunately persons with this condition are frequently the very patients in whom prostate cancer is a strong possibility. Other false-positive elevations have been observed in patients with malignancies other than prostate cancer, such as leukemia, and so interpretation of isoenzyme concentrations depends on adequate clinical information. The diag-

nostic role of PAP has been taken over largely by prostate-specific antigen (PSA; see Chapter 49). Nonetheless, levels of PAP are still considered useful when one is monitoring patients receiving treatment to assess tumor burden, the relative amount of tumor tissue that is present before treatment or that remains after treatment.

Other clinical situations in which ACP isoenzyme studies may be requested include the diagnosis of Gaucher's disease, an inborn error of metabolism, and various leukemias in which leukocyte acid phosphatase (also termed *leukocyte alkaline phosphatase*) can be measured. Total ACP and the prostatic isoenzyme associated with prostatic secretions have been used in rape cases as legal evidence of sexual assault.

Alkaline phosphatase

The value of characterizing alkaline phosphatase (ALP) isoenzymes and isoforms in serum as a diagnostic aid is becoming better established as improved methods to better differentiate the various ALP forms become available. Most often ALP fractionation is requested in order to determine whether bone or liver is the source of an elevated level of total serum ALP activity. Specific ALP isoenzyme and isoform measurements, as compared with total ALP measurements, are at least twofold more sensitive for assessment of both bone and liver diseases.

The measurement of bone and liver isoforms so far has proved clinically useful for diagnosing and monitoring certain diseases of these organs. High levels of the bone ALP isoform are seen in several bone disorders including Paget's disease, osteosarcoma, hyperthyroidism, and perhaps osteoporosis. Also, there is an increased production of liver ALP in hepatobiliary diseases. Quantitative measurements of the "bone" ALP fraction may be important for monitoring patients with bone diseases to evaluate the patient's response to therapy.

The increased expression of certain ALP genes, mainly variants of placental ALP, as well as the "Regan" and "Nagao" isoenzymes, is associated with germ cell tumors. These ALP isoenzymes are expressed predominantly in hepatocellular carcinomas or when liver is the site of a metastatic tumor. It is interesting that a significant amount of ALP is expressed in some but not all malignancies. The reasons why only some tumors express significant amounts of ALP are still unknown.

In the past, the practical implications of ALP isoenzyme and isoform analysis precluded their measurement in many cases. However, the use of improved methods for measuring bone ALP for the monitoring of Paget's disease, osteoporosis, and bone cancer may increase the future use of ALP fractionation.[26,27]

Lactate dehydrogenase

Although lactate dehydrogenase (LD) isoenzymes have been widely investigated, the clinical usefulness of these isoenzymes is mainly limited to the diagnosis of myocardial infarction (see p. 596), partly because LD is found in virtually every tissue. Although there is some relative tissue specificity for the various isoenzymes, there is considerable overlap in isoenzyme-tissue specificity with the five isoenzyme forms commonly found in serum. For example, although the LD_5 isoenzyme is frequently used to ascertain damage to skeletal muscle, LD_5 is also the predominant isoenzyme in liver. A similar situation exists for each of the other four isoenzymes, which leads most clinicians to depend on other more specific tests for primary liver, muscle, or cardiac assessment. For several decades an increase in the LD_5 isoenzyme has been observed in the sera of patients with various types of cancer; however, the association of LD isoenzymes with tumors is a nonspecific finding.

Thus, LD isoenzyme fractionation is most useful for late diagnosis of myocardial damage and muscle injury and occasionally for monitoring the progression of certain malignancies.

Other isoenzymes

Isoenzymes and isoforms of amylase, aspartate aminotransferase, and aldolase are worthy of mention because they are reported to have some clinical applications. Fractionation of these enzymes and others is performed by few laboratories because the clinical usefulness of these isoenzymes and isoforms is not well established.

Fluids other than serum

Some reports indicate that isoenzyme fractionation of several enzymes has significance in cerebrospinal fluid, pleural effusions, urine, and other fluids. For effusions, the main purpose of isoenzyme and isoform studies is usually to determine the source of the fluid. These fluids are rarely examined for quantitative isoenzyme concentration, and the methods for fractionation of fluid isoenzymes are occasionally very different from those used for serum. Because so little data exist, laboratories that are involved in analyzing these fluids generally determine their own guidelines for clinical consultation and interpretation. Comparison of results to the reference intervals in serum should be discouraged.

MODES OF ISOENZYME ANALYSIS

Most of the physical and catalytic differences among individual isoenzymes and isoforms have been utilized to determine the isoenzyme concentrations in serum (Table 55-4). All these methods depend on differences in individual subunit polypeptide and posttranslational modifications that impart detectable variations to the molecule of interest. More sophisticated methods using specific immunoassays can differentiate between the isoenzymes and isoforms based on the immunological differences of the subunit chains.

The use of substrate affinity and catalytic rates to differ-

Table 55-4   Modes of isoenzyme (isoform) analysis

Technique	Principles of analysis	Isoenzyme, isoform
Electrophoresis	Subunits have different charges; isoenzymes are separated in an electrical field.	All
Ion-exchange chromatography	Subunits have different charges; isoenzymes are separated by differential affinity for ion-exchange resin.	CK, LD
Immunoinhibition	Antibody reacts specifically with one subunit type; this property can be used to render an isoenzyme or isoenzymes catalytically inactive or to physically remove an isoenzyme or isoenzymes from solution.	CK, LD, acid phosphatase
Immunoassay	Antibody reacts specifically with one subunit type; extent of reaction is monitored by use of radioisotope, enzyme, or fluorescent tag.	CK, LD, acid phosphatase, alkaline phosphatase, amylase
Heat stability	Individual isoenzyme subunits are rendered catalytically inactive at different temperatures.	Alkaline phosphatase
Catalytic inhibition	Individual isoenzyme subunits bind low-molecular weight-inhibitors with different affinities; such binding results in different inhibition of each isoenzyme.	Acid phosphatase (L-tartrate), alkaline phosphatase (urea and L-phenylalanine), cholinesterase (dibucaine)
Substrate specificity	Each isoenzyme subunit binds a substrate with different affinities (K_m), giving each isoenzyme various rates of activity. Also each isoenzyme subunit may bind various substrates with different affinities; different isoenzymes have increased catalytic rates with certain substrates, whereas others have very low activities.	CK, acid phosphatase (α-naphthyl phosphate) LD_1

CK, Creatine kinase; *LD,* lactate dehydrogenase.

entiate between CK isoenzymes is rare today. Similarly, the use of alpha-hydroxybutyrate as a "specific" substrate for the measurement of LD_1 activity is now viewed as an inadequate and unsatisfactory method. Although methods using specific substrates for ACP measurement, such as alpha-naphthyl phosphate, are still used to discriminate between the PAP and other ACP forms, methods using L-tartrate to inhibit PAP activity are being replaced by immunoassays. Heat stability, catalytic inhibition, and wheat germ lectin precipitation methods for the differentiation of isoenzymes and isoforms with alkaline phosphatase activity are also rarely used for routine clinical analysis.

Electrophoretic techniques for fractionating CK have historically been considered the "reference" methods for CK-MB analysis. However, the widespread use of immunoassay techniques for CK-MB measurement that have greater analytical sensitivity has made use of electrophoresis as the standard for CK-MB measurement an anachronism. Measurement of the CK-MM and CK-MB isoforms is made after fractionation by high-voltage electrophoresis. Attempts at developing immunoassays for measuring the various CK isoforms have had little success.[28,29] Electrophoretic methods for the separation and quantitation of amylase, ALP, ACP, and other isoenzymes and isoforms have also been developed. Electrophoretic methods separate the liver and bone ALP forms to the extent that the technique allows a visual estimate of their relative proportions; quantitation by densitometric scanning is possible only after treatment with neuraminidase. Electrophoretic methods are based on differences in the net charge of each form (see Chapter 10). The electrophoretic methods have been popular because they provide a visual record of results and are relatively easy to use.

Newer immunoassays are based on monoclonal antibodies derived against specific recognition sites (epitopes) on isoenzyme or isoform molecules. Isoenzyme analysis based on immunological differences between isoenzymes and isoforms has become an important and widespread technique. The immunoassay methods include competitive and sandwich-immunometric techniques (see Chapters 12 and 13) and immunoinhibition techniques. Immunoassay and solid-phase immunometric "sandwich" assays are commercially available for CK-MB, bone ALP, and PAP measurement.

For additional information on isoenzyme analysis of the more commonly analyzed isoenzymes, refer to the individual technologies listed in Table 55-4.

BIBLIOGRAPHY

Foreback CC, Chu JW: Creatine kinase isoenzymes: electrophoretic and quantitative measurements, *CRC Crit Rev Clin Lab Sci* 15:187-230, 1981.

Moss DW: *Isoenzymes,* New York, 1982, Chapman & Hall.

REFERENCES

1. Wilkinson JH: *Principles and practice of diagnostic enzymology,* London, 1976, EJ Arnold & Son.

2. Moss DW: *Isoenzyme analysis,* London, 1979, The Chemical Society.

3. Markert CL: The molecular basis for isoenzymes, *Ann NY Acad Sci* 151:15-39, 1968.

4. Harris H: The human alkaline phosphatases: what we know and what we don't know, *Clin Chim Acta* 186:133-150, 1989.

5. Moss DW: Perspectives in alkaline phosphatase research, *Clin Chem* 38:2486-2492, 1992.

6. Rothe GM: A survey of the formation and localization of secondary isoenzymes in mammalia, *Hum Genet* 56:129-155, 1980.

7. Panteghini M: Serum isoforms of creatine kinase isoenzymes, *Clin Biochem* 21:211-218, 1988.

8. Wu ABW: Creatine kinase isoforms in ischemic heart disease, *Clin Chem* 35:7-13, 1989.

9. Moss DW: Alkaline phosphatase isoenzymes, *Clin Chem* 28:2007-2016, 1982.

10. Moss DW, Whitaker KB: Modification of alkaline phosphatases by treatment with glycosidases, *Enzyme* 34:212-216, 1985.

11. Perryman MB, Knell JD, Roberts R: Carboxypeptidase-catalyzed hydrolysis of C-terminal lysine: mechanism for in vivo production of multiple forms of creatine kinase in plasma, *Clin Chem* 30:662-664, 1984.

12. Fishman WH: Alkaline phosphatase isoenzymes: recent progress, *Clin Biochem* 23:99-104, 1990.

13. Russell RGG: Excretion of inorganic pyrophosphate in hypophosphatasia, *Lancet* 2:461-464, 1965.

14. Cahn RD, Kaplan NO, Levine L, Zwilling E: Nature and development of lactic dehydrogenases, *Science* 136:962-969, 1962.

15. Behrens CM, Enns CA, Sussman HH: Characterization of human foetal intestinal alkaline phosphatase: comparison with the isoenzymes from the adult intestine and human tumor cell lines, *Biochem J* 211:553-558, 1983.

16. Wilhelm A: Topochemical variation of LDH and CK isoenzyme patterns in aorta, *Artery* 8:362-367, 1980.

17. Pfleiderer G et al: Tissue enzymes in phylogenetic and ontogenetic development. In Schmidt E et al, editors: *Advances in clinical enzymology,* Hannover, West Germany, 1979, S Karger AG.

18. Verpooten GF, Nouwen EJ, Hoylaerts MF, et al: Segment specific localization of intestinal-type alkaline phosphatase in human kidney, *Kidney Int* 36:617-625, 1989.

19. Bowers GN, McComb RB, Statland BE, et al: Measurement of total alkaline phosphatase activity in human serum (selected method), *Clin Chem* 21:1988-1995, 1975.

20. Lang H, Wurzburg U: Creatine kinase, an enzyme of many forms, *Clin Chem* 28:1439-1447, 1982.

21. Schapira F: Isoenzymes and cancer, *Adv Cancer Res* 18:77-153, 1973.

22. Raymond F, Datta H, Moss D: Alkaline phosphatase isoforms in bile and serum and their generation from cells in vitro, *Biochim Biophys Acta* 1074:217-222, 1991.

23. Adams JE, Sicard GA, Allen BT, et al: Diagnosis of perioperative myocardial infarction with measurement of cardiac troponin I, *N Engl J Med* 330:670-674, 1994.

24. Mair J, Dienstl F, Puschendorf B: Cardiac troponin T in the diagnosis of myocardial injury, *Crit Rev Clin Sci* 29:31-57, 1992.

25. Christenson RH, Ohman EM, Clemmenson P, et al: Characteristics of creatine kinase–MB and the MB isoforms in serum after reperfusion in acute myocardial infarction, *Clin Chem* 35:2179-2185, 1989.

26. Kaddam IM, Iqbal SJ, Holland S, et al: Comparison of serum osteocalcin with total and bone specific alkaline phosphatase and urinary hydroxyproline : creatine ratio in patients with Paget's disease of bone, *Ann Clin Biochem* 31:327-330, 1994.

27. Garnero P, Delmas PD: Assessment of serum levels of bone alkaline phosphatase with a new immunoradiometric assay in patients with metabolic bone disease, *J Clin Endocrinol Metab* 77:1046-1053, 1993.

28. Christenson RH: Specificity of an immunochemical reagent for quantifying the isoforms of creatine kinase–MB, *J Clin Lab Anal* 7:220-224, 1993.

29. Panteghini M, Bonora R, Pagani F, Alebardi O: An immunochemical procedure for determination of creatine kinase 3_1 (serum-specific) isoform in human serum evaluated, *Clin Biochem* 23:225-228, 1990.

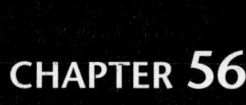

CHAPTER 56 · *Therapeutic drug monitoring (TDM)*

Wolfgang A. Ritschel
Michael Oellerich
Victor W. Armstrong

───────────────■───────────────

───────────────■───────────────

OBJECTIVES

- Describe the steps involved in the physiological processing of a drug given to a patient.
- Define therapeutic index and therapeutic range.
- Describe the rationale for therapeutic drug monitoring (TDM).
- Describe various dosing regimens and the influence these have on laboratory TDM programs.
- List the factors that may have an influence on the need to perform a TDM analysis stat.

KEY TERMS

absorption Uptake of unchanged drug into circulation.

absorption rate constant Value describing how much drug is absorbed per unit of time.

active transport Movement of drug across a membrane by binding to a carrier molecule and delivery to the opposite side with expenditure of energy.

bioavailability The amount of drug in the formulation that the system of the patient can absorb.

biophase The site of interaction between the drug molecule and its receptor.

bound drug A pharmacological agent that exists in blood complexed with another molecule (usually protein or lipid).

C_{max} Maximum plasma level of drug.

C_{av}^{ss} Average steady-state concentration.

C_{max}^{ss} Maximum steady-state concentration (peak concentration).

C_{min}^{ss} Minimum steady-state concentration (trough concentration).

compartment A pharmacokinetic term for the drug concentration, C, and the volume of distribution of that drug.

distribution Proportional division of drug into different compartments of the body, such as blood and extracellular fluid.

elimination Final excretion of an agent.

first-order kinetics The rate of change of plasma drug concentration that is dependent on the concentration itself; that is, a constant proportion of drug is removed with time, or $dC/dt = -k \cdot C$.

free drug Pharmacological agent that exists in biological fluids unbound by other molecules.

half-life ($t_{1/2}$) The amount of time required to reduce a drug level to one half its initial value. Usually it refers to the time necessary to reduce the plasma value to one half of its initial value. The term is also applied to the disappearance of the total amount of drug from the body.

LADME An acronym for the time course of drug distribution: *l*iberation, *a*bsorption, *d*istribution, *m*etabolism, and *e*limination.

liberation The process of drug release from the dosage form.

limited fluctuation method of dosing A method of dosing in which the drug given is not to exceed or to go below specified limits.

maintenance dose The amount of drug required to keep a desired mean steady-state concentration.

MEC, MIC The minimum effective concentration, or the minimum inhibitory concentration, for a drug to be active. A drug is effective at any level above this value.

metabolism The biotransformation of the parent drug into metabolites.

Michaelis-Menten kinetics A method of transforming drug plasma levels into a linear relationship using the parameters of drug concentration and a constant, K_m.

passive diffusion The transport of drug by a concentration gradient across the membrane.

peak concentration The highest concentration reached after a dosage (usually soon after the dose is given).

peak method of dosing A method whereby the drug must reach a specified maximum level to be effective.

pharmacokinetics The quantitative study of drug disposition in the body.

pharmacological effect The influence of a drug on a patient's biochemical or physiological state (such as lowering of blood pressure and bacteriostasis).

prodrug A parent compound that is usually not active and must be metabolized to the active form.

receptor The structure in the body with which the drug interacts, yielding its pharmacological effect. Most often it is located on a cell membrane or other cellular component.

slow release A dosage form of drug that allows the drug to be slowly placed into solution.

steady state A condition in which drug input and drug output are equal. This is obtained when, after multiple dosing, the peak concentration and the trough concentration after each dose oscillate within a certain range.

subtherapeutic A level of drug less than that necessary to have the desired clinical effect.

t_{max} The time of maximum drug concentration.

t Dosing interval.

terminal disposition rate constant The overall elimination of drug from the body per unit time.

therapeutic index The ratio between the plasma concentrations yielding the desired and undesired effects of a drug.

therapeutic range The relationship between the desired clinical effect of a drug and the concentration of the drug in the plasma.

therapeutic window A term describing a bell-shaped response curve of drug level versus pharmacological response.

total clearance (Cl_{tot}) A term that describes how much of the volume of distribution of a drug is cleared per unit of time.

toxic Implies poisonous or deleterious, sometimes fatal, side effects from a therapeutic agent that is present at a level that is too high.

trough concentration The lowest drug concentration reached, usually before the next dose is given.

zero-order kinetics The rate of change of plasma concentration, independent of the plasma concentration. A constant amount is eliminated per unit of time, or $dC/dt = k_0$.

zero-time blood level A hypothetical blood concentration obtained by extrapolation back to the initial, or zero, time of administration. Usually this yields a maximal value.

Part I: Basic overview of principles
WOLFGANG A. RITSCHEL

FATE OF DRUG AND NEED FOR THERAPEUTIC DRUG MONITORING
Concept of therapeutic range

For many drugs a relationship has been established between the clinical effects and the drug concentration in plasma. In general, to achieve the desired pharmacological effect (such as lowering of blood pressure, pain relief, or bacteriostasis) a certain concentration must be reached at the site of interaction between the drug molecule and the receptor (cell membrane, cell component) to elicit the clinical effect.

Currently the only qualitative measurements available to assess the drug interactions at the cellular level are measurements of serum drug levels. If the degree of clinical response to a drug is plotted against the logarithm of dose or blood concentration of that drug, one obtains a linear curve. One obtains the same semilogarithmic curve if the drug dose or blood concentration is plotted against the percentage of a given population that has a specific clinical response to the drug. Any dose or concentration that does not result in any measurable or quantifiable effect is subtherapeutic. Any dose or concentration larger than the minimum dose or concentration that gives 100% effectiveness is unwarranted and may be toxic. (Consider the box on p. 1088.)

Similar to the log dose-response curve, there usually is a log dose-toxicity curve (see Chapter 51). Often one finds an overlap between the upper portion of the log dose-response curve and the lower portion of the log dose-toxicity curve. For most drugs the therapeutic range is a concentration range somewhere in the lower third to middle portion of the log concentration-response curve. The steepness of the log concentration-response curve indicates the magnitude of the therapeutic range. Absolute toxicity is less

<table>
<tr><td>

Major Causes of Unexpected Serum Drug Concentrations Outside of the Therapeutic Range

Noncompliance of patient
Inappropriate dosage
Malabsorption
Poor bioavailability of the administered preparation
Drug interactions
Kidney and liver disease
Altered protein binding
Fever
Genetically determined fast or slow metabolism

</td></tr>
</table>

important than the ratio between the average toxic dose and the average therapeutic dose or concentration (see additional discussion on p. 1098). This ratio, called the *therapeutic index,* is narrow for some drugs (digoxin, lithium compounds) and wide for others. Hence the therapeutic range may also be narrow or wide. It is particularly desirable to monitor drug concentrations for drugs that have a narrow therapeutic range and low therapeutic index (digoxin, lithium, gentamicin), have dose-dependent elimination kinetics (phenytoin), or show great individual variability in metabolism (tricyclic antidepressants). Thus it is important for the physician to know whether the drug is present in a concentration within the therapeutic range.

The purpose of this chapter is to describe the fate of drugs once administered, to provide some insight into the type of dose regimen used to achieve the therapeutic range, and to describe some basic principles of pharmacokinetics.

LADME system to describe drug disposition

It is generally accepted that changes in drug concentrations in the body, which occur with time, are related to the course of the pharmacological effects. The change of drug concentration with time is described by the LADME system, in which the *l*iberation, *a*bsorption, *d*istribution, *m*etabolism, and *e*limination of a drug is considered in sequence.

Liberation, or drug release, from a dosage form. To be absorbed, a drug must be present in the form of a true solution at the site of absorption. Hence the active ingredient of any dosage form except those that are already true solutions (such as intravenous injection, peroral elixir, peroral syrup, rectal enema, eye drops, and nose drops) has to be released from the dosage form before the drug can be absorbed. The release or liberation is the process of the drug passing into solution. When given orally by tablets, capsules, or suspensions, the drug dissolves in gastric fluid. After intramuscular or subcutaneous injection of suspensions, the drug dissolves in tissue fluid. After rectal administration, suppositories melt in the rectum, and the drug dissolves in rectal fluid. After application of ointments, the drug dissolves in the water of perspiration at the interface

between the skin and the ointment. These are a few cases in which liberation is necessary for the drug to be absorbed.

Sustained or controlled-release dosage forms are preparations with slow release rates. These are designed for those drugs that do not remain in the body for a long time. Since the drug cannot be absorbed faster than it is released, the apparent absorption rate becomes a function of the release rate and the entire absorption process takes longer, resulting in a prolonged duration of clinical effect.

Absorption. Absorption is the process by which the drug molecule is taken up into systemic circulation. Systemic circulation is usually defined as the bloodstream. The process of absorption must occur whenever a drug is administered *extravascularly,* that is, perorally, orally, intramuscularly, subcutaneously, rectally, topically, and so on. Whenever a drug is given *intravascularly* (intravenously, intra-arterially, intracardiacly), no absorption takes place because the drug is directly introduced into the bloodstream.

There are various mechanisms of absorption, including passive diffusion, active transport, facilitated transport, convective transport, and pinocytosis. *Passive diffusion,* applicable for about 95% of all drugs, depends on the concentration of nonionized drug being higher on one side of the membrane than on the other. As long as there is a concentration gradient across the membrane, the drug will be absorbed into the region of lower concentration. For weak electrolytes, the drug's pK_a and the pH at the absorption site (such as stomach pH 1.5 to 3, intestines pH 5 to 7, rectum pH 7.8, or skin pH 5) influence the degree of ionization. The pH of blood is 7.4 and rather constant. As a general rule, ionized drug species are passively absorbed much *less* readily than nonionized species. At two pH units below an acid drug's pK_a and 2 pH units above a basic drug's pK_a, the drugs will be 99% nonionized and have maximal rates of absorption.

The next important absorption mechanism is *active transport,* which requires binding of the drug molecule to a carrier (protein) in the membrane. The carrier delivers the drug to the opposite side of the membrane by an expenditure of energy. The process moves the drug (such as cardiac glycosides, hexoses, monosaccharides, amino acids, riboflavin) against a concentration gradient. *Facilitated transport* is a similar mechanism, but facilitated transport of a substance (such as vitamin B_{12}) follows the concentration gradient. *Convective transport* is the mechanism of absorption by which small molecules (such as urea) enter systemic circulation through water-filled pores in the membrane. For all these mechanisms the drug must be in true aqueous solution at the absorption site.

A unique absorption mechanism is that of *pinocytosis* of fats and solid particles. Engulfing vesicles form in the cellular membrane and open at the intracellular side, releasing the fat droplets or particles (such as vitamins A, K, D, and E; parasite eggs; fats; and starch).

Distribution. Once drug molecules are absorbed, they distribute within the bloodstream and can (1) be confined to the blood space, (2) leave the bloodstream and enter other extravascular fluids (such as interstitial fluid), or (3) migrate into various tissues and organs. The entire process of transfer of drug from the bloodstream to other compartments is called *distribution*. This process usually takes between 30 minutes and 2 hours but may be completed within a few minutes or may take much longer than 2 hours (distribution time for methotrexate is 15 hours).

Metabolism. Metabolism is the process of biotransformation of the parent drug molecule to one or more metabolites. The metabolites are usually more polar, that is, more water soluble, and can thus be more easily excreted by the kidney. Metabolism occurs primarily in the liver and the kidney but also takes place in plasma and muscle tissue. Usually, but not always, metabolites are less active and less toxic than their parent compounds. However, at this point a group of drugs, known as *prodrugs,* should be mentioned. The prodrug as parent compound is usually not active and must be metabolized to the active form (for example, the inactive cancer drug cyclophosphamide is biotransformed to the active compound 4-hydroxycyclophosphamide). The active form of prodrugs is either unstable, not readily soluble, or poorly absorbed.

Some drugs form metabolites that are also active. For example, the active drug procainamide is biotransformed to the equipotent metabolite acetylprocainamide. The knowledge of active metabolites is particularly important for therapeutic drug monitoring to correlate the total concentration of all active forms with pharmacological effects.

Elimination. The final excretion of the drug from the body either as unchanged parent compound or in the form of metabolites is called *elimination*. The major routes of excretion are through the kidney into urine and through the liver into bile and consequently into feces. Other pathways of elimination are through skin (sweat), lungs (expired air), mammary glands (milk), and salivary glands (saliva).

The elimination half-life is the time required to reduce the blood level concentration to one half after equilibrium is obtained. After the drug is absorbed and distributed, it takes one half-life to eliminate 50% of the drug, seven half-lives to eliminate 99% of the drug, and 10 half-lives to eliminate 99.9% of the drug.

Effects of biological variation on LADME. If a drug is given in identical amounts by the same route of administration at the same time of day to identical twins, the pharmacokinetic parameters will differ only very slightly. In fraternal twins there will be larger differences. Greater differences will occur within a population group, even if this group is homogeneous with regard to sex, age, body weight, and health. These differences are genetically based variations in drug handling, which may influence absorption, dis-

tribution, metabolism, elimination, and drug-receptor interactions. Hence pharmacokinetic parameters for healthy subjects reported in the literature are means with ranges. They are actually valid only for the group studied.

Physiological and pathological factors influencing drug disposition. Apart from biological variations caused by genetic differences, many physiological and pathological factors may alter considerably a drug's disposition.[1]

The most prominent physiological factors are body weight and composition, age, temperature (hyperthermia and hypothermia), gastric emptying time and gastrointestinal motility, bloodflow rates (during rest and exercise), environment (high altitude, mountain sickness), nutrition, pregnancy, and circadian rhythm.

Among the most important pathological factors are renal impairment, liver impairment, acute congestive heart failure, burns, shock, trauma, and gastrointestinal diseases.

Blood levels as indicators of clinical response

The rationale for the use of blood levels as indicators of clinical response is based on the concept that, for those drugs that interact at a receptor site without being changed, the drug concentration at the site of action will determine the intensity and duration of the pharmacological effect. Since it is usually not possible to sample at the site of action or biophase (such as the cell membrane), the next alternative is to sample whole blood, plasma, or serum, which is the biological fluid in closest equilibrium with the receptor site that can be easily sampled. After the distribution phase is complete, the drug concentration in the central and peripheral compartments (that is, blood) will decline in parallel. At this point a pseudoequilibrium of distribution is obtained regardless of whether the site of action is in the central compartment or in any peripheral compartment. Although the total drug concentration may differ considerably between central and peripheral compartments, the concentration of *free* (unbound) drug will be the same. Hence, once the pseudoequilibrium of distribution is reached, a correlation should exist between pharmacological effect and drug concentration in blood. Usually only the total drug concentration is measured in plasma. This is quite acceptable under normal conditions because individual differences in plasma-protein binding seem to be small[2]; in some cases, however, this is not true.[3,4]

Blood levels after single dose of drug

Most graphical descriptions of a pharmacokinetic response are given as a plot of blood concentration versus time (Fig. 56-1). The shape and course of a blood level–time curve depend on the route of administration and the LADME system.

With rapid intravenous administration, each facet of the drug is instantly in the systemic circulation. If the drug is given by extravascular administration, none will be in sys-

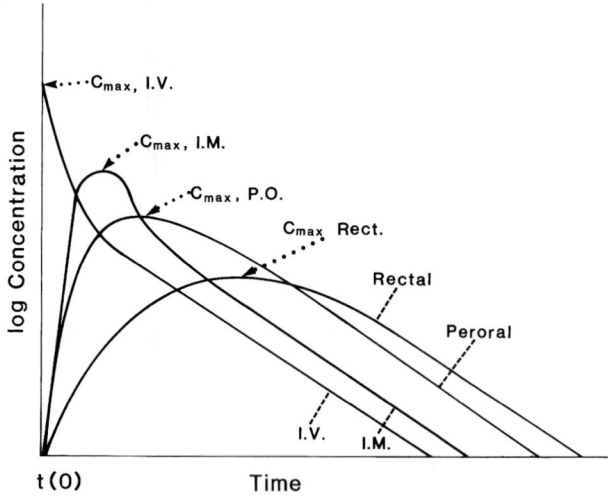

Fig. 56-1 Blood level–time curves of a hypothetical drug upon different routes of administration.

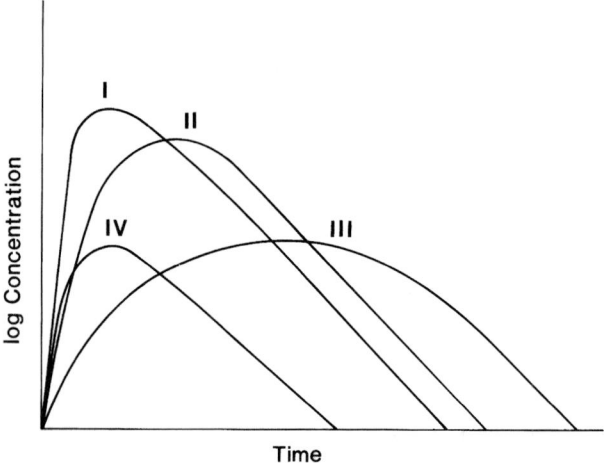

Fig. 56-2 Influence of liberation process on course of blood level–time curves. *I,* Fast-dissolving tablet; *II,* tablet with slower dissolution rate; *III,* sustained-release tablet; *IV,* tablet with poor bioavailability.

temic circulation at the moment of administration, that is, at time zero. After the drug is released from the dosage form, the blood level–time curve rises with continuous absorption. Once absorbed, a molecule is exposed to distribution, metabolism, and elimination. Since initially a greater proportion is absorbed than is distributed, metabolized, and eliminated, the blood level–time curve rises until input and output are equal. At this time (t_{max}) the peak concentration (C_{max}) is reached and the blood level-time curve declines as elimination exceeds absorption (Fig. 56-1).

Two liberation factors may change the shape of the curve: the rate and the extent of liberation. Drug products from different manufacturers may release the drug at various rates. A slow release may also be intentional, as in the case of slow-release (sustained-release) dosage forms. However, if all the drug is released, the areas under the blood level–time curves of different formulations will be the same. If the drug is not fully released, a so-called bioavailability problem might be present and the area under the curve will be reduced (Fig. 56-2). *Bioavailability* refers to the amount of drug systemically absorbed.

The absorption process can be influenced by many factors. Food (when the drug is given orally before, during, or after meals) may have no effect on the absorption, may accelerate or prolong the absorption, or may influence the extent of absorption. For example, the blood level of griseofulvin is greatly enhanced when the drug is given with fat, whereas a tetracycline blood level decreases when the drug is ingested with milk.

The volume of distribution may change in various pathological conditions. If the volume of distribution increases, the blood level decreases and vice versa. In congestive heart failure the volume of distribution for certain drugs is reduced (digoxin, quinidine). The same dose will therefore result in a higher concentration (Fig. 56-3).

For drugs that are extensively metabolized, changes in the course of blood levels may result from impaired metabolism (liver damage) or other drugs given concomitantly that either compete for metabolic pathways (enzyme inhibition) or accelerate metabolism (enzyme induction) (Fig. 56-4).

Elimination of drugs, particularly of those predominantly eliminated through the kidney, may be tremendously prolonged in case of renal failure and in aged persons. The reduced elimination can result in a manyfold prolonged elimination half-life. Classic examples are the aminoglycosides. Gentamicin's normal half-life of 2 hours may easily be prolonged to 20 hours or more (Fig. 56-5).

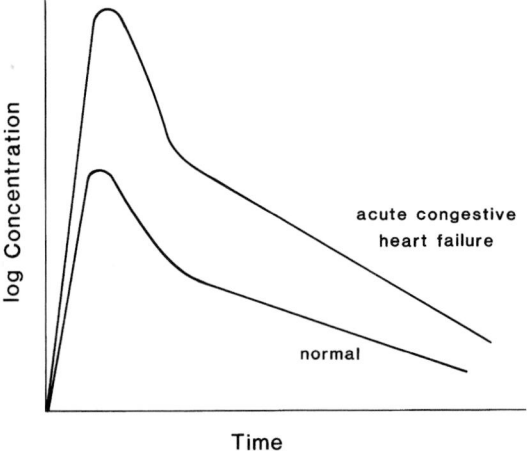

Fig. 56-3 Influence of distribution process on course of blood level–time curves of digoxin. In acute congestive heart failure a higher blood level is observed because of decreased volume of distribution.

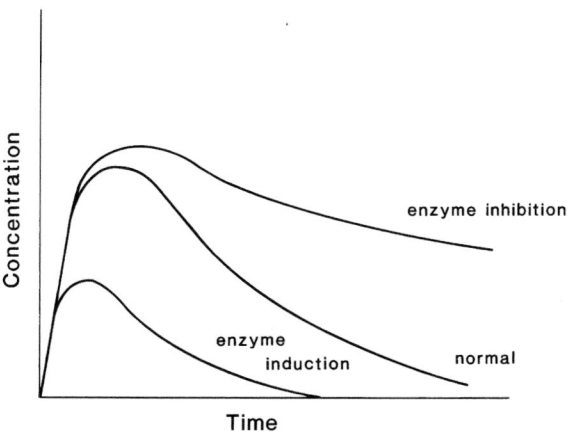

Fig. 56-4 Influence of metabolism processes on course of blood level–time curves. Enzyme inhibition and liver damage may greatly increase blood level, whereas enzyme induction may decrease it.

Effects of high levels of drugs

As stated earlier, for most drugs there is a relationship between drug concentration in the blood and the pharmacological and toxic response. Hence an increase in the blood level is usually associated with an increase in intensity not only of clinical effectiveness but also of toxicity. For most drugs it is desirable either to reach a therapeutic range with the peak concentration or to maintain the blood level throughout the dosage interval within the therapeutic range. A concentration below the therapeutic range is subtherapeutic or ineffective, and a concentration above the therapeutic range is likely to be toxic and cause side effects. However, the therapeutic and subtherapeutic range and the therapeu-

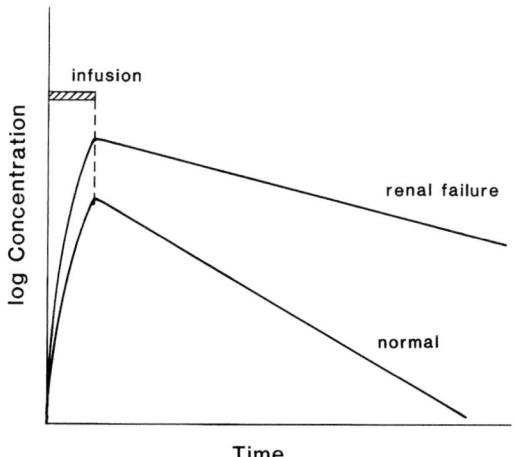

Fig. 56-5 Influence of elimination processes on course of blood level–time curve of gentamicin. In presence of renal failure, peak concentration after short-term infusion is higher and blood level remains elevated with a longer elimination half-life.

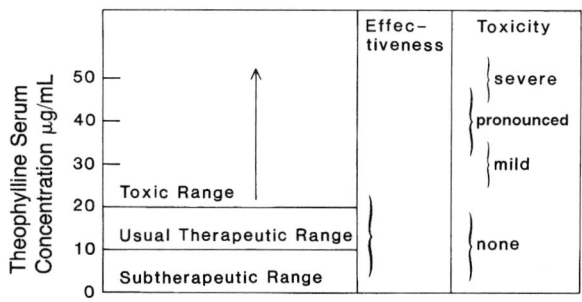

Fig. 56-6 Relationship between serum theophylline concentration and effectiveness and toxicity.

tic and toxic range often overlap (Fig. 56-6). Additionally, an established therapeutic range may be applicable for the majority of patients but may be too low or too high for an individual patient. One such example is theophylline, for which the usual therapeutic range is between 10 and 20 μg/mL. However, some patients are perfectly controlled with levels as low as 5 μg/mL. On the other hand, whereas most patients do not experience theophylline side effects with levels of 23 μg/mL, some already show toxic signs at this level.

Need for monitoring of drug therapy

Many patients, regardless of whether they are hospitalized or ambulatory, receive more than one drug during any given day,[5] which increases the probability of drug-induced diseases, drug interactions, and side effects. One of the most widely used drugs, cimetidine, has been reported to interact with 21 different drugs.[6] A definite need for drug monitoring is also indicated by the finding that 30% to 50% of dosage administrations in hospitals and nursing homes were in error.[7]

Another reason for drug monitoring is noncompliance with a prescribed dosage regimen. One report states that the percentage of patients failing to take their medication as directed ranges between 20% and 82%.[8]

Drug monitoring for all drugs and all patients is neither possible nor feasible. Furthermore, total drug monitoring is, at least at present, not relevant for all drugs. For other drugs, for which a pharmacological response is easily, quickly, and accurately measured, it is clinically more relevant to monitor directly the clinical response (such as blood pressure, blood glucose, electrolyte excretion) instead of the blood level.

If a patient is responding well to the drug therapy without any signs of toxicity, this dosage regimen should be maintained even though the blood level might be outside the usual therapeutic range. One can answer the question, "For which drugs is therapeutic drug monitoring indicated?" as follows. Monitoring is indicated for many drug groups such as antiepileptic drugs, antiarrhythmic agents, peroral anticoagulants, theophylline, tricyclic antidepressants, lithium carbonate, and aminoglycosides that either show large individual variation or are toxic above the therapeutic range. A flow chart showing the factors underlying the need for monitoring is given in Fig. 56-7.[9]

DOSAGE REGIMENS USED IN ACHIEVING THERAPEUTIC TARGET CONCENTRATION
Prediction of dosage for steady-state therapeutic levels

Most drugs are not administered as a single dose. Instead most drugs are administered in a series of doses given at specified intervals throughout the entire course of drug therapy. If the drug is administered repeatedly using dosing intervals shorter than the time required to eliminate the drug remaining in the body from the preceding dose, the drug

will *accumulate* until a steady state is achieved, that is, one in which drug input and output are equal. Steady state is obtained when, with a specific regimen of dosage, the peak concentration (C_{max}^{ss}, or maximum steady-state concentration) and trough concentration (C_{min}^{ss}, or minimum steady-state concentration) after each dose oscillate within a certain range; the goal is to achieve the therapeutic range. By obtaining a blood level–time curve after a single dose, one can derive the necessary parameters to predict the steady state and in turn the dose required to achieve a desired steady state.

The *maintenance dose* required to maintain a desired mean steady-state concentration, C_{av}^{ss}, at a given dosage interval, *t,* depends on the magnitude of C_{av}^{ss} (the required drug concentration in blood to elicit the pharmacological response), the pharmacokinetic parameters of drug disposition, and the patient's body weight. The generalized equa-

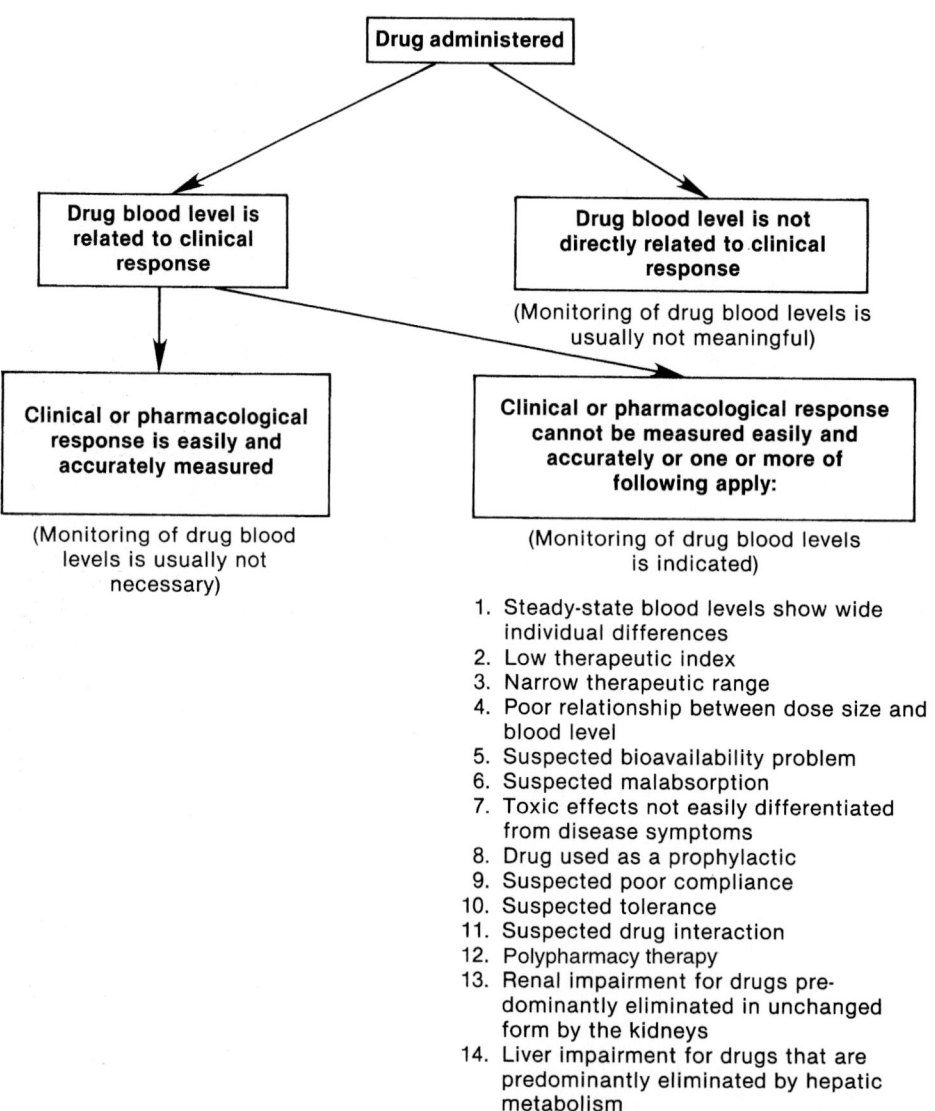

Fig. 56-7   Scheme to identify cases and situations when drug monitoring is indicated. (Modified from Pippenger CE: *Ther Drug Monit* 1:3-9, 1979.)

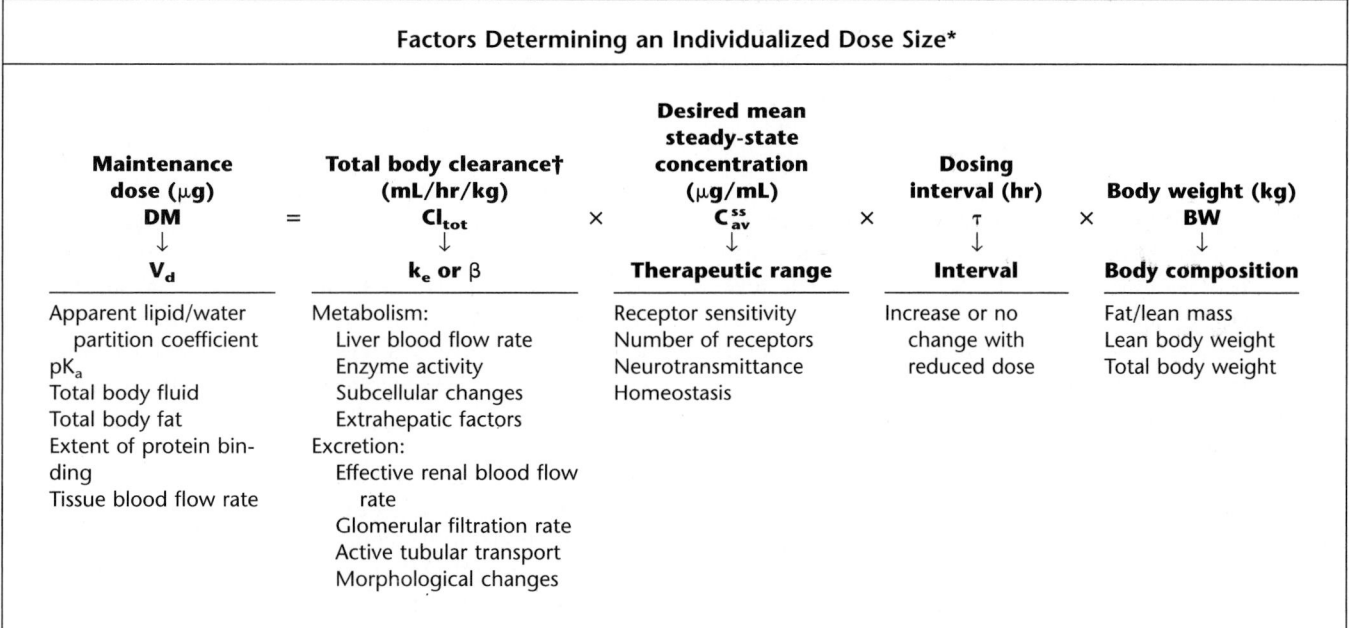

Factors Determining an Individualized Dose Size*								
Maintenance dose (μg) DM ↓ **V$_d$**	=	**Total body clearance† (mL/hr/kg) Cl$_{tot}$** ↓ **k$_e$ or β**	×	**Desired mean steady-state concentration (μg/mL) C$_{av}^{ss}$** ↓ **Therapeutic range**	×	**Dosing interval (hr) τ** ↓ **Interval**	×	**Body weight (kg) BW** ↓ **Body composition**
Apparent lipid/water partition coefficient pK$_a$ Total body fluid Total body fat Extent of protein binding Tissue blood flow rate		Metabolism: Liver blood flow rate Enzyme activity Subcellular changes Extrahepatic factors Excretion: Effective renal blood flow rate Glomerular filtration rate Active tubular transport Morphological changes		Receptor sensitivity Number of receptors Neurotransmittance Homeostasis		Increase or no change with reduced dose		Fat/lean mass Lean body weight Total body weight

*For further information see Ritschel WA: *Contemp Pharmacy Pract* 5:209-218, Washington, D.C., 1982, American Pharmaceutical Association.
†V_d, Apparent volume of distribution (mL/kg); k_e or β, overall terminal disposition rate constant (hr^{-1}); Cl$_{tot}$ = $V_d \cdot$ β.

tion for determining the correct maintenance dose is given in the accompanying box.[10]

The dosing interval, t, is freely chosen within a wide range, most often at times less than $t_{1/2}$ (half-life). It may have to be increased in renal or hepatic diseases because $t_{1/2}$ is often greatly extended in these cases. In general, at the end of four half-lives (if a dosing interval less than the half-life is chosen) a steady-state level is reached with multiple dosing (Fig. 56-8).

Dosing regimens

One can design the dosage regimen for multiple dosing maintenance therapy according to five different methods,

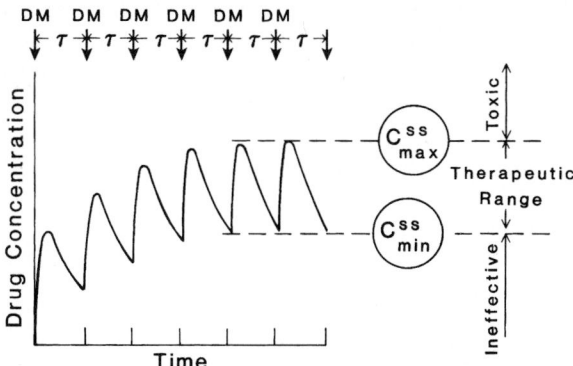

Fig. 56-8 Graph of blood-drug concentrations as function of dose and time. *DM,* Dose; *τ,* interval between doses; C_{max}^{ss}, concentration maximum at steady state; C_{min}^{ss}, concentration minimum at steady state. In this sample *τ* is chosen to be equivalent to the half-life of elimination.

depending on the desired target concentration to be achieved or maintained throughout each dosing interval. For monitoring purposes it is necessary to know which method will be used because the optimum blood sampling protocol for laboratory analysis depends on the method in question. Five methods for dosage regimen design follow:

Minimum effective concentration (MEC) or minimum inhibitory concentration (MIC) method

C_{max}^{ss}, or peak, method

C_{max}^{ss}-C_{min}^{ss}, or limited-fluctuation, method

C_{av}^{ss}, or log dose-response, method

TW, or therapeutic window, method

All methods refer to steady-state concentrations.

MEC or MIC method. For some drugs to be effective it is necessary to reach and maintain a minimum inhibitory concentration (MIC), or a minimum effective concentration (MEC), at steady state. Above the MIC or MEC the drug will be effective regardless of how high a peak level is reached as long as the entire steady-state blood level–time curve is above the required MIC or MEC. If the blood level–time curve falls below the MIC or MEC level, the drug will be ineffective as long as the concentration stays below this level. Drugs such as bacteriostatic antibiotics and other antimicrobial agents (sulfonamides) that have a relatively large *therapeutic index* are often prescribed at dosages calculated by this method.

C_{max}^{ss}, or peak, method. For some drugs it is desirable to reach a certain steady-state peak concentration during each dosing interval. However, for the remainder of the dosing interval it is not required that the drug concentration remain above a minimum level. This is particularly the case with bactericidal drugs, which act only on the proliferating microorganisms. In these cases one does not want to inhibit growth of those microorganisms that have not been killed by the previous dose. Drugs that are often given in dosage regimens based on the C_{max}^{ss}, or peak, method include penicillins, cephalosporins, gentamicin, and kanamycin.

C_{max}^{ss}-C_{min}^{ss}, or limited-fluctuation, method. For some drugs it might be desirable to maintain at steady state an MIC or MEC throughout the dosing interval but never exceed a certain peak value. This is particularly the case if the drug has a narrow therapeutic range. Drugs that might be administered using this method to compute dosage include gentamicin, kanamycin, streptomycin, isoniazid, and theophylline.

C_{av}^{ss}, or log dose-response, method. For drugs whose clinical effect follows a log dose-response curve, drug doses are selected to be in the lower portion of the log dose-response curve. The desired steady-state concentration is then usually in the lower third of the log dose-response curve. For drugs following a log dose response, the intensity of effect (and of toxicity) increases with increasing peak size. Drugs whose dosages are often based on this pattern are digoxin, lidocaine, procainamide, theophylline, quinidine, bactericidal antibiotics, analgesics, antipyretics, and hypoglycemic agents.

TW, or therapeutic window, method. With some drugs, such as antidepressants and antipsychotics, the clinical effect increases with dose size only up to a certain point and then actually diminishes as the dose size is further increased. Instead of a therapeutic range there exists a therapeutic window, showing a more or less bell-shaped log dose-response curve.

PHARMACOKINETICS

Pharmacokinetics is the quantitative study of drug disposition in the body. Pharmacokinetics permits one (1) to describe mathematically the fate of a drug after administration in a given dosage form by a given route of administration, (2) to compare one drug with others or one dosage form with other dosage forms, and (3) to predict blood levels of a drug with different dosage regimens or disease states.

Basically, in pharmacokinetics three types of kinetic processes are used to characterize the fate of drugs in the body: first-order, or linear, kinetics; zero-order, or nonlinear, kinetics; and Michaelis-Menten, or saturation, kinetics.

First-order kinetics

Most processes of drug uptake (absorption), diffusion and permeation in the body (distribution), and excretion (urinary elimination) can be described by first-order, or linear, kinetics. This means that the rate of change of concentration of drug is dependent on the drug concentration. When the concentration *versus* time data are plotted on numeric, or cartesian, graph paper, a concave curve is obtained; when plotted on semilog paper, a straight line is obtained. The relationship is expressed by Equation 56-1

$$dC/dt = -k \cdot C \qquad \textit{Eq. 56-1}$$

where C is the concentration of the drug, k is the first-order rate constant, and t is time. The minus sign indicates that the drug concentration decreases with time. Drugs are eliminated in a manner that can be described by first-order kinetics when a *constant percentage* of drug is eliminated per unit of time. Drugs exhibiting first-order elimination kinetics are antibiotics and sulfonamides, digoxin, lidocaine, procainamide, and theophylline. First-order kinetics describes the elimination of most drugs.

Zero-order kinetics

If the rate of elimination of a compound from the body is not proportional to the concentration of the drug taken, the elimination usually follows zero-order, or nonlinear, kinetics. This means that the rate of change of concentration is independent of the concentration of the particular drug. In other words, a *constant amount* of drug, rather than a constant proportion, is eliminated per unit of time (elimination depends on the amount per unit of time). When the concentration versus time data are plotted on numeric, or cartesian, graph paper, a straight line is obtained, whereas on semilog paper a convex curve is obtained. The classic example for zero-order kinetics is the disposition of alcohol (ethanol).

The relationship can be expressed by Equation 56-2

$$dC/dt = -k_0 \qquad \textit{Eq. 56-2}$$

where the rate of change of concentration, dC/dt, is equal to the zero-order rate constant, k_0, which has the units of amount per unit of time.

Michaelis-Menten kinetics

In metabolism nearly all biotransformation processes are catalyzed by specific enzyme systems with a limited capacity for the drug. Also in active transport of drugs across membranes the carriers have a limited capacity. Whenever the drug concentration present in a given system exceeds the capacity of the system, the rate of change of concentration is most precisely described by the Michaelis-Menten equation

$$dC/dt = -(V_{max} \cdot C)/(K_m + C) \qquad \textit{Eq. 56-3}$$

where C is the drug concentration, t is the time, V_{max} is a constant representing the maximum rate of the process, and K_m is the Michaelis constant, the drug concentration at which the process proceeds at exactly one half its maximal rate.

Examples of drugs that show saturation-elimination kinetics are phenytoin, high doses of barbiturates, and glutethimide.

Compartment models

To describe the quantitative processes of a drug in the organism, pharmacokinetics uses the concept of compartments. A compartment is a unit characterized by two parameters: the drug concentration, C, and the volume, V_d. By multiplying the drug concentration by the apparent volume of distribution, one obtains the amount, A, of the drug in that compartment:

$$C \cdot V_d = A \qquad \textbf{\textit{Eq. 56-4}}$$

A given compartment model is not necessarily specific for a given drug. For example, a drug given intravenously is often described by a two-compartment open model, whereas the same drug given orally or by any other extravascular route may be described by a one-compartment open model. *Open* means that there is input to and output from the compartment.

In reality the human body is a multimillion-compartment system. However, usually one has in the intact organism easy access to only two kinds of biological fluids, blood (serum, plasma), and urine. Being restricted to blood or urine specimens, the drug has a fate in the body usually described by either a one-compartment or a two-compartment open model. Clinically speaking, the concept of the one-compartment and two-compartment models is usually satisfactory for therapeutic use. The difference between a one-compartment and a two-compartment model is that in the former the distribution occurs instantly whereas in the latter the distribution process needs a measurable time before pseudoequilibrium is obtained.

Terminal disposition rate constant

In the one-compartment open model, the last or terminal portion of the straight (monoexponential) slope of a semilog blood level–time curve gives the overall elimination rate constant, k_e (metabolism, renal excretion, and other pathways of elimination). In the two-compartment model it gives β, the slow-disposition rate constant (Figs. 56-9 and 56-10).

Zero-time blood level

Back extrapolation of the blood level-time curve after intravenous administration results in the zero-time blood level C_0. After extravascular administration, the "fictitious" zero-time blood level, C_0, is the intercept of the k_e slope with the ordinate on a semilog plot in the one-compartment model, and the sum of the intercepts A + B of the α and β slopes in the two-compartment model (Figs. 56-9 and 56-10).

Absorption rate constant

The k_e slope is extrapolated back to time zero. This yields C_0, a theoretical concentration roughly equivalent to that obtained from an intravenous injection of the same amount of drug. By subtraction of the observed drug concentration during the absorption phase from the concentrations read from the back-extrapolated k_e slope, *residual points* are obtained. When plotted on semilog paper, they are described by a straight line, the slope of which is the absorption rate constant k_a (Fig. 56-9) in the one-compartment model.

Elimination half-life

Whenever a monoexponential straight line is obtained, one can calculate a drug's half-life. Notice the line describing

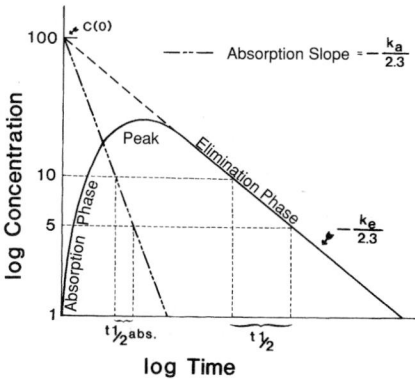

Fig. 56-9 One-compartment model blood level–time curve after extravascular administration, with monoexponential slopes for elimination, k_e, and absorption, k_a. (From Ritschel WA: *Graphic approach to clinical pharmacokinetics*, Barcelona, 1983, JR Prous.)

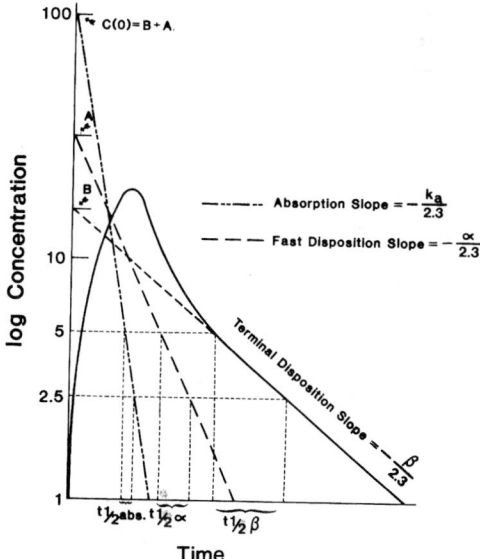

Fig. 56-10 Two-compartment model blood level–time curve after extravascular administration, with monoexponential slopes for slow disposition, β; fast disposition, α; and absorption, k_a. (From Ritschel WA: *Graphic approach to clinical pharmacokinetics*, Barcelona, 1983, JR Prous.)

the terms k_e and β in Figs. 56-9 and 56-10. Other half-lives frequently used are the absorption half-life ($t_{1/2}$abs) and distribution half-life ($t_{1/2}$).

The terms *half-time, half-life, plasma half-life, elimination half-life,* and *biological half-life* are often used interchangeably. Half-life is equal to the time required for elimination of one half the total dose of drug from the body. The elimination half-life, or plasma half-life, is the time required for the elimination of one half the amount of drug that is in the blood (plasma or serum). In those instances in which the decline of drug concentrations in all tissues does not parallel the decline of drug concentration in plasma, blood, or serum, the half-life and the elimination half-life will be different. Most statements on drug disposition refer to the elimination half-life. In Fig. 56-10 the elimination half-life ($t_{1/2}\beta$) is depicted graphically.

Volume of distribution

The volume of distribution is not a real volume and usually has no relationship to any physiological space or body fluid volume. It is simply a term to make the mass-balance equation valid. On intravenous administration the amount of drug in the body is known; however, only the blood can be sampled. Because an amount of drug, A, equals the product of concentration and volume ($\mu g/mL \times mL$), the volume of distribution is the hypothetical volume that would be required to dissolve the total amount of drug to achieve the same concentration as that found in blood.

The volume of distribution is expressed in milliliters. If this value is divided by the patient's body weight, the distribution coefficient, Δ' is obtained in mL/g (or L/kg).

Area under blood level-time curve

The integral under a blood level–time curve is a measure of the total amount of drug in the body. One can calculate the area under the blood level–time curve from time zero to infinity, AUC, or one may approximate it by plotting the curve on graph paper and cutting out the area and weighing it. The AUC is shown in Fig. 56-11.

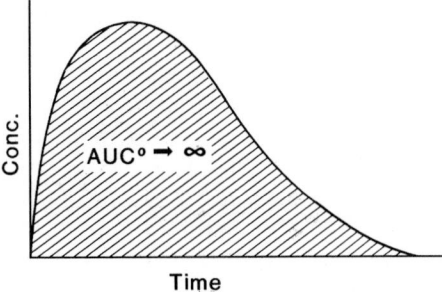

Fig. 56-11 Scheme of total area under the blood level–time curve. $AUC^{0 \to \infty}$, Area under curve from time = 0 to time = ∞. (From Ritschel WA: *Graphic approach to clinical pharmacokinetics,* Barcelona, 1983, JR Prous.)

Total clearance

The total clearance in pharmacokinetics describes how much of the volume of distribution is cleared of the drug per unit of time, regardless of the pathway for the loss of drug from the body. In effect it is the sum of all clearances by different pathways. The total clearance is the product of the apparent volume of distribution and the terminal disposition rate constant.

Steady state

Steady state refers to the accumulation of drug in the body in multiple dosing when input and output are equal within a dosing interval. The magnitude of accumulation depends on the drug's elimination half-life and the dosing interval. The smaller the dosing interval for a given dosage, the greater the accumulation and the smaller the fluctuation around the mean serum value. At steady state the drug concentration oscillates around a mean steady-state concentration, C_{av}^{ss}, with a definite maximum steady-state concentration, C_{max}^{ss}, and a minimum steady-state concentration, C_{min}^{ss}. Only in the case of an intravenous constant rate infusion are C_{max}^{ss}, C_{min}^{ss}, and C_{av}^{ss} identical.

APPLICATION OF PHARMACOKINETICS TO TDM
Clinical assessment

Clinical (physician) estimation of patient response is the first and most important task in therapeutic monitoring. One should not forget that therapy requires an approach that considers all aspects of a patient's condition, including the disease symptoms; the disease itself; other diseases present; and the patient's physical condition, age, nutritional status, and psychological aspects. Furthermore, one should not forget that clinical pharmacokinetics is only a tool that can assist with but never substitute for clinical evaluation.

Application. The clinical evaluation of patient response comprises the evaluation of vital signs and change of symptoms in response to the drug therapy, such as blood pressure, pulse rate, electrocardiogram, measurement of edema, and urinary output. Furthermore, supportive laboratory analyses may be required, such as serum glucose and electrolytes. In all these cases the pharmacological response is evaluated *clinically,* either as direct measurement of pharmacological effect or as a measurement of body constituents, but *not* by the measurement of drug concentration in biological fluid.

Limitations. Sometimes the clinical evaluation might be difficult because of the presence of two or more disease states with similar or overlapping symptoms, polypharmacy (many drugs are given simultaneously), or *unexpected* results. Unexpected results that might occur are that (1) the patient is not responding as expected, showing either no effectiveness or limited effectiveness of therapy, or (2) the patient may exhibit unexpected toxicity or side effects.

A drug may be less effective than expected because (1) the drug has a low bioavailability, (2) the patient is not complying with the prescribed drug regimen, (3) a malabsorption syndrome exists and less of the drug than expected is being absorbed. A patient may exhibit unexpected toxicity or side effects because of drug interactions, enzyme induction, enzyme inhibition, renal or hepatic impairment, edema, dehydration, and so on. In these cases it is advisable, when possible, to request drug monitoring in biological samples (see Fig. 56-7 and the box on page 1088).

Assessment by drug analysis

When the therapeutic target concentration, therapeutic range, or toxic concentration is known, therapeutic drug monitoring can be used to support the clinical evaluation. When a patient is treated with drugs of low therapeutic index, such as aminoglycosides, digoxin, and a lithium compound, or when unexpected side effects or toxicity are occurring (see Fig. 56-7), therapeutic drug monitoring should be used.

Basis for monitoring. For monitoring, it is essential to fulfill certain requirements. Otherwise, any evaluation will be in error[11]:

1. The dose size, dosage form, and route of administration must be known.
2. The dosage regimen must be followed.
3. The time between the administration of the last dose and the drawing of the blood sample must be known.
4. The blood sampling time or times must be recorded exactly.
5. The sampling times must be appropriate.

Most of the requirements listed above are self-explanatory. To understand item 5, one should remember that any samples taken during the absorption or distribution phase are useless for monitoring. Samples taken at peak time allow only an approximation of pharmacokinetic data. Samples taken at peak time and during the terminal elimination phase will result in an overestimation of the elimination rate constant and an underestimation of the elimination half-life.

The optimal sampling times for the various dosage regimen methods are shown in Fig. 56-12. Sampling times of commonly monitored drugs are listed in Table 56-1.[12]

A review of the elimination half-lives and the therapeutic ranges of 18 commonly monitored drugs also is given in Table 56-1.[13]

Limitations. The ability to monitor a specific drug in a blood sample can sometimes be limited because (1) accurate information about the times of drug administration and blood drawing is not available, (2) a reliable assay method is not available, and (3) laboratory analysis time is not reasonable. Most difficulties experienced in monitoring are caused by limited or inaccurate information. Precision of the assay must also be considered. The coefficient of variation of an assay can be important when the drug concentration is found to be either at the lower or the upper end of the therapeutic range. The therapeutic ranges reported in

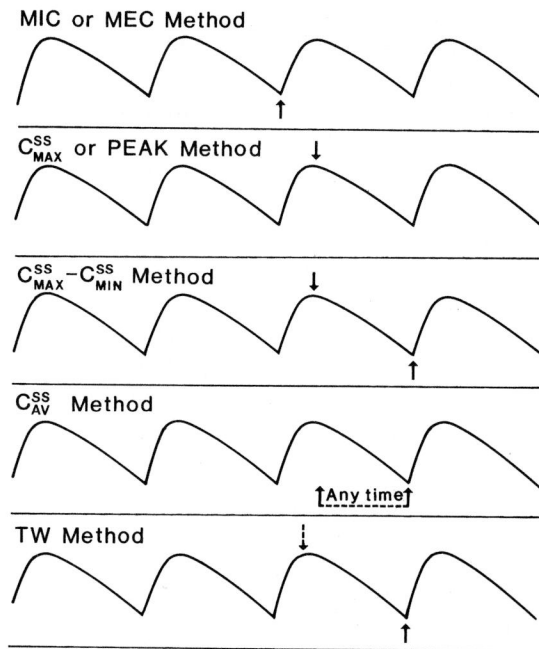

Fig. 56-12 Scheme showing optimal sampling times for monitoring for different methods used for dosage regimens.

Table 56-1 are mean values applicable to the majority of patients; the therapeutic or toxic concentration may be different for a particular patient (see Fig. 56-6).

Assessment by pharmacokinetic calculations

To evaluate blood samples pharmacokinetically, one must know whether the drug concentration is at steady state. To decide if a steady state has been achieved, one needs to know the dosage regimen (dose size and dosing interval) and how long this dosage regimen has been in effect. Usually it is assumed that a steady state is reached when the dosage regimen has been implemented for a time greater than four times the drug's elimination half-life. If the regimen has been in effect for less than $4t_{1/2}$, one should know the number of doses given before the sample was obtained. Using classic pharmacokinetic equations one can calculate what the drug concentration should be, based on mean pharmacokinetic parameters from the literature and patient information (age, body weight, sex, height, renal status, and so on). The purpose of drug monitoring is to compare the observed drug concentration to the expected or desired one. The observed concentration may be equal to, smaller than, or greater than the desired one. In the latter two cases an adjustment of the dosage regimen may be indicated and recommended.

If C_x (the measured drug concentration) differs from the desired concentration (such as $C_{av\ des}^{ss}$ or $C_{max\ des}^{ss}$), one should try to find the reason for the deviation. Some general and probable causes are presented here.

A concentration higher than the expected one could be associated with an increased bioavailability of a drug of

Table 56-1 Commonly monitored drugs, recommended sampling times, half-lives, therapeutic ranges, critical values

Drug	Recommended sampling time	Healthy $t_{1/2}$ (hours)	Therapeutic range (μg/mL)	Critical range (μg/mL)
Amikacin	0.5 to 1 hour after dose (trough) and end of dosing interval peak	0.5-3.0	Max. 20-30 Min. <5	Max. >35 Min. >10
Amitryptilin	End of dosing interval	17-40	0.120-0.250	>0.500
Carbamazepine	End of dosing interval	10-60	4-11	>15
Cyclosporine	End of dosing interval	4.7-12.7	0.1-0.3	>0.4
Digitoxin	8-24 hours after dose	72-384	0.01-0.025	>0.035
Digoxin	8-24 hours after dose	20-50	0.0008-0.002	>0.0024
Ethosuximide	End of dosing interval		40-100	>150
Gentamicin	0.5 to 1 hour after dose and end of dosing interval	0.5-3.0	Max. 5-10 Min. <2	Max. >12 Min. >2
Lidocaine	During infusion	1.2-2.3	1.5-5.0	>7
Lithium	End of dosing interval	14-33	0.3-1.3 (mmol/L)	>1.5
Phenobarbital	End of dosing interval	50-150	10-40	>50
Phenytoin	End of dosing interval	20-100	10-20	>20
Primidone	End of dosing interval	4-22	5-12	>15
Procainamide	End of dosing interval	3-5	4-10	>16*
Salicylate	1 to 3 hours after dose	3-20	150-300**	>400
Theophylline	Intravenous infusion: 4-8, 12-24 hours and 24-hour intervals after start of infusion Oral or intravenous injection; 2 hours, after dose Oral sustained release; 4-6 hours after dose	3-12, Nonsmokers 2-6, Smokers	8-20	>20
Tobramycin	0.5 to 1 hour after dose and end of dosing interval	0.5-3.0	Max. 5-10 Min. <2	Max. >12 Min. >2
Vancomycin	1 hour after dose and end of dosing interval	4-10	Max. 20-40 Min. 5-10	Max. >80 Min. >20

*Measure both parent and metabolite therapeutic range of combined; critical range >35 for both.
**Anti-inflammatory

generally low bioavailability (for example, cimetidine increases bioavailability of propranolol), patient noncompliance (such as, use of more drug or shorter dosage intervals than prescribed), or decreased total clearance (as occurs with renal or liver failure and acute congestive heart failure), or increased protein binding. A concentration lower than expected could result from decreased bioavailability (possibly drug interaction), insufficient drug dosing (longer dosing intervals, missed doses, or noncompliance), increase in the total clearance (drug interaction or enzyme induction), or decreased protein binding.

More complex pharmacokinetic analyses

The preceding equations presented are basic ones. Space and background information do not permit more detail. The purpose of this chapter is to present a general review and to transmit a general understanding of the pharmacokinetic principles involved, including dosage regimens.

Part II: Practical aspects of TDM
MICHAEL OELLERICH
VICTOR W. ARMSTRONG

THERAPEUTIC RANGE

Although therapeutic ranges have been empirically established in numerous clinical studies to assist in interpreting

drug measurements, drug concentrations must always be interpreted in the context of all clinical data. In contrast to the concept of reference intervals in clinical chemistry, there is no generally accepted concept or protocol on how to establish the therapeutic range of a drug. These therapeutic ranges, therefore, vary somewhat throughout the literature and should be used only as a general guide. They represent the range of drug concentrations within which the probability of the desired clinical response is relatively high and the probability of unacceptable toxicity is relatively low. Clinicians should never assume, however, that a serum concentration within the therapeutic range is safe and effective for every patient. Recommended therapeutic ranges for some commonly monitored drugs are presented in Table 56-1. Serum concentrations within the therapeutic range of a drug will produce a pharmacological response in the majority of patients. At concentrations above the upper limit of the therapeutic range an increased incidence of toxic side effects can be expected without as a rule any substantial improvement in the therapeutic effect. The range between the concentration of drug required to produce the therapeutic response and that which produces a toxic effect determines how carefully the dosage of the drug must be monitored. The ratio of these concentrations is called the *therapeutic index* and is expressed as the minimum concentration (or dose) that produces toxicity divided by the minimum concentration (or dose) that gives the therapeutic response in a patient population. When this ratio is 2.0 or less, the compound can be difficult to use in patients without significant toxicity being encountered. Toxic drug concentration values above which there is an enhanced or high probability of adverse effects are listed in Table 56-1.

Therapeutic ranges may require adjustment if other drugs with either synergistic or antagonistic actions are also administered to the patient. A serum concentration of phenytoin considered within the therapeutic range may produce toxic symptoms when other central nervous depressants are present. The existence of pharmacologically active metabolites and alterations in protein binding must also be taken into consideration when one is interpreting serum concentrations. When certain drugs, such as phenobarbital, are administered over a long period of time, patients may develop a tolerance to the drug, and the upper limit of the therapeutic range may then be raised.

Target concentrations for cyclosporin A depend on the indication for treatment, time after initiation of therapy, and concurrent immunosuppressive therapy.[15,16] Thus the therapeutic range for cyclosporin A can be taken only as a general guide. Most transplant centers[16] recommend higher target concentrations during the early postoperative period and then tapering of cyclosporin A doses to achieve a lower maintenance concentration range usually 3 to 6 months after transplantation (see also pp. 1013 and 1103).

For a correct interpretation of drug levels, knowledge of the time interval between the administration of the last dose and blood sampling is imperative. With long-term therapy the blood samples should be taken in the steady state. In practice samples are usually taken after 4 to 5 half-lives have elapsed when over 90% of the steady-state concentration has normally been reached (see Fig. 56-8). Depending on the clinical question either the peak concentration or the trough concentration taken directly before administration of the next dose is measured. When a drug is given by intravenous infusion, blood samples should be taken after the initial distribution phase is completed, usually around 1 to 2 hours. However, for digoxin and digitoxin the time to equilibrium after oral or intravenous administration is usually 8 to 12 hours. For serum concentrations to best reflect the effect on cardiac activity, samples should be taken when drug equilibrium has been achieved between serum and tissue.[17]

In the case of some drugs such as phenytoin or phenobarbital, the timing of the blood sampling is not important, since the fluctuations between the peak and trough concentrations in the steady state are relatively small. With other drugs such as theophylline, which have a narrow therapeutic range and a short half-life, it may be necessary to obtain blood samples at both the peak and trough levels to determine whether the correct dosage has been used. In the case of multiple daily dosing of the aminoglycosides, both peak and trough values should be monitored to prevent the administration of inappropriately high doses, which might predispose the patient to nephrotoxicity and ototoxicity.[18]

For once-daily dosing,[19] it may be necessary only to monitor trough levels or a level obtained at a defined interval after the infusion.[20]

Some of the commoner causes of unexpected serum drug concentrations observed in patients are listed in the box on p. 1088. If these factors cannot be eliminated and if an adequate compliance of the patient can be ascertained, it will be necessary to adjust the dosage of the drug.

DOSE-PREDICTION METHODS

Estimates of the dose required to achieve a drug concentration in the therapeutic range have been tabulated based on the levels found in test populations. The use of this information is termed *population-based pharmacokinetic dosing.* These estimates are in the form of tables or nomograms and allow the clinician to choose a dose based on certain features of the patient (such as age, diseases, smoking habits). Although these procedures are inexpensive, they often have a large prediction error. Therefore, prediction methods that allow one to estimate drug clearance from a few drug concentration measurements on an individual have been developed to facilitate individual dosage adaptation.

Adjustment of dosage at steady state

Clearance is the most important parameter to be considered in designing a rational dosage regimen. At steady state, one can easily estimate clearance by dividing dosing rate by the average steady-state serum drug concentration. For those drugs having a clearance linearly proportional to dosage, a new dose (DN) to achieve the desired concentration can then be calculated from the actual dosage (DA), the actual steady-state serum drug concentration (CA), and the desired serum drug concentration (CN) according to the following equation:

$$DN = \frac{DA}{CA} \times CN \qquad\qquad \textit{Eq. 56-5}$$

For practical purposes, the trough concentrations rather than the average steady-state concentrations are generally employed. The use of equation 56-5 is limited in patients whose LADME parameters are at the extremes of the usual patient range. In those cases, peak and trough levels may not change in a linear manner after a dosage adjustment and more sophisticated methods using a small number of serum concentration measurements are used to estimate the individual pharmacokinetic parameters. These estimates are used to predict the optimal dosing scheme when measurements are made under non–steady state conditions or for those drugs whose elimination cannot be described by first-order kinetics.

Three-point method of Sawchuk

The dosage prediction method of Sawchuk requires determination of (1) a predose level, (2) a drug concentration obtained 30 minutes after the end of a constant-rate IV infusion and (3) an additional concentration measured 1 hour before the next dose.[21] If one assumes a one-compartment model, the elimination-rate constant can be estimated from the slope of the concentration-time curve (see Fig. 56-9). The distribution volume, V_d, can then be calculated from the dosage, D; the duration of constant-rate infusion, t; the elimination-rate constant, k; the predose level, C_0; and the theoretical initial concentration, C, according to the equation:

$$V_d = \frac{D}{t \cdot k} \times \frac{(1 - e^{-kt})}{(C \cdot e^{-kt} - C_0 \cdot e^{-kt})} \qquad \textit{Eq. 56-6}$$

The clearance, CL, is then the product of the elimination-rate constant, k, and the distribution volume, V_d.

Bayesian forecasting

The clearance and distribution volume of an individual patient can be derived through application of the Bayes formula to pharmacokinetic parameter estimation.[22] This approach uses previously obtained information on the distribution range of pharmacokinetic parameters within the population combined with data on one or more serum drug concentrations observed on the test individual.

The estimates of the pharmacokinetic parameters in the individual patient are obtained from the Bayes formula. One can improve these estimates by taking into account patient-specific data (such as age, sex, disease, medications). Given a patient data set, a best fit is obtained for possible clearance and distribution volume values. Bayesian drug-dosing programs are now commercially available and have been applied to various drugs.[23-26] The prospective value of this Bayesian prediction model has been demonstrated[27,28] on patients receiving aminoglycosides. Use of the clinical pharmacokinetic service recommendations led to lower direct costs of hospitalization, including reduction of hospital stay, illustrating the cost-savings effect made through rational use of TDM predictive models.

CLINICAL INDICATIONS FOR TDM

For those drugs in which there is knowledge of dose response and toxicity the need for monitoring is very dependent on patient clinical status.

Clinical indications for the need to have information on drug concentrations are presented in the box. In the prophylactic application of drugs, for example, it is essential to know if the drug concentration is in the desired therapeutic range to prevent the disease symptoms. One example is determination of theophylline levels to ascertain if they are in the range that prevents asthmatic attacks.

Knowledge of drug concentrations is critical for patient management when symptoms resulting from drug toxicity and the underlying disease are similar. Premature ventricular contractions, for example, can indicate either digitalis toxicity or intrinsic heart disease. High levels of either quinidine or procainamide can induce ventricular arrhyth-

---

Clinical Settings Requiring TDM

Suspected drug overdose*
Lack of therapeutic effect
Compliance problems
Toxic effects not easily differentiated from disease-specific symptoms
Drug interaction or multidrug therapy
Drug used as a prophylactic
Disease state that alters pharmacokinetic response
Dosage optimization in the critically ill patient*
Unknown medication (as in a comatose patient)*
Leucovorin rescue therapy during treatment with high-dose methotrexate*

*Indications for measuring drug levels in the stat. laboratory.

---

mias similar to the ones controlled by these drugs. Tachycardia cannot be used in the diagnosis of a theophylline overdose, since tachycardia is present in patients with severe respiratory obstruction. Toxic doses of phenytoin can cause seizures that are symptomatic of the underlying epilepsy.

Measurement of serum drug levels is required to optimize drug dosage in cases in which drug interactions are suspected, or for those drugs that have a considerable intraindividual and interindividual pharmacokinetic variability. It must be stressed that in many severely ill patients, drug absorption, protein binding, and drug elimination can change effective drug concentration or allow potentially active metabolites to accumulate. Determination of drug concentrations is necessary when a change in bioavailability is suspected or when persistent adverse effects occur. Monitoring is also necessary to avoid toxicity such as that seen in patients undergoing high-dose methotrexate therapy, where severe adverse reactions are usually avoidable if the dosage of the antidote, leucovorin, is adjusted according to methotrexate serum concentrations.

SAMPLING AND FREQUENCY OF DRUG MONITORING
Sampling

For most drugs either plasma or serum samples are used to determine circulating levels of the drug. However, in the case of cyclosporin A[15,16,29] whole blood is the preferred matrix. Accurate and precise timing, both in administration of the drug and in obtainment of each blood sample, are of paramount importance in therapeutic drug monitoring. This one parameter, time, is often the most difficult to obtain. Quality assurance should be directed to ensuring that this information is obtained. The recommended sampling times of commonly monitored drugs are presented in Table 56-1. The specimen has to be accompanied by a request form providing demographic data on the patient as well as the collection date and time. Data on dose amount, dose interval, time of last dose, route of administration, and other medication should also be included.

Frequency of drug monitoring

In addition to the acute care cases described above, the frequency of monitoring will depend very much on the clinical situation of the patient, the experience of the physician, whether or not serum concentrations have reached steady state, and the half-life of the drug.

In the case of critically ill patients being treated with drugs, such as the aminoglycosides, that have rapid clearance changes, a daily modification of drug dosage may be necessary. For other drugs such as cyclosporin A, the variability in response and thus in dosage requirement means that blood level monitoring of this drug should therefore start immediately after the initiation of therapy. Remember that in these cases failure to achieve adequate blood concentrations can be fatal whereas overdosage can result in severe toxic effects. However, because of cost and convenience factors, monitoring can be relaxed with time. Monitoring of cyclosporin A in the early posttransplantation hospitalization period of liver, heart, and kidney transplants is done 4 to 7 times per week. After the intensive early monitoring, the measurement of cyclosporin A blood levels can be gradually reduced; for example, in renal transplant recipients with an uncomplicated course, cyclosporin A concentrations should be monitored once a month during the first year and at 1- to 3-month intervals thereafter.[16] However, there are no hard and fast rules, and measurements should be performed if the clinical signs or symptoms indicate that dosage adjustment might be necessary.

Frequent monitoring is often required when one is optimizing drug dosage or initiating drug therapy. For example, frequent serum digoxin measurement (daily) early in the course of therapy is desirable in patients with moderate to severe renal failure because of variability in both volume of distribution and elimination associated with diminished renal function. Knowledge of drug concentrations is particularly important when a loading dose is administered. Frequent measurements may be necessary to monitor the appropriateness of a modified dosage regimen or to follow the course of drug interaction–induced changes in serum digoxin concentration.

The frequency of monitoring is usually decreased for outpatients following a course of long-term drug therapy. Frequency is in part dependent on the drug. For theophylline, the narrow therapeutic index and the relationship of serum concentration to both efficacy and toxicity make measurement of serum concentrations an essential part of patient management. Serum concentrations of theophylline should be monitored during the initial phase until the steady state has been reached and then at regular intervals (such as 6 to 12 months) thereafter. Serum concentrations of phenytoin should be measured after initiation of therapy to determine if a therapeutic serum concentration has been achieved.

Drugs for Which Analyses Should Be Available in the Stat. Laboratory
Stat. analyses in suspected drug overdose Theophylline Digoxin Phenytoin, phenobarbital, carbamazepine Salicylic acid, acetaminophen Lithium, tricyclic antidepressants, barbiturates, benzodiazepines **Other analyses** Tobramycin, amikacin, gentamicin, netilmicin Cyclosporin, tacrolimus (FK506) Methotrexate

Measurements can be made 2 weeks to 1 month after initiation of therapy because a steady state is generally reached in this time.

The measured concentration should be used with relevant clinical information to decide whether an adjustment in the daily dose is required. In patients with therapeutic failure, signs of drug overdose, or suspected noncompliance, an immediate response to obtain an appropriate measurement of serum drug concentration is indicated.

High-dose methotrexate therapy requires serial monitoring of serum concentrations during the leucovorin rescue phase, since the dose of leucovorin needed depends on the serum methotrexate level. In patients with normal renal function it is usually sufficient to measure serum methotrexate levels at 24, 48, and 72 hours.

Turnaround times

For many of the drugs listed in Table 56-1 a same-day analytical service is feasible. When dosage adjustment is necessary, the results of serum drug concentration measurements will obviously be required before administration of the next dose. Since aminoglycoside levels are ordered as peaks and troughs, it is more accurate and efficient to obtain both specimens during the same dosing interval. The laboratory can then measure both peak and trough levels in the analytical batch to minimize variance. This immediate response often allows the laboratory to give results to the physician on the same day, thus allowing sufficient time to establish a new dosage regimen.

Stat. analyses

In certain clinical situations a prompt determination of serum drug levels may be necessary. Some of the most important indications for the rapid measurement of serum drug concentrations are indicated in the box, p. 1100, and the drugs most likely to require monitoring in the stat. laboratory are listed in the box above. The drugs requiring analysis in the stat. laboratory can be divided into two categories depending on the urgency of the analysis. In the case of a suspected drug overdose, that is, a potentially life-threatening situation, an immediate analysis should be carried out. One example is measurement of the tricyclic antidepressants that occur in suicide attempts. Drug levels that include parent and metabolite are useful for clarification of intoxication with these drugs.

There are occasions for which analyses outside of the usual routine laboratory working hours are necessary. Examples include aminoglycosides, where urgent determination of serum drug levels in critically ill patients for whom an individual dosage adjustment is necessary, specific treatment protocols for high-dose methotrexate with leucovorin rescue, which may require the off-hour determination of serum methotrexate concentrations, and cyclosporin A as well as tacrolimus levels, which may be required 7 days a week, particularly in patients after liver transplantation.

QUALITY ASSURANCE
Quality control

Quality control programs use commercially available quality control materials as well as proficiency-testing programs for TDM. TDM differs from other clinical chemistry testing in that the level of analyte is achieved by changing of the dose. Therefore physicians must have confidence in the concentration measurements, and for the laboratory it is important that both satisfactory accuracy is achieved and analytical precision is within acceptable limits. Performance standards based on pharmacokinetic theory and consensus strategy have been proposed.[30] More recently statistical principles for analytical goal setting have been applied to the determination of theophylline concentration in serum.[31]

Critical value callback

It is sometimes necessary to communicate urgently a critical drug concentration to the clinician or health care provider. Critical values include high concentrations associated with enhanced risk of toxicity for that particular drug (see Table 56-1), or low concentrations that are inadequate to achieve the desired therapeutic effect. The usual practice is to exclude analytical error by checking the internal quality control used in the analytical run for the assayed specimen and to exclude possible preanalytical error (such as inverted peak and trough values as the result of sample switching, inappropriate time of sampling, specimen taken from same infusion line used to administer the drug) as possible causes of unexpected serum drug concentrations.

DRUGS TO PREDICT ORGAN FUNCTION

Since drugs are not passive passengers, their metabolism has been used to measure organ function, with the argument being that the inability to metabolize is indicative of organ dysfunction. Drug metabolism has been used to determine liver function under the assumption that the quantitative measurement of capacity of the liver to metabolize certain drugs may serve as an estimate of hepatic function. One liver function test uses the metabolism of the drug lidocaine, which is converted by the hepatic cytochrome P-450 system to the metabolite monoethylglycinexylidide (MEGX). A dynamic liver-function test has been devised[32] based on the measurement of MEGX found in serum before and 15 or 30 minutes after a standardized bolus of lidocaine is given (1 mg/kg of body weight injected over 2 minutes). Loss of the ability to metabolize the drug as well as a decrease in hepatic functional blood flow lead to diminished production of MEGX. Since the metabolite can be measured rapidly, the MEGX test is of particular value in the field of liver transplantation[33-35] (see also p. 1011) and in the evaluation of liver function in children with chronic liver disease.[36] Because of its versatility, its use to monitor liver function in other diseases is being intensively studied.[37,38]

FUTURE PROSPECTS

The number of drugs that must be monitored to optimize therapy continues to grow as new agents are approved for human use. Monitoring is essential for medications with low therapeutic indices. Additional resources will be needed to monitor those drugs and clinical situations in which the measurement of "free" rather than total drug levels in serum will provide greater therapeutic benefit.[39,40] More specific analyses are required for the monitoring of drug enantiomers rather than the racemate mixtures that are currently measured.[41] Monoclonal antibodies that are used for therapeutic purposes are also potential candidates for monitoring serum concentrations. Finally, individualization of therapy based on understanding the patients' pharmacogenetics will play a more important role in drug monitoring.

METHODS OF ANALYSIS
Anticonvulsant drugs

PAUL SALM
PAUL J. TAYLOR
JULIA M. POTTER

Principles of analysis and current usage Most anticonvulsant drugs have specific ultraviolet spectral characteristics that were exploited in the initial attempts to monitor the therapeutic levels of these drugs.[42] For example, after their extraction and separation by thin-layer chromatography, quantitation of anticonvulsants was achieved by either ultraviolet scanning of the plate or by elution of the drug from the plate and recording of its ultraviolet absorption.[43]

Gas chromatographic (GC) techniques were for many years the primary technique used to analyze antiepileptic drugs in biological fluid (see Table 56-2, method 1, on p. 1104).[44] Flame ionization detection (FID) or the more sensitive nitrogen selective detection (NSD) systems were the most widely used methods for quantitation. Approximately half of the GC methods do not require derivatization of the anticonvulsant drugs,[44] but, of those procedures that use derivatization, methylation is most commonly used. Fused-silica capillary columns are preferred because of their high-temperature stability and inertness, which not only removed the need for derivatization but offered high sensitivity, selectivity, and speed as well.[46]

High-performance liquid chromatography assays (HPLC) (Table 56-2, method 2) require drug purification before analysis either by organic solvent extraction or by protein precipitation. Nearly all methods use reverse-phase chromatography with ultraviolet absorption detection.[47,48]

Immunological procedures (Table 56-2, methods 3a to 3h) developed for the measurement of anticonvulsants include radioimmunoassay (RIA), enzyme immunoassay (EIA), fluorometric enzyme immunoassay (FEIA), fluorescence immunoassay (FIA), fluorescence polarization immunoassay (FPIA), nephelometric inhibition immunoassay (NIA), cloned enzyme donor immunoassay (CEDIA), and dry-film multilayer immunoassay (DFMI).

The introduction of the enzyme-multiplied immunoassay technique (EMIT, Syva Co., Inc., Palo Alto, CA 94303) in the 1970s made possible the routine monitoring of all the anticonvulsant drugs (Table 56-2, method 3b). This homogeneous enzyme immunoassay is based on the competitive protein-binding technique, with an enzyme as the label and an antibody as the binding protein (see Chapter 13). This is the second most frequently used method according to the 1995 CAP therapeutic drug monitoring (TDM) survey.

Fluorometric enzyme immunoassay (FEIA, Baxter Diagnostics Inc. Deerfield, IL 60015) is a competitive-binding method that is based on the radial partition immunoassay principle, which combines solid-phase immunological techniques and radial chromatography (Table 56-2, method 3c).[49] In FEIA the drug of interest in the clinical sample is premixed with enzyme-labeled conjugate and placed on a glass-fiber filter paper that contains immobilized antibody. The drug and labeled drug then compete for binding sites on the antibody. After a suitable incubation period, unbound label is removed from the center of the reaction zone through radial elution when a wash solution is applied. This solution also contains the substrate for the enzyme and initiates enzymatic activity simultaneously with the wash. The enzymatic activity of the bound fraction at the center of the reaction zone is quantified by front-surface fluorescence and is inversely proportional to the concentration of drug present in the sample.[49] The automation of this technology requires specialized equipment and is used by only a few laboratories.

Fluorescence polarization immunoassay (FPIA) is based on the principle of competitive-binding assay and measures binding of fluorescein-labeled drug directly by fluorescence polarization (Table 56-2, method 3d). See Chapter 13 for a detailed description. The FPIA method can be highly automated and provide very precise results.[50] Based on data in recent TDM surveys, this has become the most widely used procedure.

The Ames Seralyzer has methods for the measurement of phenytoin and phenobarbital that employ a labeled prosthetic group assay[51] (see Chapter 13 for a detailed description, and see Table 56-2, method 3e). This assay is used for point-of-care testing in physician offices.

A rate nephelometric inhibition immunoassay is the procedure employed by the Immunochemistry Systems (ICS) of Beckman Instruments, Inc. (Fullerton, CA 92634) (Table 56-2, method 3f). In this assay the anticonvulsant drug is covalently linked to a protein. Drug from the patient's sample competes with this protein-bound drug for binding to an antibody. The rate of change of light scatter is inversely related to the drug concentration.[52] This method is used by only a small number of laboratories.

A homogeneous immunoassay technique, cloned enzyme donor immunoassay (CEDIA, Microgenics Corporation, Concord, CA 94520) utilizes genetically engineered β-galactosidase enzyme fragments (Table 56-2, method 3g).[53] The automation of this technology can be performed on many routine clinical chemistry analyzers.

The OPUS immunoassay system (PB Diagnostic Systems, Westwood, MA 02090) is based on a combination of multilayer film technology and competitive immunoassay (Table 56-2, method 3h).[54] A coated multilayer film chip is encased in a plastic test module. The serum sample is applied to the top layer in the test module. This layer contains buffer components, surfactants, and other reagents (such as antibody and labeled hapten drug) and also acts as a filter to prevent protein interference with the immunoreaction. The sample diffuses from the topcoat layer through an iron oxide screen to the signal layer. The iron oxide serves to block excitation of the label outside the signal layer. The signal layer contains a fluorescent-labeled drug bound to a monoclonal antibody specific for the drug being assayed. The sample antigen displaces the labeled-antigen from the binding sites of the antibodies. The unbound labeled-antigen then diffuses into the upper layers where it cannot be measured. Equilibrium occurs within 3 to 5 minutes, after which the fluorescent signal from the remaining antibody-bound conjugate is measured from the bottom of the test module by front-surface fluorimetry. The fluorescent intensity measured is inversely proportional to the antigen concentration in the serum sample.

Specimen   Serum is the usual specimen, though serum separator tubes are not recommended because they can adsorb drug and thus give unreliable results.

Therapeutic range   The generally accepted therapeutic ranges for the major anticonvulsant drugs that are subject to therapeutic drug monitoring are as follows:

Carbamazepine	4-12 mg/L	(17-51 μmol/L)
Ethosuximide	40-100 mg/L	(280-460 μmol/L)
Phenobarbital	15-30 mg/L	(65-170 μmol/L)
Phenytoin	10-20 mg/L	(40-80 μmol/L)
Primidone	5-12 mg/L	(23-55 μmol/L)
Valproate	50-100 mg/L	(350-700 μmol/L)

Cyclosporin A
LESTER SHAW

Principles of analysis   Measurement of cyclosporin A (CsA) is performed by one of two techniques; high-performance liquid chromatography (HPLC) and immunoassay; all the available immunoassay procedures have been shown to correlate well with HPLC. However, both the parent drug, cyclosporin A, and its metabolites are present in blood. Because the immunoassays detect cross-reacting CsA metabolites, they report higher cyclosporin A concentrations

Table 56-2   Methods for anticonvulsant analysis

Method	Principle	Matrix	Comments
1. Gas chromatography (GC)	C18 solid-phase extraction; capillary column; flame ionization detection.	Blood, plasma, serum, saliva	Can resolve all anticonvulsants simultaneously; requires simple extraction
2. High-performance liquid chromatography (HPLC)	Organic solvent extraction of drugs or protein precipitation of sample; anticonvulsants are separated by reverse-phase chromatography and monitored by ultraviolet spectroscopy.	Blood, plasma, serum, saliva	Can resolve all anticonvulsants except valproate simultaneously; commonly used
3. Competitive-binding assays			
a. Radioimmunoassay (RIA)	Competitive binding of radioactive ligand; radiolabeled hapten competes with unknown for antibody binding site.	Plasma, serum, saliva	Rarely used; all problems of radioactive usage; slower than other immunoassays
b. Enzyme-multiplied immunoassay technique (EMIT)	Competitive binding with drug attached to enzyme.	Plasma, serum, saliva	Can measure all drugs, but each must be done separately; commonly used; can use routine chemistry analyzers
c. Fluorometric enzyme immunoassay (FEIA)	Combination of competitive binding with enzyme-labeled conjugate for antibody-binding site (on a solid-phase matrix) and radial chromatography.	Plasma, serum	Measures all anticonvulsants except valproate and ethosuximide
d. Fluorescence polarization immunoassay (FPIA)	Competitive binding with fluorescein-labeled drug; fluorescent drug competes with unknown for antibody site.	Plasma, serum, saliva	Each drug assayed individually; requires specialized instrument; most commonly used
e. Labeled prosthetic group assay	Antibody binding to drug labeled with prosthetic group prevents glucose oxidase activity. Competition with endogenous drug allows prosthetic group to activate enzyme. Glucose oxidase is coupled to colorimetric reaction.	Serum	Designed for inexpensive instrument; reflectance spectrophotometer; rapid test
f. Rate nephelometric inhibition immunoassay	Competitive binding for hapten; hapten-protein competes with unknown for antibody-binding site.	Plasma, serum	Each drug individually assayed; requires specialized instrument
g. Cloned enzyme donor immunoassay (CEDIA)	Competitive binding with enzyme donor (ED)–ligand conjugate for antibody-binding site. Endogenous drug modulates enzymatic activity by influencing free ED-ligand conjugate available for complementation.	Plasma, serum	Measures phenobarbital and phenytoin; each drug assayed individually; can use routine clinical chemistry analyzers; not commonly used at present
h. Dry-film multilayer immunoassay	Combination of competitive binding with a fluorescent-labeled hapten in an agarose matrix and multilayer film technology. Labeled antigen competes with sample antigens for antibody-binding site.	Serum	Each drug assayed individually; requires specialized instrument; not widely used at present

than HPLC methods do. For example, immunoassays utilizing polyclonal antibodies have been reported to overestimate CsA concentrations by 51% to 132% when compared to HPLC.[55] Newer immunoassays that employ monoclonal antibodies have somewhat improved specificity, with measured CsA concentrations being only 8% to 48% more than HPLC.[16]

Various HPLC methods have been developed for measurement of CsA in whole blood or plasma (Table 56-3, method 1). Differences in these methods include the use of either gradient or isocratic elution conditions and the choice of solvent used for extraction of the CsA. Extraction of CsA by either diethyl ether or methylbutyl ether yield an extraction efficiency of approximately 90%. Although HPLC methods have the greatest specificity and accuracy and continue to serve as the reference method, immunoassays have largely replaced HPLC as the method of choice. Differences in the cyclosporin A concentrations measured by HPLC and the various immunoassay procedures appear to be less significant in patients with renal transplants and more significant in patients with liver disease or liver transplants.[56] This pattern is consistent with the inactivation of cyclosporin A by hepatic metabolism.[57]

Radioimmunoassay (RIA) (Table 56-3, method 2) techniques were the original immunoassay procedures used to measure CsA; both monoclonal and polyclonal RIA immunoassays have since been developed. The analytical performance of the RIA procedures are similar to the non-RIA procedures. Disadvantages of the RIA procedures, such as the handling and disposal of radiolabeled compounds and the long assay time (6 to 8 hours), have led to the increased use of immunoassay techniques that employ a nonradioactive label.

The most popular immunoassay currently in use for CsA is the fluorescence polarization immunoassay (FPIA; Abbott Diagnostics Inc., Abbott Park, Illinois).[58] The FPIA (Table 56-3, method 3) procedure is automated, providing a rapid turnaround time. Originally introduced utilizing a polyclonal antibody, the method has since been updated with use of a monoclonal antibody more selective for the parent CsA. The assay requires pretreatment of the whole blood sample before analysis.

Recently, an enzyme-multiplied immunoassay (EMIT; Syva Inc., Palo Alto, California) (Table 56-3, method 4) has been introduced. Of all the CsA immunoassays, the EMIT procedure exhibits the greatest specificity for the parent drug.[16,59] Like the FPIA assay, the EMIT procedure requires a sample pretreatment step to lyse the red blood cells, solubilize the CsA, and precipitate blood proteins; the remainder of the assay is automated.

Specimen Serum, plasma, and whole blood have all been used for the determination of CsA concentrations. CsA is found predominantly in erythrocytes (57%) and leukocytes (15%) in whole blood at 37° C.[47] However, a redistribution of CsA from plasma into cells occurs as the temperature of the sample decreases. Thus several factors have led to the general acceptance of whole blood as the sample of choice: (1) There is no effect of temperature on CsA analysis of whole blood, (2) use of whole blood eliminates the problems associated with sample separation, and (3) use of whole blood results in higher measurable CsA concentrations.[16,59] However, from a clinical perspective, no advantage of monitoring CsA in whole blood versus plasma has been reported.[59]

Both heparin and EDTA have been employed as anticoagulants for whole blood samples used for CsA measurements; however, EDTA is the recommended anticoagulant.[61] Specimens for CsA analysis may be stored for up to 1 week at 2° to 8° C. For longer periods of storage, samples should be frozen at −20° C.[60]

Therapeutic range The establishment of a therapeutic range for CsA has been difficult because the correlation between blood concentrations and immunosuppressive effect is poor.

Table 56-3 Methods of cyclosporin A (CsA) measurement

Method	Principle	Usage	Comments
1. High-performance liquid chromatography (HPLC)	Extraction of CsA from biologic matrix is followed by chromatography using reversed-phase HPLC and detection at 210 to 214 nm	Less common	Measures parent drug Labor intensive Not suitable for stat. analysis
2. Radioimmunoassay (RIA)	Competitive binding of radiolabeled CsA and nonlabeled CsA to limited amount of monoclonal or polyclonal antibody	Less common	Problems of radioactivity usage and disposal Cross reactivity with metabolites
3. Fluorescence polarization immunoassay (FPIA)	Competitive binding of fluorescein-labeled CsA and nonlabeled CsA to limited amount of antibody Amount of measured plane-polarized fluorescent light is inversely related to patient CsA concentrations	Most frequently used	Automated Cross reactivity with metabolites
4. Enzyme-multiplied immunoassay (EMIT)	Competitive binding of enzyme-labeled CsA and nonlabeled CsA to limited amount of antibody Activity of enzyme label is decreased after binding to antibody. Thus enzyme activity is directly related to patient CsA concentrations	Recently introduced	Automated Greater specificity as compared to FPIA

Overall, the incidence of organ rejection is higher at low CsA concentrations, whereas toxicity occurs more frequently at high CsA concentrations. Predose, whole blood concentrations of >400 μg/L during maintenance therapy are associated with a high possibility of toxicity. Some suggested target ranges for whole blood CsA as measured by use of HPLC in renal transplant patients on triple drug therapy are as follows: up to 3 months after surgery, 150 to 225 μg/L; after 3 months after surgery, 100 to 150 μg/L.[16] (See also Chapter 50.)

Gentamicin and other aminoglycosides

JOSEPH R. DiPERSIO

Principles of analysis Gentamicin and the other important aminoglycoside antibiotics—streptomycin, kanamycin, tobramycin, amikacin, and netilmicin—are important agents for the treatment of infections caused by aerobic gram-negative bacilli. Treatment using aminoglycosides is complicated by the fairly narrow therapeutic window that exists between effective and toxic concentrations. As a result of this narrow therapeutic window, frequent laboratory measurements are often performed to ensure that appropriate therapeutic concentrations are achieved.

The methods in use for measurement of gentamicin are also applicable to the measurement of the other aminoglycosides. Thus measurement of gentamicin serves as a prototype for the analysis of these other compounds.

The original method used to quantitate gentamicin was a microbiological assay that measured biological activity. The agar plate diffusion method was based on the extent of bacterial growth inhibition caused by the diffusion of antibiotic from a paper disk into agar containing a growing indicator bacterium. The actual procedure entails adding gentamicin standards and unknown samples to blank paper disks in carefully measured amounts. The disks are then placed on the surface of an agar plate containing the growing bacterium susceptible to the antibiotic. The plate is then left to incubate for anywhere from 4 to 18 hours. The paper disks containing antibiotic will inhibit bacterial growth in an area surrounding the paper disks. The diameter of the zone of bacterial growth inhibition is directly related to the concentration of antibiotic initially applied to the paper disk. A standard curve is created by plotting on semilogarithmic graph paper the diameter of the zones of growth inhibition for each standard against the concentration of antibiotic on each disk. The concentration of antibiotic in the unknown sample is determined by interpolation from the standard curve.

The agar plate method suffers from several drawbacks, including the presence of other antimicrobial drugs in addition to the one being measured and the long analysis time. The development of immunoassays in the early 1970s have allowed for rapid and automated analysis of aminoglycosides and have replaced the microbiological assays.

The first immunoassays used to measure gentamicin were radioimmunoassays (RIA)[62] (Table 56-4, method 1). In this procedure, gentamicin is labeled with a radioactive tag by the use of a bacterial enzyme that enzymatically transfers a radiolabeled substrate to gentamicin:

Labeled group
$$+ \text{Gentamicin} \xrightarrow{\text{(Bacterial enzyme)}} \text{Labeled gentamicin}$$

RIA has the disadvantages of disposal of radioisotopes and is also not well suited for stat. analysis. As a result, competitive-binding immunoassays that utilize fluorescent or enzyme labels have been developed and are the most popular methods currently in use.

Fluorescence polarization immunoassay (FPIA) is a homogeneous competitive binding immunoassay that measures the change in polarized fluorescence caused by gentamicin in patient's sera competing with fluorescein-labeled gentamicin for a limited number of antibody-binding sites[30] (Table 56-4, method 2). Another widely used homogeneous immunoassay procedure is the enzyme-multiplied immunoassay technique (EMIT, Syva Co., Palo Alto, Calif.)[64] (Table 56-4, method 3). This procedure is based upon the competitive binding between gentamicin labeled with the enzyme glucose-6-phosphate and gentamicin in the patient's sample to an antibody. Binding of enzyme-labeled gentamicin to antibody results in loss of enzymatic activity. Thus, increasing concentrations of gentamicin in the patient sample are directly related to enzyme activity in the reaction mixture.

Chromatographic procedures for the aminoglycosides include thin-layer chromatography, high-performance liquid chromatography, and ion-exchange chromatography. These

Table 56-4 Methods of analysis for gentamicin

Method	Principle	Usage	Comment
1. Radioimmunoassay (RIA)	Competitive binding occurs between radiolabeled gentamicin and gentamicin in patient sera.	Infrequently used	Sensitive, specific, accurate; use of radioisotopes Not suitable for stat. analysis
2. Fluorescence polarization immunoassay (FPIA)	Competitive binding occurs between fluorescein-labeled drug and drug in patient's sera. Antibody-bound labeled drug has higher fluorescence polarization than the free drug has.	Frequently used	Sensitive, specific, accurate Suitable for stat. analysis Automated
3. Enzyme-multiplied immunoassay technique (EMIT)	Competitive binding occurs between enzyme-labeled gentamicin and gentamicin in patient's sera for binding to antibody. Binding of enzyme-labeled gentamicin to antibody results in loss of enzyme activity.	Frequently used	Sensitive, specific, accurate Suitable for stat. analysis Automated

Table 56-5   Usual doses and desired serum concentrations (µg/mL) for aminoglycosides

Antibiotic	Usual dose*	Peak†	Trough‡	Toxic range
1. Gentamicin Tobramycin	3 to 6 mg/kg/day divided q8h	5-10	<2	*P*, >12 *T*, >2
2. Netilmicin	4.0 to 8.0 mg/kg/day divided q8h	6-12	<3	*P*, >15 *T*, >3
3. Amikacin	10-20 mg/kg/day divided q12h	20-30	<5	*P*, >35 *T*, >10
4. Streptomycin	15 mg/kg/day divided q12h	5-20	<5	>40-50

*For adults with normal renal function.
†Peak, *P*, concentration determined 1 hour after intramuscular dose or 30 minutes after intravenous dose.
‡Trough, *T*, determined just before next dose.

techniques are generally not used in clinical laboratories for measurement of aminoglycosides.

Specimen   Serum or EDTA-plasma are the specimens of choice for aminoglycoside analysis using any of the immunoassay procedures. Heparin is not recommended as an anticoagulant because of assay interference.[7,8] Other specimen types, including cerebrospinal fluid, synovia, and other, nonviscous, fluids, can be used in the microbiological procedure.

Therapeutic range   See Table 56-5 for the accepted reference intervals for aminoglycoside antibiotics.

Lithium
STEVEN C. KAZMIERCZAK

Principles of analysis and current usage   Lithium is not bound to plasma proteins, passing freely through the glomerular membrane, and is reabsorbed in the proximal convoluted tubule. Because lithium has a relatively narrow therapeutic index, monitoring of the blood concentration of this therapeutic agent is routinely performed.

Until recently, lithium measurements in the clinical laboratory were performed by one of two techniques: atomic emission spectrometry (AES) (Table 56-6, method 1) and atomic absorption spectrometry (AAS) (Table 56-6, method 2). AAS is the reference method for lithium.[65] With the introduction of the lithium ion–selective electrode and more recently a colorimetric assay for lithium, use of AES and AAS for measurement of lithium has declined considerably.

The general principles of AES are discussed in Chapter 4. The thermal energy of an air-propane flame vaporizes lithium salts to form free lithium atoms. The heat also causes

a small fraction of the ground-state lithium atoms to become excited, causing an electron in the 2*s* orbital to be raised to the more energetic 2*p* orbital. Because of the instability of this excited state, the electron in this higher energy orbital returns instantaneously to its original 2*s* orbital with a concomitant emission of energy in the form of light at 671 nm.

The sample is diluted with a solution containing either potassium or cesium, which serve as an internal standard. The potassium or cesium in the internal standard follows the same reaction pathway of vaporization, excitation, and return to ground state with emission of light. The emission of light, however, occurs at a wavelength different from that of lithium. Measuring the ratio of the emission of light from the internal standard to the emission of light from lithium allows for correction of possible sources of analytical error. Sources of error can be introduced by fluctuations in flame temperature, sample aspiration rate, fuel-to-oxidant ratio, and the composition of reducing gases present in the flame. Since it is the ratio of the emission of internal standard to lithium that is measured, fluctuations in instrument performance that affect both elements are essentially canceled out and measurement error is minimized.

Most AES procedures today utilize cesium as the internal standard. Unlike potassium, cesium is undetectable in serum or plasma; thus no correction for endogenous cesium concentrations needs to be performed. Also, with the use of cesium as the internal standard, sodium, potassium, and lithium can all be analyzed using the same specimen.

The use of AAS is an infrequently used means for determining lithium in body fluids. See Chapter 4 for a review of the theory and applications of AAS. Atomic absorption spectrometry is similar to AES in that ground-state lithium at-

Table 56-6   Methods of lithium analysis

Method	Type of analysis	Principle	Usage
1. Atomic emission spectrometry	Quantitative	Emission of light from unstable lithium atom at 670.8 nm.	Infrequently used Serum, plasma
2. Atomic absorption spectrometry	Quantitative	Absorption of light at 670.8 nm by ground-state lithium.	Infrequently used Serum, plasma, urine, red blood cells
3. Ion-selective electrode	Quantitative	Interaction of lithium with lithium-specific ionophore generates a voltage difference proportional to lithium concentration.	Most frequently used method Serum, plasma, whole blood Correction for endogenous sodium necessary
4. Colorimetric	Quantitative	Lithium + Crown ether dye → Dye complex (400 nm) (600 nm)	Frequently used Serum, plasma

oms are produced by the heat generated from an acetylene and air flame. Ground-state lithium atoms absorb light at 670.8 nm produced by a lithium hollow cathode lamp. The amount of light that is absorbed is proportional to the amount of lithium present in the flame. Sodium and potassium concentrations up to 180 and 8 mmol/L respectively do not interfere with lithium determinations by AAS.[66] A very small amount of lithium ions will ionize under these conditions and emit light at 670.8 nm instead of absorbing the light at 670.8 nm produced from the hollow cathode lamp. Because the lithium that ionizes can introduce error in measurement, the incorporation of an electron-donating, ionization-suppression compound such as tin chloride is sometimes used. However, since the amount of lithium that becomes ionized is small (approximately 1%), use of an ionization-suppression compound is not necessary.

The use of an ion-selective electrode (Table 56-6, method 3) has become the predominant method in clinical laboratories for measuring lithium concentrations. Unlike AES and AAS, instruments that incorporate ion-selective electrode technology are more readily automated and are less technically demanding. The ion-selective membrane incorporates an ionophore with a high specificity for lithium. However, other cations, notably sodium, but also potassium, calcium, magnesium, and ammonium, may interfere with this method.[55] Most instruments that incorporate ion-selective electrode technology for lithium determinations will correct for interference by sodium but not the other interfering cations mentioned above. Lithium concentrations determined using ion-selective electrode technology have been found to favorably compare with lithium measured using AES or isotope dilution/mass spectrometry.[67]

The most recent method developed for lithium determinations is a colorimetric method that uses a crown ether (15 available types) as the chromophore (Table 56-6, method 4). Sample is deposited on a dry reagent slide where the lithium is specifically bound by a crown ether chromophore conjugate. Because the chromophore is specific for lithium, no correction for other endogenous cations is required. As the lithium in the sample binds to the crown ether, a shift from 400 to 600 nm of the peak absorbance of the chromophore occurs. The increase in absorbance at 600 nm is proportional to the concentration of lithium in the sample. A comparison of lithium determinations performed using the crown ether procedure with the AES technique revealed a negligible bias and good correlation between results.[68]

Specimen Serum or plasma are acceptable specimens. If plasma is used, sodium heparin or ammonium heparin are the preferred anticoagulants. Interference with the ion-selective electrode technology has been observed with plasma anticoagulated with EDTA, oxalate/fluoride, and sodium citrate.[69] Use of lithium heparin must be avoided. Lithium is completely absorbed from the gastrointestinal tract within 1 to 2 hours after dosing. For routine monitoring, trough samples are usually drawn 8 to 10 hours after an oral dose.

Serum or plasma should be separated from the cells if analysis is not performed within 4 hours of collection. Once separated, lithium is stable for at least 24 hours at room tem-

perature, 7 days if refrigerated at 4° C, and for at least 6 months if frozen at −18° C.

Therapeutic range Therapeutic concentrations of lithium in serum or plasma are reported to be 0.3 to 1.3 mmol/L, whereas toxic concentrations are those greater than 2.5 mmol/L.[70] Side effects associated with lithium toxicity include vomiting, ataxia, unconsciousness leading to coma, muscular rigidity, mild pyrexia, and EEG changes.

Lithium concentrations within red blood cells may also be determined as a guide for estimating lithium concentrations within tissue and for detecting noncompliance, since equilibrium between serum and red blood cells is established only after regular usage.[71] For patients with therapeutic lithium concentrations in serum, the corresponding lithium concentrations within the red blood cells is 0.2 to 0.8 mmol/L.[71]

Theophylline and caffeine
SAEED A. JORTANI

Principles of analysis and current usage Theophylline and caffeine are pharmacologic agents that have the ability to relax bronchiole smooth muscles leading to bronchodilatation. After administration, theophylline is rapidly and almost completely absorbed, with peak plasma concentrations being reached in 2 to 3 hours. In neonates, theophylline is methylated to form caffeine. Caffeine has been found to be as effective as theophylline for the treatment of apnea in neonates. Therefore, in neonates receiving theophylline, both theophylline as well as caffeine concentrations should be monitored.

A variety of techniques have been developed for the determination of theophylline in serum. Some of these methods can also be used for measurement of caffeine as well. The earliest routine method developed for determination of theophylline was a spectrophotometric procedure (Table 56-7, method 1). Theophylline in serum is extracted by use of a chloroform-isopropanol mixture and then reextracted with dilute sodium hydroxide. The absorbance of the final extract was measured at 277 and 310 nm. The concentration of drug in the unknown sample was determined by comparison to a standard curve prepared with calibrators containing known concentrations of theophylline. The spectrophotometric method is of historical interest only and seldom if ever used today.

Determination of theophylline by high-performance liquid chromatography (HPLC) (Table 56-7, method 2) is an acceptable method; however it is rarely used today. Although HPLC methods are less costly to perform when compared to other techniques, the widespread availability of immunochemical procedures for theophylline, which are easily automated, limits its use. HPLC methods that do not require extraction of theophylline from serum and require as little as 10 μL have been reported.[72] However, several drugs including ampicillin, methicillin,[73] chloramphenicol, and some cephalosporins[76] have been found to interfere with HPLC methods. Interference from these compounds can be eliminated by use of an extraction step.[75] Acetonitrile is typically used as the mobile phase. Most HPLC procedures use 8-chlorotheophylline or 8-hydroxyethyltheophylline as the internal standard.[73,75] The concentration of theophylline is

Table 56-7   Methods for theophylline analysis

Method	Type of analysis	Principle	Usage	Comment
1. Ultraviolet	Spectrophotometric	Extraction of theophylline; absorption measurement at two wavelengths.	Serum, plasma	Historical
2. High-performance liquid chromatography (HPLC)	Chromatographic with spectrophotometric detection	Depending on the method, analysis of extracted or nonextracted specimen is by reversed-phase chromatography.	Serum, plasma	Possible reference method
3. Fluorescence polarization immunoassay (FPIA)	Competitive binding with fluorescence polarization	Bound labeled drug has higher polarized fluorescence and is inversely proportional to amount of unlabeled drug.	Serum, plasma	Commonly used
4. Enzyme-multiplied immunoassay technique (EMIT)	Competitive binding with enzyme label	Antibody binding to enzyme-hapten inhibits catalytic reactivity; competition by analyte in sample prevents inhibition.	Serum, plasma	Commonly used
5. Enzyme immunoassay using genetically engineered enzyme (CEDIA)	Competitive binding with spectrophotometric detection	Enzyme has been synthesized as two fragments (enzyme donor, ED and enzyme acceptor, EA); association of ED and EA forms an active enzyme that cleaves a substrate causing a color change; drug and drug-labeled ED compete for an antibody and increased drug allows more ED to remain free for binding to EA to create active enzyme.	Serum, plasma	
6. Enzyme-inhibition immunoassay	Competitive binding with spectrophotometric detection	Drug-inhibitor conjugate competes with drug for sites on an antibody; binding of conjugate to antibody results in reduced inhibition of enzyme; amount of product formed is inversely proportional to the concentration of drug.	Serum, plasma, whole blood	
7. Rate nephelometric inhibition immunoassay (NIIA)	Competitive binding with nephelometric detection	Hapten-protein conjugate competes with drug for binding to antibody; production of protein-antibody complexes increase light scatter; amount of free drug is inversely proportional to the rate of increasing light scatter.	Serum, plasma	
8. Turbidimetric inhibition immunoassay (PETINIA)	Competitive binding with turbidimetric detection	Particle-labeled drug competes with free drug for antibody; rate of aggregate formation is inversely proportional to amount of drug.	Serum, plasma	
9. Enzymatic inhibition	Noncompetitive inhibition and spectrophotometric detection of product	Conversion of substrate to product by beef liver alkaline phosphatase is inhibited by drug; amount of product formed is inversely proportional to amount of drug.	Serum, plasma	Thin-film technology
10. Labeled prosthetic group assay	Competitive binding with enzymatic procedure	Antibody binding to drug labeled with prosthetic group prevents glucose oxidase activity; competition with drug allows a prosthetic group to activate enzyme; the activity is coupled to colorimetric reaction.	Serum	

determined by comparison of the peak height or area of the chromatogram produced by a patient's serum to that produced by a standard. One major advantage of HPLC is that measurement of caffeine may also be performed, since it elutes as a separate peak. HPLC is a commonly used procedure for determination of caffeine concentrations in neonates.

Another chromatographic method for theophylline is gas-liquid chromatography (CLC). Because of the high degree of complexity and time required to analyze theophylline by this method, GLC is rarely used in the clinical laboratory today.

A very accurate technique for measurement of theophylline is gas chromatography with mass spectroscopy (GC/MS). This method has been recommended as a reference method for theophylline.[76] A radiolabeled internal standard, [13-^{15}N,2-^{13}C]theophylline is added to the specimen, and then the labeled theophylline and the theophylline present in the patient's sera are extracted into a chloroform-isopropanol mixture (pH 5.2). The internal standard and theophylline are then derivatized by incubation of the extracted residue with iodopentane. Gas chromatography is then used to separate theophylline from other similar compounds. A mass selective detector is then used to monitor the mass spectral profile of theophylline and internal standard ions at m/z (mass-to-charge ratio) 250 and m/z 253 respectively. The ratios of these ions is then compared against standards with known theophylline concentrations, and the concentration of theophylline in the patient's sample is calculated from the standard curve.

The most commonly used technique for theophylline determinations is fluorescence polarization immunoassay FPIA (Table 56-7, method 3). In this method, theophylline labeled with fluorescein competes with theophylline present in the patient sample for a limited amount of antibody.[77] The fluorescein-labeled theophylline bound to antibody is a much larger molecule when compared to the unbound fluorophore and, as a result, rotates much more slowly than the smaller, or unbound, fluorophore. Plane-polarized light striking a fluorescein-labeled theophylline-antibody complex will excite the fluorescein fluorophore. The fluorescence emitted from the antibody-bound fluorophore will be largely polarized when compared to that emitted from the more rapidly rotating unbound fluorophore. Thus the intensity of the emitted polarized fluorescence is inversely proportional to the concentration of theophylline in the patient's specimen.

Another popular immunoassay method for theophylline is a homogeneous enzyme immunoassay (EMIT) (Table 56-7, method 4). This technique utilizes a competitive-binding format whereby theophylline labeled with the enzyme glucose-6-phosphate dehydrogenase (G-6-PD) competes with the theophylline present in patient samples for binding to a theophylline-specific antibody. When enzyme-labeled theophylline binds to antitheophylline antibody, the resulting complex causes a reduction in G-6-PD activity. Enzyme activity that remains after an incubation period is proportional to the concentration of theophylline in the patient's serum. The amount of enzymatically active G-6-PD remaining after the incubation period is measured spectrophotometrically at 340 nm by monitoring the rate of formation of NADH. A

similar assay procedure has also been developed for determination of caffeine in serum.

Another widely used EIA procedure for theophylline is a fluorometric EIA method based on the competitive binding between enzyme-labeled theophylline and theophylline present in a patient's serum to an antitheophylline antibody conjugated onto the surface of a glass fiber paper. The enzyme label that is used is typically bacterial alkaline phosphatase (ALP). After an equilibrium has been established for binding of labeled and unlabeled theophylline to antibody, any remaining unbound theophylline-enzyme complexes are washed from the reaction zone. The substrate 4-methylumbelliferone phosphate is then added and is converted by the ALP present in the theophylline-enzyme antibody complexes to a fluorescent product. When little or no theophylline is present in the patient serum, a maximum of theophylline-enzyme complexes will be bound to the immobilized antibody resulting in maximal production of fluorescent product.

A relatively new immunoassay procedure that utilizes recombinant DNA technology is the CEDIA assay for theophylline (Microgenics Corp., Concord, CA 94520) (Table 56-7, method 5). In this assay, the enzyme beta-galactosidase is synthesized as two separate fragments; one fragment designated as the enzyme-donor (ED) portion and the other designated as the enzyme-acceptor (EA) portion. Theophylline is covalently attached to the ED portion of the enzyme.[78] The association of ED and EA results in the formation of enzymatically active beta-galactosidase. The addition of an antibody directed toward theophylline to the reagent system will inhibit the association of the ED and EA fragments to form active enzyme. Competition by theophylline present in the patient's serum will create active enzyme in direct proportion to the concentration of theophylline in sera. The amount of enzyme that is created is monitored through the hydrolysis of an enzyme substrate such as chlorophenol red–β-D-galactopyranoside.[79]

Automated methods for theophylline, based on an enzyme-inhibition immunoassay, have been developed (Table 56-7, method 6), which can utilize either serum, plasma, or whole blood as specimens.[80] In this procedure, theophylline has been conjugated to an inhibitor of the enzyme acetylcholinesterase. The theophylline present in the patient's sample competes with the theophylline–enzyme inhibitor conjugate for binding to a theophylline-specific antibody. Binding of antibody to the inhibitor complex prevents the inhibitor from binding to the enzyme, resulting in more enzymatic activity. Thus the concentration of theophylline in the patient's sample is inversely proportional to the amount of enzymatically active enzyme that remains. The activity of acetylcholinesterase is monitored by use of the substrate acetyl-β-(methylthio)choline iodide, which is hydrolyzed by the enzyme to produce free thiols. The free thiols that are formed react with 5,5'dithiobis(2-nitrobenzoic acid) to form thionitrobenzoate, which is measured spectrophotometrically.

The use of an immunonephelometric assay is utilized by some clinical laboratories for quantitation of theophylline in serum (Table 56-7, method 7).[81] In this procedure, theophylline is conjugated to a high-molecular-weight protein. Theophylline present in the patient's serum competes with the protein-theophylline conjugate for binding to a theophylline-specific antibody. Binding of the protein-theophylline conjugate to antibody results in the formation of an insoluble complex, which precipitates and causes light scatter. Binding of soluble theophylline, present in the patient's serum, to antibody does not result in light scatter. The rate of increase in light scatter is inversely proportional to the theophylline concentration in the patient's sample and is monitored by use of a nephelometer.

A method for determination of theophylline that is analogous to the immunonephelometric inhibition assay described above is the particle-enhanced turbidimetric inhibition immunoassay (PETINIA) (Table 56-7, method 8). In this procedure, theophylline that has been covalently linked to a latex particle competes with theophylline present in a patient's serum for binding sites on a theophylline-specific antibody. Binding of the theophylline-latex complex to antibody results in the formation of aggregates causing an increase in the turbidity of the solution. The rate of formation of these aggregates can be monitored spectrophotometrically at 340 nm and is inversely proportional to the concentration of theophylline in the patient's sample.

A novel approach for determination of theophylline concentrations is employed in a thin-film procedure (Johnson and Johnson, Rochester, NY 14650) (Table 56-7, method 9). This assay is based on the finding that theophylline is an inhibitor of alkaline phosphatase (ALP) obtained from beef liver. The enzyme and a suitable substrate are incorporated into the reagent slide system. The application of patient sample containing theophylline to the slide results in an inhibition of enzyme activity that is proportional to the concentration of theophylline in the sample. In the absence of theophylline, the conversion of substrate to product by the ALP occurs at the maximum rate.

Another technique that incorporates a dry film format for theophylline determinations makes use of the competitive binding between theophylline and a theophylline–enzyme–prosthetic group complex to an antibody (Bayer, Inc., Tarrytown, New York) (Table 56-7, method 10).[82] In this procedure, the enzyme glucose oxidase without its prosthetic group is incorporated into a dry film along with a suitable substrate. The glucose oxidase requires its prosthetic group (flavin adenine dinucleotide, FAD) to be bound for activity. FAD, which has been covalently linked to theophylline, is also included in the reagent system along with a theophylline-specific antibody. The application of a patient's serum containing theophylline to the system results in a competition between theophylline-FAD complexes and the theophylline in the patient's sample for binding to antibody. The greater the amount of theophylline present in serum, the less likely it is that theophylline-FAD complexes will bind to antibody and instead be available for combining with enzyme to form an active enzyme–prosthetic group complex. If no theophylline is present in the patient's sample, maximum formation of antibody-theophylline-FAD occurs with minimal theophylline-FAD complexes remaining for binding to glucose oxidase and formation of enzymatically active enzyme. The amount of glucose oxidase with enzymatic activity is monitored by the conversion of glucose and O_2 to glu-

conolactone and H_2O_2. A peroxidase uses the H_2O_2 generated to oxidize the substrate 3,3′,5,5′-tetramethylbenzene to form a colored chromogen, which can be monitored at 740 nm.

Specimen Serum or heparinized plasma can be utilized for most of the previously described analyses. For those methods that can use whole blood as specimen, the sample type should be noted when one is interpreting results because whole blood has only 82% of the theophylline concentrations that are present in serum or plasma. Saliva can also be used as a specimen if HPLC or FPIA is employed as the method of analysis.[83,84] Saliva is collected while the patient chews on paraffin wax and the sample is then centrifuged to remove sediment.

Therapeutic range The therapeutic range for theophylline in serum and plasma of children and adults is 8 to 20 μg/mL (44 to 111.0 μmol/L).[85-89] For the treatment of apnea in neonates, the therapeutic range for theophylline is 6 to 11 μg/mL (33-61 μmol/L).[86,87] Therapeutic concentrations of caffeine in these same individuals is 5 to 20 μg/mL and can cause headache, hypotension, nausea, restlessness, seizures, and tachycardia.[88,89] Caffeine concentrations greater than 30 μg/mL can produce symptoms such as insomnia, restlessness, delirium, tachycardia, and muscle tenseness and tremors.

REFERENCES

1. Ritschel WA: *Handbook of basic pharmacokinetics including clinical applications,* Hamilton, Ill., 1986, Drug Intelligence Publications.
2. Borga O, Azarnoff DL, Plym Forshell G, Sjöqvist F: Plasma protein binding of tricyclic antidepressants in man, *Biochem Pharmacol* 18:2135-2143, 1969.
3. Reidenberg MM, Odar-Cederlof I, von Bahr C, et al: Protein binding from diphenylhydantoin and desmethylimipramine in plasma from patients with poor renal function, *N Engl J Med* 285:264-267, 1971.
4. Levy G: Relationship between pharmacological effects and plasma or tissue concentrations of drugs in man. In Davies DS, Pritchard DNC, editors: *Biological effects of drugs in relation to their plasma concentrations,* Baltimore, 1973, University Park Press.
5. Stewart RB, Forgnone M, Cluff LE: Drug utilization and reported adverse drug reactions in outpatients, *Drugs in Health Care* 2:231-243, 1975.
6. Ritschel WA: Pharmacokinetics of H_2-receptor antagonists, *Sci Pharm* 50:250-259, 1982.
7. Barker KN, McConnell WE: How to detect medication errors, *Mod Hosp* 99:95-106, 1962.
8. Stewart RB, Cluff LE: A review of medication errors and compliance in ambulant patients, *Clin Pharmacol Ther* 13:463-468, 1971.
9. Bochner F, Carruthers G, Kampmann J, Stiner J: *Handbook of clinical pharmacology,* Boston, 1978, Little, Brown & Co, pp 22-25.
10. Ritschel WA: The effect of aging on pharmacokinetics: a scientists' view of the future, *Contemp Pharmacy Pract* 5:209-218, 1982.
11. Hassan FM, Pesce AJ, Ritschel WA: Pitfalls and errors in drug monitoring: analytical aspects, *Methods Find Exp Clin Pharmacol* 5:567-573, 1983.
12. Slaughter RL, Koup JR: Clinical pharmacokinetic service. In McLeod DD, Miller WA, editors: *The practice of pharmacy,* Cincinnati, 1981, Harvey Whitney Books.
13. Ritschel WA: *Handbook of basic pharmacokinetics,* ed 2, Hamilton, Ill., 1980, Drug Intelligence Publications, pp 412-427.
14. Evans WW, Schentag JJ, Jusko WJ: *Applied pharmacokinetics: prin-*

ciples of therapeutic drug monitoring, Vancouver, Wash., 1994, Applied Therapeutics, Inc.

15. Holt DW, Johnston A, Roberts NB, et al: Methodological and clinical aspects of cyclosporin monitoring: report of the Association of Clinical Biochemists task force, *Ann Clin Biochem,* 31:420-446, 1994.

16. Oellerich M, Armstrong VW, Kahan BD, Shaw L, Holt DW, Yatscoff R, Lindholm A, Halloran P, Gallicano K. Wonigeit K, Schütz E, Schran H, Annesley T: Lake Louise Consensus Conference on Cyclosporin Monitoring in Organ Transplantation: Report of the Consensus Panel, *Ther Drug Monit,* 1995. (In press.)

17. Matzuk MM, Shlomchik M, Shaw LM: Making digoxin therapeutic drug monitoring more effective, *Ther Drug Monit* 13:215-219, 1991.

18. Edson RS, Terrell CL: The aminoglycosides, *Mayo Clin Proc* 66:1158-1164, 1991.

19. Barclay ML, Begg EJ, Hickling KG: What is the evidence for once-daily aminoglycoside therapy? *Clin Pharmacokinet* 27:32-48, 1994.

20. Blaser J, Konig C, Simmen HP, Thurnheer U: Monitoring serum concentrations for once-daily netilmicin dosing regimens, *J Antimicrob Chemother* 33:341-348, 1994.

21. Sawchuk RJ, Zaske DE, Cipolle RJ, et al: Kinetic model for gentamicin dosing with the use of individual patient parameters, *Clin Pharmacol Therap* 21:362-369, 1977.

22. Sheiner LB, Rosenberg B, Melmon K: Modelling of individual pharmacokinetics for computer-aided dosage, *Computer Biomed Res* 5:441-459, 1972.

23. Yuen GJ, Taylor JW, Ludden TM, Murphy MJ: Predicting phenytoin dosage using Bayesian feedback: a comparison with other methods, *Ther Drug Monit* 5:437-441, 1983.

24. Böttger H-Ch, Oellerich M, Sybrecht GW: Use of aminoglycosides in critically ill patients: individualisation of dosage using Bayesian statistics and pharmacokinetic principles, *Ther Drug Monit* 10:280-286, 1988.

25. Hurley SF, McNeil JJ: A comparison of the accuracy of a least squares regression, a Bayesian, Chiou's and the steady-state clearance method of individualising theophylline dosage, *Clin Pharmacokinet* 14:311-320, 1988.

26. Pryka RD, Rodvold KA, Garrison M, Rotschafer JC: Individualizing vancomycin dosage regimens: one- versus two-compartment Bayesian models, *Ther Drug Monit* 11:450-454, 1989.

27. Destache CJ, Meyer SK, Bittner MJ, Mermann KG: Impact of a clinical pharmacokinetic service on patients treated with aminoglycosides: a cost-benefit analysis, *Ther Drug Monit* 12:419-426, 1990.

28. Destache CJ, Meyer SK, Rowley KM: Does accepting pharmacokinetic recommendations impact hospitalization? A cost-benefit analysis, *Ther Drug Monit* 12:427-433, 1990.

29. Bennet MJ, Carpenter KH, Worthy E, Lilleyman JS: Cyclosporin concentrations in whole blood and plasma, *Clin Chem* 30:817, 1984.

30. Fraser CG: Desirable standards of performance for therapeutic drug monitoring, *Clin Chem* 33:387-389, 1987.

31. Jenny RW: Analytical goals for determinations of theophylline concentration in serum, *Clin Chem* 37:154-158, 1991.

32. Oellerich M, Raude E, Burdelski M, et al: Monoethylglycinexylidide formation kinetics: a novel approach to assessment of liver function. *J Clin Chem Clin Biochem* 25:845-853, 1987.

33. Oellerich M, Burdelski M, Ringe B, et al: Lignocaine metabolite formation as a measure of pre-transplant liver function, *Lancet* 1:640-642, 1989.

34. Adam R, Azoulay D, Astarcioglu I, et al: Reliability of the MEGX test in the selection of liver grafts, *Transplant Proc* 23:2470-2471, 1991.

35. Oellerich M, Burdelski M, Lautz HU, et al: Predictors of one-year pretransplant survival in patients with cirrhosis, *Hepatology* 14:1029-1034, 1991.

36. Gremse DA, A-Kader HH, Schroeder TJ, Balisteri WF: Assessment of lidocaine metabolite formation as a quantitative liver function test in children, *Hepatology* 12:565-569, 1990.

37. Schroeder TJ, Gremse DA, Mansour ME, et al: Lidocaine metabo-

lism as an index of liver function in hepatic transplant donors and recipients, *Transplant Proc* 21:2299-2301, 1989.

38. Lehmann U, Armstrong VW, Schütz E, et al: Monoethylglycinexylidide as an early predictor of posttraumatic organ failure, *Ther Drug Monit* 17:125-132, 1995.

39. Oellerich M, Müller-Vahl H: The EMIT FreeLevel ultrafiltration technique compared with equilibrium dialysis and ultracentrifugation to determine protein binding of phenytoin, *Clin Pharmacokinet* 9(suppl 1):61-70, 1984.

40. Zielmann S, Mielck F, Kahl R, et al: A rational basis for the measurement of free phenytoin concentration in critically ill trauma patients, *Ther Drug Monit* 16:139-144, 1994.

41. Williams KM: Molecular asymmetry and its pharmacological consequences, *Adv Pharmacol* 22:57-122, 1991.

42. Svensmark O, Kristensen P: Determination of diphenylhydantoin and phenobarbital in small amounts of serum, *J Lab Clin Med* 61:501-507, 1963.

43. Pippenger CE, Scott JE, Gillen HW: Thin-layer chromatography of anticonvulsant drugs, *Clin Chem* 15:255-260, 1969.

44. Rambeck B, Meijer JWA: Gas chromatographic methods for the determination of antiepileptic drugs: a systematic review, *Ther Drug Monit* 2:385-396, 1980.

45. Plotczyk LL: Application of fused-silica capillary gas chromatography to the analysis of underivatized drugs, *J Chromatogr* 240:349-360, 1982.

46. Volmut J, Matisova E, Pham Thi Ha: Simultaneous determination of six antiepileptic drugs by capillary gas chromatography, *J Chromatogr* 547:428-435, 1990.

47. Meatherall R, Ford D: Isocratic liquid chromatographic determination of theophylline, acetaminophen, chloramphenicol, caffeine, anticonvulsants, and barbiturates in serum, *Ther Drug Monit* 10:101-115, 1988.

48. Ou CN, Rognerud CL: Simultaneous measurement of ethosuximide, primidone, phenobarbital, phenytoin, carbamazepine, and their bioactive metabolites by liquid chromatography, *Clin Chem* 30:1667-1670, 1984.

49. Price CP, Newman DJ, editors: Radial partition immunoassay. In *Principles and practice of immunoassay,* New York, 1991, Stockton Press.

50. Frings CS, Phillips G: Therapeutic drug monitoring of anticonvulsant drugs using fluorescence polarization immunoassay, *Clin Chem* 28:1611, 1982.

51. Tybach R: Adaptation of prosthetic-group label homogeneous immunoassay to reagent strip format, *Clin Chem* 27:1499-1504, 1981.

52. Nishikawa T, Kubo H, Saito M: Competitive nephelometric immunoassay method for antiepileptic drugs in patient blood, *J Immunol Methods* 29:85-89, 1979.

53. Engel WD, Khanna PL: CEDIA in vitro diagnostics with a novel homogeneous immunoassay technique, *J Immunol Methods* 150:99-102, 1992.

54. Jandreski MA, Shah JC, Gardinius J, Bermes EW Jr: Clinical evaluation of five therapeutic drugs using dry film multilayer technology on the OPUS immunoassay system, *J Clin Lab Anal* 5:415-421, 1991.

55. Blick KE, Melouk SH, Fry HD, Gillum RL: *Clin Chem* 36:670-674, 1990.

56. Tredger JM, Gonde CE, Williams R: Monitoring cyclosporine in liver-transplant recipients: effects of clinical status on the performance of two monoclonal antibody–based methods, *Clin Chem* 38:108-113, 1992.

57. Chou D: Therapeutic drug monitoring (immunosuppressive drugs), *Anal Chem* 65:412R-415R, 1993.

58. Yatscoff RW, Copeland KR, Faraci CJ: Abbott TDx monoclonal antibody assay evaluated for measuring cyclosporin in whole blood, *Clin Chem* 36:1969-1973, 1990.

59. Sketris I, Yatscoff R, Keown P, et al: Optimizing the use of cyclosporin in renal transplantation, *Clin Biochem* 28:195-211, 1995.

60. Lemaire M, Tillement JP: Role of lipoproteins and erythrocytes in the in vitro binding and distribution of cyclosporin A in the blood, *J Pharm Pharmacol* 34:715, 1982.

61. Shaw LM, Bowers L, Demers L, et al: Critical issues in cyclospor-

ine monitoring: report of the task force on cyclosporine monitoring, *Clin Chem* 33:1269-1288, 1987.

62. Lewis JE, Nelson JC, Wilson TN: Radioimmunoassay of an antibiotic: gentamicin, *Nature (New Biol)* 239:214, 1972.

63. Dandiker WB: Investigation of immunochemical reactions by fluorescence polarization. In Atassi MA, editor: *Immunochemistry of proteins*, New York, 1977, Plenum Publishing.

64. Bastiani RJ: The EMIT system: a commercially successful innovation, *Antiobiot Chemother* 26:89, 1979.

65. Okorodudu AO, Burnett RW, McComb RB, Bowers GN Jr: Evaluation of three first-generation ion-selective electrode analyzers for lithium: systematic errors, frequency of random interferences, and recommendations based on comparison with flame atomic emission spectrometry, *Clin Chem* 36:104-110, 1990.

66. Hansen JL: The measurement of serum and urine lithium by atomic absorption spectrophotometry, *Am J Med Tech* 34:19, 1968.

67. Bertholf RL, Savory MG, Winborne KH, et al: Lithium determined in serum with an ion-selective electrode, *Clin Chem* 34:1500-1502, 1988.

68. Bodman V, Arter T, Masiewicz F, et al: Development of the Kodak Ektachem clinical chemistry slide for lithium (Li), *Clin Chem* 38:1049, 1992 [Abstract].

69. Brzezicki J, Muirhead C, Schmitz J, et al: Acceptable anticoagulants for analysis of calcium and lithium on Beckman's Synchron EL-ISE system, *Clin Chem* 38:1023, 1992 [Abstract].

70. Platman SR, Fieve RR: Biochemical aspects of lithium in affective disorders, *Arch Gen Psychiatry* 19:659-663, 1968.

71. Rybakowski J, Strzyżewski W: Red-blood-cell lithium index and long-term maintenance treatment, *Lancet* 1:1408-1409, 1976 [Letter].

72. Rainbow SJ, Dowson GM, Tickner TR: Non-extraction HPLC method for simultaneous measurement of theophylline and caffeine in human serum, *Ann Clin Biochem* 26:527-532, 1989.

73. Orcutt JJ, Kozak PP, Sherwin AG, Cummins LH: Microscale method for theophylline in body fluids by reversed phase high performance liquid chromatography of theophylline in serum, *Clin Chem* 23:599, 1977.

74. Weidner N, Dietzler DN, Ladenson JH et al: A clinically applicable high pressure liquid chromatographic method for measurement of serum theophylline, with detailed evaluation of interferences, *Am J Clin Pathol* 73:79, 1980.

75. Soldin SJ, Hill JG: A rapid micromethod for measuring theophylline and reversed phase high pressure liquid chromatography, *Clin Biochem* 10:74, 1977.

76. Desage M, Soubeyrand J, Soun A, Brazier JL: Automated theophylline assay using gas chromatographic and a mass-selective detector, *J Chromatogr* 336:285-291, 1984.

77. Loomi KF, Frye RM: Evaluation of the Abbott TDM™ for the stat measurement of phenobarbital, phenytoin, carbamazepine, and theophylline, *Am J Clin Pathol* 80:686-691, 1983.

78. Klein G, Castineiras J, Collinsworth W, et al: Results of multicenter evaluation of the CEDIA® theophylline line assay, *Wien Klin Wochenschr* 104:31-37, 1992.

79. Henderson DR, Friedman SB, Harris JD, et al: CEDIA™, a new homogeneous immunoassay system, *Clin Chem* 32:1637-1641, 1986.

80. Chan K, Koenig J, Walton KG, et al: The theophylline method of the Abbott "vision" analyzer evaluated, *Clin Chem* 33:130-132, 1987.

81. Mordelet-Dambrine M, Baglin J, Roux A, et al: Comparison between theophylline analysis by nephelometric inhibition immunoassay and high performance liquid chromatography, *Ther Drug Monit* 8:106-110, 1986.

82. Lindberg R, Ivaska K, Irjala K, Vanto T: Determination of theophylline in serum with the Seralyzer® Aris reagent strip test evaluated, *Clin Chem* 32:613-614, 1985.

83. Sood S, Green VI, Nieva LL: Routine methods in toxicology and therapeutic drug monitoring by high-performance liquid chromatography. VI: A rapid microscale method for determination of caffeine in plasma and saliva, *Ther Drug Monit* 11:361-364, 1989.

84. Niemann A, Oellerich M, Schumann G, Sybrecht GW: Determination of theophylline in saliva, using fluorescence polarization immunoassay (FPIA), *J Clin Chem Clin Biochem* 23:725-732, 1985.

85. Jenne JW, Wyze E, Rood FS, McDonald FM: Pharmacokinetics of theophylline: application to adjustment of the clinical dose of aminophylline, *Clin Pharmacol Ther* 13:349-360, 1972.

86. Giacoia G, Jusko WJ, Menke J, Koup JR: Theophylline pharmacokinetics in premature infants with apnea, *J Pediatr* 89:829-832, 1976.

87. Aranda JV, Turmen T, Trippenbach T, et al: Effects of caffeine on control of breathing in infantile apnea, *J Pediatr* 103:975-978, 1983.

88. Rall TW: Drugs used in the treatment of asthma: the methylxanthines, cromolyn sodium, and other agents. In Gilman AG, Rall TW, Nies AS, Taylor P, editors: *The Pharmacological basis of therapeutics*, ed 8, New York, 1990, Pergamon Press.

89. Bergmeyer HU: Methods of enzymatic analysis, vol. XII, drugs and pesticides, Weinheim, III, 1986, VCH Publishers.

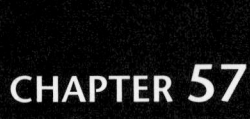
Examination of urine

G. Berry Schumann
Susan C. Schweitzer

OBJECTIVES

■ Understand the proper method of collection of urine specimen
for specific testing.

■ Discuss the important physical properties of urine and their
relationship to disease.

■ Identify the important chemical constituents of urine, how
they are quantified, and how their presence is confirmed.

■ Describe the proper methods of standardization of urine
specimens and common microscopic findings.

■ List the urine findings commonly observed in renal and lower
urinary tract diseases.

■ Understand quality control procedures for urinalysis.

KEY TERMS

acute tubular necrosis A disease that involves the destruction
of renal tubular epithelial cells and is most commonly associated with reduced blood supply to the renal tubules (ischemia)
or toxic exposures.

Addis count A quantitative urine sediment test in which the
number of erythrocytes, leukocytes, and casts are quantified in
a timed urine specimen.

albuminuria Increased albumin in urine.

aminoaciduria An excess of one or more amino acids in urine.

amorphous crystals The granular, noncrystalline precipitate of
salts with no pathological importance.

bacteriuria The presence of bacteria in urine.

bilirubinuria The presence of bilirubin in urine.

calculus An abnormal concretion, usually composed of mineral
salts, present in the urinary system or other tissues; a renal stone.

cast A molded, cylindrical structure that is formed as a result of
cell conglutination and protein precipitation in the lumen of the
distal convoluted tubule or collecting duct of the nephron. It is
extruded into the urinary sediment.

catheterization The passage of a thin, flexible, tubular instrument into the bladder or ureter for the withdrawal of urine.

crystalluria The presence of crystals in urine.

cylindruria The presence of casts in urine.

cystitis Inflammation of the bladder.

cytodiagnostic urinalysis A specialized urine test combining
both physicochemical assessments with a concentrated
Papanicolaou-stained urine sediment examination.

dipstick urinalysis A chemical urine test using test strips for the
detection of albumin, glucose, ketone, bilirubin, hemoglobin,
bacteria, leukocytes, and other chemical constituents.

diuretic An agent that promotes the secretion of urine.

dysmorphic erythrocyturia The presence of fragmented erythrocytes in urine sediment indicating renal (glomerular or tubular) hematuria.

erythrocyturia The presence of erythrocytes in urine.

funguria The presence of fungus in urine.

glitter cells Pale-staining, swollen, and degenerated neutrophils found in dilute urine, with cytoplasmic granules that exhibit a characteristic brownian movement.

glomeruli Coils of blood vessels projecting into the expanded end of the capsule of each of the uriniferous tubules of the kidney.

glycosuria The presence of glucose in urine.

hematuria The presence of blood in urine.

hemoglobinuria The presence of free hemoglobin in urine.

hyaline cast A transparent cast composed of mucoprotein.

hydrometer An instrument used for determining the specific gravity of a fluid.

ketone Any compound containing the carbonyl group, —CO—, and having hydrocarbon groups attached to the carbonyl carbon.

ketonuria The presence of ketones, which are intermediary products of fat metabolism, in urine, as in diabetes mellitus.

melanin The dark amorphous pigment of the skin, hair, and various tumors. It is produced by polymerization of oxidation products of tyrosine and dihydroxyphenol compounds and contains carbon, hydrogen, nitrogen, oxygen, and often sulfur.

myoglobinuria The presence of myoglobin, an oxygen-binding protein of muscle cells, in urine.

nephritis Inflammation of the kidney.

nephrosis A disease of the kidney.

osmolality The number of solute particles per unit mass of solvent (mOsm/kg).

Papanicolaou stain A differential stain that aids in the identification of nuclear chromatin, cytoplasmic properties (such as keratinization), noncellular entities (such as crystals and casts), and hematopoietic elements.

porphyrins A group of iron-free or magnesium-free pyrrole derivatives that occur universally in cells. They constitute the basis of the respiratory pigments in animals and plants.

proteinuria Increased protein in urine.

pyuria An abnormal number of leukocytes in urine.

reagent-strip testing The use of a chemical test strip to determine whether pathological concentrations of various substances are present in the urine.

specific gravity The weight of a substance compared with that of an equal volume of another substance taken as a standard.

Sternheimer-Malbin stain A crystal violet and safranin stain used in urinalysis. This stain provides additional contrast for some cells and casts.

urobilinogen A group of colorless compounds formed from the reduction of conjugated bilirubin by intestinal bacteria; about 1% of the total urobilinogen produced reaches the urine.

virus A self-replicating agent that consists of a core of nucleic acid enclosed by a protein coating. This microorganism can multiply only within living host cells.

wet urinalysis A screening urine test combining both physicochemical assessments and a wet unstained urine sediment examination.

yeast A unicellular nucleated microorganism that reproduces by budding.

INTRODUCTION AND CLINICAL UTILITY OF URINALYSIS

The clinical laboratory examination of urine can provide a wide variety of useful information on an individual's kidneys and the systemic diseases that may affect this excretory organ. Both structural (anatomical) and functional (physiological) disorders of the kidney and lower urinary tract may be elucidated as well as sequential information about the disease, its cause, and prognosis. Careful laboratory examination of urine often narrows the clinical differential diagnosis of numerous urinary system diseases. Usually these laboratory data may be obtained without pain, danger, and distress to the patient. Therefore, properly performed and interpreted laboratory urine tests will always remain an essential part of clinical medicine.

Currently, three types of urinalysis are performed and they include *dipstick urinalysis* for physician offices and patient home testing; *a screening, wet urinalysis,* commonly referred to as a "routine" or "basic" urinalysis; and *cytodiagnostic urinalysis,* which is a specialized, cytological approach to the urine sediment and correlative reagent-strip testing. The dipstick urinalysis is a front-line test for the detection and monitoring of patients for chemical abnormalities.[1,2] Diabetic patients often monitor their own disease for signs of glucosuria, proteinuria, and urinary tract infections by home testing of urine.[3]

Wet or routine urinalysis provides a cost-effective screening test for the detection of both chemical and morphological abnormalities present in urine. Wet urinalysis procedures depend on two major components: (1) macroscopic urinalysis, or physicochemical determinations (appearance, specific gravity, and multiparameter reagent-strip measurements of several chemical constituents), and (2) bright-field or phase-contrast microscopic examination of urinary sediment for evidence of hematuria, pyuria, cylindruria (casts), crystalluria, and so forth. With experience, a urinoscopist may detect many conditions affecting the kidneys and lower urinary tract, and many conditions can be monitored with this easily performed urine test.[4,5]

Recently, cytodiagnostic urinalysis has gained medical acceptance as a new and more sensitive pathologic test for examining urine sediment in several renal and lower urinary tract disorders.[6-8] However, this more time-consuming, permanently prepared and stained procedure should be reserved for symptomatic patients whose renal disease and lower urinary tract neoplastic conditions are being considered. In addition, this specialized urine test has replaced the quantitative Addis counts and provides sequential information regarding the progression or regression of many renal or lower urinary tract disorders.[8]

The purpose of this chapter for medical or clinical chemistry laboratories is to describe briefly common methodologies employed by most wet or routine urinalysis laboratories. Emphasis is placed on the responsibilities of the urinalysis laboratory in the following areas: (1) common procedures and equipment; (2) quality reagents; (3) sensitivity, specificity, and limitations of each procedure; (4) confirmatory tests; (5) accurate identification of urine sediment entities primarily using bright-field microscopy; and (6) quality control. The technical and diagnostic significance of urinalysis results, and the mechanism of diseases that produces urinalysis abnormalities are discussed. Be encouraged to follow the literature for advances in urine laboratory testing and to supplement your knowledge by using the reference list.

SPECIMEN COLLECTION

Careful attention to collection of the urine specimen and its prompt delivery to the laboratory are crucial for optimum information to be derived from urinalysis.[9,10] Urine should be collected in a clean, sterile container that has a tightly fitting lid to prevent spillage, evaporation, and contamination. Specimen containers should be marked with the patient's name, date, and time of collection.

The first voiding in the morning is usually the most desirable for urinalysis testing, since it provides the most concentrated urine. A clean-catch, midstream collection avoids contamination from the distal area of the urethra. The sample must be free of vaginal secretions and other extraneous debris. Kunin[11] thoroughly describes a variety of collection techniques for urinary tract diseases.

If data from the urinalysis are to be accurate, it is essential that urine be either examined within 2 hours of collection or preserved in some manner, usually by refrigeration (2° to 8° C). Appropriate fixatives or preservatives may also be used as long as their effects on the urine and its testing are well understood. If urine is allowed to sit unpreserved at room temperature, it will begin to decompose. Preservatives work by modifying urine so that chemical changes associated with decomposition do not occur and by preventing growth and metabolism of microorganisms. Toluene, phenol, thymol, and acid preservatives are commonly used for urine chemistry determinations. Other forms of preservation include adjusting pH and excluding light. Ethanol (95%) or commercially available fixatives, such as Mucolexx and Saccomanno, may be used to preserve cell structure. Laboratories should be responsible for the correct type and amount of urine preservatives used for cellular preservation.

Timed urine specimens are frequently used to quantitate various aspects of renal function. The urine must reflect excretion over a precisely measured duration of time. Timed urine specimens must not include urine in the bladder before the timed test. One would therefore obtain a 24-hour urine specimen by discarding the first-voided morning urine on the first day and collecting all subsequent urine up to and including the first-voided morning urine on the second day. Recommended types of specimens for various urine tests are listed in Table 57-1.

When a specimen is received for urine testing, the laboratory workers performing that test must make a decision as to its acceptability. Specific criteria should be established in the form of written guidelines for the rejection of urine specimens and should include criteria such as visible signs of contamination, incorrect or incomplete labeling, inappropriate type of specimen or preservatives, and time lapse since collection.

PHYSICAL EXAMINATION OF URINE

The physical examination of urine is the initial part of a routine urinalysis. This examination includes assessment of volume, odor, appearance (color and turbidity), and specific gravity or osmolality.

Volume

Urinary volume is influenced by the fluid intake; solutes to be excreted, primarily sodium and urea; loss of fluid by perspiration and respiration; and cardiovascular and renal status. Normally adults excrete 750 to 2000 mL/24 hours. Conditions that produce an increased or decreased amount of urine are discussed in Chapter 26. Although the volume of a random specimen is clinically insignificant, the volume of specimen received should be recorded for purposes of documentation and standardization.

Odor

Normal fresh urine has an inoffensive odor. An offensive odor can indicate that a specimen is too old for accurate analysis. A foul odor in a specimen that was collected (and not preserved or refrigerated) more than 2 hours earlier indicates an unacceptable specimen. Odor can also provide clues to certain urine abnormalities. An ammonia-like odor is suggestive of urea-splitting bacteria, fruity odors indicate the presence of acetone (ketone), a sweet odor is suggestive of the presence of glucose or another sugar, and a foul odor is suggestive of pus or inflammation. Odor is important in the clinical detection of maple-syrup urine disease (a congenital metabolic defect).

Appearance (color and turbidity)

The color of urine is determined to a large degree by its degree of concentration. Normal urine varies widely from colorless to deep yellow. Interpretation of color is subjective and varies with each laboratory examiner. It may be helpful to the technologist to use standardized colored objects in the laboratory as reference points and to use defined colors to describe the urine, avoiding ambiguous terms such as *straw* or *bloody*. Common colors of urine are listed in Table 57-2.

Red urine is perhaps the most clinically important discoloration; it may be a result of urinary hemoglobin or myoglobin. Intact erythrocytes, hemolyzed erythrocytes, or free hemoglobin (hemolysis) can be responsible for the red color. Hemolysis may occur intravascularly or after the urine has been formed. Myoglobinuria is rare and results from crushing damage to muscle. Urinary hemoglobin and

Table 57-1 Recommended types of urine specimens

Tests	Types of collection					Types of storage		
	Random	First morning	2-hour	12-hour	24-hour	Fresh	Refrigerated	Preserved
Addis count				×			×	
Albumin								
Qualitative analysis	×					×		
Quantitative analysis					×		×	
Aldosterone					×		×	
Amino acid-nitrogen					×		×	×
Bence Jones		×				×		
Bilirubin	×					×		
Blood	×					×		
Calcium					×		×	
Catecholamine					×			×
Coproporphyrin								
Qualitative analysis	×					×		
Quantitative analysis					×			×
Creatinine				×	×		×	
Cytological		×				×	×	
Estrogen	×				×		×	
Glucose	×					×		
17-Hydroxycorticosteroid					×		×	
17-Ketosteroid					×		×	
Ketone	×					×		
Lead		×					×	
Microbiological		×				×		
Nitrite		×				×		
Osmolality	×					×		
pH	×					×		
Phosphorus					×		×	
Porphobilinogen	×					×		
Potassium					×		×	
Pregnanediol					×		×	
Pregnanetriol					×		×	
Protein						×		
Qualitative analysis	×						×	
Quantitative analysis					×	×		
Sediment		×					×	
Sodium					×	×		
Specific gravity	×					×		
Sugar	×						×	
Urea nitrogen					×		×	
Uric acid					×	×		
Urobilinogen			× (afternoon)					×
								×
Uroporphyrin					×		×	
Vanillylmandelic acid					×			×
Volume					×			

myoglobin may not be differentiated by gross inspection or simple tests. Ingestion of beets or certain drugs may redden the urine, and thus such chromogens must be excluded as a source of urine coloration.

Urine characteristic of acute glomerulonephritis is brownish red. It is acidic and contains blood, a combination producing brownish-colored, acidic hematin. Blood in the urine also may assume a smoky appearance. One can observe this only by shaking the urine while holding it up to the light. The "smoke," or turbidity, is actually erythro-cytes suspended in solution. Centrifugation will yield clear urine with a red plug at the bottom of the tube. The smoky appearance of erythrocytes should not be confused with the faint turbidity of other suspensions (such as crystals and cells).

Normally freshly voided urine is clear. When urine is allowed to stand, amorphous crystals, usually urates, may precipitate and cause urine to be cloudy. The turbidity of urine should always be recorded and microscopically explained. Table 57-3 lists common causes of cloudy urine.

Table 57-2 Common colors of urine

Colors	Potential causes				Clinical conditions	Commonly associated diseases
	Foodstuffs	Metabolites	Drugs	Organisms		
Yellow to colorless					Polyuria	Diabetes insipidus Diabetes mellitus Chronic renal failure
Yellow	Food color	Urochrome	Quinacrine (Atabrine) Sulfasalazine (Azulfidine) Phenacetin Nitrofurantoin Riboflavin		Healthy	

Yellow-orange	Food color
	Carotene
	Rhubarb
		Urobilin	Sulfisoxazole and
			  phenazopyridine (Azo
			  Gantrisin)
			Riboflavin
			Furazolidone (Furoxone)
					Dehydration
					Jaundice
						Liver disease

Yellow-green		Bilirubin-biliverdin	Methylene blue Indican Amitriptyline (Elavil)		Jaundice	Liver disease Biliary obstruction

Yellow-red-brown	Beets
	Food color
	Rhubarb
		Hemoglobin
		Myoglobin
		Porphyrin
			Sulfisoxazole and
			  phenazopyridine (Azo
			  Gantrisin)
			Phenytoin (Dilantin)
			Pyrvinium pamoate
			  (Povan)
			Phenazopyridine
			  (Pyridium)
			Phenolsulfonphthalein
			Phenindione
			Amidopyrine
				Serratia marcescens	Hematuria
					Hemoglobinuria
					Myoglobinuria
					Porphyrinuria
					Menstrual
					  contamination
						Hemolysis
						Transfusion
						Burns
						Renal disease
						Urological disease

Brown-black		Porphyrin Melanin Methemoglobin Homogentisic acid	Chloroquine (Aralen) Levodopa		Alkaptonuria	Melanoma Ochronosis Phenol poisoning
Blue-green		Indican	Methylene blue	*Pseudomonas* species	Dysuria	Urinary tract infection

Specific gravity

Urinary specific gravity measurement serves as a partial assessment of the ability of the kidneys to concentrate urine. The normal range is 1.003 to 1.035 g/mL. A value of 1.020 or greater indicates good renal function and increased amounts of dissolved solutes excreted by the kidneys. A specific gravity greater than 1.035 represents the presence of extraneous solutes and should be investigated. Increased specific gravity greater than 1.030 is found in dehydration, diabetes mellitus, congestive heart failure, proteinuria, and adrenal insufficiency. Decreased specific gravity is found in patients with hypothermia and those using diuretics. In a patient with severe kidney disease, urine is produced with a fixed specific gravity that is identical to that of the glomerular filtrate, approximately 1.010. Sediment constituents are often poorly preserved in dilute urine. Therefore a low specific gravity indicates that microscopic examinations of urine may not yield optimally accurate results.

High-molecular-weight substances will affect specific gravity to a greater extent than simple crystalloids will. This becomes significant when urine contains abnormal amounts of larger molecules such as glucose, protein, or x-ray con

Table 57-3 Common causes of cloudy or turbid urine

Causes	Methods of clearing	Comments
Chemical		
Urates	Soluble at 60° C or alkali	Pink sediment
Phosphates and carbonates	Soluble in dilute acid	

Crystals	See specific solubility
	  characteristics (Table
	  57-11)	

Mucus	—	Sticky

X-ray contrast
  mediums
	Soluble in 10% sodium
	  hydroxide	

Lipids	Soluble in ether	Opalescent
Chyle	Soluble in ether	Milky
Cells		
Bacteria	Centrifugation	Foul-smelling odor
Fungi	Centrifugation	Sweet-smelling odor
Erythrocyte	Centrifugation	Red, smoky
Leukocyte	Centrifugation	
Epithelium	Centrifugation	
Spermatozoa	Centrifugation	

trast mediums. In cases of pronounced glucosuria or proteinuria, correction factors can be used to adjust the specific gravity to a more representative value; 0.004 is subtracted for every 10 g/L glucose and 0.003 for every 10 g/L protein. The presence of x-ray contrast mediums or preservation is often associated with values of 1.040 or greater.

A hydrometer (urinometer) and a suitable container may be used to determine specific gravity. There are several limitations to the use of hydrometers: (1) they require a large volume of urine (10 to 15 mL); (2) they are calibrated to be used at 20° C (if urine is not tested at this temperature, a temperature correction is necessary); and (3) hydrometers cannot be recalibrated. For these reasons few laboratories employ hydrometers to measure specific gravity.

Most laboratories are now equipped with refractometers that can relate density of a solution to specific gravity (see Chapter 4). There are several advantages to the use of refractometers: (1) they require only a drop or two of urine, (2) they are temperature compensated, (3) readings are less affected by density than readings by urinometers are, and (4) refractometers have a zero set screw for calibrating the instrument. The biggest disadvantage of refractometers is their expense.

In specific gravity methodology calibration is essential. Instruments should be checked with distilled water on a regular basis. Standardized salt and sucrose solutions can be used for calibration and quality control (Table 57-4).

Refractometer method

1. Clean the surfaces of the cover with a damp cloth and then dry.
2. Using two applicator sticks or a capillary pipet, apply a drop of urine at the notched bottom of the cover so that it flows over the prism surface by capillary action.
3. Point the refractometer toward a light source and read the specific gravity value directly on the specific gravity scale at the sharp dividing line between light and dark contrast.
4. For specific gravity over 1.030, dilute the urine with equal parts of water and read. Multiply the last three digits by three.[3]

Reagent-strip method. An indirect colorimetric method for estimating specific gravity is available on reagent strips. This method uses a strip that contains a pretreated electrolyte that elicits a pH change based on the

Table 57-4 Standardizing solutions for specific gravity

Solution	Specific gravity
Distilled water	1.000
3% NaCl	1.015 ±0.001
5% NaCl	1.022 ±0.001
9% sucrose	1.034 ±0.001

ionic concentration of the urine. This test for specific gravity is fast and simple and requires no additional equipment. The manufacturer states that there is no interference with glucose, protein, or radiographic dye. Sensitivity is poorer than that of the refractometer method (units of 0.005), and urines with a pH of 6.5 or greater require a correction factor.

Falling-drop method. The falling-drop method is a direct method of measuring specific gravity that is usually used with automated instruments, such as the Clinitek Auto 2000 (Ames Division, Miles Laboratories, Inc., Elkhart, Indiana). This instrument uses a silicone oil in a specially designed column. Specific gravity is related to the time it takes for a drop of urine to fall a distance defined by two optical gates. This procedure is more specific and accurate than the use of refractometry and more precise than the use of hydrometers.[9]

Osmolality

The normal kidney is capable of producing urine with a range of 50 to 1200 mOsm/kg (see Chapter 26). Urine ranges from one sixth to four times the osmolality of normal serum (280 to 290 mOsm/kg). Osmolality is measured by an osmometer (see Chapter 14).

Osmolality is determined by the number of particles per unit mass, whereas the specific gravity is a reflection of the density (size or weight) of the suspended particles. Generally, specific gravity and osmolality are directly related in a linear fashion, though there are important exceptions. For example, if iodinated dyes are administered to a patient for intravenous pyelography, the specific gravity may reach as high as 1.070 or 1.080, though the osmolality will remain within normal limits. The dye particles have a mass that is large enough to raise the specific gravity, but too few molecules are present to notably increase the osmolality.

CHEMICAL EXAMINATION OF URINE

Several chemical constituents are routinely analyzed by urinalysis. Both qualitative reagent-strip and tablet tests are used as well as quantitative methods for protein, electrolytes, and porphyrins.

Normal constituents

Urine is composed of numerous chemical substances. Table 57-5 lists common chemical constituents measured by urinalysis laboratories.

Reagent-strip testing

Reagent-strip tests have enabled urinalysis laboratories to generate valuable semiquantitative chemical results in a rapid, accurate, and efficient manner. In general, properly performed urine test strips are sensitive, specific, and cost effective.

The urinalysis laboratory is responsible for selecting the most suitable type of reagent strip for its hospital or clinical setting. The following guidelines will ensure the best results:

1. Test urine promptly; use properly timed test readings only.
2. Beware of interfering substances.
3. Understand the advantages and limitations of the test.
4. Employ controls.

Strip tests should be performed on well-mixed urine equilibrated to room temperature. Each chemical parameter must be evaluated within a specific time interval, as suggested by the manufacturer's instructions. The correct number of strips needed for immediate analysis should be removed from the container and the lid tightly replaced. Reagent strips should be stored in a cool (not refrigerated), moisture-free environment. Outdated and air-exposed urine dipsticks must never be used.[12]

After dipping the reagent strip into the urine, remove excess urine by gently tapping the strip on the edge of the specimen container. Compare individual reagent-pad reactions with the correct color chart in a properly lighted area. Automated reagent-strip readers (reflectance photometers) are widely available. Table 57-6 lists the sensitivities of two commercially available multiple test strips. Reagent-strip results that are positive may require confirmation with chemical and microscopic methods. Manufacturers' inserts should be reviewed to identify sources of inhibitors and false-positive and false-negative results. Ascorbic acid in urine can interfere with reagent-strip reactions for glucose, hemoglobin, bilirubin, and nitrite. Manufacturers have been encouraged to minimize or eliminate this interference when possible because ingestion of vitamin C supplements is so common.[13] Quality control samples are essential to verify reagent-strip results.

Confirmatory testing

Many laboratory workers equate a confirmatory test with rechecking for a given parameter. This confirms nothing; it

Table 57-6 Practical sensitivities of commercial reagent strips

Urine parameters	Chemstrip*	N-Multistix†
pH	±1 pH unit	±1.0 pH unit
Protein	60 mg/L	50-200 mg/L
Glucose	400 mg/L	750 mg/L
Ketones	50 mg/L acetoacetic acid	90 mg/L acetoacetic acid
	400-700 mg/L acetone	800-1400 mg/L acetone
Bilirubin	5 mg/L	4-8 mg/L
Blood	5 intact erythrocytes/μL or hemoglobin from 10 erythrocytes/μL	5-20 intact erythrocytes/μL or hemoglobin from 5 erythrocytes/μL
Urobilinogen	4 mg/L	2 mg/L
Nitrite	0.3 mg/L	0.6-1 mg/L
Esterase (neutrophils)	6-10 leukocytes/hpf	5-15 leukocytes/hpf

*Ames, Inc, Division of Miles Laboratories, Inc., Elkhart, Indiana.
†BMC/Biodynamics, Indianapolis, Indiana.

establishes only the precision for that parameter.[9,14] A confirmatory test is one that will establish the accuracy or correctness of another procedure. Examples of confirmatory tests are quantitative protein analysis, protein electrophoresis, bacterial cultures, and cytological appearance (Table 57-7). A confirmatory test should have either the same or better specificity, be based on a different principle, or have a sensitivity equal to or better than that of the original test.

Urinary pH

Although the standard method for pH measurements uses glass electrodes, urinary pH is usually measured with indicator paper, since small changes in pH are of little clinical significance. Most urinalysis laboratories use multitest reagent strips with two indicators—methyl red and bromthymol blue. These provide a pH range from 5.0 to 9.0 that is demonstrated by a color change from orange (acid) to green to blue (alkaline). The urinary pH range is 4.7 to 7.8. Extremely acidic or alkaline urine usually indicates a poorly collected specimen.

Table 57-5 Composition of urine from healthy subjects

Constituent	Value
Albumin	<15-30 mg/L
Calcium	100-240 mg/24 hr
Creatinine	1.2-1.8 g/24 hr
Glucose	<300 mg/L
Ketones	<50 mg/L
Osmolality	>600 mOsm/L
Phosphorus	0.9-1.3 g/24 hr
Potassium	30-100 mEq/24 hr
pH	4.7-7.8
Sodium	85-250 mEq/24 hr
Specific gravity	1.005-1.030
Total bilirubin	(Not detected)
Total protein	<150 mg/24 hr
Urea nitrogen	7-16 g/24 hr
Uric acid	300-800 mg/24 hr
Urobilinogen	<1 mg/L

Table 57-7 Useful confirmatory tests

Test	Confirmatory test	Reason
Protein	Sulfosalicylic acid (SSA) method	Increased specificity Increased sensitivity
	Protein electrophoresis	Increased specificity
Ketones	Acetest	Increased sensitivity Increased specificity Increased color stability
Bilirubin	Ictotest	Increased sensitivity
Bacteriuria	Culture	Identification Quantitation
Abnormal cells, casts	Cytological examination	Increased visualization Quantitation

Table 57-8 Common clinical conditions causing acidic and alkaline urine

Acidic urine	Alkaline urine
Protein diet	Vegetable diet
Starvation	Vomiting
Dehydration	Renal tubular acidosis
Diarrhea	Respiratory and metabolic
Diabetic acidosis	alkalosis
Metabolic and respiratory	Ammonia-producing,
acidosis	urea-splitting bacteria
Metabolism of fats	Acetazolamide therapy
Sleep	Low-carbohydrate diets
Acid-producing bacteria	Chronic renal failure

Table 57-8 lists common clinical causes of acidic and alkaline urine. The average American ingests an acid-residue diet high in protein that results in acidic urine (5.0 to 6.5). With alkaline urine (8.0 to 8.5) one should always suspect an unpreserved or old specimen with the presence of urease-producing ammonia bacteria, such as *Proteus* species. Patients with renal tubular acidosis, a clinical syndrome characterized by an inability to excrete acidic urine, may produce urine with a much higher pH than would be expected on the basis of the acidosis.

The urinary pH is important in the management of renal stones or crystals. Uric acid stones precipitate in acidic urine and are more soluble in basic urines. Alkaline urine will precipitate calcium or calcium phosphate stones, whereas acidic urine will tend to dissolve them. Alkaline urine is desirable during sulfonamide and streptomycin therapy to prevent precipitation of the drugs in the kidneys and the formation of uric acid, cystine, and oxalate stones. The alkaline pH is also maintained during treatment of transfusion reactions and salicylate intoxication. In cystitis, the pH is kept acidic to combat bacteriuria and to prevent formation of *alkaline stones*. Technologists should be aware that alkaline urine interferes with the determination of proteins and may alter the urine sediment examination.

Proteins

A healthy person will have a daily protein excretion of about 100 mg/day, a very small fraction of the plasma protein content. The majority of the urine protein is albumin that has crossed the glomerular membrane, but smaller-molecular-weight proteins such as globulins may also be present. Once filtered, proteins are almost completely reabsorbed in the proximal tubule. Proteinuria, therefore, can be the result of either increased filtration or decreased reabsorption (tubular function).

Reagent-strip tests represent a screening procedure for proteinuria. Since the specificity of strip tests is limited to the detection of albumin, it is highly recommended that the laboratory simultaneously perform both a reagent-strip test

and an acid precipitation test for the detection of all types of protein. Reagent strips are pH sensitive and depend on the presence of protein for color generation (Sørensen's protein error). The presence of protein on the strip changes the pH environment of the dye embedded in the pad, resulting in a change in color. Highly buffered, alkaline urine can result in a false-positive test:

$$\text{Tetrabromphenol blue} \xrightarrow[\text{Protein}]{\text{pH 3}} \text{Positive results } (\textit{green-blue})$$

$$\text{Tetrabromphenol blue} \xrightarrow[\text{No protein}]{\text{pH 3}} \text{Negative results } (\textit{yellow})$$

A positive or faintly positive result should be confirmed with a more specific test such as the trichloroacetic acid or the sulfosalicylic acid tests. A mildly positive test-strip result and a grossly positive turbidity test result may indicate the presence of drugs or Bence Jones proteins.

Sulfosalicylic acid test and semiquantitative turbidity method

Principle. Protein, denatured by acid, precipitates and renders the urine specimens progressively more turbid as the protein concentration increases.

Materials

Sulfosalicylic acid, 3% (30 g/L) aqueous solution
Test tubes, 13 × 100 mm

Procedure

1. Add 3 mL of sulfosalicylic acid reagent to 1 mL of centrifuged urine.
2. Mix and allow to stand for 5 minutes.
3. Observe the degree of turbidity (see accompanying unnumbered table below) and compare the test sample with the original urine specimen in a 13 × 100 mm test tube.

In urine from healthy individuals, turbidity should be absent and protein should represent less than 75 mg/L. Table 57-9 lists the sensitivities, types of proteins detected, and sources of false-negative and false-positive results for both the reagent-strip and the sulfosalicylic acid tests. Commercial SSA standards are available.

Reporting of SSA turbidity confirmation

Grade	Turbidity*	Protein range (mg/L)
None	Clear	≤75
Trace	Print can be easily seen and read when viewed through test tube	200
1+	Print can be easily seen and read with some difficulty when viewed through test tube	300-1000
2+	Print can be seen but not easily read when viewed through test tube	1000-2500
3+	Print cannot be seen when viewed through test tube	2500-4500
4+	Precipitate formed	4500

*Urine clarity when light is passed through specimen in a clear test tube.

Table 57-9   Tests for proteinuria

	Reagent strip	Sulfosalicylic acid	Results
Sensitivity	50-200 mg/L (albumin)	100 mg/L (all proteins)	
Combined use	Negative result	Negative result	No protein
	Positive result	Negative result	Clinically insignificant protein level or false-positive reagent-strip test
	Negative result	Positive result	Bence Jones proteins
			Heavy-chain proteins (electrophoresis confirmation required)
			Drug interference (penicillin)
Common urine constituents causing false-positive or false-negative results			
Urine turbidity	—	False-positive and false-negative result	
X-ray contrast mediums	—	False-positive result	
Tolbutamide (Orinase)	—	False-positive result	
Penicillin (massive dose)	—	False-positive result	
Sulfisoxazole (Gantrisin)	—	False-positive result	
Highly buffered alkaline urine	False-positive result	False-negative result	
Quaternary ammonium salts	False-positive result	—	
Tolmetin sodium (Tolectin)	—	False-positive result	

Sugars

Enzymatic tests. The reagent-strip test is an excellent test that is specific for glucose. It detects the oxidation of glucose to gluconic acid:

Glucose + Oxygen in room air $\xrightarrow{\text{Glucose oxidase}}$ Gluconic acid + Hydrogen peroxide

Hydrogen peroxide + Chromogen $\xrightarrow{\text{Peroxidase}}$ Oxidized chromogen *(blue)* + H_2O

One reagent-strip product uses *o*-tolidine as the chromogen for the indicator reaction.

Copper reduction (Clinitest, Benedict's test)

Cupric ions + Glucose (or reducing substances) $\xrightarrow[\text{Alkali}]{\text{Heat}}$ Cuprous oxide *(red)* + Cuprous hydroxide *(yellow)*

The Clinitest tablet (Ames Division, Miles Laboratories, Inc., Elkhart, Indiana) provides another test for sugar. It is a copper reduction test that measures total reducing substances. In addition to glucose, Clinitest will detect sugars such as galactose, lactose, and pentoses. It also detects ascorbic acid and certain drugs (that is, nalidixic acid [NegGram]), used to treat urinary tract infections; probenecid, used to treat gout; and cephalosporin, an antibiotic.

Clinitest is an important test in pediatric screening. A negative test-strip result (specific for glucose) but a positive Clinitest result (sensitive for any reducing sugar) may indicate the presence of an inherited metabolic disorder in the newborn.

Clinitest will detect reducing substances at a concentration of 2000 mg/L (200 mg/dL) or greater. Reagent strips will detect glucose at a concentration of 400 to 750 mg/L.

Because Clinitest is both less specific and less sensitive than the reagent strip, it cannot be used as a confirmatory test for a positive reagent-strip glucose test. Clinitest should be reserved for patient populations in whom non–glucose reducing substances need to be detected.

Sugar will appear in the urine because of an increased filtered load, as in diabetes mellitus, or because of decreased tubular reabsorption, as in renal glucosuria. The presence of ascorbic acid may lead to erroneous low results.

Ketones

The term *ketone bodies* includes three discrete but related chemicals: acetoacetic acid, β-hydroxybutyric acid, and acetone (see p. 631 and Chapter 32). Reagent-strip testing for ketones uses a sodium nitroprusside reaction that detects acetone and acetoacetic acid but not β-hydroxybutyric acid, the primary ketone body. It is important to realize that the sodium nitroprusside reagent reacts primarily with acetoacetic acid; acetone has only a 20% reactivity compared with acetoacetate:

Acetoacetic acid + Sodium nitroprusside + Glycine $\xrightarrow{\text{Alkaline pH}}$ *purple color*

Ketone determinations are important in the monitoring of diabetes and ketoacidosis and should be performed whenever sugar determinations are made.

Blood and myoglobin

As previously discussed, red urine usually indicates the presence of erythrocytes, hemoglobin, or myoglobin in the urine. Hematuria most often represents a combination of intact erythrocytes (greater than 5 per high-power field), degenerated erythrocytes, and free hemoglobin. Gross hematuria implies hemorrhage or fresh bleeding and in acidic urine results in a red to brown, turbid or smoky appearance. The reagent-strip method for hemoglobin and myoglobin uses the peroxidase-like activity of these proteins:

$$\text{Hydrogen peroxide (H}_2\text{O}_2\text{)} + \text{Chromogen} \xrightarrow{\text{Myoglobin or hemoglobin}}$$
$$\text{Oxidized chromogen } \textit{(blue)} + \text{H}_2\text{O}$$

A positive test indicates the presence of hematuria, hemoglobinuria, or myoglobinuria, and a microscopic urinalysis is needed to confirm the presence of erythrocytes. Oxidizing agents such as iodides and bromides in the urine may cause false-positive results; large quantities of ascorbic acid (used in some antibiotics) in the urine may produce false-negative results with some reagent strips.

Myoglobin is a ferrous porphyrin similar to hemoglobin that is commonly seen in urine after crush injuries and muscle trauma. When myoglobin is released in the circulatory system, it is rapidly excreted by the kidney. Like hemoglobin, its presence will produce pink to red urine. Myoglobinuria should always be confirmed with rapid immunodiffusion or radioimmunoassay procedures.

Bilirubin

Dark, yellow to brown, foamy urine is suggestive of the presence of conjugated bilirubin. Normal urine does not contain bilirubin. Jaundiced patients with hepatocellular disease, such as hepatitis, or obstructive disease, such as biliary cirrhosis, may have conjugated bilirubin in the urine. The reagent-strip method for determining bilirubin involves a diazotization reaction:

$$\text{Bilirubin glucuronide} + \text{Diazonium salt} \xrightarrow{\text{Acid}}$$
$$\text{Azobilirubin } \textit{(brown)}$$

Negative results from suspicious urines and questionably positive results, as from highly colored urines, should be confirmed by use of Ictotest tablets (Ames Division, Miles Laboratories, Inc., Elkhart, Indiana). The Ictotest employs the same diazotization reaction as the reagent strip. False-negative results may occur if the urine is not fresh because urinary bilirubin may become hydrolyzed or oxidized when exposed to light.

Urobilinogen

Urobilinogen, a colorless compound, is formed in the intestine by the bacterial reduction of bilirubin (see Chapter 27). Normal urine contains small amounts of urobilinogen. Decreased urobilinogen is found in infants, who lack reducing intestinal bacteria; in patients after administration of antibiotics that suppress intestinal flora; and in patients with obstructive liver disease. Increased urobilinogen is present in hemolytic anemia (increased bilirubin formation) and liver dysfunction.

The reagent-strip tests for urobilirubin differ with the manufacturer. Ames products use the Ehrlich reaction employing _p_-dimethylaminobenzaldehyde in a simple color reaction with porphobilinogen. The reaction is not specific for urobilinogen, and false-positive findings may result from other Ehrlich reagent–positive compounds (porphobilinogen, PAS). Boehringer Mannheim Diagnostics products employ a reaction that is specific for urobilinogen; urobilinogen reacts with a diazonium compound to form a red color. It should be noted that reagent strips will not detect the absence of urinary urobilinogen.

A fresh specimen is essential for the detection of urobilinogen because it is a light-sensitive compound. The preferred specimen for detecting or quantitating urinary urobilinogen is a 2-hour early afternoon specimen. This collection takes into account the diurnal excretion pattern of urobilinogen.

Nitrites

The nitrite test is used in urinalysis laboratories to detect bacteriuria. The reagent-strip nitrite test depends on the reduction of nitrate to nitrite by the enzymatic action of certain bacteria in the urine. Under conditions of acid pH, nitrite reacts with _p_-arsanilic acid to form a diazonium compound, which in turn couples with _N_-(1-naphthyl)ethylenediamine to produce a pink color.[11] The nitrite test should be performed on the first morning specimen or on a urine sample that has been collected at least 4 hours or more after the last voiding to allow the organisms in the bladder time to metabolize the nitrate. Stale urine may have a positive nitrite test result because of bacterial contamination after voiding. The nitrite test is specific for gram-negative organisms; however, some false-negative results will occur if organisms such as enterococci, streptococci, or staphylococci, which do not form nitrite, are present. The sensitivity of the nitrite test is about 60% when compared with microbiological procedures.[15] There are very few cases of false-positive nitrite results.

Nitrite testing is of dubious value in hospital clinical urinalysis because there is limited effective control over how and when the urine sample is collected. The nitrite test may have use in a clinic or physician's office because proper control over sampling can be better achieved.

Leukocytes

The presence of leukocytes (pyuria) is a clinically important indicator of inflammation. Reagent-strip tests for pyuria will detect both lysed and intact leukocytes and are based on the presence of intracellular esterases. These enzymes will catalyze the hydrolysis of esters, releasing components that are then used in a color reaction. The intensity of the color reaction is proportional to the number of leukocytes in the specimen. Sensitivities for the two reagent-strip manufacturers are listed in Table 57-6. False-positive results are seen with trichomonads and oxidizing agents. It has not yet been well established whether eosinophils and histiocytes will also give a positive reaction. False-negative values may be seen with high levels of protein and ascorbic acid. Several studies have documented the clinical utility of the leukocyte test as a screening test for pyuria, and many laboratory workers believe a microscopic examination for leukocytes need be performed only on urine specimens that are positive for esterase when tested with reagent strips.[16-19]

Porphyrins

Porphyrins are groups of intermediary products in the biosynthesis of heme and cytochromes, which are produced in the liver and bone marrow (see Chapter 27). Identification of various porphyrins and porphyrin precursors (especially porphobilinogen) is important in the clinical diagnosis of porphyrias, a group of genetic or metabolic disorders. Normal urinary excretion of porphyrins is approximately 2 mg/day. Increased quantities of excreted porphyrins (porphyrinuria) give urine a red or wine color. A screening urinalysis test for porphobilinogen is based on the Watson-Schwartz test (see p. 714).[20] Confirmatory and quantitative tests are available.[9]

Melanin

Normal urine does not contain melanin. Melanin is found in the urine of patients with malignant melanoma. Patients with this malignancy will excrete a colorless precursor of melanin (melanogen) that, when exposed to air, will polymerize to form the dark pigment melanin. Screening tests using ferric chloride oxidize melanogen to melanin, which turns urine brown-black.

MICROSCOPIC EXAMINATION OF URINE
Methods

Accurate microscopic identification of urine sediment is important in the early recognition of infectious, inflammatory, and neoplastic conditions affecting the urinary system.[4] It is debatable whether all routine urine specimens require the more time-consuming microscopic analysis. Instead, most laboratory workers agree that a microscopic examination should be performed when the patient is symptomatic, when the physician specifically requests this examination, and when the macroscopic urinalysis is abnormal, that is, hematuria, proteinuria, or a positive result for pyuria (positive nitrate or esterase result).[11,21]

Several microscopic procedures are available for the sediment examination. Standardized bright-field microscopy is still the most common technique employed.[22] Supravital staining can be combined with bright-field microscopy to enhance cellular detail. Phase-contrast microscopy is probably the best method for rapid urine sediment evaluations without the use of stains. Commercially available standardized slide methods are far superior to conventional glass slide and coverslip methods and a practical alternative to hemocytometer chamber counts.[23]

Currently, automation has not been widely accepted because of the need to identify and classify numerous urine sediment entities. Systems to partially automate the microscopic urinalysis, using flow cytometry or a flow cell mounted on a microscope stage are being developed.

Standardization

Standardization of the microscopic urinalysis is essential to reduce ambiguity and minimize subjectivity.[24] Aspects of the microscopic examination that should be standardized are:

1. Volume of urine analyzed
2. Length and force of centrifugation
3. Resuspending volume and concentration of sediment
4. Volume and amount of sediment examined
5. Terminology and reporting format

Bright-field microscopy of unstained urine. Unstained bright-field microscopy uses reduced light to delineate the more translucent formed elements of the urine, such as hyaline casts, crystals, and mucus threads.

Accurate identification of leukocytes, macrophages, renal tubular epithelial cells, and viral inclusion-bearing cells may be very difficult in unstained preparations. Cytological techniques, stained preparations, or both should be used to confirm results.[8,25]

Procedure. The urine specimen must be examined while fresh, since cells and casts begin to disintegrate within 1 to 3 hours. Refrigeration (2° to 8° C) for up to 48 hours usually prevents the disintegration of cells and pathological entities. Each specimen is concentrated tenfold or twentyfold for the purpose of standardization. The examination proceeds as follows:

1. Mix the specimen well.
2. Pour a fixed volume (10, 12, 15 mL) of urine into a graduated centrifuge tube.
3. Centrifuge at 1500 rpm or approximately 80 *G* for 5 minutes.
4. Remove the supernatant fluid by careful decantation or aspiration to a fixed volume; 1 mL and 0.4 mL are the most common. Resuspend the sediment by gently tapping the bottom of the tube.
5. Place a drop of resuspended sediment on one area of a standardized slide.
6. Examine with low power (100×) and subdued light. Vary the fine focus continuously while randomly scanning the area under the coverslip. During the scan, evaluate the specimen for the presence of squamous and transitional epithelial cells, crystals, mucus, bacteria, yeast, and artifacts. Report according to laboratory protocol. Further identification of casts, renal epithelial cells, erythrocytes, and leukocytes can be accomplished using high power.
7. Examine at least 10 low-power fields using subdued light. Count and report the number of casts per low-power field. Be sure to examine the edges because casts are often found along the edge of a coverslip. Abnormal crystals, when present, should also be

counted on low power. Bacteriuria, visible at low power, should be reported as at least 2+.

8. Examine at least 10 high-power (440×) fields and report numerical values for erythrocytes, leukocytes, and renal tubular epithelial cells per high-power field.

9. Report all counts (average of 10 fields) and qualitative assessments according to standardized terminology.

Bright-field microscopy with supravital staining.
Cellular detail is enhanced with stained sediments.[2,6] A crystal violet–safranin O stain is often used in the rapid assessment of certain cellular elements.[27]

Reagent (Sternheimer-Malbin stain)

Solution 1	Crystal violet	3.0 g
	Ethanol (95%)	20.0 mL
	Ammonium oxalate	0.8 g
	Distilled water	80.0 mL
Solution 2	Safranin O	1 g
	Ethanol (95%)	40 mL
	Distilled water	400 mL

Three parts of solution 1 and 97 parts of solution 2 are mixed and filtered. The mixture should be clarified by filtration every 2 weeks and discarded after 3 months. Separately, solutions 1 and 2 keep indefinitely at room temperature. In highly alkaline urine, the stain will precipitate.

Procedure

1. Add one or two drops of crystal violet–safranin O stain to approximately 1 mL of precentrifuged, concentrated urine sediment.

2. Mix with a pipet and place a drop of this suspension on a slide.

Phase and interference microscopy.
Many urinalysis laboratories recommend phase microscopy for the detection of more translucent formed elements of the urinary sediment. Sediment, notably hyaline casts, mucus, and bacteria, may escape detection using conventional, unstained, bright-field microscopy. Phase microscopy has the advantage of hardening the outlines of even the most ephemeral formed elements, making detection simple.[24] Even greater morphological detail of formed elements (notably casts and cells) is afforded by interference contrast microscopy.[28-30]

Standardized slide methods.
The KOVA system (ICL Scientific, Fountain Valley, California), Count-10 and Count-6 (V-Tech, Palm Desert, California), and the Uri-System (Fisher Scientific, Pittsburgh) offer complete standardized procedures that are technically more precise, reproducible, and reliable than conventional bright-field microscopy.[23] A comparison of standardized microscopic urinalysis systems is shown in Table 57-10. All these standardized slides are superior to conventional glass slides.

In some laboratories, the hemocytometer continues to be used for quantifying urine sediment entities. Kesson et al.[31] provide evidence that chamber counts are more reliable in detecting sediment abnormalities than conventional methods of counting cells under high-power fields.

Semiautomated urinalysis work station.
An automated urinalysis instrument called the Yellow IRIS (International Remote Imaging Systems, Chatsworth, California) combines automated microscopy with a dipstick reader and specific-gravity module. This technology may provide more accurate results over standardized manual systems when there are high volumes of test samples and very low concentrations of sediment elements.[32] Manual methods appear to be more sensitive in detecting casts.[33]

Combined cytocentrifugation and Papanicolaou stain.
A technique that combines cytocentrifugation and Papanicolaou staining has been recommended for more accurate assessment of urine sediment. This more specialized method provides a simple, reproducible, and semiquantitative method for identifying urine sediment entities. Cellular casts, mononuclear cells, tissue fragments, and neoplastic cells may be clearly identified with this method. Although not found in routine laboratories, this technique's acceptance is growing.[6-8]

Table 57-10   Physical features of urinalysis slide systems

	Conventional	Uni-Slide*	KOVA†	Count-10‡
Volume of urine sediment				
Mean amount	1 drop	16 μL	6 μL	6 μL
% Coefficient of variation		7%	6%	10%
Surface for microscopic examination				
Total area (mm²)	484	90	32	36
Number of 100× fields	144	25	9	12
Number of 400× fields	2116	420	119	49
Number of focal planes before settling	1-2	1-2	1-2	3-4
Type of coverglass	Glass	Glass	Plastic	Plastic
Cost per test	7¢	9¢	9¢	6¢
Maximum number of tests or slides	2	4	10	10

*Uni-Slide, Uri-System Slide distributed by Fisher Scientific, Pittsburgh, as part of the Fisher brand Uri-System.
†KOVA IV Slide, ICL Scientific, Fountain Valley, California.
‡Count-10 Slide, V-Tech, Inc., Palm Desert, California.

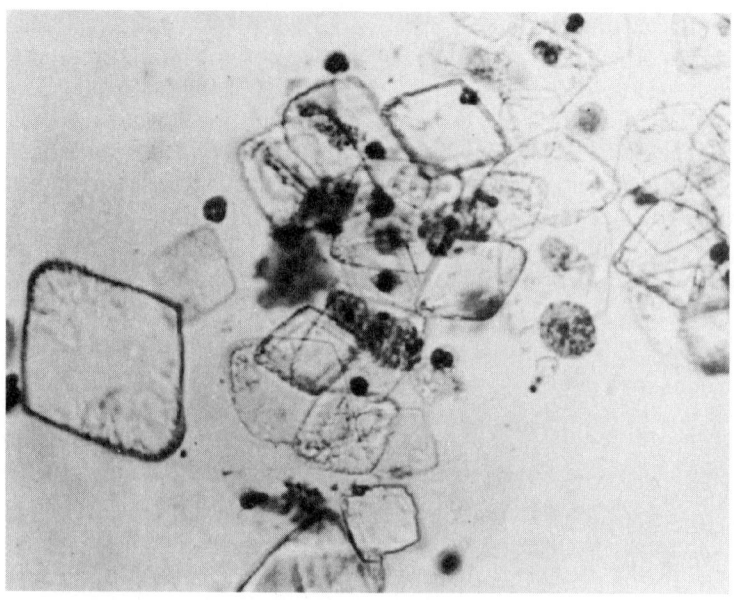

Fig. 57-1   Uric acid crystals. (Papanicolaou stain, 400×.)

Crystals

Urinary crystals (Figs. 57-1 to 57-5) are commonly seen. Usually crystals are not present when urine is freshly voided, and in general the formation of crystals should be regarded as an artifact of the system of collection. Crystal formation occurs when various chemical constituents become saturated or undergo altered solubilities when urine is stored at cooler temperatures. Certain chemical substances such as albumin prevent crystallization. When heated to 37° C, most crystals disappear. Those still present might have some diagnostic significance when correlated with clinical symptoms.[9]

The types of urinary crystals formed depend on the pH of freshly voided urine. Table 57-11 lists the common types, properties, and clinical significance of various urinary crystals. Cystine, uric acid, leucine, and tyrosine crystals are the most diagnostically important crystals to recognize.   Be-

cause of the limited clinical significance of the urinary crystals, most laboratory workers agree that time should not be wasted on their specific identification. Many crystals are induced by various medications though their clinical significance remains unclear.

Organisms

In a properly collected and processed urine specimen, the presence of organisms is clinically significant. Bacteria, fungi, parasites, and virally infected cells are frequently reported. Organisms seen in urine sediment are microscopically recognized as extracellular or intracellular structures.[25] Bright-field microscopy readily detects extracellular bacteria, fungi, and parasites. Detection of intracellular phagocytized bacteria and fungi, *Toxoplasma* organisms, and viral inclusion bodies usually requires cytological procedures.

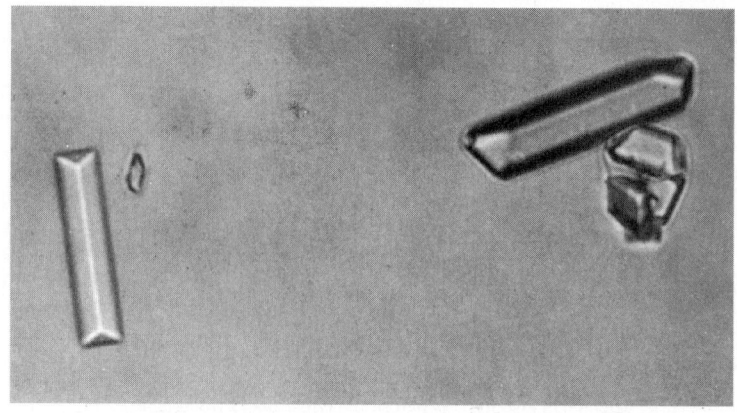

Fig. 57-2   Triple phosphate crystals. (Bright field, 400×.)

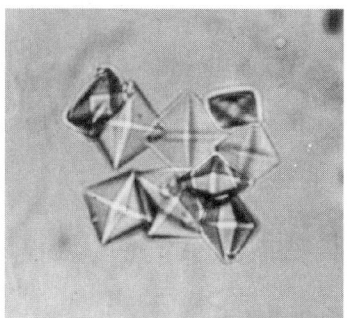

Fig. 57-3   Calcium oxalate crystals. (Bright field, 1000×.)

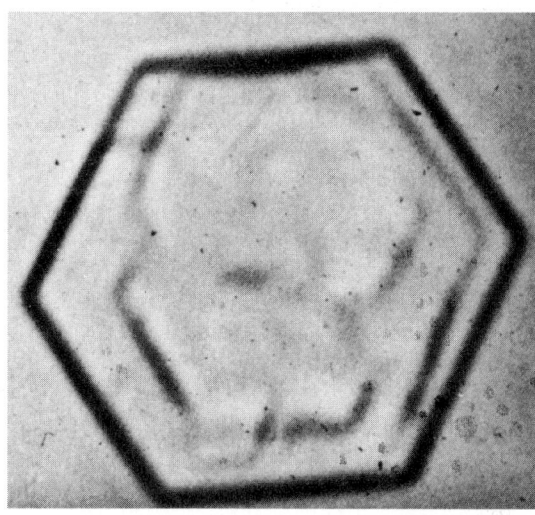

Fig. 57-4   Cystine crystals. (Bright field, 2500×.)

Accurate identification of organisms aids in the clinical differential diagnosis of urinary system infections. Stained preparations are important in the evaluation of organisms, identification of associated inflammatory cells, and assessment of epithelial exfoliation and renal cast formation for purposes of localization.[4] Microbiological techniques should be used to confirm and fully classify various urinary organisms.

Bacteria. Urine from healthy individuals is sterile and does not contain bacteria. Some bacteria may be present because of contamination during collection or prolonged stor-

age. If bacteria are seen in centrifuged specimens but not in unspun urine specimens, less than 10^5 bacteria/mL are present. Bacteria in an unspun specimen indicate that greater than 10^5 bacteria are present. The presence of 10^5 bacteria or greater is suggestive of a urinary tract infection. This number corresponds to 10 or more bacteria per high-

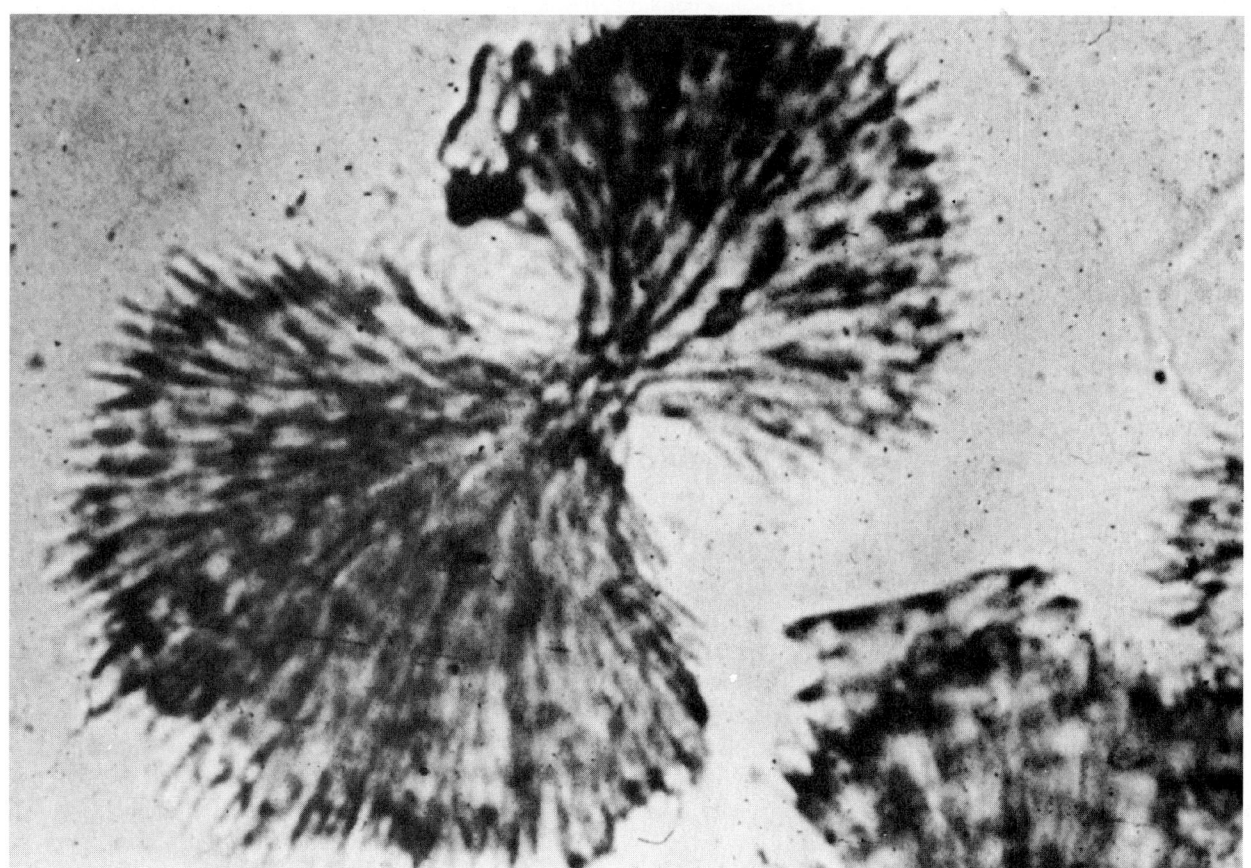

Fig. 57-5   Sulfonamide crystals. (Bright field, 2500×.)

Table 57-11   Common urinary crystals

Types	Urine pH				Diagnostic morphological appearance	Solubility characteristics	Clinical significance
	Acid	Alkaline	Neutral	Variable			
Urates	×				Colorless, amorphous, spherical, or needle shaped	Soluble in alkali or at 60° C	Healthy
Uric acid	×				Colorless to yellow brown, pleomorphic, rhombic, four-sided plates or rosettes	Soluble in alkali	Healthy, chemotherapy, gout
Calcium carbonate				×	Colorless dumbbells or spheres	Soluble in acetic acid	Healthy
Phosphates (triple phosphates)		×			Colorless, three- to six-sided prisms; "coffin lids"	Soluble in acetic acid	Healthy
Ammonium urates		×			Brown, "thorn apple"	Soluble in 60° C with acetic acid	Healthy
Calcium oxalate				×	Colorless, octahedron, dumbbell, or envelope or internal "X" forms	Soluble in dilute hydrochloric acid	Healthy, glycol poisoning
Cystine				×	Colorless, hexagonal, flat	Soluble in alkali	Cystinosis
Cholesterol				×	Colorless, flat plates with corner notched	Soluble in chloroform and ether	Renal damage
Tyrosine				×	Yellow to colorless, fine needles, in sheaves or rosettes	Soluble in alkali	Liver damage, aminoaciduria
Leucine				×	Yellow spheroids with striations	Soluble in hot alcohol	Liver damage, aminoaciduria
Bilirubin				×	Reddish brown, amorphous, needles, rhombic plates, or cubes	Soluble in alkali	Bilirubinuria
Sulfonamides				×	Cubes, globules, or sheaves	Soluble in acetone	Antibiotic therapy

power field. Identification of bacteria, cocci, or rods can readily be accomplished by bright-field or phase-contrast microscopy. Occasionally, there is difficulty in distinguishing bacteria from amorphous crystals.

Fungi. Urinary tract (fungal) infections (UTIs) are common in patients with diabetes, those taking birth control pills, or those undergoing intensive antibiotic or immunosuppressive therapy. An associated inflammatory pattern is seen in most UTIs from nonimmunocompromised patients.

Candida albicans is the most common fungus and is identified as budding yeast or mycelia (Fig. 57-6). In general the budding yeast appearance indicates that the fungi are coexisting with the host, whereas the mycelial forms appear during tissue invasion. Yeasts of *Candida albicans* are oval and highly refractile and measure 3 to 5 μm. Often they can be misinterpreted as erythrocytes (7 μm). Unlike erythrocytes, yeasts are not lysed by acids.

Parasites. The presence of parasites in urine usually indicates vaginal or fecal contamination. *Trichomonas vaginalis*, a flagellate, is the most common parasite seen in urine. The incidence of this type of parasitism is very high

in women and may be the cause of intense vaginitis. In men the parasite causes an asymptomatic urethritis. Because of the motility of this oval organism, bright-field microscopy is used for simple and rapid identification. Nonmotile trichomonads can easily be mistaken for leukocytes or epithelial cells.

Pinworm ova *(Enterobius vermicularis)* have been found in urine in children because of fecal contamination. Morphologically a pinworm ovum is surrounded by a thick two-layered transparent capsule, and a coiled embryo may be visible inside. Trematode ova, of *Schistosoma haematobium* (found in North Africa), and *Schistosoma mansoni* (found in Central America) may be found in urine.

Virally infected cells. Virus-induced cellular changes have been recognized with increased frequency in urine sediment, especially in immunosuppressed patients. Cytological techniques should be used for the accurate identification of cytomegalovirus, herpes simplex, and *Polyomavirus*, which produce diagnostic intranuclear inclusion cells and are the most common types of urinary system viral infections. Viral inclusion cells must be distinguished from nonviral sources of inclusion cells such as heavy

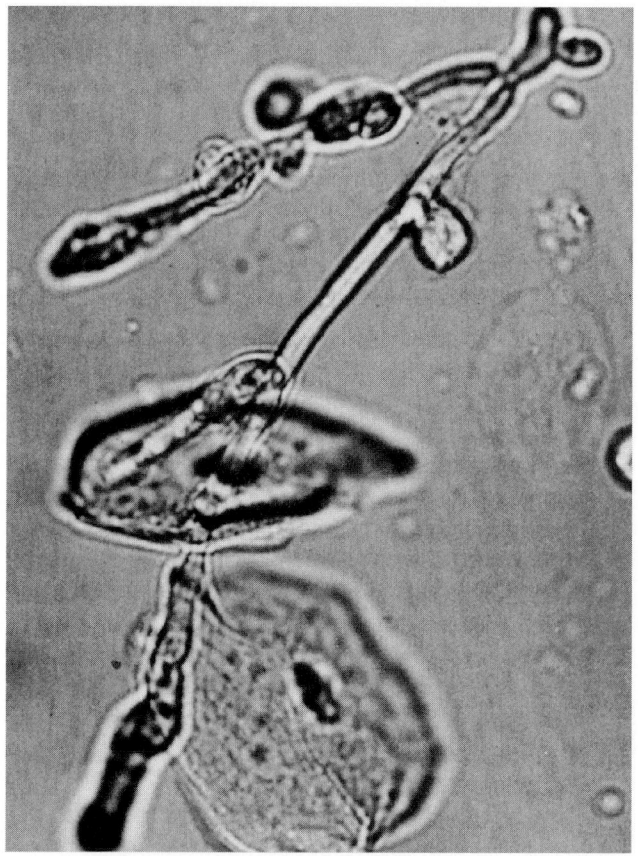

Fig. 57-6   Fungal yeast and mycelia, probable *Candida* species. (Bright field, 2500×.)

metal exposure (lead and cadmium) and nonspecific degenerative cellular changes. A detailed description of viral inclusion cells can be found in standard textbooks on urine cytology.

Cells

Microscopic identification and evaluation of cells is an important part of urinalysis. Common types of cells normally found in urine include a few erythrocytes, leukocytes, and epithelial cells of renal or lower urinary tract origin. All cells of pathological significance are usually quantified by high-power field examination.

Erythrocytes. Normal urine should never contain more than a few erythrocytes per high-power field.[3,4] They appear in the urine stream after vascular injury or disorders in the kidney or lower urinary tract. The presence of erythrocytes accompanied by blood casts or dysmorphic erythrocytes (Fig. 57-7) is suggestive of renal parenchymal or glomerular bleeding.[35] The detection of urinary dysmorphic erythrocytes, especially acanthocytes, is an important morphologic marker of glomerular or tubular bleeding.[36-38] Quantification aids in diagnosis and patient management. It is important that contamination from

menstrual flow be avoided when urine from females is to be examined.

Erythrocytes measure approximately 7 μm in diameter, have a biconcave disk shape, and often appear pale yellow when bright-field microscopy is used (Fig. 57-8). In hypertonic urine they are smaller and crenated, whereas in hypotonic urine they are larger and swollen. When erythrocytes have been in urine for a considerable time, the hemoglobin may have leaked out of the cells.

On occasion hemoglobin is detected by reagent strip testing in urine in the absence of microscopic erythrocytes in the sediment. Possible explanations for this discrepancy include hypotonic urine or an alkaline urine, both of which can cause erythrocyte lysis. The absence of these conditions is strongly suggestive that the pigment that appears in the urine (which may be hemoglobin or myoglobin) originates from filtration of these products from the blood.

Leukocytes (Fig. 57-8). The normal excretion rate for leukocytes in the urine is up to 1 leukocyte per 3 high-power fields, 3000 cells/mL, or up to about 200,000 cells/hour. Elevated numbers of leukocytes (pyuria) are associated with numerous urinary tract inflammatory and infectious conditions. Most leukocytes recognized by bright-field microscopy are segmented neutrophils. The identification of lymphocytes, plasma cells, and eosinophils requires special stains.

Little[39] has shown that leukocyte excretion rates in excess of 400,000 cells/hour virtually always indicate urinary tract infection. This rate corresponds to more than 10 neutrophils per high-power field. Patients with active upper urinary tract infections frequently have more than 50 neutrophils per high-power field or have a leukocyte excretion rate in excess of 2 or even 3 million/hour.

Renal tubular epithelial cells (Figs. 57-9 to 57-11). Various types of renal tubular epithelial cells line the nephron, and senescent or diseased cells are constantly being shed into the urine. Since they represent actual renal exfoliation, the presence of more than two renal tubular epithelial cells per high-power field indicates active renal tubular damage or injury.

Considerable difficulty exists in the accurate identification of renal tubular cells, particularly in distinguishing them from other mononuclear cells commonly found in urine. By bright-field microscopy they are polygonal and slightly larger than leukocytes. For accurate identification of various types of renal tubular cells (convoluted versus collecting duct) and sheets or fragments, cytological techniques are required.[8,25]

Oval fat bodies (Fig. 57-12). Oval fat bodies are renal tubular epithelial cells that are filled with absorbed lipids or that have undergone degenerative cellular changes. Oval fat bodies are often associated with proteinuria and lipiduria and are characteristically seen in the nephrotic syndrome and diabetes mellitus.

Transitional epithelial cells (Fig. 57-13). A few tran-

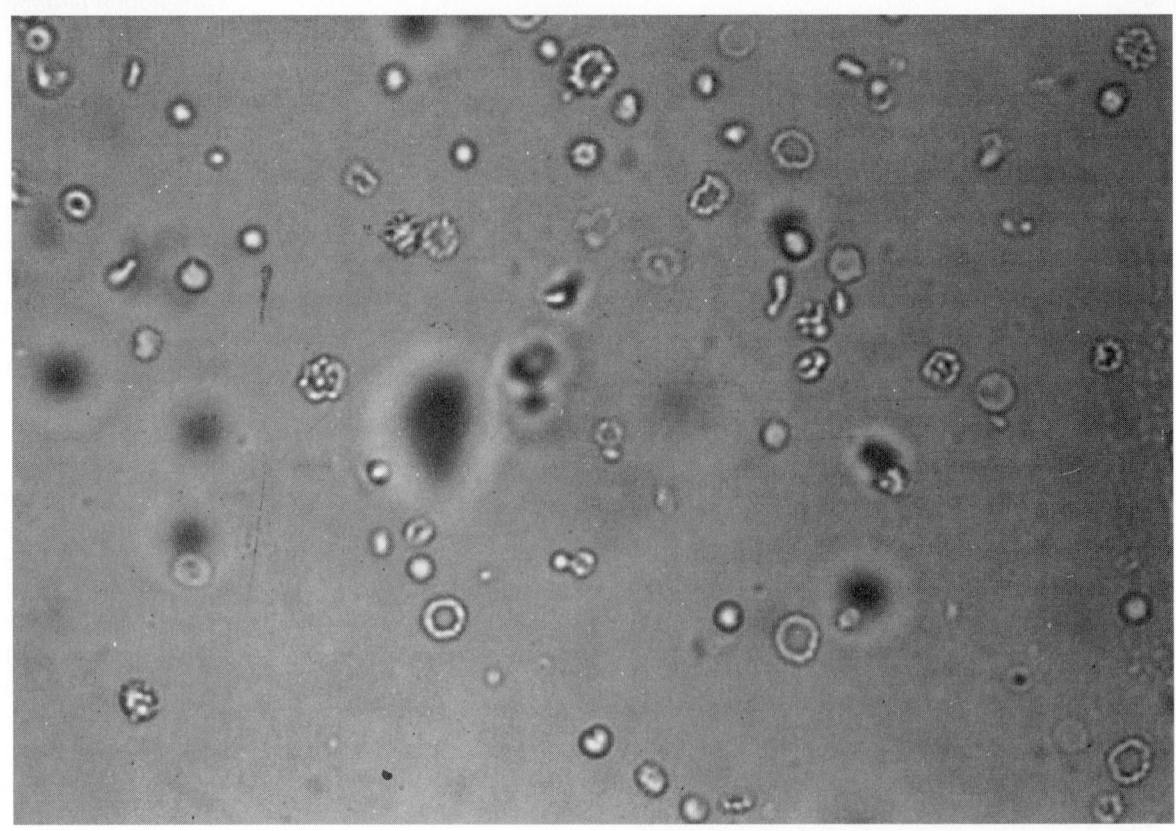

Fig. 57-7 Dysmorphic erythrocytes. (Bright field, 400×.)

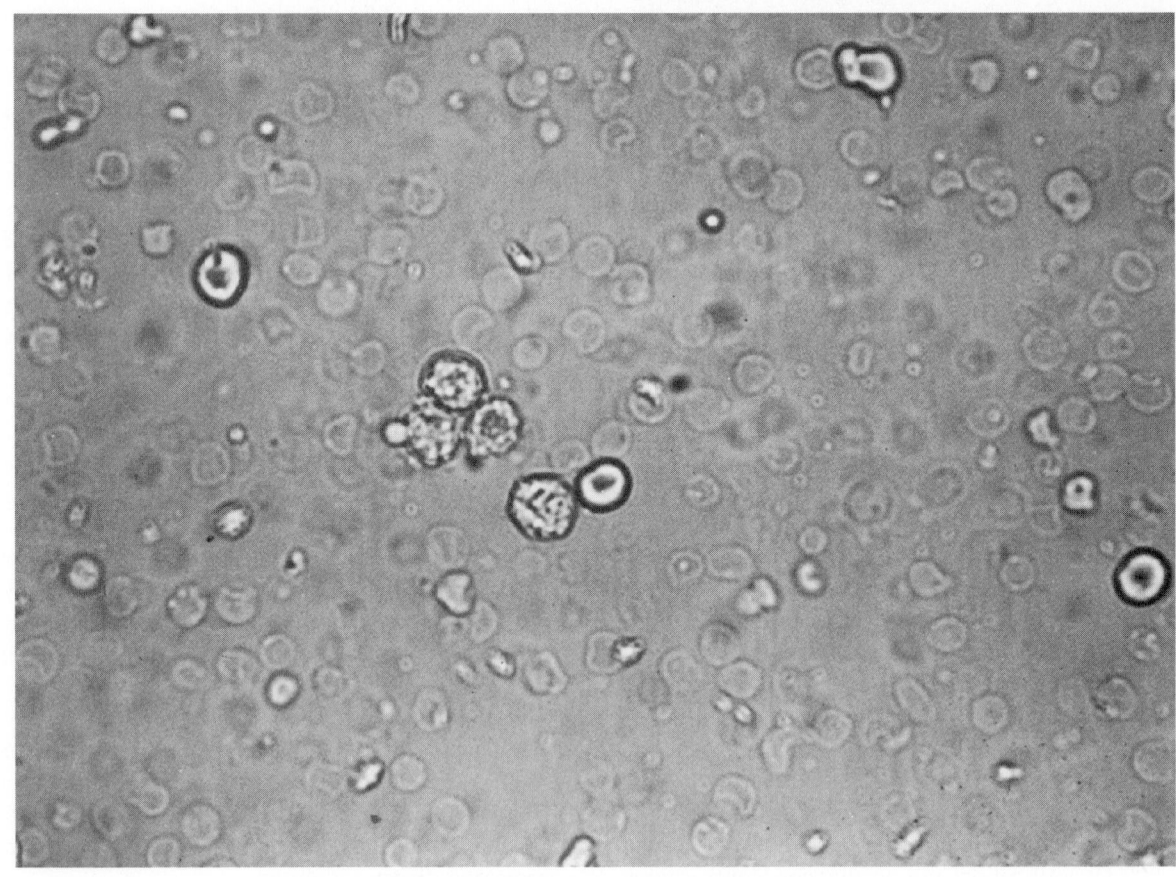

Fig. 57-8 Erythrocytes and leukocytes. (Bright field, 400×.)

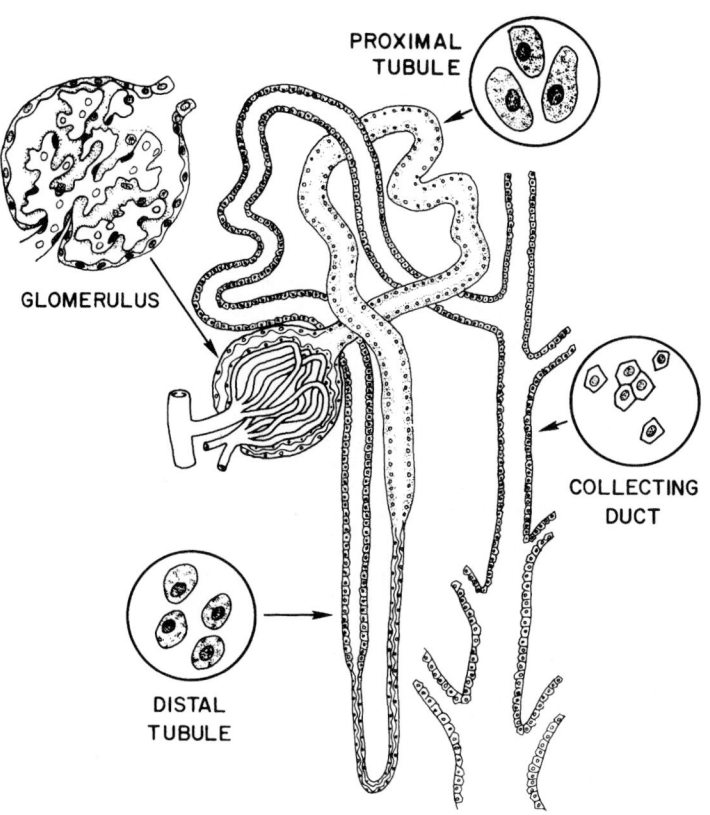

PROXIMAL
TUBULE

GLOMERULUS

COLLECTING
DUCT

DISTAL
TUBULE

Fig. 57-9   Location of renal tubular epithelial cells.

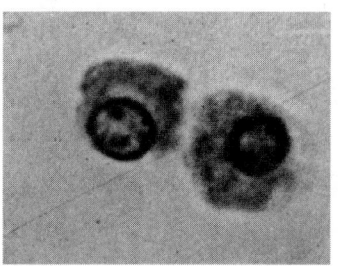

Fig. 57-10   Renal tubular epithelial cells. (Bright field, 1000×.)

sitional (urothelial) cells can be found in normal urine. In flammatory conditions in the bladder, catheterization, or a pathological process such as malignancy may be indicated by large numbers of transitional cells.

By bright-field microscopy, transitional cells appear round to oval, measure 40 to 60 μm, and have a centrally located nucleus. The cytoplasm borders of these cells appear thickened and crisp. When the nuclei of transitional cells become enlarged or irregular, cytological techniques should be suggested for the purpose of detecting a urinary system malignancy.

Squamous epithelial cells (Fig. 57-14). Squamous epithelial cells line the distal portion of the lower urinary tract and the female genital tract. Squamous cells are the largest of the epithelial cells found in urine. They have abundant flat cytoplasm with small nuclei. Frequently one or more corners of these cells may be folded. Squamous cells in urine usually indicate contamination (vaginal in women, urethral in uncircumsized men) or squamous metaplasia of the bladder and represent the least significant type of epithelial cell found in urine.

Tissue fragments in urine (Fig. 57-15). Any clumps or chunks of solid-appearing material in urine specimens should be noted. This material is identified during the initial inspection of the specimen because of its large size. It is often white or tan. Precise identification of such material is important for an accurate diagnosis. This involves transfer of the observed material to an appropriate fixative to preserve it for a cytological or histological evaluation. Renal papillary necrosis and bladder tumors are most frequently responsible for shedding large tissue fragments into the urine.

Spermatozoa. Spermatozoa may be easily recognized

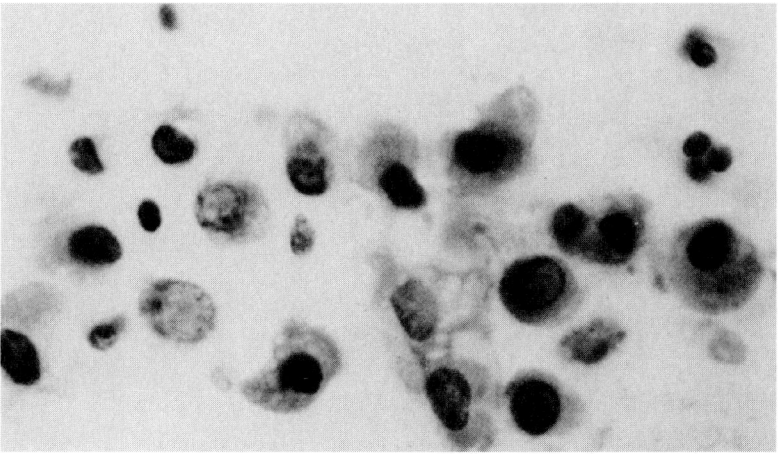

Fig. 57-11   Renal tubular epithelial cells. (Papanicolaou stain, 1000×.)

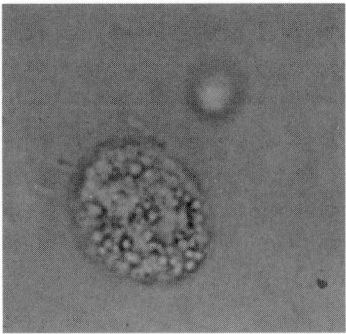

Fig. 57-12   Oval fat bodies. (Bright field, 1250×.)

in the urine of a man after ejaculation or in the urine of a woman as a vaginal contaminant after coitus. Their identification is of limited clinical significance, and the presence of spermatozoa is usually not reported.

Renal casts (Figs. 57-16 to 57-21)

Renal (urinary) casts are formed cylindrical structures that are organized in the nephron. Casts are significant because of their localizing value. Casts are composed of uromucoid (Tamm-Horsfall mucoprotein), which is always present in urine, usually in solution. Uromucoid is produced by the renal tubular epithelial cells of the ascending limb of the loop of Henle. Casts are formed as a result of urine stasis allowing uromucoid to precipitate. Other factors contributing to cast formation include an increased concentration of protein, salts, and a low urine pH. Since the precipitation

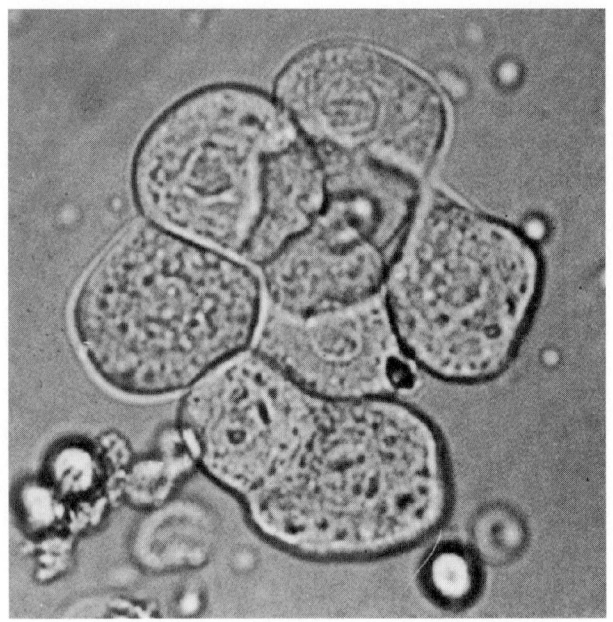

Fig. 57-13   Transitional epithelial cells. (Bright field, 1000×.)

of this protein depends on the concentration and composition of urine, casts are more likely to be formed at the distal portion of the nephron and in the collecting ducts of the kidney where the urine is more concentrated. Casts may form in the proximal convoluted tubules in patients with Bence Jones proteins (multiple myeloma).

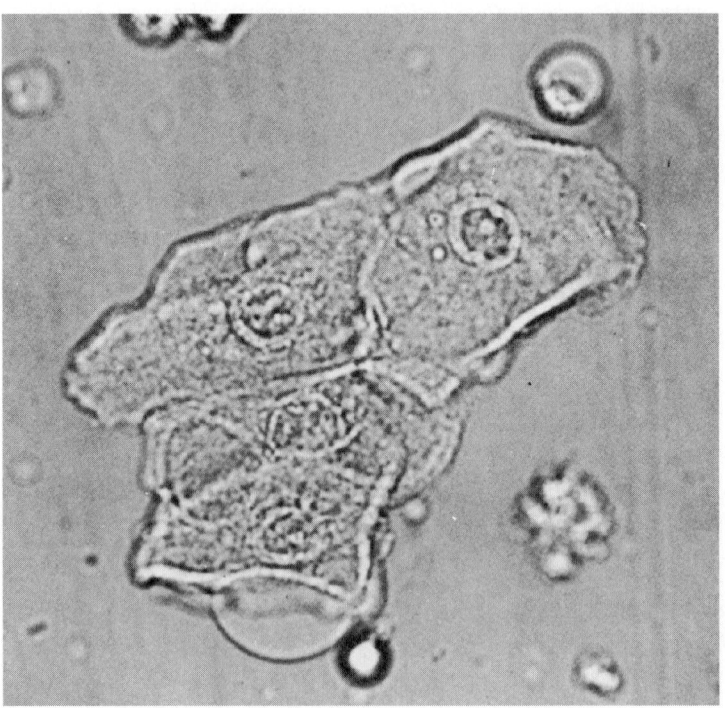

Fig. 57-14   Squamous epithelial cells. (Bright field, 1000×.)

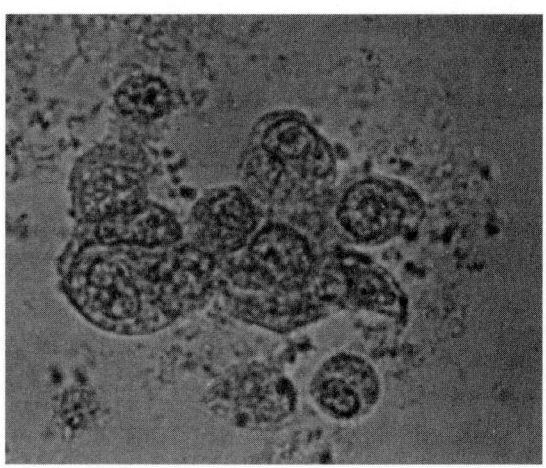

Fig. 57-15 Malignant tissue fragments in urine. (Bright field, 1000×.)

The appearance of these cylindrical formed elements in urine reflects the shapes (long versus short, straight versus convoluted) and diameter (thin versus broad) of the renal tubular lumens in which they originally were formed. Their number and measurable properties of size, form, and compositions are valuable clues to intrinsic renal parenchymal disease.

Microscopically casts are characterized by the appearance of the matrix (hyaline, granular, or waxy), the cellular constituents (erythrocytes, leukocytes, or renal tubular epithelial cells), or particulate matter embedded in the matrix (fine or coarse granules or fibrin).

Accurate identification of casts, especially the cellular types, is often difficult when unstained bright-field micros-copy (wet preparation) is used. A skilled microscopist is essential to avoid misinterpretations. Phase-contrast and interference-contrast microscopy, as well as special stains, can be used to improve visualization. The cytocentrifugation-Papanicolaou technique is a superior method for the accurate identification of casts in urine specimens of patients with renal disease.

For diagnostic purposes, renal casts are classified as *physiological* or *pathological*. Table 57-12 lists the common types, properties, and clinical significance of casts.

Fats

Fats are found in the urine of patients who have fat emboli after bone-crush injuries, fatty degeneration of the kidney, or nephrotic syndrome. Fat will appear on top of urine and is the last part of voided urine. Vacuolated epithelial cells may be found in the urinary sediment. Oil Red O or Sudan III fat stains should be used for accurate identification of fat droplets in urine.

URINE CYTOLOGY

Urinalysis laboratory workers should be able to recognize abnormal mononuclear cells suggestive of malignancy. These should be referred for urine cytology. Holmquist[26] has advocated the use of supravital stains for malignant cell detection and suggests a role for the urinalysis laboratory in cancer screening.

CALCULI (LITHIASIS)

Urinary calculi are precipitates, concretions, or crystalloids embedded in a binding substance of mucus and protein. Bacteria and epithelial cells also may be included in the calculi.[40] Although the cause of calculus formation remains

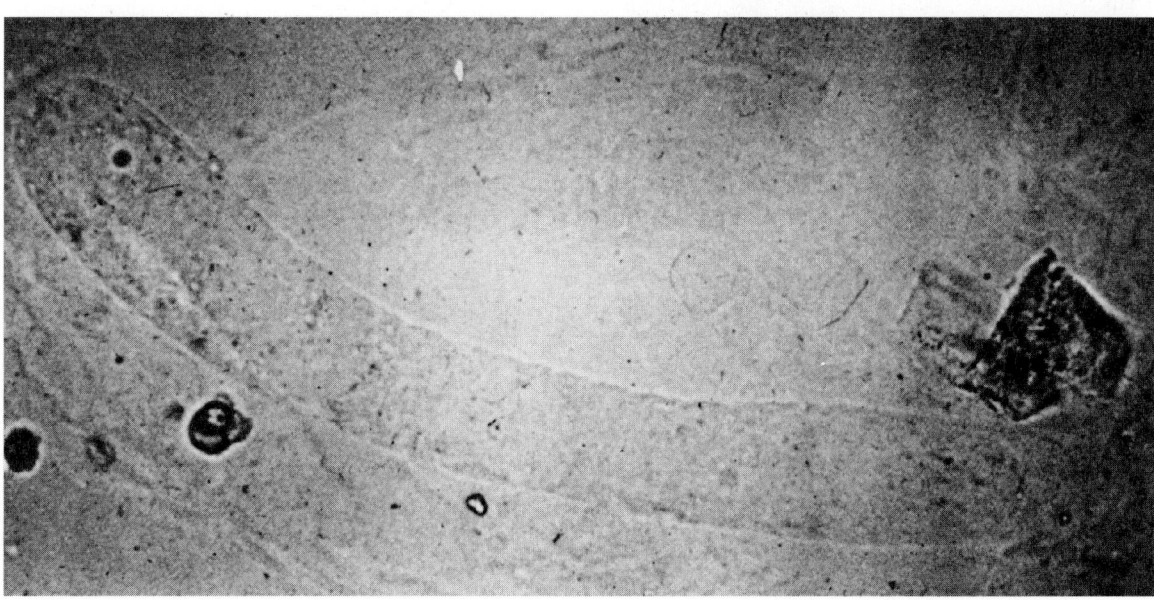

Fig. 57-16 Hyaline cast. (Bright field, 1000×.)

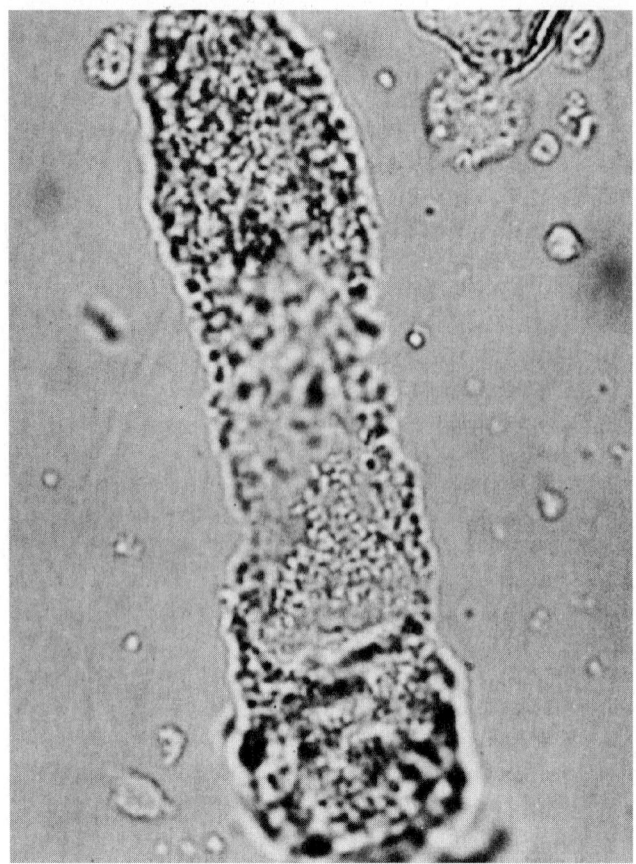

Fig. 57-17   Granular cast. (Bright field, 1000×.)

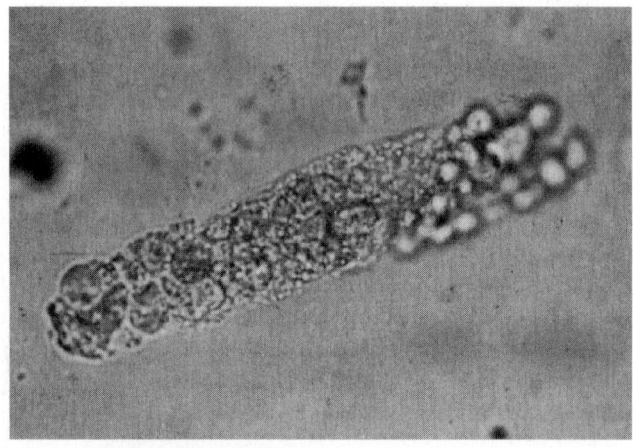

Fig. 57-18   Renal tubular cell cast. (Bright field, 400×.)

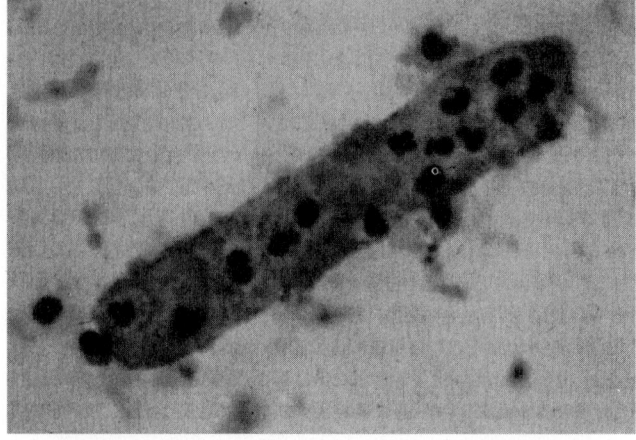

Fig. 57-19   White blood cell cast. (Bright field, 400×.)

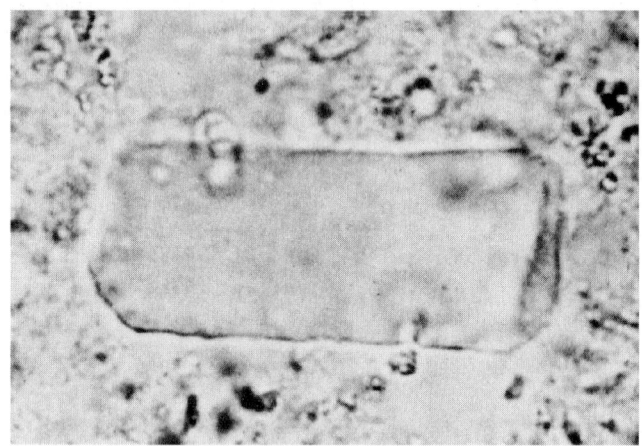

Fig. 57-20   Waxy cast. (Bright field, 1000×.)

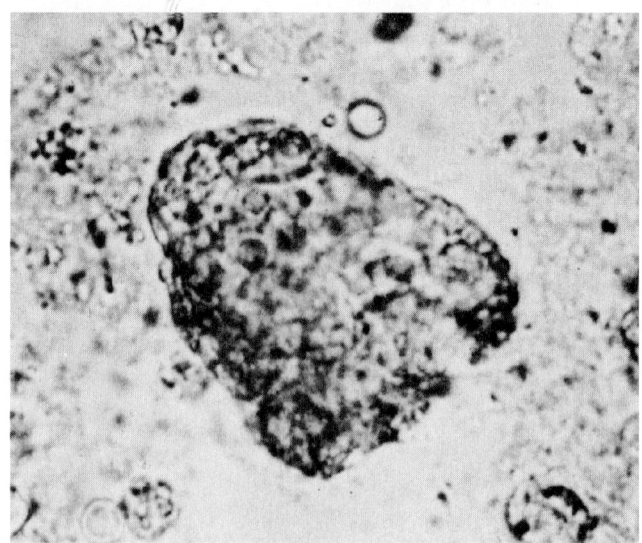

Fig. 57-21   Broad cast. (Bright field, 1000×.)

Table 57-12   Common renal (urinary) casts

Types	Characteristic morphological appearance	Significance	Associated diseases
Physiological			
Hyaline	Transparent cylinder	Exercise, dehydration, and fevers	Nonspecific
Granular (fine)	Semitransparent cylinder containing fine refractile granules	Exercise, dehydration, and fever; accumulation of plasma proteins	Nonspecific
Pathological			
Cellular			
Erythrocytic	Semitransparent or granular cylinder containing distinct erythrocyte stroma	Renal parenchymal bleeding, glomerular leakage	Glomerular disease, interstitial hemorrhage (infarction)
Blood	Red-brown granular cylinder, but intact erythrocyte stroma *not* seen	Same as above	Same as above
Leukocytic	Transparent granular or waxy cylinder containing segmented neutrophils	Renal inflammation	Tubulointerstitial inflammation (pyelonephritis), glomerular disease
Renal tubular epithelial	Semitransparent granular or waxy cylinder containing intact or necrotic renal tubular epithelial cells	Renal tubular damage	Renal tubular injury, acute tubular necrosis, acute allograft rejections, tubulointerstitial disease
Bacterial	Semitransparent or granular cylinder containing bacteria	Renal infection	Acute pyelonephritis
Fungal	Semitransparent or granular cylinder containing fungi	Renal infection, probably sepsis	Acute pyelonephritis, papillary necrosis
Noncellular			
Granular (coarse)	Semitransparent cylinder containing coarse refractile granules	Cellular degeneration, accumulation of plasma proteins	Nonspecific
Waxy	Sharply defined, highly refractile, homogenous cylinder with broken-off borders and indentations	Cellular degeneration	Nonspecific
Fibrin	Transparent or granular cylinder containing thin long fibrils	Leakage of coagulation products	Glomerular disease, thrombosis
Fatty	Semitransparent or granular cylinder containing large highly refractile vacuoles or droplets	Lipiduria	Nephrotic syndrome
Bile	Deep yellow, transparent, granular waxy cylinder	Leakage of bile salts	Liver dysfunction, tubulointerstitial disease
Crystal	Crystalline inclusion in a semitransparent or granular cylinder	Cellular degeneration and malabsorption or excretion	Nonspecific
Other			
Broad	Width of cylinder two to six times that of other casts; waxy and granular most common types	Tubular dilatation and stasis	Advanced renal disease

controversial, the detection and identification of calculi are important for diagnosis of urinary system conditions. Calculi formation in the kidney or lower urinary tract can be the source of gross hematuria and can cause serious anatomical damage and excruciating pain for the patient. Knowledge of the specific composition of a passed or surgically removed calculus may aid the physician in effectively treating lithiasis and preventing future stone formation.

Calculus (stone) analysis for chemical constituents is a complex laboratory procedure. Urinary system calculi are usually composed of calcium oxalate, calcium oxalate mixed with calcium phosphate, ammonium magnesium phosphate, uric acid, or cystine. Most laboratories refer specimens for calculi analysis to more specialized laboratories.

URINE FINDINGS IN COMMON RENAL AND LOWER URINARY TRACT DISEASES

Numerous primary and secondary conditions and diseases occur in the kidney and lower urinary tract. An accurate diagnosis of urinary system disease requires correlation of ab-

Table 57-13   Urinalysis abnormalities found in common urinary system diseases

Conditions	Diagnostic physicochemical findings (macroscopic urinalysis)	Diagnostic urine sediment findings (microscopic urinalysis)
Renal		
Acute glomerulonephritis	Decreased urine volume, increased turbidity (smoky), proteinuria (<2 g/24 hr), hematuria (often gross)	Erythrocytic and blood casts, erythrocytes (often dysmorphic), neutrophils, mixed cellular casts, renal epithelial cells, occasional leukocytic or renal tubuloepithelial casts
Nephrotic syndrome	Lipiduria, significant proteinuria (>4.5 g/24 hr)	Fatty and waxy casts, doubly refractile oval fat bodies (Maltese cross with polarized light), lipid-laden renal tubuloepithelial cells
Chronic glomerulonephritis	Occasional lipiduria, decreased and fixed specific gravity, proteinuria (>2 g/24 hr), hematuria	Pathological casts, especially broad types
Acute tubular necrosis	Decreased urine volume, decreased specific gravity, minimum proteinuria, hematuria	Intact and necrotic renal epithelial cells, renal epithelial fragments, pathological casts
Acute pyelonephritis (tubulointerstitial inflammation)	Occasional odor, increased turbidity, minimum proteinuria, positive nitrite reaction	Leukocyte casts, neutrophils, especially in clumps; bacterial, granular, and waxy casts; renal tubuloepithelial cells
Diabetes mellitus	Proteinuria, glycosuria, ketonuria	Fatty and waxy casts, oval fat bodies, renal epithelial cells, leukocytes
Systemic lupus erythematosus	Proteinuria	Pathological casts, renal epithelial cells, neutrophils, erythrocytes
Cystinosis	Minimum proteinuria or hematuria	Cystine crystals
Acute allograft rejection	Decreased urine volume, minimum proteinuria, hematuria	Renal epithelial cells, renal epithelial casts, lymphocytes, pathological casts, especially renal epithelial casts
Viral nephropathy (cytomegalic inclusion disease)	Minimum proteinuria, hematuria	Mononuclear cells (occasional giant cell forms) with prominent intranuclear or cytoplasmic inclusions
Lower urinary tract		
Bacterial urinary tract infection	Occasional odor, increased turbidity, positive nitrite reaction, occasional hematuria	Bacteria, neutrophils, reactive transitional epithelial cells, absence of cast formation
Fungal urinary tract infection	Increased turbidity, occasional hematuria	Fungi, neutrophils and lymphocytes, reactive transitional epithelial cells
Viral urinary tract infection	Occasional hematuria	Viral inclusion bodies, neutrophils, transitional cells
Eosinophilic cystitis	Hematuria	Eosinophils (numerous), reactive transitional epithelial cells, absence of cast formation
Transitional cell carcinoma	Hematuria	Increased numbers of malignant transitional epithelial cells with high nuclear-to-cytoplasmic ratio, hyperchromasia, and chromatin clumping; cells occur singly and as tissue fragments

Modified from Schumann GB: *Urine sediment examination*, Baltimore, 1980, Williams & Wilkins.

normal urine findings with the patient history, physical examination, symptoms, signs, renal function tests, and other laboratory data. To be classified as abnormal, urine sediment must meet at least one of the following criteria:

1. More than five erythrocytes or leukocytes per high-power field (400×)
2. More than two renal tubular cells per high-power field (400×)
3. More than three hyaline casts, more than one granular cast, or the presence of any pathological cast per low-power field (100×)
4. More than 10 bacteria per high-power field (400×)

5. Presence of fungus, parasites, or viral inclusion cells
6. Presence of pathological crystals (such as cystine) or a large number of nonpathological crystals (such as uric acid)

A summary of urinalysis abnormalities found in common renal and lower urinary tract disease is shown in Table 57-13. Diagnostic findings of both the macroscopic and microscopic examination are also listed for quick review.

COORDINATED APPROACH TO URINALYSIS

Urinalysis continues to be one of the most commonly requested and demanding clinical laboratory procedures.[14]

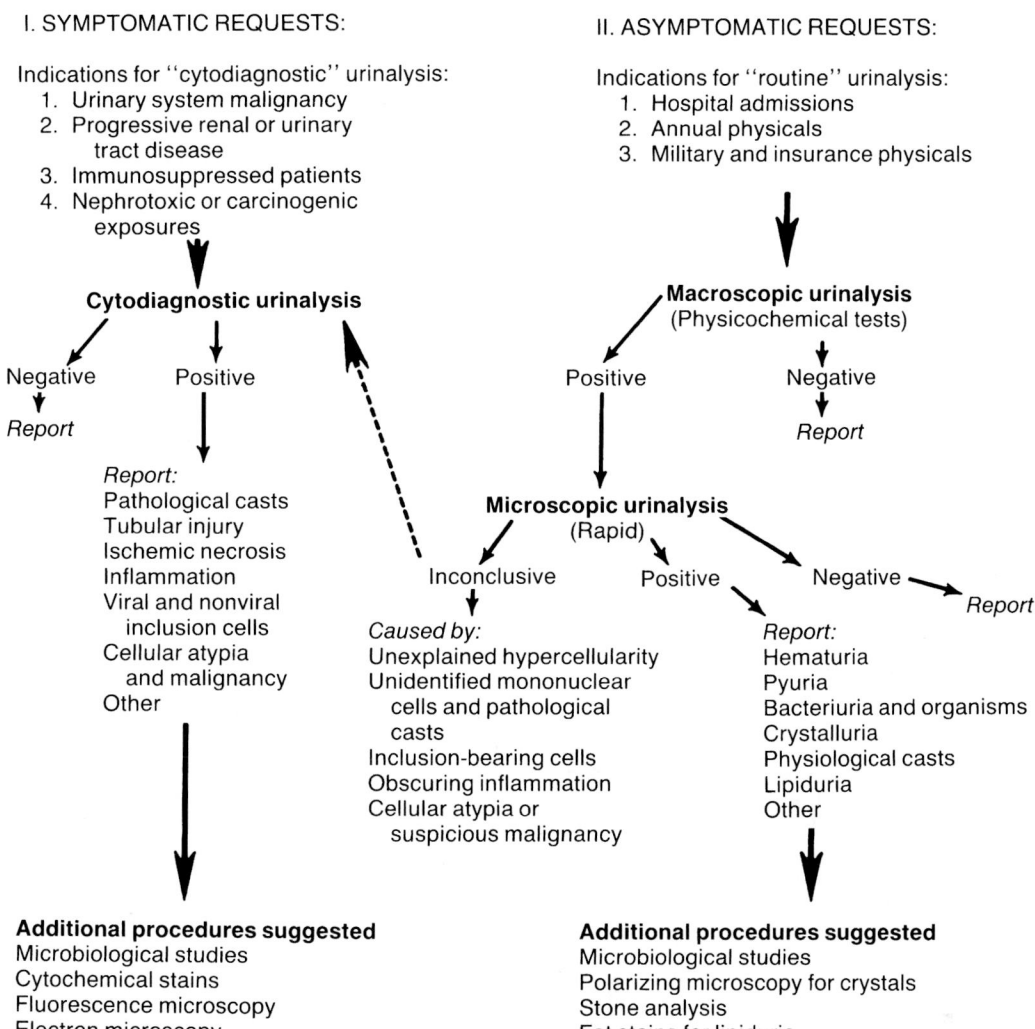

I. SYMPTOMATIC REQUESTS:

Indications for "cytodiagnostic" urinalysis:
1. Urinary system malignancy
2. Progressive renal or urinary tract disease
3. Immunosuppressed patients
4. Nephrotoxic or carcinogenic exposures

Cytodiagnostic urinalysis

Negative   Positive

Report

Report:
Pathological casts
Tubular injury
Ischemic necrosis
Inflammation
Viral and nonviral inclusion cells
Cellular atypia and malignancy
Other

II. ASYMPTOMATIC REQUESTS:

Indications for "routine" urinalysis:
1. Hospital admissions
2. Annual physicals
3. Military and insurance physicals

Macroscopic urinalysis
(Physicochemical tests)

Positive   Negative

Report

Microscopic urinalysis
(Rapid)

Inconclusive   Positive   Negative → *Report*

Caused by:
Unexplained hypercellularity
Unidentified mononuclear cells and pathological casts
Inclusion-bearing cells
Obscuring inflammation
Cellular atypia or suspicious malignancy

Report:
Hematuria
Pyuria
Bacteriuria and organisms
Crystalluria
Physiological casts
Lipiduria
Other

Additional procedures suggested
Microbiological studies
Cytochemical stains
Fluorescence microscopy
Electron microscopy

Additional procedures suggested
Microbiological studies
Polarizing microscopy for crystals
Stone analysis
Fat stains for lipiduria

Fig. 57-22 Coordinated approach to urine sediment examination. (From Schumann GB, Schumann JL, Schweitzer SC: *Lab Management* 1:47, 1983.)

Laboratories involved in the examination of urine must define new responsibilities for both the rapid, routine assessment of urine and the more time-consuming, specialized interpretive tests.[41]

Current, rapid dipstick technology and standardization of bright-field microscopy provide a quality program for the analysis of urine specimens from asymptomatic individuals. If symptomatic patients are to receive a more comprehensive urine examination, more definitive evaluation and confirmation procedures are required.

A coordinated approach to the examination of urine is depicted in Fig. 57-22. Proper use of this approach requires that the clinician and urine technologist understand the roles of both the routine laboratory, which offers basic urinalysis, and the specialized laboratory, which offers a more comprehensive sediment examination. After the collection of urine and macroscopic analysis, the physician or laboratory must differentiate between results from symptomatic and

asymptomatic patients. Emphasis must be placed on the urinalysis technologist's ability to recognize the results that require additional follow-up testing. This coordinated approach represents a flexible system in which technical responsibilities can be shared, and additional laboratory confirmation procedures can be integrated into the system (Fig. 57-22). Communication among physicians, the laboratory technologist, and the medical director is essential to resolve inconclusive results and reestablish credibility of the urine examination.

QUALITY CONTROL

An effective quality control program is essential to ensure accuracy in urinalysis. A program of quality assurance that covers all aspects of urinalysis and is similar to that used in other areas of the clinical laboratory must be implemented to achieve more reliable urinalysis results.[14]

Commercial quality control preparations are available for

Table 57-14   Suggested urinalysis quality control schedule

Areas checked	Daily	Weekly	Monthly	Semiannually or annually	As needed
Reagents and supplies					
Reagent strip	×				
Reagent tablets	×				
Remaking protein standard				×	
Equipment					
Refrigerator temperature	×				
Freezer temperature	×				
Refractometer calibration	×	×			
Urinometer calibration	×	×			
Spectrophotometer calibration		×			
Microscope maintenance				×	
Thermometers		×			
Glassware			×		
Centrifuge maintenance				×	
Education					
Revise laboratory manual				×	
Technologist's proficiency testing			×		
Update library				×	
Clinicopathological correlations					×

the assessment of specific gravity and reagent-strip testing. These preparations may be in tablet, strip, liquid, or lyophilized form. Hoeltge and Ersts[31] describe a 3-year experience using a synthetic-urine control prepared in their laboratory. Currently there is no ideal commercial preparation for urine sediment elements. Quality control of sediment evaluation should focus on standardized techniques and policies.

A suggested urinalysis quality control schedule is found in Table 57-14. It is important that reagents are dated when they are received by the laboratory and used before expiration. Urine control solutions should retain their utility if they are stored in a tightly stoppered container, refrigerated, and protected from light.[11] The new lot number should always be recorded. A laboratory manual containing operating instructions and documentation of equipment maintenance should be maintained and reviewed yearly. The importance of continuing education of technologists and the use of current references cannot be overemphasized.[42]

REFERENCES

1. Bonnardeau A, Sommerville P, Kaye M: A study on the reliability of dipstick urinalysis, *Clin Nephrol* 41:167-172, 1994.
2. Kennedy TJ, McConnell JD, Thall ER: Urine dipstick vs. microscopic urinalysis in the evaluation of abdominal trauma, *J Trauma* 28:615-617, 1988.
3. Free AH, Free MA: Rapid convenience urine tests: their use and misuse, *Lab Med* 9:9-17, 1978.
4. Schumann GB: *Urine sediment examination,* Baltimore, 1980, Williams & Wilkins.
5. Fairley KF, Birch DF: Microscopic urinalysis in glomerulonephritis, *Kidney Int* 44:9-12, 1993.
6. Eggensberger DL, King C, Gaudette LE, et al: Cytodiagnostic urinalysis: three year experience with a new laboratory test, *Am J Clin Pathol* 91:202-206, 1989.
7. Marcussen N, Schumann JL, Schumann GB, et al: Analysis of cytodiagnostic urinalysis findings in 77 patients with concurrent renal biopsies, *Am J Kidney Dis* 20:618-628, 1992.
8. Schumann GB, Schumann JL, Marcussen N: *Cytodiagnostic urinalysis of renal and lower urinary tract disorders,* New York, 1995, Igaku-Shoin.
9. Bradley M, Schumann GB, Ward PCJ: Examination of urine. In Henry JB, editor: *Todd-Sanford clinical diagnosis by laboratory methods,* ed 16, Philadelphia, 1979, Saunders.
10. Tentative Committee for Clinical Laboratory Standards: *Routine urinalysis and collection, transportation and preservation of urine specimen,* Villanova, Penna., 1992, 12(26) GP16-T.
11. Kunin CM: *Detection, prevention and management of urinary tract infections,* ed 2, Philadelphia, 1974, Lea & Febiger.
12. Cohen HT, Spiegel DM: Air-exposed urine dipsticks give false-positive results for glucose and false-negative results for blood, *Am J Clin Pathol* 96:398-400, 1991.
13. Zweiss MH, Jackson A: Ascorbic acid interference in reagent-strip reactions for assay of urinary glucose and hemoglobin, *Clin Chem* 32:674-677, 1986.
14. Schweitzer SC, Schumann JL, Schumann GB: Quality assurance guidelines for the urinalysis laboratory, *J Med Technol* 2:567-572, 1986.
15. Monte-Verde D, Nosanchuk JS: The sensitivity and specificity of nitrite testing for bacteriuria, *Lab Med* 12:755-757, 1981.
16. Shenoy UA: Current assessment of microhematuria and leukocyturia, *Clin Lab Med* 5:317-329, 1985.
17. Kusumi RK, Grover PJ, Kunin CM: Rapid detection of pyuria by leukocyte esterase activity, *JAMA* 245:1653-1655, 1981.
18. Gillenwater NY: Detection of urinary leukocytes by Chemstrip-L, *J Urol* 125:383-384, 1981.
19. Avent J, Schumann GB, Vars L: Comparison of the Chemstrip leukocyte test with a standardized Papanicolaou-stained urine sediment evaluation, *Lab Med* 14:163-166, 1983.
20. Race GJ, White MG: *Basic urinalysis,* Hagerstown, Md., 1979, Harper & Row.
21. Schumann GB, Greenberg NF: Usefulness of microscopic urinalysis as a screening procedure: a preliminary report, *Am J Clin Pathol* 71:452-456, 1979.
22. Ferris JA: Comparison and standardization of the urine microscopic examination, *Lab Med* 14:659-662, 1983.

23. Schumann GB, Tebbs RD: Comparison of slides used for standardized routine microscopic urinalysis, *J Med Technol* 3:54-58, 1986.

24. Winkel P, Statland BE, Jörgensen K: Urine microscopy: an ill-defined method examined by a multifactorial technique, *Clin Chem* 20:436-439, 1974.

25. Schumann GB, Weiss MA: *Atlas of renal and urinary tract cytology and its histopathologic bases,* Philadelphia, 1981, Lippincott.

26. Holmquist N: Detection of cancer with urinary sediment, *J Urol* 123:188-189, 1980.

27. Sternheimer R: A supravital cytodiagnostic stain for urinary sediment, *JAMA* 231:826-832, 1975.

28. Brody LH, Webster MC, Kark RM: Identification of elements of urinary sediment with phase contrast, *JAMA* 206:1777-1781, 1969.

29. Haber MH: Interference contrast microscopy for identification of urinary sediment, *Am J Clin Pathol* 57:316-319, 1972.

30. Haber MH: *Urinary sediment: a textbook atlas,* Chicago, 1981, American Society of Clinical Pathologists.

31. Kesson AM, Talbott JM, Gyory AZ: Microscopic examination of urine, *Lancet* 2:809-812, 1978.

32. Roe CE, Carlson DA, Daigneault RW, Statland BE: Evaluation of the Yellow IRIS™: an automated method for urinalysis, *Am J Clin Pathol* 86:661-665, 1986.

33. Elin RJ, Hosseini JM, Kestner J, et al: Comparison of automated and manual methods for urinalysis, *Am J Clin Pathol* 86:731-737, 1986.

34. Bard RH: The significance of asymptomatic microhematuria in women and its economic implications: a ten-year study, *Arch Intern Med* 148:2629-2632, 1988.

35. Thal SM, DeBellis CC, Iverson SA, Schumann GB: Comparison of dysmorphic erythrocytes with other urinary sediment parameters of renal bleeding, *Am J Clin Pathol* 86:784-787, 1986.

36. Kuster S, Ritz E: Fragmentocytes in the diagnosis of renal hematuria—observations in the 19th century, *Nephrol Dial Transplant* 9:569-570, 1994.

37. Stapleton FB: Morphology of urinary red blood cells: a simple guide in localizing the site of hematuria. *Pediatr Clin North Am* 34:561-569, 1987.

38. Kohler H, Wandel E, Brunck B: Acanthocyturia—a characteristic marker for glomerular bleeding, *Kidney Int* 40:115-120, 1991.

39. Little PJ: A comparison of the urinary white cell concentration with the white cell excretion rate, *Br J Urol* 36:360-363, 1964.

40. Mandel N: Urinary tract calculi, *Lab Med* 17:449-458, 1986.

41. Schumann GB, Schumann JL, Schweitzer S: Coordinated approach to the urine sediment examination, *Lab Management* 1:45-48, 1983.

42. Schweitzer SC, Schumann JL, Schumann GB: A model for educating future urine technologists, *J Med Technol* 2:251-255, 1986.

Appendix A: Buffer solutions*

Buffer solutions (or buffers) are solutions whose pH value is to a large degree insensitive to the addition of other substances. It is important to realize, however, that the pH value of a buffer solution does not change only when acids or bases are added or on dilution but also when the temperature changes or neutral salts are added. In accurate work, therefore, it is important to check the pH value electrometrically after all the ingredients have been added. The extent to which the pH values of buffer solutions vary when acids or bases are added or the temperature changes is shown in the table that follows. In general, dilution to half the concentration changes the pH value by only some hundredths of a unit (Buffer No. 1 in the table is an exception in that the change amounts to approximately pH 0.15); addition of 0.1-molar neutral salt solution may change the pH value of approximately 0.1.

In the table opposite the solutions are classified into general buffers (mostly in use for the last 50 years), universal buffers with a low buffering capacity but a wide pH range, and buffers for biological media with a moderate pH range but containing stable ingredients (phosphate and borate, for example, often undergo side reactions with biological media). An important property is often the transparency to ultraviolet light. Occasionally it is desirable to have a volatile buffer, which can be readily removed[1] (examples are buffers Nos. 20 and 21), but the use of very volatile systems makes a close control of the pH essential. Most of the pH data to be found in the literature relate to the Sørensen scale, and it should be noted that the values given in the following table of buffers are on the conventional pH scale.

Both stock and buffer solutions should be made up with distilled water free of CO_2. Only standard reagents should be used. If there is any doubt as to the purity or water content of solutions, their molarity must be checked by titration. The amounts x of stock solutions required to make up a buffer solution of the desired pH value are given in the second table in Appendix B.

*This appendix has been compiled by F. Kohler, Department of Physical Chemistry, University of Vienna, and taken from CIBA-Geigy AG, Basel, Switzerland.

REFERENCE

1. For a list of volatile buffers see Michl H: In Heftmann E, editor: *Chromatography,* part 1, New York, 1961, Reinhold, p 250.

No.	Name	pH range	Temperature	pH change per °C
General buffers				
1	KCl/HCl (Clark and Lubs)[1]	1.0- 2.2	Room	0
2	Glycine/HCl (Sørensen)[2]	1.2- 3.4	Room	0
3	Na citrate/HCl (Sørensen)[2]	1.2- 5.0	Room	0
4	K biphthalate/HCl (Clark and Lubs)[1]	2.4- 4.0	20° C	+0.001
5	K biphthalate/NaOH (Clark and Lubs)[1]	4.2- 6.2	20° C	
6	Na citrate/NaOH (Sørensen)[2]	5.2- 6.6	20° C	+0.004
7	Phosphate (Sørensen)[2]	5.0- 8.0	20° C	−0.003
8	Barbital-Na/HCl (Michaelis)[3]	7.0- 9.0	18° C	
9	Na borate/HCl (Sørensen)[2]	7.8- 9.2	20° C	−0.005
10	Glycine/NaOH (Sørensen)[2]	8.6-12.8	20° C	−0.025
11	Na borate/NaOH (Sørensen)[2]	9.4-10.6	20° C	−0.01
Universal buffers				
12	Citric acid/phosphate (McIlvaine)[4]	2.2- 7.8	21° C	
13	Citrate-phosphate-borate/HCl (Teorell and Stenhagen)[5]	2.0-12.0	20° C	
14	Britton-Robinson[6]	2.6-11.8	25° C	at low pH 0 at high pH −0.02
Buffers for biological media				
15	Acetate (Walpole)[7-9]	3.8- 5.6	25° C	
16	Dimethylglutaric acid/NaOH[10]	3.2- 7.6	21° C	
17	Piperazine/HCl[11,12]	4.6- 6.4 8.8-10.6	20° C	
18	Tetraethylethylenediamine*[12]	5.0- 6.8 8.2-10.0	20° C	
19	Trismaleate[7,13]	5.2- 8.6	23° C	
20	Dimethylaminoethylamine*[12]	5.6- 7.4 8.6-10.4	20° C	
21	Imidazole/HCl[14]	6.2- 7.8	25° C	
22	Triethanolamine/HCl[15]	7.0- 8.8	25° C	
23	N-Dimethylaminoleucylglycine/NaOH[16]	7.0- 8.8	23° C	−0.015
24	Tris/HCl[7]	7.2- 9.0	23° C	−0.02
25	2-Amino-2-methylpropane-1,3-diol/HCl[7,13]	7.8-10.0	23° C	
26	Carbonate (Delory and King)[7,17]	9.2-10.8	20° C	

From *Geigy scientific tables,* ed 8, Basel, Switzerland, 1981, CIBA-Geigy AG.
*Can be combined with tris buffer to give a cationic universal buffer (see reference 12).

REFERENCES

1. Clark and Lubs: *J Bact* 2:1, 1917.
2. Sørensen SPL: *Biochem Z* 21:131, 1909, 22:352, 1909; Ergebn Physiol 12:393, 1912; and Walbum LE: *Biochem Z* 107:219, 1920.
3. Michaelis L: *J Biol Chem* 87:33, 1930.
4. McIlvaine TC: *J Biol Chem* 49:183, 1921.
5. Teorell and Stenhagen: *Biochem Z* 299:416, 1938.
6. Britton and Welford: *J Chem Soc,* 1937, 1848.
7. Gomori G: In Colowick and Kaplan, editors: *Methods in enzymology,* vol 1, New York, 1955, Academic Press, p 138.
8. Walpole GS: *J Chem Soc* 105:2501, 1914.
9. Green AA: *J Am Chem Soc* 55:2331, 1933.
10. Stafford et al: *Biochim Biophys Acta* 18:319, 1955; Krebs, HA, unpublished, 1957.
11. Smith and Smith: *Biol Bull* 96:233, 1949.
12. Semenza et al: *Helv Chim Acta* 45:2306, 1962.
13. Gomori G: *Proc Soc Exp Biol* (NY) 68:354, 1948.
14. Mertz and Owen: *Proc Soc Exp Biol* (NY) 43:204, 1940, quoted by Rauen HM, editor: *Biochemisches Taschenbuch,* ed 2, part 2, Berlin, 1964, Springer, p 90.
15. Beisenherz et al: *Z Naturforsch* 8b:555, 1953.
16. Leonis J: *CR Lab Carlsberg, Sér Chim* 26:357, 1948.
17. Delory and King: *Biochem J* 39:245, 1945.

Appendix B: Preparation of buffer solutions

When not otherwise specified, both stock and buffer solutions should be made up with distilled water free of CO_2. Only standard reagents should be used. If there is any doubt as to the purity or water content of solutions, their molarity must be checked by titration. The amounts x of stock solutions required to make up a buffer solution of the desired pH value are given in the table in the second part of Appendix B.

| Buffer no. | Stock solutions | | Composition of the buffer |
	A	B	
1	KCl 0.2-N (14.91 g/l)	HCl 0.2-N	25 ml A + x ml B made up to 100 ml
2	Glycine 0.1-molar in NaCl 0.1-N (7.507 g glycine + 5.844 g NaCl/l)	HCl 0.1-N	x ml A + (100 − x) ml B
3	Disodium citrate 0.1-molar (21.01 g $C_6H_8O_7 \cdot 1H_2O$ + 200 ml NaOH 1-N per liter)	HCl 0.1-N	x ml A + (100 − x) ml B
4	Potassium biphthalate 0.1-molar (20.42 g $KHC_8H_4O_4$/l)	HCl 0.1-N	50 ml A + x ml B made up to 100 ml
5	As No. 4	NaOH 0.1-N	50 ml A + x ml B made up to 100 ml
6	As No. 3	NaOH 0.1-N	x ml A + (100 − x) ml B
7	Monopotassium phosphate $1/15$-molar (9.073 g KH_2PO_4/l)	Disodium phosphate $1/15$-molar (11.87 g $Na_2HPO_4 \cdot 2H_2O$/l)	x ml A + (100 − x) ml B
8	Barbital sodium 0.1-molar (20.62 g/l)	HCl 0.1-N	x ml A + (100 − x) ml B
9	Boric acid, half-neutralized, 0.2-molar (corr. to 0.05-molar borax: 12.37 g boric acid + 100 ml NaOH 1-N per liter)	HCl 0.1-N	x ml A + (100 − x) ml B
10	As No. 2	NaOH 0.1-N	x ml A + (100 − x) ml B
11	As No. 9	NaOH 0.1-N	x ml A + (100 − x) ml B
12	Citric acid 0.1-molar (21.01 g $C_6H_8O_7 \cdot 1H_2O$/l)	Disodium phosphate 0.2-molar (35.60 g $Na_2HPO_4 \cdot 2H_2O$/l)	x ml A + (100 − x) ml B
13	To citric acid and phosphoric acid solutions (ca. 100 ml), each equivalent to 100 ml NaOH 1-N, add 3.54 cryst. orthoboric acid and 343 ml NaOH 1-N, and make up the mixture to 1 liter	HCl 0.1-N	20 ml A + x ml B made up to 100 ml
14	Citric acid, monopotassium phosphate, barbital, boric acid, all 0.02857-molar (6.004 g $C_6H_8O_7$ $\cdot 1H_2O$, 3.888 g KH_2PO_4, 5.263 g barbital, 1.767 g H_3BO_3/l)	NaOH 0.2-N	100 ml A + x ml B
15	Sodium acetate 0.1-N (8.204 g $C_2H_3O_2Na$ or 13.61 g $C_2H_3O_2Na$ $\cdot 3H_2O$/l)	Acetic acid 0.1-N (6.005 g/l)	x ml A + (100 − x) ml B

From *Geigy scientific tables,* ed 8, Basel, Switzerland, 1981, CIBA-Geigy AG.

Buffer no.	Stock solutions		Composition of the buffer
	A	B	
16	ββ-Dimethylglutaric acid 0.1-molar (16.02 g/l)	NaOH 0.2-N	(a) 100 ml A + x ml B made up to 1000 ml (b) 100 ml A + x ml B + 5.844 g NaCl made up to 1000 ml (NaCl $\triangleq$ 0.1-molar)
17	Piperazine 1-molar (86.14 g/l)	HCl 0.1-N	5 ml A + x ml B made up to 100 ml
18	Tetraethylethylenediamine 1-molar (172.32 g/l)	HCl 0.1-N	5 ml A + x ml B made up to 100 ml
19	Tris acid maleate 0.2-molar (24.23 g tris[hydroxymethyl]aminomethane + 23.21 g maleic acid or 19.61 g maleic anhydride/l)	NaOH 0.2-N	25 ml A + x ml B made up to 100 ml
20	Dimethylaminoethylamine 1-molar (88 g/l)	HCl 0.1-N	5 ml A + x ml B made up to 100 ml
21	Imidazole (0.2-molar (13.62 g/l)	HCl 0.1-N	25 ml A + x ml B made up to 100 ml
22	Triethanolamine 0.5-molar (76.11 g/l) containing 20 g/l ethylenediaminetetraacetic acid disodium salt ($C_{10}H_{14}O_8N_2Na_2 \cdot 2H_2O$)	HCl 0.05-N	10 ml A + x ml B made up to 100 ml
23	N-Dimethylaminoleucylglycine 0.1-molar (24.33 g $C_{10}H_{20}O_3N_2 \cdot \frac{3}{2}H_2O$/l) containing NaCl 0.2-N (11.69 g/l)	NaOH 1-N 100 ml made up to 1 liter with A	x ml A + (100 − x) ml B
24	Tris 0.2-molar (24.23 g tris[hydroxymethyl]aminomethane/l)	HCl 0.1-N	25 ml A + x ml B made up to 100 ml
25	2-Amino-2-methylpropane-1,3-diol 0.1-molar (10.51 g/l)	HCl 0.1-N	50 ml A + x ml B made up to 100 ml
26	Sodium carbonate anhydrous 0.1-molar (10.60 g/l)	Sodium bicarbonate 0.1-molar (8.401 g/l)	x ml A + (100 − x) ml B

The table gives the amounts (x ml) of the stock solutions listed in the first part of Appendix B required to make up a buffer solution of the desired pH value.

pH	1	2	3	4	5	6	7	8	9	10	11	12	13	14	15	16a	16b	17	18	19	20	21	22	23	24	25	26	pH
1.0	54.2																											1.0
1.2	36.0	11.1	9.0																									1.2
1.4	23.2	26.4	17.9																									1.4
1.6	14.7	36.2	23.6																									1.6
1.8	9.3	43.9	27.6																									1.8
2.0	5.9	50.7	30.2									98.8																2.0
2.2	3.8	56.5	32.2									94.5	74.4															2.2
2.4		62.3	34.1	41.0								90.0	68.8															2.4
2.6		68.4	36.0	34.3								85.1	64.6	1.6														2.6
2.8		74.7	37.9	27.8								80.3	61.3	3.6														2.8
3.0		81.0	39.9	21.6								76.0	58.9	5.7														3.0
3.2		86.2	42.1	15.9								72.0	56.9	7.8														3.2
3.4		90.3	44.8	10.9								68.4	55.2	9.9		7.0												3.4
3.6			47.8	6.7								65.1	53.9	11.7		13.3	14.4											3.6
3.8			51.2	3.3								62.0	51.8	13.5	10.9	20.7	20.9											3.8
4.0			55.1	0.0								59.1	50.7	15.3	16.6	26.3	26.8											4.0
4.2			60.0		3.0							56.4	49.7	17.5	23.9	32.4	32.4											4.2
4.4			66.4		6.7							53.7	48.6	19.7	33.5	36.2	36.6											4.4
4.6			74.9		11.1							51.2	47.5	21.9	44.9	39.3	40.3	94.3										4.6
4.8			85.6		16.5							49.0	45.4	24.1	56.6	41.3	43.1	87.8										4.8
5.0			100.0		22.6		99.2					46.9	44.3	26.3	67.8	43.5	45.7	83.6	94.3									5.0
5.2					28.8	87.1	98.4					44.7	42.0	28.6	76.8	45.7	48.3	77.8	91.5	3.2								5.2
5.4					34.4	78.0	97.3					42.4	40.8	31.0	84.0	48.4	51.5	71.8	87.8	5.0								5.4
5.6					39.1	70.3	95.5					40.0	39.7	33.4	89.3	51.3	53.6	66.5	83.1	7.3	94.3							5.6
5.8					42.4	64.5	92.8					37.4	38.4	35.8		55.0	58.2	61.8	77.6	9.7	91.7							5.8
6.0					45.0	60.3	88.9					34.5	37.0	38.3		58.8	63.6	58.2	71.7	12.4	88.0	43.4						6.0
6.2					46.7	57.2	83.0					31.4	35.6	40.8		63.9	68.7	55.5	66.4	15.2	83.3	40.4						6.2
6.4						54.8	75.4					27.9	34.2	43.3		69.5	73.6		61.7	17.9	77.9	36.5						6.4
6.6						53.2	65.3					23.5	32.9	45.8		74.1	78.5		58.0	20.8	72.0	31.4						6.6
6.8							53.4	53.3				19.0	31.7	48.3		83.5	83.3		55.3	22.2	66.6	25.4						6.8
7.0							41.3	55.0				13.8	30.6	50.9		87.4	87.4			23.7	61.9	19.6	86.2	86.4				7.0
7.2							29.6	57.6				9.8	29.6	53.4		90.0	91.0			25.2	58.1	14.6	79.6	80.6				7.2
7.4							19.7	60.8				6.8	28.8	55.8		91.8	93.2			26.7	55.3	10.2	71.3	72.8	44.7			7.4
7.6							12.8	65.2				4.6	28.1	58.2		93.0	94.9			28.6		6.6	62.0	63.2	42.0	43.9		7.6
7.8							7.4	70.6	53.0				27.6	60.5		93.8	95.8			31.2			52.0	52.1	39.3	41.6		7.8
8.0							3.7	75.9	55.4				27.0	62.8			96.8			33.9			42.0	41.1	33.7	38.4		8.0
8.2								81.2	58.0	94.7			26.3	65.0					46.4	36.9			31.9	31.4	27.9	34.8		8.2
8.4								86.2	62.1	92.0			25.2	67.2					43.9	39.9			22.5	22.9	22.9	30.7		8.4
8.6								90.1	73.6	88.4			24.0	69.3				45.5	40.9	42.7	45.4		16.0	15.9	17.3	23.3		8.6
8.8								93.2	83.5	84.0			22.6	71.3				43.2	36.8		42.8		11.7	10.3	13.0	17.7		8.8
9.0									95.6	78.9			21.4	73.2				40.0	31.8		39.2				8.8	13.3		9.0
9.2										73.2	87.0		20.2	75.1				35.8	26.2		34.7				5.3	9.2	10.0	9.2
9.4										67.2	75.5		19.0	77.0				30.8	20.4		29.3					5.2	18.4	9.4
9.6										62.5	65.1		18.1	78.8				25.0	15.2		23.6					4.1	29.3	9.6
9.8										58.8	59.6		17.1	80.4				19.4	10.8		19.0					2.3	42.0	9.8
10.0										55.7	56.4		16.5	81.8				14.3	7.4		13.1						53.4	10.0
10.2										53.6	54.1		16.0	83.1				10.0			9.2						63.7	10.2
10.4										52.2	52.3		15.5	84.3				6.9			6.2						73.1	10.4
10.6										51.2			14.7	85.4													81.2	10.6
10.8										50.4			13.5	86.5													87.9	10.8
11.0										49.5			11.7	87.8														11.0
11.2										48.7			9.1	89.3														11.2
11.4										47.6			5.5	91.3														11.4
11.6										46.0			1.3	94.5														11.6
11.8										43.2				99.0														11.8
12.0										39.1																		12.0
12.2										31.8																		12.2
12.4										21.4																		12.4
12.6																												12.6
12.8																												12.8

From *Geigy scientific tables*, ed 8, Basel, Switzerland, 1981, CIBA-Geigy AG.

Appendix C: Concentrations of common acids and bases

Compound	Molecular weight	Specific gravity	Percent	Normality	mL/liter for 1N* solution
HCl	36.46	1.19	36.0	11.7	85.5
HNO_3	63.02	1.42	69.5	15.6	64.0
H_2SO_4	98.08	1.84	96.0	35.9	28.4
CH_3COOH	60.03	1.06	99.5	17.6	56.9
NH_4OH	35.04	0.90	58.6	15.1	66.5
H_3PO_4	98.00	1.69	85.0	44.1	22.7
Thioglycolic acid	92.12	1.26	80.0	10.9	91.3
HCOOH	46.03	1.21	97.0	25.5	39.2
	46.03	1.19	88.0	22.7	44.1
$HClO_4$	100.50	1.67	70.0	11.65	85.7
Pyridine	79.10	0.98	100.0	12.4	80.6
2-Mercaptoethanol	78.13	1.14	100.0	14.6	68.5

From Brewer JM, Pesce AJ, Ashworth H: *Experimental techniques in biochemistry,* Engelwood Cliffs, NJ, 1974, Prentice-Hall, Inc.
To calculate concentration *(c)* from the weight percent *(w)* of a compound, use the formula:

$$\frac{10\ ws}{M} = c.$$

M, Molecular weight; *s,* specific gravity.
*Remember, the normality *(N)* is not the same as the molarity *(M)* for sulfuric and phosphoric acid.

Appendix D: Gases in common laboratory use—technical information

| Product | Formula | State | Cylinder specifications | | | | Thermophysical properties | | |
			CGA no. valve outlet	Highest purity grade (%)	Cylinder size (cubic feet)	Approximate cylinder pressure (psi)	Molecular weight	Vapor pressure at 21.1° C (psig)	Specific gravity at 21.1° C (1 atm)
Acetylene	C_2H_2	Dissolved gas (in acetone)	510/300	99.6	3-5	250	26.04	635	0.095
Air		Compressed gas	346/677	Mixture	200-500	2200-6000	28.96		1
Carbon dioxide	CO_2	Liquefied gas	320	99.999	2-6	274-838	44.01	839	1.53
Carbon monoxide	CO	Compressed gas	350	99.99	2-6	315-1602	28.01	*	0.97
Helium	He	Compressed gas	580/677	99.9999	200-300	2200-2640	4.003	*	0.138
Hydrogen	H_2	Compressed gas	350	99.9995	2-200	323-2200	2.02	*	0.0695
Methane	CH_4	Compressed gas	350	99.992	12	780-2000	16.04	*	0.555
Nitrogen	N_2	Compressed gas	580/677	99.999	30-200	2200-2640	28.01	*	0.967
Oxygen	O_2	Compressed gas	540	99.995	30-200	2200-2640	32.0	*	1.105
Propane	C_3H_8	Liquefied gas	510	99.98	12	109	44.1	109	1.55

Data derived from the *Airco Industrial Cases catalogue,* Murray Hill, NJ, 1977.
SA, Simple asphyxiant.
*Above critical temperature at 21.1° C.

Thermophysical properties			Hazardous properties			
			Flammability			
Critical temperature (°C)	Critical pressure (psia)	Specific volume (cf/lb)	Flammable limits in air (vol %)	Ignition temperature (°C)	Physiological properties	Threshold limit value (ppm)
35.1	890	14.7	2.3-100	305		SA
		13.3			Oxidant	
31.0	1071	8.74			Inert	5000
−140.0	507.4	13.8	12.5-74	651.1	Toxic	50
−267.8	33.2	96.7				SA
−239.98	190.8	192	4-75	585		SA
−82.1	673	23.7	5-15	538		SA
−146.9	492.9	13.8			Inert	SA
−118.4	736.9	12.1			Oxidant	
96.8	617.4	8.5	2.1-9.5	468		SA

Appendix E: Major plasma proteins*

Protein	Molecular weight	Concentration, mg/100 mL	Electrophoretic† mobility	Biological function
Prealbumins				
Thyroxine binding (TBPA)	55,000	10-40	7.6	Thyroxine transport
Retinol binding (RBP)	21,000	3-6		Vitamin A transport
Albumin	66,300	3500-5500	5.92	Maintain osmotic pressure, transport of bilirubin, free fatty acids, anions, and cations, cell nutrition
α_1 Globulins				
α_1 Acid glycoprotein (α_1S)	40,000	55-140	5.7	Unknown, inactivates progesterone
α_1 Antitrypsin (α_1AT)	54,000	200-400	5.42	Antiserine type of protease
α_1 Glycoprotein (9.5S, α_1M)	308,000	3-8	α_1	Unknown
α_1 Glycoprotein B (α_1B)	50,000	15-30	α_1	Unknown
α_1 Glycoprotein T (α_1T)	60,000	5-12	α_1	Unknown, tryptophan poor
α_1 Antichymotrypsin (α_1X)	68,000	30-60	α_1	Chymotrypsin inhibitor
α_1 Lipoproteins, high density (HDL)	28,000	254-387	α_1	Lipid transport
α_2 Globulins				
G_0 Globulin (Gc)	51,000	40-70	α_2	Vitamin D transport
Ceruloplasmin (Cp)	134,000	15-60	4.6	Copper transport, peroxidase activity
α_2 Glycoprotein, histidine rich (HRG)	58,000	5-15	α_2	Unknown
Zn-α_2-glycoprotein (Znα_2)	41,000	2-15	4.2	Unknown, binds Zn^{2+}
α_2 HS-glycoprotein (α_2HS)	49,000	40-85	4.2	Unknown, binds Ba^{2+}
α_2 Macroglobulin (α_2M)	725,000	150-420	4.2	Inhibitor of thrombin, trypsin, and pepsin
Transcortin (TC)	49,500	<7	α_2	Cortisol transport
Haptoglobins (Hp)				
Type 1-1	100,000	100-200	4.1	Binds hemoglobin, prevents loss of iron
Type 2-1	200,000	160-300	α_2	Binds hemoglobin, prevents loss of iron
Type 2-2	400,000	120-260	α_2	
α_2 Lipoproteins (VLDL)	250,000	150-230	Pre-β	Lipid transport
Thyroxine-binding protein (TBG)	58,000	1-2	α_2	Thyroxine transport
β Globulins				
Hemopexin (Hpx)	57,000	50-100	3.1	Binds heme
Transferrin (Tf)	76,500	200-320	3.1	Iron transport
β Lipoproteins (LDL)	250,000	280-440	3.1	Lipid transport
C4 Complement component (C4)	206,000	40-80	β_1	Complement system
β_2 Microglobulin ($\beta_2\mu$)	11,818	Trace	β_2	Common portion of the HLA transplantation antigen
β_2 Glycoprotein I (β_2 I)	40,000	15-30	1.6	Unknown
β_2 Glycoprotein II (GGG)	63,000	12-30	β_2	C3 activator (activates properidin)
β_2 Glycoprotein III (β_2 III)	35,000	5-15	β_2	Unknown
C-Reactive protein (CRP)	118,000	1	β_2	Opsonin, motivates phagocytosis in inflammatory disease
C3 Complement component (C3)	180,000	55-180	β_2	Complement system
Fibrinogen (ϕ, Fib.)	341,000	200-600	2.1	Blood clotting
γ Globulins				
Immunoglobulin M (IgM)	950,000	60-250	2.1	Antibodies, early response
Immunoglobulin E (IgE)	190,000	0.06	2.1	Reagin of the allergy system
Immunoglobulin A (IgA)	160,000	90-450	2.1	Tissue antibodies
Immunoglobulin D (IgD)	160,000	15	1.9	Cell surface and plasma antibodies
Immunoglobulin G (IgG)	160,000	800-1800	1.2	Antibodies, long range

From Natelson S, Natelson EA: *Principles of applied chemistry,* vol 3, New York, 1980, Plenum Publishing Corp.
*Does not include clotting factors, complement factors, or enzymes except fibrinogen, C3 and C4 of complement, which occur in substantial concentrations.
†Tiselius moving boundary electrophoresis in Tiselius units ($cm^2\ V^{-1}\ sec^{-1} \times 10^5$, at 0° C, pH 8.6, and ionic strength 0.15).

Appendix F: Conversions between conventional and SI units

Conventional units		× Factor	= SI units
Gram	g/mL	$\dfrac{10^{15}}{mw}$	pmol/L
	g/100 mL	10	g/L
	g/100 mL	$\dfrac{10}{mw}$	mol/L
	g/100 mL	$\dfrac{10^4}{mw}$	mmol/L
	g/d	$\dfrac{1}{mw}$	mol/d
	g/d	$\dfrac{10^3}{mw}$	mmol/d
	g/d	$\dfrac{10^9}{mw}$	nmol/d
Microgram	μg/100 mL	$\dfrac{10}{mw}$	μmol/L
	μg/d	$\dfrac{1}{mw}$	μmol/d
	μg/d	$\dfrac{10^3}{mw}$	nmol/d
Picogram	pg	$\dfrac{10^3}{mw}$	fmol
	pg/mL	$\dfrac{10^3}{mw}$	pmol/L
Milliequivalent	mEq/L	$\dfrac{1}{valence}$	mmol/L
	mEq/kg	$\dfrac{1}{valence}$	mmol/kg
	mEq/d	$\dfrac{1}{valence}$	mmol/d

Conventional units		× Factor	= SI units
Milligram	mg/100 mL	10^{-2}	g/L
	mg/100 mL	$\dfrac{10^{-2}}{mw}$	mol/L
	mg/100 mL	$\dfrac{10}{mw}$	mmol/L
	mg/100 mL	$\dfrac{10^4}{mw}$	μmol/L
	mg/100 g	10	mg/kg
	mg/100 g	$\dfrac{10}{mw}$	mmol/kg
	mg/d	$\dfrac{1}{mw}$	mmol/d
	mg/d	$\dfrac{10^3}{mw}$	μmol/d
Milliliter	mL/100 g	10	mL/kg
	mL/min	1.667×10^{-2}	mL/s
Millimeters of mercury	mm Hg	1.333	mbar
	mm Hg	0.133	kPa
Minute	min	60	s
	min	0.06	ks
Percent	%	10^{-2}	1 (unit)
	% (g/100 g)	10	g/kg
	% (g/100 g)	10^{-2}	kg/kg
	% (g/100 mL)	10	g/L
	% (g/100 mL)	$\dfrac{10}{mw}$	mol/L
	% (g/100 mL)	$\dfrac{10^4}{mw}$	mmol/L
	% (mL/100 mL)	10^{-2}	L/L

Modified from Campbell JM, Campbell JB: *Laboratory mathematics*, ed 3, St. Louis, 1983, Mosby.
d, Day; *Eq,* equivalent; *g,* gram; *L,* liter; *min,* minute; *mw,* molecular weight; *Pa,* pascal; *s,* second. *f,* Femto (10^{-15}); *p,* pico (10^{-12}); *n,* nano (10^{-9}); μ, micro (10^{-6}); *m,* milli (10^{-3}); *k,* kilo (10^{3}).

Appendix G: Conversions between conventional and SI units for specific analytes

| Analyte | Conventional units | Multiply by | | SI unit |
		Conventional to SI	SI to conventional	
Acetominophen	µg/mL	6.61	0.151	µmol/L
Albumin	g/100 mL	144.9	0.0069	µmol/L
Ammonia	µg/100 mL	0.59	1.7	µmol/L
Anticonvulsant drugs				
Carbamazepine	µg/mL	4.32	0.23	µmol/L
Ethosuximide	µg/mL	7.08	0.14	µmol/L
Phenobarbital	µg/mL	4.31	0.23	µmol/L
Phenytoin	µg/mL	3.96	0.25	µmol/L
Primidone	µg/mL	4.58	0.22	µmol/L
Valproic acid	µg/mL	6.93	0.14	µmol/L
Bilirubin	mg/100 mL	17.1	0.059	µmol/L
Bromide	µg/mL	0.0125	80	mmol/L
Calcium	mg/100 mL	0.25	4	mmol/L
Chloride	mEq/L	1	1	mmol/L
Cholesterol	mg/100 mL	0.026	38.7	mmol/L
Cortisol	µg/100 mL	0.0276	36.2	µmol/L
Creatinine	mg/100 mL	88.4	0.0113	µmol/L
Digoxin	ng/mL	1.28	0.781	nmol/L
Estriol	µg/L	3.47	0.288	nmol/L
Ferritin	µg/L	2.2	0.445	pmol/L
Folic acid	µg/100 mL	22.7	0.044	nmol/L
Gentamicin	µg/mL	2.22	0.45	µmol/L
Glucose	mg/100 mL	0.055	18	mmol/L
Haptoglobin	mg/100 mL	0.118	8.47	µmol/L
HDL cholesterol	mg/100 mL	0.026	38.7	mmol/L
HCG	U/L	—	—	—
5-HIAA	mg	5.23	0.19	µmol
Ig A	mg/100 mL	0.0625	16	µmol/L
D	mg/100 mL	0.054	18.5	µmol/L
E	ng/mL	0.005	200	nmol/L
G	mg/100 mL	0.067	15	µmol/L
M	mg/100 mL	0.011	91	µmol/L
Insulin	pg/mL	0.174	5.74	nmol/L
	µU/mL	7.25	0.138	nmol/L
Iron	µg/100 mL	0.179	5.58	µmol/L
Ketones (acetoacetate)	mg/L	0.111	9.01	mmol/L
Lead	µg/L	4.83	0.207	nmol/L
Lithium	mEq/L	1	1	mmol/L
LDL cholesterol	mg/100 mL	0.026	38.7	mmol/L
Magnesium	mg/100 mL	0.41	2.43	mmol/L
Phosphorus	mg/100 mL	0.323	3.1	mmol/L
Phenylalanine	mg/L	6.05	0.165	µmol/L
Potassium	mEq/L	1	1	mmol/L

| Analyte | Conventional units | Multiply by | | SI unit |
		Conventional to SI	SI to conventional	
Quinidine	μg/mL	3.09	0.324	μmol/L
Salicylate	mg/100 mL	0.0724	13.8	mmol/L
Sodium	mEq/L	1	1	mmol/L
TIBC	μg/100 mL	0.179	5.58	μmol/L
Theophylline	μg/mL	5.55	0.180	μmol/L
Thyroid-stimulating hormone	mU/L	—	—	—
Thyroxine	μg/100 mL	12.9	0.078	nmol/L
Transferrin	mg/100 mL	0.11	9.09	μmol/L
Triglycerides	mg/100 mL	0.0114	87.5	mmol/L
Urea	mg/100 mL	0.166	6.01	mmol/L
Urea N	mg/100 mL	0.356	2.81	mmol/L
Uric acid	mg/100 mL	59.5	0.0168	μmol/L
Vanillylmandelic acid	mg	5.03	0.20	μmol
VLDL cholesterol	mg/100 mL	0.026	38.7	mmol/L
Vitamin B_{12}	pg/mL	0.738	1.36	pmol/L
Gases	mm Hg	0.133	7.51	kPa
Enzymes	U/L	1.67×10^{-8}	0.6×10^{8}	katal/L

Appendix H: Body surface of children

Nomogram for determination of body surface from height and mass*

Height	Body surface	Mass

From *Geigy scientific tables,* ed 8, Basel, Switzerland, 1981, CIBA-Geigy AG.
*From the formula of Du Bois and Du Bois: *Arch Intern Med* 17:863, 1916: $S = M^{0.425} \times H^{0.725} \times 71.84$, or $\log S = \log M \times 0.425 + \log H \times 0.725 + 1.8564$ (S, body surface in cm^2; M, mass in kg; H, height in cm).

Appendix I: Body surface of adults

Nomogram for determination of body surface from height and mass*

Height	Body surface	Mass

Height (cm / in):
cm 200 — 79 in, 78, 195 — 77, 76, 190 — 75, 74, 185 — 73, 72, 180 — 71, 70, 175 — 69, 68, 170 — 67, 66, 165 — 65, 64, 160 — 63, 62, 155 — 61, 60, 150 — 59, 58, 145 — 57, 56, 140 — 55, 54, 135 — 53, 52, 130 — 51, 50, 125 — 49, 48, 120 — 47, 46, 115 — 45, 44, 110 — 43, 42, 105 — 41, 40, cm 100 — 39 in

Body surface (m^2):
2.80 m², 2.70, 2.60, 2.50, 2.40, 2.30, 2.20, 2.10, 2.00, 1.95, 1.90, 1.85, 1.80, 1.75, 1.70, 1.65, 1.60, 1.55, 1.50, 1.45, 1.40, 1.35, 1.30, 1.25, 1.20, 1.15, 1.10, 1.05, 1.00, 0.95, 0.90, 0.86 m²

Mass (kg / lb):
kg 150 — 330 lb, 145 — 320, 140 — 310, 135 — 300, 130 — 290, 125 — 280, 120 — 270, 115 — 260, 110 — 250, 105 — 240, 100 — 230, 95 — 220, 90 — 210, 85 — 200, 80 — 190, 180, 75 — 170, 70 — 160, 150, 65 — 140, 60 — 130, 55 — 120, 50 — 110, 105, 45 — 100, 95, 40 — 90, 85, 35 — 80, 75, 70, kg 30 — 66 lb

From *Geigy scientific tables,* ed 8, Basel, Switzerland, 1981, CIBA-Geigy AG.
*From the formula of Du Bois and Du Bois: *Arch Intern Med* 17:863, 1916: $S = M^{0.425} \times H^{0.725} \times 71.84$, or $\log S = \log M \times 0.425 + \log H \times 0.725 + 1.8564$ (S, body surface in cm^2; M, mass in kg; H, height in cm).

Index

A

A; *see* Alanine
A (adenine), *970*
A (atomic mass number), 187
A posteriori sampling, 369
A priori sampling, 369
AAT; *see* Alpha-₁-antitrypsin
Abbé refractometers, *104,* 104-105
Abbott TDx/FLx, IMx, AXSYM, 304, 305*t*
Abdominal pain, clinical problems associated
    with, *562*
Abdominal paracentesis fluid, 821
Abell et al procedure, cholesterol, 673, 674*t*
Abetalipoproteinemia, 644, 662-663
Abnormal, 365
ABO blood groups, 239
ABP (androgen-binding protein), 895, 898
Absence, 837
Absorb, 65
Absorbance, 38, 83, 87, 425
    absorbance error versus, *426*
    background, *430*
    blank, *430*
    delta, 429
    relationship between transmittance and, *87,*
        88
    true, *88*
Absorbance detection, 146-147
Absorbance error, 425*t*
    absorbance versus, *426*
Absorbance variance, 425
Absorption, 484, 1086, 1088
    carbohydrate, 576
    fat, 576-577
    gastrointestinal function, 576-577
    iron, 577
    protein, 576
    sodium, 577
    water, 577
Absorption peak, wider, 92
Absorption process, 85-86
Absorption rate constant, 1086, 1095
Absorption spectra
    of fluorescent compound, *98*
    idealized, schema of, *93*
Absorption spectrophotometry
    errors in, 425
    limits in, 426
Absorption spectroscopy, 87-95
Absorption spectrum, 83, 86, *1065*
    of NAD and NADH, *1065*
    of oxyhemoglobin, *86*

Page numbers in **boldface** indicate structural
formulas.
Page numbers in *italics* indicate illustrations
and boxed material.
Page numbers followed by *t* indicate tables.

Absorptive fat phase, 643
Absorptivity, 83
    molar, 84, 88
Abused substances, 1017
ACA Star instrument, 296-297*t,* 301
ACA V instrument, 296-297*t,* 301
AcAc (acetoacetate), 625
Acarboxyprothrombin, 769
ACAT (acyl-CoA:cholesterol acyltransferase),
    647, 654
Accelerating voltage, 167
Acceptance regions for rank sum *T,* 358, 359*t*
Access, 306*t,* 307-308
Accession number, 327
Accreditation program, laboratory, 183
Accuracy, 342, 350, 402
    control required by CLIA '88, 398-399
Accutane (13-*cis*-retinoic acid), 764
ACE; *see* Angiotensin-converting enzyme
Acetaldehyde, 687
p-Acetamidobenzoylglutamic acid, 783
Acetaminophen, 289*t,* 513, 1020
    plasma, *1027*
    principles of analysis, 1025-1026, 1026*t*
    specimen, 1026
    spot tests for, 1027*t*
Acetate, 897
Acetest, 630
Acetoacetate (AcAc), 625
Acetoacetic acid
    methods of analysis, 631-632
    principles of analysis and current usage,
        631, 633
    specimen, 633
Acetone, 272*t*
"Acetone" bodies, 270
Acetyl coenzyme A (acetyl CoA), 508
Acetyl-L-carnitine, 786
Acetylcholine, 833
    as neuromuscular transmitter, 594-595
Acetylcholinesterase (AChE), 833, 967
N-Acetylneuraminic acid, **1054**
N-Acetylprocainamide (NAPA)
    principles of analysis, 610-611, 611*t*
    specimen, 611
Acetylsalicylic acid; *see* Salicylates
AChE (acetylcholinesterase), 833, 967
Achlorhydria, 571, 582
Acid-base balance, 468-471
    disorders of, effects on selected blood-gas
        parameters, 476*t*
    kidneys and, 489-490
    in normal cerebrospinal fluid, *832*
Acid-base control, 465-471
Acid-base disorders, 471-476
    classes of, 475*t*
Acid-base pair, conjugate, 465
Acid-base parameters, blood, 473

Acid phosphatase (ACP), 893, 990, 1080-1081
    isoenzymes, clinical significance of, 1083
    names for, 1063t
    principles of analysis, 992-993, 993*t*
    specimen, 993
    stability in storage, 1072*t,* 1073
Acid washing, 12
Acidemia, 464
Acidosis, 439, 464, 471-472, 473-475, 596,
    626
    biochemical abnormalities with, 495*t*
    metabolic; *see* Metabolic acidosis
Acids, 465
    dietary and metabolic sources of, 465
Aciduria profiles, 166
Acidurias, organic, 953-954, *954*
Acinar, 555
Acinar cells, 556
    diagram of, *557*
ACP; *see* Acid phosphatase
ACP (acyl carrier protein), 778, **779**
Acquired immunodeficiency syndrome (AIDS),
    836
Acridinium esters, 100
Acromegaly, 613, 849, 864, 867
ACS-180, 306*t,* 308
ACT (activated clotting time), 314
ACTH (adrenocorticotropic hormone), 912,
    918
    change in disease, 865
    ectopic change of analyte with, 925*t,* 927
    plasma, 926
    synthetic form of (cosyntropin, Cortrosyn),
        930
ACTH excess, 864
ACTH-producing pituitary tumors, 864
ACTH stimulation test, 912
Actin, 593, 594, 594*t,* 597
Action control limits, setting, 391-392
Action limits, 382
Action limits log book, 394
Activated clotting time (ACT), 314
Activation energy, 1056, 1060
    reduction in, *1059*
Activators, 1056, 1058, 1070
Active absorption, 484
Active agglutination, 240
Active centers, 1060
Active reabsorption, 487
Active sites, 151, 1056, 1060, *1060*
    GLC, 156
Active transport, 439, 1086, 1088
Activity, 270, 277, 278, 279*t,* 1056
    of enzymes, 1059
Activity coefficient, 277, 278
Activity unit, 1067
Acyl carrier protein (ACP), 778, **779**
Acyl-CoA:cholesterol acyltransferase (ACAT),
    647, 654